W9-ATY-534

Primary Care

The Art and Science of Advanced Practice Nursing

Primary Care

The Art and Science of Advanced Practice Nursing

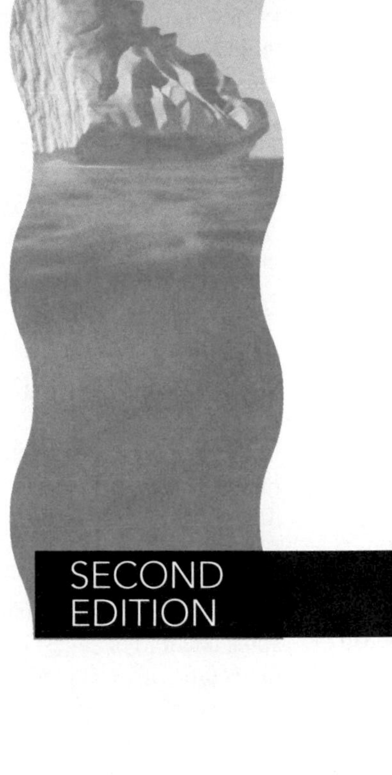

Lynne M. Dunphy, PhD, MSN, APRN, BC
Family Nurse Practitioner
Routhier Chair of Practice and Professor of Nursing
College of Nursing
University of Rhode Island
Kingston, Rhode Island

Jill E. Winland-Brown, EdD, MSN, APRN, BC
Family Nurse Practitioner
Professor
Christine E. Lynn College of Nursing
Florida Atlantic University
Port St. Lucie, Florida

Brian O. Porter, MD, PhD, MPH
Fellow in Allergy and Immunology
National Institute of Allergy and Infectious Diseases
National Institutes of Health
Bethesda, Maryland
and
Department of Internal Medicine
Department of Pediatrics
Medical College of Virginia
Virginia Commonwealth University Medical Center
Richmond, Virginia

Debera J. Thomas, DNS, APRN, BC
Family and Adult Nurse Practitioner
Assistant Dean of Undergraduate Programs and
Associate Professor
Christine E. Lynn College of Nursing
Florida Atlantic University
Boca Raton, Florida

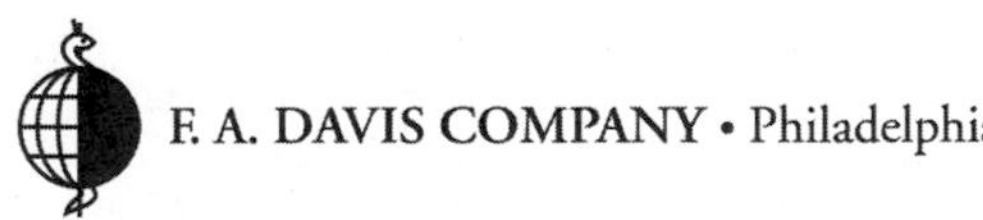
F. A. DAVIS COMPANY • Philadelphia

F. A. Davis Company
1915 Arch Street
Philadelphia, PA 19103
www.fadavis.com

Printed in the United States of America

Last digit indicates print number: 10 9 8 7 6 5 4 3

Acquisitions Editor: Joanne Patzek DaCunha, RN, MSN
Project Editor: Kristin L. Kern
Art and Design Manager: Carolyn O'Brien
Interior Design: B.J. Crim

Library of Congress Cataloging in Publication Data

Primary care : the art and science of advanced practice nursing / [edited by] Lynne M. Dunphy … [et al.]. — 2nd ed.
p. ; cm.
Includes bibliographical references and index.
ISBN-13: 978-0-8036-1487-1
ISBN-10: 0-8036-1487-X
1. Nurse practitioners. 2. Primary nursing. I. Dunphy, Lynne M. Hektor.
[DNLM: 1. Nurse Practitioners. 2. Primary Nursing Care. WY 128 P9523 2007]
RT82.8.P755 2007
610.73—dc22 2006101751

Dedications

To our families:

To my husband—you are my very special balance in life, who makes it all worthwhile! For your patience, support, and affection, which have been ENDLESS!!!!!!

To my parents, Joan and Arthur, and to my brother, Jim, for his good humor, steadfastness, and vacation-planning!!!

Lynne M. Dunphy

To my husband, Harvey, who is my soul mate.

To my parents, who instilled a sense of purpose in me and never let me give up on myself.

To my children: My sons, who have grown into wonderful friends—Ken, Nathan, Eddie, and Mason—and my daughter Cydney, for all that we've shared in the past and look forward to in the future.

Jill E. Winland-Brown

For my beautiful wife, Carolyn, and our four joyful children—Mitchel, MJ, Cheyanne, and Brennan. Your support and patience have furthered my development as a physician, educator, and researcher as much as any diploma!

Brian O. Porter

To my husband, Bob Coan, who got around to marrying me 35 years after we went to the senior prom together.... even after many nights of peanut butter sandwiches and pizza delivery as I was working on this book.

To my parents, who inspired me to believe that I could do anything.

To my dog, for his unfailing devotion and guardianship as I spent endless hours at the computer with him at my feet.

Debera J. Thomas

Preface

"We are not really in doubt about the more serious of our shared aims. Wc know what they are. Wc know they are difficult. And we know that we have not achieved them."

—John Gardner, Excellence, p. 155, as quoted by Martha E. Rogers, Reveille in Nursing, p. 1

This book grew out of a commitment to primary care practice and a love and valuing of nursing knowledge. Forty years ago, in 1964, Martha E. Rogers, Chairperson of the Department of Nursing Education, New York University, came out with a small red and white volume, soft-covered and a total of 96 pages, entitled *Reveille in Nursing,* published by F.A. Davis. It was a book, she was later to comment, ". . . that scared the pants off a lot of people" (Martha E. Rogers, personal communication, June 22, 1988). F.A. Davis continues to stand on its commitment to nursing knowledge with its publication and second edition of this text. The abandonment of nursing knowledge in some primary care nurse practitioner programs is not a trend that Martha would have favored. One can hear her saying, "Where's the *nursing* in nurse practitioner primary care practice? 'Where's the beef?'"

What we offer here is the "beef," a text that builds on the Circle of Caring, a holistic, caring-based approach to primary care practice, consistent with nursing's historic base. Unit 1 contains four chapters that provide the theoretical base to a caring-based primary care practice, which is operationalized in the remainder of the text. In this first unit, we provide a theoretical model of primary care nursing, the Circle of Caring, elaborated in Chapter 1. The caring base of primary care practice is presented by Drs. Boykin and Schoenhofer in Chapter 2, as a transformative model for our health care system. A chapter on Health Promotion by Dr. Cathy St. Pierre provides a base for primary care practice that situates the patient and family in the context of the community. Chapter 4, "The Art of Diagnosis and Treatment," by Dr. Susan Chase, describes how primary care practice in a Circle of Caring is actualized through decision-making and management plans.

Unit 2 uses the traditional system-based approach to provide the essential information necessary to provide safe and effective primary care to patients. Each chapter begins with "Common Complaints," a symptom-based approach to phenomena that lays out the associated differential diagnoses of each symptom-based complaint a patient may present with. Then each chapter develops these various differentials under "Common Problems." Each problem is defined, and the associated epidemiology and causes are outlined, as well as the pathophysiologic processes. One of the major changes made to the second edition of this text is an increased emphasis on advanced pathophysiology. Dr. Brian Porter has joined our team to provide a thorough and indepth treatment of the pathophysiology of each disorder developed within the chapters, as well as a thorough review of diagnostic processes and management plans.

The subjective and objective manifestations of each clinical problem are elaborated, as well as the associated diagnostic testing that might be used. A review of potential differential diagnoses is presented, as well as the underlying reasoning and critical thinking involved in the decision making used to reach a specific diagnosis. As consistent with our model, a holistic data-base should be established, built on each individual patient's voice and experience. Management strategies, including pharmacological and surgical therapy, when indicated, are outlined. Again, as consistent with our approach, complementary therapies and psychosocial interventions are elaborated providing a holistic plan of care. Follow-up and referral are included, along with long-term management strategies, and patient education—the important teaching/learning component of caring-based primary care practice—is also included. Dr. Debera Thomas, a frequent contributor to a wide-variety of medical surgical nursing as well as primary care practice books, also joined us on this edition. Dr. Thomas also brings expertise in the area of complementary therapies and has provided the inclusion of these modailites throughout the Unit 2 chapters.

Tables, figures, and recurring displays are provided in each chapter in Unit II: Displays include drug charts, therapeutic procedures that a clinician in primary care might be called upon to perform, risk factors, screening guidelines, differential diagnosis flowcharts, treatment standards and guidelines, as well as sidebars on focusing the history and advanced assessment techniques. Also, we provide highlights of complementary therapies and holistically-based advanced practice nursing interventions. Included are "Nursing Situations," essentially case studies, along with abstracts of nursing-based research, and anecdotes from patients, called "The Patient's Voice." The provision of this variety of information will assist any primary care provider, regardles of disciplinary background in establishing and implementing a holistic, caring-practice base. These features assist the student (or current practitioner) in linking ideas to practice, and actualizing a Circle of Caring.

Unit 3 includes a chapter on "Palliative Care," by Ms. Susan Derby of Memorial Sloan-Kettering Cancer Center in New York City, including comprehensive information on pain management. We are very pleased to provide our readers with a chapter by Dr. Marian Stuart, "The 15-Minute Hour: A Short-Term Approach to Psychotherapy in Primary Care." This content, developed specifically for primary-care practice, will provide the primary care practitioner with additional therapeutic communication skills that will enable them to "hear" the patient's true concerns, again supporting a holistic and caring practice model. "Evidence-based Practice," by Dr. Susan Folden and Dr. Shawn Kneipp, provides essential information for today's care practice environment. It is essential that all clinicians be able to provide care with a good understanding of the standard of care and the ability to meet that standard in a meaningful way. "Ethical and Legal Issues of a Caring-Based Practice" is also an essential for practice, as is an understanding of "The Business of Advanced Practice" provided in Chapter 23. We conclude with essential information: "Putting Caring into Practice: Caring for Self." Caring and holistic practice begins—and ends—with care of self.

As long-time nurse practitioner faculty, we felt the need to provide a large book, with a comprehensive and holistic approach, that could be used across the curriculum, and in a variety of different curricula. A professional doctorate for advanced nursing practice is under development: the Doctor of Nursing Practice. This text provides a high-level pathophysiologic base, evidence-based diagnostic and management strategies, and a holistic plan of care that is consistent with this level of nursing practice. The student is able to find a large amount of information in one text. Although we realize that graduate students will always need supplementary texts to provide the depth of information that they need, as well as current therapeutics we nonetheless believe that they (and their faculty!) will appreciate one large, complete text.

What we have provided is "the beef"—the "beef" of caring-based advanced practice nursing as actualized in the DNP role, in the full flowering of all that primary-care practice *could* be. We are answering the call that Jean Watson sounded in her 1995 article, "Advanced Nursing Practice . . . and What Might Be":

> Such a reform calls for nursing to shift its accountability and voice from the medical cure functional tasks and institutional demands and constraints toward making itself directly accountable to the public for its caring, healing, health knowledge, skills, and practices.
>
> —*Watson, 1995, p. 81*

It is the most exciting time for advanced practice nursing. Medicare reimbursement is a reality. The demand for new service approaches in health care is high. The professional doctorate – the DNP – is providing primary care practitioners of nursing with a well-grounded base of pathophysiology, diagnosis and management, and follow up. Consumers are informed, and powerful. Now it is time for Doctors of Nursing Practice to provide consumers with the "beef"—advanced nursing primary-care practice within a circle of caring.

Acknowledgments

There are numerous people to thank for helping this book become a reality:

Joanne P. DaCunha, our wonderful, PATIENT, always supportive, always optimistic editor, whom we have come to know well, and who is, most of all, our friend.

Kristin L. Kern, who has provided support, food, good humor and hard work, and fun.

The entire F.A. Davis production team - ALL of whom were always patient, flexible, and terrific! Berta Steiner, Director of Production, Bermedica Production Ltd. for her patience and sanity!

Dr. Anne Boykin, Dean of the Christine E. Lynn College of Nursing, who has helped us shape our vision for nursing, and provide the glue that holds it together—caring.

The entire Florida Atlantic University's Graphics Department, especially Adrien Spano, who has supported us in numerous endeavors, providing good humor, patience, and willingness to "hear" our voice!!!!

Dr. Dayle Joseph, Dean of the College of Nursing, University of Rhode Island, is thanked for her support and leadership by Lynne and Jill, a former colleague.

Our past graduate students: Nina Nolte and Joann Gruber, who created tables and charts for vitamins, minerals, and herbal therapies; Mary Jane Hopkins for her assistance with the design of flow charts; and Paula Friend and Teresa Halm, for their assistance with literature reviews.

Dr. Luz Porter, PhD, ARNP, FNP, FAAN, is thanked for her tireless commitment to the creation and dissemination of knowledge in nursing, by her son Brian, and her former student and colleague, Lynne.

Charlotte Dison, RN, MSN, Vice-President Emeritus, Baptist Health System of South Florida, Miami, FL, for her wonderful poem about nursing—"Seasons of My Life."

Christine Sanders, BSN, RN for her beautiful illustration of the patient struggling with Parkinson's disease and Jamie Castanada, BSN, RN, for his poem and drawing, *The Dementia Patient*.

All of our students, past and present, who always continue to teach us as much, if not more, than we teach them!!!!

And most of all, our patients, who taught us to "hear" their voices.

Contributors

Theresa Beckie, PhD, RN
Assistant Professor
University of South Florida Health Sciences Center
College of Nursing
Tampa, Florida
• CHAPTER 8 Respiratory Problems

Anne Boykin, PhD, RN
Dean and Professor
Christine E. Lynn College of Nursing
Florida Atlantic University
Boca Raton, Florida
• CHAPTER 2 Caring and the Advanced Practice Nurse

Susan K. Chase, EdD, APRN, BC
Associate Professor and Assistant Dean
Graduate Programs
Christine E. Lynn College of Nursing
Florida Atlantic University
Boca Raton, Florida
• CHAPTER 4 The Art of Diagnosis and Treatment

Susan Derby, RN, MA, CGNP, ACHPN
Nurse Practitioner
Pain and Palliative Care Service
Memorial Sloan Kettering Cancer Center
New York, New York
• CHAPTER 19 Palliative Care

Patricia Welch Dittman, PhD(C), RN, CDE
Assistant Professor
Nova Southeastern University
Fort Lauderdale, Florida
• CHAPTER 23 The Business of Advanced Practice

Lynne M. Dunphy, PhD, MSN, APRN, BC
Family Nurse Practitioner
Routhier Chair of Practice and Professor of Nursing
College of Nursing
University of Rhode Island
Kingston, Rhode Island
• CHAPTER 1 Primary Care in the Twenty-First Century: A Circle of Caring; • CHAPTER 7 Eyes, Ears, Nose, and Throat Problems; • CHAPTER 14 Musculoskeletal Problems; • CHAPTER 17 Psychosocial Problems; • CHAPTER 23 The Business of Advanced Practice

Margaret A. Fitzgerald, DNP, APRN, BC, NP-C, FAANP, CSP
President
Fitzgerald Health Education Associates, Inc.
North Andover, Massachusetts
• CHAPTER 9 Cardiovascular Problems

Susan L. Folden, PhD, APRN, BC
Family Nurse Practitioner
Associate Professor
Christine E. Lynn College of Nursing
Florida Atlantic University
Boca Raton, Florida
• CHAPTER 15 Endocrine and Metabolic Problems; • CHAPTER 21 Evidence-Based Practice

Mary Layman Goldstein, RN, MS, APRN, BC
Nurse Practitioner
Pain and Palliative Care Service
Memorial Sloan Kettering Cancer Center
New York, New York
• CHAPTER 19 Palliative Care

Sande Garcia Jones, PhD, ARNP, ACRN, FAAN
Professor
Florida International University
School of Nursing, College of Health & Urban Affairs
Miami, Florida
• CHAPTER 16 Hematologic and Immune Problems

Shawn Kneipp, PhD, APRN, BC
Associate Professor
College of Nursing
University of Florida
Gainesville, Florida
• CHAPTER 21 Evidence-Based Practice

Maria Leik, MSN, APRN, BC
President
National ARNP Services, Inc.
Fort Lauderdale, Florida
Family Nurse Practitioner
Countryside Medical Center
Cooper City, Florida
and
Adjunct Faculty
Florida International University
Graduate School of Nursing
North Miami, Florida
• CHAPTER 6 Skin Problems

Ruth McCaffrey, DNP, APRN, BC
Family Nurse Practitioner & Geriatric Nurse Practitioner
Associate Professor
Christine E. Lynn College of Nursing
Florida Atlantic University
Boca Raton, Florida
• CHAPTER 7 Eyes, Ears, Nose, and Throat Problems

Linda E. Moody, PhD, APRN, FAAN
Professor
University of South Florida Health Sciences Center and Institute on Aging
College of Nursing
Tampa, Florida
• CHAPTER 8 Respiratory Problems

Linda Denise Oakley, PhD, RN
Professor of Nursing
University of Wisconsin-Madison
Madison, Wisconsin
• CHAPTER 17 Psychosocial Problems

Lori Martin Plank, MSPH, MSN, APRN, BC
Family and Gerontological Nurse Practitioner
Coordinator, Family Nurse Practitioner Track

Clinical Assistant Professor, Department of Nursing
College of Health Professions
Temple University
Philadelphia, Pennsylvania
• CHAPTER 14 Musculoskeletal Problems

Brian O. Porter, MD, PhD, MPH
Fellow in Allergy and Immunology
National Institute of Allergy and Infectious Diseases
National Institutes of Health
Bethesda, Maryland
and
Department of Internal Medicine
Department of Pediatrics
Medical College of Virginia
Virginia Commonwealth University Medical Center
Richmond, Virginia
• CHAPTER 1 Primary Care in the Twenty-First Century: A Circle of Caring; • CHAPTER 6 Skin Problems; • CHAPTER 7 Eyes, Ears, Nose, and Throat Problems; • CHAPTER 8 Respiratory Problems; • CHAPTER 9 Cardiovascular Problems; • CHAPTER 11 Renal Problems; • CHAPTER 12 Men's Health Problems; • CHAPTER 13 Women's Health Problems; • CHAPTER 15 Endocrine and Metabolic Problems; • CHAPTER 16 Hematologic and Immune Problems; • CHAPTER 18 Emergency Problems

Jacqueline Rhoads, PhD, RN, CCRN, ACNP-CS
Professor
Louisiana State University
Health Science Center
School of Nursing
New Orleans, Louisiana
• CHAPTER 5 Neurologic Problems

Marcie Rutherford, PhD(C), MBA, RN
Doctorial Student
Christine E. Lynn College of Nursing
Florida Atlantic University
Boca Raton, Florida
• CHAPTER 23 The Business of Advanced Practice

Edwin W. Schaefer, ND, RN, FNP
Instructor
Rush University
Chicago, Illinois
Emergency Department Nurse Practitioner
Northwest Community Hospital
Arlington Heights, Illinois
• CHAPTER 18 Emergency Problems

Savina O. Schoenhofer, PhD, RN
Professor
Alcorn State University
School of Nursing
Natchez, Mississippi
• CHAPTER 2 Caring and the Advanced Practice Nurse

Karilee Halo Shames, PhD, RN, HNC
Private Practice
Preventive Medicine Center of Marin
San Rafael, Calfiornia
• CHAPTER 24 Putting Caring into Practice: Caring for Self

Cathy M. St. Pierre, PhD, APRN, BC
Assistant Professor
Christine E. Lynn College of Nursing
Florida Atlantic University
Boca Raton, Florida
• CHAPTER 3 Health Promotion

Marian R. Stuart, PhD
Clinical Professor
Department of Family Medicine
UMDNJ–Robert Wood Johnson Medical School
New Brunswick, New Jersey
• CHAPTER 20 The 15-Minute Hour: A Short-Term Approach to Psychotherapy in Primary Care

Debera J. Thomas, DNS, APRN, BC
Family and Adult Nurse Practitioner
Assistant Dean of Undergraduate Programs
and
Associate Professor
Christine E. Lynn College of Nursing
Florida Atlantic University
Boca Raton, Florida
• CHAPTER 1 Primary Care in the Twenty-First Century: A Circle of Caring; CHAPTER 10 Abdominal Problems; • CHAPTER 11 Renal Problems; • CHAPTER 12 Men's Health Problems; • CHAPTER 13 Women's Heatlh Problems; • CHAPTER 15 Endocrine and Metabolic Problems

Sharon Thrush, MSN, APRN, BC
Family Nurse Practioner
Palm Beach Family Physicians
West Palm Beach, Florida
and
Adjunct Faculty
Christine E. Lynn College of Nursing
Florida Atlantic University
Port St. Lucie, Florida
• CHAPTER 7, Eyes, Ears, Nose, and Throat Problems

Mary Webb, PhD, RN
Assistant Professor
University of South Florida Health Science Center
College of Nursing
Tampa, Florida
• CHAPTER 8 Respiratory Problems

Jill E. Winland-Brown, EdD, MSN, APRN, BC
Family Nurse Practitioner
Professor
Christine E. Lynn College of Nursing
Florida Atlantic University
Port St. Lucie, Florida
• CHAPTER 1 Primary Care in the Twenty-First Century: A Circle of Caring; • CHAPTER 5 Neurologic Problems; • CHAPTER 6 Skin Problems; • CHAPTER 8 Respiratory Problems; • CHAPTER 9 Cardiovascular Problems; • CHAPTER 13 Women's Health Problems; • CHAPTER 16 Hematologic and Immune Problems; • CHAPTER 18 Emergency Problems; • CHAPTER 22 Ethical and Legal Issues of a Caring-Based Practice

Contributors to the First Edition

The authors would like to acknowledge the significant contributions made to the first edition of this book without which this new edition would not have been possible. The contributors held the following positions at the time of the publication of the first edition.

Violeta Aquilar-Figuly, MSN, ARNP, ANP, PNP
Senior Associate Professor
Miami-Dade Community College
School of Nursing
Miami, Florida

Susan Barker, MSN, FNP
Nurse Practitioner
Veteran's Administration Medical Center
Savannah, Georgia

Catherine M. Berardelli, PhD, RN, CS, FNP
Associate Professor
University of New England
College of Nursing
Portland, Maine

Theresa A. Boyd, EdD, ARNP-C
Adult Nurse Practitioner
Student Health Clinic
Florida International University
North Miami, Florida

Nancie Bruce, DNSc, RN, CCRN
Emergency Department Nurse
Boca Raton, Florida

Catherine T. Brunner, MS, RN, CS, ANP, WHNP, OCN
Nurse Practitioner in Hematology/Oncology
Practice with Marc S. Zimmerman, MD
Pomona, New York

Geraldine Budd, PhD(c), CRNP, CS, FNP-C
Instructor
Pennsylvania State University
School of Nursing
University Park, Pennsylvania
Nurse Practitioner
Rural Nursing Center
Mt. Union, Pennsylvania

Sherri Lynn Coffman, DNS, APN, CPN
Advanced Nurse Practitioner
Pediatrics
Sierra Health Service
Las Vegas, Nevada

Brenda Corripio, MSN, FNP
Indian River Memorial Hospital
Vero Beach, Florida

Carol Ann Devine, BSN, MPH, APRN
Nurse Practitioner
Palm Beach County Health Department
West Palm Beach, Florida

Cynthia Dexter, MSN, RN, IBCLC
Perinatal Clinical Nurse Specialist
Maine Medical Center
Portland, Maine

Sargit Dillon, CNM, RN
Student
University of New England
Portland, Maine

Darcy Egging, MS, CS-ANP, CEN
Emergency Department Nurse Practitioner
Delnor Community Hospital
Elgin, Illinois

Margaret A. Fitzgerald, MS, RN, CS-FNP
President
Fitzgerald Health Education Associates, Inc.
North Andover, Massachusetts

Lynn Fletcher, MSN, ARNP
Nurse Practitioner
Veteran's Administration Hospital
West Palm Beach, Florida

Joan Freedman, ND, APRN
Women's Health Practitioner
Women's Health Care
Fort Lauderdale, Florida

Julia Gamble, MSN, FNP
Nurse Practitioner
Health Essentials
St. Petersburg, Florida

Wendy S. Geier, PhD, RN, CS, ANP, OGNP
Associate Professor
CW Post College at Long Island University
Department of Nursing
Brookville, New York

Shirley Countryman Gordon, PhD, RN
Associate Professor
Christine E. Lynn College of Nursing
Florida Atlantic University
Boca Raton, Florida

JoAnn Kelle Gottlieb, MS, SPRN, CS
Assistant Professor
Barry University
School of Nursing
Miami Shorés, Florida
Education Consultant
Baptist Hospital of Miami
Miami, Florida

Joann Gruber, BSN, RN
Graduate Student
Christine E. Lynn College of Nursing
Florida Atlantic University
Boca Raton, Florida

Margaret Hamilton, DNS, RN
Assistant Professor
Purdue University
School of Nursing
West Lafayette, Indiana

Valerie Hart, EdD, RN, CS
Associate Professor
University of Southern Maine
Department of Nursing
Portland, Maine

Julie Hilsenbeck, MSN, ARNP, CCRN, CNRN
Vice-President
North Ridge Medical Center
Fort Lauderdale, Florida

Mary Jane Hopkins, MSN, FNP
Assistant Professor
Indian River Community College
Fort Pierce, Florida

Elaine Kahn, MSN, ARNP
Adult Nurse Practitioner
Private Practice
Ft. Lauderdale, Florida

Kathryn Buchanan Keller, PhD, RN
Associate Professor
Christine E. Lynn College of Nursing
Florida Atlantic University
Boca Raton, Florida

Joan M. Kennedy, MN, APRN
Owner and Care Provider
Staywell, A Wellness Promotion Service
Jupiter, Florida

Kim Grosskopf Klein, MS, GNP
Savannas Hospital
Port St. Lucie, Florida

Shawn Kneipp, PhD, APRN, BC
Assistant Professor
College of Nursing
University of Florida
Gainesville, Florida

Mary S. Koithan, PhD, RN, CS
Assistant Professor
University of Arizona
College of Nursing
Tucson, Arizona

Lori L. Kondora, PhD, APNP, CS
Nurse Practitioner
Mental Health Center of Dane County
Madison, Wisconsin

Rhonda M. Kutil, PhD, RN
Assistant Professor
Illinois Wesleyan University
School of Nursing
Bloomington, Illinois

Pamela B. Lester, MSN, ARNP
Family Nurse Practitioner
Western Communities Family Practice
Associates
Wellington, Florida

Carol Gullo Mest, PhD, RN, CRNP
Assistant Professor and Director Graduate
Nursing Programs
Allentown College of St. Francis de Sales
Center Valley, Pennsylvania

Mary Miller, PhD, RN, CS
Clinical Nurse Specialist
Associate Professor
Armstrong Atlantic State University
School of Nursing
Savannah, Georgia

Nina Nolte, RN, BSN
Graduate Student
Christine E. Lynn College of Nursing
Florida Atlantic University
Boca Raton, Florida

Linda Denise Oakley, PhD, RN, ARNP
Associate Professor and Clinical Specialist
University of Wisconsin-Madison
School of Nursing
Madison, Wisconsin

Marie-Eileen Onieal, MMHS, RN, CPNP
President, American Academy of Nurse Practitioners
Health Policy Coordinator, Bureau of Health
Quality Management, Massachusetts Department
of Public Health
Lowell, Massachusetts

Barbara B. Phillips, MS, GNP, CS
Veterans Administration Medical Center
West Palm Beach, Florida

Judith Marie Pine, MS, MPH, ANP-C, FNP-C
Nurse Practitioner
Emergency Department
Mt. Sinai Hospital
New York, New York

Lori Martin Plank, PhD-c, GNP, FNP
Nurse Practitioner, PHMC Health Connection
Clinical Assistant Professor
Temple University, College of Health Professions
Department of Nursing
Philadelphia, Pennsylvania
Doctoral Student
Duquesne University
Pittsburgh, Pennsylvania

Ginger Pruden, MSN, RN
Assistant Professor
Armstrong Atlantic State University
Department of Nursing
Savannah, Georgia

Marilyn A. Ray, PhD, RN, CTN, CNAA
Professor
Florida Atlantic University
Christine E. Lynn College of Nursing
Boca Raton, Florida

Kit Sebrey Schafer, MSN, RN-C, NP
Perinatal Nurse Practitioner
Clinical Associate Professor
Purdue University
School of Nursing
West Lafayette, Indiana

Marcy Schwartz, MS, FNP, CS
Family Nurse Practitioner
South Broward Hospital District
Hollywood, Florida
Adjunct Faculty
Florida Atlantic University
College of Nursing
Boca Raton, Florida

Maria Seidel, MS, FNP
Assistant Professor
Indian River Community College
Fort Pierce, Florida

Patricia M. Siccardi, MSN, MEd, ARNP, CS
Adjunct Assistant Professor
Florida Atlantic University
Christine E. Lynn College of Nursing
Boca Raton, Florida

Lisa M. Silbert, MSN, ARNP-CS, CCRN
Neurosurgical Nurse Practitioner
Veteran's Administration Medical Center
Miami, Florida

Ann Marie Szoke-Halal, MSN, RN, CRNP, ONC
Nurse Practitioner
Geriatrics Institute
St. Luke's Hospital
Bethlehem, Pennsylvania

Ruth M. Tappen, EdD, RN, FAAN
Professor, Christine E. Lynn Eminent Scholar, and Vice President for Research
Christine E. Lynn College of Nursing
Florida Atlantic University
Boca Raton, Florida

Mary Beth Thompson, MSN, FNP, CS
Hahn and Adler Internal Medicine and Gastroenterology
Plantation, Florida

Karen Thornton, PhD, RN
Assistant Professor
Florida Atlantic University
Christine E. Lynn College of Nursing
Boca Raton, Florida

Theris A, Touhy, ND, APRN, CS
Assistant Professor
Florida Atlantic University
Christine E. Lynn College of Nursing
Boca Raton, Florida

Marian C. Turkel, PhD, RN
Assistant Professor
Florida Atlantic University
Christine E. Lynn College of Nursing
Boca Raton, Florida

Elvira Velez, MPH, APRN, C
Faculty and Associate Director of the Student Health Clinics
Florida International University
North Miami, Florida

Kathi Voege, MS, FNP
Adjunct Faculty
Florida Atlantic University
Christine E. Lynn College of Nursing
Boca Raton, Florida

Doris R. Weisman, MS, OGNP, RNC
Clinical Instructor
School of Medicine
Clinical Assistant Professor
School of Nursing
Stony Brook University Hospital
Stony Brook, New York

Gayle R. Wooley, EdD, APRN
Professor and Coordinator, Acclerated Option/Transitional RN Programs
Miami-Dade Community College
Miami, Florida

Carolyn Zaumeyer, MSN, ARNP, BC
Nurse Practitioner and President
Women's Health Watch, Inc.
West Milford, New Jersey

Joyce Zerwekh, EdD, RN, CS
Associate Professor
Florida Atlantic University
Christine E. Lynn College of Nurisng
Boca Raton, Florida

Consultants

Diane Blantz, RN, PhD, FNP-BC
Associate Professor
Ball State University
Muncie, Indiana

Theresa M. Capriotti, DO, MSN, RN, CRNP
Clinical Associate Professor
Villanova University College of Nursing
Villanova, Pennsylvania

Susan Ewing, PhD, FNP, APRN, BC
Clinical Assistant Professor
University of Arizona, College of Nursing
Tucson, Arizona

Kenneth M. Certa, MD
Clinical Assistant Professor
Director, Adult Acute Psychiatric Services
Jefferson Medical College of Thomas Jefferson University
Philadelphia, Pennsylvania

Sheila Grossman, APRN, BC, PhD
Professor & Director Family Nurse Practitioner
Program Fairfield
Fairfield University School of Nursing
Fairfield, Connecticut

Carolyn Zaumeyer, MSN, APRN, BC
Nurse Practitioner and President
Women's Health Watch, Inc.
West Milford, New Jersey

Contents

UNIT 3

Caring-Based Nursing: The Practice

Nursing—The Seasons of My Life

Nursing is the spring of my life—
Each experience is fresh and new.
There's wonderment
Like flowers washed with morning dew.
Nursing is the summer of my life—
A time to perfect all I know.
There's confidence
A world where I can grow.
Nursing is the autumn of my life—
Ablaze with experience rich and glowing.
There's compassion
From richness of caring and knowing.
Nursing is the winter of my life—
A tapestry, a mosaic of all I am.
There's challenge
To find the spring again.

—Charlotte Dison, RN

Caring-Based Nursing: The Art

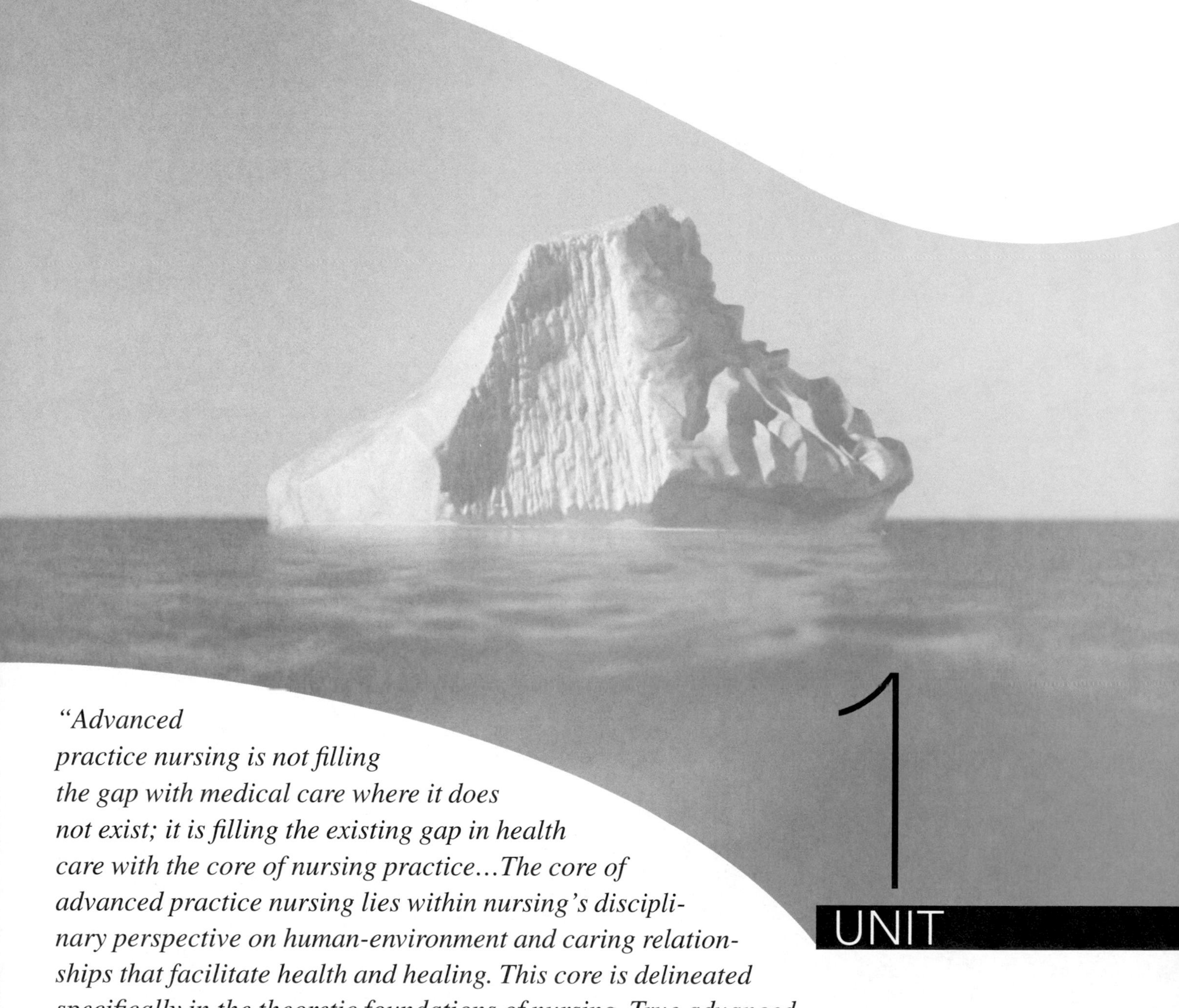

1

UNIT

"Advanced practice nursing is not filling the gap with medical care where it does not exist; it is filling the existing gap in health care with the core of nursing practice...The core of advanced practice nursing lies within nursing's disciplinary perspective on human-environment and caring relationships that facilitate health and healing. This core is delineated specifically in the theoretic foundations of nursing. True advanced nursing practice is theory-based [and] fully integrated into the nurse's way of being and practicing."

—Marlaine Smith: The core of advanced practice nursing. Nurs Sci Q 8(1):2–3, 1995

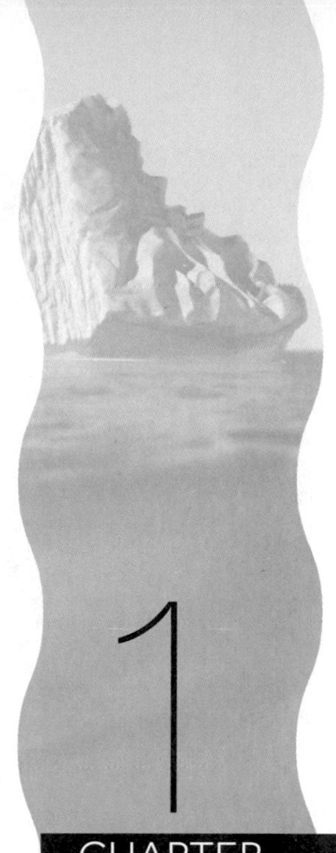

Primary Care in the Twenty-First Century: A Circle of Caring

Lynne M. Dunphy, PhD, MSN, APRN, BC
Jill E. Winland-Brown, EdD, MSN, APRN, BC
Brian O. Porter, MD, PhD, MPH
Debera J. Thomas, DNS, APRN, BC

1
CHAPTER

Where We Have Been and Where We Are Going

At present, our health-care system is struggling to come to grips with fiscal realities, managed care, continued technological advancements, an aging population, and an increasingly educated and informed consumer. Illness is often treated episodically, outside the context of home, community, and people's day-to-day lives, in isolation from the trajectory of the life of the individual. The major goals of *Healthy People 2010* of increasing quality and years of a healthy life and the elimination of health disparities are far from being met.

According to Donna Shalala, former Secretary of the Department of Health and Human Services, in a 1993 keynote address at the Centennial Conference of the National League for Nursing, patients, families, groups, and communities are calling for the appearance of the "good fairy" in health care—someone who really hears them and their concerns, the nitty-gritty of their day-to-day experiences and struggles. Patients and their families need someone to hear why they did not take the medication that their health-care provider was so quick to prescribe, but that they just could not tolerate, could not afford, could not get to the pharmacy to pick up, or that had directions for administration that they could not understand; to hear why they did not have the mammogram—because they were afraid; to hear why the baby was not immunized—because putting food on the table was more important.

The Tip of the Iceberg

The health problems encountered in day-to-day practice are merely the tip of the iceberg that our health-care system, traditionally focused on the easily visible peaks above the water, has plowed into. Reimbursement streams pay for the "tip" of this iceberg: a visit to a primary care provider that puts a diagnostic label, for billing purposes, on the symptomatology that the patient presents with, and a "treatment"—typically a pharmaceutical product—aimed at treating that symptom or underlying disease.

The multifactorial, and frequently community-situated, iceberg of the patient's life, manifested in whatever "complaint" brought him or her into that primary care setting, is what needs to be addressed. The true causality of the illness manifestations is represented by the massive, not necessarily visible structures under the surface. This "understructure" is built of various lifestyle issues, environmental, community, socioeconomic, family, and biologic–genetic factors that have an impact on health. Nurses understand that the visible alterations often represent only the tip of the iceberg. A nursing perspective is the "good fairy" in health care that Donna Shalala called for in 1993, and the need for that "good fairy" is even more critical in today's world. Nurses understand the *whole* of the iceberg (Fig. 1.1); they are educated to see both above *and* below the water and to intervene accordingly.

The classic medical model focuses on disease, meaning an abnormality in the structure and function of body organs and systems, and as such is concerned with the malfunction or maladaption of biological or psychophysiological processes in the individual. In his textbook of family practice, Robert Rakel (1995) makes a distinction between the terms "disease" and "illness." He describes "illness" as "all sensations of a patient and all the ramifications of a disorder" (p 305). "Disease," he notes, is a theoretical and taxonomic concept, a useful tool that enables the caregiver to make inferences and predictions concerning phenomena. As

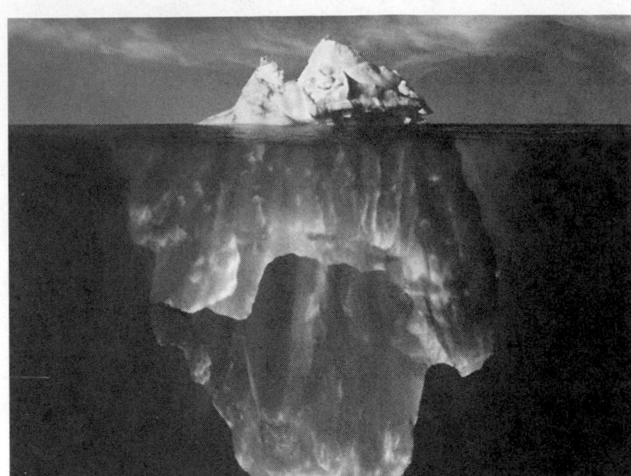

FIGURE 1.1

such, these two concepts, illness and disease, belong to two different universes of discourse: one, the world of theory; the other, the lived experience of the patient. Benner and Wrubel (1989) also distinguish between disease and the experience of disease or illness. Illness is defined as the way that the sick person and his or her social network perceive and respond to disease. Illness is inextricable from the context of the patient's life, including the intersections of social, political, economic, and cultural factors, the whole of the iceberg.

Historically, nursing has been concerned with the whole person, the promotion of health across the lifespan—what Florence Nightingale referred to as "the Laws of Health." Nurses also have historically focused on people's responses to the illness experience in the context of their day-to-day lives. Much of the challenge in the role of the advanced practice nurse (APN) has been the negotiation of seemingly disparate worlds: the reconciliation of an essentially wholistic nursing model into a health-care system still predominantly focused on episodic and fragmented, disease-oriented care, and willing to pay only for the same.

It is precisely this nexus between more discrete diagnostic categories of disease and a more wholistic view of the continuum between health and illness, of the "whole" of the iceberg, that gives nursing its identity, richness, diversity, and usefulness. Today's primary care practitioners dwell in this nexus, and must mitigate and bridge these two realities—that of the world of disease and the world of illness, including the context of the patient's life in all its complexity. The placement of APNs into primary care settings across the health-care continuum provides nursing with the opportunity to mediate and effect change on both the micro- and macrolevel—in the lives of individual patients and families and the well-being of communities, including the global community. The real-life health needs of people, lifestyle adjustments, health education, and self-care are part of a traditional domain of nursing practice as stated by Florence Nightingale, that of health promotion and disease prevention, as well as care of the sick.

Baer (1993) notes that the services demanded of primary-care providers today are broader in scope than those within the domain of medicine before the 1960s. Supportive functions, previously the domain of the clergy or multigenerational families and the like, are now within the province of the primary-care provider. Likewise, the conceptual shift to health promotion, coupled with increased knowledge about healthy lifestyles, all necessitate that primary-care providers be well grounded in the community context in which their patients live their lives as well as the day-to-day life experiences of those patients. Baer concludes, in making her case for the role of the nurse in primary care: "The best reason for nurses to provide primary care is because they are nurses. Nursing's focus on people; its blend of medical, behavioral, and social science expertise; and its commitment to caring, teaching, counseling, and supporting patients are the characteristics of nursing that make nurses so uniquely qualified to provide primary health care services" (p 114).

This text provides a nursing-based approach to the diagnosis, management, and treatment of disease. The essentials of disease pathology and management necessary for safe and satisfactory functioning in the clinical area are integrated into a view of the wholeness of persons, an understanding of human responses, and a repertoire of therapeutic options. This will enable the primary care provider, regardless of disciplinary background, to become an orchestrator of health and wellness, as well as a skilled negotiator and mediator in the space that exists between health and illness, between disease and the "lived experience of the patient" in the context of their community.

Historical Perspectives of Advanced Practice Nursing

Nursing as a discipline and a profession with a theoretical base can be traced back to Florence Nightingale. As long ago as 1860, Nightingale in *Notes on Nursing* proclaimed that there were laws of sickness and laws of health. There was not enough known, she wrote, about the laws of health. Nursing the "room," meaning the environment surrounding the patient, was as important as nursing the patient. She also wrote that nursing and medicine were like "cats and dogs" and should not be mixed.

The early public health nurses of Lillian Wald's Henry Street Settlement House at the turn of the 20th century were an autonomous lot, with their own vision of heath and illness. They took this message directly to the community. Lavinia Dock, one of the first Henry Street nurses, evolved a model, shown in Fig. 1.2, which is still applicable today.

The nurses' functions were educational and preventive as well as curative; they alleviated illness and actualized self and "other" through service to the individual, family, and community. These activities flowed from the spirit, science,

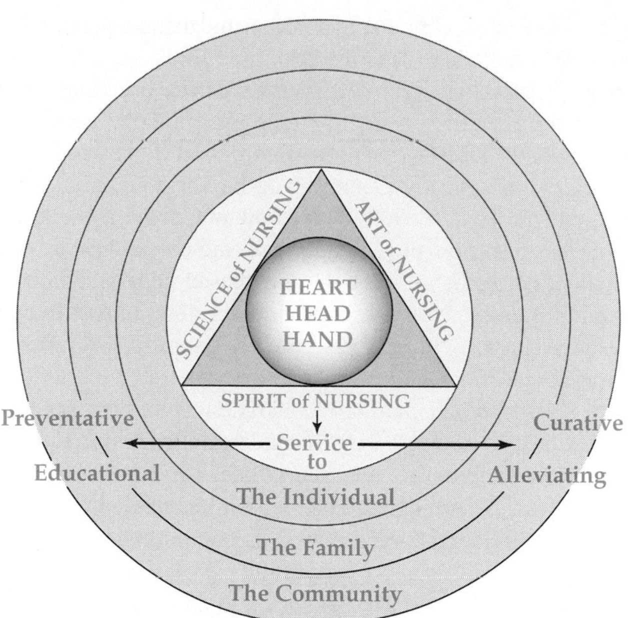

FIGURE 1.2 The professional equipment of the modern nurse and the scope of her responsibilities. *(Source: Dock, LL, and Stewart, IM: A Short History of Nursing: From the Earliest Times to the Present Day, ed 3. GP Putnam's Sons, New York, 1931, p 337.)*

and art of nursing or the "heart, head, and hand" of nursing (a phrase later popularized by Virginia Henderson [1966]). The first instances of standardized protocols evolved from the work of the early school nurses and the New York City Public Health Department. These early public health nurses enjoyed an autonomy of practice similar to that exercised by today's primary care providers. Dock and Stewart (1920) stated that "… medicine flourished in periods when scientific inquiry and experimentation were relatively active while nursing seemed to follow more closely the waves of religious awakening and of social and humanitarian effort (p 366)." She likened the relationship between nursing and medicine to workers on a team who complement and supplement each other; the relationship is based on neither independence nor subordination but on interdependence and cooperation.

Virginia Henderson formulated a theory of nursing described in her 1966 book, *The Nature of Nursing,* an attempt to provide nursing with its own explanatory model for practice. Building on her own experiences in nursing (Henderson also spent time as a public health nurse at the Henry Street settlement) and on her understanding of physiology, she tried to place nursing within a continuum with medicine. Henderson argued that nurses had to place themselves (figuratively) "inside" patients in order to become their "counterpart, alter ego, or helper."

Martha Rogers, another eminent nurse-theoretician, argued the necessity of an independent basis of nursing science, out of which autonomous nursing practice grows. According to Rogers (1972), "Primary care by nurses is as old as modern nursing," citing a number of examples rooted in her early public health nursing experiences. She was, however, in staunch opposition to the development of the nurse practitioner role in the late 1960s and 1970s. In a 1975 position statement published in the *American Journal of Nursing,* she boldly asserted, "Not all nurses have succumbed to the blandishments of euphemisms and the increasingly blatant perfidy spawned by such terms as pediatric associate, nurse practitioner, primary-care practitioner, geriatric practitioner, physician extender, and other equally weird and wonderful cover-ups—designed to provide succor and profit for the nation's shamans."

The early nurse practitioner "movement" evolved with little connection to academe and the flurry of theoretical models and theories that proliferated throughout the 1970s and 1980s. Rooted in practice, usually in a primary-care setting, and often "trained" in certificate programs, these practitioners had little patience with the abstractions of nursing theory that provided little meaning for their day-to-day practice. They needed and valued the medical model to care for their patients. And yet most remained, at heart, nurses, devoted to providing wholistic care to their patients.

Very few nursing models have addressed or attempted to make sense of the dichotomy of nurse practitioner practice. Some argue that no dichotomy exists. A number of others, however, identify the relationship between advanced nursing practice and medical practice as an issue requiring ongoing attention. Cody (1994) views medicine as still dominating nursing politically, and he states that many nurses "actually value having medical tasks delegated to them" (p 144). On a more ominous note, he points out that nursing needs to realize that what is merely delegated from another (more powerful) discipline can also be taken away. He concludes that "Only when nurses everywhere are guided by a theory base specific to nursing will nursing have achieved a parity with other scholarly disciplines." In a coauthored article (1973), Barbara Bates, MD (of physical assessment fame) and Joan Lynaugh, nurse practitioner (and Professor Emerita at the University of Pennsylvania) venture some thoughts on the relationship between nursing and medicine: Medicine, they speculate, is concerned with structure; nursing is focused on function.

In an unpublished paper, Lynaugh discusses the respective roles of nurses and physicians in greater depth. She notes that the biomedical model of disease and cure, which swept across the Western world, seemed far more compelling and promising than nursing's holism, environmentalism, and "watchful waiting" approach to illness. Nurses, she elaborates, seem to be both inarticulate in explaining their work and "touchingly confident" that altruism will eventually be rewarded. Years of medical dominance have drawn a veil over the work of nursing. Lynaugh stresses that this invisibility is serious, because it compromises the public's access to good nursing care in an era in which reimbursement for care is restricted to payment based exclusively on the phenomena of interest to physicians. The power relationships between patient, nurse, and physician are complicated by economic issues, professional territoriality on all sides, and profound questions of disciplinary identity; therefore, Lynaugh suggests, adjustments in these relationships will come slowly, step by step, but inevitably. An essential component of this process is making the "invisible" work of nurses more visible. It is the part of the iceberg that is below the water that takes up so much of nursing's time and energy, and is so un-named and un-seen. Demonstration of nursing's contribution to patient care is vital. This is accomplished, in part, through the clear articulation of nursing's theoretical base.

As nursing theory embraces the mode of mid-range theory development and testing, with real-life clinical applications for practice, the applicability to advanced practice nursing and the utilization of theory-based practice should increase. This still begs the question, however, of an underlying theoretical basis for advanced practice nursing.

Advanced Practice Nursing: Models of Practice

Expert practice domains of the clinical nurse specialist and nurse practitioner were identified by Fenton and Brykczynski (1993) and evolved from domains identified in Patricia Benner's 1984 book, *From Novice to Expert.* Because that work arose from generic nursing practice, the question remains whether this model can provide a true base for advanced nursing practice. The original seven domains identified by Benner were reduced to five by the National Organization of Nurse Practitioner Faculties (NONPF) (Zimmer et al, 1990) for use as a framework for primary-care nurse practitioner curricula:

1. Management of health/illness status in ambulatory care settings
2. Monitoring and ensuring of the quality of health-care practices
3. Organizational and role competencies
4. Helping role
5. Teaching–coaching function

In addition, this document spelled out healing role competencies. Lewis and Brykczynski (1994) elaborated on the practical knowledge and healing role competencies of nurse practitioners. This interpretive study of nurse as healer validated the competencies labeled in the NONPF (Zimmer et al, 1990) document and identified two additional competencies:

1. Using humor with sensitivity
2. Risk taking

In the discussion of their findings, the authors state that to bring about healing, nurse practitioners will go beyond the call of duty, going to schools, for example, to fight for a patient's rights, making phone calls, driving patients to appointments, and going to funerals. The practitioners in the study describe both the professional and personal satisfaction derived from their caring practices, even when the rewards of such actions were small. Lewis and Brykczynski (1994) situate their work within a caring paradigm, citing work by Gadow, Watson, and Leininger. They also cite the 1991 work of Benner, who in studying the effectiveness of expert nurses, found that mere technique and knowledge were not enough, and that caring, or a certain level of human involvement, was required for expert human practice. Expert "human practice" is a goal for all primary care providers.

Ackerman et al (1996) at the University of Rochester School of Nursing and Medical Center developed a model of advanced practice for acute-care nurse practitioners. Placing the patient in the center of their model, they delineate five domains of practice:

1. Direct, comprehensive care
2. Support of systems
3. Education
4. Research
5. Publication and professional leadership

These domains are situated in a continuum of novice to expert practice. Conceptual strands pervade the model and provide unity to its structure. These include empowerment, scholarship, and collaboration. The model, designed like a web, envisions the role of the acute-care nurse practitioner as facilitating the progression of the patient through the health-care system in an efficient and cost-effective manner with the patient always at the center. The patient's needs are the priority. A major function of the acute-care nurse practitioner is to ensure that the patient's needs are met and that nothing is missed (Ackerman et al, 1996). Although it is an elegant conceptualization of advanced practice role-functions in an acute-care setting, this model does not describe specific elements, such as advanced practice nursing interventions, that distinguish the practice.

Johnson (1993) cites clear evidence of a nursing perspective in nurse practitioner practice in primary care. According to Johnson, nurse practitioner–patient dialogue incorporates the voice of medicine and the voice of the "life-world" (of the patient). The medical management of patients is blended into the nursing role, acknowledging the importance of management but not letting it overshadow the life-world experience of the patient. One nurse practitioner said, "The medical aspect is a piece of the nursing care plan anyway." Because nurse practitioner education includes physical assessment and medical management, it "gives you a chance to make a better assessment and be a better nurse." The skilled practitioner "knows self" and how to share his or her own personal experience to either enhance the patient's progress or strengthen the provider–patient bond. An element of camaraderie was viewed as positive and not in opposition to maintaining a professional stance. Coordination, continuity, and advocacy were the major functions the nurse practitioners in this study believed they contributed to the practice. Given the nature of our current (broken) health-care system, all primary care practice would be enriched by such approaches.

Swanson (1995) proposed "A Spirit-Focused Conceptual Model of Nursing for the Advanced Practice Nurse" in which she identifies the core of every person, both patient and nurse, as the spirit, defined as an animating or vital principle held to give life to physical organisms (based on the definition of "spirit" in Webster's 9th New Collegiate Dictionary, 1987). She describes the act of nursing as a goal-directed interpersonal relationship between the patient and nurse, based on traditional nursing process components such as assessing, planning, intervening, and evaluating. Interventions are broad-based, ranging from play, music, and stories to utilization of counseling principles such as active listening and anticipatory guidance. The use of this approach in primary care practice could be adapted by any primary care practitioner.

The Schuler Nurse Practitioner Practice Model (1993) is an ambitious attempt to describe the nurse practitioner's integrated role. It is rooted in a wholistic patient database that includes physical, psychological, social, cultural, environmental, and spiritual dimensions. The database enables the nurse practitioner to accurately identify and evaluate patient needs that are categorized as either health or health-related. Health needs refer to a person's current physical and psychological health status, and health-related needs refer to those that originate from cultural and health beliefs, social support and networks, environmental or occupational conditions, and spiritual tenets.

Mutually identifying unmet patient health needs is the first step in identifying health problems in this model. The treatment plan must be mutually agreeable and oriented toward self-care; disease prevention and health promotion activities are incorporated into the treatment plan. Nonpharmacological treatments, including alternative healing practices, are also integrated into the plan. This is all framed within the concept of functioning within a multidisciplinary team.

In addition, this model is seen as enhancing both the patient and nurse practitioner's personal movement toward wellness. Patients are encouraged to examine their lives honestly and to identify areas that are not "balanced." The patient's physical and psychological ability to participate in wellness activities is assessed; creative, uninhibited problem-solving and identification of appropriate wellness activities are pursued. The model emphasizes that the primary care provider's personal commitment to wellness and health can have a direct impact on the practitioner's ability to influence positive patient outcomes.

Another interesting approach to nursing phenomena, not elaborated as unique for APNs, but yet with wide applicability to the autonomy of an advanced practice nursing role, is "symptom management." This work has evolved from the University of California, San Francisco School of Nursing Symptom Management Faculty Group (1994). Proponents of this approach note that when the underlying cause of the patient's problem and the presenting symptoms are managed concurrently, patients are more likely to benefit and remain in treatment.

The Symptom Management group proposes that symptoms be viewed as subjective experiences reflecting changes in a person's biopsychosocial function, sensation, or cognition. They contrast this view of the word "symptom" with the word "sign," which is used to mean an abnormality indicative of disease, which can be observed by another person and sometimes by the patient. The model they propose for looking at symptoms has three dimensions:

1. The symptom experience
2. Symptom management strategies
3. Symptom outcomes

The model encompasses a multidimensional approach to the experience of the symptom, ways to approach the management of symptoms (always in concert with the patient and family and cognizant of health-care system interactions), and outcomes that are gauged on a variety of axes.

Snyder and Mirr (1995) conceptualize advanced practice within a nursing paradigm around human responses as a focus for nursing interventions. Drawing on the 1980 Social Policy Statement published by the American Nurses Association (ANA), they conceptualize the following areas as a focus for advanced practice nursing:

1. Self-care limitations
2. Impaired functioning in areas of rest, sleep, ventilation, circulation, nutrition, and the like
3. Pain and discomfort
4. Emotional problems related to illness and treatment, life-threatening events, or daily experiences, such as anxiety, loss, or loneliness
5. Distortion of symbolic functions reflected in interpersonal and intellectual processes such as hallucinations
6. Deficiencies in decision-making ability to make personal choices
7. Self-image changes required by health status
8. Dysfunctional perceptual orientations to health
9. Strains related to life processes such as birth, development, and death
10. Problematic affiliative relationships

Patient problems, conceptualized in this manner, are amenable to uniquely nursing-based interventions. Attention to human responses, as such, provide the missing link to much that is absent within today's contemporary health-care system. In similar fashion, the associated interventions—often specifically "low tech"—provide a promise of improved outcomes that are meaningful to patients and not just to their providers or administrators. Our current health-care system, however, is not structured in such a way to make many of these practices sustainable: they are not coded for reimbursement. And additional outcome data are needed to make a compelling case for fee-for-service.

The 1995 Nursing: A Social Policy Statement

The 1995 Social Policy Statement published by the ANA specifically addresses advanced nursing practice (p 14). The role of the APN is defined as still rooted in traditional nursing process: that is, the APN is defined as someone who works with individuals, families, groups, and communities to "assess health needs; develop diagnoses; plan, implement, and manage care; and evaluate outcomes of care." APNs are also seen as planning and advocating care that promotes health and prevents disease and disability; directing care or managing systems of care for complex patient, family, and community populations; managing acute and chronic illnesses, childbirth, and the care of patients before, during, and after anesthesia; and prescribing, administering, and evaluating pharmacological treatment regimens.

Advanced practice registered nurses (APRNs) are defined in this 1995 policy statement as nurses who have acquired the knowledge base and practice experiences to prepare them for specialization, expansion, and advancement in practice. *Specialization* is defined as concentrating or delimiting one's focus to a particular area of practice; *expansion* refers to the acquisition of new practice knowledge and skills (including in areas that may overlap the bounds of traditional medical practice); and *advancement* involves both specialization and role expansion, characterized by integration of theoretical, research-based, and practical knowledge that occurs as part of graduate education in nursing.

Significantly, although the 1995 statement reaffirms a commitment to nursing process, it spells out the phenomena of concern to nurses as "human experiences and responses to birth, health, illness, and death." The authors note that since the 1980 statement, nursing philosophy and practice have been greatly influenced by the science of *caring*. They go on to elaborate that contemporary nursing practice attends to the range of human experiences and responses to health and illness without restriction to a problem-focused orientation: they emphasize that objective data must be situated within the context of the patient, family, group, or community's subjective experience; and that it is the provision of a caring relationship that facilitates health and healing (p 6). This has implications for all primary care practice.

Changing Models of Medical Practice

Changes are afoot in medical practice. It is commonly recognized that the educated consumer, who often has access to the Internet, in the context of a cost-conscious environment and such trends as the move from hospital to community, multiculturalism, the growing interest in holistic care and alternative therapies, an increasingly litigious environment, and increased use of technology will continue to force reexamination of traditional professional roles.

Advances in therapeutics that have occurred over the course of the 20th century, which are often taken for granted, are overwhelmingly different than any that have ever been seen earlier. Medicine is able to routinely intervene, specifically, powerfully, and radically, in the course of previously fatal diseases. No disorder, however complex, is beyond the possibility of conquest. As a result, the impact of medicine's capabilities is felt far beyond the immediacies of the patient–provider encounter. Medicine now shapes the economic, demographic, and social structure of human populations; to deny this reality would be naive.

A review of the progress of medicine in combating disease is a journey from an integrated view of illness and therapeutics to one of discrete diseases with distinct causes, and an armamentarium of ever-expanding and specific therapeutics. At one time, dating back to the ancient Greek and Roman era but persisting well into the 19th century, illness was seen as an imbalance in the economy of the whole body, which could be expressed in the relationships between input or output of food, sweat, secretions, urine, phlegm, and the like. Treatment was focused on restoring harmony and balance between body and environment (a view promulgated by Nightingale, 1860/1969). Specific symptoms were not attacked; instead, a systemic physiologic effect was sought through such methods as inducing or facilitating sweating, febrilysis, diuresis, and/or vomiting. These interventions, it was theorized, would assist the body to recover its balance.

Through the course of the 19th century, however, this integrated view of disease and therapeutics was increasingly challenged by notions of discrete disease states with specific causes. Illnesses seemed less amenable to purges, bleeding, and diuretics, the so-called holistic approaches, than was previously thought. Quite late in the modern era, the first active principles of some of the oldest, most useful botanicals were isolated, and later some were even synthesized. A new dimension was added to the emerging concept of specificity of therapeutics by the discovery of sulfonamides, in the late 1930s, and penicillin, in the early 1940s. Not only could therapy be directed at particular symptoms, but for the first time, therapeutics could become "radical," matching the powers of the surgeon's knife—that is, they could eradicate the primary cause of an illness, in this case, specific microorganisms.

Even more highly specific measures, such as the use of antisera, the isolation of blood fractions, and the synthesis of polypeptide hormones, are products of the last few decades. Advances in laboratory analysis and diagnostic techniques confer on therapeutics the capability of effecting cure at the molecular loci of disease. The era of specific and radical therapeutics has really only begun. What seems certain is the trend toward even greater specificity in diagnosis and treatment of disease, extending to the genetic level. This will continue to have profound effects on the medical profession, society, and on inherent power balances between patient, nurse, and physician.

Medicine's successes have led to a generation of physician-specialists, some of whom are far removed from the day-to-day lives of their patients. The effectiveness of modern therapeutics adds a powerful strain of reductionism and positivism to the 21st-century medical ethos. This has been useful in seeking out radically effective medical treatments. When these interventions become universalized, however, to all realms of medical practice, they become impediments to the fulfillment of the more sensitive moral and social responsibilities of medicine. Care, when defined as helping the patient and family to cope, offering reassurance, educating, and relieving worry, though not necessarily deprecated, does not require a high level of scientific sophistication. When the physician's remuneration was meager and he or she was a member of the community, issues such as those raised above may have been negotiated more successfully between doctor and patient. The doctor of today, however, is more often a stranger. This raises a fearful dilemma for patients: They must trust the physician because of his or her power to heal, but that trust is undermined by the fear of the physician's self-interest.

Medicine is not unaware of this quandary; indeed these issues are widely discussed in medical circles and beyond. An ad hoc group representing a cross section of policymakers, health-care providers, and insurance companies drafted the Pew Health Commission report, "Critical Challenges: Revitalizing the Health professions for the Twenty-First Century." According to this commission, medical schools must produce more generalists and fewer specialists; health professions should aim to promote the wellness of communities rather than to try to fill hospital beds. A loss of 60 percent of the nation's hospital beds is predicted. Richard D. Lamm, former governor of Colorado and chairman of the report, said, "Allopathic medicine does not give the country that much health. I think nine-tenths of the health of a community has to do with their habits, their lifestyles, their environment, their genetics, etc., and I think allopathic medicine only operates at the margin, yet we have put all our efforts into it."

All health professional schools are charged with expanding the scientific base of their programs to include the psychosocial–behavioral sciences, as well as population-based approaches to clinical work. Sharing of clinical teaching resources, especially in key areas of preclinical and clinical training, is mandated, as well as cross-teaching and more exploration of the roles played by various professionals. Active modeling of effective team integration in the delivery of efficient, high-quality care was seen as essential.

Many in medicine are taking note. Dacher (1995) espouses a model he calls "the Whole Healing model," which is rooted in assumptions of dynamism, holism, and purposefulness. He calls for a renewed emphasis on the quality and character of the relationships that constitute the healing process—the practitioner to himself, his or her patient, other practitioners, and the community at large—and a careful balance between reductive and holistic perspectives (p 30). This integrated model expands the diagnostic process, for example, to include a concern with psychological, spiritual, community, and environmental issues and acknowledges the uniqueness and subjectivity of a person's life circumstances.

This approach is totally consistent with a nursing-based approach. Dacher (1995) says, "Responsibility must at all times move toward the individual and away from the professional" (p 32). He theorizes that the "art" will return to medicine. And what is this art? "It is the creative capacity to enter into the experience of another human being, understand from the client's perspective that nature of that life and its forces (by empathic listening) and participate with this individual in composing a health life, involving recovery, healing, and health—the fully lived life" (p 32).

Jeanne Achterberg, senior editor of *Alternative Therapies,* at the closing plenary session of "Creating Integrated Healthcare" in 1996 elaborated seven fundamental aspects of medicine:

1. Trust, which is what imbues the caregiver with power
2. Communication, conceptualized as a dual process
3. Linkage to the divine
4. Shared worldviews of a culture
5. Rituals
6. Medicine as a holy privilege
7. A concept of caring and compassion, inseparable from cure

She also discusses qualities associated with healing and personal transformation. She suggests that *passion* for something—anything—seems to allow one to grow larger than a problem; that *creativity* can provoke healing (she goes so far as to suggest that the cessation of creativity may trigger disease). In addition, she focuses on *intentionality,* both on the part of the healer and the patient as an essential element of healing, stating that the effectiveness of any therapeutic intervention may well reside in intentionality. *Self-discovery,* defined as the process of finding one's true self, of placing circumstances—no matter how taxing or dreadful—into the appropriate chapters of one's life story, is a fourth quality associated with healing.

In *Patient-Centered Medicine,* the physician authors (Stewart et al, 1995) speak loudly to the need for a new method of patient care, founded in new paradigms. On the limitations of the current medical model, situated in the context of disease and curative, for example, radical therapeutics, the authors remind us that "A particular disease is what everyone with that disease has in common, but the illness experience of every person is unique" (p 32). *Patient-Centered Medicine* espouses a model that encourages exploring both the disease and illness experience, understanding the whole person, finding common ground, incorporating prevention and health promotion, enhancing the patient doctor relationship, and being realistic. Clearly, these components have been well established in nursing models.

In 2003 the Institute of Medicine published *Health Professions Education: A Bridge to Quality.* This report on reforming education for the health professions emphasized the relationship of high-quality and safe patient care to substantive changes in the way health professionals are educated. Five core competencies were identified:

- Provide patient-centered care.
- Work in interdisciplinary teams.
- Use evidence-based practice.
- Apply quality improvement.
- Use informatics.

These competencies no doubt sound familiar to baccalaureate- and higher-degree nursing educators. The American Association of Colleges of Nursing's (AACN) *The Essentials of Baccalaureate Education for Professional Nursing* Practice (1998) includes, to some extent, all the core competencies recommended in the Institute of Medicine report. *Healthy People 2010* encourages the rexamination of clinical education by including an objective to "increase the proportion of schools of medicine, schools of nursing and health professional training schools whose basic curriculum for health care providers includes the core competencies in health promotion and disease prevention."

Medicine recognizes the need to incorporate new perspectives of practice, essentially following long-established leads from nursing. Likewise, it is equally appropriate that nursing incorporate traditional aspects of the medical model into its continually expanding scope of practice. Patient problems, after all, are real and as such are complex, necessitating multidimensional approaches. The Circle of Caring model (discussed next) is offered as a unique approach to patient problems, one that incorporates and builds on both traditional nursing and medical approaches, as well as retaining an openness to a variety of other approaches to phenomena. This model may indeed reflect what most primary care providers intuitively "do;" it attempts to put this reality on paper, making more *visible* the so-often invisible work of nursing in the health-care encounter, "work" that is not coded and reimbursed but that is there and is often tremendously meaningful for the patient. In this sense, this model is not actually original, but rather is derived from the realities of day-to-day advanced nursing practice in primary care.

A Transformative Template: The Circle of Caring

Both the traditional medical and nursing models are predicated on a subjective and objective database, a labeling of the patient's problem and response, a therapeutic plan, and an evaluation of the outcome. The Circle of Caring model builds on these features and expands them to include:

1. A broadened and contextualized database
2. A labeling of the patient's concern that more actively incorporates the patient's responses to the meaning of illness in his or her day-to-day life, as well as standard medical diagnostic language
3. A holistic approach to an individualized, therapeutic plan that includes nursing-based interventions along with complementary therapies, as appropriate, incorporated into standardized pharmacologic, surgical, and other non-pharmacologic interventions
4. A view of outcomes based on the patient, family, group, and community perceptions of improvement as well as the more traditional, quantified outcome measures such as mortality and morbidity data

The Circle of Caring model is a synthesized view of the problem-solving methodology that may be used in a variety of settings—primary-care, acute-care, and community-based settings. A linear representation of the problem-solving method necessitated in practice was chosen for clarity of communication of the concepts of the model, and it is embedded in the middle of the schema (see Fig. 1.2).

This process is encircled by caring, a visual representation of the interpersonal process occurring between caregiver and the patient, family, group, and community. The ability to provide effective and meaningful care for the patient is predicated on the processes of care. This is what enables the nurse to hear the patient's "call" and to fashion creative nursing responses. The process of care is actualized through caring processes drawn from Mayerhoff (1971) and Boykin and Schoenhofer (1993): patience, courage, advocacy, authentic presence, commitment, and knowing.

A Broadened, Contextualized Database

A contextualized approach—the lived experience of the patient, family, group, in the context of community—is central to this model and is one that most nurses have learned in their undergraduate programs. Although the patient's subjective perception of experience is captured in the history portion of the assessment database, the Circle of Caring is predicated on hearing the patient's story in all its complexity, as well as eliciting the meaning of *health* to the patient, family, group, and community. In addition, increased attention is focused on the interplay among perceptual, psychodynamic, socioeconomic, cultural, and environmental factors that have an impact on the patient's health status.

The Nature of Patient Responses

The 1995 American Nurses Association's Social Policy Statement defines nursing as the "diagnosis and treatment of human responses to actual and potential health problems."

The Circle of Caring model may be used effectively with the traditional tool of nursing diagnosis. Boykin and Schoenhofer (1993) conceptualized the phenomenon of human responses as "calls for nursing." As such, these calls remain unique, interactional, and contextualized, and thus not amenable to any form of generic labeling. It is through coming to know people as caring persons that the nurse is able to fully hear each patient's call. There are any number of ways to label the category called "identification of patient's responses to illness." The wording on the template could be changed depending on the nursing theoretical lens utilized, but the underlying phenomenon remains the same and is instinctively, intuitively understood by nurses.

Although the use of both medical diagnosis and patient responses may seem cumbersome, as collaborative practice increases, a more generic labeling of clinical phenomena may well emerge. One example is the Agency for Health Care Policy and Research (AHCPR) guidelines, generated around clinical conditions that are often labeled in a more generic fashion, for example, low back pain, heart failure, post-stroke rehabilitation. The democratization of information and databases used by an increasingly informed consumer all necessitate such a tradition.

The importance of the labeling of the patient's problem, or "call," be it in medical or nursing diagnostic terminology or in a more generic format, is that it helps the patient responses to be addressed more effectively. Labeling thus involves the acknowledgment and knowledge of the complex interplay of perceptual, psychodynamic, socioeconomic, cultural, and environmental factors that contribute to health. APNs are especially skilled at eliciting and understanding this human phenomenon, and at fashioning nursing-based responses that are uniquely suited to the individual.

A Creative Approach to Therapeutics

Another hallmark of this model is its broadened approach to therapeutics. In reality, this is actualized in day-to-day practice by APNs, yet it remains an especially invisible piece of nursing work. This flexible nursing-based approach entails working with the individual patient to tailor interventions geared to the meaning of "health" as defined by that patient, family, group, or community. Building on current standards of medical and nursing practice, interventions are fine-tuned for each patient. Alternative and complementary therapies are considered. This requires a creative approach to therapeutics that includes holistic approaches to healing. Research in this area is proliferating as patients, families, groups, and communities are calling for alternative and complementary approaches.

In nursing as caring, the nurse is an artist who responds creatively to calls for nursing with unique nursing responses. This has, in part, contributed to the dilemma that has kept nursing invisible—that is, how to make visible and, more importantly, generalizable the aspect of care that must be unique and individualized in order to be meaningful for patients. Any taxonomy of nursing must, of necessity, have universal applicability. What distinguishes so many of nursing's interventions, however, is precisely their uniqueness, the tailoring of an individual response to each patient. This is the artistry of the APN.

Outcomes: According to Whom? Who Decides?

The Circle of Caring model also predicates a broadened view of outcomes. Outcome-based research of today demonstrates the need to incorporate patients' perceptions as measured objectively (by functional assessments and similar methods) and subjectively. Quality-of-life measures and, most importantly, the meaning of health and illness to the patient, family, group, and community must be taken more fully into consideration. Plans must be assessed according to their potential to assist patients, families, groups, and communities to meet their goals in ways that are meaningful to them, not just in terms of their potential to improve mortality and morbidity measures. The voice of an increasingly informed, information-savvy consumer demands no less.

Environmental science and the impact of multiple environmental factors on health and the experience of a healthful life are recognized as additional pieces of the health-care puzzle, that of public health. Labeled "community-oriented primary care" in current medical textbooks, these approaches, along with preventive aspects of care, were largely abandoned by medical science in the earlier parts of this century in favor of science, technology, and specialization. Medicine has awakened to the renewed need for such approaches to deal with current health-care realities such as violence, teen pregnancy, and acquired immunodeficiency syndrome (AIDS). Like medicine, nursing has renewed its emphasis on community-based approaches, reaffirming its historic roots.

The Circle of Caring

The Circle of Caring model (Fig. 1.3) has grown out of, and is rooted in, the assumption that caring is the central concept in nursing and is uniquely known and expressed in nursing. It builds on a definition of nursing as defined by Boykin and Schoenhofer (1993). Specifically, they view nursing as a discipline of knowledge and a professional service that has as its goal nurturing persons living caring and growing in caring (p 21). Further, Boykin and Schoenhofer (1993) contend that all nursing takes place within nursing situations, "shared lived experiences in which caring between the persons of nurse and nursed enhances the process of living and growing in caring (p 3)."

Watson (1988) viewed caring as an intersubjective human process, the ideal of intersubjectivity based on the belief that "persons learn from one another how to be human by identifying ourselves with others or finding their dilemmas

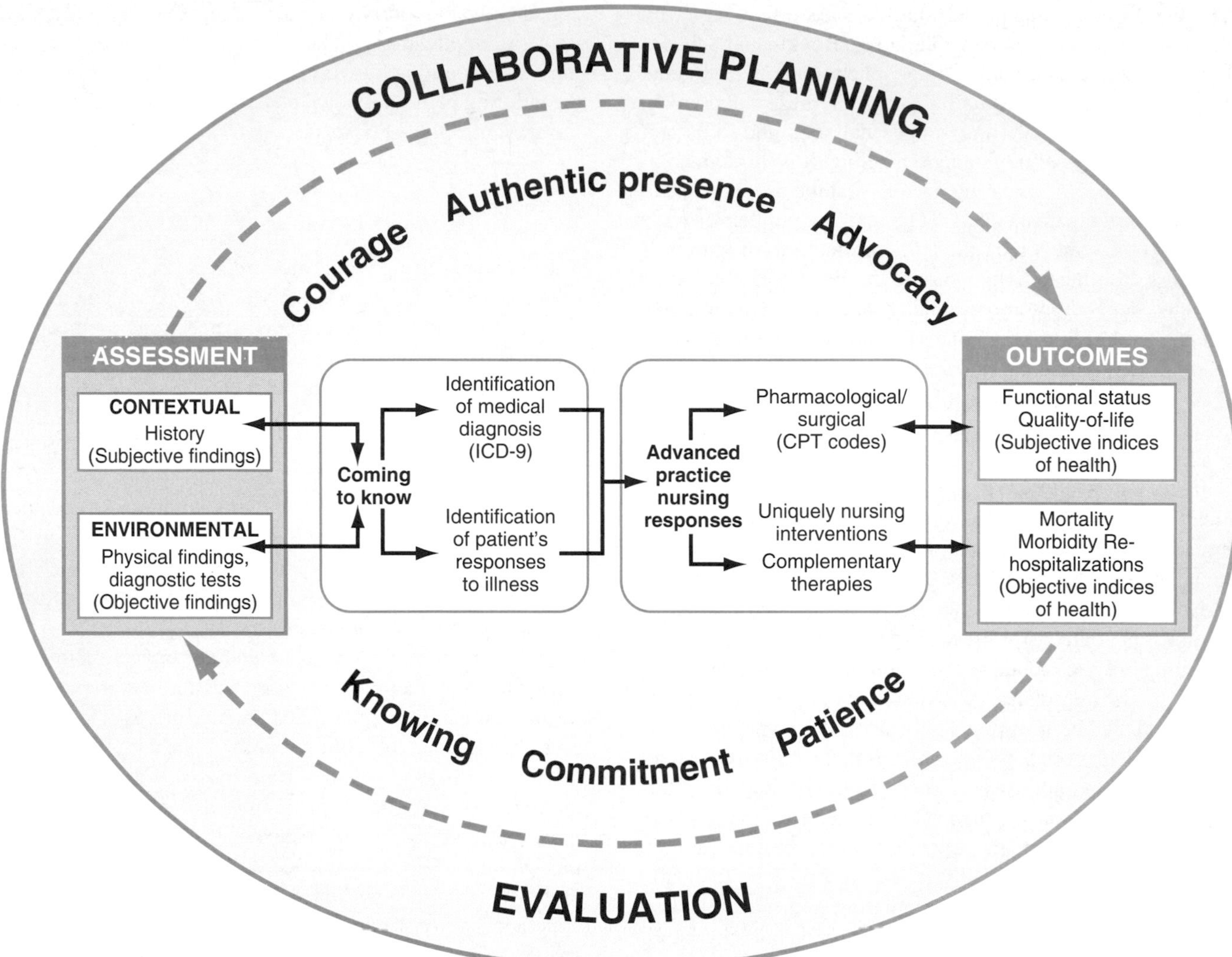

FIGURE 1.3 The Circle of Caring model.

in ourselves (p 6)." Boykin and Schoenhofer (1993) extend this and define caring in nursing as "the intentional and authentic presence of the nurse with another who is recognized as a person living caring and growing in caring (p 25)."

Mayeroff (1971) discussed the primacy of caring as a process in contrast to caring as a product, with caring viewed as an end in and of itself. Mayeroff also identified "ingredients" of caring: knowing, alternating rhythms, patience, honesty, courage, humility, and hope. Boykin and Schoenhofer viewed caring in nursing "... as a mutual human process in which the nurse responds with authentic presence to a call from another (1993, p 33)." The caring attributes of the Circle of Caring—knowing, patience, authentic presence, commitment, courage, and advocacy—are elaborated by Boykin and Schoenhofer in Chapter 2. It is the caring attributes that characterize the nurse–patient (or family, group, and community) relationship, enabling healing.

An added dimension of Boykin and Schoenhofer's (1993) conception of caring is the extension of multiple ways of knowing. Carper's (1978) analysis of the nursing literature yielded four patterns of knowing: (1) empirics, the science of nursing; (2) esthetics, the art of nursing; (3) personal knowing; and (4) ethics, the component of moral knowledge. Building on that work, Boykin, Parker, and Schoenhofer (1994) propose that "... aesthetic knowledge in nursing is the creating experience in the nursing situation, expression of the experience, and appreciation of it through encounter (p 160)." All nursing and nursing-related knowledge and activities are grounded in *nursing situations.*

Expressing nursing as an art requires an understanding of the art of nursing. The nurse artist values unique individual experiences. By being open to the aesthetic pathway, the fullness of the nursing situation is known. The aesthetic pathway fosters full realization of the interconnectedness of persons and objects. Each experience of creating and appreciating is unique and cannot be predicted; it is the experience of aesthetic knowing that is primary in nursing, rather than either the process of creating or the product. The nurse may bring science and empirics to the nursing situation yet can never exactly predict the outcomes. Nursing practice is seen not as linear but as a continual unfolding. The nurse responds to the call of the patient and responds in concert, with mutuality, consonance, and harmony of action. Examples of nursing situations are presented throughout this text, adding a dimension to practice often left unspoken.

Caring: An Integrated Approach

Neither nurses nor physicians alone can take on the undeniable challenges of the current health-care system. Neither the discipline and profession of medicine nor nursing alone can claim to heal the current problems. Both are needed more than ever in carving a healthful future. Both professions are being forced to rethink their roles, functions, and cultures. Moving away from the safety and hierarchical role structures of the hospital setting creates the opportunity for retooling the content and processes of the clinical landscape, renegotiating a new, as yet undefined space. The boundaries of practice continue to expand and contract for both disciplines. The larger questions, for both professions, include: "How will all health care professionals be accountable to their patients?" "Are physicians and APNs willing to share accountability in a responsible manner?" "How can the Institute of Medicine's *Bridge to Quality* become a reality?" And, "How can disciplines work together in a meaningful way to achieve the goals and objectives of *Healthy People 2010?"*

Lynaugh, in an unpublished paper, advocates that both disciplines can occupy the same territory to the benefit of patient care; however, she notes that tension is created by proximity, stating that "... physicians and nurses quarrel occasionally when they jostle each other in the narrow passageway of patient care (p 20)." She makes the case, however, that tension is preferable to the distrust and ignorance that stem from silence and distance between the two disciplines. She advocates a "productive tension" and social parity between the two disciplines, noting that it is the care of all patients that will benefit. Nurses and physicians are natural allies. Both are needed on the same side of the playing field for good and effective change to occur in the health-care system. Never did we need both perspectives more.

Don't Throw Out the Baby with the Bathwater

Espousing a multiparadigmatic approach, the Circle of Caring model embraces a multidisciplinary perspective. Engebretson (1997) states, "Many times the praxis of nursing is covertly, if not overtly, aligned with the medical model" (p 22). The purpose of the Circle of Caring model is to make the "jostling" more explicit. Nurses have straddled these disparate worlds, a holistic universe defined by nursing philosophy and theory, and day-to-day biomedical practice. As essential as the nurse–patient relationship, grounded in caring, is to the care of patients, it is recognized that it provides only part of the story. The APN must be conversant with the empirics of current "medical" practice, which when enacted through a nursing prism, can provide a vital and overall missing piece in today's managed care environment

The Circle of Caring is a nursing-based template superimposed on the traditional medical model to create a new whole. As such, it builds on traditional aspects of medical decision-making and therapeutics as well as on the problem-solving approach of the nursing process. The Circle of Caring model synthesizes these many strands. The Circle of Caring encompasses, in essence, a nursing situation. Each encounter is unique and is guided by the caring processes of authentic presence, knowing, courage, patience, advocacy, and commitment. Caring is seen as the way to bridge the gulf between holistic nursing theories and biomedical nursing praxis. Caring permeates the entire encounter.

Encircled by Caring

Daily in practice, primary care providers hear the frustration of patients and families in dealing with today's health-care system. Although the technology of medical care continues unabated, the interactional and collaborative aspects of care are often underdeveloped. A Circle of Caring model is needed for patients, families, groups, and communities. This is also a way to document and describe the practice of primary care providers, who respond to calls from patients and who imaginatively, creatively, and powerfully foster appropriate responses. These responses may be fashioned on the microlevel—the one-to-one clinician–patient relationship in primary or acute care, for example, or on a macrolevel, as uniquely nursing-based knowledge unites with traditional public health approaches and is applied to the care of communities and populations (see Chapter 3). These transformative models, Circles of Caring, incorporate the individual strengths of nursing, public health, and medicine, but reformulate them in a new model of care. Primary care clinicians are the appropriate providers to demonstrate the efficacy of an integrated model of caregiving, rooted in the lived experience of the patient as experienced in the context of community. This text provides the necessary tools to do this in ways that will be meaningful for patients, families, groups, and communities.

Bibliography

Achterberg, J: What is medicine? Altern Ther 2:3, 1996.

Ackerman, MH, et al: Development of a model of advanced practice nursing. Am J Crit Care 5(1):68, 1996.

American Medical Association. Physician's Current Procedural Terminology—CPT 99. Author, Chicago, 2005.

American Nurses' Association: Nursing: A Social Policy Statement. Author, Kansas City, Mo., 1980.

American Nurses' Association: Nursing: A Social Policy Statement. American Nurses' Association, Kansas City, Mo., 1995.

Baer, E: Philosophical and historical bases of primary care nursing.

In Mezey, MD and McGivern, DO (eds): Nurses, Nurse Practitioners: Evolution to Advanced Practice, ed 2. Springer, New York, 1993.
Benner, P: From Novice to Expert. Addison-Wesley, Menlo Park, Calif., 1984.
Benner, P, and Wrubel, J: The Primacy of Caring: Stress and Coping in Health and Illness. Addison-Wesley, Menlo Park, Calif., 1989.
Boykin, A, Parker, ME, Schoenhofer, SO: Aesthetic knowing grounded in an explicit conception of nursing. Nurs Sci Q 7(4):158–161, 1994.
Boykin, A, and Schoenhofer, S: Nursing as Caring: A Model for Transforming Practice. National League for Nursing Press, New York, 1993.
Carper, BA: Fundamental patterns of knowing in nursing. Adv Nurs Sci 1(1):13 – 23.
Cody, WK: Nursing theory-guided practice: What it is and what it is not. Nurs Sci Q 7(4):144–145, 1994.
Dacher, E: Reinventing primary care. J Altern Ther Health Med 1(5):29–34, 1995.
Dock, LL, and Stewart, IB: A Short History of Nursing. G. P. Putnam's Sons; New York, 1920.
Eisenberg, L: Disease and illness: Distinctions between professional and popular ideas of sickness. Cult Med Psychiatry 1:9, 1977.
Engebretson, J: A multiparadigm approach to nursing. Adv Nurs Sci 20(1):21–33, 1997.
Fenton, MV, and Brykczynski, KA: Qualitative distinctions and similarities in the practice of the clinical nurse specialists and nurse practitioners. J Prof Nurs 9:313, 1993.
Gordon, M: Nursing Diagnosis: Process and Application, ed 2. McGraw-Hill, New York, 1987.
Henderson, V: The Nature of Nursing. Macmillan, New York, 1966.
Henderson, V, and Nite, G: Principles and Practice of Nursing. Macmillan, New York, 1978.
Howie, JGR: A new look at illness in general practice: A reclassification of illness based on antibiotic prescribing. In Rakel, R (ed): Textbook of Family Practice, ed 4. WB Saunders, Philadelphia, 1995.
Institute of Medicine: Health Professional Education: A Bride to Quality. National Academy Press, Washington, D.C. 2003.
Institute of Medicine: Health Care Quality Initiative: Crossing the Quality Chasm: A New Health Care System for the Twenty-First Century. National Academy Press, Washington, D.C., 2001.
International Council of Nurses. Nurses' Next Advance: An International Classification for Nursing Practice, ICN, Geneva, 1993.
Johnson, R: Nurse practitioner patient discourse: Uncovering the voice of nursing in primary care practice. Schol Inq Nurs Pract Int J 7(3):143, 1993.
Kleinman, A, et al: Culture, illness, and care: Clinical lessons from anthropologic and cross-cultural research. Ann Intern Med 99:25, 1978.
Lewis, PH, and Brykczynski, KA: Practical knowledge and competencies of the healing role of the nurse practitioner. J Am Acad Nurse Pract 6(5):207– 213, 1994.
Locsin, RC: Technology and caring. In Boykin, A (ed): Power, Politics, and Public Policy. National League for Nursing Press, New York, 1995.
Lynaugh, J: Narrow passageways: Nurses and physicians in conflict and concert since 1875 (unpublished paper).
Lynaugh, JE, and Bates, B: The two languages of nursing and medicine. Am J Nurs 73(1):66, 1973.
Madden, M: Conceptualizations of advanced nursing practice. In Hamne AB, Spross JA, and Hanson CM (eds): Advanced Practice Nursing: An Integrative Approach. WB Saunders, Philadelphia, 1996, pp 25–41.
Mayerhoff, M: On Caring. Harper and Row, New York, 1971.
McCloskey, J, and Bulechek, GM: Standardizing the language for nursing treatments. Nurs Outlook 42(4):45, 1994.
Mishler, EG: The Discourse of Medicine: Dialectics of Medical Interviews. Ablex, Norwood, N.J., 1984.
Mitchell, G: Nursing diagnosis: An obstacle to caring ways. In Boykin, A (ed): Power, Politics, and Public Policy. National League for Nursing Press, New York, 1995.
Moore, N: PEW Commission Report: Focusing care on the community for the 21st century. Altern Ther 2:5, 1996.
Nightingale, F: Notes on Nursing: What It Is and What It Is Not. Dover, New York, 1860–1969.
Parker, M: Exploring the aesthetic meaning of presence in nursing practice. In Gaut, D (ed): The Presence of Caring in Nursing. National League for Nursing Press, New York, 1992.
Pew Health Professions Commission: Phase Two. Shifting the supply of our health care workforce: A Guide to Redirecting Federal Subsidy of Medical Education. Pew Charitable Trust Foundation, San Francisco, Calif., 1995.
Rakel, R: Textbook of Family Practice, ed 6. WB Saunders, Philadelphia, 1995.
Reed, PG: A treatise on nursing knowledge development for the 21st century: Beyond postmodernism. Adv Nurs Sci 17(3):70, 1995.
Rogers, ME: Nursing: To be or not to be? Nurs Outlook 20:42–46, 1972.
Rogers, M: The nurse practitioner movement: Pro and con. Am J Nurs 75(10):1834–1843, 1975.
St. Anthony's: ICD-9-CM: Code Book for Physician Payment, Vol 1 and 2, St. Anthony Publishing, Cincinnati, 2005.
San Francisco School of Nursing Management Faculty Group: A model for symptom management. Image J Nurs Scholar, 26(4):272 – 276, 1994.
Schuler, PA, and Davis, JE: The Schuler Nurse Practitioner Practice Model. J Am Acad Nurse Pract 5(1):11–17, 1993.
Shalala, DE: Nursing and society—The unfinished agenda for the 21st century. Nurs Health Care 14(6): 1993.
Snyder, M: Defining nursing interventions. Image J Nurs Scholar 28(2):137, 1996.
Snyder, M: Independent Nursing Intervention, ed 2. Delmar, Albany, N.Y., 1992.
Snyder, M, and Mirr, MP: Advanced practice nursing within a nursing paradigm. In Snyder, M and Mirr, MP (eds): Advanced Practice Nursing: A Guide to Professional Development. Delmar, Albany, N.Y., 1995.
Stewart, M, et al: Patient-Centered Medicine: Transforming the Clinical Method. SAGE Publications, Thousand Oaks, Calif., 1995.
Swanson, C: A spirit-focused conceptual model of nursing for the advanced practice nurse. Issues Comp Pediatr Nurs 18:267–275, 1995.
U.S. Department of Health and Human Services. Health People 2010. International Medical Publishing, McLean, VA, 2000.
University of California, San Francisco, School of Nursing Symptom Management Faculty Group: A Model for Symptom Management. Image J Nurs Scholar 26:272–276, 1994.
Watson, J: Nursing: Human Science and Human Care. Appleton-Century-Crofts, Norwalk, Conn., 1988.
Websters' 9th New Collegiate Dictionary. Merriam-Webster, Springfield, MA, 1987.
Wolf, ZR: Uncovering the hidden work of nursing. Nurs Health Care, 10, 1989.
Zimmer, P, et al: Advanced Practice Nursing: Nurse Practitioner Curriculum Guidelines. National Organization of Nurse Practitioner Faculty, Seattle, Wash., 1990.

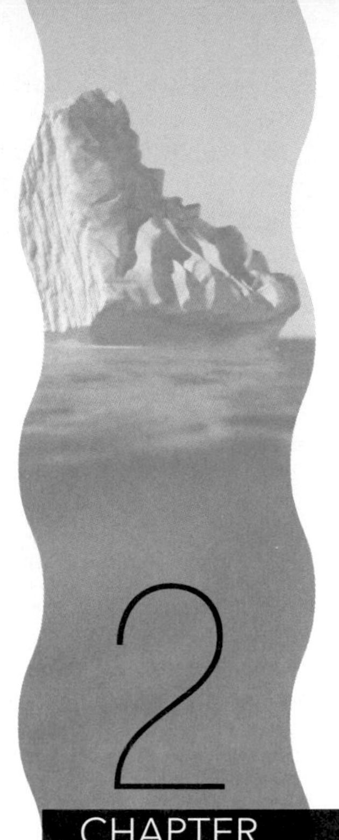

Caring and the Advanced Practice Nurse

Anne Boykin, PhD, RN
Savina O. Schoenhofer, PhD, RN

2
CHAPTER

The role of advanced practice nurse (APN) is a special way of nursing. While the role often blends elements of medical practice and generic primary care, it is also a form of nursing and is thus characterized by caring as a way of being, knowing, and doing. The prominent place of medical science knowledge and skill in master's programs to prepare APNs may have a tendency to obscure the fact that the educational program is intended to facilitate the development of advanced practice nursing.

The advanced practice of nursing must be firmly grounded in advanced knowledge and skill in caring. The framework presented in this text is intended to help students, faculty, and providers retain a nursing focus while addressing advanced practice in the interdisciplinary environment.

Dunphy's advanced practice nursing model, the Circle of Caring (see Chapter 1), introduces the term "caring process" as a pivotal element. "Process" in this model is understood to mean "unfolding" (rather than a series of cognitive or psychomotor steps or things to do, as in familiar uses such as nursing process or problem-solving process). Caring processes are ways to express your way of being and living as a caring person in the profession of advanced nursing. There is no defined set or list of caring processes; rather, there are as many caring processes as there are persons and situations.

Caring

Caring is the essence of being human, and nursing is a deeply human relationship; thus, caring is the essence of nursing. The meaning of caring as the essential nature of humanness cannot be encapsulated within a single limiting definition; however, caring can be understood, recognized, and developed both philosophically and practically. Caring expressed in nursing is the intentional and authentic presence of the nurse with another who is recognized as person who is living, caring, and growing in caring (Boykin & Schoenhofer, 2001).

All human service disciplines are based on caring. Nursing is unique, however, as caring is what most directly characterizes nursing's knowledge base and service. By contrast, in the discipline of medicine, the fundamental commitment to caring is directly characterized in the diagnosis and treatment of human structural and functional problems manifested primarily in physical terms. The nature of the APN role permits the direct focus on care and caring that is nursing while incorporating in limited ways the focus of medicine. An APN does not practice medicine but rather draws upon and transforms characteristic medical ways of practice for nursing purposes, just as the practice of holistic medicine draws upon and transforms characteristic nursing ways of practice for medical purposes.

The APN, such as the nurse practitioner, practices a specialized form of nursing practice, which means that specialized opportunities for creating situations of care call forth specialized patterns of caring. What does this mean in a practical sense? It means that the person coming for care presents with an issue that is typically viewed as being within the medical sphere. As in all nursing practice, the APN is focused on co-creating a relationship in which care is experienced and possibilities for personally meaningful ways of living unfold. Specialized patterns of caring in the role of nurse practitioner blend knowledgeable perspectives of the health situation (diagnosis) and recommendations for characteristically medical ways of ameliorating presenting issues (treatment) with generalized patterns of nursing care. Generalized patterns of nursing care are represented in the Circle of Caring model as:

- courage
- authentic presence
- advocacy
- knowing
- commitment
- patience

Specialized patterns of care are incorporated in the uniqueness of caring processes. Knowledge of general patterns of care is important; however, that knowledge must be creatively used in actual, unfolding processes of care if the situation is to be considered nursing.

Caring is the matrix, the medium, the "stuff" within which the APN–patient relationship is brought to life. The recognition of the person as caring and the intention to care moves the level from the implicit to the explicit. In this relationship, the APN lives his or her commitment to caring by facilitating a personal connection that communicates "I acknowledge you as a caring person, one who is worthwhile and deserving of my respect, my attention, my commitment, my care." That effort to create a personal connection also communicates the practitioner's acceptance of the trust being placed in him or her as a caring person, as one who is available and able to participate effectively in the life of the other. Within the caring relationship each participant has the opportunity for enhancing personhood, that is, for living life grounded in caring and for growing in one's capacity to express caring in meaningful and satisfying ways. Knowing another as a caring person requires a commitment to entering into the world of the nursed with the explicit intention of knowing the person individually and uniquely as caring. Entering into the world of another with the caring intention requires that the practitioner know himself or herself as caring and be open to growing in the relationship. A truly collaborative relationship (in contrast to one in which the collaboration is at token face value or in some way limited) emerges in the context of this caring intention.

The APN's involvement with the nursed reflects themes or qualities of caring expressed as courage, authentic presence, advocacy, knowing, commitment, and patience. These themes of caring can serve as a conceptual structure or framework to assist the practitioner in examining, recognizing, and understanding the fullness of caring in practice. Though interconnected, each individual theme will be addressed theoretically and then in action in a practice situation to illustrate caring processes.

Courage

Courage is a human act (Tillich, 1952). Courage comes to light in making deliberate choices resulting in acts that express who we are and what is important to us. Courage is the daily application of values, the living out of one's beliefs in spite of obstacles and challenging situations. Expressions of courage affirm our being.

This understanding of courage offers an ethical grounding for the practice of advanced nursing. It requires that, in each nursing situation, the nurse live the values held dear. The nurse risks entering each situation with the fullness of his or her being, willing to be rejected or not understood, or, perhaps equally risky, being accepted and known.

As part of courage, the nurse also understands and acts on the obligation to come to know that which matters to those seeking care. What shapes the moments the nurse has with people is the intention to know them as caring, to hear their stories, and to create nurturing responses reflective of the uniqueness of the situation. Courage manifests itself because of the nurse's deliberate choices to carry out, in a particular time and place, the beliefs that serve as the core of advanced nursing practice. Courage manifests itself in making one's nursing vocation a commitment to these values and beliefs that undergird caring.

Authentic Presence

Nursing is communicated through authentic presence. Authentic presence is a unique way of being with others, unique in that it is a way of ordering and balancing self so as to grow in one's beauty and spirit. Such presence with self requires trust, courage, and the desire to know. One who is authentic with self and others is able to see things from the inside that others see only from the outside. There is an inner genuine awareness that is congruent with feelings, attitudes, and actions lived moment to moment. The commitment to truly know oneself frees one to be with others in authentic presence.

Authentic presence may be understood as intentionally being with another in the fullness of one's personhood. The caring that is communicated through authentic presence is the initiating and sustaining medium of nursing within the nursing situation. Nurses are called to be authentically present in nursing situations. Stories of nursing practice portray the depth of such experiences. The degree to which one knows oneself influences one's presence with others and thus the degree of commitment possible in the situation.

Advocacy

Advocacy is a way in which nurses have traditionally expressed caring. There are many opportunities for advocacy, that is, many situations in which "speaking up for" another is an important aspect of the role. From a depth of knowledge and understanding, the practitioner speaks up for the person as unique and worthwhile, for the person as having personal hopes, dreams, intentions, and preferences that are honorable. In addition, Gadow's (1990) formulation of existential advocacy calls for the nurse to advocate for alternative interpretations of the situation that arise from experience and specialized knowledge. Existential advocacy is contrasted with advocacy that is either paternalistic or consumer oriented. Paternalistic advocacy is characterized by a sense of "as the expert, I know what is best for you and your life." Consumer-oriented advocacy takes the approach that "I'll just give you the facts and options; you sort them out by yourself."

In existential advocacy, self is brought into the situation as a full partner, sharing alternative perspectives for consideration, though not insisting upon them or imposing them. The patient enters into the relationship seeking to connect with the practitioner as a whole person, not just as a set of facts. When the practitioner takes the paternalistic stance (dismissive and overbearing, offering an all-or-none option) or the consumer-oriented stance (withdrawn to an objective distance, offering an essentially value-free set of options), the patient experiences the loss of an opportunity to connect with another assumed to be truly concerned, knowledgeable, and giving. When the nurse offers existential advocacy, the nursed feels truly known, respected, and connected in a way that affirms humanity and being.

Knowing

Knowing as an aspect of caring encompasses "knowing that," "knowing about," "knowing directly" and "unknowing." "Knowing that" and "knowing about" refer to descriptions and analyses of the patient's situation in the context of facts and information. Caring competence requires knowledge of facts and data points that are empirically and objectively derived. "Knowing directly" involves being deeply attuned to the person-as-person and comes through intentionality and authentic presence. "Unknowing" refers to an openness to unfolding, a humble sense that all is not yet known. The practitioner who truly embraces unknowing recognizes that what might be right or timely in general terms may be neither right nor timely for the particular person seeking care in a particular moment.

Carper (1978) describes patterns of knowing fundamental to nursing: personal, empirical, ethical, and esthetic knowing. The practitioner draws on the personal way of knowing as essential intuitive knowing. Empirical knowing is an avenue for drawing upon science and skilled observation. Ethical knowing prompts the practitioner to ask, "What are the personal and professional values that enter into this situation?" And thus, "what is right for this situation?" Aesthetic knowing develops as the practitioner incorporates knowing gained from the other patterns in the context of fully living the situation as she or he co-creates with the nursed an integrated understanding of the unfolding whole picture.

The Circle of Caring is developed and strengthened as the practitioner and patient communicate their unfolding knowing of self, each other, and of the situation. Knowing, as described briefly here, contributes to enhanced personhood, to the affirmation and growth of self and other as caring persons.

Commitment

Is there any greater act of courage than the commitment to another? Commitment is a sign of that which we value. Choosing to be a member of the discipline and profession of nursing speaks to the deep valuing and lifelong commitment of service to humankind. Commitment directs obligations or what "ought to be" in particular situations. Because these commitments are so internalized as values, however, one's obligation is not experienced as a burden but as a response that is right, deliberate, conscious, and caring (Roach, 2002).

Nurses in advanced practice roles frequently face challenges to commitment. Choices made in practice reflect one's devotion to particular commitments. Often the values of an economically based health-care system, of which nursing is such an integral part, do not support or seem to be in line with the substantive nature of caring and its essential relation to practice. A struggle to preserve nursing's values often results. The APN has the unique opportunity to demonstrate how a commitment to the values of nursing influence the outcomes of care.

The practice of advanced nursing must be firmly rooted in the values of the nurse. In addition to many essential knowledges and skills, he or she must be able to draw on the knowledge of nursing, especially knowledge of caring, to create environments for care that honor person-as-person and humanize care.

Nursing always occurs in a relational context. As a human science, nursing calls for the continued commitment to better understand the lived experiences of the nursed, to truly hear their stories, and to respond in ways that matter, ways that nurture and sustain persons as they live and grow in caring. Central to advanced practice is the commitment to know self and others as caring.

Patience

Patience as a key theme in caring refers to trusting people to grow in their own time and in their own way (Mayeroff, 1971). Patience is not passive but rather an active openness to "the moment alive with possibilities." Humility and courage are intimately connected to patience. The ability to remain actively engaged with the person while honoring individual circumstances and freedom of choice is an act of courage and leads to the kind of patience that communicates caring.

Caring Processes

The following story illustrates how the Circle of Caring comes to life in the caring processes of advanced practice nursing.

> *After being in a physician's practice for a few months, I came to know the "regulars." One patient, a 55-year-old woman, had hemorrhoids and slight rectal bleeding. The bleeding was typical of hemorrhoids—bright*

red upon straining, staining the water and toilet tissue red. Over time, different prescriptions for hemorrhoidal preparations were ordered and she was instructed to increase the fiber in her diet and to drink more water. This, however, did not relieve her symptoms. The doctor was getting fed up with her—feeling like "it's only hemorrhoids, you're either not using the cream or suppositories right, or not drinking enough water, etc." He had been seeing her longer than I had. After I had seen her several times, I felt that the problem should have been resolved or at least a little better. I made the decision to refer her to a gastroenterologist. I'd rather have him think I was "stupid" for referring her for hemorrhoids than to have her continue feeling pain. As it turned out, she had rectal cancer and subsequently underwent major surgery. Now when she comes to the office, she will see only me, as she credits me "for her being on this earth today." I've learned my lesson—that patients know their own bodies better than we do.

In this story, the nurse intended to participate fully in the nursing situation, to be open to unfolding possibilities, and to come truly to know the woman being nursed. She expressed caring as courage, authentic presence, knowing, advocacy, commitment, and patience.

Concern for knowing and for helping the patient established a relationship in which the nurse was willing to risk everything because she cared for and about the person being nursed. It was risky for the nurse to consider the possibility that the physician's assessment might be incorrect. Recognizing that the woman had been in his care for a long time, the nurse had to reflect on the possibility that the diagnosis and treatment were, in fact, correct.

As the nurse practitioner attentively listened, she honored the woman's personal knowing of self. The nurse trusted that the woman had followed the prescribed medical regimen and, therefore, she had the courage to step beyond this solution even though she might jeopardize her position and reputation—especially if she was wrong.

It was the nurse's broad knowledge base, patience to hear the story, and expression of compassion and commitment that provided her with the courage to advocate in new ways. The nurse knew she had to speak out, to be the voice for someone who was growing weary and frustrated with continuing to seek assistance for the same symptoms.

The commitment to advanced practice nursing directed the process of "coming to know." The value of respect for person-to-person guided this interaction. Through active patience, the nurse grew in her personal knowing of the woman and of herself as a nurse practitioner. She compassionately responded to one who was calling to be known so that patient could receive the help.

Not only did the nurse draw on personal knowing in creating the nursing response, she also trusted her past experiences, intuition, self-knowing, and sound knowledge base. In a multilayered way the nurse knew that the necessarily and appropriately personal response required in this situation was still unfolding. She *knew* there had to be something more, at least that something more had to be considered—something like consulting a specialist.

In this situation, the person being nursed presented with a set of medical symptoms. The nurse used the symptoms as ways to access and come to know the person-as-person. The nurse practitioner lived the commitment to be in the situation for nursing purposes rather than for medical purposes; thus she practiced truly advanced nursing.

This story of advanced nursing practice illustrates the use of caring processes. As situations are studied and relived, students, faculty, and providers discover the limitless ways caring is expressed. As nurses, we live out our personhood—our living grounded in caring—in unique and special ways. We bring to our practice our humanness, our expertise in caring, and our intention to participate fully in the life experiences of those we are privileged to nurse, and thus to bring the benefits of nursing to those seeking care.

Bibliography

Boykin, A, and Schoenhofer, SO: Nursing as Caring: A Model for Transforming Practice. Jones & Bartlett Publishers, Sudbury, Mass., 2001.

Carper, B: Fundamental patterns of knowing in nursing. Adv Nurs Sci 1(1):13–23, 1978.

Gadow, S: A model for ethical decision making. In Pence, T, et al (eds): Ethics in Nursing: An Anthology. National League for Nursing Publ. No. 20–2294, New York, 1990, pp. 52–55.

Mayeroff, M: On Caring. HarperPerennial, New York, 1971.

Roach, S: Caring: the Human Mode of Being. A Blueprint for the Health Professions. Ottawa, Canada, CHA Press, 2002.

Tillich, P: The Courage to Be. Yale University Press, New Haven, Conn., 1952.

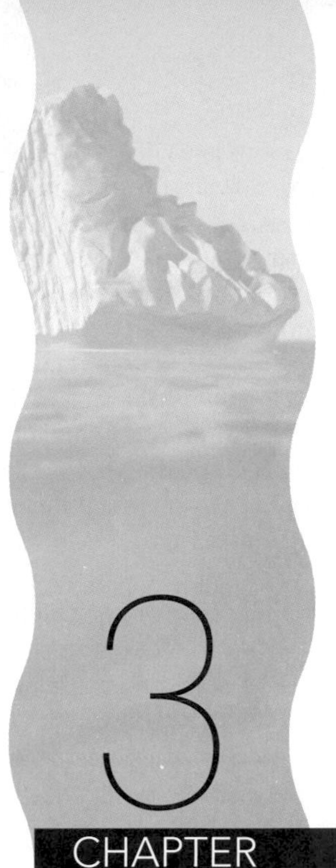

Health Promotion

Cathy M. St. Pierre, PhD, APRN, BC

Health

The ultimate goal of all health-care clinicians is to promote health to minimize illness and disease; it is also the goal of all patients with whom we work in primary care. All patients want to live long and healthy lives, and with health promotion efforts, this is an attainable goal. To help put it all in perspective, the basic tenets of health must first be explored.

What is health? Several disciplines and organizations have tried to define health, and the definition continues to evolve. A very primitive definition of health, "the absence of disease," is not comprehensive and does not account for the multidimensional characteristics integral to a human being. To define health only as the absence of disease is not enough. We must take into account the many dimensions of a person that contribute to health or disease, including physical, spiritual, social, and psychological attributes. To exclude any of these in the definition of health is not holistic. The 2005 Merriam-Webster dictionary defines health more globally as "the condition of being sound in body, mind, or spirit," but it may be difficult to clearly delineate or define what is meant by "being sound." This term is vague and contributes little to the definition of health.

In 1948, the World Health Organization (WHO) defined health as a "state of complete, physical, mental and social well-being," which provides a more holistic view of health as it incorporates the social and mental aspects of a human being as well as the physical dimension. However, this definition does not account for the spiritual dimension of a person. Health is therefore a state in which the physical, psychological, social, and spiritual attributes of a person are in balance, creating harmony within the body (Fig. 3.1).

The balance of each of these dimensions is an important parameter when considering health. A patient whom we care for may be physically healthy but the spiritual, social, and psychological dimensions may not be balanced, and therefore the patient is not truly healthy. It has been long determined that the whole is greater than the sum of its parts. We cannot determine someone's health status without evaluating all of these attributes.

Historically, the evaluation of a patient was based only on *physical* signs and symptoms of a disease. If the

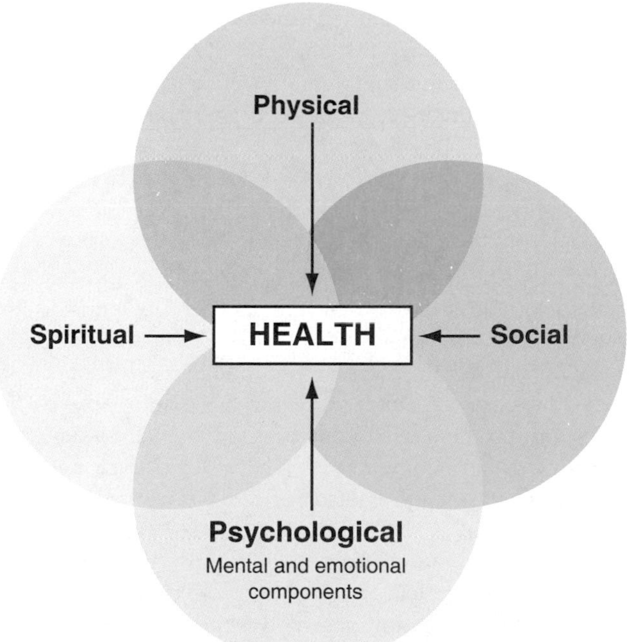

FIGURE 3.1 The components of health.

patient lacked symptoms, we considered him or her healthy. We now know that this type of assessment is incomplete and does not take into account how the other attributes of a person either contribute to or deter from heath status. We also know that many patients have medical problems that have not yet presented as signs and symptoms of a disease.

It is important in assessing the patient that we also evaluate his or social, psychological, and spiritual attributes. In performing a complete health assessment of each patient, the health-care provider needs to ask questions related to the person's social and dietary habits; current living and work situation environment; and feelings, beliefs, and satisfaction with his or her life as well as some relevant questions pertaining to his or her philosophical and spiritual beliefs.

All of these component parts of a patient's history are as important as the physical signs and symptoms that he or she may be currently experiencing. The focus on all of these attributes of a person helps to provide a more holistic view of person that will assist in making a more comprehensive assessment as to the current health status of the patient. The determination of health is based on the synthesis of all of these parameters of health and should be incorporated into all patient assessments.

Health Promotion

Health promotion as defined by O'Donnell in 1989 is "the science and art of helping people change their lifestyle to move toward a state of optimal health." Optimal health is created by a balance of all of the components of health previously described: physical, psychological, and spiritual health. Health promotion can be achieved in many ways and requires a commitment on the part of the individual patient, the health-care provider, and the community. Optimal health promotion efforts will be achieved only through the efforts of the individual, health-care provider, and community working in partnership to achieve goals that will enhance health and well-being.

Health promoton efforts should always begin with the health-care provider. The health-care provider plays a pivotal role in educating the patient and the community regarding health promoting behaviors. The health-care provider can help to provide insight for each patient as to how his or her environment will contribute to health or disease. In addition, the impact that environment can have on the individual must be understood by the community, so that efforts to promote health can be supported. Providing consultation to the community and the legislature regarding environmental health is also the role of health-care practitioners.

Consultation efforts such as this will help to develop legislation that can enforce healthy living conditions in a community. In addition, legislative efforts can help to provide funding to maintain or improve environmental health. If patients are trying to promote their own health, living conditions in the community must also be healthy to sustain and support their efforts. Basic community resources such as water, sanitation, and hygiene must be monitored for potential threats to health and well being. Efforts to maintain and support good hygiene, sanitation, and clean water become the responsibility of community and local government agencies. Healthcare practitioners and patients need to work in collaboration with these agencies to ensure that the basic elements that contribute to health, i.e., clean water and proper hygiene and sanitation, are being maintained or improved upon. To be successful, health promotion must be a group effort.

Health promotion has been viewed as an effort to prevent disease and illness,. with three levels of prevention defined in the literature (in descending order): *Tertiary prevention* is the restoration of health after illness or disease has occurred; *secondary prevention* encompasses early screening and detection of disease or illness; and ultimately *primary prevention* focuses on the prevention of illness and disease. Focusing our health-care efforts on all three levels of prevention is important to promoting health, but during the last two decades, the focus on primary prevention has become the ultimate goal of health promotion.

During the first half of the 20th century, most of the focus in health care was on the tertiary level of prevention: caring for the patient after illness or disease had occurred. The prevailing belief at the time was that patients would or should seek health care when they had developed signs and symptoms of a disease. The phrase to "seek health care" was a misnomer and should have been "seeking illness or disease care." For a patient to seek health care without any signs or symptoms of disease would have been considered inappropriate. During this time, most health-care practitioners cared for patients at the tertiary level by: (1) preventing further insult or injury after the disease or illness had occurred, by stabilizing the patient's condition to prevent deterioration; (2) helping patients to recover from the current illness or disease through treatment; and (3) whenever possible, to help restore patients to their previous state of health.

During the second half of the 20th century, with the advancement of techonologies in health care, the health-care system began to incorporate secondary health promotion strategies into health care. Providers became more savvy about the importance of screening "at risk" patients during appropriate intervals for known diseases and illnesses. A focus on secondary levels of prevention led health-care practitioners to reconsider the current view of health care (see only patients with signs and symptoms of an illness/disease) and encourage early detection and treatment. We were no longer waiting for the patient to present with the symptoms of an illness or disease but rather were screening them for potential diseases that had not presented with signs/symptoms in the patient, yet.

With this focus on early screening and detection, it was believed that early diagnosis could foster early treatment and thereby prevent some of the long-term sequelae

Box 3.1 Criteria for U.S. Clinician Handbook of Preventive Services Inclusion

1. The condition must have a significant effect on the quality and quantity of life;
2. Acceptable methods of treatment must be available;
3. The condition must have an asymptomatic period during which detection and treatment significantly reduce morbidity and mortality;
4. Treatment in the asymptomatic phase must yield a therapeutic result superior to that obtained by delaying treatment until symptoms appear;
5. Tests that are acceptable to patients must be available, at a reasonable cost, to detect the condition in the asymptomatic period; and
6. The evidence of the condition must be sufficient to justify the cost of the screening.

associated with illness and disease. For example, blood pressure would be checked in a patient with no symptoms of hypertension, and if elevated, a plan of treatment would be instituted. The goal of this focus was that the patient's blood pressure would normalize and create less strain on the heart and potentially avoid the development of stroke or myocardial infarction. Certain circumstances must exist for a screening test to be useful as summarized in the U.S. Government's Clinician's Handbook of Preventive Services (1996) (Box 3.1).

In determining whether or not screening is appropriate, health-care practitioners must keep in mind that people seek health care more frequently during midlife (40 to 65 years) than at any other age. With the exception of pregnancy; early signs of chronic disease surface in the midlife years: the earlier disease is identified, the better it can be treated and sequelae prevented. In addition, growth and development knowledge documents that individuals in the midlife years focus more on behaviors to extend life and prevent disability than do individuals in early adulthood (20 to 40 years). Adults 20 to 40 years old focus more on relationship, family, self-image, and career development, whereas those older than 65 spend much time responding to and coping with overt, established illness. As life expectancy increases and older adults anticipate living longer, more attention is focused on health enhancement.

During the last 20 years of the 20th century, the health-care industry began to include the third dimension and perhaps the most optimal aspect of health promotion: primary prevention. The focus on primary prevention enabled providers to assess patients' potential risk factors including lifestyle and genetic history, and to help patients implement a treatment plan that fostered health promotion to potentially prevent disease and disability in patients. Health-care practitioners were now aware that the focus of achieving health or wellness would best be achieved through primary prevention strategies. However, when this was not possible, secondary and tertiary levels of prevention were still employed. Each health-care interaction between a patient and health-care practitioner is an opportunity to promote health at the primary, secondary, or tertiary level of prevention, thereby working toward the goal of optimal wellness or health for all patients.

Health-care practitioners can utilize the levels of prevention in several ways: on an individual level, with small groups (families) and larger groups such as a community. Their individual encounters with patients provide an opportunity to educate patients regarding their individual risk factors with the intent of influencing change to prevent, or at the very least, delay the onset of disease(s) and the potential sequelae of disease (implementing primary and secondary prevention strategies). Incorporating family members into the educational process of health promotion can provide support and reinforcement for patients during the early phase of risk reduction. This incorporation of family may also serve the individual family members by educating them regarding their *own* risk for disease. Family members can also serve as advocates for patients by helping to sythesize the information given and providing the patient with a support system to make healthy lifestyle changes.

Health-care practitioners can also be instrumental in developing health promotion strategies on a larger scale: through community intervention. This can be accomplished by developing interventions that include identifying community groups at risk for certain diseases and developing community-wide educational programs that will educate this group about their potential risk. It is now known that health promotion or early intervention should be the goal (Fig. 3.2), and development of a community based educational program will reach a broader audience with the potential for significant impact on the health status of a community.

The evolution of knowledge has increased our awareness of the fact that many diseases today can be minimized or potentially avoided with early assessment and management. The effects of diseases such as hypertension, cardiovascular disease, and diabetes on patients' lives can be minimized or avoided with early interventions. For example, it is currently believed that most patients with diabetes are not diagnosed until the disease has been present for 5 years. Diabetes is a serious disease that impacts on multiple systems in the body and can have severe consequences on one's health, if not treated aggressively. The development of a community- wide diabetes education/screening program will help to identify patients who are at high risk for this disease, and through early identification and treatment potentially prevent the long-term complications associated with diabetes such as peripheral neuropathy, cardiovascular complications, and retinopathies.

Health-care practitioners can take a leadership position within a community by developing targeted programs for early identification and treatment. This type of wide-scale intervention can have life-saving results. Early

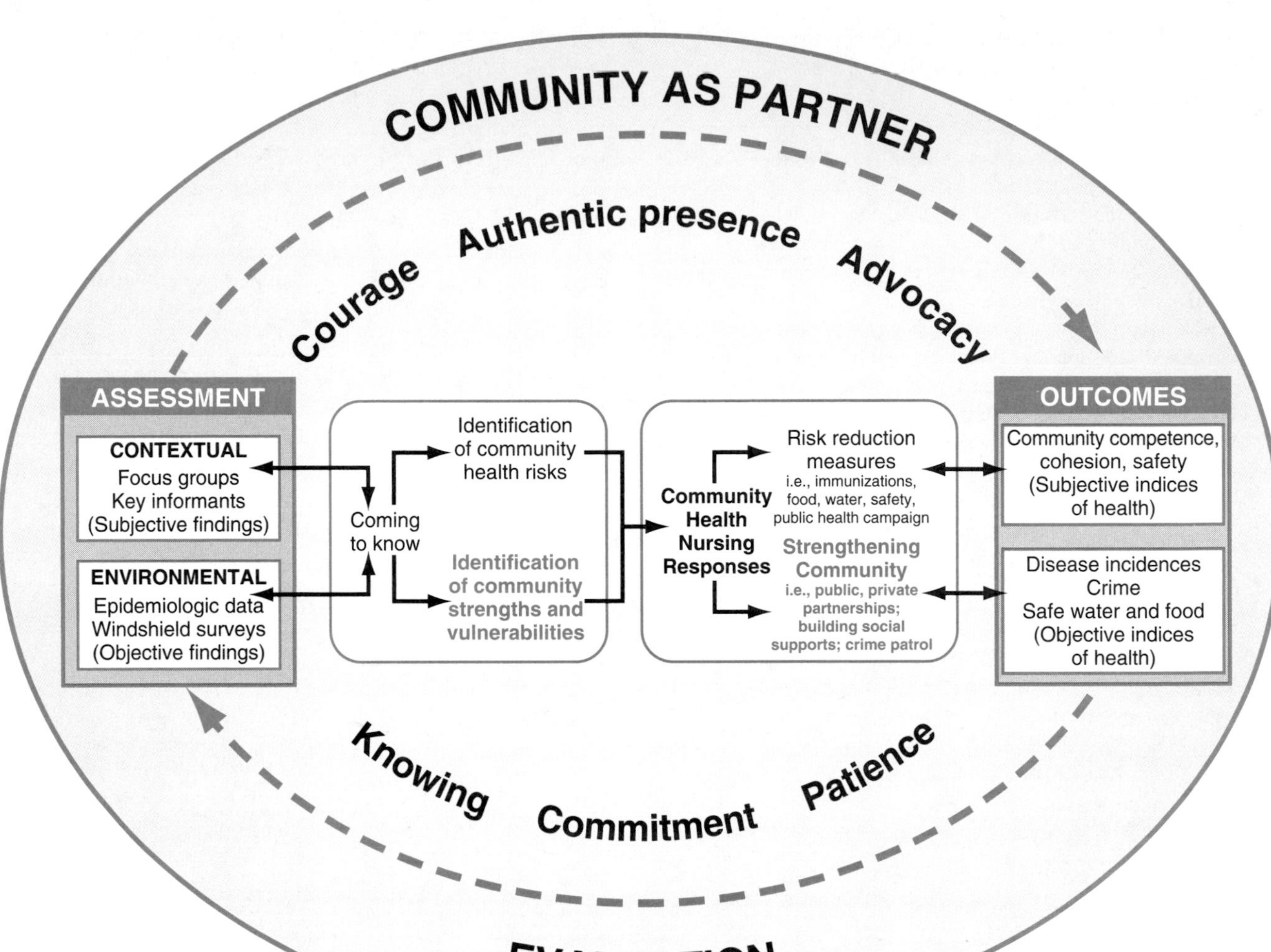

FIGURE 3.2 The Community-based Circle of Caring.

diagnosis, prior to the patient presenting with signs/symptoms of a disease, can have a significant impact on the outcomes of disease. If patients are identified early, educated about the importance of healthy nutrition and lifestyle practices, and treated aggressively treated, the outcome may be a long and healthy life without disease complications. Table 3.1 provides examples of primary, secondary, and tertiary prevention.

Risk Factors in Health Promotion

The identification of risk factors by screening is an essential component of health promotion. Not all patients have risk factors for all diseases. Some patients have no known risk factors; others have many. The key component to providing effective health promotion is to screen patients for potential known risk factors and intervene. Although we do not have the current knowledge to prevent illness and disease with certainty, the elimination or alteration of certain risk factors can impact on disease outcomes. Knowledge of risk factors is important but not all risk factors are amendable to modification.

These risk factors, known as *nonmodifiable risk factors,* include the patient's sex, age, and genetic/family history and are considered nonmodifiable because they cannot be changed in any way (at this time). Because these factors are nonmodifiable, early and aggressive identification of *all* risk factors needs to be done so that patients with nonmodifiable risk factors may still influence their future outcomes by making changes in *modifiable risk factors.*

Modifiable risk factors include items that can be effected through change such as weight, diet, social habits, lifestyle choices, and stress reduction. For example, 38-year-old Mr. Hart is being seen for a physical examination. He has not had a physical in 20 years. His past medical history is negative for any diseases, surgeries, or illnesses. His social history includes the use of alcohol and cigarettes; he works an average of 60 hours per week as a emergency medical technician (EMT) and does not exercise. His family history reveals that his father, paternal uncle, and grandfather

Table 3.1 **Examples of Primary, Secondary and Tertiary Prevention**

Primary Prevention	Secondary Prevention	Tertiary Prevention
Immunizations	Screening for:	Treatment to prevent further sequelae of:
Health education	Skin cancer	Cardiovascular disease
Skin cancer prevention measures	Oral cancer	Respiratory disease
Weight control	Lung cancer	Gastroenterology disease
Seatbelt uses	Breast cancer	Genitourinary disease
Violence prevention	Testicular cancer	Endocrine diseases
Substance abuse education on: smoking, alcohol and drugs	Prostate cancer	Immunodeficiency disease
	Diabetes	Infectious disease
	Hypertension	Dermatological disease
Environmental hazards avoidance	Cardiovascular disease	Oncology disease
Protective hearing equipment	Ovarian cancer	Gynecological disease
Protective eye equipment	Cervical cancer	Musculoskeletal disease
Safety helmets for motorcycles, skateboards and bicycles	Fecal occult blood	Neurological disease
	Sexually transmitted infections	Psychiatric disease
Nutrition counseling	Tuberculosis infection	Reproductive disease
Exercise	Pediatric developmental screening	
Stress reduction	Lead screening	
Eliminate allergen exposure	Anemia screening	
	Height, weight, and body mass index (BMI) screening	

have all had a myocardial infarction before the age of fifty. Mr. Hart's physical exam reveals the following: height, 69 inches, weight, 230 lbs., and a body mass index (BMI), 34. Lab work on Mr. Hart reveals an elevated cholesterol of 250, a high-density lipoprotein (HDL) of 30, and a low-density lipoprotein (LDL) of 160. Box 3.2 reviews the risk factors for heart disease for Mr. Hart.

Although Mr. Hart cannot change his age, sex, or family history, there are several factors that he can change. With good nutrition patterns, regular exercise, stress reduction, moderation of alcohol intake and smoking cessation, Mr. Hart may be able to reduce his risk for heart disease. This case illustrates the importance of early identification of risk factors for intervention. The biggest challenge that we face in health promotion today is that at this point in our history, we do not yet have knowledge about all of the potential risk factors that contribute to disease, and some are still unidentified.

Through research, we have made significant strides in determining the relationship between certain risks such as smoking, alcohol, and diet and the presence of disease but some factors remain unknown. For example, some of the patients that we will care for will have *no* identified risk factors for disease X and will still develop this disease. The opposite is also true; some of the patients whom we evaluate may find that they have several identified modifiable risk factors for disease Y, elect to not to take action to modify any of their risks, and yet will never go on to develop disease Y. Both of these groups of patients require further investigation. Evidence-based research needs to focus on efforts to identify other unknown risk factors or health promoting determinants, as is the case of the second patient, that could influence the outcomes for disease.

Box 3.2 **Risk Factors for Mr. Hart**

Nonmodifiable Risk Factors

- Male sex
- Age
- Family history

Modifiable Risk Factors

- Weight
- Sedentary lifestyle
- Elevated cholesterol
- Suboptimal LDL and HDL
- Alcohol consumption
- Smoking
- Stress level

Influences on Health Promotion

Several factors influence health promotion activities. Factors such as government-sponsored initiatives, community health programs, and individual factors all influence outcomes in health promotion and disease prevention. Many government-sponsored initiatives have helped to highlight the importance of health promotion and disease prevention in the past 30 years. Two major government initiatives that have had great impact on effecting change in the United States are *Healthy People 2000, 2010* and the United States Preventive Services Task Force (USPSTF). The historical evolution and current status of each of these programs, as well as their impact on health promotion and disease prevention, is described here. Other influencing factors such as immunizations, community health programs, and individual factors are also highlighted.

Healthy People 2000, 2010

Disease prevention has always been a major goal of the public health service (PHS), but this department recommitted its efforts to health promotion and disease prevention during the late 1970s as a result of the Public Health Service Act. The Secretary of Health and Human Services was commissioned by the legislature to develop an agenda for promoting the health of the nation. The result of the initiative was a landmark report: *The Surgeon General's Report on Health Promotion and Disease Prevention,* published in 1979. This document highlighted the fact that many of the diseases and injuries affecting the population at that time could be prevented or minimized with early intervention. It also stressed the importance of healthy lifestyle choices to enhance health and well-being. As a result of this report, five major goals for the nation were established and 226 objectives were developed to meet these goals (Box 3.3). The result of this initiative was the government publication of *Healthy People 2000.*

The target year to achieve these goals was 1990. Many of the federally funded primary and community care programs around this time were developed to help meet these goals. By 1987, a review of the progress on this initiative found that all of the goals had already been achieved except for no. 2—reducing the number of deaths in children by 20%. The achievement of this goal was near target. In 1990, the focus on health promotion and disease prevention continued and was expanded into what has now become known as *Healthy People 2000* (http://www.healthypeople.gov). The five overall goals from the previous initiative were reviewed and evaluated and three new goals were established. The overall goals for *Healthy People 2000*, focused

Box 3.3 Major Goals for the Health of the Nation (1980)

1. Reducing infant deaths by 35% through prevention of birth defects and low birth weight
2. Reducing deaths in children by 20% through injury prevention and screening for growth and development delays
3. Reducing adolescent deaths by 20% through prevention of motor vehicle injuries and reduction of alcohol and drug use.
4. Reducing adult deaths by 25% through early screening and prevention of myocardial infarctions, stroke, and cancer
5. Reducing the number of sick days in older adults by 20% through prevention of influenza and pneumonia as well as the maintenance of functional status.

Box 3.4 Goals of Healthy People 2000

1. Increase the span of healthy life for Americans.
2. Reduce health disparities among Americans.
3. Achieve access to preventive services for all Americans.

more on the general health of the population, are listed in Box 3.4.

These new goals established a more general view of health promotion and disease prevention without reference to specific parameters for achieving these goals. In other words, the focus was on the general improvement in health without the constraints of achieving a specific goal such as a reduction in morbidity by 25%. However, to meet these goals, 22 priority areas were developed that were divided into four areas of focus: health promotion, health protection, preventative services, and surveillance and data systems (Table 3.2). Individual objectives to meet the overall goals were also developed and categorized under one of these 22 priority areas, and included specific targets for meeting the goals such as "reduce unintentional injury deaths to no more than 29.3/100,000 people (15% decrease)." These objectives identified specific parameters that could be measured to evaluate the success of the program.

According to *Healthy People (2000), health promotion* is defined as strategies "related to individual lifestyle-personal choices made in a social context-that can have a powerful influence over one's health prospects" (p 6). *Health protection* is defined as strategies "related to environmental or regulatory measures that confer protection on a large population group" (p 6). *Preventative services* include "screening, counseling, chemoprophylactic or immunization interventions for individuals in the clinical setting" (p 7). The last priority area of surveillance and data systems is considered paramount to tracking all of the changes that would occur with programs focusing on meeting the goals of *Healthy People 2000*. Systems were set up to monitor and organize the data for this initiative. Progress toward meeting the goals was evaluated and reviewed every 5 years. The results of this review and evaluation was a report titled "midcourse reviews for *Healthy People 2000*." By the year 2000, the National Center for Health Statistics (2001) stated that 68 objectives (21%) had met the goals of *Healthy People 2000* while 41% (129 objectives) had made progress toward meeting the target goal for 2000. Eleven percent of the goals had mixed results and 15 percent of the goals had "showed movement away from the target." Although all of the major goals were not reached by 2000, more than 50 percent of the goal of eliminating health disparities (major goal 2) was achieved. The momentum for this initiative continues to grow.

During the late 1990s, the commitment to health promotion through this program was strong; the outcomes overall were positive; and the agencies involved on the local, regional, and national level still believed there was progress

Table 3.2 **The 22 Priority Areas for Healthy People 2000**

Health Promotion	Health Protection	Preventative Services	Surveillance and Data Systems
1. Physical activity and fitness	1. Unintentional injuries	1. Maternal and infant health	1. Surveillance and data systems
2. Nutrition	2. Occupational safety and health	2. Heart disease and stroke	
3. Tobacco	3. Environmental health	3. Cancer	
4. Alcohol and other drugs	4. Food and drug safety	4. Diabetes and chronic disabling conditions	
5. Family planning	5. Oral health	5. HIV infection	
6. Mental health and mental disorders		6. Sexually transmitted infections	
7. Violent and abusive behavior		7. Immunization and infectious diseases	
8. Educational and community-based programs		8. Clinical preventative services	

to made in this area. As we approached the new millenium, the goals and objectives for *Healthy People 2000* were reevaluated and the development of a new program for the next decade, *Healthy People 2010,* was established. The major goals for *Healthy People 2010* were streamlined into two major objectives: "to increase quality and years of a healthy life and to eliminate health disparities." While the *major goals* for this initiative decreased from three to two, the priority areas and objectives were expanded from 22 to 28 (Fig. 3.3). In addition to the expansion of priority areas, the targeted objectives have increased from 300 in *Healthy People 2000* to 462 objectives in *Healthy People 2010*. This next initiative, *Healthy People 2010,* was "designed to serve as a roadmap for improving the health of all people in the United States during the first decade of the 21st century."

The *Healthy People 2000 and 2010* initiatives have significantly impacted on primary health care in this country. The incorporation of health-promoting and disease prevention strategies has become mainstream for primary care providers. It is believed that all of the goals of *Healthy People 2010* are achievable with support from individual health-care practitioners, the local and national government agencies, and most importantly, the active participation of individual patients.

These initiatives also stressed the importance of each individual taking personal responsibility for his or her own health, in partnership with his or her health-care professional. This represented a shift away from the view of health care as solely the province of health-care professionals and augmented the fact that their "ways of functioning" are crucial to returning responsibility for health to the individual. For the lay public to have an effective role in illness prevention, individuals must work in partnership with professionals who have been specially educated in health promotion and prevention.

United States Preventive Service Task Force

The United States Preventive Service Task Force (USPTF) is an organization that is composed of private sector experts who make recommendations to the health-care community regarding clinical prevention strategies. This task force was first convened by the U.S. Public Health Service in 1984 and since 1998 has come under the umbrella of the Agency for Healthcare Research and Quality (AHRQ). Their mission as mandated by public law section 915 is to:

> *conduct scientific evidence reviews of a broad array of clinical preventative services, develop recommendations for the health care community and provide ongoing administrative, research and technical, and dissementation support.*

The current USPTF task force is composed of 16 health-care practitioners who represent a variety of specialties, including family practice physicians, internists, pediatricians, obstetricians/gynecologists, and nurses. This task force meets and reviews scientific evidence for each of the current health-care screening guidelines as well as preventive medications, immunizations, and counseling and makes recommendation. Through consensus, the task force assigns a grade to each recommendation based on net benefits for patients as well as the strength of evidence for each of the current recommendation. The grading criteria are listed in Table 3.3.

The result of the task force efforts is a summary book that can be utilized by health-care practitioners who provide preventive services. The guideline book, entitled *Guide to Clinical Preventive Services,* is currently in its 3rd edition(2005), is available for distribution from several sources and has its own Web site: http://www.ahrq.gov/clinic/uspstfab.htm. Providers are able to download the whole

What Is Healthy People 2010?

Healthy People 2010 is a comprehensive set of disease prevention and health promotion objectives for the nation to achieve over the first decade of the new century. Created by scientists both inside and outside of government, it identifies a wide range of public health priorities and specific, measurable objectives.

Overarching Goals:

1. Increase quality and years of healthy life
2. Eliminate health disparities

Focus Areas:

1. Access to Quality Health
2. Arthritis, Osteoporosis, and Chronic Back Conditions
3. Cancer
4. Chronic Kidney Disease
5. Diabetes
6. Disability and Secondary Conditions
7. Educational and Community-Based Programs
8. Environmental Health
9. Family Planning
10. Food Safety
11. Health Communication
12. Heart Disease and Stroke
13. HIV
14. Immunization and Infectious Diseases
15. Injury and Violence
16. Maternal, Infant, and Child Health
17. Medical Product Safety
18. Mental Health and Mental Disorders
19. Nutrition and Overweight
20. Occupational Safety and Health
21. Oral Health
22. Physical Activity and Fitness
23. Public Health Infrastructure
24. Respiratory Diseases
25. Sexually Transmilted Diseases
26. Substance Abuse
27. Tobacco Use
28. Vision and Hearing

FIGURE 3.3 *Healthy People 2010* goals and priority areas.

book from this Web site, which also has capabilities to download the information into a personal digital assistant (PDA). This guide provides several recommendations for screening, including preventive service recommendations; cancer screening and chemoprevention strategies; screening for heart and valvular disease, infectious disease, injury and violence, mental health, substance abuse; metabolic, nutritional, and endocrine screening; and pediatric screening guidelines (Table 3.4).

Table 3.3 Grading Criteria for USPSTF Guidelines (USPSTF, 2005)

Grade	Defined Criteria
A	The USPSTF strongly recommends that clinicians provide [the service] to eligible patients. The USPSTF found good evidence that [the service] improves important health outcomes and concludes that benefits substantially outweighs harm
B	The USPSTF recommends that clinicans provide [the service] to eligible patients. The USPSTF found at least fair evidence that [the service] improves important health outcomes and concludes the benefits outweighs harms.
C	The USPSTF makes no recommendations for or against routine provision of [the service]. The USPSTF found at least fair evidence that [the service] can improve health outcomes but concludes that the balance of benefits and harm is too close to justify a general recommendation.
D	The USPSTF recommends against routinely providing [the service] to asymptomatic patients. The USPSTF found at least fair evidence that [the service] is ineffective or that harms outweighs benefits.
I	The USPSTF concludes that the evidence is insufficient to recommend for or against routinely providing [the service]. Evidence that [the service] is effective is lacking, of poor quality, or conflicting, and the balance of benefits and harms cannot be determined.

Source: USPSTF, 2005.

The USPSTF makes these recommendations for screening to select populations as noted but also states "that (clinicians) give lower priority to services with "C" recommendations—they need not be done unless there are individual considerations in favor of providing the service" (USPSTF, 2005, p. 4) Thus, although guidelines are provided and recommendations are made, each health-care provider has a responsibility to assess each patient's history and risk factors and determine whether the current recommendations are appropiate for the individual patient. For example, patients who have a significant family history for a particular type of cancer may need to be screened earlier than recommended for the general population. Guidelines can be a very helpful tool to utilize in primary care. However, the individual patient's history always takes precedence over the current recommendations.

The United States Preventive Service task force is an ongoing effort to evaluate guidelines and periodically

Table 3.4 **Sample of USPSTF Guidelines**

Recommendations	Recommendation Grade	Males	Females	Pregnant women	Children
Alcohol misuse screening and behavioral counseling interventions	B	X	X	X	
Aspirin for the primary prevention of cardiovascular events	A	X	X		
Bacteruria, screening for asymptomatic	A			X	
Breast cancer, chemoprevention	B		X		
Breast cancer screening	B		X		
Breastfeeding, behavioral interventions to promote	B		X	X	
Cervical cancer screening	A		X		
Chlamydial infection screening	A-female B-pregnant	X	X		
Colorectal cancer, screening	A	X	X		
Dental carries in preschool children, prevention	B				X
Depression, screening	B	X	X		
Diabetes mellitus in adults, for type 2	B	X	X		
Diet, behavioral counseling in primary care to promote health	B	X	X		
Hepatitis B virus, infection, screening	A			X	
High blood pressure, screening	A	X	X		
Lipid disorders, screening	A-* depends On age and history.	X	X		
Obesity in adults, screening	B	X	X		
Osteoporosis in postmenopausal women, screening	B		X		
Rh (D) incompatibility, screening	A			X	
Syphilis infection, screening	A-* if at risk A-pregnant	X	X	X	
Tobacco use and tobacco-caused disease, counseling to prevent	A	X	X	X	
Visual impairment in children younger than age 5 years, screening	B				X

For full description, see references.

updates these guidelines. Some of the items that are currently being reviewed by this task force for recommendations are listed in Box 3.5.

The work of this task force continues, and it will be interesting to see what develops in the near future. Some of the current recommendations noted in Table 3.5, such as lead and iron deficiency anemia screenings, have been included as part of the well child visits in pediatrics for many years. It is important that screening programs be continued or eliminated based on the strength of scientific evidence available and not just on tradition. If the evidence is not strong enough to support current recommendations, then practices such as generalized screening for anemia and lead poisoning may need to be eliminated. This type of screening is relatively easy to do and is inexpensive but does cause trauma to the child (and often the parent), so we must base our decisions on sound evidence and not just a matter of routine. It will also be interesting to note whether or not the focus in health care, on primary prevention today, will yield more recommendations for health promotion and disease prevention practices in the near future.

Box 3.5 **Sample Topics Being Evaluated by USPSTF for Recommendations**

1. Aspirin for prevention of colorectal cancer (prevention)
2. BRCA1 and 2 (genetic testing)
3. Carotid artery stenosis (screening)
4. Coronary heart disease (screening)
5. Dyslipidemia (screening)
6. Hearing impairment in the elderly (screening)
7. Hemochromatosis (screening)
8. Hip dysplasia (screening)
9. Iron-deficiency anemia (screening)
10. Lead (screening)
11. Motor vehicle collisions prevention (counseling)
12. Delay in speech and hearing (screening)
13. Elderly vision (screening)

Source: USPSTF, 2005.

With the rapid evolution of technology in health care, it is important to stay up to date on current health care information. Resources such as *Healthy People 2010* and the USPSTF guidelines are essential tools to help health-care practitioners remain current in their practice styles. All of these initiatiaves have Web sites that provide updated editions to the current printed reports. With easy access to Internet sources, information can be updated with the click of a button. Initiatives such as *Healthy People 2010* and the USPSTF guidelines are excellent examples of well researched tools that can help to enhance health promotion and disease prevention. The end result will be comprehensive care to our patients with the goal of optimal health for all.

Immunization Practices

Immunization administration is one of the best examples of primary health promotion. Immunizations provide the patient's body with the ability to build up antibodies to a potential life-threatening illness before exposure to the offending agent. The administration of immunizations, therefore, prevents an illness or disease from developing. The guidelines for immunization continue to evolve and change over time. At present, we begin immunizations at birth and continue them throughout life. The total number of immunizations that one will receive depends on a person's longevity. During early childhood, infants and children are immunized with a wide variety of vaccines, including hepatitis B (Hep B); diphtheria, acellular pertussis, and tetanus (DtaP); inactivated polio vaccine (IPV); *Haemophilis influenzae* type B (HIBS); measles, mumps, and rubella (MMR); varicella vaccine (VZV); pneumococcal conjugate vaccine (PCV); and influenzae, pneumococcal vaccine, and menigococcal vaccine. All children will receive approximately 25 vaccines by the time they reach 5 years of age. After this point, they will continue to receive a tetanus diphtheriae (Td) every 10 years. They may also continue to receive an influenzae vaccine yearly, depending on their past medical history. The immunization schedules change rapidly, so to obtain the most current information, go to: http://www.cdc.gov/nip/ACIP/. which offers current immunization guidelines for children and adults. Table 3.5 provides a summary of immunization guidelines.

Immunizations are an effective form of primary health promotion but they are not without some problems. Over the past several years, some consumers have argued that immunizations are not safe and in fact are the cause of diseases such as autism and attention deficit hyperactivity disorder (ADHD). To date, the etiology of these diseases has not been found to be a result of immunization administration. However, there is always the potential for vaccines to cause side effects.

Each health-care practitioner must provide patients and their families with accurate information regarding immunization administration, including potential side effects as well as known contraindications to immunization, and to keep a copy of a written consent for each immunization on file. This consent must be obtained for each immunization given, prior to vaccine administerion. If, after administration of a vaccine, a patient develops a significant reaction (such as very high fever, uncontrollable crying for more than 2 hours, lethargy, coma, etc.), the patient should be evaluated in a timely manner and the potential adverse reaction to the vaccine should be reported. In 1986, the National Childhood Vaccine Injury Act required that all health-care practitioners report any severe adverse reactions to the Centers for Disease Control and Prevention (CDC). The length of time from administration to the presence of an adverse event is between 14 and 30 days, and is dependent on whether the vaccine administered is a live virus or not. When in doubt, it is best to report the event.

Table 3.5 Summary of Immunization Guidelines for Adults and Children (ACIP, 2005)

Immunizations	Pediatric	Adult
Types and number of Immunizations required	3 Hepatitis B 5 DtaP 2 Td 4 HIBS 4 IPV 2 MMR 1 VZV 5 PCV 1 Meningococcal vaccine (if at risk)	3 Hepatitis B (if at risk) Td every 10 years Influenzae every year (if at risk) Pneumococcal (if at risk) Meningococcal vaccine (if at risk)

Source: ACIP, 2005.

The information regarding potential reactions for each vaccine are available in the *Red Book* developed by the American Academy of Pediatrics (http://www.aap.org) or on the CDC Web site under the Morbidity and Mortality Weekly Reports (MMWR)(http://www.cdc.gov/mmwr) section. A report on a potential reaction is filed with the CDC by completing the Vaccine Adverse Event Reporting Systerm (VAERS) form, which can be downloaded from http://www.vaers.org. Immunizations are still one of the best methods we have for preventing illness and disease or the serious sequelae that can develop from specific diseases such as polio, diptheriae, *Haemophilis influenzae*, etc. It is an example of primary prevention at its best.

Individual Influences on Health Promotion

The key to successful health promotion is the commitment of the individual patient. Without the patient's willingness to participate in lifestyle changes, health promotion will not be realized. The health-care practitioner needs to provide patients with health education that informs them of their current risk factors, the possibility of reducing or eliminating any modifiable risk factors by lifestyle changes, and the potential benefits of implementing these changes. Once the health-care practitioner has accomplished this task, the decision to take action now rests with the patient. An ideal scenario for health promotion would involve both patient and health-care provider working in partnership toward mutually agreed on health goals. However, the choice to engage in this partnership is predominately the patient's decision. For example, 36-year-old Kathleen is being seen for a physical examination. She reveals that she has smoked a pack a day of cigarettes for 20 years. It is well known that smoking is a significant risk factor for several illness and diseases. Kathleen is counseled regarding her smoking habit with the associated risk for diseases such as cardiac, respiratory, and peripheral vascular disease. Kathleen states that she understands that smoking is not good for her health but currently is not willing to give up the habit. This scenario illustrates that despite the best efforts of the health-care practitioner, the individual (Kathleen), still has the right to *not* engage in health-promoting behaviors.

Many factors can influence a patient's willingness to engage in health promotion activities, such as willingness to alter current lifestyle practices, belief patterns as to whether or not making these changes will impact on one's health, and as well as a belief that promoting health can prevent disease. All of these factors will influence whether or not a patient decides to make lifestyle changes. Several health models have been developed to identify factors that influence a patient's willingness to take action and make changes. Nola Pender's 1997 health belief model provides a framework for health-care practitioners to utilize in assessing patients' readiness to make lifestyle changes to promote their own health. Pender's model describes and defines several factors impacting on the patient's decision to take action (Fig. 3.4). Pender divides these factors into two types: cognitive–perceptual factors and modifying factors.

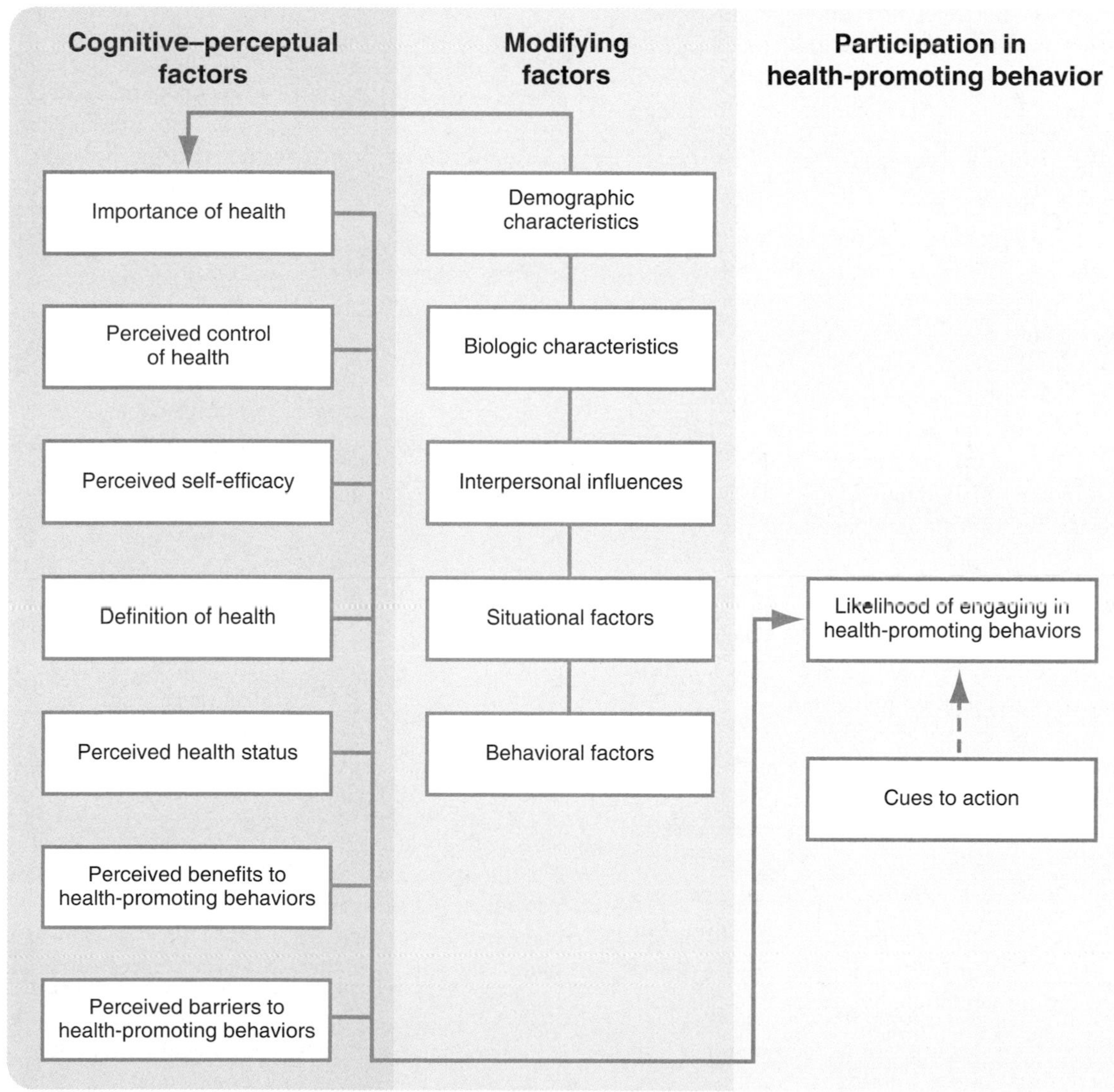

FIGURE 3.4 Health Promotion Model. (From Pender, N: Health Promotion in Nursing Practice, ed 2. Appleton & Lange (Prentice Hall)).

Cognitive–perceptual factors include items such as importance of health, perceived control of health, and perceived barriers to health-promoting behaviors. *Modifying factors* include biologic characteristics, situational factors, and demographic characteristics.

Pender states that all of these factors will impact on a patient's willingness to take action (which she terms "cues to take action"). For example, 17-year-old Jonathan has not consistently been wearing a seat belt while riding in or driving a car until 2 months ago. His friend Kyle was involved in a motor vehicle accident (MVA) in which Kyle was seriously injured. Kyle's parents have informed Jonathan that Kyle's injury could have been prevented if Kyle had been wearing a seat belt. In this situation, Jonathan has changed his perception (cognitive–perceptual factors) about the importance of wearing a seat belt (health-promoting behavior) based on interpersonal influences (his friend's involvement in a MVA). His "cue to action" was hearing that the injuries incurred by Kyle could have been avoided had Kyle being wearing his seat belt.

This scenario illustrates that although various factors can influence positive health changes, the "cues to action" for patients may vary. In the above scenario, it would be interesting to find out if the MVA caused Kyle to change his behavior regarding seat belt use. It is important that health-care practitioners strive to offer patients a variety of scenarios to promote health.

As health-care practitioners, our responsibility is to screen patients, identify known or potential risk factors, educate our patients regarding their risk factors, provide health education about making positive lifestyle changes, and discuss how these lifestyle changes can impact on one's health. The optimal outcome of this process would be a joint partnership between patient and health-care provider to work toward the goal of enhancing the patient's health. This type of partnership provides for optimal balance, as the burden for outcomes rests equally with both patient and health-care provider.

Today's focus on primary prevention is empowering for patients, in contrast to the situation 20 years ago, when most patients were not given the option of actively participating in their health care. Health care today provides many opportunities for patients and health-care practitioners to optimize health through health promotion and disease prevention.

THE PATIENT VOICE 3.1

The Promise

If you could just lose weight
Your blood pressure would go down
Your diabetes would clear up
You could get off all those pills you take
Your joints wouldn't ache
You could climb the stairs
Run after the bus
Carry the groceries
Pick up the baby
The swelling in your legs would go down
You could reach all the way to your aching feet
You could breathe again

You could find clothes to fit
Get out of those slippers and into real shoes
Who knows but what your old man would come back
You'd get more respect from your children
A decent job
Your son would kick drugs
Your daughter wouldn't get pregnant again
You'd live to see your last one grown

Your neighbors wouldn't talk about you
The toilet would flush
The roof wouldn't leak
There'd be food enough at the end of the month
They wouldn't cut off your check
Jack up the rent
You'd hit the number
Go off for two weeks in Aruba

Jesus would save the world from sin
Those who mourn would be comforted
The poor would enter the Kingdom of God
Your hunger would be filled.

Venetta Mason (1999)

Community Influences on Health Promotion

Community efforts can also substantially enhance health promotion efforts. As described previously, the burden of responsibility regarding sanitation, hygiene, and clean water supplies rests with the local community government. A person who lives in a community that lacks appropriate waste disposal, air pollution controls, or law enforcement is exposed to greater health risks than does an individual who lives in a community in which each of these environmental issues has been effectively addressed. Local government needs to play an active role in promoting the health of its citizens.

Health-care practitioners need to work in partnership with local government to ensure that healthy living condiitons are a right for each citizen and not geographically dependent. Health-care practitioners can provide education and expertise for local community government and agencies in understanding the connection between effective sanitation measures and health. Each health-care provider can also alert the local community to possible outbreaks of illness and disease that can affect the greater community at large.

Working with local community and government agencies can provide momentum and power to getting the

> Over the years, it has become clear that individual health is closely linked to community health –the health of the community and environment in which individuals, live, work and play. Likewise, community health is profoundly affected by the collective behaviors, attitudes, and beliefs of everyone in the community. Indeed, the underlying premise of *Healthy People 2010* is that the health of the individual is almost inseparable from the health of the larger community and that the health of every community in every State and territory determines the overall health status of the Nation. That is why the vision for *Healthy People 2010* is "Healthy People in Healthy Communities"
> *Healthy People 2010* (2000,Vol 1, p 3)

message out: improving the health of our nation through health promotion. Community agencies and local health-care practitioners can utilize each other's expertise to develop and carry out community-wide initiatives to improve the health status of the local community. The major goal of health promotion and disease prevention should be a shared one for community government and health-care practitioners, and it . can be achieved in many ways.

One of the major transitions that occurred from the earlier initiatives of *Healthy People* to *Healthy People 2000, 2010* was the encouragement from national governmental agencies to local and community agencies to become actively involved in meeting the goals of *Healthy People 2010*. The intent was to shift the activities in meeting the goals of *Healthy People 2010* from a large national effort to local community efforts. It was believed that this shift in responsibility would result in a more significant impact in meeting the goals of the initiative.

Community programs aimed at providing health information are one way that local communities can assist with this initiative. Offering forums for dialogue between health-care practitioners and community citizens is an excellent way to educate a broader audience. If these types of efforts are supported by community leaders, it will impact on the number of community members that the message of health promotion can reach. The development of health-promoting legislation is another way that local communities can help effect change. For example, the passage of "no smoking" restrictions in public areas is an excellent example of how local efforts can improve the health of the communities they serve. Legislative policies and interventions that affect the health of individuals and communities, such as housing, labor, energy, transportation, education, justice, and so forth can be initiated by local and regional agencies . *Healthy People 2010* encourages the active participation of all civic and community agencies to help meet the goals for 2010.

Communities can also respond to the "call for action" from *Healthy People 2010* by ensuring that its citizens have equal access to health care, which . is a priority for *Healthy People 2010,* but it is often difficult for indigent populations to access health-care services in their communities. Many communities do not have systems in place to support the efforts of patients who have language or financial barriers to seek care in their community. Often, a disadvantaged patient's only access to care is when he or she is taken to the hospital for emergency care. At that time, tertiary measures of prevention are employed and are very costly. Many community hospitals can work together with local government agencies to develop health programs/settings that will provide access to health care for all citizens, not just those who have health insurance or whose primary language is English. The long-range goal of establishing these types of health programs is a reduction in direct hospital costs as well as an improvement in the quality of life for all citizens. Saving money is a major concern for most hospital settings and local communities, and improving access to health care can provide significant savings to hospitals. Providing access to health-care services to groups of people who lack the means to access care in traditional settings will do much to improve the health disparities currently affecting our nation. "An ouncc of prevention is worth a pound of cure" is certainly true when it comes to issues of access to care. When patients have access to health-care practitioners for their care, primary, secondary, and tertiary prevention strategies can be implemented and. significant cost savings can be and optimal health promotion can be realized. When access issues continue to be a problem, we are forcing disadvantaged populations to seek care only after an illness or disease has already occurred (which becomes very expensive) and the chance for improvement in health is minimized.

Other Influences

Many other influencces also impact on health promotion efforts. Health promotion strategies can be effective only when we are cognizant of the known diseases affecting our population. With this knowledge in hand, individual health-care practitioners, community partners, and governmental agencies can work together to alleviate or minimize the impact of disease on patients. The evaluation of current health indicators is important if we want to change the course of illness and disease. We must learn from our history. Evaluating and reviewing the current leading causes of death for our nation is one way to learn from our "history." Once we determine what these indicators are, we can then try to determine whether the causes of the diseases are amenable to lifestyle changes. The leading indicators of death in this country are tabulated and recorded every 5 years by the National Center for Health Statisics. The most recently published, in 2003, top 10 causes of death in the United States are listed in Table 3.6. Our current knowledge regarding all of the top 10 causes of disease indicates that healthy lifestyles can indeed impact on their outcome. For example, heart disease has been the number 1 cause of death

Table 3.6 Top 10 Causes of Death (National Vital Statistics Report, 2005)

Cause of Death	Statistics	Amendable to Intervention
Heart disease	725,192	Yes
Malignant disease	549,838	Some
Cerebrovascular disease	167,366	Yes
Chronic lower respiratory disease	124,181	Yes
Unintentional injuries	89,703	Yes
Diabetes mellitus	68,339	Yes
Influenza and pneumonia	63,730	Yes
Alzheimer's disease	44,536	?
Nephritis, nephrotic syndrome	35.525	Yes
Septicemia	30,680	Yes

in the United States for many years. We have gained knowledge about many risk factors that can influence a patient's risk for heart disease. The previously discussed health scenario of Mr. Hart is an excellent example of risk factors for heart disease. As you recall, Mr. Hart had several lifestyle factors that put him at risk for heart disease: smoking, alcohol consumption, overweight, and elevated cholesterol and LDL levels. All of these lifestyles choices, if modified in a more positive direction, could potentially help Mr. Hart to control his heart disease so that he lives a long and healthy life, without the devastation of experiencing a myocardial infarction or possibly even death from heart disease.

Every one of the current top 10 causes of death could be modified with healthy lifestyle choices, providing hope for our patients' future health status. With early health assessment and screenings, we can intervene by helping patients to make healthier life choices that may increase the quality of their lives and potentially help them to avoid the devastation of a disease.

The United States Census Bureau has predicted that the average life expectancy from birth for the year 2005 is 77.7 years. Women are predicted to live an average of 2 years longer than men (79.9 vs. 74.5). Over the past 10 years, life expectancy for men has increased from 72.5 to 74.5 years while the rates for women have remained essentially the same (78.9 to 79.9). The gaps in life expectancy rates in women and men have been attributed to many factors including earlier age at onset for heart disease in men, unhealthier lifestyle choices by men, and the fact that women's hearts do not lose "strength" as they age, in comparison to men's. Researchers in an English study on the strength of hearts in men and women found that men's hearts lose 20 percent to 25 percent of their power from age 20 to 70 while the power of women's heart essentially remains unchanged. These researchers found that 70-year-old men who did regular aerobic exercise had the same functioning power of the heart as 20- year-old men. The study helps to illustrate the fact that although men's hearts can, with aging, lose some of their power or strength, aerobic exercise can help to prevent this loss. This is another example of how encouragement of healthy lifestyle choices (i.e., regular aerobic exercise) can enhance or preserve health.

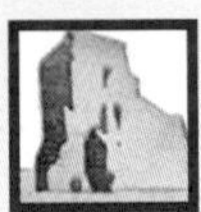

CASE STUDY 3.1

Delia, a 41-year-old woman, comes in to be seen for a complete physical examination. She states that she has completed the questionnaires that were sent to her in anticipation of this appointment. She shows you the completed primary health promotion questionnaire (see Box 3.6) and tells you that she has never had any health-care provider in the past ask her so many in-depth questions about her own health and well-being. She states that she realizes, after completing this assessment form, that there are many factors in her life that contribute to her health status. She relates that completing this survey has made her take a personal inventory of her patterns on a emotional, social, and psychological level and has begun to see how they either contribute or deter from her current physical health. She indicates she is willing to work with her health-care provider to begin to change some of her current health and lifestyle patterns to enhance her own health and well-being. She states that completing this questionnaire has been a very enlightening exercise for her and she is excited to begin "her journey" to balancing her life for better health and harmony.

Practical Epidemiology

As health-care practitioners, it is important for us to closely monitor trends in health and disease that may impact on our patients' health. Research efforts have been numerous in this regard, and the data often yield a multitude of facts and statistics. To make sense of the data, we need to be familiar with basic epidemiological terms that will enhance our ability to understand these facts and statistics and their impact on health promotion and disease prevention.

The definition of epidemiology is the evaluation of distribution patterns and determinants of health and disease in populations. The focus of epidemiology is to study the trends of disease occurrences in groups rather than in individuals. Epidemiological studies are interested in discovering and evaluating the trends of illness or disease in

Box 3.6 Primary Health Promotion Assessment Form

Identifying Information:
Name:
Date of Birth
Current Medical History
Past Medical History

Current Medication History

	Name(s)	Dosage(s)	Frequency
Prescription meds			
Non-prescription med			
Vitamins			
Supplements			
Alternative/complementary meds			
Home remedies			
Other			

Describe your current health status: ______________________________

____

Has your health status changed in the past two years? (If yes, describe) ______________________________

____

What are your own personal health goals? ______________________________

____

Current weight ______________________________ BMI ______________________________

Current height ______________________________

Current Social Habits

Type	Amount	Frequency	Date of most recent use
Cigarettes/cigars			
Alcohol			
Illicit drug use: Type:			
Other :_________			

(continued)

Box 3.6 Primary Health Promotion Assessment Form (continued)

Current Health Promotion Activities

Do you currently wear a seat belt?
Consistently?

Use of sun screen protection: lotions? sun protective filter (SPF) no. ____________

Clothing

How many times/week are you out in direct sunlight? ____________

Duration of time in sun per week? ____________

Helmet Use

Do you currently wear a helmet when using a bike, scooter, motorcycle, etc? ____________

Do you consistently wear a helmet? ____________

Have you ever sustained a head injury/fall related to use of a bike, scooter, motorcycle, etc? (describe) ____________

Home Hazards

Do you have lights to help you to see where you are going outside of your home? ____________

Do you have paved sidewalks to your home/apt/condo? ____________

Are there smoke detectors in your home? ____________

Electric? ____________ battery operated? ____________

Other (describe) ____________

Where do you store chemicals in your home? ____________

Any guns/weapons in the home? ____________

If yes, type and where are they stored? ____________

Work Hazards

Type of work that you do? ____________

Are you currently aware of any hazards to your health at work? ____________

____

Environmental Hazards

Do you currently feel safe where you are living? ____________

Are you aware of any hazards/toxic exposures in your neighborhood? ____________

Gas exposure

Chemical exposure

Lead exposure

Current Exercise Patterns

Do you currently exercise? ____________

Type of exercise: ____________

How often do you exercise? ____________

Duration of exercise? ____________

Injuries related to exercise: ____________

Leisure Time Patterns

Type of activity	Time spent doing activity	How often	Last time you engaged in activity?	
Reading				
Crafts				
Woodworking				
Playing sports				
Watching television				
Listening to music				
Meditating				
Journaling				
Knitting				
Sewing				
Playing a musical instrument				
Gardening				

Religious/Spiritual Affiliations

Do you participate in any religious/spiritual programs?
Type:
Frequency:

Current Emotional Health

Describe your current emotional status: ____________________

____

____

Who are your current social supports?

When was the last time you felt happy? ____________________

When was the last time you felt sad? ____________________

When was the last time you felt angry? ____________________

What do you do when you are upset? Angry? ____________________

(continued)

Box 3.6 Primary Health Promotion Assessment Form (continued)

Dietary health habits:

How many meals do you eat/day?

Do you follow any special type of diet?

Describe:

Duration of time on this diet?

Do you currently have any food allergies/sensitivities?

Describe:

Onset of time for each allergy?

Daily servings of: ______ meats/protein ______ fruits ______ vegetables ______ fats ______ sugar ______ other

What is your favorite beverage of choice? (check all that apply)

______ water ______ how much/day Type: ______ (bottled, filtered, tap)
______ milk ______ how much/day Type: ______ (% of fat)
______ coffee ______ how much/day
______ tea ______ how much/day
______ soda ______ how much/day
______ other (describe) ______ how much /day ______

Do you have any concerns about your current weight? ______

Immunization Health

When was your last : ______ Tetanus
______ Flu Shot
______ Measles, Mumps and Rubella
______ Hepatitis B
______ Pneumococcal vaccine
______ Tuberculosis Screen
______ Other (describe) ______

Current Life Stressors

Which of the following do you consider current stressors in your life (check all that apply):
______ home ______ school ______ work ______ health ______ family
______ friends ______ other (describe)

Please provide more detail regarding each of the identified stressors: ______

What do you do for yourself when you feel stressed?(check all that apply)
______ overeat ______ avoid food ______ use alcohol and/or drugs
______ yell/scream ______ cry ______ become depressed
______ become physically aggressive ______ isolate myself
______ talk with family and friends ______ talk with no one
______ seek counseling ______ journaling ______ use exercise as an outlet
______ meditate ______ listen to music
______ other (describe) ______

What is the best thing that you do for yourself? ______

What is the worst thing that you do to yourself? ______

______

Add any other comments that you would like:

______

______

______

groups of people in order to delineate a cause and effect to try and prevent further disease. For example, one case of West Nile virus is a concern but not the focus of epidemiology. Rather, increasing numbers of cases of West Nile virus become an epidemiological study when they take place in close proximity of time and place. When susceptible populations are studied for the presence of a particular infection or disease, distribution patterns and symptoms may begin to emerge.

It is important to understand the meaning of certain epidemiological terms when reading and evaluating health and disease trends in research studies. When most disease statistics are given, they often refer to the *prevalence* and *incidence* rates of a certain disease. The *prevalence rate* refers to the number of cases of a particular disease at a particular point in time divided by the percentage of the population at a point in time (Table 3.7). The prevalence rate does not distinguish between *new* and *old* cases. For example, the current prevalence rate of type 2 diabetes in the United States is approximately 18.2 million. This number indicates the number of new and old cases of type 2 diabetes in the current population. It also predicts that during the following year, 1.3 million people who are 20 years of age or older will develop diabetes (new cases only). This is the *incidence rate,* which is the number of *new* cases of diabetes diagnosed at a point in time (e.g., 1 year). Prevalence and incidence rates are commonly used terms to describe disease trends, and the formula is provided in Table 3.7.

Additional common terms utilized to study trends include morbidity, mortality, sporadic, endemic, pandemic, and epidemic. Morbidity and mortality rates are often described together and help to define the number of people who have been diagnosed with a disease (*morbidity*) divided by the number of total population at risk vs. the number of people who have died from a particular disease (*mortality*) divided by the total population (Table 3.8).

To understand the difference between morbidity and mortality, consider human immunodeficiency virus (HIV). During 2003, the estimate for the number of persons living with HIV/AIDS in the United States was 1,185,000 (*morbidity rate*). During the same year, the total number of deaths from AIDS was 17,934 (*mortality rate*). The current rates for HIV infection indicate that significant strides have

Table 3.7 Prevalence and Incidence Rate

Prevalence Rate	Incidence Rate
New and old cases of "B" disease at a specific point in time No. of total population at a specific point in time	New cases of "C" disease at a specific point in time No. of total population at a specific point in time

Table 3.8 Morbidity and Mortality Formulas

Morbidity Formula	Mortality Formula
No. of new cases of "D" disease divided by total population at risk	No. of deaths from "E" disease divided by total population at risk

been made in improving prevention of HIV, which has in turn influenced the incidence, prevalence, morbidity, and mortality associated with the disease. More people are also living longer with the HIV as a result of significant advances in its medication and management.

Certain illnesses will affect the population during annual predictable cycles. Terminology regarding these cycles includes epidemic, endemic, sporadic, and pandemic. For example, influenzae virus is known to be prevalent during the winter season and can cause significant morbidity and mortality. The ability to predict the active cycle of this virus helps health-care practitioners to educate and inoculate patients before predicted outbreaks. These health promotion efforts are effective means of decreasing the prevalence and incidence of the influenzae virus or the "flu." Each year, predictions are made regarding the number of patients who, without health promotion efforts, will experience the "flu." In the past, there have been years in which the number of patients experiencing the flu was significantly higher than expected. This would be termed an "*epidemic,*" defined as the presence of an event (illness or disease) at a much higher than expected rate projected on the basis of past history.

Although the common cold appears to have some variation, it is known to be present throughout the year. Because it is considered to be present consistently throughout the year, it would be considered an *endemic* outbreak. *Endemic* is the term used when the presence of an event is constant at or about the same frequency as expected based on past history. A *sporadic* outbreak occurs when there are occasional cases of an event unrelated in space or time. For example, a gastrointestinal virus may be present in 3 patients this month, 20 patients 2 months from now, and 100 patients in 6 months. The virus is present but is not causing illness at a specific time and place. It is rare to hear of a patient having the "flu" during the summer season. The last epidemiological term that it is important to understand is **pandemic**, defined as the presence of an event in epidemic proportions affecting many communities and countries in a short period of time. For example, at this time, there is grave concern regarding avian or "bird" flu. It has been found in several countries in a short period of time, and there is concern that it will soon reach pandemic proportions by affecting many people in many countries. All of these epidemiological terms help to clarify the sig-

Table 3.9 **Epidemiological Terms**

Term	Definition
Sporadic	Outbreaks of an illness/disease that occur occasionally and are unrelated in space and time
Epidemic	Presence of an event (illness or disease) at a much higher than expected rate based on past history
Endemic	Presence of an illness/disease constantly present or present at a rate that is expected based on history
Pandemic	Presence of an event in epidemic proportions affecting many communities and countries in a short period of time

nificance of a current illness or disease at a point in time (Table 3.9).

The CDC generally monitors and reports the incidence, prevalence, morbidity, and mortality rates of diseases and specifically monitors the rates of infectious diseases. This information is distributed weekly in a report titled *The Morbidity and Mortality Weekly Report (MMWR)* which is available online at http://www.cdc.gov/mmwr. It informs health-care practitioners about current infectious diseases that are a threat to our local and global community and provides them with the latest guidelines for treatment of infectious diseases. It is a helpful tool to utilize for current infectious disease trends and potential health promotion practices that may minimize or eliminate the threat of infectious disease.

Conclusion

Health promotion is one of the most powerful tools that we have today to prevent disease and disability. Health-care practitioners need to utilize health promotion strategies on the primary, secondary, and tertiary levels of prevention. Each level of prevention is important but our ultimate goal should be to focus efforts on the area that can have the most significant impact on health, which is primary prevention. Actively engaging in primary prevention strategies such as health promotion creates a wonderful opportunity for patients and health-care practitioners to work together as a team with the common goal of wellness and the prevention of disease. When primary prevention strategies are not feasible, *Healthy People 2010* and the *U.S. Preventive Service Task Force* provides health-care practitioners with guidelines to initiate secondary prevention strategies such as early screening and detection of illness and disease. The utilization of these guidelines and health-focused initiatives will help to improve the health of our nation and enable new threats, such as the bird flu, recurrent and severe hurricanes, and bio-terrorism to be anticipated and dealt with as expeditiously as possible. With all of the current health promotion strategies in place and a continued effort to focus on disease prevention, it may be possible to eliminate or minimize the most expensive level of health promotion: tertiary prevention. As we advance further into the 21st century, we should continue to build momentum on primary health promotion strategies with the goal of ensuring optimal wellness for all of our nation's citizens. This goal, if met, would help to achieve the goals of *Healthy People 2010* and perhaps eliminate the need for developing a future *Healthy People 2030*!

References

Agency for Healthcare Research and Quality. Guide to Clinical Preventive Services, 2005. AHRQ Publication No. 05-0570, June 2005. Rockville, Md. http://www.ahrq.gov/clinic/pocketgd.htm (Accessed June 30, 2006).

Masson, Veneta. Rehab at the Florida Avenue Grill. B& B Printing. Richmond. 1999, 18–19.

National Center for Health Statistics. Healthy People 2000: Final Review. Hyattsville, Md., Public Health Services. 2001. http://www.cdc.gov/nchs/data/hp2000/hp2k01.pdf (Accessed June 30, 2006).

O'Donnell, M. Definition of health promotion: part iii; Expanding the definition. Am J Health Promot 3(3):5, 1989.

Pender, N. Health Promotion in Nursing Practice, 5th ed. Prentice Hall, Upper Saddle River, N.J., 2006.

U.S. Department of Health, Education and Welfare, Public Health Service. The Surgeon General's report on health promotion and disease prevention. U.S. Department of Health and Human Services. U.S. Government Printing Office, Washington, D.C., 1979.

U.S. Department of Health and Human Services: Healthy People 2000. U.S. Government Printing Office, Washington, D.C., 1996.

U.S. Department of Health and Human Services: Healthy People 2010 (Conference Edition, in Two Volumes). U.S. Government Printing Office, Washington, D.C. January 2000. http://www.healthypeople.gov

U.S. Department of Vital Statistics. National Center for Health Statistics World Health Organization. Official Records of the World Health Organization. No. 2, p. 100. http://www.cdc.gov/nchs/index.htm

The Clinician's Handbook of Preventative Services. International Medical Publishing, Alexandria, Va., 1996.

Webster's College Dictionary. Random House, New York, 1995.

Bibliography

Edelman, C., and Mandle, C: Health Promotion Through the Lifespan, 5th ed. C.V. Mosby. St. Louis, 2002.

Fitzgerald, F: Preventive medicine and the "road to hell." Consultant 8 (August) 2003. 1055–1056.

Hitchcock, J, Schubert, P., and Thomas, S: Community Health Nursing—Caring in Action, 2nd ed. Thomson-Delmar. Australia.

Jerzak, L: The role of dietary calcium in promoting health and preventing chronic disease across the lifespan. Am J Nurse Pract 9(3):21–28, 2005.

Murphy, D., and Istenes, N: Strategies to promote successful aging: Part 2, the physician's role. Consultant 5:653–658, 2005.

Resources

Agency for Health Care Policy and Research
http://www.ahcpr.gov/
American College of Nurse Practitioners
http://www.nurse.org/acnp
American Academy of Family Physicians
http://www.aafp.org
American Academy of Nurse Practitioners
http://www.aanp.org
American College of Sports Medicine
http://www.acsm.org
http://www.physsportsmed.com
Centers for Disease Control and Prevention
http://www.cdc.gov/cdc.html
Food and Drug Administration
http://www.fda.gov
National Institutes of Health
http://www.nih.gov/
National Institute of Nursing Research
http://www.nih.gov/ninr
National Library of Medicine
http://www.nlm.nih.gov
Occupational Safey and Health Administration
http://www.osha.gov
U. S. Department of Health and Human Services
http://www.hhs.gov

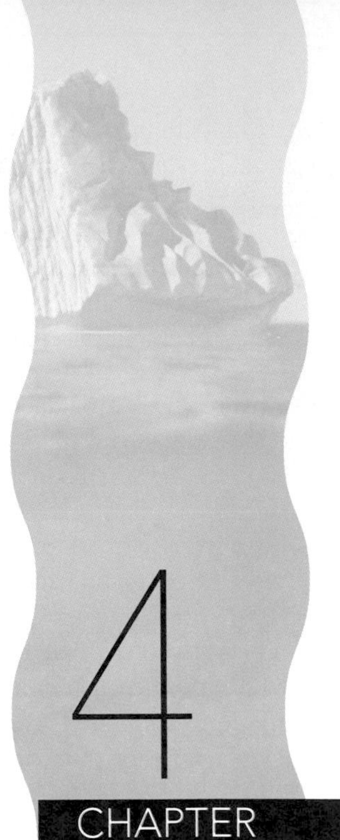

The Art of Diagnosis and Treatment

Susan K. Chase, EdD, APRN, BC

Advanced practice nurses (APNs) are able to offer unique services in primary care for several reasons. First, they bring a nursing perspective of whole person care to patient encounters that in some settings have been more disease centered than person centered. A correct diagnosis is required, but there is more to do than focus on the diagnosis. Second, as clinicians work with patients to plan how to improve health, they take into account more than a plan for prescription medications. They include considerations of each individual's life situation when choosing regimens that may include medication, but will also include diet, activity, rest, stress management, and health promotion. There is more to do in a primary-care visit than set up a treatment plan. Learning to practice primary care in an artful way such as this requires a certain kind of thinking. The kind of thinking that clinicians engage in is the subject of this chapter.

The Context of Clinical Judgment in Primary Care

Clinical Judgment and the Circle of Caring

The Circle of Caring model, introduced in Chapter 1, provides a framework for advanced practice nursing. It includes aspects of the more traditional medical model approaches within a model that has nursing as its origin. The Circle of Caring incorporates elements of the patient's experience, including the context of that experience and the environment in which care is delivered. It includes traditional modes of assessment, such as history taking, that are similar to those of the medical model, as well as a database for a nursing perspective, the functional health patterns, or other more holistic measures. Objective findings include physical assessment data, laboratory test data, and functional measures. The Circle of Caring demonstrates that the clinician takes these data as part of a data collection process that leads to the identification of both medical diagnoses as listed in the International Classification of Diseases, 10th Revision (ICD-10) and the human responses to those specific diagnoses or nursing diagnoses as listed in taxonomies such as the North American Nursing Diagnosis Association (NANDA). The NANDA list includes consideration of problem prevention and wellness promotion and goes beyond a narrow problem-solving framework. A full understanding of the patient situation provides a basis for planning interventions. Especially here, patient preferences are considered as the patient and provider together design a treatment plan that may include pharmacologic measures, but will also include lifestyle choices and complementary modalities to approach healing and wellness. The Circle of Caring reflects that outcomes of APN practice include improved mortality and morbidity statistics for aggregates of patients; optimized use of the health-care system that provides early, relatively inexpensive treatments to prevent more expensive problems later; and improved functional status and quality of life, as judged by the patient.

Not only is the Circle of Caring an expanded way of thinking of both the nursing and the medical clinical process but it also denotes the way in which the APN and patient relate to each other within this model. The APN is able to make appropriate diagnosis and intervention selections on the basis of knowing the patient, being committed to finding acceptable treatment options, and having patience when working with the patient, who may be required to make substantial lifestyle change as a result of illness or risk factors. In addition, both patient and nurse exhibit courage in that they engage in this most human of endeavors, that of caring. Throughout the assessment, diagnosis, and treatment, the APN brings an authentic presence, which is in itself humanizing and healing, and is willing to be an advocate for the patient in personal or professional realms. The Circle of Caring requires a balance among the consideration of the attention that the nurse together with the patient can generate in forming a workable treatment plan and follow-up support. The Circle of Caring depicts a complex yet rewarding practice that enriches both patient and nurse.

This chapter focuses on the process aspects of the model. The Circle of Caring model includes the medical model perspective that nurses with baccalaureate degrees may not have learned in an academic setting or practiced in hospital or community settings. It also includes a broader sense of nursing than practice at the baccalaureate level allows. The APN role includes elements from the medical realm, but it also functions from an expanded nursing basis.

Essential to high-quality clinical judgment is the ability of the nurse to form a link between the patient's experience of his or her health concerns and the range of diagnostic and therapeutic choices available to achieve a range of possible outcome states. The nurse must be expert at eliciting the true story of the patient and in recognizing patterns that are presented in the data so as to arrive at an appropriate diagnosis and therapeutic plan. This chapter focuses on merging the results of research with diagnostic reasoning and clinical judgment to facilitate their application by the APN.

Purpose and Goal of Diagnostic Reasoning

From the patient's point of view, the purpose of some visits to clinicians may be to solve a physical problem. Beyond problem solving, the practitioner must always keep in mind that every visit is an opportunity for disease prevention, for screening for high-risk problems, and for health promotion. The patient must know that his or her initial concerns are taken seriously and are not ignored. The APN can establish a tone that attends to body, mind, and spirit in every visit. Diagnostic reasoning to solve problems, to promote health, and to screen for disease or illness all require a sensitivity to complex stories, to contextual factors, and to a sense of probability and uncertainty. At times, the patient will schedule a visit stating one concern, but during the visit other issues arise that become more important. Headache might be caused by a stressful job or family situation, or the patient might not want to tell the scheduler that domestic violence or a sexual concern is really what is bothering them. Clinicians learn to pay attention to the "By the way, I was wondering about……" lead-ins to real concerns.

The mental tasks of eliciting and sorting through large amounts of data, of clustering those data elements into meaningful patterns, of connecting patterns to reasonable diagnostic statements, of considering risk factors, and of selecting appropriate interventions require the highest order of cognitive processes. It is these analytical functions that distinguish advanced practice nursing and are the reason patients seek our services. The human element of caring helps elicit rich data and establish the trust necessary to encourage patients to adjust their living patterns in the short or long range.

Primary Care and Its Uniqueness

Many students come to advanced practice programs with extensive experience in acute- or critical-care nursing. They are committed to learning an expanded mode of practice but may be overwhelmed by the amount of new material that must be mastered. Even students with community health experience find that the issues faced in primary care are different from those encountered in their previous practice and require new knowledge and skills. Primary care is a new world with a different set of problems to be solved, different kinds of constraints on choices, and a different culture of care. Entering this world with sensitivity to its differences can help reduce anxiety for new advanced practice students and can explain other reactions to this new nursing setting that might arise.

The types of problems that are solved in primary care are different from those encountered in acute- or critical-care settings. Upper respiratory infections, common abdominal complaints, skin rashes, and vaginal discharges are problems not often encountered in acute-care settings. Even chronic conditions present differently in primary care. Hypertension, congestive heart failure, arthritis, or diabetes present with day-to-day management problems that are different from the crises that acute-care nurses must respond to in tertiary-care settings. Patients with psychosocial problems such as anxiety and depression frequently present with vague, nonspecific somatic complaints.

The pace of care is different in primary care. Nurses who are seeking refuge from busy acute-care duties will be surprised by the mental fatigue that comes from diagnosing and treating up to 30 different patients or families in a day. The sheer variety of possible problems faced in a day's time is exciting and interesting, but it is also challenging. The office visit allows for focused attention with an individual patient, but the former staff nurse will realize that an organized approach to obtaining and processing information is necessary because the patient will not be available to fill in missing pieces of information at the end of the day. On the other hand, the relationship with a growing family or the treatment of patients with chronic conditions will continue over years. This long-term relationship is very rewarding to both the APN and the patient and family.

Primary care includes more than problem solving and symptom management. It involves screening for problems as yet undetected as well as supporting health promotion and disease and injury prevention at every opportunity. Teaching patients of all ages about how their bodies work, about risk reduction, and treatment options helps patients assume more responsibility for their own wellness.

Uncertainty

Primary care and the increased autonomy that advanced practice clinicians enjoy also bring an increase in uncertainty. Patient problems are not already labeled when the nurse practitioner sees the patient. Many different conditions present in similar ways. Even the "hard numbers" of laboratory tests must be evaluated for their reliability. Once a diagnosis is made, multiple treatment approaches are available even for simple problems. Furthermore, patients do not always carry out recommended treatment plans. Many problems require life-long lifestyle adjustment. At the end of the day, the clinician may have nagging doubts about the decisions that were made on many levels. As a support for new practitioners, preceptors and new employers are available to encourage the development of confidence in diagnostic and treatment planning, but even experienced practitioners describe learning to live with the uncertainties involved in primary care. Intellectual honesty and humility are important aspects of thoughtful practice and can be cultivated, but they must be balanced with confidence that is based on experience; this serves to increase the effectiveness of the provider.

Nursing versus Medical Model

APNs perform in both the nursing and the medical domain. The nursing domain contains consideration of individual and family responses to actual or potential threats to health. It involves helping patients cope with disease processes that may be occurring, and it anticipates human distress and works on the level of what an illness experience means to the patient. By becoming an APN, nurses do not leave their nursing model of practice. As APNs gain skill in the medical domain of practice, they learn new diagnostic reasoning possibilities and new treatment options for specific medical problems. These new skills are built upon the nursing framework; they do not replace the nursing basis for practice. APNs have been proved to be effective and efficient care providers for patients with acute and chronic health problems. Though much of this textbook is designed to provide a background for managing medical problems, all that the nurse has learned in caring for patients still applies. An APN's approach to patient problems is often very individualized and, therefore, less easy to summarize in a textbook. Nevertheless, the nursing model supports and nurtures the APN's practice. It provides the basis for the Circle of Caring.

Patient-Advanced Practice Nurse Linkages

A model for how the provider and patient work together in a clinical encounter is presented in Fig. 4.1. Clinical judgment is not a process that happens in the mind of the practitioner

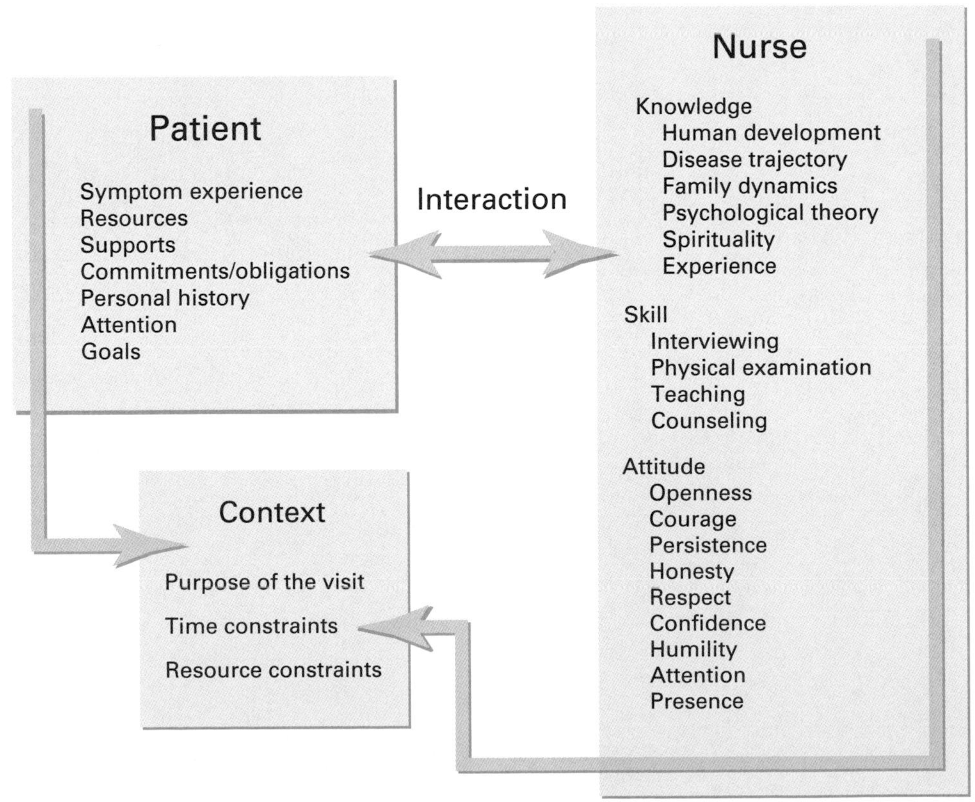

FIGURE 4.1 Patient-advanced practice nursing linkages. (From Chase, SK: Clinical Judgment and Communication in Nurse Practitioner Practice. FA Davis, Philadelphia, 2004.)

alone: It happens in a dialogue that occurs between patient and provider. The quality of communication and the agreement about what the encounter is meant to accomplish will improve both effectiveness and satisfaction with the patient encounter for both parties. The model includes patient factors, provider factors, and environmental factors, all of which have an influence on the clinical judgment process (Chase, 2004).

The Patient-Advanced Practice Nurse linkage model is based on research in diagnostic reasoning in general and the particulars of the primary-care encounter. Johnson (1993) described the discourse between patient and nurse as having several phases: establishing the agenda for the encounter; eliciting information from the patient, including being alert to cues and helping to problem solve; conducting the physical examination, including attending to comfort level, preparing and informing, and developing a plan of care and using a teachable moment. Teaching in this case is not content-centered but patient-centered, based on understanding the perspective of the patient. Finally, the APN personalizes solutions based on knowing the patient. Investigating overall satisfaction with care, a large quantitative study has shown that patients are equally satisfied with care access and overall care experience when care is provided by a nurse practitioner or physician assistant as compared to a visit managed by a physician in both adult and pediatric settings. Patients were more satisfied, however, with nurse practitioner and physician assistant care when rating the quality of practitioner interaction (Roblin, Becker, Adams, Howard and Roberts, 2004). The personal relationship between APN and patient within which this work is done is unique.

The Clinical Process and Its Limitations

Human Memory Limitations

One of the most useful models available to understanding diagnostic reasoning is that of the information processing model. This model is built on the premise that the human brain has both short- and long-term memory and that these forms of memory are different from each other. Short-term memory is the processing space that can hold new pieces of information and elements of the patient history as well as physical data. It has the limitation of only being able to hold approximately seven "bits" of information. Much of the mental activity used in diagnostic reasoning is done to maximize the active processing space and to cluster or "chunk" cues into collections of data that can be managed together to maximize processing capacity. In contrast, long-term memory is practically unlimited. It can hold vast quantities of facts, sensations, and experiences. To bring these facts or experiences to bear on a given situation, long-term memories must be accessible. Research has shown that the ability to retrieve a fact depends on the frequency with which the fact is brought forward for use. This is why in some cases repetitive exercises assist in cementing long-term memory. Another factor that affects retrievability of facts from long-term memory is the organization structure with which the fact is associated. Body systems and functional health patterns are systems of data organization that help busy clinicians retrieve relevant bits of information as needed.

In actuality, although the information processing model is a useful starting point, the human brain functions differently from a computer. The brain is able to sense patterns of data and to include emotional responses to experiences with human beings. The ability to empathize with a patient, to be available personally, and to be invested with the patient in maximizing health make the human decision-maker much more valuable than any computer or protocol system could ever be. If protocols were enough for effective management, then the Internet or other computer system would be sufficient to provide health care to anyone with access to the system. Patients come to a health-care provider for more than a diagnosis, however. They come for a human connection. The human aspect of the nurse–patient relationship adds to, rather than detracts from, diagnostic accuracy.

Critical Thinking

Diagnostic reasoning can be seen as a kind of critical thinking. Critical thinking has been defined as reflective thinking, because the process involves questioning one's thinking to determine if all possible avenues have been explored and if the conclusions that are being drawn are based on evidence. This kind of thinking supports clinical judgment in several ways. First, it becomes a habit of mind to have humility about one's thought processes and to know that even the most experienced thinker can be mistaken. Second, it becomes a systematic way of generating creative ways of thinking about problems. Third, critical thinking returns one to an examination of the strength of evidence for a given conclusion. "Evidence" in this context means more than "hard" data such as laboratory values. Even laboratory values must be examined critically when they are used to assist diagnostic reasoning. The type of evidence that is useful includes subjective impressions of the ways patients present themselves. The patient's initial complaint may be fatigue, but any patient who describes a bone-chilling inability to generate energy for daily living (compared with a fulfilled fatigue that comes after a challenging situation is completed) is providing data the APN can use to investigate potentially serious health problems.

Critical thinking can include creative thinking—in this sense, the APN is creative in developing potential problem lists. A patient may complain of abdominal pain. The pattern is unclear or may indicate irritable bowel syndrome. The creative APN will explore stress management issues as a way of generating diagnostic and therapeutic choices that could include a diet and symptom log, increased fiber in the diet, a walking program, or a quick follow-up visit to check on symptoms. Creativity may also be required in developing goals with patients for their short- or long-term problems. In addition to creative processing, critical thinking includes systematic thinking that evaluates each new piece of data as it either supports some diagnostic hypotheses or reduces the likelihood of others.

Intuition

Another kind of thinking that develops with experience is that of intuition. Research on intuition shows that it develops after long experience in the particular setting and that it is based on unconscious thought that is probably an exquisite pattern matching. The experienced clinician is reminded of a situation that occurred in the past when presented with a certain new situation. Past experience provides a picture of what will likely happen. The experienced clinician often could not list the specific data points that led to the conclusion. In fact, in some studies of computerized "artificial intelligence," experienced clinicians were asked to "think aloud" as a research device aimed at identifying the steps involved in reaching a diagnosis. Experienced clinicians reported that being asked to do that kind of thinking changed their thought process and slowed them down.

Developing Expertise

Benner (1996) has done extensive work describing differences in clinical judgment based on experience. APN students, even those who are experts in hospital or specialty care, find it disconcerting to enter a world where they feel like novices again. Even skills that were a part of their old practice feel awkward. Their minds often do not generate ideas smoothly, and they focus on their own performance of skills more than on the patient's situation. With the experience of the clinical practicum, however, the student gains skill and by graduation is probably functioning at the advanced beginner level. Features of diagnostic reasoning used in the various stages of expertise are summarized in Table 4.1.

Table 4.1 Skill Acquisition in Advanced Nursing Practice

Skill Level	Features of Clinical Judgment
Novice	Rule-based actions, unaware of context
Advanced beginner	Sensitive to aspects of the situation, able to formulate principles, needs help setting priorities
Competent	Goal-directed actions, feeling of mastery based on experience, deliberate planning
Proficient	Sees situation as a whole, immediate grasp of meaning, recognizes patterns of normalcy or aberrance, uses maxims to guide action
Expert	Transcends rules, intuitive grasp of the wholeness of situation, creative response to particularities of situation, flexible response to situations

Diagnostic Process Overview

Diagnostic reasoning is a process of data generation and clustering, hypothesis generation, probabilistic reasoning, pattern matching, planning, problem solving, and critical reflection. These processes are commonly summarized by describing the steps in the nursing process or the clinical reasoning process. Research has shown that many clinicians, physicians, nurses, occupational and physical therapists, dentists, and others use a similar method. Although research that uses simulated case studies to examine methods of clinician reasoning tends to oversimplify what happens in real life, it is helpful to review a simplified description of the diagnostic process as outlined here.

Data Collection

Research has shown that expert clinicians generate a list of possible diagnoses or diagnostic hypotheses early in the clinical encounter. Further, the likelihood that the diagnostic choice will be correct is higher if the correct diagnosis is included in the initial hypothesis list. In generating hypotheses, the APN considers a number of labels that could be associated with the initial complaint and considers potential problems for each patient based on the patient's age and demographics and the setting of the practice.

For experienced clinicians, data acquisition in history taking and physical examination is most effective if it is hypothesis driven—that is, when the information selected and gathered is related to the list of possible diagnoses. For common problems, the data collection approach becomes routine and, therefore, takes less active processing space in short-term memory. In contrast, novices tend to use a "shotgun" approach and ask a little bit about everything that might be possible, not considering which diagnoses are most likely. Hypothesis-driven data collection means that data that would confirm or disprove a specific hypothesis that is being considered is specifically sought and recorded. It is not enough to note only those data that fit with one possible problem. Competing hypotheses must be ruled out by seeking nonconfirmatory data. In doing this, the clinician must be open to changing the priority list of hypotheses based on new information. For example, rhinitis may present like a viral infection, but if, when asked whether the symptoms have occurred before, the patient says, "Yes, I had the same thing two weeks ago," this decreases the likelihood of viral illness and increases the likelihood of allergy.

An approach to data collection that is completely symptom driven, however, can result in leaving out important concepts. The agenda for the visit includes not only the patient's agenda but also expands the visit to provide health promotion.

Hypothesis Evaluation

Data are clustered together into meaningful "chunks" of information that explain and account for the different elements of the history. Clinicians are alert to any data bits that do not fit the pattern of what is expected. They are alert to the feeling in themselves that "something is just not right here." This can indicate that the problem is more serious than initially appeared or that there are data bits that are not yet accounted for. Diagnosticians are persistent in trying to fit the pieces of data into a coherent picture. One must be on guard not to ignore discrepant data. Research has shown that "we see what we expect to see" in many cases, so an openness to the patient situation must be maintained in order to continue "seeing" all the data present.

A maxim of practice is that "common things occur commonly." Students are frequently excited to make a diagnosis for the rare or exotic condition. This can be the result of a rich experience in acute- or critical-care settings where the most serious cases were seen. In primary care, common problems predominate. The maxim that "when you hear hoofbeats, think horses, not zebras" applies. In real life, "zebra" diagnoses are rare. Rare conditions can be considered with the differential list, but their lower probability must be taken into consideration.

Experienced clinicians keep their antennae raised for the most serious conditions. Abdominal pain could be from gas, but if it is from a ruptured ectopic pregnancy, a dissecting abdominal aortic aneurysm (AAA), or a ruptured appendix, then immediate surgical consultation is necessary. The clinician must first collect and document data that rule out any potentially life-threatening condition.

Diagnoses are frequently interrelated. Obesity, hypertension, hyperlipidemia, and type 2 diabetes frequently occur together. When evaluating competing hypotheses, the APN can cluster related problems together. The lifestyle recommendations for all these conditions are the same. The medication approach might differ. For nursing diagnoses, many occur together. Try to approach the core diagnosis, which, if managed appropriately, will ameliorate all the others. For instance, ineffective coping with stress can result in an array of symptoms including altered sleep patterns, constipation, difficulty concentrating, and interpersonal tension. By dealing with the underlying problem, the other problems might not need direct intervention. If the APN focuses only on the superficial problem level, the problems may still remain. Table 4.2 summarizes habits that promote effective clinical judgment. Table 4.3 describes common errors in diagnostic thinking that are made even by experts.

Clustering history data into a likely problem list helps to focus the physical examination, laboratory test evaluation, and initial management plan. Physical examination for a problem-focused visit serves to rule in or rule out com-

Table 4.2 Habits That Support Clinical Judgment

Phase of Diagnostic Reasoning	Habits That Support Clinical Judgment
Data acquisition	Use systematic or hierarchically organized approach (general to specific) Review multiple systems (selective)
Hypothesis formulation	Generate hypotheses early in encounter Develop competing hypotheses Consider life- or function-threatening problems Consider "zebras" but recognize them as such
Hypothesis evaluation	Recognize interrelation of diagnoses Consider probabilities in context Consider likelihood of altering course of problem with treatment Rule out life- or function-threatening problems
Problem naming	Choose most fundamental problem Include multiple perspectives (biopsychosocial, spiritual; medical, nursing) Include illness prevention and health promotion
Goal setting	Include patient in goal setting Make goals explicit and realistic
Therapeutic option consideration	Include modalities from multiple paradigms Consider patient preferences Consider context and cost in economic and human terms
Evaluation	Plan for follow-up visit or phone call Consider symptom or treatment logs or diaries Measure and document the outcome of your practice for the individual Report the effectiveness of your practice in the aggregate

Source: Chase, SF: Clinical Judgment and Communication in Nurse Practitioner Practice. FA Davis, Philadelphia, 2004, p 43.

Table 4.3 Errors in Diagnostic Reasoning

Phase of Clinical Judgment	Diagnostic Errors
Data collection	Not obtaining all relevant cues Misjudging importance of cues Overemphasizing cues that favor top hypotheses Ignoring data that disconfirm working hypothesis Forgetting that some data are unreliable Ignoring pertinent negative findings
Hypothesis generation	Not generating enough competing hypotheses Oversimplifying Not generating hypotheses early Not including correct diagnosis on hypothesis list Failing to revise hypothesis list (premature closure) Selecting "favorite" hypotheses Generating too many hypotheses and getting lost Overestimating low-probability situations Underestimating high-probability situations

Source: Chase, SF: Clinical Judgment and Communication in Nurse Practitioner Practice. FA Davis, Philadelphia, 2004.

peting diagnostic hypotheses. A new hypothesis rarely emerges during a physical examination, but this might occur for a problem that the patient cannot see or that causes no symptoms such as a skin lesion. Laboratory tests also provide information that is not available any other way.

Finally, a working diagnosis is reached, even though there might still be some uncertainty. A management plan is discussed with the patient in light of mutually shared goals. Honest conversation about the patient's ability and willingness to follow treatment recommendations will result in more realistic plans. Written instructions often help patients implement complicated treatment directions. Part of the treatment plan always includes a plan for follow-up. Patients need to know when to return for a visit and under what circumstances they should telephone. Documenting these plans in the patient record reduces the possibility of misunderstanding and places appropriate responsibility with the patient.

The Diagnostic Process in Action

A simple encounter for a self-limiting acute illness might proceed like this:

A patient requests an appointment for a "sore throat." The patient is known by the APN as a resourceful, independent young adult. Before even entering the room, the clinician draws from experience with other patients who have complained of sore throat and begins to generate a list of hypotheses. Contextual factors enter into the reasoning: it may be allergy season in that particular area, or the clinician may have seen a large number of other patients with similar complaints who have tested positive for *Streptococcus* infection. The clinician enters the room and notes the general appearance of the patient. Is the patient ill appearing, flushed, fatigued, or mildly irritated? These observations may serve to adjust the hypothesis list. The patient's story is elicited, beginning with history of present illness, along with a review of data already present in the record regarding past medical history and medications. Further questions regarding current life stresses and exposures may also serve to adjust the hypothesis list. The history narrows the hypothesis list to a short one, although experienced clinicians have ways of preventing the common diagnostic error of premature closure and work to consider alternative conditions that could also be represented by the same cluster of symptoms.

The physical exam serves to verify hypotheses and to screen out unlikely, though troubling alternative diagnoses. The hypothesis list is narrowed further as data are weighed to see whether they fit the pattern of the highest favored hypothesis; disconfirming data are also elicited, to avoid leaping to conclusions too early. Finally, diagnostic tests may be chosen to firm up the diagnosis if the findings of the tests will have a bearing on how the patient is to be managed. Once findings of relevant tests have been obtained, treatment decisions are considered, including patient factors such as resources, reliability, and the risk of the patient not following through on instructions. For example, insufficiently treated strep throat could result in rheumatic heart disease. Besides prescribing medication, consider comfort measures that are likely to assist the patient and judge the appropriateness of health promotion and educational opportunities at the moment. For example, is this a good time to give the patient smoking cessation materials? Finally, a plan to evaluate the treatment plan is made. Is a follow-up appointment necessary? Would a telephone call be useful? For which date should the next "well" visit be scheduled? The list of decisions made in this rather simple example is long. Given a few data or situational changes, the management of the patient could be quite different, and a new-patient visit requires deeper background data collection. Patients who present with more complex, long-term problems require even more complex decision-making by the clinician.

Focus on Elements of Clinical Judgment

A more detailed examination of each step in the diagnostic reasoning process follows.

Focus on Data Collection: History

History of Present Illness

Taking a history is the first step in the diagnostic reasoning process. Problems cannot be found, strengths identified, or appropriate direction known without a real grounding in the life experience of the individual patient. If the patient's visit is for "episodic" care or one in which a new complaint is being addressed, the history begins with a history of present illness (HPI). There are a number of mnemonics that can help the clinician remember the essential data elements. The elements of the "OLD CART" mnemonic are listed in Box 4.1.

Immediately on hearing the chief complaint, the clinician begins to sort out diagnostic possibilities. The list of possibilities helps to generate questions to follow up on the HPI and in other areas of the history. Specific questions are asked that help distinguish between competing diagnostic hypotheses. For example, the question, "Do you feel the pain more often on an empty stomach or several hours after eating?" helps distinguish between ulcer and gall bladder disease. In general, asking open-ended questions helps the patient give his or her perspective and provides a richer database. An open-ended question is one that cannot be answered by a Yes or No response. Eliciting the patient's story will assist the APN in understanding the illness experience from the patient's point of view.

The APN continues to clarify the patient's story until a clear picture of the illness appears. This can require patience, because patients do not know which facts "fit together" to support diagnostic hypotheses. Patients may get the chronological order confused or not recall the exact onset of their problems. They may also have more than one problem and may not be able to distinguish which symptoms cluster together. At times, the picture is not completely clear at this point of history taking, but other areas of history can fill in some gaps. Periodically, the APN can restate the emerging understanding of the story to clarify and summarize it. This summary allows the patient to clarify any misunderstandings. One important issue to address as part of the HPI is what the *patient* thinks may be wrong. Patients know their own bodies better than anyone and may have important insights to share. On the other hand, when patients share their fears, the APN can also explain reasons why many of those fears may be unfounded. A recurring headache does not necessarily indicate a brain tumor.

Visits for periodic health screening, to establish a new patient–provider relationship, or to follow on an existing problem do not use the HPI in the same sense unless a new problem is also identified. The APN can ask, "What do you want to accomplish today?" or "What is the most important issue for us to deal with today?" This is particularly useful for the patient with a long list of problems or complaints. Be sure to make a plan for follow-up on other problems. Other elements of patient history are discussed in detail during the visit.

BOX 4.1 Old Cart Mnemonic

Onset	When did this problem start? How did it start? Has it changed over time? For an injury, exactly how did the injury occur (the mechanism of injury)?
Location	Where exactly are the symptoms experienced? Can a specific location be identified, or is the problem more generalized? Has the symptom moved?
Duration	Are the symptoms constant, fluctuating, getting better or worse?
Characteristics	How are the symptoms experienced? Dull ache, sharp pain, heat, or electrical?
Aggravating factors	What makes the symptoms worse?
Relieving factors	What makes the symptoms better?
Treatment	What have you done so far to try to help the problem?

Past Medical History

Past medical history helps to refine the hypothesis list by offering new explanations for symptoms or by ruling out others. The history also gives suggestions of risk factors for other problems that are being considered. If a patient reports that his or her gall bladder was removed 10 years ago, cholecystitis is now off the hypothesis list. Past medical history is frequently divided into childhood and other illnesses, surgical history, other hospital admissions, history of trauma, pregnancies, and psychiatric diagnoses. Travel outside the United States and any possible exposure to infectious or toxic agents can be explored.

The history includes information regarding all medications that patients take, including prescription and over-the-counter medications, as well as vitamins and herbal remedies. Patients also need to be asked if they take any medications that have been prescribed for other members of the family. Even for patients who are well known to the practice and whose medications are listed on the chart, by asking the patient what medications he or she is currently taking, the clinician learns what the patient remembers about the medication regimen. For patients with multiple prescriptions, it sometimes helps to use the "brown bag" method: Ask the patient to bring in all the medications he or she is taking, then go over them one by one. This helps to determine if the medications that have been ordered are really being taken. This review of medications also gives the clinician information about the patient's understanding of his or her medications and helps to determine any difficulties he or she is having with the prescribed regimen. Immunization status is part of the history. Many parents bring their child's immunization cards with them to office visits. This allows any additional immunization series to be documented. Adults often forget that they need immunizations for things such as tetanus or pneumonia.

Allergies can be discussed at this time and reviewed. The kind of reaction the medications or food caused can help to distinguish an adverse effect from a true allergy. By noting the adverse effect one can avoid confusing it with an allergy, which is characterized by rash, hives, wheezing, or other hypersensitivity reactions.

Health maintenance practices can be questioned, as well as risk reduction techniques such as seat belt use and exercise habits.

Family History

Family history provides information for a part of the risk factor pattern for this patient. The most efficient way to represent the family history is to draw a genogram (Fig. 4.2). This method of representation can be used to record family patterns of births, ages at death, and causes of death. The genogram can also record family members with whom the patient currently lives. Try to include information for at least two generations back as well as for any children and their health status. The genogram can be used to map difficulties such as alcoholism or the quality of relationships in the family by drawing slashes across the relationship lines that are troubled or by using thick lines to represent relationships that are strongly supportive. Judgment is required to determine if this level of information is useful. If there is no room in the patient's record for a genogram, list the major diseases that have familiar patterns, such as diabetes, heart disease, arthritis, psychiatric problems, alcoholism, and cancer.

Social History

Social history in a medical model interview includes such things as work patterns. Even if the patient is retired, the type of work in which the patient had engaged in is important because worksite exposures can be risk factors for many potential problems. Work background also gives the clinician a sense of how the person might handle new information and what kind of resources they might have at their disposal. Medical model histories also include the use of alcohol, tobacco, and illegal drugs. Nursing histories are more expanded in this area. Include such information as leisure time activities, risk factors and exposures, and the patient's resources and activity level. If a full functional health pattern is collected, much of this information can be recorded there. If the documentation system in use in a particular setting does not accommodate functional health patterns, then expand the social history section to reflect nursing issues.

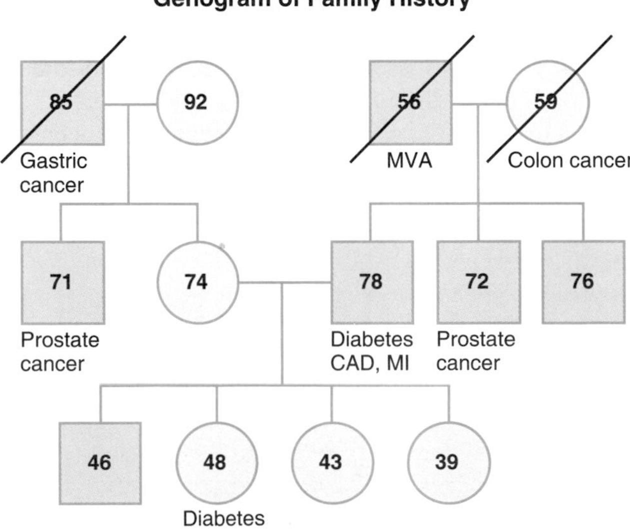

FIGURE 4.2 Genogram of family history. (Source: Chase, SK: Clinical Judgment and Communication in Nurse Practitioner Practice. FA Davis, Philadelphia, 2004.)

Review of Symptoms

This section of the history is often completed by the patient immediately before the physical exam. It is organized by body systems and makes an introduction to the body. In some settings, the patient completes a questionnaire that reflects these data before they enter the examination room. Advanced Assessment 4.1 presents sample questions that can be used during the review of systems. Whenever the review is completed, it can include symptoms that are current or related to past medical history and prompt the patient to report any past difficulties. This also helps remind patients of conditions they may have forgotten and can help to refine the hypothesis list further or to screen out potential new problems. When introducing a body system, start questions in general terms and then proceed to more specific items. When documenting this section, students frequently forget these data are appropriately recorded as subjective data because it is reported from the patient's point of view.

Functional Health Patterns

Functional Health Patterns, developed by Marjory Gordon, serve as a database for determining nursing diagnoses. APNs engage in some activities that require making medical diagnoses, but their practice base is always nursing. The value that APNs bring to a practice is an enhanced ability to assist patients with lifestyle changes and an ability to support patients as they cope with illness. The openness and thoroughness that patients report when cared for by an APN are dependent on the APN practicing from a database that is broader and more personal than that of the traditional medical model. Even in practice settings using a medically dominated model, the nurse has an obligation to represent nursing's contribution to care; the type of data recorded in the functional health pattern in the medical record can reflect a nursing approach.

For episodic visits, some patterns are more important than others, and the list can be prioritized accordingly. For example, for a patient with a sore throat, important data are nutrition (Is he able to eat and drink sufficiently?), sleep and rest (Is sleep interrupted?), activity and exercise (Does he

ADVANCED ASSESSMENT 4.1

Review of Systems Sample Questions

System	Sample Questions
General	How is your general health? Are you sleeping restfully? Is your appetite good? Have you had any recent weight changes? Any fever, chills, or night sweats?
Skin	Any rashes, moles, itching, changes in color, easy bruising, changes in hair?
Head	Any headache, dizziness, fainting, history of head trauma?
Neurologic	Any weakness or paralysis? Any feeling of needles and pins or other loss of sensation? Any trouble walking, any seizures? Any trouble with memory or speech? Any nervousness or depression?
Eyes, ears, nose	Any eye problems, blurring, loss of vision? Any trouble hearing, ringing in ears, pain, and throat discharge, or itching? Any problem with runny nose, change in ability to smell, nosebleeds, or sinus trouble? Frequent sore throats, trouble swallowing, hoarseness?
Mouth	Any mouth sores, dental problems?
Neck	Any pain, swelling or stiffness in the neck?
Lymph nodes	Any swelling or painful lymph nodes in armpits, groin, neck?
Breasts	Any lumps, pain, or discharge? Do you check your breasts regularly?
Chest	Any chest pain, cough, difficulty breathing, shortness of breath? How far can you walk before becoming breathless?
Cardiovascular	Any chest pain, palpitations?
Gastrointestinal	Any stomach pains, indigestion, nausea, or vomiting? Any blood in your stool? Have your bowel movements changed? Any diarrhea or constipation? Any rectal itching, pain?
Endocrine	Any intolerance of heat or cold? Frequently thirsty?
Urinary	Any trouble passing urine, burning, itching, odor, frequency, loss of control or pain?
Female genitalia	Any vaginal discharge, itching, or odor? When was your last menstrual period? What is the length of your cycle, the length and amount of flow? Do you engage in sexual relations with men, women, or both? What method of contraception is used? Is your sex life satisfying?
Male genitalia	Any urethral problems such as discharge, burning? Do you do testicular self-exam? Do you engage in sexual relations with men, women, or both? What method of contraception is used? Is your sex life satisfying?
Extremities	Any leg pain or cramping, joint pain, or stiffness? Do your feet get cold easily? Do you have vein problems? Any back pain?

feel fatigued?), and role relationship (Is he able to work? Are there children in the home?). Inability of the patient to carry out any normal day-to-day function is often a "red flag"—an indicator for the APN of a potentially serious disease process that may be developing.

The purpose of the functional health pattern is to determine the extent to which illness is affecting the person's ability to live his or her "normal" life. What accommodations must be made, even for a self-limiting condition? This is nursing's central question. What is the human response to the health problem? Advanced Assessment 4.2 presents the 11 functional health patterns and sample questions that can be used to elicit data for each functional pattern area.

At this phase of history taking, the hypothesis list is taking shape. The initial diagnostic possibilities generated are weighed as each new piece of information is gathered. Some data serve to support one hypothesis in favor of another; some data are noncontributory. Some data serve to rule out specific hypotheses. The problem list may contain physical disorders with signs or symptoms that are visible, along with other physical disorders that are presumed to be present based on the patient's story, emotional distress related to specific disorders, general emotional disorders, family or social disorders, or even spiritual distress. The patient's problem list may contain more than one diagnosis from any of the biological, psychosocial, or spiritual realms. Further data are available to help refine the hypothesis list by performing the physical examination and ordering diagnostic tests.

Focus on Data Collection: Physical Examination

The physical examination serves to clarify diagnostic hypotheses and to detect unanticipated problems of which the patient is unaware. In primary care, there is a wide range of ways of performing the examination. Textbooks of physical assessment outline a general head-to-toe model that is useful for an initial visit with a full physical examination or a periodic reassessment. In most practices, an initial patient visit is scheduled for more time, and in coding schemes, the visit may be reimbursed at a higher level because of its compre-

ADVANCED ASSESSMENT 4.2

Functional Health Patterns: Questions to Elicit Data

Pattern	*Sample Questions*
Health perception	Do you have a regular health-care provider? Health Management How often do you go to your health-care provider? What do you do to stay healthy?
Nutrition/metabolic	What did you eat yesterday or on a typical day? What do you drink? How is your appetite? Any skin problems?
Elimination	What are your bowel and bladder elimination patterns? Do you have unexpected loss of control?
Activity/exercise	How far can you walk before feeling tired? Do you have energy to do the things you want? Do you need any assistance with feeding, bathing, toileting, dressing, getting around (activities of daily living)? Do you need any help with cooking, or shopping, cleaning (instrumental activities of daily living)?
Sleep/rest	How many hours do you sleep? Any trouble falling asleep or with early wakening? Do you feel rested?
Cognitive/perceptual	Any hearing or vision problems? Any memory changes? How do you like to learn new things? Any pain or discomfort?
Self-perception/self-concept	How would you describe yourself? Do you feel good about yourself? Any changes in how you feel about your body? Do you get angry or down at times?
Role relationship	Who lives with you? Do you have friends? What kind of work do you do? Do you have other responsibilities?
Sexuality/reproductive	Any problems with your sexuality? Any changes? If sexually active, do you practice safe sex? Do you use birth control? What mode of birth control do you use?
Coping/stress tolerance	How do you cope with stress? Any use of alcohol, drugs? Do you have someone to talk things over with?
Value/belief	What is most important to you in your life? Are you religious? Any values about life that health-care providers should know? Do you have a health-care proxy or living will?

hensiveness. Students in nursing or medical school learn to perform the head-to-toe exam in an organized way. In actual practice, however, clinicians must learn to focus their physical assessment skills and make the examination appropriate to the patient's complaint and history. If the patient complains of headache, then a review of head, eyes, ears, nose, and throat and a neurologic examination are indicated, as well as a skin survey. For joint pain, a review of musculoskeletal tenderness, range of motion, and strength might be indicated. The body systems that are examined depend on the working hypothesis list that the clinician has generated. Examination skills need to be organized at a surface, general screening level, with subroutines of examination techniques that can be adapted to specific findings and complaints. Positive or negative findings that serve to refine the hypothesis list must be noted and recorded in the documentation system that is in use. At times, a condition is in evolution and the symptoms may not be clear when the patient comes for a visit. Nonetheless, the rich data reporting from that visit—even though the diagnosis is not clear—can serve to make the diagnosis more accurate later, when the condition evolves further. Full documentation serves to protect both patient and provider. The physical examination can also be a time to provide feedback and teaching about findings and about self-care.

Ordering Diagnostic Tests

Diagnostic tests can be used to confirm or to rule out diagnostic hypotheses, or as screening devices for conditions with subtle presentations that need to be picked up early, such as lead poisoning in children. Diagnostic tests vary in their usefulness based on their sensitivity, specificity, and their predictive value. When considering or evaluating a test, consider that there are patient, test, and disease factors that affect the interpretation of the tests. The prevalence of a condition is the number of cases present in a given population at a particular point in time. The incidence of a condition reflects the total number of cases during a specified time period. For example, the number of cases of flu in a year (incidence) is greater than the number of people who have the flu on a given day (prevalence). Both incidence and prevalence rates are important considerations in making accurate diagnoses. Laboratory tests and radiographic or other imaging can assist in screening for conditions and in making diagnoses. For chronic conditions, tests are used to monitor progress in managing the condition.

No test is perfect. In a given population, a positive reading is found for some people who have the condition and as well as for some who do not. When a patient who does not have the condition has a positive reading on a test, it is called

Table 4.4 Tests: Characteristics and Diseases

Test Reading	Disease Present	Disease Absent	Total
Positive	True positive (TP) A	False positive (FP) B	All positives A+B
Negative	False negative (FN) C	True negative (TN) D	All negatives C+D
Totals	All diseased A+C	All healthy B+D	Grand Total

Source: Chase, SF: Clinical Judgment and Communication in Nurse Practitioner Practice. FA Davis, Philadelphia, 2004.

a "false positive." On the other hand, a negative test is found with people who do not have the condition and some who do. A negative test result that occurs when the patient does have the condition is referred to as a "false negative." The sensitivity of a test is greater when it has few false negatives. Sensitivity equals the number of true positives for a test divided by the number of tested individuals who truly have the disease. The specificity of a test is greater when it has few false positives. The specificity of a test equals the number of true negatives divided by the number of all tested individuals who do no have the disease. Table 4.4 represents the relationship between test results and actual conditions.

In clinical practice, the predictive value of a test is the important consideration. Given a positive test result, what is the likelihood that the patient actually has the condition? Positive predictive value equals true positives divided by all positives. Negative predictive value equals true negatives divided by all negatives. Predictive value is in part dependent upon the prevalence of the condition. If a condition is highly likely, then a positive test result is more likely to be accurate. If a condition is very unlikely, then a positive test result needs to be questioned, perhaps with different tests.

When deciding whether to order a test, cost, convenience, sensitivity and specificity, and risk of missing a condition are considered. One can ask whether the test result would affect the potential treatment plan. If not, then the test might not be necessary. Tests are not appropriately ordered to increase the clinician's confidence and comfort. Appropriate screening for life-threatening or life-altering conditions must be considered. Clinicians can use the Clinical Preventive Services Guidelines or other research-based guidelines for deciding on screening tests for specific patients. Always consider the individual patient's situation. For example, at the age for first mammogram has changed over the years based on research data and is dependent, in part on a strong family history of breast cancer.

Differential Diagnosis

A differential diagnosis list is the list of possible diagnoses, usually in priority order. When clinicians discuss a case, the list of differential diagnoses is usually considered. Supports for developing a rich differential diagnosis list include several guides. One approach suggests considering the problem from the "skin in." This means that if the patient complains of chest pain, the clinician can consider all the possible causes of chest pain, beginning at the skin, and visualize all the structures in the area that could possibly be affected. For example, chest pain at skin level could indicate early herpes zoster sensitivity and pain. Below the skin, the musculoskeletal system (including the rib cage) could be causing pain, from costochondritis or from muscle strain. The clinician can consider pain below the rib cage as a source of pain. Could the patient have pneumonia, pneumothorax, or pulmonary embolus? Next is the esophagus. Could the pain be from esophagitis, gastric esophageal reflux, or hiatal hernia? Next consider the pericardium as a possible source of pain, as with pericarditis. Finally, consider cardiac pain. This "skin in" approach keeps the student from jumping to early conclusions without considering a wide range of problems. It thus avoids the common diagnostic error of premature closure.

An evolving problem list can become quite long, even on an initial visit. The Patient's Voice 4.1 describes one approach to differential diagnosis. The Patient's Voice 4.2 illustrates how the diagnosis often involves more than medical problems.

Developing a Management Plan

The definition of advanced practice nursing is linked to the expansion of the therapeutics that are available to be used. In addition, a specialized clinical area, graduate education, and certification by the profession are criteria (Hanson and Hamric, 2003). Once the problem list has been clarified, clinical judgment about how best to manage those problems is addressed. Although APNs bill for services in the medical realm, they also operate in the nursing domain. One expectation for APN students is learning to "present the patient" to their preceptor in the clinical area. This skill involves taking all the data collected in history and physical assessment, organizing the content, and presenting the major findings in a coherent way to the preceptor so that the preceptor can review with the student what the treatment options are so that when the preceptor sees the patient he or she can verify and clarify the data collection and move to treatment planning. Initially, students may need to use a template to ensure that they are organized as they begin this process. With experience, the organization of patient data will become more obvious. This same skill of organizing patient data is useful when communicating with consulting providers. They need a clear summary of the case for efficient consultation.

Selection of interventions for APNs is broader than a consideration of prescription medications. The discussion in Chapter 1 of Engebretson's (1997) contribution is useful to consider here. In addition, Eisenhauer (1994) has argued that

THE PATIENT'S VOICE 4.1

An Advanced Practice Nurse's Approach to Differential Diagnosis

An APN describes her approach to a new patient.

> My initial diagnosis at that time, just by speaking with him, without any labs and examining him physically, was this: His diabetes was in poor control. His hypertension was in poor control. He had some rhinitis, probably allergic, but he was not having a problem. He has known unequal pupils since he had surgery and had damage to the pupillary musculature, but it does not affect his vision; if you did not happen to know that, you might be very concerned about it, you know? It is real important to put that in the problem list. He had a TUR for BPH. He had a real bad pars planes with secondary hip pain, and he kept going to people with back pain and nobody ever stood him up and looked at his feet. He also had seborrheic dermatitis. The guy is an Irishman with pale skin and washed-out blue eyes, and he never used sunscreen. He had lots of skin cancers. The doctor kept calling him back to cut out the skin cancers but never told him to use sunscreen.

For this patient, the APN goes on to describe her approach to ordering diagnostic tests. Note that the hypotheses precede the test consideration. She describes her initial treatment plan:

OK, first thing you need is your laboratory parameters to check the problems that you have just defined. I would do blood counts, chemistries, thyroid function, glycohemoglobin, urines, PSA [prostate-specific antigen]. The first time I see a patient I always do the whole gamut. This guy also had had a bilateral total hip replacement, so I reviewed the subacute bacterial endocarditis prophylaxis because he had never been told about it. I started him on Prinivil, an ACE [angiotensin-converting enzyme] inhibitor, because he has diabetes and had previously been on Hytrin, but it was not doing the trick, and it was not protecting his kidneys. I started him on Glucotrol. He had not been on anything other than Micronase, which he quit using because he really did not know how to use the stuff. I also talked to him about his seborrhea and sunscreen.

The APN sees the wholeness of the patient's situation. This is a different approach than treating discrete problems as they come up. The APN's description of her approach to this patient continues:

He had had previous health care and he thought he was doing fine. He just had never had it all put together. As far as he was concerned, he happened to have some elevated blood pressure and some elevated blood glucose, but nobody had ever put it all together in terms of the effects on the whole body. He went to someone for his glucose and he went to somebody for his blood pressure. The guy was not a train wreck, but he had a number of problems that had been overlooked until he saw me and somebody (me) made a list. For example, he had not had a recent eye exam. For any patients with diabetes, I make sure they get an eye exam every single year. And that is how I started. His wife is also a patient of mine—a great cook, which is a tragedy for a diabetic—and he, like most husbands, will eat what he is given. So she needed some education as to what is the proper thing to eat and when and how they could cheat.

The APN is able to pull all of this patient's concerns and problems together in a way that honors his wholeness and his family dynamics. Her concern is for preventing future problems that are likely to develop, given his pattern of risk factors. Her method of collecting data and clustering it together to form a comprehensive picture of his life results in an effective, personal plan.

The differential diagnosis list should always include any conditions that are life-, organ-, or function-threatening. An APN describing a different patient situation stated: I always think in terms of the most dangerous or the most serious thing first—not necessarily the most catastrophic, but the most serious problem. If I know somebody has an AAA [aneurysm] and he comes in with abdominal pain and it's sensitive, well, he probably has diverticulitis, but if I blow the diagnosis and go that way and it turns out that his aneurysm is dissecting, then he is dead. So I will treat his diverticulitis but I will get the abdominal ultrasound right away. I consider the most urgent, deadly thing first. Cancer can be deadly, but it usually is not an emergency. It will kill you, but it is not going to kill you tomorrow. But an AAA can blow at any time. I had someone with an aneurysm blow in here once while I had the surgeon and the OR team waiting for him in the ER. We knew we had an aneurysm that was about to blow because I put my hand on his belly and it was throbbing and the patient was hypotensive and he was sweating. He had come in to the hospital because he was ready to go on vacation and just wanted to check this out before he left. So, you think of the most life-threatening situation first.

different levels of nursing interventions are useful when dealing with patient problems. At the most basic level, interventions deal with symptom relief, such as heat application for strained muscles or a prescription for pain medication. At a higher level of complexity, interventions address functional patterns, such as stress and coping. The provider could schedule a follow-up visit to determine if a stressful condition is being managed more successfully after a brief teaching or counseling session. At yet another level, an intervention could be concerned with life patterns, such as recommending a course of rehabilitation to help a patient to regain confidence in exercising after a cardiac event. Finally, at the highest level, interventions such as spiritual support could be chosen to help patients and their families cope with

THE PATIENT'S VOICE 4.2

An Advanced Practice Nurse's View of Nursing

One pediatric APN described her interaction with an immigrant father who brought in a 3-year-old girl with a runny nose. The father was not disciplining the child, even though she was being difficult, because he had been reported to Human Services for hitting this child previously and for hitting a well baby 8 months of age.

> I see myself making a dual diagnosis—a nursing diagnosis as well as a medical diagnosis. If the father does not discipline his child at the appropriate time in an appropriate way, that is a knowledge deficit. So I made a nursing decision there and I intervened on the basis of that nursing decision, but I also made a medical decision, in that the child had an upper respiratory infection and I prescribed what I thought to be the appropriate medication for that. So, I see myself making nursing diagnoses as well as medical diagnoses and trying to somehow mesh these two to care for the family holistically, because there is no way you can care for a child without caring for the family. That is my belief.

When asked if her full response was documented in the treatment plan, she responded:

Yeah, well, it sure does not fall under "upper respiratory infection." In this case, I did not know when the family was going to apply for insurance, so I certainly did not want to put "behavior disorder" down. Instead, I put down under my diagnosis, "knowledge deficit, re: discipline." In my treatment plan, I noted that I discussed discipline and that I gave the father 'time out' guidelines and how to reward good behavior. I also noted that the father is coming back to me in 2 weeks to report differences in his approach to discipline and how it worked out. Nobody ever leaves my office without knowing when he or she needs to come back, and I document when I tell them to come back in my treatment plan.

life processes such as a terminal condition. This typology of intervention is useful to consider when selecting an approach to a problem. If, for example, a patient has been unable to lose weight using simple diet instruction, a higher order intervention such as counseling may be required to address the source of the problem at a deeper level.

Evidence-Based Practice

There is a push in health care today to promote evidence-based practice. In a just society, patients have equal access to the most up-to-date treatment approaches, and are also able to make informed choices about their treatment. To justify a treatment approach, proponents of evidence-based practice argue that there must be evidence, either from clinical trials or from case studies, that the approach is likely to benefit the patient. Obviously, it is easier to demonstrate the benefit of a certain drug that has been tested on a large number of individuals than it is to demonstrate the effectiveness of individual counseling. Be on guard that your own practice is not limited to medicine based on clinical trials alone. This may require clinical research to demonstrate case studies of creative nursing intervention success. A research study that investigated how clinicians used guidelines in day-to-day practice showed that practitioners seldom referred directly to guidelines when planning care. They did, however, use internalized guidelines and could discuss what they were and how they were formed. Their own and colleagues' experience were also part of forming this knowledge in practice (Gabbay and LeMay, 2004). Guidelines for practice are available from government agencies (http://guidelines.gov), or from specialty/disease-related groups such as the American Heart Association. These guidelines can form the basis for protocol development and for peer evaluation.

Outcome Considerations

In many instances, the patient's and provider's chosen outcomes for an encounter are clear. The simple, acute health problem is to be resolved. The screening measures recommended for the person's age group are to be ordered to rule out the presence of nascent disease. When dealing with more chronic problems or problems that provide the patient with what may be reduced quality of life, then the APN must be more sensitive to outcome determination.

Different settings prompt a different set of concerns. The Patient's Voice 4.3 presents an APN's approach to outcome considerations.

Documentation

Preparing concise, comprehensive, and meaningful documentation of one's thoughts and activities as a provider of primary care is a skill that takes time to develop. The purposes of documentation are to record the patient's report of symptoms, past medical history, lifestyle and family factors, positive and negative findings on physical exam, and the clinician's decisions and actions. An accurate record is essential to remind the clinician of findings and actions for the next follow-up visit. In a large practice, other providers will be seeing the patient and will need the benefit of the clinician's observations and actions during previous visits. The effectiveness of a treatment plan can be judged only if the plan has been adequately described. For example, if teaching about diet was provided at one visit but not recorded, then the same teaching might be repeated at the next visit, to the frustration of the patient for whom it did not work the first time. This frustration might be misunderstood by the next provider as a lack of cooperation with the treatment plan. Finally, docu-

THE PATIENT'S VOICE 4.3

An Advanced Practice Nurse's Approach to Outcome Considerations

One gerontological APN described doing an initial evaluation on an elderly client in a residential hospice situation.

> Well, I think in terms of triage—comfort is the priority for me. Is there pain? I try to address that issue, and if the patient is anxious, I try to put that on the same level as psychic pain and physical pain. I try to give my patients as much information as they can tolerate—partly what the plan is, and what we are going to do to relieve their pain and try to make their living more comfortable. So then I work from there. What are some of the problems I see in my patients? Skin problems, incontinence, risk for falls, risk for aspiration—all those kinds of things.

One APN was treating an 85-year-old patient who had suffered a CVA [cardiovascular accident stroke]—and was unable to communicate. The patient also had dysphagia, which meant that she needed a feeding tube. The APN took time to ask a pertinent question: What would this patient want?

[This patient] would occasionally have bedsores and sometimes she had a urinary tract infection and occasionally a rash from the urination [she was incontinent]. She also had frequent respiratory infections and it appeared that she had a very poor quality of life. She could not express herself at all and every few months, her PEG [percutaneous endoscopic gastrostomy] tube would have to be replaced, which happens with most patients. So after we had replaced about the fourth one, I called the family member and I posed the question to her this way: 'Would it be her wish to continue this way?' I did not ask the family member what she wanted. I asked, 'What do you think would be her wish? [emphasis added]' This was the first time I had ever talked to this woman and she acted as if no one had ever posed that question to her before. She said, 'Well, I want the tube back in.' And I said, 'Well, I understand that, but what do you think would be her wish?' It was as if she had never thought about that before. And after she thought about the situation from that perspective, it was very easy for her to come to the answer that her relative's wish would be that her tube not be replaced and that she be allowed to die. She recognized that the patient's wish would not be at all to live like that. After she thought about it and talked it over with her family members, they agreed that the tube should not be replaced, and that is what happened. Without the feeding tube, the patient died in peace. She had a peaceful death.

This APN asked the question that made everyone consider the meaning of the experience from the patient's point of view. In this case, the outcome of the care was a peaceful death, an outcome that can be prized.

mentation can serve as protection for the provider or the practice in the rare case in which litigation is brought by the patient or family. In addition, third-party payers may be auditing the patient's record to determine whether the level of the visit that was billed was justified and whether the interventions billed were actually delivered. Additional detail on billing and coding can be found in Chapter 23. In the student situation, the depth and comprehensiveness of documentation can assist the preceptor or faculty in determining the student's progress in learning judgment.

SOAP Format

General principles for documentation are commonly applied using the "SOAP" format—Subjective, Objective, Assessment, and Plan—of charting. If other systems of charting are used, the principles still apply.

Subjective

The subjective portion of the record includes all data from the patient's report: the HPI (history of present illness), past medical history, family history, social history, functional health patterns data, and review of systems. The clinician can include here, in an easily visible way, current medications, immunization status, allergies to foods or medications, past hospitalizations (if appropriate), and for women, the last menstrual period and menstrual cycle information. Even when a woman is being treated for simple problems, her pregnancy status must be known before certain medications are prescribed. It is an error to confuse physical findings noticed during the exam with subjective data from the patient. If the patient's particular way of describing a problem seems important, then use exact words and include quotes. This is not necessary if the description is simple and without nuance. Develop an outline form for your documentation that includes all essential data elements in a way that is retrievable. Writing in full sentences and paragraphs does not allow for easy retrievability of data by other providers. An outline template also serves as a memory tool for the new APN. This template is useful in organizing patient presentation for the preceptor.

Objective

The objective section of the record includes all data obtained through objective means. This is not limited to numeric data. Begin the objective portion of the record with a brief description of the overall impression of the patient. Such phrases as "tired-looking," "energetic," or "worried" can convey much of the patient impression that is useful in diagnostic reasoning. Include vital signs and pertinent findings from the physical examination as well as laboratory data. Do not record diagnostic judgments in this section—think of this part of the record as "just the facts."

At first, students are unable to focus on which pieces of data are significant to a problem and tend to include every piece of data available. All data need not be recorded, but "pertinent negatives" need to be recorded. These include data that by being normal tend to rule out a possible diagnosis. Recording pertinent negatives helps to show that a diagnosis was considered and why it was ruled out. It does not take long, however, for both the subjective and objective sections to be recorded with reasonable skill, even for advanced beginner students. When following patients over time, flow sheets can be useful for tracking data. A flow sheet can show the effect of a change in medication management of hyperlipidemia or weight or blood pressure over months or years.

Assessment

The assessment portion is an area of documentation in which much variability can be found. The assessment must include active problems that are being managed in this visit. It can also include chronic problems that may have an impact on the treatment plan. Many practices always include a health promotion line on the problem list to remind each clinician that the visit should reflect the preventative focus of that practice. For the list to serve both patient and practitioner well, a simple diagnostic label may not be enough. For example, if the patient has hypertension that is being managed by lifestyle change and medication, the effectiveness of control of the problem can be recorded in the assessment section. Assessment is ongoing in the management of health problems. For example, a patient's problem list might read as follows: (1) hypertension stage 1, well controlled, (2) type 2 diabetes mellitus, poorly controlled, (3) obesity, unchanged. This documentation directs evaluation and intervention adjustment much more clearly than a simple list of "HTN, DM, obesity." Many practices maintain an active problem list near the front of the patient record or in a part of the electronic record. This is particularly useful when dealing with chronic conditions and is recommended. The clinician can initiate such a tool in any practice, even if a blank progress note sheet is filed at the beginning of that section of the patient's record.

When reviewing the assessment part of the record, students can evaluate their own thinking by asking themselves if all data that were used to justify the naming of a problem are included in the subjective and objective section of the note. Furthermore, one can ask whether all data were accounted for in the assessment section. In some cases, a clear problem cannot be identified. Abdominal pain that does not fit a clear diagnostic pattern can be reported in the problem list by simply naming the complaint. The clinician can reflect diagnostic hypotheses by writing "abdominal pain, R/O irritable bowel syndrome." Or "cough, viral bronchitis vs. allergy." Students are often reluctant to admit that they cannot name the problem. It is a mistake, however, to name a problem in error, simply to have a problem on the list. The patient will not be well served if the record fails to reveal competing diagnostic hypotheses. In primary care, uncertainty is reasonable and expected. Even if the problem is not completely specified, the problem list is the basis for the intervention schedule in the treatment plan, as usual.

Plan

The plan for treatment is most effective if it is described in detail, including specific directions for each intervention. Three general sections are included in planning: First, any diagnostic testing that is to be conducted is be listed. The results of these diagnostic tests will help to clarify the assessment but, of course, are not yet available to the provider. Second, educational approaches are to be laid out. Every visit is a teaching opportunity. Patient education might include specifics of the problems being managed, such as symptom control for upper respiratory infections, medication teaching, diet and activity recommendations, and risk reduction, such as smoking cessation information or a discussion of seat belt usage. The documentation of the plan includes details regarding any therapeutic plan that is to be carried out—including prescriptions, various therapies, counseling, activity promotion or restriction, dietary changes, or any of the therapeutics discussed earlier. When recording prescriptions, be sure to include all the data that were written on the prescription list, including number or volume of doses to be dispensed and number of refills allowed. This is important because patients may call for refills before they are due, and if a different provider takes the call, he or she may have an unclear idea of how you managed the patient. It is especially important when prescribing drugs that are prone to abuse.

Finally, the treatment plan is not complete without clear plans for follow-up. When will the patient be seen again, and under what circumstances is the patient instructed to call back? For example, when treating a viral infection, remind the patient to call back if not better in 2 days or if fever develops. By documenting your instructions for follow-up, other providers will be able to manage the patient better if the patient calls in when you are not available.

Plans are most effective when they include a sense of the goal of treatment. If the condition is simple and self-limiting, the goal of treatment may be obvious and need not be stated. For chronic or complex problems, however, the short- and long-term goals of therapy need to be discussed and recorded. By engaging the patient in this discussion, the choices that the patient makes in altering lifestyle and in following a treatment plan may be made more clear. For example, the patient with hypertension, diabetes, and obesity might have as a goal to lose four pounds in a month. The planned intervention to help the patient achieve this goal might be walking three times a week and one less restaurant meal a week. The feedback on the short-term goal at the next visit can help to keep the patient motivated to sustain lifelong change.

Finally, when reviewing the documentation for personal or peer evaluation, the clinician must consider whether the note written conveys the scope and tone of the visit. Does it reflect the type of visit that occurred? If the patient were to ask to see the record, would the information be clear? The APN can write the note in such a way that the patient could agree with what has been stated. Discussions of sensitive issues such as family problems can be left in general terms. This is a useful approach when one considers that other parties such as third-party payers or lawyers might have access to the record in the future. If the provider and the patient disagree on a treatment plan, for example, on the use of medications, the record can reflect the disagreement in nonjudgmental terms, such as "Patient requested prescription for muscle relaxants, which was discussed as being unlikely to benefit the shoulder pain described." This kind of note can assist in determining patterns of behaviors or difficulties.

Documentation is an opportunity for clinicians at all levels to review the level of their thought. In general, APNs document visits more completely and less often have charts refused for payment by third-party payers (Chase and Leuner, 1996). It is best to develop a system for maintaining current accurate records. Saving up quick scratches of notes and writing all formal patient notes at the end of a busy day is not the recommended approach. Dictation and computer systems allow for complete recordkeeping and help to keep time spent on the task more manageable.

All documentation systems are invented by each practice. If you find that elements of your care are invisible in the record because of restrictive coding or limited space, then plan a meeting with the head of the practice or clinic to discuss what you feel is missing in the record that you are providing. Most systems in which APNs work are dominated by the medical model. APNs can ensure that their contributions that come from a nursing model are not invisible by claiming credit and billing for the care actually provided.

Reduction of Medical Error

The reduction of medical error and the support of patient safety are important in the health-care arena. The Institute of Medicine has called for attention to the processes and systems of care (Kohn, Corrigan, and Donaldson, 2000). A study of reported medical error in primary care showed that the largest number of errors were considered administrative, such as information filed in the wrong place or time, charts not being available at the time of the visit, and lack of documentation. Errors also occurred in obtaining or processing a laboratory specimen. Some errors were reportedly due to lack of clinical knowledge or skills such as wrong or missed diagnosis or wrong treament choices (Dovey et al., 2005). Attention to decision making and follow-through is important to all primary-care providers.

Telemedicine

The use of electronic media in all facets of the health-care process is becoming more and more of a reality. Patients have access to information about health promotion and about specific health care concerns from the Internet. Patients can also communicate with health-care providers through e-mail or Web sites. Health records can be maintained electronically and made accessible to providers throughout a care delivery system. The Veterans Administration in the United States has been a leader in electronic medical records. Telemedicine has the capacity to open access to health care for people at remote sites, but it also has the potential to exclude persons who do not have access to computers or the Internet. Health insurance companies are beginning to reimburse practices for telemedicine services, which will likely increase its availability (Reed, 2005). Some practices send a weekly e-mail to their patients with health related information. This can be good for marketing as well as for providing information.

Ethics

Every clinical judgment is an ethical judgment. Clinical judgment begins with respect for persons and supports each individual's autonomy. Some decisions call upon balancing such principles as beneficence against autonomy, for example, as when a patient chooses not to follow a treatment plan. Truth telling by the clinician can do much to establish trust and to develop a plan the patient can accept. Ethical judgments are involved in the allocation of scarce resources, the most prominent for APNs being time. If one patient constantly requires more time than is allotted, other patients are made to wait or are given less time for their visits. Being a patient advocate to ascertain that the health-care system provides for each patient everything that is reasonable to which the patient is entitled is a role of the APN. A survey of nurse practitioners in one mid-Atlantic state showed that 61 percent agreed that they sometimes weighed the needs of the patient against the interests of the managed care organization (Ulrich, Soeken, and Miller, 2003). Fidelity to the patient until the problem has been determined or solved is another aspect of APN practice that is based on ethical principles.

The privilege of being an APN and entering as a partner into patients' lives to support their health and wholeness is one that requires true human presence, clear clinical judgment, and a commitment to do one's best. The Circle of Caring includes patient and nurse together as they enter a relationship that has the potential to enhance the humanity of both.

Bibliography

American Medical Association: CPT 2005: Current Procedural Terminology. Chicago: American Medical Association, 2005.

American Medical Association Physician International Classification of Diseases-9: Clinical Modification. Chicago: Author, 2005.

Benner, P: From Novice to Expert: Excellence and Power in Clinical Nursing Practice. Addison-Wesley, Menlo Park, Calif., 1984.

Benner, PE, et al: Expertise in Nursing Practice: Caring Clinical Judgment and Ethics. Springer, New York, 1996.

Billings, JA, and Stoeckle, JD: The Clinical Encounter: A Guide to the Medical Interview and Case Presentation, ed 2. CV Mosby, St. Louis, Mo., 1999.

Brykczynski, KA: An interpretive study describing the clinical judgment of nurse practitioners. Schol Inquiry Nurs Pract 3(2):75, 1989.

Chase, SK: Clinical judgment and communication in nurse practitioner practice. FA Davis, Philadelphia, 2004.

Chase, SK, and Leuner, JD: Documentation by nurse practitioners: Challenges and opportunities. In Proceedings of the Twelfth Conference. NANDA, Philadelphia, 1996.

Davis, S, et al: Teaching strategies used by expert nurse practitioner preceptors: A qualitative study. J Am Acad Nurse Pract 5:27, 1993.

Dovey, SM, Meyers, DE, Phillips, RL, Green, LA, Fryer, GE, Galliher, JM, Kappus, J, and Grob, P: A preliminary taxonomy of medical errors in family practice. Qual Safe Health Care 11:233–, 2005.

Dunphy, LM, and Winland-Brown, JE: The circle of caring: A transformative model of advanced practice nursing. Clin Excell Nurs Pract 2:241, 1998.

Eisenhauer, LA: A typology of nursing therapeutics. Image J Nurs Schol 26:261, 1994.

Elstein, A, et al: Medical Problem Solving. Harvard University Press, Cambridge, Mass., 1979.

Engebretson, J: A multiparadigm approach to nursing. Adv Nurs Sci 20:21, 1997.

Gabbay, J, and leMay, A: Evidence based guidelines or collectively constructed "mindlines?" Ethnographic study of knowledge management in primary care. Br Med J 329(7473):1013, 2004.

Gordon, M, et al: Clinical judgment: An integrated model. Adv Nurs Sci 16(4):55, 1994.

Hanson, CM, and Hamric, AB: Reflections of the continuing evolution of advanced practice nursing. Nurs Outlook 51:203.

Johnson, R: Nurse practitioner-patient discourse: Uncovering the voice of nursing in primary care practice. Schol Inquiry Nurs Pract 7:143, 1993.

Kohn, LT, Corrigan, JM, and Donaldson, MS (eds): To Err Is Human: Building a Safer Health System. National Academy Press, Washington, D.C., 2000.

Lewis, PH, and Brykczynski, KA: Practical knowledge and competencies of the healing role of the nurse practitioner. J Am Acad Nurse Pract 6:207, 1994.

North American Nursing Diagnosis Association: NANDA Nursing Diagnoses: Definitions and Classification, 1997–1998. NANDA, Philadelphia, 1996.

Radwin, LE: Research on diagnostic reasoning in nursing. Nurs Diag 1(2):70, 1990.

Reed, K: Telemedicine: Benefits to advanced practice nursing and the communities they serve. J Am Acad Nurse Pract 17:176, 2005.

Roblin, DW, Becker, ER, Adams, EK, Howard, DH, and Roberts, MH: Patient satisfaction with primary care: Does type of practitioner matter? Med Care 42:579, 2004.

Rogers, JC, and Biggs, WS: Problem solving in family medicine. In Rakel, R (ed): Essentials of Family Practice. WB Saunders, Philadelphia, 1999.

Rubin, RH: Primary Care. WB Saunders, Philadelphia, 1995.

Shuler, PA, and Davis, JE: The Shuler nurse practitioner practice model: A theoretical framework for nurse practitioner clinicians, educators and researchers, Part 1. J Am Acad Nurse Pract 5:11, 1993.

Snyder, M, et al: Defining nursing interventions. Image J Nurs Schol 28:137, 1996.

Tanner, CA, et al: The phenomenology of knowing the patient. Image J Nurs Schol 25:273, 1993.

Ulrich, CM, Soeken, KL, and Miller, N: Ethical conflict associated with managed care: Views of nurse practitioners. Nurs Res 52:168, 2003.

Weed, LL: Medical Records, Medical Education and Patient Care. Press of Case Western Reserve, Chicago, 1971.

White, JE, et al: Content and process in clinical decision-making by nurse practitioners. Image J Nurs Schol 24:153, 1992.

Caring-Based Nursing: The Science

2 UNIT

"The march of professionally educated nurses onto the panoramic scene in the nation's health services re-defines the boundaries of nursing practice.... Inter-professional collaboration is imbued with the essence of conjoined learning to provide a higher degree of service than could be offered by one profession."

—Martha E. Rogers: Reveille in Nursing. F.A. Davis, Philadelphia, 1964, p 77.

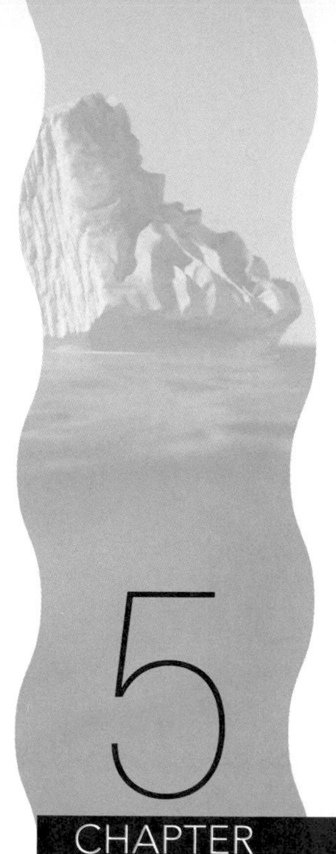

Neurologic Problems

Jill E. Winland-Brown, EdD, MSN, APRN, BC
Jacqueline Rhoads, PhD, RN, CCRN, ACNP-CS

Common Complaints

Confusion

Confusion is described not as a disease process or disease state but rather as a symptom of the presence of a particular disease process or its progression. *Confusion* is an inability to think quickly or coherently. A confused patient is disoriented as to time, place, or person and usually demonstrates impairment of cognitive functioning, which is usually demonstrated by inappropriate reactions to environmental stimuli and can arise suddenly or gradually and may be either temporary or irreversible. Confusion may be precipitated by stressful events, lack of sleep or food, or sensory deprivation. Age is not a reliable predictor of confusion; however, older adults are most at risk because of polypharmacy (multiple prescription drugs), the aging process, and the presence of chronic disease.

Differential Diagnosis

Confusion is one of the key signs of neurologic disorders, and the clinician must be diligent in determining its cause. The physical examination will provide clues. The Mini-Mental State Examination (MMSE) can help the clinician determine the degree of confusion, which helps to isolate possible causes. Once the disease has been identified and treatment started, the symptom of confusion often disappears. Differential diagnoses for confusion involve almost all body systems (Differential Diagnosis Flowchart 5.1). Common causes are presented next.

Dementia

An acute transient disturbance in thought process can be a result of delirium, whereas persistent or more severe confusion, with or without psychomotor hyperactivity, may be caused by dementia. *Dementia* is a decline in mental functioning, which affects memory, cognition, language, and personality. Clinically significant confusional states in older patients would lead the practitioner to suspect dementias such as Alzheimer's disease (AD; in 56.8 percent of patients in one study); multi-infarct dementia as a result of cerebrovascular accident (CVA) (in 13.3 percent); and depression (in 4.5 percent), which can coexist with dementia, or excessive consumption of alcohol (in 4.2 percent) or drugs (in 1.5 percent of patients studied).

Patients with dementia present with an inability to focus or sustain attention span. There is a significant alteration in memory, personality, and affect, accompanied by disorientation and often language disturbances. These signs and symptoms develop over a short period of time and tend to fluctuate over the course of a day. Patients may experience disturbances in the sleep–wake cycle, anxiety, fear, or depression. The history and physical examination along with diagnostic studies will reveal the presence of a medical condition or drug toxicity. The MMSE and computed tomography (CT) scan have the greatest usefulness in the diagnosis of dementia. Routine laboratory studies may also be performed. Treatment for dementia should be disease specific. Antipsychotic drugs such as haloperidol (Haldol) and thioridazine (Mellaril) can be used to reduce agitation or anxiety. Carbamazepine (Tegretol) is an anticonvulsant that may control impulsivity and aggression. Patients with panic

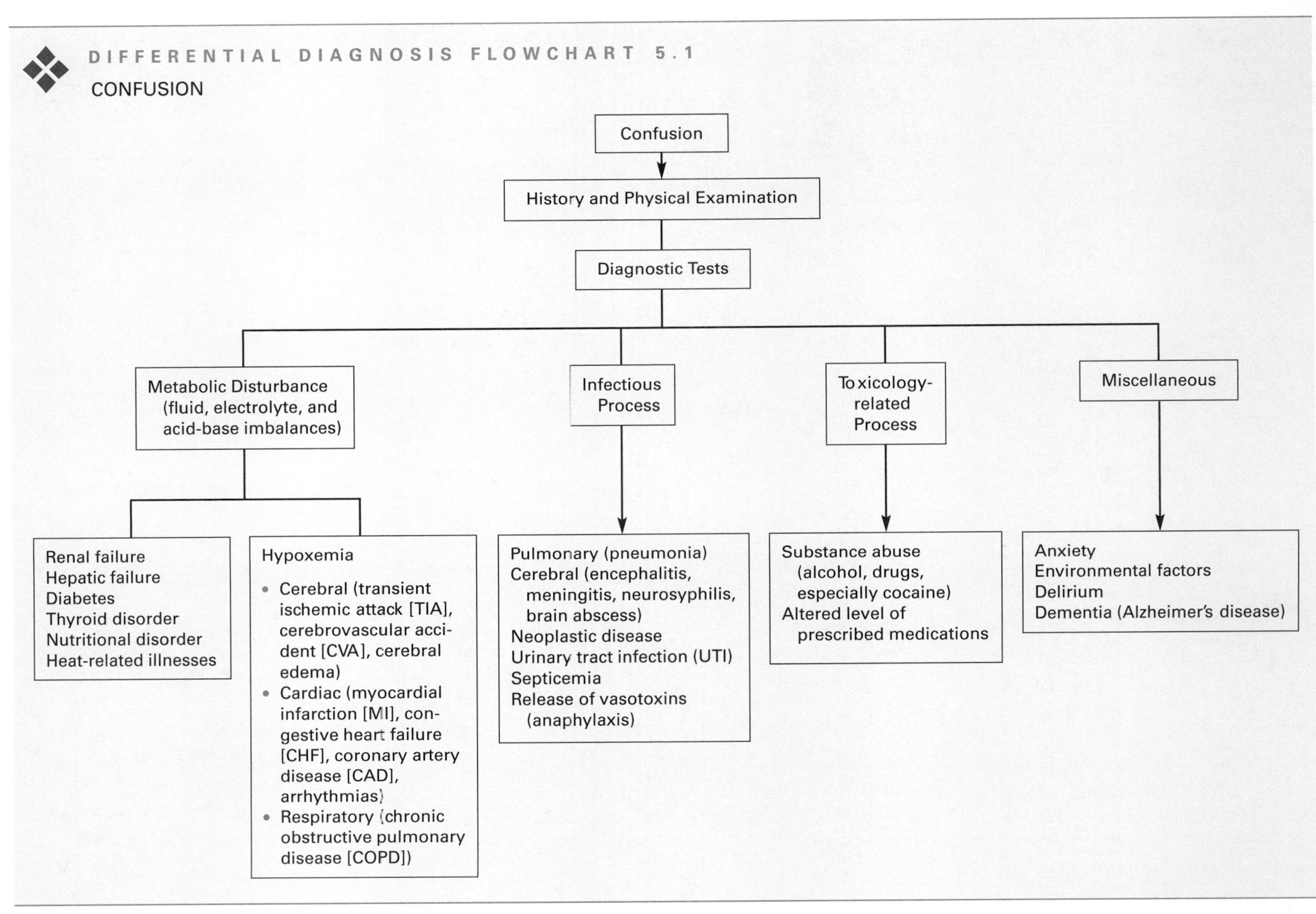
DIFFERENTIAL DIAGNOSIS FLOWCHART 5.1
CONFUSION
Confusion
History and Physical Examination
Diagnostic Tests
Metabolic Disturbance (fluid, electrolyte, and acid-base imbalances)
Infectious Process
Toxicology-related Process
Miscellaneous
Renal failure
Hepatic failure
Diabetes
Thyroid disorder
Nutritional disorder
Heat-related illnesses
Hypoxemia
• Cerebral (transient ischemic attack [TIA], cerebrovascular accident [CVA], cerebral edema)
• Cardiac (myocardial infarction [MI], congestive heart failure [CHF], coronary artery disease [CAD], arrhythmias)
• Respiratory (chronic obstructive pulmonary disease [COPD])
Pulmonary (pneumonia)
Cerebral (encephalitis, meningitis, neurosyphilis, brain abscess)
Neoplastic disease
Urinary tract infection (UTI)
Septicemia
Release of vasotoxins (anaphylaxis)
Substance abuse (alcohol, drugs, especially cocaine)
Altered level of prescribed medications
Anxiety
Environmental factors
Delirium
Dementia (Alzheimer's disease)

disorders may respond to lorazepam (Ativan) or oxazepam (Serax). Referral to a psychiatrist may also be indicated. Management goals for the family and caregivers should be supportive, specific, and consistent.

Metabolic Disturbances

Fluid, electrolyte, and acid–base imbalances may be the result of metabolic problems, which can alter a patient's level of consciousness, producing confusion. The extent of the imbalance determines the severity of the patient's confusion. Typically, the patient is dehydrated and has poor skin turgor, dry skin, and a low-grade fever. Additional signs and symptoms such as dizziness, confusion, altered level of consciousness, hypotension, and coma, when evaluated with an extensive history and physical, will usually lead the clinician to a diagnosis. Routine laboratory tests, including electrolytes, urinalysis (UA), chest x-ray exam, and electrocardiogram (ECG), may be performed. Treatment should be focused on restoration of appropriate fluid and electrolyte balance—specifically, correction of the primary metabolic disorder.

Infectious Process

Confusion may also be the result of an infectious process that can cause extensive tissue and organ impairment through the release of vasotoxins and histamine, the presence of edema and compression, and the loss of electrolytes. Ischemia often occurs, producing cell injury and death if the infectious process is allowed to continue. Severe generalized infections (such as septicemia or bacteremia) often produce symptoms suggestive of delirium, whereas infections that affect the nervous system (such as meningitis) cause confusion, headache, and nuchal rigidity. Specific signs and symptoms of infections include fever, tachycardia, tachypnea, decreased blood pressure (BP), confusion, and irritability. Diagnostic studies should include routine tests as well as those associated with the suspected infectious agent. Treatment should focus on managing the primary cause of the infection.

Tissue Hypoxia and Ischemia

Cardiovascular disorders can cause confusion as a result of tissue hypoxia and ischemia. Confusion may be insidious and may come and go, as is frequently the case. The patient typically appears ill and has significant changes in vital signs (decreased blood pressure, elevated and/or irregular pulse, and tachypnea), edema, cyanosis, reduced level of consciousness, confusion, severe headache, agitation, vomiting, and motor deficits. Diagnostic examinations should include routine laboratory testing, arterial blood gases (ABGs), chest x-ray, and ECG. Treatment depends on the problem or disease identified.

Neoplastic diseases that can cause confusion include systemic cancers and intracranial lesions to the brain secondary to the extensive tissue and organ destruction caused by the invading cancers. Signs and symptoms depend on the areas of the body where the cancer is located. Extensive cerebral edema, compression, and cell injury produce ischemic states and result in death to cells and tissue. This destruction impairs the circulation of oxygen, increases intracranial pressure, and results in confusion, headaches, disorientation, tremors, seizures, memory loss, gait disturbances, dehydration, changes in levels of consciousness, vomiting, sensory, and motor deficits. Diagnostic studies should include basic routine tests. Additional studies and treatment measures will vary depending on the type and characteristics of the cancer.

Dizziness and Vertigo

Dizziness is the sensation of unsteadiness and a feeling of movement within the head. *Vertigo* is the sensation of rotation or movement of the patient or of the patient's surroundings. The terms are often used synonymously, but they do not have the same meaning. Vertigo may result from an inner ear disease or a disturbance of the vestibular center or pathway in the central nervous system (CNS). Dizziness is described as a feeling of lightheadedness, weakness, or faintness. Loss of consciousness rarely occurs, but the feeling of faintness encourages the patient to lie down, which usually causes the feelings to disappear. It is important to distinguish between vertigo and dizziness. Episodes of dizziness are brief and may be mild or severe, with an abrupt or gradual onset. Dizziness is often accompanied by nausea, vomiting, nystagmus, and unsteady gait; it occurs as a result of inadequate blood flow and oxygen supply to the brain and spinal cord.

Differential Diagnosis

Differential diagnoses for dizziness are classified into four categories: peripheral vestibular disease, systemic disorders, CNS disorders, and anxiety states (Differential Diagnosis Flowchart 5.2). The history and physical examination are essential to pinpoint a diagnosis. Key questions to ask a patient regarding dizziness during a history are those pertaining to duration, severity, and nature of the episodes and about associated symptoms such as hearing loss and weakness. Key points to assess during the physical examination include physical examination of the ear, to rule out cerumen impaction or otitis media; hearing tests, including whisper, Weber, and Rinne; a thorough neurologic assessment; and the Hallpike maneuver, to distinguish between benign vertigo and vertigo resulting from a CNS lesion. The Hallpike maneuver is performed by rotating the patient's head to one side and then lowering it slowly to 30 degrees below the bodyline. The patient should be observed for nystagmus during head rotation and vertical positioning. In patients with benign vertigo, there is rotational nystagmus and possible severe vertigo, which usually occurs on one side. This resolves quickly and cannot be reproduced after two to three

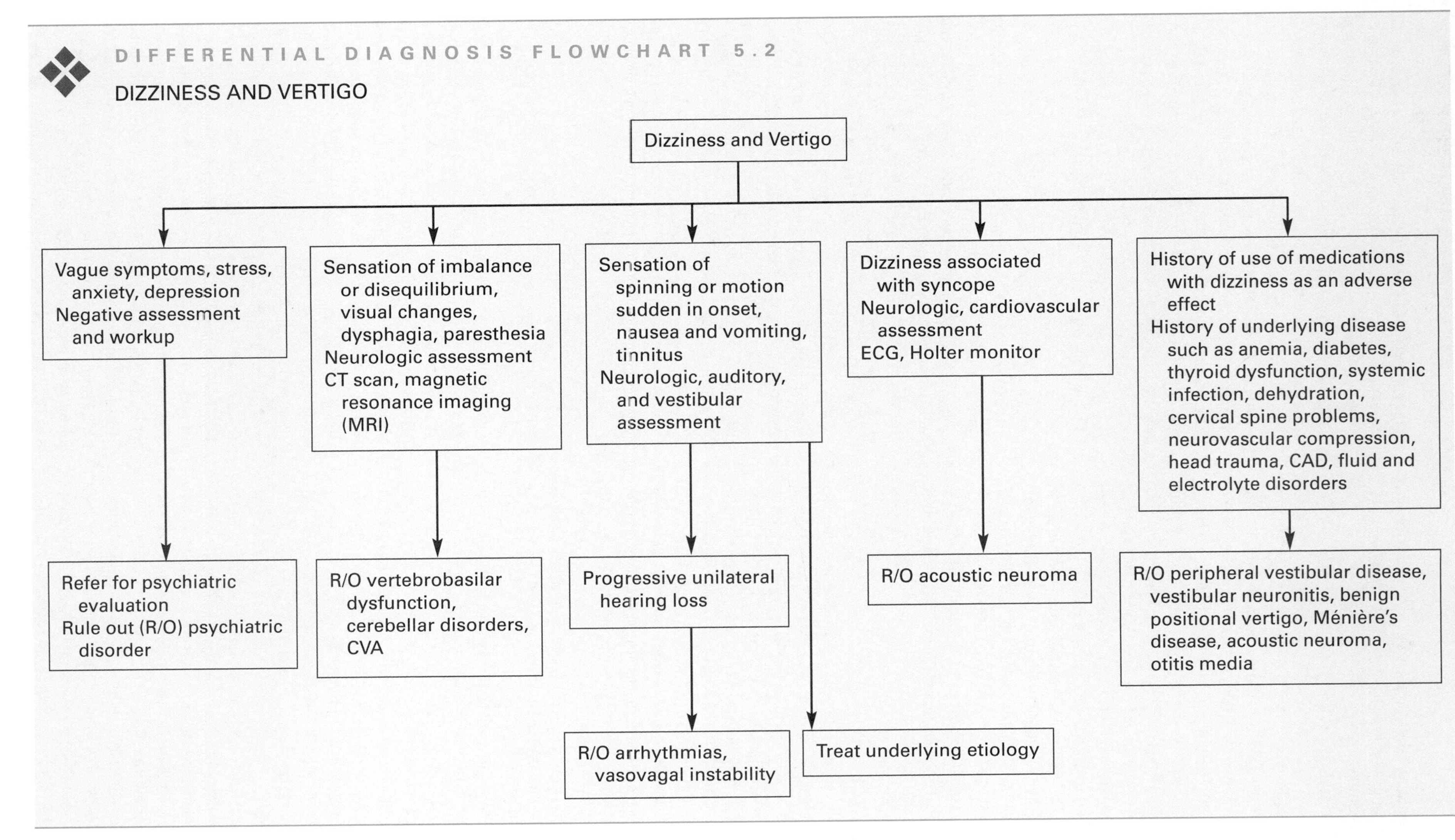
DIFFERENTIAL DIAGNOSIS FLOWCHART 5.2
DIZZINESS AND VERTIGO
Dizziness and Vertigo
Vague symptoms, stress, anxiety, depression
Negative assessment and workup
Sensation of imbalance or disequilibrium, visual changes, dysphagia, paresthesia
Neurologic assessment
CT scan, magnetic resonance imaging (MRI)
Sensation of spinning or motion sudden in onset, nausea and vomiting, tinnitus
Neurologic, auditory, and vestibular assessment
Dizziness associated with syncope
Neurologic, cardiovascular assessment
ECG, Holter monitor
History of use of medications with dizziness as an adverse effect
History of underlying disease such as anemia, diabetes, thyroid dysfunction, systemic infection, dehydration, cervical spine problems, neurovascular compression, head trauma, CAD, fluid and electrolyte disorders
Refer for psychiatric evaluation
Rule out (R/O) psychiatric disorder
R/O vertebrobasilar dysfunction, cerebellar disorders, CVA
Progressive unilateral hearing loss
R/O acoustic neuroma
R/O peripheral vestibular disease, vestibular neuronitis, benign positional vertigo, Ménière's disease, acoustic neuroma, otitis media
R/O arrhythmias, vasovagal instability
Treat underlying etiology

repetitions. The clinician should suspect a central lesion when the vertical nystagmus is of a longer duration and continues with each repetition.

Peripheral Vestibular Disease

Peripheral vestibular disease accounts for up to 36 percent of all cases of dizziness and vertigo. Many patients who experience dizziness may have a diseased vestibular nerve away from the brain stem, the point of origin. Most often the problem is located in the labyrinth of the middle ear. Signs and symptoms of vestibular disease include dizziness, nausea and vomiting, diaphoresis, difficulty with balance, vertigo, tinnitus, fluctuating hearing loss, feelings of pressure in the ear, and diplopia. Diagnostic studies include audiologic evaluation, electronystagmography, brain stem–evoked responses, and basic laboratory screening as guided by history and physical examination. Treatment is centered on supportive therapy. Patients and their families should be instructed that whenever the patient experiences vertigo, he or she should lie down in a darkened room and avoid head movement, which may help prevent some of the accompanying nausea and vomiting. Antihistamines are the most commonly prescribed medication for vertigo because they suppress the vestibular end organ receptors and inhibit activation of vagal responses. Patients are instructed to take the medication for a week, then to try to taper the drug slowly. Meclizine (Antivert) 25 mg q4 to 6h or diphenhydramine (Benadryl) 50 mg q4 to 6h may be tried. Antiemetics should be considered when nausea and vomiting are severe. These agents suppress central vestibular pathways, which activate the vagal stimulus. Prochlorperazine (Compazine) 5 to 10 mg q6h PO or by suppository 25 mg bid, or trimethobenzamide (Tigan) 250 mg PO q8h or 200 mg suppository q6h usually will bring relief to the patient. Vestibular exercises can help the patient cope with the symptoms of vertigo. These exercises have been shown to decrease the duration of vertigo or produce longer symptom-free periods. The patient is instructed to reproduce the feelings of vertigo by placing the affected ear down, then to assume a supine position and hold that position until the vertigo disappears. The vertigo will return when the patient sits up. The patient must repeat these maneuvers at least five times a day or until the vertigo no longer returns. Patients with persistent symptoms should be referred to an ear specialize for assessment of nerve function. Surgery may be indicated when all else fails to relieve the vertigo.

Systemic Disorders

Systemic disorders may cause dizziness. Patients typically complain of lightheadedness or feelings that they are about to faint or pass out. Dizziness may be aggravated by postural changes or exertion; pallor, dyspnea, tachycardia, bounding pulse, weakness, hypotension, blurred vision, decreased breath sounds, headache, diaphoresis, and agitation suggest systemic problems. These symptoms should prompt the practitioner to look for signs of anemia, cardiovascular disease, hyperventilation, drug reactions, endocrine disorders, fluid and electrolyte imbalances, and psychiatric problems. Systemic diseases require diagnostic examination and treatment that is specific for the cause of the dizziness.

Central Nervous System Disorders

CNS disorders that disrupt the pathway between the vestibular apparatus and the brain may cause dizziness. Facial numbness, hemiparesis, diplopia, dysarthria, headache, nausea, and vomiting are some common signs and symptoms suggesting CNS dysfunction. Diagnostic examination and treatment depend on the underlying disorder.

Headache

The most common of all human ailments is the headache. Headache may be localized or generalized and may produce mild to severe pain. About 90 percent of all headaches are without pathological cause.

Differential Diagnosis

Headaches may be classified into four types: muscle contraction (tension) headaches, vascular (migraine and cluster) headaches, mixed headaches (a combination of muscle contraction and vascular), and traction or inflammatory headaches. Muscle contraction headaches, often referred to as tension headaches, are either primary (without underlying pathology) or secondary (the result of pathology such as trauma, infection, arthritis, or tumor). They occur in 20 to 25 percent of all new cases of headaches. More than 50 percent of all headaches seen in primary care are muscle contraction headaches. These headaches can occur at any age but are most common in young adults. Females present with the most severe cases, with underlying causes of generalized anxiety or depressive disorders. Forty percent of all patients with muscle contraction headaches have a positive family history of headaches. Any headache that is abrupt, explosive, severe, and described as the worst headache of the patient's life is suggestive of a traction or inflammatory headache and is most often due to intracranial hemorrhage.

The clinician should ask questions to determine the following factors: onset; location of the headache; frequency; duration; severity; character, such as throbbing versus constant; presence of an aura; an association with sleep patterns; emotional factors; precipitating and alleviating factors; and family history. This information is essential to delineate the diagnosis and rule out other problems. Differential Diagnosis Flowchart 5.3 presents common characteristics, associated symptoms, and precipitating factors of common disorders that present with a complaint of headache. Additional information about headaches is provided later in this chapter; different types of headaches, along with their associated signs and symptoms, diagnosis, and treatment, are compared in Table 5.6.

DIFFERENTIAL DIAGNOSIS FLOWCHART 5.3

HEADACHE

Headache

- Location: temporal/occipital; unilateral
  - Characteristics: aching or burning; possible temporal artery pulsations
    - Associated symptoms: possibly loss of vision
      Precipitating factors: none
      - R/O temporal arteritis
- Location: variable
  - Characteristics: variable frequency and intensity; may awaken at night
    - Associated symptoms: papilledema, nausea, projectile vomiting, altered mental status
      Precipitating factors: none
      - R/O brain tumor
  - Characteristics: hypertensive; possible retinopathy
    - Associated symptoms: possibly signs and symptoms of TIA, CVA, hypertensive encephalopathy
      Precipitating factors: none or possibly discontinuation of hypertensive medications
      - R/O hypertension
- Location: generalized
  - Characteristics: intense, sudden onset, "worst headache I've ever had"
    - Associated symptoms: nuchal rigidity, altered level of consciousness
      Precipitating factors: none or possibly head trauma
      - R/O subarachnoid hemorrhage/bleeding
  - Characteristics: variable severity; may be worse in the neck
    - Associated symptoms: fever, nuchal rigidity, altered level of consciousness, positive Kernig's and/or Brudzinski's signs
      Precipitating factors: none or possibly exposure to infection
      - R/O meningitis

Paresthesia and Paresis

Paresthesia and paresis are abnormal sensations described as numbness or tingling, cramping, or pain without a known stimulus, felt along peripheral nerve pathways. Although the terms are used interchangeably, *paresis* is really a slight or incomplete paralysis, whereas *paresthesia* is the abnormal sensation of burning or prickling. Paresis may develop suddenly or gradually and may be permanent or transient. Feelings associated with paresthesia are annoying "pins and needles" sensations that often cause the patient to touch or rub the affected area. Paresthesia is a common complaint, especially in patients with certain systemic diseases or those on certain drugs.

Differential Diagnosis

Paresthesia is usually due to damaged or irritation to the parietal lobe, thalamus, spinothalamic tract, or to the spinal or peripheral nerves that are the usual pathways for transmission and interpretation of sensory stimuli. It is important to explore the symptom of paresthesia by asking the patient

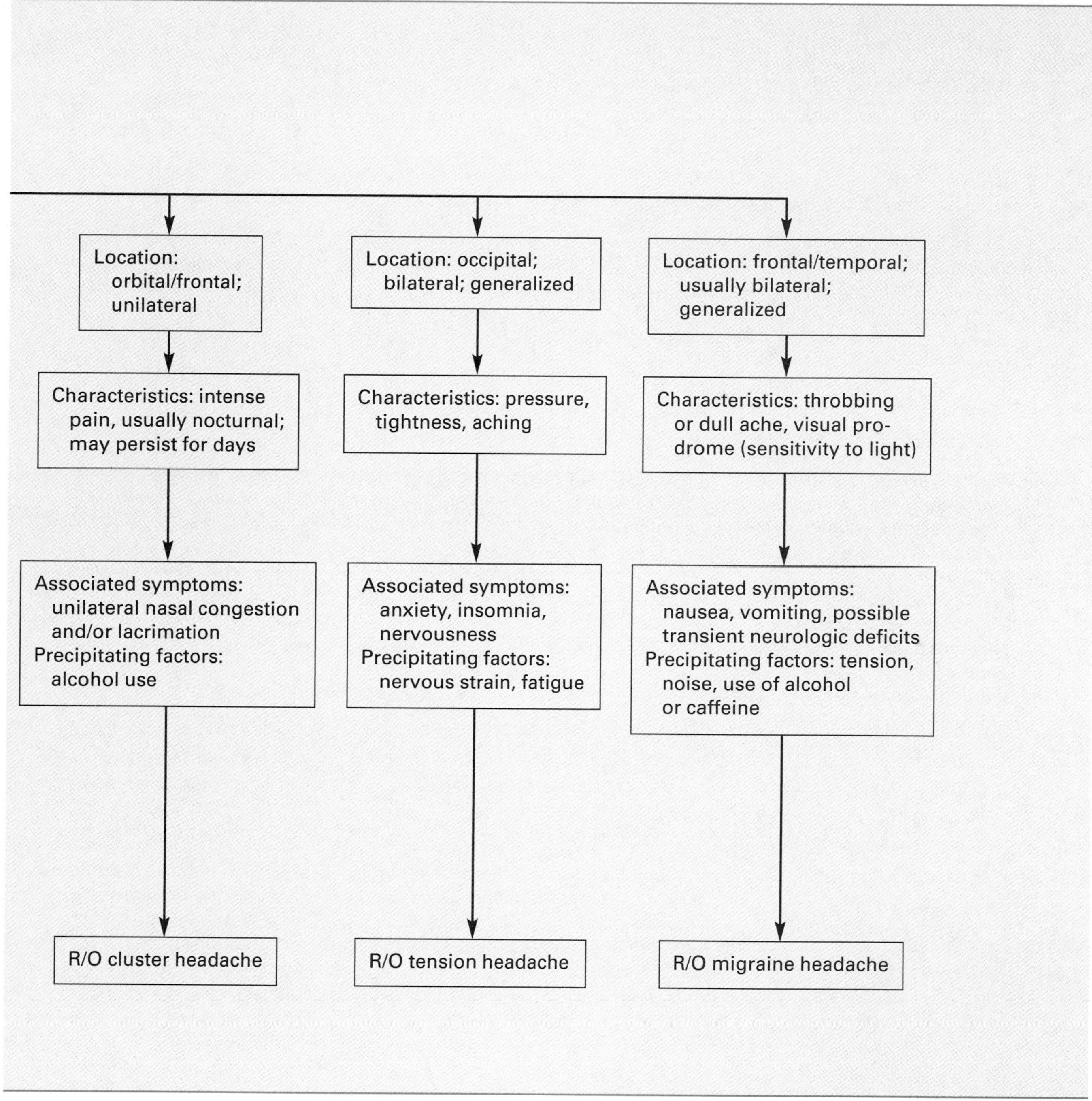

to describe when it first began; the character, duration, and distribution of the paresthesia; as well as any other associated signs and symptoms such as sensory or motor loss. A medical history will reveal any neurologic, cardiac, vascular, endocrine, renal, or inflammatory diseases the patient may have had or still has. Recent trauma, surgery, or invasive procedures may reveal possible causes of peripheral nerve injury. The physical examination should focus on the neurologic system, assessing level of consciousness; cranial nerve function; reflexes; motor strength; and touch, pain, and temperature sensations. Skin color and the quality of all pulses should also be noted. If the patient has diabetes, symptoms of diabetic neuropathy such as a bilateral loss of pain sensation and diminished touch, temperature sensation, and proprioception may be present.

The most common diagnoses associated with paresthesia symptoms are arterial occlusion, arteriosclerosis obliterans, nerve entrapment syndrome, neuropathy, transient ischemic attacks (TIAs), and herpes zoster (Differential Diagnosis Flowchart 5.4).

Arterial occlusion is a surgical emergency. An acute occlusion may be either an arterial embolism or a

DIFFERENTIAL DIAGNOSIS FLOWCHART 5.4

PARESTHESIA AND PARESIS

Paresthesia and Paresis

- Sudden paresthesias, coldness, mottling of extremities, absent pulses distal to occlusion
  - Doppler studies, arteriography, electromyogram (EMG), nerve conduction studies, labs (serum B12, iron, ferritin, folate, Schilling's test, complete blood count (CBC), blood urea nitrogen (BUN), creatinine, calcium, bicarbonate), MRI (R/O multiple sclerosis)
  - Arterial occlusion
  - Refer to vascular specialist, possible embolectomy, anticoagulant therapy
- Intermittent claudication, diminished or absent pulses, pallor, coldness, mottling of affected limb, pain at rest, extremity ulcers
  - Doppler studies, ankle/arm systolic BP index (AAI), angiography
  - Arteriosclerosis obliterans
  - Treatment: Lifestyle modifications (diet, exercise, weight reduction, smoking cessation, control of diabetes and hypertension, management of hyperlipidemia), pentoxifylline (Trental) 400 mg tid or cilostazol 100 mg bid, surgical intervention (last resort)
- Weakness, paresthesia sensations (numbness, tingling, cramping, pain)
  - EMG, Tinel's sign and Phalen's sign (to evaluate for carpal tunnel syndrome)
  - Nerve entrapment syndrome
  - Treatment: Refer to neurologist or orthopedic surgeon (will usually try splints, braces, or other musculoskeletal support options), possible steroid injections, surgical decompression

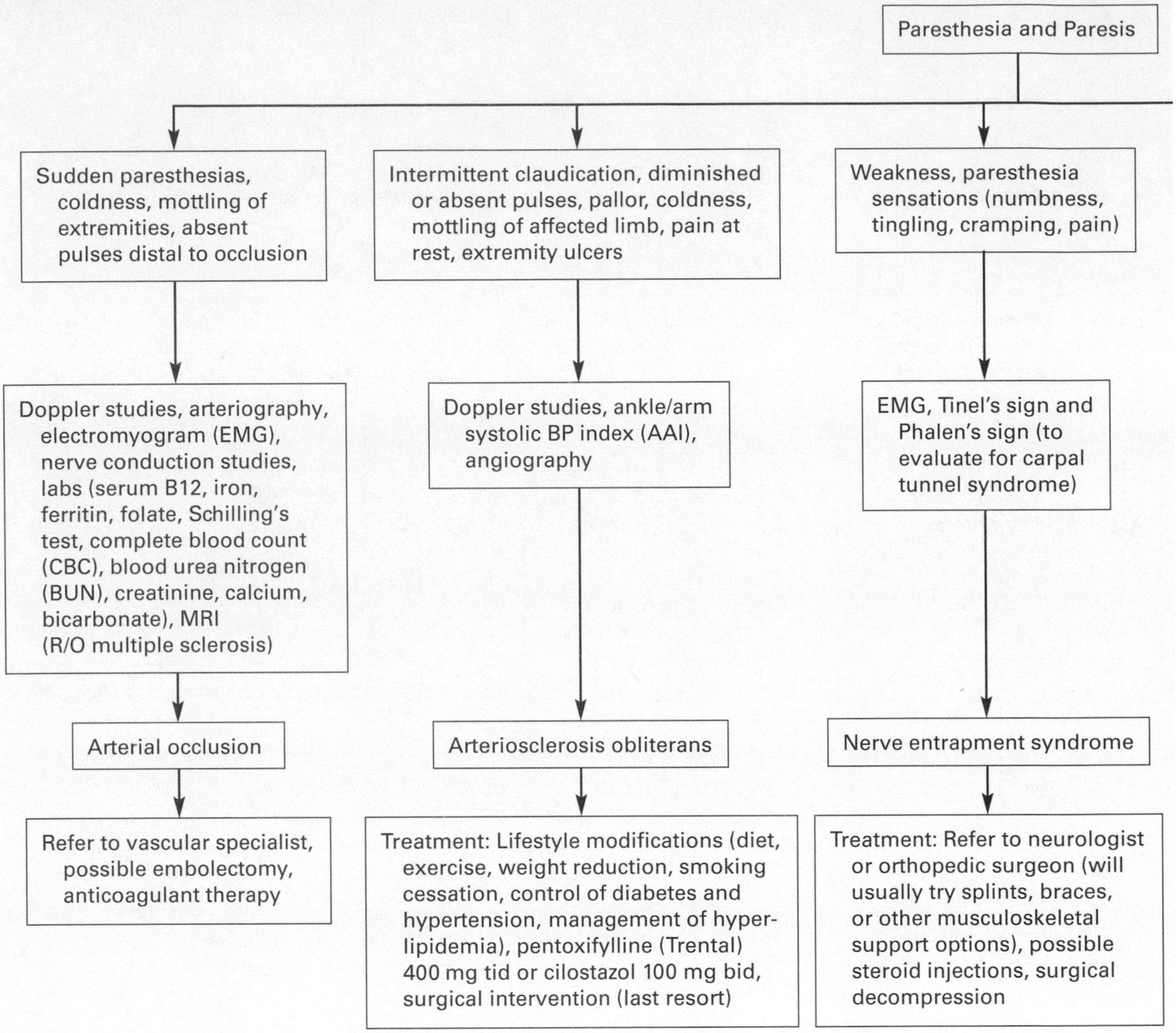

thrombosis. Immediate embolectomy is the treatment of choice in early emboli in the extremities and is preferably performed within 4 to 6 hours of the embolic event.

Arteriosclerosis obliterans is a disorder that involves the pathological process of atherosclerosis, which causes progressive narrowing of the arteries with subsequent obstruction of blood flow, resulting in diminished or decreased flow of blood to the legs and feet.

Nerve entrapment syndrome results from compression of a nerve pathway along the root of the nerve, which results in paresthesia or weakness. Trauma causing compartmental syndrome or bruising, rheumatoid arthritis, edema, infection, prolonged standing or sitting, and tight clothing can all cause entrapment of the nerve. The compression diminishes blood supply and can result in cellular changes to the nerve pathway.

Neuropathy is usually the result of underlying diseases such as diabetes, renal failure, multiple sclerosis, cancer, collagen disease, vasculitis, thyroid disease, or ingestion of toxins or nutritional deficiency. Afferent nerve fibers conduct impulses from the skin to the brain. Alterations along these nerve pathways because of disease pathology can

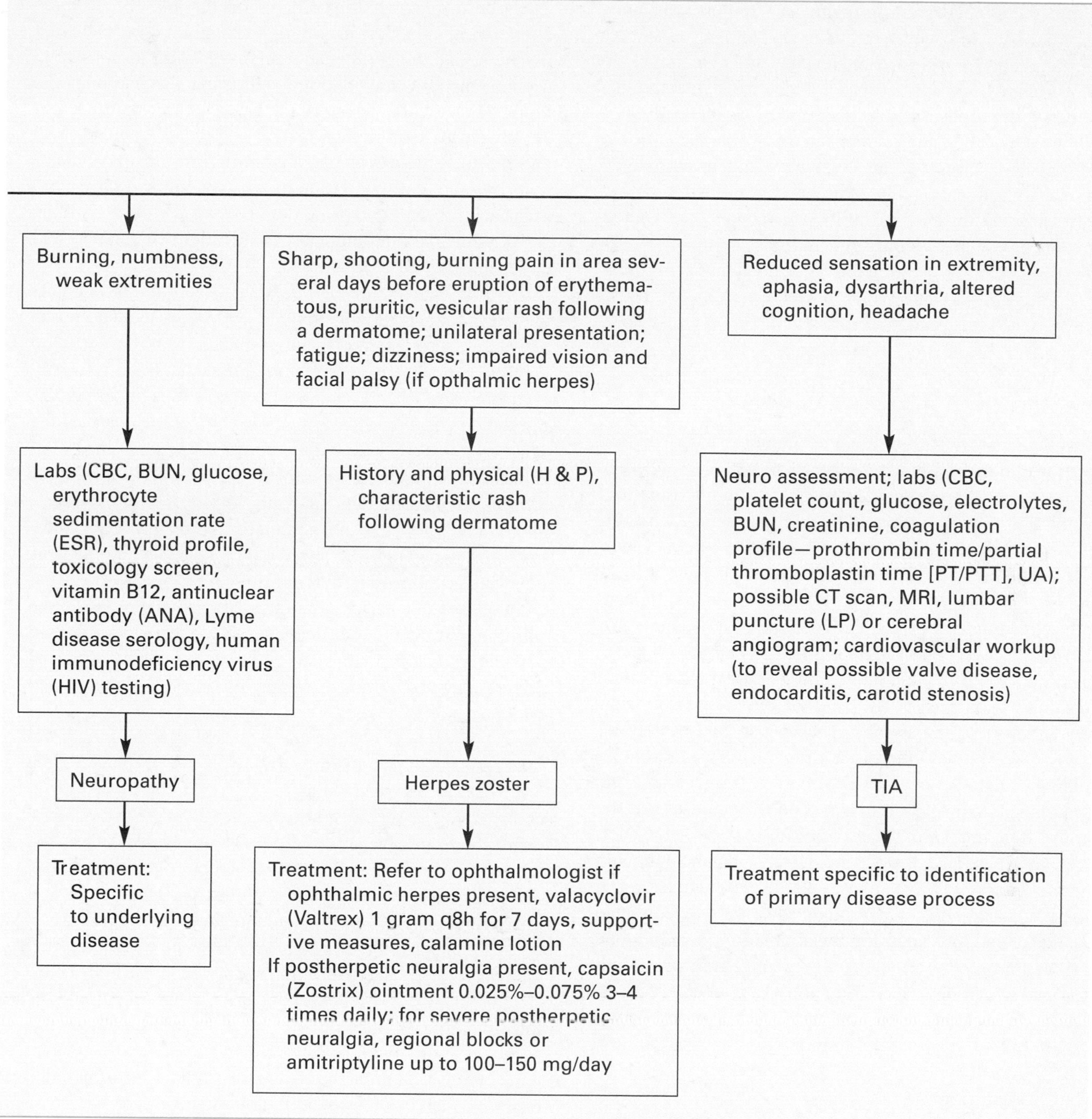

cause paresthesia. The majority of the diseases listed involve peripheral nerves and can alter their function.

Herpes zoster is caused by the varicella-zoster virus, which causes an acute vesicular eruption in adults and immunocompromised patients. An early symptom of herpes zoster is paresthesia, which occurs as a result of inflammation and compression of the dermatome, which is supplied by the spinal cord.

A TIA is a sudden transient loss of neurologic function caused by impaired blood flow to the brain. The loss of function can last from a few minutes to 24 hours; after a TIA, normal function returns. If some residual weakness remains, the patient has had a stroke. TIAs are discussed in detail later in this chapter.

Tremors

Tremors are rhythmic involuntary muscle movements that result from alternate contraction and relaxation of opposing muscle groups. They are typically evident in patients with cerebellar or extrapyramidal disorders and are also seen as side effects with certain drug regimens. Tremors are sometimes classified into seven groups: physiologic, essential, toxic, cerebellar, Parkinsonian, resting, and intentional. A *resting tremor* occurs in a relaxed and supported extremity and ends with purposeful movement, whereas an *intentional tremor* occurs when the patient attempts voluntary movement. Essential tremors are typically underreported, as many persons do not seek treatment for mild tremors. It is estimated that at least 10 million persons in the United States have essential tremor. As the most common movement disorder, it is apparent in 1 in 20 Americans older than the age of 40, and 1 in 5 over the age of 65. These patients, when they do present, should be referred to a neurologist.

Differential Diagnosis

A complete history and physical examination are necessary to obtain important subjective data that will provide information on the tremor's characteristics, including duration, onset of action, progression, alleviating factors, and associated symptoms (such as memory loss, agitation, and nausea). It is important to note when the tremor is present (e.g., with rest or activity), what part of the body is affected, whether it is bilateral or not, and the type of movement produced by the tremor (e.g., flexion or extension, pronation, supination, or pill rolling, and so on). The patient's muscle tone should also be assessed: Is it normal or increased (cogwheel rigidity)? The patient's speech, gait, and posture all must be assessed. A thorough drug history is essential, including a list of any over-the-counter (OTC) drugs the patient is taking. The clinician should note whether the tremors affect the patient's activities of daily living (ADLs) and if there is any history of family members having tremors. A review of systems will disclose a history of endocrine, metabolic, or neurologic disorders. A complete musculoskeletal and neurologic examination must be done to assess range of motion (ROM), mental status, strength and sensitivity, cranial nerve function, deep tendon reflexes, and gait. Differential Diagnosis Flowchart 5.5 presents common differential diagnoses of tremor.

Common Problems

Seizure Disorders

The terms *seizure disorder, convulsive disorder,* and *cerebral seizures* are synonymous with the term "epilepsy." They all refer to recurrent paroxysmal episodes of brain dysfunction manifested by stereotypical alterations in behavior. *Epilepsy,* by definition, is a condition in which an individual is predisposed to three or more recurrent seizures because of a CNS disorder. Seizure disorders referred to in this chapter include the diagnosis of epilepsy.

A *seizure* is a sudden, involuntary, time-limited alteration in behavior, including a change in motor activity, in autonomic function, unconsciousness, or in sensation, accompanied by an abnormal electrical discharge in the brain. The major behavioral feature that distinguishes seizures from usual activity is that seizures are stereotypical and repetitive. For example, a *clonic seizure* involves maximal contraction of one group of muscles followed by relaxation, with the cycle repeated three times per second. Table 5.1 presents the international classifications of seizures and epilepsies (ICES).

Partial seizures are those in which the first clinical and electroencephalographic (EEG) changes indicate initial activation of a system of neurons limited to one part of the cerebral hemisphere. A partial seizure is classified primarily on the basis of whether or not consciousness is impaired during the attack. When there is no loss of consciousness, the seizure is classified as a *simple partial seizure.* When consciousness is impaired, the seizure is classified as a *complex partial seizure.* In patients with impaired consciousness, aberrations of behavior (automatisms) may occur. Automatisms are distinguished by symptoms: eating automatisms (chewing, swallowing); automatisms of mimicry, expressing emotional state; gestural automatisms, crude or elaborate (directed toward either the subject or his or her environment); ambulatory automatisms; and verbal automatisms. A partial seizure may not terminate; it may progress to a generalized motor seizure instead.

There is considerable evidence that simple partial seizures usually have unilateral hemispheric involvement and only rarely have bilateral hemispheric involvement; complex partial seizures, however, frequently have bilateral hemispheric involvement. Partial seizures can be classified into three fundamental groups: simple partial seizures, complex partial seizures, and complex partial seizures that evolve into generalized tonic–clonic convulsions.

Generalized seizures are those in which the first clinical changes indicate initial involvement of both hemispheres of the brain. Consciousness may be impaired, and this impairment may be the initial manifestation of the seizure. Motor manifestations are bilateral. The EEG patterns are bilateral, and presumably reflect neuronal discharge, which is widespread in both hemispheres.

The hallmark of an *absence seizure* is a sudden onset, interruption of ongoing activities, a blank stare, and possibly a brief upward rotation of the eye. If the patient is speaking, speech will be slowed or interrupted; if the patient is walking, he or she will stand transfixed; if eating, the food will be stopped on the way to the mouth. The attack may last from a few seconds to a half a minute.

Tonic–clonic, or *grand mal, seizures* are the most frequently encountered generalized seizures. There is a sudden, sharp tonic contraction of muscles, stridor, or a cry, and the patient falls to the ground in the tonic state. The patient lies rigid; during this state, tonic contraction inhibits

Table 5.1 International Classification of Epileptic Seizures (ICES)

Seizures	
I. Partial (focal, local) seizures	
A. Simple partial seizures (consciousness not impaired)	1. With motor symptoms 2. With somatosensory or special sensory symptoms 3. With autonomic symptoms 4. With psychic symptoms
B. Complex partial seizures (with impairment of consciousness)	1. Beginning as simple partial seizures and progressing to impairment of consciousness a. with no other features b. with features as in simple partial seizures c. with automatisms 2. With impairment of consciousness at onset a. with no other features b. with features as in simple partial seizures c. with automatisms
C. Partial seizures evolving to secondarily generalized seizures	1. Simple partial seizures evolving to generalized seizures 2. Complex partial seizures evolving to generalized seizures 3. Simple partial seizures evolving to complex partial seizures to generalized seizures
II. Generalized seizures (convulsive or nonconvulsive)	
A. Absence seizures (petit mal)	1. Absence seizures 2. Atypical absence seizures
B. Myoclonic seizures	
C. Clonic seizures	
D. Tonic seizures	
E. Tonic–clonic seizures (grand mal)	
F. Atonic seizures (astatic seizures)	
III. Unclassified seizures	1. Includes all seizures that cannot be classified because of inadequate or incomplete data and some that defy classification as already described. This includes some neonatal seizures, such as rhythmic eye movements, chewing, and swimming movements.
Epilepsies	
I. Localization-related epilepsies	1. Idiopathic (age-related) a. benign childhood epilepsy with centrotemporal spikes b. benign childhood epilepsy with occipital paroxysms 2. Symptomatic a. epilepsies involving the limbic system b. epilepsies not involving the limbic system (frontal, temporal, central, parietal, occipital)
II. Generalized epilepsies	1. Idiopathic (age-related) (benign neonatal familial convulsions, benign neonatal convulsions West's syndrome [idiopathic cases], epilepsy with myoclonic-astatic seizures [idiopathic and familial cases of Lennox–Gastaut–Dravet syndrome], childhood absence epilepsy [pyknoepilepsy], epilepsy with [myo]clonic absences, juvenile absence epilepsy, benign juvenile myoclonic epilepsy [impulsive mal], epilepsy with generalized tonic–clonic seizures on awakening) 2. Symptomatic a. nonspecific cause (age-related) (neonatal seizures, early myoclonic encephalopathy, West's syndrome [infantile spasms, Blitz–Nick–Salaam–Krampfe], Lennox–Gastaut–Dravet syndrome) b. specific cause (progressive myoclonus epilepsies such as Lafora's disease, Unverricht's disease, Unverricht–Lundborg–Hartung disease, Kufs'disease, Zeman's disease) 3. Epilepsies undetermined whether focal or generalized 4. Special syndromes

DIFFERENTIAL DIAGNOSIS FLOWCHART 5.5

TREMORS

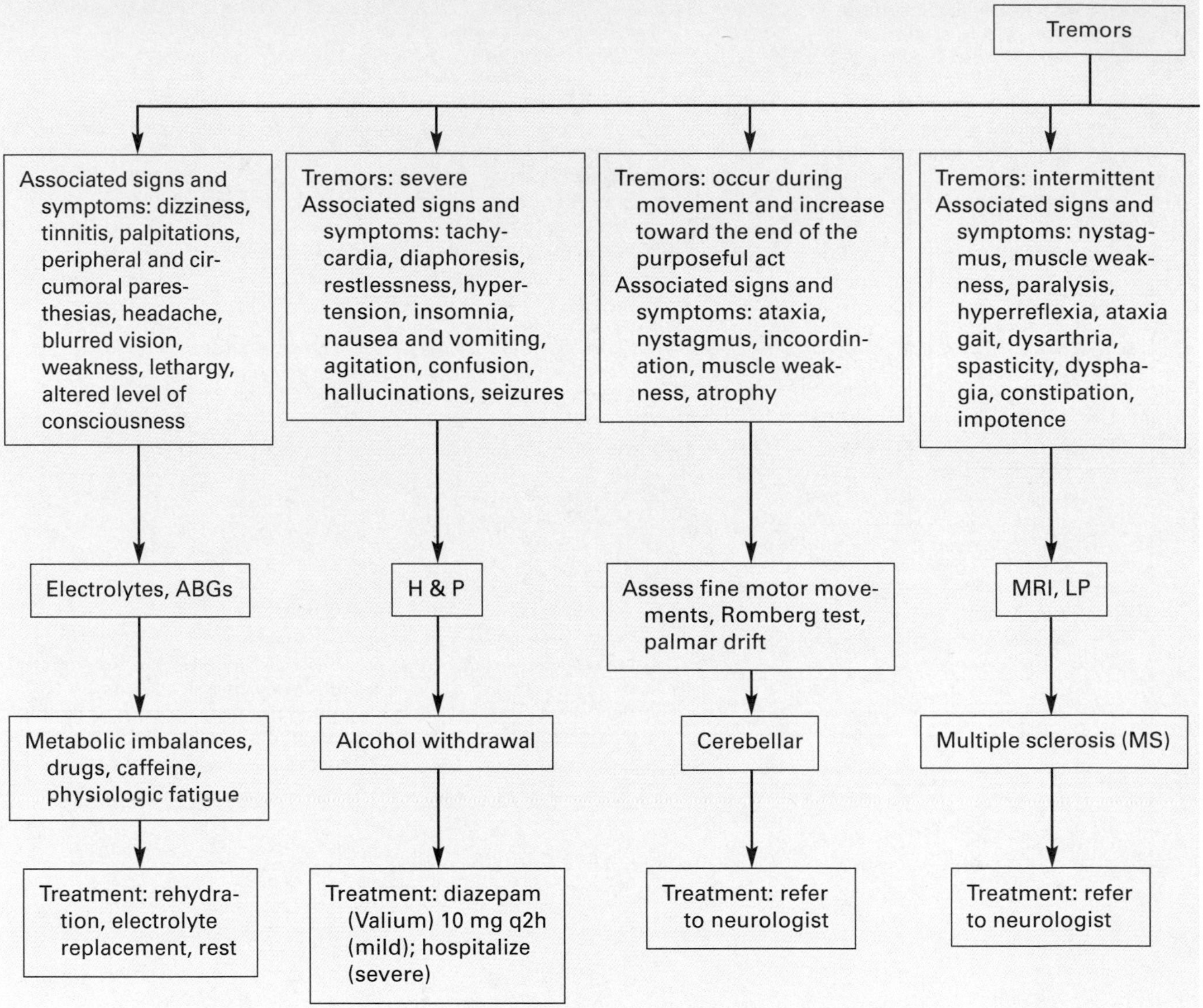

respiration and cyanosis may occur. The tongue may be bitten and urine may be voided involuntarily. This tonic stage then gives way to clonic convulsive movements lasting a variable period of time. At the end of this stage, deep respiration will occur and all muscles will relax, after which the patient will remain unconscious for a period of time. After this type of seizure, the individual frequently goes into a deep sleep and may have a significant headache when awakened.

Myoclonic jerks are sudden, brief shock-like contractions, which may be generalized or confined to the face and trunk or to one or more extremities. They may occur predominantly during sleep.

Epidemiology and Causes

Seizure disorders are among the most common neurologic conditions, affecting more than 2 million people in the United States. Each year about 300,000 individuals in the United States seek medical attention because of a newly recognized seizure, representing an incidence of about 120 per 100,000. The majority of patients (75,000 to 100,000) presenting for treatment of seizure are younger than age 5 and have experienced only convulsions associated with a febrile illness. Each year 50 per 100,000 individuals in the United States are diagnosed as having a seizure disorder, which

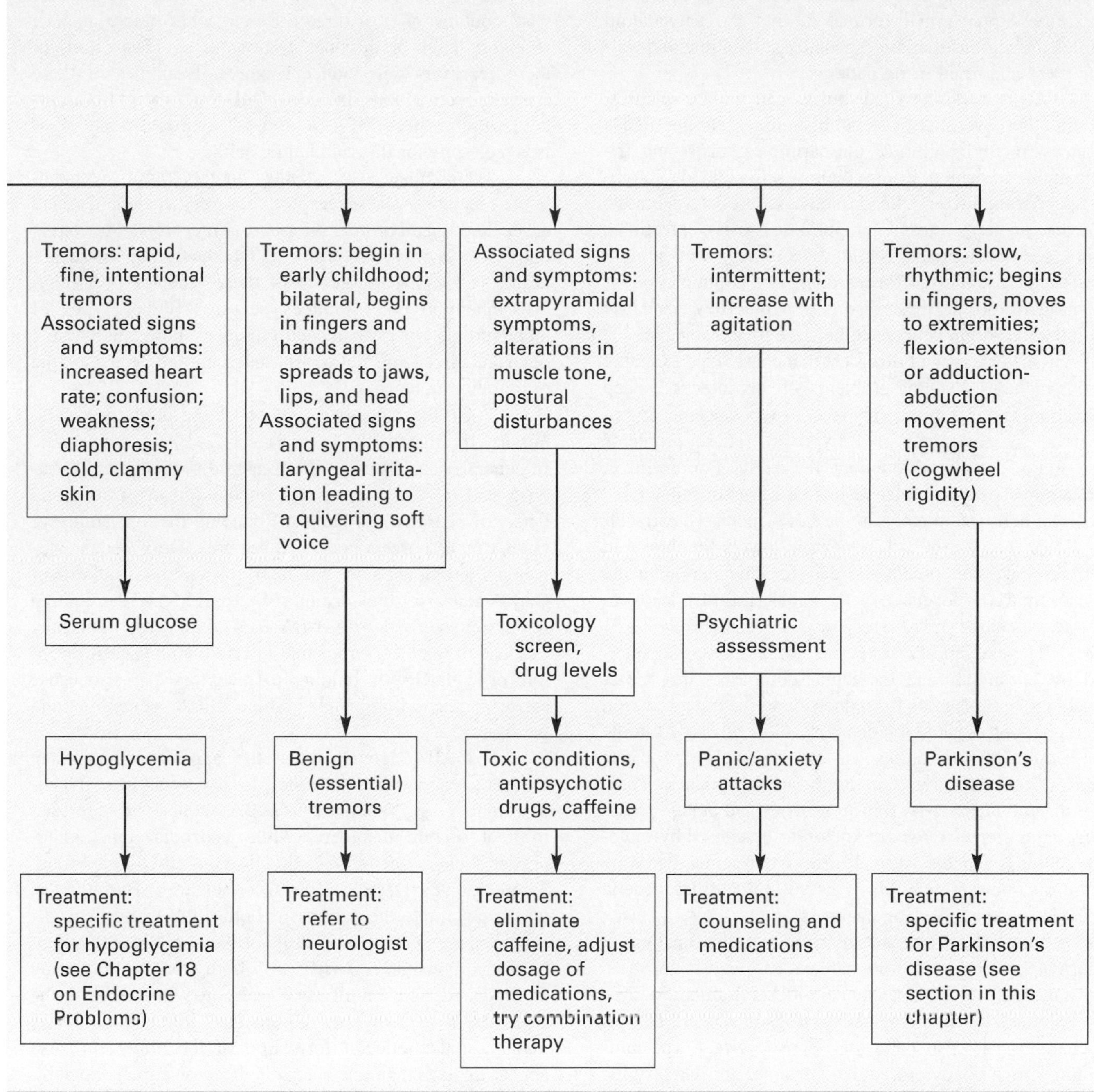

is approximately 125,000 new cases each year. Although seizure disorders may start at any age, the highest incidence of seizure is among children younger than age 2 and persons older than age 65.

Men are more likely to have a seizure disorder than women. In most newly diagnosed cases, no specific cause is identified. Many factors have been implicated in the etiology of seizure disorders, such as severe head trauma, CNS infections, and stroke. Children with motor disabilities present from birth, such as cerebral palsy or mental retardation, have an increased risk for a seizure disorder. When both conditions coexist, 50 percent or more of patients affected can be expected to develop a seizure disorder by age 20. In addition, children who experience febrile seizures are at increased risk for developing a seizure disorder during their lives.

Seizure disorders frequently occur in families. The parents, siblings, and offspring of a patient with a seizure disorder are more likely (3 to 5 percent) than the general population to have a seizure as a result of both genetic and environmental causes.

Pathophysiology

A seizure is an uncontrollable paroxysm that often includes muscular convulsions. The paroxysm is the bodily effect of abnormal repetitive firing of neurons in the brain. The motor cortex, the hippocampal formation, and the amygdaloid complex are regions that are especially susceptible to developing these abnormal firing patterns.

A great variety of disorders can initiate seizures, including drug overdose (e.g., antihistamines, cholinesterase inhibitors, methylxanthines, muscarinic agonists, and tricyclic antidepressants), drug withdrawal (e.g., alcohol, hypnotics, and tranquilizers), head trauma, strokes, degenerative brain disease (e.g., mesial temporal sclerosis), infections, tumors, and developmental brain defects (e.g., cortical dysgenesis and vascular malformations). The common epileptogenic feature of all these disorders is that they can cause populations of brain neurons to become hyperexcitable.

One category of disorders that cause hyperexcitable neurons includes systemic problems—fever, infection, sleep deprivation, and metabolic imbalances (hypocalcemia, hypoglycemia, hyponatremia, and hypoxia). These problems cause ionic changes throughout the body. For example, hyponatremia causes a relative increase in extracellular K^+ concentrations systemically. In the CNS, increased extracellular K^+ at the neuron cell membrane lowers the threshold for triggering axon potentials, and for this reason, acute hyponatremia (at levels less than 115 mEq/L) leads to seizures.

The excitability of neuron cell membranes is regulated by intramembrane molecular complexes that either actively move molecules from one side to the other (i.e., ion pumps) or control gated ion channels. Genetic defects in the manufacture of ion pumps or ion channels can cause seizures. Some of the uncommon heritable epilepsies (e.g., *generalized epilepsy with febrile seizures* and *benign familial neonatal convulsions*) are known to be caused by mutations in ion channels. It is believed that other heritable seizure disorders are caused by as yet unidentified genetic defects in ion pumps or ion channels.

Similarly, drugs that interfere with the functioning of normal ion pumps or ion channels can lead to seizures; for instance, the potassium channel blocker 4-aminopyridine is a potent seizure-inducing drug. Drugs that interfere with ion channels can also have the opposite effect. The anti-epileptic drugs phenytoin, carbamazepine, and lamotrigine reduce the hyperexcitability of neuron cell membranes by slowing the activation of Na^+ channels, and ethosuximide decreases the activity of certain Ca^{2+} channels.

Much of the excitatory activity throughout the brain is via glutamatergic synapses, and increasing the amount or the effect of glutamate in the brain predisposes a person to seizures. Normally, the amount of extracellular glutamate in the brain is minimized by astrocytes, which selectively take up glutamate. Experimental studies have shown that a brain will have seizures if its astrocytes cannot efficiently clear extracellular glutamate from the vicinity of synapses.

Glutamate depolarizes neurons by activating specific receptors that open channels for small cations, such as Na^+ and K^+. These are called *ionotropic receptors*, and the CNS contains at least three different ionotropic glutamate receptors. High brain concentrations of agonists of any of these receptors will induce seizures. Examples of these types of convulsants include NMDA (*N*-methyl-D-aspartate), quinolinate, AMPA (a-amino-3-hydroxyl-5-methyl-4-isoxazole-propionate), and kainic acid.

Glutamate also activates another family of membrane receptors. These receptors alter cell metabolism and are called *metabotropic glutamate receptors*. Activating one variety of metabotropic glutamate receptors depolarizes cells, and an agonist of these receptors, 3,5-dihydroxyphenylglycine, induces seizures. Other types of metabotropic glutamate receptor agonists, however, have the opposite effect—activating these receptors decreases the excitability of synapses.

On the other hand, much of the inhibitory transmission throughout the brain is via GABAergic synapses. In general, neurons using the transmitter gamma-aminobutyric acid (GABA) act to prevent the spread of abnormal bursts of neuronal discharges. Reducing the availability of GABA predisposes a person to seizures. Drugs, such as 3-mercaptopropionic acid, that interfere with the synthesis of GABA cause seizures. Vitamin B_6 (pyridoxine) is required for the biosynthesis of GABA, and vitamin B_6 deficiency can lead to seizures. Drugs that interfere with GABA receptors or with GABA binding to receptors can also cause seizures; such drugs include bicuculline, penicillin, and picrotoxin.

GABA agonists have the opposite effect—they counteract a person's tendency to have seizures. Benzodiazepines (e.g., Valium) are GABA agonists and are used to treat seizure disorders, while benzodiazepine antagonists, such as methyl-6,7-dimethoxy-4-ethyl-b-carboline-3-carboxylate (DMCM), produce seizures. Barbiturates, which potentiate the actions of both GABA and benzodiazepines, are anti-epileptic drugs. Likewise, the anti epileptic drugs tiagabine and vigabatrin both work by enhancing GABA-mediated inhibitory circuitry. Besides the GABAergic pathways, noradrenergic circuits (originating mainly in the reticular formation of the brainstem) also appear to play an anti-seizure role, because damage to noradrenergic pathways can predispose a person to seizures.

During a seizure, brain metabolism accelerates in the affected areas. Oxygen consumption, glucose use, and lactate levels go up, free fatty acids are released into the blood, extracellular concentrations of neurotransmitters rise, and cerebral blood flow increases. Between seizures, metabolism in the affected areas drops below normal. Prolonged seizures increase the local transcription of certain genes and the synthesis of certain proteins (although the synthesis of most proteins declines). The abnormal metabolic activities associated with repeated seizures produce long-term changes in brain circuitry that make further seizures more likely. One reason for controlling epilepsy is to prevent these lasting increases in neural sensitivity.

Clinical Presentation

Subjective

The patient may or may not be aware of a seizure. He or she may wake up, slightly confused, on the floor, or in a different position. The patient may have been incontinent. If an aura was present, the patient will know that a seizure took place.

Objective

The most difficult decision in evaluating a presumed seizure is determining if it was a seizure or another type of condition (such as syncope, a pseudoseizure, or a panic attack). Not all events associated with abnormal body movements are seizures. Some events may be mistaken for seizures on initial presentation but must be differentiated from them because their treatment is different. Careful and detailed history taking remains the cornerstone of accurate diagnosis of a seizure disorder. A diagnosis of seizure disorder is primarily a historical diagnosis, and the initial assessment and approach to management is based on the patient's clinical history, especially on an accurate description of the event in question.

It is often very useful to ask the patient for a description of specific attacks. This should include the last attack actually witnessed as well as the first seizure. The setting in which the attacks occurred may be significant for differential diagnosis. A careful review of the events occurring days before the seizure is important. Points of particular interest include relation of events to the sleep–wake cycle. It is important to determine if there is a stimulus regularly associated with an attack and if the seizure was provoked or unprovoked. Many things can provoke a seizure such as extensive sleep deprivation or use of stimulants. Questions need to be asked to determine if there is an aura associated with the seizure. The regular presence of an aura indicates that the seizure is probably localized. Obtaining a history of the patient's life, including social, behavioral, and cognitive functioning, as well as a previous health history and family history of seizure disorders or neurologic disorders, is crucial. History of postictal behaviors should be elicited—how long did it take to recover to normal function? Other important questions should address any history of neonatal seizures or febrile seizures, or history of previous brain injury. The clinician should also ask whether there is a personal or family history of other neurologic, mental, or system disease.

The physical examination should take into account the interval since the patient's most recent seizure. If the exam is performed within minutes or hours of an attack, the practitioner should look for postictal signs, even of a minor grade. When the examination is performed after some time has elapsed since the last seizure, the practitioner's main objective is to determine whether there are signs of permanent nervous system dysfunction, favoring a diagnosis of symptomatic epilepsy, and if there is evidence of a focal brain lesion. The clinician should look for signs of increased intracranial pressure, although this is rather uncommon. Additional neurologic signs of interest include language difficulties and possible evidence of drug toxicity, such as nystagmus, ataxia, diplopia, or tremor.

An eye and visual examination should aim to detect papilledema and visual field cuts associated with focal brain lesions. Ocular motor abnormalities may suggest involvement of the brain stem or floor of the third ventricle. Cranial nerves should be assessed to determine if neurologic signs or symptoms are present. The findings on the patient's motor exam should be symmetrical. Weakness could indicate a brain lesion. A cardiovascular exam should also be performed to detect the presence of a heart arrhythmia or murmur, which may suggest a syncopal episode rather than a seizure.

Diagnostic Reasoning

Diagnostic Tests

Initial tests should be done to rule out other non-neurologic causes of the seizures. Tests may include complete blood count (CBC) with differential, blood glucose, serum electrolytes, liver function tests (LFTs), serum calcium, urinalysis (UA), a drug screen or blood alcohol level, if appropriate, and blood levels to assess target levels if the patient is on antiseizure medications.

Subsequent tests that may lead to the cause of the seizure disorder are EEG, CT scan, or magnetic resonance imaging (MRI); lumbar puncture (LP), if CNS infection is suspected; and ECG, if warranted.

Differential Diagnosis

The patient should be reevaluated to confirm the diagnosis and to exclude others in several situations. If the attacks are uncontrolled despite rigorous treatment and if the diagnosis of a seizure disorder has never been supported by EEG or other tests, review and repeat testing are indicated. Drug-seeking behavior, dramatic presentations with multiple attacks in public, and repeated visits to the emergency room should also invite skepticism. Common disorders such as migraine, panic attacks, and sleep apnea can develop in addition to a seizure disorder. Additional differential diagnoses are included in Table 5.2.

Management

The main principle of seizure management is to prevent the recurrence of seizures with anticonvulsant medications while avoiding adverse effects from the drugs. The clinician should refer the patient to a neurologist, who should make the decision to start treatment after a complete review of the risk of further seizures is discussed with the patient. Some structural lesions are clearly associated with recurrent seizures. These include brain tumor and arteriovenous malformation (AVM). When these conditions are diagnosed after a single seizure, there should be no hesitation in

Table 5.2 **Differential Diagnosis: Seizure Disorder**

Diseases/Disorders	Possible Causes
Cerebrovascular disorders	TIAs (carotid artery, vertebrobasilar), CVA (paramedian thalamic nuclei, fusiform gyrus, right parietal lobe), Moya moya disease
Diencephalic and brainstem disorders	Decorticate and decerebrate posturing, diencephalic attacks, nonepileptic paroxysmal laughter, peduncular hallucinosis, Kleine-Levin syndrome
Headaches	Classic migraine (with aura), basilar artery migraine, cluster headache, chronic paroxysmal hemicrania, ice-pick headache, trigeminal neuralgia
Infant and pediatric disorders	Jitteriness, shuddering, esophageal reflux (Sandifer's syndrome), breath-holding attacks, alternating hemiplegia
Miscellaneous disorders	Idiopathic drop attacks of older adults, transient global amnesia, flumazenil-responsive recurring stupor, paroxysmal attacks in MS
Movement disorders	Habit spasm, tic, paroxysmal kinesogenic choreoathetosis, paroxysmal dystonia, paroxysmal ataxia, tremor, chorea, segmental dystonia
Nonepileptic myoclonus	Hypnic jerks, myoclonus (spinal, reticular, palatal, essential), myoclonus and asterixis in toxic-metabolic states
Psychiatric disorders	Psychogenic seizures, depersonalization, psychogenic amnesia, psychogenic fugue, panic attacks, hyperventilation anxiety attacks, intermittent explosive disorder (episodic dyscontrol), schizophrenia
Sleep disorders	Pavor nocturnus, jactatio capitis nocturna, confusional arousals, somnambulism, periodic leg movements of sleep (PLMS) or nocturnal myoclonus, sleep apnea syndrome, narcolepsy, other hypersomnias, rapid eye movement (REM) behavior disorder
Startle disorders	Startle reaction, startle disease (hyperekplexia), jumping Frenchman, Malay latah, etc.
Syncope disorders	Vasovagal syncope, convulsive syncope, cardiac syncope (Stokes-Adams attack, tachyarrhythmias, prolonged QT syndrome, aortic stenosis, hypertrophic cardiomyopathy), orthostatic syncope (idiopathic orthostatic hypotension, Shy-Drager syndrome, autonomic neuropathy), deliberate syncope ("fainting lark"), syncope in specific situations (micturition syncope, tussive syncope, carotid sinus hypersensitivity, glossopharyngeal neuralgia)
Toxic-metabolic or infectious disorders	Alcoholic blackouts, hallucinogens (LSD, mescaline), strychnine and camphor poisoning, tetanus, rabies, hypoglycemia, porphyria, pheochromocytoma, carcinoid syndrome, mastocytosis

Source: Adapted from So, N, and Andermor, F: Differential diagnosis. In Engel, J, and Pedley, T (eds): Epilepsy: A Comprehensive Textbook. Lippincott-Raven, Philadelphia, 1998.

initiating pharmacologic treatment; however, a much more common situation is the one in which the initial evaluation fails to reveal a specific causative factor for the seizure. Then the neurologist must carefully evaluate the risk of subsequent seizures.

Some patients have only one seizure. For these patients, the probability of a second seizure is less than 10 percent in the first year following the seizure and approximately 24 percent by the end of 2 years after the first seizure. The impact of a second seizure depends on the patient's lifestyle. Treatment may be indicated for patients who need to be able to drive or for those who face significant risk of injury or loss of self-esteem from a second seizure. The risk of recurrence is greatest in the first 2 years, so if treatment is initiated, it probably can be halted after this highest risk period passes.

If the decision to treat is made, accurate identification of the seizure type is very helpful in choosing the drug for the best outcome. Drugs Commonly Prescribed 5.1 presents suggested medications based on the different types of seizures. While only the first-line medications are listed, there are many drugs given in combination with these medications. These are not included here because a patient will initially be prescribed medications by the neurologist. Some neurologists choose to begin long-term therapy with anticonvulsant medications after a single seizure in the following situations: if the single seizure is rapidly followed by a second seizure; if an MRI or EEG shows evidence of a structural lesion such as a brain tumor, arteriovenous malformation, or infection; if there is a history of a seizure disorder in a sibling; or if there is a history of a brain injury or stroke.

Once the appropriate drug has been chosen based on the seizure type, serum levels should be assessed for baseline hematologic and hepatic parameters. Blood levels should be checked two to three times in the first 6 months of

Drugs Commonly Prescribed 5.1: Seizures

Type of Seizure	Drug	Adult Daily Dose	Doses per Day	Comments/Selected Adverse Effects
Absence seizures (petit mal) and myoclonic seizures	Valproic acid (Depakene)	1500–2000 mg	In three divided doses	Optimum drug level is 50–100 mcg/ml.
	Divalproex sodium (Depakote)	15 mg/kg per day		Take with food. Max: 60 mg/kg per day. Headache, unsteadiness, blood dyscrasias, urticaria may occur.
	Clonazepam (Klonopin)	0.04–0.2 mg/kg; also comes in wafers	In two divided doses	Optimum drug level is 20–80 mg/ml Potentiates CNS depression with alcohol.
Partial or generalized seizures	Phenytoin (Dilantin)	200–400 mg	Once	Optimum drug level is 10–20 ng/ml. Ataxia, blood dyscrasias, peripheral neuropathy
	Carbamazepine (Tegretol)	600–1200 mg	bid	Dysarthria, ataxia; may exacerbate myoclonic seizures.
	Valproic acid	See above.		
	Phenobarbital (Luminal)			
	Primidone (Mysoline)	750–1500 mg	tid	Sedation, nystagmus, irritability, megaloblastic anemia
Partial seizures	Oxcarbazepine (Trileptal)	Initially 600 mg/day; increase by 300 mg every third day to 1.2 g/day.	bid	Potentiates CNS depression with alcohol. Potentiates action of phenobarbital and phenytoin, ataxia, fatigue, GI upset

Several adjunctive meds are available. The drugs listed above are for first-line therapy.

therapy to determine if target levels have been attained and are being maintained.

Follow-Up and Referral

If the seizures are controlled and blood levels are adequate, the clinician can monitor them every 6 months (twice each year) for the duration of treatment. If the seizures are not controlled with adequate doses and levels of the medication, the clinincian should refer the patient to a neurologist for a second opinion and possible combination therapy.

Patient Education

Education about seizure disorders can provide the patient with an understanding and a sense of control over the illness. It is necessary to recognize that to the affected individual, this condition is more than seizures. The impact of the condition comprises many facets, which are different for each individual, that contribute to disability and impaired quality of life. For example, such factors as age at onset, duration of seizure activity, frequency, seizure type, associated neurologic abnormalities, and associated environmental factors contribute to the degree of disability in each patient. Education is ongoing and should be constantly reinforced. Patients and their families should be referred to seizure literature available through the Epilepsy Foundation of America as soon as they are diagnosed, because the well-informed patient is the best advocate for his or her own care. Using the Circle of Caring Model and coming to know the patient and what matters most to him or her will assist in helping the patient reach his or her highest potential.

A patient with a seizure disorder lives with a constant fear that a seizure may strike at any moment. Persons with a seizure disorder fear dying during a seizure. They also fear personal injury. This fear is justified; therefore, health-care providers need to counsel patients regarding common sense safety issues. Persons with a seizure disorder should take showers instead of baths and only when someone else is home. Automatic safety devices that adjust water temperature and shut off water when the shower drain is blocked can be installed. Persons with a seizure disorder

Table 5.3 Seizure First Aid

Partial Seizures

The patient may resemble an intoxicated or drugged person. He or she may stare without focusing or speaking, appear to be fidgeting, make chewing movements, or smack the lips.

During the seizure:

- Do not attempt to restrain the patient.
- Gently move the patient away from dangerous objects.

After the seizure:

- Stay with the patient until the patient is fully alert.
- Reassure others that the behavior was medically caused.

Generalized Seizures

The patient may have a warning sign, cry out or scream, then fall down and rhythmically jerk arms and legs in a strong movement that cannot be stopped.

Before or during the seizure:

- Remove the patient's glasses (if wearing) and help the patient lie down in a prone position, but do not restrain.
- Clear the area of dangerous objects.
- Loosen tight clothing around the patient's neck.
- Do not force any object into the patient's mouth.

After the seizure:

- Turn the patient to one side to allow the patient's mouth to drain.
- Stay with the patient until he or she is fully awake.
- If the patient has a known seizure disorder, it is not necessary to call for medical help unless an injury has occurred, the seizure lasts longer than three minutes, a second seizure occurs, or the patient requests help.

should use an occupied sign on the bathroom door rather than locking it. They should swim only with a buddy who is aware of their diagnosis and knows what to do if a seizure occurs while the individual is swimming. When cooking, patients should be instructed to use the microwave or back burners on the stove and keep pot handles turned inward. They should be encouraged not to smoke, but if they must, they should never smoke when alone. Their home should be evaluated to identify any safety hazards and to develop a risk-reduction plan. Families, friends, and co-workers need to know what to do in case of a seizure and should be taught "seizure first aid" (Table 5.3).

Patients with a seizure disorder and their caregivers should be apprised of the risks of harm. In comparison with the general population, children and adolescents with seizure disorders have a 1000-fold greater risk of drowning during bathing and a 70-fold greater risk of drowning while swimming. Burns tend to occur in the home and are most commonly associated with cooking, showering, and use of space heaters. Driving needs to be discussed at length. The loss of driving privilege is very serious because it restricts a patient's mobility and, therefore, independence. Each state has different laws governing the granting of driver's licenses for individuals with a seizure disorder. At the federal level, the U.S. Department of Transportation (DOT) has regulations that bar anyone with a history of seizures from being licensed to drive in interstate trucking. The purpose of the driving restrictions is obvious—to protect the public. Although only six states require health-care providers to report patients who have been diagnosed with seizure disorder, all practitioners have the responsibility to advise their patients of the medical risks, legal requirements, and recommendations regarding driving. Educational and support materials are available through the Epilepsy Foundation of America.

Degenerative Disorders

Multiple Sclerosis

Multiple sclerosis (MS) is a chronic, potentially disabling, and demyelinating disease of the CNS that begins most commonly in young adulthood and is associated with periods of relapse and remission. MS is the most common cause of disability in young adults. Multiple areas of CNS or white matter inflammation, demyelination, and glial scarring or gliosis characterize MS.

There are four types of MS, each with its own course and progression. The *relapsing–remitting* type of MS is characterized by acute attacks, with either a full recovery or some residual deficits between episodes. The *primary progressive* type of MS has a steady disease progression of, with possibly some plateaus and remissions. *Secondary progressive* MS is a combination of the first two types, beginning as a relapsing–remitting disease but then slowly acquiring the primary progressive characteristics. The *progressive–relapsing* type of MS is a progression of the disease (including relapses and remissions, with or without recovery) on a steady downhill course, as compared to the relapsing–remitting variety, in which the disease progression may stop at any point.

The clinical course of MS varies. Prognosis is a common concern. Although there are no definitive prognostic indicators, the following are general guidelines. Good prognostic indicators include minimal disability after 5 years of onset, complete and rapid remission of initial symptoms, onset at age 35 or younger, only one symptom during first year, acute onset of the first symptoms, brief duration of most recent exacerbation, long first remission, optic neuritis, or sensory symptoms. Poor prognostic indicators include late onset, chronic progressive course, motor symptoms, polysymptomatic onset, and vertigo. Patients are concerned about disability. After 15 years, 50 to 60 percent of patients with MS remain ambulatory, 10 to 20 percent need assistance devices to ambulate, and 15 to 30 percent are bedridden.

Epidemiology and Causes

MS occurs worldwide, but there are differences in both incidence and prevalence on the basis of race, sex, genetics, geographic location, and age at the time of environmental exposure to a virus or other infectious agent. Onset of MS peaks between ages 20 and 30. It is rarely seen before age 10 or after age 60. The disease affects two to three times more women than men. The geographic distribution is on a nonrandom, north to south gradient. The disease increases in frequency with latitude in both Northern and Southern hemispheres, and the rates tend to decrease at about 65 degrees north or south of the equator. Epidemiologic studies have focused on prevalence of the disease. Areas with a prevalence rate of 30 per 100,000 population are considered high-risk areas for MS. Low-prevalence areas have fewer than 5 cases per 100,000 population. Some of the geographical distribution may be explained by racial differences. White populations are at the greatest risk and Asian and black populations are at lower risk.

Environmental factors may also play a role in pathogenesis. Studies suggest that age during time of immigration to another latitude may play a role. Studies have suggested that individuals who immigrate before age 15 tend to be subject to the risk level of the new (adopted) country, whereas individuals who immigrate after age 15 years tend to retain the risk level associated with the country of origin.

Some epidemiologic findings suggest a relationship between MS and an unknown environmental factor, possibly a viral exposure during childhood. This exposure may lead to the entry of immune cells into the CNS, where a population of T cells becomes sensitized to a CNS antigen. After years of latency, an environmental trigger may lead to an upregulation of circulating mediators or T-cell activation that may set off an episode of demyelination and clinical disease.

The cause of MS is unknown. There are many theories on possible causes, including genetic susceptibility, autoimmune mechanisms, viral infections, and environmental factors. One leading hypothesis is that of a cell-mediated immunopathologic response directed against myelin in genetically predisposed persons.

Studies have suggested that susceptibility to MS is inherited. The higher incidence in twins and in certain families provides support for this genetic susceptibility. The major histocompatibility complex on chromosome 6 has been identified as one genetic determinant for MS. Although genetic factors may contribute to an individual's susceptibility, they are neither sufficient nor necessary for development of MS. Clinical expression of the disease is likely to require additional exposure to one or more environmental factors, which are as yet undefined.

There is evidence of autoimmune mechanisms in the pathogenesis of MS. In a normal immune response, foreign antibodies are processed and presented to T-cell helpers by antigen-presenting cells and macrophages. These T-helper cells recognize foreign peptides bound to major histocompatibility complex (MHC) molecules, become activated, and release various cytokines, tumor necrosis factor (TNF), and interleukins that augment the immune response to a particular antigen. These particular class II MCH molecules are usually found only on cells involved in an immune response. In MS, class II MHC induction has been shown to occur in CNS tissue. In peripheral blood of patients with MS, several nonspecific changes are seen that are similar to those in other autoimmune diseases. Suppressor T-lymphocytes are decreased in both function and number. Excessive immunoglobulin is present, especially high levels of IgG. Suppressor cell inducers are decreased in many patients with progressive disease.

Pathophysiology

Multiple sclerosis (MS) is a disease of the central nervous system (CNS) stemming from the progressive patchy demyelination of axons. In MS, local immune reactions destroy CNS myelin and cause the death of oligodendrocytes. Astrocytes react to these injuries by proliferating. At the same time, many of the axons remain intact.

MS is characterized by neurologic problems that periodically flare up and then abate. The symptoms reflect repeated episodes of demyelination in new parts of the white matter throughout the CNS. The specific neurologic deficits of an MS patient depend on the regions of the CNS that have been affected. For example, lesions in the optic nerve produce blindness, lesions in the corticospinal tracts produce weakness or paralysis, lesions in the posterior columns produce unusual sensations or numbness, lesions in the medial longitudinal fasciculus produce double vision, and lesions in the vestibular pathways produce dizziness.

Areas of MS damage form sharply defined plaques, which are typically found around venules. MS plaques tend to be large (greater than 6 mm diameter) and oval-shaped, and over time, the plaques become more and more widely distributed. Newly forming plaques, in which demyelination is not yet complete, are filled with lymphocytes, plasma cells, and macrophages. Older plaques have no myelin in their centers and contain only fibrous astrocytes and unmyelinated axons. Axon damage inevitably follows, but this appears to be a secondary phenomenon and occurs slowly. Between the plaques, myelin is also affected, although here the damage is not as dramatic.

MS plaques are the result of immune reactions, and the state of the disease is reflected in the immune indicators in the cerebrospinal fluid (CSF). When the disease flares up, the CSF has an increased number of lymphocytes (although usually less than 50/μL). The CSF will also contain elevated levels of immunoglobulins, the majority of which are IgGs. As MS progresses, specific oligoclonal bands are found in the CSF, regardless of the current state of the disease symptoms.

It is likely that MS is an autoimmune disease, but the triggers for the immune destruction of myelin are unclear. Evidence suggests that genetically susceptible individuals develop the disease many years after exposure to certain environmental factors. One hypothesis is that these factors are viruses that happen to consist of molecules with shapes similar to regions of certain myelin molecules. Alternatively, the initial trigger may be a less specific infection that causes leakage in the blood–brain barrier and thus sensitizes peripheral lymphocytes to normal but previously unseen CNS myelin antigens.

Clinical Presentation

Subjective

The most common presenting symptoms in MS include sensory disturbances of the extremities, spasticity and weakness of legs, bladder and bowel dysfunction, ataxic gait, paresthesias in the extremities, fatigue, optic neuritis, and trigeminal neuralgia. Exacerbations and remissions occur frequently and signs and symptoms may indicate more than one lesion. The clinical course is variable and usually occurs in two phases, relapsing–remitting and chronic progressive. In the early phase the patient presents with symptoms that may last from days to months and may disappear abruptly. The patient most often presents with the same chief complaint during the exacerbation, but some of the events will involve new symptoms. After several years, many patients enter the chronic progressive phase of MS, with a mean time from onset of the initial symptom to this phase from 6 to 7 years. In approximately 20 percent of patients the disease begins in this phase and 50 percent of patients enter the phase within 10 years.

Objective

Clinical manifestations of MS may be transient. The patient may experience unusual sensations and have difficulty describing these. Signs and symptoms may be diverse and appear to include all the symptoms that can occur from injury to any part of the spinal cord and cerebral cortex. Symptoms tend to vary in nature and severity. Frequently, complete remission of the first symptoms occurs, but with subsequent attacks, remissions are incomplete or do not occur. The clinical manifestations depend on the areas of the CNS involved. The brain stem, spinal cord, optic chiasm, and cerebellum are commonly involved.

The clinician should assess the patient for common visual symptoms, including diplopia, blurred vision, diminution or loss of visual acuity unilaterally or bilaterally, and visual field defects. These symptoms may begin to manifest over a period of hours to days. Involvement of the fifth cranial nerve causes pain sensation impairment and diminished or lost corneal reflex. The diagnosis of MS should be considered whenever a young adult develops trigeminal neuralgia.

Limb weakness is a common sign of MS, presenting as monoparesis, hemiparesis, or tetraparesis. Fatigability out of proportion to muscle weakness is common. Fatigue may be persistent, easy fatigability related to physical activity or mental exertion. Fatigue interferes with ADLs in 75 percent of patients with MS. There may be concomitant ataxia and spasticity. Cerebellar involvement causes dysarthria, scanning speech, tremor, gait ataxia, and incoordination of limbs and trunk. Spasticity limits activities and leg stiffness may interfere with walking or transferring. In patients with severe spasticity, there may be extensor or flexor spasms either spontaneously or on attempted movement. Spasticity may cause pain, interfere with sleep, or prevent movement.

Bladder symptoms are common, including incontinence and frequency or urgency. Patients may have small capacity, spastic bladder or a large flaccid bladder with overflow incontinence. Loss of libido and erectile dysfunction are common in men with MS; in women with MS, sexual dysfunction most commonly involves lack of lubrication and failure to reach orgasm. Although bowel symptoms are uncommon, constipation may occur.

Sensory impairment and paresthesias are common. Patients may complain of tingling or numbness in the face, limbs, or trunk. A sensation of "electricity" down the back after passive or active neck flexion is called Lhermitte's sign and is indicative of a lesion in the posterior column in the cervical spinal cord. Pain is also recognized as a symptom of MS. Pain may be associated with trigeminal neuralgia, flexor–extensor spasms, tonic spasms of the limbs, and local pain syndromes such as constricting pain around a limb, burning pain, pseudoradicular pain, foreign body sensation, headache, neuralgic pain, and pain caused by pressure sores.

Patients may experience depression, euphoria, subtle aphasic manifestations, or cognitive changes. Patients may have difficulty with tasks that require processing new information rapidly, recalling newly acquired knowledge, and problem solving. Attention deficits may be present early in MS, even before the onset of physical symptoms. In general, the longer the history of MS, the greater the attention impairment. Memory and abstract reasoning may be affected, as well as the capacity to direct attention (CDA). CDA is critical to the management of a chronic illness, and a strong CDA is necessary to learn new information, implement therapeutic self-care, and handle necessary and difficult adjustments in daily life. This problem may be a result of demyelination.

Diagnostic Reasoning

Diagnostic Tests

There is no specific test for MS. The diagnosis must be based on multiple signs and symptoms with a history of remissions and exacerbations. The diagnosis is also based on the ability to demonstrate, on the basis of patient history, neurologic examination, and diagnostic tests, the existence of lesions involving different parts of the CNS. An initial clinical neurologic examination focused on the patient's signs and symptoms is necessary. Tests should be done to assess for increased muscle tone in legs, decreased motor strength, changes in visual acuity, bilateral clonus of ankles and knees, positive Babinski's sign, and a decreased appreciation of vibration or position sense in arms and legs. There are several instruments available to assess functional status. An MMSE may be administered to screen for global and focal cognitive impairment.

For a diagnosis of MS to be made, two or more parts of the CNS must be involved and signs of MS must consist predominantly of dysfunction of the optic nerve (affecting vision) or dysfunction of the corticobulbar system (affecting speech, swallowing), the corticospinal system (affecting strength), the cerebellar system (affecting gait, coordination), the medial longitudinal fasciculus system (affecting internuclear ophthalmoplegia [INO], with diplopia and nystagmus), the spinocerebellar system (affecting balance), and the long-tract sensory system (causing position and vibratory disturbances). In addition, CNS involvement must occur in one of the following patterns: two or more episodes of exacerbations, separated by 1 month or longer and lasting more than 24 hours, with subsequent recovery (i.e., relapsing–remitting MS); a slow or stepwise progression of signs and symptoms over a period of at least 6 months (i.e., primary progressive MS); a clinical history of clearly defined exacerbations and remissions, with or without complete recovery, followed by a slow progression of signs and symptoms over a period of at least 6 months (i.e., secondary progressive MS); progression in signs and symptoms and occasional attacks (i.e., progressive relapsing MS); or no relapse or progression of attacks in the past 18 months (i.e., stable MS).

A lumbar puncture with an evaluation of CSF for the presence of immunoglobulins, lymphocytes, and oligoclonal IgG bands may provide supportive data for a diagnosis of MS. Immunoglobulin synthesis within the CSF can be expressed by formulas that adjust for passive transfer of proteins across a damaged blood–brain barrier. Oligoclonal IgG bands can be detected by electrophoresis of CSF and are present in the CSF of 90 percent of patients with MS, but this finding is not specific to MS. An increase in CSF basic myelin protein may confirm that an acute MS exacerbation has occurred. Elevated values (>9 ng/mL) suggest demyelination.

Cortical-evoked responses or evoked potentials are of value in demonstrating clinically unsuspected lesions. Visual responses are abnormal in 75 to 97 percent of patients with MS. Somatosensory responses are abnormal in 72 to 87 percent and brain stem responses are abnormal in 50 to 70 percent of patients with MS.

MRI is a sensitive, objective measure of plaques and is used to measure the outcomes of treatment. Periodic recording of the volume and number of lesions detected in the brain by MRI can assist the clinician in monitoring the extent of the disease. Pathologically, areas of contrast enhancement observed by MRI correlate with active perivascular inflammatory damage.

The advent of some technologies such as MRI has added the ability to document lesions to support the diagnosis of MS. A clinically definitive diagnosis of MS requires either (1) evidence from history of two episodes at least 1 month apart, signs of one lesion on examination, and evidence from evoked responses or MRI of other lesions or (2) evidence from both history and neurologic examination of more than one lesion. A laboratory-supported definitive diagnosis of MS requires evidence from two lesions in either history or neurologic examination. If only one lesion is evident on examination or history, at least one more lesion must be evident in MRI or evoked response testing. The CSF IgG pattern and content should also be abnormal. A clinically probable diagnosis of MS requires that either history or examination, but not both, provides evidence of more than one lesion. If only one lesion is evident by history or neurologic examination, MRI or evoked responses may provide evidence of additional lesions. If the collaborating physician is uncertain of the MS diagnosis, reevaluation of the patient may be performed.

Differential Diagnosis

Other CNS diseases may resemble MS clinically or radiologically. These are lymphomas and gliomas of the hemispheres, spinal cord, and brain stem; collagen vascular disease such as systemic lupus erythematosus (SLE); human T-cell lymphotrophic virus type I (HTLV-I); HIV infection; encephalopathy; Lyme disease; peripheral neuropathy; Behçet's disease; and sarcoidosis.

It is important to consider Lyme disease as a differential diagnosis because chronic CNS infection with *Borrelia burgdorferi* can cause spastic paraparesis, cerebellar signs, and cranial nerve palsies. Patients with Lyme disease will have a history of erythema migrans plus arthralgias or evidence of cardiac manifestations, as well as positive Lyme titers.

Patients with systemic lupus erythematosus (SLE) will have a positive antinuclear antibody (ANA) and anti-DNA antibody titers as well as joint or renal involvement.

Patients with suspected MS should be tested for HIV, HTLV-I, and syphilis (human T-cell lymphoma virus) because these diseases may mimic MS. Vascular disease, tumors of the brain and spinal cord, arteriovenous malformations, and arachnoid cysts may have relapsing and remitting signs that mimic MS. MRI is usually the definitive test to rule out these causes.

Management

The principles of management include three major goals: to delay the progression of the disease, manage chronic symptoms, and treat acute exacerbations. There is no known cure for MS. Therapeutic regimens are either disease specific or symptomatic (immunosuppressive or immunomodulatory). Disease-modifying therapy should be considered early in the course of treatment, before neurologic deficits have persisted for more than 6 months. Treatment decisions on individual patients should be made based on both the probability of severely disabling disease and the course of disease. Follow-up should be based on progression of disease, and the treatment of symptoms and exacerbations. Patients with benign or very slowly progressing disease do not need disease-specific treatment.

Drugs commonly prescribed for the management of MS are described in Drugs Commonly Prescribed 5.2.

Corticosteroids are the mainstay of treatment for acute exacerbations. Corticosteroids have both immunomodulatory and anti-inflammatory effects, which restore the blood–brain barrier, decrease edema, and may improve axonal conduction. If symptoms of an exacerbation are severe enough to require treatment, methylprednisolone (Depo-Medrol) IV followed by an oral taper is given.

The treatment of choice for patients with relapsing–remitting MS is interferon beta. This cytokine halts disease progression and inhibits the accumulation of inflammatory lesions in the CNS white matter as evidenced by MRI; it also reduces the number and severity of clinical relapses.

Physicians who prescribe these medications initially must be thoroughly familiar with dosage, possible adverse effects, and management of those adverse effects. Patients must be taught the adverse effects, injection techniques, storage, and care of the medications. Once appropriate drug therapy has been stabilized, the clinician may monitor the patient as described under Follow-Up and Referral later.

Two types of antibodies occur in patients treated with interferons: binding antibodies and neutralizing antibodies (NAbs). Binding antibodies develop at some time in 97 percent of treated patients and are measured by enzyme-linked immunosorbent assays (ELISA) or the Western blot technique. Many of these antibodies do not impair therapeutic effectiveness and have no known function. NAbs are formed in a minority of treated patients but are capable of reducing or abrogating the normal biologic treatment effects of interferons. They are measured by a viral cytopathic effect reduction assay. There is no evidence that NAb-positive patients fare significantly worse than placebo-treated patients.

Symptomatic management and therapy are important in MS. Spasticity is a major cause of disability in 55 percent of patients with MS. Antispasmodics are listed in Drugs Commonly Prescribed 5.2. If other noninvasive therapeutic measures for spasticity have failed, the patient may be referred to a neurosurgeon for evaluation as a candidate for an implantable drug infusion pump to administer baclofen (Lioresal) intrathecally. This is highly effective because the drug can cross the blood–brain barrier. Adverse effects are minimal, and a test dose is administered intrathecally before implantation as part of the screening process for candidates.

Selective chemodenervation may be beneficial for localized spasticity in a single muscle or limb. This may be accomplished through administration of botulin (*Clostridium botulinum*) toxin type A (Botox). Only a specialist familiar with the use, adverse effects, and injection sites for botulinim toxin should administer this medication.

The tremors associated with MS are usually cerebellar outflow tremors. Medications recommended for the treatment of tremor are included in Drugs Commonly Prescribed 5.2.

Fatigue is a common problem in patients with MS. The existence of sleep apnea, pain, spasms, restless leg syndrome, ability to sleep, and pattern of sleep should all be investigated. Other medical problems that may cause fatigue should be excluded. Patients should be instructed to take a daytime nap and remain in a cool environment, and should be educated in energy conservation techniques. A referral for occupational therapy may be beneficial for this.

Many patients with MS experience pain in the form of unpleasant sensations or overt pain. This pain can assume many forms and the cause of new pain should be established. Acute pain includes trigeminal neuralgia, Lhermitte's sign, paroxysmal burning, extremity pain, and painful tonic spasms. Acute pain may be treated with carbamazepine (Tegretol) or phenytoin (Dilantin). Chronic pain includes dysesthetic pain in extremities, chronic back pain, and painful leg spasms. Amitriptyline (Elavil), carbamazepine, and phenytoin may be given for chronic pain.

Providers should be aware of issues relating to complementary therapies that may be raised by patients with MS. These therapies have become so widely used that the National Institutes of Health (NIH) has established an Office of Alternative Medicine. The following are frequently used complementary therapies for patients with MS: acupuncture, hypnotherapy and imagery, massage, biofeedback, tai chi, and chiropractic therapy. If referring a patient with MS to complementary therapy providers, it is important to list those who have an understanding of MS.

Follow-Up and Referral

Follow-up and referral should occur soon after diagnosis and should be repeated initially at monthly intervals or more

Drugs Commonly Prescribed 5.2: Multiple Sclerosis (MS)

Drug	Indication	Dosage (Adult)	Comments
Methylprednisolone (Depo-Medrol)	Exacerbation	1 g IV daily for 7–10 days, then taper (see under prednisolone)	Masks infection. Adverse effects: glaucoma, cataracts, secondary infections, hypokalemia, hypocalcemia, hypernatremia, hypertension, psychotic disorders, myopathy, osteoporosis, peptic ulcer, dermal atrophy, increased intracranial pressure, carbohydrate intolerance.
Prednisolone (Deltasone)	Taper after IV therapy	80 mg qid for 4 days; then 60 mg qid for 4 days; then 40 mg qid for 4 days; then 20 mg qid for 4 days; then 10 mg qid for 4 days; then 5 mg qid for 4 days; then 5 mg every other day for 4 doses	As above.
Interferon beta, Interferon 1a (Avonex)	Relapsing–remitting MS	30 mcg IM once weekly self-injection	Adverse effects: flulike symptoms for 24–48 hours after injection (subsides after 2–3 months); treat with acetaminophen or nonsteroidal anti-inflammatory drugs (NSAIDs).
Interferon 1b (Betaseron)	Relapsing–remitting MS	8 million units SC every other day	As above.
Azathioprine (Imuran)	Depression of cell-mediated and humoral immunity	1–2 mg/kg per day	May reduce rate of relapse; has no effect on progression of disability.
Glatiramer acetate (Copaxone)	Relapsing–remitting MS resistance to interferon beta neutralizing antibodies	20 mg SC daily	Adverse effects; reaction at injection site, flushing, sweating, shortness of breath, palpitations, chest tightness, anxiety.
Methotrexate (Rheumatrex)	Progressive MS	7.5 mg PO every week	Do not give in chronic liver disease, pregnancy or nursing women, or in the presence of blood dyscrasias.
Baclofen (Lioresal)	Symptomatic treatment for spasticity	Initial dose: 5 mg bid with 5 mg increases every 5 days; once 10 mg is reached, it may be given qid; may be increased to 80 mg total daily dose; then 100–200 mg daily	May cause drowsiness and confusion.
Tizandine (Zanaflex)	Spasticity	4 mg PO hs; titrate gradually to a maximum of 12 mg tid	May cause drowsiness. Do not use with clonidine (Catapres).
Dantrolene (Dantrium)	Spasticity	25 mg qd; maximum dose: 100 mg qd	Use with caution in patients with impaired hepatic, pulmonary, or cardiac function.
Diazepam (Valium)	Spasticity	2–10 mg three to four times daily	Contraindicated with acute narrow-angle glaucoma; potential for abuse.
Carbamazepine (Tegretol)	Tremors	400–600 mg tid	Take with food; use with caution in patients with history of cardiac, hepatic, renal, or hematopoietic dysfunction.

(continued)

Drugs Commonly Prescribed 5.2: Multiple Sclerosis (MS) (continued)

Drug	Indication	Dosage (Adult)	Comments
Clonazepam (Klonopin)	Tremors	0.5 mg bid–tid	Contraindicated with liver disease or acute narrow-angle glaucoma; withdraw gradually; potential for abuse.
Primidone (Mysoline)	Tremors	125–250 mg bid–tid	Potentiated with alcohol and other CNS depressants; antagonizes oral anticoagulants, contraceptives, and steroids.

often as symptoms appear, to assess level of functioning, effectiveness of medications, and make dosage adjustments if needed. The patient should be instructed to contact the clinician immediately for the appearance of symptoms, which may signal an exacerbation. Referral to a neurosurgeon may be necessary for extreme spasticity.

Patient Education

Patients should be educated in all aspects of the disease, medications, adverse effects, complications, progression, fatigue management, pain management, diet, and exercise. The weakness that results from MS may be amenable to strengthening exercises. ROM exercise is important to prevent contractures and joint restriction. Referral to a physical therapist who has experience in the treatment of patients with MS may be beneficial. Regular exercise may change the course of the patient's response to illness by minimizing the deconditioning process and maintaining optimal levels of physical activities and functioning. The beneficial effects of prolonged activity are well documented; it can help prevent muscular atrophy and weakness, fatigue, loss of flexibility, cardiovascular deficits, depression, and sleep disturbances. It is important to balance activity and exercise to prevent fatigue. There is no conclusive scientific evidence that any diet or nutritional therapy affects the course of MS. Many of the diets available are not harmful but may be tiring because of the attention to detail required, while offering no benefit. A generally well-balanced diet is recommended.

Patients who have been diagnosed with MS may experience a wide range of emotions ranging from euphoria to depression, including helplessness, lack of hope, mental confusion, stress, and anxiety. These emotions can affect marital relationships and increase child-rearing stress. The chronic nature of MS and the inability to predict level of dysfunction contribute to difficulty in coping with chronic illness and symptoms disruptive to daily living. Patients may also experience lack of employment, embarrassment, exhaustion, and the feeling of making no contribution to society. It is important to teach patients health promotion behaviors to emphasize emotional and social well-being.

Patients and families should also be educated in coping with possible behavior changes and mood swings. Patients with MS have reported feelings of hopelessness, loss of control, conflict, fear, loss, and uncertainty. Education in the management of problems related to sexual dysfunction may also need to be addressed. Caregivers should be educated not to neglect their own health, because coping with a chronic illness may change and stress the dynamics both within a family and within other individual relationships.

Parkinson's Disease

Parkinson's disease (PD) is a chronic, progressive, degenerative disorder of the basal ganglia in the CNS. The disease usually begins insidiously and eventually leads to disability. PD is the second most common neurodegenerative disorder in the elderly after AD. Affecting 1 percent of the population older than age 65, there are approximately 1 million people in the United States suffering from Parkingson's disease with 60,000 new cases diagnosed each year. It affects people in middle to later life, with the mean age at onset of age 57. The incidence is slightly greater in men, with a 3:2 ratio of men to women. People in all ethnic groups, all countries, and all socioeconomic classes are affected.

A *parkinsonian syndrome* (parkinsonism) is any disorder that manifests the symptoms of PD. Parkinsonism is divided into four categories: idiopathic, symptomatic, Parkinson-plus syndromes, and other heredodegenerative diseases in which parkinsonism is a manifestation. Patients with idiopathic Parkinson's disease (IP) make up the largest subgroup, which represents 78 percent of the affected population. Symptomatic and Parkinson-plus syndromes are often referred to as secondary parkinsonism when there is a known cause for the disorder such as cerebrovascular disease, drugs, infections, trauma, or exposure to toxins. Parkinsonian syndromes include heredodegenerative disorders such as Huntington's disease and other acquired degenerative diseases.

Epidemiology and Causes

The cause of PD is unknown. The pathogenesis is thought to be multifactorial, resulting from a combination of genetic

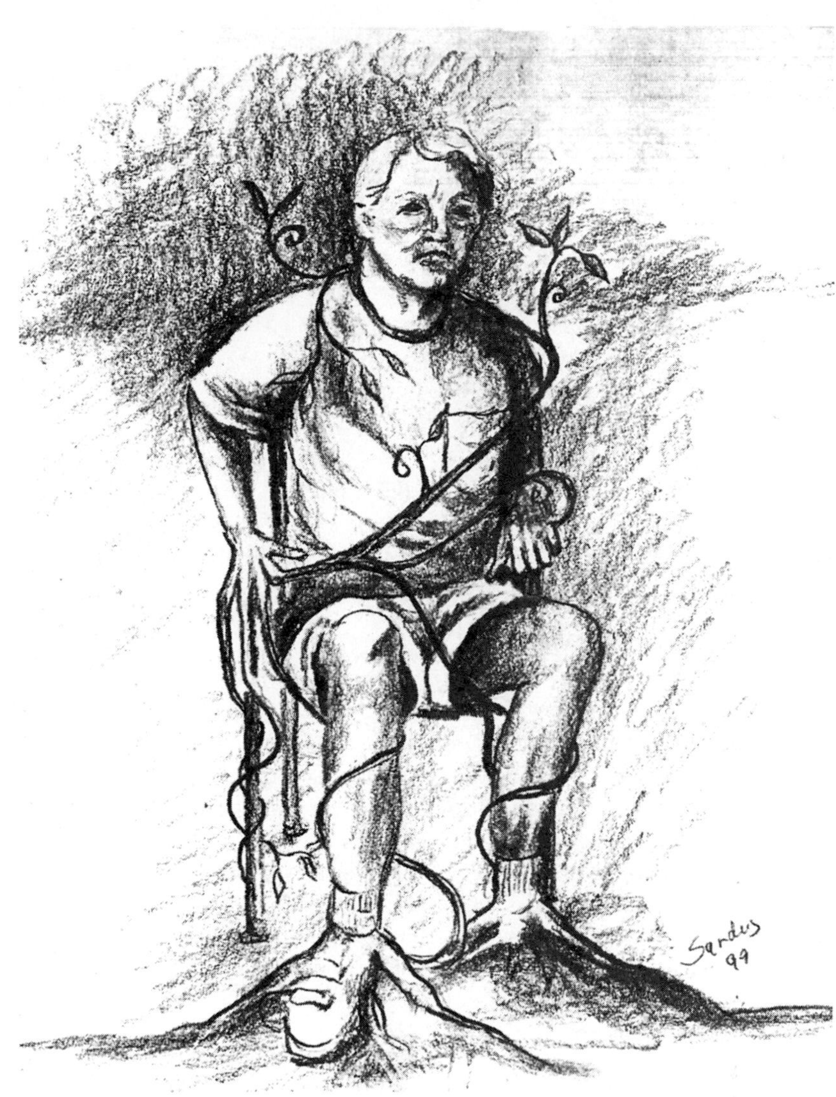

One man's depiction of being a victim of Parkinson's disease. (Illustration by Christine Sanders.)

predisposition, exogenous toxins, and endogenous toxins. The evidence regarding the role of heredity is conflicting. A positive family history is reported in approximately 15 percent of cases. It has also been reported that a higher prevalence of familial PD is revealed when an informative history is obtained.

There are many theories regarding the role of environmental factors in the development of PD. One theory has suggested increased vulnerability of "old" (i.e., aging) neurons to environmental toxins. There are also theories that have identified the following factors in the development of PD: drug-induced parkinsonism (antipsychotics, lithium), rural living, infections, exposure to heavy metals, and free radical–oxidative stress. Oxidative mechanisms are believed to be important in the pathogenesis of PD. In a normal individual, oxidative stress is balanced by antioxidative protective mechanisms naturally occurring in the brain. In patients with PD, the balance is thought to be tilted toward the oxidative stress side. Other influences, including drinking well water, farming, and industrial exposure to heavy metals, have also been associated with increased prevalence of PD.

The role of normal aging needs to be considered. During aging, pathways lose neurons. Aging is also associated with a loss of catecholamine-containing neurons and an increase in monoamine oxidase (MAO), types A and B. In addition, there is a progressive loss of more than 60 percent of the dopaminergic neurons in the substantia nigra. This normal process begins at approximately age 30. There is also a decline in the striatal concentration of dopamine, an increase in the turnover of striatal dopamine, and a loss of striatal D_2 receptors. Compensatory mechanisms are thought to be responsible for the absence of PD before a decrease of 80 percent in striatal dopamine.

The morbidity and mortality rate for PD is high, with an estimated 9 percent of patients being disabled or dead within 1 to 5 years, 21 percent in 6 to 10 years, and almost 38 percent in 11 to 15 years.

Pathophysiology

PD is a degenerative disease of the motor systems of the brain. Its neurologic effects include symmetrical tremor at rest, muscular rigidity, slow movements, and difficulty maintaining a steady posture. Characteristically, the motor problems of PD improve when a patient is treated with levodopa.

PD slowly kills neurons in the substantia nigra, an adjunct to the basal ganglia. The full basal ganglia complex—the striatum, the globus pallidus, the subthalamic nucleus, and the substantia nigra—comprises a set of interconnected nuclei deep inside the cerebral cortex. The basal ganglia are a critical part of the motor system, with which they interact through the motor nuclei of the thalamus. The main output of the basal ganglia is a GABAergic inhibitory circuit from the internal segment of the globus pallidus to the ventral anterior and ventral lateral nuclei of the thalamus. This GABAergic circuit is itself inhibited (indirectly) by dopaminergic axons from the substantia nigra. PD depletes the substantia nigra of dopaminergic axons. As a result, the globus pallidus output remains unchecked, resulting in a blanket inhibition of the motor activity passing through the thalamus.

Besides depopulating the substantia nigra, PD kills dopaminergic neurons in the adjacent ventral tegmental area, noradrenergic neurons in the locus coeruleus and the dorsal and medial raphe nuclei in the brain stem, and cholinergic neurons in the nucleus basalis of Meynert. In the process, PD produces a typical intracellular abnormality called a Lewy body inside degenerating neurons. Lewy bodies are spherical insoluble clumps of neurofilaments, tubulin, synphilin, α-synuclein, and ubiquitin. Ubiquitin is normally used in a major intracellular degradative pathway, and evidence suggests that one metabolic abnormality underlying PD is a selective defect in this particular degradative pathway.

Clinical Presentation

Subjective

Presentation of the disease is variable. The patient may present with one or more of the six cardinal features of PD: tremor at rest, rigidity, bradykinesia or hypokinesia, flexed posture, loss of postural reflexes, and the freezing phenomenon. The major manifestations of tremor, rigidity, akinesia or bradykinesia, and postural disturbances form the mnemonic "TRAP."

A tremor may be the reason the patient or family is seeking care and is recognized as the first symptom of PD in 70 percent of patients at initial diagnosis. The tremor almost always appears distally in the extremities when the extremity is motionless and as a result is termed a "resting tremor." This resting tremor disappears with action but reemerges as the limbs maintain a posture. A resting tremor is common in the chin, lips, and tongue. The resting tremor of the hands increases when the patient is walking and may be an early sign of PD before other signs are visible. Stress worsens the tremor, but resting tremors are absent during sleep. A classic presentation of PD is a characteristic motion of the thumb and forefinger called "pill-rolling."

A common subjective complaint in patients with PD is fatigue, which may be related to rigidity or bradykinesia. Progressive bradykinesia may contribute to slowness and difficulty in the performance of ADLs. Patients may also suffer from sleep disturbances contributing to fatigue. Swallowing may be impaired in advanced disease, causing aspiration and choking.

Objective

The four common manifestations of PD may be objectively observed and evaluated by the clinician: tremor, a weak and clumsy limb, a stiff and aching limb, and a gait disorder. Rigidity is a state of increased resistance in muscle tone elicited when the clinician moves the patient's neck, trunk, or limbs. The muscle feels stiff and is difficult to move. This can appear as though the patient is having difficulty initiating movement. Rigidity is equal in all directions and is usually manifested by "cogwheeling," a ratchet-like, rhythmic contraction, especially in the hand, on passive stretching. Cogwheeling can be caused by an underlying tremor in the absence of a visible tremor. When another limb is engaged in voluntary movement, rigidity of the passive limb increases.

The patient with PD often has a flexed posture that involves the entire body. The head is bowed, the trunk is bent forward, and the back posture is kyphotic. The elbows, hips, and knees are flexed. The hands are held in front of the body. There may be hand deformities, including ulnar deviation (fingers flexed at the metacarpal phalangeal joints) and striatal hand (extension of interphalangeal joints). Striatal toe (big toe dorsiflexion) and inversion of the feet may be present, along with a lateral tilting of the trunk.

The most common features of PD are slowness of movement, difficulty initiating movement, loss of automatic movement (bradykinesia), and reduction in the amplitude of movement, particularly with repetitive movement (hypokinesia). Bradykinesia has many facets depending on the body parts affected. In addition, walking is slow; patients have a tendency to shuffle, with a shortened stride length. Truncal bradykinesia causes difficulty when a patient attempts to arise from a deep chair, get out of an automobile, or turn in bed.

Loss of postural reflexes may lead to falling; some individuals are unable to stand unassisted. As postural reflexes become impaired, the patient will collapse into a chair on attempting to sit. The *freezing phenomenon,* also called "motor block," is the transient inability to perform active movements. Most often, the legs are affected, but it may also involve eyelid opening, speaking, and writing. Freezing is transient and occurs suddenly. It typically occurs when the patient begins to walk (start-hesitation), attempts to turn while walking, or approaches a destination (target-hesitation). The patient may be fearful about the inability to handle perceived barriers such as elevator doors and heavily trafficked streets.

Other common manifestations of PD are drooling as a result of decreased frequency of swallowing, dysphagia secondary to the neuromuscular incoordination of the hypopharyngeal musculature, excessive perspiration as a result of a disorder of the hypothalamic heat-regulating mechanism and impairment of perspiration controls, constipation secondary to hypomotility of the gastrointestinal (GI) tract, orthostatic hypotension as the result of deterioration of the peripheral autonomic nervous system, and urinary hesitation secondary to autonomic dysfunction. The patient may also demonstrate a "mask-like" face (hypomimia), soft speech (hypophonia), slurred speech (dysarthria), and small, slow handwriting (micrographia).

The clinician may also perform the pull test in which the examiner stands behind the patient, gives a sudden, firm pull on the patient's shoulders, and checks for retropulsion. Obtaining a specimen of the patient's handwriting and comparing it with previous samples may assist in the diagnosis. Most patients with PD exhibit behavioral changes. Personality changes become apparent as the patient becomes fearful, dependent, and anxious. Passivity, lack of motivation, and decreased attention span are common. There may also be confusion, agitation, hallucinations, and mania related to activation of dopamine receptors in nonstriatal regions. More than 50 percent of patients with PD experience depression, and this may precede motor symptoms.

Patients with PD commonly experience cognitive decline. The MMSE is a simple means of measuring this impairment. This exam assesses temporal and spatial orientation, digit span, and the ability to express and understand language, to follow commands, and to remember complete simple instructions. The severe type of dementia seen in patients with AD is exhibited in approximately 15 to 20 percent of patients with PD.

The patient may be slow to answer questions and may be unable to change mental set rapidly. There may also be sensory and autonomic dysfunctions such as pain, burning, and tingling. The patient may report that these sensations diminish or disappear on moving. Autonomic dysfunctions such as cool skin, constipation, inadequate bladder emptying, difficulty in obtaining an erection, and orthostatic hypotension may be present.

Diagnostic Reasoning

Diagnostic Tests

Usually the history and physical examination leads the clinician to the diagnosis of PD. The major features of bradykinesia and akinesia; temor with the limb at rest or resistance to passive movement of the joints (rigidity) or both of these usually lead the clinician to the diagnosis. CT scan and MRI of the brain may be performed to exclude structural brain lesions but not to demonstrate pathologic changes indicative of PD. A serum calcium level may be drawn to exclude hypoparathyroidism. A positron emission tomography (PET) scan with 18F-6 fluorodopa can be used to assess changes in striatal dopamine and to detect subclinical nigral pathology.

There are clinical and laboratory clues, which suggest that a patient with parkinsonism may have some form of the syndrome other than PD itself. PD often manifests with unilateral symptoms, whereas symptomatic parkinsonism or Parkinson-plus syndromes usually have symmetrical symptoms. Levodopa may be given on a trial basis and one of the most important diagnostic aids is the patient's response to levodopa. Patients with PD usually have a satisfactory response to levodopa while other forms of parkinsonism are most likely if there is no response to levodopa.

Differential Diagnosis

Diagnosis is based on the clinical features of PD. These include insidious onset; slow progression; and lack of other findings to explain the symptoms, or history, examination, or laboratory tests that point to some other cause of parkinsonism. PD is commonly mistaken for *essential tremor,* which is characterized by postural and kinetic tremor, not resting tremor. The most common diagnostic difficulty is recognizing progressive supranuclear palsy (Steele-Richardson-Olzewski syndrome), when the PD like symptoms are accompanied by a supranuclear disorder of eye movements, pseudobulbar palsy, and axial dystonia. Another diagnostic error is confusion with multiple system atrophy, Shy-Drager syndrome, where there are additional symptoms of autonomic insufficiency leading to postural hypotension, and widespread neurologic deficits. Reversible parkinsonism may be caused by dopamine-blocking or dopamine- depleting medications such as antipsychotics, metoclopramide (Reglan), and reserpine (Serpasil). PD must be differentiated from cerebrovascular accidentss, dementia, Wilson's disease, and Huntington's disease. Wilson's disease may be recognized by its onset at an earlier age than PD, the presence of other abnormal movements, gray-green Kayser-Fleischer rings in the cornea, chronic hepatitis, and increased concentrations of cpper in the tissues. Patients with Huntington's disease also present with rigidity and bradykinesia, but the family history and accompanying dementia will differentiate it from PD.

Management

The principle of management is to control the symptoms of PD, because no drug or surgical approach prevents the progression of the disease. PD costs are estimated at $25 million per year in the United States, counting medications, treatment, hospitalzization, loss of productivity, and disability. As PD is one of the most expensive neurologic diseases, clinicians need to work closely with families to monitors patients' conditions to help them obtain the best quality of life of which they are capable. Each patient has a unique set of signs, symptoms, and responses to medications, so treatment must be individualized. Patients also have social, occupational, and emotional needs to be considered. Treatment is lifelong; the goal is to keep patients functioning independently as long as possible.

The decision of when to initiate symptomatic treatment for PD is controversial. When the diagnosis of PD is made, it is appropriate to consider the introduction of a neuroprotective agent. Neuroprotection can be defined as an intervention that protects vulnerable neurons. It may also slow or stop disease progression. Some practitioners advocate early treatment to provide maximal clinical benefit. Others advocate treatment delay, to minimize the risk of developing motor complications or accelerating disease progression because of an increased concentration of oxidant radicals from levodopa metabolism. The major decision is when to introduce levodopa. The most common issues providers consider important in deciding to use symptomatic agents are threat to employability; threat to performance of ADLs; threat to the abilities to handle domestic, financial, or social affairs; and appreciable worsening of gait or balance.

Medications commonly prescribed for the management of PD are presented in Drugs Commonly Prescribed 5.3. Levodopa, a dopaminergic agent, is considered the most effective antiparkinsonian agent and has been shown to improve the symptoms of PD by 40 to 50 percent.

Once levodopa therapy is started, the rule of thumb is to administer the lowest dosage that brings adequate symptom reversal. A trial period of 3 months should be given before it may be determined that the patient does not respond to the medication. Ninety percent of patients with true PD respond to levodopa. Patients may also experience the "on–off" phenomenon. After 2 to 5 years of treatment, more than 50 percent of patients experience fluctuations in their response to levodopa. They may also experience dyskinesia, freezing, and mental and behavioral changes. Selegiline (Eldepryl [L-deprenyl]) is a MAO-B inhibitor and considered a neuroprotective agent. It has fewer side effects than levodopa but the effects tend to be only moderate and provide inadequate symptomatic therapy and thus is not used typically as monotherapy.

Dopamine agonists presumably act directly on striatal dopamine receptors and do not require metabolic conversion to an active product in order to exert effects. They are slightly less effective than levodopa, but are alternative first-line agents for PD. These are independent of degenerating dopaminergic neurons. Anticholinergic agents are centrally acting drugs and have been used to treat PD for a long time. These drugs are typically used in patients age 70 or less in whom tremor is the dominant clinical feature but in whom cognitive function is preserved. These agents are useful for treating resting tremors; however, adverse effects—including memory impairment, hallucinations, and confusion—are common with these drugs. Adverse CNS effects of drugs used to treat PD include dysphagia, sedation, and dyskinesias. These drugs should always be discontinued gradually.

Peripheral catechol O-methyltransferase (COMT) inhibitors such as tolcapone (Tasmar) and entacapone (Comtan) have been studied as adjunctive therapies to levodopa. These drugs are thought to increase the bioavailability of levodopa, thereby extending the duration of levodopa's effect. COMT inhibitors have been shown to be effective in both nonfluctuating and fluctuating patients.

Patients with severe symptoms such as tremor that are refractory to medications may require referral to a movement disorder neurologist or neurosurgeon for evaluation. Options of thalamotomy, pallidotomy, and deep brain stimulation may be discussed with these patients. Thalamotomy and thalamic stimulation are best for intractable tremors and drug-induced kinesias. Pallidotomy is helpful in some patients for relief of bradykinesias, tremor, and dyskinesias. All of these procedures except deep brain stimulation are destructive in nature. Deep brain stimulation is considered nondestructive and reversible. High-frequency thalamic stimulation may be effective in suppressing the rest tremor of PD. Chronic bilateral stimulation of the subthalamic nuclei or globus pallidus shows promising results as a nondestructive treatment for relief of bradykinesias, tremors, and dyskinesias. Surgical implantation of adrenal medullary tissue or fetal substantia nigra tissue is still under investigation because of mixed results.

Follow-Up and Referral

The frequency of follow-up and visits is based on the patient's response to treatment, adverse effects of medications, and disease progression. Follow-up should be early and repeated initially, especially during the introduction of a new medication or dose change. The decision for referral to a specialist should be made based on the practitioner's knowledge level and comfort treating PD and on the severity of symptoms. As the disease progresses, especially in the area of tremor, it may become necessary to refer the patient to a movement disorder neurologist or to a stereotactic neurosurgeon.

Rating scales are frequently used to evaluate and monitor a patient's response to medications. The Unified Parkinson's Disease Rating Scale (UPDRS) is a comprehensive evaluation tool, which assesses mental, historical, and motor features and the complications of dopaminergic therapy. A subscale of the UPDRS is the Activities of Daily Living Scale, which assesses speech, salivation, swallowing, handwriting, cutting food, handling utensils, hygiene, turning in bed, falling, freezing, walking, tremor, and sensory symptoms.

Patient Education

The impact of Medicare's new prescription drug benefit will greatly improve the quality of life of many seniors who have been unable to purchase all the PD medications that are prescribed for them. As of November 2005, a new presciption drug plan under a new Part D benefit of Medicare reduced

Drugs Commonly Prescribed 5.3: Parkinson's Disease

Class	Drug	Dosage	Comments
MAO Inhibitors	Selegiline (Eldepryl L-deprenyl)	5 mg before breakfast and lunch Maximum: 10 mg/day	After several days, levodopa dosage may be reduced 10%–30%. Adverse effects: nausea, dizziness, confusion, hallucinations, dry mouth. Do not give with meperidine (Demerol) or narcotic analgesics. When given with levodopa, selegiline can increase dopaminergic effects and contribute to dopamine toxicity.
Dopaminergics	Carbidopa/levodopa (Sinemet, Sinemet CR, Atamet)	25/100 mg tid 50/200 mg bid	Gradually titrate to relief of symptoms; may go up to 300–500 mg/day. Monitor for orthostatic hypotension.
	Amantadine (Symmetrel)	Initially 100 mg qd; gradually increase to bid	Adverse effects: dizziness, ataxia, insomnia, leg edema. Do not give hs. May cause postural hypotension.
Dopamine Agonists	Bromocriptine (Parlodel)	2.5 mg qd; increased over several weeks Maximum: 30–50 mg bid–tid	Potentiates alcohol and other CNS depressants. Monitor BP and mental status. Adverse effects: fluctuation of symptoms, dyskinesia, dystonia.
	Pergolide (Permax)	Initially, 0.1 mg qd; usually 2–4 mg qd	As above.
	Pramipexole (Mirapex)	Initially, 0.125 mg tid, to 1.5 mg tid	As above. Titrate over 7 weeks.
	Ropinirole (Requip)	Initially, 0.25 mg tid to maximum of 1 mg tid	As above. Taper dose over 7 days to discontinue.
Anticholinergics	Trihexyphenidyl (Artane)	1.0–5.0 mg tid	Adverse effects: memory impairment, dysphagia, rigidity. Discontinue drug gradually.
	Benzotropine (Cogentin)	0.5–4.0 mg tid	As above.
COMT Inhibitors	Tolcapone (Tasmar)	100 mg tid; increase to 200 mg tid	With carbidopa/levodopa, discontinue if no substantial benefit after 3 weeks. Increases dopaminergic side effects. Perform baseline transaminase levels, then recheck every 2 weeks for 1 year, then every 4 weeks for 6 months, then every 2 months; monitor for liver disease. Adverse effects: dyskinesias, nausea, sleep disorders.
	Entacapone (Comtan)	200 mg; max eight tablets/day	Each dose of carbidopa/levodopa increases dopaminergic side effects: nausea and vomiting, dry mouth, postural hypotension.

the out-of-pocket expenditures for prescription drugs by an average of 83 percent for seniors who are eligible for this low-income subsidy and 34 percent of all other seniors. As it is a voluntary program, the clinician should make sure that patients are aware of this and put them in touch with appropriate persons to assist them in acquiring the benefit.

Speech therapy may be beneficial to increase the voice volume; effect the speech pattern modification; and assist with breathing, memory, and vocal ROM exercises. Occational swallowing assessments and therapies may be needed tdo assist with problems of dysphagia and drooling.

Patients should be educated on all issues of the disease, medications, adverse effects, complications, progression of the disease, diet, sleep, and exercise. Patients with PD should be encouraged to exercise regularly. This should be focused exercise, and a referral to physical therapy may be indicated. Patients should be observed for fatigue. Exercises should include swimming, stretching, and walking. These activities can slow the secondary effects of PD. Nutrition in patients with PD is an important component in care. The patient should also be assessed for physical and psychological problems, which may interfere with eating and nutrition. Functional capacity may be limited, hindering the patient's ability to prepare meals. Special table cutlery is available with large non-slip handles that may help with eating. Fiber and fluid may need to be increased. Protein may be taken in the evening to avoid interactions between dietary protein and levodopa.

Patients must also be instructed to continue routine health maintenance and screenings. In addition, both patient and caregiver must be educated to the risk for falls in patients with decreased mobility, as well as other home safety issues. There is an increase in mortality from influenza and pneumonia among patients with PD, so guidance for immunizations must be given. Patient and caregivers may benefit from referral to a support group. Resources are listed at the end of this chapter.

Alzheimer's Disease

Alzheimer's disease (AD) is a progressive, neurodegenerative condition and the most common form of dementia in the older population. It is characterized by an insidious onset, slow progressive cognitive decline, and an array of emotional and behavioral problems that result from the cognitive decline. AD accounts for about $100 billion per year in medical and custodial expenses, with approximately $27,000 per year for each patient for medical and nursing care.

According to the American Psychiatric Association, AD is characterized by the impaired ability to learn new information or recall previously learned information and one or more additional cognitive disturbances in language (aphasia), function (apraxia), perception (agnosia), or executive function. Once considered an inevitable result of old age, recent advances in understanding AD have modified both diagnostic and treatment choices. There is a familial as well as a sporadic form of the disease. Most clinicians treat patients with the sporadic form of AD.

Epidemiology and Causes

The incidence of the sporadic form of AD in the general population rises rapidly with age, from 0.6 percent at ages 60 to 69 to 2.0 percent at ages 70 to 79; and 10.2 percent at ages 80 to 89 It is projected to reach nearly 16 million cases in 2050 from 4.5 million cases in 2000. This equates to 60 percent of people in 2050 with AD will be older than 85. Additional risk factors that have been identified include lower educational and occupational levels, family history, head injury, Down's syndrome, and decreased estrogen levels. Because onset is often undetected, it is difficult to accurately predict duration or survival time with the disease. For 60- to 70-year-old patients with AD, the average life expectancy is 7 to 10 years after diagnosis.

The relatively rare familial form of AD is considered a straightforward genetic disease. Onset is typically earlier than in the sporadic form of AD. For example in an extended St. Louis family with the familial form of AD, the typical age at onset is 26 to 28 years. The physically fit but demented individuals in this family are considered evidence that the disease is not entirely due to age. Members of another large family from villages outside Medellín, Colombia, exhibit symptoms of AD in their early 30s. Many patients complain of severe headaches before onset of familial AD, but the progression is otherwise similar to that of the sporadic form. If a parent has the familial form of AD, offspring have a 50–50 chance of developing the disease

See Nursing Research-Based Practice 5.1 for information on variability of familial risk of AD across the late life span.

Pathophysiology

AD is a progressive and irreversible cortical disconnection syndrome. The disease depletes the cerebral cortices of neurons, causing generalized cortical atrophy, widened cortical sulci, and enlarged ventricles. Neurons that use the neurotransmitter acetylcholine are especially susceptible to the disease; for example, the nucleus basalis (the basal nucleus of Meynert), a set of large cholinergic neurons in the telencephalon beneath the basal ganglia, is selectively depopulated of neurons. Cortical areas that are especially hard hit include the hippocampus (which loses most of its inputs and outputs), the amygdala (which shrinks as it becomes depleted), the temporal cortex, the olfactory system (including the primary sensory epithelium in the nose), and corticocortical (intercortical) connections.

Two pathologic lesions are found in large numbers throughout the brain of an Alzheimer's patient: neuritic plaques (also called "senile plaques") and neurofibrillary tangles. Neuritic plaques are macroscopic spherical lesions found throughout the cortex (although they are relatively

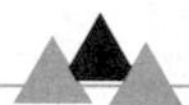

NURSING RESEARCH-BASED PRACTICE 5.1

Variability of Familial Risk of Alzheimer Disease Across the Late Life Span

Silverman, JM, Ciresi, G, Smith, CJ, Marin, DB, and Schnaider-Beeri, M:
Arch Gen Psychiatry (May) 62:565–573, 2005.

Context: The role of genetic factors in Alzheimer's disease (AD) varies across the late life span, complicating efforts to quantify the risk of AD for relatives of probands with AD.

Objectives: To visualize the changing levels of familial risk according to proband onset age and the age of at-risk relative and to determine the familiality of the age at onset in AD.

Design: A retrospective, informant-based family study.

Setting, Patients, and Other Participants: Siblings and parents of probands with AD (relatives = 4687; probands = 904), ascetained at geriatric clinic and nursing home settings, and of elderly probands without dementia (relatives = 7649; probands = 1525) who were spouses of probands, participants at senior centers, or nursing home residents without dementia.

Main Outcome Measures: Informant-based assessments of AD in the relatives were used to generate three-dimensional surfaces representing the patterns of risk of AD across the late life span depending on the specific onset age of the proband with AD (or assessment age of the elderly proband without dementia). We then constructed a three-dimensional, age-specific, 10-year hazard rate ratio (HRR) surface representing the relative risk of AD in relatives of probands with AD with smoothly shifting levels of onset age compared with relatives of elderly probands without dementia.

Results: The HRR surface peaked (HRR, 13.0) for younger sexagenarian relatives related to probands with AD with onset age in their early 60s. The HRRs dropped sharply both as the proband age at onset and the age of the relative increased. For relatives in their late 80s, the HRR fell lower than 2.0 regardless of proband onset age and their lower-limit 95% confidence intervals were less than 1.0.

Conclusions: The role of genetic risk factors decreases with increasing onset age of the proband with AD regardless of the age of the relatives themselves. The familiality of onset age is greatly reduced at later ages. The role of environmental risk factors in AD likely increases with onset age.

sparse in the primary motor and sensory areas), the hippocampus, and the amygdala. Each plaque has a core of β-amyloid, an insoluble peptide. The core is surrounded by swollen and degenerating neurites, and these are encased in a layer of microglia and astrocytes. Excess β-amyloid is also found diffusely throughout the cerebral cortex, the cerebellar cortex, and the basal ganglia, especially in and around blood vessels.

Neurofibrillary tangles are microscopic collections of intertwined cytoskeletal fibers that form inside neurons. The tangles are best seen in silver stained tissue, and their density correlates with the degree of the patient's dementia. One major protein in these tangles is an aberrant form of *tau* protein (which, in its normal form, stabilizes microtubules), and patients with AD have elevated concentrations of *tau* proteins in their cerebrospinal fluid. The formation of neurofibrillary tangles immobilizes or otherwise deactivates the neuron's normally dynamic cytoskeleton and leads to the cell's death. The tangles are insoluble and remain after the neurons have degenerated.

The central biochemical problem in AD appears to be a defect in the metabolism of *beta-amyloid precursor protein.* Normally, many types of cells, including neurons, make beta-amyloid precursor protein, the function of which is not yet fully understood. When this protein is broken down by specific secretases, the byproducts include beta-amyloid peptides. There are four different forms of beta-amyloid peptide. The form identified as beta-amyloid-42 is insoluble, readily forms fibrils, and is found in neuritic plaques.

In AD, beta-amyloid peptides accumulate excessively in the brain. It is thought that abnormalities in the functioning of the secretases cause the overproduction of beta-amyloids. One current theory proposes that beta-amyloid deposition is the primary problem in AD and that intracellular neurofibrillary tangles are the consequence of the toxic effects of beta-amyloid on neurons.

Clinical Presentation

Subjective

The patient usually presents initially with complaints of memory problems. The boundary between the benign forgetfulness of age-associated memory impairment (AAMI) and the onset of AD is unclear. A complaint of memory problems must be thoroughly explored to distinguish not only AAMI but also emotional disorders, other physical insults to the brain, and early AD. Recognition of cognitive difficulty on the part of the patient or family is often related to a change in pattern: getting lost in familiar places, inability to accomplish a demanding task at work, or increasingly slow response to any cognitive challenge. Word-finding difficulty (anomia) usually occurs. Trouble balancing the checkbook, preparing dinner, traveling alone, or maintaining employment are frequent problems reported by family members when the disease has progressed to the point where it is noticeable to others. As the disease progresses to the middle stage, family members report difficulty with simpler tasks: choosing clothes, doing housework, and finishing chores. These behavior difficulties worsen with cognitive decline. In the later stages, the person needs help dressing, bathing, and staying continent. Eventually, the person loses capacity to converse, walk, sit, or hold up the head. Eighty percent of patients in nursing homes with AD have behavioral problems. These may include hostility, aggression, suspiciousness and paranoia, delusions, agitatin, sundowning, incontinence, and inappropriate or impulsive sexual behavior.

Objective

The Agency for Health Care Policy and Research (AHCPR) Guidelines for Early Identification of Alzheimer's Disease and Related Dementias asserts that there is no support at present for assessing dementia in asymptomatic individuals. However, if concern about cognitive decline is expressed by the patient or family or changes in behavior or cognition are noted, this should trigger an initial assessment for dementia (Advanced Assessment 5.1).

The often heard rule of thumb that if a patient reports memory loss, he or she is not demented, has been refuted. Routine social conversation and questions that can be answered automatically will not elicit symptoms of early AD. Instead, ask the person such questions as "Do you remember what you did last Sunday?" or "What did you have for breakfast this morning?" The AHCPR Guidelines emphasize the importance of maintaining the patient's dignity by examining the patient alone before interviewing others. The patient should be informed if others are to be interviewed. It is also important to be alert to the possibility that family members at times may minimize or exaggerate their report of symptoms depending on their motives. Family members can report on the patient's ability to perform the independent activities of daily living using the Functional Activities Questionnaire (Advanced Assessment 5.2).

The clinician should get a focused history documenting signs and symptoms related to the dementia, chronology of the problem (including onset, duration, and stepwise versus continuous progression), family history, and any condition or medications that may mimic or contribute to cognitive impairment. The physical examination should include a neurologic evaluation and evaluation of any factors contributing to delirium and evidence of neglect or abuse. Neuropsychological testing can pinpoint the types and severity of impairments in language, reasoning, and visuospatial and memory deficits.

ADVANCED ASSESSMENT 5.1

Alzheimer's Disease: Triggers for Further Assessment

Learning and retaining: Is more repetitive; has trouble remembering recent conversations, events, new information appointments; frequently misplaces objects

Handling complex tasks: Has trouble following a complex train of thought or performing tasks that require many steps such as balancing a checkbook or cooking a meal

Reasoning ability: Is unable to respond with a reasonable plan to problems at work or home, such as knowing what to do if the bathroom is flooded; shows uncharacteristic disregard for rules of social conduct

Spatial ability and orientation: Has trouble driving, organizing objects around the house, finding his or her way around familiar places

Language: Has increasing difficulty with finding the words to express what he or she wants to say and with following conversations

Behavior: Appears more passive and less responsive; is more irritable than usual; is more suspicious than usual; misinterprets visual or auditory stimuli

SOURCE: US Department of Health and Human Services: Early Identification of Alzheimer's Disease and Related Dementias. US Department of Health and Human Services, Rockville, Md., 1996, AHCPR Publication 97-0703.

The MMSE (Advanced Assessment 5.3) is a well-known, easily administered test of cognition. It should be the initial test done when trying to diagnose AD. Within the possible scoring range of 0 to 30, the median score for adults aged 18 to 59 is 29, but the median score drops to 25 for age 80. A score of 20 to 25 indicates early-stage AD, a score between 10 and 19 indicates middle-stage ADg, and a score below 10 indicates late-stage AD. Age, visual, auditory, and other physical impairments and educational level must be taken into consideration in interpretation of test results. The Functional Activities Questionnaire (FAQ) if not already used, may be performed by the practitioner. It is also a useful measure that is reported to discriminate well at higher functional levels. These tests are appropriate for initial assessment. The results also provide a baseline from which any further decline can be noted quantitatively. The APN should refer the patient to a memory disorder center or a specialist in dementing diseases if the initial assessment is suggestive of AD, particularly when atypical presentation, severe impairment, or complex comorbidities are present.

ADVANCED ASSESSMENT 5.2

Functional Activities Questionnaire

The Functional Activities Questionnaire (FAQ) is an informant-based measure of functional abilities. Informants provide performance ratings of the target person on 10 complex, higher-order activities. *Individual items of the FAQ:*

1. Writing checks, paying bills, balancing a checkbook
2. Assembling tax records, business affairs, or papers
3. Shopping alone for clothes, household necessities, or groceries
4. Playing a game of skill, working on a hobby
5. Heating water, making a cup of coffee, turning off the stove
6. Preparing a balanced meal
7. Keeping track of current events
8. Paying attention to, understanding, discussing a TV show, book, or magazine
9. Remembering appointments, family occasions, holidays, medications
10. Traveling out of the neighborhood, driving, arranging to take buses

The levels of performance assigned range from dependence to independence and are rated as follows:

- Dependent = 3
- Requires assistance = 2
- Has difficulty but does by self = 1
- Normal = 0

Two other response options can also be scored:

- Never did [the activity], but could not now = 0
- Never did and would have difficulty now = 1

A total score for the FAQ is computed by simply summing the scores across the 10 items. Scores range from 0 to 30; the higher the score the poorer the function, i.e., the greater the impairment. A cutpoint of "9" (dependent in three or more activities) is recommended.

SOURCE: Pfeffer, RI, et al: Measurement of functional activities of older adults in the community. J Gerontol 37(3):323, 1982, with permission.

Diagnostic Reasoning

Diagnostic Tests

Laboratory tests (CBC, electrolytes, blood glucose, serum calcium, and a thyroid-stimulating hormone [TSH] level at a minimum) are used to rule out other conditions that may impair brain function. CT scans and MRI of the brain may be performed to exclude structural lesions. Genetic testing is available, but its value remains controversial in most cases. EEGs are not routinely performed and the pupillary drug test is considered unreliable.

Differential Diagnosis

To some extent, the diagnosis of AD is still a process of excluding other causes of cognitive impairment (Fig. 5.1).

Medical conditions and drug-related adverse effects need to be ruled out in patients suspected of AD. Infection, structural CNS conditions, traumatic conditons, metabolic organic failure, and anemia need to be considered. In addition, depression, drug and alcohol abuse, drug-induced delirium, and psychosis need to be ruled out.

The patient should be assessed for deterioration from a higher level of function. Mental retardation should be ruled out. If there is no alteration in consciousness, delirium should be ruled out. Amnesia and aphasia need to be considered if multiple cognitive functions are impaired. If the course of the disease is chronic rather than subacute, the following should be excluded: Creutzfeldt-Jacob disease, tumor, nutritional deficiency, drug intoxication, metabolic disorders, and so on. If there is a steady versus stepwise decline, vascular dementia should be ruled out. If there is primarily cortical dysfunction, Parkinson's dementia, Huntington's disease, trauma, vascular dementia, and so forth should be ruled out.

Many patients present with more than one problem. Delirium or depression may be superimposed on AD; PD, vascular problems, or other dementia can also coexist with AD, complicating diagnosis.

Depression can mimic AD and is frequently mistaken for AD in older adults. Information from multiple sources—patient self-report, family members, health provider observations, and patient history—should be used in drawing conclusions.

The Alzheimer's Disease Management Council (ADMC) Clinical Consensus Panel and Scientific Roundtable propose that the following are highly suggestive of the diagnosis of AD:

- ▲ absence of a precipitating medical illness
- ▲ absence of a drug-related phenomena
- ▲ presence of objective, well documented, progressive and worsening deficits in new learning and memory
- ▲ signs of functional impairment.

Management

The principle of management of AD is directed toward slowing progression of the disease pharmacologically, protecting physical health, providing emotional support and maintaining maximum possible function through prevention or reduction of excess disability. Maintaining as much normality as possible in relationships and everyday activities may be the most effective way to prevent the development of excess disability, defined as the difference between the observed function and the actual underlying impairment.

Family members have reported that sensitivity to their distress, acknowledgment of their contributions and information about the disease and its management have not always been dealt with adequately in encounters with

MiniMental LLC

THE ANNOTATED MINI MENTAL STATE EXAMINATION (AMMSE)

NAME OF SUBJECT __________ Age _____
NAME OF EXAMINER __________ Years of School Completed _____
Approach the patient with respect and encouragement. Date of Examination _____
Ask: Do you have any trouble with your memory? ☐ Yes ☐ No
May I ask you some questions about your memory? ☐ Yes ☐ No

SCORE	ITEM
5 ( )	**TIME ORIENTATION** Ask: What is the year _____ (1), season _____ (1), month of the year _____ (1), date _____ (1), day of the week _____ (1)?
5 ( )	**PLACE ORIENTATION** Ask: Where are we now? What is the state _____ (1), city _____ (1), part of the city _____ (1), building _____ (1), floor of the building _____ (1)?
3 ( )	**REGISTRATION OF THREE WORDS** Say: Listen carefully. I am going to say three words. You say them back after I stop. Ready? Here they are...PONY (wait 1 second), QUARTER (wait 1 second), ORANGE (wait 1 second). What were those words? _____ (1) _____ (1) _____ (1) Give 1 point for each correct answer, then repeat them until the patient gets all three.
5 ( )	**SERIAL 7's AS A TEST OF ATTENTION AND CALCULATION** Ask: Subtract 7 from 100 and continue to subtract 7 from each subsequent remainder until I tell you to stop. What is 100 take away 7? _____ (1) Say: Keep going, _____ (1), _____ (1), _____ (1), _____ (1).
3 ( )	**RECALL OF THREE WORDS** Ask: What were those three words I asked you to remember? Give 1 point for each correct answer _____ (1), _____ (1), _____ (1).
3 ( )	**NAMING** Ask: What is this? (show pencil) _____ (1). What is this? (show watch) _____ (1).

OVER

primary-care providers. Both patient and family need assistance in understanding and coping with a diagnosis of AD. Most patients are eager to try approved and research-stage drugs. Support group attendance can be very helpful but must be relevant to the stage of the disease. Anxiety and depression should be recognized and treated vigorously because they probably are responsible for much of the disturbing behavior associated with AD. Legal and financial planning and discussion of future care options should take place early in the disease course.

Pharmaceutical agents may improve cognitive function or lesson some of the dementia in mild to moderate AD. Acetylcholinesterase inhibitors may also show effects on self-care function and behavior. (See Drugs Commonly Prescribed 5.4.) The doses for these drugs: donepezil (Aricept), galantamine (Reminyl), and rivastigmine (Exelon) are adjusted gradually as tolerated. A *N*-methyl-D-aspartate (NMDA) receptor antagonist, memantine (Namenda) has been effective in moderate to severe AD by improving cognitive function and has additive effects to

MiniMental LLC

1 ( ) **REPETITION**
Say:
Now I am going to ask you to repeat what I say. Ready? No ifs, ands, or buts.
Now you say that. ______________________________ (1)

3 ( ) **COMPREHENSION**
Say:
Listen carefully because I am going to ask you to do something.
Take this paper in your left hand (1), fold it in half (1), and put it on the floor. (1)

1 ( ) **READING**
Say:
Please read the following and do what it says, but do not say it aloud. (1)

Close your eyes

1 ( ) **WRITING**
Say:
Please write a sentence. If patient does not respond, say: Write about the weather. (1)

____

____

1 ( ) **DRAWING**
Say: Please copy this design. (1)

TOTAL SCORE ______

Assess level of consciousness along a continuum.

Alert — Drowsy — Stupor — Coma

	YES	NO
Cooperative:	☐	☐
Depressed:	☐	☐
Anxious:	☐	☐
Poor Vision:	☐	☐
Native Language:	☐	☐

	YES	NO
Deterioration from previous level of functioning:	☐	☐
Family History of Dementia:	☐	☐
Head Trauma:	☐	☐
Stroke:	☐	☐
Alcohol Abuse:	☐	☐
Thyroid Disease:	☐	☐

FUNCTION BY PROXY
Please record date when patient was last able to perform the following tasks.
Ask caregiver if patient independently handles:

	YES	NO	DATE
Money/Bills:	☐	☐	______
Medication:	☐	☐	______
Transportation:	☐	☐	______
Telephone:	☐	☐	______

Source: "Mini-mental state." A practical method for grading the cognitive state of patients for the clinician. J Psychiatr Res 12(3):189-198, 1975, with permission.

acetylcholinesterase inhibitors. Antidepressant drugs have shown effect in patients with depressive symptoms. Anxious and agitated behavior may respond to anxiolytic drugs, however, use of pharmaceutical agents for noncognitive symptoms such as anxiety, depression, and insomnia should be reserved for instances where behavioral intervention is ineffective.

Antipsychotics should be used only for patients who exhibit persistent disruptive or dangerous behavior. Precautions include avoidance of drugs that have even a moderate anticholinergic effect and drugs that sedate, affect balance, or are known to cause confusion in older individuals. Atypical antipsychotic medications, risperidone (Risperdal). Olanzapine (Zyprexa), and quetiapine (Seroquel), are usually well tolerated. Risperidone should be avoided in patients with vascular risk factors as it may as it may increase the risk of stroke. Federal regulations require that if antipsychotic agents are used in nursing homes, that an effort be made to reduce the dosage at least every 6 months. α-Tocopherol (vitamin E) may help to slow pro-

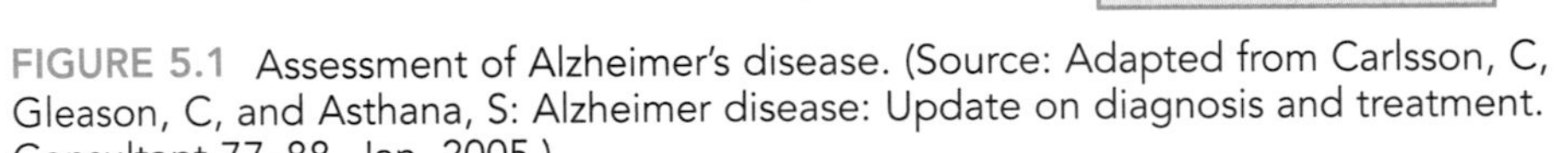

FIGURE 5.1 Assessment of Alzheimer's disease. (Source: Adapted from Carlsson, C, Gleason, C, and Asthana, S: Alzheimer disease: Update on diagnosis and treatment. Consultant 77–88, Jan. 2005.)

gression of AD, and an herbal extract of *Ginkgo biloba* has also been reported to have modest beneficial effects, with few adverse effects.

The failure to institute pharmacologic management in patients with AD may result in possibly a more rapid need for institutionalization, an increase in aggression, further difficulty with ADLs, and further cognitive decline.

Given the advanced age, compromised brain function, and frequent presence of other chronic conditions in most patients with AD, close monitoring of response to any drug regimen is advisable. In addition, as the patient becomes less able to communicate physical or emotional distress, more careful observation of general health and well-being is needed.

Vigilance in regard to good nutrition, exercise, and preventive care (immunizations, dental, vision and hearing care) should not be reduced. Patients and their families also need continued support and assistance related to continuing changes that occur as the disease progresses. Recognition and respect for the patient's humanity is difficult for some caregivers in the face of declining cognition, leading to the unfortunate temptation to care for family members while ignoring the patient.

Follow-Up and Referral

Referral to a memory disorder center is usually warranted. These centers offer multidisciplinary services ranging from

Drugs Commonly Prescribed 5.4: Alzheimer's Disease

Drug	Starting Dose	Maximum Dose	Comments
Acetylcholinesterase inhibitors			For mild to moderate AD. Side effects include diarrhea, nausea, anorexia, and weight loss.
Donepezil (Aricept)	5 mg PO daily at bedtime	10 mg daily	
Galantamine (Reminyl)	4 mg PO bid with food	12 mg twice daily	
Rivastigmine (Exelon)	1.5 mg PO bid at the end of a full meal	6 mg twice daily	Rivastigmine has shown fewer side effects than the other drugs in this category.
N-Methyl-D-aspartate (NMDA) receptor antagonist			For moderate to severe AD. Can be used in conjunction with acetylcholinesterase inhibitors.
Memantine (Namenda)	5 mg PO daily with or without food	10 mg twice daily	Contraindicated with renal impairment.
Anxiolytics			Requires several weeks to show efficacy.
Buspirone (Buspar)	5–7.5 mg bid	30 mg daily	
Atypical antipsychotics			Avoid in patients with vascular dementia or vascular risk factors. Avoid alcohol.
Risperidone (Risperdal)	2–3 mg daily	6 mg/day	
Olanzapine (Zyprexa)	5 mg daily	20 mg/day	
Quetiapine (Seroquel)	25 mg bid	800 mg/day in divided doses	

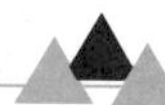

NURSING RESEARCH-BASED PRACTICE 5.2

Vitamin E and Donepezil for the Treatment of Mild Cognitive Impairment

Petersen, RC, Thomas, RG, Grundman, M, Bennett, D, Doody, R, Ferris, S, Galasko, D, Jin, S, Kaye, J, Levey, A, Pfeiffer, E, Sano, M, van Dyck, CH, and Thal, LJ: N Engl J Med 352:2379–2388, 2005.

Background: Mild cognitive impairment is a transitional state between the cognitive changes of normal aging and early Alzheimer's disease (AD).

Methods: In a double-blind study, we evaluated subjects with the amnestic subtype of mild cognitive impairment. Subjects were randomly assigned to receive 2000 IU of vitamin E daily, 10 mg of donepezil daily, or placebo for 3 years. The primary outcome was clinically possible or probable AD; secondary outcomes were cognition and function.

Results: A total of 769 subjects were enrolled, and possible or probable AD developed in 212. The overall rate of progression from mild cognitive impairment to AD was 16% per year. As compared with the placebo group, there were no significant differences in the probability of progression to AD disease in the vitamin E group (hazard ratio, 1.02; 95% confidence interval, 0.74–1.41; $P = 0.91$) or the donepezil group (hazard ratio, 0.80; 95 percent confidence interval, 0.57–1.13; $P = 0.42$) during the 3 years of treatment. Prespecified analyses of the treatment effects at 6-month intervals showed that as compared with the placebo group, the donepezil group had a reduced likelihood of progression to AD during the first 12 months of the study ($P = 0.04$), a finding supported by the secondary outcome measures. Among carriers of one or more apolipoprotein $\epsilon 4$ alleles, the benefit of donepezil was evident throughout the 3-year follow-up. There were no significant differences in the rate of progression to AD between the vitamin E and placebo groups at any point, either among all patients or among apolipoprotein $\epsilon 4$ carriers.

Conclusions: Vitamin E had no benefit in patients with mild cognitive impairment. Although donepezil therapy was associated with a lower rate of progression to AD during the first 12 months of treatment, the rate of progression to AD after 3 years was not lower among patients treated with donepezil than among those given placebo.

differential diagnosis and access to experimental medications to counseling and support groups. They are excellent sources of accurate information on AD. Most cities have local chapters that usually offer referrals and support groups as well. Respite, both at home and overnight in participating health-care facilities, and adult day centers provide social outlets for people with AD and a break in the constant care demands for family members. Family members must be cared for as well and if the clinician is unable to support them, it is essential to find social service agencies that will be able to help.

Patient Education

Both patient and family members need to understand the disease, its ramifications, its future course, and treatment options. Memory aids and environmental modifications can prolong independent function. Specialized communication techniques, memory training, exercise, training in the independent and basic ADLs, and therapeutic recreational activities can all contribute to improved function and quality of life as the disease progresses. Patients need information on legal and financial issues related to capacity to make decisions, including end-of-life decisions. Driving and living alone are safety issues that arise in the earlier stages; wandering and falls become issues in the later stages. Emotional issues are often ignored: both patient and family must deal with changes in ability, lifestyle, and relationships with others. Finally, family members need to learn how to help the patient while taking care of themselves as well.

Many patients with advanced disease are taking as many as six to eight medications daily. Many of these medications have side effects that affect cognition and result in falls. Fall precautions need to be taken at home as well as in long-term care facilities and clinicians should educate families regarding these at every visit.

Neurovascular Disorders

Cerebrovascular Accident

Cerebrovascular accident (CVA), commonly referred to as a stroke, is the rapid onset of neurologic deficits as a result of decreased blood flow to a focal or localized area of brain tissue. Although the incidence of CVA has decreased in the past 20 years because of risk-factor management and improved treatment, it has continued to be a significant public health problem in terms of both mortality and permanent disability. A CVA is the leading cause of disability in adults, incurring major economic burdens on the patient, family, and the public as a result of direct medical costs and cost in lost employment. Its impact as a major health problem with demands on health-care and other support systems will continue to grow as the number of CVA survivors living with disabilities increases, the proportion of African-Americans increases, and the population continues to live longer. The need for continued improvement in the control of risk factors and the prevention of CVAs is critical.

There are two different kinds of CVAs—*hemorrhagic* and *ischemic*. Hemorrhagic CVAs are most often caused by intracerebral hemorrhage from ruptured aneurysms, arteriovenous malformation, hypertensive arteriolar disease, and amyloid deposition. The obstructions that cause ischemic CVAs can be caused by atherosclerosis, embolus, thrombus, hemorrhage, or vasospasm. Up to 85 percent of CVAs are due to ischemia. Thirty-three percent of all cases of CVAs are caused by atherosclerotic lesions and thrombosis; another 31 percent are attributed to emboli.

A transient ischemic attach (TIA) serves as a warning of serious underlying atherosclerotic vascular disease. It is defined as an episode of temporary, focal cerebral dysfunction due to vascular disease that lasts less than 24 hours and usually less than 10 minutes. Because most people know the seriousness of a heart attack and the necessity for early treatment, many are referring to a CVA as a "brain attack" for similar reasons.

Epidemiology and Causes

CVAs are the third leading cause of death in the United States, after heart disease and cancer, and are highest in the southeastern United States. Although there are approximately 158,000 deaths from CVAs (1 in every 15 deaths), an estimated 700,000 people suffer a CVA each year. Every 53 seconds, someone has a CVA. More women than men (about 3:2) die from a CVA. This is attributed to the fact that whereas more men have CVAs (19 percent), women live longer and thus are more prone to them. In reviewing long-term survival, 25 percent of people who have an initial CVA die within a year and two-thirds die within 12 years. Health costs are significant. The average health-care costs per person (inpatient and outpatient) for CVAs have been estimated to be between $8,000 and $16,500. These impressive numbers do not include the additional costs of morbidity—related expenses (lost time from work, additional nursing care, etc). The direct and indirect costs to the nation are an estimated $53 billion. Age, sex, race, ethnic origin, and heredity have been identified as nonmodifiable risk factors for CVAs, helping to identify those at greatest risk. Compared with whites, young African-Americans are two to three times at greater risk of a CVA as well as being 2.5 times more likely to die of one. A higher incidence of CVAs is also noted in Hispanics, Asians, particularly Chinese and Japanese, than in white Americans. For people older than age 55, the incidence of a CVA more than doubles in each successive decade. Twenty-eight percent of people who suffer a CVA are younger than age 65. An increased incidence of CVAs in some families has been noted, probably because of a genetic tendency and familial exposure to similar environmental or lifestyle risks.

Important modifiable risk factors for a CVA include hypertension, cardiac disease, diabetes, hypercholesterolemia, smoking, illicit drug use, and lifestyle factors. There is a fourfold increase of a CVA when a patient is hypertensive with a BP over 160/95 mm Hg. Studies show that with treatment for hypertension, there is a 38 percent reduction in CVAs and a 40 percent reduction in mortality from CVAs. Atrial fibrillation is associated with a three- to fivefold increased risk for a CVA. Other cardiac diseases are cardiac valve abnormalities, such as mitral stenosis or mitral annular calcification. Cardiac structural abnormalities, such as patent foramen ovale and atrial septal aneurysm, increase CVA risk. Myocardial disease, left ventricular hypertrophy, and cardiac failure also increase the risk of a CVA. People with diabetes are more prone to develop atherosclerosis, thus increasing the risk of a CVA.

Although the risk of ischemic stroke that can be attributed to lipids is uncertain, cigarette smoking increases the risk two times. Moderate use of alcohol may actually reduce the risk of a CVA, whereas heavy consumption increases the risk. Drug abuse involving substances such as cocaine, heroin, amphetamines, and marijuana has been linked to CVAs. Lifestyle factors associated with CVAs are obesity, physical activity, diet, and emotional stress. Recently, studies have shown there is no increase in risk of ischemic stroke with use of low-dose oral contraceptives. Migraine is also associated as a minor risk factor in men older than age 40. Studies have shown a link between high blood levels of homocysteine (produced from the essential amino acid methionine) and CVAs. However, treatment did not lower the incidence of a CVA. The risk of a CVA may be higher in patients with a progressing and severe stenosis of the carotid artery or in patients who have experienced a TIA. A CVA is an important complication in patients suffering an anterior myocardial infarction (MI) or in patients treated with long-term oral anticoagulants. Complicated atherosclerotic plaques in the aortic wall may contribute to a source of a CVA.

Pathophysiology

Pathologically, there are two distinct categories of cerebrovascular accidents: ischemic and hemorrhagic.

Cerebral Ischemia

Neurons will stop functioning after less than 10 seconds of insufficient blood flow, but they will recover fully if local circulation is restored within a few minutes. After a few minutes without oxygen and glucose, however, neurons begin to die. Cerebral ischemia is caused by a reduction in blood flow that lasts for more than 4 or 5 minutes.

Transient Ischemic Attacks. A brief bout of ischemia will produce neurologic deficits. If the ischemia is short-lived, the neurologic signs and symptoms usually resolve within an hour. When the neurologic problems take more than 4 hours to improve, some neuron death has probably occurred. Sudden neurologic deficits that resolve in less than 24 hours are usually the result of TIAs, fleeting occlusions of cerebral arteries. People who have suffered a TIA are likely later to have a stroke.

Arterial Occlusions. Neurologic deficits lasting longer than 24 hours indicate that there has been significant neuron death. When the deficits are focal, the ischemic injury is probably due either to atherothromboses or to emboli. Atherosclerosis produces atheromatous plaques, gummy bulges that protrude from the inner walls of arteries. Atheromatous plaques are masses of lipids, cell debris, collagen, fibrin, platelets, and blood cells, covered by smooth muscle cells, macrophages, and lymphocytes. Plaques that fragment send embolic debris downstream, occluding smaller arteries and arterioles and producing areas of ischemia. Plaques that erode can also initiate local blood clotting. When the clot sticks to the plaque, it often grows, occludes the arterial lumen, and leads to ischemia downstream. The specific neurologic deficits caused by atherosclerotic plaques reflect the locations of the areas of ischemia.

Occlusive emboli can be generated upstream some distance from the cerebral arteries. Clots and fragments of atherosclerotic plaque in the internal carotids or the vertebral arteries can dislodge and be carried into brain arteries, which then become occluded. Cardiac arrhythmias (atrial fibrillation and sick sinus syndrome), valvular diseases, prosthetic heart valves, and myocardial infarcts can generate emboli. Clots and clumps of platelets formed during angiography and cardiac surgery can become occlusive emboli. Hypercoagulability syndromes, elevated levels of blood platelets, calcified fragments of plaque and tissue, air, fat, cholesterol crystals, tumor fragments, bacterial vegetations, and foreign material (such as talc and cornstarch injected with illicit drugs) can all clog brain arteries. The occluding emboli are sometimes pushed distally in the affected arteries. This abrades the vessels walls. The injured vessels then bleed and add hemorrhagic damage to the ischemic infarction.

Decreased Brain Perfusion. Low cerebral blood flow causes syncope (fainting). If brain perfusion remains low, neurons begin to die in the areas farthest from the main arteries, i.e., at the borders between regions supplied by the major cerebral arteries. Hypoperfusion ischemia leads first to loss of vision, decreased alertness, and weakness in shoulder, hand, and thigh muscles. In addition, certain hippocampal neurons are especially sensitive to a temporary loss of cerebral perfusion, and this may explain the memory defects that occur after the hypoperfusion caused by even a brief cardiac arrest.

Cerebral Hemorrhage

The neurologic symptoms of a cerebral hemorrhage result from the pressure of the hematoma. Sometimes, this pressure causes infarcts in the compressed tissue. Other times, however, there is less cell death so that when the hematoma is resorbed, the neurologic deficits resolve to some degree. As a rule, the larger the hematoma, the greater and more permanent is the damage.

Epidural Hematomas. Epidural bleeding is caused by severe head injuries. Epidural hematomas are most common along the temporal cranial wall and result from tears in the middle meningeal artery. The leaking arterial blood rapidly creates a hematoma between dura and bone. This increases the overall intracranial pressure, which in turn reduces the cerebral blood perfusion. As the hematoma enlarges, it presses on adjacent brain tissue, causing contralateral hemiparesis. Next, the increasing pressure affects the diencephalon, and the patient gets lethargic and drowsy. When the midbrain becomes compressed against the dural rim of the tentorium, patients develop ipsilateral oculomotor nerve palsy and an enlarged pupil. Continued expansion of the hematoma compresses the contralateral cerebral peduncle, leading to ipsilateral hemiplegia. Eventually, the diencephalon and ipsilateral temporal lobe can be pushed down through the tentorial notch—such herniations compress the posterior cerebral arteries, press on the brainstem, and can be fatal.

Subdural Hematomas. Subdural bleeding is usually caused by blunt trauma that knocks the brain against the skull. Movement of the brain relative to the skull tears the thin superior cerebral veins (the bridging veins), which drain the external cerebral veins into the superior sagittal sinus. Minor repeated injuries can cause chronic venous leakage.

Venous subdural hematomas expand more slowly than the higher pressure arterial epidural hematomas. Small, self-limited subdural hematomas are often absorbed spontaneously, but subdural hematomas can also continue to enlarge slowly without severe or clear-cut neurologic symptoms, especially in the elderly. An untreated subdural hematoma will lead to permanent severe neurologic deficits or death.

Subarachnoid and Intraparenchymal Hemorrhages. The remaining two classes of intracranial hemorrhages, subarachnoid bleeding and intraparenchymal bleeding, can be caused by trauma and can coexist with epidural and subdural bleeding. They can also happen without apparent external provocation.

Subarachnoid hemorrhages are caused by tears in the arteries running along the subarachnoid space at the surface of the brain. Ruptured arterial aneurysms are the most common source of subarachnoid bleeds. In the brain, these aneurysms usually occur at branch points of the large arteries, especially in the circle of Willis. A less common nontraumatic cause of subarachnoid bleeding is the rupture of a congenital arteriovenous malformation.

Cerebrospinal fluid (CSF) circulates through the subarachnoid space, and blood from a subarachnoid hemorrhage will spread quickly throughout the CSF surrounding the brain and spinal cord. In such cases, a lumbar puncture will produce CSF that contains red blood cells. Ruptures of arteries in the subarachnoid space cause a sudden increase in intracranial pressure and produce severe headache, vomiting, and drowsiness.

Sudden rises in cerebral blood pressure or cerebral blood flow can rupture intraparenchymal arteries, especially when the arteries have been weakened by chronic hypertension, aneurysms, or vascular malformations. Clotting disorders, low platelet counts, anticoagulant drugs, vasoconstrictors, and eclampsia during pregnancy increase the risk for intraparenchymal bleeds. Intraparenchymal hemorrhages most often develop from ruptures of arteries to the basal ganglia and the thalamus, although hematomas also form elsewhere in the cerebral lobes, the cerebellum, and the pons. The first neurologic symptoms of an intraparenchymal hemorrhage will reflect the specific location of the hematoma—for example, a basal ganglia hematoma pressing on the internal capsule will first cause contralateral motor weakness.

Clinical Presentation

Subjective

A CVA should be suspected when a patient presents with an acute onset of specific signs and symptoms. Patients presenting in the primary-care setting usually complain of weakness, numbness, or paralysis of one or both extremities on one side of the body. In addition, they usually complain of a severe headache. Impairment is seen in cognitive abilities, level of consciousness, speech, visual fields, extraocular muscle functioning, motor functioning, and gait. Cognitive changes that are exhibited by patients may indicate denial of the illness, neglect syndrome or hemiparesis, spatial and proprioceptive (awareness of body position in spaces) dysfunction, impairment of memory, judgment, problem-solving or decision-making abilities, and decreased ability to concentrate and attend to tasks. The patient may experience emotional lability, especially if the frontal lobe is involved. Aphasia, alexia (reading problems), and agraphia (difficulties in writing) may be apparent.

Objective

Information obtained during the history and physical examination assists in identifying the area of the brain involved, the etiology of the CVA, and in determining whether the CVA is hemorrhagic or ischemic. Aspects of the history that are relevant are the nature of the onset; the nature, timing, and duration of the neurologic deficit; and whether the deficit is static, improving, or worsening. It is important to specifically inquire about the patient's activity when the CVA began, how the symptoms progressed, the severity of the symptoms, and whether they have worsened, improved, or remained the same. Likely findings for ischemic CVAs caused by thrombus would show that symptoms began during the day, occurred gradually, and the patient had periods of improvement between episodes of worsening. On exam, no seizures are noted and the patient is awake but confused. Prodromal symptoms are those associated with a TIA. Deficits increase during the first few weeks. Likely symptoms are slight headache, speech deficits, and visual problems. Patients with CVAs caused by embolus typically reveal that their symptoms began during sleep, occurred abruptly, and have progressed steadily. The patient is awake.

Maximum neurologic deficits occur at the onset with paralysis and expressive aphasia. Symptoms with a hemorrhagic stroke commonly occur during the day with activity and are abrupt in onset, with level of consciousness possibly worsening after the initial onset. Other indicators are vomiting, seizures, severe headaches, coma, and focal deficits. Symptoms also associated with a CVA are seizures or syncope. The patient may complain of feeling "drowsy and dull." The foot on the affected side may be externally rotated, a frequent finding of hemiparesis.

It is important to determine if the symptoms are transient and last no longer than 1 hour, the typical pattern in TIAs. Most TIAs last less than 1 hour. Information can be obtained from the patient as the practitioner observes and interviews the patient for the first time. To assist in differentiating a TIA from a CVA, the patient should describe the event, what precipitated it, and the associated symptoms (vision loss, diplopia, paresthesia, aphasia), and how long the event lasted. Table 5.4 presents the different pathologies of TIAs, symptoms, and diagnostic tests.

Patients with carotid atherosclerotic disease are identified by the detection of a carotid bruit or through screening examinations. Detecting the presence of a bruit is significant. Not only does it indicate atherosclerosis and ischemic heart disease, but it may also increase the risk for a CVA. In caring for a patient with asymptomatic carotid bruit, the practitioner should begin with a thorough history for the presence of coronary and peripheral vascular occlusive disease. Most importantly is the identification and management of CVA risk factors. A flattened nasolabial fold and

Table 5.4 Pathologies of Transient Ischemic Attacks (TIAs)

Type of TIA	Signs and Symptoms	Physical Examination	Diagnostic Tests
Carotid Artery Pathology	Paresthesia Weakness of hand, arm, face Aphasia Dysarthria Unilateral neglect Transient blindness or blurred vision in one eye Cognitive/behavioral changes (rare)	Neurologic exam Assess for carotid bruits Assess for retinal emboli (refer for complete ophthalmologic exam) Assess for temporal artery tenderness	• Laboratory tests: CBC, platelets, electrolytes, ESR, ANA, syphilis serology, toxicology screen, coagulation studies (antiphosphid antibodies, PT/PTT, Russell's viper venom time for lupus anticoagulant) • CT scan of the head (10%–20% or patients with TIA have existing infarction) • MRI (more sensitive than CT) • Vascular evaluation: Doppler studies of temporal and carotid vessels, transcranial Doppler studies of intracranial vertebrobasilar system, magnetic resonance angiography • Echocardiography and Holter monitoring to R/O cardiac sources of emboli • Transesophageal echocardiography • LP
Small Cerebral Vessel Pathology	Motor hemiparesis Hemibody sensory loss or paresthesia	As above	As above
Vertebrobasilar System Pathology	Ataxia Dizziness, vertigo Dysarthria Confusion Diplopia, hemianopia, or bilateral vision loss Unilateral or bilateral sensory or motor systems (rare)	As above	As above

widened palpebral tissue on the same side as the hemiparesis raises the suspicion of a supratentorial lesion. The patient may be confused, agitated, or unresponsive. Difficulties may be noted in speech and cognitive abilities as well as an increased incidence of incontinence. The practitioner should inquire about a history of similar dysfunctions, especially within the last 2 weeks, or coexistence of cardiovascular diseases, such as hypertension, coronary artery disease (CAD), cardiac valvular disorders, atrial fibrillation, recent MI, or related disorders, such as coagulation and bleeding disorders or diabetes mellitus. A list of current medications should be obtained, including prescribed, OTC, and recreational (illicit) drugs. The practitioner should be attentive to the use of anticoagulants, aspirin, vasodilator, and illegal drugs, which may provide clues to the cause of the stroke or affect treatment. To complete the history, data should be obtained regarding stroke risk factors, both modifiable and nonmodifiable, with particular focus on gender, ethnic origin, age, familial history, lifestyle (obesity, physical activity, diet), and use of alcohol or cigarettes.

Assessment of visual fields may identify deficits such as horizontal defect, blindness, bitemporal hemianopsia, homonymous hemianopsia, or homonymous quadrant defect. A review of the cranial nerves may indicate difficulties with chewing (nerve V), facial paralysis or paresis (nerve VII), dysphagia (nerves IX and X), an absent gag reflex (nerve IX), or impaired tongue movement (nerve XII).

The degree of infarction following a CVA varies depending on the severity of the reduction in blood flow, the duration of ischemia, and the adequacy of cerebral circulation.

Signs and symptoms exhibited by the patient may be localized to a particular area of the brain (see Table 5.5).

Bruits become audible when the distal lumen is narrowed to approximately 3 mm or less (about 50 percent stenosis). The higher the pitch of the bruit, the higher the degree of stenosis. A high-pitched bruit that fades into diastole indicates a hemodynamically important stenosis of the proximal internal carotid artery (ICA) with a residual lumen of less than 1.5 mm (75 percent stenosis or more). The atherosclerotic plaque commonly forms at the origin of the ICA and at the posterior aspect of the bifurcation of the carotid. The plaque narrows the lumen in a concentric fashion. Occasionally, a thrombus may form near this restricted lumen or blood may penetrate the plaque, creating an ulcer that becomes the source of formation of a thrombus.

Diagnostic Reasoning

Diagnostic Tests

The initial assessment of the patient with a possible CVA should include a CBC with platelet count, prothrombin time (PT)/partial thromboplastin time (PTT), electrolytes, blood urea nitrogen (BUN), creatinine, glucose, calcium, magnesium, sedimentation rate, ECG, and chest x-ray study.

Table 5.5 Signs and Symptoms of Occlusion of Specific Areas of the Brain

Specific Areas	Part of Brain Supplies	Signs and Symptoms of Occlusion
Internal carotid artery (carotid system)	Anterior cerebral surfaces (2/5 of CBF)	Unilateral sensory and motor disturbances Hemiparesis, numbness, or paresthesia Visual disturbances (mononuclear blindness [amaurosis fugax], complete unilateral blindness or homonymous hemianopsia) Aphasia with left-sided lesions
Branches from subclavian into vertebral and basilar arteries (vertebrobasilar system)	Posterior cerebral surfaces (1/5 of CBF)	Ipsilateral visual field deficits Contralateral hemiplegia Bilateral motor, sensory, and visual complaints Vertigo Diplopia Dysphagia
Vertebral arteries	Parts of medulla	Contralateral impairment of pain and temperature sensation Ipsilateral Horner's syndrome (sunken eyeball, ptosis of upper eyelid, slight elevation of lower lid, constriction of pupil, narrowing of palpebral fissure, anhidrosis) Dysphagia Vertigo
Basilar artery branches	Occipital and temporal lobes, dorsal surface of thalamus, upper part of cerebellum, midbrain	Limb paralysis Nystagmus Vertigo Nausea Slurred speech Cerebellar ataxia

A decreased platelet count and prolonged PT/PTT may indicate a bleeding disorder or use of anticoagulants, respectively, leading to a hemorrhagic stroke. Elevated blood glucose levels are sometimes seen in patients with hemorrhagic strokes. An elevated glucose level may be found in patients with diabetes mellitus, a contributing factor toward the development of atherosclerosis. An ECG will detect the presence of a recent MI, atrial fibrillation, or left ventricular hypertrophy, risk factors increasing the probability of a CVA. Left ventricular hypertrophy may be seen on a chest x-ray film. In addition, a high platelet count (>1 million) leads to hypercoagulability, contributing to the development of a thrombus. A hematocrit (Hct) greater than 60 causes increased viscosity, resulting in decreased perfusion, and can contribute to cerebral ischemia.

Practice guidelines of the American Heart Association Stroke Council recommend the use of noncontrast CT of the head in patients with suspected acute CVA to exclude a nonvascular lesion as the case of the manifestations and determine whether the CVA is an ischemic infarction or an intracranial hemorrhage. It is also recommended for early evaluation of young adults with acute CVA.

MRI is generally recommended for patients with CVAs because it is more sensitive than CT for identifying small ischemic lesions. It also can identify hemorrhagic features, including mass effect. Echoplanar MRI defusion and perfusion MRI may document changes within minutes, whereas conventional high-field MRI shows changes in 90 percent of patients after 24 hours. The changes produce increased signals in T2-weighted sequences, indicating the presence of an intraluminal clot. Other signs consist of an absence of flow void in the intracranial arteries, suggestive of occlusion. These signs can be detected almost immediately after onset. Hemorrhage can be detected through high-signal changes in T1-weighted sequences. There is no consensus regarding a method to measure the degree of stenosis from x-ray exams because of the difficulty involved with differentiating one type of lesion from the other (e.g., an atherosclerotic plaque from a thrombus or artery occlusion). Angiography is considered the test of choice. Magnetic resonance angiography (MRA), color duplex ultrasound, and transcranial Doppler (TCD) are acceptable, noninvasive techniques to screen patients with suspected lesions.

Ideally, a neurologic consultation should also be available within 30 minutes of the patient's arrival. In the practitioner's physical and neurologic examination and management of the CVA, the time at onset of symptoms is particularly important to determine the proper use of thrombolytic therapy. It is strongly recommended that emergency CT be the initial brain imaging study for the emergency evaluation of a suspected ischemic CVA. Other important information can be obtained from laboratory tests, including CBC, blood chemistry, and coagulation profiles; pulse oximetry; and cranial CT scan without contrast. Other imaging techniques or ultrasonography can help with diagnosis, but not if treatment might be delayed. Laboratory data are used to guide intervention as well as to determine the etiology of the CVA.

Ischemic CVA caused by embolus has a high incidence in pregnant women. In these women, there are no specific imaging recommendations other than those related to radiation precautions. There is a potential risk of radiation-induced defects during the first trimester, when the patient may be unaware of pregnancy. Detection of an acute ischemic CVA by CT depends on the location and extent of the infarct. Large infarcts are often not documented until 3 hours after onset, but nearly 60 percent can be detected by 24 hours and 100 percent by 7 days. In hemorrhagic stroke, the CT demonstrates an irregularly hyperdense, "mottled" infarct. These signs, though subtle, can be seen within 5 hours of onset of symptoms. The most common early signs are anatomic changes, an "obsuration" of the lentiform nucleus, and especially the loss of the "insular ribbon."

In hemorrhagic CVAs, an early mass effect in cerebral or cerebella infarcts can be detected on CT within hours from onset. These effects develop before the hypodensity and are indicative of massive infarction. Calcified or hyperdense, cordlike areas in a major artery are suggestive of embolic CVAs. The use of CT with contrast for the evaluation of acute stroke is controversial and does not increase the yield. A concern exists over promoting cerebral "toxicity" when the blood-brain barrier has been disturbed in large infarcts.

An ESR may be warranted in cases of unexplained CVA. If anemia is present and the history suggests ethnic or genetic predisposition to thrombosis, a hemoglobin electrophoresis may be performed. An LP may be an additional test indicated to confirm a diagnosis of subarachnoid hemorrhage if blood is detected in the CSF when the CT is negative. Contraindications to this procedure include papilledema, thrombocytopenia, coagulation disorders, and focal neurologic deficit. When common risk factors are not evident, an immune electrophoresis or fibrinogen level may be obtained. Since increased fibrinogen levels appear in early CVAs, as well as increased viscosity, this particular test can help to confirm the diagnosis. All other tests should exhibit normal findings. No laboratory test will definitively confirm the diagnosis of a CVA.

Though it is not meant to be used as a screening tool for CVA, panoramic radiography can also identify asymptomatic patients with carotid calcifications, also revealing a significant correlation with obesity.

Differential Diagnosis

CT scanning and MRI assist in the differential diagnosis of CVA. A subarachnoid hemorrhage may present with a severe headache of abrupt onset with a decreased level of consciousness. In subdural hematoma, headache is the single most common symptom and is more common in older adults; however, the headache is generalized and often bitemporal. Neurologic signs are usually not present for a long period of time. In most patients with a brain abscess a headache is present, as well as neurologic signs of altered level of consciousness and focal deficit, most often hemiparesis. Nausea and vomiting are frequent, along with a fever. Idiopathic intracranial hypertension (pseudotumor) shows symptoms of papilledema and diplopia, along with a headache and normal CT scan. Transient visual symptoms are present. Headache is present in most patients with brain tumor, along with seizures, weakness, and subtle cognitive changes; however, vomiting and papilledema may be present. No focal neurologic signs are seen.

Arterial dissection, although occurring frequently in young adults, has an extremely important symptom of cephalic pain or headache of sudden onset, often preceding retinal or hemispheric ischemic symptoms. Carotid dissection appears initially with occipital headache or acute neck pain and is followed by ischemic symptoms of diplopia, syncope, and amaurosis fugex. Unilateral neck pain that is sudden and radiates to the ipsilateral face or eye is usually present. The headache is related to cervical manipulation, sustained exertion, or trauma. A symptom of new onset, progressive headache appears as a major feature in temporal arteritis with some cranial symptoms of diplopia and mental sluggishness. Other symptoms are local swelling; tenderness and pulselessness of the temporal artery; and systemic symptoms of fever, anorexia, weight loss, and chills. Systemic markers of inflammation also are present. Because a headache occurs commonly in cerebral venous thrombosis and often is the only initial symptom, cerebral venous thrombosis can be differentiated easily from a CVA. No neurologic deficits are seen, and it usually occurs in isolation. Common causes associated with this type of thrombosis are pregnancy and oral contraceptive use. In meningeal irritation, headache is often the most prominent feature, along with lethargy. Encephalitis is associated with a generalized headache of rapid onset, particularly when it is accompanied by confusion, altered level of consciousness, focal neurologic signs, or seizures. Fever, meningism, and signs of myalgia and fatigue are present. Changes associated with these conditions can be detected by either CT or MRI. In addition, a hemorrhagic CVA can be identified via CT, thus differentiating it from an ischemic CVA. Initial diagnostic studies should also rule out other conditions that can masquerade as a CVA (e.g., recent seizures, delirium, syncope, intoxication, suicide attempts, conversion disorders, and possible recent cocaine or amphetamine use).

Management

The main principle in the management of CVAs today is CVA prevention and early recognition and treatment. Much remains to be done in order for CVAs to be recognized and managed as a medical emergency.

Patients with symptoms of a possible stroke require immediate referral to a physician for evaluation, CT scanning of the brain, and possible use of thrombolytic therapy. In patients with a cardioembolic source of stroke, a referral to a neurologist is recommended for hospitalization and consideration of the use of heparin anticoagulant therapy. Patients with a high-grade carotid artery stenosis ipsilateral to the side of a TIA should also be considered for hospitalization and may benefit from carotid endarterectomy if they are good surgical candidates or from anticoagulant therapy if they are not. An emergency neurosurgical consult is indicated in the presence of an intracranial lesion, caused by hemorrhage, mass effect, or an increase in intracranial pressure. Patients experiencing TIAs with negative echocardiograms and carotid Doppler ultrasounds and no other need for hospitalization may be discharged from the emergency department (ED) and referred to a physician for further evaluation as an outpatient.

Initial management of a CVA is focused on maintaining adequate tissue oxygenation. Anaerobic metabolism with depletion of energy stores can increase the extent of brain injury and worsen the outcome. In the prehospital setting, special attention is given to monitoring of the patient's oxygen status through pulse oximetry and the use of supplemental oxygen as needed. Intubation and mechanical ventilation are initiated when there is decreased level of consciousness. An adequate airway is maintained. Hypotension is treated to maximize CBF and minimize complications. Hypertension, on the other hand, is not treated in the prehospital setting because the lowering of BP may exacerbate hypoperfusion and injury. Prehospital evaluation and transport time account for significant delays in initiation of thrombolytic therapy for patients with acute CVA who require it. Aggressive CVA protocols and educational programs keyed to emergency medical services can markedly reduce the time from CVA onset to initiation of treatment.

Once the clinical presentation, the laboratory data, and the results of the CT scan are completed, if they point to a diagnosing of acute ischemic stroke, thrombolytic agents must be considered. The patient and/or family should understand that thrombolytic therapy carries at least a 6.4 percent risk of intracerebral hemorrhage. Intravenous thrombolytic therapy is effective in reducing the neurologic deficit in some patients without CT evidence of intracranial hemorrhage if administered within 3 hours after the onset of an ischemic stroke. A cerebral hemorrhage is a contraindication of this therapy.

It would be important for the practitioner to treat and reduce sources of fever, which can accompany an infectious complication of a CVA, with antibiotics and antipyretics; to prevent recurrent seizures with anticonvulsants; and to prophylactically administer heparin, low-molecular-weight heparin or heparinoids to prevent deep vein thrombosis. The use of corticosteroids is not indicated in the management of cerebral edema and increased intracranial pressure due to CVA.

Once a patient's condition has deteriorated, including development of a herniation syndrome as a result of increased intracranial pressure, osmotherapy and hyperventilation are used. Surgery is indicated to decompress and evacuate a large cerebellar infarction that compresses the brain stem, although survivors may have severe residual neurologic deficits. Early ambulation with preventative measures against aspiration, malnutrition, pneumonia, deep vein thrombosis, pulmonary embolism, decubitus ulcers, contracture, and joint abnormalities are important goals in managing the patient with a CVA.

Although heparin is the drug most commonly prescribed following an ischemic CVA, most clinicians wait for 2 to 3 days after the attack thereby verifying with a repeat CT that the stroke was not hemorrhagic in nature. Certain patients with TIAs may benefit from hospitalization and IV heparin because of an increased risk of a CVA. Included are patients with at least four TIAs within 2 weeks before presentation, TIAs with a probable cardioembolic source, crescendo immediate effect on TIAs, severe deficits, and anterior circulation deficits with high-grade stenosis. Aspirin, with its platelet aggregation at doses of 325 mg, is very useful in acute CVA (once a hemorrhagic CVA has been ruled out).

One of the most significant approaches to the medical management of patients with CAD with respect to CVA risk reduction has been the use of antiplatelet drugs, principally acetylsalicylic acid (ASA). Ticlopidine (Ticlid), have shown some improvement over the effects of ASA. Combination therapies, such as ASA plus dipyridamole (Persantine), are no better than ASA alone. The optimal dose of ASA is as follows: thromboembolic disorders: 325 to 650 mg once or twice daily; TIA prophylaxis—650 mg bid, and for MI prophylaxis—81 to 325 mg/day. This is very controversial and clinicians disagree as to whether high or low doses are efficacious. Clopidogrel (Plavix), 75 mg daily may be used in patients with TIAs to reduce the likelihood of thrombosis and microemboli who are scheduled for elective surgery.

Although ticlonipine (Ticlid) is more effective than ASA in decreasing the risk of CVA, the cost and adverse effects are higher. Studies have shown adverse effects such as rash or diarrhea, and thus poor patient compliance. Neutropenia has been known to occur between 3 weeks and 1 month after starting treatment. CBCs should be monitored every 2 weeks for the first 3 months, with therapy continuing for a period of no longer than 6 months.

The recommended dosage for ticlonipine is 250 mg bid. Because a significant portion of patients with carotid artery disease have concomitant CAD, serum cholesterol in patients with CAD should be evaluated and treated. The hydroxymethylglutaryl-coenzyme A (HMG-CoA) reductase inhibitors, or statins, reduce the risk of nonfatal and fatal CVAs, demonstrating a significant protective effect similar to that conferred by antiplatelet agents.

Follow-Up and Referral

Follow-up and rehabilitation focus on the return of the patient's optimum level of functioning. The patient may be assessed for the potential for rehabilitation and transferred to a rehabilitation unit. The rehabilitation process involves six major areas of focus: (1) preventing, recognizing, and managing comorbid illness and medical complications; (2) training for maximum independence; (3) facilitating psychosocial coping and adaptation by the patient and family; (4) preventing secondary disability by promoting community reintegration, including resumption of home, family, and vocational activities; (5) enhancing quality of life in view of residual disability; and (6) preventing recurrent CVAs and other vascular conditions, such as MI, that occur with increased frequency in patients with CVAs.

Patient Education

Adjustments may need to be made in the home environment before discharge, such as building a ramp or removing a door to accommodate a wheelchair. Specific areas of teaching involve exercise and ambulation techniques, dietary requirements, recognition of symptoms of another CVA, and an understanding of the emotional lability and depression that commonly accompany a CVA. Also important are knowledge of appropriate use of medications as well as the time, place, and frequency of occupational and physical therapy activities. To help prevent caregivers at home from becoming overburdened and thus ill themselves, clinicians should teach caregivers to plan for respite or time away from caregiving activities on a regular basis. Information regarding community, state, and national resources can be a welcome source of support to patients and their families. The National Stroke Association has resource information, including referral services as well as a quarterly newsletter. The American Heart Association provides a large variety of information regarding risk factors and referrals for assistive devices. The Easter Seal Society also may provide assistance with wheelchairs or other assistive devices. Additional listings of resources for the patient and the practitioner appear at the end of the chapter. Some communities have organizations to help with meals or transportation, along with self-help groups. Education regarding the modification and reduction of risk factors plays a significant role toward the reduction in the incidence of CVAs and TIAs. The most relevant risk factors are the control of hypertension, the use of ASA for prophylaxis in patients with a moderate to high risk of CVA or TIA, and the use of anticoagulants in patients with atrial fibrillation. In a summary of 17 treatment trials of hypertension throughout the world with nearly 50,000 patients, there was a 38 percent decrease in all strokes and a 40 percent decrease in fatal CVAs after treatment of hypertension. In the Framingham study, smoking cessation promptly reduced the risk of a CVA, with the major risk reduced within 2 to 4 years. Heavy use of alcohol also should be avoided. Moderate and heavy levels of physical activity have been associated with a decrease in chronic incidence of CVA. The physical activity is believed to exert a beneficial influence on the risk factors for atherosclerotic disease by decreasing BP, weight, and pulse rate; raising high-density lipoprotein (HDL) cholesterol and lowering low-density lipoprotein (LDL) cholesterol; decreasing platelet aggregability; increasing insulin sensitivity and improving glucose tolerance; and promoting a lifestyle conducive to changing diet and promoting a cessation of cigarette smoking. A diet low in fat, sodium, and cholesterol and high in fiber, fruits, and vegetables should be encouraged. Patients should also be encouraged to exercise modestly, to avoid weight gain, and to use stress reduction techniques. If the patient has atrial fibrillation, anticoagulant therapy should be initiated to prevent pooling of the blood in the atria that could promote potential microemboli.

Because treatment within 3 hours of onset of a stroke is critical, successful treatment depends on educating the patient and the family to recognize CVA symptoms and to contact and secure access to medical care by calling 911. Delay in treatment has been known to occur for patients who call their primary-care physician instead of 911, live alone, have onset of CVA while asleep, have onset at home rather than work, and who experience a milder severity of a CVA. Studies have documented that 38 percent of patients and their families did not know a single warning sign of a CVA and 28 percent could identify only one sign of seizures. Thus, mild tingling or numbness of the fingers or mild gait clumsiness is attributed to a problem with the arm or leg. Patients may also feel they have dust in their eyes, when in fact, they are experiencing amaurosis fugax. Patients may think such symptoms are trivial and may not seek attention, or if they do, they may not mention those symptoms to their practitioner. Older adults may simply forget that any symptoms occurred.

Education of the patient and family should include the importance of reporting any symptoms of graying, darkening, or fogging of vision; a shadow coming over the visual field; or a sudden decrease in vision. In addition, patient and family should be instructed to notify the practitioner if any episodes of peripheral numbness, tingling, or clumsiness in the upper or lower extremities (e.g., leg giving way suddenly or being weak for a short period of time) occur. Thorough teaching high-risk patients and their families of the warning signs of a CVA, along with frequent evaluation and a careful review of symptoms by the practitioner, will assist in detecting symptomatic carotid artery stenosis and initiating treatment as soon as possible.

Headaches

Headaches are a pain or ache in the head, sometimes restricting activity, reducing the level of functioning, and decreasing work performance. The prevalence of headaches greatly impacts society because of lost or reduced effec tiveness at home, work, or school. Individual burdens result from pain, suffering, and the disabling effects of various headache syndromes. It remains difficult to gain a measure of control over headaches. Headaches pose a challenge to the practitioner to avoid underestimating their significance as an early manifestation of serious neurologic disease.

Headaches may be classified into four general categories: muscle contraction headaches (tension); vascular headaches (migraines and cluster headaches); mixed headaches (a combination of muscle contraction and vascular); and traction or inflammatory headaches. A *tension headache* presents as a mild to moderate bilateral, nonpulsating, tightening pain that is not aggravated by routine physical activity. It is usually not accompanied by nausea and vomiting or photophobia. A *migraine headache* may last for 4 to 72 hours and may or may not be precipitated by an aura. It is usually of moderate to severe intensity with a pulsating quality, aggravated by routine physical activity, and accompanied by nausea, vomiting, and photophobia. A *cluster headache* usually occurs at night and may last from 15 to 180 minutes. There is usually severe unilateral orbital, supraorbital, and/or temporal pain that is accompanied on the same side of the face with sweating, lacrimation, nasal congestion, ptosis, rhinorrhea, eyelid edema, and/or conjunctival injection. A *traction or inflammatory headache* is an acute new-onset headache that has an increasing intensity; this type of headache is a medical emergency. Table 5.6 presents a comparison of the four categories of headaches.

Epidemiology and Causes

Headache is one of the most common symptoms people experience, affecting anyone of any age. In the United States, some researchers estimate the annual cost, including costs of direct medical care and lost productivity to exceed $17 billion. More than 18 million Americans of all ages visit a health-care provider with complaints of headaches annually, with the incidence decreasing with age. Headaches affect women two to three times more than men across all age groups, with its incidence in women increasing during adolescence and peaking at menarche.

Muscular traction or a tension-type headache is a highly prevalent condition that can be disabling. It is found more often in women (86 percent) than men (65 percent). Its prevalence peaks at about age 30 to 38. It occurs more frequently in whites (40.1 percent), especially with increasing educational levels (48 percent). Although few people who suffer tension-type headaches lose time from work, more than 40 percent of people affected reported decreased effectiveness at work, home, or school because of this type of headache.

Eighteen percent of women and six pecent of men are affected by migraine headaches. During the reproductive years, 25 percent of women have migraine headaches. Racial differences in migraine prevalence are striking: African-Americans and nonwhites of Hispanic or other nonspecified ethnic origin are at least twice as likely as whites or Asians to be migraine sufferers. An inverse relationship exists between migraine and age. Prevalence of migraine is

Table 5.6 **Headaches: A Comparison of the Different Types**

Type	Muscle Contraction (Tension)	Vascular (Migraine, Cluster)	Mixed	Traction or Inflammatory (Acute Headache)
Signs and symptoms	Nausea and vomiting Bilateral throbbing pain	**Migraine:** Unilateral pulsating episodic pain Nausea and vomiting Photophobia Confusion Disorientation **Cluster** (associated with alcohol use): Periorbital night-time unilateral nonpulsatile pain Photophobia Tearing Nasal stuffiness	Combination of muscular and vascular headache	New onset Usually older than age 35 Acute, constant, progressive pain that prevents sleep "Worst headache of my life"
History and physical examination findings	Sleep cycle Disturbances Depression Appetite changes Relationship Difficulties Recent or remote memory loss Limited neck ROM with crepitus	May be similar	May be similar	Acute onset
Diagnostic tests	MRI: lesions, trauma, hematomas CT: hemorrhage LP: to determine presence of organisms	Same	Same	Same
Treatment	Support Biofeedback Stress management Drugs: aspirin, acetaminophen (Tylenol), NSAIDs, muscle relaxants Preventive treatment	**Migraine:** Avoidance education Drugs: beta-blockers, ergot alkaloids, NSAIDs, antiemetics, selective serotonin receptor agonists (sumatriptin [Imitrex]), tricyclic antidepressant (amitriptyline) **Cluster:** 100% oxygen by mask Drugs: inhaled ergotamine Preventive treatment (propranolol, amitriptyline, valproate, or lithium)	Combined approach of counseling, migraine prevention, drugs, antidepressants, and stress reduction	Refer to neurosurgeon

highest in adults younger than age 40 and lowest in those older than age 60. Migraine headaches occur in 4 to 5 percent of school-age children. It is not unusual for migraine headaches to begin during childhood. Migraine syndromes are painful and often disabling, accounting for a loss of more than 157 million workdays to headache pain each year. In one study of patients who met the International Headache Society criteria for migraine, fewer than half had actually received a diagnosis of migraine.

Migraine headaches are often hereditary and can be traced to hormonal shifts in women. In familial migraine headaches, the cause is associated with mutations in calcium-channel genes. The causes of menstrual migraine are explained by hormonal fluctuations either before, during, or after menstruation. Falling estrogen levels can trigger a migraine that is either endogenously or exogenously induced (e.g., by a week-off [21-day] oral contraceptive pill or by hormonal replacement therapy). There are multiple and varied precipitating factors or "triggers" of migraine headaches. A migraine headache may occur shortly after or just before a period of stress. One type of migraine sometimes known as an exertional migraine is associated with strenuous physical activity, but in general, women who regularly exercise are less likely to get migraines or at least experience them with less severity. Some sports, however, may actually precipitate a headache, resulting in common phrases, such as "swimmer's migraine" or "runner's headache." Weight lifting, cycling, and hockey have been identified as other possible culprits. Researchers believe that the relationship between exercise and sports activities and migraine is associated with increased pressure on the head or a strained neck muscle. Physical activity at high altitudes is another factor that may trigger a migraine between 6 hours and 4 days after arrival. Other factors associated with exercise may be an inadequate warmup or dehydration. Certain foods containing tyramine or phenylethylamine are known triggers of migraine. These vasoactive substances cause both vasodilation and vasoconstriction of the cerebral vessels. Examples of vasodilator agents include alcohol and sodium nitrate. Sodium nitrate is used as a preservative and is present in processed meats and food coloring. Vasoconstrictor agents, on the other hand, stimulate the release of noradrenalin and adrenalin, causing vascular constriction of the cerebral vessels. Caffeine is known to cause a headache after six cups of coffee are consumed. Although consuming smaller amounts of coffee may protect a person from a headache, sudden caffeine withdrawal may trigger a migraine as a result of rebound vasodilation. MSG (monosodium glutamate) can also produce a migraine. Table 5.7 presents common triggers of migraine headaches.

Cluster headaches, another form of vascular headaches, are named for their particular pattern of occurrence: They usually come in groups over the span of several weeks or months, then disappear for months or even years. They occur in middle-aged men and typically cluster on a seasonal basis, with anywhere from 3 to 18 months between headaches. A dysfunction of the hypothalamus may account for the periodicity and clocklike regularity of cluster headaches.

Older adults have fewer headaches overall. Unfortunately, about a third of those that occur are traction or inflammatory headaches that are secondary to systemic disease or primary intracranial lesions such as subarachnoid hemorrhages resulting from AVM or intracranial aneurysms. Other causes may be temporal arteritis and subdural hematoma.

Temporal arteritis affects men equally with women and predominantly occurs in adults older than age 60. Its incidence increases with age and is rare in the young. The headache from a subdural hematoma is of venous origin, typically resulting from a head injury that is usually mild and easily forgotten by the patient. It predominantly occurs in persons older than age 50 and is more common in men. The abuse of alcohol and use of anticoagulants contribute to its occurrence. It rarely is associated with a fractured skull.

The headache from subarachnoid hemorrhage commonly occurs from a ruptured intracranial aneurysm, such as a "berry" aneurysm or dissecting arterial aneurysm of the carotid or vertebral vessels. A berry aneurysm, or berry-shaped aneurysm, results from a congenital abnormality of intracranial vessels, primarily at the circle of Willis. Ruptured intracranial aneurysms are the primary cause of hemorrhagic stroke. Less often, a subarachnoid hemorrhage is caused by an AVM or bleeding disorder. An AVM is a congenital disorder that results in the formation of a tangled collection of dilated arteries and veins. Symptoms are usually seen in persons between 20 and 40 years of age. Two-thirds of people affected by a subarachnoid hemorrhage are between the ages of 40 and 60; women are affected slightly more frequently because of the higher incidence of hypertension among women. In the United States, 10 to 15 cases occur per 100,000 population per year. Activities such as lifting, straining, intercourse, or emotional excitement can precipitate a hemorrhage. However, subarachnoid hemorrhage has been known to occur during sleep.

Table 5.7 Common Triggers of Migraine Headaches

Hormonal
- Low estrogen level, increased prostaglandin level

Environmental
- High-pitched noises, excessive sun, bright lights, weather changes, strong odors, video display terminals

Diet
- Vasodilating agents: alcohol, sodium nitrate
- Vasoconstricting agents: caffeine, tyramine (bananas, ripe cheese, nuts, pods of broad beans [Italian pole, lima, or butter beans]), chicken livers, yogurt, avocado, sour cream

Phenylethylamine
- Some cheeses, red wine, chocolate

MSG
- Chinese food, canned soups, frozen dinners

Artificial sweeteners

Lifestyle
- Stress, sports, swimming, cycling, hockey, weight lifting, running, inadequate warmups

Physical activity at high altitudes
- Cycling, climbing, skiing

Fatigue

Changes in sleep schedule
- Excessive sleep, too little sleep

Cigarette Smoking

Dehydration

Primary Headache Syndromes

Pathophysiology

Head Pain. Inside the skull, only certain structures are sensitive to pain; these include the fold of dura between the cerebral hemispheres (the falx cerebri), the middle meningeal artery of the dura, the dural venous sinuses, and the extraparenchymal regions of the larger pial arteries. Increased pressure on and inflammation of the meninges will cause pain, and distention of or traction on the arteries will cause pain. Head trauma usually causes headaches through all these pain-inducing mechanisms.

Besides head trauma, many other medical problems can initiate a headache secondarily—cerebrovascular accidents (hematomas, hemorrhages, and thrombi); intracranial infections, tumors; metabolic disorders (hypercapnia, hypoglycemia, and hypoxia); sudden hypertension; changes in intracranial pressure; drugs and drug withdrawals; cranial nerve pain; and eye, ear, nose, sinus, teeth, and jaw disorders. On the other hand, in certain disorders headaches are considered to be the primary problem. The three primary headache syndromes are chronic tension-type headaches, migraine headaches, and cluster headaches.

Pain signals are transmitted from most structures in the head by branches of the trigeminal nerve (Fig. 5.2), although pain from the back of the head and the posterior fossa of the skull are transmitted by branches of the first three cervical spinal nerves. First order pain fibers from these nerves synapse in the brain stem and upper spinal cord, and from there, the second-order pain fibers project to sensory nuclei in the thalamus. Regardless of its cause, headache pain is the result of activating these trigemino-thalamic and cervico-thalamic pain circuits.

The primary headache syndromes, however, are not caused simply by the normal activation of trigeminal or cervical pain receptors inside the skull. Instead, primary headache syndromes require hypersensitization of the trigemino-thalamic or cervico-thalamic circuitry at one or more points along their route from the primary afferent axons to the thalamic sensory nuclei.

One part of this circuitry on which many headache studies have focused is the thalamus. When pain stimuli pass through the thalamus, the signals are modulated by serotonergic axons coming from the dorsal raphe nuclei in the midbrain. It is thought that an abnormal reduction in serotonergic activity in the thalamus is a part of the hypersensitization in primary headache syndromes. Among the observations consistent with this idea are:

- ▲ Serotonin agonists (ergotamine, dihydroergotamine, and triptans) can reduce the pain and frequency of migraines and can reduce the duration and frequency of cluster headaches.
- ▲ Increasing the effectiveness of serotonergic synapses with a selective serotonin reuptake inhibitor can reduce the frequency of tension-type headaches.
- ▲ Reserpine, a drug that depletes CNS synapses of serotonin, can precipitate migraine headaches.

Chronic Tension-Type Headaches. Chronic tension-type headaches produce mild to moderate pain that feels like a constant, bilateral head tightness and that lasts from a half hour to a week. These headaches do not pulsate, do not cause nausea, and usually are not made worse by physical activity. Chronic tension-type headaches happen repeatedly (typically many times a month), they come on gradually during the day, and they are more common in people with depression.

Although patients with chronic tension-type headaches have muscle tenderness, their headaches seem not to be caused by unusual muscle tension or contraction. Instead, in patients with this type of primary headache, the

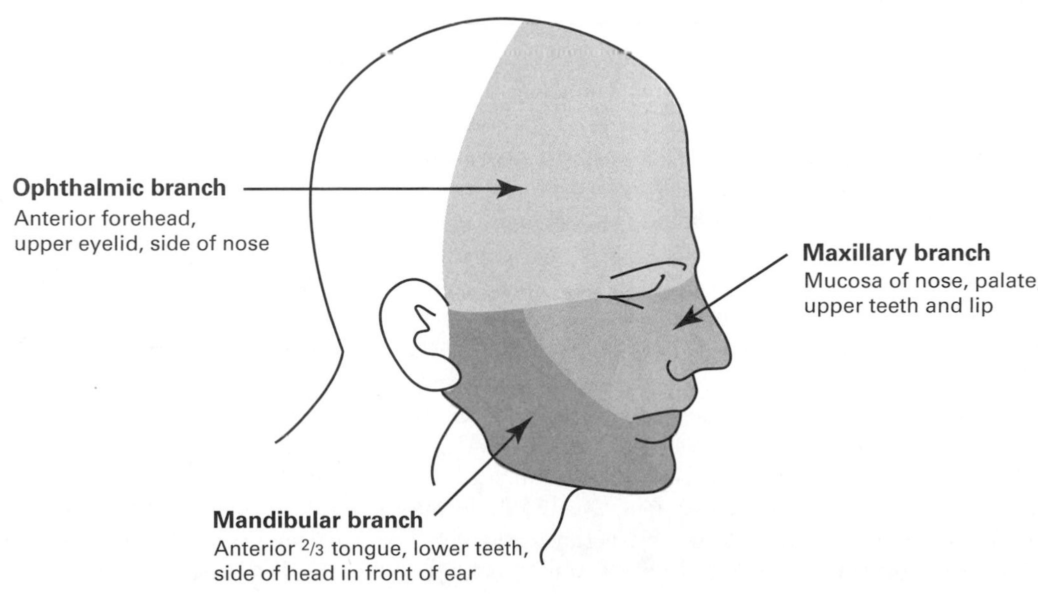

FIGURE 5.2 The three branches of the trigeminal nerve.

head and neck pain circuitry is hypersensitized, so that normal stimuli and typical muscle strains lead to headaches. The basic cause of the hypersensitization is not known, although it is thought that chronic tension-type headaches result from abnormalities in the serotonin, norepinephrine, or dopamine pathways that originate in the brain stem and that modulate the trigemino-thalamic or cervico-thalamic pain circuits.

Migraine Headaches. Migraine headaches produce moderate to severe unilateral pain lasting from four hours to three days. These headaches throb, cause nausea, and are made worse by activity. Migraine headaches happen repeatedly (typically one to three times per month) and can be triggered by certain stimuli, most commonly alcohol, stress, menstruation, or diet.

Migraine headaches come as a set of events that unfold in a predictable pattern. First there is a prodrome, which begins hours or days before the headache. The prodrome is a often a psychological change—it can be drowsiness, depression, euphoria, hyperactivity, difficulty concentrating, irritability, or increased sensitivity to noises, lights, or smells. The prodrome is thought to reflect disturbances in the hypothalamic-limbic system.

Patients with the most common type of migraine then develop a unilateral throbbing headache, which is accompanied by anorexia and nausea (with vomiting in a third of the cases) and by a heightened sensitivity to noises, lights, and smells. The basis for the pain is a hypersensitized trigemino-thalamic circuit, which makes the normally innocuous pulsing of cerebral blood flow feel painful. The hypersensitivity can carry over to all trigeminal nerve stimuli on the same side of the head, so that normal pressures (caused by, e.g., combing, shaving, taking a shower, or wearing glasses or earrings) on the skin of the face and scalp also feel painful.

In an experimental model, migraine-like headaches can be initiated by electrical stimulation of areas in the midbrain. In this region, focal stimuli set off a cascade of specific reactions including an increase in local blood flow and a hypersensitization of the trigemino-thalamic pain circuits.

In a less common type of migraine (classic migraine), the headache is preceded by sensory phenomena called an aura. An aura is usually either a set of patterns in the visual fields or a sequence of strange feelings moving from the hand, up the arm, and onto the face. The aura coincides with a slowly spreading wave of chemical and metabolic changes that moves across the cerebral cortex from initial foci in the occipital lobe(s). As the wave reaches a region, it briefly activates the local neurons and increases the local blood flow. After the wave passes, it leaves the neurons refractory and the local blood flow decreased. It is thought that this wave contributes to the hypersensitization of the trigemino-thalamic circuits and that the wave also elicits the headache pain that follows the aura. Experimentally, it has been found that drugs that reduce migraine headaches (specifically, the adrenergic agonist norepinephrine, the α_2-agonists yohimbine and clonidine, and the β-blocker propranolol) also stop or slow this wave of cortical depression.

Like epilepsy sufferers, patients with migraine headaches have cortical neurons that are permanently hyperexcitable. Even between migraine attacks, migraine patients experience other headaches with unusual frequency, and they can get headaches and perceptual distortions from minor visual stresses such as patterns of glare. The neuronal hyperexcitability underlying this continuous sensitivity can be inherited, and there are indications that it is due to abnormalities in certain ion channels in nerve cell membranes.

Cluster Headaches. Cluster headaches give severe unilateral pain behind the eye or temple lasting from a half hour to longer than an hour. The pain is constant, deep, and piercing and can radiate to the forehead, neck, or shoulder. These headaches do not pulsate, do not cause nausea, and usually are not made worse by physical activity. Together with the pain, there are eye or nose symptoms, such as tearing, swollen conjunctivae, runny nose, nasal congestion, eyelid droop, eyelid edema, facial sweating, or pupillary constriction. Cluster headaches come in groups that last 2 to 3 months. During one of these periods, headaches can occur as often as eight per day or as few as one every other day. Typically, a sufferer has one or two clusters of headaches per year.

Cluster headaches appear to be triggered by an abnormality in the ipsilateral circadian pacemaker, which is located in the ventral hypothalamus. The headache pain is caused by a hypersensitized ophthalmic nerve (the ophthalmic branch of the trigeminal nerve). The autonomic symptoms are caused by concurrent excitation of parasympathetic fibers running with the ophthalmic nerve. It is not known what causes these nerve problems.

Clinical Presentation

Subjective

Patients with episodic tension headaches rarely seek health care. Patients with chronic tension headaches present with symptoms of anxiety and depression but do not attribute their headaches to these symptoms. It is the astute clinician who can relate patients' subjective comments to the stress and anxiety that they are experiencing in their lives and help each patient to attribute his or her headache to that cause, thereby encouraging patients to seek treatment for the underlying stress, anxiety, and/or depression.

Two basic types of migraine headaches occur—those with aura and those without. A typical migraine without aura (previously called "common migraine") is often unilateral but may become generalized. The headache lasts 2 to 72 hours or longer and is of pulsating quality. Most patients describe the pain as intense, throbbing, or pulsating. It is moderate to severe in intensity, inhibiting or prohibiting daily activities. It can be aggravated by routine physical activity and is often relieved by sleep. During the attack, nausea and vomiting, photophobia, and phonophobia are common. Adults often experience both photophobia and phonophobia, whereas children are more likely to have one or the other.

In migraine with aura (previously called "classic migraine"), the aura develops over 4 minutes and usually lasts an hour. Following the aura may be a pain-free period lasting no longer than 1 hour before the headache pain begins. The headache may also start before or at the same time as the aura. Patients typically have one or more symptoms associated with the aura that are characteristically neural in nature, such as unilateral numbness or paresthesia of the face or extremity and speech difficulties. Visual symptoms are common and usually occur 20 to 40 minutes before the headache. These symptoms include scotoma (blind spots), photopsia (flashing lights), fortification spectra (zigzag pattern), and diplopia. The aura phase may include additional symptoms of euphoria or depression, fatigue, hunger, and hyperosmia.

Migraine attacks may occur sporadically, with just a few headaches per year, or may be more frequent, with eight or more occurrences each month. Other symptoms may be associated with migraines, such as anorexia, constipation, pallor, dizziness, tremors, or diaphoresis. Some patients complain of cold hands or feet or experience polyuria, hunger, diarrhea, or body aches following the migraine.

The patient with a headache from a subarachnoid hemorrhage presents a picture of a sudden, abrupt, and unrelenting headache. Associated symptoms include nausea and vomiting, photophobia, and decreased level of consciousness. With small "warning leak" hemorrhages, the patient may complain of severe hemifacial pain spreading to the neck or back. The headache may have begun after exercise or intercourse.

Objective

Careful attention to the headache history is essential, including such particulars as onset, location, character and severity of headache, frequency and duration, associated signs and symptoms, prodromal symptoms, and precipitating factors. The practitioner should explore the patient's family and social history. Information should be sought regarding other family members who suffer from headaches, the type of headache, and the age at occurrence.

Patients with migraines usually have a parent who suffers from migraines. Information regarding the age of onset with migraines is also important because frequently, migraine starts before age 20. A social history may elicit stressors or precipitating factors for the headache. Identifying the possible precipitating factors for the migraine can assist the practitioner in developing an individual prescription plan for the patient to decrease the severity or frequency of the attacks. The patient's lifestyle, dietary habits, possible job-related stress, and environmental factors should be explored. In women, information should be sought regarding the relationship of the migraine to the menstrual cycle. Headaches usually occur after ovulation and before and during menstruation. Migraines that occur before menses are considered premenstrual and associated with the premenstrual syndrome (PMS). Women are more likely to have their first migraine in the year of menarche and often cease to have migraine headaches during pregnancy. The use of oral contraceptive pills or hormonal replacement therapy should be explored. Initially, the cycle is more haphazard because of unstable blood estrogen concentration. Their use for the first time may precipitate a migraine and cause the migraine to become more frequent or to be preceded by auras. Most women who suffer from migraines do not experience an aura. Discontinuing the oral contraceptive does not always resolve the problem. In patients with gynecologic disorders, migraines often become more frequent and can improve when the disorder is corrected. Practitioners may consider postponing a complete medical history to a more pain-free period for the patient once more serious disorders have been ruled out. The final step of the medical history is obtaining a record of all previous work-ups and past treatment performed, including their effectiveness.

In contrast to migraine, the patient with a cluster headache experiences severe, unilateral, orbital, supraorbital, or temporal pain lasting 15 minutes to 3 hours. The pain is most commonly unilateral and is sharp and burning in quality. Frequently, the headache occurs at night, awakening the patient. No aura is present, and it is rare to find nausea and vomiting. Attacks commonly occur in "clusters" or groups and can last up to several weeks or even months. One of the following can be demonstrated on the affected side: conjunctival injection, miosis, ptosis and eyelid edema, nasal congestion, rhinorrhea, and forehead and/or facial sweating. Physical findings to detect a headache resulting from a subarachnoid hemorrhage are visual blurring, diplopia, fever, slight decrease in awareness, asymmetrical pupillary response, equivocal extensor plantar response, and pronator drift. Other findings from a subarachnoid hemorrhage may include decreased level of consciousness and nuchal rigidity.

Frequently, a headache is seen in patients with temporal arteritis. Its intensity is severe with the quality of the pain described as deep and burning, sometimes throbbing. A symptom specific to temporal arteritis is "claudication" of the muscles of mastication. Because of ischemia of the muscles, the patient complains of pain in the jaw on prolonged chewing. Localized tenderness of the affected artery is found. The practitioner should be alert to the potential complication of blindness. Diplopia is a common sign seen before visual impairment. Once visual impairment occurs, however, it can progress quickly to blindness in several hours. On physical examination, few abnormalities are revealed. A low-grade fever may appear. The temporal arteries may be tender and more visible or pronounced on palpation but have absent or decreased palpations.

The single, most commonly occurring symptom with a subdural hematoma is headache. It is subacute and usually progresses. Characteristically, the headache is generalized, temporal, and worsens with changes in posture. It can occur during the night and may cause the patient to awaken in the morning. Associated symptoms are nausea, vomiting, confusion, seizures, or weakness. The practitioner should be alert to changes in personality, decreasing level of consciousness, excessive sleepiness, or sensory changes. Less common findings are focal neurologic signs, such as hemiparesis or pathologic reflexes. Papilledema rarely occurs because of the large volume of CSF.

Diagnostic Reasoning

Diagnostic Tests

An electroencephalogram (EEG) is not useful in the routine evaluation of a patient with a headache and is not recommended to exclude a structural cause for headache. Neither a CT scan nor MRI is warranted in adult patients whose headaches fit with the broad definition of tension or migraine headache and who have not demonstrated any recent substantial change in headache pattern, occurrence of seizures, or presence of focal neurologic signs or symptoms.

A CT scan or MRI study is recommended if the patient's headache pattern is atypical, has changed in pattern or character, or is accompanied by seizures, personality changes, or an abnormal neurologic finding. Patients with migraines commonly have normal physical findings between attacks. Extensive diagnostic testing for a patient with a migraine is not warranted. A CBC, chemistry profile, and urinalysis may be obtained to rule out a systemic illness for the patient with typical migraine with no change in pattern and a normal physical examination. Nonspecific EEG abnormalities can occur; however, some of these findings are normal and others often do not require treatment.

The Headache Classification Committee of the International Headache Society has a headache classification system and operational diagnostic criteria for the 129 different headache syndromes, divided into 13 categories. This system was designed to describe and identify headaches to allow for more accurate diagnosis and research. For example, a diagnosis of migraine with aura must include the presence of one or more fully reversible neurologic (visual, motor, or sensory) symptoms. For migraine without aura, two of the following characteristics are required: unilateral location, pulsating quality, moderate to severe intensity, and exacerbation by physical activity. In addition, at least one of the following must be present: nausea or vomiting, photophobia, or phonophobia.

In an older adult patient with late-onset migraines, it is recommended that a CT scan be done, just in case, even in the presence of a typical migraine with normal physical exam, to rule out organic disease. In a patient who has a history of migraines, the presentation of migraines can often change as the patient ages and a headache can easily be mistaken for a migraine, overlooking a TIA. In older adults, a good indication of the need for imaging studies is an unusual presentation or change in symptoms associated with migraine.

Physical examination of patients with cluster headaches usually reveals normal physical findings. If there has been no change in the pattern or pain of the cluster headache and a normal physical examination is found, then a CBC, chemical profile, and urinalysis may be completed to rule out a systemic illness.

Headaches from a subarachnoid hemorrhage should be identified quickly and an immediate CT scan performed. In a few patients with a small hemorrhage, the result may be negative. The benefit from the CT scan diminishes with time, that is, there is less sensitivity if the scan is obtained more than 7 days after headache onset. If the results are positive, an immediate neurosurgical referral is initiated.

With temporal arteritis, the ESR may be strongly elevated, from 50 to 100 mm, but it may also be normal. In this case, referral is essential, and a biopsy of the temporal artery is recommended along with excision of a long segment of the artery because lesions typically are not present along the entire artery. Other laboratory findings may include anemia and an elevated alkaline phosphatase level.

A subdural hemorrhage is best evaluated by CT, which has a greater sensitivity to early hemorrhage. The CT reveals the bleeding as hyperdense, isodense, or hypodense. If bleeding is isodense, there may be a shift of midline structures without any further evidence of abnormalities on CT. MRI or angiography may be utilized to determine if a hematoma is present.

Differential Diagnosis

A complete history is paramount in order to distinguish and diagnose headaches and to rule out life-threatening events, such as subarachnoid hemorrhage and a TIA that could lead to a CVA. Patients may have more than one headache, so each event must be identified. A thorough history should be explored, including the family, social, and medical history. A family history may reveal migraine headaches in other family members. A social history may identify stress or other precipitating factors for the headache. A general medical history, including a review of systems, may lead to a diagnosis other than migraine headache. The clinician should explore any recent or past history of head or neck traumas and previous medical procedures contributing to a headache, such as LP, spinal anesthesia, or surgeries. Following an LP, for example, a bilateral headache may develop after seven days. It typically worsens in 15 minutes upon standing and once the patient is recumbent, the headache is relieved within 30 minutes. Possible causes of headache might be related to current medical conditions, especially hypothyroidism, hypertension, and asthma. Identifying current medications, both prescription and OTC agents, would help in distinguishing the headache. Chronic daily headaches are frequently associated with the daily use of nonprescription "pain killer" drugs, especially compounds containing 50 to 75 mg of caffeine per tablet.

Sudden onset of pain may suggest serious pathology such as subarachnoid hemorrhage, meningitis, or brain tumor. A headache that has been present over a period of years is more likely to be associated with migraine cluster or tension-type headaches. The character of pain in migraines also is helpful in distinguishing a migraine headache from a tension-type headache. A tension-type headache is dull and nonpulsating; it changes in intensity. Its duration may be 30 minutes to 7 days and it is not associated with nausea or vomiting. Patients with tension-type headaches may report phonophobia or photophobia, but not both. Though tension-type headaches may limit some activities, these are generally not aggravated by physical activity and will not incapacitate the individual. Testing should include motor and sensory function to detect serious organic disease. A diagnosis of migraines with aura requires the presence of one or more fully recoverable neurologic symptoms (visual, motor, or sensory). This finding helps the practitioner distinguish migraine from a progressive, organic disorder that requires further assessment. An aura that is rapid in onset and short in duration, atypical of migraine, may be caused by a paroxysmal event or specific cardiovascular disease. Prodromal signs (aura) can be differentiated from signs of a stroke by the length of the aural event, which is usually less than 60 minutes. Differentiating a migraine with aura from a TIA may be difficult. Age, for instance, may play a role in the differential diagnosis, since a TIA is rare in the young.

Management

Immediate hospitalization is required for the person with a severe headache occurring suddenly with signs of meningeal irritation. Possible causes are intracranial hemorrhage or meningeal infection. If examination reveals evidence of symptoms or signs of increased intracranial pressure or severe intractable migraine, urgent hospitalization is indicated.

Because the majority of headaches (tension-type and migraines) can be recurrent and chronic, the principle of management is to design an individual treatment plan that identifies therapeutic goals for the patient. Goals would include strategies to avoid possible triggers, the ability to abort an attack, to obtain relief from pain and associated symptoms, and to decrease the frequency and severity of attacks.

Management for a tension-type headache is focused on the use of nonsteroidal anti-inflammatory drugs (NSAIDs), cool compresses, and stress reduction techniques.

Migraine treatment can be divided into four methods: nonpharmacologic, abortive therapy, pain relief, and prophylactic treatment. Nonpharmacologic measures are useful for minor migraines or as an adjunct to pharmacologic treatment to prevent or decrease the severity of a headache. These methods include identifying and eliminating known triggers. Maintaining a strict schedule for sleep and meals can prevent a headache related to fatigue and hunger. It is critical to keep from getting too much or too little sleep. If exercise precipitates an attack, an adequate warmup before working out is recommended. Biofeedback, relaxation techniques, and regular aerobic exercise are encouraged. Deep breathing, massage, and hot or cold therapy sometimes ease the pain, but excessive cold (e.g., icepacks) or caffeine can backfire.

Most migraine attacks vary in the effect on the patient's ability to function. In mild attacks, the effect is minimal. In moderate attacks, visual activities are moderately impaired. In severe attacks, however, the patient is unable to continue normal activities or can continue them only with severe discomfort. In some severe attacks, the patient is incapacitated, requiring treatment in the provider's office or emergency department.

Drug therapy should be added when these measures are not completely effective. It is appropriate for the practitioner to take a trial-and-error approach to identify medications most successful in the relief of headaches and associated symptoms with the fewest adverse effects and minimal costs and a return to normal functioning for each patient. Some patients may require three different medications: a triptan as an abortive medication, a rescue medication for breakthrough or residual pain, and a daily preventive medication.

Drugs Commonly Prescribed 5.5 presents a listing of medications commonly used to treat headaches. Complementary Therapies 5.1 presents other measures that may be taken to help treat headaches.

Follow-Up and Referral

A neurologic referral should be considered in any patient with episodes of transient neurologic deficits, increasing frequency and severity of unilateral headaches, atypical auras, as well as changes in personality, excessive sleepiness, and new onset of progressive deficits suggesting a mass lesion, hemorrhage, or structural disorder. The possibility of ischemia must be carefully considered in a middle-aged or older patient with vascular risk factors who presents with a new and unexplained headache. The patient should be monitored regularly with follow-up examinations. Surgical referral may be necessary for a temporal artery biopsy and definitive diagnosis or possible use of chronic steroid therapy.

Patient Education

The management of migraine is a team effort in which the patient plays an equal role. Patients must be convinced of the practitioner's interest in their complaints and commitment to their treatment. Realistic outcomes should be discussed because treatment is often ineffective or can be used

Drugs Commonly Prescribed 5.5: Headaches: Adults

Drug	Dose	Comments
Abortive		
Triptans (serotonin receptor agonists)		
Almotriptan (Axert)	6.25 or 12.5 mg once; may repeat in 2 hours. Max two doses in 24 hours.	Side effects: paresthesias, asthenia, nausea, dizziness, chest or neck tightness, heaviness, somnolence. Contraindicated in ischemic heart disease or other significant CVD, or cerebrovascular disease. There is a risk of rebound headache if triptans are used more than twice a week.
Eletriptan (Relpax)	20 or 40 mg once; may repeat in 2 hours. Max 80 mg/day.	
Frovatriptan (Frova)	2.5 mg with fluids; may repeat in 2 hours. Max 7.5 mg/24 h.	
Naratriptan (Amerge)	1 or 2.5 mg with fluids; may repeat in 4 hours. Max 5 mg/24 h.	
Rizatriptan (Maxalt)	5 or 10 mg once; may repeat in 2 hours. Max 30 mg/day.	
Sumatriptan (Imitrex)	Injection: 6 mg SC; may repeat in 1 hour. Max two doses/24 h. Tablets: 25–100 mg once with fluids; may repeat in 2 hours. Max 200 mg/day. Nasal spray: 5, 10, or 20 mg once. May repeat in 2 hours. Max 40 mg/day.	
Zolmitriptan (Zomig)	2.5 mg once; may repeat in 2 hours. Max 10 mg/day.	
Ergot derivatives		
Ergotamine 1 mg/ Caffeine 100 mg (Cafergot)	Two tablets at onset of attack, then one tablet every 6 hours prn. Max 6 tablets per attack. Max 10 tablets/week.	Contraindicated in peripheral vascular disease, coronary heart disease, hypertension, and hepatic or renal disease.
Ergotamine 2 mg/ Caffeine 100 mg (Cafergot supp)	One supp rectally at onset of attack, then one supp after 1 hour. Max two supp per attack. Max five supp/week.	
Dihydroergotamine (DHE 45, Migranal)	IV/IM/SC 1 mg; may repeat at 1-hour intervals for a total of 3 mg IM or 2 mg IV/SC. Max 6 mg/week. Intranasal spray: One spray (0.5 mg) in each nare; may repeat in 15 minutes. Max 4 sprays per attack. Max 8 sprays/24 h. Max 24 sprays/week.	IV route preferred when rapid relief is desired.
Prophylactic Medications		
Beta-blockers		
Propranolol (Inderal)	80 mg daily in divided doses. Usual range 160–240 mg/day.	Contraindicated in asthma, sinus bradycardia, second or third AV block. Potentiated by alcohol.
Timolol (Blocadren)	10 mg bid, 20 mg as a single dose. Max 30 mg in divided doses.	
Tricyclic antidepressants		Adverse effects: blurred vision, weight gain, dry mouth, constipation, cardiovascular effects, urinary retention.
Amitriptyline	10–100 mg PO hs	
Nortriptyline (Pamelor)	10–100 mg PO hs	
Fluoxetine (Prozac)	10–40 mg daily	
Calcium channel blockers		May take several months to be effective. Contraindicated in pregnancy. Adverse effects: extrapyramidal effects, bradycardia, fatigue, weight gain, constipation, nausea, edema, muscle pain.
Verapamil (Calan)	120–480 mg/day	
Antiepileptic agents		
Divalproex (Depakote)	250 mg–1500 mg/day	Adverse effects: asthenia, back pain, diarrhea, nausea, vomiting, dizziness, somnolence, tremor, weight gain. Has teratogenic effects.

Drug	Dose	Comments
Gabapentin (Neurontin)	90–2400 mg/day	Adverse effects: somnolence, dizziness, asthenia.
Topiramate (Topamax)	Up to 200 mg/day	As above plus paresthesias, diarrhea, altered taste, diminished appetite, weight loss
Rescue Medications		
Triptans (see previous section)		
Ergot derivatives (see previous section)		
NSAIDs		For mild to moderate attacks. Increased risk of GI bleed with alcohol. Adverse reactions: GI upset, GI bleed.
Ibuprofen (Advil, Motrin)	400–2400 mg	
ASA (aspirin)	500–1000 mg	
Naproxen sodium (Aleve, Naprosyn)	825 mg initially, then 550 mg after 1 hour	
Combination analgesics		For tension or muscle contraction headache. Potentiation with alcohol. Adverse effects: drowsiness, dizziness, GI disturbances.
Butalbital 50 mg/ Acetaminophen 325 mg/ Caffeine 40 mg (Fioricet)	One to two capsules q4h. Max six capsules daily.	
Butalbital 50 mg/ ASA 325 mg/ Caffeine 40 mg (Fiorinal)	One to two tablets or capsules q4h. Max six capsules daily.	
Analgesic		Avoid alcohol. Monitor for respiration, depression. Adverse reactions: sedation, lightheadedness, nausea, tingling sensation to skin, urticaria, difficulty urinating.
Butorphanol (Stadol)	IM: 1–4 mg q3–4h prn. Max 4 mg/dose. IV: 0.5–2 mg q3–4h prn Intranasal: 1 mg (one spray) in one nare; may repeat in several minutes, then may repeat these two doses q3–4h.	

for only a short period of time. Patients should be educated about the nature of migraine and given additional literature. Patients should keep a diary of any events that may be associated with an attack. This helps to identify and avoid triggers associated with a single episode and distinguish them from triggers that lead to an increase in the frequency and severity of attacks. While clinicians may not help patients deal with endogenous triggers: endocrine factors; genetic tendencies; and psychological depression, they may help the patient identify other triggers. Exogenous triggers include foods, e.g. red wine, alcohol, aged cheese, monosodium glutamate, aspartame (dietary sweetener), and chocolate; the frequency and pattern of light; and oral contraceptives. Environmental triggers include stress and stressful family events; air travel; weather changes; odors (bad and good); and meteorologic depression. Having an awareness of the triggers may help the patient avoid them which should diminish the frequency and intensity of the attacks. The clinician should explain the importance of warming up before exercise and avoiding tight-fitting goggles, sunglasses, helmets, or other headgear, and that regular exercise may prevent or decrease the headaches. If exercise is found to trigger an attack, discuss the importance of adequate nutrition and fluids before and after such activities.

Stress management strategies and relaxation techniques are commonly taught to patients to manage frequently unavoidable family- or work-related stress and emotional problems. When pharmacologic treatment is necessary, the family should fully understand the treatment. Impaired judgement may occur with severe attacks, and the patient may not remember what drugs or dosages were used. The patient should understand the type, its proper use, and adverse effects of the medications, including interactions with other medications and any contraindications such as pregnancy. Ask the patient to record in a headache diary the medications used (including any over-the-counter or other medications being used), dosages, response to medication, and evaluation of treatment, including adverse effects. Clinicians should advise patients not to take headache medications other than those prescribed. Excessive use of other analgesics may reduce their effectiveness. Using ergotamine and analgesics frequently can lead to rebound headaches or chronic daily headaches. Adverse effects are common, and the patient must keep the practitioner informed in case

COMPLEMENTARY THERAPIES 5.1

Headaches

Acupuncture/acupressure
Aroma and herbal therapy
- Apply lavender oil to the temples (women)
- Apply peppermint oil to the temples (men)
- Use eucalyptus for sinus headaches
- Drink rosemary tea or mix the essential oil in hot water and inhale
- Take evening primrose oil 500 mg
- Apply cold black tea bags to the eyes for 15 minutes
- Take feverfew *(Tanacetu partnenium)* 50 mg (or 1.2 g of leaf powder) daily for migraine headache (may interact with thrombotic medications, aspirin, and warfarin [Coumadin])
- Take *Ginkgo biloba* 120–240 mg of dried extract in 2–3 doses daily.
- Take valerian *(Valeriana officialis)* 2–3 g 1–3 times per day.

Biofeedback
Diet Therapy
- At the first sign of a migraine, drink 1–2 cups of strong coffee to prevent vessel dilation (effective for some individuals) or a glass of carrot or celery juice
- To reduce throbbing and contractions, eat foods high in magnesium such as dark, leafy greens, fresh seafood, sea vegetables, nuts, whole grains, molasses
- Eat vitamin C-rich foods such as broccoli, hot and bell peppers, sprouts, cherries, citrus
- Drink green tea or products such as Crystal Star Green Tea Cleanser or Be Well juices (as a prevention)
- Avoid foods known to trigger headache:
- Additive and chemical-based foods (MSG, sulfites [red wine], condiments, nitrates [aged and smoked meats]; pickled fish and shellfish; caffeine-containing foods, including chocolate; cultured foods [e.g., yogurt]; refined sweeteners); red meats; dairy products (cheese); soft drinks (the phosphorous binds up magnesium); alcohol; salty, sugary, and wheat-based foods

Exercise
Massage or chiropractic manipulation
- Massage the temples for 5 minutes
- Do 10 neck rolls
- Pull ear lobes for 5 seconds
- Rub back and all around ear shell
- Apply an ice pack to the back of the neck to reduce vasodilation or put feet in a cold water bath

Poultices
- Rub capsaicin (Zostrix) cream on the forehead
- Apply onion or horseradish poultices to the nape of the neck or soles of the feet

Reflexology
- Apply pressure to the inside base of the foot and big toe 3 times for 10 seconds each

Relaxation Therapy
- Perform deep breathing

Vitamin Therapy
- Take magnesium citrate 800 mg daily
- Take niacin 100–500 mg daily

Other
- Avoid smoking and second-hand smoke.
- Take a coffee enema to stimulate the liver and normalize bile activity. (Bowel movements may relieve vomiting.)

changes in medicine are needed. Patients should discuss with the practitioner if they desire to become or are pregnant.

Infectious and Inflammatory Disorders

Meningitis

Meningitis is an inflammation of the meningeal membranes surrounding the structures of the CNS and/or the CSF. Although meningitis is typically depicted as an acute process, syndromes of both chronic and subacute nature have been found. The common factor shared by all types of meningitis is an abnormality in the number of white blood cells (WBCs) in the CSF.

Purulent forms of acute meningitis are usually caused by three types of bacteria: *Neisseria meningitidis, Haemophilus influenzae* type B, and *Streptococcus pneumoniae.* Subacute or chronic manifestations occur with fungus, mycobacteria, spirochete, HIV, and neoplasms. Aseptic meningitis (no bacteria found in CSF) is usually associated with a virus or noninfectious causes such as a brain tumor or CVA. Table 5.8 reviews the types of meningitis.

Epidemiology and Causes

The incidence of meningitis is 15 per 100,000 with a prevalence of 5 cases per 100,000. Since the initiation of the widespread use of antibiotics in the 1950s, the mortality figures have remained steady at 14 percent, and those who do survive may experience chronic neurologic problems. Susceptibility differs with the causative organism, but generally young people, elderly people, and immunocompromised patients are at greatest risk.

Table 5.8 Types of Meningitis

Major Type	Description	Organism	Diagnostic Tests	Treatment
Bacterial (purulent)	Rapid onset: hours or days after exposure	**Age 3 months–18 years:** *H. influenza, N. meningitidis, S. pneumoniae* **Age 18–50:** *S. pneumoniae, N. meningitidis* **Age: 50 or older:** *S. pneumoniae, N. meningitidis, L. monocytogens,* Gram-negative bacilli	CSF Gram's stain analysis Culture	**Age 3 months–18 years:** Cefotaxime (Claforan) IV 50 mg/kg q6h Ceftriaxone (Rocephin) IV 50–100 mg/kg q12h **Age: 18 or older:** Cefotaxime 2–3 g q6h IV Ceftriaxone 2 g q12h IV plus Vancomycin 10 mg/kg Ampicillin 2 g IV q4h
Chronic (subacute)	Symptoms develop over months; less acutely ill	*M. tuberculosis* Atypical mycobacteria Fungi Spirochetes	CSF analysis Culture	**Mycobacteria:** INH (Isoniazid) IV 10 mg/kg/day Rifampin (Rifadin) IV 600 mg/day **Fungi:** Amphotericin (Fungizone) IV 0.3–0.6 mg/kg per day Flucytosine (Ancotil) IV 150 mg/kg per day **Spirochetes:** Penicillin G IV 12–18 million units over 21–24 days Acyclovir (Zovirax) IV 30 mg/kg per day
Aseptic (viral)	More benign type; self-limited syndrome caused primarily by viruses	Mumps virus Echo virus Herpes virus	Increased immunoglobulins in CSF	Rest, fluids, acetaminophen or ibuprofen

The majority of cases of meningitis are attributed to bacteria and viruses, with a much smaller occurrence caused by fungi or parasites. Among the viral causative agents, enteroviruses are leading in incidence. Seasonal occurrence shows a higher incidence of meningitis in the spring and fall. Infants and young children are particularly susceptible because of a lack of immunity and also because of the higher fecal to oral transmission that takes place in this age group. Arboviral infection is another common source during warm months when insect vectors are in abundance. The mumps virus can also be a causative factor in unimmunized populations. Various herpes viruses have been associated with meningitis, although the incidence is low.

Meningitis caused by bacterial sources is predominantly from the organisms *H. influenzae, N. meningitidis,* and *S. pneumoniae. H. influenzae* occurs primarily in infants and young children, usually in conjunction with or following otitis media, epiglottitis, or pneumonia. *N. meningitidis* is found as a cause of meningitis in children and young adults and is significant because of its rapid progression and high mortality (50 percent of patients affected die within 24 hours of symptom onset). *S. pneumoniae* is more frequently observed in adults with concurrent conditions such as pneumonia, sinusitis, otitis media, or endocarditis. *S. aureus* can be a causative factor of meningitis in patients who have undergone invasive neurologic instrumentation or trauma and in those with shunting of CSF.

Other organisms may be responsible for chronic meningitis syndromes and are generally rarer in occurrence than acute forms. *Mycobacterium tuberculosis* (tuberculosis) and *Treponema pallidum* (syphilis) sometimes produce indicators of meningitis in addition to their primary symptomatology. Other rare forms include fungal meningitis, parasitic meningitis, and rickettsial meningitis.

Pathophysiology

Meningitis is an infection that produces inflammation of the brain's meningeal membranes. Viruses, fungi, and parasites can cause meningitis, but the serious meningitides are most often caused by bacteria. Bacterial meningitis is an acute purulent infection that develops within the subarachnoid space. In adults, its signs and symptoms are fever, headache, and stiff neck, usually accompanied by vomiting, lethargy, confusion, or coma.

In the developed countries, adult bacterial meningitis is usually caused by *Streptococcus pneumoniae* (gram-positive cocci) or *Neisseria meningitidis* (gram-negative diplococci). Both types of bacteria first colonize the nasopharynx. From the infected nasopharyngeal epithelium, bacteria then get into the underlying blood vessels. *S. pneumoniae* and *N. meningitidis* are both encapsulated bacteria, and their capsules protect them from phagocytosis in the bloodstream.

From the circulation, bacteria enter the CSF through the choroid plexuses in the ventricles and through injured or leaky areas of the blood–brain barrier. Bacteria can multiply rapidly in the subarachnoid space because normal CSF has few white blood cells, no IgM antibodies, and low concentrations of the complement components C3 and C4.

As the number of bacteria increases, they come in repeated contact with the brain and the meninges. Local monocytes, macrophages, astrocytes, and microglia react to components in the bacterial cell walls by making and releasing inflammatory molecules, such as cytokines, interleukin-1, and tumor necrosis factor. These molecules increase the permeability of the blood–brain barrier and attract polymorphonuclear leukocytes from the systemic circulation. Large numbers of white cells enter the CSF and form a purulent exudate in the subarachnoid space. The exudate reduces the flow of CSF. Meningeal irritation from the exudate causes nuchal rigidity (meaning that the neck will resist passive flexion), and lumbar punctures in bacterial meningitis produce CSF with a high white cell count.

The invading leukocytes add to the concentration of inflammatory molecules, and the blood–brain barrier becomes sufficiently permeable to cause cerebral edema and significantly increased intracranial pressure. Increased intracranial pressure causes a number of neurologic and systemic signs, including: a depressed level of consciousness, a triad of bradycardia, hypertension, and irregular breathing, dilated nonreactive pupils, weakness in the abductors of the eyes, papilledema, nuchal rigidity, hiccupping, projectile vomiting, or decerebrate body postures. In addition, under significantly increased intracranial pressure, the mechanisms that regulate intracranial blood flow become ineffective, and systemic hypertension and hypotension will both have disproportionate effects on cerebral blood flow. Lumbar punctures of patients with bacterial meningitis yield high CSF pressures.

Clinical Presentation

Subjective

Subjective symptoms of meningitis include headache, photophobia, and neck pain and stiffness (nuchal rigidity).

Objective

Objective signs include fever (usually high, greater than 103°F [39°C]) with accompanying chills, tachycardia, and tachypnea. Signs of meningeal irritation such as Brudinski's sign (hip and knee flexion when the neck is flexed) and Kernig's sign (inability to fully extend the legs) are often present. Occasionally, opisthotonus (severe back spasm, causing arching) is observed. Altered level of consciousness is present and may include confusion, progressive lethargy, stupor, and coma. Cranial nerve dysfunction can occur, resulting in possible diplopia, deafness, facial weakness, and pupillary abnormalities.

History-taking may yield clues to possible causative agents or risk factors for meningitis. Major areas to emphasize in taking the history include pertinent exposures (contacts, food consumption, sexual practices, drug use), history of extraneural disease (especially respiratory), evidence of immunocompromise, underlying systemic disorders, and travel history.

Diagnostic Reasoning

Diagnostic Tests

Initially, routine blood studies may show marked elevation of WBCs (neutrophils) in bacterial meningitis or mild elevation in viral meningitis. In addition, electrolytes, especially sodium, are evaluated for a common complication of meningitis, the syndrome of inappropriate antidiuretic hormone secretion (SIADH).

If the clinical signs and symptoms indicate the possibility of meningitis, the collaborating physician will probably refer the patient to a neurologist for LP and CSF studies. Bacterial infection is indicated by cloudy appearance of CSF, increased CSF pressure greater than 20 mm H_2O, protein levels greater than 15 mg/dL, increased neutrophils, and reduced glucose content. Gram stains and cultures of CSF may assist in detecting causative organisms. An LP should not be performed if increased intracranial pressure is suspected because cerebral herniating may occur.

Imaging studies such as MRI may reveal meningeal enhancement, basilar exudate, hydrocephalus, and possible focal lesions as indicators of meningitis. Any other contributing abnormalities such as skin, lung, or sinus lesions should be investigated.

Differential Diagnosis

Many infectious and noninfectious conditions may mimic meningitis. It is also important to establish the specific type of meningitis. Some differential diagnoses include encephalitis, giant-cell arteritis, metabolic or toxic encephalopathy, SLE, and thrombotic thrombocytopenic purpura. Similarities in symptoms include headache and visual disturbances (encephalitis, arteritis), fever (encephalitis, SLE), nuchal rigidity (encephalitis), and headache (encephalopathy). Other diverse processes may also cause changes in CSF (e.g., increased neutrophils or glucose) resembling those caused by meningitis.

Management

Meningitis can be a life-threatening problem. If meningitis is suspected, the clinician should refer the patient to the collaborating physician for immediate hospitalization for extensive diagnostic examination and treatment. The principal goals for managing meningitis include eliminating infection, symptomatic care, and prevention or treatment of complications.

The first goal and priority is to eliminate infection. This is achieved through the judicial use of specific antimicrobial therapy if the meningitis is bacterial in origin. Initial IV antibiotic therapy is chosen based on CSF Gram stain results. The CSF culture results show the most effective antimicrobials that can be used to prevent further progression of the disease. These antimicrobials may be adjusted to achieve the most effective drug level therapy. The usual course of IV antimicrobials is 10 to 14 days. Specific treatment regimens are included in Table 5.8. Although the concomitant use of corticosteroids has been reported in the care of children with meningitis, this strategy has not been studied thoroughly in adults and is not recommended. Use of these treatment regimens is thought to decrease inflammation and enhance circulation of the antibiotic.

Chronic meningitis may require prolonged intrathecal and/or IV antimicrobial therapy. Symptomatic treatment includes reduction of fever with acetaminophen and headache management with an analgesic such as codeine. The literature strongly recommends the use of acetaminophen q4 to 6h. If nausea and vomiting are present, an antiemetic such as prochlorperazine (Compazine) may be used. Oversedation should be avoided, as it may mask increasing intracranial pressure. Other supportive treatment includes bed rest in a quiet, darkened room, adequate liquids, and a soft, nutritious diet appropriate for the patient's age.

Several vaccines are available for the more common forms of meningitis or contributing infections. In some cases, chemoprophylaxis is advised for documented exposure. The most common preventative measures for meningitis, including vaccine for the unexposed and chemoprophylaxis if exposure has occurred, are listed in Table 5.9.

Of major concern as a complication of meningitis is increasing intracranial pressure caused by cerebral edema brought on by the inflammatory process. Early signs include drowsiness, episodes of confusion, and pupillary changes. Later signs include decreasing levels of consciousness, increase in pulse pressure, bradycardia, and respiratory changes. This serious complication requires ventilatory support, oxygen therapy, close monitoring of circulatory and respiratory status, and careful management of IV fluid replacement. Techniques such as hyperventilation and use of osmotic diuretics, such as mannitol (Osmitrol), and anti-inflammatory agents, such as dexamethasone (Decadron), help reduce intracranial pressure.

Follow-Up and Referral

All patients who are suspected of having any form of meningitis should be referred to a neurologist for more definitive care. When the patient's condition is stable, the neurologist will release the patient back to the care of the primary health-care provider to continue follow-up care consisting of completion of antibiotic regimen and monitoring of blood work. Any indication of a complicated course warrants close follow-up and neurologic referral. Cases of uncomplicated acute meningitis such as aseptic meningitis may require only home IV antibiotic therapy after discharge. The total course of antibiotics is about 10 to 14 days. Patients with

Table 5.9 Prevention of Meningitis

Type	Vaccine	Indications	Chemoprophylaxis
Meningococcal	Monovalent serogroup A Monovalent serogroup C Bivalent A-C Quadrivalent A/C/Y/W-135	Epidemics Military personnel or travelers to epidemic locations College students living in dorms	**Adults:** Rifampin (Rifadin) IV 1200 mg/day; Ciprofloxacin (Cipro) IV 500–750 mg/day For close contacts to known cases
Pneumococcal	Pneumovax: provides immunity up to 5 years	All older than age 2 who are immunosuppressed or with chronic disease Elderly especially those in chronic care facilities	None recommended
H. influenza	HbOC (Hib titer) PRP-OMP (Pedvax Hib)	Children from age 2 months to 5 years, especially with chronic illness and over 18 months attending day care Children older than age 5 according to risk	Rifampin (Rifadin) IV 20 mg/kg per day for 4 days For household or daycare contacts, especially if younger than age 6 years

chronic meningitis, or with neurologic deficits require rehabilitation and continuous follow-up. The facility for this depends on the individual nature of the patient's needs and family resources.

Patient Education

Education regarding prevention of meningitis through available immunization or chemoprophylaxis, as well as observance for clues to impending complications, should be provided. Home management following hospital discharge should emphasize the need for assistance with routine activities for a period lasting up to several weeks to allow for complete recovery. The patient should be encouraged to have frequent rest periods and to gradually increase activities while looking for signs (e.g., shortness of breath, increased pulse) that the activity is too strenuous. The diet should be well balanced to ensure nutrients such as protein and vitamin C. Soft foods may be better tolerated. Plenty of fluids should be encouraged unless other conditions are present, such as congestive heart failure or kidney disease. Two tablets of acetaminophen (Tylenol) may be given q4 to 6h for pain or headache. The patient may feel more comfortable initially in a darkened, quiet room, which will prevent discomfort related to photophobia. The importance of completing the full course of antibiotic or antiviral medications exactly as prescribed must be stressed to the patient and family. To protect the family and others, the patient needs to avoid close contact with others who may transmit germs orally. The patient needs to be taught about potential complications and when it is necessary to call the healthcare provider, for example, if he or she has any signs of an upper respiratory infection (URI), any change in alertness or awakeness, any recurrent fever, or any other sign of a worsening illness.

Encephalitis

Usually of viral causation, encephalitis is an acute inflammation of brain tissue, which produces inflammation, hyperthermia, altered levels of consciousness, and other focal neurologic signs. Often referred to as "sleeping sickness," encephalitis may on rare occasions be caused by nonviral agents. Table 5.10 presents the types of encephalitis.

Epidemiology and Causes

With more than 25 viral organisms causing the inflammation, encephalitis is relatively common, with an incidence of 15 cases per 100,000 and prevalence of 10 per 100,000. Arboviruses (carried by arthropods such as mosquitos) can occur in epidemic fashion during warm-weather months. With overall mortality due to encephalitis averaging between 5 and 20 percent and with residual neurologic deficits occurring in up to 90 percent of cases, treatment and supportive care become important. Although most cases of encephalitis are viral, there are many nonviral agents responsible for the other few cases of encephalitis. These include tertiary syphilis, *Rickettsia rickettsii* (responsible for Rocky Mountain spotted fever), *S. aureus, S. pneumoniae, H. influenzae, Bacteroides frugilis, Brucella* species, *Leptospira* species, *Cryptococcus neoformans,* and *M. tuberculosis.*

Encephalitis may occur at any age, but very young children and older adults are at the highest risk. There is no significant ethnic predisposition, and encephalitis occurs equally among men and women.

Pathophysiology

Encephalitis is an infection of the brain parenchyma. Typical symptoms include fever and confusion or drowsiness, which

Table 5.10 Types of Encephalitis

Major Type	Description	Organism	Diagnostic Tests	Treatment
Viral	Most common type; progressive altered level of consciousness, seizures, motor weakness, headache	More than 25 viral organisms, including arboviruses	Primarily diagnosed from the clinical picture	Symptomatic treatment Supportive care Acyclovir 15 mg/kg q8h
Herpes simplex virus (HSV)	Sudden development of olfactory or gustatory hallucinations, prominent memory loss, bizarre behavior	HSV	CSF analysis EEG CT MRI	Foscavir (Foscarnet) 20 mg/kg IV bolus, then 120 mg/kg IV q8h Acyclovir 15 mg/kg q8h
Microbial	Selectively attacks CNS cells; varied signs and symptoms	Multiple bacterial organisms	Gram stain of CSF Serum antibody levels	Penicillin 20 million units/day Chloramphenicol (Chloromycetin 75–100 mg/kg per day divided q6h)

sometimes progresses to stupor and coma. Encephalitis is usually accompanied by inflammation of the meninges; therefore, headache and nuchal rigidity are also frequent symptoms. A bout of encephalitis can produce a range of specific neurologic problems, including seizures, muscle weakness or paralysis, isolated cranial nerve palsies, heightened or depressed deep tendon reflexes, and papilledema. Sometimes the infection disrupts the hypothalamic-pituitary axis, and this can lead to diabetes insipidus, inappropriate antidiuretic hormone secretion, or the inability to maintain a normal body temperature. When the infective agent is the herpes simplex virus, the encephalitis can cause personality changes, hallucinations, and aphasia.

Encephalitis is usually caused by a virus—in the United States, the most common cause is herpes simplex virus—and the neurologic signs and symptoms of encephalitis are usually preceded by other signs of viral infection, such as fever, malaise, muscle aches, rashes, gastrointestinal disturbances, or respiratory symptoms. Encephalitis viruses get into the body through a number of routes: herpes simplex viruses are transmitted through person-to-person contact; enteroviruses are swallowed and invade through the gut; arboviruses are introduced by bites of insects, other arthropods, birds, and rodents; rabies enters through bites of mammals; and varicella-zoster viruses are inhaled. In most cases, the viruses replicate, a viremia develops, and virus particles get into the CNS from the bloodstream. Some viruses (rabies, herpes simplex, and varicella-zoster), however, are carried into the CNS retrogradely inside axons.

A typical case of viral encephalitis comprises a mix of parenchymal inflammation, meningitis, cerebral edema, and hemorrhage. Throughout the brain and meninges, there is perivascular inflammation with local collections of lymphocytes, brain monocytes, microglia, and a lesser number of polymorphonuclear leukocytes. Capillary endothelial cells are injured, especially in the gray matter, causing small hemorrhages. There are areas of neuron cell death. In addition, ependymal cells can be damaged, contributing to the brain swelling.

The brain areas suffering the most damage vary from case to case. Some patients develop seizures, which can be either generalized or focal. Sometimes oligodendroglia are selectively infected and the main damage is demyelination, which leads to focal neurologic deficits. When the brainstem becomes infected, coma or respiratory failure can result. Generalized cortical edema decreases consciousness. The direct cause of these and other major symptoms of encephalitis seems to be the inflammation and immune reactions themselves, because when these host responses subside, patients often recover dramatically.

Clinical Presentation

Subjective

A common presentation of viral encephalitis includes alteration in level of consciousness related to parenchymal swelling. The manifestations are usually progressive from lethargy to coma with the swelling and resultant increased intracranial pressure. Other focal neurologic signs may develop, including seizures and motor weakness. Generalized headache with abrupt onset often accompanies other signs as a result of intraparenchymal bleeding and swelling.

Encephalitis caused by HSV may be heralded by bizarre behavior, aphasia, or hallucinations as the temporal and frontal lobes are selectively attacked by this organism. Other types of infectious agents (other herpes viruses, Lyme disease [*B. burgdorferi*], varicella-zoster virus, *R. rickettsii*) may produce a cutaneous rash in addition to neurologic signs such as headache, seizures, or nuchal rigidity. The rash is a typical feature of many viral diseases.

Objective

Physical examination may reveal a fever, nuchal rigidity, paralysis, and hyperresponsive deep tendon reflexes, and possibly, a viral rash.

Diagnostic Reasoning

Diagnostic Tests

A lumbar puncture (LP) is essential for the diagnosis. When encephalitis is suspected, the patient should be referred to the collaborating physician as well as a neurologist. CSF testing reveals increased WBC (especially mononuclear) and an increased protein level. A Gram stain of CSF may be useful for bacterial infection to provide early guidance for appropriate antibiotic treatment. Serum antibodies taken early in the infectious course and compared with a specimen drawn 1 to 3 weeks after onset of illness will reveal significant antibody increase. This may be helpful clinically to provide confirmation of a viral cause and further therapy guidance. With encephalitis caused by HSV, extensive hemorrhagic necrosis is demonstrated on CT scan and MRI. Occasionally cell damage occurs that does not demonstrate abnormality on a CT scan or MRI.

Because changes in the CSF may not be apparent at the beginning of the infection, a repeat LP may be indicated. An EEG taken in the presence of herpes simplex encephalitis often is abnormal because of localized hemorrhage and edema. An MRI may indicate areas of demyelination or edema.

Differential Diagnoses

Because encephalitis often produces signs of meningeal irritation, the differentiating factor to consider encephalitis over meningitis is usually alteration in level of consciousness. Meningitis has an abrupt onset, and although the condition may show signs of parenchymal damage that are seen in encephalitis (e.g., memory difficulties, confusion, hallucinations, dysphasia, seizures, and focal motor/sensory deficits), these signs are usually seen late in the course of the disease as compared to encephalitis, in which these signs are exhibited from the beginning. Photophobia and severe headache may point to acute meningitis rather than encephalitis. A preceding viral illness such as measles or mumps points to encephalitis occurring as a complication. Patient history of an animal bite in the presence of the typical symptoms may lead suspicion regarding encephalitis caused by rabies. In addition, seasonal factors may point to an arboviral cause of encephalitis by mosquito or tick bite.

Management

A suspicion of encephalitis requires referral and patient hospitalization for definitive neurologic diagnosis and treatment. The principles of treatment include inactivating and eliminating the causative organism, providing supportive care, and preventing complications.

Viral causation is treated with antiviral agents such as acyclovir (Zovirax). Antivirals are most effective when used early in the course of illness, especially before changes in level of consciousness occur. Antivirals act by suppressing replication of the virus. Vigorous supportive care for unconscious patients is necessary to prevent complications of ventilator support, catheters, IV lines, or other invasive treatment. Handling invasive equipment aseptically is essential in preventing infection. It is crucial to be alert for IV infiltration and phlebitis. The patient on a mechanical ventilator must be observed to prevent pressure necrosis, atelectasis, infection, and barotrauma.

Seizure control is achieved by the use of phenytoin (Dilantin), with dosage up to 600 mg per day for adults. Safety must also be a consideration with these patients. Padding should be used to prevent seizure injury. Although some fever can be beneficial, occasionally extreme hyper thermia can cause seizure activity. Acetaminophen (Tylenol) is used to reduce hyperthermia and may be given as a rectal suppository indicated. Dosage is 650 mg q4h. Cerebral edema resulting in increased intracranial pressure is another ominous complication of encephalitis. An osmotic diuretic such as mannitol (Osmitrol) 250 mg to 2 g/kg IV over 60 minutes is chosen first to reduce edema, but glucocorticoids, such as dexamethasone (Decadron) 4 mg q6h, may be added if necessary. Agents used for the treatment of encephalitis are listed in Table 5.10.

Follow-Up and Referral

Patients suspected of having encephalitis are referred to a neurologist for definitive care and follow-up. When the patient is stabilized, the neurologist will release the patient's care to the primary-care provider. The relative degree of neurologic deficit determines the nature of follow-up care. Complete convalescence can take weeks.

Patient Education

Prevention of infection vectors through mosquito control and insect repellants should be one important focus of patient and community education. Early detection and proper removal of ticks is another important aspect. For convalescence, the importance of bed rest, fluids, and nutrition is emphasized, as well as clues to impending complications. The patient should be encouraged to take frequent rest periods and to increase activities gradually while looking for signs that the activity is too strenuous, for example, shortness of breath and increased pulse. The patient should be instructed to eat a balanced diet to ensure the inclusion of nutrients such as protein and vitamin C. Fluids should be encouraged unless contraindicated. Acetaminophen may be used for pain or a headache. The patient may feel more comfortable in a darkened, quiet room if photophobia is present. The importance of taking the antibiotics or antiviral medications exactly as prescribed should be stressed to the patient. Patients should be instructed to avoid close contact with others who may be harboring germs. If they notice any signs of an upper respiratory infection, they should seek help from their health-care provider immediately. Patients and families should be instructed to inspect the skin for ticks and how to remove them intact. They should wear protective clothing to prevent tick bites. Lastly, the patient should be instructed when to call the health-care provider, for example, if there are any changes in their level of consciousness, recurrent fever, or any other signs of a worsening illness.

Herpes Zoster

Herpes zoster, commonly known as shingles, is a viral infection by varicella zoster occurring along dermatomal pathways and resulting in a vesicular skin rash, especially in the intercostal areas.

Epidemiology and Causes

Varicella-zoster virus is thought to become latent after primary infection of chickenpox, then reactivates, usually in persons who are immunocompromised, as herpes zoster (shingles). The incidence rises to 5 to 10 cases per 1000 in adults older than age 60 and is thought to be caused by immunosuppression that often accompanies the aging process. Four percent of patients with herpes zoster may experience a second episode but rarely a third episode. Immunocompromised patients also have a higher incidence of complications because of their impaired ability to thwart the infectious process. In adults who have no previous history of chickenpox, exposure to the virus (usually transmitted by respiratory route or by direct contact with vesicular fluid) causes herpes zoster.

Pathophysiology

Varicella-zoster virus, which causes chickenpox, is also responsible for a number of neurologic disorders, including encephalitis, meningitis, polyneuritis, multiple cranial neuropathies, and Reye's syndrome. Varicella-zoster virus initially infects people through the mucosa of the upper respiratory tract or the conjunctivae of the eyes. Within a week, the virus has spread throughout the body via the bloodstream, and about a week later, infections of the capillaries of the skin produce the vesicular lesions of chickenpox.

At this point, virus particles are retrogradely transported inside sensory axons to dorsal root ganglia, where the viruses remain latent for the life of the patient. Varicella-zoster virus is most often found in the sensory ganglia of the ophthalmic division of the trigeminal nerve and in the dorsal root ganglia of the mid to lower spinal cord (ganglia T3 to L2). If viruses in a ganglion are reactivated, they replicate, destroy ganglion nerve cells, and migrate through the nerves to the innervated dermatomes where they again produce vesicular skin lesions.

The destruction of sensory neurons in a ganglion produces pain in the innervated dermatome. This pain usually precedes the skin lesions by a few days, although sometimes pain is the only symptom. Typically, viruses are reactivated in only a single ganglion at a time; therefore, the symptoms are unilateral and affect a single dermatome. When the pain does not resolve within a few weeks, the syndrome is called postherpetic neuralgia (PHN). The pain of PHN can be either constant or intermittent and worsens at night and during temperature changes. Varicella-zoster that has been reactivated in the ophthalmic division of the trigeminal nerve can cause eye problems including lesions of the cornea.

It is not known what triggers the reactivation of latent varicella-zoster viruses. The likelihood of developing this reactivation syndrome (called "herpes zoster" or "shingles") increases as a person ages and when a person's immune system becomes compromised. Herpes zoster is a frequent complication of HIV infections.

Clinical Presentation

Subjective

Initially, the patient with herpes zoster may present with unexplained pain. The pain is described as constant or intermittent, with a stabbing quality. The pain occurs along the involved dermatome and usually occurs 48 to 72 hours before eruption of the classic vesicular skin rash. Pain acuity differs among individuals, but many patients say the pain becomes progressively worse at night or with changes in temperature. When herpes zoster is manifested along the branches of the fifth cranial nerve, herpes zoster ophthalmicus results. This condition can cause blindness and requires immediate referral to an ophthalmologist for evaluation and treatment. If the site of infection is along the trigeminal nerve, lesions will occur on the inside of the mouth, and occasionally in the external ear opening. Lesions on the eighth cranial (acoustic) nerve can cause vertigo, hearing loss, and ear pain.

Another major characteristic of the disease is the occurrence of acute neuritis along the path of the rash dermatome. PHN occurs in approximately 25 to 50 percent of patients older than age 60. The constant or intermittent stabbing pain worsens at night or with temperature changes.

Objective

Herpes zoster is characterized by a unilateral vesicular rash along a dermatome, most commonly a thoracic or lumbar dermatome. The rash begins as erythema, then changes to papular lesions that rapidly form vesicles. The vesicles rupture releasing infectious fluid, and then form scabs. Occasionally the vesicles coalesce to form bullae. The skin lesions usually continue to develop for 3 to 5 days, and the entire disease course usually lasts 10 to 15 days. In some individuals, the skin lesions and pain can persist for 30 days.

Diagnostic Reasoning

Diagnostic Tests

Diagnosis is made after careful review of data obtained from the history and physical examination. The characteristic appearance and distribution of the lesions along with a history of neuritis helps establish the diagnosis of herpes zoster. Usually the history and physical examination is all that is needed to make a definitive diagnosis.

If the diagnosis is questionable, a polymerase chain reaction (PCR) assay, which detects the DNA sequence of the virus, may be done, along with antibody titer (which requires more than one test for comparison).

Differential Diagnosis

Other conditions with similar rashes need to be ruled out. Impetigo may present as vesicles around an area of broken skin. The scrapings of these lesions can be sent for a Gram stain, which will reveal a gram-positive cocci if herpes zoster is present. Viral cultures may be done to rule out HSV or coxsackie viral infections that can appear with a dermatomal pattern.

Management

The principal goals are to manage the healed vesicles, obtain pain relief, and prevent secondary infection and other complications. Initial management of herpes zoster involves the use of antiviral agents. They reduce the impact of herpes zoster by diminishing neuritis and speeding the healing of the skin lesions. Early intervention in the treatment of herpes zoster produces the best results. Famciclovir (Famvir), acyclovir (Zovirax) or valacyclovir (Valtrex) may be used. Famciclovir is prescribed as 500 mg tid; acyclovir as 800 mg five times a day for 7 to 10 days; and valacyclovir as1 g q8h for 7 days. Systemic corticosteroids such as prednisone starting at 60 mg a day and tapering over 3 weeks may assist in reducing acute pain when given in conjunction with the antiviral therapy. Lotions such as calamine and dressings soaked with Burrow's solution may be used on the lesions to soothe the lesions and prevent scratching or rubbing, thereby improving healing time, decreasing pain, and preventing secondary infection. Some patients find that corticosteroid cream helps as well. Some report that the pain of lesions in the thoracic area can be diminished by using a tight wrap of the chest to produce a splinting effect. The practitioner should use this method with care, especially in older adult patients or those with pulmonary disease, because the restriction (splinting) of normal breathing patterns could promote pulmonary stasis of secretions and increase the incidence of pulmonary infections. Patients with ophthalmic herpes affecting the first branch of the trigeminal nerve must be referred to an ophthalmologist as this condition may result in blindness. The patient with ophthalmic herpes will usually have a lesion on the tip of the nose.

Analgesics (from nonnarcotic to narcotic agents in doses individualized for the patient) are supportive in reducing neuritis and PHN. If postherpetic neuralgia is present, the use of tricyclics such as amitriptyline 25 to 75 mg taken each night may help if simple analgesics are ineffective. For additional pain relief, gabapentin (Neurontin) starting at 300 mg tid up to 3600 mg daily may help. If pain is persistent, chronic postherpetic neuralgia may respond to a regional block with or without corticosteroids. Ideally, the patient should be referred to a pain center because PHN can have devastating effects. (See The Patient's Voice 5.1.)

Follow-Up and Referral

It is essential that any patient with ophthalmic herpetic lesions be referred to an ophthalmologist. Other follow-up would include a return visit if skin lesions become infected or if PHN is present. Referral to a neurologist may be required at any time if the patient does not respond to primary treatment plans. Patients should be referred to a pain center if PHN results in chronic persistent pain.

Patient Education

Because herpes zoster is usually treated on an outpatient basis, patient and family education is important. The clinician should encourage patients to complete the course of the antiviral agent, even if they feel the disease has abated, or especially if they feel the treatment is not as effective as they had hoped it would be. Patients should be informed that elimination of the disease could take longer than anticipated and careful medication administration and follow-up care could mean fewer complications in the long run. Patients should be instructed that the medication may be better tolerated if taken with food. If adverse effects from the treatment plan occur, patients need to keep the practitioner informed, so adjustments can be made. Education on the potential for spread of the herpes zoster virus via fluid from ruptured vesicles is important. Patients should be instructed that before the rash crusts, it can release fluid that will cause an infection in others. Patients must be careful in handling dressing, linens, towels, and clothes that they have used. They should not be around children who have not been vaccinated for chickenpox or those who have not had chickenpox yet; contact with pregnant women should also be avoided. Because patients will have a low resistance to infection, they should not be around those who may have an infectious illness, such as a cold. Patients need to know that scratching the rash can lead to an infection. The clinician should pursue ways to relieve the pruritus, as mentioned previously. Patients should be instructed about the nature of the rash so that when they see it in varying stages of progression, they will not think that it is not healing. Again, the importance of completing all prescribed medications needs to be stressed. Patients need to know the reason they are taking other medications, e.g., antidepressants (which may help prevent PHN), so they will continue taking them.

THE PATIENT'S VOICE 5.1

Postherpetic Neuralgia

My mother died of postherpetic neuralgia (PHN).

My mother was 80 years old and had recently won the golf championship at her club. She had been a widow for 25 years and decided that she wanted to move in with me, her daughter with her only granddaughter (age 3). We lived 4 hours away. At first she was very independent—driving around by herself and going shopping while I worked. That only lasted a few months. Then the decline began. First, she broke a wrist, which incapacitated her, and then she got pneumonia, which weakened her. Then she got "shingles" [herpes zoster], which did her in. She was diagnosed at the earliest onset of pain, yet treatment wasn't started until the vesicles erupted. She had ophthalmic herpes so her vision was affected. She developed PHN very early and due to the persistent pain, she became a reclusive. She stopped going out, retreating to her room and eventually wouldn't get out of bed. Nothing helped the pain. I'm convinced it was because preventive treatment wasn't started early. As she became more depressed and stayed in bed, she got weaker and weaker and just gave up. She complained of shooting pain over half of her head that was worse at night so she'd be awake all night and sleep all day. Nobody could help; her primary-care provider, neurologist, ophthalmologist, psychologist, nor me. She died in her sleepg, and I'm convinced it was the result of PHN.

I've learned two things from this experience. First, if older persons are optimally functioning, don't move them out of their familiar supportive environment. Second, treat all cases of herpes aggressively, as you don't know who is going to develop PHN. As my mom used to say, "An ounce of prevention is worth a pound of cure."

Trigeminal Neuralgia

Trigeminal neuralgia is a distressing, painful idiopathic disorder of the trigeminal nerve (cranial nerve V). It is also known as tic douloureux (unbearable painful twitch). This excruciating facial pain is paroxysmal and lasts usually less than 3 seconds. For many individuals the severity of the pain is disabling, and patients will do almost anything to prevent triggering an episode.

The lancinating, sharply cutting pain occurs along one or more of the three branches of the trigeminal nerve. Characteristically, the painful episodes occur when specific trigger zones are stimulated by touch, chewing, talking, shaving, or environmental temperature changes. Patients often describe the pain as "electric" or "stabbing" and penetrating. The pain of trigeminal neuralgia is chronic. Although patients may experience periods of spontaneous pain remission that may last weeks or months, the pain returns with the same or greater intensity.

Epidemiology and Causes

Trigeminal neuralgia occurs more frequently in women than men and more often in late middle age. The incidence is 4.3 per 100,000 of the general population. A higher incidence of risk occurs in individuals with hypertension and MS. These at-risk individuals are much younger than the characteristic age of patients with trigeminal neuralgia.

Most often with trigeminal neuralgia there is involvement of the muscles of the right side of the face where two or three branches of the trigeminal nerve are affected. The lower and center portions of the face are most commonly affected, and it is rare to have pain in the forehead and scalp areas.

Pathophysiology

Trigeminal neuralgia, which produces episodic paroxysms of sharp facial pain, is caused by demyelination of axons in the fifth cranial nerve, the trigeminal nerve. The trigeminal nerve has three main branches: V_1, the ophthalmic branch, transmits sensation from the eye region and forehead; V_2, the maxillary branch, transmits sensation from the midface and upper jaw; and V_3, the mandibular branch, transmits sensation from the lower jaw. The neuron cell bodies for the sensory axons in these nerves are located in the trigeminal (gasserian) ganglion, which is inside the skull along the floor of the middle cranial fossa.

Trigeminal neuralgia most often affects the mandibular or the maxillary branches of the trigeminal nerve. The problem tends to occur in middle-aged and elderly people. Patients with multiple sclerosis, another demyelinating syndrome, get trigeminal neuralgia with a higher frequency than the rest of the population.

Although it is extremely painful, trigeminal neuralgia produces no obvious neurologic deficits. On the other hand, patients with trigeminal neuralgia have a general sensory hypersensitivity of the face, and 90 percent of sufferers have trigger points on their faces that will set off paroxysms of pain.

Trigeminal neuralgia is caused by focal demyelination of axons in the affected nerve, ganglion, or roots. Biopsy specimens of affected nerves show patches of demyelination but no significant inflammation. It has been hypothesized that, due to demyelination, axons come in direct contact with neighboring axons so that signals in one axon spread laterally to adjacent axons. A modest stimulation of the nerve will then be amplified into a massive excitation, which is interpreted by the brain as a sudden burst of pain.

Clinical Presentation

Subjective

The patient with idiopathic trigeminal neuralgia presents with complaints of severe paroxysmal pain, most commonly on one side of the face. The pain lasts for a few seconds, with no ache or pain between occurrences, and follows the trigeminal nerve distribution. The patient's history includes the onset of a painful event after trigger points have been stimulated by chewing, talking, brushing teeth, touching the face, or in some cases, after intense physical activity, lowering of the head, and wind touching the face. The patient's history may include periods of remission with or without medical treatment.

During periods of exacerbation, the patient may be totally disabled by the severity of the pain. Patients may report refraining from eating, sleep deprivation, depression, and even suicidal tendencies, which reflect their willingness to go to great extremes to escape the severe paroxysmal pain.

Objective

On physical examination, the cranial nerves, specifically the trigeminal nerve, have normal motor and sensory function and facial muscle strength and reflexes are normal. Clinically, the cardinal signs of idiopathic trigeminal neuralgia are elicited when a facial trigger point is stimulated; the patient experiences a sharp, electric-type pain that follows the distribution of the trigeminal nerve and lasts for only a few seconds, and the patient's face grimaces. After the painful attack, there is no residual ache or pain. Facial pain, however, that is continuous and varies in intensity must be further evaluated for atypical trigeminal neuralgia that is caused by trauma, tumor, or previous facial surgery. Because of the many pathological and etiological theories regarding trigeminal neuralgia, the clinician must be alert to the characteristic symptoms of typical (idiopathic) trigeminal neuralgia. These are short periods of paroxysmal pain associated with trigger zones, pain limited to the distribution of the trigeminal nerve branches, and negative neurologic findings.

Diagnostic Reasoning

Diagnostic Tests

Idiopathic trigeminal neuralgia can often be diagnosed based on clinical history that describes paroxysmal pain episodes triggered by specific activities in patients characteristically older than age 50.

Patients who have prolonged episodes of pain that increases in intensity and occurrence and are younger need to be further evaluated for pathology-related tumors, trauma, MS and vascular compression. The tests most frequently used for the diagnosis of atypical trigeminal neuralgia are a CT scan and MRI. The MRI is the method of choice in differential diagnoses of trigeminal nerve pathology.

Another diagnostic method for typical trigeminal neuralgia is the administration of carbamazepine (Tegretol). Carbamazepine causes pain relief, and because of this effect, it may be used to diagnose this disorder.

Differential Diagnosis

There are many causes for the general presentation of orofacial pain; and these conditions can be generally categorized as inflammatory (e.g., dental pathology, sinusitis, parotitis, sialolithiasis, temporal arteritis, HSV type I), neurologic (e.g., trigeminal, glossopharyngeal, or partrigeminal neuralgia; cluster or migraine headaches; meningiomas; posterior fossa tumors), or musculoskeletal (e.g., temporomandibular joint [TMJ] pain, myofascial pain dysfunction syndrome). It is important, therefore, to identify whether the clinical presentation is either typical trigeminal neuralgia or some other orofacial pain cause.

Management

The major principles in the management of trigeminal neuralgia are to elicit a remission by drug therapy, to prevent untoward effects in patients resulting from prescribed medications, and to help the patient avoid triggering painful episodes. Trigeminal neuralgia is a chronic condition that results in the need for the patient's chronic pain to be managed. In addition to interventions related to establishing a remission and avoidance of painful episodes, the patient's psychological needs—related to depression, isolation, and possible suicidal tendencies—are significant areas in the plan of care.

Initially, pharmacologic management is to try to initiate remission of the pain. Carbamazepine (Tegretol) is the drug of choice and is started at a dose of 100 mg bid to avoid nausea and somnolence. The dose is increased in increments up to the maximum of 1200 mg/day or until pain is relieved. Pain control is usually reached between 400 and 800 mg/day. A blood level of 12 mg/mL is considered therapeutic. The patient experiencing pain relief must stay on that dose for at least 6 months before tapering the dose. Serial blood counts and liver function studies should be done while being treated with this drug. The adverse effects of carbamazepine; ataxia, dizziness, confusion, rash, sleepiness, and blood dyscrasias require a change in drug treatment. If carbamazepine cannot be tolerated or is ineffective, phenytoin (Diliantin) 200 to 400 mg daily may be tried. The initial dose of phenytoin is 100 mg tid with a maximum dose of 800 mg daily to achieve a therapeutic level of 10 to 20 mg/mL. Baclofen (Lioresal), started at 5 mg tid and increased up to 10 to 20 mg three to four times per day (not to exceed 80 mg per day) may be helpful either alone or in combination with carbamazepine or phenytoin.

Patients who are taking oral contraceptives should be cautioned that they may not be reliable when these analgesic drugs are being prescribed. The patient should also be warned about the hazard of driving a motorized vehicle when on these drugs.

Follow-up for complications of drug therapy with anticonvulsants is essential in the pharmacologic management of typical trigeminal neuralgia. If carbamazepine and baclofen become ineffective after prolonged use, or if adverse effects develop, the dosage must be gradually decreased to prevent withdrawal symptoms. Carbamazepine has many adverse effects, including nausea, vomiting, mouth ulcers, dizziness, diplopia, skin rash, blood dyscrasias (aplastic anemia, agranulocytosis, thrombocytopenia, and leukopenia), fever, and chills.

In patients refractory to conventional medical therapy, gabapentin (Neurontin) up to 2400 mg day in divided doses, may be useful for pain, especially in patients with multiple sclerosis.

Fluoxetine (Prozac) may be prescribed for patients who experience psychological depression and difficulty coping with the pain associated with performing normal ADLs. Periods of remission and exacerbation that occur as pharmacologic intervention becomes less effective are also very stressful for the patient.

Other therapies for trigeminal neuralgia include acupuncture, transcutaneous electrical nerve stimulation (TENS), and topical application of capsaicin (Zostrix). Patients with trigeminal neuralgia who have fewer or no periods of remission should be referred for surgical intervention.

The unrelenting paroxysmal pain associated with trigeminal neuralgia is frequently associated with compression of the trigeminal nerve root. Surgical intervention is performed to relieve the compression, although reoccurrence in 1 to 2 years is common after surgery, regardless of the surgical method chosen.

Follow-Up and Referral

Because of the intense and chronic pain associated with trigeminal neuralgia, the patient may experience depression, social isolation, and suicidal tendencies. The clinician must recognize these effects of the disease and reinforce coping mechanisms the patient may use during periods of exacerbation. Referral for counseling may be required if the patient is not able to cope with the chronicity and severity of the pain. The patient experiences pain when eating and washing the face and frequently avoids these and other activities. The patient begins to lose weight and becomes dehydrated, and hygiene becomes a problem.

Patient Education

The goals of patient instruction are the avoidance of triggering painful events, pharmacologic management, and coping with chronic, severe pain. Nutritional counseling should encourage intake of soft or pureed, high-caloric foods, along with increased fluids. For hygiene, the use of soft washcloths and mouthwashes should be encouraged. Patients should be educated about adverse reactions (e.g., dizziness, sleepiness, ataxia, nausea and vomiting) to their medications and about the necessity for follow-up blood studies to detect any blood dyscrasias. Intense counseling and supportive education is a continuous process in caring for the patient with trigeminal neuralgia. Recognition of the patient's educational needs, based on their coping mechanisms, search for pain treatment, and the status of the neuralgia will direct the clinician in establishing an individualized plan.

Bell's Palsy

Bell's palsy (prosopoplegia) is a condition with an acute onset of flaccid paralysis, usually occurring on one side of the face in an otherwise healthy person. The peripheral facial palsy is self-limiting and complete recovery usually occurs in a few weeks or months in 80 to 86 percent of patients. Initially, the facial paralysis may be incomplete and then worsen within 48 hours after onset. The sudden experience of facial paralysis is very frightening to the patient, who usually seeks medical care immediately.

Epidemiology and Causes

The specific cause of Bell's palsy is unknown. Theories of etiology include viral infections such as herpes simplex virus type I, respiratory infections, and heredity. The incidence worldwide is 20 per 100,000 each year, with no prevalence associated with gender, facial side, season, or age. A higher incidence is seen in individuals with diabetes, hypertension, trauma, toxin exposure, Lyme disease, and pregnancy.

A complete recovery from facial paralysis usually occurs in 4 to 6 months or no longer than 12 months. Persons at risk for incomplete recovery are those older than age 55, hypertensive, with pain other than ear pain, with complete facial paralysis, and those who have changes in lacrimation, such as involuntary shedding of tears.

Pathophysiology

Cranial nerve VII—the facial nerve—comprises both motor and sensory axons. Its efferent motor axons innervate the muscles of facial expression and its preganglionic parasympathetic axons innervate the lacrimal and nasopalatine glands and all the salivary glands except the parotid. Its afferent axons carry sensation from the taste buds of the anterior two-thirds of the tongue and from cutaneous sensory receptors of the external ear.

The various classes of axons in the facial nerve peel off group by group as the nerve makes its way through the bony canals of the skull; therefore, pressure on or lesions of the nerve at different locations will produce different deficits. Inside the skull, the facial nerve runs with cranial nerve VIII, the vestibulocochlear nerve, and pressure on the facial nerve here (such as from an acoustic neuroma) will usually cause hearing loss and vestibular problems in addition to deficits in all the motor and sensory components of the facial nerve.

Within the skull wall, the facial and vestibulocochlear nerves separate. After this, the first components to leave the facial nerve are the lacrimal and nasopalatine axons; therefore, damage to the facial nerve distal to this juncture will not affect a patient's ability to produce tears. The next components to leave the facial nerve are the taste axons and the axons to the salivary glands; therefore, damage to the facial nerve distal to this juncture will cause unilateral paralysis of all the muscles of facial expression but will not affect taste or the production of saliva.

Damage to the facial nerve inside the skull wall can be caused by skull fractures, hemangiomas, tumors, and inflammation. When the facial nerve is damaged and no structural problems are found, the condition is called Bell's palsy. Bell's palsy always produces unilateral facial paralysis, and depending on the location of the nerve lesion(s), it may also include deficits in functions of the other components of the facial nerve.

The majority of cases of Bell's palsy are preceded by systemic symptoms of a viral infection. Most cases are thought to be caused by a reactivated herpes simplex infection of the geniculate ganglion, which this leads to inflammation and swelling of the nerve inside its restrictive bony canal. Reactivated varicella-zoster virus can also cause Bell's palsy; these cases probably involve demyelination of the nerve and include severe pain and sometimes hearing loss. In addition, a Bell's palsy-like facial paralysis is the most common neurologic problem caused by Lyme disease.

Clinical Presentation

Subjective

Patients with Bell's palsy present with an acute onset of partial or total facial paralysis on one side of the face, usually involving lower motor neurons. The patient has normal ocular movements and facial sensation and often complains of loss of taste (dysgeusia), postauricular pain, abnormal sensitivity to sound (hyperacusis), and a heavy feeling in the face.

Objective

On physical examination, the motor and sensory functions along the entire facial nerve should be assessed. Bell's palsy can be diagnosed because of its acute onset and the fact that no other CNS symptoms exist. The physical assessment characteristically reveals on the affected side the absence of forehead wrinkles, wider palpebral fissure of the eye, decreased corneal reflex, Bell's phenomenon (the eyeball turns upward when the patient tries to close the eyelid), open eyelid, flattening of the nasolabial fold, narrowed lips, and loss of taste on the anterior two-thirds of the tongue. Lacrimation may or may not be affected.

A patient with Bell's palsy typically is unable to make these movements on the affected side on request: raise the eyebrow, wrinkle the forehead, close the eyelid, whistle, or retract the muscles of the mouth or chin. When talking, the patient's cheek puffs out and there is an inability to clearly pronounce words that require pursing of the lips. There appears to be a deviation of the tongue because of mouth paralysis on the affected side. The patient is unable to suck or hold fluids in the mouth but is able to swallow.

During the history, it is important to ask about pregnancy, diabetes, any recent infection such as URI or HSV, and any stress.

Diagnostic Reasoning

Diagnostic Tests

Diagnosis is based primarily on patient history and clinical examination. If the history and physical examination are inconclusive for Bell's palsy, the patient should be referred for further diagnostic workup, to include a CT scan or MRI. Evoked electromyography or electroneurography can assess the extent of nerve involvement. These tests are helpful when the patient is not recovering from the Bell's palsy as expected.

Documentation of the extent of facial function at the time of initial diagnosis and at subsequent assessments is critical to evaluate the course of the disease. Several methods to assess and document facial function are available to the clinician. Photographs, an automated computer-assisted clinimetric system, or a facial grading system may be used. Regardless of what method is used to assess facial functioning, the progression or lack of progression of the symptoms is important to differentiate Bell's palsy from other pathology.

Differential Diagnosis

Tumors, infections, trauma, drug ingestion, TIAs, CVAs, and trigeminal neuralgia may appear similar to Bell's palsy. The history and physical examination will usually provide conclusive data to support the diagnosis of Bell's palsy. Close inspection of the patient's ears and skin is done to assess for herpes simplex lesions that would indicate Ramsey Hunt syndrome, which is herpes zoster affecting the facial and auditory nerves, causing facial palsy and cutaneous herpes zoster lesions of the external ear and/or tympanic membrane. Associated symptoms include tinnitus, vertigo, and deafness.

Management

Sixty percent of patients with Bell's palsy totally recover without treatment since the lesion is mild and a a result of a conduction block. Therefore, management of a patient with idiopathic Bell's palsy is primarily directed at preventing eye injury. Loss of the ability to blink and close the eyelid subjects the cornea to drying and ulceration.

The patient is instructed to keep the eye moist by topical application of artificial tears every 30 minutes during the day and use of an ocular lubricant ointment at night. Wearing wraparound sunglasses, and using a moisture shield (self-adhesive eye bubble, cellulose wrap) are ways to provide eye protection. An eye patch may be necessary if eye closure is not possible. An ophthalmologist should be consulted if the patient experiences any signs of corneal irritation or injury.

Pharmacologic management of Bell's palsy is controversial because the disorder is a self-limiting condition. Some practitioners recommend treatment with acyclovir (Zovirax); others recommend prednisone (Deltasone). If drug treatment is chosen, the medication should be started as soon as Bell's palsy is diagnosed.

Ear pain control is essential during the first few weeks after onset of symptoms. The patient may try a variety of OTC drugs, such as acetaminophen (Tylenol) and ibuprofen (Advil). Rest and decreased auditory stimulation may lessen the effects of hyperacusis.

Follow-Up and Referral

The patient should be examined at regular intervals to assess for resolution or deterioration of Bell's palsy symptoms and adverse effects of medication, if prescribed. Special attention should be given to effectiveness of eye care by the patient. If the patient's symptoms have not resolved in 6 months or if other neurologic signs are evident, the patient should be referred to a neurologist. In some cases, though rarely, the patient may be advised to have surgery. Surgery may be indicated for cases in which paralysis is progressive and when incomplete involvement of some branch of the facial nerve is evident.

Patient Education

The patient with Bell's palsy is experiencing a physical and psychological crisis. The clinician provides essential teaching that supports the recovery process. The patient is in a state of shock and disbelief at the change in self-image and concern about the causes of the symptoms. Reassurance that Bell's palsy is usually a short-term condition will allay some anxiety.

To help the patient cope with self-esteem issues, the clinician may advise the patient to use cosmetic interventions to decrease objective symptoms. For example, combing hair over the affected side of face, using make-up to emphasize the unaffected side, growing a beard or mustache, and wearing sunglasses can lessen the appearance of facial paralysis. Drinking from a plastic, spouted bottle may be easier than drinking from a cup or glass, because liquid can be squeezed into the back of the mouth.

In addition to meticulous eye care, the patient should be taught to perform oral hygiene vigorously because food becomes trapped, there is a reduced amount of saliva, and chewing is impaired. The patient should be instructed to use a soft-bristled toothbrush, mild mouth rinses, dental floss, and an oral water-jet machine to remove food particles after each meal. Foods may also need to be spicier than normal to compensate for loss of taste. The clinician should encourage the patient to eat soft foods of high nutritional value because patients often avoid eating because of difficulty chewing and holding food in the mouth.

When muscle strength returns, facial massage and exercise can be started for 15 to 20 minutes at least twice a day. Using a cream or oil, the affected side of the face from forehead to chin should be massaged. The patient should also be encouraged to perform facial exercises, including opening and closing of eyes, winking, smiling, and showing teeth in front of a mirror.

Bibliography

General

Kasper, DL, Braunwald, E, Fauci, A, Hauser, SL, Longo, DL, and Jameson, JL: Harrison's Manual of Medicine, ed 16. McGraw-Hill, New York, 2005.

Deglin, JH, and Vallerand, AH: Davis' Drug Guide for Nurses, ed 9. FA Davis, Philadelphia, 2005.

Folstein, MF, Folstein, SE, and Fanjiang, G: "Mini-Mental State": A practical method of grading the cognitive state of patients for the clinician. J Psych Res 12(3):189, 1975.

Goetz, GG, and Pappert, EJ: Textbook of Clinical Neurology, ed 2. WB Saunders, Philadelphia, 2003.

Hess, DC, and Hughes, MD: Multiple sclerosis: When to suspect—keys to diagnosis. Consultant 45(8):844, 2005.

Jagoda, A, and Riggio, S: What you forgot about the neurologic exam, Part I: History, mental status, cranial nerves. Consultant (Dec.):1773, 2004.

Khouzam, HR, El-Gabalawi, F, and Donnelly, NJ: Tremors: Diagnostic clues, treatment options. Consultant (Sept.):1429, 2004.

Mandell, GL, Bennett, JE, and Dolin, R: Principles and Practice of Infectious Diseases, ed 6. Churchill Livingstone, Philadelphia, 2005.

McElhaney, JE: Memory problems in the elderly: What's significant—what's normal? Consultant (Aug):1153, 2003.

Tierney, LM, McPhee, SJ, and Papadakis, MA: Current Medical Diagnosis and Treatment, ed 44. Lange Medical Books. McGraw-Hill, New York, 2005.

Victor, M., and Ropper, AH: Adams & Victor's Principles of Neurology, ed 8. Mc-Graw-Hill, New York, 2005.

U.S. Preventive Services Task Force: Screening for dementia: Recommendations and rationale. AJN 103(9): 87, 2003.

Alzheimer's Disease

Alzheimer's Disease Management Council (ADMC) Clinical Consensus Panel: Primary Care Consensus Reports, Clinical Update, June, 2004

Bender, KJ (ed): Slowing the progression of Alzheimer's disease: The role of cholinesterase iinhibitors. Consultant 45(3):53, 2005.

Bryan, RH: Therapy for Alzheimer's. Adv Nurse Pract 38:38, 2004.

Carlsson, CM, Gleason, CE, and Asthana, S: Alzheimer disease: Update on diagnosis and treatment. Consultant (Jan.):77, 2005.

Murphy, DP, and Kasper, J: Behavioral symptoms in Alzheimer dementia: A guide to evaluation and management. Consultant (Aug.): 1265, 2004.

Murphy, DP, and Cleveland, M: Alzheimer disease: A commonsense approach to evaluation and management. Consultant (Mar.):388, 2004.

Peskind, ER, Tangalos, EG, and Grossberg, GT: A case-based approach to Alzheimer's disease. Clin Advisor 8(6):32, 2005.

Silverman, JM, Ciresi, G, Smith, CJ, Marin, DB, and Schnaider-Beeeri, M: Variability of familial risk of Alzheimer disease across the late life span. Arch Gen Psychiatry 62: 565, 2005.

Wheldon, M: Untangling the confusion. Adv Nurse Pract. May: 47, 2005.

Wider, J: Alzheimer cases expected to skyrocket over next fifty years. Women's Health Care 2(9):31, 2003.

Cerebrovascular Accident

Fair, D, and Story, D: Acute ischemic stroke—evaluation and treatment. Clin Rev 14(10):42, 2004.

Fisher, M., and Bardutzky, J: Stroke: Update on new therapies— and the implications for primary care. Consultant (Jan.):60, 2004.

Headaches

Cady, R: Better, faster therapies for migraine headache. Clin Advisor: 21, 2004.

Diamond, S: Prevention and symtomatic relief of migraine: Which drugs to choose? Clin Advisor (Suppl) 9, 2005.

Diamond, S, and Pepper, BJ: Severe migraine: Options for acute therapy in the emergency department. Consultant (Mar.):325, 2002.

Glassroth, CH: Successful migraine management—patient-customized care. Clin Rev 14(5):56, 2004.

Loder, S., and McAlvary, P: Women with migraine: Treatment opportunities and pitfalls. Wom Health Primary Care 7(1):19, 2004.

Ruoff, GE: Headache: Benign or worrisome? Keys to making the diagnosis. Consultant (Oct.):1581, 2004.

Ruoff, GE: Effective pharmacologic strategies for prevention and treatment. Consultant (June):969, 2004.

Tepper, SJ: Alternative medicine in migraine: Is it ever a good alternative? Consultant (May):662, 2005.

Wright, W: Serotonin agonists target the pathogenesis of migraine. Clin Advisor (Suppl) 15, 2005.

Wright, W: Practitioners on the front line: Assessing patients for migraine. Clin Advisor (Suppl) 3, 2005.

Parkinson's Disease

Nutt, JG, and Wooten, GF: Diagnosis and initial management of Parkinson's disease. N Engl J Med 353(10):1021, 2005.

Penna, P: Epidemiology, economics and effective practices in managed care. Schwarz Pharma Parkinson's Report for Managed Care, Neurology & Senior Care Decision-Makers. 1(1):11; 4, 2005.

Stefanacci, RG: Managing Parkinson's disease. Schwarz Pharma Parkinson's Report for Managed Care, Neurology & Senior Care Decision-Makers. 1(1):1-15, 2005.

Resources

Alzheimer's Disease
Alzheimer's Association
1-800-272-3900
http://www.alz.org
Alzheimer's Foundation of America
1-866-232-8484
http://alzfdn.org

Cerebrovascular Accident
The National Stroke Association
1-800-STROKES
http://www.stroke.org
American Stroke Association
1-800-242-8721
http://www.strokeassociation.org
The American Heart Association
1-800-242-8715
http://www.americanheart.org

Epilepsy
Epilepsy Foundation 1-800-EFA-1000
http://www.epilepsyfoundation.org
Multiple Sclerosis
Multiple Sclerosis Foundation
1-800-225-6495
http://www.msfacts.org
National Multiple Sclerosis Society
1-800-FIGHT-MS (1-800-344-4867)
http://nmss.org
Parkinson's Disease
Parkinson's Disease Foundation
1-800-457-6676
http://www.pdf.org
The National Parkinson Foundation, Inc.
1-800-327-4545
http://www.parkinson.org/
United Parkinson Foundation
833 West Washington Blvd.
Chicago, IL 60607
1-312-733-1893
Headache
National Headache Foundation
1-888-NHF-5552
http://www.headaches.org

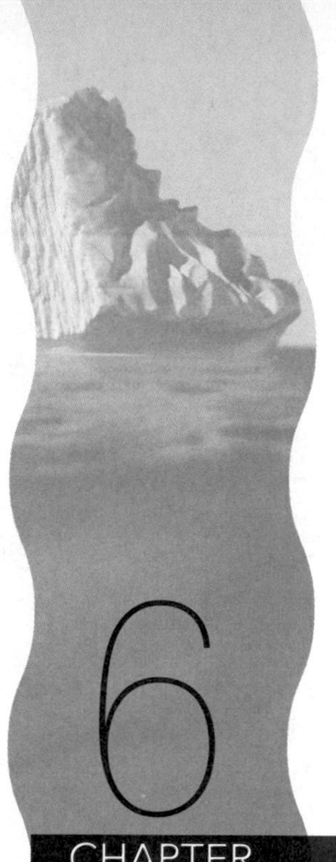

Skin Problems

Jill E. Winland-Brown, EdD, MSN, APRN, BC
Brian O. Porter, MD, PhD, MPH
Maria Leik, MSN, APRN, BC

Common Complaints

Alopecia

Alopecia (baldness) can occur anywhere on the body where hair is present, although it is commonly associated with absence of hair on the scalp area. Scalp hair loss can occur in patches (*alopecia areata*) or over the entire scalp (*androgenetic alopecia*). Hair loss can occur on the eyebrows, beard area, or on the entire body (*alopecia universalis*), and it can be either a temporary or permanent condition.

Hair loss is a gradual process; up to 50 percent of scalp hair can be lost before the loss becomes clinically apparent. Alopecia is associated with emotional distress even if the hair loss is temporary (alopecia areata). The most common cause of permanent hair loss is androgenetic alopecia or male-pattern baldness (common baldness). Androgenetic alopecia has a polygenic inheritance pattern: It is inherited from both parents, not only through maternal genes—a common myth. Another common misconception is that androgenetic alopecia is more common in men; in reality, it occurs equally between both sexes.

Factors that influence normal hair development and cycling include estrogens, growth hormone, glucocorticoids, thyroid hormone, retinoid, prolactin, and androgens, and they can be adversely affected by certain medications. The most important hair growth factors are the androgens testosterone and its active metabolite, dihydrotestosterone. During puberty, when androgen secretion starts, hair follicles become enlarged in certain areas of the body such as the beard area, the chest, and the extremities. Androgens have the opposite effect on the hair follicles of the scalp region: They cause a decrease in the size of the hair follicles (miniaturization) and can alter the hairline on the bitemporal region and the vortex areas. Three cycles of scalp hair growth exist. The growth phase (*anagen*) of scalp hair is the longest cycle, lasting from 2 to 6 years. The majority of hair on the scalp (90 to 95 percent) is in the anagen phase. The latent or involution phase (*catagen*) is the shortest cycle, which lasts only 2 to 3 weeks. The resting phase (*telogen*) lasts from 2 to 3 months. Hair is shed during the resting phase (50 to 150 hairs daily) and the cycle is repeated. Both topical and systemic medication for hair loss affects some or all of the cycles of hair growth.

In reversible cases of nonscarring alopecia, regrowth of hair usually takes several months. Patients who are reassured of this important fact will have lessened anxiety over their condition. Two important factors that the practitioner should address in the evaluation of alopecia are (1) whether it is scarring or nonscarring alopecia and (2) whether hair loss is in a small, well-circumscribed area (alopecia areata or trichotillomania) or generalized (androgenetic alopecia). Based on these two general categories, the differential diagnosis is made easier for the clinician. Scarring alopecia (*cicatricial alopecia*) causes permanent hair loss and is not reversible. Hair loss from nonscarring alopecia (*noncicatricial alopecia*) can be either temporary or permanent.

Differential Diagnosis

A thorough history is important in the evaluation of alopecia. Information regarding family members—both male and female—with hair loss should be elicited. Because some medications affect hair growth factors, a review of the patient's medication history is important and should not be missed. Drugs that cause hair loss include hormones, anticonvulsants, anticoagulants, oral contraceptives, beta-blockers, antimetabolites, antithyroid drugs, and excessive amounts of vitamin A or of topical Retin-A.

A potassium hydroxide (KOH) and Wood's light exam is helpful in the diagnosis of tinea capitis in cases of patchy hair loss. Although most cases of tinea capitis do not fluoresce, a fungal culture can provide definitive proof of fungal infection and should be done if suspicion is high. Some dermatologists utilize the telogen count, which is done by removing 100 hairs from different areas of the scalp and counting how many hairs are in telogen. Telogen hairs are recognized because of the large white club on the end of each hair.

The appearance of the skin on the scalp will give the practitioner a clue to the type of alopecia that is involved. In nonscarring alopecia, the scalp will have normal texture and color. In contrast, the scalp of a patient with scarring alopecia has no visible hair follicles (or no follicular openings) and is atrophied and smooth. The affected area of the scalp (or the entire scalp) is sometimes hypo- or hyperpigmented. Obvious scarring is seen in some patients and some have erythema and scaling (in these cases, it is important to rule out fungal infection).

Both systemic and nonsystemic causes are seen in nonscarring alopecia. Nonsystemic causes of alopecia include hair pulling (*trichotillomania*), excessive traction of the frontal and temporal area of the scalp (from tight cornrows or tight ponytails), trauma (both physical and chemical), radiation therapy of the head, local bacterial infection, and local fungal infection. Trichotillomania (compulsive hair pulling) is more commonly seen in children and teens.

Systemic causes of nonscarring alopecia include alopecia areata, telogen effluvium, androgenetic baldness (common baldness), systemic lupus erythematosus (SLE), hypothyroidism or hyperthyroidism, secondary syphilis, severe herpes zoster of the scalp, drug-induced alopecia, common in patients on cyclophosphamide therapy, iron-deficiency anemia, and pituitary insufficiency.

Telogen effluvium—excessive shedding of scalp hair as a result of an increased number of hair follicles entering the resting stage (telogen)—can be caused by fever and certain drugs; therefore, a search for these possible causes should be included in the history taking. The classic signs of androgenetic baldness are thinning hairs of various diameters and lengths ("miniaturized" hairs) located in typical areas, which differ in men and women. In men, hair loss usually starts on the hairline and around the temple (bitemporal) area and the vortex or top of the head. In women, hair loss is much more diffuse and occurs mostly on top of the head. Hair loss is sometimes harder to recognize in women because of hairstyles that are used to camouflage the problem.

Alopecia areata is not an uncommon condition in primary-care practice. The cause of alopecia areata is still unknown, although an immunologic mechanism is suspected. The typical patient will present with well-circumscribed patches of hair loss on the scalp, or sometimes on the face, in areas such as the eyebrows or the beard area. Occasionally only one patch is seen; sometimes multiple patches of hair loss are apparent. Alopecia areata can occur once in a lifetime, or it can be a recurrent problem. Some cases become recalcitrant and are best treated by specialists. In alopecia areata, when the scalp is examined closely with a magnifying lens, short, stubby hairs with tapered ends (so-called exclamation point hairs) are seen on the periphery of the bald patch (or patches). Alopecia areata is associated with autoimmune endocrinopathies such as Hashimoto's thyroiditis, Addison's disease, and pernicious anemia.

Hair regrowth occurs after several months, with new hairs that look thinner and finer than the original hair. There is no cure for alopecia areata, but in most patients hair usually regrows spontaneously after several months. The prognosis for alopecia areata is good if it occurs after puberty: Studies have found that up to 80 percent of these patients will regrow hair. Occasionally, a case of persistent alopecia areata that is unresponsive to treatment is seen; these cases are best referred to dermatologists for management.

Etiology of scarring or cicatricial alopecia can include trauma (physical or chemical), severe bacterial or fungal infections of the scalp, scleroderma, discoid lupus erythematosus, lichen planopilaris, and excessive radiation. Early recognition and treatment of bacterial or fungal infections can help prevent or minimize the incidence of scarring. Severe local infection with either bacteria or fungi can permanently damage hair follicles and cause a patchy (and scarring) alopecia that is permanent.

When an autoimmune disease is suspected, laboratory tests include antinuclear antibodies (ANA—to rule out lupus or autoimmune disorders), the rheumatoid factor, and the erythrocyte sedimentation rate (ESR—a nonspecific marker for inflammation). The rheumatology or arthritis profile is a panel of tests specific for autoimmune disorders that may help in the diagnosis of autoimmune disorders that can cause alopecia, such as SLE and scleroderma. Scleroderma (progressive systemic sclerosis) is a multisystemic inflammatory disorder associated with sclerotic changes in the body, including the skin. The skin becomes diffusely thickened with telangiectasia. A scalp biopsy is reserved for difficult and recalcitrant cases of alopecia. For the differential diagnosis of alopecia, see Table 6.1.

In addition, serum testosterone, dehydroepiandrosterone (DHEAS), iron, total iron-binding capacity, and thyroid function tests, along with a complete blood count (CBC), will identify most other causes of hair thinning in premenopausal women.

A biopsy is useful in diagnosing scarring alopecia but specimens must be obtained from the active border rather than from the scarred central zone.

Table 6.1 Differential Diagnosis: Alopecia

Type of Alopecia	Differential Diagnosis
Scarring alopecia (Cicatricial alopecia)	Trauma (chemical, physical, heat) Kerion formation in tinea capitis Chronic discoid lupus erythematosus Scleroderma Excessive radiation to scalp Lichen planopilaris Bacterial infection of scalp
Nonscarring alopecia (Noncicatricial alopecia)	Alopecia areata Drug-induced hair loss Trichotillomania (hair pulling) Telogen effluvium (after pregnancy, major surgery, major emotional stress) Androgenetic baldness Tinea capitis (with no kerion formation) Hypothyroidism (Hashimoto's thyroiditis) Systemic lupus erythematosus Addison's disease

Treatment

Medical treatment is available but is not a permanent solution for alopecia. Patients should be educated that total return to previous levels of hair growth is not possible, but cosmetically acceptable hair coverage is possible. Medical treatments must be used daily to maintain regrown hair. Stopping treatment will result in shedding of hair and a return to the previous levels of alopecia. Hair shedding is seen rapidly in a matter of days after stopping minoxidil (Rogaine), but is more gradual over several months with finasteride (Propecia). Propecia is for men only. Nonmedical options include hair weaves, toupees, and wigs. Wigs are either worn on top of the head or are interwoven into existing hair. As the existing hair (that the wig is anchored to) grows, the wig must be readjusted periodically. The only currently available permanent treatment for alopecia is scalp surgery with hair transplantation.

Topical treatment includes minoxidil 2 percent solution (Rogaine for Men or Rogaine for Women), and minoxidil 5 percent solution (Rogaine Extra Strength for Men), which are both available over the counter (OTC). The mechanism of minoxidil in inducing hair growth is still unknown. At a higher dose, oral minoxidil (Loniten) is a vasodilator and is used to treat hypertension. Topical minoxidil has not been found to cause lowering of systolic or diastolic blood pressure and pulse rate. The best candidates for treatment with topical minoxidil are patients with recent onset of alopecia (less than 5 years), those younger than age 50, and patients with smaller areas of hair loss. Up to 40 percent of patients who use topical minoxidil for a period of 1 year or more will experience moderate to dense hair regrowth. Even more effective is minoxidil 5 percent solution, but it is indicated for use by men only. Rogaine is used twice daily on the affected scalp area. Adverse effects include irritation, itching, dryness, scaling, and redness of the scalp; sometimes minoxidil can cause contact dermatitis. An adverse effect that is more common in women is *hypertrichosis* (excessive hair growth on the body).

Systemic treatment for alopecia with finasteride (Propecia) should not be used in women of reproductive age, because this drug can cause abnormalities of the external genitalia of male fetuses. Finasteride (Propecia), 1-mg tablet once daily, is used for the treatment of androgenetic baldness in men only. Finasteride is metabolized in the liver and should be used with caution in patients with liver disease. In men age 60 or older, finasteride may not be as effective as in younger men because of reduction in alpha-reductase activity. Adverse effects seen in clinical trials include decreased libido (1.8 percent), erectile dysfunction (1.3 percent), and ejaculatory dysfunction (1.2 percent). In most men, these sexual side effects gradually resolve with prolonged treatment.

The treatment choice is determined by the patient's age and the severity of the hair loss. For patients with hair loss of less than 50 percent, treatment options include corticosteroid intralesional injections, anthralin, minoxidil solution, or topical corticosteroid creams. Topical treatment with a potent topical steroid is preferred by primary-care practitioners because it is not invasive and is simple to use, although it is not as effective as intralesional injections. Small amounts of triamcinolone acetonide 5 mg/mL (Kenalog) are injected intralesionally into the mid-dermal layer approximately 1 centimeter (cm) apart on bald patches. Hair growth is usually seen in 4 weeks. One side effect of steroid use that patients and practitioners should monitor for is atrophy of the skin.

Pigmentation Changes

The skin is the largest and most visible organ of the body. For most people, skin color is an important part of their identity as an individual. Because of the skin's visibility, conditions affecting the skin cause not only physical discomfort, but also have emotional overtones. Pigmentation disorders seen in primary care include both hyperpigmentation and hypopigmentation. Either condition can be a sign of disease, or it can be considered a normal finding, depending on the rest of the clinical picture.

Melanin is skin pigment produced by melanocyte cells that determines skin color. Although there is no difference in the number of melanocytes among the different ethnic groups, the ability of the melanocytes of darker-skinned people to produce and retain melanin (from melanosomes) is much greater than in people with lighter skin. Research has found that melanosome size is directly related to skin color: The larger the size of the melanosomes, the darker the skin color. Asians and whites have fewer and smaller melanosomes, whereas in individuals with darker skins, especially in blacks or people of African descent, melanosomes are much larger and more numerous. Darker skin gives protection from ultraviolet (UV) radiation. Studies of people with darker skin have shown that dark skin has a sun protection factor (SPF) between 5 and 13. Because of the protective aspect of darker skin, the incidence of nonmelanoma skin cancer in blacks or people of African origin is much less than in whites. Studies have shown that basal cell carcinomas are extremely rare in individuals with darker skin.

Pigmentation disorders that can be clinical manifestations of disease include endocrine, genetic, metabolic, or nutritional problems, or a malignancy. Pigmentation disorders seen in primary care include normal variations in color as a result of ethnic differences (i.e., oral hyperpigmentation in darker skins). *Vitiligo,* or the total loss of skin color in patchy areas of the body (rarely over the entire body) is recognized clinically as extremely white macules or patches that are usually located on exposed areas like the face and the hands. More than half the cases of vitiligo occur between the ages of 10 and 30; vitiligo occurs equally in both sexes. It is relatively common and affects up to 1 percent of the population. Vitiligo is an autoimmune disorder in which the body produces antibodies against its own melanocytes. Vitiligo is associated with a higher risk of other autoimmune disorders such as thyroid disease and diabetes mellitus type 1 but not with diabetes mellitus type 2.

Differential Diagnosis

Differential diagnoses to consider in oral hyperpigmentation include Peutz-Jeghers syndrome, pigmented tumors such as melanoma, Addison's disease, heavy metal exposure, and a history of taking antimalarial medications. Peutz-Jeghers syndrome is an inherited disorder that presents with pigmented (dark brown-colored) macules on the lips and inside the mouth, on the mucous membranes. It is associated with multiple polyps in the stomach, the small intestine, and large bowel, causing abdominal pain and other gastrointestinal symptoms. Patients who are suspected of having this disease need to be referred to a gastroenterologist for further evaluation.

Normal variations in pigmentation are commonly seen in the clinical area in patients with darker skin. In patients with dark skin or those of African descent, oral hyperpigmentation is considered a normal variant, but underlying pathology should be ruled out. The exception is newborn infants—oral pigmentation should not be present at this early time. The most common site of involvement is the gingivae (the gums), but other sites, such as the inside of the cheeks (buccal mucosa) and the tongue, can be involved as well. The hyperpigmented areas can range from bluish black to a deep brown in color. Another pigmentation change that is considered a normal variant in blacks or people of African descent is hypopigmentation of the midsternal area. It is more common in males; this type of hypopigmentation is seen in up to 70 percent of black children and in one-third of adults.

Voigt's or Futcher lines are seen in up to one-fourth of blacks or people of African descent and less frequently in Asians. These distinct lines appear down the length of each arm symmetrically, dividing lighter-colored skin anteromedially from the patient's darker skin color (the lighter shade of skin is touching the trunk). The nails of people with darker skin can be pigmented, with involvement of the entire nail plate or in longitudinal bands of streaks of darker color. Normal nail pigmentation should be bilateral and symmetrical. Any asymmetry or new onset of pigmentation should arouse the clinician's suspicion for disease, including acral melanoma. Pigmentation changes in people with darker skin do not necessarily point to pathology, but the clinician should not neglect the possibility of a disease process either.

A physiologic hyperpigmentation called *melasma* or *chloasma* ("the mask of pregnancy") is caused by increased levels of estrogen, progesterone, and of melanocyte-stimulating hormone during pregnancy. Chloasma may also occur in 30 to 50 percent of women taking oral contraceptives Areas commonly affected include the face, the nipples, the genitals, and the linea nigra extending midline on the abdomen from the umbilicus to the pubis. The hyperpigmentation is worsened by exposure to sunlight and patients should be cautioned to decrease sun exposure at this time. Treatment for severe melasma includes the use of hydroquinone and sunscreen combinations such as Solaquin and Solaquin Forte. A 24-hour skin patch test to rule out an allergy to the agent should be done prior to use. The cream can be applied twice a day for 2 months. The patient should be advised to avoid the eye area and to use the cream cautiously in sensitive areas such as the nose and the lips. Unfortunately, hydroquinone is labeled pregnancy category C, so the patient should be referred to an obstetrician for management. Certain drugs that are known to cause a diffuse hyperpigmentation (melanosis) include zidovudine and cyclophosphamide. Skin discoloration has also been reported in patients who have been taking amiodarone, chlorpromazine, and certain antimalarials. Photosensitivity reactions resulting in hyperpigmentation following sun exposure can be caused by citrus oils that are present in fruit or certain perfumes.

Addison's disease is caused by inadequate secretion of corticosteroids as a result of partial or complete destruction (70 percent of cases are due to an autoimmune mechanism) of the adrenal glands. It can cause a diffused generalized hyperpigmentation, especially on skin creases, because of increased levels of adrenocorticotropic hormone (ACTH) from the pituitary. Classic areas where hyperpigmentation is seen are skin folds; palmar creases; pressure points such as the elbows, knees, or knuckles; inside the mouth on the cheeks (buccal area); and on scars. Symptoms of Addison's disease include generalized weakness, amenorrhea, and loss of axillary hair in women. Laboratory findings in Addison's disease include elevated serum potassium and calcium, low serum sodium, anemia, and an elevated ACTH level. Screening laboratory tests to detect autoimmune diseases include thyroid-stimulating hormone (TSH), ANA, sedimentation rate, random blood glucose levels, vitamin B_{12} level, rheumatoid factor (RF), and a CBC.

In patients with pigmented nevi (moles), the presence of certain unusual colors on nevi, such as blue, gray, pink, white, and black (or a variegation of color) should arouse suspicion in the clinician. Benign moles are usually a small size (less than 5 mm)—smaller than a pencil eraser—and have a well-defined border. Benign moles should be only a single shade of color—either brown, beige, or pink.

When evaluating nail pigmentation changes, symmetry and bilateral involvement of the nails and a history of no change is reassuring. A variegated color or very dark color on one solitary nail should arouse suspicion for acral melanoma. Melanomas in people with darker skin are more likely to present on the extremities (or acral area) rather than on the trunk area. The nail beds, the palms, and the soles are sites where acral melanoma is more likely to be seen in darker-skinned people. The differential diagnoses of nail pigmentation change include acral melanoma, Peutz-Jeghers syndrome, a subungual nevus, gold therapy, Addison's disease, hemachromatosis, and a history of taking antimalarial medications. If acral melanoma is suspected, referral to a dermatologist for a nail biopsy and definitive diagnosis is imperative.

Malignant melanoma, the deadliest of all skin cancers, requires a high index of suspicion. Factors that can precipitate the appearance of acquired melanocytic nevus (AMN) include immunosuppression, pregnancy, puberty, and sun exposure. Any asymmetry and changes in pigmentation, size, or surface of a mole require referral to a dermatologist. Moles that are larger than 5 mm are more likely to be atypical. Persons at higher risk for skin cancer include patients with numerous moles (50 or more countable moles), atypical and large (more than 5 mm) moles, and a family history of melanoma. The American Cancer Society mnemonic to help detect skin cancer is ABCDE: A—Asymmetry, B—Border (irregularity), C—Color (variegation), D—Diameter (greater than 6 mm), and E—Elevation. Any patient with a suspicious mole should be referred to a dermatologist for definitive diagnosis and treatment.

Pruritus

Pruritus—the sensation of itching—is perceived as unpleasant; therefore, people often seek help for this problematic symptom. Pruritus is a frequent symptom of dermatologic disease; it can be acute or chronic and is sometimes so severe as to interfere with sleep and daily life activities.

Pruritus is generally caused by either local (e.g., insect bite) or systemic (e.g., uremia) etiology. In Hodgkin's disease, the incidence of pruritus is between 10 and 25 percent. Rashes or other skin lesions generally accompany the sensation of itching on the skin, although in some cases of systemic etiology, no external findings on the skin are ever located. Therefore, the finding of skin lesions or rashes is most useful in classification of the differential diagnosis of pruritus.

Differential Diagnosis

A thorough and careful history is an important step in the evaluation of pruritus. If skin findings (such as the linear shape characteristic of contact dermatitis) suggest an external causation, then the history should be directed toward eliciting an external etiology. If the patient complains of generalized itching with no skin lesions, then an internal or systemic causation is more likely. The presence of a generalized rash should also arouse the clinician's suspicion to drug reactions. Some systemic causes of pruritus include conditions such as allergies, drug reactions, malignancy (lymphomas and leukemias), uremia of chronic renal disease, and pruritus from obstructive biliary disease, as a result of elevated blood levels of unconjugated bilirubin. (See Focusing the History 6.1.)

Pruritus is a symptom and should elicit an investigation of the possible causation. External causes of pruritus include insect bites, insect infestation (scabies, pediculosis), pinworms (more common in children), larva migrans, contact dermatitis, fiberglass dermatitis, seabather's eruption, and bacterial folliculitis. It is not uncommon for patients to deny the knowledge of insect bites (especially if the event occurred during sleep), because some insects do not have painful bites. The patient should be asked about any history of medication use, including prescriptions, hormones, vitamin supplements, and the use of nutritional and protein supplements. A history of alternative medicines, including herbals, homeopathic remedies, and oils for aromatherapy should also be included. Many young women who take oral contraceptives forget that these drugs are prescription drugs and therefore do not mention them unless the practitioner makes a special effort to elicit information about oral contraceptive use. The use of recreational substances, including chewing tobacco, marijuana, and illicit drugs, should be considered as a potential cause of pruritus. Psychiatric illness as a cause of pruritus is a diagnosis of exclusion. Skin markings are seen more often on extremities; the urge to scratch even in the absence of itch is sometimes reported. The clinician should search for symptoms of depression or mood disorder. There is frequently a history of increased stress because of personal, financial, or familial problems.

The most predominant and disturbing symptom of scabies is pruritus, especially nighttime pruritus. The clinician needs to have a high index of suspicion for scabies,

FOCUS ON HISTORY 6.1

Pruritus

History	Questions to Ask
Insects	Have you had any exposure to mosquitoes, fleas, sand flies, ticks, or spiders? (brown recluse and black widow bites have necrotic centers)
Outdoors	Have you been to the beach, at a picnic, gone camping or swimming, or attended a sporting event?
Plants	Have you been in contact with plants or done any gardening?
Jewelry/metals	Any new watches, belts/belt buckles, earrings, necklace? Any contact with metals?
Occupation	What is your occupation? (gardeners and employees of prisons, day-care centers and schools have the potential for scabies, pediculosis, or impetigo exposure) Have you been exposed to fiberglass?
Hobbies and sport participation	Any exposure to hobby paints and glues? Do you participate in any sports? (weight lifters, athletes are prone to fungal skin infections)
Chemical exposure	Any use or exposure to pesticides, herbicides, fertilizers, household cleaners?
Medications	Any use of topical medications such as neosporin ointment, benadryl topical lotion, anti-itch lotion or spray? (contact dermatitis) Any prescription medicines, over-the-counter, herbs, vitamins
Family history	Any family members or intimate friends with the same symptoms? (scabies, pediculosis, tinea capitis)

because it frequently does not manifest in its classic presentation. If the clinician is looking for the mites' burrows, which the patient can obliterate by scratching, then the diagnosis can easily be missed. Frequently, the rash has secondary changes, including excoriation, scaling, lichenification, and occasionally nodules (nodular scabies) because of the intense inflammatory response from the mite. Even if skin lesions do not resemble those associated with scabies, the clinician should consider the diagnosis if the location of the rash is on the axilla, under the breast, on the waistline, on the penis, or between the fingers. The clinician should not assume a lack of scabies infection if the classic rash on the interdigital webs is not seen. Scabies is more common in group homes and nursing homes. The management and treatment of scabies are discussed in depth later on this chapter, under Parasitic Infestations.

If a pruritic rash does not respond to symptomatic treatment, then a work-up for systemic diseases is in order. Laboratory tests that should be ordered if systemic disease is suspected include CBC with differential; ESR; fasting blood sugar, liver, and renal function tests; a thyroid profile or a TSH level; and a hepatitis profile. If the pruritic area is in the anus, a search for external hemorrhoids should be done. In children or in adults with small children (when pinworm infestation is suspected), then a stool sample to check for ova and parasites, or a Scotch tape test, is recommended.

Dry skin, or *xerosis,* is a common finding in the elderly. It is also seen in young adults who have dry skin and are overly meticulous with personal hygiene. Use of strong deodorant soaps or daily hot baths can precipitate dry skin and worsen pruritus. Systemic causes of pruritus to consider include atopic dermatitis (eczema), psoriasis, drug reactions, urticaria (from exposure to any substance, including airborne allergens), urticarial eruptions of pregnancy, lichen planus, and a malignancy, such as Hodgkin's lymphoma, cutaneous T-cell lymphoma (mycosis fungoides), and leukemia. A history of similar pruritic lesions in the past (especially if on the same location) should bring to mind an atopic history or urticaria. Atopic skin diseases that present predominantly with pruritus include atopic dermatitis (eczema) and psoriasis. The presence of hives or a history of hives is sufficient to diagnose urticaria. It is often seen with dermatographism, which can be elicited by rubbing a blunt object or finger on the skin firmly. An immediate response is seen, with formation of whealing that resolves within a few hours.

Lichen planus can mimic psoriasis; its cause is unknown. The lesions appear with shiny flat tops that are a red to violaceous color (red violet-tinged). Other presentations include small, flat-topped papules and a netlike lesion on the buccal mucosa (reticular lichen planus). Malignant oral lesions occasionally occur, but oral carcinoma is rare. Lichen planus may have several presentations and locations: Lesions may be generalized, or they may be located on the arms, the trunk, the mouth, and the genitalia. This disease may last for months to years; it does not have a cure and is best managed by a dermatologist. See Table 6.2 for the differential diagnoses of pruritus.

Treatment

The treatment of pruritus depends on making the correct diagnosis. Symptomatic treatment for dry skin consists of

Table 6.2 **Differential Diagnosis: Pruritus**

Type of Pruritus	Differential Diagnosis
Pruritus—rash present	Insect bites/pediculosis Burrowing insects/larvae (scabies) Tinea (corporis, pedis, cruris) Contact dermatitis Atopic dermatitis (eczema) Drug eruptions Urticaria (hives) Malignancy (cutaneous T-cell lymphoma) Pregnancy-induced Psoriasis Milaria (heat rash) Folliculitis Seborrheic dermatitis Lichen planus Prurigo nodularis
Pruritus—no rash present	Uremia from chronic renal disease Cholestatic liver disease Hyperparathyroidism Hodgkin's lymphoma Polycythemia vera Delusions of parasitosis

avoidance of strong soaps, taking shorter, tepid showers (10 to 20 minutes) instead of hot baths, and the use of good emollients. Mild bland soaps such as Dove, Basis, Purpose, and Neutrogena are recommended. The patient should be educated to gently towel dry the skin after showering, because rubbing the skin stimulates pruritus. To seal in the moisture in the skin, applying a bland emollient such as Eucerin, Lubriderm, or Alpha-Keri immediately after dabbing the skin with the towel is helpful. Waiting too long (more than 5 minutes) after finishing a bath or shower allows moisture to evaporate. The strongest emollients are ointments that are petrolatum-based, followed by creams (oil in water), and then lotions (powder in water). Gels are alcohol-based; they should not be used for pruritus associated with dry skin because of their drying effect. Pruritus of the scalp caused by seborrheic dermatitis (with dandruff and fine scales at the hairline, by the nares, and the ears) should be treated with ketoconazole 2 percent shampoo (Nizoral shampoo). The rash of seborrheic dermatitis on the hairline, nares, and ears is best treated with hydrocortisone 1 percent (OTC) used twice to three times a day (bid to tid). Fluorinated topical steroids should not be used on the face because of the risk of skin atrophy. If the etiology is an irritating external agent (such as fiberglass insulation), then elimination of irritating external agents may provide clinical relief of pruritus. Treatment of scabies infection is discussed later in this chapter.

Symptomatic treatment of generalized pruritus includes classic oral H_1 antihistamines such as hydroxyzine (Atarax, Vistaril) 10 to 25 mg, one of the most effective treatments for pruritus, given tid to qid. Cyproheptadine 4 mg (Periactin) is used bid to tid. Over-the-counter antihistamines include loratadine (Claritin) 10 mg once a day, diphenhydramine (Benadryl) 25 to 50 mg, brompheniramine maleate (Dimetapp Allergy) 4 mg, and chlorpheniramine maleate (Chlor-Trimeton) 4 mg; all can be taken every 4 to 6 hours (q4 to 6h) as needed (prn). Prescription antihistamines do not cross the blood–brain barrier and cause less (or no) sedation. These include cetirizine (Zyrtec) 5 to 10 mg daily, fexofenadine (Allegra) 60 mg bid, and desloratadine (Clarinex) 5 mg once daily.

Any patient who is on antihistamines should be warned of possible drowsiness and should be warned against driving or operating dangerous machinery until the effects of the antihistamine are known. Alcohol and other central depressants worsen this effect. In addition, topical steroids may be helpful for pruritus.

For anogenital pruritus, treatment includes the use of hydrocortisone and pramoxine cream 1 or 2.5 percent (Pramosone) on the anogenital area. Pramoxine preparations are very effective and have a low incidence of sensitivity reactions compared to topical antihistamines and benzocaine. They are effective not only for anogenital pruritus but also for short-term relief of urticaria, insect bites, pruritus vulvae, and nummular eczema. Use of fluorinated and potent topical steroids on the anogenital area is not recommended, because it can lead to atrophy and striae. Lichen planus is treated with topical and systemic steroids and retinoids, cyclosporine, and PUVA (Psoralens with ultraviolet A) photochemotherapy; the treatment of this disease is best managed by dermatologists.

If Hodgkin's lymphoma is suspected, the clinician should perform a thorough physical exam and should especially look for painless and enlarged lymph nodes and constitutional symptoms such as generalized pruritus, weight loss, night sweats, and fever. Cutaneous T-cell lymphoma (mycosis fungoides) is a malignancy of the helper T cells of the immune system. Onset of lesions may take many years; sometimes intractable pruritus may be the only presenting symptom. The lesions are sometimes misdiagnosed as psoriasis or as nummular dermatitis (eczema) because of their similar appearance. The lesions go through several stages and can present as red and scaly plaques that mimic the appearance of psoriasis. Nodules and tumors can be present, sometimes with ulceration. Diagnostic laboratory testing for suspected malignancy can include a CBC with differential, a peripheral smear, liver and renal function tests, ESR, a chest x-ray film, and computed tomography (CT) scan. Patients with suspected malignancy should be referred to cancer specialists.

Rash

The word *rash* refers to any pink or red-colored skin eruption. Words that are synonymous with rash include *exan-*

them and *eruption*. Rashes are clinical manifestations of inflammation and have multiple etiology.

Skin cells (keratinocytes) originate in the basal layer of the epidermis. These cells take approximately 28 days to mature and migrate to the surface (*stratum corneum*). The epidermis has no blood supply of its own and is dependent on the dermis for its circulation. It is stratified into two main layers—the inner viable layer (*stratum germinativum*) and the outer layer of dead, anucleated cells, called the *stratum corneum* or the horny layer. The stratum corneum consists of up to 25 layers of flat and tightly packed anucleated cells filled with keratin. Keratin, a tough and durable protein, limits the passage of molecules in and out of the skin. Thus, this tough outer layer is relatively impermeable to many external substances and also acts to prevent the evaporation of bodily fluids. It is a protective barrier against numerous microorganisms. When the stratum corneum is damaged by inflammation (rash), it becomes more permeable to external substances, including microorganisms and chemicals. Not only do these substances and microorganisms have a greater chance of gaining entrance into the body, but therapeutic topical creams and ointments applied to inflamed skin also are more likely to be absorbed and thus increase the chance of toxicity.

The dermis, which gives the skin its elasticity and strength, is made up primarily of a complex network of collagen and elastic fibers interspersed with blood vessels, cutaneous nerves, apocrine glands, eccrine glands, the lymphatics, and the pilosebaceous units of the skin. The *dermoepidermal junction* (the topmost section of the dermis) is the interface between the epidermis and the dermis. A defect in the dermoepidermal junction results in separation of these layers and bullous formation. Inherited autoimmune diseases of the skin resulting from abnormalities of the dermis include bullous pemphigoid and epidermolysis bullosa.

Gram-positive bacterial infections such as *Staphylococcus aureus*—the causative agent of toxic shock syndrome (TSS)—present with systemic symptoms such as fever, malaise, and an erythematous rash. Drug reactions can also present with a rash (e.g., erythema multiforme, urticaria). Autoimmune disorders that can cause a rash include SLE (butterfly rash), erythema nodosum, and Kawasaki disease (seen in children).

Viruses are responsible for many cases of rash and are usually self-limiting in patients with intact immune systems. Viral infections that manifest with rash and systemic symptoms such as fever and malaise include measles, rubella (German measles), hand–foot–mouth disease, erythema infectiosum, herpes simplex infection, herpes zoster, varicella-zoster (chickenpox), and roseola infantum (also known as exanthema subitum) in children.

Rashes are more difficult to see in patients with darker skins because the red to dark pink color that is associated with rash becomes less visible. Instead of the pink to red color, a rash in a person of African descent might appear as a dark brown color. Rashes on patients with darker skin can sometimes go unnoticed unless the patient complains of the problem to the clinician. The clinician must learn to use other dermatologic clues besides skin color to differentiate rashes in this population. These include the history of the rash and associated symptoms, the type of lesions present (macule, papule, pustule), the texture of the lesions (flat, raised, rough), and the pattern of distribution (central versus on the extremities). (See Focusing the History 6.2 and Table 6.3 Skin Lesions.)

Differential Diagnosis

Because the differential diagnosis of rash is so numerous, this section focuses on rashes that are associated with serious health consequences. Primary-care clinicians should become familiar with these rashes because of the potential for serious sequelae (including death) if the diagnosis is missed.

Cancers such as mammary Paget's disease present with a rash that looks like eczematous dermatitis of the nipple and areola. The onset is very gradual, ranging from several months to years. Early in the course of the disease, it is asymptomatic except for a rash. During the later stages, it is accompanied by symptoms such as pruritus, discharge, bleeding, and ulceration. The sizes of lesions can range from less than 1 cm in diameter to several centimeters. Sometimes an underlying breast mass is palpable during the later stages of the disease—a worse prognosis is associated with this ominous finding. Patients with suspected mammary Paget's disease should be referred to a breast specialist.

The usual location of the classic rash of mammary Paget's disease is on one nipple (or areola); rarely is it seen on both breasts. The skin lesion appears as an oval-shaped, erythematous scaling plaque with sharp margins. Because of the similarity in the appearance, this lesion can be misdiagnosed as eczema, psoriasis, contact dermatitis, or impetigo. Usually, the lesions of eczematous dermatitis involve both breasts and will last from 2 to 3 weeks; the lesions respond to treatment with topical steroids. Contact dermatitis usually involves only one breast (sometimes both); again, the rash usually resolves in 2 weeks and responds to topical steroids. If a rash on the nipple or areolar region lasts longer than 2 weeks and does not resolve with topical steroids, then a high index of suspicion is imperative and the patient should be referred to a breast specialist for further evaluation.

Toxic shock syndrome (TSS) is an acute illness caused by toxin-producing *Staphylococcus aureus*. In the United States, while TSS is seen in both male and female patients, the incidence of TSS among childbearing women represents 90 percent of the cases of TSS. Risk factors for menstrual TSS include use of superabsorbent tampons. In these cases, symptoms begin in nearly all patients within days of the onset of a menstrual period in women who have used tampons. Risk factors for nonmenstrual TSS (NMTSS) include surgical wounds, nasal packs, burns, catheters, postpartum period, and use of birth control methods such as the

FOCUS ON HISTORY 6.2

Rash

Onset of skin lesions:
- When did the skin lesion(s) first appear?
- How did the skin lesion appear at onset?
- Where did the skin lesion first appear?

Spread of skin lesions:
- Have the skin lesions spread? Where?

Change in skin lesions:
- Has the appearance of the skin lesions changed over time?
- Have the skin lesions gotten better or worse?

Symptoms associated with the skin lesions:
- Are there any associated symptoms, such as itching, burning, or pain?
- Are there any systemic symptoms such as fever, anorexia, malaise, pharyngitis, or myalgia?

Treatment:
- What type of self-treatment has the patient attempted?
- Has the patient seen another health-care provider for the skin lesions? What type of treatment was given? Was it effective?

Foods:
- Does the patient have any food allergies or sensitivities, such as dairy, seafood, peanuts, other nuts, strawberries, tomatoes, alcoholic drinks (such as red or white wine, beer, or mixed drinks)

Medications:
- Is the patient taking any prescription medications (e.g., antibiotics such as penicillin or sulfa drugs or pain medications such as codeine) and/or OTC medications such as aspirin, NSAIDs, cold medicines, or vitamins?
- Do any of these medications contain artificial color or preservatives?

Alternative medicines:
- Is the patient taking any herbal medicines or teas, homeopathic remedies, aromatherapy, juices, or other alternative medicines?

Atopic history:
- Does the patient have a history of the same rash before? What was the diagnosis? How was it treated?
- Does the patient have a family history of skin conditions or rash?
- Has the patient or family member ever been diagnosed with eczema, psoriasis, skin allergies, asthma or allergies?

Infectious disease exposure (any exposure up to 2 weeks before onset of rash):
- Does the patient have any exposure to other people with the same symptoms?
- Does the patient have any exposure to small children, day care, or schools?
- Has the patient had any sexual activity with a new partner (known for less than 3 months)?

Systemic symptoms (infectious, autoimmune, malignancies, metabolic):
- Does the patient have any systemic symptoms, such as sore throat and rhinitis (viral etiology) fever, fatigue, myalgia, joint pain, nausea, night sweats, weight loss (malignancy) or weight gain (diabetes mellitus)?

sponge and the diaphragm. The mortality rate for nonmenstrual cases is 18 percent, 5 percent for menstrual-related TSS. Severe group A beta-hemolytic *Streptococcus* (GABHS) infection can mimic TSS (except GABHS is associated with necrotizing fasciitis) and has a higher mortality rate (30 percent).

TSS presents with a sudden onset of high fever (fever higher than 102°F [38.8°C]) and vomiting. It is associated with a tingling sensation of the hands and feet, myalgia, weakness, headache, and diarrhea. In severe cases, it is associated with confusion, hypotension, and shock. It is accompanied by bright red, fine maculopapular (scarlatiniform) rash and is sometimes accompanied by petechiae and bullae. The skin on the palms of the hands and the soles of the feet is very erythematous, and in 1 to 2 weeks the palms and soles start to desquamate. Abnormal laboratory results include leukocytosis, thrombocytopenia, abnormal liver function tests, elevated levels of creatinine, and abnormally low levels of platelets (thrombocytopenia).

Complications of TSS include multisystem failure, including adult respiratory distress syndrome, acute renal failure, metabolic acidosis, disseminated intravascular coagulation (DIC), septic shock, and death. A high index of suspicion and early recognition of serious causes of rash is important in order to avoid potential sequelae. Patients with suspected TSS should be referred immediately to a physician or to an emergency room. Treatment consists of hospitalization in the intensive care unit for aggressive systemic antibiotic therapy and systemic supportive therapy.

Urticaria

Urticaria (hives or wheals) is a common problem seen in primary care. It affects from 10 to 20 percent of the population at least once in a lifetime. *Urticaria* is defined as a sudden generalized eruption of pale, evanescent wheals or papules

Table 6.3 Skin Lesions

Primary skin lesions: 1 cm or less in diameter	*Mucules* Nonpalpable; caused by changes in skin pigmentation. Example: Freckles. *Papules* Elevated and palpable lesions on top of the skin. Example: Nevi (moles). *Nodules* Elevated and palpable lesions that are deeper than papules and feel harder. Example: Acne nodule.
Primary skin lesions: Larger than 1 cm in diameter	*Patches* Nonpalpable; caused by changes in skin pigmentation on a larger area than macules. Example: Cafe-au-lait stain. *Plaques* A superficial lesion—flat-topped, firm, and elevated; palpable, with a firm to rough surface. Example: Psoriasis. *Tumor* An elevated solid mass with a hard texture; shape and borders can be regular or irregular. Can be benign or cancerous. Examples: Neoplasms. *Wheal* Transient elevated wheal (hive-like); pink to red color from local edema and inflammation. Borders can be regular or irregular. Example: Mosquito bite, urticaria.
Primary skin lesions: Fluid-filled lesions	*Vesicle* Superficial elevated lesion with distinct borders; filled with serous fluid. Example: Herpes simplex. *Bulla* A vesicle larger than 1 cm in diameter. Example: Blister. *Pustule* Sizes vary. Superficial elevated lesion filled with purulent fluid. Example: Acne pustule. *Cyst* Sizes vary. An elevated encapsulated lesion that is deeper than a pustule, with distinct borders. Skin on top of a cyst can be moved. Filled with fluid or semi-solid material. Example: Sebaceous cyst.
Secondary skin lesions	*Atrophy* A thinning of skin (epidermis and dermis); appears white or translucent. Example: Striae. *Lichenification* An increase in skin markings; feels rough and thickened. Frequently caused by chronic scratching or rubbing. Example: Atopic dermatitis (eczema). *Scale* Shed epithelial cells in variable sizes. Can be flat or flaky in texture; color ranges from white to yellow. Example: Seborrheic dermatitis. *Excoriation* A loss of epidermis. Shapes and sizes vary and depend on the cause. Example: Abrasion. *Crust* Dried exudate from blood, serum, or pus. Elevated and rough with colors ranging from gold, brown, red or brown. Example: Scab from an abrasion. *Fissure* A linear crack extending from the epidermis to the dermis. Example: cheilosis. *Erosion* A loss of parts on all the epidermis; appears moist and thick, but more shallow than an ulcer. Example: Rupture of a blister caused by a burn. *Ulcer* Depressed lesion due to loss of the epidermis and dermis; appears as a moist pink to red lesion with exudate. Example: Decubitus ulcer. *Scar* Fibrous tissue that forms as skin trauma heals, extending beyond the epidermis. Color can be red, pink or white; scars can be hypertrophic (thickened) or keloidal (more common in darker skins). *Keloids* Sharply elevated bulky scar tissue that appears shiny and smooth. Formation of keloids may have a genetic component.

Vascular lesions	*Ecchymosis* Bleeding into the skin layers and surrounding tissue as a result of trauma or coagulation defects. Example: Bruise. *Hematoma* A large collection of blood as a result of trauma or coagulation defects. It is frequently tender and discolored; colors change from dark blue (when new) to green, then yellow. A hematoma usually resolves in a few weeks but may take several months. If it occurs in a vital area (brain), causing increased pressure, it is drained surgically or locally. Example: Hematoma on the thigh after a car accident. *Purpura* Skin discoloration, ranging from dark pink to purple to blue. Does not blanch with pressure. Purpura can be punctate (capillaries) to larger-sized lesions. Almost all causes of palpable purpura are serious and vasculitis must be ruled out. Example: Large bruise.

that is associated with severe itching. *Angioedema* is urticaria that involves not only edema of the dermis, as in plain urticaria, but the subcutaneous tissues as well. Angioedema and urticaria can be part of a life-threatening immunoglobulin E (IgE)-dependent anaphylactic reaction, which involves bronchospasm, laryngeal edema, and shock. If anaphylaxis is not treated and reversed immediately with subcutaneous (SC) epinephrine, it can be fatal. Angioedema associated with chronic urticaria is rarely life-threatening. In these cases, the patient will report a history of angioedema without any compromise of the throat or airway.

Urticarial wheals (hives) and angioedema are produced by the degranulation of mast cells when an offending allergen to which the patient has been sensitized is encountered. Degranulated mast cells release inflammatory factors, including histamines that increase vascular permeability and cause pruritus. On microscopic exam, the edema on the dermis is manifested by the wide separation of dermal fibers in cells from urticarial lesions, along with dilation of the venules and lymphatics. Urticaria is also associated with non-IgE–dependent reactions involving the complement cascade of the immune system. Chronic urticaria may be a symptom of an autoimmune condition.

Differential Diagnosis

The typical patient with urticaria will present with a complaint of numerous intensely pruritic hives or wheals that appear regularly at certain times of the day, then spontaneously resolve within a few hours, only to reappear again the next day. The wheals typically enlarge and coalesce, forming round to irregular shapes. Most cases of acute urticaria spontaneously resolve in 1 to 2 weeks. Because most cases of acute urticaria resolve spontaneously in 2 weeks, some authorities recommend waiting at least 2 weeks before initiating an extensive (and expensive) laboratory work-up. Laboratory results are usually normal when testing is done.

Urticaria that lasts longer than 6 weeks is classified as *chronic idiopathic urticaria.* Studies of patients with chronic urticaria have found changes in the quality of life, including sleep deprivation, social isolation, and mood changes that are on the same level as in patients with ischemic heart disease.

Urticaria is classified into several categories. *Cholinergic urticaria* accounts for one-third (34 percent) of all cases of physical urticarias. Factors that trigger cholinergic urticaria include exercise, anxiety, elevated body temperature (e.g., fever, exercise, sweating) or hot baths or showers. The lesions usually resolve within 30 minutes after the offending activity is stopped. The hives are small (2 to 4 mm), very pruritic, are surrounded with erythema, and appear on the upper trunk and arms. *Physical urticaria* accounts for 17 to 20 percent of all urticarias; it occurs immediately or shortly after exposure to physical stimuli such as pressure, cold, heat, exercise, sunlight (solar urticaria), water (aquagenic urticaria), vibration, or in response to increased body temperature. Urticarial episodes resulting from exposure to these stimuli are usually of short duration; most last only 2 hours. Dermatographism occurs in 2 to 5 percent of the normal population and can occur with other forms of urticaria. A dermatographic reaction can be elicited by applying friction with a dull object to the skin and watching for wheal formation. The wheal (hive) lasts for a few hours, then resolves.

Some pregnant women develop an extremely pruritic eruption known as pruritic urticarial papules and plaques of pregnancy (PUPPP). These lesions appear as erythematous urticarial papules and plaques (striae distensae) that usually start on the striae of the abdomen and spread to the thighs, buttocks, and, occasionally to the arms. The lesions can start anytime during the third trimester, but they are frequently seen during the last 2 to 3 weeks of pregnancy. The cause is unknown—PUPPP is not associated with increased maternal or fetal morbidity and usually resolves after delivery of the fetus. Treatment during the last trimester of pregnancy involves the use of a moderate potency topical steroid such as triamcinolone acetonide cream 0.1 percent (Aristocort, Kenalog) applied bid to tid on the skin lesions. With topical treatment, improvement of the lesions should be seen in a few days. Topical steroids should not be applied to rashes that are suspected to be of viral etiology (such as herpes simplex or varicella-zoster) because steroids can worsen them. Severe cases are best referred to an obstetrician for possible treatment with systemic steroids. There are no antihistamines that are considered absolutely safe in pregnancy, and their use should be avoided.

Treatment

The treatment for urticaria is to find the cause and to stop exposure to the sensitizing allergen. Certain drugs, such as aspirin, angiotensin-converting enzyme (ACE) inhibitors and nonsteroidal anti-inflammatory drugs (NSAIDs) should be avoided in patients with urticaria. Tight clothing should be avoided, because wheals tend to occur in areas with increased pressure or friction. Showering or bathing with hot water should be avoided because this worsens itching. Cool environmental temperatures in the home are helpful and aid in inducing sleep.

Allergens that can cause both acute and chronic urticaria include drugs, foods, food preservatives, insect bites, and bacterial, fungal, viral, or parasitic infections. If the patient is taking vitamins, herbs, and supplements that are not necessary, they should all be stopped: Even natural vitamins and herbs are not exempt. The patient can start a trial of eliminating certain highly allergenic foods such as eggs, strawberries, tomatoes, chocolate, citrus fruits, peanuts and other nuts, all vinegars and wines (sulfites), alcoholic beverages, and shellfish, although this is cumbersome and bothersome for most patients. Chronic urticaria can be caused by food dyes or food additives such as sulfites (found in dried fruit, wines, vinegar, and salad bars). Food allergens can be occasionally confirmed by the radioallergosorbent test (RAST) or by skin-prick tests done by allergists. Viral infections that have been implicated in causing urticaria include herpes, hepatitis, acute mononucleosis, and rubella. Bacterial infections such as sinusitis and fungal infections have also been implicated.

In chronic urticaria, the clinical evaluation should look for underlying disease, although the etiology in most cases of chronic urticaria is never found. A careful history (including history of travel abroad) and a thorough physical exam should search for signs of chronic disease such as chronic sinusitis, a tooth abscess, a low-grade fungal infection (candidiasis), intestinal parasites, chronic hepatitis, and so on. Some screening tests that are helpful (depending on the history) include stool sample for ova and parasites, sinus x-ray films or CT scan, ESR or a C-reactive protein, CBC, liver function test, a hepatitis profile, urinalysis, and urine sample for culture and sensitivity. In most cases of chronic urticaria (which is more common in adult women in their thirties to fifties), the cause is never uncovered. Up to half of the cases of chronic urticaria and angioedema may resolve spontaneously after a period of 5 years.

The main drugs used to treat urticaria are the H_1 antihistamines, which are available both OTC (diphenhydramine [Benadryl]), loratidine (Claritin), or by prescription (hydroxyzine [Atarax, Vistaril], fexofenadine [Allegra], desloratidine [Clarinex], cetirizine [Zyrtec], and cyproheptadine [Periactin]). The timing of administration of the antihistamine is very important—it should be tailored individually so that the bloodstream levels of the drug will peak during the times when the urticarial lesions do occur, which will differ among individuals. All antihistamines, even the so-called nonsedating prescription antihistamines, have the potential for sedation. Susceptible patients, especially elderly patients, are at higher risk for sedation and somnolence. Patients should be educated regarding drowsiness as a potential adverse effect of antihistamine use and should be warned against driving or operating dangerous machinery until the effects of the medication on the patient are known. The combination of antihistamines with other central nervous system (CNS) depressants such as alcohol, tranquilizers, and certain antidepressants will increase the risk of sedation.

Different classes of H_1 antihistamines should be tried on patients with chronic urticaria: Some patients will respond better to one type of antihistamine than to another. A combination of H_1 and H_2 antihistamines is used by some clinicians, but studies have shown only a very small increase in effectiveness. Some antihistamines (such as Benadryl) tend to cause more sedation than others; diphenhydramine is the main ingredient in OTC sleep aids. For patients who can tolerate its sedating effects (or avoid a problem by taking it at bedtime), diphenhydramine (Benadryl) can be taken at 25 to 50 mg qid (maximum 300 mg daily). The classic prescription antihistamine used for pruritus and urticaria is hydroxyzine (Atarax, Vistaril) 10 to 25 mg bid to tid. Hydroxyzine can be given as a bedtime dose of 50 mg at night to reduce risks associated with daytime sedation. Cetirizine (Zyrtec) is less sedating (13 percent) than hydroxyzine and has a rapid onset of action. The dose of cetirizine is 10 mg once daily given at bedtime. Cetirizine has been found to be especially useful for delayed pressure urticaria. Cetirizine does not cause cardiac toxicity when it is combined with other drugs such as erythromycin, imidazole antifungals, or other hepatically metabolized drugs. Fexofenadine (Allegra), a nonsedating antihistamine, is given as 60 mg every 12 hours. For treatment of cold urticaria, cyproheptadine (Periactin) is given as 4 mg tid. The use of cyproheptadine is contraindicated in angle closure glaucoma, concurrent use of monoamine oxidase (MAO) inhibitor, prostatic hypertrophy, and in elderly or debilitated patients. Because of its atropine-like actions, caution should be taken in patients with asthma, increased intraocular pressure, heart disease, hypertension, or hyperthyroidism.

Types of urticaria that should be referred to a specialist include urticaria associated with angioedema of the tongue or throat, peanut allergy, latex allergy, and urticaria that persists beyond 6 weeks (chronic urticaria).

Common Problems: Parasitic Infestations

Scabies

Human *scabies* is a highly contagious infestation that occurs mainly in children, young adults, and institutionalized persons of all ages. It is characterized by generalized intractable pruritus, often with minimal cutaneous manifestations. The diagnosis of scabies infection is easily missed and should be considered in patients of any age with persistent and severe pruritus. Scabies can develop into a chronic condition.

Epidemiology and Causes

Human scabies is caused by the itch mite *Sarcoptes scabiei* var. *hominis* which infects human skin. The adult female measures 0.3 to 0.5 mm long and has a rounded body with four pairs of short legs. Scabies infestations occur worldwide and are endemic in most parts of the world. Epidemics are historically associated with war, conditions of poverty, overcrowding, poor hygiene, malnutrition, and sexual promiscuity. Close personal contact is the major mode of transmission for scabies, although casual contact such as nursing care may be sufficient for transmission to occur. Institutional epidemics have been reported in which caregivers were infested. Live mites have been discovered in dust samples from the homes of infested persons, suggesting fomite transmission as a possibility.

Pathophysiology

The scabies itch mite is an aerobic organism and thus requires exposure to surface air to survive. The male mite dies shortly after mating, but the female mite may live up to 4 to 6 weeks. As an obligate parasite, the scabies mite burrows into the skin shortly after contact. It both resides and reproduces in human skin. The female mite can lay 2 to 3 eggs per day (up to 10 to 25 total) in burrows created at the base of the stratum corneum of the epidermis, traveling up to 2 mm per day. Burrows average 5 mm in length allowing for continued exposure to surface air, but soon after egg-laying is completed, the female mite dies. Eggs hatch, and larvae emerge in 72 to 84 hours, molting at least three times before reaching adulthood. Mating of these new mites thus occurs after approximately 17 days.

Interestingly, sensitivity to *Sarcoptes scabiei* must take place for pruritus to occur. Initial sensitivity takes several weeks to develop after primary infection and is caused by a foreign body inflammatory reaction to either the mite itself or its feces. In persons who are experiencing re-infestation, pruritus may occur within 24 hours, as the immune system has been previously sensitized. Individuals who are immunocompromised or have been diagnosed with a neurologic disorder such as Down's syndrome, stroke, dementia, neuropathy, or spinal cord injury may be predisposed to a variant of scabies known as crusted scabies (scabies crustosa; previously known as Norwegian scabies). Scabies crustosa is characterized by scaly lesions at the sites of invasion that soon become warty and encrusted, creating a protective barrier for these mites. The number of mites infesting a patient with scabies crustosa can exceed more than a million, whereas infestation with classic scabies is usually limited to 10 mites or fewer. Half of patients with crusted scabies do not experience pruritus, reflecting the absence of key inflammatory mediators seen in classic scabies. A nodular form of scabies also exists in which firm, erythematous, dome-shaped lesions roughly 0.5 cm in size develop over the groin, buttock, and axillary areas. Histamine-mediated urticarial lesions may accompany this rash, which is intensely pruritic. In all forms of scabies, if rashes go untreated, bacterial superinfection by *Staphylococcus* species may result, worsening acute inflammation.

Clinical Presentation

Subjective

The typical patient usually presents with complaints of intense itching that is usually described as being more severe at night. Mothers may report changes in feeding patterns of children and that they are more tired and irritable than usual. Itching may be widespread but is commonly located in the interdigital web spaces, wrists, anterior axillary folds, periumbilical skin, pelvic girdle, penis, and ankles. The palms, soles, face, neck, and scalp are more frequently involved in small children. The pruritus is usually described as not responding to treatment. Many patients will complain of a rash, whereas others experience itching for months with no apparent rash. Patients are often aware of similar symptoms in family members and/or in sexual contacts. Patients presenting with the symptoms described above should be screened for possible scabies infestation. (See Focusing the History 6.3.)

Objective

The earliest physical sign of scabies are small, 1 to 2 mm red papules, located in areas of the body that are most attractive to mites. Because of the intense itching, excoriations from repeated scratching, with crusting and scaling, may also be present. Skin lesions occur at the sites of mite infestation or result from a hypersensitivity reaction to the scabies mite. Secondary skin lesions including lichenification and excoriations are the result of chronic rubbing or scratching of lesions. Secondary bacterial infections present with increased symptoms, pruritus, and crusting of lesions (secondary impetigo).

The classic scabies skin lesion is the intraepidermal burrow. Each female mite produces one burrow. In light-skinned people, burrows have a whitish color with black specks caused by fecal particles. The female mite resides at the blind end of the tunnel. She can burrow 2 to 3 mm per day. Burrows are usually distributed in areas where there are

FOCUS ON HISTORY 6.3

Scabies

If scabies is suspected:

- Do you work in a nursing home or group home, in a school or prison?
- Do you have any family members or sexual partners that have similar symptoms?
- Are young children displaying increased signs of fatigue or irritability?
- Have the eating patterns of children changed?

If patient is complaining of pruritus:

- Where is the itching the worse?
- What part of your body is itching?
- Is the itching worse at night?
- Does itching interfere with your ability to sleep?
- How long have you been itching?
- Is the itching relieved by anything? If so, what?

few or no hair follicles and where the stratum corneum is thin and soft.

Burrows are sometimes seen on the top of early scabetic nodules that occur in 7 to 10 percent of patients with scabies. Nodules vary in color from pink to brown and are 5 to 20 cm in diameter. They may become more visible after treatment.

Diagnostic Reasoning

Clinical diagnosis of scabies is almost never made until hypersensitivity has occurred. The diagnosis is based on epidemiological history, occurrence of intractable itching, and assessment of the distribution of lesions and pruritus.

Diagnostic Tests

The practitioner should search for the presence of mites. The highest yield of mites is in burrows located on the finger webs, penis, or wrists. The Burrow Ink test can be easily performed. To do so, rub a felt-tip pen over the suspected burrow. (Blue and green markers work best because they do not interfere with microscopic results.) Remove the excess ink with an alcohol wipe. The remaining ink concentrates in the tunnel and indicates the location of the burrow.

Once a burrow has been located, the clinician should place a drop of mineral oil over it, then scrape off the burrow using a number 15 scalpel blade. The scrapings should be placed on a slide with a drop of oil, then sealed with a cover slip. The identification of the *S. scabiei* mite, its eggs, or fecal pellets is diagnostic of scabies. There are no serological tests currently available for scabies.

Failure to identify mites or their eggs or burrows does not rule out scabies infestation. If scabies infestation is suspected because of clinical symptoms, then empiric treatment should be tried. Resolution of symptoms within a few days is indicative of previous scabies infection.

Differential Diagnosis

The diagnosis of scabies can be easily missed. Although there are common skin findings (e.g., burrows), the clinical picture of scabies can be extremely variable, depending on the duration of the infection and the severity of the sensitivity reaction. Variants of scabies in immunocompromised persons and persons with neurologic disorders further cloud the diagnosis. Accurate diagnosis is essential for effective treatment. Table 6.4 lists some differential diagnoses for scabies. It should be noted that it is possible for patients to have preexisting skin problems in addition to scabies. A thorough history can help minimize diagnostic pitfalls.

Management

With proper adherence to treatment regimens, cure rates for scabies approach 100 percent. However, application of medicated creams or lotions is insufficient for an affected person if the entire household is not treated and if all environmental reservoirs of the scabies mite (such as bedding, clothing, or towels) are not sufficiently cleaned with hot water and detergents. Therefore, effective care of patients with scabies involves treating the patient, his or her close personal contacts, and environment. Treating the source of the infestation and any secondary complications such as bacterial infection (secondary impetigo) or dermatitis should also be included in the management plan.

Initial management of the patient diagnosed with scabies is directed at killing all live mites. Lotions contain-

Table 6.4 Differential Diagnosis: Scabies

Pruritus	Acutaneous drug reaction Atopic dermatitis Contact dermatitis Fiberglass dermatitis Dyshidrotic eczema Dermatographism Physical urticaria Pityriasis rosea Dermatitis herpetiformis Animal scabies (sarcoptic mange) Pediculosis corporis Pediculosis pubis Lichen planus Metabolic pruritus
Pyoderma	Impetigo Ecthyma Furunculosis
Nodular scabies	Urticaria pigmentosa (in young child) Insect bites Darier's disease Prurigo nodularis Secondary syphilis
Crusted scabies	Psoriasis Eczematous dermatitis Seborrheic dermatitis Erythroderma

ing scabicides (such as permethrin, lindane, crotamiton, or sulfur) are commonly used. Antihistamines and topical steroids are helpful for pruritus. Of the products containing scabicides, lindane is the most toxic. It is rapidly absorbed through the skin and has been associated with CNS symptoms such as irritability, seizures, and in cases of ingestion or overdose, death. Older patients, young children, and pregnant and lactating women have the greatest risk of toxicity. Therefore, the choice of scabicide should be based on the age of the patient, pregnancy status, resistance patterns, degree of toxicity, and severity of infestation. High mite populations, presence of crusts, and decreased immune status of the host make treating crusted scabies more difficult. It may be necessary to remove crusts that would protect mites from scabicides before treating.

The majority of patients require only medical treatment with a topical scabicide. A number of patients experience hypersensitivity to the mite and mite products, however, and may require the use of systemic corticosteroids to provide relief from severe pruritus. When ivermectin 200 micrograms (mcg) per kg is used as a single dose it is followed by another dose 1 to 2 weeks later. This should be used in conjunction with a topical cream/lotion. Some patients may delay treatment until a secondary bacterial infection has occurred, necessitating the additional use of an antistaphylococcal antibiotic. Cephalexin (Keflex) 500 mg PO q12h for 7 to 10 days or dicloxacillin (Dynapen) 500 mg PO tid for 7 to 10 days may be prescribed.

In addition, patients with extensive dermatitis lesions may obtain relief with topical corticosteroids. Fluorinated steroids must not be used on the face or on skin folds (intertriginous areas) because of the increased risk of skin atrophy. (See Drugs Commonly Prescribed 6.1.) Management must include a strict isolation protocol for scabies crustosa.

Follow-Up and Referral

Uncomplicated scabies infestations should be followed up 1 week after the initial treatment. If generalized itching persists, hypersensitivity to remaining dead mites and mite products should be considered. It may be necessary to repeat the scabicide treatment, however. Patients who experience persistent scabetic nodules or crusted scabies may require advanced management and should be referred to a dermatologist.

Patient Education

Patient education is an integral part of successfully treating scabies. Patients should be instructed to trim their fingernails, to reduce the possibility of harboring mites and reinfesting themselves and others. Safety information regarding the use of scabicides should be stressed, such as not exceeding recommended exposure times, toxicity symptoms that should be reported, and the safe storage of treatment products, to prevent accidental ingestion in children. Patients should be informed that itching may continue for up to a week after successful treatment due to local irritation.

Patients should also receive instruction about treating their home environment to avoid reinfestation; they should be reminded that the scabies mite lives on humans, so environmental spraying of pesticides is not effective and therefore not recommended. Bedclothes and clothing should be washed in hot soapy water. Except in cases of crusted scabies, extensive decontamination of the environment is not necessary. Children in day care or school can return following treatment.

Pediculosis

Pediculosis (infestation by lice) in humans has been documented for thousands of years. It is difficult to document the number of lice cases occurring annually in the United States because most states are not required to report it. It is estimated that 6 to 10 million American children are infested with head lice alone each year.

Epidemiology and Causes

Pediculosis infestations occur worldwide and are endemic in most parts of the world. Only three species of lice are known to infest humans: *Pthirus pubis* (the crab louse), *Pediculus humanus capitis* (the head louse), and *Pediculus humanus corporis* (the body or clothing louse). Lice infestations occur in people of all ages. Head lice are commonly seen in school-age children, whereas pubic lice are most often seen in sexually active young adults. Lice are blood-obligate parasites, that obtain all their nutritional requirements from the host. Both the *pediculus capitis* and *Pthirus pubis* lice reside and reproduce on the human host. The *pediculus humanus corporis* louse feeds on the human host but resides and lays its eggs in the fibers of the clothing. Body lice are increasingly rare in the United States but can be seen in communities of the homeless or among people who live in crowded conditions without the ability to wash and change clothing. Body lice are the only lice associated with disease transmission. Infected feces of the body louse can transmit typhus, trench fever, and relapsing fever. Lice-borne outbreaks of these diseases have not been seen for many decades in the United States.

Epidemics of pediculosis in the United States are relatively rare. Outbreaks of head lice are common in elementary school settings; outbreaks usually occur at the start of the school year and after winter and spring breaks. Close personal contact is the major mode of transmission for all types of pediculosis.

Pathophysiology

Pediculosis infestation can be asymptomatic or can cause few symptoms early in the disease. Sensitivity to lice must take place before pruritus can occur. Therefore, in

Drugs Commonly Prescribed 6.1: Scabies

Drug	Indication	Dosage	Comments
Topical Permethrin cream 5% (Elimite)	Presence of live mites (scabicide)	Apply to all areas of body from the neck down. Leave on for 8–12 hours. Repeat application in one week. May repeat a third time one week later.	Mite resistance has been reported. Safe for use in children 2 months and older. May also need to treat head and neck.
Lindane 19% (gamma-benzone hexachloride)	Presence of live mites (scabicide)	*Adults:* Apply thinly to all areas of body from neck down. Wash off thoroughly after 8 hours.	Potential CNS toxicity. Rapidly absorbed through skin. Do not use on infants or young children, pregnant or lactating women, or if history of seizures. Should not be used following a bath or shower, or by persons with extensive dermatitis. Mite resistance has been reported May also need to treat head and neck.
Crotamiton cream 10% (Eurax)	Presence of live mites (scabicide)	Apply to all areas of body from the chin down for 2 consecutive nights. Change clothing and bed linen after 24 hr. Wash 48 hours after second application.	Reported failure rates up to 50%. Long- and short-term toxicity has not been studied. Shake well before using.
Sulfur ointment 6%–10%	Presence of live mites (scabicide)	Adults: Apply to all parts of the body from neck down for 2–3 days Children: May need to treat head and neck also	Extensive use suggests it is safe to use on pregnant and lactating women and young children. Malodorous and stains clothing.
Systemic Ivermectin (Stromectol)	Presence of live mites (scabicide)	"Off-label" use 200 mcg/kg PO single dose followed by another dose in 1–2 weeks	Reported to be effective for common scabies refractory to topical treatment, and crusted scabies in conjunction with topical cream/lotion
Others Antihistamines	Eczematous dermatitis	Hydroxyzine, diphenhydramine: 25 mg at bedtime	Helps patient to sleep at night
Topical corticosteroid ointment	Extensive dermatitis	Apply to areas of extensive dermatitis	For mild to moderate pruritus
Systemic corticosteroid	Severe hypersensitivity reaction	Prednisone: Tapered course 1–2 weeks	For severe pruritus
Systemic and topical antibiotics	Secondary bacterial infection	*Systemic:* 7- to 10-day course	Staph and strep common pathogens. Risk of acute poststreptococcal glomerulonephritis in severe cases

individuals who have never had lice infestation before, it can take several weeks before clinical symptoms (e.g., pruritus) develop during the initial infection. A foreign body inflammatory reaction ensues from the lice saliva which is injected into the skin during the insect's bite. In individuals who are experiencing re-infestation, pruritus occurs rapidly, within 24 to 48 hours, due to key inflammatory mediators including histamine.

Lice infestation averages about 10 lice per patient. They are transmitted through close contact rather than by fomites and can survive just over 2 days off a human host, at which time they die from dehydration. Both males and females are equipped with specialized mouth parts adapted for sucking blood, as well as legs capable of adhering to human hairs. Each female scalp louse may lay from 7 to 10 eggs per day for a month. Pubic lice ("crab lice") lay relatively fewer eggs (up to three per day) which incubate for 1 week before hatching. Severe lice infestations may be complicated by bacterial superinfection from *Staphylococcus* species that normally colonize the skin.

Clinical Presentation

Subjective

Patients may present with complaints of intense itching in areas of the body preferred by the particular type of infesting louse. The itching is usually described as being more severe at night. Mothers may report changes in feeding patterns, and that children are tired and irritable. School-age children may become inattentive and restless in class, with frequent scratching of the scalp. Some cases of pediculosis are asymptomatic or present with few symptoms.

Objective

The earliest physical signs of lice infestation are small (2 to 3 mm), red erythematous macules or papules that are pruritic. Skin lesions may appear within minutes or several days after initial infestation. Some patients develop an allergic, hive-like reaction, with typical wheal and flare formation following lice infestation.

Pruritus is the hallmark of all types of pediculosis. Because of the intense itching, excoriations on the scalp, body, or pubic area (depending on the type of lice) with crusting and scaling may also be present. Fresh nits (lice eggs) on hair shafts are deposited closer to the scalp. As the hair grows (0.5 mm daily on the scalp), the nit moves further away from the scalp. Therefore, if nits are found at varying distances on the hair shafts, the infestation has been present for several weeks to months. Individual lice are difficult to see on the scalp: They appear as six-legged, wingless insects from 1 to 4 mm in length that move extremely fast. When engorged with blood, the insect's abdomen appears dark red.

Nits (eggs) are much easier to see than live lice: The teardrop-shaped eggs are attached securely to the hair shaft by the female louse. Newly laid eggs may be tan to coffee-colored and are difficult to see. Hatched lice eggs are whitish in color and appear shiny. The cap (operculum) of the egg faces away from the scalp. Distribution of lice, itching, and lesions provides clues to the type of louse present on the host. Head lice (*P. h. capitis*) prefer the scalp and crab lice (*P. pubis*) infest the pubic and perianal region. Crab lice and their nits can also be found in such areas as the eyelids, mustache area, axillae, or on the scalp.

Diagnostic Reasoning

Clinical diagnosis of pediculosis, body lice, or pubic lice is based on both the history of pruritus (because of a hypersensitivity reaction to the lice) and the finding of white nits or lice on the hair shaft. Sometimes, lice infestation may be picked up during a routine physical exam.

Diagnostic Tests

The practitioner should search for lice and/or nits on the area of the body where the patient is complaining of pruritus. Lice and their nits can be seen with the naked eye or with a magnifying hand lens. Gloves should be worn during this procedure. Microscopic examination is generally not required. A Wood's light exam can be done in a darkened room for mass screening (or individual screening) of school children. When the light is directed at the scalp, live nits appear with a pearl-like fluorescence, whereas empty nits do not fluoresce. If secondary bacterial infection (impetigo) is suspected, then bacterial cultures should be done with a standard culturette.

Failure to identify the presence of lice or nits does not rule out lice infestation. When suspicion is strong, based on the history and clinical presentation, the patient should be treated empirically; the relief of signs and symptoms is indicative of lice infestation. Because pubic lice is considered a sexually transmitted disease (STD), patients with this type of infestation should be screened for other STDs, by a rapid plasma reagin (RPR) and VDRL (Venereal Disease Research Laboratory) tests for syphilis as well as laboratory tests for human immunodeficiency virus (HIV) infection.

Differential Diagnosis

The diagnosis of pediculosis is easily made. However, "pseudonits" (hair casts, dandruff, or sebaceous plugs) can be mistaken for nits, resulting in inappropriate treatment. A hallmark of nits is that they are extremely hard to remove from the hair shaft, compared to dandruff scales. Sebaceous plugs result from plugged oil glands on the scalp and (unlike nits) do not originate on the hair shaft. Secondary bacterial infection can also complicate the diagnosis. Secondarily infected skin lesions resemble impetigo lesions, with crusting and erythema. Table 6.5 lists some differential diagnoses for pediculosis.

Management

Effective care of patients with pediculosis involves treating not only the patient, but also his or her close personal contacts. Treating the source of the infestation (if identified) and

Table 6.5 Differential Diagnosis: Pediculosis

Pruritus	Contact dermatitis Dandruff Lichen simplex chronicus Scabies Neurotic excoriation
Pyoderma	Impetigo

any secondary complications such as secondary bacterial infection (impetigo) or dermatitis should also be included in the management plan. Patients need to be reevaluated after 1 week. If lice or fresh eggs (nits) are seen close to the scalp, then re-treatment is necessary.

Initial management of patients who are diagnosed with pediculosis is directed at killing or removing lice and their nits. Shampoos and cream rinses containing permethrin, lindane, and pyrethrin are commonly used to kill lice. (See Drugs Commonly Prescribed 6.2.)

Of these products, lindane is the most toxic. As noted previously in the section on scabies, lindane is rapidly absorbed through the skin and has been associated with CNS symptoms such as irritability, seizures, and—in cases of ingestion or overdose—death. Lindane should not be used on older patients, any patient with a history of seizure, infants and younger children, or on pregnant or lactating women because of an increased risk for toxicity. The pediculicide of choice should be based on the age of the patient, resistance patterns, degree of toxicity, treatment history, and in reproductive-aged females, pregnancy status.

Manual delousing and nit removal using a fine-toothed comb is gaining popularity in the face of increasing reports of resistance to available pediculicides. In children with respiratory allergies, asthma, or compromised immune status, manual delousing methods should be considered as an initial form of treatment.

Numerous nonpesticidal treatment options have recently become available. There is limited empirical evidence, however, to support their efficacy and safety. Practitioners should caution patients against the use of home remedies that include kerosene and agricultural-grade pesticides—such remedies are unsafe and potentially fatal.

The majority of patients with pediculosis require only pediculicide treatment or manual delousing. Some patients may delay treatment until secondary bacterial infection has occurred, necessitating the use of a topical or systemic antibiotic. Complicating *Staphylococcal* bacterial superinfection my be treated by cephalexin (Keflex) 500 mg PO q12h for 7 to 10 days or dicloxacillin (Dynapen) 500 mg PO tid for 7 to 10 days.

Drugs Commonly Prescribed 6.2: Pediculosis

Drug	Indication	Dosage	Comments
Topical			
Permethrin 1% cream rinse OTC (Nix)	Presence of lice/nits	Apply to towel dried, affected area–leave on 10 minutes, wash off.	May need to reapply in 7–14 days. Do not use cream rinse. Use nit-remover products before application of permethrin.
Pyrethrin 33% with piperonyl butoxide shampoo or gel OTC (RID, R&C shampoo)	Presence of lice/nits	Apply to dry hair until wet–leave on 10 minutes, wash off.	May need to reapply in 7–14 days. Use shampoo for head or pubic lice, gel for body lice. Contraindicated in persons sensitive to ragweed.
Lindane 1% shampoo	Presence of lice/nits	Apply to dry hair–leave on 4 minutes, wash off thoroughly.	Possible CNS toxicity. Not recommended for children under 12 years of age or pregnant or lactating women.
Malathion 0.5%	Presence of live head lice. Not approved for other lice species	Apply to dry hair. Use sufficient amount to thoroughly wet hair and scalp. Allow to air dry. Shampoo hair after 8–12 hours.	No reported resistance. Contraindicated in neonates and infants. Safety and efficacy in children younger than 6 years not well established. Product contains 78% isopropyl alcohol and is flammable.
Systemic			
Ivermectin (Stromectol)	Resistant pediculosis	200 mcg/kg PO single dose followed by another dose in 1–2 weeks.	For cases resistant to permethrin and malathion.

Children who present with pediculosis pubis (infestation by *Phthirius pubis*) in their eyelashes or hair should alert the practitioner to the possibility of sexual abuse, although intimate contact is not the only mode of transmission. Eyelash infestation can be treated by applying petroleum jelly to the eyelid margins bid for 10 days. Pediculosis ciliaris (eyelash infestation) may also be treated with physostigmine ophthalmic ointment 0.25 to 1 percent bid for 8 to 10 days, but this treatment may cause eye spasms in younger adults. Lice and nits should also be manually removed from the eyelashes by gently holding and sliding them off the eyelashes.

Follow-Up and Referral

Uncomplicated pediculosis infestations do not require a follow-up. In some areas, however, the American head louse has demonstrated resistance to pyrethrin and permethrin as well as to lindane, resulting in increased treatment failures. Follow-up in 1 week is recommended if symptoms persist; the patient or the parent can call the office to report any further symptoms. The National Pediculosis Association recommends manual delousing methods at the first sign of medical treatment failure. Because of toxicity concerns and known resistance patterns, lindane should be used only as a last resort and prescriptions should not be refilled. Referrals for pediculosis infestations are usually not required.

Patient Education

Patient education is an integral part of successfully treating pediculosis. Patients and parents should be instructed not to share hats, combs, scarves, headsets, towels, and bedding. Combs and brushes can be soaked in rubbing alcohol for 1 hour.

Safety information regarding the proper use of pediculicides should be stressed, including information on not exceeding recommended exposure times, possible toxicity symptoms that should be reported, and the safe storage of treatment products in order to prevent accidental ingestion by young children. Patients should be informed that itching may continue after successful treatment for up to a week because of the slow resolution of the inflammatory reaction caused by the lice infestation.

Patients should also receive instruction in personal hygiene. With the exception of the body louse, lice live only on humans. Excessive decontamination of the environment is not necessary. Environmental spraying of pesticides is not effective and therefore is not recommended. Bedclothes and clothing should be washed in hot soapy water. Normal vacuuming of carpets, rugs, upholstery, mattresses, cars, and car seats should be sufficient. Parents should devote their energy to removing nits. Children in day care or school can return following treatment. Some schools have initiated a "no-nit" policy that requires parents to remove all lice and nits before a child may reenter the classroom. Parents should be instructed to screen children once a week for head lice as part of their regular hygiene routine. Early detection results in fewer transmissions and easier treatment regimens.

Fungal Infections

Candidiasis

Candida, an opportunistic pathogen, causes not only superficial mucocutaneous infections but also serious disease that can be fatal, especially to the immunocompromised host. *Candida* belongs to the yeast family of fungi. It is part of the normal flora of both the oropharynx and gastrointestinal tract. In addition, up to 20 percent of women who are asymptomatic yield a positive culture for vaginal *Candida.* Favorable environmental factors and a weakened immune system are the two most important factors contributing to candidal infections. Certain areas of the body are also more prone to infection. Areas where there is increased heat and moisture are more likely to become infected with candidal organisms. Other synonyms for candidiasis include moniliasis and candidosis.

Risk factors for serious disease include conditions that alter cellular immunity, such as acquired immunodeficiency syndrome (AIDS), diabetes mellitus, corticosteroid treatment, bone marrow transplant, chemotherapy, and invasive parenteral catheterization (parenteral feeding catheters are considered high risk). Broad-spectrum antibiotic therapy, including antibiotics following major surgery in normal hosts, can increase the risk of candidal infection. Only superficial cutaneous infections are discussed in this chapter.

Cutaneous infections caused by candida include:

- Thrush, diaper dermatitis (infants)
- Oral infections: candidiasis (thrush), angular cheilitis
- Genital infections: vulvovaginitis, balanitis
- Intertriginous (skin-fold) infections: inframammary area, groin, axillae, web spaces of the fingers or toes, perianal area
- Other infections: folliculitis, candidal paronychia, subungual candidiasis (beneath the nail)

Epidemiology and Causes

Although *Candida albicans* is the most common (60 to 90 percent) of all yeast isolates found on the oropharynx and the genitalia, other types of *Candida* coexist in the body, including *C. tropicalis, C. glabrata, C. krusei, C. rugosa,* and other yeast strains. Unfortunately, some candidal species (*C. krusei, C. glabrata*) are less responsive to imidazoles and have developed resistance. *Candida* infection can occur at any age and in either gender. A higher incidence of thrush is seen among patients with AIDS and in infants. No ethnic predisposition to *Candida* has been noted. Areas in the body where there is skin-to-skin contact are more prone to candidal infection. These include areas under the breast (inframammary candidiasis), between the fingers (interdigital candidiasis), between the toes, the groin, the axillae, and the genital areas. Infections in these areas are collectively called *intertrigo* or intertriginous infections.

Cellular immunodeficiency states increase the risk of mucocutaneous disease. Conditions such as AIDS, diabetes mellitus, corticosteroid therapy, and immunosuppressive therapy increase an individual's susceptibility to infection to *Candida albicans*. Infants, who have immature immune systems, can easily become infected with *Candida* through the birth canal or through oral contact with an infected caregiver. In infants (as opposed to adults), oral candidiasis (thrush) and diaper candidiasis are considered benign findings. In adults, however, mucocutaneous candidiasis is the most common AIDS-defining condition seen. In women with AIDS, one of the earliest and most frequent opportunistic infections seen is vaginal candidiasis. Frequent episodes of vaginal candidiasis that are not accompanied by an underlying condition (e.g., diabetes, use of antibiotics, pregnancy, or oral contraceptive use) should prompt the clinician to consider HIV infection in the differential diagnosis, although most cases of candidal vaginal infections occur in normal hosts.

Vaginal infection with *Candida albicans* is very common; it occurs in up to 75 percent of women at some point in their lifetime (pregnant women and patients with diabetes are at increased risk). If left untreated, candidal vaginitis will either resolve spontaneously or will become a chronic low-grade infection. Men with diabetes, especially if uncircumcised, are at higher risk for candidal infections of the glans penis (balanitis). The uncircumcised foreskin holds heat and moisture and increases the risk of candidal overgrowth. Males become infected with *Candida* organisms from their female partners through sexual intercourse or through oral sex. In candidal paronychia, the patient will report a history of a hangnail or of minor trauma on the cuticle area before the infection. Dishwashing or frequent water exposure is sometimes the culprit.

Pathophysiology

Candida organisms cause an intense inflammatory response on the skin; this accounts for the intense erythema and pruritus commonly seen with this infection. Once *Candida* has taken hold in the skin, microscopic lesions reveal a pseudomembrane composed of masses of yeast organisms that invade the superficial layer of the epithelium. Satellite lesions are small colonies of *Candida* that have spread beyond the main lesion, which eventually enlarge and become confluent, resulting in large erythematous patches. Normal commensal flora as well as intact cellular immunity mediated primarily by cytotoxic T cells are the body's primary defenses against fungal overgrowth and invasive candidal infection. The use of systemic antibiotics has the potential for clearing normal microbial skin flora, while both oral and inhaled steroids, HIV infection and AIDS, malignancy, chemotherapy and other immunosuppressive drugs, diabetes mellitus, and senescence all contribute to decreased helper and cytotoxic T-cell function, increasing the likelihood of candidal skin infection.

Clinical Presentation

Subjective

Oral Candidiasis (Thrush). The patient will complain of a severe sore throat. Pain or difficulty is noted during swallowing (dysphagia), especially with acidic foods such as citrus.

Vaginal Candidiasis. The patient, ranging in age from adolescence to middle age, typically complains of burning, itching, and irritation, either on the vulva or in both the vulva and vagina (vulvovaginitis). Sometimes, burning is noted during intercourse (dyspareunia) and during urination (dysuria). The vaginal discharge is reported as white in color, with a "cottage-cheese" or thick texture.

Balanitis. The typical patient is a sexually active adult male who complains of a reddish rash and itching on the glans penis. It is sometimes accompanied by penile burning after intercourse. No burning is associated with urination (dysuria). Some patients will report having a female partner who is being treated for a yeast infection or who has irritative vaginal symptoms.

Intertriginous Candidiasis. The typical patient is an obese adult who complains of a red, itchy rash that is occasionally "weepy" and moist. It is sometimes accompanied by burning. The location is either the inframammary area, the groin, the perianal area, or the interdigital spaces of both the hands and feet.

Candidal Paronychia. The typical patient is an adult who complains of an extremely painful fingertip that is red, hot, and swollen. A history of frequent water immersion of the hands is common.

Subungual Candida. No pain or itching is associated with this infection. The typical patient is an adult who reports one or several discolored yellow fingernails for several weeks to months. Some of the nails are deformed or separate from the nail bed. A history of excessive contact with water from dishwashing, bartending, or other occupations is frequently present.

Objective

A cardinal sign of cutaneous candidal infections is a bright red rash with macules or satellite lesions seen on the borders. A cardinal symptom is pruritus and sometimes burning.

Oral Candidiasis (Thrush). The anterior and posterior pharynx (including the tongue) is frequently involved. White creamy patches are seen and can be easily scraped off with a tongue blade, leaving behind erythematous patches. The affected areas are tender to palpation and may bleed with minor trauma. In adults, the buccal mucosa, tongue, and lips may also be involved and may extend to the angles of the mouth (perlèche).

Vaginal Candidiasis. The vulvar area and in some patients, the surrounding area, appear erythematous and irritated. During speculum exam, the vaginal tissue appears erythematous, with white, curd-like patches pasted on the vaginal walls. The posterior fornix of the vagina may be full of thick white discharge.

Balanitis. The glans penis has small, erythematous eroded patches that are tender to touch. A different presentation is small, white round lesions on a red base on the glans.

Intertriginous Candidiasis. Any area of skin on the body where there is maceration (or skin rubbing against skin) or increased heat and moisture can become easily colonized by *Candida.* These areas include the inframammary area, the axilla, the groin, the perianal area, and the interdigital areas between the fingers and toes. In some extremely obese patients, macerated skin may occur in other areas as well. The lesions appear as bright red patches with satellite lesions. The skin will appear eroded and moist and is tender to touch.

Candidal Paronychia. The area around the nail (the paronychium) is bright red, swollen, and extremely tender. A purulent pocket of discharge is sometimes present; when fluctuant, this abscess will rupture and drain purulent pus.

Subungual Candida. The nail is discolored and a yellow color. It can be partially or totally separated from the nailbed. No pain is associated with this condition, in contrast to candidal paronychia.

Diagnostic Reasoning

Diagnostic Tests

Skin infections caused by *Candida* yeast are generally diagnosed by their classic appearance. *Candida* yeasts are normally present in the mouth, vagina, sputum, or the stool. Candidal cultures can be obtained from skin or mucous membranes with a culturette. Because *Candida* is part of the normal flora, a positive culture from the mouth or vagina is of limited value unless confirming signs and symptoms accompany it. For vaginal candidal infections, a saline wet mount, pH paper, and KOH test are helpful in the diagnosis. (See Advanced Assessments 6.1 and 6.2.) The whiff test will be negative and the vaginal pH is acidic at 4.5 or less.

Differential Diagnosis

The location of the skin lesions determines the differential diagnoses to be considered. Contact dermatitis lesions can appear similar to candidal lesions. Fungal infections caused

ADVANCED ASSESSMENT 6.1

Candidiasis

When assessing for candidiasis, a saline wet mount (vaginal discharge) or KOH (potassium hydroxide) examination may be performed. The KOH slide exam is necessary to see candida and tinea fungus; KOH is not necessary to see yeast forms in vaginal infections. The saline wet mount works very well and is faster to prepare. (For information on performing the KOH exam, see Advanced Assessment 6.2.)

Performing a saline wet mount examination:

- Take a small amount of vaginal discharge from the posterior fornix of the vagina with either a long, cotton-tipped applicator or from the end of the speculum.
- Place a small amount of the vaginal discharge in the middle of a clean, dry glass slide.
- Add 1 to 2 drops of normal saline solution to the vaginal discharge and stir/mix to produce a thin, milky mixture.
- Add a cover slip.
- View the specimen first under low power, then at 40× magnification. Look for pseudohyphae, spores and leukocytes.

Microscopy tips–saline wet mount and KOH examinations:

- Do not confuse a piece of hair or thread on the slide with pseudohyphae. Hairs or threads will appear as black opaque lines, whereas hyphae are translucent and colorless.
- Pseudohyphae or hyphae (the stems) have thin translucent walls that have septa dividing each segment (like a bamboo stem).
- Spores are small and oval to round in shape, seen either alone or in clusters.
- Leukocytes are round to oval and are the size of nuclei in epithelial cells.
- A large number of leukocytes are seen in candidal and trichomonal infections because of inflammation.
- Few leukocytes are seen in bacterial vaginosis (does not cause inflammation) unless there is concurrent infection with *Candida* of *Trichomonas.*
- Epithelial cells are the largest cells found on the slide. Superficial epithelial cells are the most numerous (about 90%) and appear like rounded squares.
- The presence of immature epithelial cells (from the basal and parabasal layer) indicates severe inflammation. The immature cells are smaller and have larger nuclei than superficial (mature) epithelial cells.
- Bacteria are too small to be seen on a regular microscope (They will appear as extremely small dark "specks" on the slide, under both low and high power.)

ADVANCED ASSESSMENT 6.2

Potassium Hydroxide (KOH) Examination

The KOH (potassium hydroxide) examination is employed to determine the presence of mycelial fragments or budding yeast cells in a skin lesion. The test involves adding KOH solution on a glass slide, covering the slide and applying gentle heat. The slide is examined microscopically for the fungal elements.

Procedure for microscopic examination for fungus:

- Scrape an area of the rash with the edge of a clean glass slide or a #15 sterile scalpel blade moistened with tap water to contain scales. Transfer the scraped tissue onto a slide and add a small droplet of plain water.
- Add 1 or 2 drops of KOH 10% solution onto the specimen slide, put on a cover slide and warm the slide carefully for 15–30 seconds, using a match, small candle, or Bunsen burner.
- Examine the specimen under low power with minimal illumination.
- Look for pseudohyphae and/or spores. Identify hyphae—thin tubular structures, often branching strands of uniform diameter.
- Switch to high dry (40×–43×) magnification to confirm findings.

NOTE: While a positive exam establishes the diagnosis, a negative test does not rule out the disease.

by dermatophytes in other sites include nails (tinea unguium)—onychomycosis, groin (tinea cruris), scalp (tinea capitis), foot (tinea pedis), and body (tinea corporis)—"ringworm." For a review of the differential diagnosis of cutaneous candidiasis, see Table 6.6.

Management

Most cases of mucocutaneous and vaginal candidal infections (and tinea infections) respond well to topical treatment with antifungal creams that are available OTC or by prescription. The formulation of the topical antifungal used will depend on the site of the infection and whether the rash is moist or dry. Powders work well with moist, macerated lesions. Creams work well in drier lesions. Solutions and sprays are alcohol-based and cause burning on inflamed or macerated skin; therefore, they should be avoided on these areas. Preparations in ointment form are far more adherent than liquid, lotion, or cream forms and tend to work best for intertriginous areas. Oral formulations include suspensions and troches.

Pharmacologic Therapy

Topical antifungals such as nystatin (Mycostatin), clotrimazole (Lotrimin), miconazole, Monistat-Derm, naftifine

Table 6.6 Differential Diagnosis: Cutaneous Candidiasis

Type of Candidiasis	Differential Diagnosis
Thrush (oral candidiasis)	Milk curd (infants) Pharyngeal exudate (bacteria/viral)
Intertrigo (skin folds)	Contact dermatitis Bacterial intertrigo (erythrasma)
Vaginal candidiasis	Trichomoniasis Bacterial vaginosis Contact dermatitis
Balanitis (glans of penis)	Flat genital warts Erythroplasia of Queyrat (Bowen's disease of the penis) Contact dermatitis Balanitis plasma cellularis (Zoon's balancitis)
Candidal paronychia (tissue surrounding the nail)	Bacterial paronychia (*Pseudomonas, Proteus*) Herpetic whitlow
Subungual *Candida* (under nail)	Tinea unguium (onychomycosis)

(Naftin), and ciclopirox (Loprox) are effective. Most topical antifungal creams are applied bid for at least 2 weeks (and up to 4 weeks). The patient should be instructed to apply creams sparingly, because too much cream will cause skin maceration, especially in intertriginous areas. The cream is massaged gently into the rash and the surrounding area. The patient is advised that some mild improvement in the rash is sometimes seen in a week, but frequently it takes 2 to 4 weeks until the rash is cleared. Adverse reactions are usually mild; they include erythema, local irritation, itching, burning, and dryness. In some patients, sensitization occurs and a true contact dermatitis results. (If so, medication should be discontinued.)

For topical treatment of severe cases of candidal vulvovaginitis, cream formulations often will yield better results than vaginal suppositories. Vaginal suppositories can become dislodged from the vagina when the patient is voiding or during defecation. For mild to moderate cases, suppositories work well and are now available for 3-day treatment. In recurrent candidal vaginitis, both partners may need treatment. Both partners should abstain from sexual intercourse until both have finished treatment. If the patient does not have symptoms, then treatment is not necessary. Treatment recommendations for vaginal candidiasis are listed in Table 6.7.

Some experts discourage the use of systemic therapies for cutaneous candidiasis because of the potential for adverse effects and an increase in resistance. Studies have found that the increased use of imidazoles for systemic therapy has been associated with an increase in the strains of the *Candida* species resistant to fluconazole (Diflucan). Less

Table 6.7 Treatment of Vaginal Candidiasis

1-Day treatment	Clotrimazole 500 mg vaginal tablet for one single dose Oral fluconazole 150 mg in one single dose
3-Day treatment	Miconazole 200 mg vaginal suppository for 3 days Terconazole 0.8% cream one applicatorful intravaginally for 3 days Terconazole 80 mg suppository intravaginally for 3 days
7-Day treatment	Miconazole 2% vaginal cream intravaginally for 7 days Miconazole 100 mg vaginal suppository for 7 days Clotrimazole 1% vaginal cream daily for 7 to 14 days Clotrimazole 100 mg vaginal tablet for 7 days Terconazole 0.4% cream one applicatorful intravaginally for 7 days

common candidal species such as *C. glabrata* and *C. tropicalis* are also more likely to be resistant to treatment with topical imidazoles. If the patient is immunocompromised, or in some cases of severe vaginal or perianal candidiasis, or in cases that are unresponsive to topical medications, then systemic antifungal therapy may be justified. Drug reactions may occur with many oral systemic antifungals that are available by prescription, including coumadin, phenytoin (Dilantin), and rifampin. Serious adverse events that occur with oral systemic antifungals include hepatotoxicity, angioedema, and anaphylaxis. For significant skin infections resistant to extended topical therapy, systemic anti-fungal treatment includes fluconazole (Diflucan) 200 mg PO × 1 dose on the first day of treatment followed by 10 to 14 days of 100 mg qd or itraconazole (Sporanox) 100 mg PO bid or 200 mg PO qd for 2 to 3 weeks. Skin infections resistant to this treatment should be reevaluated for a nonfungal or non-candidal etiology, or infection by a fluconazole-resistant candidal strain in need for alternative oral or even IV anti-fungal treatment such as voriconazole, amphotericin B, or caspofungin. These treatments would never be prescribed in the primary-care setting, as they require highly specialized care and observation.

Oral candidiasis (thrush) is treated with nystatin, which is available in suspension, pastilles, or troches. Nystatin (Mycostatin) 100,000 units/mL suspension 4 to 6 mL (or 1 teaspoon) is given (1/2 dose at each side of the mouth) four to five times daily. The patient should be advised to retain the suspension inside the mouth as long as possible before swallowing. Nystatin (Mycostatin) is available in pastille form (200,000 units); the patient should be told to allow one or two pastilles to dissolve slowly inside the mouth 5 times a day for 14 consecutive days. An alternative is clotrimazole (Mycelex) 10-mg troches; the patient should be told to dissolve one troche inside the mouth 5 times daily for 14 consecutive days. Mycelex troches are also indicated for prophylaxis of thrush; the dose is one troche tid. Itraconazole (Sporanox) oral solution (10 mg/mL) is indicated for oral candidiasis that is unresponsive to fluconazole (Diflucan); it is available in cherry or caramel flavor. The patient is instructed to swish 10 mL (100 mg) at a time twice daily in the mouth for several seconds before swallowing; treatment should continue for 2 to 4 weeks. Itraconazole (Sporanox) oral antifungal medications are rated as pregnancy Category C. Relapse frequently occurs after treatment of thrush in immunocompromised patients.

In candidal paronychia, a warm compress on the affected fingertip will enhance drainage of purulent discharge and help relieve the pain. Candidal infections of the nail (subungual candida) are best treated with systemic antifungals.

Follow-Up and Referral

The patient should be seen in 2 weeks to monitor response to treatment. If there is no response to treatment, then the initial diagnosis should be reconsidered or the patient should be referred to a dermatologist. If partial response is seen, then treatment can be continued for another 1 to 2 weeks and the patient reevaluated. If there is poor response at that time, the patient needs a referral to a dermatologist.

Patient Education

Patients must be taught to decrease favorable environmental conditions for *Candida* such as moisture, warmth, and poor air circulation. To prevent diaper rash, the infant should be kept dry as much as possible and the use of rubber or plastic pants should be discouraged. Baby powder with cornstarch should not be used because it will worsen the infection (*Candida* can utilize the cornstarch as food).

For obese patients, one method of keeping deep folds of skin apart is by using clean dry white tissues between the folds of skin. Educate the patient on the importance of keeping the affected area dry to assist in healing and to prevent future candidal infections. Patients may be instructed to use a hair dryer but stress that it must be kept in the "low" setting Patients with candida paronychia should be advised to minimize exposure of hands to water and the prolonged use of rubber gloves. If a fluctuant abscess is present, the patient should apply a warm compress to the involved finger two to three times per day to assist in drainage.

Dermatophytoses

Dermatophytoses, or *tinea,* are superficial skin infections caused predominantly by three fungal species:

Trichophyton, Epidermophyton, and *Microsporum.* Transmission occurs primarily through direct contact with an infected person or animal (dogs, cats). Other modes of transmission include contact with asymptomatic carriers who can infect family and intimate friends, or contact with soil (which is full of fungal spores). Although this route of transmission is controversial, fomites (shared objects such as combs or hats) have been implicated in spreading tinea infections. It is not uncommon to find two (or more) tinea infections in one patient. Tinea pedis ("athlete's foot") can occur simultaneously with both tinea unguium (onychomycosis) and tinea corporis (ringworm), as well as with other combinations. Multiple tinea infections are caused by spreading infection from one area of the body to another through scratching.

Environmental and host factors play an important role in the development of tinea infections. Favorable environmental factors that increase the chances of tinea infection include heat, moisture, and poor air circulation. Host factors include age, broken skin, broken hair shafts, and excessive moisture on the skin or nails. Tinea infections are classified by their location on the body; different types include:

- Tinea capitis, or ringworm of the scalp
- Tinea corporis, or ringworm of the body—also known as tinea circinata
- Tinea cruris, or "jock itch"—ringworm of the groin
- Tinea pedis, or "athlete's foot"
- Tinea manuum, or tinea of the hands
- Tinea versicolor—also known as pityriasis versicolor
- Tinea unguium (onychomycosis—covered in a separate section—see p 161

Although tinea versicolor is caused by a yeast *Pityrosporum orbiculare* (*Malassezia furfur*) and is not considered a dermatophytosis, it will be included in this section.

Epidemiology and Causes

The estimated lifetime incidence of tinea infections is between 10 and 20 percent. Tinea infections are more common in warmer climates. Individuals with diabetes are at higher risk for tinea and yeast infections. Tinea pedis, or "athlete's foot," is the most common fungal infection in the United States. Acute tinea pedis is caused by *Trichophyton mentagrophytes* var. *interdigitale* while chronic tinea pedis is caused by *Trichophyton rubrum* which is more common. Tinea cruris (jock itch) is more common in men and *Trichophyton rubrum* is the common agent. Tinea capitis (ringworm of the scalp) is more common in children until puberty when, for unknown reasons, the incidence markedly decreases. Tinea unguium (onychomycosis) is seen more frequently in adults and elderly patients.

The most contagious of all dermatophytoses is tinea capitis (scalp ringworm). It has been known to cause epidemics in crowded conditions such as schools and group homes, as well as outbreaks among family members. Tinea capitis infections are more common in toddlers and school-aged children from urban areas. The reason why tinea capitis is very contagious is because of the propensity of *Trichophyton tonsurans* to produce large numbers of infectious spores called arthroconidia. *Trichophyton tonsurans* causes up to 90 percent of all cases of tinea capitis in the United States and Western Europe. Minor causes of tinea capitis in this country include *Microsporum canis,* a zoophilic fungi from dogs. Less common causes are *Microsporum andounii* and *Trichophyton rubrum.*

Tinea barbae, an infection of the beard area, is more common in men who work with animals. Tinea manuum (tinea manus), or tinea of the hands, is relatively rare compared to all other tinea infections. Tinea manuum infection frequently occurs with tinea pedis infection. The patient infects the hand by touching or scratching an infected foot. Unlike tinea pedis, in which both feet usually become infected, in tinea manuum infection, only one hand is usually involved. Tinea versicolor (pityriasis versicolor) infection is caused by the yeast *Pityrosporum orbiculare* (which causes round lesions) or *Pityrosporum ovale* (which produces oval lesions); it is more common in the summertime. Tinea versicolor becomes more obvious during the summer, when tanning exposes hypopigmented macules that do not tan.

Pathophysiology

Three types of parasitic fungi are implicated in causing dermatophytic or tinea infections. *Microsporum* and *Epidermophyton* species both cause infections of the skin and nails. *Trichophyton* species cause infections not only of skin and nails, but also of the hair. These fungal infections are superficial, as all three types have the ability to metabolize keratin, the protein that comprises the top-most layer of body surface epithelium that normally serves as a protective barrier against microbial infection. The clinical presentation of tinea infections depends on the anatomic location and the species of fungi. Asymptomatic carriers do not show symptoms of disease but infect susceptible hosts through direct contact or by depositing spores onto fomites such as combs, brushes, or hats. Acute tinea pedis is usually caused by *Trichophyton mentagrophytes* var. *interdigitale* while chronic tinea pedis is caused by *Trichophyton rubrum* and is more common. For tinea cruris (jock itch), *Trichophyton rubrum* is the most common agent.

Microscopic exam of tinea lesions reveals either acute or chronic inflammation and a sponge-like texture in the infected tissue, appropriately termed "spongiosis." Fungal hyphae are seen on the superficial keratin layer of the epidermis. In tinea capitis, infection of the hair shaft occurs either inside (endothrix) or outside (ectothrix) of the hair shaft. In ectothrix infections, fungal hyphae and spores invade the hair shaft, leading to destruction of the hair cuticle. Ectothrix infections are caused by *Microsporum* species (*M. canis* and *M. andounii*). In contrast, endothrix infections are caused by the *Trichophyton* species (*T. tonsurans* in North America) and occur inside the hair shaft, leaving the hair cuticle intact. Spores (also called arthroconidia) are found inside the hair shaft, rather than on skin scrapings of surface scale, in endothrix infection, also known as "black dot" tinea capitis. As this type of infection is most common in African-American children, coiling of the hair shaft may play some role in infection susceptibility.

Kerion formation sometimes results from an endothrix infection and is associated with severe inflammatory changes of the scalp consisting of nodules and boggy, exudative tissue. Secondary staphylococcal infection may complicate kerion, causing purulent drainage, with infection possibly spreading to draining lymph nodes, causing painful lymphadenitis. When it heals, it results in scarring and alopecia. A variant of endothrix infection that is uncommon in North America but more common in South Africa and the Middle East is favus infection, a severe form of tinea capitis that results in extensive hair loss and scarring.

Clinical Presentation

Subjective

Tinea Capitis. The typical patient with tinea capitis is a toddler or school-aged child. The parent often reports a painless bald spot. If kerion formation accompanies the infection, the child will show signs of discomfort or will complain of pain. No systemic symptoms such as fever or malaise are associated with kerion formation.

Tinea Corporis. The typical patient will report a history of an erythematous round and elevated pruritic lesion that grows in size and starts to clear in the center—the classic shape of "ringworm." Sometimes, there is a history of another family member with the same infection. Some patients report a history of prior infection. The clinician should inquire about possible exposure through close contact with domesticated animals such as cats or dogs.

Tinea Cruris. The typical patient is an adult or obese male who complains of a pruritic rash on the groin that is spreading to the medial inner aspect of the upper thigh. Sometimes, the rash is not associated with pruritus.

Tinea Pedis. The typical patient with tinea pedis is usually a male teenaged athlete or an adult who comes to the clinic complaining of "athlete's foot" and strong foot odor. Most patients do not have pain with this infection unless it gets secondarily infected with bacteria, causing cellulitis. The patient reports areas of macerated soft, whitened skin between the toes. Some patients will complain of concurrent infections on the hand (tinea manuum), on the body (tinea corporis), and the toenails (tinea unguium).

Tinea Versicolor. Most cases of tinea versicolor are seen in the summer because the hypopigmented spots become more visible at that time of year; they do not tan. Tinea versicolor is asymptomatic and has a very gradual onset. Rarely, a patient will complain of some mild pruritus. The typical patient is a teen or young adult, although tinea can occur at any age. People of African descent with tinea will complain of either light colored (hypopigmentation) or dark-colored spots (hyperpigmentation). In adults, the usual sites are on the back, upper chest, arms, and sometimes the neck and face. In children, the rash is more likely to be on the face or forehead.

Objective

Tinea Capitis. Three clinical presentations are seen with tinea capitis infections. One presentation is the "black dot" tinea capitis caused by *T. tonsurans.* The child with "black dot" tinea capitis will present with painless patchy alopecia (either single or multiple patches). The skin on the scalp does not have erythema; the "black dot" appearance results from broken hair stubbles that remain on the scalp.

Another presentation is called "gray patch" tinea capitis. The child with this condition also presents with patchy alopecia, but the bald patches are covered with fine gray-white scales. The patch is made up of thick, keratinized skin that is grayish white in color. Broken hair shafts of different lengths are present on the surface. Because the inflammatory response is so minimal in both "gray patch" and "black dot" tinea capitis, pain, erythema, nodules, and kerion are not present.

An extremely painful and inflammatory presentation of tinea capitis is known as the kerion. The kerion looks like a bright red, boggy large "bump" on the scalp with alopecia. Purulent drainage can be expressed out of the kerion by gentle pressure and pus can be seen oozing out of its tiny follicular openings. Kerion formation can result in scarring alopecia. The affected hair follicles atrophy and become permanently damaged; hair does not grow back, even when the scalp is healed. A permanent bald patch can result from this tinea infection if it is not treated aggressively or if the patient does not present early enough during the course of the disease.

Tinea Corporis. This infection presents as the classic "ringworm" infection—it is easy to recognize in the clinical setting. The patient will present with ringlike lesions with a bright red elevated border (collarette) that is covered with scales. Tinea corporis can occur in any age group from child to adult, and the size of the lesions can range from small to large. The patient or parent will report that the lesion has been getting bigger. Some patients have only one lesion, whereas others have numerous lesions. The lesions are very pruritic, but sometimes they are asymptomatic.

Tinea Cruris. Tinea cruris ("jock itch") is more common in men; it is more common in the summer or during warm weather. It is usually extremely pruritic and most lesions will show some lichenification from chronic scratching. The typical lesion is round to a half-circle; lesions will spread to the inner medial upper thigh but spare the scrotum. In contrast, candidal intertrigo can infect not only the groin and thigh but also the penis and the scrotum. The color of the lesion, depending on whether it is chronic or acute, can vary from a bright red to a dull discoloration. The lesions can become macerated from infection and scratching; they may become secondarily infected with bacteria or with *Candida albicans.*

Tinea Pedis. This infection can be seen in the clinical area in up to five different presentations. Tinea pedis is usually asymptomatic, although sometimes the patient will complain of pain from a secondary bacterial infection. The most common cause of tinea pedis is *T. mentagrophytes.* The infection usually starts in the third or fourth interdigital web space and sometimes spreads to all toe webs and the soles. Other fungi that cause tinea pedis (but are less common) include *T. rubrum, C. albicans,* and *E. floccosum.*

The most common presentation of tinea pedis is macerated white skin between the web spaces of the toes; the infection is pruritic with occasional painful fissures and can be accompanied by a concurrent unpleasant foot odor. If it becomes infected with bacteria (usually *Staphylococcus aureus*), then a tender cellulitis with redness and ulceration can develop on the web space. This condition is called ulcerative tinea pedis. Moccasin-type tinea pedis is seen more often with *T. rubrum* infection. Scaling and thickening of the skin is seen in a moccasin distribution on both feet.

Another presentation of tinea pedis is with an "id" eruption—a dermatophytid. Acute "id" eruptions are caused by a hypersensitivity reaction to the fungus. The "id" eruption presents as vesicles on the sides of the fingers and/or the palms of the hands. The vesicles do not contain fungus, but are sterile vesicles. The patient may or may not be aware of a concurrent tinea pedis infection.

Another vesicular type of tinea pedis (*T. mentagrophytes*) is associated with burning pruritus and sometimes pain. It is more likely to flare up during warm weather, forming multiple vesicles and bullae. It can become secondarily infected with bacteria, resulting in cellulitis or even lymphangitis.

Tinea Versicolor. Tinea versicolor is usually asymptomatic; it is not associated with any pruritus. The patient will present with oval to round, hypopigmented or hyperpigmented macules, located mainly on the back, the chest, arms, and sometimes the neck and face. Tinea in children is more likely to present on the face, especially on the forehead. Sometimes very fine scales are visible, especially if the patient has not showered or bathed for several days; otherwise, daily bathing usually eradicates the scales.

Diagnostic Reasoning

Diagnostic Tests

Tinea infections are usually diagnosed by their clinical presentation. The classic "ringworm" lesions are fairly easy to recognize. The diagnosis can be confirmed by microscopy in the clinical area (or a specimen [skin scraping] can be sent to the laboratory in a sterile plastic cup). Fungal culture is usually not necessary except in cases where the diagnosis is in doubt or in resistant cases. The exception to this rule is for the treatment of onychomycosis (tinea unguium) Because of the length of treatment and the potential for adverse reaction from systemic antifungals, positive proof by fungal culture is necessary. Fungal cultures can take up to 2 weeks for results to become available, although if done on Sabouraud's agar or with dermatophyte test medium, results may be obtained in 3 days.

A fungal culture is recommended for onychomycosis (tinea unguium) and for tinea capitis. Because these two tinea infections are treated by long-term therapy with systemic antifungals (with a high potential for serious side effects), physician consultation is recommended. Proof of the causative agent must be provided by a positive fungal culture. Fungal cultures are also useful if the clinician is unsure of the diagnosis or if the infection does not respond to treatment. Hair bulbs and broken hair, along with scales from the active lesion, should be cultured. Specimens from the affected site should include scales and hair roots. It is important to look for spores and hyphae on the hair shaft, inside the hair shaft (endothrix), and outside the hair shaft (ectothrix) using microscopy.

To obtain a fungal culture for suspected tinea capitis, the clinician should use a dry toothbrush to brush the areas of alopecia, then impregnate the culture media with the bristles. Another method is by using a wet cotton swab and wiping it over the areas of alopecia and then implanting it on the media. Growth is usually seen in 10 to 14 days of culture.

Systemic antifungals can cause hepatotoxicity and physician consultation is recommended. A baseline liver function test (LFT) performed initially and again in 4 weeks is recommended. Thereafter, LFTs can be done at 6- to 8-week intervals. Griseofulvin can cause leukopenia and granulocytopenia. A baseline CBC and another one in 4 weeks is recommended. Thereafter, a follow-up CBC can be done at 4- to 6-week intervals.

Microscopy is the most useful diagnostic tool to use for tinea in the primary-care setting. A small piece of skin is scraped from the active edge of the lesion and placed on a glass slide. A drop of 10 percent KOH is placed on the sample, which is then heated gently with a lighter or match. The slide should not be placed too close to the flame or the KOH will get too hot and boil off. The heating accelerates the effect of the KOH on the keratinized cell's walls. When the sample is ready, the hyphae will be easier to see because the cell walls have already been lysed by the KOH. If KOH is not used in this test, the examiner will not be able to see the hyphae because the keratinized cells are too thick. (See Advanced Assessment 6.2.)

A Wood's light exam should be used on any area of alopecia and hypopigmentation. Some fungi fluoresce when examined under Wood's light, which emits ultraviolet (UV) light (black light). The examining room should be darkened for this exam. A characteristic color that is associated with two minor causes of tinea capitis is a blue-green or bright green color from *Microsporum canis* or *Microsporum andounii. Trichophyton tonsurans,* the most common cause of tinea capitis, does not fluoresce under a Wood's light exam.

If the tinea infection is resistant to treatment, a fungal culture is mandatory. If a secondary bacterial infection is suspected, then a sample of the exudates must be taken for culture and sensitivity using a sterile culture tube.

Differential Diagnosis

Almost all tinea infections tend to have a slow and gradual onset, producing low levels of inflammation. Low levels of inflammation do not produce bothersome symptoms such as pruritus and pain. Some tinea infections have been present for months to years before the patient reports them to a health-care provider. Sometimes, tinea infections are an incidental finding during a routine physical exam.

Some tinea infections, such as tinea manuum and tinea unguium (onychomycosis), are usually asymptomatic and are tolerated by the patient for many years. Tinea infections such as tinea cruris and tinea corporis tend to be more symptomatic—the severe pruritus associated with this infection usually drives the patient to seek medical care. The differential diagnosis of various tinea infections is presented in Table 6.8.

Table 6.8 Differential Diagnosis: Tinea Infections

Location	Differential Diagnosis
Scalp (tinea capitis, tinea of the scalp)	Psoriasis, seborrheic dermatitis Alopecia areata
Body (tinea corporis, "ringworm")	Atopic or contact dermatitis Psoriasis
Hands (tinea manuum)	Atopic dermatitis Dyshidrotic eczema
Groin (tinea of the groin, "jock itch")	Erythrasma Contact dermatitis Candidal or bacterial intertrigo Psoriasis
Feet (tinea pedis, "athlete's foot")	Candidal intertrigo Contact dermatitis Dyshidrotic eczema Impetigo
Nails (tinea unguium, onychomycosis)	Candidal nail infection Psoriasis of the nail Pseudomonal nail infection
Tinea versicolor (Pityriasis versicolor)	Vitiligo Pityriasis alba Pityriasis rosea

Management

Most cases of tinea infections (except tinea infections of the scalp and nails) respond very well to a 2-week course of topical treatment with *azole*-class drugs such as miconazole 2 percent (Lotrimin AF), clotrimazole 1 percent (Mycelex, Lotrimin-OTC), ketoconazole 2 percent (Nizoral), econazole (Spectazole), and sulconazole (Exelderm). Other classes of topical antifungals that are used to treat tinea include terbinafine 1 percent (Lamisil), naftifine (Naftin), tolnaftate (Tinactin-OTC), and ciclopiroxolamine 1 percent (Loprox). These topical agents should be continued for at least 1 week after the lesions have cleared up. They should be applied a few centimeters beyond the edges of the skin lesions.

As noted previously, for all patients who are on systemic antifungals, physician consultation is recommended. A baseline liver function profile and CBC should be done and repeated again in 4 weeks and periodically thereafter during course of treatment. The patient should be told to report symptoms like anorexia, nausea, vomiting, malaise, dark urine, jaundice, and rash to the clinician. If the clinician suspects hepatoxicity, the offending drug should be stopped and consultation with the supervising physician is recommended. For a list of antifungals frequently prescribed for tinea infections, see Drugs Commonly Prescribed 6.3.

Tinea Capitis

In tinea capitis, a kerion that looks like a honeycomb may be observed. It is an inflammatory boggy mass containing broken hairs and oozing purulent material from follicular orifices. It is a rare, delayed hypersensitivity to fungal antigens and may result in permanent hair loss. Kerion rarely needs to be treated with concurrent antibiotics because a noninfected kerion can itself look exudative. It needs to be treated only if a secondary staphylococcal infection is obvious. Tinea infections of the hair and nails do not respond to topical treatment at all, unlike the other tinea infections. Tinea capitis should be treated with oral systemic antifungals, along with a topical antifungal for the local scalp lesions. A Wood's light exam should be done on all cases of alopecia on the scalp. Although some infections will fluoresce, others (*T. tonsurans, T. violaceum*) do not. *Microsporum canis* and *Microsporum andounii* are fluorescent. A fungal culture is necessary not only to help in the diagnosis but also to classify the species of fungi. It is important to examine the

Drugs Commonly Prescribed 6.3: Tinea Infections

Drug	Indication	Dosage	Comments
Topical Agents Miconazole nitrate 2% (Monistat-Derm cream) (Lotrimin AF spray and powder)	Tinea: pedis, cruris, and corporis Cutaneous candidiasis	2 times/day (bid) for 2 weeks	Tinea pedis needs longer treatment—for 4 weeks
Clotrimazole 1% (Mycelex, Lotrimin) cream and solution	Tinea: pedis, cruris, and corporis Tinea versicolor	bid for up to 4 weeks	Tinea pedis—treat for 4 weeks
Betamethasone 0.05% and clotrimazole 1% cream (Lotrisone)	Fungal skin infections	Apply sparingly bid for 2 weeks Maximum: 2 weeks	Contraindications: varicella, herpes, vaccinia, other viral infections Do not use on face. Can cause steroid atrophic changes if used too long.
Terbinafine 1% cream (Lamisil AT)	Tinea: cruris, corporis, pedis Moccasin-type tinea pedis (or plantar tinea pedis)	Tinea cruris/corporis: 2 times/day for 1–2 weeks Plantar tinea pedis: 2 times/day for 2 weeks	Improvement may continue to be seen for up to 2–6 weeks post-therapy.
Terbinafine 1% solution (Lamisil solution)	Tinea: versicolor (pityriasis), pedis, cruris, corporis)	Versicolor/pedis: bid for 1 week Tinea cruris/corporis: Once a day for 1 week	Alcohol-based solution Use only for 1 week. Apply on dry skin. Do not use spray on face, mucous membranes; avoid broken or irritated skin.
Ciclopiroxolamine (Loprox) 0.77% cream, lotion	Cutaneous candidiasis and fungal skin infections (tinea pedis, corporis, cruris, versicolor)	bid from 2 to 4 weeks	Do not use on children younger than age 10. Avoid occlusion.
0.77% gel	Seborrheic scalp dermatitis	Apply and massage into affected areas twice/day up to 4 weeks	
Loprox shampoo 1%	Seborrheic scalp dermatitis	Shampoo and leave on for 3 minutes, then rinse. Repeat twice weekly at least 3 days apart.	Not recommended for those younger than 16 years of age. Avoid eyes and mucous membranes.
Ciclopirox 8% topical solution (Penlac nail lacquer)	Onychomycosis of fingernails and toenails	Apply thin coat once daily at bedtime	Remove with alcohol once per week. Repeat for up to 1 year. Do not use nail polish.
Ketonazole 2% (Nizoral) cream, shampoo	Tinea pedis, cruris, corporis, versicolor Cutaneous candidiasis Seborrheic dermatitis	Once daily to twice daily for 2–4 weeks or until clinical clearing	Contains sulfites. Treat tinea pedis for 6 weeks. Seborrheic dermatitis: Use shampoo or cream for 2 weeks or till clear. Tinea versicolor: Use shampoo (1 application) Apply to damp scalp, leave in place for 5 minutes, rinse.
Tolnaftate (Tinactin-OTC) 1% cream, powder, solution, aerosol powder. Liquid	Tinea: pedis, cruris, corporis	>2 years of age: twice daily for up to 4 weeks.	For maintenance or prophylactic therapy, apply once daily. Apply powder in socks and shoes.
Econazole nitrate 1% cream (Spectazole)	Tinea: pedis, cruris, corporis, versicolor	Tinea: once a day; others: 2 times/day	Treat tinea pedis for 4 weeks, others for 2 weeks

Drug	Indication	Dosage	Comments
Sulconazole (Exelderm) 1% cream, solution	Tinea: cruris, corporis, versicolor. cream only: tinea pedis	Tinea pedis: twice daily for 4 weeks; others: once or twice daily for 3 weeks	Reevaluate if no improvement within 4–6 weeks.
Naftifine 1% cream gel (Naftin)	Tinea: pedis, cruris, corporis	Cream: once/day Gel: bid for up to 4 weeks	If no improvement is seen in 4 weeks, reevaluate. Wash hands after application. Not recommended for children
Chloroxine 2% shampoo (Capitrol)	Dandruff, seborrheic scalp dermatitis	Use 2 times/week	Not for use on acutely inflamed lesions Massage into wet scalp, wait 3 minutes; rinse, and repeat
Nystatin cream (Mycostatin)	Cutaneous candidiasis (intertrigo)	Twice daily (bid) for 2–4 weeks	Apply liberally to affected area.
Nystatin powder (Mycostatin powder)	Candidiasis, especially moist lesions (under breast, groin, shoes, feet, body folds)	Two to three times a day (bid to tid) for 2–4 weeks	Good for weeping lesions under breast, in groin, body folds Irritation rare
Mycostatin suspension	Thrush (oral candidiasis)	4–6 mL (1 tsp.) 4 times/day (qid) for at least 2 weeks	Retain in mouth as long as possible before swallowing.
Systemic Agents			
Itraconazole (Sporanox PulsePak) (Sporanox)	Onychomycosis of toenail or fingernail, histoplasmosis, blastomycosis Tinea: capitis, corporis; recalcitrant tinea pedis infections	Toenail: 200 mg daily for 12 consecutive weeks Fingernail: total of 2 "pulses"; 400 mg bid for 1 week, then 3 weeks off; repeat pulse. Repeat 200 mg 2 times/day again for 1 week Recalcitrant tinea pedis: 200 mg daily for 2 weeks, or 400 mg daily for 1 week Tinea corporis/severe cruris: 200 mg once daily for 1–2 weeks	Take with food; suspension form better absorbed Hypoglycemia with oral hypoglycemics Numerous drug interactions; check before prescribing. Check liver function before, during, and after treatment.
Terbinafine (Lamisil)	Onychomycosis of toenail or fingernail due to tinea unguium Tinea: capitis, corporis, cruris, pedis	Toenail: 250 mg once daily for 12 weeks Fingernail: 250 mg once daily for 6 weeks Tinea corporis: 250 mg once daily for 1 month Tinea pedis: 250 mg daily for 2–4 weeks	Check liver function/renal function. Use with caution in patients with liver/renal disease. Clinical cure not apparent for months.
Fluconazole (Diflucan)	Oropharyngeal, esophageal, systemic candidiasis	All doses once daily: Thrush: 200 mg on day 1, then 100 mg/day for at least 2 weeks Esophageal: 200 mg on day 1, then 100 mg/day for at least 3 weeks	Check liver function test. Contraindicated in patients with liver disease.
Griseofulvin (ultramicrosized) Grifulvin V, Grisactin	Tinea capitis, onychomycosis, severe/recalcitrant tinea cruris, pedis, corporis	Tinea capitis: 500 mg once daily for 2–4 weeks Tinea corporis: 500 mg daily for 2–4 weeks Severe: 250–500 mg bid for 1–2 weeks Onychomycosis: 750 mg daily for 6 months Maximum: 1 g/day	Ultramicrosize formulation better absorbed High rate of resistant strains of tinea capitis Use with caution in patients with liver and renal disease. Monitor renal, hepatic, and hematopoietic function. Decreases effectiveness of oral contraceptives, oral anticoagulants, barbiturates.

patient's close contacts, including family members (especially other children) and schoolmates. Fungal cultures on close contacts are recommended, if possible. Asymptomatic cases of tinea capitis can be treated with selenium sulfide shampoo (e.g., Selsun Blue). There is no need to wait for results of the fungal culture (which takes 2 weeks) before initiating treatment, especially if there is kerion formation.

The treatment of choice for tinea capitis is griseofulvin (Grifulvin V) 250 to 500 mg PO bid to tid for severe cases or 20 to 25 mg/kg for children. Treatment duration is from 2 to 4 months or at least 2 weeks after negative cultures are obtained. Some authorities recommend against griseofulvin as the first-line drug because of its potential adverse effects. Other effective alternatives used to treat tinea capitis are oral terbinafine (Lamisil) 250 mg PO every day for 2 weeks, or itraconazole (Sporanox) 200 mg PO qd to bid. Male patients on griseofulvin should be advised that this drug affects sperm (it is teratogenic) and to avoid fathering a child for at least 6 months. Concurrent treatment with selenium sulfide shampoo 3 times per week is used as adjunctive therapy to systemic antifungals

Tinea Corporis

Topical therapy generally works well with tinea corporis. The patient must be reminded to apply the topical agent for at least 1 week after the resolution of the lesions and to apply the cream a few centimeters beyond the edges. Concomitant short-term treatment with a mild corticosteroid such as hydrocortisone 1 percent (available OTC) is effective in helping to relieve itch and inflammation. In severe cases, systemic antifungals such as itraconazole (Sporanox) 200 mg daily, or terbinafine (Lamisil) 250 mg daily are effective.

Tinea Cruris

Topical antifungal therapy is very effective for treatment of jock itch. Concomitant short-term treatment with a mild corticosteroid such as hydrocortisone 1 percent (OTC) is effective in helping to relieve itch and inflammation. If weeping areas are present, compresses made from Burow's solution are helpful. Use of OTC antifungal powders is helpful for prevention of future recurrences. For severe cases, a short course of a systemic antifungal such as itraconazole (Sporanox) or terbinafine (Lamisil) is effective.

Tinea Pedis and Tinea Manuum

Tinea pedis and tinea manuum are both treated with topical antifungals. Treatment of tinea pedis should emphasize moisture control: Use of drying foot powders (miconazole, tolnaftate) is very helpful. If weeping areas are present, compresses made from Burow's solution are helpful. The feet should be exposed to air as much as possible—during warm weather, the use of airy sandals or going barefoot is helpful. If socks are worn, cotton or a synthetic "wicking" blend is the best material. Socks should be changed once a day, or twice a day, if the patient's feet become wet in 4 hours or less. An antiperspirant spray on the soles of the feet (to be applied on normal skin only) can help patients who are afflicted with excessively sweaty feet. Severe tinea pedis can be treated with oral agents such as itraconazole (Sporanox) 200 mg daily or terbinafine 250 mg daily. After a short course of systemic therapy, the patient should be placed on maintenance topical therapy with a powder or a spray (miconazole, tolnaftate) to prevent recurrences.

Tinea Versicolor

Tinea versicolor is treated with topical selenium sulfide lotion (Selsun), applied from neck to waist daily and then lathered for 10 minutes before rinsing thoroughly for 7 days. Treatment is then done once a week for 1 month, and then once a month for maintenance. Ketoconazole (Nizoral) shampoo can also be used weekly for maintenance. The clinician must not forget to advise patients that treatment will get rid of the infection but not of the hypopigmented spots, which take longer to resolve. Patients should also be warned of the high rate of recurrence, because *Malassezia furfur* is a normal inhabitant of the skin. Exposing the hypopigmented lesions to sunlight can speed up the process in some patients. For patients who want more aggressive treatment, oral ketoconazole 200 mg daily for 1 week or 400 mg in a single dose or at weekly or monthly intervals is effective but does not prevent recurrence. Patients on oral ketoconazole should be advised not to shower for at least 12 to 18 hours because the drug is delivered to the skin by the sweat after it has been absorbed into the bloodstream. The patient should be advised that there is a risk of hepatotoxicity from oral ketoconazole. Because tinea versicolor is a superficial benign disease, this fact should be given serious consideration.

Follow-Up and Referral

The patient should be seen for initial follow-up 2 weeks after initiation of therapy. For resistant cases, the clinician should make sure a fungal culture is done or the diagnosis should be reevaluated. Resistant cases should be referred to a dermatologist for reevaluation or for more aggressive treatment with systemic antifungals. If the patient is on topical therapy only, then systemic therapy can be considered. Severe tinea corporis and tinea pedis respond well to oral terbinafine (Lamisil) or to itraconazole (Sporanox).

Some tinea infections have higher recurrence rates than others. Tinea versicolor (pityriasis versicolor)—although not a true tinea (because it is caused by a yeast)—has a very high recurrence rate because *P. orbiculare* and *P. ovale* are normal colonizers of the skin. Tinea pedis also tends to reoccur, so meticulous attention should be given to eradicating favorable environmental conditions by the patient (see discussion of tinea pedis for preventive measures). Maintenance therapy in tinea pedis with topical OTC agents in powder or spray form (miconazole, tolnaftate) is very effective in helping prevent recurrences.

If the clinician suspects that a secondary infection (cellulitis) is complicating tinea infection, a culture should be done on the purulent discharge. Empiric therapy for mild cellulitis, which is usually caused by gram-positive bacteria such as staphylococci or group A beta-hemolytic *Streptococcus*, includes oral antibiotics such as cephalexin 250 mg (Keflex) or dicloxacillin 250 mg qid for 7 to 14 days. For patients with penicillin allergy, either erythromycin 250 mg qid or clarithromycin (Biaxin) 250 mg bid is a good alternative. Toe web infection (ulcerative type) can be due to gram-negative bacterial (*Pseudomonas aeruginosa, E. coli,* and *Proteus*) infection and must be treated with systemic fluoroquinolones (i.e., Ciprofloxacin). Moderate or severe cellulitis should be referred to a physician for more aggressive treatment, including IV antibiotics.

Patient Education

Patients who are on systemic antifungals must be informed of the risk of hepatotoxicity and educated on the signs and symptoms of acute hepatitis, such as anorexia, nausea, vomiting, malaise, dark urine, jaundice, and rash.

For all patients on systemic antifungals, consultation with a physician is recommended. A baseline liver function profile and CBC should be done before and repeated again in 4 weeks and periodically thereafter. The patient should be told to report symptoms such as anorexia, nausea, vomiting, malaise, dark urine, jaundice, and rash. Griseofulvin decreases the effectiveness of certain drugs, such as oral contraceptives, oral anticoagulants, and barbiturates. Any woman of reproductive age who is on oral contraceptives and is prescribed griseofulvin should be warned that the contraceptive will become less effective and therefore her risk of pregnancy will be increased. The patient should be advised to see her gynecologist about using another effective method of birth control. If a patient who is on a barbiturate or an oral anticoagulant feels strongly about starting antifungal treatment, then the patient should consult the physician who prescribed the original medication before starting treatment with systemic antifungals. Terbinafine is potentiated by cimetidine (Tagamet) and is antagonized by rifampin. Itraconazole (Sporanox) is contraindicated if the patient is taking any of a number of drugs, cisapride (Propulsid), anticonvulsants, or any drug that is metabolized in the liver by the CYP3A system. Itraconazole increases the blood levels of triazolam (Halcion), diazepam (Valium), digoxin, dihydropyridine class of calcium channel blockers (Norvasc, Procardia), and several other drugs. Adverse reactions to these agents include gastrointestinal (GI) upset, abdominal pain, dizziness, headache, hepatotoxicity, rash, and taste disturbance (associated with terbinafine). Blood dyscrasias including granulocytopenia and leukopenia, a lupus-like syndrome, and proteinuria are also possible adverse effects of griseofulvin. Ketoconazole (Nizoral) is contraindicated in patients who are currently taking cisapride (Propulsid) or triazolam (Halcion).

The following measures should be recommended to help prevent spread or recurrence of tinea infections:

- Tinea capitis: The parent and the child should be advised not to share combs, hats, or any headgear.
- Tinea corporis: The patient should be advised to control excessive sweat and body moisture by wearing looser clothing, and to change clothing when it becomes wet or damp. After bathing, a hair dryer on the low setting may be used to dry intertriginous skin folds.
- Tinea cruris: Cotton boxer shorts are better than tight briefs. The patient should avoid wearing tight jeans, pantyhose, or tight biker shorts.
- Tinea corporis: Some patients (especially children) may think that an actual worm is the cause of "ringworm" infections. Reassuring these patients that the infection is a fungus goes a long way in allaying anxiety.
- Tinea pedis: The patient should be advised to avoid scratching the feet because the infection can spread to the hands and to the body (tinea corporis). The patient should also avoid tight shoes and moist socks, especially socks made out of synthetic material, unless they are designed to wick away moisture. Patients who are prone to "athlete's foot" should change socks twice or three times a day and expose their feet to air—they should use sandals if possible in warm weather. Absorbent nonsynthetic socks are preferred. Feet should be washed daily and dried thoroughly (a hair dryer on a low setting is helpful). Use antiperspirant spray on the soles to decrease sweating. Patients should also be advised to clean their showers with bleach and wash all white sheets with bleach. When showering away from home, shower shoes should be worn.
- Tinea versicolor: Advise the patient that exposure to sunlight will help in repigmentation of hypopigmented areas.

Onychomycosis

Onychomycosis (*tinea unguium*) is a benign superficial and cosmetic infection of the toenails and fingernails. Most patients tolerate tinea infections for many years. Patients who seek treatment are usually younger adults who are disturbed about the cosmetic effects of the infection. The most common etiology for onychomycosis is infection with dermatophytic fungi, but molds, yeast, and nondermatophytic fungi may be causative agents as well. Risk factors that place one at risk for onychomycosis include wearing occlusive shoes, diabetes mellitus, participation in sports, increasing age, and poor circulation of the lower extremities.

Epidemiology and Causes

Onychomycosis, or tinea unguium, is more common in adults and in elderly patients than in children. The combination of poor circulation in the lower extremities as a result of peripheral vascular disease and increasing age makes this a common problem in older adults. Toenails are more likely to become infected than fingernails. Onychomycosis is a common infection worldwide; the incidence of disease is variable and is dependent on many factors. In the United States, 20 percent of all adults have onychomycosis. Onychomycosis is sometimes caused by the yeast *Candida albicans*. Dermatophytic species of fungi commonly implicated in this tinea infection are *Trichophyton* species: *T. rubrum, T. mentagrophytes, T. shoenleinii,* and several others. A zoophilic fungi that is normally found in animal species that cause onychomycosis is *T. verrucosum.*

Like many infections, onychomycosis frequently has a multifactorial etiology. *Candida albicans* can be part of the normal flora of the mouth, the gastrointestinal (GI) tract, and sometimes the vagina. The cause cannot be attributed solely to the presence of the offending organism, because most of the yeasts and fungi are ubiquitous to our environment. Molds, for example, are plentiful in soil. The soil mold *Scopulariopsis brevicaulis* is the most common nondermatophytic cause of onychomycosis. Other molds implicated in onychomycosis include the *Aspergillus* and *Alternaria* species.

Pathophysiology

Onychomycosis is classified as either primary or secondary. *Primary onychomycosis* involves invasion of the healthy nail plate. In *secondary onychomycosis,* diseased nails (e.g., from psoriasis or trauma) are involved. Factors that increase the risk of onychomycosis include a decrease in circulation, resulting from either a chronic process such as peripheral vascular disease or from an acute traumatic process, such as a fracture of the lower extremity. Abnormal enervation during spinal trauma has also been implicated. Tinea unguium can result from an extension of an infection with tinea pedis, tinea manuum, or tinea corporis.

Nail invasion can proceed in several ways. In proximal subungual onychomycosis, the pathogen enters the nailbed through the posterior nail and cuticle area, then migrates to the proximal nailbed. This form of onychomycosis is most commonly seen in immunocompromised individuals who exhibit suboptimal T-cell function. In distal and lateral subungual onychomycosis, infection starts on the distal or the lateral margins of the nail. The infection then moves toward the center of the nail until the entire nail is affected. Distal subungual onychomycosis is almost always caused by *Trichophyton rubrum.* Superficial white onychomycosis involves infection of the nail surface only and is caused mainly by *Trichophyton mentagrophytes*. Total dystrophic onychomycosis is associated mostly with chronic candidiasis, which is seen in immunodeficiency states such as AIDS.

Clinical Presentation

Subjective

The typical patient who seeks treatment for onychomycosis is either a young or middle-aged adult who is bothered greatly by the cosmetic effects of the infection. The duration of the infection can range from a few weeks to many years. Onychomycosis is an asymptomatic infection and there should be no pain involved. Some patients will report having tried several OTC remedies with no result. The patient will complain of thickened nails, or nails with cloudy, white-colored patches. Some will report nail discoloration, ranging from yellow to green or brown to black. Some patients will complain of nails that are partially detached from the nailbed (onycholysis).

Objective

Onychomycosis has several presentations. In some patients, two types can occur simultaneously. Superficial infections are more responsive to treatment with prescription topical antifungals (naftifine gel) than subungual types. (Onychomycosis infections with "subungual" as part of their name denote infection beneath the nail.) Superficial white onychomycosis involves only the nail surface but can occur with either distal or lateral subungual onychomycosis. Subungual onychomycosis can include distal, lateral, and proximal sites of infection. The first or fifth toenail is more likely to become infected than the other toes. The infected nail appears dry and has an opaque white patch with sharp borders that start on the distal, lateral, or proximal subungual portion, or occurs only on the surface (superficial white onychomycosis). As the infection persists, the nail becomes brittle and thick. The area underneath (the nail) accumulates chalky material made up of hyperkeratotic debris that can be scraped off easily for fungal cultures. In some patients, the white opaque areas become discolored—either yellow or brown. A green-black color indicates a bacterial *Pseudomonas* infection.

Diagnostic Reasoning

Diagnostic Tests

All cases of presumed onychomycosis must be confirmed by laboratory findings. A positive result on the fungal culture (which includes proper identification of the fungus species involved) is necessary to start treatment with systemic antifungals. Findings on the classic KOH exam indicating fungal infection are hyphae and spores, or the classic "spaghetti and meatballs" appearance. Under the microscope, hyphae appear like translucent long tubes with septae (separate sections), and spores are small round to ovoid shapes.

Fungal Culture. Fungal cultures done on Sabouraud's agar or with Dermatophyte test medium produce results faster in up to 3 days. The area where the samples are to be taken should be cleansed with 70 percent alcohol before specimen collection. Skin should be taken from the active border of the lesion. Nail samples should be taken from the subsurface of the infected nail. To obtain samples from underneath the nail, a scalpel can be used to scrape the underside of the infected nail. In proximal subungual onychomycosis, the affected part of the nail is on the proximal fold, and cannot be sampled without nail removal. Nail removal is done with a bilateral digital nerve block and is contraindicated in any bleeding disorder. The patient should be referred to a podiatrist for nail removal and treatment.

KOH Exam. A laboratory exam, potassium hydroxide (KOH) is necessary for diagnosis, as only 50 percent of dystrophic nails are due to dermatophytosis. A drop of 10 percent KOH is placed on the sample of nail clippings and is heated gently with a lighter or match. The slide should not be placed too close to the flame, or the KOH will get too hot and boil off. The heating accelerates the effect of the KOH on the keratinized cell walls. When the sample is ready, the hyphae will be easier to see, because the cell walls have already been lysed by the KOH.

Differential Diagnosis

Differential diagnosis of onychomycosis includes psoriasis of the nail, Reiter's syndrome, trauma to the nail, and congenital nail abnormalities. Onychomycosis accounts for only 50 to 60 percent of abnormal appearing or dystrophic nails. Lichen planus, eczematous conditions, and senile nail bed ischemia all may result in similarly appearing nails; however, fungal infection does not underlie such conditions, and antifungal medications would be inappropriate.

Management

Traditionally, onychomycosis of the toenail required long-term treatment with systemic antifungals and had a high recurrence rate. With the advent of other antifungals (fluconazole, itraconazole, terbinafine) the cure rates for onychomycosis have greatly improved. Fluconazole (Diflucan) has consistently been shown to be less effective than either itraconazole or terbinafine and is not typically recommended.

Fingernail infection is easier to cure and has a lower rate of recurrence. The decision to treat onychomycosis aggressively must be considered carefully, because it is a benign cosmetic infection. The patient's desires for treatment and health history are probably the strongest determinants in deciding whether or not to treat with systemic antifungals. Other important factors include the presence of any preexisting medical problems and the past medical history. Patients who have liver disease should never be on any systemic antifungal drugs because of the high risk of hepatoxicity and liver failure. A history of infection with viral hepatitis can result in chronic infection with hepatitis B and C. A history of excessive alcohol use can result in cirrhosis of the liver or elevations in liver function tests (LFTs).

Medication interactions are also problematic. Drugs metabolized by the cytochrome P450 3A enzyme system (CYP450) interact with systemic antifungals. Itraconazole potentiates the effects of many common prescription drugs, among them diazepam (Valium), digoxin (Lanoxin), triazolam (Halcion), anticoagulants (coumadin), HIV protease inhibitors (i.e., indinavir, ritonavir), methylprednisone, and verapamil. Patients who are taking Vinca alkaloids (used in cancer chemotherapy) should not take itraconazole.

In addition, itraconazole requires a low gastric pH (acidic) to be absorbed. Therefore, H_2 blockers (ranitadine, cimetidine, famotidine, lansoprazole) and antacids must be avoided within 2 hours of taking the drug.

Topical Therapy

Topical treatment of onychomycosis is generally not very effective (10 percent or less), but it is worth a try because it is not associated with any serious side effects. Good candidates for topical treatment are motivated patients with only mild involvement or with surface involvement (superficial white onychomycosis). A topical solution such as ciclopirox nail laquer 8 percent (Penlac) or naftifine gel 1 percent (Naftin) applied twice daily may be effective when it is applied religiously to toenails for at least 6 to 18 months and to the fingernails for 4 to 6 months. Ciclopirox 8 percent (Penlac) is indicated for mild to moderate onychomycosis of the fingernails and toenails (without lanula involvement). Initial improvement may take up to 6 months, treatment can continue up to 48 weeks. Penlac should be applied evenly on the affected nail and surrounding 5 mm of skin once daily, preferably at bedtime. It should be applied over previous coats, then removed with alcohol once a week. Nail polish should not be used during treatment.

Systemic Therapy

For patients who desire treatment for onychomycosis, most authorities recommend systemic therapy. If concurrent tinea pedis, tinea manuum, or tinea corporis is present, it should be treated with topical antifungals, so that the source of infection is eradicated. Fingernails are easier to treat than toenails and have a higher cure rate. For fingernails, ultramicrosize oral griseofulvin (Grifulvin V) (which allows much better absorption) can be given at 750 mg daily for at least 6 months. The success rate is a cure rate of 50 to 70 percent for fingernails. Other alternatives for fingernail infection include itraconazole (Sporanox) 200 mg bid for 1 week of each month for 2 months ("pulse" therapy). This approach has good compliance because of its convenient schedule. Terbinafine (Lamisil) 250 mg can be given daily for 6 to 8 weeks for treatment of the fingernails.

Itraconazole (Sporanox) or terbinafine are better choices for toenail infections, which are more difficult to treat. Terbinafine (Lamisil) 250 mg PO can be given daily for 3 months and has better efficacy than oral itraconazole for toenail involvement. Patients who are on H_2 blockers (ranitadine, cimetidine, famotidine, lansoprazole) can also take this drug. The dose for itraconazole (Sporanox) to treat toenail infection is 200 mg daily for 3 months. Itraconazole can also be taken as "pulse" therapy at 200 mg bid for the first 7 days of each month for a period of 3 months. There is no role for griseofulvin in the treatment of toenail onychomycosis, because up to 80 to 90 percent of patients will relapse with this drug.

Follow-Up and Referral

After initiation of therapy, liver function tests should be rechecked every 4 weeks. The first follow-up visit is scheduled during the fourth week to monitor for symptoms of hepatoxicity, adverse reactions, and compliance to treatment, and to obtain a liver function panel. Thereafter, the patient should be seen for follow-up every 4 to 6 weeks and liver function tests done. Resistant cases of onychomycosis should be referred to a dermatologist. Nail growth should be monitored until the nails become clinically normal.

Patient Education

The patient should avoid tight, ill-fitting shoes because they traumatize nails, especially the first toenail. Cotton socks that become moist should be changed. Patients should be encouraged to air dry their feet and wear open-toed slippers or sandals.

Patients on itraconazole and terbinafine should be advised that although mycologic curc has been achieved, normal nails might not be clinically apparent until regrowth in 3 to 12 months.

Bacterial Infections

Impetigo

Impetigo is a highly contagious and superficial vesiculopustular infection of the skin that is commonly seen in infants and children. Impetigo spreads easily through direct contact among family members and from one child to another in the classroom or in play groups. Impetigo infection in adults is not as contagious as impetigo infection in infants and younger children. Impetigo infection typically demonstrates a mixed flora of Gram-positive bacteria that includes *Staphylococcus aureus* and group A or group B beta-hemolytic *Streptococcus*. Two forms of impetigo are seen in the clinical area—bullous and nonbullous (vesiculopustular) forms.

Epidemiology and Causes

Impetigo affects primarily infants in nurseries and young children (5- to 7-year-olds), especially those with poor hygiene and who are in day-care groups. Impetigo is more prevalent in hot, humid weather, when biting insects and mosquitoes are most pervasive. The trauma caused by their bites favors bacterial growth on moist skin. There is an increased incidence of impetigo in lower socioeconomic groups because of several factors, including overcrowding, lack of good personal hygiene, a higher incidence of anemia, and malnutrition. In addition, any preexisting skin disease that goes untreated (e.g., atopic dermatitis) may also be predisposed to secondary infection. Staphylococcal impetigo may be associated with immunodeficiency disease.

Pathophysiology

The infectious process in impetigo is limited to the stratum corneum. The presence of numerous neutrophils within the blister (subcorneal blister) and the presence of gram-positive cocci are characteristic of impetigo infections. The etiologic agents may be found alone or in combination. If a combination of gram-positive bacteria is causing the impetigo infection, symbiosis promotes the growth of both bacteria and produces more rapid spread.

Staphylococci bacteria are usually noted during the very early stage of the lesions, whereas S*treptococci* bacteria tend to predominate in the later stages. In recent years, epidemiologists have noted an etiologic shift in which *Staphylococcus aureus* either alone or in combination with group A *Streptococcus* has replaced the latter as the most common causative organism. Thus, chronic skin colonization with either *Staphylococcus aureus* or group A *Streptococcus* predisposes to impetigo. Infected lesions typically result from sites of previous injury, such as insect bites. The blisters are the result of local separation (acantholysis) of the keratinocytes in the underlying epidermal layer forming the floor of the blister. Blister formation is caused by the action of epidermolytic (exfoliative) exotoxins produced by the bacteria. Group A *Streptococci* are the primary etiologic agent for a particularly severe, albeit rare, ulcerative form of impetigo known as ecthyma. Ulcer formation is also aided by coagulase-positive *Staphylococci*.

Finally, bullous impetigo is caused by *Staphylococcus aureus* infection in newborns and young children. In this condition, exfoliative toxin A causes loss of cellular adhesion in the superficial epidermis normally mediated by the protein desmoglein. This results in large blistering lesions known as bullae, which eventually drain, leaving thin, nonpurulent crusts over the entire affected skin area.

Clinical Presentation

Subjective

The most common symptom of both types of impetigo is pruritus from the lesions. The parent of a young or school-aged child will complain of a red, crusty rash that is spreading or getting larger in size. The rash is usually located on the face or on the extremities. Some parents or the child will report that a close friend or classmate of the patient has the same rash.

The provider should ask about the location, onset, and duration of the lesions and any associated symptoms. The clinician should also inquire if any other family member has been affected and if treatment has been effective. Fever is unusual in impetigo but if present, it should prompt investigation for a deeper infection.

Objective

The plaques of impetigo begin as vesicles whose roofs break down, leaving shallow erosions with yellowish crusts. The lesions may be discrete or confluent in their distribution and are usually seen on the face. Early impetigo may resemble many vesicular skin conditions, such as herpes simplex. Two forms of impetigo are commonly seen in the clinical area are bullous impetigo and nonbullous impetigo.

The bullous type of impetigo may present with bullae that begin as small (1 to 2 mm) superficial vesicles with a fragile roof. The roof on each bulla is very fragile and ruptures easily. Sometimes the parent or patient will deny seeing bullae because they rupture quickly thus are not easily and quickly recalled by the patient or the parent. The serous fluid inside the ruptured vesicles develops into a thin, transparent, and varnish-like crust. Hence the vesicles become pustular in a matter of hours. The bullous type of impetigo is usually caused by *Staphylococcus* bacteria; it commonly occurs on the face, elbows, and knees.

In the nonbullous or vesiculopustular type, the lesions are characterized by thick, adherent, dirty yellow-colored crusts that have erythematous margins. This type of impetigo occurs more often in older children. Both bullous and nonbullous types produce symptoms such as burning and pruritus. In addition, regional lymphadenopathy is seen: When the face is involved, the cervical nodes (and sometimes the preauricular and submandibular nodes) are enlarged; when the lesions are on the upper extremities, the axillary nodes become enlarged.

A variant of bullous impetigo that is caused exclusively by *Staphylococcus aureus* is known as *staphylococcal scalded skin syndrome* (SSSS). Exotoxins produced by the bacteria lead to bullous, sheet-like necrosis of the epidermis and cause the epithelium layer of the skin to peel off in large pieces. The "scalded skin" thus mimics a thermal burn. This serious infection is more commonly seen in children and usually begins in the intertriginous areas.

A less common form of impetigo that is ulcerative in nature is known as *ecthyma.* This form of impetigo is seen predominantly on the feet, ankles, legs, and thighs. It afflicts mostly homeless people, sewage and garbage workers, alcoholics, and neglected elderly individuals. It is a deeper version of impetigo and often results from a neglected or poorly treated superficial abrasion, or from infected insect bites. Itching is common, and auto-inoculation from scratching may cause satellite lesions that are annular in form. Ecthyma presents as pruritic and tender red vesicles or pustules that are surrounded by erythema and eventually ulcerate. Because this process is very superficial, healing often occurs spontaneously in the center of the lesion and results in scarring. The inflammatory process involves both dermal and epidermal layers (Table 6.9).

During physical assessment, a thorough examination of the skin should search for erosions that are covered with moist, honey-colored crusts. Any firm and dry or dark crusts with surrounding erythema characterize a deeper form of impetigo called ecthyma. The physical assessment should include an examination of the head, ears, pharynx, the neck, and the regional lymph nodes should be noted for lymphadenopathy.

Diagnostic Reasoning

Diagnostic Tests

Initial testing for impetigo includes a culture and sensitivity from the moist crusts of the lesions. The results of the culture and sensitivity help to assess for antibiotic resistance of

Table 6.9 Types of Impetigo

Types of Impetigo	Causative Agent	Clinical Presentation
Bullous impetigo	*Staphylococcus aureus*	Lesion starts as about 1–2 mm superficial vesicle with fragile roof, easily ruptured; ruptured vesicle forms thin, transparent, varnishlike or classic "honey-colored" crust. Becomes pustular in matter of hours; pruritic; burning sensation.
Staphylococcal scalded skin syndrome (SSSS)	*Staphylococcus*	Variant of bullous impetigo: Epidermal necrosis caused by bacterial exotoxins, resulting in the epithelial layer peeling off in large, sheetlike pieces; mimics scalded-skin thermal burn.
Non-bullous impetigo	*Streptococcus, Staphylococcus aureus*	Lesions are thick, adherent; recurrent with dirty yellow-colored crusts with erythematous margins; pruritic and burning sensation.
Ecthyma	*Staphylococcus, Streptococcus;* other infective organisms may be observed	Pruritic tender, red vesicles or pustules surrounded by erythema; rash eventually ulcerates. Deeper impetigo resulting from inadequately treated or neglected skin infections; also seen in infected insect bites or abrasions.

the responsible pathogen. In addition, a Gram stain can be obtained; if the lesions are caused by impetigo, the stain will reveal gram-positive cocci. If herpes simplex is suspected, a viral culture can be obtained. If the patient is febrile or has systemic symptoms, a CBC with differential should be obtained.

Differential Diagnosis

The typical dirty-looking, honey-colored crust is almost pathognomonic of bullous impetigo, so much so that cultures are not necessary before treatment is started. Bullous impetigo should be differentiated from other vesicular and pustular skin conditions. Many skin diseases with weepy lesions may resemble impetigo, such as varicella-zoster virus, herpes simplex virus, eczematous dermatitis (atopic dermatitis), and contact dermatitis. The history, distribution, and morphologic features of the primary skin lesions provide the best information to help in the differential diagnosis of other skin conditions.

Varicella-zoster infection (herpes zoster or chickenpox) produces a rash with widely distributed papules and vesicular lesions. The onset of the rash typically starts on the head and neck area. The lesions of herpes zoster follow a dermatomal pattern that consists of a group of uniform 2- to 3-mm vesicles on an erythematous base.

A localized group of vesicles located on a single anatomic site, with a clear to cloudy fluid on an erythematous and edematous base, helps to characterize herpes simplex lesions. These lesions are usually preceded by a prodrome of burning and tingling before the lesions erupt.

Acute nummular eczema manifests as pruritic, coin-shaped plaques or papulovesicles on an erythematous base; the lesions may become exudative and crusted. Candidiasis lesions are bright red; this rash forms satellite lesions along with macerated moist patches. Candidiasis is often accompanied by pruritus and sometimes by burning in the macerated areas.

Management

There are two principles of therapy in the management of impetigo: (1) Nonpharmacologic measures are employed to enhance resolution and to reduce bacterial colonization on the skin surface and (2) antibiotics are prescribed to help to eradicate the responsible pathogen and to prevent recolonization and complications.

Nonpharmacologic Management

Nonpharmacologic management of impetigo involves the use of solutions or substances to débride the impetiginized lesions and to expose the skin surfaces where the bacteria are present. Exudative impetigo lesions may benefit from drying compresses to remove thick crusts and desiccate (dry out) the lesions. Saline, plain tap water, or Burow's solution may be applied for 10 to 20 minutes tid to qid. While the dehydrating effect of the compresses may help to improve the appearance of the skin lesions, disinfectant solutions are not particularly effective.

Pharmacologic Management

Pharmacologic treatment of impetigo includes the use of both topical and oral antibiotics. Mild cases of nonbullous impetigo can be treated effectively with a topical antibiotic, combined with cleansing and débridement. The best topical agent is mupirocin 2 percent (Bactroban cream) applied tid for 10 days. This is equivalent in efficacy to oral erythromycin. Washing with chlorhexidine (Hibiclens) is a valuable adjunct because of its bactericidal properties. The patient should be instructed to wash the affected skin areas with the bactericidal soap two to three times a day before the mupirocin cream is applied. Antibiotic creams and ointments containing neomycin may be used, although neomycin can produce contact dermatitis in sensitive individuals. Sensitization usually develops after long-term use on denuded skin and is not recommended.

Systemic antibiotics are indicated when there are systemic symptoms such as fever or toxicity, if a large area is involved, or if there is possibility that a nephrogenic strain of *Streptococcus* is causing the infection. Penicillin therapy used to be the standard for impetigo, but with increasing beta-lactamase expression by *Staphylococcus*, this is no longer the treatment of choice. Bullous impetigo should be treated with oral antistaphylococcal drugs for a total of 10 days. Antistaphylococcal drugs include dicloxacillin (Dycill, Dynapen) or cephalexin (Keflex) 250 mg PO qid or 500 mg PO bid which are both effective for staphylococcal impetigo. Patients with penicillin allergy can be treated with erythromycin 250 mg qid. (See Drugs Commonly Prescribed 6.4.) Erythromycin, however, has not been shown to be superior to topical mupirocin cream, As oral antibiotics have far more gastrointestinal and systemic side effects than topical therapy; topical therapy is often preferred for mild to moderate infections.

Follow-Up and Referral

The patient with an uncomplicated case of impetigo should be followed up in 10 days to 2 weeks after initiation of therapy. Patients who are toxic or have fever should be followed closely; consultation or referral to a physician is recommended. Development of acute glomerulonephritis (acute nephritic syndrome) requires referral to a kidney specialist. Symptoms of this disease include the abrupt onset of proteinuria, hypertension, edema, azotemia, and red blood cells (RBCs) in the urine.

The majority of cases of both types of impetigo resolved uneventfully after 10 days of treatment. Patients with recurrent impetigo should be tested for nasal carriage of *Staphylococcus aureus* bacteria (culture the anterior nares). If the culture is positive, treatment of the nares with topical muciprocin 2 percent (Bactroban) bid for 5 days is effective.

Drugs Commonly Prescribed 6.4: Impetigo

Drug	Indication	Dosage	Comments
Topical			
Mupirocin 2% (Bactroban) cream	Nonbullous impetigo Impetigo caused by *S. pyogenes* or *S. aureus*	Apply three times daily for 10 days	Wash with bactericidal soap prior to applying cream
Systemic			
Dicloxacillin (Dycill, Dynapen)	Bullous staphylococcal impetigo	250 mg four times/day or 500 mg two times/day Children (<40 kg) 12–25 mg/kg per day in four divided doses	
Cephalexin (Keflex)	Bullous staphylococcal impetigo	250 mg four times/day or 500 mg bid Children: 25–50 mg/kg per day in divided doses	Discontinue if colitis occurs.
Erythromycin (EryPed, e-mycin)	For penicillin allergy	250 mg four times/day for 10 days or 500 mg bid for 10 days Children: 30–60 mg/kg per day divided in four doses for 10 days	

Bullous impetigo typically resolves even without antibiotic treatment. Nonbullous impetigo generally has a good prognosis, although poststreptococcal glomerulonephritis is a possible complication of this infection.

Patient Education

The clinician plays a pivotal role in the treatment and prevention of this highly contagious skin infection through patient education and counseling. Good hand washing and personal hygiene are strongly recommended to reduce the likelihood of spread. The fingernails should be kept short, so that there is less likelihood of spread to other areas of the body through self-inoculation.

Children and family members should be educated of the contagious nature of impetigo. They should be informed to refrain from participation in any contact sport or activity that might spread the infection. Family members should not use or share personal effects such as towels, robes, razors, shavers, and so on. Bed linens should be washed with soap and hot water.

The patient should be instructed to gently clean the crusts from the lesions with antibacterial soap before applying mupirocin 2 percent cream. Application at nighttime is also advised. If occlusive dressings are used, they should be discarded carefully to prevent spread of infection. If the patient is on oral antibiotics, the side effects and potential adverse reactions of the drug should be explained, as well as the importance of completing the course of antibiotic therapy to prevent the possible complication of streptococcal glomerulonephritis. Patients should be informed that good personal hygiene and cleanliness, along with prompt attention to skin trauma, will help to prevent future breakouts of impetigo.

Folliculitis

Folliculitis is a superficial to deep skin infection of the hair follicles. Lesions can range from minute white-topped pustules in newborns to large, yellow-white tender pustules in adults. Bacteria infect the hair follicle at a superficial level, leading to erythematous papules and pustules. While the main pathogens are gram-positive bacteria, occasional cases are caused by a fungus or by gram-negative bacilli. Folliculitis represents the start of a continuum of skin infections. Deeper infections (as complications of folliculitis) can include the furuncle (boil) or carbuncle (multiple boils), which are covered in depth further in this chapter.

Epidemiology and Causes

Folliculitis is often caused by bacteria; in particular, it is frequently caused by coagulase-negative *Staphylococcus* bacteria. Predisposing factors include the following: diabetes, obesity, a chronic carrier state of *Staphylococci* (present in the nares, axillae, or perineum), poor hygiene, hyperimmunoglobulin E (Job's syndrome—an immunodeficiency disorder), exposure to chemicals and solvents (cutting oils), and chronic skin friction. However, folliculitis may have other etiologies, as well. Gram-positive resident flora of the nasal mucosa and adjacent facial skin become suppressed by long-term oral antibiotic therapy and are replaced by gram-negative rods, namely *Klebsiella* and *Escherichia coli*. Thus, gram-negative folliculitis may develop in patients who are on long-term tetracycline therapy for acne (or rosacea), as well as in older men who are suffering from seborrhea. Patients who have become colonized by gram-negative bacteria in the sebaceous follicles of the perioral and perinasal areas can become infected due to trauma (e.g., from shaving), resulting in a suppurative process within the hair follicle. This type of folliculitis is usually seen on the upper lip in men. In addition, antibiotic use also increases the risk of candidal folliculitis, due to clearance of the normal bacterial skin flora. Exposure to wet environments such as whirlpools or inadequately chlorinated pools which contributes to *Pseudomonas aeruginosa* infection also predisposes to folliculitis. In addition, chronic steroid use which compromises T-cell immunity contributes to folliculitis by *Candida albicans*.

Folliculitis most commonly occurs among middle-aged individuals (aged 40 to 60 years) and children, especially if they are immunocompromised or spend an extended amount of time in a prone position due to impaired mobility. Studies have found that folliculitis may be spread by fomite transmission. Intensive care units (ICUs) are the frequent origin of nosocomial outbreaks in the hospital setting. The higher incidence of folliculitis in the ICU is the result of trauma from invasive procedures performed on immunocompromised or severely ill patients. Impairment of host resistance increases a patient's risk of contracting folliculitis in the presence of virulent pathogens such as gram-negative coliform bacilli. In addition, the presence of *Malassezia furfur* (a yeast that is part of the normal skin flora in animals) has been seen among infected ICU patients. One study found the same fungus on the stethoscopes and patient care instruments of the ICU staff who had touched their pets from home.

Folliculitis may occur anywhere on the skin as a result of trauma or damage to the hair follicle from chronic irritation due to friction from clothing or blockage of the hair follicle. Occlusion of the skin with tight-fitting nylon clothing promotes infection, and symptoms may occur abruptly within 1 to 3 days. Occlusive therapy (plastic wrap) used for other diseases such as severe psoriasis allows for significant bacterial multiplication in a moist environment, which can also lead to folliculitis. Spread of bacterial infection to the surrounding skin may develop from exudative or transudative discharge from wounds, abscesses, or any type of draining lesion.

A new form of sterile folliculitis called *eosinophilic folliculitis* (EF) was originally identified in an 8-month-old HIV-positive Japanese infant. On histologic exam, the hair follicle in EF is invaded by eosinophils and lymphocytes. Clinically, it presents in patients with HIV as intensely pruritic papules and pustules that appear over the entire body. Successful treatment of EF with interferon-alpha 2b has been reported, but the management of this form of folliculitis requires hospitalization and patient isolation. The presence of HIV with EF lesions is a marker for advanced HIV disease, and death from opportunistic infection usually occurs within 6 months of the onset of cutaneous lesions.

Pathophysiology

Infection of the hair follicle with *Staphylococcus* or *Streptococcus* is marked by suppuration and liquefaction necrosis of the follicular base, thus termed a pyodermal infection. It is usually localized and results in abscess formation. Liquefaction necrosis develops when lytic enzymes released by polymorphonuclear leukocytes (PMNs) digest bacteria and cellular material. Thus, a competent immune system is required for such a response, as large numbers of PMNs are found in the central area of the abscess, along with necrotic debris. As this inflammatory response is localized, however, folliculitis rarely causes systemic manifestations in the immunocompetent individual. Interestingly, HIV-positive patients do not display this neutrophilic response, as they typically experience an eosinophilic perifollicular pustular folliculitis, as described above.

Clinical Presentation

Subjective

Generally, the patient will present with a "bumpy rash," which can appear on any area of the body. The rash can be located on the hair follicles of the face, forehead, back of the earlobes, the neck, the shoulder, the buttocks, the torso, or the extremities. Usually, the rash is not accompanied by itching. Often there is no history of previous skin eruptions or of pertinent medical history like diabetes. The patient is usually concerned about the cosmetic effect of the lesions. The patient may report a history of hot tub use, or of borrowing a shaver or razor from a friend. The clinician should inquire about the onset, duration, and locations of the rash, its appearance, and whether purulent drainage was present. The patient should also be asked about any associated systemic symptoms of fever and chills.

Objective

The primary lesions in folliculitis are small pustules surrounded by 1 to 2 mm of erythema located over the pilosebaceous orifice or the ostium of the hair follicle. There is no involvement of the surrounding skin. The eyelids, face, scalp, and extremities are the most typical sites. A hair on the center of the pustule sometimes perforates the lesion. This presentation is a hallmark for diagnosis. The pustules resolve into red macules, which fade to leave postinflammatory hyperpigmented scars in susceptible persons. Folliculitis is usually asymptomatic, but it can be very pruritic and is sometimes accompanied by burning. During the physical examination, checking the vital signs, including the temperature, is important to help rule out systemic involvement. The practitioner should inspect the lesion for signs of inflammation and suppuration (erythema, swelling, pustules) and palpate the surface of the pustule for fluctuance. It is also important to palpate the adjacent lymph nodes.

Folliculitis is divided into two main types—*superficial folliculitis* and *deep folliculitis*. Follicular impetigo (Bockhart's impetigo) is a superficial form of folliculitis that presents as small, dome-shaped pustules that occur over the opening of the hair follicle. It is more common on the scalps of children. When follicular impetigo becomes chronic, it may lead to follicle destruction and consequent permanent patchy alopecia.

The distinctive forms of deep folliculitis include barber's itch, pseudofolliculitis barbae, and *Pseudomonas* follicilitis. In addition, newer diagnoses have been established based on the histologic characteristic of the skin eruption, such as eosinophilic folliculitis (HIV-EF) and nosocomial folliculitis.

Barber's itch (sycosis barbae) is a chronic and recurrent staphylococcal infection of the hair follicles on the bearded area of the face in men (usually the upper lip). It is aggravated by shaving and is most commonly seen in black men. It is usually propagated by the autoinoculation of bacteria caused by shaving. A differential diagnosis of tinea barbae is similar to barber's itch, but the tinea infection is caused by a fungus. Pseudofolliculitis barbae, another differential diagnosis for sycosis barbae, is caused by hair in the beard area that curls toward the skin, causing an inflammatory reaction that can mimic folliculitis. This can become a chronic problem; the hair follicles involved can become infected with any variety of bacteria.

Pseudomonas folliculitis presents as follicular erythematous papules, pustules, or vesicles over the back, buttocks, and the upper arms. Associated features include pruritus, malaise, low-grade fever, sore throat and eyes, and axillary lymphadenopathy. This type of folliculitis resolves spontaneously within 10 days.

Folliculitis decalvans is a rare disease that tends to occur in individuals who have coarse and bristle hair. The predisposing factors of this disease are still unknown. The infection begins as a localized area of follicular pustules or papules. Exudation or suppuration soon follows and as the crust accumulates, the hairs are shed. New follicles become involved at the periphery, while at the center the process eventually subsides, with scarring and permanent hair loss.

Hot tub folliculitis is caused by *Pseudomonas aeruginosa. Pseudomonas aeruginosa* is able to withstand temperatures of up to 107°F (41.6°C) and chlorine levels of up to 3 mg/L. The lesions of this variant of folliculitis are found on the trunk and lower extremities of patients who have a recent history of hot tub use. Superhydration of the stratum corneum softens this protective layer and allows the bacteria to cause infection.

There are documented cases of superficial actinic folliculitis characterized by recurrent skin eruptions occurring within 6 to 24 hours after sun exposure. Histologically, there is perivascular lymphocytic infiltration and intrafollicular accumulation of neutrophils in the upper infundibulum of the follicle; these findings indicate the presence of inflammatory response and a suppurative process.

Diagnostic Reasoning

Diagnostic Tests

A Gram stain and culture of purulent discharge is obtained by rupturing a pustule and getting samples of the exudate. The culture is useful to distinguish *Staphylococcus* infection from other bacterial or fungal infections, as well as from epidermal and pilar cysts that are sterile lesions. The Gram stain is usually positive for clusters of gram-positive cocci (*Staphylococcus aureus*) along with a large number of PMNs. With deeper forms of folliculitis, the presence of systemic symptoms and positive blood culture require referral to a physician for hospitalization and IV antibiotics.

If fungal infection is suspected, a fungal culture or KOH microscopic exam is helpful; if results are positive, treatment should change to an antifungal agent.

Differential Diagnosis

Superficial folliculitis is differentiated from tinea barbae by using the KOH examination (see Advanced Assessment box in the section on Dermatophytoses) of the affected hair or by a fungal culture. Acne vulgaris and bullous impetigo may occasionally mimic folliculitis, but the patient's age (i.e., nonadolescent) and the absence of comedones (blackheads or whiteheads) suggests a diagnosis of folliculitis. The lesions of bullous impetigo are usually larger and rupture easily, and the exudate is serous, not purulent. About 50 percent of HIV-infected persons with scabies have coexistent *S. aureus* folliculitis.

Occasionally, follicular lesions extend more deeply, forming abscesses. Rarely, follicles several centimeters across become infected, forming large violaceous plaques. The plaque may be studded with pustules and have deep sinus tracts connecting infected follicles. Rarely, an abscess of the muscles (pyomyositis) may occur due to extension of the infectious process.

Management

Patients rarely consult a health-care provider for this minor problem except for infections that become recurrent and persistent. The goal of treatment of superficial and deep folliculitis is to make the skin inhospitable to pathogens. This includes both nonpharmacologic and pharmacologic approaches.

Gentle cleansing by the simple method of washing the skin twice a day with antibacterial soap (for example, Lever 2000, Safeguard, Dial) is as important as prescription antibacterial medicines. Large pustular lesions with necrotic areas should first be cleansed with a weak soap solution, followed by soaking (or the use of compresses) of the affected skin with saline or aluminum subacetate twice daily. When the skin is softened, the clinician can gently open the large pustules and trim away necrotic tissue. A triple antibiotic ointment (containing polymyxin B, bacitracin, and neomycin) or simply mupirocin 2 percent (Bactroban) can be effective when applied bid to qid for 10 days. Clearance of nasal colonization of *Staphylococcus aureus* by mupirocin treatment twice daily for 5 days has been shown to significantly reduce the incidence of recurrent folliculitis. (See Drugs Commonly Prescribed 6.5.) Systemic antistaphylococcal antibiotics may be ordered if the infection is resistant to local treatment or if the scalp is involved. Usually,

(Text continued on page 172)

Drugs Commonly Prescribed 6.5: Folliculitis, Acne, and Rosacea

Drug	Indication	Dosage	Comments
Topical			
Mupirocin 2% (Bactroban cream)	Folliculitis and impetigo due to *Staphylococcus aureus*	Apply 3 times/day for 10 days	
	Bactroban nasal 2% ointment: for nasal colonization of MRSA	Apply twice daily for 5 days	Spread ointment by closing and releasing the nostrils repeatedly for 1 minute after applying.
Sulfacetamide 10%, sulfur 5% (Clenia)	Rosacea	Once or twice daily after cleansing	Comes as a foaming face wash and emollient cream. Avoid mucous membranes.
(Rosula) also contains urea 10%		Rosula—apply gel 1–3 times/day; as cleanser: 1–2 times/day	
Metronidazole 0.75% gel (Metrolotion) 0.75% lotion (Metrocream) 0.75% emollient cream	Rosacea	Twice daily after cleansing	Avoid eyes. May potentiate oral anticoagulants.
Metronidazole 1% cream (Noritate) 1% cream	Rosacea	Once daily Once daily	
Benzoyl peroxide (Benzac AC gel)	First-line therapy for acne	2.5%	Available in 5 concentrations but 2.5% as effective as 10% and less irritating. Use water-based rather than alcohol-based.
Topical antibiotics			
Erythromycin 2% (A/T/S solution or gel) Clindamycin 1% (Cleocin-T) solution, gel, or lotion	Folliculitis, inflammatory acne and rosacea	Applied once or twice daily	Both may cause mild erythema and burning. Lotion less irritating than solution and gel. May cause diarrhea, colitis. Contraindicated in patients with a history of colitis.
Ciprofloxacin (Cipro)	*Pseudomonas*, folliculitis	500 mg twice daily for 5 days	
Combination therapy			
Benzoyl peroxide 5% and erythromycin 3% (Benzamycin) Benzoyl peroxide 5% and clindamycin 1% (BenzaClin, Duac)	Acne vulgaris	Apply twice daily	More potent than either agent used alone. Requires refrigeration. May bleach clothing and bed linens. Caution in pregnant or breast-feeding patients.
Topical retinoids			
Tretinoin (Retin-A)	First-line therapy for all acne variants	Begin with 0.025% cream twice weekly at night, build to every evening. Tretinoin available in 6 strengths as a cream, gel, or liquid	Original tretinoin formulation unstable in sunlight—apply at bedtime. Newer microencapsulated formulation is more photostable. Pregnancy category C.
Tazarotene (Tazorac)	First-line therapy for all acne variants	0.1%	Pregnancy category X. Erythema and burning are the most common adverse effects. Possibly more effective and faster acting than Retin-A.

Drug	Indication	Dosage	Comments
Adapalene (Differin)	First-line therapy for all acne variants	0.1% once daily at bedtime	Less sun sensitivity than Retin-A. Pregnancy category C.
Other topical treatments			
Azelaic acid (Azelex) (Finacea 15%)	20% cream approved for mild to moderate acne vulgaris 15% gel indicated only for rosacea	Apply twice daily; may decrease to once daily	As with all topical agents, wash hands after use. May cause hypopigmentation in patients with dark complexions.
Systemic therapies			
Oral antibiotics			
Erythromycin (E-mycin, Ery-Tab)	Folliculitis Severe rosacea Moderate to severe acne vulgaris	Rosacea: 250 mg qid Acne: 250 mg bid initially; therapeutic dose: 500 mg bid, may taper back to 250 mg when skin is clear.	Mild GI distress—coadminister with food. Pregnancy category B. *Propionibacterium* acnes quickly becoming resistant to erythromycin.
Tetracycline (Achromycin, Sumycin)	Severe rosacea Moderate to severe acne vulgaris	Acne: 500 mg bid; when skin is clear, taper to 250 mg Rosacea: 250–500 mg bid for 3–4 weeks	Must take 1 hour before or 2 hours after meals. Not for age 9 and younger.
Doxycycline (Doryx, Vibra-Tabs, Vibramycin)	Moderate to severe acne vulgaris Severe rosacea	Acne: 100 mg bid Rosacea: 50–100 mg bid	Photosensitivity may occur.
Minocycline (Minocin, Arestin)	Moderate to severe acne vulgaris Severe rosacea	Rosacea: 50–100 mg bid Acne: Start at 100 mg in the evening for 4–7 days, then 100 mg daily (decreases incidence of vertigo); may taper to 50 mg	Rare but severe side effects—hyperpigmentation, drug-induced lupus, autoimmune hepatitis
Isotretinoin			
(Accutane, Claravis, Amnesteem, Sotret)	Severe nodulocystic and/or inflammatory acne	40–80 mg daily	Causes severe birth defects and possibly depression. Must follow prescribing program from the manufacturer.
Hormonal therapy			
Norgestimate/ethinyl estradiol (Ortho Tri-Cyclen) Norethindrone acetate/ethinyl estradiol (Estrostep)	Moderate acne vulgaris in females over 15 years of age	1 tablet daily for 28 days, repeat	See Chapter 13 on women's health problems for all the precautions that accompany someone taking birth control pills.
Other			
Ketoconazole (Nizoral)	Fungal forms of folliculitis	200-mg tablets daily for 7–14 days	Monitor hepatic function before and during therapy.

however, systemic antibiotics are not helpful or advantageous over topical treatments.

Follow-Up and Referral

A patient who does not respond to therapy should be evaluated for possible diabetes mellitus or for chronic carriage (in the nares, axillae, or perineum) of *Staphylococcus aureus*. Cultures of the anterior nares, axillae, and perineum are recommended. Topical mupirocin 2 percent (Bactroban) should be applied bid for 5 to 7 days to the sites that yielded a positive culture.

More severe forms of folliculitis and rare skin eruptions such as the HIV-EF should be referred to the physician. Systemic IV antibiotics may be necessary. Referral is in order for patients with recurrent or persistent infections that do not respond to the treatment regimen.

Patient Education

The clinician should emphasize to the patient that good hygiene is essential in treating this condition. Good handwashing technique is the best approach in preventing the spread of folliculitis. Patients who are prone to folliculitis can be advised to use an antibacterial soap and to wash the affected areas twice a day with antibacterial soaps before applying topical agents. Patients should also be informed that any source of friction can predispose them to recurrence of folliculitis.

In hospitals (especially the ICU), an emphasis on proper handwashing and proper disposal of cleaning supplies can help to prevent the spread of bacteria on fomites.

Men who arc prone to recurrent sycosis barbae should be advised to grow a beard (if possible) during treatment to allow complete healing. A preventive approach is the best treatment for this condition. When shaving is resumed, an electric shaver may cause fewer breaks in skin than a razor. Patients should be cautioned to avoid borrowing or using old razor blades when shaving infected areas. The patient needs to know that the disease can only be cured by the complete cessation of shaving.

Furuncles and Carbuncles

A *furuncle* (*boil*) is a deep bacterial infection of a hair follicle with abscess formation. Furuncles are caused almost exclusively by gram-positive *Staphylococcus aureus*. Furuncles are extremely tender to touch and appear a bright red color. The most common locations for furuncles are the scalp, neck, axilla, buttocks, groin, and thighs. Furuncles frequently become fluctuant. With the application of warm compresses, most furuncles drain pus and resolve spontaneously.

A *carbuncle* is a large, multiloculated abscess that is made up of multiple furuncles in a contiguous area. Carbuncles, which are less common than furuncles, appear as large, red painful lumps on the skin, with multiple follicular openings. Some carbuncles can get quite large—up to 10 cm in size. Eventually, a carbuncle will spontaneously drain pus.

Epidemiology and Causes

Furuncles and carbuncles are usually caused by *Staphylococcus aureus* and rarely by other pathogens. In some patients, especially the immunocompromised, infection can be due to methicillin-resistant *Staphylococcus aureus* (MRSA). Conditions predisposing patients to formation of furuncles and carbuncles include diabetes mellitus, poor hygiene, obesity, and immune system defects. Chronic staphylococcal carriage in the anterior nares, axilla, and perineum also increase the risk of infection and should be explored in cases of recurrent infections. Favorable environmental conditions that predispose the individual to furuncle and carbuncle formation include areas of moisture, friction, or occluded skin. Any area of skin that is subject to friction, such as the axilla, buttocks, groin, or thighs, is at increased risk of infection.

Pathophysiology

Both furuncles and carbuncles evolve from superficially infected hair follicles (folliculitis), mediated primarily by *Staphylococcus aureus*. Thus, all factors which contribute to folliculitis also predispose to furunculosis and carbuncle formation. As this superficial infection extends along the hair shaft, a small, painful inflammatory nodule is formed at the follicular base which is termed a furuncle. Eventually, a series of abscesses form along the hair shaft involving dermal and subcutaneous layers, ultimately coalescing into a fluctuant, subcutaneous mass which develops a soft, pointed necrotic center. When the furuncle ruptures, it results in the extrusion of pus and a necrotic plug at the entrance to the follicle. A small opening or cavitation remains which eventually heals with scarring. Thus, the affected hair follicle is destroyed and does not regenerate, resulting in destruction of the hair itself.

Carbuncles ("boils") undergo a similar process, except on a larger scale. Carbuncles are made up of several furuncles that form into a large, multi-loculated abscess with multiple follicular openings that eventually drain pus. Carbuncles are significantly larger than furuncles, typically involving deeper skin layers. They are more likely to occur on thicker skin, in areas such as the nape of the neck and upper back. A systemic response including fever resulting from the production of pyrogenic cytokines is more common with carbuncle formation than furunculosis.

Certain risk factors are particularly associated with furunculosis and carbuncle formation. Obesity results in thick skin folds which are closely approximated. This creates a moist environment in which bacteria are prone to reproduce. Impaired immune function from chronic steroid use, underlying systemic disease such as HIV or diabetes mellitus, or impaired neutrophil function also predispose to this condition. In particular, the presence of a bacterial virulence factor known as the Panton-Valentine leukocidin in certain strains of *Staphylococcus aureus* has been associated with particularly aggressive skin infections.

Clinical Presentation

Subjective

The typical patient will complain of a hot and tender, bright red bump or "boil" of several days duration that is getting larger. Some furuncles will come "to a head" or become fluctuant and will drain spontaneously on their own. Some patients will report a history of manipulation of the furuncle or carbuncle, either by squeezing it or by puncturing it with a heated needle. Some patients will report a past history of boils and other skin infections.

Objective

Both furuncles and carbuncles are extremely tender to touch and are a bright red color. A furuncle initially appears as a small (0.5 to 1 cm) red, indurated nodule. As the nodule grows in size, it starts to develop a yellow-colored central plug. It begins to appear conical, with a central "nipple" that is covered by thinning skin. The pus, which is a yellow to green color, gives the "nipple" its characteristic color. Most furuncles eventually spontaneously rupture and drain pus, which hastens their resolution. As the necrotic material and pus are discharged, a small cavitation is left that heals with minimal scarring. Carbuncles initially appear as multiple furuncles that develop into a large, erythematous lump that eventually starts to drain pus from multiple follicular openings. Patients with darker skin can have permanent hyperpigmentation changes as a result of severe inflammation.

Diagnostic Tests

Although most cases of furuncles and carbuncles are caused by *S. aureus,* a culture of the fluctuant lesion is still recommended. Occasional cases of MRSA are sometimes found. A CBC with differential is not necessary unless the patient has a severe case with an underlying disease like diabetes, or shows systemic symptoms such as fever.

No subsequent testing is necessary unless a patient is a staphylococcal carrier. The nares and anogenital region should be recultured after treatment with topical muciprocin (Bactroban) is finished. In resistant cases where no response is seen after 1 week of therapy, a repeat culture should be done.

Differential Diagnosis

Some skin conditions to consider in the differential diagnosis of furuncles include an epidermal inclusion cyst that is acutely inflamed. Epidermal inclusion cysts are usually located in areas of the body where there is thicker skin and a large amount of sebaceous glands, such as on the back and upper shoulders. The patient with an epidermal inclusion cyst will report a history of the cyst on the same site for months to years. In contrast, furuncles are an acute process, taking only several days to form. Another characteristic of an epidermal inclusion cyst is a cheesy white discharge with a strong odor that is present when it is expressed. A furuncle or carbuncle will have a purulent yellow to green-colored discharge when it ruptures.

Another differential diagnosis for a furuncle is a deep fungal infection of the soft tissue called *sporotrichosis.* It is more common in gardeners and other agricultural workers, and is usually seen on the hands or arms. It is caused by injury from a thorn or wood splinter that has been contaminated with the common soil fungus *Sporothrix schencki.* Because it is usually asymptomatic, patients tend to ignore it.

If the furuncle or carbuncle is located on the axilla, a differential diagnosis to consider is hidradenitis suppurativa. The lesions of hidradenitis suppurativa are also extremely tender and inflamed. Patients with this condition report a chronic history of recurrent infection in the axilla. It is a chronic disease of the apocrine glands of the axilla and is associated with severe hypertropic scarring and pilonidal sinuses, which are not seen in furuncles or carbuncles. The classic finding in hidradenitis suppurativa that would tend to differentiate it from a furuncle or carbuncle is the numerous hypertropic scars that are found on both axilla.

Management

Application of warm compresses will promote the localization and spontaneous rupture and drainage of a furuncle. No treatment with systemic antibiotics is necessary for a healthy host if no surrounding cellulitis is present. Treatment with topical antibiotics with good gram-positive coverage (e.g., mupirocin [Bactroban] or neomycin–polymyxin B [Neosporin]), applied bid until resolution, is satisfactory in those cases.

For furuncles or carbuncles on an immunocompromised patient (or one who is at risk for bacteremia because of a preexisting condition), systemic antibiotics are always mandatory and physician referral is recommended. In addition, incision and drainage will speed up resolution of the infection. Preexisting conditions such as diabetes or chronic steroid use (or any condition affecting the immune system) predispose a patient to more complications. These patients should be monitored very closely or referred to a physician. A furuncle (especially if it is located on the upper lip or the central area of the face) or a carbuncle located on the neck, face, or scalp should be treated with physician consultation or referred to a physician for management. Because of its proximity to the cavernous sinus, a furuncle located on the central face can spread via the venous drainage to the cavernous sinus and result in cavernous sinus thrombosis or meningitis. An occasional patient with furuncles or carbuncles will have bacteremia as a complication, with possible hematogenous spread to the heart valves (endocarditis), the kidneys (perinephric abscess), joints, spine, and long bones (osteomyelitis).

If a furuncle has not come to a head by the time the patient is seen, the patient should be instructed to apply warm compresses to it bid to tid until it becomes fluctuant. Systemic antibiotics are often used to treat and hasten the resolution of furunculosis. However, randomized controlled trials have failed to consistently show the benefit of such treatment. In theory, however, systemic antibiotics should lessen the risk of bacteremia. Fluctuant furuncles are ideally treated with incision and drainage. A sterile 18-gauge needle can be used to puncture the thin skin on top of a small furuncle, to allow for adequate drainage of pus. For larger furuncles that are fluctuant, incision and drainage is indicated. The cavity formed by the furuncle should be packed with iodoform or Vaseline (petroleum jelly)-impregnated gauze. After a furuncle has been incised, the patient should be instructed to use warm compresses bid in order to hasten the drainage of pus.

Carbuncles frequently need incision and drainage as well to aid in recovery. Systemic antibiotics and physician referral are always indicated for the treatment of carbuncles. Systemic antibiotics with adequate gram-positive bacterial coverage (except for MRSA) include dicloxacillin (Dynapen) 250 mg to 500 mg PO qid for 10 days, cephalexin (Keflex) 250 mg to 500 mg PO qid for 10 days, or amoxicillin–clavulanate (Augmentin) 500 mg to 875 mg PO bid for 10 days. For patients with penicillin allergies, erythromycin ethylsuccinate (EES) 250 mg to 500 mg PO qid for 10 days, clindamycin (Cleocin) 150 mg PO qid for 10 days, clarithromycin (Biaxin) 250 mg to 500 mg PO bid for 10 days, or azithromycin (Zithromax) 250 mg PO daily for 5 to 7 days may be used. Many strains of community-acquired MRSA are susceptible to trimethoprim sulfamethoxazole (Bactrim) 1 double strength tablet PO bid to tid plus rifampin 600 mg PO qd, both for 10 days, clindamycin (Cleocin) 300 mg PO qid for 10 days, doxycycine 100 mg PO bid for 10 days, or minocycline 100 mg PO bid for 10 days. However, particularly aggressive or extensive infections with MRSA or Panton-Valentine leukocidin–expressing strains of *Staphylococcus* may require inpatient IV antibiotic therapy (e.g., vancomycin) to ensure adequate treatment. The antibiotic linezolid 600 mg PO bid for 10 to 14 days is also approved for the treatment of MRSA. However, this antibiotic is typically used only under close physician supervision, given its potential for inducing thrombocytopenia, anemia, and neutropenia. Thus, antibiotic susceptibility testing is critical in these cases to most appropriately direct therapy.

If a patient has a history of frequent infections, a search for staphylococcal carriage is recommended. Cultures should be taken from the patient's nares, the perineum, and the anogenital region. If a patient is found to be a *Staphylococcus aureus* carrier, a daily shower with an antibacterial or benzoyl peroxide soap is recommended. Mupirocin ointment (Bactroban) should be applied tid to the anatomic sites where *S. aureus* was cultured (nares, body folds, perineum, anogenital region) for 1 week. A repeat culture should be done to document clearance of the bacteria. This program will eliminate the staphylococcal carrier state and reduce the incidence of recurrence. There is some evidence that Vitamin C supplementation (1 g/day for 4 to 6 weeks) may also help prevent recurrent skin infection in persons with impaired neutrophil function.

Follow-Up and Referral

The patient should be seen for initial follow-up within a few days to 1 week, to monitor response to therapy, compliance with treatment, and any adverse reactions. Subsequent visits can be scheduled in 7 to 10 days to monitor for continuing progress and resolution of the lesions. For carbuncles or multiple furuncles on immunocompromised patients (or patients at risk for bacteremia because of preexisting disease), a physician referral is recommended.

If a patient has systemic signs such as fever or looks toxic, physician consultation or referral is recommended. These patients frequently need multiple laboratory tests, including blood cultures, which can be done in a hospital setting, in addition to treatment with parenteral antibiotics.

Patient Education

The patient should be warned not to pop, squeeze, or to manipulate furuncles in any way, especially those that are located on the mid- to upper lip or near the border of the nasolabial folds because of the risk of serious cavernous sinus thrombosis which is sometimes fatal.

Cellulitis

Cellulitis is a deep bacterial infection of the skin involving both the dermis and subcutaneous tissue, which in certain cases may result in fatality. Most cases of cellulitis are caused by group A beta-hemolytic *Streptococcus* or by *Staphylococcus aureus* (gram-positive bacteria). Other less common bacteria that can cause cellulitis include *Haemophilus influenzae* (more common in children), *Eikenella corrodens* (human bites), *Pasteurella multicoda* (cat bites), *Capnocytophaga canimorsus* (dog bites), and the *Vibrio* species (seawater-exposed injuries).

The typical lesion of cellulitis is a wide, diffuse area of erythematous skin that is warm and tender to palpation. Infection is occasionally accompanied by severe edema. Systemic symptoms such as fever, chills, and malaise may accompany some cases as well. A cellulitic infection can occasionally result in the loss of a limb.

Cellulitis may become a life-threatening event that is heralded by shock, hypotension, and toxicity. Toxic shock syndrome (TSS) and multiple organ failure resulting from both streptococcal and staphylococcal infections have been reported. The clinician must learn to differentiate between a severe case of cellulitis that is potentially life-threatening and an uncomplicated case that can be treated on an outpa-

Table 6.10 Types of Cellulitis

Erysipelas	Erysipelas is a streptococcal infection of the superficial layers of skin that does not involve the subcutaneous layers, unlike more typical cellulitis. An older name for erysipelas is "St. Anthony's fire." Despite the superficial nature of this infection, erysipelas should not be taken lightly, because it can be fatal if it is not treated promptly (especially in the very young and the elderly). Before the advent of antibiotics, a high rate of fatality was associated with this infection. Most cases of erysipelas are caused by group A beta-hemolytic *Streptococcus*. Erysipelas is sometimes seen after an episode of strep throat. The most common sites of involvement are the face (especially the cheeks) and the lower legs. Patients usually have systemic symptoms like high fever, chills, and malaise. Erysipelas on the face first appears as a bright red lesion by the nares that can spread rapidly within a few hours to days. An enlarging shiny, bright red, indurated plaque develops that is very warm to touch and has very sharp and distinct borders, as opposed to cellulitis, which has more diffused, flat borders. The affected skin appears shiny because of the edema from the infection.
Necrotizing fasciitis	The hallmark of this infection is its rapid progression and the severity of the symptoms. The progress of the infection is measured in terms of hours instead of days, and the border can be seen to literally spread in just a few hours. This infection is the dreaded "flesh-eating bacteria" and loss of life or limb is a potential complication. During the early phase of the infection, the lesion appears a bright red color with edema that progresses to purpuric changes (indicated by purple color), including gangrene (indicated by black color). The patient will usually complain of severe pain at the affected site, which seems to be out of proportion to the appearance of the skin lesion. This pain is due to involvement of the fascia around the muscle and sometimes of the muscle itself (myositis). Pressure on the skin sometimes reveals crepitus due to gas production by the anaerobic bacteria *Clostridium perfringens.* Gangrene can present in a few hours, with hypotension and mental status changes regarded as particularly ominous signs.
Periorbital cellulitis	Periorbital cellulitis is a potentially life-threatening form of cellulitis that should be treated as an emergent condition. The typical patient is a young child with erythema and edema over the affected periorbital area. The edema can be severe enough so that the entire affected side of the face is puffy. Symptoms include pain with certain eye movements because of inflamed extraocular muscles. Other symptoms include high fever, tachycardia, lethargy or mental status changes, and other systemic symptoms. On physical exam, the involved eye will lose the ability to move into certain quadrants (i.e., lateral or downward gaze) and will have an abnormal exam of cranial nerves III, IV, and VI (EOMs).

tient basis. Special types of cellulitis that have potentially serious consequences discussed in this chapter include erysipelas, necrotizing fasciitis, and periorbital cellulitis (Table 6.10). Severe cases of cellulitis, such as necrotizing fasciitis, must be treated with surgical débridement in addition to parenteral antibiotics to stop the spread of rapid tissue destruction; these patients require hospitalization. Periorbital cellulitis, an emergent condition, should also be treated aggressively with parenteral antibiotics and hospitalization to prevent permanent vision loss and extension of infection into deep cranial structures.

Epidemiology and Causes

There is usually an obvious portal of entry into the skin or mucous membranes, such as an insect bite or a wound, although in some cases there is no obvious point of entry (this is more common with recurrent cellulitis). Cellulitis may occur at any age, but some organisms are more common in certain age groups. *Haemophilus influenzae* type B (Hib) infections are more common in children. In adults and elderly patients, *Staphylococcus aureus* and *Streptococcus pyogenes* are more common. In patients with diabetes mellitus or who are otherwise immunocompromised unusual bacterial pathogens may include *Escherichia coli* and other enteric species (*Enterobacter*), as well as *Proteus mirabilis, Pseudomonas aeruginosa, Acinetobacter, Mycobacterium fortuitum,* and *Cryptococcus neoformans.*

Any break on the skin or mucous membranes is a potential portal of entry for bacterial pathogens. Skin breaks can be caused by surgical incisions, wounds, trauma, insect bites, animal or human bites. Preexisting skin conditions such as stasis ulcers, dermatitides (eczema, psoriasis, contact dermatitis), viral skin infections (herpes simplex, herpes zoster, or varicella-zoster), superficial bacterial infections (acne, folliculitis) and bullous diseases (bullous pemphigoid, pemphigus vulgaris, burns) all have the potential for secondary bacterial infection. The likelihood and severity of cellulitis infection is affected by three important factors: (1) virulence of the pathogen, (2) host immune status, and (3) depth of infection.

Risk factors that predispose an individual to cellulitis include conditions that affect cellular immunity and lymphatic drainage:

- ▲ Diabetes mellitus
- ▲ Lymphatic blockage
- ▲ History of recurrent cellulitis
- ▲ Postmastectomy and postsaphenous vein grafting
- ▲ HIV infection and AIDS
- ▲ Chronic steroid use
- ▲ Cancer chemotherapy
- ▲ Drug or alcohol abuse
- ▲ Peripheral vascular disease

Pathophysiology

The skin and subcutaneous tissue respond to bacterial invasion with an acute inflammatory process. An increase in vascular permeability of the microcirculation of the skin allows protein-rich fluids to leak into the interstitial tissue. This results in tissue edema which may become chronic in recurrent cellulitis. Agents that are released into the tissue increasing vascular permeability include histamine, cytokines, platelet-activating factor, bradykinin, complement proteins, and arachidonic acid metabolites including leukotrienes and prostaglandins. Vasodilation also occurs, giving cellulitis its characteristic bright red color and indistinct borders. In addition, during the cellular phase of inflammation, leukocytes accumulate at the site of injury and engulf particulate material such as bacteria, cellular debris, and antigen–antibody complexes. Engulfed bacteria and other cellular debris are digested inside phagolysosomes by potent hydrolytic enzymes. Interestingly, the bacterial burden in cellulitis may be low, except in cases where abscesses or skin ulcers are present.

The most predominant leukocyte during the cellular inflammatory phase is the polymorphonuclear leukocyte (neutrophil or PMN) and, to a lesser extent, basophils, mast cells, and platelets. PMNs express at least three types of granules containing proteolytic enzymes. Necrosis of normal tissue may occur during the inflammatory process due to these proteolytic enzymes, as well as reactive oxygen metabolites. Some aggressive cases of cellulitis may progress to TSS in which certain strains of *Staphylococcus* and *Streptococcus* release toxins that stimulate a massive release of inflammatory cytokines. This in turn can result in shock, multiple organ failure, and ultimately death if untreated. In addition, bacterial exotoxins have been shown to potentiate hypersensitivity responses to fungal antigens such as *Trichophyton*, the primary agent involved in tinea pedis or "athlete's foot" infection. Such responses have been shown to contribute to the pathogenesis of cellulitis in certain individuals.

Clinical Presentation

Subjective

The typical adult patient with cellulitis will complain of a tender, warm, and erythematous area of skin that is usually located on the face, neck, or the extremities. The patient will usually report a history of a precipitating condition like an insect bite or a small cut that "got infected." The patient might already have a preexisting skin condition like acne, tinea pedis, or chronic eczema with breaks in the skin that can become the portal of entry for bacteria, although at times this is not apparent to the patient. In cases of recurrent cellulitis of the lower leg, the patient will frequently deny any trauma or injury but will report a history of repeated infections on the same leg. The size of involvement can vary from a few centimeters to a larger area, such as an entire limb. The patient will report a history of the lesion or plaque getting progressively larger over several days, but in the case of necrotizing fasciitis, the border will literally be seen to spread in just a few hours. Some patients will complain of tender and enlarged lymph nodes near the affected area. Patients with more severe cases of cellulitis or with special types such as necrotizing fasciitis, erysipelas, and periorbital cellulitis are more likely to complain of systemic symptoms such as fever and chills, lethargy, and malaise.

Objective

In adults, the lower leg is usually the most common site of infection. In cases of lower extremity cellulitis, the clinician should search for signs of tinea pedis. The clinician should look for areas of macerated or peeling skin on the interdigital area of the toes. A chronic tinea pedis ("athlete's foot") infection can become the point of entry for bacteria. In children, and occasionally in adults, the cheeks and the periorbital area are more common sites of involvement. In lighter-skinned patients, the area of skin that is infected will have a bright red color that is warm and tender to touch. (In darker-skinned patients, the color will be a darker red.) Sometimes extensive edema will be present, especially if an arm or leg is involved.

The red borders seen in cellulitis are flat and diffused, compared to the distinct raised border seen on an erysipelas infection. Serious signs of systemic toxicity to look for include high fever, hypotension, tachycardia, marked leukocytosis, and associated lymphangitis. If these signs are present, the patient must be treated aggressively with hospitalization and parenteral antibiotics. Referral to a physician is recommended for severe or special cases of cellulitis.

Diagnostic Reasoning

Diagnostic Tests

Most cases of mild to moderate cellulitis are diagnosed by clinical presentation and history. In the majority of cases of acute cellulitis, there is usually no discharge or obvious wounds present; therefore, obtaining cultures is very difficult. Some studies have only shown a 20 percent positive rate from cellulitis cultures. If an open wound or purulent discharge is present, then a culture and Gram stain should be obtained. For patients who appear ill or have systemic symptoms like fever, a CBC and consultation with a physician is necessary. If periorbital cellulitis is suspected (swelling and redness of eyelids, limited EOMs, fever), testing for extraocular eye movements (EOMs) should be done, along with other tests for cranial nerve function. Leukocytosis is seen in periorbital cellulitis as well as in necrotizing fasciitis and erysipelas.

Differential Diagnosis

The site of the infection helps to guide the clinician in searching for a differential diagnosis. If a lower limb is affected, deep vein thrombosis (DVT) should be considered. Sometimes it is hard to make the distinction between the two conditions: DVT presents as a swollen and warm limb with erythema that is tender to touch and can be very similar in presentation to acute cellulitis. A history of recent surgery, bedrest, or prolonged immobility points more toward DVT; however, DVT can occur after cellulitis, although rarely. There are usually no systemic symptoms like fever associated with DVT. If fever is present, it points more toward the presence of cellulitis. If crepitus is noted on palpation, or if violaceous bullae and intense pain are present, the clinician should rule out necrotizing fasciitis. Serious systemic symptoms that point to severe infection include hypotension, lethargy (or any change in mental status), nausea and vomiting, severe pain (points to possible fascial involvement), and a toxic appearance. If these signs are present, immediate consultation with a physician or referral to the emergency room is necessary.

Management

Treatment of cellulitis should take into consideration several factors: the severity of the infection, the site of the infection, the presence of underlying disease, and the virulence of the pathogen. Patients with diabetes are known to have a higher incidence of complications from skin infections because of chronic high levels of glucose that adversely affect the immune system and the microcirculation. Patients who are under long-term treatment with steroids and chemotherapy are also at increased risk because of immune system depression. Previous surgical procedures, such as a mastectomy or saphenous vein grafts, predispose the affected limb to cellulitis because of defective lymphatic drainage. Some sites of the body, such as the hands, feet, and the face, must be treated more aggressively to prevent any potential loss of future function. Particular care must be taken with soft tissue infections of the hand because a compartment-like syndrome can ensue in addition to destruction of complex structures.

Human bite wounds are known to have a higher rate of infection because of the large amount of anaerobic bacteria present in the mouth. Because of increased vascularity, the face and neck areas are less likely to become infected than the hands and feet. Closed-fist injuries are more likely to become infected, probably because exposed tendons and tissue that become contaminated with oral flora retract back into the skin under anaerobic conditions and allow bacteria to proliferate. Cat bites (30 to 50 percent) are more likely to become infected (with *Pasteurella multicoda*) than human bites. To a lesser extent, some dog bites (only 5 percent) become infected with *P. multicoda* or *Capnocytophaga canimorsus*. The clinician must remember that any injury that occurs in salty or brackish water has potential for infection with *Vibrio* species of bacteria. Periorbital cellulitis is potentially life-threatening and should be regarded as an emergent condition. It is seen more commonly in children than in adults.

Although *Streptococcus* and *Staphylococcus* cause the majority of skin infections, it is still important to establish the specific etiology of any infection. If purulent discharge or an open wound is present, then culture and Gram stain should be obtained. Because it is difficult to culture most cases of cellulitis, diagnosis is based mostly on clinical presentation. Empiric treatment for cellulitis must provide good coverage for both staphylococci and streptococci. Good choices for uncomplicated cases of cellulitis that are not associated with human or animal bites include dicloxacillin 500 mg qid for 10 days, or cephalexin (Keflex) 500 mg qid for 10 to 14 days.

Patients with severe penicillin allergy are prescribed erythromycin 500 mg qd. Infected human and animal (cat or dog) bites are best treated with amoxicillin–clavulanic acid (Augmentin) 500 to 875 mg q12h for at least 2 weeks. Physician consultation or referral is recommended in complicated cases of cellulitis. Prophylaxis (not treatment) for fresh, uncomplicated human and animal bites (less than 6 hours old) is amoxicillin–clavulanic acid (Augmentin) 500 to 875 mg q12h for 3 to 5 days.

Management of cellulitis infection of the lower extremities requires bedrest (with bathroom privileges) and elevation of the infected leg. Patients who are at increased risk of thrombus formation should be referred to the physician for possible anticoagulation therapy.

Erysipelas is treated in the hospital with parenteral antibiotics. The drug of choice is penicillin 2 million units IV given q4h, along with elevation of the affected area. Necrotizing fasciitis must be treated aggressively in the hospital with parenteral antibiotics, surgical debridement, and fluid replacement.

Patients with underlying disease such as diabetes, neuropathy, arterial insufficiency, lymphatic drainage abnormalities, intermittent claudication, and a history of recent trauma on the same leg are more prone to complications and infection with unusual bacterial pathogens (gram-negative bacteria, anaerobes) and must be treated more aggressively. These cases frequently require referral and consideration for hospitalization. Unusual pathogens that may cause cellulitis include *E. coli, Klebsiella,* and *Pseudomonas,* which are more common in patients with impaired immune systems.

Cellulitis of vital structures such as the hand, feet, or the face requires close follow-up to monitor for possible complications. Patients who are at higher risk for complications, including those with severe cellulitis and associated crush injuries, should be referred to a physician. Other patients who have a higher risk of complications include patients with preexisting diseases or conditions that affect the immune system such as diabetes, AIDS, immunosuppression, chronic steroid or IV drug use, alcoholism, a history of arterial insufficiency, and chemotherapy.

Patients who are suspected of having a complicated case of cellulitis such as possible bacteremia (fever, chills) or urgent cases such as periorbital cellulitis, necrotizing fasciitis, or erysipelas need immediate consultation with a physician or referral to the emergency room. The clinician should not rely solely on certain laboratory results such as leukocytosis before considering the seriousness of cellulitis infection. Clinical presentation and symptoms are more helpful in guiding the management of cellulitis than any laboratory test result.

The type of IV penicillin to use for beta-hemolytic group A *Streptococcus* is Penicillin G. Inpatient IV antibiotic treatment is done with nafcillin 2 g IV q4h or cefazolin 1 to 2 g IV q8h for up to 2 weeks, depending on the severity of infection. Clindamycin 600 mg IV q8h is used in penicillin allergic patients, especially in all cases of TSS or other conditions in which pathogenic exotoxins are elaborated, because this is a bacteriostatic antibiotic that prohibits bacterial protein synthesis. For oral therapy, cefuroxime (Ceftin) 500 mg PO bid can be used when *Haemophilus influenzae* is suspected. Azithromycin or clarithromycin is preferred as a macrolide over erythromycin for penicillin-allergic patients if *Haemophilus* flu is suspected. If gram- negative microorganisms are suspected, fluoroquinolones are typically chosen for adult patients such as levofloxacin (Levaquin) 500 mg PO qd which is approved for complicated skin infections. Clindamycin 300 mg PO qid may be added to extend the spectrum of gram-positive coverage. Importantly, however, *Clostridium difficile* (Cdiff) colitis is particularly associated with clindamycin usage. *Vibrio* infections from seawater associated injuries are best treated with tetracyclines, while cellulitis related to fresh water injuries must cover *Aeromonas* infection and include a fluoroquinolone such as ciprofloxacin (Cipro) 400 mg IV q12h combined with cefazolin. Diabetics are typically treated with Augmentin, although this may produce significant GI effects such as loose stools. Other broad-based regimens for hospitalized patients include clindamycin plus either ceftriaxone or nafcillin, along with a fluoroquinolone. If tinea pedis infection is concurrent with cellulitis, treatment for this must be initiated using terbinafine or itraconazole (see previous section on dermatophytoses). Regarding community-acquired MRSA infection, refer back to the discussion under Furuncles and Carbuncles, regarding selected oral agents such as Bactrim. For significant MRSA infection, vancomycin 1 g IV q12h can be used.

Follow-Up and Referral

Most cases of uncomplicated cellulitis resolve with adequate antibiotic treatment. Improvement is usually obvious within 48 hours, although some cases might take 72 hours before some improvement is seen. If the patient is responding to treatment, then follow-up can be done on an outpatient basis. Recurrent infections of cellulitis on a lower extremity can result in a chronic nonpitting edema. (The patient should be advised of this potential complication.) Diabetic patients should be advised to adhere to dietary and lifestyle changes (in addition to medication) to control levels of blood glucose. Several studies have shown that good diabetic control is associated with fewer and less serious complications, including potential vascular, kidney, and eye damage.

Initial follow-up for cellulitis should be done within 48 hours or earlier for sicker patients. Improvement in signs and symptoms should be seen, including a decrease in swelling, erythema, and pain of the affected area. The borders of erythema should be be receding and getting smaller. The clinician can use a marking pen (with the patient's permission) to mark some of the borders during the initial visit: This will make any changes in size easier to notice. If the patient's response is satisfactory, then the next follow-up visit is usually done in 1 week (or sooner, if closer follow-up is necessary). Thereafter, the patient can be seen on a weekly basis until the cellulitis is resolved.

If the patient does not respond to treatment with oral antibiotics after 48 to 72 hours or starts to look toxic, then a CBC and consultation with a physician (or referral to the emergency room) is necessary.

Patient Education

The clinician should instruct the patient to call his or her health-care provider if the infection worsens or if fever persists despite antibiotic treatment for at least 48 hours. The patient should also call the office in 3 days to report progress of simple cellulitis infection. The patient should be advised to elevate the affected limb as much as possible to decrease swelling. If the patient has chronic tinea pedis ("athlete's foot"), an OTC antifungal powder or spray should be used daily to prevent a recurrence of secondary infection with bacteria.

Viral Infections

Warts

Warts (verruca vulgaris, plantar warts, flat warts) are skin tumors formed by infected keratinocytes, usually initiated by the human papilloma virus (HPV). Warts are identified based on their morphology (flat, mosaic, digitate, or filiform) and location on the body (e.g., the plantar, anogenital, and palmar areas).

Epidemiology and Causes

HPV is a small, double-stranded DNA virus that infects epithelial cells and causes hyperproliferation of these cells. HPV is species specific and affects only humans, with a particular tropism for epithelial cells and the mucous membranes. There are at least 150 genetically distinct human papilloma viruses (including HPV subunits). HPV type 1 typically causes plantar warts, while types 6 and 11 cause anogenital warts. Certain HPV serotypes are also associated with anogenital malignancies, including cervical intraepithelial neoplasia (CIN) and invasive cervical cancers. Oncogenicity of HPV appears to be determined by the viral gene products E6 and E7 proteins, which are necessary for host cell immortalization. HPV types 6 and 11 are considered either inactive or weakly capable of transformation, whereas E6 and E7 proteins in HPV types 16 and 18 are capable of producing progressive squamous epithelial neoplasia in experimental studies with mice.

In general, HPV and resultant warts can be transmitted by touch or by trauma to skin tissue such as from nail biting or shaving. Plantar warts occur at points of maximum pressure (e.g., at the heads of metatarsal bones and heels), as a thick painful callus forms in response to the pressure. In contrast, anogenital warts are usually sexually transmitted, but the route of transmission does not necessarily have to include penetrative intercourse (e.g., heavy petting, genital to genital contact, etc.). HPV enters through breaks in the skin or mucosa. Viral particles contained within skin cells serve as the vehicle for person-to-person transmission.

Pathophysiology

Warts (verruca vulgaris, plantar warts, flat warts) are skin tumors formed by infected keratinocytes, usually initiated by human papilloma virus infection. Infected keratinocytes form a mass that remains confined to the epidermis. A common misconception is that warts have roots. In reality, the underside of a wart is usually smooth and round. Although the wart appears to infiltrate the dermis and the subcutaneous layers, it is actually limited to the epidermis. Several types of warts form tightly fused cylindrical projections resulting in a uniform mosaic pattern that is unique to warts. This pattern is a useful diagnostic sign. The black dots seen on the surface of common warts are thrombosed capillaries which become trapped in the cylindrical, finger-like projections.

Clinical Presentation

Subjective

Patients typically complain of a wart or small "bump" (or group of bumps) that has been present for the past several weeks to many months, sometimes for years. Some patients report the same wart being treated before and then recurring on the same area. Most adult patients with common warts attempt self-treatment with OTC wart remedies, with limited to no success. Warts are usually asymptomatic. Occasional plantar warts can cause pain on weightbearing.

Objective

Warts are small or large, fleshy or firm growths or lumps, which can be raised, fairly flat, single, or multiple, isolated, or clustered together to form a cauliflowerlike shape. There are no skin lines crossing the surface and examination with a hand lens reveals centrally located capillaries (black dots) that bleed with paring.

Common warts initially begin as smooth, flesh-colored papules. As they evolve, they become dome-shaped, gray-brown hyperkeratotic masses with black dots on the surface. Although common warts can be found on any part of the body, the hands are the most frequent site of involvement.

Filiform and digitae warts are fingerlike, flesh-colored projections that protrude from a narrow or broad base.

Flat warts (verruca plana) are small (0.1 to 0.3 cm), slightly elevated, flat-topped papules. They are usually numerous and involve the forehead, mouth, beard, eyes, back of hands, and shaved areas. Scratching may produce a line of flat warts in the shaved areas. Flat warts range in color from pink or light brown to light yellow.

Cutaneous HPV infections (types 1, 2, 4, and 7) are more likely to be seen in children and young adults and have an incubation period of 2 to 6 months. As an individual reaches adulthood, the prevalence of cutaneous warts decreases, probably because of improved host immunity. Because these infections are usually benign, they are rarely brought to the attention of health-care providers. HPV types 5 and 8 are closely linked with a rare form of hereditary skin cancer (epidermodysplasia verruciformis).

Plantar warts occur at the heads of metatarsal bones and heels (points of maximal pressure) and appear as thick, painful calluses. This may lead to repositioning the foot while walking, causing distortion in posture, as well as producing pain in other parts of the foot, leg, or back.

Diagnostic Reasoning

Diagnostic Tests

If the clinician is unable to distinguish the lesion as a wart, a small specimen can be sent to the laboratory for identification.

Differential Diagnosis

Corns may be mistaken for warts and can be differentiated from warts by paring them with a number 15 scalpel blade. Skin lines are absent and the black dots that are interspersed in the center of the wart will bleed with additional paring. Its mosaic pattern can be easily identified under a hand-held lens. Although corns have a painful hard, translucent core, warts do not. The pain in corns is relieved when the hard central kernel is freed from the corn.

It is important to differentiate between the surface of the foot that is healing from a recent trauma and warts (black warts) that are undergoing spontaneous resolution. The black dots (thrombosed capillaries) seen on the plantar surface of a foot that has sustained a shearing injury may be confused with the black color of warts that are healing. It is hypothesized that the black color of the warts that are spontaneously healing may be part of the process of regression, and may represent a specific cell-mediated immune response to HPV-infected keratinoctyes.

Corns (*clavi*) may be confused with plantar warts. The pain caused by corns can be relieved by paring and removing the core kernel. Also, pinching a plantar corn does not cause pain, whereas lateral pressure on a wart will elicit pain.

Management

It is important to remember that most HPV lesions resolve without treatment. Therefore, initial management should be geared toward relieving pain and pressure and to minimize skin trauma and scarring caused by available therapies. Although filiform and digitate warts are relatively easy to treat, flat warts present a unique therapeutic challenge. Their duration is prolonged and they may be resistant to treatment. Because flat warts may be located in areas that are cosmetically important, treatment modalities that produce scarring should be avoided. It is important to note that therapies for HPV are usually contraindicated in pregnant women.

Therapy must be individualized, because available therapies may produce unwanted effects such as pain, hyperpigmentation, scarring, damage to normal tissue, sun sensitivity, chemical sensitization, toxicity, and potential harm to pregnant women. In addition, it is important to identify previous treatment failures and successes as well as the patient's risk factors (such as immunosuppression or lapses in therapy compliance) that may account for the failure of first-line therapy. Treatment intervals usually range from 1 to 2 weeks, but other patients may require prolonged therapy in order to eradicate more resistant lesions.

Simply covering warts with silver duct tape for 6 days at a time, then uncovering the wart, débriding it with an emery board or pumice stone, and covering it back up again a day later for repeated cycles lasting up to a month has been shown to be just as effective as pharmacotherapy. In other words, applying salicylic acid is not critical. This is an effective and inexpensive alternative therapy and might be suggested as first-line treatment.

Pharmacologic Treatments

Keratolytic therapy in the form of salicylic acid plasters (Mediplast) or solution (e.g., DuoPlant, Occlusal) is a safe, nonscarring, moderately effective and low-cost (OTC) treatment of common warts, specifically for plantar and palmar surfaces. Once the wart is pared with a number 15 scalpel blade, pumice stone, or emery board, the area is soaked in warm water to soften the surface and to facilitate penetration of the solution. In the case of salicylic acid solution, one drop or more is applied with an applicator to cover the surface of the wart. The surface is allowed to dry and covered with a piece of adhesive tape or bandage. This will enhance the penetration of the solution.

Tape occlusion may precipitate inflammation and soreness, and may necessitate periodic interruption of treatment. The patient may prefer to apply the solution at bedtime. Within a few days, a soft white keratin layer will form; this layer should be pared or abraded until pink skin is exposed. This procedure may be better accomplished by an occasional office visit. When applying keratolytic plasters (40 percent salicylic acid), the patient may use the same procedure outlined in the preceding text. The plaster is more useful when treating mosaic warts (a large cluster of warts). Once the plaster is cut to the size of the wart, the backing is removed and the adhesive surface is attached to the wart and secured with adhesive tape. The plaster should be removed in 24 to 48 hours, and the surface should be pared or abraded as outlined earlier, then a new plaster should be applied to the area. Although this treatment may take a few weeks, it is less irritating than the salicylic acid solution.

Chemicals such as bichloracetic acid (BCA) or trichloracetic acid (TCA) are caustic agents that destroy warts by chemical coagulation of the proteins. These chemicals are frequently used for recurrent warts or at times as initial therapy. The clinician should pare the excess calloused skin and apply petrolatum to the surrounding area before coating the lesion with the acid. BCA or TCA should be applied sparingly, because both are caustic agents that can damage adjacent normal tissue. Sodium bicarbonate (e.g., baking soda), talc, or soap can be used to neutralize or remove unreacted acid when an excess amount is applied. Repeat applications may be necessary every 7 to 10 days. A change of therapy should be considered if the patient has not improved substantially after three provider visits, or if the warts have not cleared after 6 treatments.

Verruca plana (flat warts) are especially difficult to treat because their duration may be lengthy and resistant to treatment. Treatment includes applying tretinoin cream 0.025 percent, 0.05 percent, or 1 percent (Retin-A) at bedtime, over the entire area. Frequency of application should be adjusted to elicit a fine scaling and mild erythema. If other treatment options fail, 5-fluorouracil (Efudex 5 percent) can be applied one or two times a day for 3 to 5 weeks. Hyperpigmentation and recurrent warts at the site of inflammation are the limitations of this therapy.

Podophyllin resin 10 to 25 percent in a compound tincture of benzoin can be used for external warts. Because of the potential complications associated with systemic absorption and toxicity, it is recommended that the area of therapy be limited to 0.5 mL or less of the solution, or to no more than 10 cm of warts per session. To minimize irritation, the area should be allowed to dry and then washed off 1 to 4 hours after therapy. Podophyllin is not used for cervical warts or dysplasia and is primarily reserved for exophytic lesions. Its safety during pregnancy has not been established, so it is contraindicated for use by pregnant women.

Surgical Treatments

Although cryosurgery is very effective for common and genital warts, it may produce severe pain around the palms, feet, and nail areas. Thermal injury to nerve tissue, epithelial cells, and melanocytes can occur and cause changes in pigmentation. Therefore, light applications of liquid nitrogen are preferable. Liquid nitrogen can be stored in 1- to 2-gallon tanks for approximately 10 days. Applications can be repeated every 1 to 2 weeks. It is preferable to spray the lesion with the nitrogen or to use a contact probe with an autoclavable tip because cotton swabs may transmit viral particles.

Surgical techniques such as blunt dissection or electrosurgery usually render patients wart-free with a single visit. Additional clinical training, equipment, and longer patient visits are necessary for these procedures. Blunt dissection is relatively painless if performed on areas other than the plantar or palmar surface. After preparation with local anesthesia, a plane of dissection is established by inserting the tip of a blunt-tipped scissors between the wart and normal skin. The wart is cut circumferentially and the lesion is separated from the normal tissue with short, firm strokes. After the lesion is removed, the blunt dissector is moved firmly back and forth over the area of excision, to ensure that no tissue fragments remain.

Table 6.11 summarizes the treatment strategies for warts.

Follow-Up and Referral

For the majority of common wart cases, a satisfactory response occurs after several treatments. For warts that are unresponsive or are recalcitrant to treatment, other, more aggressive treatment options are available—these are best done by dermatologists.

Interlesional administration of interferon (natural or recombinant) is more effective than systemic treatment. The CDC does not recommend this treatment as first-line therapy because of the need for frequent office visits and the high frequency of systemic side effects. The cure rate (efficacy) is similar to that of the other therapies available. When all other treatments fail, intralesional bleomycin sulfate may be considered. Bleomycin is mixed (with 5 mL of sterile water and 10 mL of lidocaine) to form a solution, and then this solution is reconstituted with normal saline. Using 30-gauge needle, the solution is injected into lesion to achieve blanching. The size of wart will determine the amount of solution injected. Larger warts may require repeat injections. Leakage of the solution is unavoidable during procedure. The cure rate is 48 percent (for plantar warts) to 71 percent (for periungal warts). A multiple-puncture method can result in a 92 percent cure rate. Responsive warts produce hemorrhagic eschars that heal without scarring.

Need for referral to a specialist (dermatologist) is determined by several factors, including lack of response to treatment; possible cosmetic consequences (especially with warts on the face and eyelids); and the clinician's knowledge, experience, and comfort in identifying and treating specific types of warts. If the clinician is unsure of the diagnosis, or if the wart is resistant to multiple treatments, the patient should be referred to a dermatologist.

Patient Education

The clinician should educate the patient on means of prevention of self-inoculation and the routes of transmission of the common warts. These measures include limiting shaving in the affected area until warts are eradicated, strategies to control nail biting, and avoidance of scratching and rubbing on the wart (Table 6.12).

Herpes Simplex Infections

Herpes simplex viruses (HSV) are part of the Herpesviridae family and the Alphaherpesvirinae subfamily. *Herpes simplex virus* infections are caused by two different types of viruses: HSV-1 and HSV-2. HSV-1 is primarily associated with oral infections, whereas HSV-2 is associated mainly with genital infections. Interestingly, HSV-1 genital infections are becoming more common, as are HSV-2 oral infections, probably due to oral–genital sexual contact (Table 6.13).

Epidemiology and Causes

Both types of HSV produce identical patterns of infection. More than 85 percent of people worldwide are HSV-1 seropositive; however, only 20 to 40 percent of these individuals have a history of lesions. The National Institutes of Health (NIH) estimates that one out of four (or 45 million) Americans has genital herpes. NIH estimates that 500,000 new cases may occur each year.

Pathophysiology

The majority of HSV-1 and HSV-2 infections are asymptomatic, so that only elevated IgG antibody titer shows evidence of previous infection. Herpes infections can occur anywhere on the skin. HSV infection has two phases: primary infection and secondary or recurrent infection. During the primary infection, the virus enters keratinocytes in the epidermis, eventually migrating to nerve endings. The virus then ascends via peripheral nerves to the dorsal root ganglion, where it enters a latent stage without active viral replication, which can last for days to years. The trigeminal ganglia are the targets of oral viral strains, whereas the sacral ganglia are the targets of genital herpes strains. Infection of the ganglia may occur within 24 hours of initial viral exposure and is essentially life-long.

The majority of primary infections are subclinical and asymptomatic and can be detected only by an elevated IgG antibody titer. In the past several years, it has been recognized that although HSV infection is largely asymptomatic, most transmission occurs during periods of asymptomatic viral shedding. The severity of the viral infec-

Table 6.11 **Warts and Their Treatment**

Type of Wart (HPV)	Description	Treatment
Common warts	Small, hardened growths of keratinized tissue. Warts usually grow around nails, on fingers and back of hands; can appear anywhere on the body	• Silver duct tape therapy for 6 days, then repeat (see text) • Salicylic acid solution/plasters • Freezing with liquid nitrogen • Surgical excision
Flat warts (Verruca plana)	Pink, light brown or yellow; slightly elevated papules: 0.1–0.3 cm. Numerous sites: mouth, forehead, backs of hands, shaved areas (e.g., legs or beard area); may recur despite treatment. Frequently can undergo spontaneous remission. Avoid potentially scarring therapies.	• May resolve without treatment • Tretinoin cream, 0.025%, 0.05%, or 0.1%. Apply to involved areas daily; adjust treatment to produce fine scaling and mild erythema; may require weeks to months • Freezing with liquid nitrogen • Use of 5-fluorouracil (Efudex 5%) once daily or bid for 3–5 weeks produces dramatic results; may produce persistent hyperpigmentation (use ointment to minimize this adverse effect)
Filiform/digitate warts	Fingerlike, flesh-colored projections emanating from a narrow or broad base; sites: mouth, eyes, and ala nasi	• Easiest to treat, but recurs • Shaving spreads the lesions • Retract skin and use curette drawn across base to remove wart • May use light electrocautery • Cryotherapy
Plantar warts	Lesions appear at maximum point of pressure (e.g., heads of metatarsal bones or heels) or anywhere on plantar surface; thick, painful callus forms around lesion; pain elicited on indirect pressure	• More refractory to treatment • Remove surrounding callus with pumice stone or paring after soaking feet in warm water to soften skin • Daily application of salicylic acid liquid, film, or plaster after soaking
Black warts	Warts become black when spontaneously healing; black heel caused by sheared capillaries usually associated with trauma	• Differential diagnosis for black heel: normal skin lines present; when area is pared with #15 blade, skin underneath is soft, and bleeds
Condyloma accuminata	Cauliflower-like wart Usually found in anogenital region and usually sexually transmitted	• 10%–25% podophyllin solution • Bichloracetic acid • Imiquimod cream • Cryotherapy • Intralesional injections • Laser vaporization • Refer to specialist for management of warts on anal mucosa
Oral warts	Can be located in hard/soft palate, oral mucosa. Usually transmitted through oral-genital contact	• Cryotherapy with liquid nitrogen • Surgical excision
Dysplastic cervical lesions	Lesions are usually subclinical. Colposcopy and biopsy for diagnosis; HPV DNA probes; PCR assays	• CIN stages II & III: cryotherapy—lesions are frozen with liquid nitrogen every 2 weeks • Loop electrical excision • Laser vaporization • Suspicion of invasive disease: cone biopsy
HPV/koilocytosis	Pap smear indicates HPV or koilocytosis	Refer for colposcopy and possible biopsy
Atypical squamous cells of undetermined significance (ASCUS)		Treat any underlying infections. Follow up with Pap smears every 4–6 months; if ASCUS recurs on repeat Pap smear, consider referral for colposcopy and biopsy

Table 6.12 Patient Education: Warts

About the disease

- Warts are small growths or tumors produced by infection of normal skin tissue by the human papilloma virus. The most common areas where warts can be found include the planter and palmar surfaces, nailbeds, hands, face, mouth, penis, vulva, cervix, and anus.
- One in 4 people are infected with human papilloma virus. Despite treatment, most warts will recur. Broken or abraded skin may facilitate the transport of the virus. These lesions can be spread by skin-to-skin contact, including touch, vigorous rubbing, shaving, nail biting, and sexual intercourse.
- Contrary to popular belief, warts do not have roots. The underside of a wart is smooth and round. The black dots found in the center of a wart represent broken small blood vessels (capillaries).
- Immunosuppression caused by diseases such as HIV or cancer and by organ transplants and some medications may reduce the efficacy of treatment. Cigarette smoking affects the immune system and enhances the expression of the viruses. Therefore, smoking should be discontinued.

About treatments

- See text for information on "silver duct tape therapy."
- Treatment often involves more than one session, at 1- to 2-week intervals, and therapy may be prolonged.
- To minimize inflammation, do not apply medicated solutions, ointments, gels, creams, or plasters beyond the recommended time.
- To improve efficacy, plasters should be cut to the size of the wart and kept in place with an adhesive for 24–48 hours. Pare or use a pumice stone to abrade the area and then reapply the plaster. The process may take a few weeks before you see results.
- Podophyllin is applied only to external warts and the area of application should be limited to 10 cm per session. To minimize irritation, the area should be allowed to dry and washed off 1–4 hours after therapy.
- Caustic acids such as bichloracetic acids or trichloracetic acid are very effective but may damage normal tissue if not allowed to dry properly. Repeat applications may be necessary every 7–10 days.
- Wash the treated area after the recommended waiting period. Always check for any signs and symptoms of infection, such as pus, severe pain, heat, redness, and swelling.
- For mild to moderate pain, take over-the-counter analgesics.
- Pursue stress reduction activities, such as exercise, imagery, biofeedback, meditation, and yoga, and maintain a healthy diet. Decreasing stress will boost the immune system and improve healing, as well as reduce the desire to smoke, overeat, or nail bite.

tion increases with age. Herpes infection may markedly compromise nutritional intake in the elderly. HSV is spread by direct contact with active lesions, saliva, semen, or cervical secretions. In addition, HSV can be spread by patients without active disease, in whom subclinical or asymptomatic viral shedding occurs. Viral replication in the gingival epithelia facilitates oral shedding of the virus.

Symptoms may occur from 2 to 21 days after exposure. Tenderness, pain, mild paresthesias, or burning can occur prior to the onset of lesions at the site of inoculation. Headache, fever, muscle aches, localized pain, and tender lymphadenopathy may occur as part of the prodrome. Some patients have no prodromal symptoms. After several days, grouped vesicles on an erythematous base appear, followed by ulcers or erosions which crust over. Eventually there is a loss of crusts and re-epithelialization occurs. In the moist genital region, crusts may not form; however, exudate may accumulate. Lesions typically heal in 7 to 10 days without

Table 6.13 Herpes Simplex Infections

Infection	Location	Commonly Affected Age Group
Oral-labial herpes simplex	Lips, oral cavity	Children age 2–5, adults
Herpetic keratoconjunctivitis	Eyelids, periorbital area, cornea	Newborns, adults
Herpetic tracheobronchitis	Pharynx, trachea, bronchi	Older adults
Herpes simplex encephalitis	Temporal lobe of the brain	Any age, primarily adults who are immunocompromised
Herpes gladiatorum	Shoulder, neck, knuckles, areas of contact	Age 14 and older (commonly seen in wrestlers)
Herpetic whitlow	Fingertip	Age 1 and older
Lumbosacral herpes	Trunk or back	Adult
Herpes simplex of the buttocks	Buttocks	Adult women
Genital herpes	Labia minora, labia majora, vagina, cervix, urethra, penis, rectal area	Young and older adults, 1% of pregnant women
Eczema herpeticum	Face or any area of active or recently healed atopic dermatitis	Infants and older, commonly with a history of atopic dermatiti
Erythema multiforme	Extremities, palms, soles of feet	Age 20–30; more commonly seen in men than women

scarring but may last up to 6 weeks or longer if they become secondarily infected with bacteria. Vesicles in primary HSV infection are more numerous and scattered than in recurrent infection.

Tissue destruction in HSV infection is mediated directly by viral replication within keratinocytes and other epithelial cells. A mononuclear cell and lymphocytic infiltrate occurs at sites of infection, consisting primarily of CD4+ T cells early on, but eventually involving equal numbers of CD8+ T cells, as well as macrophages and cytotoxic natural killer cells that attempt to clear infected host cells. The cytokines interferon-gamma and interleukin-6 are primary mediators of cytotoxic killing mechanisms. Interestingly, in animal models, non-classical T cells endogenous to the skin and mucosal surfaces which express gamma–delta rather than alpha–beta antigen receptors have been shown to protect against severe mucocutaneous and encephalitic HSV infection.

Recurrent disease typically occurs at or near the same site of primary infection. Physical and emotional stress, fever, exposure to ultraviolet light, chapping or abrasion of the skin, immune suppression, menses, or fatigue may cause reactivation of the virus, which descends spontaneously along sensory nerve axons to the skin surface. The anatomic site of infection and virus type affect the frequency of recurrence. Genital herpes recurs six times more frequently than oral–labial herpes. Genital HSV-2 infections recur more frequently than genital HSV-1 infections. Interestingly, oral–labial HSV-1 infections recur more often than oral HSV-2 infections.

Clinical Presentation

Subjective

The most common manifestation of HSV infection is oral–labial herpes. Primary infection with HSV may present as herpetic gingivostomatitis in children and young adults, though most commonly children between the ages of 2 and 5 years are affected. The patient may present with fever, sore throat, hypersalivation, painful vesicles and ulcers on the tongue, palate, gingiva, buccal mucosa, and lips. In genital herpes, early symptoms may include pain in the legs, buttocks, or genital area; genital burning or itching; vaginal discharge; and lower abdominal pressure. Within a few days, lesions appear at the site of infection. With the first episode of genital herpes, fever, headache, muscle aches, painful or difficult urination, and inguinal lymphadenopathy may also occur. HSV infections are usually oral or genital; however, any area of the body can be infected.

In elderly patients, primary infection or reactivation of oral–facial HSV-1 can be extensive. Painful oral lesions make eating difficult and can compromise nutritional status. Sometimes, superinfection with bacteria or *Candida* can further complicate HSV infection in the elderly. Of major concern in older adults is autoinoculation of the eye, causing keratoconjunctivitis, which is the most frequent cause of corneal blindness. Signs and symptoms include unilateral excessive lacrimation, edema, chemosis, photophobia, and purulent exudate. Decreased visual acuity is a bad prognostic sign.

Herpetic whitlow is an HSV infection of the fingertip. This disorder was common among health-care practitioners prior to the use of universal precautions. Now, herpetic whitlow is commonly found in children with a recent history of gingivostomatitis and women with genital herpes. Transmission apparently results from autoinoculation. Vesicles with a red halo may erupt on the finger. Besides generalized symptoms, a red streak may appear up the arm.

A patient with a history of atopic dermatitis who presents with vesicles on the face or areas that have recently healed is likely to have eczema herpeticum. Although a patient who recently had an HSV infection but now presents with iris-shaped lesions on the palms and the soles of the feet most likely has erythema multiforme, HSV lesions on the back are often misdiagnosed as varicella-zoster virus (VZV). Often the correct diagnosis is not made until there is a recurrence. The primary difference on clinical evaluation is that HSV vesicles are uniform in size, whereas varicella-zoster lesions vary in size.

Both types of HSV infection can cause encephalitis. The patient presents with altered level of consciousness, personality changes, fever, and seizures. The patient may also experience smell and taste hallucinations and aphasia. Herpetic encephalitis requires immediate hospitalization and treatment with IV acyclovir (Zovirax). Herpes infections in immunocompromised patients are more severe—frequent HSV recurrences often result in chronic and nearly continuous ulcerations. Focusing the History 6.4 lists some questions for eliciting information on HSV infection.

Objective

The lesions must be examined for characteristic location, appearance, and distribution. Depending on the site of lesions, the anterior and posterior cervical chains submental or the inguinal nodes should be checked for lymphadenopathy. Grouped vesicles on an erythematous base occurring in the mouth or on the face or the genitals are most likely the result of HSV infection. Vesicles on the eyelid, chemosis, or the presence of corneal dendrites require prompt referral to an ophthalmologist.

Diagnostic Reasoning

Diagnostic Tests

Viral culture is the standard method of diagnosis. HSV can be cultured from vesicle fluid or from scrapings from the base of erosion. Sampling must be done early (during the first 72 hours) in the course of the outbreak. The initial viral culture may be negative but clinical evaluation and subsequent recurrence with early culture can verify HSV infection. Viral culture differentiates between HSV-1 and HSV-2 with high sensitivity. The Tzanck smear is rapid and easily

FOCUS ON HISTORY 6.4

Herpes Simplex Virus Infections

General:

- When did the sores first appear?
- Have you ever had sores on the same area before?
- Prior to appearance of the sores, did you experience burning, tingling, pain or numbness?
- Do you have muscle aches, fever, and/or weakness?
- Are you able to swallow?
- Have you ever had this happen to you before? If so, when and how was it treated?
- Have you been around any person who may have had these symptoms?
- Do you have a history of any skin problem?

Specific questions for genital herpes:

- How old were you at first sexual intercourse?
- How many total sex partners have you had?
- How long have you been with your present partner?
- Have you ever had a sexually transmitted disease?
- Do you use latex condoms? If so, do you use them consistently?
- Do you engage in: oral sex? Vaginal sex? Anal sex?
- Have you ever had an abnormal Pap smear?

NOTE: Initiate therapy at earliest symptom.

performed and can be used to identify multinucleated giant cells in vesicular fluid. The Tzanck smear does not differentiate between HSV-1, HSV-2, or varicella-zoster virus (VZV), however. HSV antibodies can be detected in blood, but the serum analysis does not differentiate between HSV-1 or HSV-2. Enzyme-linked immunoabsorbent assay (ELISA) and complement fixation are available serologic techniques that detect circulating antibodies with 90 percent sensitivity but only 50 percent specificity. The Western blot (currently not available in doctors' offices) is another serologic technique that distinguishes between HSV-1 and HSV-2 with high sensitivity and specificity (greater than 99 percent). Viral culture remains the "gold standard" for diagnosis of HSV infection.

Differential Diagnosis

History and clinical presentation are the best guide to diagnosis. Aphthous stomatitis differs from HSV infection in that ulcerations of nonkeratinized mucosa occur. Therefore, lesions rarely appear on gingiva or hard palate, as do herpetic ulcers. Also, no fever or lymphadenopathy occurs. In addition, an aphthous stomatitis ulcer is usually solitary and larger than a herpetic ulcer. Herpangina can also mimic HSV infection. Herpangina is seen predominantly in children and infrequently seen in adults. Treatment is symptomatic for both infections. Hand-foot-and-mouth disease presents with red macules that progress to vesicles on an erythematous base. However, the extremities, in particular the hands and feet, as well as the mouth, develop lesions. Erythema multiforme can result from HSV or *Mycoplasma* infection or a drug reaction. Treatment is based on the underlying cause. Pemphigus is an autoimmune disorder that usually occurs in middle-aged patients (age 40 to 60). Erosions of the oral mucosa are followed by bullae over the body.

Management

No cure for herpes exists; however, recurrences tend to be milder and of shorter duration than the primary infection. Therapy is primarily symptomatic and supportive. Nutritional intake is important especially in elderly patients, who may benefit from using anesthetic mouth rinses. The goals for management include reduction or elimination of pain, decreased viral shedding, and healing of tissue. In cases of frequent recurrence of herpetic lesions, suppressive therapy may be needed.

Initial therapy is palliative and promotes healing. Herpetic keratoconjunctivitis requires immediate referral to an ophthalmologist to prevent blindness. For other forms of HSV infection, the practitioner can initiate management with pharmacotherapy and self-help techniques based on the location and extent of HSV infection. Acetaminophen (Tylenol) can be used to control fever and pain. Lesions on the lip (if small) may require nothing more than applications of ice and lip ointments such as Blistex. If lesions are more extensive, penciclovir 1 percent cream (Denavir) applied to the affected area q2h while awake for 4 days promotes healing, shortens the course of the illness by several days, and substantially decreases viral shedding. Extensive oral lesions may require the use of oral anesthetics such as viscous xylocaine 2 percent (Lidocaine) or dyclonine hydrochloride 0.5 to 1 percent (Dyclone) to control pain. In addition, acyclovir (Zovirax) suspension 200 mg/5 mL can be used to directly treat the lesions by rinsing the mouth with 1 teaspoon and swallowing five times a days for 7 days.

Initial treatment of genital herpes requires the use of oral antiviral drugs. Valacyclovir (Valtrex) and famciclovir (Famvir) have greater bioavailability and require less frequent daily dosing than acyclovir. This type of regimen makes these drugs preferable to acyclovir, but they are far more expensive to the patient. Comfort measures such as warm compresses or an oatmeal sitz bath several times a day can relieve pain and promote healing. A patient with genital or urethral herpes may find it easier to urinate into the warm bath water. Every patient with HSV infection benefits from an increased fluid intake and rest.

Any necessary subsequent management is based on the recurrence of symptoms. A patient with an initial negative viral culture can be told to return to the practitioner for another viral culture within the first 72 hours if symptoms recur. This procedure is important within an initial negative culture of genital herpes. A patient with genital herpes, after the first occurrence, can be given a prescription for an antiviral drug and instructed to take the medication should he or she experience the beginning of symptoms such as tingling or burning at the site. A patient with genital herpes who experiences 6 or more recurrent episodes per year should be placed on suppressive therapy. According to the Centers for Disease Control and Prevention (CDC), valacyclovir (Valtrex) 500 mg every day is not as effective as other viral suppressive therapies. Acyclovir has been used for over 5 years for suppressive therapy without major side effects. On the other hand, famciclovir and valacy-clovir have been used for only 1 year for suppressive therapy. The practitioner may consider stopping suppressive therapy after 1 year and monitoring the rate of recurrence. Practitioners who are uncomfortable with prescribing suppressive therapy can refer the patient to an infectious disease specialist or gynecologist. (See Drugs Commonly Prescribed 6.6.)

Follow-Up and Referral

Follow-up should be early and repeated depending on the extent of disease. Lesions confined to the lip area may not need to be seen unless they do not resolve. Extensive oral

Drugs Commonly Prescribed 6.6: Herpes Simplex Infection

Drug	Indication	Dosage	Comments
Topical therapy Docosanol 10% cream (Abreva)	Herpes labialis	Apply 5 times daily until healed.	Begin therapy at first indication of lesion. Avoid mucous membranes and eyes.
Penciclovir 1% (Denavir)	Herpes labialis	Apply every 2 hours while awake for 4 days.	Begin at first sign of sore. Avoid mucous membranes and eyes.
Systemic therapy Valacyclovir (Valtrex)	Herpes labialis Herpes zoster Genital herpes (initial) (recurrent) (suppression) with 9 or fewer recurrences/year more than 10 recurrences/year (immunocompromised patients)	2 g q12h for 1 day 1 g 3 times/day for 7 days 1 g twice daily for 10 days 500 mg twice/day for 3 days 500 mg q48h 500 mg q24h 500 mg bid for 5–10 days	Medication does not prevent spread of herpes labialis to others. Precautions should be taken around others who have not had chickenpox or varicella vaccine, or are immunocompromised until all lesions are crusted.
Famciclovir (Famvir)	Herpes labialis Herpes zoster Genital herpes (initial) (suppression) (immunocompromised patients)	500 mg bid for 7 days 500 mg q8h for 7 days 125 mg q12h for 7–10 days 250 mg q12h for up to 1 year 500 mg q12h for 10 days	Start within 72 hours of onset of rash.
Acyclovir (Zovirax)	Herpes labialis Herpes zoster Genital herpes (initial) (recurrent) (suppressive) (immunocompromised patients) Herpetic whitlow	400 mg 5 times/day or q4h for 5 days 800 mg q4h for 7–10 days 200 mg q4h for 10 days 800 mg tid for 2 days 400 mg twice daily for up to 12 months 400 mg 5 times/day for 14–21 days 400 mg tid for 10 days	Safety not established in pregnancy and lactation. 5 times/day is the equivalent of q4h. In addition to Valtrex during second episode Suppurative inflammation at tip of finger or toe due to herpes simplex virus. Painful and accompanied by lymphadenopathy.

lesions and genital lesions should be seen on a weekly basis until resolution. As previously mentioned, herpetic lesions of the eye must be referred to an ophthalmologist immediately. Patients with herpes zoster opthalmicus should be instructed to return to the practitioner if they experience a recurrence, until they feel comfortable in handling subsequent episodes on their own. A patient with genital herpes may benefit from referral to a local herpes organization for information and emotional support.

Patient Education

Patient education is an integral component of the management of HSV infection. Most patients achieve relief of symptoms within 4 to 7 days of beginning therapy. Self-care techniques and instructions on the proper use of pharmacotherapy are vital. Table 6.14 provides guidelines for patient education on herpes infection.

Acne

Acne Vulgaris

Acne vulgaris (commonly called "acne") is one of the most common skin conditions that the clinician will see in primary care. Acne is derived from the Greek word *acme* meaning "prime of life" because it is a disease primarily of adolescence, although it may continue into adulthood. Acne is an inflammatory disorder of the sebaceous gland and its accompanying hair follicle (or a pilosebaceous unit), with the highest incidence seen in teens and younger adults. There are approximately 5000 pilosebaceous units on the human body. Most of them are located on the face, back, chest, and upper arms, the most common sites for acne. Acne lesions include comedones, papules, nodules, and cysts. Painful nodules and cysts are found in severe forms of acne.

Although acne is not a life-threatening illness, it has the potential for resulting not only in physical scars but in emotional trauma as well. The primary-care provider should not ignore the impact of acne on self-esteem and identity, which are closely tied to physical appearance during the adolescent period. Most cases of acne can be treated safely in the primary-care arena. Treatment options should be offered to both the parent and the teen during routine wellness visits as well as during episodic visits.

Common misconceptions regarding acne abound in the community. Many patients and their parents think that antibiotic treatment can result in a "quick cure." In reality, antibiotic treatment can take up to 4 to 6 weeks before visible results are seen. No connection has been found between ingestion of certain foods (fried foods, chocolate) and acne. The response rate from acne treatment tends to be slow compared to most infections treated with antibiotics. Good education regarding acne can help prevent disappointment in angry and discouraged patients who might become noncompliant because of a loss of trust in both the treatment and provider.

Table 6.14 Patient Education: Herpes Simplex Infection

- Fever, stress, sunlight, and menses can trigger reoccurrence of lesions.
- Burning and tingling at the site may signal reoccurrence of the infection. If antiviral therapy was prescribed, begin it at the first sign of infection.
- If symptoms persist beyond 10 days, see your health-care provider.

Treatment

General:

- Apply penciclovir (Denavir) 1% cream to affected area every 2 hours while awake for 4 days, or until symptoms resolve.
- Frequent handwashing, rest, and increased fluid intake are needed during any herpetic outbreak

Lip lesions:

- Apply ice to lip lesions for 10–15 minutes as needed to relieve pain and decrease swelling.
- Lip balms (such as Blistex) may be used on the lips to prevent drying of sores and reduce pain.
- Apply lip balm sunscreen (such as Chapstick) with an SPF of 15 to lips prior to sun exposure.

Oral lesions:

- Apply a dental protective paste (such as Orabase) 4 times a day to prevent irritation of the lesions by the teeth.
- An equal mixture of diphenhydramine (Benadryl) syrup (12.5 mg/5 mL) and unflavored Maalox can be used as an oral rinse every 2 hours, then expectorated. Viscous xylocaine 2% (Lidocaine) 5 mL can be added to the mixture or used alone as an oral rinse before meals to decrease pain and facilitate eating.
- For those with orolabial lesions, there should be no sharing of towels, silverware, or glasses, or kissing until lesions are healed.

Genital, anal, and/or buttocks lesions:

- To soothe lesions, apply warm compresses or take a warm oatmeal sitz bath for 20 to 30 minutes as needed.
- A blowdryer placed on the cool setting can be used to thoroughly dry genital lesions.
- No sexual intercourse until lesions are healed. A latex condom must be used consistently to decrease viral spread.

Epidemiology and Causes

Acne vulgaris has the highest incidence among 12- to 25-year-olds; up to 85 percent of this age group is affected at one time or another. More than 17 million Americans are affected every year by acne vulgaris. The incidence of acne markedly decreases as people get older. Acne occurs equally in both males and females, although it can be more severe in males. The average age of onset for girls is age 11 and for boys, age 12. There are some racial differences. The average age of onset is 16 for Hispanics, 19 for Asians, and 20 for African Americans. Hispanic teenagers have both the highest incidence of acne and resultant scarring. Acne can recur again during adulthood and is called *adult-onset acne*. Adult-onset acne is more commonly seen in women who are in their mid-20s to 40s. Fifty percent of adult women have premenstrual flares of acne, while many women have their first flare, or worsening of existing acne, during pregnancy. The etiology of acne is interdependent upon several factors, which include:

- An increase in production of sex hormones (androgens) in puberty and adolescence
- An increase in sebum production resulting from activation of the sebaceous glands (during puberty and adolescence) and genetic factors
- A disorder of epithelial cell "stickiness" (keratinization) and shedding (desquamination), leading to plug formation
- Proliferation of *Propionibacterium acnes* bacteria inside the hair follicles
- The host's inflammatory response

Pathophysiology

Comedones are the basic lesions of acne and are caused by a defect in desquamation at the opening of the pilosebaceous follicle. Instead of regular cellular shedding, desquamation is reduced and shed epithelial cells become "sticky," forming plugs that block follicular openings, in a process known as retention hyperkeratosis. It takes about 2 months for the accumulated shed epithelial cells, sebum, and keratin to finally produce a comedone. *Comedones* are non-inflammatory lesions and are classified into two types—*closed* comedones ("whiteheads") and *open* comedones ("blackheads"). Open comedones get their black color from melanin and not from dirt, as the black color results from the oxidation of tyrosine to melanin. Tyrosine, an amino acid precursor of melanin, is a substance that is normally present in the plug material.

Enlargement of the sebaceous glands and increased sebum production triggered by adrenarche during adolescence provides a rich growth medium for the overgrowth of *Propionibacterium acnes* bacteria within the pilosebaceous follicles. *P. acnes* is an anaerobic diphtheroid that is part of the normal skin flora in humans and is responsible in large part for the inflammatory response observed in acne vulgaris. *P. acnes* utilize triglycerides as their primary source of nutrients by breaking down the sebum inside the affected hair follicle into its basic units—fatty acids and glycerol. Free fatty acids act as irritants and produce a sterile inflammatory response inside the sebaceous follicles. *P. acnes* itself also causes a direct inflammatory response by releasing proteolytic enzymes such as hyaluronidase, as well as chemotactic factors that attract neutrophils to the site of infection.

These neutrophils extrude lysozyme which further degrades surface epithelia, leading to rupture of the previously closed comedone. When a comedone ruptures, its contents, which include sebum, bacteria, keratin, and free fatty acids, enter the dermis and elicit a severe inflammatory response. This results in the formation of deep abscesses, which present on the skin surface as nodules and cysts. Although androgen excess may lead to acne formation (e.g., dehydroepiandrosterone sulfate), most acne sufferers do not overproduce androgens. However, their pilosebaceous glands are likely hypersensitive to these hormones and more prone to retention hyperkeratosis. Some studies have shown that the production of sebum is increased in patients with acne compared to controls of similar age, thus suggesting a possible genetic predisposition for acne vulgaris.

Clinical Presentation

Subjective

The typical patient is an adolescent male or female who has already tried self-treatment for several months with OTC products without much success. The patient might present to the clinician's office not only with numerous acne lesions but also with dry, irritated skin, a common side effect of many topical acne medications. Female patients are more likely to verbalize emotional distress over their appearance. Male patients are more likely to wait until their acne is severe before they will seek treatment from the clinician. Some patients with severe acne complain of pain and tenderness from multiple deep pustules, nodules, and cysts. Mild to moderate acne normally does not cause pain.

Objective

Mild Acne. Mild acne is composed mainly of noninflammatory comedones with occasional small papules. Commonly, there is a mixture of both types of comedones. The location of the comedones and papules will vary, from a predominantly facial involvement to other locations, such as the chest, back, and the upper outer arms. Closed comedones are small papules from 1 to 3 mm in size that are the same color as the surrounding skin, sometimes with a visible white plug. Occasionally, a closed comedone can get irritated from trauma (e.g., scratching) and become inflamed. Open comedones have a black-colored central plug. The hard plug on some comedones can be removed easily by putting firm pressure on the sides of the lesion.

Moderate Acne. Moderate acne is composed mainly of inflammatory lesions such as papules and pustules. The papules range in size from a few millimeters to half a centimeter. The color of the acne papules in light-skinned patients ranges from light pink to bright red. Papules in darker-skinned patients can be red to shades of brown. Pustules are easier to recognize: They appear like pointed papules, with yellow to green-colored tops. When pustules become fluctuant, they rupture spontaneously, providing relief from pain. Resolution of a pustule is usually rapid after rupture. Scarring is more likely with larger and deeper pustules. Hyperpigmentation can be problematic, especially in patients with darker skin. (Patients with olive-toned complexions and darker tones are more likely to have this problem.) Patients who are prone to hyperpigmentation should be advised to avoid prolonged sun exposure to the face and to use oil-free sunblock on the face.

Severe (Nodulocystic) Acne. Severe acne, or nodulocystic acne (consisting mostly of nodules and cysts), always results in scar formation. The severity of acne scars is variable, from numerous atrophic pits ("pockmarks") to large, depressed scars. In patients with darker skin, keloids and hypertropic scars can result. Severe acne is more common in males. Occasionally, fistula formation is seen in some patients. Nodules are inflammatory lesions that appear bright to dark red (or brown), depending on the patient's shade of skin. Nodules are smaller and feel harder than acne cysts. In addition, some darker-skinned patients often end up with permanent hyperpigmentation changes secondary to severe inflammation. Not all hyperpigmentation changes on the skin will fade; some patients will end up with permanent brown to black-colored macules on skin.

Acne conglabata is severe cystic acne in which nodules, cysts, and abscesses develop; lesions are predominantly located on the trunk area instead of the face. Females with acne conglabata should be evaluated for polycystic ovary syndrome. Acne fulminans is rare and is seen in young adolescent males. An acute onset of multiple painful, ulcerated acne lesions is seen, along with systemic symptoms such as fever, chills, malaise, and generalized joint and muscle aches.

Diagnostic Reasoning

Diagnostic Tests

Acne is diagnosed by its classic location and characteristic lesions. A complete history is crucial to the diagnosis and supplants the importance of most diagnostic tests, which are really only needed when an underlying condition is suspected or for cases refractory to standard treatments. For acne fulminans, a CBC, blood chemistry panel, urinalysis, and erythrocyte sedimentation rate (ESR) can be helpful. Abnormal lab results, however, seen in cases of acne fulminans include an increase in white blood cell (WBC) count (leukocytosis), an elevated ESR, anemia, and hematuria.

If an endocrine disorder such as polycystic ovaries is suspected (e.g., in a hirsute overweight female with moderate to severe acne and amenorrhea or irregular menses), then an evaluation for excessive androgen production should be done. A complete physical exam, along with laboratory tests that include serum total and free testosterone and dehydroepiandrosterone sulfate, is recommended. A pelvic ultrasound should be ordered to look for enlarged ovaries.

Differential Diagnosis

Rosacea used to be called "acne rosacea" and needs to be ruled out. Rosacea is more common in adults and older patients and is located more centrally on the face, cheeks, chin, and nose. There is a tendency for easy flushing in response to alcohol or heat. Telangiectasia, a dilatation of a small group of blood vessels, may be present. It can be accompanied by eye complaints such as excessive dryness and irritation. It is more common in patients from an Irish, Scottish, or English ethnic background. Chronic rosacea can result in rhinophyma (hyperplasia of nasal tissue) and is seen more often in older men.

"Hot-tub" folliculitis (folliculitis lesions caused by staphylococci) appear within 1 to 4 days after hot tub use (because of inadequate temperature and chlorination). Patients will complain of small red pustules that can be occasionally pruritic. Folliculitis is located on the areas of the body that have been immersed in the water, such as the lower torso, buttocks, and the legs. Perioral dermatitis appears as small, erythematous papules that occur only around the mouth area. The main diagnostic clue is the location: It is seen only on the perioral area and is more common in adult females (usually 20 to 30 years old). Treatment is similar to that for acne rosacea.

Management

The primary goal of acne treatment is to prevent and or to minimize scarring and permanent pigmentation changes. Patient education is very important in acne management and should not be neglected. Mild acne is treated with topical medications only (see discussion that follows). Systemic antibiotics may be used in moderate cases of acne that are unresponsive to topical agents and are used in severe cases.

A combination of several types of acne lesions is not uncommon, but the most predominant lesions present will help in the determination of treatment choices. Other factors that help determine treatment include a higher risk of pigmentation changes (more common in patients with darker skin), a patient's refusal of systemic antibiotic treatment, and severity of the acne. Parental permission is necessary to treat patients younger than age 18. The popular media has suggested tretinoin has been associated with psychotic or suicidal behavior in teens, but this has never been substantiated by rigorous epidemiologic data.

Topical Treatment of Comedonal Acne

Comedones respond well to topical retinoids. Synthetic retinoids such as tretinoin (Retin-A) and adapalene gel (Differin) decrease comedone formation by increasing cell turnover and decreasing epithelial cell cohesiveness. Adapalene gel seems better tolerated on sensitive skin than tretinoin, but patients with extremely sensitive skin can still develop skin irritation. Mild adverse effects include dryness, erythema, scaling, and burning. Azelaic acid (Azelex) is the least likely to irritate sensitive skin (compared to retinoids) and does not cause photosensitivity, but practical results in the clinical area have been disappointing. Patients who are unable to tolerate topical retinoids may be good candidates for this drug.

Tretinoin has been shown to thin out the top epidermis during the first 4 weeks of treatment, and thus can be very drying and irritating. At this time, patients might notice

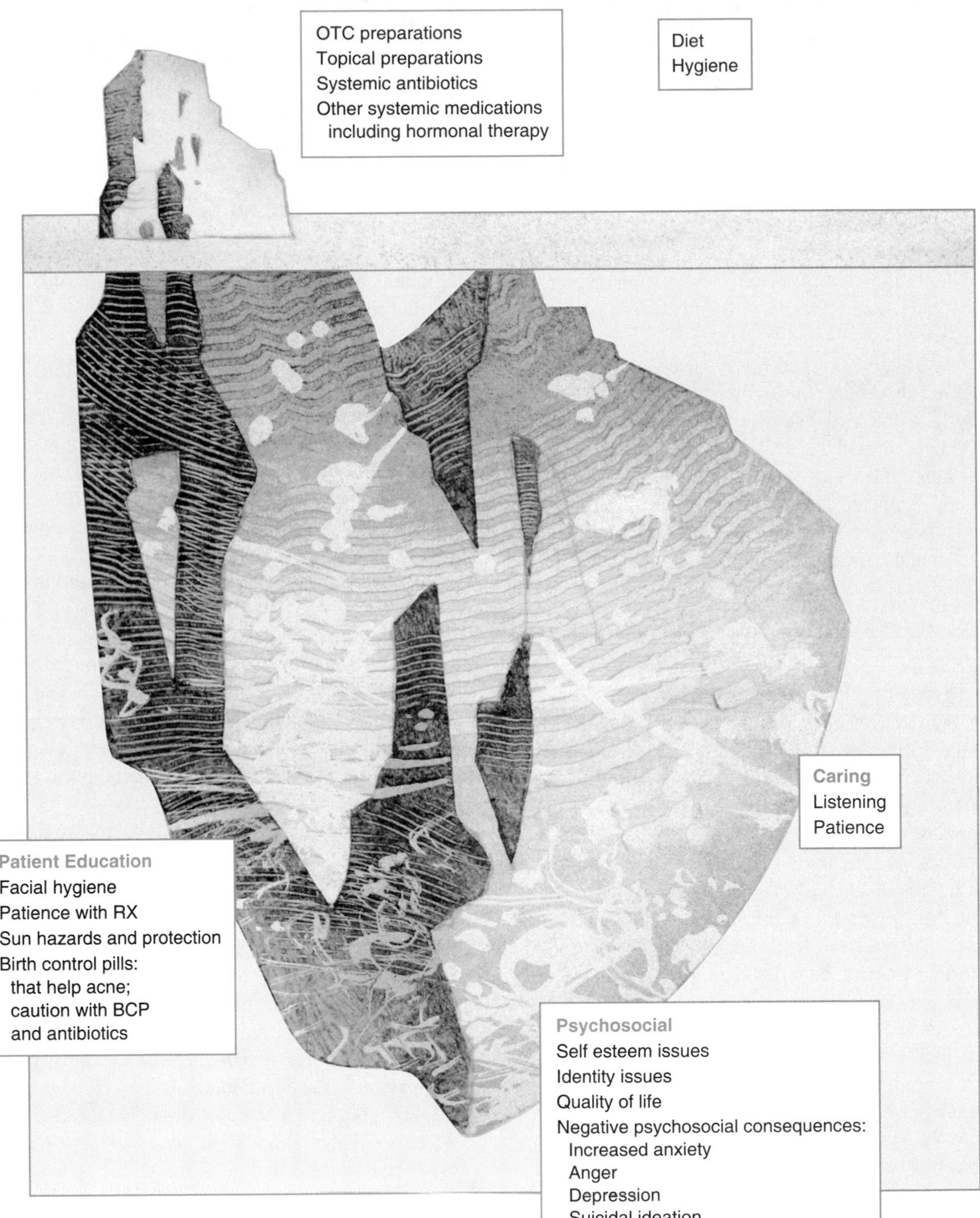
The Iceberg of Acne
OTC preparations
Topical preparations
Systemic antibiotics
Other systemic medications including hormonal therapy
Diet
Hygiene
Caring
Listening
Patience
Patient Education
Facial hygiene
Patience with RX
Sun hazards and protection
Birth control pills: that help acne; caution with BCP and antibiotics
Psychosocial
Self esteem issues
Identity issues
Quality of life
Negative psychosocial consequences:
Increased anxiety
Anger
Depression
Suicidal ideation

more skin sensitivity to the elements (cold air, wind, sun) and an increase in skin photosensitivity. Sunscreen or sunblock should be used during the entire treatment period, especially during this time. The thickness of the epidermis returns to normal after 4 to 6 weeks. Topical retinoids are derivatives of vitamin A and are available in multiple vehicles in a wide variety of concentrations. They are rated as pregnancy Category C and should not be used in pregnant women or on children.

It is important to warn patients and parents that tretinoin, and to a lesser extent, adapalene gel, will cause a worsening of acne lesions during the first 4 to 6 weeks of treatment, because preexisting comedones will continue to surface during this time. Improvement should become visible by 6 to 8 weeks, however. A trial period of 2 months is generally recommended for topical retinoids, unless the patient develops contact dermatitis or other problems with the medicine. To avoid excessive skin irritation, the patient should wait for at least 20 to 30 minutes after washing and should allow the skin time to dry before applying topical acne agents. Patients with a history of eczema or with sunburned skin should not use this medicine. The patient should avoid the eyes, mouth, angles of the nose, and mucous membranes when applying this medicine. Adverse reactions include excessive skin irritation, an apparent exacerbation of symptoms, transient pigmentation changes, stinging on application to the skin, and dry skin. The effects of other topical acne agents, such as benzoyl peroxide, sulfur, resorcinol, and salicylic acid, should be allowed to subside before the application of topical retinoids. (See Advanced Practice Nursing Interventions 6.1.)

ADVANCED PRACTICE NURSING INTERVENTIONS 6.1

Initiating Tretinoin Therapy

Start with tretinoin 0.025% (Retin-A) *cream* (the least irritating). Apply 3 to 4 times per week at bedtime for the first 2 weeks until the patient can tolerate a daily dose. Give this dose a trial of 6–8 weeks.

- Gradually increase to a 0.05% cream or 0.025% gel if patient can tolerate the above regimen and needs a stronger dose (if no reduction in acne lesions seen after 8 weeks).
- If there is still breakthrough of acne lesions, increase to the 0.1% cream.

NOTE: The most potent and irritating dose of tretinoin is the 0.05% liquid formulation. Remind the patient that acne breakout expected effect at weeks 4–6 of treatment, then skin will start to clear up. Tretinoin 0.05% (Renova) has been shown to decrease the effects of solar damage and is approved by the FDA for the treatment of fine wrinkles, mottled hyperpigmentation, and tactile roughness of the skin.

Topical Treatment of Inflammatory Acne

Patients with predominantly inflammatory lesions may respond well to topical antibiotics such as erythromycin or clindamycin (Cleocin-T), benzoyl peroxide (Benzac, Benzagel), or a combination of benzoyl peroxide and erythromycin (Benzamycin). Topical erythromycin is available as a solution of 1.5 percent (Staticin) or 2 percent (T-Stat, Erycette) and in gel form (A/T/S, Emgel). Other good candidates for nonretinoid topical acne therapy include patients who cannot tolerate tretinoin or adapalene gel, or patients who have concurrent eczema. All topical antibiotics are applied once or twice daily. The most common side effects include mild erythema or burning. Because topical antibiotic solutions use an alcohol base, they can cause excessive skin dryness. To avoid this problem, the clinician should tell the patient to start gradually on a once-a-day basis for 2 weeks. Monotherapy with topical antibiotics may lead to bacterial resistance with a resultant slower therapeutic effect, so switching the patient to a combination of antibiotics and benzoyl peroxide has shown an increased efficacy and reduction of the antibiotic resistance to *Propionibacterium acnes*. The antibiotics must be stored in the refrigerator. The combination products, available in gel form include 1 percent clindamycin–5 percent benzoyl peroxide (BenzaClin, Duac) and 3 percent erythromycin–5 percent benzoyl peroxide (Benzamycin). Azelaic acid (Azelex), a dicarboxylic acid with bacteriostatic and keratolytic properties is approved for acne in the 20 percent cream formulation. It is particularly effective in treating patients with postinflammatory hyperpigmentation or concomitant melasma.

Systemic Antibiotic and Hormone Treatment of Moderate to Severe Acne

Topical acne medicines are a much safer alternative than oral antibiotics and have less potential for adverse effects. Topical therapy has its limitations, however. Oral antibiotic treatment should generally be continued for 4 to 6 months, and maximal clinical results may not be evident before 3 to 4 months.

Good candidates for oral antibiotic treatment include patients who:

- ▲ have a lack of response to topical medications after a trial of at least 2 to 3 months.
- ▲ have the inability to tolerate topical acne treatment.
- ▲ have large numbers of inflammatory lesions after several months on topical treatment.
- ▲ have severe nodulocystic acne.
- ▲ have large numbers of inflammatory lesions located on the back or upper outer arms (hard to reach areas).
- ▲ want quick relief from inflammatory acne.
- ▲ are at increased risk of pigmentation changes or scarring.

Oral antibiotics can be used alone or in combination with topical therapy. Oral antibiotics used in the treatment of inflammatory acne include the tetracyclines (tetracycline, doxycycline, minocycline) and erythromycin. Both tetracyclines and erythromycin exert not only an antibacterial effect against *Propionibacterium acnes* but a direct anti-inflammatory effect as well. Minocycline is reserved for tetracycline-resistant cases of acne because of its higher cost and its relatively frequent adverse effect of vertigo.

Tetracyclines are preferred as the first-line oral antibiotic treatment for acne because of their efficacy and lower cost. Tetracyclines should not be used on pregnant women and patients under age 9, however, because of the risk of tooth discoloration and inhibited skeletal growth. Another important factor to keep in mind is that tetracyclines are labeled by the FDA as potentially reducing the effectiveness of oral contraceptives (a potential medico-legal risk). Patients on oral contraceptives should use a reliable second method of birth control, such as condoms. For patients who are good candidates for tetracycline therapy, the starting dose is 500 mg orally bid. In a patient who is unable to tolerate this dose, a smaller dose of 250 mg bid can be given. After results are seen in a few weeks, the dose of tetracycline can be decreased to 250 mg, then to once-daily dosing after another 6 to 8 weeks; the usual maintenance dose is 250 mg once a day. Response to therapy is seen in approximately 70 percent of patients in 4 to 6 weeks. Adverse reactions to tetracyclines include nausea, dizziness, rash, blood dyscrasias, pseudotumor cerebri, photosensitivity, and hepatotoxicity. Antacids, dairy products, and iron or magnesium-containing vitamins will inactivate tetracyclines because of their propensity for binding with those substances. Tetracyclines should be taken on an empty stomach or 2 hours after a meal.

Doxycycline and minocycline are more lipophilic and can be taken with food without affecting most of the drug's activity. Doxycycline is an alternative antibiotic for patients who develop erythromycin-resistant *Propionibacterium acnes infection.* The starting dose of doxycycline is 100 mg PO bid. Doxycycline is tapered to 100 mg daily for a maintenance dose after 4 to 6 weeks. Doxycycline should be taken with a full glass of water (if it becomes lodged in the esophagus it can cause ulceration). Adverse reactions to doxycycline include photosensitivity, GI upset, enterocolitis, rash, blood dyscrasias, and hepatotoxicity. If the patient's occupation or hobbies include plenty of sun exposure, then another drug besides doxycycline should be considered. The patient must use strong sunscreen or sunblock while on this drug in addition to avoiding excessive sun exposure.

One study found treatment with minocycline resulted in faster resolution of inflammatory acne lesions than tetracycline. The starting dose of minocycline (for tetracycline-resistant acne) is 50 mg at bedtime for 1 week; then the dose is gradually increased to 100 mg at bedtime. The usual dose is 100 mg once or twice a day depending on the severity of the patient's acne. Continue this dose until improvement is seen at 4 to 6 weeks, then start decreasing the dose of minocycline gradually by 50 mg every 6 to 8 weeks. The maintenance dose of minocycline is 50 mg once a day. Adverse effects include vertigo, dizziness, and ataxia (this antibiotic affects the vestibular apparatus of the inner ear). This effect can be avoided or decreased by starting the patient on a lower dose. Rare cases of blue-gray discoloration of the skin are sometimes seen in minocycline use. Other adverse effects associated with tetracyclines include serum sickness, hepatitis, and a lupus-like syndrome.

Erythromycin is a macrolide antibiotic that prevents the production of bacterial proteins. While the therapeutic dose is usually 500 mg twice daily, a dose of 250 mg twice daily is usually initiated, and then adjusted. Adverse reactions to erythromycin include nausea, GI upset, abdominal pain, anorexia, candidal vaginitis, hepatic dysfunction, rash, superinfection, and pseudomembranous colitis (rare). As *Propionibacterium acnes* is quickly becoming resistant to erythromycin, this is usually considered a second-line agent.

Ortho Tri-Cyclen (norgestimate and ethinyl estradiol) and Estrostep (norethindrone acetate/ethinyl estradiol) are oral contraceptives that are indicated for moderate acne in females who are 15 years of age or older and have acne that is unresponsive to topical medications. The female patient should have no known contraindications to hormonal therapy such as a history of thrombophlebitis or thromboembolic disorders, cerebrovascular or cardiovascular disease, breast or other estrogen-dependent neoplasms, hepatic tumor, or undiagnosed genital bleeding. In addition, Estrostep should be prescribed only for the patient who also desires an oral contraceptive for birth control and plans to stay on the medication for at least 6 months.

Severe Acne

Severe acne should be referred to the dermatologist for aggressive treatment with isotretinoin (Accutane, Claravis, Amnesteem, Sotret), a vitamin A derivative that is indicated for severe recalcitrant nodular acne that has not responded to conventional therapy (including oral antibiotics). Isotretinoin induces sebocyte atrophy, normalizes follicular keratinocytes, reduces *Propionibacterium acnes* colonization, and has direct anti-inflammatory effects. It is one of the most potent teratogens known today (Category X) and carries huge medico-legal implications for the clinician when it is prescribed to females of reproductive age. The manufacturer of Accutane, Roche, requires all prescribers to join a program called SMART (System to Manage Accutane Related Teratogenicity). Manufacturers of generic isotretinoin have similar programs. The clinician should refer any female of potential reproductive age who is a candidate for isotretinoin therapy to the dermatologist for management. If a clinician decides to prescribe this drug to a reliable female of child-bearing potential (physician consultation is recommended), then the criteria for the SMART program must be adhered to. The risk and the benefits of therapy should be discussed with the female patient, including the possibility of pregnancy and contingency plans if she gets pregnant (including termination of the pregnancy).

Two negative pregnancy tests must be obtained within 1 week of prescribing the medication, and two forms of reliable contraception must be used (unless abstinence is the chosen method). Monthly pregnancy tests must be ordered thereafter. The patient must have maintained effective contraception for at least 1 month before, during, and after therapy. The most frequent adverse effect is cheilitis, which occurs in up to 90 percent of patients. Other adverse effects commonly seen during therapy (in up to 80 percent of patients) include dry skin, dry nose, dry mouth, pruritus, epistaxis, and an increase in skin fragility. The link between isotretinoin and depression rermains controversial. Some state that it has been known to cause depression, psychosis, and rarely, suicide. Because of this, the clinician may not want to prescribe this in patients with a history of these conditions. Patients who complain of headache should be evaluated for pseudotumor cerebri or benign intracranial hypertension. Corneal opacities and decreased night vision have also been reported while patients are on this medication. The incidence of hypertriglyceridemia is very high (1 patient in 4). Some patients develop elevated liver transaminases, and elevated blood sugar levels have been seen in patients with diabetes. Baseline laboratory testing, such as fasting lipids and liver function tests, should be done before treatment and follow-up testing should be done weekly (or biweekly) thereafter until the patient's response to therapy is known; then it can be done monthly.

The dose of isotretinoin is initially 0.5 to 1.0 mg/kg per day in two divided doses for 20 weeks. Maintenance dose is 0.5 to 1 mg/kg per day in two divided doses for 15 to 20 weeks. The maximum dose is 2 mg/kg per day. Only 1 month's supply of the drug should be prescribed for each visit. Isotretinoin should be taken with food. The medicine can be discontinued early if the acne nodule count is decreased by 70 percent or more. If the patient complains of moderate to severe myalgias, then the medication must be discontinued immediately and follow-up laboratory tests must be done. After a period of 2 months or more off therapy, if persistent or recurrent severe nodular acne recurs, then referral to a dermatologist is recommended. Isotretinoin will induce long-term remissions of acne in up to 40 percent of patients. Patients with acne fulminans should be referred and treated with prednisone, the drug of choice for this condition. For other drugs listed above, see Drugs Commonly Prescribed 6.5.

Other Medical Therapies

There are therapies other than or in conjunction with medications that may assist in the overall treatment of the patient with acne. The surgical procedure of comedo extraction is common for the treatment of comedomal acne and may be used with topical retinoids. This extraction may be done manually or with light electrocautery. Chemical peels may also be effective against comedonal acne. To reduce acne scarring, laser resurfacing, dermabrasion, and subcision or punch grafting may help. In addition, dermal augmentation with autologous or nonautologous tissue may improve the appearance of atrophic scars.

Photodynamic therapy with the use of a blue light or a mixed red and blue light may be given once to twice weekly and clinical improvement is usually seen within a few weeks.

Follow-Up and Referral

Patients should be reevaluated in 4 to 6 weeks to monitor response and potential adverse effects of acne medication. Noncompliance issues should be addressed. Topical retinoids frequently cause skin dryness and irritation if not started gradually or if used incorrectly. The role of patient education is very important in the use of topical retinoids. Most patients are not willing to try it again after they experience skin irritation and the temporary flare-up of acne seen within 4 weeks of starting therapy. Female patients on oral antibiotics or isotretinoin should be monitored for continued use of reliable methods of birth control. There is no need to wait until the acne becomes severe enough before considering referral to a dermatologist. Severe acne or moderate acne that is unresponsive to conventional treatment should be referred to dermatologists for more aggressive treatment to minimize scarring.

By the third month of treatment, clinical improvement of acne lesions should be visible. If no improvement is seen or if the acne worsens, then topical treatment with two agents or systemic therapy should be considered. The chances of skin irritation are increased when two topical agents are combined; therapy should be started slowly to minimize these effects. Systemic oral antibiotic treatment should generally be continued for a period of 4 to 6 months. Without treatment, acne lesions can last months to years.

Patient Education

Patient education is a vital and important component in acne treatment because of the long duration of treatment and potential for adverse effects (some serious). Patients and parents (if younger than 18 years) should be warned of potential adverse effects of oral acne medication (as discussed in the Management section). Table 6.15 presents patient education information. Patients should be encouraged to read product labels and only use noncomedogenic (non-acne-causing) products make-up, moisturizers, sunscreens, etc.

Patients on oral contraceptives for acne therapy should be aware of potential drug interactions which include decrease in their efficacy when used in conjunction with certain antimicrobials, including the tetracyclines. Oral contraceptives should not be used in breast-feeding patients.

Table 6.15 Patient Education: Acne

- Wash the face gently at least twice a day with an antibacterial soap (Dial, Lever 2000) or with a very mild soap (Dove soap).
- Wait at least 30 minutes after washing their face before applying topical acne medications in order to minimize the chance of skin irritation.
- Topical acne medications should not be used on sunburned or irritated skin, abrasions, cuts, or on eczematous skin. If these conditions are present, the medication can be temporarily stopped for a few days.
- Avoid contact with eyes, lips, angles of the nose, and the mucous membranes when applying topical acne medicines.
- Sunscreen should be used with all acne medications, especially in sunny climates and during the summer.
- Avoid oily makeup or oily hair conditioners or scalp products.
- Avoid excessive handling of the face and cradling phones on the chin.
- Avoid excessive scrubbing of the face.

Rosacea

Rosacea is a chronic and progressive skin disorder in middle aged and older adults that resembles acne. It is characterized by flare-ups which include three cutaneous components that may occur individually or concurrently. The first component is vascular in nature with persistent erythema primarily involving the central face. This may be followed after a period of time by the development of telangiectasia or clusters of small, superficial blood vessels. Flushing episodes may occur spontaneously. The second cutaneous component involves recurrent acneiform erythematous papules and pustules around the central face. The third component consists of connective tissue hyperplasia around the central face with discrete sebaceous gland hyperplasia (rhinophyma), consisting of persistent yellow papules particularly around the nose. Blepharoconjunctivitis may result if there is ocular involvement.

Rosacea is a life-long condition that is usually exacerbated by sun exposure. Other environmental triggers include the following: hot or cold weather and wind; overheating during exercise; excessive alcohol ingestion or hot beverages; spicy or aged food products such as cheese; emotional stress; irritating cosmetics; hot baths, saunas, or hot tubs; smoking; caffeine; and excessive washing of the face. Rosacea and acne often look similar, may respond to the same treatments, and may coexist in the same patient.

Epidemiology and Causes

While rosacea affects nearly 14 million Americans, fewer than 10 percent are diagnosed because patients confuse the symptoms with acne, sunburn, flushing, or a temporary rash. Rosacea is most common between the ages of 30 and 60 years in fair-skinned persons of Irish, English, Scottish, Welsh, or eastern European ancestry. Women are three times more likely to develop rosacea than men, particularly the first cutaneous component. Patients sometimes have one or more close relative with the condition. Rosacea is idiopathic with no recognizable causes other than certain triggers that exacerbate the condition. Several researchers have suggested that *Helicobacter pylori*, an organism found in the stomach, may possibly be a cause, as well as the *Demodex* species of mite, which has been found in the hair follicles of patients with rosacea.

Pathophysiology

At present, the underlying pathogenesis of the vascular dilatation characteristic of rosacea is not fully characterized. Inflammation, rather than infection, appears to be the primary mechanism, as shown through several lines of indirect evidence. For example, studies have failed to show consistent differences in *Helicobacter pylori* seropositivity between patients with rosacea and unaffected controls. Moreover, the ability of amoxicillin–metronidazole–bismuth treatments to clear *Helicobacter* infection and improve rosacea symptoms has been attributed to the anti-inflammatory effects of metronidazole. This was similarly shown with tetracycline treatment of rosacea associated with *Demodex* mite infestations. Mite counts were not decreased with this treatment, although symptomatic improvement was evident. Moreover, the anti-inflammatory effects of tetracycline antibiotics have been well documented in the treatment of acne vulgaris.

Clinical Presentation

Subjective

Patients with rosacea usually do not seek out care because they think they have acne, sunburn, or a temporary rash. They usually present because they become intolerant of the persistent burning, itching, or stinging sensations. Patients with ocular rosacea complain of watery, irritated or bloodshot eyes.

Objective

Initially the patient's forehead, cheek, nose, or chin may have a rosy hue without comedones. This is the central third of the face and is referred to as the "flush/blush" area. There may be inflammatory papules, pustules, and telangiectasias. Scarring is usually inapparent unless the patient also has concomitant acne. While the lesions tend to be symmetric bilaterally, they may also appear on only one side. Seborrhea may also be seen. If there has been ocular involvement resulting in blepharoconjunctivitis, there will be redness of the eyelids and conjunctiva.

With pre-rosacea, the clinician will note a rosy-cheeked ruddy complexion on a patient who never develops the full clinical spectrum of the disease. There is no effective treatment for pre-rosacea, nor is any needed. Patients should just be observed for signs of developing rosacea and encouraged to use sunscreen.

In middle-aged men with rhinophyma, the clinician will note disfiguring sebaceous hyperplasia on the nose, resulting in a large, bumpy, and bulbous appearance. In addition, they may have typical facial and/or ocular rosacea.

Diagnostic Reasoning

Diagnostic Tests

There is no diagnostic test for rosacea, as physical assessment is the key to diagnosis. While there is no cure for rosacea, if treatment is started early, some of the cutaneous manifestations may be prevented.

Differential Diagnosis

Differential diagnoses include adult acne, perioral dermatitis, seborrheic dermatitis, the "butterfly" rash of systemic lupus erythematosus (SLE), and steroid-dependent facial dermatoses. Acne may be a concomitant condition along with rosacea, but acne is characterized by the presence of comedones, a lack of facial flushing and telangiectasias, and a broader distribution around the face than the limited central distribution of rosacea. Perioral dermatitis is typically seen in young women, although it may occur in women 15 to 40 years of age. Multiple acneiform papules are seen around the mouth with a clear area spared directly around the lips. The small erythematous papules or pustules of perioral dermatitis lack telangiectasias. Seborrheic dermatitis usually has a scaly appearance not seen in rosacea. The erythema is without acneiform lesions and may be distributed throughout the nasolabial area, eyebrows, and scalp. The "butterfly" or malar rash of systemic lupus erythematosus lacks papules and pustules, and laboratory evaluation typically verifies the presence of antinuclear antibodies. Long-term topical steroid use on the face can result in burning erythema, sometimes associated with erythematous papules and/or scaling. When topical steroids are abruptly discontinued, a rebound flare-up of this condition typically occurs.

Management

The key to management is early diagnosis and avoidance of triggers as rosacea is a chronic condition with no known cure. Topical treatments should be the mainstay of therapy, with oral antibiotics used only for breakthrough flare-ups. Potent topical steroids should be avoided as they may worsen the condition.

Topical Therapy

Metronidazole (Flagyl) cream is the mainstay of therapy but may take up to 6 to 8 weeks for a therapeutic response. If metronidazole (0.75 or 1 percent) is not effective, topical clindamycin 1 percent lotion or erythromycin 2 percent solution may be tried. (See Drugs Commonly Prescribed Table 6.5 for Rosacea.) The same therapy is used for perioral dermatitis and topical steroid-induced rosacea.

Systemic Therapy

Antibiotics should be reserved for flare-ups or when initiating therapy with topical medications, and then antibiotics should be discontinued. Clinicians should taper the dose as soon as possible; typically patients readily learn how to taper the dosage at home. Treatment with tetracycline or erythromycin usually delivers a rapid therapeutic response. Antibiotic therapy is usually effective in reducing acneiform lesions, and this helps confirm the diagnosis of rosacea. These antibiotics typically work more as anti-inflammatory agents rather than antibiotics. The flushing of rosacea and the flat telangiectasias tend to persist and do not respond well to antibiotic therapy.

Other Therapies

Electrocautery with a small needle may be used to destroy small telangiectasias. Larger telangiectatic vessels may require pulse dye laser therapy. For men with rhinophyma, surgical reduction may be used to reduce the bulbous appearance of the nose.

Follow-Up and Referral

Patients should be referred to a dermatologist if rosacea results in telangiectasias for electrodesiccation or laser treatment for cosmetic purposes. A dermatologist may also help patients with diffuse facial erythema due to rosacea with pulsed light therapy.

Patient Education

Patients should be taught about the events or circumstances that can trigger a rosacea flare-up and learn how to avoid them. Sunscreen with at least a sun protection factor (SPF) of 15 should be used on all skin exposed surfaces when outdoors. Patients should stay cool on hot days and protect their face from cold air and wind by using a scarf. Caution should be used when exercising, and patients should be encouraged to exercise for shorter, more frequent intervals, using a cool towel around the neck and taking frequent water breaks. Gentle cleansing with fragrance-free facial cleansers should be encouraged. Proper use of topical creams and lotions should be stressed, along with the use of minimal antibiotics.

Dermatitis

Atopic Dermatitis

Atopic dermatitis (eczema) is not considered a distinct disease entity, but it is a descriptive term for a group of skin disorders (characterized by pruritus and inflammation of the skin) whose cause is unknown. *Eczema* is a superficial pathological process of the skin. Early in its presentation, it is erythematous, with papulovesicular lesions that ooze and crust. At its later stages, the rash becomes a red-purple color and develops scaling and lichenification. The use of the term "eczematous rash," although indistinct, is helpful both diagnostically and therapeutically. Currently, the terms *eczema* and *dermatitis* are used synonymously in the clinical area. Eczematous dermatitis is classified into two major etiological categories—contact dermatitis and atopic dermatitis.

Epidemiology and Causes

Atopic dermatitis is a constitutional and inherited reaction, which usually begins in infancy. For unknown reasons, the prevalence of atopic disease has risen steadily over the past 30 years, and the prevalence is now estimated at 7 to 24 persons per 1000. About 10 percent of the U.S. population will have atopic dermatitis at some point in their lifetime. Atopic eczema presents more severely in childhood. Onset during the first year of life occurs in up to 50 percent of all patients; in 85 percent, onset is before age 5. Up to 5 percent of all children are affected by atopic eczema. Most cases (40 percent) resolve by adulthood, however. The remainder of patients with atopic eczema are affected with a chronic course of the disease that is characterized by acute exacerbation (often during times of stress) and intermittent remissions.

No ethnic predisposition has been found for atopic dermatitis; it occurs equally in both sexes. The cause of atopic dermatitis is unknown. Family history is positive for atopy in two-thirds of all cases. Genetic predisposition may be the most important etiologic factor in all atopic conditions. A personal or family history of all or part of the "atopic triad"—asthma, allergic rhinitis, and eczema—is often present. It has been proposed that individuals with any of these three conditions have preferential production of allergen-specific IgE, and that the presence of such antibodies should be a mandatory criterion for the diagnosis of atopic dermatitis. Such a diagnostic test, however, only establishes the diagnosis of *atopic syndrome,* not atopic dermatitis. Any patient with a history of hives (urticaria), hay fever, or rashes should be considered to have an atopic history.

All atopic individuals seem to have itchier skin, yet what seems to be unique about the atopic patient's skin is its hypersensitivity. Many factors that do not make non-atopic individuals itch will make the atopic person feel itchy. Atopic patients are known to itch seconds after experiencing a stressful event. This type of reaction is thought to be caused by neuropeptide-induced vasodilatation, which produces a rise in skin temperature and erythema. Symptoms are triggered or exacerbated through the interaction between genetic predisposition and environmental factors. Environmental factors that trigger atopic dermatitis include dust mites, animal dander, pollen, microbes, pollutants, climate, and emotional stress.

Excessively hot or cold climates or excessively dry or moist environments are particularly suitable for setting the stage for the atopic process. Anything that dries the skin can aggravate symptoms: Common triggers include excessive bathing, hand washing, lip licking, sweating, or swimming. Contact with irritants, such as solvents, detergents, deodorants, tobacco, cosmetics, and soap can precipitate an exacerbation of atopic dermatitis (as well as contact dermatitis—see p 201). Heat may also be an aggravating factor for atopic dermatitis. Factors that generate an increase in body temperature include hot showers or baths, overdressing, use of heating pads, and electric blankets. Patients with atopy are intolerant of heat, have difficulty with thermal sweating, and are more likely to develop heat exhaustion. It is thought that perspiration retention might be a complicating factor in atopic patients. Excessive humidity is, therefore, a problem, because it interferes with normal evaporation of sweat from the body. Improperly fitting clothes can create friction and irritate the skin; and contact with certain fabrics, most notably wool, can precipitate a flare-up. Other skin conditions or infections can also lead to an exacerbation of atopic dermatitis (eczema).

Pathophysiology

The inflammatory process in eczema causes erythema of the skin as a result of dilated blood vessels that are surrounded by inflammatory cells that migrate into the epidermis, resulting in edema both inside and in between the epidermal cells (spongiosis). The epidermal cells malfunction as a consequence, resulting in thickening of the epidermis (acanthosis), excess production of keratin, and scaling. The outer epidermal layer of the skin, the stratum corneum, normally forms an impermeable barrier that protects the living cells beneath from environmental irritants and toxins. In atopic dermatitis, this outer barrier is impaired. There is an increase in the water loss and a decrease in water binding, which leads to a brittle outer barrier. This condition is made worse by environmental factors such as physical trauma from scratching, cycles of wetting and drying, and from the chemical erosion that is caused by detergents and solvents. In addition, superinfection of eczematous skin by bacterial (e.g., *Staphylococcus aureus*) or fungal (e.g., *Malassezia furfur*) species and irritation from dust mites and their dung is an important factor which worsens atopic dermatitis by potentiating the immune response. Superinfection is also much more likely in atopic dermatitis than in other forms of dermatitis such as psoriasis. Thus, infection may be though of as both a trigger as well as a complication of atopic dermatitis.

Immunologic abnormalities are key to the pathophysiology of the atopic response. These abnormalities can include elevated serum IgE levels which are seen in 85 percent of affected individuals, hypereosinophilia, reduced cell-mediated immunity and antibody-dependent cellular cytotoxicity, slowed chemotaxis of neutrophils and monocytes, relative increase in the number of CD4-positive

(CD4+) T helper cells that secrete interleukin (IL)-4, and a decrease in CD4+ T helper cells that secrete IL-2. Interestingly, however, in later stages of the immune reaction, Th1 T helper cell activity which enhances cell-mediated immunity appears to play an increasing role. Moreover, impairment of essential fatty acid metabolism has also been implicated as a causative factor of atopy.

Clinical Presentation

Subjective

Atopic dermatitis is characterized by an extremely low threshold for pruritus. It is referred to as "the itch that rashes." The cardinal sign is severe pruritus, which is often extremely distressing in both the acute and chronic stages. The diagnosis of atopic dermatitis cannot be made without the history of pruritus. The patient may report a personal or a family history of other atopic conditions (asthma, allergic rhinitis). The patient usually reports a history of episodic exacerbation of similar symptoms or of a childhood rash or eczema. The clinician should inquire about any exposure to known or unknown common antigens and irritants, regardless of the history. Individuals with atopic dermatitis are not immune to contact dermatitis; in fact, they are more susceptible to irritant reactions because of their impaired epidermal barrier layer. Often, the rash is reported as better in the warmer months and worse in the fall and winter.

Objective

Atopic dermatitis usually begins as infantile eczema, with lesions affecting the cheeks, face, and upper extremities. Erythema is often seen before pruritus. The acute lesions are often excoriated, maculopapular, and inflamed. In infancy and early childhood, oozing and crusting usually characterize the erythema. As the child becomes older, the disease can go into remission or change to a flexural distribution (antecubital fossae and neck area). Flexural eczema usually lasts until about age 4 to 10 years, but may continue into adulthood.

In adults, eczema presents with symmetrical lesions that are crusting and excoriated. In the early stages, lesions may be erythematous, papulovesicular, edematous, and weeping. Later the rash becomes crusted, scaly, thickened, and lichenified. Intergluteal involvement is uncommon and should raise suspicion of another diagnosis. The classic locations for lesions are noted to correspond to areas that are most accessible to rubbing and scratching. In addition, the typical flexural sites are more susceptible, because they are areas that are more likely to be hot and moist. (See Advanced Assessment 6.3.)

ADVANCED ASSESSMENT 6.3

Atopic Dermatitis

Distribution

Infants: Trunk, face, extensor surfaces, scalp
Children: Antecubital fossae, popliteal fossae
Adults: Face, neck, upper chest, genital area, hands

Stages

Acute
- Erosions with serous exudate
- Intense pruritus
- Papules and vesicles on an erythematous base
- Pain, heat, tenderness

Subacute
- Scaly, excoriated
- Pruritus (may be intense)
- Papules or plaques over an erythematous base
- Secondary infection possible

Chronic
- Lichenification, pigmentary changes (increased or decreased)
- Pruritus
- Excoriated papules and nodules
- Dryness, fissuring

Other Clinical Manifestations

Keratosis pilaris ("chicken skin"): asymptomatic follicular papules, particularly on the posterolateral aspects of the upper arms and lateral thighs
Lichenification of the skin: predilection for flexural creases
Icthyosis vulgaris: hyperlinear palms and soles and fishlike scales, especially on the lower legs
Dennie's sign/Morgan line: infraorbital fold
Excessive fissuring under the ear lobes, palms, soles, and fingers
Pityriasis alba: hypopigmented asymptomatic areas on the face and shoulders
Allergic "shiners": facial pallor and infraorbital darkening
Anterior capsular cataracts
Keratoconus: a cone-shaped cornea may develop in the second or third decade of life (in severe cases)
Facial erythema, dry skin, history of wool intolerance, nonspecific hand dermatitis, and a tendency for skin infection (commonly impetiginization of excoriated skin)

Diagnostic Reasoning

Diagnostic Tests

Laboratory tests are usually not useful in the diagnosis of atopic dermatitis, but they can be helpful in ruling out other disorders or to confirm that a patient is prone to atopy (allergic reactions). If viral etiology (HSV) is suspected, a viral culture should be done on the exudate and moist parts of the rash. If atopy (allergy) is suspected, the radioallergosorbent test (RAST) is done on serum. The RAST test is usually available to primary-care clinicians, unlike the scratch (skin prick) tests that must be done by allergists. The RAST test panel includes testing for allergy to dust mites, mold, ragweed, animal dander, tree pollen, and many other allergens.

RAST testing also exists for food allergens which are often highly relevant in pediatric patients; however, true IgE-mediated food allergies are far less common in adults. The RAST test is useful for patients who are suspected of having an atopic history. An atopic or allergic tendency is manifested by chronic or recurrent symptoms (in addition to the dermatitis), which might include a history of allergic rhinitis (nasal congestion, chronic postnasal drip, sneezing, itchy nose) and asthma during childhood. Some patients will deny any allergic tendency but will report a history of frequent "sinus problems." The RAST test is usually positive in patients with a history of symptoms of atopic dermatitis, but it often does not correlate well with clinical symptoms. Results appear to vary with the type of allergen being tested.. Another potentially helpful marker for atopy is serum IgE (immunoglobulin E) levels. Serum IgE levels are usually elevated during acute periods of dermatitis but may decrease during periods of remission.

In addition, delayed-type hypersensitivity responses to epicutaneously applied antigens (used in scratch or skin-prick tests) are blunted in atopic skin during periods of disease activity, so scratch tests should be avoided at this time, to avoid false-positive results. Patients should be advised to stop all antihistamines for at least 2 weeks before the test as this will interfere with skin test results. This hypersensitivity may help explain the increased susceptibility of atopic patients to cutaneous viral infections, such as HSV, vaccinia, and molluscum contagiosum. Atopic patients should be warned of their increased risk to these infections, so future exposure can be avoided.

If the diagnosis is confusing or if serious pathology (mycosis fungoides) is suspected, a skin biopsy can provide important information. The skin biopsy of atopic skin will reveal a thickened and hyperkeratoid epidermis, along with and perivascular inflammation of the dermis. Patients with pustular superinfection should have their lesions cultured for antibiotic sensitivities if they do not heal in response to empiric therapy.

Differential Diagnosis

Both common and rare skin disorders can mimic atopic dermatitis. Common disorders include contact dermatitis, tinea infections (dermatophytosis), seborrheic dermatitis, and the early stages of mycosis fungoides (cutaneous T-cell lymphoma). In contact dermatitis, the characteristic linear or asymmetric distribution of the skin lesions helps to distinguish this condition from atopic dermatitis. The location and characteristic ringlike, erythematous lesions with central clearing distinguish tinea corpora infections ("ring worm") from atopic dermatitis. Mycosis fungoides skin lesions do not respond to topical steroids; therefore, lesions that do not respond to topical steroids after a minimum of 2 weeks of treatment should be referred for skin biopsy.

If none of the common skin disorders apply, rare systemic diseases and skin disorders that can mimic atopic dermatitis include gluten-sensitive enteropathy, acrodermatitis enteropathica, phenylketonuria, hyper-IgE syndrome, Wiskott-Aldrich syndrome, X-linked agammaglobulinemia, selective IgA deficiency, and Letterer-Siwe disease (Table 6.16).

Table 6.16 Differential Diagnosis: Atopic Dermatitis

Scabies
Seborrheic dermatitis
Allergic contact
Tinea
Psoriasis
Ichthyosis
Dermatitis herpetiformis
Mycosis fungoides (cutaneous T-cell lymphoma)
Netherton's syndrome
Wiskott–Aldrich syndrome
Acrodermatitis enteropathica
Neurodermatitis
HIV infection (especially in children)
Phenylketonuria (if symptoms appear during the first year of life)
Hyper-IgE syndrome
Dermatomyositis

Management

The primary aim in the management of atopic dermatitis is to control the disease, because no cure exists at present. Management of dermatitis embodies the fundamental principles of dermatology: Precipitants should be eliminated, wet lesions should be dried, dried lesions should be hydrated, and inflammation should be treated with corticosteroids. The goals of management are to decrease pruritus, prevent secondary infection, and to educate patients so that they can control the disease themselves. Crucial to management is a careful and systematic assessment of trigger factors.

Nonpharmacologic Management

Errors in bathing and moisturizing are by far the most common causes of persistent atopic dermatitis. To avoid excessive irritation and skin dryness, the patient should use mild emollients that are soap substitutes (e.g., Cetaphil) instead of soap. Some patients may insist that soap is necessary for cleanliness; they can be informed of recent studies showing that Dove soap is the least irritating among 18 soaps and detergent bars that were tested in a soap chamber test (Arndt). Reducing exposure to water will minimize the drying effects to the skin; if soap is used, it should be limited only to the axilla, groin, and feet. No other national population bathes as much as Americans and this practice has become more ritualistic than purposeful.

Personal habits such as excessive bathing can be detrimental, because bathing is an effective way to remove the skin's protective oils. Older patients should take short, lukewarm showers and avoid long, hot baths, which are extremely desiccating. The use of bubble baths and fragrance-containing oils should be discouraged. Bath oils are of minimal benefit, because whatever oil remains on the skin is wiped off with toweling. Minimizing contact with cosmetics, deodorants, detergents, and solvents should be stressed. Moisturizers are useful in helping to prevent water loss and are most effective when applied immediately after patting the skin partially dry after a short shower. Atopic dermatitis patients should be cautioned against using lotions and gels, because they contain alcohol, preservatives, and fragrance. Patients with atopic dermatitis should not use agents that contain lactic acid or other alpha-hydroxy/glycolic acids that can aggravate the condition.

Ointments (which contain petroleum jelly) form an occlusive layer and are more effective in preventing water loss than lotions. For less severe conditions or in hot, humid areas, creams that do not contain fragrance and have few preservatives are acceptable (e.g., Cetaphil cream, Eucerin, Dermabase, Unibase). Humidifiers are most helpful in cold and dry climates, but they can provide an environment that is conducive to increased dust mite and mold populations. Acaricide is an insecticide that is effective against dust mites; it can be used on all fomites (pillows, beds, sofas, etc.). After application, a thorough vacuuming, preferably with a high-efficiency particulate air (HEPA)-filtered apparatus, must be done to remove the insecticide. Antifungal cleaners for wet and damp areas are recommended for patients who are sensitive to mold. Acaricide and other pesticides/chemical treatments have not been shown to be consistently helpful and are NOT first-line preventive treatments.

Pharmacologic Management

If the skin lesions are wet, inflamed, or have exudate, wet soaks or compresses with cool tap water, Burow's solution (1:40 dilution), saline (1 teaspoon per pint), or silver nitrate solution (25.5 percent) can be used to dry out the lesions and provide comfort. Aluminum acetate solution (Burow's solution) can be applied as a compress for 20 to 30 minutes four to six times throughout the day. Topical steroids should be immediately applied to inflamed areas following the soak. Petrolatum or other emollients, for example, Aquaphor healing ointment, Eucerin cream, Keralac lotion, should be applied to all noninflamed areas. Colloidal oatmeal baths (Aveeno) are soothing and may be helpful with more generalized lesions.

Although antihistamines are often used to relieve pruritus, they are usually ineffective in atopic dermatitis, because histamine is not the only factor responsible for the mediation of pruritus in atopic dermatitis. The sedative effect of antihistamines may be more beneficial than its antipruritic properties. Individuals with atopic dermatitis have a tendency to scratch in their sleep, so sedation at bedtime may decrease the amount of scratching during sleep. If the patient does not obtain relief from antihistamines, the older sedating types of H_1 blockers, for example, ethanolamines (diphenhydramine) and phenothiazines (promethazine) are very sedating. Some tricyclic antidepressants, such as doxepin (Sinequan), have potent antihistaminic activity and are useful in urticaria and other forms of pruritus. An added benefit to using an antidepressant agent is the relief of depression that is not uncommonly seen to accompany atopic dermatitis. Older generation sedating antihistamines are NOT recommended in children. These have been shown to impair school performance in many cases and have a paradoxical hyperactivating effect in others. Sedating patients for urticaria and other forms of pruritis only applies to adults.

Corticosteroids are effective anti-inflammatory agents and usually are considered first-line therapy for atopic dermatitis. The additional use of emollients (e.g., petroleum jelly, Eucerin, Lubriderm) will enhance the absorption and effectiveness of topical steroids. Applying topical corticosteroids after hydrating the skin (after a shower or bath) will increase their absorption tenfold. A weak coal tar preparation applied over the steroid ointment can reduce itching at night.

Acute exacerbations can be treated with a potent to mid-strength topical steroid for a few days, to quickly control acutely inflamed skin lesions, but the patient should switch to a weaker strength when the lesion is under control. Medium- to high-potency topical steroids should not be used on the face or neck area because of potential adverse effects such as local irritation, atrophy of the skin, and telangiectasia. Skin atrophy is more likely to occur when potent topical corticosteroids are applied repeatedly to thin and highly absorptive inflamed skin. In rare instances, hypopigmentation has been associated with the use of topical corticosteroids, especially in blacks. Most cases of pigmentary changes are related to the underlying dermatitis, however, rather than the use of topical corticosteroids. Topical corticosteroids may complicate treatment by masking underlying bacterial or fungal infections. Topical steroids should never be used on ulcerated skin.

Systemic corticosteroids are rarely necessary for the treatment of chronic atopic dermatitis, but they may be useful for an acute and incapacitating exacerbation or when large numbers of weeping lesions are present. The patient may benefit from a short course of oral prednisone (40 to 60 mg per day for adults and 1 mg/kg per day for children). Short-term therapy with prednisone does not require tapering if it is limited to 5 to 7 days and the patient does not have a history of recent oral prednisone use. As the lesions dry, topical steroids may be started.

When the acute inflammation subsides after 2 to 3 weeks, the patient should decrease the frequency of the topical corticosteroids and use more emollients such as petroleum jelly or Eucerin cream. The chronic use of topical corticosteroids (mid- to low strength) should be limited to twice-weekly applications to any given area.

Aggressive treatment of atopic dermatitis may include cyclosporine A (CyA), an immunomodulatory drug, which may be as effective as corticosteroids, with fewer adverse effects. It is indicated for patients who have failed to respond to at least one systemic therapy, or in patients for whom other systemic therapies are contraindicated or are intolerable. Its use can be highly beneficial in severe cases, but renal function must be closely monitored and treatment courses must be restricted to 8 to 12 weeks. Montelukast sodium (Singulair) at 5 to 10 mg/day may also be effective. Singulair is a leukotriene-receptor antagonist and inhibits eosinophil infiltration, a major histiologic factor in atopic dermatitis. Azathioprine (Imuran) may also be used for maintenance therapy but hematologic and hepatic function must be followed.

Topical tacrolimus (Protopic) and the related pimecrolimus (Elidel), applied twice per day are effective for short-term or intermittent long-term treatment of moderate to severe atopic dermatitis when conventional therapies are inadvisable, ineffective, or not tolerated. These are the second-line therapies for steroid-refractory eczema flares. These are immunomodulating calcineurin inhibitors. They should not be used indiscriminately or for long periods of time, however, as the FDA is investigating the link between these immunomodulators and an increased propensity for lymphoma and cutaneous cancers in animal studies as well as in a series of human cases ($n = 29$ as of 12/04). The FDA has an advisory warning out against these agents, specifying their use only for refractory flares and as second-line therapy (and only in persons older than 2 years of age and in those with a competent immune system), although final results on ongoing studies may not be available for another 10 years, the FDA suggests. Omalizumab (Xolair), an anti-IgE antibody which has been developed as an immunotherapeutic has shown benefit in reducing atopy in highly allergic individuals and is available through referral to a specialist such as an allergist or pulmonologist. In severe cases of eczema, phototherapy with ultraviolet B radiation or PUVA photochemotherapy (psoralens with ultraviolet A radiation) may be used as an adjunct therapy. Some patients have reported beneficial results with the use of NSAIDs because of their antiprostaglandin effect. (see commonly prescribed drugs in the psoriasis section). Patients with pustular superinfection should have their lesions cultured for antibiotic sensitivities if they do not heal in response to empiric therapy. Bacterial or fungal superinfections must be treated appropriately.

Complementary Therapy

Studies published in literature indicate that certain herbs may be of value in the treatment of dermatologic conditions. These include chamomile, arnica, calendula, hamamelis (witch hazel), aloe vera, cardiospermum, *Mahonia aquifolium,* oak bark, bittersweet stalk, and capsaicin. Use of these herbs should be reserved for experienced practitioners in alternative health medicine because of the potential for allergic reactions.

Follow-Up and Referral

If basic management of atopic dermatitis fails, referral to a dermatologist should be prompt. More aggressive treatment by a dermatologist is necessary for patients who have severe and extensive lesions or do not respond to usual treatment with topical and or systemic corticosteroids. Atopic skin is very susceptible to bacterial and viral infections. These patients may develop widespread herpes infections of the skin (eczema herpeticum, which may be life-threatening in children), and they should be protected from people with active herpetic lesions. During an exacerbation, patients may contract secondary bacterial infections, and empirical therapy with erythromycin or penicillinase-resistant penicillins is sometimes necessary.

Patient Education

Patients with atopic dermatitis should be educated to be vigilant in watching for the signs of secondary bacterial infection. The patients should be told to report it immediately so that an oral antibiotic can be prescribed. Education about the importance of environmental measures in the prevention of disease exacerbation should be emphasized. House dust mites, animal dander, and pollen are all identified as potential triggers based on IgE antibodies in the bloodstream of some patients and should be addressed when educating patients. Patients can be assisted in discovering ways to reduce sweating, such as reducing the amount of bedclothes at night; avoiding occlusive, hot garments; and keeping the living areas cool. Patients should be encouraged to recognize their stress “triggers” and to find measures to reduce their stress level, such as exercise.

As *Staphylococcus aureus* colonizes the skin of more than 90 percent of patients with atopic dermatitis (as compared to only 5 percent of persons without the disease), fingernails should be kept short, smooth, and clean. This may prevent the scratching which exacerbates the inflammation that may allow microbes to be introduced into the skin. Patients should be informed that a change in seasons will cause exacerbations of their disease, especially during the fall. Patients can be reminded to use extra care in taking care of their skin at this time by upgrading to stronger moisturizers (from lotions to petroleum jelly). Refills of their medication should be ordered before recurrence of symptoms. The provider can assist the patient in developing a simple regimen of topical steroid therapy for acute exacerbations. Patients with frequent exacerbations of skin lesions on their hands should avoid occupations that require repeated handwashing, immersion in water, or other wet conditions.

Food allergies are a common aggravating factor in up to 20 percent of patients with atopic dermatitis and are more common in children. A dietician should be consulted when patients are eliminating foods from their diet as unsupervised food restriction may lead to malnutrition.

Contact Dermatitis

Contact dermatitis is a common condition categorized as either *irritant dermatitis* or *allergic dermatitis.* Although both of these conditions can have similar presentations, the etiology of each disease is what differentiates between the two dermatitides. *Allergic contact dermatitis* is immunologically mediated, whereas *irritant contact dermatitis* is the result of repeated "insults" to atopic skin from caustic, irritant, or detergent-type substances.

Epidemiology and Causes

Almost any substance may induce a cutaneous reaction depending on its concentration, the duration of contact, and the condition of the contacted skin. The etiology of allergic contact dermatitis may be from antimicrobials such as neomycin, antihistamines, anesthetics such as benzocaine, hair dyes, preservatives, latex, or adhesive tape. The etiology of irritant contact dermatitis may be from soaps, detergents, or organic solvents.

Delayed-type hypersensitivity reactions are immunologic responses to contact allergens that occur in sensitized individuals. One of the most frequent causes of allergic contact dermatitis is from plants in the *Rhus* genus, which includes poison ivy, poison oak, and poison sumac. Other common topical sensitizers include ragweed pollen, dust mites, ethylenediamine (a stabilizer in many topical creams), potassium dichromate, paraphenylenediamine (dyes), nickel (10 percent of females are allergic to nickel found in jewelry), rubber compounds, and benzocaine (an OTC topical anesthetic for itching or pain). It is estimated that there are more than 6 million chemicals in the environment and that approximately 3000 of them are potential sensitizers.

Contact dermatitis accounts for 4 to 7 percent of all dermatology consults. Hand dermatitis affects 2 percent of the population at any given time, and 20 percent of female patients will be affected at least once in their lifetime. Contact dermatitis is more common in adults than in children, and effects are more extreme in elderly patients. Women are twice as likely as men to develop dermatitis and are at highest risk following childbirth. White Americans are affected more frequently and fair-skinned redheads are the most vulnerable population.

Pathophysiology

Contact dermatitis if considered either allergic or irritant-induced. A delayed type hypersensitivity response (type IV immune reaction) elicits a non-IgE–mediated allergic response to specific antigens when applied to the skin, producing a local reaction characterized histologically by epidermal changes including intracellular edema, spongiosis, and vesiculation. Upon initial contact with the offending agent, the antigen is taken up and processed by epidermal antigen-presenting cells known as Langerhans cells. These cells present antigens to naïve, antigen-specific CD4+ and CD8+ T lymphocytes, located in regional lymph nodes which drain the affected areas of skin. Over approximately 10 to 14 days, sensitized T cells migrate from the lymph nodes to sites of antigenic exposure, where subsequent reexposure to the same antigen results in an allergic reaction mediated by cytokine release. This response with notable skin surface changes typically occurs within 12 to 48 hours of reexposure to antigen.

Irritant contact dermatitis is the result of a direct cytotoxic effect of an irritant to the cells of the epidermis, with a subsequent inflammatory response in the dermis. The main pathologic feature of contact dermatitis is intracellular edema of the epidermis, which may result in intraepidermal vesicles and bullae formation in the acute phase. In chronic cases, papules, scaling, and lichenification occur. Irritants penetrate and disrupt the stratum corneum and injure the underlying epidermis and dermis, as various immune cells congregate around dilated capillaries, contributing to the inflammatory process.

Rubber glove dermatitis demonstrates the spectrum of pathophysiologic mechanisms involved in contact dermatitis. Chemical irritants used in the glove manufacturing process (e.g., thiram, mercapto derivatives) may cause an allergic dermatitis via a delayed-type T cell-mediated hypersensitivity reaction. In addition, rubber glove components may result in a direct irritant effect on the moist skin of glove-wearers. Finally, the natural rubber protein *latex*, once widely used in medical products, may elicit a profound IgE-mediated immediate hypersensitivity response, leading to systemic anaphylaxis and even death.

Interestingly, people with venous stasis (i.e., impaired venous return with pooling of blood in distended veins, particularly in the lower extremities) are more susceptible to irritant contact dermatitis, particularly from wood alcohols such as lanolin, fragrances, topical antibiotics such as neomycin, and methylparaben preservatives. Correctly diagnosing this condition is often difficult because contact dermatitis is often indistinguishable from stasis dermatitis.

Clinical Presentation

Subjective

The cardinal symptom of contact dermatitis is a pruritic erythematous rash. Often, the patient is not aware of a previous history, but there may have been periodic episodes of pruritic rash that resolved spontaneously. The patient may or may not be able to describe the conditions or substances contributing to the dermatitis, but exposure history to known or unknown common antigens and irritants should be sought by the clinician. In allergic contact dermatitis (in contrast to atopic dermatitis), the inflammatory reaction on the skin occurs much faster, typically within 6 to 12 hours of reexposure. In contrast to allergic contact dermatitis, irritant reactions do not always occur immediately following contact with the offending substance. The response time between the initial contact with the irritant and the symptoms is variable, and the severity of the reaction depends on the concentration, amount, and length of exposure to the offending irritating substance.

Objective

Contact dermatitis presents with inflammation of the epidermis and is manifested by erythema (as in all types of dermatitis), but it does not present with the smooth, intact epidermal surface that characterizes hives (urticaria). The epidermal inflammation seen in acute contact dermatitis results in rough, reddened patches but without the thickening and discrete demarcation of psoriasis. The acute lesions of contact dermatitis are characterized by weeping lesions with numerous tiny vesicles on an erythematous base that is pruritic or has a burning or stinging sensation. The surrounding area in severe cases is also erythematous, with edema and increased heat in the area, making it difficult to rule out secondary bacterial infection in some cases.

Lesions in nonallergic and delayed-type hypersensitivity contact dermatitis present in similar fashion, but the typical distribution and the lack of an atopic history are the most helpful factors in the diagnosis. A clothing- or detergent-related cause should be suspected if the lesions are generalized and primarily affect the borders of the axillae, waist, and upper thighs. Reactions to toxic plants (e.g., *Rhus* or *Toxicodendron* species) follow a history of exposure. The characteristic rash is vesicular and linear (or asymmetric) and is frequently found on the hands and ankles. *Rhus* dermatitis lesions are sometimes found on the facial area if the patient has inadvertently scratched the face with contaminated fingers. Lesions in an area where jewelry has been worn recently (e.g., neck, wrist, ear lobes) may indicate a hypersensitivity to nickel. Usually, the area of skin that has been the most heavily contaminated will break out first, followed by areas of lesser exposure. The location of the rash gives the clinician the best clues to the possible etiologic agent. For example, a patient with a rash on the scalp and the back of the neck might report a history of the use of a new shampoo, a new hair dye, or other scalp or hair treatments. (See Advanced Assessment 6.4.)

ADVANCED ASSESSMENT 6.4

Contact Dermatitis

Stages

- Acute
  - Erythema and edema
  - Clear, fluid-filled vesicles or bullae
  - Exudate, clear fluid
  - Distinct margins
- Subacute
  - Lessening edema
  - Formation of papules
  - Less distinct margins
- Chronic
  - Minimal edema
  - Scaling skin
  - Lichenification
  - Minimal erythema

Diagnostic Reasoning

Diagnostic Tests

Contact dermatitis is diagnosed based on the history of exposure to an irritant or allergen and the subsequent appearance of a rash on the exposed skin, either immediately or later on (delayed hypersensitivity). If scabies is suspected, skin scrapings can be examined under a microscope to rule out that condition. If tinea (corporis, cruris, pedis, manuum) infection is suspected, skin scrapings should be treated with potassium hydroxide (KOH) and gently heated. A microscopic exam for tinea infection should search for hyphae and spores. If bacterial infection (impetigo) is suspected, cultures should be taken from the moist areas of the rash or from the discharge. Viral cultures can be done to rule out suspected viral etiology (herpes simplex, herpes zoster).

Laboratory tests that are done by specialists (allergist) include the scratch and intradermal tests. Scratch (skin-prick) tests should not be done during an acute episode of contact dermatitis because of an increased rate of false-positive reactions. The Patch test performed by a dermatologist is useful to identify specific irritants in patients with histories that are suggestive of acute contact dermatitis. Allergens that are commonly responsible for such reactions are fixed in dehydrated gel layers and taped against the skin of the patient's back for 48 hours and then removed. A final reading done in 96 hours will usually show any evidence of contact dermatitis. In some patients, a CBC with differential will show eosinophilia, but this blood test is neither sensitive nor necessary for the diagnosis. Skin biopsy is rarely necessary for diagnosis.

Differential Diagnosis

The differential diagnosis of contact dermatitis is similar to that for atopic dermatitis and includes both common and rare disorders. Common disorders that have a similar presentation to contact dermatitis include seborrheic dermatitis, impetigo, and herpes zoster. Seborrheic dermatitis rashes, although erythematous, have a greasy and scaly appearance and appear only in certain areas of the body such as the hairline, the ears, the scalp, and the face. Impetigo, which is caused by gram-positive *Staphylococcus* or *Streptococcus* bacteria is more common in children. A honey-colored crust is seen on top of the erythematous lesions; impetigo also does not have a linear appearance like contact dermatitis. Herpes zoster is more common in older patients and the lesions appear as multiple small vesicles on an erythematous base. Although herpes zoster has a linear distribution, it is more likely to occur on the trunk area (contact dermatitis occurs more often on the hands or face) and will follow the path of a dermatome.

Management

The clinical challenge in the treatment of contact dermatitis is to provide symptomatic relief to the patient while attempting to identify the underlying allergic precipitant. Identifying the antigen or irritant in contact dermatitis is critical, both to eliminate or minimize the current contact and to avoid future exposure. The responsible irritant should be identified and eliminated to prevent the cycle of itching, scratching, and skin disruption, which can lead to chronic changes in the skin. A careful history of exposures is key, in addition to a thorough skin examination. The effects of *Rhus* dermatitis (from poison ivy, poison oak, or poison sumac) may be lessened if the exposed skin is thoroughly rinsed in soap and water or with isopropyl alcohol, as soon as possible after exposure. Exposed clothing should be discarded.

For localized contact dermatitis with weeping lesions, treatment with moist compresses and simple drying agents or anti-pruritic lotions (e.g., Burow's aluminum acetate solution, Calamine lotion) applied several times a day is usually effective. For more extensive and severe cases, potent topical steroids in cream form (avoid the use of ointments on wet lesions because they can cause skin maceration) can be applied bid for the first few days to help decrease pruritus and inflammation. If treatment is necessary beyond 2 weeks, a less potent (mild or moderate) topical steroid may be used bid until the rash resolves. High-potency steroids should not be used on the face or in bodily folds (intertriginous areas) because of their ability to thin the skin and cause hypopigmentation.

Oral systemic steroids may be indicated in acute and particularly severe cases of contact dermatitis. Relatively high doses of oral prednisone can be given for 10 to 14 days (or up to 21 days in the most severe cases). One popular regimen is to give prednisone 40 mg PO qd for 4 days followed by 20 mg PO qd for 4 more days. A longer steroid taper for more extensive cases would call for prednisone 60 mg for 4 to 7 days, then tapered to 40 mg for 4 to 7 days, then 20 mg for 4 to 7 days, and finally 10 mg for 4 to 7 days. Abrupt cessation of high-dose systemic corticosteroids that are given for more than 5 days duration should be avoided. Potential adverse effects of oral prednisone therapy are more likely with long-term use and may include any of the following: suppression of the hypothalamic–pituitary–adrenal axis, hypokalemia, hypocalcemia, masking or worsening of infection, increased likelihood of secondary infection, carbohydrate intolerance and worsening of diabetes, glaucoma, cataracts, osteoporosis, dermal atrophy, skin hypopigmentation, and psychiatric disorders including depression, euphoria, or even acute psychosis. It should also be noted that even systemic steroids will likely prove ineffective if exposure to the offending allergen or irritant is not limited.

Follow-Up and Referral

Follow-up and referral are determined by the patient's condition and response to therapy. Severe cases should be referred to a dermatologist or allergist.

Patient Education

The provider should teach the patient and family about the disease and the appropriate use of medications, as well as adverse effects or exacerbations that should prompt the patient to contact the health-care provider. The mainstay of prevention is to help the patient identify the agents causing the dermatitis and teaching them about the avoidance of exposure or use of protective clothing and gloves.

Seborrheic Dermatitis

Seborrheic dermatitis is one of the most common skin conditions seen in primary care; it is most commonly seen in adults and the elderly. It is a chronic condition that is marked by remissions and exacerbations. Seborrheic dermatitis is one of the most common skin manifestations of patients with HIV infection. A severe or resistant case on a patient should prompt investigation for risk factors of HIV infection. The rashes of *seborrheic dermatitis* are seen on skin that is rich in sebaceous glands. (It is associated with an increased production of sebum.) The affected skin is pink, edematous, and covered with yellow to brown scales and crusts. These rashes are most easily seen on the scalp, the forehead, the eyebrows, and the area surrounding the nose and the ears.

Epidemiology and Causes

Seborrheic dermatitis affects approximately 2 to 5 percent of the adult population. Seborrheic dermatitis runs in families and has a known genetic component. It may be an inflammatory reaction to Malassezia furfur yeasts. The occurrence of seborrheic dermatitis is most common during early infancy on the scalp ("cradle cap"), after the second decade of life, and in the elderly or immunocompromised patients. A strong association with HIV infection and AIDS is well established.

Pathophysiology

This type of dermatitis was originally defined by excess oil secretion from the sebaceous glands and is thus found on areas of the body where such glands are most concentrated, that is, in decreasing order, the scalp, face, chest, upper back, pubic area and axillae. Interestingly, however, overproduction of sebum is not seen in all cases of seborrheic dermatitis, nor is the composition of the sebum the main factor in this condition. Skin biopsies typically reveal parakeratotic scale heaped around hair follicles, as well as an inflammatory lymphocytic infiltrate. Thus, mild epidermal hyperproliferation has been cited as a contributing factor. However, it is not known whether this occurs in response to infection by saprophytic skin fungi or vice versa.

Malassezia furfur commonly colonizes affected individuals. Recurrence of symptoms has been linked to an increase in the number of *Malassezia furfur* organisms found on the skin surface. Fungal-specific stains of affected skin reveal large numbers of *Malassezia furfur* spores within the stratum corneum, the uppermost skin layer.

Clinical Presentation

Subjective

The typical patient is an adult male who complains of a pink, scaling rash that is usually located on the face and scalp. It can also be an incidental finding; some patients, especially elderly patients, are not bothered by the cosmetic effect of the rashes. The lesions are usually asymptomatic in most patients but pruritus may be present (and is aggravated by perspiration), especially in scalp lesions.

Objective

Seborrheic dermatitis presents as scaly patches that may be slightly papular; each patch is surrounded by erythema. The lesion borders are poorly defined, and the scales may be greasy and appear yellow. The most frequently involved area is the scalp, and the condition is differentiated from common dandruff (pityriasis sicca) by the appearance of erythema, which may be minimal or moderate. The affected areas may include the forehead at the hairline, eyebrows, nasal folds, and the retroauricular and presternal areas. In more severe cases, intertriginous areas, as well as the external ear canal and umbilicus are involved. The rashes may be more difficult to recognize in fastidious patients, because daily bathing removes some of the scale.

Diagnostic Reasoning

Diagnostic Tests

Diagnosis of seborrheic dermatitis is based on clinical findings and the history. Dermatologists and allergists can test for *Malassezia furfur* using antigen-specific skin-prick or serum RAST testing. Fifteen to 65 percent of patients with seborrheic dermatitis have positive responses to skin-prick tests with *Malassezia* extracts. *Malassezia* antibodies have also been found in young adults with head and neck dermatitis. Fungal-specific periodic acid Schiff and Gamori Methenamine Silver stains identify hyphae and spores in skin scraping or biopsy samples; however, these specialized stains typically require specialist referral and are not commonly used in the primary-care setting. Rather, the diagnosis of seborrheic dermatitis is most commonly based on the characteristic appearance and distribution of the rash, as well as its response to empiric therapy.

Differential Diagnosis

Skin conditions that mimic seborrheic dermatitis include impetigo, atopic dermatitis, psoriasis, scabies, and Langerhans cell histiocytosis. A history of the same rash recurring at characteristic locations on the body (e.g., the scalp and hairline, sides of the nose and upper lip, eyebrows and eyelashes, cheeks, or ears) will give the clinician the best clues to correctly identify seborrheic dermatitis. Impetigo, a bacterial infection of the skin caused by *Staphylococcus* or *Streptococcus* bacteria, has an acute onset and tends to occur on the extremities (a location not seen in seborrheic dermatitis) or on the face. The most useful distinguishing feature between atopic dermatitis and seborrheic dermatitis is the increased number of lesions on the forearms in the former, as compared to the increased number of lesions in the axillae in the latter. The erythema of seborrheic dermatitis typically has a pinkish hue, rather than the bright-red appearance of psoriasis.

Seborrheic dermatitis is also associated with several chronic conditions, including Parkinson's disease, HIV infection and AIDS, phenylketonuria, cardiac failure, zinc deficiency, and epilepsy. Other dermatologic disorders, such as acne vulgaris, rosacea, and psoriasis may also be associated with these diseases, however. Importantly, florid manifestations of seborrheic dermatitis may be an early cutaneous indicator of HIV infection, and these patients may demonstrate extensive symptoms that are often resistant to therapy.

Management

The high incidence and the chronic benign nature of seborrheic dermatitis presents a therapeutic challenge. Mild to moderate cases does not seem to bother some patients, especially elderly patients. These patients frequently refuse treatment or are noncompliant. Younger patients who are bothered by the cosmetic effects of the rashes on the face frequently request treatment. The therapeutic approach is aimed at managing symptoms and reducing the yeast count on the skin.

The regular use of an OTC dandruff shampoo is sufficient to control most scalp symptoms. The preparations must remain on the scalp for at least 5 to 7 minutes to be effective. Commonly used ingredients in these products include selenium sulfide, zinc pyrithione, tar, salicylic acid, sulfur, or ketoconazole. Zinc pyrithione and selenium sulfide are classified as keratolytic agents. They appear to be both fungicidal and cytostatic. The combination of sulfur and salicylic acid has keratolytic, antifungal, and antiseptic actions. Coal tar agents must be used with caution in fair-haired persons because they may cause an undesirable change in color.

Resistant seborrheic dermatitis may require a prescription shampoo. A 2.5 percent selenium sulfide shampoo, a ketoconazole shampoo (Nizoral shampoo), and a detoconazole shampoo are available. Keratolytic or oil-based lotions are recommended to soften heavy crusts.

A topical corticosteroid may be necessary when significant erythema is present. Hydrocortisone cream 0.5 to 1.0 percent (OTC) for the face, or betamethasone valerate 0.1 percent for the scalp, should be applied after cleansing. Facial application and long-term use of topical corticosteroids should be avoided because of the risk of telangiectasia and dermal atrophy. These risks are not present with the topical use of ketoconazole. Exudative lesions may require compresses of Burow's solution applied for 30 minutes tid. Ketoconazole shampoo every other day is recommended for resistant cases. Ketoconazole 2 percent cream may be applied to the affected areas bid when there is facial or chest involvement.

Once symptoms resolve, maintenance therapy may be required with a once to twice a week application. The prophylactic use of a ketoconazole shampoo (Nizoral) once a week is safe, easy, and at times very rewarding. For a list of antiseborrheic topical preparations, see Table 6.17.

For a superinfection for coverage for gram-positive skin bacteria (e.g., Cephalexin (Keflex) 250 to 500 mg PO qid for 7 to 10 days) is required.

As a strong association with HIV infection and AIDS is well established, treating the underlying HIV infection with effective antiretroviral therapy is often the key to resolution of the patient's skin findings.

Follow-Up and Referral

Repeated secondary infections or resistance to standard management require a prompt referral to a dermatologist.

Table 6.17 Antiseborrheic Topical Preparations

Availability	Preparation	Trade Name
Over-the-counter	Zinc pyrithione	Danex DHS Zinc Head & Shoulders Sebulon Zincon ZNP bar
	Selenium sulfide	Selsun Blue
	Sulfur and Salicylic acid	Sebulex Ionil Vanseb
	Coal Tar	Sebutone Pentrax T-Gel Zetar
	Oil-based lotions	Derma-Smoothe P & S liquid
Prescription	Selenium sulfide	Exel Selsun
	Chloroxine	Capitrol
	Ketoconazole	Nizoral
	Keratolytic	Sebizon
	Lotion	Sebucare

Patient Education

Patients should be reassured that seborrheic dermatitis is not contagious or progressive. They must, however, understand the chronic nature of the condition and the need for continued management. The role of emotional stress in acute flare-ups should be explained. If topical steroids are utilized, the patient needs to be instructed in the proper application and the potential adverse effects. A list of effective OTC preparations should be provided, so each patient can select one that meets his or her personal preferences. Daily shampooing of oily hair is recommended for the first week, decreasing to two or three times a week as maintenance therapy.

Psoriasis

Psoriasis is a chronic relapsing disorder of keratin synthesis that is characterized by well-circumscribed, raised, erythematous papules and plaques, covered with silvery-white scales, usually involving extensor areas in adults such as the elbows and knees, the scalp, and in some forms, the flexural surfaces of the body. The "heartbreak of psoriasis" was coined because of the physically and emotionally disabling effects of the disease. The more commonly seen variants of psoriasis are plaque, guttate, inverse, pustular, and erythrodermic psoriasis. Arthritis may complicate this condition in 10 percent of cases. Plaque psoriasis is the most common form in young adults, which presents are erythematous lesions with well-demarcated margins, topped with a thick, silvery scale. Guttate psoriasis is more common in children, presenting as an acute eruption of multiple, smaller plaques (less than 1 cm). Inverse psoriasis is characterized by localization of psoriatic plaques to flexural (intertriginous) surfaces. Pustular psoriasis is the most serious form characterized by widespread scaling with sheet of superficial pustules. Erythrodermic psoriasis is the most severe form of pustular psoriasis which may be life-threatening and is associated with chronic immunosuppression (e.g., HIV disease); bright-red erythema is the most prominent feature, with variable keratotic scale.

Epidemiology and Causes

Psoriasis affects almost 3 million Americans annually and 1 to 3 percent of the population worldwide. Psoriasis is universal in occurrence but the prevalence varies according to geography, race, and ethnicity. Geographic variations in prevalence (including 0 percent in the South American Andes and 2.9 percent in Denmark) reflect the influence of both genetic and environmental factors. Psoriasis is uncommon among Asians and among North and South American native peoples. It is also infrequent among West Africans, which may help explain the low prevalence of psoriasis among African Americans. Prevalence is highest among Scandinavians. The prevalence of psoriasis is slightly higher in northern rather than in southern Sweden, further supporting the role of climate and sunlight in the expression of the disease. Prevalence of the disease in the United States is about 2 to 3 percent.

Adult men and women are affected with equal frequency. The two peak ages at onset are during the late teens to early 20s and in the late 50s to early 60s. Women and adolescent girls tend to have earlier onset. Earlier onset is associated with a more severe disease. There is little to no epidemiological evidence that psoriasis is an infectious disease.

Psoriasis has a strong genetic influence. One-third of patients with psoriasis report having a relative with the disease. In family studies, when one parent is affected, 8 percent of offspring develop psoriasis and tend to have earlier onset. When both parents have psoriasis, the percentage increases to 41 percent. The mode of genetic transmission is not yet defined, however.

Environmental factors are known to precipitate the disease among genetically predisposed patients and include trauma to normal skin that results in psoriasis in the area (Köbner's phenomenon), infections (upper respiratory infections, *Streptococcus pyogenes,* HIV), stress, fatigue, warm humid climate, sunlight, and certain drugs (systemic corticosteroids, lithium, beta-adrenergic blockers, NSAIDs, and antimalarials). Risk factors for psoriasis are listed below (see Risk Factors 6.1).

Despite intensive investigation, the cause of psoriasis remains unknown, but it is deemed to be a multifactorial disease, with genetic, environmental, biochemical, and immunologic origins. Psoriasis, formerly theorized as an idiopathic skin disease, is now known to be a genetically controlled, immune system–modulated chronic disease. Because cutaneous lesions of psoriasis were thought to result from unregulated hyperproliferative activity in the epidermis, for decades, treatment for psoriasis was primarily suppressive and was directed toward normalizing the hyperkeratinocytic activity.

Currently, the speculation is that genetically predisposed persons may experience clonal T cell activation in response to antigenic stimulation. Proponents of this theory advance this view based on evidence that affected persons have an increase of various human leukocyte antigens (HLAs), particularly certain class I HLA antigens such as HLA B27, which is seen in patients with psoriatic arthritis. In addition, psoriatic plaques are rich in activated T lymphocytes that are capable of both cellular proliferation and inflammation.

Current research is focused on the role of the T cell and the ability of cytokines to influence the dermal immune response to an as-yet-unidentified antigen. This focus is based on the finding that the immune-modulating agent cyclosporin is capable of improving psoriatic symptoms, which led to the rethinking of disease pathogenesis. The genetic component of the disease has been clarified. One genetic region linking susceptibility to psoriasis in some individuals has been isolated to chromosome 6, while the first non–chromosome 6 gene marker for psoriasis has been identified on chromosome 17q. Others have identified possible DNA loci on chromosomes 4, 8, and 16. Thus, a primary goal of current psoriasis research is to elucidate fully the interplay of genetic and environmental influences on the errant cellular effects seen in the disease.

RISK FACTORS 6.1

Psoriasis

Trauma to normal skin (in patients with preexisting psoriasis) that develops into new psoriatic lesions (Köbner's phenomenon)
Physical, chemical, electrical, surgical, infective, or inflammatory insults

Infections
HIV, streptococcal
Endocrine and metabolic factors
Postpartum period
Hypocalcemia (e.g., after dialysis and parathyroidectomy)

Weather-related factors
Extreme cold weather
Prolonged exposure to sun* or hot, humid weather (more exacerbations occur in summer)

Medications
Systemic corticosteroids
Lithium
Beta-adrenergic blockers
Antimalarial drugs
NSAIDs

Psychogenic factors
Psychological factors, e.g., stress, depression

Other factors
Fatigue
Alcoholism
Smoking

***NOTE:** Controlled exposure to sun/ultraviolet light can be therapeutic—see discussion in text.

Pathophysiology

Microscopic examination of psoriatic plaques typically reveals thickened stratum corneum with hyperplasia of epidermis and little inflammation. The basic pathology of psoriasis is the uncontrolled hyperkeratinization of the stratum corneum layer of the skin. Hyperproliferation of keratins 6 and 16 (common to reactive and healing skin) predominates, while expression of keratins 1 and 10 (typically found in normal skin) is reduced. The psoriatic process occurs in varying degrees and results in a wide range of clinical symptoms. If increased mitosis or hyperkeratinization predominates, the result is a thick, silvery scale because of the separation of corneocytes and the presence of air in between. Despite this epidermal hyperplasia and parakeratosis, however, the granular layer of the epidermis is significantly thinned or absent. In contrast, if vasodilatation predominates, the result is a diffused red and hot, slightly scaling skin. Of note, these two processes may coexist.

There are three stages to the psoriatic process: (1) an increased mitotic rate that results in rapid cellular turnover and shortened transit time for the basal layer to the stratum corneum or epidermis (3 to 4 days, versus a normal 28 days); (2) dilatation of upper dermal capillaries with intermittent extravasation of T cells and polymorphonuclear neutrophils into both the dermis and epidermis, leading to (3) the faulty keratinization and accumulation of the stratum corneum, which clinically presents itself as raised papules and plaques covered with white, silvery scales. Multiple growth factors (e.g., epidermal growth factor, transforming growth factor-alpha) and cytokines (e.g., interferon-gamma, IL-2, -6, and -8) are overexpressed in psoriatic skin. Moreover, in plaque-type psoriasis, the T cells localized to the epidermis appear to express specific clonalities with regard to their antigenic receptors, implicating unrestrained T cell replication in the pathogenesis of the disease. Interestingly, however, psoriasis is also associated with many causes of chronic immunosuppression and may be the presenting finding in newly diagnosed HIV infection—particularly the erythrodermic form.

Drug-exacerbated psoriasis offers some insights into disease mechanisms. Lithium is believed to act by enhancing the release of inflammatory mediators from neutrophils. Beta-blockers lead to psoriasis by decreasing cyclic AMP-dependent protein kinase—an inhibitor of cellular proliferation. Nonsteroidal anti-inflammatory drugs (NSAIDs) cause a buildup of the pro-inflammatory mediator arachidonic acid by inhibiting the enzyme cyclooxygenase. Antimalarials, the antifungal terbinafine, and angiotensin-converting enzyme inhibitors are also associated with exacerbation of psoriasis, although these mechanisms are unclear. Drug-induced exacerbations can be unpredictable and severe. Importantly, they are often delayed and may occur months after the start of drug use.

Clinical Presentation

Subjective

Patients with psoriasis usually present to the practitioner with concern over "itchy, red, inflamed and dry, scaly plaques that have gotten worse." Statements about the onset and course of the disease are highly variable for each individual. Symptoms usually begin gradually and are confined to only a few areas (one or both elbows, knees, buttocks, or scalp), but psoriasis can also be explosive in onset. One cause of an explosive onset is a preceding streptococcal throat infection, which can lead in 2 to 3 weeks to multiple, small, guttate lesions with a generalized distribution over the body. Once the disease appears, it follows an irregular, chronic, unpredictable course. It may remain localized to a few areas, or it may cause intermittent or continuous generalized lesions. Itching is usually not a problem in psoriasis, but it may be severe in some patients. These patients often notice blood stains on the bed linens from traumatic, inadvertent scratching of the plaques during sleep. Lesions often occur at sites of trauma (Köbner's phenomenon). A family history of psoriasis is elicited in one-third of patients, and 50 percent of these patients have an affected parent.

Objective

Physical examination reveals lesions that are erythematous and plaques surrounded by thick, silvery scales (which are not easily removed) resembling mica. When these micaceous scales are traumatically removed, multiple small bleeding sites appear (Auspitz's sign). In intertriginous areas, maceration and moisture prevent dry scales from accumulating, but the lesions remain red and sharply defined.

Lesions usually are distributed symmetrically over areas of bony prominences such as elbows and knees. Scaly plaques also occur frequently on the trunk, scalp, intergluteal cleft, and umbilicus. The latter three areas are frequently overlooked by the patient and clinician, but are important in the diagnosis, especially in patients with associated psoriatic arthritis and limited skin lesions. The nature of the arthritis becomes apparent only after the typical skin lesions are recognized.

A thorough examination of the entire skin is crucial, therefore, to the diagnosis and treatment of a patient with suspected psoriasis. Another helpful diagnostic feature is the Köbner's phenomenon, in which intense trauma induces formation of new skin lesions. Such isomorphic lesions can also be induced on the palms of patients whose hands are exposed to friction.

Nail involvement may include stippling or pitting of the nail plate, or a yellow to red-brown coloring ("oil-staining") of the nails. An accumulation of yellow debris under the nails, simulating a tinea infection (tinea unguium), is seen in some patients. Swelling, redness, and scaling of the paronychial margins occur often and are associated with arthritis of the distal interphalangeal joints. The clinical course of this disease is characterized by chronicity and seasonal fluctuations, with improvement in the summer (due to sun exposure) and worsening in the winter, as dry skin leads to epidermal injury.

Some patients with psoriasis (10 percent) may suffer from arthritis, although this association of symptoms is uncommon. Psoriatic arthritis may occur when the skin lesions are present or may precede the initial skin manifestation. The arthritis involves the distal interphalangeal joints of the hands and feet, or the vertebrae of the spine (ankylosing spondylitis).

Several variations of psoriasis have been classified: plaque psoriasis, inverse psoriasis, erythrodermic psoriasis, pustular psoriasis, and guttate psoriasis (Table 6.18).

Table 6.18 **Differential Diagnosis: Psoriasis**

Type of Psoriasis	Clinical Presentation	Differential Diagnosis	Key to Diagnosis
Plaque psoriasis	• Plaques with white silvery scales • Seen on knees, elbows, neck, scalp, between buttocks, or on back • Usually bilateral involvement • Intertiginous areas may be involved, but scales are absent • Positive Auspitz's sign and Köbner's phenomenon • Gradual onset, chronic course	Seborrheic dermatitis	Sharply marginated yellowish red patches with sharp borders and greasy scales. Seen on scalp, central face, eyebrows, eyelids, nasolabial folds, and external ear. Can be pruritic.
		Nummular eczema	Pruritic, coin-shaped plaques or papulovesicles on an erythematous base and uniform scaling; may become exudative and crusted. Typically seen on legs, upper extremities, and trunk.
		Lichen planus	Pruritic, flat, irregular purple papules with fine white lines and scales. Commonly seen on flexor surfaces, nails, and scalp.
		Pityriasis rubra pilaris	Generalized erythematous, red-orange lesions with diffuse thickening interspersed with areas of normal skin; the palms and soles are usually affected.
		Mycosis fungoides	Sharply demarcated, scaly, raised plaques to violaceous nodules that may ulcerate. Also known as T-cell lymphoma.
		Atopic dermatitis	Severe pruritus; palmar markings; infraorbital folds increase, red cheeks in infancy; sides of neck, hands, and flexural surfaces most commonly affected after age 12.
Pustular psoriasis	• Lesions may be localized, appearing on the hands and feet (Barber's disease), or involve the entire skin (Von Zumbusch's disease) • Accompanying systemic symptoms	Pustular dermatitis	Persistent or recurrent dry red and scaly rash; first appearance in infancy; history of dry skin since birth. Onset is sudden. Pustules appear on the edges of existing psoriatic plaques and on the palms. Pruritus and intense burning sensation are present. Patient may have a fever and systemic symptoms. Systemic complications include pneumonia, congestive heart failure, and hepatitis.
Guttate psoriasis	• Characterized by small, red papules (<1 cm in diameter) • Discrete lesions, seen in a raindrop- or showerlike distribution, usually on the trunk and extremities • Triggered by streptococcal infection • May see Köbner's phenomenon	Secondary syphilis	Base of lesion (ulcer) is clean and smooth; edges are raised and well circumscribed. Usually occurs in genital region or on lips.
		Pityriasis rosea	Peripheral scaling, well-demarcated, salmon-colored patch, forming a fine collarette (herald patch); followed by other lesions on trunk and proximal extremities. Christmas-tree distribution on exposed areas
Inverse psoriasis	• Involves the flexural area (e.g., armpit, groin)	Candidiasis	Erythematous; macerated patches with sharp, scaling border. Satellite papules and pustules that are tender and pruritic are common.
Erythrodermic psoriasis	• Severe form of pustular psoriasis • Generalized distribution • Erythema with variable scale with fluid and electrolyte loss; chills	Drug eruption	Massive superficial dermal edema lifts the epidermis, forming necrosis, appearing as violaceous plaques or bullae; then heal with postinflammatory hyperpigmentation; e.g., Stevens-Johnson syndrome (SJS), toxic epidermal necrosis (TEN)
		Pityriasis rubra pilaris	Fine to thick scales on palms or soles; orange-red with diffuse thickening
		Eczematous dermatitis, mycosis fungoides	See nummular eczema and atopic dermatitis

Diagnostic Reasoning

Diagnostic Tests

Initial laboratory studies include routine laboratory testing (CBC with differential and blood chemistry profile) plus serum uric acid level, antinuclear antibody (ANA) titer, or rheumatoid factor. Throat culture is appropriate if *Streptococcus pyogenes* infection is suspected as the precipitating factor (such as in guttate-type psoriasis). Often, the laboratory values are generally within normal limits except for the serum uric acid level, which may show elevation (hyperuricemia). In more severe variants of psoriasis, other specific tests may be ordered. An elevated erythrocyte sedimentation rate (ESR) and decreased albumin levels, along with anemia, can be observed in chronic disease. Immunoglobulins are generally normal, but selective IgA and IgG deficiency are observed in some patients. In pustular psoriasis, leukocytosis and hypocalcemia are seen.

X-ray studies of the hands are sometimes helpful to search for associated psoriatic arthritis in patients who complain of joint pains in their hands. X-rays of patients with psoriatic arthritis will show extensive erosion and luxation of distal interphalangeal or metatarsophalangeal joints bilaterally.

Only in unusual circumstances (severe or unusual forms of the disease) are histologic studies necessary to diagnose psoriasis. Biopsy is seldom necessary because the clinical features of psoriasis are so distinctive. At times, an invasive biopsy may be necessary for questionable diagnoses. Biopsies should be planned to yield maximal information. When biopsying patients, intact, nonexcoriated lesions should be sampled. If there are lesions at different stages of eruption, more than one sample is necessary. Biopsies can include partial dermal thickness procedures such as shave or curettage biopsy, or full-thickness sampling with punch or excisional biopsy.

A skin biopsy is done with the use of a local anesthetic to obtain sufficient tissue for accurate diagnosis. Skin biopsy is a "clean" procedure and should be done very simply and quickly. The standard 4 mm punch biopsy is often used and is recommended. Minimal scarring is the desired end result. A biopsy should not be performed on infected skin on any patient with a bleeding disorder or on any individual who is allergic to local anesthetics. The key to a good biopsy is good selection of the sample. It is often useful to take two to six samples at the first examination of complex cases. Experience is invaluable in performing good biopsies. Clinicians who are not experienced in this procedure should refer the patient to a dermatologist. (See Therapeutic Procedures 6.1.)

Differential Diagnosis

Often, psoriasis is mistaken for other dermatologic conditions. It is not uncommon to see a patient with more than one variant of psoriasis at the same time, and the pattern may also change over time. Other skin diseases should be ruled out, especially in atypical cases that are complicated by other systemic disorders.

Differential diagnosis for psoriasis includes the following: atopic dermatitis, nummular eczema, cutaneous T-cell lymphoma, tinea corporis, lichen planus, seborrheic dermatitis, drug eruptions, and secondary syphilis. Hyperkeratotic eczema of the palms is a common cause of misdiagnosis.

Atopic dermatitis frequently has its first presentation in infancy or childhood. The patient has a persistent or recurrent dry, red, scaly rash and a history of dry skin since birth. Nummular eczema has a characteristic morphology that helps to distinguish it from other eczematous eruptions. Initially, nummular eczema presents with tiny papules and vesicles and then assumes its characteristic clinical appearance of coin-shaped plaques. It is typically seen on the legs, but it can also appear on the upper extremities and trunk; the lesions are pruritic, erythematous, and surrounded with uniform scaling.

Cutaneous T-cell lymphoma (CTCL) can be difficult to diagnose in its early stages. Early on, the rash may appear as single or multiple erythematous, scaly macules. In its subsequent stage, which may occur anywhere from 6 months to 6 years later, the development of sharply demarcated, scaly, elevated, red to violaceous plaques known as mycosis fungoides occurs. These plaques may coalesce to form larger plaques with annular, circinate, or serpiginous

THERAPEUTIC PROCEDURE 6.1

The Skin "Punch" Biopsy

- Prep the area around the lesion that has been carefully selected.
- Inject 1% lidocaine slowly and superficially at several sites around the lesion, for rapid effect and minimal injury. Epinephrine may be used to control bleeding except at certain sites (nose, ears, fingertips, toes, penis).
- Punch into the skin around the lesion at a 90-degree angle to the plane of the skin, with a quick back-and-forth twisting motion, reaching in fast.
- Carefully lift out the plug and snip it at the base with sharp tissue scissors.
- Place the tissue plug in a formalin solution.
- Apply pressure with sterile gauze for hemostasis.
- Close with two sutures (4.0 or 5.0 size). (Suture removal will be determined according to the location—sutures on the face should be removed sooner than those on the extremities.)

NOTE: Nerve damage can occur in areas where they are very superficial, such as the lateral aspects of fingers and the ulnar groove of elbows. Any lesions in these areas (including the face for cosmetic reasons) should be referred to a dermatologist.

borders, or may completely regress. The disease may further progress to brown or purplish red dermal nodules (tumors). The nodules often occur in the face, body folds, and the inframammary area in women. The tumors can progress further to exfoliative erythroderma. Through much of the process, CTCL may resemble atopic dermatitis with diffuse erythema and scaling; a definitive diagnosis can be made by skin biopsy.

Tinea corporis ("ringworm") presents as erythematous patches and plaques with central clearing and peripheral scales, crusts, vesicles, and pustules. It may spontaneously resolve or worsen with topical steroid treatment. In seborrheic dermatitis, the lesions are lighter in color, less well defined, and are covered with a dull yellow scale. Lesions commonly occur in similar psoriatic distribution, including face, scalp, and central chest. Eczema at times develops a psoriasiform appearance, especially on the legs. Lichen planus gives rise to diagnostic difficulty if it presents as hypertrophic lesions on the legs, as penile lesions, or on the hands. It results from excessive scratching. In pityriasis rosea, a single herald patch occurs first; subsequent smaller eruptions follow skin lines in a Christmas-tree pattern. Pityriasis rubra pilaris consists of generalized erythematous lesions with areas of normal skin; the palms and soles are usually affected.

Drug eruptions resulting from beta-blockers, methyldopa, and gold can produce psoriatic-type lesions. Intertriginous psoriasis may appear similar to candidiasis but in most cases would be distinguishable through Wood's light and KOH testing. Mycosis fungoides lesions progress to violaceous, indurated plaques and nodules; begins on thighs, buttocks, and trunk. Sudden onset of psoriasis may be associated with HIV; its presence must be investigated, if unknown (Table 6.18).

Management

The goal of therapy for psoriasis is to control the disease so that the patient no longer feels physically or psychologically hindered by the skin lesions. For sparse or mild lesions that do not bother the patient, no treatment is needed. When treatment is indicated, the disease is controlled by decreasing epidermal proliferation and underlying dermal inflammation with topical steroids and other agents, along with phototherapy in some patients. Systemic agents are reserved for severe or recalcitrant cases. The chronic course of psoriasis and the lack of cure can be both discouraging and challenging for the patient and the clinician. Patients should be reassured that the therapeutic options today are much broader than even in the recent past. Several therapeutic approaches and medications have become available, along with improvements in phototherapy.

Some patients find the presence of even a few small plaques highly objectionable because the location of the plaques in more visible areas of the body is disfiguring or hinders physical activity. Other patients are willing to accept the condition as bothersome but not overly impairing, particularly when they realize there is no cure. A long-term plan of disease management is helpful for patients with psoriasis, to help deal with exacerbation, which frequently can cause frustration or discouragement.

Topical Therapy

Topical agents are the first line of pharmacotherapeutics for psoriasis and are usually effective. If less than 20 percent of the body (e.g., no more than the elbows, knees, and ears and scalp) is involved, topical agents are very effective. But if more than 20 percent of the body is involved, then systemic therapy may be required and referral to a dermatologist is recommended. For stubborn, persistent, and widespread lesions, ultraviolet (UV) light treatment should be strongly considered. Systemic therapy in psoriasis is usually used as the last resort.

Topical agents that are popularly used are available both as OTC and in prescription form. Emollient creams or ointments (OTC products) applied on the skin twice a day are helpful in preventing cracking and fissuring of lesions, especially those on palms and soles. Keratolytic agents, such as salicylic acid preparations (1 to 5 percent concentration) may be combined with any of these preparations to enhance absorption of other drugs such as topical steroids through thick lesions. These agents may be applied twice daily.

Topical corticosteroids are widely used because they are relatively easy to apply. Those with intermediate and strong potency should be applied once or twice a day. Topical steroids are appropriate in cases involving 10 percent or less of body surface (e.g., the face, neck, flexures, and genitalia). The plaques usually blanch and thin in response to the treatment. The more potent steroids are applied to achieve complete clearing of psoriasis and are helpful in treating exposed areas of the body. However, caution is needed in steroid usage, because steroids can cause skin atrophy and suppression of the hypothalamic–pituitary–adrenal (HPA) axis, resulting in a Cushing-like syndrome.

The effective treatment approach for exacerbations of psoriasis is to initially use "superpotent" topical corticosteroid preparations (e.g., Diprolene, Psorcon, Temovate, Ultravate) for 2 weeks and then decrease to a lesser potency for maintenance therapy. Superpotent corticosteroids should not be used for more than 2 weeks. Once symptoms are under control, other topical agents or a weaker steroid may be substituted after gradually tapering the dose (Table 6.19).

The penetration and absorption of topical steroids will increase with occlusive dressing, but some superpotent steroids should not be used with occlusion because of increased risk of HPA suppression. Ointment preparations are preferred over creams or lotions if the psoriatic scale is thick. When heavy scaling is present, gentle brushing of the psoriatic scales after warm soaks or during warm baths before applying the topicals will increase the absorption. Hard scrubbing should be avoided, because skin trauma can exacerbate the psoriasis.

Table 6.19 **Potency of Topical Corticosteroids for Atopic Dermatitis**

Potency	Topical Corticosteroids (Generic Name)	Trade Name
Highest	Betamethasone dipropionate 0.05%	Diprolene (oint, gel)
	Clobetasol propionate 0.05%	Clobex (lotion, shampoo)
		Olux (foam)
		Temovate (cream, gel, oint scalp application)
		Temovate-E (emollient crm)
	Diflorasone diacetate 0.05%	Psorcon (oint)
	Flurandrenolide 4 mcg/cm^2	Cordran (tape)
	Halobetasol propionate 0.05%	Ultravate (cream, oint)
High	Amcinonide 0.1%	Cyclocort (crm, lotion, oint)
	Betamethasone dipropionate 0.05%	Diprolene AF (emollient)
		Diprolene (lotion)
	Desoximetasone 0.05%	Topicort (gel)
	Desoximetasone 0.25%	Topicort (emollient, oint)
	Diflorasone diacetate 0.05%	Psorcon (emollient crm and oint)
	Fluocinonide 0.05%	Lidex (crm, gel, oint, soln)
		Lidex-E (emollient)
	Halcinonide 0.1%	Halog (crm, oint, soln)
	Triamcinolone acetonide 0.5%	Aristocort A (crm)
		Kenalog (crm)
Medium	Betamethasone valerate 0.12%	Luziq (foam)
	Clocortolone pivalate 0.1%	Cloderm (crm)
	Desonide 0.05%	DesOwen (crm, lotion, oint)
	Desoximetasone 0.05%	Topicort-LP (emollient)
	Fluocinolone acetonide 0.01%	Derma-Smoothe/FS (oil)
		Capex (shampoo)
	Fluocinolone acetonide 0.025%	Synalar (crm, oint)
	Flurandrenolide 0.025%	Cordran-SP (crm)
		Cordran (oint)
	Flurandrenolide 0.05%	Cordran-SP (cream)
		Cordran (lotion, oint)
	Fluticasone propionate 0.005%	Cultivate (oint)
	Fluticasone propionate 0.05%	Cultivate (crm)
	Hydrocortisone probutate 0.1%	Pandel (crm)
	Hydrocortisone butyrate 0.1%	Locoid (crm, oint, soln)
	Hydrocortisone valerate 0.2%	Westcort (crm, oint)
	Mometasone furoate 0.1%	Elocon (crm, lotion, oint)
	Prednicarbate 0.1%	Dermatop (emollient, oint)
	Triamcinolone acetonide 0.1%	Aristocort A (crm, oint)
		Kenalog (crm, lotion)
	Triamcinolone acetonide 0.2%	Kenalog (spray)
Low	Alclometasone dipropionate 0.05%	Alcovate (crm, oint)
	Flucocinolone acetonide 0.01%	Synalar (soln)
	Hydrocortisone base or acetate 0.5%	Cortisporin (crm)
	Hydrocortisone base or acetate 1%	Cortisporin (oint)
		Hytone (crm, lotion, oint)
		Vytone (crm)
		U-cort (crm)
	Hydrocortisone base or acetate 2.5%	Anusol-HC (crm)
		Hytone (crm, lotion, oint)
	Triamcinolone acetonide 0.025%	Aristocort A (crm)
		Kenalog (crm, lotion, oint)

Topical steroid therapy has its shortcomings. Remission periods are often relatively short. Prolonged use produce striae and thinning of skin (atrophy) and the rebound effect is much worse, possibly converting a "stable" disease to an "unstable" one if the dose of steroid is suddenly discontinued. Prolonged use of steroids has been associated with suppression of the HPA axis and a Cushing-like syndrome, as noted previously.

Topical tar and anthralin are agents that can be used once a day in combination with topical steroids. Scalp involvement may benefit from use of a tar shampoo (Zetar, Sebutone, Pentrax) before the application of a topical steroid. The tar shampoo is gently massaged on the scalp and left on for a few hours and then rinsed off. Softened scales are gently removed. The scalp should be gently dried before application of the steroid lotion. Wearing a shower cap after steroid application enhances absorption and improves results. Excessive combing after washing the hair should be avoided, to prevent trauma.

Anthralin (0.1 and 3.0 percent ointment) belongs to the class of trihydroxyanthracene compounds; it is used topically for psoriasis. Anthralin is an antimitotic agent capable of inhibiting DNA synthesis. Anthralin is applied in high concentrations from once to twice a day and should be washed off after 10 to 30 minutes. It produces quick remission of plaques after several weeks of use but has a tendency to irritate and stain adjacent skin and clothing, making it less preferable than other treatment options. Paradoxically, if topical steroids are added to an anthralin program, there is an earlier relapse.

A newer topical treatment includes calcipotriene (Dovonex). This is a vitamin D derivative that is available as an ointment. Calcipotriene produces keratinocyte differentiation and controls proliferation. It is superior to a superpotent steroid and is the best treatment for mild to moderately severe disease. It is likely to become a major alternative to topical steroid therapy for plaque-type psoriasis. Study have found it to be effective in nearly three quarters of patients with plaque psoriasis, with relatively minor side effects.

Another topical agent with similar action to calcipotriene is tazarotene (Tazorac). It interferes with excessive differentiation and proliferation of epidermal cells and also limits the migration of inflammatory mediators to the areas of hyperkeratinization. It achieves a 60 to 70 percent rate and long remissions (up to 12 weeks). It is available as an ointment, cream, or lotion preparation. Like other receptor-selective retinoids, tazarotene is considered teratogenic and should not be used by pregnant women.

Topical tacrolimus (Protopic) and the related pimecrolimus (Elidel), calcineurin inhibitors, appled twice per day may be effective. These treatments have been particularly helpful for pssoriasis in the facial and intertriginous areas where topical cortisone treatments (other than low potency steroids) should be avoided, given the tendency for dermal atrophy. They should not be used indiscriminately or for long periods of time, however, as the FDA is investigating the link between these immunomodulators and an increased propensity for lymphoma and cutaneous cancers. The FDA has an advisory warning out against these agents, specifying their use only for refractory flares and as second-line therapy (and only in persons older than 2 years of age and in those with a competent immune system), although final results on ongoing studies may not be available for another 10 years.

Exposure to natural sunlight improves psoriasis and permits a more enduring remission than does the use of topical steroids. In some patients, topical steroids may even be suspended during the summer. Although sun exposure to the point of mild erythema is helpful, sunburn exacerbates psoriasis and should be avoided.

In 1925, W.H. Goeckerman, a physician at Mayo Clinic, achieved encouraging results with experimental use of mid-range ultraviolet B (UVB) light and coal tar ointment for patients whose psoriasis did not respond to topical therapy. With some modifications of the sunbeam spectrum and combined with topicals, the traditional Goeckerman program is still being utilized. Crude coal tar of 1 to 2 percent in gel or ointment form is applied at night to the psoriatic plaques and is followed by UVB treatments. UVB treatment is continued for 4 to 6 weeks and causes remission (for up to 4 months) in 60 to 90 percent of patients without evidence of increased risk of skin cancer. Guttate psoriasis, in particular, responds well to UVB therapy.

A more aggressive treatment approach used by dermatologists (since 1971) is the combination of oral psoralens and long-wavelength (320 to 400 nm) UV light, commonly referred to as PUVA therapy. It has been reported to achieve an 80 to 90 percent rate of remission on otherwise recalcitrant severe psoriasis, such as the pustular form. The treatment inhibits mitosis by stopping DNA replication and is given two to three times per week. PUVA involves ingestion of an oral psoralen compound (methoxsalen) prior to light exposure. (Psoralen may be taken orally, or it can be added to a bath.) "Bath PUVA therapy" is not widely used in this country. Psoralen is inactive in the body, but on the skin it is activated by UVA (long-wavelength ultraviolet A light). The eyes must be protected during and after exposure to UVA light because of the potential for cataract formation. Because of the significant occurrence of nausea, body malaise, phototoxic erythema, premature aging of the skin, and pruritus following administration of psoralens, the attrition rate of this treatment is high. Although it can clear chronic plaque psoriasis in 6 to 8 weeks, overexposure to UVA light can cause acute sunburn in the short term; in the long term, it can cause non-melanoma cancer. Since the mid-1980s, the use of phototherapy has been shown to be associated with squamous cell carcinoma. In 1991, some cases of melanoma began to surface among patients who had gotten more than 250 courses of treatment. Therefore, careful follow-up of patients who have had PUVA therapy is crucial. Patients considered to be at increased risk for skin cancer (those with fair skin who are easily sunburned, or individuals who have had previous x-ray therapy to skin) should not receive PUVA.

Systemic Therapy

Systemic therapy is reserved for those patients with severe incapacitating disease—pustular, guttate, and/or arthritic psoriasis. It is administered only by expert specialists such as rheumatologists or dermatologists, who regularly utilize systemic antimitotic agents, including methotrexate, etretinate, and cyclosporine.

Methotrexate is a folic acid antagonist and a cytotoxic agent that inhibits cellular proliferation. It is used in chemotherapy for cancer but is also useful in patients with severe psoriatic arthritis. The drug is given in low doses of 5 to 25 mg per week. Oral regimens include every other day and once-weekly dosing. If nausea is significant, intramuscular administration can be used. A therapeutic response is usually seen within 2 to 3 weeks, at which time the dose or interval should be reduced. With prolonged use, accumulative doses of methotrexate could result in hepatotoxicity, nephrotoxicity, and bone marrow depression. Coadministration of folic acid 1 mg PO qd effectively protects against many of the minor side effects associated with this treatment, such as stomatitis. Methotrexate is contraindicated in patients with cirrhosis of the liver or diabetes, or with a history of alcohol or IV drug use.

Monitoring of blood counts, including platelets, should be done weekly, followed by monthly testing. Renal and liver function tests (baseline and follow-up) should be done. Intermittent liver biopsies are recommended, because hepatic fibrosis may occur with prolonged use. Methotrexate is teratogenic and should not be given to those who are pregnant or who want to become pregnant.

Cyclosporine is an immunosuppressant that was originally used for prevention of organ rejection in organ transplant patients. Its efficacy in severe erythrodermic and psoriatic arthritis was discovered serendipitously while the drug was being tested for rheumatoid arthritis. Significant improvement and even total clearing of psoriasis becomes evident within days in some patients. Withdrawal of cyclosporine is associated with relapse within weeks. Hypertension and nephrotoxicity can develop during cyclosporine treatment, although in the vast majority of patients, renal function subsequently returns to normal. Treatment with cyclosporine for more than 1 year is not recommended because it may cause prolonged immunosuppression and myalgias. Serum creatinine levels should be monitored throughout the duration of treatment, because cyclosporine can cause interstitial fibrosis and tubular atrophy.

Other systemic immunosuppressants such as hydroxyurea, azathioprine (Imuran), and tacrolimus may be used if patients do not tolerate more common systemic therapies. The newest immunomodulatory drugs now used for moderate to severe plaque psoriasis, psoriatic arthritis, and refractory disease include etanercept (Enbrel)-a tumor necrosis-α (TNF-α) inhibitor, alefacept (a recombinant CD2 antagonist which inhibits T-cell activation), efalizumab (a monoclonal antibody against CD11A), and infliximab (Remicade) another TNF-α inhibitor). These agents have been revolutionary in the treatment of refractory psoriasis, according to most rheumatologists. These treatments do require an increase in immune monitoring, however (e.g., CD4+ T cell counts). As these agents are very expensive, they are considered second-line therapy when UV light therapy fails. (See Nursing Research-Based Practice 6.1.)

An oral systemic agent, etretinate (Acitretin) is a vitamin A derivative that can be beneficial for patients with moderate to severe pustular and erythrodermic variants of psoriasis. In severe cases, etretinate can be used in combination with PUVA. About 50 percent of patients who are refractory to PUVA alone improve when a retinoid is added. Female patients who are treated with etretinate should be advised not to get pregnant for 3 years after ceasing treatment, because retinoids are teratogenic. Careful monitoring of blood counts, plasma triglycerides, and LFTs is required.

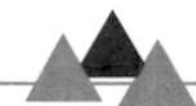

NURSING RESEARCH-BASED PRACTICE 6.1

Use of Etanercept (Enbrel) in the Dermatology Setting: A Review

Lebwohl, MG: Am J Clin Dermatology 6(1):49–59, 2005.

As psoriasis and psoriatic arthritis are chronic in nature, ideal treatment should have sustained efficacy, with minimal short- and long-term toxicities to allow lifelong treatment. Traditional therapies such as phototherapies and systemic agents do not satisfy these criteria. Most patients are not satisfied with their treatment options.

The tumor necrosis factor (TNF) antagonist etanercept (Enbrel) has been shown to play a fundamental role in the inflammatory processes underlying psoriateic arthritis and psoriasis, as well as in other inflammatory, immune-mediated diseases, such as rheumatoid arthritis (RA). Etanercept prevents initiation of the proinflammatory cascade by competitively binding TNF. First indicated for RA, etanercept is also approved for the treatment of psoriatic arthritis, juvenile RA, ankylosing spondylitis, and most recently psoriasis.

Etanercept is a safe, effective, and convenient treatment option for patients with psoriatic arthritis and psoriasis, which can be used continuously with or without traditional therapies. The self-administered injections provide a distinct advantage over traditional therapies that often require frequent office visits and laboratory monitoring, and other biologic agents that require administration in the doctor's office. Ongoing research is continuing with etanercept in psoriasis and other dermatologic conditions.

Follow-Up and Referral

Newly diagnosed patients and patients who have moderate to more extensive skin involvement or severe disease (e.g., pustular psoriasis) should be referred to a dermatologist or psoriasis specialty center. Support groups are of great psychological help. Patients with recalcitrant and frequent flare-ups should be referred to a dermatologist for UV light therapy and systemic treatment. An ophthalmology consult is necessary prior to ultraviolet therapy, to rule out any presence of cataracts.

Patients with severe psoriasis are usually followed up every 2 months by a specialist, or more often as necessary. Patients who exhibit symptoms of depression or poor coping skills will benefit from referral to a psychiatrist for psychological evaluation and therapy.

Patient Education

Psoriasis presents many challenges to both the patient and the health-care provider. For patients with disfiguring and uncontrollable psoriasis, education and support are central to the treatment process. The patient should be informed of available community resources and support groups. Explanation of the disease process and treatment, including potential adverse effects of medications, is very helpful. The new patient and his or her family should be reassured that the disease is not contagious or infectious.

The genetic aspect of the disease follows classic mendelian law, however, and should be explained to the patient, especially to a concerned parent. If neither parent has psoriasis, the chances are less than 10 percent that another child will display the disease. If one parent is affected, the chance of developing psoriasis increases to 15 percent; if both parents are affected, the chances rise up to 59 percent that one or more children will have the disease.

The clinician should educate the patient that there are several ways of remaining in remission: Patients with psoriasis should avoid skin trauma and should keep the skin relatively dry, to decrease pruritus, scratching, and scaling. They should avoid photosensitizing medications such as tetracyclines, sulfa drugs, or phenothiazines. If drugs of these types are necessary, the patients should be advised to inform the prescribing physician of their psoriasis and to ask for a possible alternative. Although photosensitizing drugs should be avoided, controlled sun exposure during the summer is beneficial. The patient should be advised to use a high-SPF sunscreen to prevent sunburn. Patients should be informed to seek treatment for streptococcal infections (skin infections, sore throats) immediately. Aggravating factors for psoriasis include increased stress and alcohol.

The clinician should explain to the patient that dietary manipulations do not play a role in treating psoriasis. However, healthy eating habits support a good immune system. Nutritionists recommend a low-fat, high-fiber diet for patients. Naturopaths recommend many herbal medicines to improve psoriasis and to control or provide relief from the disturbing effects of the flare-ups. (See Complementary Therapies 6.1.) An active support group for psoriasis is the National Psoriasis Foundation, 6600 SW 92nd Avenue, Suite 300, Portland, OR 97223-7195, 1-800-723-9166, http://www.psoriasis.org.

Skin Lesions: Benign

Seborrheic Keratosis

Seborrheic keratoses are benign, warty-appearing growths that are commonly seen in the older adult. These growths are usually found on the trunk, but they may also be seen on the hands and face. They develop in sun-exposed as well as in protected areas. See Table 6.20 for information about other skin lesions, including nevi, skin tags (acrochordons), and lipomas.

Epidemiology and Causes

The tendency to develop seborrheic keratosis is an autosomal dominant trait. Seborrheic keratosis is extremely common; it has been found in 88 percent of persons older than age 65. Of this group, approximately 50 percent often develop 10 or more lesions. In fact, for some individuals, lesions may number into the hundreds. The lesions found on sun-exposed areas rarely increase in size, whereas seborrheic keratotic lesions in protected areas tend to be darker, have a more crumbly appearance, and may enlarge in size.

Seborrheic keratosis is more prevalent in persons with white skin. The lesions are raised, brownish gray, and appear "stuck on."

Pathophysiology

Seborrheic keratosis lesions originate from the horny layer of the epidermis and are the result of a benign proliferation of immature keratinocytes. Inspection of the lesions may reveal dark keratin plugs or firm, horny cysts on their surface. A predisposition for seborrheic keratosis appears to be inherited in an autosomal dominant pattern. These are epidermal tumors, but they are not considered malignant or premalignant, as they do not undergo transformation into cancerous lesions. However, a phenomenon known as the sign of Leser-Trélat exists which is characterized by the sudden development of multiple seborrheic keratotic lesions, along with skin tags, and acanthosis nigricans (a darkening and mild thickening of the skin in characteristic intertriginous areas). While the skin lesions in this condition are not considered malignant, the sign of Leser-Trélat is associated with various types of underlying malignancies, including lung and gastrointestinal cancers and, thus, is considered a neoplastic syndrome. Moreover, seborrheic keratosis has also been observed in associated with certain skin malignancies such as basal cell carcinomas, occurring at different skin sites.

COMPLEMENTARY THERAPIES 6.1

Acne

Herb	Comments
Marigold (*Calendula officinalis*)	Topical application Available as a soap Has anti-inflammatory properties
Tea tree oil (*Melaleuca alternifolia*)	Topical application twice daily

Excema

Herb	Comments
Chamomile (*Bertholettia* excelsa)	Topical application Anti-inflammatory Contraindicated in patients with ragweed allergy
Evening primrose (*Oenothera biennis*)	Dose is six capsules daily. Should not be taken with phenothiazines.
Marigold (*Calendula officianalis*)	Topical application—ointment or cream Has anti-inflammatory properties
Goldenseal (*Hydrastis canadensis*)	Used topically by Native Americans Powdered root mixed with water to make a paste and applied to rash
Licorice (*Glycyrrhiza glabra*)	Topical application Anti-inflammatory properties
Turmeric (*Curcuma longa*)	Topical application; anti-inflammatory

Fungal Infections

Herb	Comments
Tea tree oil (*Melaleuca alternifolia*)	Topical application; antifungal properties Apply twice daily.

Psoriasis

Herb	Comments
Angelica (*Angelica archangelica*)	After ingestion, expose affected area to mild sunlight Contains photosensitizers (furocoumarin) Possible interaction with anticoagulants and aspirin
Avena (*Avena sativa*) "Oatmeal"	Applied as an oatmeal paste
Avocado (*Persea americana*)	Cooling, soothing effect Mashed avocados are rubbed into scaling patches
Bishop's weed (*Ammi visnagae*)	Topical application Inhibits cell division Treatment may irritate the skin
Brazil nut (*Bertholettia excelsa*)	Soothing; relieves itching Contains an oil rich in vitamin E and selenium
Chamomile (*Bertholettia excelsa*)	Topical application Anti-inflammatory Contraindicated in patients with ragweed allergy
Flax (*Linum usitatissimum*)	Need to ingest about 10–12 grams (5–6 tsp.) May add flaxseeds to salads
Licorice (*Glycyrrhiza glabra*)	Topical application; may be more effective than hydrocortisone
Milk thistle (*Silybum mariannum*)	Anti-inflammatory Taken as a tea, tincture, or in capsules
Oregon grape (*Mahonia aquifolium*)	Antioxidant
Red pepper (*Capsicium*)	Contains capsaicin Reduces scaling and redness, but can cause burning and stinging Wash hands thoroughly after applying, avoid getting in the eyes or on mucous membranes
Omega-3 fish oil	Clinical trials (Mayser et al.) have shown fish oils to decrease symptoms and severity of chronic plaque psoriasis and acute guttate psoriasis.

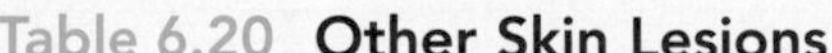

Table 6.20 **Other Skin Lesions**

Lesion	Description	Clinical Presentation	Management
Lipoma	A lipoma is a benign subcutaneous tumor that consists of adipose tissue. Lipomas are most commonly found in older adults; usually asymptomatic. Cause is unknown.	• Rubbery smooth and round mass of adipose tissue that is compressible and has a soft to very firm texture • May have symptoms of irritation, such as redness and tenderness • Commonly occurs on back of the neck, trunk, and forearms	• Observe for changes, rapid growth • Excision or liposuction • Referral to dermatologist if indicated
Nevi	Nevi (moles) are circumscribed areas of pigmentation. Types include congenital, acquired, or atypical or dysplastic (>5 mm, in diameter, with color variation and irregular borders)	• Flat or raised circumscribed area of pigmentation • Assess for suspected melanoma (check ABCDEs: asymmetry, irregular borders, variations in color, diameter >6 mm, elevation above the surface of the skin)	• Excision • Referral to dermatologist if melanoma is suspected
Skin tags	Skin tags (acrochordons) are benign overgrowths of skin, commonly seen after middle age. Cause is unknown.	• Overgrowths of normal skin that have formed soft, polyplike lesions that have a stalk • Usually found on the neck, axilla, groin, upper trunk, and eyelid	• Usually none unless patient is bothered by the cosmetic effect or irritation • If treatment is required, may include snip excision, electrocautery, or cryosurgery • Referral to dermatologist if skin tag is located on the eyelids or face or if patient has a history of keloids, diabetes, or infection, or is on high-dose steroid therapy, or if there is the possibility of a malignant lesion

Clinical Presentation

Subjective

The typical patient is an older white woman who complains of the cosmetic effects of the lesion. The patient typically complains of the unsightliness of the lesion, itching, and constant irritation from friction or clothing.

Objective

Seborrheic keratotic lesions are benign, superficial epithelial growths that appear as well-defined scaly, hyperpigmented lesions with a warty or "stuck-on" appearance. They are most often found on the trunk, face, and arms. Lesions look as if they could literally be "picked off" the skin surface. Seborrheic keratotic lesions tend to grow slowly and are round to oval in shape. The lesions occasionally appear as smooth papules. The color of the lesions can range from flesh tone to dark brown in white patients. In black women, the lesions also appear as smooth, round to oval black papules on the upper part of the face (dermatosis papulosa nigra).

Diagnostic Reasoning

Diagnostic Tests

No laboratory testing is necessary to diagnose seborrheic keratosis. However, if the patient presents with an atypical lesion, diagnosis should be confirmed with a biopsy.

Differential Diagnosis

The diagnosis of seborrheic keratosis is based on the appearance of the lesion and on patient demographics (especially age). Skin lesions that can mimic seborrheic keratosis include any pigmented papule or nodule. The differential diagnoses for seborrheic keratosis include benign pigmented nevi, pigmented basal cell carcinoma, and malignant melanoma.

Pigmented nevi appear as smooth round macules or papules that do have a warty appearance. Nevi (moles) are also seen in younger patients as well as in adults, unlike seborrheic keratosis, which appears mostly in patients who are age 30 and older. Pigmented basal cell carcinomas usually have a waxy surface with dilated blood vessels. They may be ulcerated during later stages—a feature not seen in seborrheic keratosis. Malignant melanomas can appear in younger patients; melanomas may be nodular but usually do not have a warty, stuck-on appearance. A malignant melanoma's borders can be irregular, and it can have a variegation (inconsistency) of color. Most patients with melanoma will also report a history of a changing mole.

Management

If the diagnosis is uncertain, especially if melanoma cannot be ruled out, the patient should be referred to a dermatologist for further evaluation. A skin biopsy can be done for a more definitive diagnosis.

Treatment is warranted for those lesions that are symptomatic or are unsightly to the patient. Seborrheic keratosis may be removed using liquid nitrogen therapy or mechanical methods. Results obtained with cryosurgery (liquid nitrogen) are slightly superior to those obtained using electrodesiccation with curettage; however, the choice is generally the practitioner's preference. Liquid nitrogen may produce transient hyper- or hypopigmentation. Mechanical methods of removal include curettage and snip or shave excision. (See Therapeutic Procedures 6.2.)

Follow-Up and Referral

A follow-up visit is generally not necessary unless the liquid nitrogen does not completely remove the lesion. Any keratosis that fails to respond to liquid nitrogen should be biopsied. Should the removal of a lesion by cryotherapy from the dorsa of the hands result in blistering, the patient should return to have the blister drained. This is accomplished by puncturing one edge of the blister with a sterile needle or with a number 11 scalpel. The top of the blister should not be removed. Infection following the application of liquid nitrogen is rarc.

A biopsy or referral to a dermatologist should be done if the diagnosis is unclear and the clinician wants to rule out a pigmented basal cell carcinoma or malignant melanoma. A high index of suspicion is necessary in the diagnosis of melanoma because of its aggressive and malignant nature. Any pigmented lesion in which the clinician suspects melanoma should be evaluated by a dermatologist.

Patient Education

The clinician should inform the patient that seborrheic keratoses are a harmless and common occurrence as people age. Some people develop many lesions, whereas others will have only a few. These lesions are not caused by chronic exposure to sunlight and may develop on any exposed or protected area of the body. Color changes in these lesions are harmless, but if the clinician is unsure about the exact nature of the lesion, referral to a dermatologist is recommended.

THERAPEUTIC PROCEDURE 6.2

Removal of Seborrheic Keratoses

Liquid nitrogen

- Spray the area with liquid nitrogen or apply the liquid nitrogen with rayon–wool tipped applicators. Special care must be taken not to contaminate the reservoir of liquid nitrogen. If using applicators, dip the applicator into the reservoir only once, apply, and discard.

NOTE: It is generally preferable to lightly freeze (underfreeze) the lesion than to freeze too deeply and risk scarring. A second application may be applied at a follow-up visit if necessary. Hyper or hypopigmentation are possible sequelae of liquid nitrogen treatment (cryotherapy). (Reactive hyperpigmentation is more common in Asians.)

NOTE: Care must be taken in treating areas where the nerves are relatively superficial and can be damaged, such as the lateral aspects of the fingers and the ulnar groove of the elbows.

Currettage

- Anesthetize the area with 1% lidocaine and cleanse the area.
- Stretch the skin surrounding the lesion with the fingers of one hand.
- Using a 5-mm or 6-mm curette, scrape off the base of the keratosis with short, clean strokes.

NOTE: If the lesion is in a critical area like the face, lateral aspects of the fingers, ulnar groove in elbow (superficial nerve present), or if diagnosis is uncertain, referral to a dermatologist is recommended. If the lesion is in the hairline or groin, styptics or aluminum chloride may be used to control bleeding.

Snip or shave excision

- Anesthetize the area with 1% lidocaine and cleanse the area.
- Using iris scissors, snip off the lesion, or, using a #11 or #15 scalpel, shave off the lesion.

NOTE: Control bleeding using pressure, gel foam, styptic, or aluminum chloride, if needed.

NOTE: Treatment is for patient comfort or for cosmetic reasons only.

Skin Lesions: Premalignant

Actinic Keratosis

Actinic keratosis is the most common precancerous skin lesion found in the white population. *Actinic keratoses* are premalignant lesions that are also known as senile or solar keratosis. They are found on sun-exposed areas of skin that have been damaged from cumulative sun exposure. Left untreated, actinic keratosis can progress to squamous cell carcinoma with a latency period of 10 years. Estimates of progression to squamous cell carcinoma range from 0.25 percent to 20 percent. Another estimate is that only 1 in 1000 actinic keratotic lesions may progress to squamous cell carcinoma. However, up to 25 percent of actinic keratoses spontaneously regress without treatment. Therefore, aggressive treatment of these premalignant lesions currently remains controversial.

Epidemiology and Causes

Actinic keratosis is caused by the accumulation of damage to epithelial skin cells caused by chronic sun exposure. These keratoses are more common in men, probably as a result of occupational exposure (working outdoors). The most susceptible individuals are fair-skinned, with a history of frequent sun exposure and evidence of other signs of sun damage, such as freckles, senile lentigines (liver spots), wrinkles, and uneven pigmentation. Actinic keratosis lesions are found predominantly in older adults (older than age 50); however, occasionally they are seen in young adults with fair skin. Renal transplant patients have also been found to have an increased tendency to develop actinic keratoses.

Pathophysiology

Cumulative damage from ultraviolet radiation in sunlight causes damage to the DNA in epithelial cells. The primary lesions of actinic keratosis consist of macules or plaques that are poorly circumscribed. Secondary lesions appear erythematous and scaly. Areas of skin that have actinic keratosis feel rough to the touch due to hyperkeratosis and have been likened to feeling like sandpaper. With further ultraviolet light exposure, continued cumulative DNA damage may lead to malignant transformation of epidermal cellular clones. Actinic keratoses that progress to squamous cell carcinoma tend not to be very aggressive unless they occur on the lip.

Clinical Presentation

Subjective

The typical patient is a middle-aged or older adult who complains of an irritated rough or scaly rash. Some patients also complain of pruritus, tenderness, or a stinging sensation in one or several lesions. Some patients are asymptomatic and will only complain of cosmetic concerns or uneasiness about a potential malignancy. The lesion is also typically found on a fair-skinned patient. These patients usually have some Celtic background (Irish, Scottish, English) and are light-haired (blond or red-haired) and blue-eyed. They also tend to freckle easily and sunburn.

Objective

The lesions of actinic keratosis appear reddened, scaly, rough, or have an uneven surface. The hyperkeratosis of these lesions is characteristically hard or spiny. Actinic keratoses are found in areas of skin that have been chronically exposed to the sun, such as the face, ears, back of the neck, neckline, dorsum of the arms, and (in women) the dorsum of the legs. Palpation is generally the best diagnostic tool to use because of the typical sandpaper-like texture of the lesions. Actinic keratoses are small (0.2 mm to 5 mm) papules that can be flesh-colored or slightly hyperpigmented. Actinic keratosis lesions are predominantly found on the cheeks, forehead, forearms, and dorsal surface of the hands. In older men, they are also predominant on the ears and balding scalp.

Diagnostic Reasoning

Diagnostic Tests

Diagnosis is by history and physical examination; laboratory testing is generally not indicated. Palpating the lesions is key to the diagnosis by feeling for the texture. Lesions are better recognized by palpation than inspection.

Differential Diagnosis

Skin lesions that can mimic actinic keratosis include squamous cell carcinoma, seborrheic keratosis, and verruca plana (flat warts). Squamous cell carcinoma is characterized by an indurated plaque or nodule that is eroded or ulcerated and has a thickened scale. The lesion is also found on sun-exposed skin, as is actinic keratosis. What differentiates squamous cell carcinoma from actinic keratosis is the induration and ulceration. Seborrheic keratosis lesions are highly pigmented (brown to black) and have a warty, stuck-on appearance. They can appear on both sun-exposed and protected skin. Verruca plana is caused by the human papilloma virus (HPV) and appears as multiple flesh-colored to light brown warts that are from 1 to 5 mm in size. Their color and smaller size distinguish them from actinic keratosis.

Management

There is no solid evidence that removal of all actinic keratosis lesions on a patient is effective in the prevention of skin cancer. Indeed, only 1 in 1000 actinic keratosis lesions will progress to squamous cell carcinoma. However, it is standard dermatologic practice to remove most actinic keratosis lesions. Because the lesions reside in the epithelium, therapies that separate the epidermis from the dermis are most effective and do not leave scars.

Two methods are currently available to the primary-care provider—topical therapy and cryosurgery. Treatment may also include a combination using both methods. The dermatologist may also perform superficial or tangential surgical removal of the lesions.

Topical Therapy

Topical application of 5-fluorouracil (5-FU) cream (Efudex, Carac) is the treatment of choice for eradicating actinic keratoses on the face and for patients with multiple lesions. 5-Fluorouracil is selective for affecting only sun-damaged cells and causing little to no damage of surrounding healthy skin. The cream is applied to the lesion bid for an average treatment time of 3 weeks. (The eyelids, folds of the nose, and lips should be avoided.) Healing takes from 2 to 4 weeks and is accomplished by the replication of epidermal and adnexal cells. Patients treated with 5-FU frequently become noncompliant because the inflammatory effect (destruction of the lesion) leaves raw, tender, reddened skin in its place. If the lesion or lesions do not respond to one treatment with 5-FU, then these lesions must be evaluated for potential carcinoma with a skin biopsy. Some new evidence is showing that tretinoin (Retin-A) when used in combination with 5-FU may increase effectiveness and shorten the length of therapy. Use of 5-FU during pregnancy has not been established.

Imiquimod 5 percent cream (Aldara) may be used on face and scalp lesions and is applied three times weekly for 8 weeks. Other topical treatments which have been used include topical chemotherapies such as diclofenac 3 percent in 2.5 percent hyaluronan gel (Solaraze) applied bid for 60 to 90 days, and topical retinoids such as adapalene 0.1 to 0.3 percent gel (applied to lesions qd for 4 weeks, and then increased to bid). More extensive outcome data is needed to fully establish these agents as treatment options. Moreover, side effects include erythema, pruritis, rash, and xerosis (dry skin). Some topical chemotherapeutic treatments have even been used in conjunction with phototherapy, such as aminolevulinic acid (Levulan Kerastick) in conjunction with either blue or red wavelength light. These specialized treatments typically give improved cosmesis over the more commonly used method of cryosurgery and may be preferred for facial lesions. In addition, they only require a 2-day course.

Cryosurgery

Before cryosurgery is done, informed consent must be obtained from the patient. Cryosurgery with liquid nitrogen is used most frequently for patients with solitary or few lesions. (See Therapeutic Procedures 6.3.)

With cryosurgery, the practitioner must rely entirely on clinical diagnosis, because tissue is destroyed by freezing—therefore, there is no specimen available for pathology analysis. Liquid nitrogen is a rapid and effective treatment for eradicating actinic keratoses, especially in patients with one to few lesions. The liquid nitrogen probe should be applied firmly to the lesion for 10 to 15 seconds and repeated twice in one visit. The lesions will crust over and generally disappear in 10 to 14 days. A possible drawback to this procedure is the potential for hypopigmentation: In some patients a white spot appears at the treated site.

THERAPEUTIC PROCEDURE 6.3

Performing Cryosurgery for Actinic Keratoses

- Liquid nitrogen using a cotton-tipped applicator, which is preferred as it causes minimal damage to the dermis.
- Using liquid nitrogen, freeze each lesion for 10–15 seconds. It may be necessary to repeat the freezing cycle a second time. The more pressure is applied to the cotton swab, the deeper the "freeze ball."
- The "freeze balls" should be approximately one and a half times as wide as they are deep.
- If in doubt, it is better to underfreeze and to retreat lesions than to overfreeze them and leave a scar or hypopigmentation (if damage to the dermis is avoided, scarring will not occur).
- Any lesion that does not respond to liquid nitrogen must be biopsied.

NOTE: If diagnosis of skin lesion is in doubt, refer to dermatologist for possible skin biopsy. The treated area will become red and swollen a few hours after treatment. A serous or blood-filled blister forms and will crust and disappear in 10–14 days. The patient should be advised not to cover the blister with any bandages, and to leave the blister alone. The blister will protect the treated area until it is healed.

Curettage

Finally, lesions which are isolated and thick may be amenable to surgical curettage or shave removal, particularly when located on the dorsal surfaces of the upper extremities. However, there are very little data which speak to the efficacy of this approach, and it is typically not considered first-line intervention. Importantly, however, this is the only method of actinic keratosis removal that produces an intact biopsy sample available for histologic examination and diagnostic confirmation. In addition, this method may be more appropriate for immunocompromised patients.

Follow-Up and Referral

Patients on 5-FU should be followed up in 2 to 3 weeks, or during completion of treatment. Adverse effects of the medication, compliance issues, and effectiveness of treatment should be noted at this time. Any skin lesions that remain after treatment with 5-FU cream for 2 to 3 weeks must be biopsied for pathologic examination. Patients treated with cryosurgery are reevaluated in 2 weeks. Patients who have had excision biopsy by a dermatologist are usually seen again in 2 weeks.

Any actinic keratosis lesion that does not respond to treatment should be referred to a dermatologist for further evaluation, including the need for a skin biopsy, even for superficial lesions. A dermatologist may remove multiple superficial lesions with an acid followed by pulsed light laser therapy or photodynamic therapy. This is effective on the face and does not result in the hypopigmentation that may result from cryotherapy. An added benefit is one of aesthetic skin rejuvenation.

Patient Education

Regardless of the method of treatment, the patient should be educated regarding the need for using sunscreen and wearing of protective clothing such as a hat or a shirt with long sleeves. The hallmark of actinic keratosis management must actually center around prevention—avoidance of excessive sun exposure is key to avoiding development of these premalignant lesions and their cancerous sequelae. In addition, the patient can also be taught the signs and symptoms of melanoma by using the ABCDE mnemonic: A = asymmetry, B = irregular borders, C = color change, D = diameter larger than a pencil eraser, E = elevation from a flat lesion to a raised one.

Patients treated with 5-FU should be warned that exposure to sunlight during treatment can exacerbate the inflammatory effect of the medicine. The clinician should instruct the patient that if erosions develop while using 5-FU cream, petroleum jelly can be applied to provide comfort, but the treatment must be continued for a total of 10 to 14 days. Patients should be warned to avoid prolonged sunlight exposure during and after treatment. A good quality sun block should be worn after treatment to prevent future damage to the skin.

Patients treated with cryosurgery should be informed that bandages are not necessary after treatment and actually impede healing. If blister formation results, the patient should be instructed to return to the office so the blister can be drained. The patient should be advised to avoid irritation of the treated lesion with clothing or jewelry. Showering and the use of makeup are permissible. The patient should be taught the signs and symptoms of infection (e.g., redness, purulent discharge, heat). Infection is a rare occurrence after cryosurgery.

Skin Lesions: Malignant

Malignant Melanoma

Malignant melanoma is the most deadly of all skin cancers. *Melanoma* is malignancy of the skin that arises from epidermal melanocytes. Melanocytes produce *melanin,* a brown-black pigment that is responsible for skin, hair, and eye color. Almost all melanomas arise from the skin (more than 90 percent), but a few melanomas originate from the eye (uveal melanoma), and very few (less than 4 percent) do not have a primary site.

Types of melanoma are *superficial spreading* (70 to 85 percent—characterized by extensive lateral or radial growth prior to vertical invasion), *nodular* (15 to 30 percent—characterized by vertical growth only), *lentigo maligna* (5 percent—an in situ form that may persist for years prior to vertical extension), and *acral lentiginous* (2 to 8 percent—a particularly aggressive form most common in darker-skinned patients, especially when appearing on the hands or feet).

Although the majority of skin cancers in this country are basal cell carcinoma (the most numerous type) and squamous cell carcinoma, melanoma is responsible for 75 percent of all skin cancer deaths Melanoma, if discovered early enough, is a highly curable malignancy, but if the melanoma extends beyond 4 mm in depth, then prognosis is extremely poor. A 75 percent mortality rate is associated with this stage. Therefore, the role of primary-care clinicians in screening for this dreaded skin cancer is important and cannot be overemphasized. Screening programs that result in early diagnosis are important weapons in the armamentarium against this dreaded disease, both by health-care professionals and the public. The American Cancer Society's ABCDE mnemonic (Table 6.21) is an easy tool for the clinician to remember and use to teach patients how to recognize potential melanomas and dysplastic nevi, the precursor lesion of melanoma, at an early stage.

Epidemiology and Causes

The incidence of melanoma in this country has been rising rapidly over the past few years. Melanoma is uncommon in blacks and Asians. It is estimated that almost 8000 patients die of invasive melanoma annually. It is estimated to be the fifth most common cancer in men and the seventh most common in women.

Several factors have been identified that increase an individual's risks of melanoma (see Risk Factors 6.2). Exposure and sensitivity to sunlight remains one of the most widely recognized risk factors. A disproportionate number of melanoma deaths occur among whites, particularly fair-skinned individuals who sunburn easily. Whites (Caucasians) who are at highest risk come from Celtic (Irish, Scottish, English) backgrounds and have light hair (espe-

Table 6.21 The ABCDEs of Assessing Skin Cancer

A	Asymmetry
B	Borders are irregular
C	Color change or color variegation
D	Diameter larger than a pencil eraser (>6 mm)
E	Elevation from a flat lesion to a raised one

RISK FACTORS 6.2

Malignant Melanoma

Age	Risk increases with age
Skin, eye, hair color	Fair, blue eyes, red or blond hair
Personal history	History of skin cancer
	History of dysplastic nevi; congenital nevi >20 mm
	History of blistering sunburn before age 20
	History of immunosuppression
Family history	History of melanoma
Environmental history	Excessive exposure to ultraviolet radiation

cially red hair), light eyes, and freckles. The ability of the skin to freckle in response to sun exposure is thought to be a marker of susceptibility to melanoma, although stronger risk factors for melanoma exist.

Recent research into the genetic component of melanoma as well as the presence of dysplastic nevi has found a relationship between dysplastic nevi, family history, and the development of melanoma. The finding of dysplastic nevus (one or more atypical moles) or any other type of skin cancer (such as basal cell carcinoma or squamous cell carcinoma) is thought to increase one's risks of melanoma. The number of nevi (moles) normally peaks during young adulthood (ages 20 to 25), then gradually decreases after age 50. Large numbers of nevi on an individual who is older than age 50 is considered to be a strong marker for increased risk of melanoma. It is estimated that 7 percent of the white population has at least one atypical nevus; many individuals have numerous nevi that should be monitored closely.

The combination of a history of a first-degree relative with melanoma, combined with the presence of one or more dysplastic nevi, increases the chances of developing melanoma by up to 50 percent compared to the general public. Individuals in this population tend to develop multiple primary lesions at a younger age than individuals with other melanomas. In addition, large-sized nevi (more than 20 mm) are believed to be associated with increased melanoma risk. Currently, lifetime risk among all populations is estimated at 1 in 75, with fully one-third of all cases occurring in persons younger than age 45.

Pediatric overexposure to UV rays, especially a history of one or more blistering sunburns before age 20, has been linked to a dramatic increase in lifetime risk of developing melanoma. The effect of accumulated sunburn in addition to genetic predisposition may not be seen until years later, as the incidence of malignant melanoma in children is low. Intermittent intense exposures (e.g., those that may occur in occupational groups such as farmers) that result in blistering sunburn appear to be associated more with increased melanoma risk than chronic exposure.

Pathophysiology

A combination of UV exposure and genetic susceptibility are believed to be the most common mechanisms for developing melanoma. Studies have linked UV radiation, particularly UVB rays, to genetic mutations in DNA in susceptible individuals, resulting in the development of abnormal pigmented lesions (dysplastic nevi). Genetic predisposition to melanoma appears to be the result of the presence of a mutated or absent tumor suppressor gene. Abnormalities have been mapped to chromosomes 1 and 9. In particular, mutations in chromosomal region 9p21 which encodes the tumor suppressor gene *CDKN2A* that produces the protein p16 have been observed in a large proportion of both familial as well as spontaneous melanomas. Germline mutations in the gene *CDK4* have also been observed. Individuals in these susceptible groups tend to develop melanoma at multiple primary sites at an earlier age. Another strong genetic association is observed in the autosomal recessive condition xeroderma pigmentosum. Persons affected with this inherited disorder lack a critical DNA repair mechanism which corrects UV light-associated cross-linked DNA nucleotides. This results in multiple DNA breaks in response to cumulative UV light exposure and a resultant high level of sun-associated skin cancers.

Atypical nevi are precursors to malignant melanoma. They differ histologically from benign nevi in that they are disorganized and carry higher potential for transformation into malignant tissue. Initially, the tumor remains confined to the epidermis. If left untreated, it spreads into the subcutaneous fat. Metastasis occurs into the regional lymph nodes and occasionally into distant sites such as the lungs, liver, bone, brain, and other viscera. Microscopic lesions of superficial spreading-type melanoma have large, atypical pigmented cells of variable colors in the epidermis and the papillary dermis, and lymphocytes. Nodular melanoma lesions have multiple tumor cells that form a nodule in the dermis, with invasion to the deeper dermal layers. Metastases to distant sites result when tumors invade through dermal lymphatics or blood vessels. The most commonly affected target organs are the lung, liver, and brain.

In the absence of metastasis, the four primary prognostic factors for melanoma are patient age and gender, tumor thickness, and tumor location. Worse prognoses are seen in older men with thicker tumors located in an axial distribution, as opposed to on the extremities. In addition, the relative importance of certain prognostic factors also depends on tumor stage. In earlier disease limited to the skin, tumor thickness and the presence of ulceration are key.

However, in more advanced disease, along with the presence of ulceration, the degree of nodal involvement is the most important factor.

Clinical Presentation

Subjective

The typical patient is an adult who is concerned about a large mole that has changed in appearance. A change in characteristics of a mole is a frequent observation made by melanoma patients. Some patients who come in do so in response to a concerned family member, typically a spouse, who has advised them to have the mole checked. The patient typically will report having had the same mole for many years. A family history of melanoma or skin cancer may be reported by some patients. There are usually no symptoms associated with the majority of cases of melanoma; however, some patients present with a pruritic, ulcerated, or bleeding mole.

Objective

Most melanomas appear on sun-exposed areas of skin. The back and the neck are the most common sites in men, and the legs are more common in women. In blacks and Asians, the feet, fingers, the nailbed, the eye (uveal tract), and mucous membranes are more common sites.

Melanoma often presents as an asymmetric lesion with an irregular border, notching, and a diameter greater than 6 mm. The tumor often exhibits variegation in color, with admixtures of blue, red, tan, brown, black, and white. Rarely, tumors appear as amelanotic. Early nodular tumors, for example, are typically flat and may lack most of the typical characteristics of melanoma. As the tumor advances, an increase in thickness causes elevation into a firm nodule (in nodular melanoma). Atypical nevi bear many of the same characteristics of a true melanoma, including irregular, ill-defined borders; color variegation; and large size (more than 6 mm). The emphasis on larger lesion size as an increased risk factor for melanoma is not always accurate, because early melanomas can be smaller than 6 mm in diameter. Distinguishing between malignant melanoma and benign nevi can be difficult and often requires a skin biopsy.

Nail bed or subungual melanoma may be observed in older patients and is most commonly found on the thumb or great toe. This variant of acral lentiginous melanoma may present similarly to an ungual fungal infection, as discoloration of the nail bed known as longitudinal melanonychia may distort the nail itself. Posterior nail bed involvement called Hutchinson's sign is an ominous physical finding associated with advanced disease.

Diagnostic Reasoning

Diagnostic Tests

Suspicious lesions should be biopsied under local anesthesia by a dermatologist. Excisional biopsy is the preferred method if melanoma is suspected, because measurement of thickness can be made along with staging (using Clark's level of invasion) and prognosis. If the pathology report indicates only atypical nevi, removal of the lesion by excisional biopsy is sufficient treatment. A patient who has dysplastic nevi should receive regular skin surveillance. Skin exams are usually done at 6-month intervals by the dermatologist. A patient diagnosed with melanoma should be referred to a dermatologist or oncologist for excision of the melanoma and its margins.

Subsequent testing may include a lymph-node biopsy via computed tomography (CT)-guided needle aspiration. Sentinel node biopsy and lymphatic drainage mapping have been shown to identify more occult metastasis, employing a technique that identifies the lymph node that specifically drains the area of skin that contains the melanoma. This node, called the *sentinel node,* is excised and examined for melanoma cells. If any cancer cells are present, the remaining nodes in the area are dissected. If biopsy of the sentinel node is negative, metastasis is unlikely and recurrence rates are very low. If metastatic disease is suspected, a thorough physical exam, laboratory tests, x-ray films, and CT scans are done to identify distant sites of metastases.

Differential Diagnosis

Differentiating between melanoma and benign or premalignant lesions can prove challenging, even for dermatologists. Although the majority of atypical nevi and melanomas fit the ABCDEs of melanoma, an occasional lesion will escape early detection. The differential diagnosis for melanoma includes pigmented skin lesions such as benign nevi, solar lentigines, and seborrheic keratoses. Seborrheic keratoses are benign lesions that are common in elderly and older adult patients. The lesions are light to dark brown and appear as soft, wart-like growths, located mainly on the trunk. In contrast, melanoma is usually located on sun-exposed areas such as the neck, the back, or the legs. Solar lentigines (liver spots) are pigmented (light to dark brown) macules that appear on sun-exposed areas like the dorsum of the hands and arms. Benign nevi (moles) are round to oval, with regular borders; most are less than 5 mm in diameter. The color is evenly distributed in a benign nevus; it is asymptomatic.

Management

A high index of suspicion is necessary because it is often hard to distinguish atypical nevi from melanoma or from normal nevi. If a clinician suspects possible melanoma or dysplastic nevi, then referral to a dermatologist is necessary. If the melanoma lesion is discovered early enough (at less than 4 mm in diameter and with superficial involvement only), the chance of a complete cure with excision is good. Management will depend upon the staging of the lesion. (See Table 6.22 for classification systems.) In situ melanomas require excisional margins of at least 0.5 cm. Melanomas measuring less than 2 mm in thickness require

Table 6.22 Skin Cancer Classification

The American Joint Committee on Cancer (AJCC) has an ongoing collaborative staging system in process. (http://www.cancerstaging.net)
The TNM (tumor, node, metastasis) system adopted by the AJCC uses both Clark and Breslow's methods to clinically stage malignant melanomas (MM). The extent of the tumor is determined only after excision.
The presence or absence of lymph node involvement is the most important predictor of survival.

Two different classifications used to describe tumors

Clark's Levels—describes the lesion based upon the invading depth into the dermis and subcutaneous fat and is related to the metastatic potential of the lesion

Level I (in situ)	Does not penetrate the basement membrane
Level II	Extends through the basement membrane and into the papillary dermis
Level III	Extends into the reticular dermis
Level IV	Extends into the subcutaneous fat

Breslow's method—describes tumor thickness by measuring the distance from the dermis to the deepest level of involvement. The thicker the lesion, the higher the incidence for metastasis. Measured in millimeters (mm).

at least a 1 cm circumferential surgical margin, while thicker tumors need at least 2-cm margins. Lymph node dissection is required when there is evidence of draining lymph node involvement on clinical exam, but its ability to improve outcomes is unclear when performed empirically.

In addition to excision of the lesion with its margins, patients with metastatic disease are treated with several modalities. One of the main treatments is chemotherapy with dacarbazine, cisplatin, and vincristine, or a combination of these agents. Only 15 to 30 percent of patients respond to chemotherapy with a reduction in tumor size. Unfortunately, the response to chemotherapy is typically short term. Less than 5 percent of patients will experience a remission of their disease. If the melanoma is located on a limb, then high-dose chemotherapy via isolated limb perfusion is available. In this technique, the circulation of the affected limb is isolated by tourniquet at the root of the limb. High-dose chemotherapy is infused and is limited to the affected limb only, minimizing adverse systemic effects from the chemotherapy.

External beam radiation to treat melanoma is usually reserved for palliative treatment. For metastatic lesions of the lung, brain, or viscera that cause pressure on tissue, radiation therapy is used to reduce the tumor's size and provide relief from pain.

Research trials into the effectiveness of adjuvant therapies to prevent recurrence of melanoma have demonstrated mixed results. Administration of biologic therapy such as high-dose interferon and interleukin in high-risk patients (to prevent recurrence) has shown some promise. Combination therapy with both biologic therapy and chemotherapy is also being studied.

Recent advances in the knowledge on the mechanisms of immune function have provided new and innovative ways to combat cancer of all types. Currently, therapies to correct gene mutations that often lead to cancer are being explored. It is hoped that targeting specific mutated genes responsible for tumor suppression (or growth) will provide promising therapies for all cancers. In addition, vaccines that stimulate immune function against tumors are being developed and tested. Despite chemotherapy, the patient with extensive metastasis has a life expectancy of about 6 to 8 months.

Follow-Up and Referral

The patient identified as at increased risk for developing melanoma should be referred to a dermatologist for increased surveillance. The patient who wishes to participate in clinical trials for melanoma can obtain information on current studies from the oncologist. Hospice and palliative care should be offered for consideration to the patient and his or her family.

Patient Education

Prevention of all skin cancers should start early during infancy, especially in individuals with Celtic backgrounds or with a positive family history for skin cancer. Early detection is made easier to remember with the ABCDE mnemonic. The patient should avoid staying out in the sun at the hottest part of the day, sun block or high-factor sunscreens should be worn, and hats or headgear are useful in helping to protect the scalp and the back of the neck. Wearing loose-fitting long-sleeved shirts and pants provides some protection from the sun and is equivalent to wearing a sunscreen.

Survivors of melanoma need to be informed of their increased risk of a second primary tumor or of recurrence of the previous lesion. Any change or any new pigmented skin lesion should be reported to the patient's primary-care clinician and dermatologist. Likewise, patients should be urged to report any swelling in the lymph nodes of the neck, axilla, or groin area.

Non-melanoma Skin Cancers

Basal cell carcinoma is a malignant tumor of the skin that originates from the basal cells of the epidermis. It is a slow-growing and locally invasive tumor that rarely metastasizes. It represents the beginning of a continuum of skin cancers in both severity and mortality. *Squamous cell carcinoma,* a malignant tumor originating from the keratinocytes, can invade the dermis and occasionally metastasize to distant sites. Together, basal cell and squamous cell carcinoma are the most common non-melanoma skin cancers in humans. Avoidance of excessive sun exposure is an important factor in preventing these skin cancers. In addition, screening programs are important in the early recognition and diagnosis of these skin cancers because they are highly curable when discovered in their early stages.

Epidemiology and Causes

The incidence of basal and squamous cell carcinoma is expected to rise in the United States during the next decade because of the increase in the size of the older adult population and longer life expectancy. The exact incidence of basal cell and squamous cell carcinoma is not yet known, because physicians are not required to report cases of non-melanoma skin cancers. It is estimated that 900,000 new cases of basal and squamous cell carcinoma were diagnosed in 1998, with 1900 deaths attributed to non-melanoma skin cancers.

Basal cell carcinoma is the most common malignancy seen in humans, accounting for approximately 75 percent of all skin cancers and 25 percent of all cancers. Rarely, basal cell carcinoma results from basal cell nevus syndrome, an inherited autosomal dominant disorder. Patients with this disorder tend to have multiple sites of basal cell carcinoma at a younger age; it is associated with bone cysts, palmar pits, and frontal bossing.

Squamous cell carcinoma is the second most common skin cancer, accounting for an estimated 20 percent of all skin cancers. Bowen's disease is an intradermal squamous cell carcinoma that can be induced by exposure to inorganic trivalent arsenic or inhaled mustard gas, in addition to chronic sun exposure. It affects mostly older white males.

The most important risk factor for both basal cell and squamous carcinoma is chronic accumulated sun exposure. Therefore, these skin cancers are typically seen in older adults and elderly patients. In particular, mid-range ultraviolet light in the UVB part of the spectrum is believed to be more cancer-inducing than UVA rays. Individuals most at risk are those patients of Celtic background (Irish, Scottish, English) who are fair-haired (red-haired or blond), blue-eyed, freckled, and sunburn easily. In addition, men are twice as likely to develop basal cell carcinoma and three times as likely to develop squamous skin cancers compared to women. Other conditions that increase the risk of squamous skin carcinoma include immunosuppression, a history of exposure to ionizing radiation, exposure to arsenic and polycyclic aromatic hydrocarbons (paint thinners, organic solvents), treatment with psoralens and UV light (PUVA therapy, used for psoriasis), and infection with oncogenic human papilloma virus (HPV). Squamous cell carcinomas are also seen with increased frequency in areas of damaged skin resulting from chronic inflammation, burns, old scars, or chronic ulcers. (See Risk Factors 6.3.)

Pathophysiology

The majority of basal and squamous cell carcinomas are the result of DNA damage in skin cells that have been exposed to many years of UV radiation from sunlight. The damage is cumulative and is mediated primarily by defects in DNA repair mechanisms in response to mutational cross-linking by UV light. Such cumulative damage is particularly important in the development of basal cell carcinoma, particularly within skin containing a high concentration of sebaceous glands. Several forms of basal cell carcinoma are seen clinically, including nodular, sclerosing, and superficial forms. The nodulo–ulcerative type is the most common, with well-differentiated tumor cells which may extend from the dermal–epidermal interface into the dermis and subcutaneous fat. Superficial basal cell carcinoma appears similar to dermatitis with erythema and scaling bordered by a fine rim. The origins of these tumors appear to be multifocal, with multiple small nodules arising from different epidermal foci. The sclerosing or morpheaform type of basal cell carcinoma

RISK FACTORS 6.3

Non-Melanoma Skin Cancer

Age	Risk increases with age
Gender	Male
Skin, eye, hair color	Fair; tendency to tan poorly and burn quickly Blue eyes, red or blond hair
Personal history	History of skin cancer History of basal cell nevus syndrome History of precancerous lesions, including actinic keratosis History of burn scars or areas of skin damaged by chronic inflammation or ulcers History of immunosuppression
Environmental history	Excessive exposure to ultraviolet radiation Exposure to arsenic, polycyclic aromatic hydrocarbons, or radiation

is highly aggressive with a high rate of recurrence, presenting as a white plaque with palpable fibrosis and poorly circumscribed margins. Histologically, these tumors consist of spindle cells invading the dermal skin layer. If left untreated, basal cell carcinomas continue to grow and invade surrounding cartilage, bone, and soft tissues. Basal cell carcinomas rarely metastasize to distant sites, however.

In contrast, squamous cell carcinoma is considered more dangerous than basal cell carcinoma because of its faster rate of growth and its more aggressive tendency to metastasize. The precursor lesion of most squamous cell carcinomas is a skin lesion called actinic keratosis, a relatively common finding in older white patients. Actinic keratosis results from accumulated chronic sun exposure and is found only on sun-exposed skin. Actinic keratoses are premalignant lesions involving the uppermost layer of the epidermis and have a very low potential for malignancy (estimated at 1 to 5 percent chance). In situ squamous cell carcinoma (Bowen's disease) involves the full thickness of the epidermis and is the earliest form of squamous cell carcinoma. Interestingly, in contrast to basal cell carcinoma, more recent excessive UV light exposure, rather than cumulative lifetime exposure, correlates best with the development of squamous cell skin cancer, particularly in areas with few sebaceous glands. Invasive squamous cell carcinoma is characterized by penetration through the epidermis and into the dermis, with a rate of metastasis of approximately 5 percent, primarily to the regional lymph nodes. Lesions that metastasize at a higher rate include those located on the lips, the ear, or at sites of trauma such as old scars and chronic wounds (ulcers). Larger lesions (more than 2 cm in diameter or more than 4 mm in depth) and patients on immunosuppressive therapy also have a higher rate of metastasis.

As observed in melanoma, any underlying condition affecting the capacity for DNA repair increases the risk of developing basal cell and squamous cell carcinoma, for example, the rare autosomal recessive condition xeroderma pigmentosum in which individuals lose the ability to repair UV light-induced DNA cross-linking damage, resulting in multiple DNA breaks and malignant transformation of skin cells. UV light exposure has also been correlated with mutations of specific oncogenes and tumor suppressor genes, including *p53* (seen in more than half of all basal cell carcinomas and up to 90 percent of squamous cell carcinomas) and the human patched gene. Such mutations result in dysregulated programmed cell death (apoptosis) and uncontrolled proliferation of epidermal cellular clones.

Several other mechanisms also contribute to the development of keratinocyte and basal cell skin cancers. Epidermal antigen-presenting Langerhans cells suffer direct damage from UV radiation, compromising the ability of the immune system to recognize and clear tumor antigen-expressing cancer cells. Systemic glucocorticoids also contribute to immunosuppression and have been shown in some studies to more than double the risk of non-melanoma skin cancer. In fact, intact immunosurveillance is key to the prevention of cutaneous carcinomas, as basal cell carcinoma is 10 times more likely to develop in chronically immunosuppressed organ transplant recipients, while squamous cell carcinoma is up to 250 times more likely to occur. Although these tumors tend to develop after at least 2 years post-transplant, they are more aggressive, more likely to occur at multiple sites, and begin to develop at a younger age than in nontransplanted, immunocompetent individuals.

Several types of proinflammatory cytokines have been identified in affected skin including TNF-α and IL-10. Prostaglandin synthesis also appears critical to this process, and selective cyclooxygenase-2 (COX-2) inhibitors have been shown to confer a protective effect against basal cell and squamous cell carcinoma in mouse models. Infection by the human papilloma virus (HPV) is well associated with the development of anogenital squamous cell carcinoma—particularly by serotypes 16 and 18. In immunosuppressed individuals, the development of cutaneous warts and non-melanoma skin cancers appears to be correlated. In addition, keratoacanthoma (a fast-growing hyperkeratotic nodular lesion indistinguishable from well-differentiated squamous cell carcinoma) has also been associated with HPV infection. However, the specific role of HPV in additional forms of keratinocyte skin cancers remains controversial, and further research to explore this relationship is ongoing.

Clinical Presentation

Subjective

A typical patient with non-melanoma skin carcinoma is an adult or elderly patient who presents with complaints of a spot or a bump that is getting larger or a sore that is not healing. The skin lesion may be pruritic or asymptomatic.

Objective

Basal cell carcinomas typically appear in areas of skin that are chronically exposed to the sun, such as the face, ears, cheeks, nose, and the neck. Nodulo–ulcerative basal cell carcinomas are characterized by elevated papules that have a pearly appearance, with some crusting. When the crusts are removed, a small amount of bleeding ensues. On close examination, telangiectatic blood vessels are seen on the border of the lesion. A central ulceration is seen during the later stages of basal cell carcinoma lesions. Basal cell carcinoma lesions may be the same color as the patient's skin or have areas of variegated color like blue, black, or brown.

Squamous cell carcinomas are typically found on sun-exposed areas, such as the lips, the tips of ears, nose, the upper cheeks, the scalp (in bald men), the dorsa of the hands and forearms, and the shins in women. Smokers are prone to cancerous lesions on the lips and tongue. The most common presentation of squamous cell carcinoma is a firm papule with a scaly (keratotic) rough surface with irregular borders. These lesions may even present as cutaneous horns, with columnar hyperkeratosis atop an erythematous base. Later on, the surfaces of squamous cell carcinoma lesions tend to bleed easily (become friable) with minor trauma and appear eroded with ulcerations. The typical lesion of Bowen's disease appears as a solitary, slowly enlarging erythematous, red-brown hyperkeratotic plaque that has a slight scaling and minimal crusting. Similar lesions in the anogenital region known as Bowenoid papulosis have been associated with oncogenic HPV strains.

The presence of actinic keratosis lesions on patients is considered a marker for excessive sun exposure. Recognition of actinic keratosis, a precancerous skin lesion, is important because treatment during this stage is very simple (see p 217). Typical actinic keratosis lesions appear on sun-exposed surfaces and are pink to red or sometimes brown. In contrast to basal cell carcinomas, where only one or a few lesions are present at a time in most patients, actinic keratosis lesions typically are present in greater numbers. Lesions vary in size from 2 mm to 1 cm in diameter. These numerous lesions are also located on chronically sun-exposed areas such as the face and the head, the back of the neck, the dorsum of the hands and arms, and the upper shoulders.

Diagnostic Reasoning

Diagnostic Tests

Suspicious lesions (if not located on the face) can be biopsied by an experienced primary-care clinician or referred to a dermatologist. Because basal cell carcinomas rarely metastasize, staging of the lesions is not necessary. Squamous cell carcinomas, however, have a higher rate of metastasis and may require staging based on the pathologist's report. Other important factors that determine staging include tumor characteristics, spread to regional lymph nodes, and metastasis to other organs (Table 6.23).

Differential Diagnosis

The differential diagnosis of non-melanoma skin cancer includes seborrheic keratosis, eczema, solar lentigo, and actinic keratosis. In contrast to squamous and basal cell carcinoma, seborrheic keratosis lesions predominantly appear on nonexposed areas such as the trunk in older adult patients and do not appear erythematous or scaly. A patient with eczema will report an atopic history and recurrence of lesions on the same location that resolve with treatment on steroid creams in 2 weeks. Solar lentigo are found in older adults on sun-exposed areas of skin; these "liver spots" appear as multiple smooth, flat brown macules (like enlarged freckles) that are from 1 cm to 3 cm in size.

Table 6.23 Staging of Non-melanoma Skin Cancers

Stage	Criteria
0	Squamous cell carcinoma in situ, or Bowen's disease Involves only the epidermis
I	Less than 2 cm deep No spread to lymph nodes or organs
II	More than 2 cm deep No spread to lymph nodes or organs
III	Spread to muscle, bone, or cartilage, and/or regional lymph nodes No spread to organs
IV	Spread to organs, e.g., lungs or brain

Management

Management of non-melanoma skin cancers is dependent on several factors: size and depth of the invasion, location, cosmetic concerns, and metastasis to other sites. Squamous cell carcinoma has an overall rate of remission of up to 90 percent after therapy.

Almost all cases of basal cell carcinoma and most cases of squamous cell carcinoma require only simple excision under local anesthesia. Some primary qcare practitioners and dermatologists elect excisional biopsy at the time of initial diagnosis; this procedure is both diagnostic and curative. Alternative methods for removal of small basal and squamous cell carcinomas include electrodesiccation and curettage, cryosurgery (liquid nitrogen), and laser surgery.

Mohs microsurgery has the highest cure rate for both basal and squamous cell carcinomas. This precise technique involves the surgical removal and simultaneous microscopic examination of small layers of skin, with removal of only the smallest amount of tissue necessary to eradicate the tumor. This technique involves less scarring and is particularly suited for treatment of tumors in places of cosmetic importance, such as the face. Skin grafting may be necessary in addition to tumor removal.

In addition to surgical excision, lymph node dissection and systemic chemotherapy are used to treat large and invasive squamous cell carcinomas that have metastasized. External beam radiation is used as the primary treatment on tumors that are large or located in areas of skin that make surgery difficult, or in elderly or debilitated patients who are poor surgical candidates. External beam therapy is also used as adjuvant therapy in lesions with high risk of recurrence or in cancers that have metastasized.

Topical therapies are also used for superficial forms of basal cell carcinoma, including imiquimod cream (used five times weekly), topical 5-fluorouracil (5-FU), and photodynamic treatment (used for both nodular and superficial forms) utilizing a photosensitizer with blue wavelength phototherapy to create reactive oxygen species. Similar approaches are being used for squamous cell carcinoma, for example, imiquimod for in situ Bowen's disease. Premalignant actinic keratosis is also typically treated with top-

Table 6.24 Patient Education: Skin Self-Exam

Once a month, perform a skin self-exam. Record your initial exam, then note any changes with each subsequent exam. Use the table below as a guide for your exam.

Head	Looking in a mirror, carefully inspect your head. Using a comb or hair dryer, carefully part your hair and inspect your scalp.
Face and neck	Looking in a mirror, carefully inspect your entire face and neck, including the nose, lips, and ears
Arms and hands	Holding up each arm, carefully inspect each arm and hand, including the underarms and back of your upper arms (a mirror may be needed). Holding up each hand, carefully inspect the front and back of each hand and wrist, including the areas between each finger and the fingernails.
Chest, torso, and front of the legs	Standing and looking in a full-length mirror, carefully inspect your chest (including breasts), torso, and front of the legs.
Back, buttocks, and back of the legs	Standing and looking a full-length mirror, turn so that you can carefully inspect your full back, buttocks, and back of the legs (a hand mirror may also be needed).
Ankles and feet	Sitting and propping each foot on a chair or stool at a comfortable height, carefully inspect the tops and bottoms of both ankles and feet, including the areas between the toes and the toenails.
Genitalia	Sitting and using a hand mirror, carefully inspect the genitalia.

ical chemotherapy (e.g., 5-FU cream) or cryotherapy with liquid nitrogen. Other treatment options include dermabrasion, shave excision, electrodesiccation and curettage, and laser therapy.

Recurrence rates for both basal cell and squamous cell carcinomas after treatment range from 5 to 50 percent. Rates vary with tumor characteristics and treatment modality, and most recurrences occur within 3 years post-treatment. Mohs microsurgery is an option for recurrent lesions; it has a particularly high curative rate in lesions that have recurred after other types of treatment.

Follow-Up and Referral

Referral to a dermatologist or oncologist is necessary for all suspicious skin lesions, including non-melanoma skin cancers. The majority of patients require only simple excision of the skin lesion, with follow-up to monitor skin healing by the dermatologist or practitioner who performed the procedure. Subsequent follow-up includes complete physical exams with skin exams every 6 to 12 months or more often if there is any sign of new or changing skin lesions or recurrence at the primary site. The patient who has been diagnosed with any type of skin cancer is at increased risk of developing more skin lesions in the future or of recurrences of the primary lesion.

Patient Education

The American Cancer Society recommends annual skin examinations for all adults age 40 and older. The importance of careful examination of the skin on an annual basis in certain patients cannot be overemphasized. This includes patients with a family history of melanoma, multiple nevi, history of sunburns and frequent sun exposure, and persons who work in certain occupations or avocations, such as farmers, gardeners, and sailors. Unfortunately, research has shown that a large proportion of primary-care practitioners do not routinely document findings related to the skin on physical exams. Patients of all ages should be taught the importance of monthly skin self-examinations and to report any changes in preexisting skin lesions (Table 6.24).

The patient should be instructed to report any changes in existing moles or the development of new or rapidly growing lesions. Survivors of non-melanoma skin cancer should be informed of increased risk of developing a second lesion or of recurrence of the original lesion. Approximately 80 percent of lifetime exposure to UV radiation occurs before the age of 20 in the majority of patients. Strategies to avoid sun exposure should be discussed with all patients at every physical exam, particularly with parents of infants, young children, and adolescents. Patients and their families should be advised to:

- ▲ Avoid sun exposure from 11 A.M. to 4 P.M.—the time of the most intense UV radiation.
- ▲ Wear protective clothing (a tight-weave fabric, long-sleeve shirt and a wide-brimmed hat.)
- ▲ Wear large-framed, wraparound sunglasses with 99 percent to 100 percent UV absorption.
- ▲ Apply a sunscreen with an SPF (sun-protective factor) of at least 15 as directed, even on hazy days; reapply sunscreen as needed.
- ▲ Avoid the use of tanning beds and sun lamps.

Bibliography

General

Chow, AW: In Dombro, MR (ed): Griffith's 5-minute Clinical Consult. Lippincott Williams & Wilkins, Philadelphia, 2000, pp 1094–1095.

Colyar, MR, and Ehrhardt, C: Ambulatory Care Procedures for Nurse Practitioners. FA Davis, Philadelphia, 1999.

Deglin, JH, and Vallerand, AH: (2005). Davis's Drug Guide for Nurses, ed 9. FA Davis, Philadelphia.

Goodheart, HP: Common dermatologic diagnoses (part 2). Womens Health Primary Care 6(7):319–322, 2003.

Joseph, MG: Dermatology for Clinicians—A Practical Guide to Common Skin Conditions. CRC Parthenon, New York.

Kasper, DL, Braunwald, E, Fauci, AS, Hauser, SL, Longo, DL, and Jameson, JL: Harrison's Manual of Medicine. McGraw Hill, New York, 2005.

Nicol, NH: Managing atopic dermatitis in children and adults. Nurse Pract 25(4):58–79, 2000.

Norman, R, and Wallace, K: A quick guide to five common skin diseases. Clin Advisor 24–30, March 2005.

Odom, RB, James, WD, and Berger, TB: Andrew's Diseases of the Skin, ed 9. WB Saunders, Philadelphia, 2000.

Papadakis, MA, and McPhee, SL:Current Consult Medicine. Lange Medical Books/McGraw-Hill, New York, 2005.

Nurse Practitioners' Prescribing Reference: 12(1). Prescribing Reference, New York, 2005.

Powell, J, Stone, N, and Dawber, RPR: An Atlas of Hair and Scalp Diseases. CRCParthenon, New York, 2002.

Tierney, LM, McPhee, SJ, and Papadakis, MA: Current Medical Diagnosis & Treatment. Lange Medical Books/McGraw Hill, New York, 2005.

Weiss, BD: 20 Common Problems in Primary Care. McGraw-Hill, New York, 1999.

Acne

Goodheart, HP: Acne and related disorders in women, part 3: Treatment modalities for acne. Womens Health in Primary Care 3(3):167–172, 2000.

Goodheart, HP: Acne and related disorders in women, part 5: Rosacea. Womens Health Primary Care 3(7):499–505, 2000.

Lewis, ZA: Acne in adult women: It doesn't always resolve with age. Womens Health Primary Care 6(7):333–343, 2003.

McMichael, AJ, Hancox, J, Careccia, R, and Cayce, K: Choosing the opti mum treatments for acne. Clin Advisor 24–38, October, 2004.

Odom, RB, James, WD, and Berger, TG: Acne. In Andrews' Diseases of the Skin, ed 9. WB Saunders, Philadelphia, 2000, pp 284–295.

Photoclinic—Foresee your next patient. Refractory acne vulgaris. Consultant 417, March 2002.

Tierney, LM, et al: Acne vulgaris. In Current Medical Diagnosis and Treatment, ed 39. Lange Medical Books/McGraw-Hill, New York, 2000, pp 153–155.

Cellulitis

Chan, PD, Winkle, CR, and Winkle, PJ: Family Medicine. Year 2000 Edition. Current Clinical Strategies Publishing, Laguna Hills, Calif., 2000, pp 51–52.

Jacobs, RA: General problems in infectious diseases. In Tierney, LM, et al: Current Medical Diagnosis and Treatment, ed 39. Lange Medical Books/McGraw-Hill, New York, 2000, pp 1250–1251.

Dermatitis

Odom, RB, et al: Atopic dermatitis, eczema, and noninfectious immunodeficiency disorders. In Andrews' Diseases of the Skin, ed 9. WB Saunders, Philadelphia, 2000, pp 69–85.

Folliculitis

Archer-Dubon, C, et al: An epidemic outbreak of *Malassezia* folliculitis in three adult patients in an intensive care unit: A previously unrecognized nosocomial infection (report). Int J Dermatol 38(6):453–456, 1999.

Melanoma

Balch, CM, et al: An evidence-based staging system for cutaneous melanoma. CA Cancer J Clin 54:131–149, 2004.

Psoriasis

Goodheart, HP: Psoriasis, Part 4: Generalized plaque psoriasis, exfoliative dermatitis due to psoriasis, psoriatic arthritis, Womens Health Primary Care 5(3):147–149, 2002.

Pearce, DJ, and Feldman, SR: New developments in the treatmen tof psoriasis: Beginnings of the biologic era. The Female Patient 29:pp 31–34, September 2004.

Scheinfeld, N, and Mikhail, M: Biologics revolutionize psoriasis management. Clin Advisor 39–42, July 2004.

Tinea

Grin, C: Tinea: Diagnostic clues, treatment keys. Consultant 214–216, February 2004.

Urticaria

Frank, MM: Urticaria and angioedema. In Cecil Textbook of Medicine, ed 21. WB Saunders, Philadelphia, 2000, pp 1440–1444.

Resources

American Academy of Dermatology
http://www.aad.org
American Cancer Society
http://www.cancer.org
Centers for Disease Control and Prevention
http://www.cdc.gov
National Alopecia Areata Foundation
(415) 472–3780
http://www.alopeciaareata.com
National Cancer Institute
http://www.nci.nih.gov
The National Eczema Society
http://www.eczema.org
Online resource for herpes and HPV
Herpes.org
National Institute of Allergy and Infectious Disease
http://www.niaid.nih.gov
National Institutes of Health
http://www.nih.gov
National Pediculosis Association
http://www.headlice.org
National Psoriasis Foundation
Suite 300, 6600 SW 92nd Ave.
Portland, OR 97223
(503) 244–7404, (800) 723–9166
http://www.psoriasis.org
Others
Information on dermatological drugs
http://www.nsc.gov.sg/brochures.html
American Society of Dermatology
http://www.asd.org

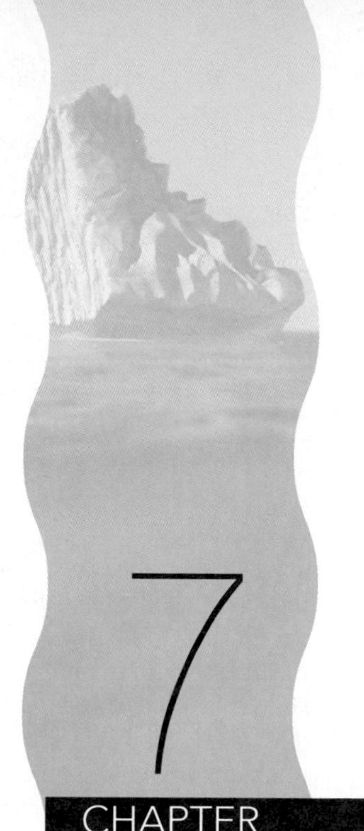

Eyes, Ears, Nose, and Throat Problems

Ruth McCaffrey, DNP, APRN, BC
Sharon Thrush, MSN, APRN, BC
Lynne M. Dunphy, PhD, MSN, APRN, BC
Brian O. Porter, MD, PhD, MPH

Common Complaints

Dry Eye

Dry eye is a syndrome in which tear production is inadequate. It occurs as a result of (1) mechanical abnormalities that interfere with the spread or maintenance of tears over the eyeball surface, (2) lacrimal gland malfunction, or (3) mucin deficiency. Mechanical abnormalities include abnormalities of eyelid structure and function and protrusion of the eyeballs, and may result from the misuse of contact lenses. Lacrimal disorders may be acquired or congenital. Acquired disorders may be systemic, such as Sjögren's syndrome, may reflect a more local infectious process, as in some forms of conjunctivitis, or may be related to trauma, such as in facial nerve (cranial nerve [CN] VII) palsy. It has been shown that patients with chronic dry eye experience increased activation of T cells. These T cells produce cytokines that may result in a neural signal to the lacrimal gland that disrupts production of natural tears, leading to a decrease in the patient's own tears, tissue damage in lacrimal glands and ocular surface, recruitment of additional T cells, and increased cytokine production

Certain medications, such as anticholinergic agents, beta-adrenergic blockers, and antihistamines, decrease tear production, because the lacrimal gland is stimulated by the parasympathetic system. Mucin deficiency may also be caused by certain medications, such as those listed here, as well as by vitamin A deficiency, by certain forms of chronic conjunctivitis, or as a result of the aging process. Consequently tear production decreases with aging, especially in women during menopause, so this is a frequently encountered complaint. In addition, patients may have a diminished blink rate.

Differential Diagnosis

Dry eye commonly affects both eyes and is often described as "a feeling of sand in the eyes," especially when blinking. The eyes feel hot, irritated, and gritty and may become reddened. The patient may present with complaints of blurred vision, lack of tears, burning, itching, foreign body sensation, sensitivity to light, and loss of glossy appearance of cornea. The triad presentation of burning, itching, and a foreign body sensation in the eye is sometimes referred to as *keratoconjunctivitis sicca* (KCS). This symptom is frequently associated with the diagnosis of Sjögren's syndrome, a systemic disorder affecting all secretory glands that is often associated with rheumatoid arthritis. Approximately 1 percent of the United States population is affected with Sjögren's syndrome; it affects 15 percent of patients with rheumatoid arthritis.

Untreated or severe KCS may result in inflammation, erosion, and eventually keratinization of the cornea and/or conjunctiva, and may even cause blindness. A correlation does not always exist, however, between the failure of tear production, leading to dry eye, and inflammatory or degenerative changes to the surface of the eye. Accessory glands in the palpebral conjunctiva may secrete sufficient tears to prevent corneal damage.

Careful history taking, including inquiries about current medication usage and past medical history, should allow the clinician to determine the cause of the disorder. Close physical examination should reveal any mechanical, infectious, and/or traumatic cause. Once this is treated, the

Table 7.1 Ocular Self-Care

Keep home humidity between 30% and 50%
Wear wraparound sunglasses, especially on windy days
Wear goggles when swimming
Use a preservative-free artificial tears preparation or bathe your eyes in an herbal therapy solution made with Eyebright *(Euphrasia officinalis)*
Avoid blowing hot air from a hair dryer in the eyes
Replace eye makeup every 6 months

dry eye should resolve. The patient's contact lens prescription may need to be altered, or the self-care regimen may need to be addressed (Table 7.1). Elimination of systemic medications that may have contributed to the condition should be considered. A patient with chronic conjunctivitis may need to be referred to an ophthalmologist. Reports in the literature have associated the relief of dry-eye symptoms with the institution of estrogen replacement therapy in postmenopausal women. Most cases of dry eye are best managed symptomatically.

The principles of treatment for dry eye involve tear restoration or stimulation. Wearing wraparound sunglasses to keep wind from drying the eye surface, using a humidifier in the home, and avoiding rubbing the eyes are methods patients can use to overcome dry eye. Specific pharmacologic measures include ocular lubricants such as Alcon (Duratears Naturale), an ophthalmic ointment of petrolatum, lanolin, and mineral oil to be applied as needed (prn), which is especially helpful for use with soft contact lenses, or 1 percent polyvinyl alcohol (HypoTears®), a preservative-free ophthalmic solution that can be used one to two drops prn. Sodium chloride (MURO 128) 2 percent or 5 percent ophthalmic solution may be used (one to two drops) every 3 to 4 hours, reducing frequency as inflammation subsides. Transient stinging may occur on instillation. Occasionally, surgical intervention, such as a surgically induced punctal occlusion, may be warranted. Cyclosporin ophthalmic emulsion (RESTASIS®) is used to treat chronic dry eye. It contains a very small concentration of cyclosporine, which is believed to inhibit the activation of T cells. T cells disrupt normal tear production in the lacrimal glands. Improving lacrimal gland function is believed to result in increased tear production.

Dysphagia

Dysphagia means inability or difficulty swallowing and is differentiated from *odynophagia,* or painful swallowing. Although dysphagia may accompany odynophagia, classic dysphagia is not usually accompanied by pain. The prevalence of the problem increases with age, and the symptom is not uncommon in older adults.

The swallowing process is divided into four phases: (1) the *oral preparatory phase,* involving voluntary mastication and preparation of food into a bolus; (2) the *oral phase,* which encompasses the voluntary movement of the food bolus from the tip of the tongue to the anterior tonsillar pillars; (3) the *pharyngeal phase,* which includes the reflexive passage of the bolus from the oral cavity into the upper esophagus; and (4) the *esophageal phase,* which encompasses the reflexive passage of the bolus through the esophagus into the stomach. Often, a combination of underlying factors causes dysphagia.

Differential Diagnosis

Eighty percent of esophageal-phase abnormalities are mechanical in nature, such as strictures, erosions, infections, or carcinomas, whereas 80 percent of oral preparatory-, oral-, and pharyngeal-phase abnormalities are neurologic in origin. The neurologic problems may be fixed defects, such as post-stroke dysfunction, or part of progressive disorders such as multiple sclerosis, Parkinson's disease, and amyotrophic lateral sclerosis (ALS). Sometimes the dysphagia may be the first sign of such an underlying disorder. Psychological conditions may also cause the symptom: the term "globus hystericus" refers to a manifestation of acute anxiety disorders and panic attacks. Dysphagia may also be associated with underlying depressive disorder. Other factors contribute to abnormal bolus presentation, such as poor dentition, dysgeusia (use of medications or vitamin and mineral deficiencies may lead to abnormal taste and smell perception in some patients), and chronic diseases, such as congestive heart failure (CHF) and chronic obstructive pulmonary disease (COPD), which create increased metabolic demands but are accompanied by anorexia. Often a combination of factors occurs that results in dysphagia and malnutrition.

The patient may present with the specific complaint of dysphagia, or it may manifest as weight loss, often accompanied by fatigue, poor wound healing, and a variety of other indications of nutritional deficiencies.

Weight loss may be caused by any number of problems and must be evaluated accordingly. If it is associated with dysphagia, the patient or his or her caretakers may have noted signs of aspiration, dribbling, and so on related to food intake. Early detection and diagnosis of the underlying physiologic mechanism causing the dysphagia is important, so that significant nutritional deficiencies and consequences may be avoided. Problems with swallowing are best evaluated by observation of food and fluid intake. Serial weight measures are one of the best ways to monitor nutritional status, especially of elderly patients, who can be "subclinically" malnourished, meaning that they have normal serum albumin levels but apparent weight loss or low body weight.

Alterations of the swallowing process may manifest differently depending on the underlying pathology. For example, the oral preparatory phase is characterized by problems of spillage, dribbling, pocketing of food in the mouth, and aspiration. The pharyngeal phase is the first reflexive, or involuntary phase; problems during this phase may be characterized by nasal regurgitation, aspiration, and/or altered voice. This is the phase in which aspiration most commonly occurs during a swallow. Aspiration may occur before a swallow, from spillage posteriorly, or after a swallow, from regurgitation. A normal gag reflex is insufficient evidence of a safe swallow. Problems in the esophageal phase are characterized by neck pain, heartburn, and the sensation of food becoming "stuck" below the sternum.

Videofluoroscopy is considered the "gold standard" for evaluation of swallowing. This imaging technique allows observation of an outline of the structures from the oral cavity to the stomach, as well as an assessment of the velocity and range of movement of oral and hypopharyngeal structures and their temporal relationship to each other. Through observations of ingestion of various food consistencies, such as thin liquids, thick liquids, semisolids, and solids, the patient's tolerance of oral intake and thus the safest diet plan can be determined. (See Nursing Research–Based Practice 7.1.)

Treatment

A number of approaches will help the patient improve safe food intake, including positioning (usually sitting upright, with the head tilted slightly forward and downward) and food-consistency modification (no thin liquids, mechanical soft diet) during food intake, along with exercises and rehabilitation to improve oral motor control. If the risk of aspiration is severe, the clinician may have to consider limitation or elimination of food intake PO. The position of the American Society for Enteral and Parenteral Nutrition is "…if the gut works, use it." Thus parenteral feeding should have limited indications.

If parenteral nutrition is indicated, nasogastric tubes are generally recommended for short-term use of 2 to 4 weeks. Patients who are likely to require a longer course should be referred to a gastroenterologist or invasive radiologist for percutaneous endoscopic gastrostomy (PEG) tube placement. PEG placement and parenteral feedings often are incorrectly thought of as irreversible decisions, but in fact, patients may be withdrawn easily from PEG feedings if no longer indicated. Another common misconception is that artificial (parenteral) feeding is an all-or-nothing decision. Many patients have indications for both oral intake and supplementation via tube feeding; thus, partial support is not uncommon, nor is it necessarily contraindicated. In decisions regarding artificial feedings, one must consider the indications, the patient's prognosis, and treatment preferences, in order to avoid imposing unwanted therapy or life prolongation.

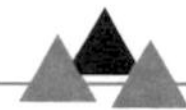

NURSING RESEARCH-BASED PRACTICE 7.1

Siegel, RM, Kiely, M, Bein, JP, et al: Treatment of otitis media with observation and a safety-net antibiotic prescription. Pediatrics 112(3):527–532, 2003.

J. S. is a 2-year-old child who presents to the pediatrician's office with a temperature of 101.8°F. Her mother reports that for the past 2 days she has been tugging on her right ear, producing a moderate amount of yellow nasal drainage, and has been very irritable. On physical examination you discover that the tympanic membrane is erythematous, bulging, and has decreased motility. The mother states that the child's appetite is normal, and denies any vomiting or diarrhea. The child's history is negative for previous ear infections, congenital syndromes, and prematurity. Immunizations are up to date and no one else in the family has experienced these symptoms. The mother states that the child has started attending day care 2 weeks ago.

Your diagnosis is acute otitis media (AOM). What treatment plan would you develop for this patient? How would you explain your diagnosis and treatment plan to the mother? What instructions would you give the mother to assist her in caring for her child?

A quasi-experimental study design was conducted to evaluate the treatment options of AOM. The aim of the study was to determine if parents in the United States would wait at least 48 hours before deciding whether to fill a safety-net antibiotic prescription (SNAP) for the treatment of uncomplicated acute otitis media in children aged 1 to 12. Pain control was the treatment of choice for all 194 participants in the Cincinnati Pediatric Research Group's study. After criteria had been met and consent forms were signed by the parents, the SNAP was given with instructions to wait 48 hours before filling the prescription and to treat the symptoms with acetaminophen, ibuprofen, and anesthetic otic drops. Patients were contacted on day 10 with a telephone interview and were questioned about the treatments given. Initial data and the 10-day telephone interview information were entered into the researcher's Internet Web site. The findings showed that 175 participants completed the 10-day interview. Of the 175 participants, 31 percent had filled the SNAP and 78 percent of the parents were satisfied with paracetamol treatment alone. Sixty-three percent of the parents were willing to treat future acute otitis media episodes with pain mediation rather than with immediate antibiotics.

Excessive Snoring

Excessive snoring—often referred to as *obstructive sleep apnea syndrome* (OSAS), or upper airway collapse during sleep—results from a complex interaction of neuromuscular and anatomic factors. A pharyngeal airway that is congenitally small or has become narrowed as a result of obesity is more likely to collapse than a large airway. In adults, OSAS seems to be primarily related to an imbalance between the activity of the chest-wall muscles and the upper airway dilators. Adequate activity of the upper airway-dilating muscles is necessary to maintain airway patency; otherwise, the negative pressure produced by the chest-wall musculature will obstruct the upper airway. In addition, nasal obstruction and abnormal arousal thresholds during sleep may influence the incidence and severity of OSAS.

Excessive snoring is a common complaint, especially in men. It affects anywhere from 4 to 8 percent of the adult population, depending on the criteria used for diagnosis. OSAS is commonly a disorder of middle age; the incidence of excessive snoring tends to increase as a person ages. It is more prevalent in certain races, especially African Americans, even after adjustment for other risk factors. Patients with OSAS may present with complaints of daytime sleepiness, or the patient's partner may report loud snoring and long breathing pauses by the patient during the night. Another common presenting complaint is falling asleep during sedentary daytime activity, such as reading a book. Some patients fall asleep while driving a car, and there is a sevenfold increase in the risk of auto accidents among persons with OSAS. These patients may also report restless sleep, morning headaches, and cognitive difficulties.

Risk factors for OSAS include obesity, family history, craniofacial abnormalities, increased age, alcohol consumption, smoking, supine sleeping position, hypothyroidism, and use of certain medications such as benzodiazepines, muscle relaxants, and testosterone. Upper airway narrowing from an enlarged tongue or tonsils may also contribute to the disorder.

Differential Diagnosis

The complaint of excessive daytime sleepiness may stem from a variety of differential diagnoses, such as depression, other sleeping disorders (such as narcolepsy), hypothyroidism, inadequate sleep, and periodic limb movement during sleep (restless leg syndrome). When this complaint is associated with excessive snoring, the clinician should strongly consider the diagnosis of OSAS. The clinician should elicit any associated risk factors during the history: For example, is there a history of witnessed episodes of apnea? Reports of loud snoring punctuated with gasps and snorts? Any accidents due to sleepiness? In addition, a neck size greater than 16 inches in women and 17 inches in men, or a body mass index (BMI) higher than 28 may be present in those with this disorder.

Nocturnal polysomnography (sleep apnea study) is the "gold standard" for the diagnosis of OSAS, although a normal result does not always exclude the diagnosis of OSAS. The apnea–hypopnea index (AHI) is the most commonly used criterion to establish the diagnosis of OSAS and quantify its severity. An AHI above 5 and complaints of daytime hypersomnolence are usually sufficient to establish a definitive diagnosis of OSAS.

Treatment

The first line of action is to identify the precipitating and predisposing factors for OSAS, such as obesity, alcohol, smoking, and medication usage. Nearly all patients with OSAS will benefit from weight loss, usually in approximate proportion to the amount of weight lost, as well as from cessation of smoking. Abstaining from or limiting alcohol intake before sleep, as well as avoiding use of narcotics, barbiturates, and muscle relaxants before sleep have proved to be helpful. Sometimes the simple intervention of adjusting the patient's sleeping position to a side-lying one, or sleeping on several pillows to prevent upper airway collapse may be sufficient. Some sources report using an old trick of taping a marble to the patient's back to discourage him or her from lying supine. The patient should be counseled to avoid excessive neck flexion by using a cervical pillow only (placed under the nape of the neck), or by elevating the entire head of the bed, as in the management of reflux esophagitis. Any nasal obstruction from chronic rhinitis should be treated.

For patients whose symptoms are refractive to these lifestyle changes, nasal continuous positive airway pressure (nasal CPAP) continues as a mainstay of therapy for OSAS. In some patients, oral devices may be helpful, or a gravity-activated position monitor that will ring if the patient stays on his or her back for longer than 15 minutes. Occasionally, surgical intervention, such as nasal reconstruction or laser-assisted uvulopalatoplasty, may be necessary. A variety of other surgical techniques may be employed, depending on the underlying etiology.

Excessive Tearing

Excessive tearing is often a case of paradoxical tearing, that is, a response to dry eye. It is an especially common complaint in elderly patients and in individuals with allergies.

Differential Diagnosis

The complaint of excessive tears is often related to dryness of the eye. The eye attempts to compensate or waters secondary to irritation; this condition is frequently related to allergy. Eyes can also water as a result of eyestrain that may be sustained, for example, with prolonged computer use, which can also lead to pain that spreads to the neck, shoulders, and back. The patient may complain of "excess tears," when in reality the tears are a discharge secondary to some form of red eye. Sensitivity to preservatives in certain eyedrops and contact lens solutions can also cause this relatively common problem. Excessive tearing may also occur secondary to a blockage in the drainage system. Frequently, excess tearing will lead to increased irritation and even more tearing, so it is necessary to break this cycle to treat the symptom effectively.

Eye Pain

The most important thing for the clinician to know in the case of eye pain, and in dealing with eye problems in general, is when to refer the patient to an ophthalmologist. The liability and potential for human suffering related to damage to vision is high. Table 7.2 presents conditions associated with any eye pathology that require immediate referral to an ophthalmologist.

Because of the subjective nature of the pain experience, the presentation of eye pain might mean a variety of things. In addition, it is important to differentiate whether the pain is coming from the eye itself or from one of the surrounding structures. The most common cause of eye pain is trauma.

Differential Diagnosis

Focusing the History 7.1 presents important items to cover when taking an ocular history in general. Advanced Assessment 10.1 presents the important items to assess as part of the physical exam. In the case of eye pain, the clinician must determine whether the eye pain is coming from the eye itself or whether it is referred pain from another structure.

Eye pain that is referred may be either from contiguous structures or from structures that are innervated by the recurrent meningeal branches of the ophthalmic nerve. The possible causes of referred eye pain are numerous; they include trauma; headache; sinusitis; temporal arteritis; temporomandibular joint (TMJ) pain; herpes zoster ophthalmicus prodrome or postherpetic neuralgia (see Chapter 5); very occasionally orbital tumors, both primary and metastatic; or a locally invasive paranasal tumor. Increased intracranial pressure may cause a penetrating sensation of eye pain associated with vomiting and papilledema; this pain increases with Valsalva maneuver. Trigeminal neuralgia, occipital neuralgia, and stroke, specifically parieto-occipital or thalamic infarct, are all potential sources of referred eye pain.

The ophthalmic nerve innervates the eyelid, the conjunctiva, the cornea, and the uveal tract, so all these areas are quite sensitive to pain. The retina, the vitreous humor, and the optic nerve, by comparison, are less richly innervated and thus are seldom a source of pain. This knowledge can be of assistance diagnostically.

Eye pain with a foreign body sensation is most likely to be attributable to conjunctivitis; it may also be associated with corneal abrasions (from ingrown lashes, contact lens overuse, or trauma); or corneal ulcers, which always require referral to an ophthalmologist; or it may be caused by foreign matter on the lid or surface of the eye; or, occasionally, overexposure to ultraviolet light. This pain is usually referred to the outer portion of the upper eyelid, regardless of the location of the lesion.

To differentiate pain from mild abrasions and foreign objects from trauma to deeper structures, the clinician should place a drop of local anesthetic in the conjunctival sac; this will alleviate pain from superficial causes but not pain from deeper structures.

Pain accompanied by burning or itching is usually attributable to conjunctivitis; allergy; dry eyes, sometimes secondary to collagen vascular disease (sicca syndrome); chemical injury; and infrequent blinking related to overexposure to video display terminals.

Pain with swelling around the eye can be attributable to a number of causes, the most serious of which is orbital cellulitis. This must be treated with parenteral anti-

FOCUS ON HISTORY 7.1

Eye Complaints

Onset of symptoms (sudden or gradual)
Change in vision (sudden or gradual)
Pain
Photophobia
Mechanism of injury (if pertinent)
Use of contact lenses (type, wearing schedule, and care)
Current medications
Past history of eye problems/eye surgery
Exposure history (e.g., use of new cosmetics, contact with person with an eye infection, travel, etc.)
Systemic complaints (e.g., fever, genital discharge, rash, etc.)

Table 7.2 Conditions Requiring Immediate Referral to an Ophthalmologist

Patient complaint
- Severe and sudden vision loss

Clinical presentation
- Corneal ulceration
- Suspected herpes zoster ophthalmicus
- Hazy cornea
- Irregular pupil
- Elevation of fundus on fundoscopic exam
- Papilledema
- Limal flush
- Muscle paresis

Management
- Conditions requiring steroid therapy
- Patient not improved with conservative treatment

biotics and computed tomography (CT) may be required to differentiate it from preseptal cellulitis. Swelling on the lid margin usually is a *stye,* or hordeolum, and is secondary to inflammation of the glands of Zeis or Moll; a chronically inflamed meibomian gland usually manifests as swelling pointing away from the lid margin (a *chalazion*). There may be inflammation of the lacrimal system also. Trauma can also cause pain with swelling.

Pain on eye movement may indicate a posterior scleritis, which presents also with decreased vision and disk edema; there is an idiopathic orbital inflammatory syndrome that presents with pain, lid edema, chemosis, and proptosis. A myositis of the orbital muscles presents with pain and diplopia. Some loss of central vision and a swollen disk may indicate a retrobulbar optic neuritis. All patients suspected of having these disorders should be referred to an ophthalmologist and/or neurologist.

Deep pain in the eye is usually indicative of a more ominous etiology; a patient with deep pain usually should be referred to an ophthalmologist for diagnosis and treatment. This type of pain may indicate an anterior uveitis, with purplish red vessels around the limbus of the cornea, miotic pupils, and blurred vision. Glaucoma can present with eye pain; this is an ophthalmologic emergency. Purplish red vessels are apparent around the limbus of the cornea, which may appear "steamy"; the pupils assume a fixed midposition. Scleritis presents with severe pain and may perforate; episcleritis may be confused with conjunctivitis, but dilated vessels are typically more purplish in episcleritis and do not disappear with topical decongestants.

Eye pain on movement with no other specific signs may indicate eye strain, astigmatism, or a tonic pupil.

Hoarseness

Hoarseness is a common complaint; the term describes a voice with harsh quality and low pitch. Use of the term can also include weakness, raspiness, or simply a change from the usual voice quality. Hoarseness suggests an abnormality in voice production at the level of the larynx. It is a common symptom that may occur in both men and women at any age. Changes in the voice are part of the natural process of aging. In elderly men, the voice becomes weaker and higher in pitch, as a result of muscle atrophy and increased stiffness of tissues. In women, the same changes occur, but the pitch of the voice becomes lower, because during menopause, mucoid edema accumulates in the submucosa of the vocal folds. More severe edema and polyps may occur in women who smoke. Hoarseness is a cardinal sign of laryngeal cancer, which is most commonly seen in men 50 to 70 years of age.

Vocal sound is produced when exhaled air causes passive vibration of the vocal folds (usually referred to as vocal cords). For normal voice tones, adequate breath support, adequate laryngeal closure, healthy vocal-fold mucosa, control of vocal-fold length and tension, and normal resonance are all required. Most often, hoarseness is caused by an intrinsic pathologic process in the larynx. If the vocal folds cannot be brought close enough together, there will be a sizable air leak and the voice will sound breathy. If the vocal folds are pressed together too tightly, or if the vocal folds are swollen and edematous, more expiratory effort is required, so that speech becomes strained.

Differential Diagnosis

Hoarseness may be acute and self-limiting. It may arise from an infectious or inflammatory process in the larynx, or it may be a result of a more serious, usually more chronic problem, such as compression or disruption of the vocal cords from polyps, nodules, and tumors. It may also result from vocal cord paralysis or from muscle atrophy related to aging. Gastroesophageal reflux may also cause laryngeal irritation that can lead to hoarseness, as can chronic allergies. Table 7.3 presents differential diagnoses for hoarseness.

Onset of the problem is an important key to diagnosis. A 1-day complaint is unlikely to be caused by cancer, whereas hoarseness persisting for 1 year is unlikely to be the result of an acute infection. Associated conditions should be ascertained. Sore throat and otalgia often accompany hoarseness in malignant tumors of the larynx or pharynx. Chronic pain often suggests more serious underlying disease than acute-onset pain.

Dysphagia or odynophagia accompanying hoarseness indicates the presence of disease affecting the pharynx or esophagus. Cough suggests irritation of the endolarynx or pulmonary disease. Hemoptysis is more serious, suggesting a malignant process of the pharyngeal, laryngeal, or pulmonary areas. Fever and oral, nasal, or otalgic discharge suggest an infectious process.

Table 7.3 Differential Diagnoses: Hoarseness

- Infectious
  - Viral laryngitis
  - Bacterial tracheitis or laryngitis
  - Papillomatosis
- Neurologic
  - Dystonia
  - Neuromuscular disease
  - Laryngeal nerve involvement by thyroid, pulmonary, or esophageal causes
- Traumatic
  - Vocal cord nodules or polyps
  - Smoke inhalation
  - Esophageal reflux
  - Chronic cough
- Neoplastic
  - Vocal cord cancer
  - Supraglottic cancer with muscle invasion

Voice use and lifestyle should be reviewed. A professional singer or weekend football fan can suffer voice overuse and abuse. An individual who smoked two packs of cigarettes per day for 45 years may have irritation or malignancy. A scratchy throat the morning after eating spicy foods suggests a diagnosis of gastroesophageal reflux.

A complete examination of the head and neck is necessary. Nasal drainage and excess mucus may indicate sinusitis. Tonsillar erythema or exudate indicates viral or bacterial infection. If otalgia is present, an ear examination should be performed. Ear canal erythema or exudate suggests infection. A normal ear exam despite pain may be seen in patients with cancer of the pharynx or larynx.

The clinician should palpate the oral cavity, tongue, neck, and lymph nodes for masses. Infections such as abscesses often feel warm, tender, tense, or fluctuant. Malignancies typically are hard masses that may be fixed to underlying tissue.

Infections cause elevated white blood cell (WBC) counts. Culture and sensitivity of oral, nasal, or otalgic discharge can reveal the organism responsible for the infection and guide antibiotic therapy. If hoarseness persists for more than 2 weeks and is clearly not caused by an infection, then referral to an otolaryngologist for a laryngoscopy is required. An adequate laryngeal exam should visualize the base of the tongue, epiglottis, pyriform sinuses, false vocal cords, subglottic larynx, and true vocal cords. Use of stroboscopy improves detection of small lesions by "freezing" the vocal cords (making them appear immobile) during vibration. Adequate examination of structures may require general anesthesia, which is usually necessary for palpation and biopsy of any abnormalities. Routine use of CT scanning is neither cost-effective nor necessary. If vocal-cord paralysis is seen, CT scans from the skull base to the aortic arch are required to assess the recurrent laryngeal nerves. Thyroid tumors are the most common cause of bilateral vocal-cord paralysis; esophageal and pulmonary tumors are common causes of left-sided vocal-cord paralysis.

Treatment

Treatment for hoarseness may be pharmacologic or surgical, or it may consist of lifestyle adjustments. In the case of acute hoarseness, or laryngitis, voice rest, cough suppression, gastric acid suppression, hydration, and management of rhinitis are the principles of therapy, with administration of antibiotics as appropriate. In cases where "the show must go on," so to speak, and voice rest is impossible, if laryngeal examination rules out vocal-fold hemorrhage or abrasion, it is usually safe to manage vocal-fold edema temporarily with oral or parenteral steroids. A long-acting topical vasoconstrictor such as oxymetazoline (Afrin) may be applied directly to the laryngeal mucosa to reduce edema further. These measures do not promote healing, nor do they prevent further damage to the vocal cords.

For repeated and recurrent episodes of hoarseness, vocal hygiene and voice therapy should be considered, especially in professionals who must rely on their voice. Screening for contributing conditions (such as underlying allergies, chronic sinusitis, or gastroesophageal reflux) should be pursued. As noted earlier, if hoarseness persists for more than 2 weeks, further evaluation is warranted.

Impaired Hearing

Hearing loss is the decreased ability or complete inability to hear. It may involve the middle ear, which indicates a mechanical or conductive problem (usually implying a reversible problem), or the inner ear, which indicates a nerve, or sensorineural problem. Hearing loss may have both conductive and sensorineural components. Often cerumen (ear wax) impaction is present. Many types of hearing loss can be improved with hearing aids; however, only 10 to 15 percent of patients who could benefit from a hearing aid actually use one.

The prevalence of hearing loss increases after age 40. Hearing loss affects approximately 25 percent of all adults 65 to 74 years of age, and 50 percent of all adults older than age 85. Sensorineural hearing loss increases with age. The degenerative decline starts at age 20. Ethnicity and gender are not significant. Hearing loss is a universal phenomenon of aging, with an increased incidence in individuals with a family history of hearing loss.

Exposure to loud noises, either occupationally or recreationally, is a risk factor for hearing loss, as are ototoxic drugs (such as aminoglycoside antibiotics, aspirin, and quinine, to name a few). Allergies and other causes of eustachian-tube obstruction may also contribute to hearing loss. Risk factors for cerumen impaction specifically are ear canal hairs, hearing aids, bony growths secondary to osteophyte or osteoma, as well as previous episodes of impacted cerumen. Chronic middle ear infections (otitis media) also are a contributing factor in the development of hearing loss.

Sensorineural hearing loss is defined as a lesion in the organ of Corti or in the central pathways, including the eighth cranial nerve (CN VIII) and auditory cortex. Age-related hearing loss, termed *presbycusis,* is a form of sensorineural hearing loss. After age 50, hair cells in the organ of Corti tend to degenerate. A capillary-fed layer of stratified epithelium known as the *stria vascularis* that secretes endolymph and promotes the sensitization of hair cells in the cochlea may atrophy. This first affects perception of high-frequency sounds and then progresses to affect hearing of lower-frequency tones. Sensorineural loss may also be a result of Ménière's disease (discussed later in this chapter) or be noise-induced. Other causes of hearing loss include tumors, genetic predisposition, ototoxicity to a variety of drugs, syphilis, and metabolic disorders such as hypothyroidism. Hearing loss also may be secondary to an inner ear fistula, usually secondary to pressure changes or trauma. Viral syndromes, especially mumps, may also affect hearing.

Conductive hearing loss is a lesion involving the outer and middle ear to the level of the oval window that may result from a variety of structural abnormalities. Cerumen impaction, a reversible form of hearing loss, is a common cause in all age groups. Perforation of the tympanic membrane, middle ear fluid, damage to the ossicles from trauma or infection, otosclerosis, tympanosclerosis, cholesteatoma, middle ear tumors, temporal bone fractures and injuries related to trauma, or congenital problems may all cause conductive hearing loss.

Differential Diagnosis

Hearing loss is not a distinct clinical entity; it is a symptom or sign of multiple medical conditions. Patient complaint terminology is more diversified than for many other medical conditions. A patient may report having "difficulty hearing," which may be associated with pain, pressure, discomfort, vertigo, or loss of balance. Or the patient may complain of tinnitus, dizziness, blockage, popping, pressure, crackling, distant sounds, or stiffness. The clinician should question the patient as to how long he or she has noticed a hearing loss, and whether it is partial or complete. Does the patient think both ears are affected? Is there a family history of hearing loss? The clinician should inquire whether the patient has ever had any injury or surgery to the ears, and if he or she has had any serious illnesses or tuberculosis (which might have required treatment with ototoxic drugs). The review of systems should focus on the neurologic system, including cranial nerve function (e.g., facial weakness or tingling, loss of taste, or dysphagia). The social and occupational history should include specific questions regarding noise or toxin exposure and any blast-related injuries. A complete history of prescription and over-the-counter (OTC) medication use should be obtained.

The physical exam should include otoscopic examination to inspect the external auditory canal and middle ear. The clinician should note any redness, foreign objects, discharge, scaling, lesions, and cerumen (ear wax). There may be a significant accumulation of cerumen, especially in elderly patients. The tympanic membrane should have no perforations and should be a translucent pearly gray. Changes in the tympanic membrane may be consistent with conductive hearing loss.

The clinician should perform Weber, Rinne, and Schwabach tests to determine whether hearing loss is primarily conductive or sensorineural. Unexpected findings from the three tuning fork tests must be integrated to differentiate clinically what is occurring. Conductive hearing loss occurs when sound transmission is impaired through the external or middle ear. Sensorineural hearing loss occurs because of a defect in the inner ear that leads to distortion of sound and misinterpretation of speech.

For office testing, utilize the Weber test first. A vibrating 512-Hz (or higher frequency) tuning fork is placed midline on the patient's skull. Normally, the sound should be equal in both ears. In sensorineural loss, the sound in the unaffected (or less affected ear) is louder. In conductive loss, the sound is louder in the affected ear.

The Rinne test can also be done in the office. A vibrating tuning fork is placed on the mastoid process. When the sound fades away, the fork is promptly placed (without restriking it) over the external auditory meatus. Normally, via air conduction, the sound can be heard for twice as long as in bone conduction. In sensorineural loss, the ratio remains the same, whereas in conductive loss, the ratio is closer to 1:1, or even reversed.

In the Schwabach test, a vibrating tuning fork is placed over the mastoid process of the patient and the examiner and the results are compared. In sensorineural loss, the patient's bone conduction is present for a shorter time than the examiner's; in conductive loss, the patient's bone conduction persists for a longer time.

Often, the patient needs to be referred for audiometry. Audiometry includes pure tone and speech testing, as well as impedance (middle ear pressure) testing. Both types of hearing loss may fluctuate, making audiometric results variable from test to test. Marked conductive loss on one ear may be difficult to exclude (mask) when testing the opposite ear. CT and magnetic resonance imaging (MRI) scans are used to detect tumors such as acoustic neuromas and glomus tumor, as well as damage from traumatic injuries.

The most important task, and frequently a difficult one, is to determine whether the hearing loss is sensorineural (which is usually irreversible), or conductive (which is often reversible). Another important piece of data is whether the loss is unilateral or bilateral. Presbycusis produces a typical high-frequency loss that is bilaterally symmetrical. Ménière's disease causes fluctuating hearing loss, usually unilateral, associated with tinnitus and vertigo. Acoustic neuroma (schwannoma), a rare tumor of cranial nerve VIII, causes unilateral constant or progressive hearing loss, possibly associated with headache. With a tumor of the acoustic nerve, there will most likely be neurologic changes such as facial weakness and tingling and loss of taste and dysphagia in addition to hearing loss.

The various mechanical obstructions, be they wax or tumor, or fluid associated with infection/inflammation, that lead to conductive hearing loss may be visualized. CT scan and/or MRI may be needed to demonstrate tumors and cholesteatoma. Cholesteatoma may sometimes be identified by perforation that is located near the margin of the eardrum.

Treatment

To treat hearing loss properly, the underlying cause must be identified properly. Many types of conductive loss are reversible; sensorineural causes tend to be irreversible. In cases of conductive hearing loss caused by cerumen buildup, cerumen disimpaction may be necessary. The recommended procedure is as follows: Use a 1:1 mixture of 3 percent hydrogen peroxide and mineral oil. Place three drops in the external ear and wait 1 hour. Then attempt to lavage the ear with warm saline. Direct the saline toward the canal wall, not toward the drum. An alternative method is to put three drops of warm olive oil in each ear to soften the wax, then flush with warm 3 percent hydrogen peroxide cerumenolytic agents such as 6.5 percent carbamide peroxide (Debrox); docusate sodium liquid may also be used. These agents should not be used in the presence of a perforated tympanic membrane or infection. Press gently but firmly behind the ear, then in front of the ear. Pull the lobe up and down to work the wax out. Dry ear canal following irrigation with alcohol or low heat hair dryer. Consider steroid/antibiotic otic solution (Cortisporin otic), four drops tid to qid for 5 to 7 days following prolonged irrigation and trauma to the canal. Consider cerumenolytic installation bid for 5 days monthly in recurrent, resistant cases. Do not disimpact the ear if tympanic membrane perforation is present. If perforation is present, referral to an ear, nose, and throat specialist is indicated. If hearing loss is caused by infection, treat as appropriate (see section on otitis media/externa under Common Ear Problems). In cases of damage to ossicles, tympanosclerosis, otosclerosis, tumor, and temporal bone injury, referral is indicated.

The cause of the hearing loss in cases of sensorineural loss must also be identified correctly in order to treat it properly. Noise damage is a common cause of hearing loss in the United States. Although this type of hearing loss is not reversible, it is preventable, and patients should be referred to an audiologist. Hearing loss related to the use of ototoxic medications (especially certain antibiotics) needs greater recognition. This etiology should be suspected when hearing loss, dizziness, and tinnitus occur during course of treatment with certain medications. In this case, the patient should stop the medications. Salicylate toxicity, for example, is reversible. In cases resulting from metabolic causes, such as hypothyroidism, the underlying disorder should be treated. Patients who are suspected of having Ménière's disease should be referred for appropriate diagnostic testing and treatment. In the case of perilymphatic fistula, diagnosis should be based on evidence or history of injury to the ear (including barotrauma during diving) and referral to a specialist is indicated. Acoustic neuromas should be referred for surgical treatment.

For cases of sudden, sensorineural hearing loss with no apparent cause, high doses of steroids (80 mg per day of prednisone or equivalent) are sometimes used. Any patient who presents with this type of acute hearing loss should be referred to an audiologist for treatment, however.

In cases of presbycusis, although no specific treatment will reverse the process, it is important to educate and support the patient so that no further damage will occur; for example, exposure to excessive noise and ototoxic drugs should be avoided. Teach the patient lip-reading when appropriate, and instruct family members to speak clearly. Consult a telephone equipment company about special audio equipment that is available.

Permanent hearing loss is common in cases of sensorineural hearing loss, and may also occur with conductive hearing loss. Patients need to be counseled about follow-up with audiometry and the need to use hearing aids. If not performed properly, cerumen removal may cause damage to the external auditory meatus, perforation of the tympanic membrane, and/or otitis media. Middle ear problems may progress to chronic ear problems such as perforations and/or cholesteatoma, which will adversely affect hearing. Severe nerve deafness, particularly when associated with tinnitus, may produce severe depression and isolation and, occasionally, even lead to suicide.

In cases of occupational or recreational hearing loss, the patient must be counseled to utilize protective devices. Teach the patient to equalize ear pressure when diving and to chew gum while in airplanes. Decongestants might be indicated. If an upper respiratory infection (URI) is present, the patient should avoid flying and/or diving. Avoid prescribing drugs, especially for elderly patients.

Mouth Sores

Problems of the oral cavity and throat account for approximately 20 percent of visits to primary-care providers. Although the mouth may be thought of as merely a receptacle for food and a vehicle for speech, several anatomic structures within the oral cavity may be the foci of disease. The oral cavity is lined by the buccal mucosa, which is rich in mucous glands. The mucous glands of the lips open into the oral cavity. The mouth cavity communicates with the pharynx posteriorly. The floor of the mouth contains the tongue and the openings of submandibular and sublingual salivary glands.

Specific lesions of the oral and buccal mucosa are immunogenic, inflammatory (most commonly aphthous ulcers), traumatic, or may be caused by a localized malignancy. Painful inflammatory lesions may occur in isolation, or they may be associated with a generalized disorder of other mucous membranes or skin. The patient's history is important, because it indicates whether the lesions are acute or chronic, single or multiple, and primary or recurrent. Pain is frequently related to ulceration of the lips or tongue. Although cancer is not the most common cause of oral cavity ulceration, it should always be considered.

When a patient complains of ulceration, the clinician should ask the following questions: Has this occurred before? Are there multiple lesions? How long have the lesions been present? Are there lesions anywhere else on the body (e.g., vagina, urethra)? Are the lesions painful? The clinician should investigate the patient's smoking history, alcohol intake and pattern, as well as any history of sexually transmitted diseases (STDs). Sexual habits should be queried. Smoking and drinking are important risk factors for precancerous lesions of the oral cavity, such as leukoplakia and erythroplakia. Does the patient have dentures and how well do they fit? Is there a history of allergies, or ingestion of hot and spicy foods?

Inflammation of the oral mucous membranes or mouth sores may be characterized by erythema and/or vesicular or ulcerative lesions. Glossitis may accompany mouth sores, and clinicians often group the two conditions together under the designation of stomatitis. In general, both disorders are classified according to etiology, which is variable.

Types of mouth sores seen in adults include oral candidiasis, aphthous stomatitis (aphthous ulcers, "canker sores"), secondary herpetic stomatitis/herpes labialis, Vincent's stomatitis (acute necrotizing ulcerative gingivitis, also referred to as "trench mouth"), allergic stomatitis, nicotinic (cigarette-related) stomatitis, denture-related stomatitis, angular stomatitis, pseudomembranous stomatitis, candidiasis, and parasitic glossitis (black hair tongue, anthracosis linguae).

Differential Diagnosis

In general, excessive dryness of the oral cavity; food and drug allergies; chemical irritation; mechanical or thermal injury; bacterial, fungal, and viral pathogens; host immunosuppression; and nutritional deficiencies of iron, folate, riboflavin (B_2), niacin, and cyanocobalamin (B_{12}) are all causative factors of mouth sores. If complicated by human immunodeficiency virus (HIV) infection and left untreated, the condition may progress to necrotizing stomatitis. Nicotinic stomatitis results directly from the chemical irritants in tobacco. Denture-related stomatitis results from the mechanical injury caused by ill-fitting dentures. Angular stomatitis is symptomatic of the aforementioned vitamin deficiencies, and pseudomembranous stomatitis has been associated with numerous chemical irritants and bacterial pathogens. Parasitic glossitis is caused by several mycoses (fungal infections) of the tongue, including *Cryptococcus linguae-pilosae* and *Nocardia lingualis* coinfection. Erythema multiforme may be caused by different types of infections, drug allergies, and collagen disorders, whereas the etiology of pemphigus vulgaris is unknown.

In the United States, herpes simplex virus (HSV) infection is widespread. Up to 20 percent of the adult population may be secreting herpes simplex type 1 or type 2 viruses at any given time. The prevalence of HSV-specific antibodies indicative of past or dormant HSV infection is up to 30 percent among individuals in higher socioeconomic strata; prevalence may even approach 100 percent in lower socioeconomic groups. Prior HSV infection is the primary risk factor for all secondary manifestations of herpes simplex infection. In addition, any factors that can lead to immunosuppression, such as fever, physical and/or emotional stress, excessive sun exposure, menstruation, common colds, gastrointestinal upset, and other underlying systemic illnesses, may be considered precipitating factors for HSV lesions (mouth sores).

Mouth sores may affect adults of all ages. Oral candidiasis (thrush) most commonly occurs in immunosuppressed adults, such as patients with HIV infection or patients with cancer status post chemotherapy and/or radiation therapy. Nicotinic stomatitis and denture-related stomatitis are very common; most other forms of stomatitis are rare among adults. Specifically, Vincent's stomatitis is prevalent among adolescents and adults 20 to 40 years of age, whereas denture-related stomatitis affects primarily older adults.

The most common forms of mouth sores seen regularly in the primary-care setting are secondary HSV/herpes labialis and aphthous stomatitis, both often recurrent in nature; recurrent aphthous stomatitis is referred to as recurrent aphthous stomatitis (RAS). As mentioned previously, oral candidiasis is seen primarily in immunosuppressed patients. The patient's history can assist in distinguishing these disorders.

Red Eye

Red eye, a common ophthalmic problem encountered in the acute and primary-care settings, is a nonuniform redness of the conjunctiva from hyperemia, which can be diffuse, localized, or peripheral, or may encircle a clear cornea. The most common condition is viral conjunctivitis, which is benign; other causes of red eye include bacteria, allergies, chemical irritations or minor eye irritation from inadequate sleep, overuse of contact lenses, environmental irritants, or excessive rubbing. Some conditions are benign; others may threaten vision and require the immediate attention of an ophthalmologist.

An accurate history from the patient is essential for diagnosis and should include the following inquiries, if there is a history of disease or trauma to the eyelid, globe, or head: Has there been any acute loss of vision or blurring vision? Does the patient complain of pain, and if so, when did it begin, where is it located, and is it constant or intermittent? Are there any complaints of photophobia, halo vision, or excessive tearing? The clinician should also ask about burning, itching, or a foreign body sensation in the eye.

The next step is an accurate examination. The clinician should always record the patient's visual acuity in both eyes as well as in each eye (when tested separately) and should ask the patient if his or her vision has been affected. The clinician should determine the amount of inflammation involved. When looking at the patient's eyes, it is important to note where the inflammation is in relation to the pupil, whether it is localized or diffuse, whether it is symmetric or asymmetric in one or both eyes, and whether the eyelids are swollen. The clinician should inspect the eyelids, lashes, and surrounding skin and lymph nodes for abnormalities and determine the type of conjunctival discharge. The following steps should also be part of the exam: (1) Inspect for corneal opacities and abrasions with the use of a slit lamp and with fluorescein staining. (2) Determine any corneal epithelial defect or abnormality. (Trauma and inflammation of the cornea are the two most common causes of epithelial defects.) (3) Assess pupillary response for equality and reactivity to light and accommodation. (Failure to react appropriately is indicative of a more serious problem and should be referred to an ophthalmologist.) (4) Determine intraocular pressure, unless there is an obvious external infection.

Differential Diagnosis

Differential diagnoses for red eye include conjunctivitis, chalazion, hordeolum (stye), cataracts, glaucoma, and retinopathies. Table 7.4 presents a comparison of the selected differential diagnoses for red eye.

Signs and symptoms of *bacterial conjunctivitis* include itching and tearing, either bilaterally or unilaterally, with a moderate amount of mucopurulent (yellow-green) discharge. There is a moderate amount of conjunctival hyperemia, with a shiny red appearance to the lower lids. There is no pain, nor are there any visual disturbances. The cornea is clear; there is no preauricular adenopathy. Bacterial conjunctivitis most commonly occurs in the winter and fall.

Allergic conjunctivitis is another differential diagnosis for red eye. There is bilateral itching, with a watery discharge. The patient may have a history of atopy. The conjunctiva and lids are swollen and reddened. This is a seasonal occurrence, most common in fall and spring, and may be accompanied by sneezing, rhinorrhea, and throat itching.

Viral conjunctivitis should also be ruled out. The patient with this type of conjunctivitis typically complains of itching, burning, and increased tearing. The conjunctiva is brilliant red, diffuse, and peripheral. There is a watery mucoid discharge, with a moderate amount of mucoid debris. The patient may also have conjunctival edema, follicles on the palpebral conjunctiva, and lid edema. There are usually signs of a upper respiratory tract infection or a history of recent contact with another person with red eye.

Iritis is another differential diagnosis. The patient presents with marked conjunctival injection, mainly around the cornea; it is unilateral, without discharge. The patient has moderate to severe pain and photophobia. The vision is blurred, pupils are constricted, and pupillary response to light is poor. Iritis requires a referral to an ophthalmologist.

Keratoconjunctivitis—in which the lack of an adequate tear film to cover and protect the cornea and conjunctiva causes a nonspecific irritation, with burning redness, dryness, the sensation of foreign body, and generalized eye pain—should also be ruled out.

Blepharitis is an inflammation involving the structures of the lid margin, with redness, scaling, and crusting. It commonly affects older adults, and is usually secondary to either chronic staphylococcal infection or seborrheic der-

Table 7.4 Differential Diagnosis: Red Eye

Assessment	Bacterial Conjunctivitis	Allergic Conjunctivitis	Viral Conjunctivitis	Iritis	Acute Glaucoma
Discharge	Purulent, thick	String mucoid	Watery	Rare	None
Visual acuity	Normal	Normal	Normal	May be decreased if iritis is severe	Decreased
Pain	Sandiness, crusted lids in morning	Itching and burning	Itching, burning, and tearing	Moderate pain	Severe pain
Conjunctival injection	Moderately heavy, diffuse	Mild, diffuse	Moderate, diffuse	Moderate, around cornea	Moderate, around cornea limbus
Corneal abnormalities	None	None	None	Punctate lesions on lower half of cornea	Anterior chamber may appear narrow with penlight exam
Pupillary abnormalities	None	None	None	Poor light reflex	Mid-dilated, nonreactive, or sluggish
Photophobia	No	No	No	Yes	Mild
Bilateral involvement	Sometimes	Usually	Often (highly contagious)	No	Sometimes
Intraocular pressure	Normal	Normal	Normal	Normal	Increased
Preauricular lymph nodes	Not palpable	Not palpable	Palpable	Not palpable	Not palpable
Other	Occurs in fall and winter	Rhinorrhea, sneezing Occurs in fall and spring	URI (upper respiratory infection)	May have connective tissue disease	Nausea, vomiting, headache

matitis. Treatment includes warm eyelid compresses and eyelid scrubs with dilute baby shampoo two to four times per day. Chronic cases may require antibiotic ointment.

Pterygium, a conjunctival degeneration that results in an opacity that partially covers the cornea, is most commonly seen at the 3 and 9 o'clock positions. There is conjunctival injection and tear filming; the opacity is usually slow growing and may obstruct the vision. Pterygium is most commonly seen in persons with excessive exposure to ultraviolet light, windy conditions, or dusty surroundings. Treatment includes artificial tears to alleviate irritation, protective eyewear to be worn when outside, and surgical removal of the opacity if visual disturbance occurs.

Subconjunctival hemorrhage—the sudden onset of painless red eye without any other associated symptoms—is usually caused by trauma, excessive straining, coughing, or hypertension. No treatment is needed if the cause can be found. The patient should be reassured that resolution will take place in 2 to 4 weeks.

The signs and symptoms of *herpes zoster ophthalmicus* include eye pain (which may be severe), tearing, photophobia, mucoid discharge, and moderate conjunctival hyperemia. The cornea may be clear or cloudy. Vesicles may or may not be present. Symptoms are usually the result of reactivation of latent zoster infection because of stress or infection. Patients with herpes zoster ophthalmicus should be referred to an ophthalmologist.

Signs and symptoms of *corneal abrasion* include pain, foreign body sensation, photophobia, tearing, and conjunctival hyperemia. The patient will usually have a history of scratching the eye, contact lens irritation, or actual trauma. The clinician should stain the eye with fluorescein and use cobalt blue filter light to inspect the eye for foreign objects or scratches. Treatment includes antibiotic drops or ointment for 5 days. Patching is not usually necessary. The patient should avoid wearing contact lenses until the abrasion heals. The clinician should follow up daily until symptoms are resolved.

With acute closed-angle *glaucoma,* the patient will have a sudden onset of severe pain and blurred vision, with nausea and vomiting. The patient will report seeing rainbow halos around lights. There will be corneal cloudiness, with diffuse conjunctival hyperemia. The pupil of the affected eye will be moderately dilated and completely unresponsive to light. Any patient with glaucoma should be referred to an ophthalmologist immediately.

A *hordeolum* (stye) is a swollen, tender, erythematous lesion located on the eyelid margin, lasting less than a few weeks. It is caused by a blocked meibomian or Zeis gland. Treatment includes warm, moist compresses three to four times per day, with topical antibiotic drops or ointment.

A *chalazion* is a hordeolum that does not resolve and eventually forms granulation tissue. A chalazion is usually not reddened; it may be minimally painful but is usually more irritating than painful. Chalazia usually do not affect the vision. They may spontaneously resolve after several years. If visual disturbances or cosmetic problems occur, the patient should be referred to an ophthalmologist.

With *dacryocystitis,* the patient has a large, diffuse conjunctival injection, pain over the temporal part of the eye, considerable lid swelling, and may have a purulent discharge and fever. The cause is an obstruction due to infection or inflammation of the lacrimal sac, which may result from overgrowth of normal skin flora, trauma, congenital obstruction, or nasal or sinus surgery. The common pathogens are *Staphylococcus aureus* or *S. epidermidis;* the discharge should be cultured. Dacryocystitis may lead to cellulitis. Mild cases can be treated with oral antibiotics. Patients should use topical antibiotic drops, massage the ductal area, apply warm moist compresses, and be monitored closely for 24 to 48 hours.

Tinnitus

Tinnitus is a subjective perception of noise when in reality no environmental noise is present. It may be intermittent, continuous, or pulsatile (synchronous with heartbeat). It has been variously described as the sound of escaping air, running water, or the sound heard inside a large seashell, or as a buzzing, ringing, or humming noise. Tinnitus also has been described as a roaring or musical sound. It may be unilateral or bilateral.

Recent estimates suggest that as many as 40 million Americans are affected by tinnitus. Approximately 90 percent of patients with hearing loss experience some tinnitus, and approximately 1 percent of the population suffers from chronic tinnitus. Risk factors include hearing loss, labyrinthitis, Ménière's disease, otitis media or externa, otosclerosis, ear-canal blockage (from ear wax or a foreign body), a history of high or low blood pressure, head trauma, anemia, hypothyroidism, hyperthyroidism, or allergies. Chronic exposure to noise, especially high-pitched sounds, may damage the cilia and auditory hair cells, causing tinnitus. Certain medications may contribute to tinnitus; some (salicylates, quinine, alcohol, and indomethacin [Indocin]) with reversible effects, and others with irreversible effects (kanamycin, streptomycin, gentamicin, and vancomycin).

Differential Diagnosis

Tinnitus may arise from cardiovascular and system disorders (hypertension and anemia). Nonpathologic causes include acute anxiety and presbycusis. The patient experiencing tinnitus may also present with multiple symptomatology; those symptoms may alert the practitioner to the underlying cause. For example, hearing loss and tinnitus accompanied by vertigo, facial paralysis, headaches, nausea, vomiting, and papilledema may occur with acoustic neuroma. An early symptom of acoustic nerve (CN VIII) tumor is unilateral tinnitus. Occasionally, anemia may produce mild, irreversible tinnitus. In this case, the patient may complain of dim vision, syncope, and the associated signs of anemia, such as fatigue, weakness, exertional dyspnea, and tachycardia that accompany the tinnitus.

Other presentations commonly seen include a stiff neck and pain aggravated by activity that produces the tinnitus, accompanied by vertigo, nystagmus, hearing loss, and pain that radiates down the arms. Weakness, confusion, and feelings of unsteadiness (orthostatic hypotension) may also occur, especially when the patient stands up quickly. These symptoms may be indicative of atherosclerosis as a causative factor.

Complaints of ear fullness, itching, and hearing loss along with the tinnitus may be caused by a foreign body obstruction, such as cerumen (ear wax) impaction, and this should always be ruled out. Bilateral, high-pitched tinnitus may occur with severe hypertension (diastolic blood pressure exceeding 120 mm Hg). The patient may have associated symptoms of headache, numbness, nausea, and vomiting.

The patient may describe a sudden onset of vertigo, unilateral or bilateral hearing loss, dizziness, nausea or vomiting, and nystagmus. Labyrinthitis may be considered. In Ménière's disease, low-pitched tinnitus, along with vertigo, and fluctuating hearing loss, may occur. Tinnitus accompanied by bleeding from the ear canal can be caused by trauma. Purulent drainage and pain with tinnitus may be caused by infection. Other presenting symptoms of tinnitus may be fever, chills, and dizziness.

Laboratory studies are necessary to confirm possible underlying causes of tinnitus. A complete blood count (CBC) should be done to rule out anemia or infection. If drainage from the ear canal is evident, a culture should be obtained. Serum electrolyte readings and thyroid studies should also be ordered.

A thorough otologic exam should be done. Auscultation of the upper part of the neck near the ear of the affected side may detect a bruit and palpation may reveal a weak pulse. Vascular studies may need to be considered. MRI may reveal pathology in detail; this is currently the diagnostic procedure of choice. If the patient cannot tolerate this, CT scan with dye enhancement is an alternative. Special tests to determine the presence of middle ear fluid may be considered, such as tympanometry, acoustic reflex measurement, or acoustic reflectometry.

Treatment

Tinnitus usually cannot be treated successfully. Treatment of the underlying disorder (if one can be identified) may help, but overall, learning to cope with the tinnitus is the only approach. Avoidance of risk factors such as excessive noise whenever possible is advised.

Protective earplugs may need to be worn. Tinnitus-masking devices can match the frequency range and intensity of the tinnitus, producing a level of noise that will help block out the tinnitus without interfering with hearing. The device fits in the ear like a hearing aid and presents a more pleasant sound. Regular relief may be obtained by masking the tinnitus with background noise. Hearing aids are also helpful in tinnitus suppression: they help to amplify environmental sounds, thereby obscuring tinnitus. For patients who find the noise intolerable, biofeedback may be needed to help with psychological problems that can develop from the near-constant feeling of distress.

Although there is no medication to help tinnitus, oral antidepressants have proved to be effective. Nortriptyline (Elavil), at an initial dose of 50 mg orally at bedtime, may be considered. Meclizine HCl (Antivert, Bonine) is the most commonly used vestibular suppressant. Diazepam (Valium), usually in low doses such as 2 mg, may be a valuable adjunct therapy to treat an acute attack of vertigo, as well as being effective for those with anxiety. If chronic vertigo and dizziness accompany the tinnitus, vestibular rehabilitation should be considered.

Patients with tinnitus related to otitis media or other infections should be treated with antibiotics for an adequate duration, with careful monitoring of serum peak and trough levels. This will also prevent loss of vestibular function and deafness from antibiotic therapy with aminoglycosides. If medical management does not resolve ear infections, surgical intervention—with myringotomy and possible tube placement—may need to be considered. Referral to an otorhinolaryngologist should be initiated.

Referral to an audiologist should be initiated for a patient with tinnitus and hearing loss. If vertigo, nausea, and vomiting accompany the tinnitus, the patient should be referred to an otorhinolaryngologist.

General measures might include playing background music during the daytime and before sleep. Patients should be advised to quit smoking and to cut back on caffeine, chocolate, and salt intake. Fatigue may increase tinnitus; therefore, patients need to be encouraged to rest during the course of the day. Chewing gum or swallowing should be encouraged during descent on airplanes to promote eustachian tube opening with deglutition (swallowing)

Visual Disturbances and Impaired Vision

Common visual disturbances include "floaters" and flashing lights. These subjective complaints usually have different causes. The visualization of floaters is usually due to contraction of the vitreous, which is a common sequela of the aging process (degenerative vitreous changes, or syneresis). This may also result from tear-film debris, or material in the vitreous. Floaters are usually unilateral and are often seen when looking at a bright background. Floaters that appear gradually and become less noticeable over time are usually benign and require no treatment. Floaters that appear suddenly, especially if bilateral, may warrant further evaluation.

Photopsia, or flashing lights, is the subjective sensation of sparks or flashes of light induced by mechanical or electrical retinal stimulation. Any patient who complains of seeing flashing lights should be evaluated immediately for retinal tear or detachment. Monocular photopsia may occur secondary to cataracts, migraine headaches, epilepsy, vertebral basilar insufficiency, retinitis, retinal hole, detachment of the retina, or retinal microembolization. In addition, a condition seen especially among women 55 to 65 years of age is vitreous detachment, causing a fluid-filled optically empty space between the vitreous and the retina. A number of medications, such as clomiphene (Clomid) and many antibiotics, may cause this symptom, and more rarely, certain substances, such as hallucinogenic mushrooms, cannabis, mescaline, myristica (nutmeg), and gasoline. Static light and stars that appear bilaterally arise from the occipital cortex; bilateral photopsia with visual formed or unformed images is usually of cerebral origin.

Patients often come to the primary-care setting with symptoms related to changes in their vision. The list of differential diagnosis of impaired vision is quite lengthy; however, a number of conditions occur commonly and should be well known to the clinician. Light must pass through the cornea, aqueous humor, lens, and vitreous humor, and a clear image must be projected on the retina. All those structures must be clear to provide a clear retinal image. The optic nerve and retina must be healthy to transmit an accurate image to the visual cortex in the occipital lobe. Essentially parallel rays of light must enter the cornea, which are then bent by the cornea and lens to converge on the retina. The macula of the retina is responsible for central visual acuity and thus is the most important portion of the retina. This region of the retina distinguishes details and is used in reading. The patient perceives a blurred image when the light rays do not come to a point on the retina. Light-ray convergence in front of the retina causes myopia, or nearsightedness. If the light rays converge posterior to the retina, the patient is hyperopic, or farsighted. If the light rays focus on two lines rather than a single point, the patient has astigmatism. Corrective lenses must be ordered to correct refractive errors.

Differential Diagnosis

Refractive errors that are incompletely corrected or not corrected are the most common cause of visual impairment. Approximately 45 percent of the population have some form of refractive error. Often, if the refraction occurs in only one eye, no problem is perceived unless something happens to the other eye. Refractive errors have a gradual onset, are not usually accompanied by pain or redness, and improve with pinhole.

Another common cause of impaired vision is cataracts, commonly associated with aging, although these may also occur related to trauma, congenital defects, or secondary to medication usage. Opacities are usually visible on the lens. Cataracts have a slow onset and are not accompanied by redness or pain.

Glaucoma is another cause of impaired vision. In the population older than age 40, the prevalence of glaucoma is approximately 4 percent; more than 90 percent of these cases are chronic open-angle glaucoma (COAG). The other 10 percent of cases represent acute angle-closure glaucoma. Acute angle-closure glaucoma has a sudden onset and is extremely painful because of the rapid rise in intraocular pressure and resulting corneal edema.

Diabetic retinopathy is the leading cause of blindness in patients 20 to 60 years of age. It is a slow, progressive process of microangiopathy characterized by small vessel damage and occlusion. Background diabetic retinopathy reflects the incompetence of the vascular walls.

Microaneurysms form as well as retinal hemorrhages. Leaking capillaries cause edema of the retina and a decrease in central vision if the macula is involved. In areas where the fluid is reabsorbed, a lipid precipitate called hard exudate is left behind.

Acute monocular visual loss with sudden floaters in a person with diabetes suggests a vitreous hemorrhage.

Macular degeneration, or low vision, as it is sometimes referred to, is a disease of aging and is the leading cause of blindness in patients older than age 60. Risk Factors 7.1 presents the risk factors associated with macular degeneration. Approximately 25 percent of all Americans older than 60 years of age are affected by macular degeneration, a condition characterized by a slow, progressive atrophy and degeneration of the retina. This condition is termed "dry" macular degeneration. Occasionally, new blood vessels develop under the retina in the macula, causing a sudden distortion or loss of central vision. This condition is known as "wet" age-related macular degeneration; it presents as a sudden decrease in vision that should be referred immediately to an ophthalmologist.

There is often a progression from dry to wet macular degeneration. The macula is the most sensitive and central portion of the retina, a nerve-rich area essential for sight. For largely unknown reasons, after age 60, the macula begins to break down. As it degenerates, central vision and

RISK FACTORS 7.1

Macular Degeneration ("Low Vision")

- Caucasian race
- Female gender
- Age over 60 years
- Cigarette smoking
- Other risk factors that are unproved, but documented in some studies include:
  - High serum cholesterol
  - Low serum carotenoid levels
  - Exposure to ultraviolet lights
  - Thin build
  - Light-colored eyes
  - Farsightedness

fine-detail perception deteriorate. Patients typically cannot read print well (if at all), see facial details, read signs, or carry out ordinary daily visual activities.

The main task is to determine if the problem is an acute one, needing referral and immediate treatment, or a more routine one. Determining whether the onset of the visual impairment has been acute or gradual will assist the clinician in making this determination. Likewise, the severity of the visual loss is also important. Severe and sudden visual loss should be referred immediately to an ophthalmologist. Vitreous hemorrhage, retinal detachment, uveitis, retrobulbar optic neuritis, and vascular occlusion generally present in this manner. A gradual progressive change is more indicative of changing refractive error, cataract, glaucoma, diabetic retinopathy, and macular degeneration.

Another distinguishing feature is whether the vision loss is monocular, or whether the deficit affects both eyes. Retinal detachment, vitreous hemorrhage, acute glaucoma, and central retinal artery or vein occlusion are more likely to be acute and monocular. If both eyes are affected, the problem is more likely at or distal to the optic chiasm rather than a problem affecting the globe or optic nerve. No afferent defect is present if both eyes are similarly affected. Some examples include a *homonymous hemianopia,* in which the same half of the visual field is lost in both eyes, or *bitemporal hemanopsia,* in which the temporal fields of both eyes are affected. The effect of the fields of vision produced by lesions at various points along the optic pathway is shown on the right. Testing of visual fields will help localize the problem.

Although ophthalmologic problems may often need to be referred, examination in the primary-care office with a slit lamp and fundoscopic exam may assist in making the diagnosis.

First, visual acuity must be evaluated, with the patient wearing any assistive lenses. If vision is less than 20/20, it should be checked with a pinhole. Vision that corrects with a pinhole implies an uncorrected refractive problem. Then the clinician should conduct an external evaluation of the eye and its structures: The lids, conjunctiva, pupils, and extraocular movements should be checked. Acute angle closure glaucoma presents with an unreactive pupil, for example. A Marcus Gunn pupil implies damage to the optic nerve. In addition, conjunctival injection is present with trauma, corneal problems, iritis, acute angle closure, glaucoma, and hyphema.

The fundoscopic exam is normal in patients with refractive error. Cataracts, if dense, may make it difficult to visualize the retina, but otherwise the exam is unremarkable. Patients with glaucoma have increased cupping of the optic disk (a normal cup-to-disk ratio is 0.5 or less, meaning that the cup should be one-half the size of the disk or less). Increased cupping is cause for referral to an ophthalmologist. Retinal hemorrhages, hard exudate, "cotton wool" spots, or neovascularization indicate diabetic retinopathy. If the fundus is difficult or impossible to view in a patient with diabetes, suspect vitreous hemorrhage, especially in diabetic patients with sudden visual loss. Yellowish round spots (drusen) may be indicative of early macular degeneration; clumps of pigment irregularly interspersed with depigmented areas of atrophy in the macula are more typical of a later phase of the disorder. Analysis of central vision may be done with an Amsler grid to locate macular blind spots and areas of distortion and wavy lines. Measurement of contrast sensitivity with specially designed tests for low vision may reveal the degree of loss of retinal sensitivity (contrast) and indicate the potential success (or failure) of optical magnifying devices.

Patients with suspected optic nerve disease or neurologic disorders require visual field testing and referral to an ophthalmologist and/or neurologist. Often these patients have diminished color vision, easily tested with Ishihara's color plates.

A comparison of the differential diagnoses of impaired vision is provided in Table 7.5.

Treatment

All patients with sudden, severe vision loss should be referred to an ophthalmologist. Similarly, all patients who complain of seeing flashing lights should be evaluated immediately for retinal tear or detachment. Refer any case of suspected glaucoma if intraocular pressure is above 30 or if the presentation is acute. Sudden visual loss, especially in a patient with diabetes, should be referred immediately. Sudden visual loss or distortion of vision in a patient with macular degeneration also requires immediate referral.

Patients with diabetes should be monitored by an ophthalmologist yearly (including a dilated fundoscopic exam) and their blood glucose should be controlled. Patients with refractive error should be referred for nonemergent care. Patients with glaucoma and macular degeneration should be followed by an ophthalmologist. Importantly, all patients with HIV infection or AIDS should have a retinal exam every 6 months.

In cases of macular degeneration, treatment options, for example, laser treatment, have not proven to be very effective. A number of clinical trials are investigating potential alternative treatment for macular degeneration, such as submacular surgery, photodynamic therapy, and irradiation. Experimental pharmacologic interventions include antibodies against vascular endothelial growth factor, angiostatin, batimastat, tissue plasminogen activator, and thalidomide (Synovir), for its anti-angiogenetic properties.

Instead of telling the patient that nothing can be done, however, refer him or her to a rehabilitation source where the outcome of the disease can be evaluated, daily living needs can be assessed, and visual aids may be offered. Sources may include ophthalmologists who provide low vision services in their practice, optometrists who are trained to offer low vision remediation, agencies for visually impaired individuals (either private or state-supported),

Table 7.5 Differential Diagnosis: Impaired Vision

Diagnosis	Patient Age	Subjective Assessment	Objective Assessment	Urgent Treatment Required?
Refractive error				
Myopia	Teenager	Painless progressive loss of vision (PPLV)	No change in fundus exam	No
Presbyopia	Over 40	PPLV May have blurred vision Gradual onset	No change in fundus exam	No
Cataracts	Older adults	PPLV	Vision decreased Opacity may be apparent Cloudy lens Decreased view of fundus	No
Macular degeneration	Older adults	PPLV Decreased central vision	Decreased in central vision Blood, lipid exudates on fundal exam	Usually not
Diabetic retinopathy	Related to length of time patient has had diabetes and any comorbid conditions	PPLV	Vision will usually not improve with pinhole Varies with stage of retinopathy Dot-blot hemorrhages Microaneurysms Lipid exudates Infarcts in nerve fiber layer	Usually not
Chronic glaucoma	Usually over 40, but may occur in younger patients	PPLV Halo around lights	Decreased peripheral field vision Decreased central vision is a later sign Increased intraocular pressure Increased cup-to-disk ratio Normal chamber angle	Usually not
Acute glaucoma	Usually 50–85	Sudden onset Severe eye pain Vomiting Headache	Conjunctiva may be injected Steamy corneas Pupil may be fixed, partially dilated Narrow chamber angle	Yes

institutions that offer services for veterans, and organizations such as the American Academy of Ophthalmology, the American Optometric Association, the National Eye Institute, and the Lighthouse. A team approach is useful in rehabilitation, and the primary-care provider is part of that team.

Optical aids include spectacles with and without prisms, hand magnifiers, stand-mounted magnifiers, and telescopes. As with any type of rehabilitation, time and patience are needed to determine the appropriate remedial lens for the patient. Working with the patient until he or she understands how to use the device is an important part of patient education. In addition, patients may be taught practical skills such as folding money in such a way that the denomination is more apparent, as well as techniques for grooming and identifying medications. The goal is to use "whatever works" for each patient.

Antioxidants and other plant chemicals (phytochemicals) have also been shown to protect against the development of macular degeneration.

Common Eye Problems

Blepharitis

Blepharitis is an inflammation of the eyelids and margins. There are two forms of blepharitis: a nonulcerative form associated with seborrhea of the face and scale and an ulcerative form that may involve the lash follicle and the meibomian glands of the eyelid. Secondary infections may develop with either form, and recurrences are common and frequently persistent. Both types may coexist.

Epidemiology and Causes

Blepharitis is the most common ocular disease, affecting males and females equally. Nonulcerative blepharitis is occasionally seen in those with trisomy 21, and tends to affect people with psoriasis, seborrhea, eczema, allergies, and lice infestations. Poor hygiene is implicated, as well as poor nutritional status, immune suppression, acne rosacea, and yeast infections. Exposure to chemical or environmental irritants may contribute to the development of this disorder, as well as the use of eye makeup and contact lenses.

Pathophysiology

Although difficult to discern without a full ophthalmologic exam, the localization of blepharitis speaks to the differentiation of affected structures. Anterior blepharitis typically affects the eyelash hair follicles along the eyelid's anterior lamella, while posterior blepharitis involves inspissation and inflammation of the meibomian gland orifices (meibomianitis) along the tarsal plate. Seborrheic gland dysfunction along with accelerated shedding of skin cells appears to be the primary insult resulting in inflammation in the nonulcerative form, in which an oily crust envelopes individual eyelash cilia (seborrheic blepharitis). The inflammatory, noninfectious skin disorder known as acne rosacea, which commonly affects the central face, is another common etiology of blepharitis in young adults younger than 30 years of age. Blepharitis may also be a manifestation of an allergic process such as a contact dermatitis, if a foreign irritant comes into contact with facial skin. In contrast, underlying infection by skin flora, most notably *Staphylococcus aureus*, produces an ulcerative form that may become chronic, extending to the conjunctivae and cornea, known as blepharoconjunctivitis—a condition with a strong potential to affect eyesight.

Clinical Presentation

Subjective

Both forms of blepharitis may present with complaints of itching and burning, and foreign body sensation in the eye. Sensitivity to bright lights and tearing may also be present. Presentation may be unilateral or bilateral.

Objective

Lid margins are edematous and erythematous. Inspection with a magnifying glass may reveal scaling, erythema, and ulcers. Nonulcerative blepharitis may present with scales along the lid margins that are easily removed. With ulcerative blepharitis, there may be pustules at the base of the hair follicles that may crust and bleed. The lashes become thin and break easily. Use gloves to palpate the lid margins and lid for masses and palpate for preauricular lymphadenopathy.

Diagnostic Reasoning

Diagnostic Tests

With any eye problem, it is vital to evaluate visual acuity. Any alteration in visual acuity may indicate a potentially serious underlying problem that warrants further investigation. If there is a discharge, a culture and sensitivity should be considered. Referral for patients with blepharitis should occur in the following situations: visual loss, moderate to severe pain, chronic redness of the eye, corneal involvement, recurrent blepharitis, and when patients fail to respond to therapy. Any lesion in or around the eye that does not respond to conventional therapy in one month should be referred to a specialist for possible biopsy. Persistent inflammation and thickening of the eyelid margin may indicate squamous cell, basal cell, or sebaceous cell carcinoma. Sebaceous cell carcinoma has a 23 percent fatality rate; up to one-half of potentially fatal sebaceous cell carcinomas resemble chronic, benign inflammatory disease, particularly chalazions and blepharoconjunctivitis.

Differential Diagnosis

Persistent inflammation and thickening of the eyelid margin may indicate squamous cell, basal cell, or sebaceous cell carcinoma masquerading as blepharitis. Carcinoma may also mimic styes or chalazions. Any swelling or inflammation of the eyelid that does not resolve promptly (within 1 month) with treatment should be evaluated further. Management Table 7.1 describes the management of various forms of blepharitis.

Follow-Up and Referral

The clinician should reevaluate the patient in 2 weeks; if symptoms are improving, the patient should be reevaluated every 2 months or when symptoms return. As noted, if there is no resolution in a month, the patient should be referred to an ophthalmologist. Vision changes and pain in the eye also warrant referral. Blepharitis may be difficult to resolve and recurrences are common. Hordeolum, loss of lashes, or misdirection of the eyelashes (trichiasis), scarring, and corneal infection may occur.

Patient Education

Patients should be encouraged to wash their hands often and dry them with clean towels to prevent reinfection or transfer of bacteria or virus to other persons. In addition, patients should be advised to avoid environmental irritants; to use hypoallergenic soap and makeup; and to exercise care in use of contact lenses. The clinician should educate the patient as to the chronic and recurrent nature of this disorder and the need for vigilance in adherence to the treatment plan until the blepharitis is completely resolved. Long-term eyelid hygiene—gently cleansing with baby shampoo daily—is required to control this disorder. Eye makeup should not be used until resolution of the disorder, and then the patient should switch to hypoallergenic makeup. A blepharitis fact sheet is available from the American Academy of Ophthalmology.

Hordeolum/Chalazion

A *hordeolum,* also known as a *stye,* is an acutely presenting, erythematous, tender lump within the eyelid. This condition involves an inflammation/infection of the eyelid margin involving the hair follicles of the eyelashes (external hordeolum), or the meibomian glands (internal hordeolum) and

Management Table 7.1 Blepharitis

Type	Description	Treatment
Initial treatments for nonulcerative blepharitis	This type of blepharitis may be persistent and treatment is aimed at improved hygiene.	Warm compresses Eyelid hygiene with no tears shampoo—patients should be advised that eyelid hygiene may be required for life, and that symptoms may recur if treatment is discontinued. Warm, moist compresses may also be used to provide comfort and facilitate distribution of antibiotic ointment. The patient should apply soaks for 20 minutes, then rest for at least an hour. The patient should also discontinue the use of eye makeup and contact lenses.
Staphylococcal blepharitis ulcerated lesions	Infectious blepharitis should be treated with topical antibiotic ointments that adhere to the eyelid margins more effectively than drops.	Bacitracin or erythromycin 0.5% ointment can be prescribed and applied on the eyelids one or more times daily or at bedtime for one or more weeks. The frequency and duration of treatment should be guided by the severity of the blepharitis. For resistant staphylococcal infections a quinolone antibacterial ointment.
Severe blepharitis	Associated with rosacea	Doxycycline 100 mg PO twice daily (bid) or tetracycline 250 mg PO qid. These are usually prescribed for several weeks and tapered.

may evolve into a chalazion. A chalazion is a granulomatous infection of a meibomian gland, presenting in the form of painless swelling on the eyelid. Initially, a chalazion may be tender and erythematous before evolving into a nontender lump. Blepharitis is frequently associated with chalazia.

Epidemiology and Causes

These are all common eyelid disorders that affect men and women equally. The cause is often a blockage in a duct of the meibomian gland leading to the eyelid surface; secondary infection may be present, again, commonly with *Staphylococcus.* This obstruction results in inflammation that may manifest as a hard mass (chalazion); infection of the sebaceous glands of the eyelash (external hordeolum); or infection of posterior margin of the eyelid (internal hordeolum). Previously unresolved blepharitis, poor hygiene, immunosuppression, and underlying chronic diseases all contribute to the development of eyelid disorders. Again, skin conditions such as acne rosacea or seborrheic dermatitis may also predispose the individual toward the development of a hordeolum.

Pathophysiology

Hordeolums and chalazia are various manifestations of the inflammatory response at the eyelids, exhibiting both microscopic (accumulation of fluid and cells at the inflammatory site) and macroscopic (redness, swelling, heat, pain, and loss of function) hallmarks of inflammation. An internal hordeolum is a suppurative infection of the oil-secreting meibomian glands within the tarsal plate of the eyelid that may evolve into a chalazion. An external hordeolum occurs with infection of the more superficial anteriorly located Glands of Zeis or Moll found at the eyelid margin. With a stye (hordeolum), the eyelid may manifest a classic inflammatory reaction; however, a chalazion results from an obstruction of the meibomian gland with a granulomatous response and is typically painless. The blockage of the gland's duct at the eyelid margin results in the release of the gland's contents into the surrounding eyelid soft tissue, and a lipogranulomatous reaction ensues, producing a pea-sized nodule within the eyelid. Occasionally, a chalazion may also become secondarily infected with *Staphyloccocus aureus.*

Clinical Presentation

Subjective

Hordeolum presents as a localized inflammation of the eyelashes (external) or redness at the margin of the eyelid, with swelling (internal). In addition, patients may experience itching or scaling of the eyelid, chronic redness, and eye irritation, leading to localized tenderness and pain.

Chalazion commonly presents as a slow-developing, painless hard mass, with inflammation and possible involvement of the surrounding tissue.

Objective

The clinician should evaluate visual acuity. With chalazion, inversion of the eyelid will reveal a red, elevated mass that may become quite large and press against the eye, causing nystagmus. The clinician should also palpate for preauricular adenopathy.

Diagnostic Reasoning

Diagnostic Tests

Hordeolum and chalazia are usually diagnosed by their appearance. If drainage is present, culture the drainage. If the conditions persist, referral for biopsy may be indicated.

Differential Diagnosis

As noted previously, any inflammation or swelling that does not resolve within a month with treatment should be referred. Squamous cell, basal cell, or sebaceous cell carcinoma may mimic other disorders of the eyelid. Sebaceous cell carcinoma, according to some reports, has a 23 percent fatality rate. Up to one-half of these potentially fatal carcinomas may resemble benign inflammatory disorders. A concurrent and predisposing blepharitis may be present. Management Table 7.2 describes the various treatments of hordeolum and chalazion.

Follow-Up and Referral

Any patient with visual change or pain should be referred to an ophthalmologist. Recurrence of hordeolum/chalazion is likely without proper lid hygiene.

Patient Education

The clinician should explain the recurrent nature of the disorder and the need for vigilance, and begin treatment at the first sign of recurrence. The practitioner should explain that staph (*S. aureus*) infections are contagious and instruct the patient and family members not to share towels or washcloths. The patient should use clean cloths for each warm compress to the eye, and be sure to wash his or her hands frequently.

Conjunctivitis

Conjunctivitis is an inflammation of the conjunctiva (mucous membrane) covering the front of the eye. The conjunctiva protects the eye against foreign materials and microorganisms. "Pink eye" refers to non-*Neisseria* bacterial conjunctivitis. Although most conjunctivitis is self-limiting, a few types may lead to permanent vision impairment if not promptly diagnosed and treated. It is essential for the clinician to be able to distinguish between types of conjunctivitis.

Epidemiology and Causes

Conjunctivitis is the most common of all eye disorders, affecting all ages. Males and females are equally affected; there are no specific ethnic predispositions. Risk factors are numerous; including trauma from wind, heat, smoke, cold, chemicals, and foreign bodies. Common causes of conjunctivitis include infectious agents (which may be bacterial, viral, or fungal) as well as toxicity (from an inciting agent of some sort) and allergy. Sexual transmission and ophthalmia neonatorium (transmission from passage down the birth canal) are associated with *Chlamydia, Neisseria gonorrhoeae,* and herpes simplex (HSV) I. The disorder, depending on the organism, may be transmitted by contaminated towels, washcloths, or from the patient's own hands. Noninfectious conjunctivitis may be drug-induced as a result of chronic irritation from use of eye medications over a long period of time. A chronic inflammatory conjunctivitis may develop similarly, secondary to irritation from contact lens use, seen most commonly with soft lenses but occasionally with hard lenses. A family history of atopy is a risk factor for certain types of allergic conjunctivitis.

Pathophysiology

A hallmark of conjunctival inflammation is hyperemia of the ocular and palpebral surfaces, with injection of this cell layer by engorged, superficial capillaries. Contact with viruses, bacteria, or allergens is the most common cause of

Management Table 7.2 Hordeolum/Chalazion

Initial treatment	The stye should not be squeezed. At the first sign of problem, warm compresses to the area should be applied to reduce inflammation and may increase blood supply and potentiate spontaneous drainage. Gently scrub the eyelids with diluted baby shampoo two to four times daily, or directly apply baby shampoo with a cotton-tipped applicator and then rinse. Blepharitis, if present, should be treated.
Infection or inflammation	Erythromycin ophthalmic ointment or sulfacetamide sodium (Sulamyd) ophthalmic ointment four times daily (qid) may be applied thinly to the lid margin with a cotton-tipped applicator.
Resistant or Reoccurence	Aminoglycoside ophthalmic ointment such as gentamicin
Prevention of secondary infection	Antibiotic eyedrops
Unresolved chalazia—Persists for more than 4 weeks.	Refer to an ophthalmologist for incision and drainage, biopsy, or injection directly with glucocorticoids. An internal hordeolum, if untreated, may lead to a generalized cellulitis of the lid.

inflammation of the conjunctiva. There is also an idiopathic form of conjunctivitis associated with certain systemic diseases such as thyroid disorders and infectious monoarthritis (formerly known as Reiter's syndrome). The most common causative bacterial agents include *Staphylococcus aureus, Streptococcus pneumoniae,* and *Haemophilus influenzae. Neisseria gonorrhoeae* and *Moraxella catarrhalis* are responsible for a particularly virulent hyperacute bacterial conjunctivitis. Viral agents implicated are adenovirus serotypes 3, 4, 7 (which cause pharyngitis with conjunctivitis), adenovirus serotypes 8 and 19 (which cause epidemic keratoconjunctivitis), adenovirus 11, coxsackie virus A24, enterovirus 70 (which causes acute hemorrhagic conjunctivitis), primary or recurrent HSV (usually type I), herpes zoster (which spreads down the optic nerve), as well as molluscum contagiosum. *Chlamydia trachomatis* (trachoma) causes adult inclusion conjunctivitis as well as ophthalmia neonatorum. *Chlamydia oculogenitalis* (which causes inclusion conjunctivitis) and *Chlamydia lymphogranulomatis* (which causes lymphogranuloma venereum) are also sexually transmitted causative agents.

Allergic (atopic) conjunctivitis may be linked to a systemic humoral or local histaminic response to an inciting environmental allergen. Certain autoimmune phenomena such as Sjögren's syndrome or Wegener's granulomatosis may also be involved. The conjunctivitis may be (1) seasonal, also called hay fever conjunctivitis, which is usually caused by grass pollens in May and June and by ragweed pollen in August and September; (2) vernal keratoconjunctivitis, which usually occurs in childhood and youth in individuals with a family history of atopy, is recurrent in warm weather, and is associated with large "cobblestone" papillae lining the posterior pharynx in those with a history of chronic atopy; or (3) an atopic keratoconjunctivitis that usually occurs in the late teen years.

Clinical Presentation

Subjective

Symptoms will vary with the cause, but cardinal symptoms of conjunctivitis are itching, watering, and redness of the eye. There may be a foreign body sensation and/or a sense of fullness around the eyes. Bacterial infections such as *S. aureus* may produce significant thick, yellow, sticky exudate of the eyelids. This profuse exudate occurs especially in the morning and the patient may complain that their eyelids "are stuck together" when they wake. Bacterial infections usually begin unilaterally whereas viral infections often appear in both eyes at once. Adenovirus conjunctivitis causes a foreign body sensation and minimal pruritus and exudate but profuse tearing. This type of conjunctivitis is often bilateral; preauricular adenopathy is common, along with systemic symptoms typical of a virus, such as fever, myalgia, and the like. Other family members may be affected. Associated upper respiratory tract infection symptoms may point to a viral cause. Visual loss, photophobia, and severe eye pain may suggest corneal involvement. The clinician should ask the patient about any history of allergens and potential contacts, including mention of symptoms of sexually transmitted diseases. Chlamydial causality tends to present bilaterally, with minimal pruritus and moderate to profuse tearing and exudate. Allergic conjunctivitis also presents bilaterally, with severe pruritus, moderate tearing, and no exudate.

Objective

Use gloves when examining the eyes of a patient with suspected conjunctivitis. On inspection, there will be hyperemia and tearing. If exudate is present and is thick and copious, the cause is probably bacterial or chlamydial. There may be eyelid swelling. Areas of lymphoid tissue hyperplasia that appear as dome-shaped elevations with blood vessels on their surface are called follicles; these are present in many types of conjunctivitis. If follicles are prominent in the upper tarsus, this is usually indicative of a viral etiology such as adenovirus, or *Chlamydia.* Minute elevations with vascular cores that may coalesce to form large papillae occasionally form secondary to inflammatory process. These may be present on the superior tarsal plate in cases of vernal keratoconjunctivitis, adenovirus, or HSV.

Preauricular nodes often represent a viral etiology, such as HSV or adenovirus, chlamydial infections, and in *N. gonorrhoeae.* The nodes are less prominent and more tender to palpation in patients with conjunctivitis of bacterial etiology. Subconjunctival hemorrhage may be seen in bacterial conjunctivitis or enterovirus 70 conjunctivitis.

Corneal involvement, which often manifests as eye pain, decreased visual acuity, and photophobia, may be present; it may manifest as punctate epithelial lesions. The potential for corneal involvement is increased in cases of adenovirus, vernal keratoconjunctivitis, and *N. gonorrhoeae.* The presence of a membranous film that covers and adheres to the entire surface of the conjunctival epithelium is usually associated with epidemic keratoconjunctivitis, HSV, *S. pneumoniae,* and *N. gonorrhoeae.* If the membrane is removed, a bleeding surface is left behind.

Diagnostic Reasoning

Diagnostic Tests

The clinician should always check visual acuity first. Additional testing in routine cases of conjunctivitis is usually not necessary. A dilated pupil exam should be performed in patients with hyperemia accompanied by proptosis, optic nerve dysfunction, decreased visual acuity, diplopia, or anterior chamber inflammation. Fluorescein staining may be indicated to rule out corneal involvement or keratitis. Use blue penlight illumination to observe for corneal scratches, corneal dendrites (which represent HSV), or corneal ulceration. The practitioner should use anesthetic drops before staining the eye. If *N. gonorrhoeae* is suspected, or if conjunctivitis has failed to respond to treatment, or in cases of ophthalmia neonatorum, membranous conjunctivitis, and prolonged, severe conjunctivitis, Gram stain and culture should be done. In cases of suspected *Chlamydia* or herpes, the clinician should do specific cultures and/or perform a fluorescent antibody test.

In persistent cases of conjunctivitis, referral to an ophthalmologist is essential so that scrapings, cultures, and smears can be taken. Conjunctival biopsy is occasionally useful in refractory or atypical conjunctivitis and is always done in cases of suspected neoplasm. When a hypopyon (a layer of white blood cells) or hyphema (a layer of red blood cells) in the anterior chamber is detected on examination an immediate referral to an ophthalmologist is required as this may reflect infectious keratitis/endophthalmitis or penetrating eye trauma.

Differential Diagnosis

Corneal disease or foreign body may be ruled out with fluorescent staining. The patient who presents with acute glaucoma is usually older; more visual loss is present, pain is more severe, and there may also be headache and nausea. Uveitis (iritis, iridocyclitis, choroiditis) usually presents with more severe eye pain, photophobia, blurred vision, injection in the limbus area, and deposits in the cornea. All of the above are ocular emergencies; patients should be referred to an ophthalmologist immediately to avoid permanent vision loss.

The more typical task for the clinician is to decide which type of conjunctivitis is involved, an essential task before treating the patient.

Management

Treatment will depend on etiology. In general, visual acuity should be tested and recorded. Do not patch the eye, although steroids sometimes help with irritation. Clinicians should not order topical steroids, but rather refer the patient to an ophthalmologist if there is an ulcer, keratitis, suspected herpes, or if the conjunctivitis worsens in 24 hours. Any purulent material or debris should be removed from the conjunctival area. Lubrication of the eye with artificial tears is recommended, or frequent cleansing by lavage. The patient should clean the lid margins with a no-tears shampoo and discontinue wearing contact lenses (if any). Compresses are often effective for local relief; they should be warm in cases of infective conjunctivitis, and cold in cases of allergic or irritative conjunctivitis. The patient should be cautioned to avoid spreading the conjunctivitis (or persistent reinfection) through autoinoculation. Pharmacologic therapy will depend on the identified or suspected causative agent (see Management Table 7.3).

Patient Education

The clinician should teach the patient to instill medication to the inner aspect of the lower lid. It may be best to use ophthalmic solution during the daytime and then to apply a thin film of ointment before sleep. The practitioner should explain that secretions may remain infectious for at least 48 hours after the start of treatment. Conjunctivitis is highly contagious; therefore the patient should take care when coming in contact with other members of the household, especially infants, children, older adults, and pets. Spread of conjunctivitis may be prevented by using good hand washing, not touching eyes, and not sharing towels and washcloths. The clinician should teach the patient to avoid autoinoculation: The patient should not touch the medication applicator to the eye, and should use separate eyecups for each lavage. No contact lens usage is allowed until the infection is resolved.

Cataracts

A *cataract* is any opacity of the natural lens of the eye. It may or may not be associated with visual impairment or functional consequences, and may be localized or generalized. More than 90 percent of cataracts are age-related. Other causes of cataracts include congenital, metabolic, and traumatic etiologies, such as excessive exposure to sunlight (ultraviolet B rays) without protective lenses over time. In the United States, cataract surgery is the most common surgical procedure performed under Medicare, is most commonly done in an outpatient setting, and is effective in improving vision in 95 percent of patients treated.

Epidemiology and Causes

Cataracts remain one of the leading causes of blindness worldwide. An estimated 17 million people have become blind from cataracts, mainly in third-world countries. More than 50 percent of all people between ages 65 and 75 have cataracts; 92 percent of all patients older than age 75 have some opacities, and 46 percent of this group have significant vision loss, defined as 20/30 or worse. These percentages are equally distributed between males and females, as well as across ethnic groups.

Risk factors for cataract formation include aging and predisposing diseases such as diabetes, uveitis, intraocular tumor, medication usage (such as corticosteroid usage) over time, excessive exposure to sunlight (ultraviolet B rays) over time, trauma (blunt or penetrating), excessive exposure to heat (e.g., glass blowers, welders), radiation exposure, and electrical injury. Smoking has been identified as a risk factor for cataracts, along with family history, excessive alcohol intake, poor dietary habits (lack of antioxidants), and atopic dermatitis.

Pathophysiology

The transparency of the human lens results from the highly ordered nature of its composite stratified epithelia, which contain a high density of cytoplasmic proteins called crystallins. Normally, the lens is a naturally clear, biconvex structure located behind the cornea and supported by zonules.

Management Table 7.3 Types of Conjunctivitis and their Treatments

Type of Conjunctivitis	Treatment
Allergic conjunctivitis	Supportive treatment including lubricants and cold compresses for symptomatic relief. Medications: Topical antihistamines, topical nonsteroidal antiinflammatory drugs, topical mast-cell stabilizers, and systemic antihistamines
Bacterial conjunctivitis	Acute bacterial conjunctivitis may be prevented with meticulous hand washing and good hygiene. Patients should be advised to avoid sharing eye drops, towels, washcloths, makeup, and pillows. Antibiotic drops that may be used include: norfloxacin 0.3%; ciprofloxacin 0.3%; ofloxacin 0.3%; lomefloxacin 0.3%; levofloxacin 0.5%; chloramphenicol 0.5%; sulfacetamide sodium 10%; erythromycin 5 mg/g; gentamicin sulfate 0.3%; trimethoprim sulfate-polymyxin B 10,000 U/1 mg/1 mL; fusidic acid 0.1%; and tobramycin 0.3%. Most cases are self-limiting however, the addition of steroids with antibiotic treatment can lessen the patients' inflammation and duration of disease. The practitioner MUST distinguish between viral, hyperacute, and bacterial conjunctivitis before prescribing topical steroids to prevent further damage. Refer to a specialist if no improvement within the first 24 hours after initiating therapy or if patient develops moderate to severe ocular pain, develops severe purulent discharge, if there is diminished visual acuity or loss of vision, when conjunctivitis is associated with a sexually transmitted disease, or when infection proves to be resistant to conventional antibiotic therapy.
Viral conjunctivitis	Supportive therapy—cold compresses, lubricants, and ocular decongestants. Topical antibiotics or steroids are not recommended unless there is a secondary bacterial infection because of potential side effects and minimal benefit. Herpes simplex conjunctivitis requires systemic or topical antiviral agents. Topical steroids are specifically contraindicated for treating herpes simplex. Herpes zoster conjunctivitis–use systemic antiviral treatment to reduce duration of viral shedding and postherpetic neuralgia. Start therapy within 72 hours of symptoms.
Chlamydial conjunctivitis	Systemic antibiotics as topical therapy alone is not adequate. Single-dose azithromycin 1 g or doxycycline 100 mg twice daily for 7 days. Patients' sexual partners should be evaluated for the presence of the infection and treated as indicated.
Contact lens-related conjunctivitis	Discontinue the use of contact lenses. Causes include solution allergy, hypoxic conditions, giant papillary conjunctivitis, bacterial infection, or trauma. Cause should be corrected before resuming contact lens use.
Mechanical conjunctivitis	Removal of the offending trauma inducing agent (eye lash, exposed suture) and lubrication are usually adequate. If significant epithelial disruption occurs consider lubricants and broad-spectrum antibiotic ophthalmic drops.
Traumatic conjunctivitis	Resolving the trauma. Treat abrasions with antibiotics, cycloplegia, and patching. Oral analgesics for pain. For chemical injuries aggressive treatment is required with copious irrigation using normal saline or a balanced salt solution.
Toxic conjunctivitis	These result from overuse of topical medications or cosmetics or both. Stop all offending medications. Removing the offending agent is the cornerstone of treatment. Cold compresses, topical ophthalmic antibiotic/corticosteroid combination.
Neonatal conjunctivitis	Should be evaluated by a neonatologist or pediatric infectious disease specialist. Treatment should be initiated immediately upon diagnosis.
Parinaud's oculo-glandular syndrome	Usually self-limiting. Requires symptomatic relief. Mild topical vasoconstrictor and warm soaks. In severe cases a biopsy may be required
Phlyctenular conjunctivitis	Treatment directed at removing underlying cause which includes chronic eye lid diseases caused by *Staphylococcus aureus.* This should be treated with topical antibiotics and corticosteroids.
Secondary conjunctivitis	Identification and treatment of underlying cause.

Over time, the crystalline lens becomes fibrotic, hardened, and dehydrated, in turn, progressively opacifying and transforming into a cataract. Contained within the lens capsule is a central nucleus surrounded by a cortex. The lens is avascular, deriving its metabolic needs from the aqueous and vitreous humors. Early in life, the lens is pliable and can change its shape as connecting zonules anchored to ciliary bodies place varying degrees of stress on the lens through involuntary contraction and relaxation. These changes in lens shape result in accommodation, allowing objects to come into focus at varying distances.

Aging alters the biochemical and osmotic balance required for lens clarity, as does the hyperglycemia of uncontrolled diabetes mellitus. Fluctuating visual acuity and rapid-onset nearsightedness known as a "myopic shift" caused by alterations in the glucose, electrolyte, or water balance within the lens are early symptoms of diabetes mellitus. Moreover, unlike the other endothelia in the body, the lens cannot shed nonviable cells. Thus, as the lens ages, it loses both its pliability as well as its clarity. These changes are thought to occur because of damage from oxidation, a biochemical process set in motion when a highly reactive form of oxygen (an oxygen radical) forms within the cells of the lens itself. Although antioxidants have not been shown to definitely delay or treat cataracts, in addition to senescence, several other cataract risk factors are thought to increase oxidative damage, including alcohol consumption, sunlight (ultraviolet B) exposure, and tobacco smoking, which has been attributed to more than 20 percent of the cataracts in the United States. Additional well-recognized risk factors include excessive lead exposure and systemic corticosteroid use. Moreover, healing fibrosis from ocular trauma is a primary etiology of acquired cataracts, while secondary cataracts may also result from other forms of ocular inflammation that extend to the lens, including uveitis, topical anticholinesterase preparations, and radiation therapy used to treat ocular tumors.

There are three subtypes of cataracts, categorized by anatomic localization: nuclear sclerotic, cortical spoking, and posterior subcapsular. Many patients have a combination of these subtypes. The size, density, and location of the cataract determine its effect on vision and the most appropriate method of surgical intervention/lens replacement. Nuclear cataracts are characterized by significant nearsightedness and a slow, indolent course. In contrast, cortical cataracts do not significantly impair vision. Posterior cataracts, on the other hand, create a subcapsular haze and a severe glare in bright light. They are strongly associated with systemic steroid use and progress much faster than the nuclear form (months rather than years). Regardless of anatomic type, immature cataracts are those that do not obscure the red retinal light reflex on funduscopy. In contrast, mature cataracts obscure the red reflex with significant visual impairment, while hypermature cataracts are characterized by liquefaction of the cortical lens with mobility of the nucleus.

Clinical Presentation

Subjective

The patient with cataracts may or may not present with visual changes and/or functional impairment. Cataracts produce a gradual, painless, progressive loss of vision and many patients are unaware of vision problems. For example, with monocular (asymmetric) cataracts, reduced vision may only be apparent when the less affected eye is covered. Age-related cataracts tend to be bilateral in nature and may manifest as blurred or distorted vision, with complaints of a glare when driving at night or in bright light, or the patient may present after a fall, injury (e.g., hip fracture), or accident. Because of the increase of yellow-brown pigment in the lens, color perception is also affected.

The increased density of the lens nucleus results in nearsightedness that may require frequent eyeglass prescription changes. Myopia, or nearsightedness, may result from nuclear cataracts. The term "second sight" refers to older adults who abandon their reading glasses related to this phenomenon; however, as the cataract worsens, so does their vision. Mononuclear diplopia (double vision in one eye) is a cardinal refractive error associated with cataracts. Cataracts in patients younger than age 60 should raise suspicion of an underlying systemic or localized eye disease.

Objective

In some patients, an opacity will be apparent on inspection, but this is not always the case. Decreased visual acuity, often manifested as asymmetry, is the most common objective finding associated with cataracts. Mature or "ripe" cataracts eventually produce a gray or white pupillary reflex known as leukoria, although a dense posterior subcapsular cataract may produce reduction in vision without altering the pupillary reflex. Cataracts are best evaluated by slit-lamp evaluation after pupillary dilation, a procedure that should be performed by an ophthalmologist.

Diagnostic Reasoning

Diagnostic Tests

A visual acuity of 20/30 or worse that is not corrected with glasses, with concurrent observation of opacity, confirms the diagnosis of cataracts. In family practice cataract should be classified according to types based on visual impairment using the Snellen's far and near visual testing. Cataracts are classified as follows:

- Type I is characterized by visual acuity better than 20/40 in the affected eye/eyes.
- Type II is characterized by visual acuity of 20/40 or worse in the affected eye/eyes.

No cataract will produce an afferent pupillary reaction (Marcus Gunn pupil); if abnormal pupillary reactions are present, other ocular pathology must be ruled out. In these cases, biomicroscopic (slit lamp) examination or careful ophthalmoscopic exam should make the diagnosis.

Visual quality assessment tests such as the Glare test may assist in the diagnosis, or assessment of retinal/macular function. Increased intraocular pressure and/or an increased cup-to-disk ratio with significant cupping should raise the suspicion that glaucoma is contributing to the vision loss.

Differential Diagnosis

Cataracts remain the most common cause of decreased visual acuity in adults. Among patients suspected of having cataracts, the following causes of visual impairment should be ruled out: (1) error of refraction, (2) corneal opacities, (3) glaucoma, (4) retinopathy, and (5) age-related macular degeneration. Any sudden change in vision should be referred to an ophthalmologist and sudden vision loss should be treated as an emergency and referred immediately. Cataracts are gradual in onset; they develop over time. Macular degeneration usually presents as a slow, progressive loss of central vision, but may also manifest with symptoms of acute vision loss and distortion (metamorphopsia) resulting from leakage from abnormal subretinal vessels. Open-angle glaucoma produces a slow, painless visual field loss that usually begins peripherally, and often (although not always) presents with increased intraocular pressure and/or an increased cup-to-disk ratio and cupping. Diabetic retinopathy may also contribute to vision loss; funduscopic exam will usually reveal dot-and-blot hemorrhages, microaneurysms, exudates, dilated and torturous vessels, and neovascularization of the disk and retina. Cataracts often obscure the fundus, however, making assessment difficult.

Opacities may be a surface opacity of the cornea (scarring), lens opacities, tumor, retinal detachment, or gliotic retinal scars. In elderly patients, visual impairment is usually the result of multiple factors, including cataracts and macular degeneration, to name a few. Cataracts develop sooner in diabetic patients because metabolic imbalances predispose the lens to cataract formation.

Management

The role of the clinician will involve referral to an ophthalmologist. While surgery is the only definitive treatment for cataracts, the patient may manage at first with monitoring and frequent eyeglass prescription changes. The decision regarding at what point to have surgery should be determined by the patient and the ophthalmologist together. Surgery may be indicated when the cataract interferes with the optic nerve and retina, not allowing evaluation in cases of patients with diabetes, macular degeneration, and glaucoma. Surgery should be discussed when changes in eyeglasses no longer help, when quality of life is jeopardized, and when it is felt that the surgery will be effective. Current cataract surgery is a relatively safe outpatient procedure.

Patients who are scheduled for cataract surgery may be referred to their primary health care provider for a preoperative health assessment. However, among healthy adult patients scheduled for cataract surgery under local anesthesia, no routine preoperative medical testing is necessary. For patients with risk factors or comorbid conditions a physical exam, electrocardiogram (ECG), electrolytes, and urinalysis may be required. Causes for concern are the presence of diabetes mellitus, hypertension, ischemic heart disease, certain pulmonary disorders, and the use of anticoagulants. Any patient with uncontrolled diabetes runs the risk of postoperative vision loss related to diabetic macular edema, which causes the retinal vessels to leak, leading to swelling of the visual center. If possible, anticoagulant therapy should be discontinued prior to surgery. Systemic hypertension may place the patient at risk for intraocular hemorrhage during or after surgery. All medications, intolerances, and allergies should be reviewed, especially in elderly adults, who make up the bulk of patients who undergo this procedure.

Two surgical techniques are currently used—phacoemulsification and extracapsular cataract extraction. In both surgeries, an incision is made into the eye and the central anterior lens capsule is removed. In phacoemulsification, the surgeon makes a 2- to 4-mm incision and inserts an ultrasonic vibrating needle through a small incision, which breaks the cataract into small pieces, which are then aspirated through the needle's central bore. The smaller incision and smaller sutures used in phacoemulsification make it the preferred method for cataract removal. In extracapsular surgery, the surgeon makes a 10- to 14-mm incision and the entire lens nucleus is loosened from the cortex and removed through the incision. In both cases, the surgery continues with removal of the residual lens cortex and insertion of an intraocular lens. The incision may be self-sealing or closed with sutures. More than 95 percent of patients achieve visual acuity of 20/40 or better after surgery.

After surgery, the patient should have a protective eye shield in place, and topical antibiotic and steroid ophthalmic medications. Lifting and bending should be avoided for several weeks, until cleared by an ophthalmologist. Bilateral cataract surgery is common and often indicated because of better visual acuity outcomes, although optimal timing of the second surgery remains controversial. Cataract surgery has been shown to be highly cost-effective, given the reduction in comorbidities and injury associated with progressive visual impairment.

Follow-Up and Referral

As noted, these patients need early referral and monitoring by an ophthalmologist. The most important job for the clinician is to rule out any acute threat to vision, and to encourage referral for more gradual cases of deteriorating vision loss. Education about the advances in surgical techniques and reassurance may be important aspects of care prior to referral. Comprehensive preoperative assessment is important, including psychosocial aspects of care, such as who will drive the patient to and from the surgery and assist him or her during the postoperative period.

Patient Education

Some of the educational and adaptive measures have been mentioned previously. In addition, the patient will need to have his or her vision reevaluated several weeks after the surgery for a new prescription for corrective lenses. Use of wraparound ultraviolet protecting glasses in sunny climates may slow progression of cataracts. Evidence supports the benefits of an antioxidant diet, as well as the use of multivitamin supplements, along with additional vitamin C (500 mg per day minimally), vitamin E (400 international units [I.U.]), and beta-carotene (15 mg [25,000 I.U.]) daily. Carrots contain carotenoids, which have been documented to provide preventive effects against cancers, cardiovascular diseases, and cataracts. Vegetables that are rich in antioxidant nutrients such as beta carotene and vitamins C and E—any yellow, orange, or dark green, leafy vegetables—help prevent the oxidation process that can contribute to and worsen cataracts. Likewise, the trace minerals magnesium and manganese appear to play a role in cataract prevention. Enzymes containing these minerals help dispose of proteins damaged by oxidation that contribute to eye clouding. Catnip and other mints contain both these essential trace minerals, as well as flavonoids (see Complementary Therapies 7.1).

Glaucoma

Glaucoma is defined as a group of diseases characterized by progressive damage to the optic nerve, resulting in optic nerve atrophy and blindness, most typically associated with elevated intraocular pressure. Glaucoma is classified as *open-angle* and *angle-closure* (classically referred to as *closed angle,* or *narrow-angle* glaucoma). These classifications are made based on the anatomy of the anterior chamber. Both types of glaucoma may be present in the same eye (referred to as combined-mechanism glaucoma). Glaucoma is further differentiated as *primary* or *secondary* (associated with an ocular condition or a systemic process). There is also a congenital form of glaucoma seen in infants. Open-angle glaucoma is more commonly seen and is characterized as a chronic form of the disorder which, prior to loss of peripheral visual fields, is strikingly asymptomatic. It has an excellent prognosis if treated early and appropriately. Angle-closure glaucoma, on the other hand, may have subacute and chronic components, but it is most associated with acute episodes of significant eye pain, redness, and acute visual loss, which if untreated, may rapidly lead to permanent blindness.

Epidemiology and Causes

Glaucoma affects approximately 4 percent of all individuals older than age 40. Primary open-angle glaucoma (chronic glaucoma) is the most prevalent form of glaucoma and accounts for 90 to 95 percent of all cases. Angle-closure glaucoma (acute glaucoma) is not as common; it affects approximately 100 per 100,000 of the population (approximately 0.1 percent). Glaucoma is the second-leading cause of blindness among white Americans and the most common cause of blindness in African Americans. Chronic open-angle glaucoma usually occurs after age 40, but can occur at any age. Angle-closure glaucoma tends to occur between the ages of 55 and 70. African Americans have a higher incidence of chronic open-angle glaucoma. Angle-closure glaucoma is more prevalent in people of Asian descent, especially among the Inuit, as well as in those with Eskimo ancestry. Chronic open-angle glaucoma occurs equally in males and females. Angle-closure glaucoma occurs more frequently in females.

Increasing age, a positive family history, myopia (nearsightedness), and diabetes may all contribute to the development of chronic open-angle glaucoma. Glaucoma may develop secondarily as a result of a number of ocular and systemic diseases. Risk factors that have been identified in angle-closure glaucoma are family history, hyperopic (farsighted) eyes, and a small cornea. The use of steroid therapy (either topical, inhaled, or systemic) may lead to increased intraocular pressure. Antidepressant drugs, or other anticholinergic drugs, and emotional stress may contribute to an acute episode, as well as childbirth, sneezing, laser therapy or surgery, and intravenous overhydration. Increased pressure in the anterior chamber that is uncorrected will over time result in impaired peripheral visual fields, destroy central vision, and ultimately destroy the optic nerve. Increased intraocular pressure, optic nerve atrophy, and visual field loss make up the classic triad of glaucoma.

Pathophysiology

The ciliary body of the eye produces aqueous humor, which circulates from the posterior chamber to the anterior chamber and then exits through the trabecular meshwork. In primary open-angle glaucoma (in which no secondary cause is identified), elevated intraocular pressure is almost always caused by obstruction of the outflow channels, especially the trabecular meshwork; however, overproduction of aqueous humor may also occur. The manner in which the trabecular meshwork is obstructed is a matter of debate, but it probably involves changes in the biochemical makeup of the cells lining this meshwork. These changes appear to often occur with aging. In addition, secondary glaucoma may result from increased intraocular pressure caused by ocular trauma or inflammation such as uveitis, chronic steroid use, vasoproliferative retinopathy, and recurrent retinal hemorrhages.

The specifics regarding how intraocular pressure leads to optic nerve atrophy are also debated. One theory is that intraocular pressure causes direct mechanical damage and loss of retinal ganglionic cell axons known as "cupping." Others theorize that intraocular pressure impairs the small-vessel circulation that provides nutrients to the optic nerve and extracellular matrix. Glutamate toxicity and processes involved with runaway apoptosis leading to axonal loss are also currently being investigated. It is critical to recognize, however, that optic atrophy may occur in the absence of

COMPLEMENTARY THERAPIES 7.1

Problem	Supplement	Dosage	Comments
Cataracts	Bilberry (*Vaccinium myrtillus*)	80–160 mg (standardized extract) bid-tid	Boosts oxygen and blood delivery to the eye. There are no known drug interactions or adverse effects.
	Vitamin C	500–1500 mg qd (may cause diarrhea at higher doses)	Prevents lens damage from cigarette smoke and UV light.
	Beta-carotene	25,000 IU qd	The body converts beta-carotene to vitamin A which maintains a healthy lens.
	Vitamin E	400 IU qd	Research has shown that people taking vitamin E supplements cut their risk of cataracts in half.
	Zinc	30 mg qd	Boosts effectiveness of vitamin A.
	Quercetin	125–250 mg qd	*Quercetin* blocks an enzyme that leads to sorbitol accumulation that contributes to cataract formation.
	Alpha-lipoic acid	100 mg bid	Increases effectiveness of vitamins C and E in protecting the lens from UV damage.
Macular degeneration	Bilberry	80–160 mg (standardized extract) bid-tid	Protects cells in the eye from free radical damage and boosts oxygen delivery to the retina.
	Vitamin E	400 IU qd	Protects against free radical damage and decreases risk or late-stage macular degeneration.
	Zinc	30 mg qd	Critical in the functioning of the retina and macula and slows vision loss in those with macular degeneration.
Otitis externa	Rubbing alcohol Vinegar	Equal parts rubbing alcohol and vinegar mixed then one dropper full instilled in each ear after swimming.	Prevents otitis externa. May also treat it by changing the pH in the ear canal making it less hospitable to *Pseudomonas*.
Sore throat	Bilberry	80–160 mg (standardized extract) bid–tid	Decreases mild inflammation in mucous membranes.
	Slippery elm (*Ulmus rubra*)	Lozenge 1q4h (dissolve in mouth) or 1 tsp slippery elm bark powder in 2 cups boiling water let stand at least 10 minutes then drink 1–2 cups daily. (may add sugar)	Mucilage is the major chemical compound that restores the mucous coating of irritated mucous membranes.
Oral herpes simplex and mouth sores	Lemon balm (*Melissa officinalis*)	Tea: 1–2 tsp dried leaves in 1 cup boiling water; steep 5 minutes. Available in a cream: Herpilyn or Herpalieve apply to sores tid–qid	Mechanism of action unknown, but may keep herpes virus from attaching to cells. May potentiate barbiturates and may increase intraocular pressure in people with glaucoma. Do not use in pregnancy
	Lysine	1000 mg L-lysine tid with meals at the first sign of outbreak for as long as outbreak lasts. (for those prone to herpes outbreaks maintenance dose is 500 mg qd)	Lysine competes with arginine (needed for herpes replication) thereby inhibiting replication of herpes.

Sources: Bascom, A: Incorporating herbal medicine into clinical practice. FA Davis, Philadelphia, 2002.
http://www.wholehealthmd.com
Blumenthal, M, Goldberg, A, and Brinckmann, J (eds): Herbal medicine expanded Commission E monographs. Austin, TX: American Botanical Council; Newton, Mass: Integrative Medicine Communications, 2000.

increased intraocular pressure. Traditionally, elevated intraocular pressure has been defined as greater than 21 mm Hg, but ocular hypertension has also been identified in the absence of optic nerve atrophy. Thus, other pathophysiologic processes leading to progressive, irreversible vision loss also function in primary open-angle glaucoma, and increased intraocular pressure by itself, must only be considered a risk factor, rather than the definitive glaucomatous etiology. Work is also underway to identify the gene products and functions associated with inherited forms of open-angle glaucoma which typically occur before the age of 40 years, known collectively as juvenile glaucoma.

Angle-closure glaucoma, which may be either acute or chronic, is less common than open-angle glaucoma and is caused by anatomic narrowing of the anterior chamber angle, a factor that is fundamentally determined by genetics and becomes more likely with advanced age. This narrowing is primarily related to the size of the eyeball and lens. Specifically, angle-closure glaucoma results from the forward displacement of the iris toward the cornea, with narrowing of the iridocorneal angle resulting in an obstruction of outflow from the anterior chamber. Acute angle-closure glaucoma occurs when there is an acute closure of the iridocorneal angle, with a sudden, severe rise in intraocular pressure often well above 40 mm Hg, which is highly symptomatic. Permanent vision loss may result if this condition is not treated within 24 hours of onset.

Screening, Diagnosis, and Treatment

One of the most important aspects of glaucoma in primary care is screening. The United States Preventative Services Task Force has found good evidence that early treatment of adults with increased intraocular pressure detected by screening reduces the number of persons with small, visual field defects, and that early treatment of those with asymptomatic glaucoma decreases the number of persons whose visual field defects progress.

In general, tonometry readings are recommended as part of every eye exam. This should be done every year after age 40. Follow-up with an ophthalmologist should be sought for visual changes.

The diagnosis of glaucoma is not made on the basis of a single test but on the finding of characteristic degenerative changes in the optic disc and defects in visual fields.

Increased intraocular pressure, family history, older age, and being of African American descent place an individual at increased risk for glaucoma. Older African Americans have a higher prevalence of glaucoma and a more rapid progression of the disease.

Tonometry to measure intraocular pressure is essential. Multiple testing methods requiring specialized equipment and training are available, including pneumotonometry which uses a puff of air against the eyeball or the more accurate method of applanation tonometry in which the cornea is directly observed while pressure is placed against it. Normal intraocular pressure is typically considered to be 8 to 21 mm Hg. In all chronic forms of glaucoma (open- or closed-angle), intraocular pressure may or may not be elevated, whereas in an acute exacerbation of angle-closure glaucoma, symptomatic pressures occur as high as 40 to 80 mm Hg. However, increased intraocular pressure in and of itself is not diagnostic, because many patients with open-angle glaucoma consistently have intraocular pressure within the normal range.

Testing of visual fields using confrontational finger motions to test where the patient's fields are compared to the examiner's is unreliable for diagnosing glaucoma. There are specialized tests that can be performed by an ophthalmologist or optometrist, including perimetry, tangent screen testing, or Goldmann perimetry. Pachymetry, which is a method of measuring corneal thickness, may be done by an ophthalmologist. Thinner corneas are at higher risk for the development of primary open-angle glaucoma.

Clinical Presentation

Subjective

Generally, patients are asymptomatic until optic nerve damage is quite advanced. Chronic open-angle glaucoma has a gradual onset, with slow, painless bilateral peripheral vision loss and poor night vision. Frequent changes in refractory prescription may be a common presenting symptom. In later stages, symptoms may include seeing halos around lights and further visual loss. Acute angle-closure glaucoma has a rapid onset, with unilateral pain and pressure, blurred vision, seeing halos around lights, and photophobia, followed by loss of peripheral vision, subsequently followed by central vision loss. A headache may be present and possibly nausea and vomiting. Chronic angle-closure glaucoma is as insidious in onset as open-angle glaucoma. Its fundamental mechanism relates to the anatomic narrowness of the anterior chamber angle. Often patients have a history of vague discomfort about the eyes and intermittent blurring of vision.

Objective

The physical exam in most patients with chronic glaucoma will most likely be unremarkable. In later stages, the eyeball may be hardened. Visual acuity may or may not be affected. Visual field abnormalities to confrontation will be present only in very late, profound cases. A Marcus-Gunn pupil (afferent pupillary defect) may be present.

In acute angle-closure glaucoma, intraocular pressure rises rapidly to very high levels. The eye becomes red and painful, the cornea may have a "steamy" appearance, and vision is severely blurred. There may be a pupil that is mid-dilated and immobile. Findings on fundoscopic exam may show a pale optic disk with excavated cupping and a shallow anterior chamber; there may be an increased cup/disc ratio related to atrophy, and asymmetry on comparison with the other eye. Visual acuity is severely affected because visual field defects are common. In many cases, the primary-care provider can detect a shallow anterior chamber and narrow angle with the flashlight test: In this test, a penlight is held at the temporal limbus of the eye and the degree of illumination is noted. A narrow angle is suggested if the nasal half of the iris is in the shadow. Dilation of the pupil with mydriactic agents tends to further narrow the angle, which can lead to an acute attack, as can dim light or darkness, and physical or emotional stress.

Physical diagnosis relies on gonioscopic evaluation of the angle by an ophthalmologist. However, the clinician, as the primary-care provider, should closely monitor patients with a family history of angle-closure glaucoma or hyperopia accompanied by a history of eye ache, headache, and blurred vision.

Diagnostic Reasoning

Diagnostic Tests

Tonometry to measure intraocular pressure is essential. In chronic, closed-angle glaucoma, there may or may not be elevation of intraocular pressure. Normal intraocular pressure is 10 to 20 mm Hg. In chronic, open-angle glaucoma, you may see a normal or elevated pressure, whereas in an acute exacerbation of angle-closure glaucoma, you may see pressure as high as 40 to 80 mm Hg. However, increased intraocular pressure in and of itself is not diagnostic, because many patients with open-angle glaucoma consistently have intraocular pressure within the normal range.

Gonioscopy determines the angle of the eye's anterior chamber and thus enables the examiner to differentiate between open-angle and angle-closure glaucoma; the angle is normal in open-angle glaucoma, although this often narrows with aging. This is determined by visual inspection of the angle using a special lens (goniolens) at the slit-lamp biomicroscopy. The two primary types of disease—open-angle glaucoma and angle-closure glaucoma—are classified according to the anatomy of the anterior chamber angle. Both types of the disease may be present in the same eye.

The appearance (e.g., color and contour) of the optic nerve and findings on visual field examination are the most important clues to diagnosis. Pathognomonic changes indicate glaucoma. Funduscopic examination of the optic nerve reveals changes in the cup and neuroretinal rim relatively early in the disease, indicating the possibility of open-angle glaucoma. Particularly significant are the size of the cup relative to the optic nerve, any thinning or nicking of the disk rim, and the presence of disk hemorrhages. Visual field examination, which requires specialized equipment, detects defects in the field of vision that are characteristic for glaucomatous damage to the optic nerve relatively early in the disease.

Differential Diagnosis

Conjunctivitis and uveitis may be ruled out related to the other symptomatology the practitioner will observe in cases of glaucoma, specifically visual changes. Vascular disease may also produce funduscopic changes; however, these will be more hemorrhagic in nature. Medications such as steroids, amphetamines, and chlorpromazine can all increase intraocular pressure. Many ocular and systemic conditions are associated with the development of glaucoma; in addition, the use of topical, systemic, and inhaled corticosteroids may increase intraocular pressure, depending on dose and duration of treatment.

Management

Once nerve damage has occurred, it is irreversible; thus, the goal of treatment is to prevent progression of damage and to protect the optic nerve from pressure. Glaucoma is a disease of pressure; adequate lowering of intraocular pressure by one means or another almost always stops optic nerve damage.

Traditionally, open-angle glaucoma is managed pharmacologically for as long as possible, with laser or surgical treatment reserved for glaucoma that cannot be controlled by medication alone. The choice of medication regimen is usually made by an ophthalmologist. The goal of pharmacologic therapy is to decrease and control intraocular pressure. Each type of medication has a different color top. Therefore, if the patient is not sure what type of glaucoma medication he or she is taking, but can describe the color of the cap, the clinician will know what class of glaucoma medication the patient is taking (see Management Table 7.4).

Beta-blockers are usually first line therapy, but sometimes prostaglandin analogs may be used first line or added soon after beta-blockers are started. Treatment compliance with multiple doses of eye drops daily is often poor in open angle glaucoma; however, newer topical agents require less frequent dosing (once daily for prostaglandins). If medications do not control pressure, surgical options include laser or external trabeculectomy. Laser therapy is often effective only in the first several years after surgery and then the pressure begins to build again. The timing of surgery has not been shown to influence visual outcomes and surgery imparts greater risk for future cataracts; therefore, medications should be tried first. Target intraocular pressure that therapy attempts to achieve must be decided on an individual basis for functions associated with inherited forms of open-angle glaucoma which typically occur before the age of 40 and have become collectively known as juvenile glaucoma.

Angle-closure glaucoma may be either acute or chronic and is less common than open-angle glaucoma. Angle-closure glaucoma is caused by anatomic narrowing of the anterior chamber angle, a factor that is determined by genetics and becomes more likely with advancing age. The narrowing is primarily related to the size of the eyeball and lens. Specifically, angle-closure glaucoma occurs when there is an acute closure of the iridocorneal angle, with a

Management Table 7.4 Medications used to treat Glaucoma

Type of Medication	Mechanism of Action	Contraindications	Names of Drugs in this Category
Cholinergic agent	Pupillary constriction to open the angle and allow aqueous to escape.	Conditions in which pupillary constriction is contraindicated	Pilocarpine, Isopto, Pilocar, Pilostat
Beta-blocker	Reduce the production of aqueous fluid	Additive effect in patients who are on an oral beta-blocker Contraindicated in patients with asthma, sinus bradycardia, second or third degree AV block, overt CHF	Timolol, betaxolol, levobunolol, carteolol, metipranolol
Prostaglandin analog	Decrease intraocular pressure by increased ureoscleral outflow (drainage)	Can cause conjunctival hyperemia, iris pigment color changes, uveitis, and macular edema.	Bimatoprost, latanoprost, travoprost, Xalatan
Carbonic anhydrase inhibitor	Reduce aqueous production	Caution in patients with nephrolithiasis, diabetes, hepatic disease, and a history of sulfonamide sensitivity	Brinzolamide, dorzolamide, echothiophate physostigmine
Alpha-adrenergic agonist	Prescribed for their inhibitory effect on aqueous production	Avoid in patients with grade 2 or 3 heart block, CHF, COPD, asthma, or pulmonary edema	Epinephrine and dipivefrin, apraclonidine, brimonidine
Systemic medications	Reduce production of aqueous		Acetazolamide (Diamox), dichlorphenamide (sulfonamide) and metazolamide (sulfonamide)

sudden, severe rise in intraocular pressure often well above 40 mm Hg, which is symptomatic. Acute angle-closure glaucoma requires emergency treatment or total blindness with follow-up within 2 to 5 days. Medications are administered during the acute attack to lower intraocular pressure, so that surgical intervention can occur. Acetazolamide (Diamox) and intravenous (IV) mannitol with a topical miotic such as pilocarpine may be administered, followed by laser iridotomy or peripheral iridectomy. Bedrest should be maintained until the attack is broken.

Follow-Up and Referral

Patients with glaucoma should be referred to and followed by an ophthalmologist. Nonetheless, as the primary-care provider, the clinician needs to understand the medications that the patient is on, as well as how often the patient should be monitored by an ophthalmologist (every 3 to 4 months for life). The clinician needs to be alert to possible signs and symptoms of exacerbation. There is always potential for loss of vision and possible blindness if acute glaucoma attacks are not treated promptly and consistently.

Patient Education

Careful and lifelong follow-up is essential for patients with glaucoma, especially periodic checks of intraocular pressure and eye exams. The need to take medications as ordered, to be aware of adverse effects of medications prescribed, and to recognize changes (such as sudden changes in vision) that warrant a call to the health-care provider is essential for all patients with glaucoma. Any sign of eye infection, especially fever, should be reported. In addition, the knowledge that certain medications, such as systemic steroids, may interfere with glaucoma control is essential. Support and counseling may also be necessary. In the case of open-angle glaucoma, patients need to know that they will most likely need bilateral treatment, because the second eye is at risk for the same disease process.

Diabetic Retinopathy

Diabetic retinopathy is a noninflammatory disorder of the retina developed in patients with diabetes mellitus. It is typically divided into three stages: (1) background diabetic retinopathy, (2) preproliferative diabetic retinopathy, and (3) proliferative diabetic retinopathy. The initial evaluation for a patient with diabetes mellitus should include a referral to an ophthalmologist for a comprehensive eye evaluation, with particular attention to those aspects relevant to diabetic retinopathy.

Epidemiology and Causes

Approximately 6.6 percent of the population between the ages of 20 and 74 have diabetes mellitus; approximately 25 percent of those individuals with diabetes have some form of diabetic retinopathy. Most patients with diabetes will eventually develop some form of retinopathy. Diabetic retinopathy accounts for approximately 10 percent of new cases of blindness each year, and is the leading cause of new cases of legal blindness among Americans between the ages of 20 and 64.

The peak incidence of type 1 diabetes mellitus is between ages 12 and 15; the peak incidence of type 2 diabetes mellitus is between ages 50 and 70. The incidence of diabetic retinopathy is directly related to the duration of time that the patient has had diabetes. Almost all patients with diabetes will develop background diabetic retinopathy after they have had diabetes for at least 20 years. Two-thirds of patients with type 1 diabetes who have had the disease for at least 35 years will develop proliferative diabetic neuropathy, and one-third will develop macular edema. The proportions are reversed for patients with type 2 diabetes.

Diabetes mellitus type 1 occurs about equally in males and females, whereas type 2 is more common in women. Predilection for type 1 diabetes is higher among Anglo Americans (African Americans have the lowest incidence); however, certain groups, such as the Pima Indians, have a 35 percent incidence rate of diabetes mellitus type 2.

The longer the patient has had diabetes mellitus, the greater the likelihood that he or she will develop retinopathy. In addition, poor glycemic control translates into end-organ damage, including retinopathies, in patients with either type 1 or type 2 diabetes. Pregnancy, renal disease, systemic hypertension, smoking, and elevated serum lipid levels (associated with an increased risk of retinal lipid deposits) are all risk factors for the development of retinopathy.

Pathophysiology

The key insult driving diabetic retinopathy is uncontrolled hyperglycemia. The precise mechanism by which this causes retinal damage is unclear, but there are several prevailing hypotheses that likely contribute to varying degrees. Hyperglycemia is known to contribute to the dysregulation of retinal blood flow. In the setting of systemic hypertension, increased shear stress on retinal blood vessels drives the release of vasoproliferative factors (e.g., vascular endothelial growth factor, insulin-like growth factor-1, basic fibroblast growth factor, hepatocyte growth factor) which stimulate neovascularization of the retina, optic nerve, and iris. The buildup of sorbitol (a by-product of glucose metabolism by the enzyme aldose reductase) in retinal cells is believed to increase intracellular osmolality, causing fluid shifts (cellular edema) and subsequent retinal damage. In hyperglycemic states, free amino acids, serum and tissue proteins may all become irreversibly glycosylated. These end products are thought to cross-link with collagen fibers within the extracellular space, initiating microvascular complications. Retinal microthromboses composed of platelets and fibrin have also been proposed to stimulate neovascularization, as the body attempts to compensate for decreased retinal blood flow. Moreover, several other risk factors have been identified, including certain genetic predispositions and enzymatic allelic variants, serum hypertriglyceridemia, anemia, and hormonal fluctuations associated with pregnancy.

In the case of background diabetic retinopathy, retinal pericytes and the microvascular endothelium are damaged early in the disease process, leading to vascular permeability and basement membrane thickening (similar to the histopathologic changes seen in diabetic nephropathy). This predisposes retinal capillaries to microaneurysms and the retinal surface to thickening with deposits of proteinaceous and lipid material (hard exudates). If the macula is affected (i.e., macular edema), vision may gradually blur and progress to profound visual loss if left untreated. In the pre-proliferative phase, multiple cycles of cellular death and renewal lead to venous beading, tortuous venous dilation, and intraluminal cellular proliferation along with platelet, erythrocyte, and fibrinogen aggregation which ultimately results in vascular occlusion. Upstream of such lesions, flame-shaped and blot hemorrhages occur, while downstream microvascular infarcts present as "cotton wool spots" or soft exudates on funduscopy. Finally, the proliferative phase is characterized by neovascularization on the retinal surface, optic nerve, and iris. These fragile vessels may be venous or arterial in origin and may extend into the vitreous chamber, attaching to the posterior pole of the vitreous in a fine fibrous mesh. This network places stress on the retinal surface as the fibers contract. As a result, hemorrhage into the vitreous body and even retinal detachment may occur, requiring both vitrectomy and laser photocoagulation.

Clinical Presentation

Subjective

The patient will complain of visual changes as the disease progresses but is usually asymptomatic in the early stages.

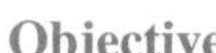

Objective

Changes will be noted on funduscopic exam. In background diabetic retinopathy, microaneurysms, intraretinal hemorrhage, macular edema, and lipid deposits may be apparent.

As the disease progresses, nerve fiber layer infarctions ("cotton wool" spots), venous beading and dilation, edema, and, in some cases, extensive retinal hemorrhage will be noted. In the proliferative form of diabetic retinopathy, new blood vessel proliferation (neovascularization) may be seen on the retinal surface, optic nerve, and iris.

Diagnostic Reasoning

Diagnostic Tests

A thorough eye examination should be done, including an assessment of visual acuity and documentation of the status of the iris, lens, vitreous, and fundus. Fluorescein angiography will demonstrate retinal nonperfusion, retinal leakage, and proliferative diabetic retinopathy.

Differential Diagnosis

A history of diabetes, especially if present for more than 10 years, correlated with observable changes on funduscopic exam, establishes the diagnosis. Other causes of retinopathy include hypertensive retinopathy, radiation retinopathy, and retinal venous obstruction.

Management

The first goal for patients at risk for microvascular complications, including diabetic retinopathy, is prevention. Risk is significantly increased for patients with blood sugar levels above 200 mg/dL. The most significant preventative measure is to keep blood sugar under control. The American Diabetes Association sets an acceptable level of glycated hemoglobin or HgbAIC at less than 7 percent. In patients who have their blood sugar under adequate control the incidence of diabetic retinopathy is far lower and the onset in those who do develop this disease is later.

Similarly, patients with diabetes and hypertension should strive to maintain as normal a blood pressure as possible, to prevent the development of end-organ damage. Because many patients have both disorders, vigilance is especially important I this subset of patients..

The only pharmacologic agent that has been found to slow the progression of diabetic retinopathy is Lisinopril, an angiotensin-converting enzyme (ACE) inhibitor.

Laser surgery is recommended for patients with proliferative diabetic retinopathy and for patients with clinically significant macular edema.

Diabetic retinopathy patients should be followed by an ophthalmologist, who can decide when to treat the disorder with laser treatment (focal and panretinal photocoagulation); in certain cases, cryoretinopexy can be used to decrease the neovascular stimulus and to treat proliferative diabetic retinopathy. Vitrectomy may be considered for patients with severe proliferative diabetic retinopathy, traction retinal detachment involving the macula, and nonclearing vitreous hemorrhage (this surgical option should be considered after 1 month for a vitreous hemorrhage that has decreased the vision to the 5/200 level or worse).

Follow-Up and Referral

All patients with diabetes mellitus should be monitored annually by an ophthalmologist. The patient with background retinopathy should be followed at least every 6 months, and patients with proliferative retinopathy should be seen at least every 3 to 4 months. Patients with active proliferative retinopathy should be seen approximately every 8 weeks.

Glaucoma, cataracts, retinal detachment, vitreous hemorrhage, and disk edema (papillopathy) are all common in patients with diabetic retinopathy, even in its early stages. Cataracts, especially, are common in patients with diabetes. If the patient has retinopathy, he or she should try to postpone the cataract surgery as long as possible, because cataract surgery can sometimes cause diabetic retinopathy to worsen.

Patient Education

Obviously, this is a critical area. Patients with diabetes, as well as those with hypertension, need to be educated regarding the need to keep their disease under maximal control to decrease the incidence of complications. Creating an alliance with the patient and family is essential in encouraging lifestyle changes. Working with the patient overtime and being there for the patient is essential. Patients should be educated about the importance of ophthalmologic evaluation and follow-up. Patience, advocacy, and commitment are all important qualities in working with these patients. Optimism and emphasis on the possibility for change, even if just to prevent further disease progression, are essential characteristics.

Common Ear Problems

Otitis Externa

Otitis externa is an inflammation of the membranous lining of the auditory canal and/or contiguous structures of the outer ear. The term refers to a wide spectrum of both acute and chronic inflammatory processes that may be diffuse, localized, or invasive in nature. This disorder is largely benign and self-limiting, albeit painful. Invasive otitis externa (malignant otitis externa, necrotizing otitis externa) is a potentially life-threatening disease, however, if left untreated.

Epidemiology and Causes

Ear pain, in general, is a common clinical complaint, accounting for 2 to 3 percent of all family practice office visits. Specifically, otitis externa is 10 to 20 times more likely to occur during the warmer summer months than in cooler seasons. Adults older than 50 years of age are at the greatest risk of developing invasive otitis externa, particularly if they are immunocompromised from medications or if they have chronic diseases such as cancer or diabetes mellitus. No ethnic predispositions to otitis externa have been documented. Men and women are affected equally.

Immunocompromised persons on steroid therapy or individuals with chronic conditions such as diabetes mellitus are at a greater risk for developing infectious otitis externa and, in particular, invasive disease. Deep tissue invasion may be related to decreased polymorphonuclear neutrophil function and/or microvascular disease associated with diabetes. Steroid use specifically increases the likelihood of otomycosis, which is significantly more prevalent in the tropics and southeastern United States, but as a whole, environmental changes are the most common risk factors for otitis externa. When the pH of the auditory canal shifts from acidic to alkaline or an increase in temperature and/or humidity occurs, the auditory canal becomes conducive to pathogenic colonization. In fact, excess moisture from any cause may predispose the external ear to infection. *Pseudomonas* infections, in particular, commonly result from the mild ear canal trauma associated with excessive swimming in hot, humid weather, especially in polluted water; hence, the common name "swimmer's ear." Highly chlorinated pool water can also contribute to this disorder, because it can dry out the ear canal, creating a potential portal of entry for bacteria and fungi. Inadequate cerumen (ear wax) production removes another critical nonspecific barrier to infection. In addition, patients with seborrhea have an increased risk of otitis externa resulting from seborrheic dermatitis caused by their excess sebum production. Manual picking of the ear, foreign bodies in the auditory canal, and the prolonged use of ear plugs, hearing aids, or cotton swabs may all contribute to local irritation of the external ear, as well. Other risk factors include previous ear infections, as well as skin allergies, particularly those to hair sprays and dyes that may enter the ear canal and cause contact dermatitis. In fact, dermatitic processes often precede microbial infection of the auditory canal, because they create a potential portal of entry through the skin for pathogens.

Pathophysiology

Inflammation of the external ear is most commonly caused by microbial infection. Pathogenic colonization of the external ear is prevented by a number of immune and anatomic mechanisms. The keratinizing squamous epithelia of the ear canal continually sloughs, while the hair follicles that line the outer third of the canal rhythmically sweep laterally, acting as a natural cleansing mechanism and mechanical barrier to the accumulation of matter in the auditory canal. The production of viscous, hydrophobic cerumen in the auditory canal maintains an acidic pH and repels moisture, both of which antagonize bacterial growth. In addition, the presence of competing, nonpathogenic endogenous microbial flora inhibits the overgrowth of more virulent bacteria along the auditory canal. If any of these protective mechanisms are compromised, pathogenic colonization by bacteria or fungi normally found in the auditory canal may occur, resulting in acute otitis externa.

Bacterial agents of infectious otitis externa include *Pseudomonas aeruginosa,* which is the most common cause of diffuse infection and accounts for nearly all cases of invasive otitis externa, and *Staphylococcus aureus,* which typically causes a localized lesion stemming from an infected hair follicle, although it may cause the diffuse form as well. In addition, group A *Streptococcus pyogenes* is associated with localized disease, presenting as a folliculitis, or more frequently as outer ear erysipelas. Polymicrobial infection has also been noted in up to one-third of cases of diffuse disease, while the anaerobic bacteria *Bacteroides* and *Peptostreptococcus* have been cited in up to one-fourth of cases. Commonly identified fungal agents include *Aspergillus niger* (which typically causes focal lesions but may occasionally lead to invasive disease with bony involvement in immunocompromised patients), *Pityrosporum,* and *Candida albicans.* Hyperkeratotic processes such as eczema, psoriasis, and contact or seborrheic dermatitis can also lead to outer ear inflammation. Chronic otitis externa may result from inadequately treated otitis media with continuous serous or exudative drainage from the middle ear into the auditory canal.

Additional risk factors, if not direct causes of otitis externa, include local skin maceration and traumatic injury. The anatomy of the outer ear, which includes the tragus and conchal cartilage, serves as a physical barrier to foreign body entry into the outer ear canal. However, excessive cleaning of the ear with cotton swabs or other devices may leave small pieces of foreign matter in the canal where they eventually disintegrate due to the canal's acidic pH, serving as a nidus of infection. This irritation in turn leads to pruritus, and excessive scratching of the ear canal only aggravates this cycle of epithelial damage and infection by creating physical access through this protective barrier. Excessive moisture in the external canal, particularly associated with swimming or humid environments, acts in a similar manner, leading to maceration and breakdown of the skin with subsequent bacterial infection.

Finally, necrotizing otitis externa (formerly known as malignant otitis externa) is the most severe infectious form of external otitis in which bacterial infection extends from the skin of the auditory canal into the soft tissues, cartilage, and bone in the temporal region or base of the skull (i.e., skull osteomyelitis). Multiple cranial nerves may become involved, increasing morbidity, and death may result from septic thromboemboli to vessels of the brain if inadequately treated. *Pseudomonas aeruginosa* remains the most common infectious agent in such severe disease, although invasive fungal disease in immunocompromised individuals may also extend to multiple tissues.

Clinical Presentation

Subjective

The most common presenting complaint of patients with otitis externa is an acute, often severe otalgia of sudden or gradual onset, which may present bilaterally. Pain may worsen at night and disturb sleep, and it is exacerbated by pulling the pinna or earlobe, or by applying pressure to the tragus. In severe cases, chewing may also elicit otic pain. Severe pain is common in invasive disease. In its early stages, the affected ear may feel full or obstructed, and a temporary conductive hearing loss related to luminal occlusion on the affected side is common if edema is severe. The affected ear may also be pruritic. A purulent discharge may be evident in bacterial disease, and systemic symptomatology such as fever or chills, although rare, may accompany cases of infectious etiology. Chronic otitis externa usually presents with dryness and pruritus of the ear canal. The ear canal may be slightly red and edematous, and there is usually an absence of cerumen.

Objective

A classic sign of acute otitis externa is tenderness on traction of the pinna and/or pain on applying pressure over the tragus. The clinician should instill several drops of Auralgan otic solution (a combination analgesic and anesthetic) before attempting examination in patients in acute distress. This solution should not be used in cases of suspected ruptured tympanic membrane, however.

On otoscopic examination, the auditory canal typically appears edematous and erythematous, with accumulation of purulent drainage in cases of bacterial infection. Diffuse cases present with nearly complete involvement of the auditory canal, whereas localized processes are recognized as focal lesions (pustules or furuncles) anywhere along the auditory canal or external ear structures. Sebaceous secretions in the ear canal are usually evident in patients with seborrhea, but cerumen production among patients is variable, depending on etiology. Fluid may be apparent in infectious cases. *Pseudomonas* infection produces a copious green exudate, whereas *Staphylococcal* infection presents as a yellow crusting in the midst of a purulent exudate. Fungal infections present as a fluffy, white, or black malodorous carpet of growth, and allergic reactions are characterized by scaly, cracked, and/or weepy tissue. Granulation tissue spreading out from the primary site of infection and eroding into the temporal bone, outer auricle, or through a perforated tympanic membrane is indicative of frank invasive disease.

Except in invasive disease or cases related to chronic otitis media, head and neck lymphadenopathy typically is not detected. Invasive disease may also be accompanied by tenderness of the temporomandibular joint (TMJ).

Diagnostic Reasoning

Diagnostic Tests

Laboratory tests are rarely needed if symptomatology clearly fits the classic clinical picture of otitis externa. However, any fluid from the ear may be cultured and, if microorganisms are detected, tested for antibiotic sensitivity. This may be particularly important in determining alternative treatment approaches for patients who do not respond promptly to empirical antibiotic therapy or those with chronic otitis externa, particularly with purulent exudates indicative of bacterial infection. Cultures and antibiotic sensitivity testing are also important for immunocompromised patients, because their disease may be caused by rare pathogens or even by endogenous, typically nonpathogenic microbial flora. Fungi and mycobacteria should be ruled out, in particular. The erythrocyte sedimentation rate (ESR) may be elevated, although this finding has not been thoroughly studied. Soft tissue or bony involvement in malignant disease may be assessed by CT and MRI scans. Plain films and gallium or technetium-99 bone scans may also detect bony involvement, but these imaging techniques are less desirable because they lack specificity and, in the case of x-ray films, sensitivity.

Differential Diagnosis

In the absence of visible changes in the auditory canal and tympanic membrane, otalgia from referred pain associated with other disorders must be ruled out. These disorders include TMJ dysfunction, dental disease, neurologic disorders such as trigeminal and glossopharyngeal neuralgia, parotitis (paramyxoviral infection) secondary to mumps, or rarely, tumors of the middle ear and auditory meatus. Chondrodermatitis chronicus helicis may cause an otalgia similar to otitis externa in elderly patients, manifesting as an extremely tender nodule of the inner ear helix. TMJ dysfunction and dental disease may be specifically ruled out via dental x-ray films to demonstrate alterations in joint morphology or dentition. Mumps may be diagnosed serologically by measuring antibody titers, but in general, a thorough head and neck examination, complete with cranial nerve testing, typically will differentiate between the aforementioned causes of ear pain.

Otitis media may be distinguished from otitis externa by changes in the tympanic membrane that are characteristic of middle ear infection, including erythema, edema, and a significant lack of mobility on insufflation with a pneumatic otoscope. Moreover, movement of the tragus fails to elicit pain in middle ear infection. Otitis media should be suspected if continuous discharge from the middle ear is evident for more than 10 days, and x-ray films may aid in ruling out this diagnosis. Otitis externa and otitis media may occur concurrently. A systemic dermatologic condition, such as seborrheic dermatitis, psoriasis, or erythroderma, may manifest as otitis externa.

Alternative pathologies to rule out through otoscopic examination include other dermatologic disorders such as impetigo, herpes zoster infection, and even insect bites. Serious cranial infections requiring aggressive therapy must also be considered. Mastoiditis is characterized by fever, spontaneous rupture of the tympanic membrane, tenderness, edema, and erythema posterior to the auricle, as well as by palpable preauricular and anterior cervical lymph nodes. The mastoid process is exquisitely painful in mastoiditis, unlike otitis externa. Meningitis typically presents with fever, diffuse headache, altered mentation, vomiting, and cervical stiffness. A recent history of URI may be a clue to these and other infectious processes, including sinusitis and otitis media. Blood in the auditory canal may indicate temporal bone fracture or the presence of an invasive tumor. Carcinoma should be ruled out if invasive disease is suspected through the biopsy of apparent granulation tissue, which in otitis externa will demonstrate necrotizing vasculitis with no evidence of malignant cells. Other noninfectious diagnoses that may be ruled out through biopsy include primary skin and cartilage disorders such as sarcoidosis, discoid lupus, and trauma-related perichondritis of the pinna. Perichondritis may also be of infectious origin caused by *P. aeruginosa,* as confirmed by culture. Excessive cerumen buildup may also lead to a feeling of fullness or stuffiness in the ear, as well as pain and hearing loss. Otoscopic examination before and after irrigation of the auditory canal should rule out this disorder, known as cerumen impaction. Gouty tophi may also affect the external ear, but they are usually painless. Rarer infectious conditions that should be ruled out by special stains, cultures, and antigen/antibody tests in refractory cases include tuberculous otitis (diagnosed by acid-fast stain for *Mycobacteria*), leprosy (diagnosed by acid-fast stain for *Mycobacteria*), and syphilitic otitis (diagnosed by rapid plasma reagin [RPR] and Venereal Disease Research Laboratory [VDRL] tests, and dark-field microscopy to identify the causative agent *Treponema pallidum*).

Management

Because the predominant symptom of otitis externa is pain, alteration in comfort is a primary focus of care. Medical management of the disease should focus on alleviating pain promptly.

- ▲ Local application of heat to the outter ear can offer some relief of pain.
- ▲ Some patients get relief with application of an ice pack to the outer ear.
- ▲ Nonprescription pain reliever such as aspirin or acetaminophen (300 to 600 mg PO q4h prn) or an NSAID such as ibuprofen (400 to 600 mg PO q4h to q6h prn to a maximum dose of 1.8 g/day).
- ▲ In cases of extreme pain, Tylenol with codeine no. 3 or acetaminophen/hydrocodone 5 mg q8h may be prescribed for the first 24 to 48 hours.
- ▲ Keep the ear dry. No swimming or submerision of the ear under water for 4 to 6 weeks.
- ▲ Treatment of otitis externa involves three basic steps:
  1. Gentle cleaning of the ear canal to remove all cerumen, exudate, and epidermal debris using a cotton pledgette or irrigation with warm tap water. (Irrigation should be done cautiously until tympanic membrane perforation has been ruled out.)
  2. Evaluation of otic discharge and edema of the auditory canal and tympanic membrane.
  3. Selection of an appropriate local medication once the etiology has been identified.
- ▲ Occasionally, the pustules or furuncles associated with localized otitis externa may require surgical drainage prior to initiating pharmacotherapy.

Diffuse bacterial otitis externa may be treated empirically. Several preparations are available for use (see Management Table 7.5).

In addition, liquid ophthalmic preparations of gentamicin and tobramycin may actually be used otically to cover both *Pseudomonas aeruginosa* and *Staphylococcus aureus*. If the ear is edematous, a small cotton plug soaked in otic solution (either an antibiotic solution of choice or Domeboro astringent solution) should be inserted. An absorptive 1-inch cotton wick or sponge may be inserted into a highly edematous ear canal by gentle twisting if luminal occlusion prevents the passage of otic preparations. Antibiotic drops may then be placed on the wick for the first 2 to 3 days of treatment, until swelling sub-sides. After this, drops should be placed directly into the ear canal.

Cases that are refractory to initial therapy or involve auricular cellulitis require systemic antibiotic treatment covering both *Staphylococcus* and *Pseudomonas*. Diffuse and localized otitis externa may be treated for 7 to 10 days with multiple empiric choices:

- ▲ First-generation cephalosporins or penicillins with relatively narrow coverage such as cephalexin (Keflex) 250 to 500 mg PO qid and dicloxacillin 250 to 500 mg PO qid
- ▲ Second-generation cephalosporins such as cefuroxime (Ceftin) 250 to 500 mg PO bid, Omnicef 300 mg PO bid, or beta-lactamase resistant penicillins such as amoxicillin/clavulanate (Augmentin XR) 1000 mg PO bid based on the amoxicillin component, which have broader spectrum coverage
- ▲ Fluoroquinolones such as ciprofloxacin (Cipro) 500 mg PO bid or levofloxacin (Levaquin) 500 mg PO qid with similarly broad coverage.

Patients who are immunocompromised from steroid therapy or who have chronic disorders such as diabetes, as well as patients with invasive bony involvement, may require surgical débridement of the affected area to drain abscesses and remove sequestered collagen. This therapy is usually followed by 4 to 6 weeks of IV antipseudomonal therapy.

- ▲ Ceftazidime (Ceftaz, Fortaz) 2 g IV q8h to q12h or a combination of tobramycin (1 to 1.5 mg/kg IV q8h with dosage adjusted by monitoring serum levels and renal function) and ticarcillin (3 g IV q4h). These regimens, however, carry a significant risk of nephrotoxicity, ototoxicity, and bleeding diatheses. An alternative to IV therapy is the oral quinolone ciprofloxacin 750 mg bid, which is generally well tolerated and has a high cure rate in complicated disease.

Management Table 7.5 Preparations available to treat diffuse Bacterial Otitis Externa

Drug Name	Ingredients	Dose	Safe with Perforated TM
Cipro HC otic Antibiotic and steroid	Ciprofloxin 0.2% Hydrocortisone 1%	< 1 year not recommended > 1 year 3 gtts in affected ear bid × 7 days	No
Ciprodex Antibiotic and steroid	Ciprofloxin 0.3% Dexamethasone 0.1%	< 6 months not recommended > 6 months 4 gtts affected ear bid × 7 days	Yes
Cortane B aqueous antibacterial/antifungal + Topical anesthetic + steroid	Chloroxylenol 1 mg Parmoxine HCl 10 mg Hydrocortisone 10 mg Per ml	Children 3 gtts affected ear tid × 7 days Adults 4–5 gtts affected ear tid × 7 days	No
Cortic −ND Antibacterial + antifungal + antiinflammatory + anesthetic	Hydrocortisone 10 mg, Pramoxine 10 mg, Chloroxylenol 1 mg, Benzalkonium chloride 0.10 mg	Children 3 gtts to affected ear tid Adults 4–5 gtts to affected ear tid	No
Floxin otic Antibiotic	Ofloxacin 0.3%	6 months to 13 years 5 gtts to affected ear daily × 7 days Adults 10 gtts to affected ear daily for 7 days	Yes
Zoto-HC Antibacterial/antifungal + topical anesthetic	Chloroxylenol 1 mg, pramoxine HCl 10 mg, hydrocortisone 10 mg Per ml	Children 3 gtts 4 times/day Adults 4–5 gtts 4 times/day	No

In the overwhelming majority of patients who present with chronic otitis externa, the condition is caused by persistent fungal infection. The ears are often dry and scaling. The treatment of fungal infections differs mainly in the choice of antimicrobials.

- ▲ Careful cleaning of the auditory canal. Then a single dusting of sulfanilamide powder is applied, followed by an otic suspension such as VoSol (2 percent nonaqueous acetic acid plus hydrocortisone), or Otic Domeboro (2 percent acetic acid plus astringent). Four drops are placed in each affected ear qid for 7 to 10 days.
- ▲ Topical fungicide preparations containing nystatin or clotrimazole are increasing accepted, although these agents are not available solely as otic preparations. If this treatment is planned then a referral to an ENT specialist should be considered. In chronic cases of otitis externa from fungal infection, systemic antifungals such as fluconazole, ketoconazole, or griseofulvin may be considered. Clotrimazole solution is available over the counter and should be used as 4 drops in each ear qd. Ketoconazole cream may be placed into the external canal by a trained specialist using an operating microsope and a syringe with a blunt needle. About 1 inch of cream is needed to fill the canal, and it should be removed a week later.
- ▲ Steroidal therapies such as 0.1 percent triamcinolone solution or cream may be applied tid or qid to relieve eczematous or psoriatic lesions.
- ▲ When otitis externa has been determined to be secondary to otitis media, therapy should be directed toward the underlying middle ear infection.
- ▲ Finally, pharmacotherapy for chronic otitis externa is directed by extensive antibiotic sensitivity testing after the infectious organisms have been cultured and identified in the laboratory.

Follow-Up and Referral

Acute otitis externa is commonly cured after 7 to 10 days of treatment. A follow-up appointment to assess the effects of treatment may be scheduled after 1 week of therapy for uncomplicated cases. If an ear wick has been placed, the patient should return in 2 days for removal and canal cleaning. The patient should be instructed to call if symptoms do not begin to subside in 48 hours.

Immunocompromised patients with invasive disease and any patient receiving IV antibiotic therapy require daily follow-up during hospitalization, and periodic appointments are recommended for up to 1 year following the discontinuation of treatment. Otherwise healthy patients with invasive disease who do not respond to treatment promptly should also be monitored closely; these patients should undergo further evaluation and diagnostic procedures as necessary. CT and MRI scans remain abnormal for many months following clinical resolution of invasive disease; thus, serial nuclear medicine scans (gallium scans) may be preferable in evaluating treatment efficacy during follow-up, because recurrence of infection may be as high as 10 percent within 6 months posttreatment.

A common complication in the management of otitis externa is dermatitis medicamentosa. Neomycin, an antibiotic commonly found in otic preparations, is known to cause skin reactions and ototoxicity; however, these complications may be minimized by limiting the duration of pharmacotherapy. The use of neomycin-containing agents in cases in which the tympanic membrane is ruptured is controversial, because neomycin may be toxic to middle ear structures if applied directly. Otitis externa may also lead to severe furunculosis (boil formation) or cellulitis (deep-tissue infection) within the ear canal. Invasive otitis externa is a potentially life-threatening complication of poorly treated diffuse and localized disease that must be detected early. Fever, excruciating pain, and the presence of friable granulation tissue are ominous signs of this sequela. Other serious cranial infections may result from inadequately treated otitis externa, including meningitis, mastoiditis, parotitis, and osteomyelitis of either the temporal bone or the base of the skull. Cranial nerve (CN) palsies affect 20 to 30 percent of patients with invasive disease, most commonly involving CN VII and, if disease progresses unchecked, CN IX, X, XI, and XII.

Invasive otitis externa, cellulitis, bony involvement, and all complicating cranial infections must be referred to a specialist for immediate treatment. Patients who are immunocompromised from steroid therapy, diabetes, or other chronic illnesses should be referred to an otorhinolaryngologist to fully evaluate the extent of disease.

Patient Education

Patients should avoid getting water in the ears for at least 4 to 6 weeks after symptoms subside, because moisture from any source can trigger a recurrent episode of infection. Shower caps or ear plugs should be worn when bathing, and swimming should be prohibited entirely for at least 1 month following an acute episode (cotton balls impregnated with petroleum jelly may be used as temporary ear plugs). For persons who are particularly susceptible to repeated infections, a 2 percent acetic acid solution may be used prophylactically to acidify the ear canal (2 to 3 drops in each ear, bid and after any contact with water in which the ears become wet).

Patients should be instructed in the proper method of cleaning the ears (with a soft cotton pledget) and warned never to use swabs, sticks, or chemical agents to clean the auditory canal. Patients should understand that a small amount of ear wax is necessary to prevent infection in the auditory canal and that excessive cleaning can be harmful. The importance of keeping the ear canals dry for at least 4 to 6 weeks, both during and after an acute episode, should also be stressed. The clinician should also discuss the importance of avoiding strong jets of water from showerheads or dental water-jet systems.

Otitis Media

Otitis media (OM) is an inflammation of the structures within the middle ear. Otitis media with effusion (OME) involves the transudation of plasma from middle ear blood vessels, leading to chronic effusion in the absence of the signs and symptoms of acute infection. Acute otitis media (AOM), also referred to as suppurative otitis media or purulent otitis media, denotes the presence of fluid in the middle ear in association with local or systemic illness, including otalgia, otorrhea, and fever. Recurrent otitis media is characterized by the clearance of middle ear effusions between acute episodes of otic inflammation. Lastly, chronic otitis media is present when inflammation persists more than 3 months, typically related to tympanic membrane perforation with either intermittent or persistent otic discharge. Seventy-five percent of children experience at least one episode of otitis media by their third birthday. Almost half of these children will have three or more episodes of otitis mediaduring their first 3 years. Although otitis media is primarily a disease of infants and young children, it can also affect adults.

Epidemiology and Causes

Ear pain, in general, is a common clinical complaint, accounting for 2 to 3 percent of all family practice office visits. Specifically, the incidence rate of otitis media increases during the winter months, when the climate is colder. Although AOM is most common in very young children, elderly adults also have a significant risk of devel-oping disease, because of decreases in natural immunity. Native Americans and Alaskan Eskimos, particularly Navajos, have higher prevalence rates than the general population. A smaller increase in rate is also seen in white Americans of European descent. Men and women are affected equally, although otitis media tends to be rare in adults.

Factors contributing to eustachian tube dysfunction, leading to OME include allergies, sinusitis, rhinitis, and pharyngitis, all of which cause swelling of the membranous lining of the eustachian tube. However, the most significant precipitating event is a recent or concurrent URI, attributed most often to influenza type A (*Influenzavirus* in family Orthomyxoviridae), respiratory syncytial virus (*Pneumovirus,* in family Paramyxoviridae), or adenovirus. URI is thought to contribute to host immunosuppression and the loss of ciliated epithelium in the eustachian tube; in turn, bacterial adherence to the membranous lining is increased. Anatomic abnormalities that can lead to direct blockage of the eustachian tube include hypertrophy or chronic inflammation of the adenoids (pharyngeal tonsils), cleft palate, deviated nasal septum, and nasopharyngeal tumors. Perforation of the eardrum from direct blunt trauma, swimming or diving accidents, or sudden outward pressure or suction (such as from a kiss over the ear), may create a portal of entry for bacteria directly into the middle ear. Certain genetic conditions such as Down's syndrome (trisomy 21) also predispose an individual to middle ear infections. Both active and passive smoking have been associated with an increased risk of all forms of otitis media, and crowded or unsanitary living conditions, along with a family history of otitis media (particularly in the same household), are also contributing factors.

Pathophysiology

AOM results when bacterial infection by nasopharyngeal microorganisms follows eustachian tube dysfunction in which the narrowest portion of the tube (the isthmus) becomes obstructed. Inflammation results primarily in response to bacterial products, including endotoxins and cell-wall components, creating in effect a middle ear abscess. Pressure from this buildup of pus may impinge on the fine blood vessels supplying the tympanic membrane, weakening its structure, reducing tensile strength, and eventually causing perforation or rupture of the ear drum to facilitate draining of inner ear fluid. Fortunately, in the absence of underlying immunocompromise, this structure typically begins to heal spontaneously within hours and may be fully healed by 1 or 2 weeks with complete restoration of baseline hearing capacity. OME is caused by a transudation of plasma fluid through engorged blood vessels resulting from the loss of eustachian tube patency, caused either by swelling of the membranous lining or direct anatomic blockage of the eustachian tube. Swelling of the mucosa is particularly common in the presence of an antecedent viral upper respiratory infection or acute allergy attack. Effective drainage of middle ear fluid is thus prevented, and negative pressure develops in the middle ear cavity, further drawing in fluid.

Streptococcus pneumoniae (implicated in 40 to 50 percent of AOM cases) is the most frequent pathogen isolated from middle ear effusions in adults, as the currently available polyvalent *Streptococcal* vaccines cover only 60 to 70 percent of these isolates. In turn, the increasing administration of the childhood pneumococcal vaccine covering 7 serotypes (Prevnar), as well as the separate 23-serotype Pneumovax vaccine used in high-risk and elderly patients, has yet to impact incidence rates of AOM. Other common organisms include non-typable *Haemophilus influenzae* (10 to 30 percent of cases) which are not covered by the *Haemophilus influenzae* type b (Hib) vaccine and *Moraxella (Branhamella) catarrhalis*, the vast majority of which express the beta-lactamase gene and are resistant to first-line penicillin and cephalosporin antibiotics. These organisms are thought to reach the middle ear from the upper respiratory tract via aspiration or reflux. *Staphylococcus aureus* and *Streptococcus pyogenes* are far less common causative agents, particularly since the introduction of sulfonamide antibiotics such as trimethoprimsulfamethoxazole (Bactrim).

Up to half of AOM cases are attributed to viral infections originating in the nasopharynx and extending to the middle ear via the eustachian tube, including rhinovirus, adenovirus, coronavirus, influenza, and respiratory syncytial virus. In fact, nearly 40 percent of documented influenza cases in children younger than 3 years of age are complicated by AOM, adding to the impetus for widespread flu vaccination. *Mycoplasma* and *Chlamydia pneumoniae* are also rare causes of otitis media. *Chlamydia trachomatis* is typically only seen in infants younger than 6 months, while in developing countries, unusual agents such as *Mycobacteria tuberculosis*, *Diphtheria*, parasites (*Ascaris*) or fungi (*Blastomycoses, Candida, Aspergillus*) may be identified.

OME may be viral in origin but is usually attributed to beta-lactamase–producing bacterial strains that are resistant to first-line antibiotic therapies. Importantly, middle ear effusions often last for weeks to months after an AOM clears; thus, OME may simply reflect part of the naturally history of a resolved episode of AOM. Recurrent otitis media typically results from bacterial infection due to anatomic abnormalities that repeatedly compromise eustachian tube patency. Chronic otitis media may also be caused by any of the bacteria associated with AOM, as well as *Escherichia coli* and *Proteus*, but *Pseudomonas aeruginosa* and *Staphylococcus aureus* are the most commonly isolated pathogens in the chronic suppurative form.

Clinical Presentation

Subjective

The patient with OME will typically complain of stuffiness, fullness, and a loss of auditory acuity in the affected ear only. Pain is rare, but patients may describe popping, crackling, or gurgling sounds when chewing, yawning, or blowing the nose. Very rarely, patients may experience vertigo (a sense of whirling or spinning in space) or ataxia, if inner ear complications such as labyrinthitis are present. Although patients are typically afebrile, a recent history of viral URI or either allergic or vasomotor rhinitis is common.

In contrast, acute otitis media (AOM) usually presents with marked "deep" ear pain and fever, as well as unilateral hearing loss, otic discharge, and a recent history of URI. Some patients may also experience dizziness (space disorientation), vertigo, tinnitus (ringing in the ears), vomiting, or nausea. Pain typically subsides if the tympanic membrane ruptures, as this relieves middle ear pressure. In these cases, patients also usually complain of otic discharge. Recurrent otitis media is characterized by the clearance of middle ear effusions between acute episodes of inflammation.

Chronic otitis media typically presents with a history of repeated bouts of acute otitis media, followed by a period of continuous or intermittent otorrhea lasting for more than 3 months. Pain is seldom a complaint, as hearing loss (related to tympanic membrane perforation) is the primary concern. Risk factors for AOM include enrollment of a child in daycare, presence of tobacco smoke in the home, and residing in communities where antibiotic-resistant forms of *Streptococcus pneumoniae* are endemic.

Objective

Examination of the external ear in patients with OME is typically unremarkable; however, the mucous membranes of the nasal and oral cavities may be injected or edematous, confirming a recent history of URI. The eardrum may be dull but usually is not bulging, and eardrum mobility typically decreases on pneumatic otoscopy. When examining a patient with AOM, the use of Auralgan otic solution (a combination analgesic and anesthetic agent—contraindicated in cases of perforated eardrum) may be needed to facilitate the examination if the patient is experiencing pain. The tympanic membrane may be amber or yellow-orange, or the membrane may be injected and pinkish gray to fiery red in color. The tympanic membrane is typically full or bulging in acute cases, with absent or obscured bony landmarks and cone light reflex.

Although the auditory canal usually shows no abnormalities, a discharge from the middle ear may be present if the tympanic membrane has perforated as a result of the collection of middle ear fluid and subsequent inflammatory response. Otorrhea may be purulent or mucoid, depending upon the stage of inflammation; polymorphonuclear neutrophils are prominent in the early stages of bacterial infection. Otoscopic examination in chronic otitis media usually reveals a perforated, draining tympanic membrane and possibly invasive granulation tissue. Chronic, foul-smelling otorrhea is typically of anaerobic bacterial infection, and a chronic, grayish-yellow suppuration may indicate the development of a cholesteatoma from the degenerative products of invasive epithelialization (involuted squamous epithelia and keratin debris) at the site of infection. Bullae formed between layers of the tympanic membrane (bullous myringitis) are seen in rare cases caused by certain viruses or *Mycoplasma pneumoniae,* and multiple perforations of the tympanic membrane are characteristic of tuberculous otitis.

On palpation, in cases of acute infection, lymphadenopathy of the preauricular and posterior cervical nodes is common. If otitis media is complicated by an acute mastoiditis, tenderness over the mastoid will be elicited, because the bony architecture of the middle ear is continuous with the mastoid process.

Diagnostic Reasoning

Diagnostic Tests

Laboratory tests are rarely needed if symptomatology clearly fits the classic clinical picture of otitis media. However, if confirmation is desired, pneumatic otoscopy will demonstrate decreased or absent tympanic membrane mobility in serous, acute, or chronic otitis media with effusion. Tympanometry may be useful if fluid buildup behind the middle ear is suspected in the absence of other clinical signs; a flat tympanogram is consistent with restrictive disease of the middle ear cavity. A CBC is usually not indicated; however, patients with AOM may demonstrate a leukocytosis, particularly if they are febrile. Cultures of tympanocentesis fluid are not indicated in serous otitis media and are of little practical value in acute disease, unless the patient is immunocompromised or infectious complications such as mastoiditis are evident. In subacute, recurrent, or chronic cases of otitis media, however, cultures and antibiotic sensitivity testing are helpful in guiding alternative treatment approaches. If cultures are obtained, fungi and mycobacteria should be specifically ruled out. Conventional sinus x-ray films and CT scans (which can reveal mucosal thickening in the middle ear space) may be helpful in evaluating patients with effusion and particularly patients with recurrent infection.

Pure tone audiometry may be helpful both pre- and posttreatment, and Weber and Rinne tuning-fork tests typically will reveal conductive, as opposed to sensorineural, hearing loss. Sound lateralization to the affected ear occurs when a 512-Hz tuning fork is placed midline on the top of the head (Weber test), and bone conduction is superior in duration and volume to air conduction (negative Rinne test).

Differential Diagnosis

Otitis media must be distinguished from otitis externa, which is inflammation of the auditory canal and/or external ear, including the pinna and tragus. These structures are usually not affected in otitis media, and otitis externa typically does not involve the tympanic membrane. Otitis externa resulting from furunculosis, local skin maceration, or trauma from a foreign body or direct blunt force must be ruled out. Exacerbated pain on manipulation of the tragus, pinna, or earlobe is a telltale sign of external ear inflammation. Barotrauma may also mimic otitis media, with transient middle ear effusion resulting from air travel or drastic increases in altitude, such as when driving up mountains. TMJ syndrome pain is similar to the pain of OAM. Patients may complain of ear pain when in fact the pain is being referred from the TMJ. Mastoiditis presenting without middle ear infection should be considered when no physical signs of middle ear involvement are evident. Referred otalgia from TMJ dysfunction or dental abscesses may be ruled out by dental x-ray films. Parotitis secondary to mumps (paramyxoviral infection) may be ruled out via serology studies (antibody titers), if suspected. Nasopharyngeal neoplasm must be ruled out through biopsy in cases of unilateral recurrent, chronic, or refractory otitis media. Rarer infectious conditions, which should be ruled out by special stains, cultures, and antigen/antibody tests, include tuberculous otitis (order an acid-fast stain for *Mycobacteria*), leprosy (order an acid-fast stain for *Mycobacteria*), and syphilitic otitis (order rapid plasma reagin [RPR] and Venereal Disease Research Laboratory (VDRL) tests, and dark-field microscopy to identify the causative agent *Treponema pallidum*). Excessive ear wax buildup (cerumen impaction) with or without infection may also lead to a feeling of fullness or stuffiness in the ear, as well as pain and hearing loss. Otoscopic examination before and after irrigation of the auditory canal should rule out this disorder.

Management

Although uncomplicated cases of otitis media are likely to be self-limited and require no specific intervention other than pain relief, treatment of complicated or recurrent otitis media is indicated to prevent permanent anatomic changes of the middle ear and subsequent hearing loss. Changes in characteristics of auditory stimuli related to middle ear pathology lead to sensory or perceptual alterations. In the unfortunate instance when middle ear infection leads to permanent comorbidity, loss of auditory perception may impact a patient's lifestyle, communication patterns, socialization, and self-concept. Other identifiable clinical problems include alteration in comfort and an increased potential for injury related to hearing loss. Interventions should focus on moving the patient toward acceptance, identifying effective communication patterns, and recognizing support mechanisms and resources for coping with hearing loss. Fortunately, the vast majority of otitis media cases never reach this advanced stage.

In cases of OME, watchful waiting is indicated, with monthly exams to monitor for resolution. If the effusion persists past several months, a 14- to 28-day course of an antibiotic such as amoxicillin/clavulanate (Augmentin), cefaclor (Ceclor), or trimethoprim-sulfamethoxazole (Bactrim) is indicated at the therapeutic doses listed below. Some studies suggest the addition of prednisone 1 mg/kg/day for 7 days increases the potential for resolution. Studies have not borne out the effectiveness of decongestants or antihistamines, although these may be of benefit in patients with comorbid allergic rhinitis.

Although there is an increasing trend to observe uncomplicated AOM in children for the first 72 hours rather than prescribe early antibacterial treatment in the hopes of self-limited resolution, antimicrobial therapy in adults is largely the norm. Selection of an agent to treat AOM requires consideration of several factors including the patient's age, otitis media history, drug hypersensitivity, prior antimicrobial response, and associated illnesses (see Management Table 7.6).

Follow-Up and Referral

Patients with OME should be reevaluated 4 to 6 weeks post-treatment, because the disease's full clinical course may last up to several weeks. Monthly otoscopic or tympanometric exams should be done at intervals as long as OME persists. Patients with AOM should be seen for follow-up in 72 hours if symptoms have not resolved. Otherwise, a follow-up appointment may be scheduled several days after the completion of pharmacotherapy. Most patients experience spontaneous closure of a ruptured tympanic membrane and recovery of normal hearing within 4 weeks of treatment. Otoscopic exam should be done 4 weeks after diagnosis. If symptoms persist, consider changing the antibiotic regimen to cover beta-lactamase–producing organisms. Chronic otitis media requires monthly follow-up to assess the efficacy of treatment and monitor for recurrence of infection.

OME can lead to irreversible conductive hearing loss if middle ear structures are permanently damaged from effusion-related pressure changes. If AOM is poorly treated or is present in an immunocompromised patient, it may lead to OME, chronic otitis media, otitis interna (labyrinthitis), vertigo, ataxia, or several acute, subacute, and chronic infections of adjacent cranial structures, including mastoiditis, petrositis, meningitis, and epidural, subdural, or brain abscesses. Other complications include perforation of the tympanic membrane, cholesteatoma, facial nerve palsies, lateral sinus thrombophlebitis, and otitic hydrocephalus.

Although the clinical course of OME may last for several weeks, patients should be referred to a specialist for impedance audiometry testing and further evaluation to rule out nasopharyngeal tumors and other anatomic eustachian tube obstructions if hearing loss persists beyond 6 weeks, extends bilaterally, or reaches more than 20 decibels. Patients with AOM may require referral to a specialist if vertigo or ataxia develops, if a ruptured tympanic membrane fails to close, if symptoms worsen after 3 to 4 days of treatment, or if significant hearing loss is present.

If subacute, recurrent, or chronic otitis media fails to clear after two to three courses of antibiotics, immediate referral to an otorhinolaryngologist is appropriate. All infectious sequelae of contiguous cranial structures, as well as invasive complications requiring excision, such as a cholesteatoma, require referral to a specialist.

Patient Education

Swimming should be avoided until the infection clears, because immersion in water may lead to otitis externa, complicating the middle ear infection. The ear canal should be kept as dry as possible. Tympanic membrane perforation can be avoided by not using cotton swabs or sharp objects of any kind to clean the ears. Traumatic injuries to the middle ear should be avoided as well to prevent perforation. In all cases, especially those in which the tympanic membrane is perforated, blowing of the nose should be avoided. If the nose must be blown, it should be done as gently as possible.

All patients and their families should be encouraged to stop smoking, because this aggravates all forms of

Management Table 7.6 **Types of AOM and their Treatment Options**

Type of AOM	Treatment Options
AOM without rupture of tympanic membrane	Systemic antibiotics for 5–7 days Amoxicillin (Amoxil) Children: 90 mg/kg per day divided into bid or tid doses (40 mg/kg per day if first time infection in girls with no risk factors) Adults: 250–500 mg bid
Children with tympanostomy tubes	Ofloxacin (Floxin otic drops 5–10 drops bid)
Beta-lactamase resistant AOM	Augmentin (amoxicillin/clavulanate) 875 mg to 2000 mg bid. Second-Generation cephalosporin such as Cefaclor (Ceclor) 40 mg/kg/day divided bid Third-Generation cephalosporin such as cefixime (Suprax 8 mg/kg/day bid for children or 400 mg qd for adults). Rocephin 50 mg/kg IM injection—effective for children but painful.
Patients with penicillin allergy	Azithromycin (Zithromax) 500 mg first day then 250 mg daily for four days. Clarithromycin (Biaxin) 250–500 mg daily Neither of these medications are effective against *Moraxell catarrhalis* or *Haemophilus influenzae.*
Treatment for otalgia	Heat Antipyretics such as acetaminophen or ibuprofen Codeine (15–60 mg q4h for severe pain) Topical agents–Auralgan otic solution (antipyrine, benzocaine, and glycerin; 4 to 5 drops q 1–2 h) Cortisporin otic suspension (polymyxin B, neomycin, hydrocortisone) 4 drops in affected ear qid 7–10 days.
Recurrent and chronic AOM No therapeutic response after 2–3 days of treatment	Another 14 days of antibiotic therapy or alternative antibiotic therapy. Systemic steroid–prednisone Nasal spray with cromolyn, beclomethasone, fluticasone to decrease inflammation
Surgical treatment—inflammation persists after two full courses of antibiotic therapy.	Myringotomy–to relieve fluid buildup in middle ear. Tympanostomy–tubes placed in inner ear to drain pus or serous fluid. Tonsillectomy and/or adenoidectomy as secondary prevention

otic inflammation. Folk remedies such as "sweet oil" should also be avoided. Patients should be instructed to return to the clinic for further evaluation after 48 hours, if symptoms of AOM have not ameliorated. Explain that otitis media per se is not contagious, but that predisposing URIs may be passed from person to person. Bed rest or reduced activity may be suggested in severe cases until fever and pain subside, and the importance of completing the full regimen of all antibiotic therapies should be emphasized. Instruct patients to keep the ear canal dry during the course of infection, and demonstrate the proper method of cleaning the ear canal without chemical agents, sharp objects, cotton swabs, or a finger.

Ménière's Disease

Ménière's disease (Ménière's syndrome, endolymphatic hydrops) is a peripheral sensory disorder of both the labyrinth (semicircular canal system) and cochlea of the inner ear. Endolymphatic volume and, in turn, pressure are increased due to unknown etiology, resulting in both vestibular (proprioceptive, balance-related) and auditory dysfunction, characterized by recurrent attacks of tinnitus (ringing or buzzing in the ears), vertigo (a sense of whirling or spinning in space), and progressive hearing loss. Although Ménière's disease is not life-threatening, if untreated, acute attacks typically recur over the course of many years.

Epidemiology and Causes

Well-documented incidence figures for Ménière's disease are not available, but it is estimated that 46 new cases per 100,000 occur annually in the United States. Prevalence is estimated at 1,150 per 100,000. Age of onset is anywhere from 30 to 60 years, with most cases developing during the fifth decade of life. The disease is rare both in young children and in adults older than age 70. Some studies indicate that white Americans of European descent are at an increased risk of developing the disease. Both sexes are affected nearly equally, but some studies have reported slightly higher rates in women.

Stress, allergies, high salt intake, and exposure to high noise levels for periods of many years have all been cited as risk factors.

Pathophysiology

The precise cause of Ménière's disease is not fully established, but marked edema of the membranous labyrinth is typically observed at autopsy, and endolymphatic hydrops has been established as the defining pathologic finding in the disease. Theories have implicated the inflammatory response of the inner ear to a variety of insults including blunt trauma; viral infection; allergies; reduced or negative middle ear pressure; and various vascular, endocrine, and lipid disorders. Migraine headache and autoimmune conditions including systemic lupus erythematosus, rheumatoid arthritis, and certain thyroid disorders also predispose to Ménière's disease. A genetic predisposition has also been identified in 8 percent of people affected.

Dilation of the endolymphatic system may lead to rupture of the membranous labyrinth. This engorgement has been associated with excessive endolymph production, decreased resorption of fluid in the endolymphatic sac, as well as hypoplasia of the vestibular aqueduct. Resultant mixing of the endolymph and perilymph is thought to cause degeneration of both vestibular and cochlear neuroepithelial sensory hair cells which are particularly sensitive to ionic changes from the potassium-rich endolymph, resulting in vertigo, tinnitus, and hearing loss. Compression of the vestibular portion of cranial nerve VIII (CN VIII) by an enlarged blood vessel is yet another etiologic theory.

Clinical Presentation

Subjective

Acute episodes of Ménière's disease last anywhere from 20 minutes to 3 hours and are characterized by sudden attacks of nausea, emesis, pallor, diaphoresis, dizziness (spatial disorientation), vertigo, roaring tinnitus, and increased pressure, fullness, and hearing loss in the affected ear. Patients typically refer to any vestibular symptomatology as "dizziness." Rapid movement aggravates all proprioceptive symptomatology, and patients often report a history of falls or accidents during acute episodes. The frequency and severity of attacks may decrease over time, and hearing may improve immediately following an acute attack. However, some episodes have been known to last for more than 24 hours. Overall, low-frequency hearing loss is typically progressive, with bilateral involvement in 10 to 50 percent of cases. Patients may also experience motion-related imbalance without vertigo between acute attacks. Complete hearing loss in advanced cases of Ménière's disease is associated with a cessation of vertiginous episodes.

Objective

On inspection, otoscopic examination typically demonstrates no apparent abnormalities, unless underlying otitis media is present. Dilation of the inner ear endolymphatic system is apparent only at autopsy. Spontaneous nystagmus is often observed after preventing eye fixation by having the patient wear 40-diopter glasses (Frenzel lenses) during the period of observation.

Diagnostic Reasoning

Diagnostic Tests

Ménière's disease is diagnosed based upon a careful history, neurotologic assessment, and response to empiric therapy, as no specific diagnostic testing exists. The American Academy of Otolaryngology and Head and Neck Surgery has established diagnostic criteria requiring two distinct episodes of rotational vertigo lasting at least 20 minutes each, along with sensorineural hearing loss and either tinnitus or a perception of aural fullness. Thus, both the Weber and Rinne tests typically elicit findings characteristic of a sensorineural hearing defect. Sound lateralization to the nonaffected ear occurs when a 512-Hz tuning fork is placed midline on the top of the head (Weber test), and air conduction is superior in duration and volume to bone conduction (positive Rinne test). Audiometry also demonstrates low-frequency sensorineural hearing loss, as well as impaired speech discrimination. Both cold and warm caloric responses are typically reduced in the affected ear, as demonstrated by electronystagmography (ENG) or direct patient observation (while wearing 40-diopter Frenzel lenses), and the direction of the fast phase of nystagmus is variable. These findings are not diagnostic for Ménière's disease, however. Vestibular function tests are used to evaluate CN VIII function; however, these findings are questionable in patients taking sedative drugs of any kind.

Differential Diagnosis

Ménière's disease is a diagnosis of exclusion. Thus, numerous disorders that mimic its clinical picture must first be ruled out. OM is evaluated through otoscopic examination and culture of otic fluid. If middle ear infection is present, the tympanic membrane is typically erythematous and either edematous or retracted, with altered bony landmarks and a diminished cone light reflex. Bubbles or an air/fluid level may be seen directly behind the membrane, and mobility is reduced or absent upon insufflation with a pneumatic otoscope. OM and Ménière's disease are not mutually exclusive conditions, however, because negative middle ear pressure associated with serous otitis media may be a contributing factor to Ménière's disease. OM may also precipitate a viral infection of CN VIII known as vestibular neuronitis (benign recurrent vertigo), which presents as recurrent vertiginous episodes lasting several hours, which may be accompanied by severe vomiting and nausea. Vestibular neuronitis may also be idiopathic, but in these patients (unlike those with Ménière's disease), auditory impairment is rarely noted. Secondary or tertiary syphilis can also affect CN VIII and is ruled out via a variety of immunological tests specific for its causative agent *Treponema pallidum,* such as the microhemagglutination (MHA), fluorescent treponemal antibody (FTA), and treponema immobilization (TPI) assays. Acute viral or bacterial infection of the labyrinth may also present with similar symptoms; however, pathogenic microorganisms are not associated with Ménière's disease, because it is not of infectious etiology. Discrete lesions of the CNS, such as tumors or infarcts of the brain and cerebellum, as well as degenerative nervous disorders including Parkinson's disease, multiple sclerosis, and Alzheimer's disease, may be ruled out via CT and MRI. Hypothyroidism may also mimic Ménière's disease and is ruled out through measurement of both free and protein-bound thyroid hormone levels (thyroxine [T4] and triiodothyronine [T_3]), as well as pituitary thyroid stimulating hormone (TSH).

Benign positional vertigo (benign paroxysmal vertigo) is a more common diagnosis than Ménière's disease of vestibular dysfunction in elderly patients who complain of dizziness. It is characterized by paroxysmal vertigo accompanied by nystagmus when lying down, turning over in bed, or tilting the head backward. The Nylen-Bárány maneuver is used to make this diagnosis: The patient is reclined rapidly from a sitting to supine position with the head tilted to one side and the neck is hyperextended 30 degrees below the horizontal for at least 10 seconds, off the end of the examination table. The maneuver is then repeated with the head tilted to the opposite side. In this benign condition, nystagmus lasting between 15 and 45 seconds is observed after each maneuver, following a brief 1- to 5-second latent period. In contrast to Ménière's disease, benign positional vertigo does not present with hearing loss or tinnitus.

Presbycusis, the most common cause of sensorineural hearing loss in the elderly, is distinguished by high-frequency rather than low-frequency hearing loss as revealed by audiometric testing. Serum glucose levels should be evaluated to rule out hypoglycemic disorders, and hemoglobin/hematocrit are measured to assess anemic conditions, if suspected. Lipid disorders affecting cerebral blood flow and, in turn, vestibulocochlear function, may be ruled out via serum lipid studies. Other cerebro- and cardiovascular disorders, such as transient ischemic attacks, vertebrobasilar ischemia, or subclavian steal syndrome, may lead to CNS ischemia and vertigo, thus mimicking Ménière's disease. However, syncope (fainting) and generalized weakness are also usually observed. Angiography is used to rule out such disorders, if suspected. Another common cause of a vestibular and auditory dysfunction is iatrogenic, drug-induced ototoxicity from many commonly used drugs, including aspirin; potent diuretics; quinine; tetracyclines (especially minocycline); many cancer chemotherapies such as *cis*-platinum; and aminoglycoside antibiotics, including gentamicin, neomycin, kanamycin, and streptomycin. If use of these medications is not prolonged, ototoxicity may be reversible once drug intake has stopped. Sedative side effects of many medications, as well as undesirable multidrug interactions, are a common cause of dizziness, especially in elderly patients, who are at an increased risk of polypharmacy-related sequelae. In the adult patient, acoustic neuroma, causing compression of the auditory portion of CN VIII, is one of the most important diagnoses of auditory dysfunction to rule out, because these tumors may be life-threatening if untreated. MRI and auditory brainstem response (ABR) audiometry are used to detect such neoplasms. Finally, psychiatric diagnoses should be a major consideration if examination and laboratory findings rule out systemic disease and specific organ involvement as the cause of vestibulocochlear dysfunction. Psychiatric illness is the second most common etiology of dizziness in elderly patients, following peripheral nervous system disorders. Common conditions include depression, anxiety, panic attacks, somatization disorders, alcoholism, and other forms of substance abuse. A proper psychiatric evaluation, which may include drug screens of the urine and blood, is necessary to rule out such illnesses.

Management

Acute attacks are best treated by calm bed rest with the eyes closed and protection from falling. Attacks rarely last longer than 4 hours. Pharmacotherapy, if necessary, is directed at symptomatic relief, because no medications are known to affect this nonspecific disease process. A low-salt diet (less than 1000 mg/day) is considered first-line therapy to reduce endolymphatic pressure and volume, along with a mild diuretic such as chlorothiazide (Diuril) 500 mg/day PO and potassium supplements to counter diuretic-induced hypokalemia. Caffeine avoidance and tobacco cessation are also suggested to avoid vasoconstriction of the labyrinthine system. However, as with salt restriction, the efficacy of these therapies is based primarily on anecdotal evidence.

Acute attacks are managed with a combination of antimuscarinics or anticholinergics and vestibulosuppressive histamine (H_1)-blockers from various classes. The muscarinic antagonist atropine 0.2 to 0.4 mg IV or the anticholinergics scopolamine (Transderm Scop 0.33 mg/24 hours—1 transdermal disc or portion thereof applied behind the affected ear for at least 3 days) or glycopyrollate (Robinul) 2 mg PO bid may be used to relieve vertigo, nausea, and emesis. Other agents with antihistaminic, antimuscarinic, and sedative effects used for acute attacks include Betahistine 8 to 16 mg PO tid (not currently available in the United States), promethazine (Phenergan) 12.5 to 25 mg IV given slowly, diphenhydramine (Benadryl) 50 mg IV given slowly, and droperidol (Inapsine) 1.5 to 2.5 mg IV given slowly. GABAergic anxiolytics such as diazepam (Valium) 5 to 10 mg given slowly IV may also be used to sedate patients during severe episodes, but it should be noted that sedatives will affect the outcome of all vestibular function tests. Oral maintenance therapies include meclizine (Antivert, Bonine) 25 to 100 mg at bedtime or in divided doses, promethazine (Phenergan) 12.5 to 25 mg PO q4 to 6h, dimenhydrinate (Dramamine) 50 mg PO tid or qid, metoclopramide (Reglan)

10 mg PO bid, or diphenhydramine (Benadryl) 25 to 50 mg PO q4 to 6h, not to exceed 100 mg/day. Of note, these treatments are most effective for vertiginous symptoms, while tinnitus and hearing loss are less impacted.

If conventional treatment fails, intratympanic perfusion with dexamethasone may prove effective, especially if an underlying autoimmune disorder is present. As a last resort, if Ménière's disease progresses bilaterally, streptomycin or gentamicin ablation therapy may be appropriate to reduce unbearable vestibular symptoms. An aminoglycoside antibiotic is administered over a course of several days to weeks, to intentionally damage the neuroepithelium of the vestibular centers in the inner ear, thus reducing related symptomatology. However, hearing must be carefully monitored both during and after this treatment to avoid damage to auditory structures. Disabling symptoms of Ménière's disease may require surgical intervention, typically used in 5 to 10 percent of all cases. For patients with normal hearing ability, decompression of the endolymphatic sac may be accomplished by surgically draining excess endolymph into the mastoid or subarachnoid space. Alternatively, the vestibular nerve may be transected intracranially. For patients whose hearing ability has degenerated and is deemed unsalvageable, the cochlea itself may be decompressed (via cochleocentesis) or directly perfused with streptomycin. A more radical surgery is labyrinthectomy of the affected ear, a procedure that entirely ablates vestibular function.

Follow-Up and Referral

If symptoms do not worsen, patients may return for follow-up in 3 to 6 weeks. However, patients should return for reevaluation immediately if disabling symptoms such as tinnitus, vertigo, nausea, or emesis persist. Hearing loss, in particular, must be carefully monitored for progression, because this is a telltale sign of an underlying, potentially life-threatening acoustic neuroma. Patients often report that previously consulted clinicians failed to take this condition seriously when they first presented with symptoms. Thus, close follow-up care of the patient with Ménière's disease provides emotionally beneficial validation, as well.

Progressive bilateral hearing loss may result from Ménière's disease, leading to chronic tinnitus, deafness, and disabling vertigo. Accidental injuries related to vestibular dysfunction may occur in the work or home setting, and patients often report an increasing inability to function productively at their present jobs in the face of progressive disease. Failing to diagnose an underlying acoustic neuroma is a potentially life-threatening complication.

Referral to a specialist is necessary if symptoms worsen with treatment. Advanced diagnostic procedures such as ENG or specialized vestibulocochlear function tests require referral to a neurologist. A physician consult is also needed in cases involving persistent emesis, convulsions or seizures, syncope, or fever. New, unexplained symptoms (which are often due to multidrug interactions or adverse effects of medications) also require referral to a specialist for diagnosis and treatment. Streptomycin ablation therapy and surgical interventions should be directed by a qualified specialist only, as the risk of serious sequelae is significant, including permanent hearing loss.

Patient Education

Patients must be encouraged to stop smoking, because this aggravates all otic disorders. Stress levels and salt intake should also be reduced (to a maximum of 1 g/day) to lessen the severity of future attacks. All ototoxic medications should be avoided, and polypharmacy (multiple prescription drug usage) should be reevaluated with the aid of a specialist. The ears must also be protected against loud noises.

Patients should be instructed to return for further evaluation if symptoms worsen or acute episodes increase in frequency. The importance of following a low-salt diet should also be stressed. Patients should understand the difficulty in treating Ménière's disease pharmacologically and that acute attacks are often best managed with quiet bed rest and careful protection from falls. To avoid accidental injuries and minimize symptoms, patients should not drive, climb ladders, work near dangerous machinery, walk without assistance, read, or look at glaring lights during these episodes . Food intake should also be reduced during acute attacks to lessen nausea and vomiting.

Common Nose and Throat Problems

Rhinitis

Rhinitis (coryza) is an inflammation of the nasal mucosa characterized by nasal congestion, rhinorrhea, sneezing, pruritus, and/or postnasal drainage. Its etiology is varied, but in general, it is categorized as either allergic or nonallergic rhinitis. Allergic rhinitis may be either seasonal or perennial. Nonallergic rhinitis may be (1) infectious; (2) irritant-related (often in the workplace); (3) vasomotor; (4) hormone-related; (5) associated with medication use or overuse (rhinitis medicamentosum); or (6) atrophic (seen primarily in geriatric patients). It may be acute or chronic, but the most common forms are viral rhinitis and perennial or seasonal ("hay fever") allergic rhinitis.

Although rhinitis is often a benign and self-limited disorder, poorly controlled allergic rhinitis may contribute to sleep loss, absenteeism from work or school, secondary daytime fatigue, learning impairment, decreased overall cognitive functioning, decreased long-term productivity, and decreased quality of life. In addition, poorly controlled rhinitis may lead to the development of other related disease processes, such as sinusitis, nasal polyps, otitis media with effusion (OME), hearing impairment, aggravation of underlying asthma, and sleep apnea.

Epidemiology and Causes

Although the actual prevalence of acute rhinitis is undocumented, it is extremely common, occurring at least as frequently as the common cold. Moreover, an estimated 40 to 50 million American adults suffer from some form of chronic rhinitis; some sources quote cumulative frequencies of 42 percent of the population of the United States by age 40. Specifically, the incidence of seasonal allergic rhinitis parallels pollen production, increasing in the fall and spring and peaking in the winter. Other forms of rhinitis may last year-round if they are caused by perennial allergens such as dust or house mites. Allergic rhinitis occurs in all age groups, most commonly in adults between 30 and 40 years of age, but it is rare in adults older than age 50. Onset of symptoms typically occurs between the ages of 10 and 20.

Nonallergic infectious rhinitis may be acute or chronic. Acute rhinitis is usually viral and self-limiting, whereas chronic rhinitis may be associated with bacterial sinusitis and may have associated allergic or mucociliary disturbances as predisposing factors. Rhinitis medicamentosum affects primarily young to middle-aged adults (correlating with medication use), and atrophic rhinitis affects primarily older adults, although the onset of symptoms may begin as early as puberty.

Most forms of rhinitis appear to have no ethnic predispositions. Hispanics, Asians, and African Americans seem to be particularly susceptible to atrophic rhinitis, however. In contrast, the incidence of this form is low in natives of equatorial Africa. Viral and atrophic rhinitis affect women more often than men, whereas most other forms affect both sexes equally.

Viral URIs occur more frequently in families with young children, whereas exposure to offending allergens is the primary risk factor for allergic rhinitis. The most common irritants implicated in the seasonal form are pollen and mold spores, and dust, mites, insect debris (cockroaches, locusts, fish food), tobacco smoke, animal dander, dried saliva, and urine for the perennial form of allergic rhinitis. Immunosuppression secondary to illness or drug/medication use and a family history of allergic disease (e.g., eczema and/or asthma) are also risk factors for allergic rhinitis. Vasomotor rhinitis is aggravated by low humidity, sudden temperature or pressure changes, cold air, strong odors, emotional stress, cigarette smoke, and other nasal irritants. Use of nasal decongestants more frequently than every 3 hours or for periods longer than 3 weeks is the primary risk factor for the development of rhinitis medicamentosum. In some patients, certain drugs may precipitate rhinitis: Antihypertensive agents are the most fre-quently cited culprits. ACE inhibitors, beta-adrenergic antagonists, certain anti-inflammatory agents, guanethidine (Ismelin), clonidine (Catapres), hydralazine (Apresoline), prazosin (Minipress), chlordiazepoxide (Librium), amitriptyline (Elavil), or even aspirin can be a contributing factor. Oral contraceptive use and estrogen replacement therapy have also been implicated as risk factors for rhinitis, along with a family history of rhinitis and septal/anatomic obstruction. In addition, ingestion of certain foods may precipitate rhinitis in susceptible individuals.

Pathophysiology

Viral rhinitis stems from an acute catarrhal response caused by viral replication in the nasopharynx, resulting in varying degrees of nasotracheal inflammation. Strongly associated with viral upper respiratory tract infection (URI or the "common cold"), the primary etiologic agents of viral rhinitis include rhinovirus, influenza virus, parainfluenza virus, respiratory syncytial virus, coronavirus, adenovirus, echovirus, and coxsackievirus. When viral sinusitis is also present, the condition is collectively referred to as rhinosinusitis. The vast majority of rhinosinusitis is due to viral infection, but bacterial superinfection may complicate a small percentage of these cases. Anatomic defects or obstructions anywhere along the nasopharyngeal tract may predispose to infection by impairing physiologic nasal drainage.

In contrast, allergic rhinitis results from immunoglobulin E (IgE)-mediated type I hypersensitivity to airborne irritants affecting the eyes, nose, sinuses, throat, and bronchi. IgE antibodies, elicited by repeated allergen exposure, bind to eosinophils and basophils in the bloodstream and their mucosal counterparts known as mast cells. These leukocytes subsequently degranulate, releasing chemoinflammatory substances including histamine, leukotrienes, prostaglandins, slow-reacting substance of anaphylaxis, and erythrocyte chemotactic factor, which result in increased vasodilation, capillary permeability, mucus production, smooth muscle contraction, and eosinophilia. On rare occasions, food allergies may be the cause. In addition, chemical or particulate airborne irritants may cause direct mucosal inflammation in the absence of IgE production or immune hypersensitivity.

Vasomotor rhinitis is a chronic, noninfectious process of unknown etiology without accompanying eosinophilia, characterized by periods of abnormal autonomic responsiveness and vascular engorgement unrelated to specific allergens. Fluctuations and reductions in estrogen associated with menses, hormonal birth control preparations, pregnancy, and menopause may all predispose to nonallergic rhinitis. Rhinitis medicamentosum is a rebound condition secondary to medication overuse. In some patients, it is caused by certain antihypertensive medications via undefined mechanisms, but most often mucosal inflammation results from the use of topical nasal decongestants such as phenylephrine (Neo-Synephrine) for greater than 3 to 4 days, which leads to secondary vasodilation, repeated small-vessel coagulation, and eventual fibrosis. Bacterial infection is thought to play a role in the development of atrophic rhinitis, in which the nasal epithelia and bones progressively atrophy, resulting in distinct morphologic changes.

Clinical Presentation

Subjective

Viral rhinitis is typically accompanied by malaise, headache, substernal tightness or burning, and occasionally fever. Patients with allergic rhinitis usually complain of itching in the nasal passages, conjunctivae, and roof of the mouth, as well as epiphoria (stringy, watery ocular discharge). Sneezing, coughing, and a sore or burning throat commonly present in both viral and allergic rhinitis.

In contrast, patients with vasomotor rhinitis (noninfectious rhinitis without eosinophilia) rarely display any of the aforementioned symptoms. However, watery rhinorrhea, nasal congestion, "nasal" speech, and forced mouth-breathing are common complaints of patients with viral, allergic, vasomotor, or medication-related rhinitis. The onset of congestion is rapid in vasomotor rhinitis; patients typically complain of a pronounced, watery postnasal drip, as well as persistent nasal obstruction that may switch sides with each attack. Rhinitis medicamentosum patients may present with increased heart rate and elevated blood pressure because of the effects of sympathomimetic decongestants. Patients with atrophic rhinitis may complain of nasal congestion, a thick postnasal drip, frequent clearing of the throat, anosmia (impaired olfaction), a constant foul odor in the nose, and severe epistaxis (nosebleeds).

Objective

On inspection, the nasal mucosa typically appears erythematous in viral rhinitis, and throat inspection may reveal pharyngitis or laryngitis, characterized by erythematous and edematous pharyngeal mucosa or vocal cords. If the viral rhinitis is complicated by a secondary bacterial infection, the nasal discharge may be greenish yellow, which is indicative of purulence. In allergic rhinitis, the mucosa are pale, boggy (edematous), and may take on a bluish hue. Yellowish, gray, or erythematous mucosa may also be seen. Gray-blue to yellow-tan nasal polyps may present with chronic perennial rhinitis. The conjunctivae are usually inflamed (allergic conjunctivitis), with the palpebral conjunctiva being particularly edematous (chemosis) and "cobblestoned" in appearance, owing to chronically injected blood vessels. Dark circles under the eyes ("allergic shiners") may be apparent, along with excess wrinkles under the lower eyelid (Dennie lines). In both viral and allergic rhinitis, the external nose may appear erythematous, with a transnasal crease resulting from repeated upward wiping and nose wrinkling. The nasal turbinates and palatine or pharyngeal tonsils (adenoids) may also be enlarged. The nasal mucosa in patients with vasomotor rhinitis will range from bright red to bluish in hue, and again, the nasal turbinates may be swollen. The mucosa in patients with rhinitis medicamentosum are also injected and edematous. In contrast, the mucosa in patients with atrophic rhinitis usually appear crusted with dried mucus or blood from repeated bouts of epistaxis, although the nasal passages typically remain patent.

On palpation, the nasal mucosa in patients with viral rhinitis appears particularly friable. If present, nasal polyps are typically soft, edematous, and nontender. The external nose may be tender from repeated sneezing in patients with viral and allergic rhinitis. Some patients with rhinitis medicamentosum may present with dry and rubbery mucosa. On auscultation, wheezing breath sounds may reflect concurrent asthma associated with allergic rhinitis.

Diagnostic Reasoning

Diagnostic Tests

Laboratory tests are not typically indicated for uncomplicated cases of viral rhinitis, allergic rhinitis, or rhinitis medicamentosum. However, if an exudate is present in a colored or translucent nasal discharge, a Giemsa- or Wright's-stained smear should be prepared, along with a CBC to characterize the disease process. Leukocytosis or the presence of polymorphonuclear neutrophils in the discharge reflects an infectious disorder other than a typical viral URI. Eosinophilia in the discharge is indicative of allergic rhinitis. Peripheral eosinophil count and serum IgE levels have low predictive values; however, intradermal skin testing of minute amounts of allergens may be helpful if the diagnosis of allergic rhinitis is in doubt. Vasomotor rhinitis tends to be a diagnosis of exclusion, because nasal smears and skin tests are typically negative, and no family history of allergic disorders is expected. Hormonally related rhinitis and rhinitis medicamentosum are diagnosed primarily through patient history, once other common forms of rhinitis have been excluded. Finally, atrophic rhinitis may be confirmed by nasal mucosal biopsy. Histopathology will demonstrate transformation of ciliated pseudostratified columnar epithelia into the stratified squamous form. In addition, the lamina propria will be decreased in thickness and vascularity, while bacterial culture of nasal secretions may also be helpful.

Differential Diagnosis

Acute or chronic sinusitis resulting from bacterial infection of the facial sinuses may also inflame the nasal mucosa. Sinus x-ray films demonstrating mucosal thickening, air-fluid levels, or opacification are effective at ruling out this disorder, as are cultures or smears of sinus aspirates to identify the infectious organisms present. Physical examination may rule out nasal foreign bodies, nasal polyps, or a deviated septum as causes of mucosal inflammation or congestion. Cocaine snorting, inhalant abuse (sniffing), and other forms of substance abuse should also be ruled out through a detailed patient history and, if appropriate, serum drug screens. Chronic inflammatory conditions such as sarcoidosis may be ruled out via biopsy, which would reveal granulomatous (histiocyte/macrophage) inflammation of the nasal mucosa. Hormonal changes associated with pregnancy and hyper- or hypothyroidism may also lead to nasal vasodilation and inflammation. Such conditions are ruled out through a careful physical examination, detailed patient history, and hematologic hormone screens.

Management

With all types of rhinitis, much of the treatment regimen will center around relief of symptoms and self-care measures, while environmental issues must also be addressed.

Viral rhinitis is treated symptomatically, as viral URIs are predominantly self-limited.

- ▲ Fever and headache may be treated with acetaminophen 325 to 650 mg PO q4h prn. Aspirin is not recommended because it may increase viral shedding.
- ▲ Rhinorrhea may be treated with oral decongestants such as pseudoephedrine (Sudafed) 30 to 60 mg PO q3h to q4h prn or topical preparations such as phenylephrine (Neo-Synephrine) 0.25 to 0.5 percent nasal spray one to two sprays in each nostril q3h to q4h prn for no more than 3 to 4 days.
- ▲ Persistent coughs may be treated with dextromethorphan 15 to 30 mg PO q3h to q4h prn, but prescription codeine 10 to 15 mg PO q3h to q4h prn usually proves to be the only consistently effective cough suppresant.

For allergic rhinitis, avoidance or reduced exposure to offending allergens is the primary method of treatment, because acute attacks are typically self-limited if not continually aggravated by allergen. Newer-generation oral antihistamines designed to be less sedating are now the first-line short-term treatment of choice for allergic rhinitis:

- ▲ Fexofenadine (Allegra) 60 mg bid or 180 mg qd
- ▲ Loratadine (Claritin, Alavert) 10 mg qd
- ▲ Desloratadine (Clarinex) 5 mg qd
- ▲ Cetirizine (Zyrtec) 5 to 10 mg qd
- ▲ Also available is the intranasal antihistamine azelastine (Astelin) two sprays in each nostril bid.

These work best for early symptoms of allergy such as sneezing, watery eyes, and ocular pruritus. However, intranasal corticosteroids have traditionally been considered the best means of controlling the longer-term symptoms of allergic rhinitis including nasal congestion and discharge. In fact, meta-analyses have suggested that intranasal corticosteroids are the best overall first-line treatment for allergic rhinitis. It should be stressed, however, that intranasal steroid therapy may require 2 or more weeks of continuous daily use before symptomatic relief is apparent.

- ▲ Fluticasone 0.05 percent (Flonase), mometasone (Nasonex), or triamcinolone (Nasocort), all at two sprays in each nostril qd.

Systemic steroids have significant side effects and tend to be discouraged for such a common condition.

A newer class of medication, leukotriene receptor antagonists, have been approved for allergic rhinitis. Randomized controlled studies have shown Singular to be as effective as Loratadine in the symptomatic relief of allergic rhinitis.

- ▲ Singulair 4 to 10 mg PO daily.

Vasomotor rhinitis is also treated symptomatically, albeit at times unsatisfactorily, with environmental humidification using a vaporizer or humidified central heating system. Congestion may also improve with topical saline nasal sprays. Thorough cleaning of the nose and restoration of nasal patency may be achieved using powered devices such as a Grossan nasal irrigator. Intranasal ipratropium (Atrovent) 0.03 percent two sprays in each nostril bid to qid prn or azelastine (Astelin) two sprays in each nostril bid may also relieve symptoms.

Rhinorrhea may be treated with systemic oral decongestants such as:

- ▲ Pseudoephedrine (Sudafed) 30–60 mg tid or qid prn
- ▲ Intranasal steroid preparations (as described for allergic rhinitis) may also be helpful if other treatments are ineffective.

Rhinitis medicamentosum is remedied by immediately stopping all topical decongestant use. The condition typically resolves after 2 to 3 weeks.

- ▲ Oral antihistamine-decongestant preparations or short courses of topical nasal steroids may provide symptomatic relief. A short course of systemic steroids such as prednisone 30 mg PO daily for 5 days may be needed if other treatments prove ineffective.

Atrophic rhinitis may be treated with bacitracin ointment intranasally bid or tid until the nasal crusting and foul odor are eliminated. Expectorants such as guaifenesin 400 mg PO q4h prn, physiologic saline solutions, or electric nasal irrigators (e.g., Grossan) may provide symptomatic relief, while menopausal women may be helped by systemic estrogens. See Drugs Commonly Prescribed 7.1 for more information.

Desensitizing immunotherapy may be an option for allergic rhinitis that is refractory to pharmacologic treatment. Patients receive subcutaneous injections of purified allergen weekly at a dosage that increases with each treatment. The interval between injections is lengthened once a maintenance dose is reached. This treatment regimen may last up to 3 to 5 years, but it should not be continued past 12 months if symptoms are not improving, as cure rates may be as low as 20 percent. In addition, to reduce the risk of anaphylactic reactions, antigen injections must never be given intravenously. Occasionally, surgery is recommended if the etiology of refractory or recurrent rhinitis is anatomic,

Drugs Commonly Prescribed 7.1: Rhinitis

Drug	Indication	Dosage	Comments
Antihistamines—First Generation			
Diphenhydramine (Benadryl)	Allergic rhinitis	25 to 50 mg PO q4–6h; maximum 300 mg/day	Must use 3–5 h prior to anticipated exposure or on a regular basis as long-term therapy. *Adverse effects:* CNS sedation, GI upset, anticholinergic effects (dry mouth, blurred vision), additive CNS depressant effects of alcohol, sedative, hypnotics Use with caution in older adults.
Chlorpheniramine maleate (Chlortrimeton)	Allergic rhinitis	204 mg PO q4–6h	Must use 3–5 h prior to anticipated exposure or on a regular basis as long-term therapy. *Adverse effects:* CNS sedation, GI upset, anticholinergic effects (dry mouth, blurred vision), additive CNS depressant effects of alcohol, sedative, hypnotics Use with caution in older adults.
Promethazine HCl (Phenergan)	Allergic rhinitis	25 mg PO q hs	Must use 3–5 h prior to anticipated exposure or on a regular basis as long-term therapy. *Adverse effects:* CNS sedation, GI upset, anticholinergic effects (dry mouth, blurred vision), additive CNS depressant effects of alcohol, sedative, hypnotics Use with caution in older adults.
Azelastine HCl (Astelin)	Seasonal rhinitis	(137 μg/spray) two sprays/nostril bid	Intranasal *Adverse effects:* Bitter taste, somnolence, CNS sedation, GI upset, anticholinergic effects (dry mouth, blurred vision), additive CNS depressant effects of alcohol, sedative, hypnotics Use with caution in older adults.
Antihistamines—Second Generation			
Astemizole (Hismanal)	Rhinitis	10 mg PO qd	Not as effective as first generation; use in patients who cannot tolerate sedation. *Adverse effects:* Headache, mild drowsiness Arrhythmias and adverse cardiac effects may occur.
Loratidine (Claritin)	Rhinitis	10 mg PO qd	*Adverse effects:* Headache, mild drowsiness Not as effective as first generation; use in patients who cannot tolerate sedation.
Cetirizine (Zyrtec)	Rhinitis	5–10 mg PO qd	Somewhat more sedation than others, but less than first generation Not as effective as first generation; use in patients who cannot tolerate sedation
Fexofenadine (Allegra)	Rhinitis	60 mg bid	Not as effective as first generation; use in patients who cannot tolerate sedation
Decongestants			
NSAID and sympathomimetic (Advil Cold and Sinus)	Rhinorrhea, sinusitis, flu	1 to 2 tablets q4–6h; maximum 6 tablets/day	Should not be used for longer than 3–4 days. Take with food. Use with caution in patients with hypertension, diabetes, glaucoma, BPH, and those taking beta-blockers.

(continued)

Drugs Commonly Prescribed 7.1: Rhinitis (continued)

Drug	Indication	Dosage	Comments
Diphenhydramine HCl 25 mg and pseudo-ephedrine HCl 60 mg	Rhinorrhea, nasal congestion	1 tablet q4–6h	Should not be used for longer than 3–4 days. Do not use with MAO inhibitors, bron-chospasm, hypertension, diabetes, BPH. Potentiates the effects of alcohol, sedatives.
Loratidine 10 mg and pseudoephedrine 50 mg (Claritin-D 24 Hour)	Rhinitis, sinusitis with conges-tion, allergic rhinitis	1 tablet daily	Should not be used for longer than 3–4 days. Do not crush or chew. Contraindicated in patients with glaucoma, BPH, hypertension, CAD Use with caution in elderly patients and those taking beta-blockers.
Pseudoephedrine HCl (Sudafed)	Nasal congestion	30 to 60 mg PO q4–6h; maximum 4 doses/day	Should not be used for longer than 3–4 days. Decongestant only Can cause CNS excitation, hypertension, palpitation. Use with caution in elderly patients and those taking beta-blockers. Contraindicated in patients with diabetes, BPH, hypertension, MAO inhibitors, car-diac disease.
Fexofenadine HCl 60 mg and pseudoephedrine 120 mg (Allegra-D)	Seasonal rhinitis with nasal con-gestion	1 tablet bid	Should not be used for longer than 3–4 days. Extend tab. Avoid giving with food. Antihistamine and sympathomimetic Avoid other sympathomimetics. Contraindicated in patients with glau-coma, BPH, hypertension, MAO inhibitors *Adverse effects:* Palpitations, hypertension
Clemastine fumanate 1.34 mg and phenyl propanolamine HCl 75 mg (Tavist-D)	Rhinorrhea, nasal congestion, common cold	1 tablet q12h	Should not be used for longer than 3–4 days. Sustained release tablets Do not crush or chew. Use with caution in patients with hyperten-sion, CAD, diabetes and those taking MAO inhibitors, beta-blockers, and CNS depressants, as well as in older adults.
Intranasal corticosteroids			
Beclomethasone dipropi-onate (Beconase, Vance-nase [pocket-haler], Vacanase AQ (aqueous solution), Vacanase AQ DS (double strength))	Decrease nasal inflammatory reaction	(42 μg/spray) one or two sprays/nostril bid (Vacanase AQ DS 84 μg/spray—two sprays/nostril)	Available in aerosol and metered pump May eliminate need for antihistamines or decongestants. Must be used regularly; onset of action in 2 or more days; use decongestant prior to application if necessary. *Adverse effects:* Local irritation, increased rhinorrhea, local-ized fungal infection
Budesonide (Rhinocort)	Decrease nasal inflammatory reaction	(32 μg/spray) two sprays/nostril bid or four sprays/nostril qid	Aerosol May eliminate need for antihistamines or decongestants. Must be used regularly; onset of action in 2 or more days; use decongestant prior to application if necessary. *Adverse effects:* Local irritation, increased rhinorrhea, local-ized fungal infection

Drug	Indication	Dosage	Comments
Dexamethasone sodium phosphate (Pex A-Cort)	Decrease nasal inflammatory reaction	(100 μg/spray) two sprays/nostril bid or tid	Aerosol May eliminate need for antihistamines or decongestants. Must be used regularly; onset of action in 2 or more days; use decongestant prior to application if necessary. *Adverse effects:* Local irritation, increased rhinorrhea, localized fungal infection
Flunisolide (Nasarel, Nasacide)	Allergic rhinitis	(25 μg/spray) two sprays/nostril bid to tid	Available in aerosol or metered pump
Fluticasone propionate (Flonase)	Allergic rhinitis	(50 μg/spray) two sprays/nostril once a day or one spray bid	Available in metered pump
Triamcinolone acetonide (Nasacort)	Allergic rhinitis	(55 μg/spray) two sprays/nostril once a day	Available in aerosol or metered pump Maintain regular regimen
Memetasone furoate (Nasonex)	Allergic rhinitis	(50 μg/spray) two sprays/nostril once daily	Begin 2–4 weeks prior to start of pollen season.
Anticholinergic			
Ipratropium bromide nasal spray 0.03%, 0.06% (Atrovent)	Prevention of rhinorrhea	(21 μg/spray) two sprays/nostril bid to tid (42 μg/spray) two sprays/nostril bid to tid	Does not relieve itching or nasal blockage. Use cautiously in patients with BPH, glaucoma.
Mast cell stabilizer			
Cromolyn sodium (Nasalcrom)	Prevention and relief of nasal allergy symptoms	(5.2 μg/spray) one spray/nostril tid to qid; maximum	Regular use required. Do not use to treat sinus infection or asthma.

including nasal polypectomy for obstructing lesions or septoplasty if septal deviation is significant enough to interfere with the benefits of medication.

Follow-Up and Referral

A return visit should be scheduled in 2 to 3 weeks to review patient education, adherence to the treatment plan, and effectiveness of prescribed treatments. After this, quarterly or biannual visits are recommended, depending on the patient's comfort level and general state of health.

Complications of most forms of rhinitis include serous otitis media (extension of nasal infection into the ear), acute or chronic sinusitis, and repeated or disseminated respiratory infections. Allergic rhinitis may lead to restless sleeping and chronic fatigue, and asthma may complicate allergic attacks. Rhinitis medicamentosum may be complicated by physical addiction to topical nasal decongestants, as relief periods shorten and severity of rebound congestion increases with each use. Thus, stopping the use of these drugs becomes especially difficult for the addicted patient.

Physician referral may be necessary for allergen skin testing, immunotherapy, or nasal irrigation. The diagnosis and treatment of certain sequelae such as chronic sinusitis or high fever may also require physician referral. Surgical referral is necessary if anatomic obstructions of the nasal cavity (e.g., nasal polyps or a deviated septum) are etiologic or complicating factors.

Patient Education

Viral rhinitis is best avoided by limiting exposure to persons with an acute URI. Allergic flare-ups are best prevented by avoiding exposure to environmental irritants. Many preventive steps may be taken. Windows and doors should be kept closed to reduce pollen entry into the household, and high-efficiency particle air (HEPA) filters are helpful in removing allergens from ambient air. Pet traffic from outside should be minimized because this may transport pollen indoors, and patients should avoid being outside on excessively sunny or windy days. Allergic attacks to mold spores can be prevented by avoiding piles of leaves during the fall months, by wiping down household surfaces where mold grows with bleach solutions, utilizing HEPA filters, and reducing ambient humidity to 30 to 40 percent. Allergic attacks caused by perennial antigens such as dust or mites can be minimized by thoroughly cleaning or removing all carpets, drapes, curtains, and fabric-covered or stuffed furniture from the house, as well as by damp mopping, floor waxing, and dusting of all surfaces with a damp cloth. Stuffed animals, feather pillows, rubber mattresses, and box springs should either be covered with plastic or removed and replaced with synthetic materials, such as polyester. Chenille bedspreads, quilts, or comforters should be avoided, and bedding should be washed weekly. The use of air conditioning with frequent filter changes, rather than open windows, to cool automobiles or homes is recommended. Patients who are allergic to animal dander should bathe their pets often and restrict them from the bedroom or the entire house altogether. Prophylactic use of 4 percent cromolyn sodium nasal spray (one spray in each nostril 3 to 6 times/day at regular intervals) prior to known antigen exposure may prevent allergic flare-ups but is ineffective once an attack is underway. Ophthalmic cromolyn sodium preparations are also available (one to two drops can be instilled in each eye four to six times/day). Vasomotor rhinitis is also best avoided by limiting exposure to environmental triggers, and rhinitis medicamentosum can be prevented by diligently monitoring topical nasal decongestant use.

Patients with allergic rhinitis should be taught to avoid allergens and to observe the onset, duration, and progression of symptoms, so they can correlate their flare-ups to environmental conditions and thus better guide self-treatment. Emphasize all preventative and prophylactic measures, particularly the importance of keeping bedrooms allergen-free. Patients with all forms of rhinitis should understand the reasoning behind limiting nasal decongestant use, as well as the appropriate use of prophylactic cromolyn sodium sprays. It is also critical to explain that symptomatic relief from topical nasal steroid preparations may not be evident until 2 weeks into therapy. All patients should be instructed to arrange for further evaluation if clear rhinorrhea becomes purulent.

Epistaxis

Commonly called a "nosebleed," *epistaxis* is a hemorrhage of the nasal mucosa resulting from the traumatic or spontaneous rupture of superficial veins and/or arteries, located most often on the anterosuperior portion of the nasal septum known as Little's area (Kiesselbach's triangle or Kiesselbach's plexus). Epistaxis is a physical sign rather than a disease. Therefore, following the initial management of bleeding, a thorough evaluation is essential to determine its underlying cause.

Epidemiology and Causes

Although actual prevalence statistics for epistaxis are undocumented, it is an extremely common condition. Approximately 10 percent of the population experiences at least one significant nosebleed over a lifetime. Epistaxis most commonly occurs in children younger than 10 years of age and in adults older than 50 years. Minor, self-limited epistaxis is twice as common in children as it is in adults. In contrast, posterior epistaxis is more common in elderly patients. No ethnic predispositions are apparent. Men and women are affected equally by nosebleeds, although some predisposing clotting disorders such as hemophilia may be expressed predominantly in males.

Excessive dryness of the nasal mucosa in poorly humidified environments or at high altitudes weakens nasal vessels, predisposing them to rupture. Septal deviation may thus contribute to epistaxis through the disproportionate exposure of one side of the nose to dry environmental air. Primary coagulopathies such as von Willebrand's syndrome, thrombocytopenia, and clotting-factor deficiencies may also predispose an individual to epistaxis, although epistaxis is rare in hemophiliacs unless it is related to trauma. Coagulopathies may also be associated with chronic disorders such as cirrhosis, renal disease, cancer (especially Hodgkin's disease), and hypertension. As a whole, however, coagulopathies and neoplasms are associated with only 10 percent of cases of epistaxis. Vascular diseases such as hereditary hemorrhagic telangiectasia and arteriovenous nasal malformations are also risk factors. Medications that prolong bleeding time (e.g., warfarin, aspirin) contribute to all types of bleeding disorders, as does cocaine abuse (snorting), which leads to septal perforation. Prolonged use of nose drops is also a risk factor, because it may lead to reflex nasal inflammation, known as rhinitis medicamentosum. In an elderly patient, arteriosclerosis is a contributing factor, specifically for posterior hemorrhage epistaxis. Many nutritional deficiencies and febrile infectious disorders may also predispose an individual to nosebleeds, including scurvy (extreme vitamin C deficiency), and rheumatic, scarlet, or typhoid fever.

Pathophysiology

More than 90 percent of nosebleeds result from local irritation related to trauma or inflammation, occurring most often in the absence of any anatomic abnormality. Trauma to both nasal polyps and the well-vascularized watershed area of the nasal mucosa known as Kiesselbach's plexus is perhaps the most common direct cause of nosebleed, particularly from picking of the nose (epistaxis digitorum) or forcible injury related to blunt trauma. Kiesselbach's plexus marks the anastomosis of three major blood vessels of the nasal cavity: the septal branch of the anterior ethmoid artery, the septal portion of the superior labial branch of the facial artery, and the lateral nasal branch of the sphenopalatine artery. Similarly, posterior epistaxis most commonly originates from rupture of the posterior wall and choanal branches of the sphenopalatine artery. Vascular disease accounts for up to one-fourth of posterior bleeds, while rupture of an intracranial or cervical vascular aneurysm must also be considered as a potentially life-threatening etiology.

Spontaneous rupture of weakened vessels may also result from acute or chronic sinusitis, upper respiratory infection, and drying or crusting of the nasal mucosa from viral or allergic rhinitis. Foreign bodies lodged in the nasal airways are another common source of vessel injury, while inhaled drugs of abuse (e.g., cocaine and heroin snorting) chronically dry and aggravate friable nasal mucosa, predisposing to epistaxis. Anticoagulant medications such as warfarin (Coumadin) and heparin may also predispose to nose bleeds by inhibiting natural clotting pathways, and alcohol intake has been implicated as an independent, albeit far from universal, epistaxis risk factor. Malignant growths in the nasal cavity or paranasal sinuses may erode into blood vessels and present with epistaxis as their sole manifestation. An exceedingly rare cause of nasal bleeding is the presence of nasal ectopic endometrium (nasal endometriosis). Familial blood dyscrasias such as hemophilia A (Factor VIII deficiency), hemophilia B (Factor IX deficiency or Christmas disease), and von Willebrand disease (the most common genetic bleeding disorder), as well as hereditary hemorrhagic telangiectasia (Osler-Weber-Rendu disease) are examples of inherited conditions that may be complicated by significant epistaxis.

Clinical Presentation

Subjective

The patient with recurrent minor anterior epistaxis typically presents with a history of several episodes over several weeks. If blood loss has been extensive, patients may report lightheadedness or shortness of breath. In addition, a rapid heartbeat may be detected, and the patient may report blackened stools (melena) that are discolored from clotted, swallowed blood. Posterior epistaxis may be asymptomatic or may present with hemoptysis (coughed-up blood), nausea, hematemesis (blood-streaked vomitus), or melena.

Objective

Prominent blood vessels are typically seen traversing the anterior septum, and a small amount of clotted blood may be visible. If the patient is actively bleeding from the front of the nose, blood is typically bright red, and localizing the bleeding source may be difficult. The second most common site of hemorrhage (after Little's area) is the anterior end of the inferior nasal turbinate. Epistaxis originating deeper in the nose may produce either bright red or dark blood. Usually only one bleeding site exists, but if multiple sites or a diffuse ooze are evident, an underlying systemic bleeding disorder is likely. If the source of hemorrhage is located in the posterosuperior nasal cavity, the bleeding is termed posterior epistaxis. In these cases, blood loss will extend into the pharynx as well, and clotted blood and brown to red throat discoloration may be evident. The most common sites of posterior bleeding are just under the posterior half of the inferior nasal turbinate or the roof of the nasal cavity. Patients with significant blood loss may demonstrate pallor, particularly in the face. Palpation of the paranasal sinuses may reveal tenderness if underlying sinusitis or malignancy is present. Likewise, percussion of the paranasal sinuses may demonstrate tenderness in sinusitis-related or malignancy-related cases.

Diagnostic Reasoning

Diagnostic tests are rarely called for when bleeding can be managed, and most episodes of epistaxis are not recurrent. A variety of diagnostic tests are helpful in determining the underlying cause of nasal hemorrhage. Lab tests exist for deficiencies of most clotting factors, but Factor VIII and Factor IX deficiencies are clearly the most commonly observed and tested for. In the past, bleeding times were monitored to help diagnose platelet-related coagulopathies. Because of labor intensity of the test and variation on results by lab technician this test is rarely performed. Today a more sophisticated test called platelet function assay detects the ability of the platelets to work not just the number of platelets. A prolonged bleeding time (more than 7 minutes) may reflect platelet-related coagulopathies (e.g., von Willebrand's syndrome or thrombocytopenia), whereas a prolonged prothrombin time (PT) or partial thromboplastin time (PTT) is characteristic of clotting factor disorders. Hemophilia A (Factor VIII deficiency) and hemophilia B (Factor IX deficiency) produce a prolonged PTT, whereas disorders of the extrinsic clotting pathway (Factor VII deficiency) result in a prolonged PT. A CBC, including hemoglobin, hematocrit, and mean corpuscular volume may offer insight into the chronicity of the condition. Radiologic (x-ray) examination of the nasal cavity and paranasal sinuses may identify masses including neoplasms or foreign bodies, as well as sinusitis if mucosal thickening or air–water levels are apparent. CAT Scan of the head may also be done with greater sensitivity for detecting structural and soft tissue abnormalities.

Differential Diagnosis

For the patient with recurrent minor epistaxis, bleeding of nasal cavity origin must be distinguished from bleeding due to chronic sinusitis. In addition, nasopharyngeal or paranasal sinus tumors should be ruled out with x-ray films, as previously described. Differentiation between posterior epistaxis, hemoptysis, and hematemesis is critical if signs of anterior nasal bleeding are inapparent. In the absence of respiratory or gastrointestinal findings, a diagnosis of posterior epistaxis can be assumed if visual evidence exists for a posterior source of bleeding, if the majority of bleeding has occurred into the pharynx, or if anterior nasal packing fails to control hemorrhage.

Management

Specific treatment should be based on the underlying cause of epistaxis. If etiology is undetermined, interventions should be geared toward alleviating anxiety related to symptoms of an unknown etiology as well as stopping the bleeding. If the cause of epistaxis is found to be traumatic injury from nose picking and/or dry and cracked mucosa, advanced practice nursing interventions should be focused on educating the patient in self-care.

No pharmacologic treatments to control acute nasal bleeding are available; however, any medication regimen that prolongs bleeding time should be reevaluated in the light of recurrent epistaxis. Initial treatment of uncomplicated anterior epistaxis consists of applying firm, continuous pressure for 10 to 15 minutes to both sides of the nose, immediately superior to the nasal alar cartilages. Patients should breathe through the mouth during this treatment period and must not release pressure to "sneak a peek" at the bleeding nares. To reduce vascular pressure, the patient should be seated upright with the head bent forward. Patients with no underlying medical problems may be treated at home, with directions to sit upright, minimize physical activity, and rest with the head elevated 45 to 90 degrees at night. Elderly or debilitated patients with epistaxis may require inpatient care, however, because of the increased risk of both immunosuppression and anemia.

Recurrent minor epistaxis can be treated between episodes of active bleeding with vasoconstricting agents and/or chemical cauterization. A small piece of cotton or nasal pledget soaked in a topical vasoconstricting agent (such as 0.25 percent phenylephrine, 1:1000 epinephrine, 0.1 percent xylometazoline, or 4 percent cocaine solution) should be applied to the nasal vestibule and pressed against the bleeding site for 5 to 10 minutes. Epinephrine should be avoided in hypertensive patients or those with coronary artery disease, and cocaine should be avoided in children. An ice pack may also be placed over the nose. Almost all venous anterior nosebleeds are stopped in this manner, but the treatment may need to be repeated. If this treatment fails, chemical cauterization of the bleeding site may be necessary. The mucosa should first be anesthetized with a cotton ball soaked in 4 percent cocaine, 4 percent lidocaine, or 2 percent lidocaine viscous preparation, held over the bleeding site for several minutes. Alternatively, a 2 percent lidocaine jelly may be used. A bead of chromic acid, 25 to 50 percent trichloroacetic acid solution, or silver nitrate stick is then applied directly onto the bleeding vessels with firm pressure for 30 seconds, which will allow for limited, shallow cautery of the bleeding site. Thermal or bipolar electrocautery may be required in cases of deeper lesions involving larger vessels; however, indiscriminate cauterization of a large area should be avoided.

If bleeding does not stop, anterior nasal packing should be placed to fill the entire nasal fossa. Layers of 1/2 in. × 72 in. gauze impregnated with petroleum jelly should be inserted in folding layers with a nasal speculum and bayonet forceps, extending as far back as possible to the posterior nasal choanae, while retaining the gauze ends at the nares. Each layer should be pressed firmly against the preceding one without disturbing the walls of the nasal cavity, with the folded ends alternating front and back in an accordion pattern. Typically, the entire 72-in. strip will be accommodated, if properly placed. A 2 in. × 2 in. gauze pad is then taped over the nostrils to prevent the anterior packing from dislodging and to catch dripping blood. Anterior packing should be removed within 2 to 3 days. The gauze inserts may be impregnated with an antibiotic cream or ointment to minimize bacterial growth and reduce odor. In addition, oral antibiotics may be administered if infection is suspected; however, the benefit of systemic antibiotics as a prophylactic measure (while quite common in practice) has not been confirmed by well-designed clinical trials. Recently, user-friendly nasal tampons have entered the market that are simply inserted in the nares in desiccated form and rehydrated by bathing them in 10 to 20 mL of saline or an antibiotic-containing solution (e.g., bacitracin). Posterior sources of bleeding require more complex treatment by a qualified specialist, because this type of bleeding is usually more severe and difficult to control. Treatments include posterior nasal packing, sphenopalatine ganglion nerve block, and even surgical ligation of the compromised vessels. Nasal balloon-packing systems are an alternative to nasal packing, but they must not be overinflated and should be removed within 24 to 36 hours. Importantly, any form of nasal packing tends to be particularly painful for the patient once local anesthetic has worn off, and oral or parenteral opioid analgesics should be considered. OTC analgesics such as acetaminophen may not be potent enough, while nonsteroidal anti-inflammatory drugs (NSAIDs) are best avoided because of their tendency to impair platelet function which may lead to further bleeding.

All underlying medical conditions that might contribute to epistaxis should also be appropriately treated (e.g., platelet transfusions or clotting factor administration for coagulopathies). Iron supplements may be given if significant blood loss has occurred. If leukemia or another source of bone marrow immunosuppression is suspected as a causative factor of epistaxis, nasal packing should be avoided because of the increased risk of infection. In these cases, topical thrombin or hemostatic substances (Oxycel cotton or Gelfoam) should be first-line treatment.

Follow-Up and Referral

Follow-up is not indicated for minor cases of nosebleed from local trauma or inflammation; however, the treatment of recurrent epistaxis should be monitored for effectiveness. Hemodynamics and blood loss should also be monitored in severe cases that require hospitalization. In the event of severe hemorrhage, anemia or even hypovolemia may develop. Various treatment modalities for epistaxis may also have important sequelae: Cocaine and lidocaine always present risks of toxicities when these therapies are used. In addition, prolonged nasal packing may lead to infection of the nasal cavity, sinusitis, or impaired gas exchange, if poorly monitored. Excessive trauma during nasal packing or cauterization can result in septal hematoma, abscess, or perforation. External nasal deformities may also result from pressure necrosis from the anterior portion of nasal packing. Balloon-packing systems may result in mucosal pressure necrosis if the balloons are overinflated. Likewise, if the anterior portion of a two-balloon system breaks, the posterior balloon may migrate posteriorly down the airway and cause obstruction. Some patients experience vasovagal episodes during nasal packing and may pass out.

All cases of anterior epistaxis that are recurrent, particularly severe in blood loss, or refractory to vasoconstrictive or cauterization therapy should be referred to a specialist or Emergency Department, as appropriate. Hypovolemic or anemic patients require physician referral to evaluate the need for transfusion. Electrocautery for recurrent epistaxis caused by deep lesions should be performed only by a qualified specialist. Any elderly or debilitated patient who requires hospitalization for epistaxis should also be referred to a specialist. The management of posterior epistaxis requires a specialist, because treatment modalities may include ganglionic nerve blocks, posterior nasal packing, and vessel ligation. Coagulopathy-related and malignancy-related epistaxis require specialized treatment related to the underlying disorder. Finally, infections resulting from nasal packing may necessitate referral to a specialist, especially if the patient is febrile.

Patient Education

Patients who have been treated for epistaxis should not blow their nose and should avoid sneezing for at least 12 hours after an acute episode, to avoid dislodging the protective blood clot. Increased environmental humidity in the home also helps to prevent acute attacks, especially during the winter months. Petroleum jelly applied liberally to the nares promotes mucosal hydration, which helps prevent drying and cracking of the nasal mucosa. If nasal probing is persistent, the patient's fingernails should be cut to avoid mucosal trauma. Proper nasal pinching techniques should be demonstrated to enable patients to administer self-care at home for minor episodes of epistaxis. The importance of maintaining nasal mucosal hydration should be stressed, as well as the need to avoid nasal probing and vigorous blowing of the nose. The ability of certain medications to contribute to bleeding disorders (e.g., antiplatelet effects of aspirin, anticoagulant therapies such as warfarin) should also be discussed. Patients should be told not to swallow blood, because this may upset the stomach, resulting in nausea, vomiting, or "gagging" (inhalation of blood into the trachea and bronchi). Patients should not talk during episodes of active bleeding for the same reason, and alcohol and hot liquids should be avoided following an acute attack.

Sinusitis

Sinusitis is an inflammation of the mucous membranes of one or more of the paranasal sinuses: frontal, sphenoid, posterior ethmoid, anterior ethmoid, and maxillary, with the latter two sinuses most often affected. This inflammation may be classified as (1) acute, characterized by an abrupt onset of infection and post-therapeutic resolution of symptoms lasting no more than 4 weeks, (2) subacute, in which a purulent nasal discharge persists despite therapy, lasting from 4 to 12 weeks, or (3) chronic, which occurs with episodes of prolonged inflammation with repeated or inadequately treated acute infection lasting greater than 12 consecutive weeks.

Epidemiology and Causes

The frequency of upper respiratory tract infections (the "common cold") accounts for the frequent occurrence of sinusitis in the general population. Researchers have estimated that 0.5 percent of all colds are complicated by bacterial infection of one or more of the paranasal sinuses. Acute bacterial sinusitis accounts for 16 million clinical visits annually, whereas chronic sinusitis is classified by the U.S. Public Health Service as the most common chronic disease in the United States and is estimated to account for more than 2 billion dollars a year in health-care costs. Sinusitis affects adults of all ages, males and females equally, with no specific ethnic predisposition.

Mucosal inflammation and congestion from a viral URI that lasts more than 7 to 10 days is a primary risk factor for sinusitis (especially for maxillary sinus involvement), particularly during the autumn, winter, and spring seasons. Smoking, exposure to air pollution, persistent coughing, sneezing against a closed mouth, exposure to cold, damp outdoor weather or dry indoor heat, sudden changes in temperature, injury to the nose or sinuses from foreign bodies (e.g., nasogastric tubes or nasotracheal intubation) or trauma, nasal polyps, and chronic use of OTC or prescription decongestants may all impair mucociliary function, which can lead to mucosal inflammation, blockage of the sinus ostia, hypo-oxygenation of the sinuses, and transudation of fluid because of negative sinus pressure. Dental abscesses with oroantral fistulae extending into the paranasal sinuses can introduce pathogenic microorganisms; this etiology is associated with 10 to 15 percent of acute sinusitis cases. In addition, particularly during the summer months, airborne allergens, as well as swimming, diving, and jumping into contaminated water without holding the nose, are also common mechanisms for sinusitis to develop; allergic rhinitis is seen in 25 percent of sinusitis cases. Traveling in an airplane while suffering from a URI may predispose an individual to develop sinusitis. Recurrent or persistent bacterial infection resulting from blockage of nasociliary sinus drainage via the sinus ostia has been particularly associated with subacute and chronic sinusitis. Mechanical blockage may result from anatomic abnormalities such as a deviated septum, adenoidal hypertrophy, nasal polyps, reduced ostial diameter, and sinus or nasal neoplasms. Half of all asthmatic patients suffer from some form of sinusitis as a result of their inflammation-prone, hypersensitive airways. Furthermore, mucosal immunoglobulin A (IgA) deficiency, immobile cilia syndrome (Kartagener's syndrome), and cystic fibrosis also contribute to decreased mucociliary clearance and persistent sinus infection resulting from stasis. Chronic inflammatory diseases such as sarcoidosis and Wegener's granulomatosis also predispose patients to mucosal inflammation. In particular, diabetic, HIV-infected, malnourished, or other chronically immunocompromised patients may develop severe invasive sinus disease.

Pathophysiology

Infection by nonendogenous pathogens or bacterial invasion of the sinuses by normal nasal or pharyngeal microbial flora are the primary causes of acute sinusitis. The vast majority (more than 95 percent) of acute sinusitis cases are caused by the same viruses associated with uncomplicated URIs. However, many of these patients do not seek primary-care interventions. Viral sinusitis (more accurately termed viral rhinosinusitis) is most commonly caused by the following five viruses, which collectively account for 80 percent of all URIs: rhinovirus (30 percent), coronavirus, adenovirus, echovirus, coxsackievirus, as well as respiratory syncytial virus, parainfluenza virus, and influenza virus.

Viral rhinosinusitis is the main predisposing factor for acute bacterial sinusitis, which complicates about 2 percent of all cases. During these episodes, mucosal secretions from sinus goblet cells increase in volume and viscosity. The nasal mucosa also swells in response to viral replication, creating an anatomic barrier to the steady outflow of nasal secretions. Nasal polyps, foreign bodies, allergen-induced mucosal swelling, and altered sensorium affecting nasal clearance and coordinated swallowing reflexes are other potential mechanisms of impaired nasal outflow. Moreover, the act of sneezing creates a tremendous pressure in the nasopharynx up to 60 to 80 mm Hg, capable of forcing fluid not only out the nares, but from the nasal cavity into the sinuses as well, transporting viruses and bacteria into these ideal environments for microbial replication. Here the normally ciliated pseudostratified, columnar epithelium lining the sinuses is eroded as infecting organisms proliferate, resulting in a loss of mucociliary clearance through sinus ostia (bony openings) and the ostiomeatal complex located in the anterior ethmoid region, which serves as a common drainage pathway for the frontal, maxillary, and ethmoid sinuses. Blockage of the osteomeatal complex and/or impairment of ciliary function is thought to underlie all forms of sinusitis.

The only consistently reliable method of identifying causative organisms in acute sinusitis is direct sinus aspiration, which typically is performed only in controlled research trials because of its invasive nature. The most common bacterial pathogens isolated in acute sinusitis are *Streptococcus pneumoniae,* seen in nearly 40 percent of all cases, particularly during the summer and fall, *Haemophilus influenzae,* implicated in nearly 30 percent of all cases, especially in winter and spring, and, to a far lesser extent, *Moraxella (Branhamella) catarrhalis* (a far more common pathogen in children). Thus, the infectious agents of sinusitis closely pattern those of acute otitis media. *Streptococcus pyogenes* (especially group A beta-hemolytic *Streptococcus*) and *Staphylococcus aureus* have each been identified in 5 percent of sinusitis cases studied, with *Staphylococcus aureus* most frequently isolated in intracranial complications. The specific role of bacteria, fungi, and viruses in chronic sinusitis is hotly debated. *Staphylococcus aureus,* Gram-negative rods, and, in up to half of cases, anaerobic bacteria including *Peptostreptococcus* and *Bacteroides* are most often implicated. Polymicrobial infection is also more common in chronic than acute sinusitis. *Staphylococcus aureus* and *Pseudomonas aeruginosa* are the most common causes of cystic fibrosis-related and nosocomial sinus infection associated with nasal or endotracheal intubation and nasogastric feeding tubes.

In the immunocompromised host, gram-negative aerobic bacteria must be considered, as well as the fungi *Aspergillus fumigatus* and *Mucor* species, both of which may cause severe, rapidly invasive sinusitis in diabetic or otherwise chronically immunocompromised patients. More common than invasive fungal sinusitis, however, is allergic fungal sinusitis occuring in atopic individuals in which the nasal and sinus mucosa undergo an IgE-mediated Type I hypersensitivity response to airborne fungal spores or fungal proliferation facilitated by obstructed sinus outflow. Dematiaceous brown-pigmented molds account for more than 75 percent of these cases, while *Aspergillus* is implicated in 10 to 20 percent of cases. The sinuses become filled with allergic mucin consisting of necrotic cellular debris, eosinophils, and fungal hyphae. Finally, if neither a hypersensitivity response nor an invasive sinusitis ensue, fungal colonization may result in unilateral chronic sinusitis characterized by formation of a dense fungal ball with sclerosis of the surrounding bone.

Clinical Presentation

Subjective

During the early stages of sinusitis, patients typically report a gradual onset of symptoms, including recurrent or chronic dull, constant pain over the affected sinuses (because of expanding purulent inflammation); as sinusitis progresses, pain increases and becomes characteristically throbbing. Typically, pain over the cheeks and upper teeth is correlated with maxillary sinus involvement; pain over the eyebrows indicates frontal sinus involvement; and pain over or behind the eyes indicates ethmoid sinusitis. Pain is exacerbated by coughing and sudden head movements. Specifically, frontal sinus pain may worsen with recumbency, whereas maxillary sinus pain may worsen when the patient is erect. Ethmoidal sinusitis is associated with retro-orbital pain. Notably, however, subacute and chronic sinusitis are often painless, as are some cases of acute sinusitis. These cases typically develop after at least 2 weeks of viral URI symptoms (such as a cough from postnasal drip, purulent nasal discharge, and headache). All types of sinusitis may present with nasal congestion (stuffiness), mucopurulent rhinorrhea (runny nose), a feeling of pressure inside the head, cough (in some cases), sore throat (in some cases), eye pain from ethmoid involvement, malaise, and fatigue. In particular, acute sinusitis is strongly predicted by maxillary toothache, a poor response to nasal decongestants, and a colored nasal discharge. Such patients usually report yellow-green or even blood-stained rhinorrhea, voice nasality, anosmia because of edematous nasal turbinates, early morning periorbital edema, fever and chills (in 25 to 50 percent of cases), and a headache that is worse in the morning or when bending forward. These patients also sometimes report a nonproductive cough and disturbed sleep. Subacute or chronic sinusitis patients typically report a persistent cough or cold-like symptoms that may last from several weeks to several months, as well as a headache or feeling of pressure specifically across the cranial midline. Fever is less common, and most patients have a past history of responding poorly to sinusitis pharmacotherapy. Other symptoms include a thick postnasal discharge (postnasal drip), "popping" ears, excessive tearing, toothache-like cheek pain, difficulty chewing, and halitosis. Immunocompromised patients may present with more subtle signs and symptoms, since leukopenia may limit the inflammatory response to infection. (See The Patient's Voice 7.1.)

THE PATIENT'S VOICE 7.1

Sinusitis

In the fall, Tina had a cold that wouldn't retreat. For weeks her nose was so stuffy she could hardly catch her breath. A jagged cough broke up her sleep. Her head pounded, the pressure increasing whenever she dipped her chin, and she constantly felt on the verge of losing her balance.

"I was mincing my steps like a 75-year-old woman," said Tina, age 50, a college professor. "I was just croaking my words out. I had to tell my students, Sorry, I can't look at your papers because my head will explode if I look down." Despite her agony, Tina was taking the same tactic most of us do when faced with a head cold: stock up on tissues and muddle through, especially since doctors are quick to point out that antibiotics won't diminish a viral infection. Tina stocked up on green tea and juice, and tried to take a few more naps. "I'm a big believer in the body's power to heal itself. Why rush to see a doctor about a cold?"

Objective

On inspection, purulent nasal secretions (recognized by polymorphonuclear neutrophils in a Giemsa-stained nasal smear) and total opacification of affected sinuses on transillumination (e.g., through the supraorbital or maxillary bony ridges) are strongly predictive of acute sinusitis. Although only one in four patients with decreased transillumination typically has a sinus infection, complete light transmission rules out an active sinus infection. A nasal speculum should be used to examine the anterior nasal passages. A red, swollen nasal mucosa indicates infection; a pale mucosa that appears swollen, with watery secretions, points to allergic sinusitis or rhinitis. Purulent secretions seen coming from inside the middle meatus are characteristic of sinusitis. Black or necrotic material may be seen in mucormycosis-related rhinorrhea in immunocompromised patients. Ethmoid sinus involvement may result in chemosis (eyelid mucous membrane edema), proptosis, conjunctival injection, extraocular muscle palsy, or orbital fixation.

On palpation, the affected sinuses may be exquisitely tender to palpation. Sphenoid sinusitis presents as tenderness over the vertex or mastoids, ethmoid sinusitis as retro-orbital or nasal bridge tenderness, maxillary sinusitis as cheek or dental tenderness, and frontal sinusitis as tenderness of the forehead. On percussion, if the area over the affected sinus is tapped, for example, with a tongue blade, the teeth and gums are particularly tender in cases of maxillary sinusitis that are related to dental abscesses.

Diagnostic Reasoning

Diagnostic Tests

Although no laboratory tests or x-ray films are routinely needed for typical presentations of sinusitis, anteroposterior, lateral, and particularly occipitomental sinus x-ray films are usually sufficient if an early, cost-efficient confirmation of diagnosis is needed, or if symptoms show no improvement after 4 to 5 days of pharmacotherapy. Air-fluid levels, mucosal thickening beyond 4 mm, or complete opacification of the sinuses on any of these views is strongly suggestive of sinusitis. However, it should be noted that such mucosal thickening as well as impaired sinus transillumination on physical exam have both been observed in healthy, asymptomatic individuals who do not meet the criteria for acute sinusitis. In turn, the positive and negative predictive value of these diagnostic tests has consistently been questioned in the literature.

A CBC to detect leukocyte elevation may be indicated if an infectious etiology is suspected in acute sinusitis; however, leucocytosis is rarely observed in chronic sinusitis. Stains or cultures of nasal and throat secretions do not correlate with the causative agents of sinusitis, because the nasopharyngeal mucosa is widely colonized by a diverse array of endogenous, nonpathogenic microbial flora. However, the presence of at least 10,000 organisms/mL on Gram stain of sinus aspirates may confirm the presence of local sinus infection. Allergic skin testing may be necessary if the patient history suggests allergic disease (e.g., allergen exposure, seasonal attacks), and these patients often demonstrate peripheral eosinophilia and elevated total or allergen-specific IgE levels. Culture and microscopic examination of sinus aspirates, sinus mucosal biopsy, or flexible fiberoptic rhinoscopy by a well-trained specialist is typically needed only for subacute, chronic, or suspected fungal sinusitis cases that are refractory to several courses of empiric pharmacotherapy or when intracranial extension is suspected. Chronic sinusitis, in particular, is characterized by a morphological change of the ciliated sinus epithelia to a hypertrophied, stratified squamous form that is evident upon biopsy.

Although sinus computed tomography (CT) scans may demonstrate mucosal thickening and osteomeatal occlusion in a large number of people with uncomplicated viral URI, this type of imaging may be helpful in cases of chronic sinusitis, infection that has spread into orbital or intracranial regions (e.g., orbital cellulitis or brain abscess), or for an immunocompromised host, to fully evaluate the disease process. Sinus magnetic resonance imaging (MRI) is superior for soft tissue discrimination but is poor at visualizing bony structures. Thus, MRI tends to be reserved for suspected sinus neoplasia or extension of sinus disease into intracranial soft tissues.

Differential Diagnosis

Myofascial pain that is unrelated to infectious causes may mimic the pain from acute sinusitis, but pain from other myofascial disorders is typically more diffuse and does not progressively worsen. Uncomplicated dental abscesses may produce a similar pain, but the pain will not extend into the maxillary sinus upon physical examination. Patients with migraine, cluster headache, or trigeminal neuralgia also present with fascial and cranial pain, but, again, the sinuses will be nontender to palpation and the accompanying signs and symptoms of inflammation will not be observed in these patients. Allergic rhinitis, vasomotor rhinitis, rhinitis medicamentosa, mechanical nasal airway obstruction, acute viral URI (persistent viral rhinitis), and chronic inflammatory conditions such as sarcoidosis or Wegener's granulomatosis, may all present with nasal congestion or pain. If these cases are uncomplicated by sinusitis, no signs of sinus inflammation will be detected on examination.

If a patient has had an URI for at least 7 days, the presence of two or more of the following signs and symptoms will confirm the diagnosis of sinusitis: colored nasal drainage, poor response to decongestant, facial or sinus pain, particularly if aggravated by postural change or Valsalva maneuver, and headache. In addition, a documented history of prior episodes of sinusitis, a fever higher than 102°F (38.9°C), and tooth pain accompanying these findings all support a diagnosis of sinusitis. Viruses may produce all of the clinical manifestations described; however, patients who meet the 7-day criteria described in the preceding text are more likely to have bacterial sinusitis than a viral URI.

Management

It is important to realize that because the vast majority of acute sinusitis cases are caused by viruses rather than bacteria, antibiotics are largely unhelpful. Their indiscriminate use for symptom complexes failing to meet the aforementioned diagnostic criteria for bacterial sinusitis offers no medical benefit, wastes financial resources, and is potentially harmful in that it encourages widespread antibiotic resistance in common nasopharyngeal flora. With this in mind, antimicrobial therapy usually cures acute uncomplicated bacterial sinusitis, although recurrence is not uncommon. Adjunctive measures may also be used to enhance mucociliary clearance, countering the main risk factor for the development of sinusitis. Saline nose drops may be helpful in improving sinus drainage, but dedicated sinus irrigation two or more times a day with an adequate volume of saline to fully flush the sinuses has been shown to significantly relieve symptoms even without antimicrobial therapy. Patients are instructed to infuse their sinuses using a warm isotonic or hypertonic saline-filled bulb syringe expressed into each nare, followed by immediate drainage of the liquid over a sink to remove both infectious organisms and excess mucous. Homemade preparations may be made by mixing 1 teaspoon of salt with 8 ounces of warm water, but noniodized salt should be used, as iodine is a known mucosal irritant. A cool-mist, ultrasonic humidifier (cleaned daily) may also assist in thinning sinus secretions and facilitating drainage. Smoke and other environmental pollutants should be avoided. Fluid intake should be increased, and heated mist from a facial sauna, steam bath, shower, or hot, moist towels wrapped around the face may help relieve sinus and nasal pain by liquefying secretions.

Oral analgesics may also be used for pain (e.g., ibuprofen [Motrin, Advil] 400 to 600 mg q6h to q8h prn, acetaminophen [Tylenol] 650 mg q4h to q6h prn, or a stronger combination of acetaminophen 300 mg/codeine 30 mg [Tylenol 3] 1 to 2 tablets q4h to q6h prn). In general, non-prescription medicated nose drops and sprays should be avoided, while prescription nasal sprays should be taken no longer than 3 to 4 days at a time, because long-term use can lead to rebound nasal congestion (rhinitis medicamentosum) and addiction. Phenylephrine (Neo-Synephrine; one to two upright sprays in each nostril tid to qid prn) or the stronger oxymetazoline (Afrin; 1 to 2 upright sprays in each nostril bid to tid prn) may be helpful in adults. Pseudoephedrine (Sudafed) 30 to 60 mg q4h to 6h prn is an oral alternative but tends to be less effective than topical preparations. Expectorants such as guaifenesin 200 to 400 mg q4h prn and iodinated glycerol 30 to 60 mg PO qid prn are used to liquefy sinus secretions and facilitate drainage. Anti-inflammatory topical steroids in nasal spray preparations such as fluticasone 0.05 percent (Flonase), mometasone (Nasonex), or triamcinolone (Nasacort), all at two sprays in each nostril qd, used for 2 to 3 weeks are becoming increasingly popular; however, randomized controlled trials have been inconsistent with regard to their effectiveness. In fact, steroid therapy has actually been shown to increase viral load in acute viral rhinosinusitis. Oral antihistamines should be avoided unless an allergic component is evident, because they tend to dry the mucosa, thicken purulent sinus fluids, and slow mucosal drainage, although some studies have suggested their efficacy in symptomatic relief of uncomplicated viral URIs.

Although localized sinus infection may be self-limited, antibiotic and symptomatic therapy may be considered appropriate for suspected bacterial sinusitis to prevent disease progression and complications. Empiric antibiotic therapy for 7 to 10 days covering the most common etiological agents should be instituted prior to the identification of causative organisms, because symptoms may progress while waiting for laboratory confirmation. In adults, common choices include narrow-spectrum antibiotics such as amoxicillin (Amoxil) 500 mg to as high as 1 g PO tid, trimethoprim/sulfamethoxazole (Bactrim) 160 mg/800 mg one Double Strength tablet PO bid, or doxycycline 100 mg PO bid. In light of increasing resistance of *Streptococcus pneumoniae, Haemophilus influenza* (up to 50 percent of strains), *Moraxella catarrhalis,* and virtually all *Staphylococcus aureus*, beta-lactamase resistant alternatives of varying dosing schedules include clarithromycin (Biaxin XL) 1000 mg PO daily, cefaclor (Ceclor; second-generation cephalosporin) 500 mg PO q6h, cefpodoxime (Vantin; third-generation cephalosporin) 200 mg PO bid, cefdinir (Omnicef; third-generation cephalosporin) 600 mg PO qd, levofloxacin (Levaquin) 750 mg PO qd, moxifloxacin (Avelox) 400 mg PO qd, gatifloxacin (Tequin) 400 mg PO qd, and amoxicillin/clavulanate (Augmentin XR) 1000 mg/125 mg (2) PO bid. Penicillin-allergic or cephalosporin-allergic patients are usually steered toward an oral quinolone or trimethoprim/sulfamethoxazole as first-line therapy. Immunocompromised hosts typically require broad-spectrum coverage for Gram-positive and Gram-negatives organisms, and possibly empiric antifungal therapy. Tetracyclines do not cover *Streptococcus pneumoniae,* however; and erythromycin, penicillin, and first-generation cephalosporins do not cover *Haemophilus influenzae.* Acute infections that fail to clear after one course of antibiotic therapy are often treated with a second course from a separate antibiotic class for 14 days.

Antibiotics against anaerobic organisms such as *Peptostreptococcus* and *Bacteroides* are typically required for subacute and chronic sinusitis, with regimens lasting up to 3 to 4 weeks or even as long as 6 weeks for refractory chronic cases (e.g., amoxicillin/clavulanate [Augmentin XR] 1000 mg/125 mg PO bid or cefuroxime [Ceftin; second-generation cephalosporin] 500 mg PO bid); for penicillin-allergic patients, clarithromycin (Biaxin XL) 500 mg (2) PO bid or clindamycin (Cleocin) 300 mg PO tid; and for documented Gram-negative infection, one of the fluoroquinolones at the doses mentioned previously (e.g., levofloxacin, moxifloxacin, or gatifloxacin). Patients requiring three or more antibiotic courses will likely benefit from referral to an otorhinolaryngologist for further diagnostic work-up. Similarly, serious invasive fungal sinusitis often requires surgical débridement and inpatient intravenous antifungal therapy with amphotericin B (1 mg/kg IV qd) or, if not tolerated due to rigors, chills, or hypotension, a liposomal amphotericin preparation (Abelcet; 5 to 7.5 mg/kg IV qd). In contrast, allergic fungal sinusitis calls for sinus drainage and systemic corticosteroids for 2 to 4 weeks followed by topical steroid therapy, as the benefits of antifungal therapy have not been clearly demonstrated. Fungal balls associated with sinus colonization must be removed surgically, as neither steroids nor antifungals have been shown to be effective in relieving obstruction.

Maxillary sinus puncture and aspiration may be needed to relieve pain in any form of sinusitis that fails to subside following pharmacotherapy, and patients with subacute or chronic sinusitis may require surgery to remove damaged mucosal tissue or to correct anatomic obstructions of the sinus ostia such as recurrent nasal polyps. In addition, complementary therapies may be considered in the treatment of patients with chronic sinusitis. Several studies indicate that vigorous exercise, for example, has been shown to improve nasal function (through vasoconstriction and decreased nasal resistance) in healthy patients, as well as those with allergic rhinitis. The same benefits may also result in patients with chronic sinusitis. Some patients with particularly severe chronic disease have reported trying acupuncture, herbal therapies, biofeedback, and self-help groups. (See Complementary Therapies 7.2.)

COMPLEMENTARY THERAPIES 7.2

Yoga for Postnasal Drip

To ease postnasal drip, try neti, a yogic nasal wash. The wash can help reduce sinus flow.

- Fill a 4 oz. Paper cup halfway with warm water.
- Add a half a teaspoon of salt.
- Put a small crease in the lip of the cup so that it forms a spout.
- Tilt the head back slightly and to the left.
- Slowly pour the water into the right nostril. The water will flow out of the left nostril or down the back of the throat if the left nostril is clogged. Spit out the water or wipe the face if water is flowing out of the left nostril.
- Fill the cup again, and repeat the procedure on the other side.

It is suggested that this be done daily to relieve post-nasal drip and to keep the sinuses clear.

Prompt treatment of all respiratory infections can prevent acute sinusitis complications, and surgery to correct anatomic blockages of the sinus ostia (e.g., deviated septum or nasal polyps) may prevent chronic sinusitis. When sinus inflammation is connected with an allergy, desensitization by a trained allergist should be considered. Recurrent attacks of sinusitis can sometimes be prevented by the routine use of a humidifier and/or air conditioner. Nose droppers or sprays should be discarded after use during an acute episode, however, and should never be shared to avoid person-to-person transmission of infectious organisms. (See Nursing Research–Based Practice 7.2.)

Follow-Up and Referral

Patients should be reevaluated for symptomatic improvement in 48 to 72 hours, and a return visit should be scheduled for 10 to 14 days from the initial assessment. If symptoms fail to improve with pharmacotherapy, the patient should be evaluated for antibiotic resistance, allergic contributions, or immunologic abnormalities. Sinus x-ray films may remain abnormal for up to 2 months following the resolution of acute sinusitis, so follow-up films to document improvement are not usually indicated until at least 6 weeks following initial therapy. Immunocompromised patients with sinusitis should be monitored daily in an inpatient setting.

Although complications are relatively uncommon, visual impairments, ophthalmoplegia, orbital or facial cellulitis, severe fever, aphasia, abducens palsy (CN VI deficit), seizures, altered mental status, and osteomyelitis of the frontal or maxillary bones, and focal swelling over the frontal bone are all reflective of localized extensions of bacterial infection. Rare but potentially life-threatening complications that require a high index of suspicion include meningitis, subdural empyema, epidural abscess, cavernous sinus thrombosis, and other CNS complications.

Patients should be referred to a specialist if their sinusitis is allergic or immunologic, refractory to antibiotic therapy, recurrent, or associated with unusual opportunistic infections, or when the infection is adversely affecting their quality of life. In addition, when sinusitis is associated with chronic otitis media, bronchial asthma, nasal polyps, recurrent pneumonia, immunodeficiency, allergic fungal disease, granulomas, or multiple antibiotic resistances, the patient should be referred to an allergist or an otolaryngologist.

Patient Education

Patients should be instructed to be wary of worsening symptoms after the institution of pharmacotherapy. Patients should also be informed of potential complications and should be instructed to contact the practitioner at once if telltale signs such as periorbital swelling develop. The APN should stress the importance of avoiding contact with all contributing factors (e.g., cigarette smoke or airborne allergens), as well as the exacerbating side effects of nonprescription antihistamine use. Patients should make sure that OTC decongestant preparations do not contain antihistamines, and they should drink plenty of fluids, to thin nasal secretions.

Pharyngitis and Tonsillitis

Pharyngitis and *tonsillitis* denote generalized inflammatory processes of both infectious and noninfectious etiology, involving the pharynx and pharyngeal tonsils, respectively.

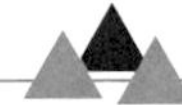

NURSING RESEARCH-BASED PRACTICE 7.2

Complementary Therapeutic Practices in Patients with Chronic Sinusitis

Krouse, HJ, and Krouse, JH: Clinical excellence for nurse practitioners. Int J NPACE 3(6):346, 1999.

The purpose of this study was to understand patient use of alternative and complementary health practices in self-care of patients with chronic sinusitis. It was established that 60% of patients used conventional medications; 81% of patients with chronic sinusitis in this sample engaged in exercise for symptom relief. Additional complementary therapies utilized included herbal therapy (32%), chiropractic therapy (16%), biofeedback (16%), acupuncture (11%), and chelation therapy (7%). In addition, self-help groups were utilized (approximately 0.5%). The sample of 84 was drawn from a pool of 340 patients with a diagnosis of chronic sinusitis in a community-based otolaryngology practice in Florida. The median age was 65. Three instruments were utilized: the Sinus Treatment Follow-Up Scale (STFS), the Rhinosinusitis Disability Index (RDDI), and the Sinus Information Scale (SIS). Thise study found that the more severe the sinus disease, the more likely the patient was to incorporate alternative modalities; in more severe cases, it is common for patients to blend both conventional and complementary therapies. Overall, patients rated physicians, nurses, and other health-care provides as their primary source of health-care information for their sinus disease.

This study demonstrates the importance of a holistic approach to the patient in the primary-care setting. The authors conclude, "By incorporating a more holistic view of . . . disease processes and their treatments, APNs can be most effective in helping patients adapt to their chronic rhinosinusitis" (p 351). Practicing within a Circle of Caring enables the APN to effectively do this.

Most virally related cases are self-limiting, with spontaneous recovery, although other infectious cases may require antibiotic or antifungal therapy. Pharyngitis and tonsillitis may occur independently of one another; however, they often co-occur, sharing a common etiology, clinical course, and treatment regimen. Many cases of pharyngitis and virtually all cases of tonsillitis are contagious.

Epidemiology and Causes

About 8 percent of all patient visits in the ambulatory care setting each year are for complaints of sore throat. Viral pharyngitis related to respiratory tract pathogens occurs most often in the colder fall and winter months. Influenza infection typically occurs in epidemics between December and April. The incidence of group A beta-hemolytic streptococcal infection pharyngitis typically increases from 10 percent of cases reported in the fall to 40 percent in the winter and spring. Herpangina is known to peak in the summer and fall. Allergic pharyngitis may also peak seasonally during the summer months. Although infectious (bacterial and viral) pharyngitis and tonsillitis tend to occur most frequently in young children age 5 to 10, both conditions may occur at any age. Streptococcal infection most frequently affects patients younger than age 25; however, it may occur sporadically in older adults. Infectious mononucleosis (primarily caused by Epstein-Barr virus [EBV]) is also most common in adolescents and young adults and is rarely seen in the elderly. Pharyngitis associated with the postnasal drip of sinusitis most often affects adults. No ethnic predispositions have been reported for either pharyngitis or tonsillitis.

Men and women are affected equally by both conditions. URI is a common predisposing factor for the development of viral pharyngitis. The postnasal drip associated with URI or sinusitis may also contribute to irritant-related pharyngitis. The risk of all forms of infectious pharyngitis (viral, bacterial, and fungal) is increased in immunocompromised persons who are afflicted by chronic illnesses, including diabetes mellitus and WBC dyscrasias such as agranulocytosis or acute leukemia. Work-related stress and excessive alcohol consumption have also been implicated as a cause of decreased resistance to throat infection. In general, close living quarters, such as military barracks, schools, and daycare centers, increase the risk of person-to-person transmission of the infectious agents causing both pharyngitis and tonsillitis. Epstein–Barr virus (EBV) transmission typically requires intimate person-to-person contact between susceptible persons and symptomatic viral shedders (hence, its nickname of "kissing disease"). Young adults and adolescents from higher socioeconomic backgrounds in developed countries who have not been exposed to EBV in their childhood are most susceptible. Persons with pharyngitis related to *Neisseria gonorrhea, Treponema pallidum* (syphilis), *Chlamydia,* or herpes usually have a history of receptive oral intercourse with an infected sexual partner. Sexual abuse may be a factor in these cases as well. Bisexual and homosexual men and patients with anogenital gonorrhea are the groups most frequently affected by gonorrheal pharyngitis. Adult cases of *Corynebacterium diphtheria* occur almost exclusively in nonimmunized individuals. Recent contact with a wild animal (especially through a bite) is the major risk factor for the development of *Francisella tularensis* infection. Excessive antibiotic use has been associated with candidal infection and an overgrowth of *Candida* (thrush) in the oropharynx; tobacco and particularly marijuana smoking have also been implicated.

Pathophysiology

In up to 40 percent of pharyngitis cases, no causative agent is identified. Definitive diagnosis of an infectious agent is difficult, as the nasopharynx is a nonsterile environment normally colonized by an array of nonpathogenic flora. However, the current literature suggests that in adults, upper respiratory tract viruses are the most common cause of infectious pharyngitis, accounting for 30 to 50 percent of all cases: rhinovirus, coronavirus, adenovirus, influenza viruses A and B, parainfluenza virus, coxsackievirus (herpangina and hand-foot-and-mouth disease), enterovirus, and respiratory syncytial virus. Rhinoviruses and influenza viruses inflame the oral and nasopharyngeal mucosa via direct invasion and colonization, but the specific pathogenic mechanisms of other viruses is not well understood. Members of the herpes family of viruses are also common causative agents, including EBV and, in immunocompromised hosts, cytomegalovirus (CMV), herpes simplex virus (HSV), and reactivated herpes zoster. EBV, which infects pharyngeal B-lymphocytes and disseminates throughout the entire lymphoreticular system, is the primary causative agent of infectious mononucleosis, accounting for 1 to 2 percent of all pharyngitis cases. However, CMV causes up to 20 percent of all infectious mononucleosis cases. Primary infection with human immunodeficiency virus (HIV) may also cause pharyngitis owing to rapid retroviral replication; thus, HIV risk factors should always be assessed.

Bacterial agents typically cause an exudative pharyngitis, which represents roughly 20 percent of all cases of sore throat. Group A beta-hemolytic *Streptococcus pyogenes,* which accounts for 10 to 20 percent of adult pharyngitis cases, invades and multiplies within the pharyngeal mucosa, causing an intense inflammatory response known as "strep throat." Collectively, *Streptococcus* bacteria are characterized into groups based on cell-wall antigenicity. Clinically relevant groups include A, B, C, D, and G. Group A is the most important cause of pharyngitis because it may lead to the most serious complications, including heart valve damage which may occur many years following systemic infection known as acute rheumatic fever. More than 80 serotypes of *Streptococcus* have been identified. The most clinically significant strain is based on the M protein, which is the major virulence factor of group A beta-hemolytic *Streptococcus pyogenes.* M protein is antiphagocytic, as it blocks activation of the alternative complement pathway. An immune response to bacterial M protein stimulates long-lasting type-specific anti-M antibodies that adhere to individual bacteria and facilitate their phagocytosis (i.e., opsonization), protecting patients against subsequent exposure to bacteria of the same M-protein serotype. The amount of time needed for patients to mount a protective immune response is unclear. In the past, it had been suggested that treatment of group A *Streptococcus* be delayed, so that a protective immune response could be mounted, but this practice has since been refuted, and rapid treatment is now the standard of care. Importantly, *Streptococcus pyogenes* strains are becoming increasingly virulent, and the incidence of subsequent acute renal insufficiency due to postinfectious glomerulonephritis has increased over the past 15 years. Reports of bacteremia, deep tissue cellulitis, and systemic toxic shock-like syndrome mediated by *Streptococcal* exotoxins are also well characterized, with pharyngitis often recognized as the presenting complaint.

Other bacterial agents of pharyngitis include *Neisseria gonorrhea* (especially in young, sexually active adults), *Haemophilus influenzae, Streptococcus pneumoniae, Treponema pallidum, Staphylococcus aureus,* and both *Corynebacterium diphtheria* and *hemolyticum* (often associated with epiglottitis and a potentially obstructive fibrinous gray membrane adherent to the posterior pharynx). The relative importance of atypical organisms known to cause bronchitis including *Chlamydia pneumoniae, Chlamydia trachomatis,* and *Mycoplasma pneumoniae* as pharyngitic agents is controversial. Studies have demonstrated markedly varied prevalence rates (0 to 20 percent), and nasopharyngeal colonization by these organisms may be asymptomatic.

Noninfectious etiologies of pharyngitis may include trauma, allergies, collagen vascular diseases such as Kawasaki's syndrome, autoimmune blistering diseases such as pemphigus, chemical or drug-induced damage, and severe dehydration. Tobacco, and particularly marijuana smoking, is a major contributing factor to noninfectious pharyngitis related to chemical irritation, while exposure to allergens such as dust and pollen increases the risk of allergic pharyngitis, typically associated with a past history or family history of atopy. Severe drug reactions mediated by both type I immediate hypersensitivity and type III antibody–antigen immune complex reactions may extend in their most serious form to the oropharynx, as well as other mucosal sites. Both low humidity and mouth-breathing may contribute to dehydration-induced mucosal inflammation.

In contrast, tonsillitis (which may involve the posterior pharyngeal tonsils as well as the more anterior adenoid glands) is foremost a disorder of infectious etiology. It is characterized by inflammation, swelling, and purulent exudation of these lymphoid tissue collections that directly drain the colonized or infected nasopharynx. The spectrum of causative agents in this disorder is similar to that described for pharyngitis, including bacteria and upper respiratory tract viruses. Acutely, it is most often caused by group A *Streptococcal* infection, while a chronic form may also result from repeated *Streptococcal* infections. *Streptococcal* tonsillar infection always has the potential for progressing to peritonsillar or tonsillar abscess requiring aggressive management (incision and drainage followed by antibiotic therapy).

Clinical Presentation

Subjective

Most patients with pharyngitis and/or tonsillitis report mild to severe throat pain or the sensation of a "tickle" or pruritus in the throat. Infectious mononucleosis, adenovirus, and especially group A *Streptococcus* pharyngitis ("strep throat") tend to cause the most painful sore throats, with fever. Many patients also describe their throats as feeling swollen, with a "lump" in the back of the throat that persists despite repeated swallowing. A history of dysphagia (difficulty swallowing) is also common with throat inflammation, particularly from *H. influenzae* infection, and hoarseness is often associated with *Chlamydia pneumoniae*. Laryngitis and cough are commonly associated with viral infection, although fever occurs only occasionally. In contrast, chills and fever are common with bacterial infection, although cough and rhinorrhea are rarely present. Group A *Streptococcus* infection usually produces a fever higher than 101°F (38.3°C); the patient may be tachycardic, and there is usually pharyngeal exudate. As with viral infections, streptococcal symptomatology is rapid in onset; although in contrast to viral disease, systemic symptoms are few. Allergic pharyngitis, on the other hand, does not present with fever, but is recognized most readily by a persistent postnasal drip, paroxysmal sneezing, itchy, watery eyes, rhinorrhea, and a mild sore throat that typically worsens with recumbency. Malaise, generalized aches and pains, and headache may also be reported in both conditions. Infectious mononucleosis is famous for its gradual onset of low-grade fever and marked fatigue. Anorexia and nausea may also be present. Influenza infection is characterized by an abrupt onset of fever ranging from 100°F to 104°F (37.8°C to 40°C), myalgias, and headache, which last for about 3 days, followed by 3 to 4 days of cough, rhinorrhea, and pharyngitis, and finally a 1- to 2-week convalescent period with persistent cough and malaise. Geriatric patients with influenza may also present with gastrointestinal symptoms such as nausea, vomiting, and diarrhea. Reactivated herpes zoster infection is characterized by painful prodromes prior to active flare-ups. In contrast, HSV infection does not usually cause a sore throat. Moreover, primary or secondary syphilitic lesions tend to be painless. Gonococcal pharyngitis may be asymptomatic. Severe cases of tonsillitis may also present with ear pain and sometimes with cough or vomiting.

Objective

On inspection, the inflamed throat typically appears erythematous, although color may vary. Conjunctivitis is often associated with adenovirus and other respiratory viruses, whereas mucosal exudates and enlarged tonsils occur only occasionally. EBV-related infectious mononucleosis, however, may present with an exudative tonsillitis (in about 50 percent of cases), in addition to palatal petechiae and exanthem. The 1- to 2-mm vesicular lesions of herpes simplex infection may extend from the pharynx to the lips, gingivae, buccal mucosa, and tongue. Reactivated herpes zoster infection typically presents with 2- to 4-mm vesicular lesions unilaterally on the tongue, lip, and buccal mucosa. Herpangina presents as 1- to 2-mm oral vesicles or ulcers on the pharynx, tonsils, soft palate, pillars, uvula, and posterior buccal mucosa. Hand-foot-and-mouth disease presents with oral lesions co-occurring with exanthem on the hands and feet. Maculopapular rashes on the extremities of young adult patients may be indicative of many types of infection, including *C. hemolyticum,* HIV, enteroviruses, or *T. pallidum* (syphilis).

Exudates and enlarged tonsils are common findings in bacterial infections. Streptococcal infection produces a characteristic white to yellow exudate and may be accompanied by a sandpaper-like, scarletiniform rash. *Mycoplasma*-related cases may be clinically indistinguishable from streptococcal infections. *C. diphtheria* presents with a characteristic grayish pseudomembrane overlying the pharyngeal mucosa, tonsils, epiglottis, uvula, or even the nasal cavity. The nonvesicular lesions of primary syphilis are 5 to 15 mm in size and appear indurated or "healed up," extending to the lips, tonsils, or tongue. Secondary syphilitic nonvesicular lesions (2 to 10 mm) arise symmetrically on all parts of the oropharynx and mouth. Candidal infections produce thin, white, nonvesicular, diffuse or patchy (3 to 11 mm) exudative ulcers on all parts of the oropharyngeal mucosa. In most inflammatory conditions of the throat, the pharyngeal mucosa and tonsils are edematous, particularly with group A beta-hemolytic streptococcal infection. This is true of allergic pharyngitis as well, although erythema of the pharynx is minimal. Tonsillitis presents with readily noticeable swollen lymph glands located bilaterally between the fauces of the posterior pharynx.

Bacterial pharyngitis commonly presents with significant tender lymphadenopathy of the draining anterior cervical lymph nodes. This finding also occasionally occurs in viral infections such as infectious mononucleosis or primary HIV infection. However, 90 percent of infectious mononucleosis cases present with posterior cervical lymphadenopathy. Hepatosplenomegaly is also a common finding. Tonsillitis usually presents with swollen lymph glands on either side of the jaw.

Diagnostic Reasoning

Diagnostic Tests

Inasmuch as most cases of pharyngitis and tonsillitis are self-limited, laboratory workup and identification of causative organisms through culture is unnecessary if the patient's clinical picture is consistent with influenza, the common cold, or irritant-induced throat inflammation. However, bacterial and viral cultures of throat swabs may be appropriate for more complicated cases or those requiring pharmacotherapy such as with herpes virus or streptococcal infection. Herpangina and hand-foot-and-mouth disease are diagnosed by coxsackie-positive viral cultures and positive serologies. For exudative cases of pharyngitis, the Rapid (10-minute) Streptococcal Antigen (Rapid Strep) Test is used to detect group A streptococcal antigens and diagnose infection. Increased anti-streptolysin O (ASO) titers are also observed, but treatment may blunt this antibody response. Rapid Strep Tests are highly specific (90 percent) and sensitive (80 to 90 percent) when used judiciously. A Rapid Strep Test to guide antibiotic therapy is considered appropriate for any patient with two or three of the following criteria: fever above 100.5°F (38.1°C), tonsillar exudate, tender anterior cervical lymphadenopathy, and the absence of cough. Patients meeting three or four of these criteria may be empirically diagnosed with group A *Streptococcus* and treated immediately. Throat swab cultures of the posterior pharynx and tonsils—the current "gold standard" test for the diagnosis of *Streptococcal* infection—are sent rather than the Rapid Strep Test for patients meeting fewer criteria and considered to have a low pretest likelihood of infection (less than 20 percent). Patients with an intermediate pretest likelihood of *Streptococcal* infection (20 to 50 percent) who present with sore throat and only two of the associated criteria are given the Rapid Strep Test first and, if positive, may avoid a throat culture. However, if the result is negative, it must be followed up by a throat culture which typically displays greater sensitivity than the Rapid Strep Test. During the summer and fall, the false-positive rates of Rapid Strep Tests may approach 50 percent. In turn, the recommended diagnostic approach is less aggressive at this time than during the winter or spring. During the summer and fall, no testing is recommended for patients with a sore throat who meet only one of the associated criteria unless the patient is at high-risk for *Streptococcal* infection due to immunocompromising illnesses such as diabetes mellitus or human immunodeficiency virus (HIV), has a history of rheumatic fever, or is presenting during a community outbreak of *Streptococcus*. If possible, household members should also be screened, since treated patients may be reinfected via contact with asymptomatic carriers in the home.

Immunofluorescence staining or viral throat swab cultures are used to detect herpes virus infection. A special Tzanck smear of any ulcerative exudative lesion is used to diagnose HSV and herpes zoster; multinucleated giant cells with ballooning degeneration represent a positive finding. Infection by the many types of herpes viruses (including HSV, EBV, and CMV) may also be diagnosed by serological tests detecting virus-specific antibodies. Convalescent titers may be necessary for proper interpretation. Pharyngeal, endocervical, and urethral cultures on Thayer-Martin agar can specifically detect gonorrheal growth, if suspected in high-risk patients. Syphilis is diagnosed via serology and, if disease is in its secondary stage, by dark-field microscopy of lesional scrapings that demonstrates *T. pallidum* spirochetes. *Chlamydia pneumoniae* and

Chlamydia trachomatis are typically evaluated via serology, although cultures and titers are not recommended initially, because the relative contribution of these pathogens to throat inflammation remains highly controversial. Suspected *Candidal* infections are diagnosed with a potassium hydroxide (KOH) wet mount or Gram stain of pharyngeal exudates, which will demonstrate spores and budding hyphal yeast forms, as well as by yeast cultures for speciation if needed. Nonspecific heterophile antibody tests, such as the Monospot test, are used to diagnose infectious mononucleosis related to EBV, although this tests decreases in sensitivity when used at the extremes of age. A CBC may be done in any case of infectious pharyngitis. An increase in granulocytes indicates bacterial infection and a documented lymphocytosis (50 percent lymphocytes, of which at least 10 percent show atypical morphology) strongly supports a viral etiology. The presence of eosinophils in a Gram stain of nasal secretions or a nasal mucosal scraping is strongly indicative of allergic pharyngitis. Radiologic evaluation of the posterior pharyngeal wall may be appropriate to detect retropharyngeal processes if abscess formation is suspected.

Differential Diagnosis

Although the entire oropharynx may be involved during many infectious processes, certain microorganisms have a greater propensity for affecting the oral cavity, resulting in stomatitis, prior to pharyngeal involvement. Pharyngitis from postnasal drip secondary to rhinitis or sinusitis may be ruled out via nasal cavity examination and sinus x-ray films. Epiglottitis due to *C. diphtheria* is an important consideration in nonimmunized (or inadequately immunized) individuals; it should be ruled out carefully by gentle physical examination, which in no way risks dislodging the pseudomembrane from the posterior pharynx. Pharyngeal or tonsillar malignancy requiring surgical removal of the affected tissues must be ruled out via biopsy if malignancy is suspected.

Infection with group A *Streptococcus* causes intense mucosal inflammation because of bacterial extracellular factors such as pyrogenic exotoxin and streptolysin O. A major virulence factor is the streptococcal cell-wall M protein (with 80 serotypes), which has antiphagocytic properties; particular serotypes appear to correlate with the occurrence of rheumatic fever and glomerulonephritis, which can lead to acute renal failure. Patients may be sicker and more febrile with bacterial infection, but this is not always the case. When challenged with an infectious agent, numerous factors are brought into play, including the host's defense mechanisms, microbial virulence, quantity of infectious inoculum, and the host's susceptibility.

Management

Pharmacologic Management

Most cases of pharyngitis and tonsillitis in otherwise healthy patients are entirely manageable with home care and/or antibiotics. For allergy-related forms of throat inflammation, contact with environmental irritants including tobacco smoke should be minimized, and patients may be treated symptomatically with a combination of antihistamines and decongestants as described for allergic rhinitis. In general, for infectious forms patients should limit their physical activity until symptoms of pharyngitis and tonsillitis have subsided. Daily fluid intake should be increased to 8 to 12 glasses (2 to 3 quarts) of fluids such as water or nonacidic juices. Bedrest is recommended if fever is present, and regular physical activity should be resumed only after 2 to 3 days of normal temperature readings. Viral pharyngitis requires only symptomatic care and antibiotics are never indicated (other than selected antiviral therapies). In fact, many cases of bacterial pharyngitis are self-limited as well (such as those caused by atypical organisms). However, cases of group A *Streptococcus* and *Neisseria gonorrhoeae* merit rapid antibiotic treatment to prevent significant sequelae in both the short and long term. In addition, cases caused by *Corynebacterium diphtheriae, Haemophilus influenzae,* or influenza virus may require hospitalization because of the risk of life-threatening complications. Fungal infections also typically require antimycotic therapy.

Throat pain may be significantly relieved by:

- Voice rest
- Ambient humidification, saline nasal sprays, viscous xylocaine
- Various types of gargles taken as needed, including hot or cold double-strength tea or a warm saltwater solution (1 teaspoon of noniodinated salt in 8 ounces of water).
- A regularly cleaned cool-mist, ultrasonic humidifier to increase ambient air moisture may also be useful in relieving feelings of dryness or tightness in the throat.
- Nonprescription throat lozenges or sprays (e.g., Cepastat, Chloraseptic) containing topical anesthetics such as phenol may also alleviate minor pain.
- Nonprescription analgesics such as acetaminophen or aspirin (325 to 650 mg q4h to q6h prn) may be used to relieve intermediate pain, and codeine preparations (30 to 60 mg PO q4h to q6h prn) may relieve more severe pain.
- Enlarged, tender cervical lymph glands may be relieved with warm, moist compresses applied qid for at least 30 to 60 minutes at a time.

Viral infections tend to be treated symptomatically, as described previously. Influenza symptoms may be relieved within the first 2 days of symptoms by prescribing amantadine (Symmetrel; 100 mg PO bid) for documented cases of Influenza A, but this drug may also cause insomnia, dizziness, drowsiness, or difficulty concentrating. Thus, the dosage for elderly patients is reduced to once a day. Oseltamivir (Tamiflu; 75 mg PO bid for 5 days) may be similarly given within the first 48 hours of symptom onset to reduce duration of illness and symptom severity, as well as prophylactically in high-risk individuals during peak flu season at once daily dosing.

Antibiotic therapy for group A streptococcal pharyngitis has been shown to shorten the clinical course of disease and reduce lymphadenopathy, fever, and pain (after 1 to 3 days of therapy), prevent suppurative complications and autoimmune sequelae such as rheumatic fever, and decrease person-to-person spread of infection. Empiric antibiotic therapy may be instituted prior to receiving culture results in certain clinical situations to prevent rheumatic fever, cardiac sequelae, and acute renal insufficiency due to post-streptococcal glomerulonephritis. Studies have demonstrated, however, that delaying treatment for 48 hours in anticipation of culture results does not significantly impact the reduction in autoimmune sequelae provided by antibiotic therapy. In cases of fever under 100.5°F (38.1°C) without an associated tonsillar exudate or anterior cervical lymphadenopathy, neither throat swab culture nor antistreptococcal therapy are recommended, because a false-positive culture may lead to unnecessary antibiotic therapy. If fever greater than 100.5°F (38.1°C) accompanies a tonsillar exudate and tender anterior cervical adenitis, anti-streptococcal therapy should be instituted immediately, because a false-negative culture could delay critical treatment. This is especially important for patients younger than 25 years of age. If a similar fever occurs with only one of the other two physical signs, antibiotic therapy should be instituted only for culture-positive patients. High-risk factors favoring immediate empiric treatment include a past history of acute rheumatic heart fever or related cardiac damage, a scarlatiniform rash, a diabetic or other immunocompromised state, a documented exposure to group A *Streptoccocus* within the past week, or the presence of a known epidemic within the community.

Adults are typically given a 10-day course of penicillin V potassium (Pen-Vee K; 500 mg PO bid or 250 mg PO qid) or benzathine penicillin (Bicillin; 1.2 million units IM once) as an alternative to prolonged oral medication. If the patient is allergic to penicillin, erythromycin (250 mg PO qd) is recommended. If the patient fails to respond to antibiotic therapy, tests for infectious mononucleosis and streptococcal antibiotic sensitivity should be performed. A 10-day course of amoxicillin/clavulanate (Augmentin; 40 mg/kg PO daily based on the amoxicillin component divided bid), erythromycin ethyl succinate (50 mg/kg PO daily divided tid), or erythromycin stearate (1 g PO qd) have all been shown to be effective for penicillin-resistant beta-lactamase-producing organisms, whereas tetracycline or trimethoprim-sulfamethoxazole preparations (Septra, Bactrim) should be avoided.

Neisseria gonorrhoeae infection calls for ceftriaxone (Rocephin; 125 mg IM once), along with empiric treatment for *Chlamydia trachomatis* (azithromycin (Zithromax) 1 g PO once or doxycycline 100 mg PO bid × 7 days), given its propensity for coinfection. Extensive throat infection with *Candida albicans* (thrush, pharyngitis, esophagitis) requires antifungal treatment such as fluconazole 200 mg PO qd once, followed by 100 mg PO qd × 2 weeks total. *Mycoplasma pneumoniae* and *Chlamydia pneumoniae* are both treated with erythromycin 250 to 500 mg PO qid × 10 days, depending on the specific preparation.

Surgical Management

Surgical removal of the pharyngeal tonsils (tonsillectomy) and/or adenoidectomy is absolutely indicated if tonsillar inflammation leads to airway obstruction associated with any of the following: cor pulmonale (right-sided cardiac hypertrophy), dysphagia, or weight loss. Tonsillectomy may also be indicated if active flares recur more than three times a year, if the patient experiences mild dysphagia, if the tonsils remain chronically hypertrophied after a bout of infectious mononucleosis, or if the patient has a history of rheumatic fever with heart damage due to recurrent tonsillitis. However, in these situations, the indication for surgical intervention is relative and must be evaluated further, because the risk of postoperative complications increases with age. It should also be noted that lymph glands normally swell during episodes of active inflammation as part of the body's normal immune response. In turn, tonsillectomy is not indicated for colds, asthma, allergic rhinitis, focal infections, fever of unknown origin, cervical lymphadenopathy, or enlarged tonsils without obstructive symptomatology.

Follow-Up and Referral

Most cases of pharyngitis and tonsillitis are usually self-limiting, and symptoms tend to improve in 2 to 3 days. If symptoms fail to improve within this time, patients should return for a follow-up appointment. Throat cultures for *Streptococcus* may be repeated on completion of therapy to confirm resolution of any infectious processes. This is not recommended, however, for asymptomatic patients who have completed a 10-day therapeutic regimen for streptococcal infection or for patients whose symptoms improve within 5 days of antibiotic therapy, because clinical resolution is typically the best measure of therapeutic success.

Group A *Streptococcus* pharyngeal or tonsillar infections may lead to scarlet fever or autoimmune rheumatic fever if not treated with antibiotics or if antibiotic therapy is discontinued before a full 10-day course. These patients should be referred to a specialist. In areas where group A streptococcal infection is endemic, the probability of developing rheumatic fever is 0.3 percent. With epidemic pharyngitis, the risk increases to 3 percent. Rheumatic heart disease may develop following rheumatic fever in an adult patient with recurrent streptococcal infection or a history of poorly treated streptococcal pharyngitis as a child or young adult. This may lead to severe sequelae such as calcification of the mitral and/or other heart valves, as well as to the destruction of cardiac myocytes, which is attributed to cross-reacting antistreptococcal antibodies. Even when acute rheumatic fever is treated appropriately with prophylactic antibiotic therapy, 4 percent of patients may develop debilitating cardiac sequelae and 1 percent may develop severe class IV rheumatic heart disease. Chest pain is a key indicator of cardiac complications. Hematuria resulting from poststreptococcal glomerulonephritis may occur 1 to 3 weeks following acute pharyngeal or tonsillar infection, because antibiotic therapy has not been shown to protect against this immune complex-mediated complication.

Cases caused by *Corynebacterium diphtheria,* if left untreated, may lead to epiglottitis, which can obstruct breathing and may prove fatal if the pseudomembrane dislodges and chokes the patient, as it is inadvertently swallowed. Spread of infectious organisms from the pharynx to the lungs may lead to pneumonia and severe respiratory complications. Infections of the posterior oropharynx may also ascend to the nasopharynx, leading to sinusitis and rhinitis—inflammation of the mucous membranes of the sinus and nasal cavities. The middle ear is another possible target of disseminated pharyngeal infection, because the nasopharyngeal (eustachian) tube acts as a conduit for the spread of microorganisms. OM may occur in more than 20 percent of adenovirus infections. A less common complication of bacterial pharyngitis is septic jugular vein thrombophlebitis, which may occur several days following the initial sore throat. Patients with this complication are typically teenagers or young adults who experience an increase in neck pain and tenderness, as well as swelling of the jaw angle.

Liver function tests (e.g., serum aspartate aminotransferase [AST], serum alanine aminotransferase [ALT], serum bilirubin, platelet count, and the Coomb's autoantibody test) should be performed for all cases of suspected infectious mononucleosis to diagnose serious sequelae, including hepatitis (ALT or AST levels of more than 1000 U/L; bilirubin levels of more than 10 mg/dL), hemolytic anemia, granulocytopenia, and thrombocytopenia. Airway obstruction may also occur in patients with infectious mononucleosis as a result of pharyngeal swelling. Such complications may require treatment with a corticosteroid such as prednisone (60 to 80 mg PO daily in divided doses, tapered over 1 to 2 weeks). Splenic rupture related to trauma is also a serious risk for all patients with infectious mononucleosis who have marked hepatosplenomegaly (liver and spleen enlargement).

Tonsillitis that goes untreated or fails to resolve with treatment may lead to grossly swollen, suppurative cervical adenitis, otitis media, or a peritonsillar abscess of the surrounding throat area, characterized by increasing unilateral ear and throat pain ipsilateral to the affected tonsil, dysphagia, drooling trismus, erythema, and edema of the soft palate with fluctuance upon palpation. Suppurative sequelae such as these may require surgical drainage and/or tonsillectomy. Repeated attacks of acute tonsillitis may lead to a chronic condition with a recurrent sore throat and greatly enlarged tonsils, which may complicate breathing and become potentially life-threatening; these cases also require surgical intervention.

All patients developing suppurative or retropharyngeal sequelae should be referred to an otolaryngologist. The physical examination and treatment of *C. diphtheria* infection is also highly risky and must be supervised by a qualified specialist. Surgical interventions such as tonsillectomy or abscess drainage require surgical referral.

Patient Education

Both pharyngitis and tonsillitis may be prevented by avoiding contact with persons with actively inflamed throats, particularly with URIs. Throat swabs from household members of patients should also be cultured, to identify and treat carriers simultaneously in an effort to prevent the development of clinical disease and prevent reinfection. Toothbrushes should be replaced as soon as a sore throat develops, because they may harbor causative microorganisms, and all eating and drinking utensils should be cleaned thoroughly and should not be shared. Food and washcloths also must not be shared during a period of active infection. It is critical to keep all immunizations up to date, particularly the diphtheria-pertussis-tetanus (DPT) vaccine that confers immunity against *C. diphtheria.* If a sexual partner is suspected of being infected with a sexually transmitted agent, sexual contact should cease until a proper diagnosis and any applicable treatment have been completed. In general, oral intercourse between persons of either gender should be performed only using a form of latex barrier protection, such as a condom during fellatio or a dental dam during cunnilingus, to avoid orogenital transmission of infectious organisms. Environmental irritants such as tobacco and marijuana smoke, pollution, dust and other allergens, and low-humidity environments should be avoided to prevent noninfectious forms of pharyngitis.

Warm compresses applied to relieve enlarged, tender cervical lymph nodes are most effective if kept warm; however, patients must be cautioned not to burn the skin inadvertently. Although the use of aspirin during viral infections in adults has not been linked to the development of Reye's syndrome (as is the case in children), nonsteroidal anti-inflammatory drugs should be used cautiously if patients suffer from ulcers or other gastrointestinal disorders. Heavy lifting and contact sports must be prohibited for all patients with infectious mononucleosis, as these activities carry a high risk of splenic trauma and rupture. Patients must be instructed to finish their entire course of antibiotics or antifungals to avoid complications from latent infection such as glomerulonephritis or myocarditis. In cases involving dysphagia, patients may be instructed on how to maintain a healthy liquid or soft food diet (e.g., milkshakes, soups, and high-protein diet or instant breakfast drinks) for a few days until the pain subsides. Patients who demand prescriptions for antibiotics in the absence of a throat culture confirming disease of bacterial origin should understand the rationale for using antibacterials versus other types of medication.

Stomatitis and Glossitis

Stomatitis is a generalized inflammation of the oral mucous membranes characterized by erythema and/or vesicular or ulcerative lesions. *Glossitis* is an acute or chronic inflammation of the tongue that shares many of the same etiologies as stomatitis. Either of the two may present alone, although glossitis often accompanies stomatitis, and clinicians often group the two conditions together under the latter designation. In general, both disorders are classified according to their etiology, which is extremely variable.

Epidemiology and Causes

A variety of types of stomatitis are seen in adults and include oral candidiasis, aphthous stomatitis (aphthous ulcers, or "canker sores," often reoccur, and may be referred to as recurrent aphthous stomatitis, or RAS), secondary herpetic stomatitis/herpes labialis, Vincent's stomatitis (acute necrotizing ulcerative gingivitis, or "trench mouth"), allergic stomatitis, nicotinic (cigarette-related) stomatitis, denture-related stomatitis, angular stomatitis, pseudomembranous stomatitis, candidiasis, and parasitic glossitis (black hairy tongue, anthracosis linguae). Glossitis is also a common symptom of systemic skin diseases such as erythema multiforme (Stevens-Johnson syndrome) and pemphigus vulgaris. Herpetic stomatitis and RAS occur commonly, as do nicotinic and denture-related stomatitis. Other causes are less commonly seen.

HSV infection in the United States is widespread. According to recent estimates, up to 20 percent of the adult population may be secreting herpes simplex type 1 or 2 viruses at any given time. The prevalence of HSV-specific antibodies indicative of past or dormant HSV infection is up to 30 percent in higher socioeconomic strata and may even approach 100 percent in lower socioeconomic groups. In general, prevalence of infection is estimated to be between 20,000 and 70,000 per 100,000. Oral candidiasis most commonly occurs in immunocompromised adults, such as patients with HIV infection, or in cancer patients status post chemotherapy and/or radiation therapy. Nicotinic stomatitis and denture-related stomatitis are very common. Most other forms are rare among adults. Mouth sores may affect adults of all ages. Specifically, Vincent's stomatitis is seen among adolescents and adults age 20 to 40, whereas denture-related stomatitis affects primarily elderly patients.

Chronic mouth-breathing dries the tongue and oral mucosa, and hot foods or beverages may lead to thermal injury. Chemical irritation may result from spicy, acidic, or salty foods such as potato chips and pickles, as well as from peroxide-containing mouthwashes, toothpaste, and other dental care products. Viral, bacterial, and fungal infections, prolonged radiation or chemotherapy treatments, long-term corticosteroid or antibiotic use, chronic metabolic diseases such as diabetes, emotional or physical stress, anxiety, depression, premenstrual tension, advanced age, low socioeconomic status, and malnourishment may all contribute to host immunosuppression, and in turn, to the development of stomatitis/glossitis. Systemic autoimmune or inflammatory diseases also predispose patients. Pregnancy has been associated with erythema multiforme. Tobacco smoking and chewing (dipping, snuff) clearly can lead to nicotinic stomatitis, whereas ill-fitting dentures, recent dental work, repeated biting during convulsive seizures, and poor oral/dental hygiene contribute to mechanical injury-related inflammation of the oral cavity and tongue. Occupational or domestic exposure to chemical irritants or allergens are risk factors as are resective gastrointestinal surgery involving the ileum and malabsorptive disorders of the ileal mucosa such as sprue (villous atrophy), both of which impair B12 absorption, contributing to angular and other vitamin deficiency-related forms of stomatitis. In fact, anemia of any type is a risk factor. Repeated emesis secondary to anorexia and bulimia may inflame the oral mucosa and erode the posterior (lingual) surfaces of the teeth, because of repeated exposure to stomach acid in the vomitus. In addition, anorexia, bulimia, and off-and-on, "yo-yo" fad dieting may lead to malnourishment, vitamin deficiencies, or immunosuppression.

Most importantly, prior HSV infection is the primary risk factor for all secondary manifestations of herpes simplex infection. In addition, any factors that lead to immunosuppression may be considered contributing factors. Specifically, fever, physical and/or emotional stress, excess sun exposure, menstruation, common colds, gastrointestinal upset, and dental work that excessively stretches the mouth, as well as other underlying systemic illnesses, may be considered precipitating factors. Intercourse with multiple sexual partners and unprotected sex (failure to use barrier protection, e.g., condoms during intercourse or latex dental dams during oral sex) increase the likelihood of HSV transmission from infected sexual partners.

Pathophysiology

In general, excessive dryness of the oral cavity; food and drug allergies; chemical irritation; mechanical or thermal injury; bacterial, fungal, and viral pathogens (e.g., coxsackie virus causes hand-foot-and-mouth disease, varicella-zoster virus causing oral and lingual vesicular lesions, primary HIV infection); host immunosuppression; and nutritional deficiencies of iron, folate, riboflavin (B_2), niacin, pyridoxine (B_6), and cyanocobalamin (B_{12}) are all risk factors that can cause stomatitis and glossitis. Aphthous ulcers, one of the most common types of oral lesions, yet their pathogenesis is poorly defined. Stress, hormonal fluctuations, inflammatory bowel disease, and anti-metabolite chemotherapies all predispose to aphthae. Specifically, the spirochete *Borrelia vincentii* is strongly associated with Vincent's stomatitis (which bears its name), as well as certain fusiform *Bacillus* bacterial species, although some cases are of indeterminate etiology. If complicated by HIV infection and left untreated, this condition may progress to necrotizing stomatitis. Nicotinic stomatitis results directly from the chemical irritants in tobacco. Denture-related stomatitis results from the mechanical injury caused by ill-fitting dentures. Angular stomatitis is symptomatic of the vitamin deficiencies discussed in the preceding text, and pseudomembranous stomatitis has been associated with numerous chemical irritants and bacterial pathogens.

Parasitic glossitis is caused by several mycoses of the tongue, including *Cryptococcus linguae-pilosasae* and *Nocardia lingualis* co-infection. The use of systemic antibiotics is well known to clear normal microbial flora from the oral cavity and, in fact, the entire gastrointestinal tract, thus facilitating fungal overgrowth caused by the lack of endogenous microbial competition. In addition, both oral and inhaled steroids are known to compromise cellular immunity within the oral cavity—the main defense mechanism against fungal overgrowth and infection. HIV infection and AIDS, malignancy, chemotherapy, diabetes mellitus, and age-related decreases in natural immunity may all contribute to immune suppression as well, increasing the likelihood of fungal overgrowth and viral reactivation of HSV. Erythema multiforme is a widespread immune-mediated inflammatory reaction of the skin and in its advanced stages, the mucous membranes including the oral cavity, which may be caused by different types of infection (e.g., HSV, *Mycoplasma*, *Streptococcus pyogenes*), drug allergies (e.g., anticonvulsants, sulfonamides, allopurinol), and collagen vascular disorders. However, oral involvement in erythema multiforme, as well as its extreme forms (Stevens-Johnson syndrome, toxic epidermal necrolysis) which cause severe sloughing of the skin and mucosa, will never be isolated to stomatitis, as these are systemic, life-threatening conditions. In contrast, the etiology of pemphigus vulgaris is unknown, but flaccid bullae typically begin in the oropharynx as superficial epidermal layers separate from their base. A similar appearing blistering disorder, bullous pemphigoid, only rarely presents with isolated oral lesions, but as this disease progresses, roughly one-third of individuals may demonstrate oral involvement. A number of inherited disorders of the epidermis and dermis known collectively as epidermolysis bullosa may also involve the oral mucosa in their moderate and severe forms. Finally, a wide array of autoimmune disorders such as systemic lupus erythematosus may also present with mucosal ulcerative lesions.

Clinical Manifestations

Subjective

In general, patients with stomatitis may complain of excessive dryness of the mouth (or excess salivation, with Vincent's stomatitis); halitosis; difficulty speaking or swallowing; minor to severe oral pain; or bleeding, swollen, or erythematous gums; as well as constitutional symptoms (including fever, malaise, headache, and weight loss) that may be secondary to infection or malnourishment. Patients with secondary herpetic stomatitis usually report a 24- to 48-hour prodrome consisting of a burning sensation in the mouth, followed by the appearance of 1- to 2-mm vesicular lesions, initially fluid-filled bullae, which then evolve into ulcerated lesions, which eventually crust over the course of several days. These frequently appear around the lips. Although most patients report only one to two recurrences per year, 5 to 25 percent of patients suffer more than one attack per month. Patients may also report itching and burning in the mouth, particularly in cases of allergic stomatitis. In contrast, parasitic glossitis is usually painless, whereas anemia and niacin deficiency lead to lingual pain.

Objective

The mouth, and the tongue (if also inflamed), often appear bright red and swollen, either at the tip and edges (from vitamin deficiencies or mechanical injury) or over the entire glossal surface. Depending on the cause of inflammation, the tongue may be ulcerated (from niacin deficiency, streptococcal infection, erythema multiforme, or pemphigus) or smooth and pale (from iron, folate, or B_{12} deficiencies). Vincent's stomatitis causes necrotic ulceration of the interdental gingival papillae and oral mucous membranes, characterized by a purulent, gray exudate. Allergic stomatitis causes intense, shiny erythema and slight swelling of the mucosa and tongue. Nicotinic stomatitis presents with centrally erythematous white nodular elevations, and pseudomembranous stomatitis produces a membrane-like exudate coating the oral mucosa. Inflammation and external fissuring of the corners of the mouth are characteristic of angular stomatitis. Parasitic glossitis presents with hypertrophied (1-cm) filiform papillae that color the dorsum of the tongue dark brown or black. In contrast, syphilis and mouth-breathing result in white patches on the tongue. Erythema multiforme presents with polymorphous disseminated macular, papular, nodular, vesicular, bullous, and target (bull's-eye–shaped) lesions of the skin and mucous membranes. Pemphigus is also characterized by disseminated thin-walled bullae throughout the skin and mucosa which, when ruptured, leave raw patches. The lesions of pseudomembranous stomatitis cannot be scraped off with a tongue blade, whereas the lesions of parasitic glossitis are easily broken. Anterior cervical or jaw lymphadenopathy may be felt in cases that are related to autoimmune or systemic inflammatory disease.

Inspection of the oral mucosa of patients with HSV infection reveals individual or groups of 1- to 2-mm vesicular lesions that evolve into ulcers, apparent after the prodromal period (24 to 48 hours, characterized by pain, tingling, burning, and itching preceding vesicle formation), particularly on the gingivae, hard palate, buccal mucosa, and tongue. If observed at a later stage of healing (4 to 10 days following vesicle formation), oral lesions may appear ulcerated but crusted over. Herpes labialis presents as similar clusters of open vesicular lesions in the labial area, particularly at the mucocutaneous border, with erythematous bases and possibly crusting, if the lesions are in an advanced stage of healing. Palpation of the oral mucosa may demonstrate edema or tenderness, aiding in the identification and characterization of oral lesions. Anterior cervical or jaw lymphadenopathy may be felt in both conditions.

Although not directly related to HSV infection, back percussion to the posterior lungs may reveal the dull tones of pulmonary consolidation characteristic of lung infections (e.g., tuberculosis) common to HIV infection, AIDS, or other immunocompromising disorders that often underlie the reactivation of HSV infection. Likewise, chest auscultation may reveal signs such as crackles, crepitus, or wheezing, which may indicate the presence of systemic inflammatory disease or pulmonary infections secondary to an underlying immune disorder.

Oral candidiasis may exhibit diverse clinical patterns, and some patients exhibit more than one form. Factors that affect clinical presentation are the immune status of the host, such as the presence of HIV or a history of organ transplant, as well as the oral mucosal environment, for example, the impaired salivary function seen in Sjögren's syndrome, postradiation xerostomia, or of age-related atrophy, and whether the person is dentate or edentulous (more common) and a nonsmoker or smoker (more common). Pseudomembranous candidiasis, also known as "thrush," is recognized by the development of creamy white plaques that resemble cottage cheese or curdled milk. When these plaques are scraped off, an erythematous mucosa is exposed. There is also an erythematous candidiasis, in which the oral mucosa appear fiery red and the mouth feels like it has been "scalded with a hot beverage." This form often follows broad-spectrum antibiotic therapy but is also associated with immunosuppression and xerostomia. Breath mints, cinnamon gum, mouthwash, or toothpaste can cause allergic reactions that mimic this form of candidiasis, so the patient's history is very important in differentiating the clinical picture, because treatment will vary accordingly.

Chronic hyperplastic candidiasis, or candidal leukoplakia, is the least common form of oral candidiasis. Patients have a white patch (leukoplakia) that cannot be scraped off. Some researchers believe that this is a candidiasis superimposed on a preexisting leukoplakia lesion. Hairy leukoplakia is associated with EBV. These white mucosal lesions do not rub off and may appear as faint vertical streaks or thick, furrowed areas of leukoplakia. *Candida* is present without the tissue's normal inflammatory reaction to the fungus. Hairy leukoplakia has been reported in organ and bone marrow transplant recipients and, on rare occasions, in immunocompetent patients. However, its presence strongly suggests HIV infection in an individual with no other signs of immune suppression. HIV patients with hairy leukoplakia frequently develop AIDS within 2 years of the lesion onset.

Diagnostic Reasoning

Diagnostic Tests

Stomatitis or glossitis may result from multicausal phenomena. However, detecting the primary underlying problem is key to effective management. A complete blood count (CBC) may reflect bacterial infection if polymorphonuclear neutrophils are elevated or viral infection if lymphocytes and mononuclear leukocytes predominate. Biochemical tests, special cellular stains, and cultures are used to identify most causative microorganisms, along with specific serologies such as the Rapid Plasma Reagin (RPR) test for the syphilitic agent *Treponema pallidum.* Serum levels of iron, folate, riboflavin, niacin, or cyanocobalamin may reveal nutritional deficiencies that can cause stomatitis and glossitis. Autoimmune disorders are diagnosed through a wide array of serologies (e.g., antinuclear antibody test for systemic lupus erythematosus).

Herpetic stomatitis caused by HSV may be ruled out via serum levels of anti-HSV antibodies, viral culture, or a Tzanck smear of lesional scrapings which will present as multinucleated giant cells with intranuclear inclusions. Concurrent genital lesions are common in herpetic infection, as is also the case with Behçet's disease, a neutrophilic inflammatory disorder treated with topical and systemic steroids, which does not appear infectious. Non–*Candida*-related pseudomembranous stomatitis may be distinguished from oral candidiasis by negative findings for the fungus on Gram stain or more appropriately 10 percent potassium hydroxide wet mount of lesional scrapings. Oral candidiasis, as well as lichen planus, may resemble nicotinic stomatitis. Lichen planus may be ruled out by biopsy, which demonstrates hyperkeratosis, irregular acanthosis, and lymphocytic dermal band-like infiltrates.

Other conditions leading to an inflamed appearance of the oral mucosa include systemic or local vasculitis and oral neoplasia; the latter (oral or glottic cancer) often presents as a single, painless lesion. Biopsy is needed to rule out these conditions if lingual or mucosal lesions are chronic or recurrent. Measles (roseola paramyxovirus infection) also leads to erythematous patches with bluish white centers on the lingual and buccal mucosa, known as Koplick's spots. However, this systemic infection is accompanied by a skin rash, cough, and coryza 24 to 48 hours following the appearance of these distinctive oral lesions. Viral culture and serologic tests may rule out measles and other viral infections, including infectious mononucleosis (EBV infection), warts (papillomaviruses), prodromal primary HIV infection, and severe cases of chickenpox (varicella–zoster infection), which may also present with vesicular lesions of the oral cavity, pharynx, and larynx.

Differential Diagnosis

The primary goal of the differential diagnosis for mouth sores is to determine their precise cause, because etiology of these lesions is so variable. Although the aforementioned hematologic screens (CBC and nutrient levels) and serologic tests may be used to detect specific pathogens or nutritional deficiencies, the signs and symptoms elicited from patient history and physical examination provide the most useful information in determining the cause of mouth sores. For example, self-induced vomiting associated with bulimic or anorexic dieting disorders should be ruled out through a careful patient history. Similarly, physical examination can rule out aphthous stomatitis, which, unlike the other forms listed, produces characteristic shallow, grayish, nonvesicular ulcers surrounded by a ring of hyperemia and covered with a fibrinous yellow membrane. Pregnancy epulis (pregnancy gingivitis) results from hormonal changes, and may be confused with other forms of stomatitis. However, hyperplasia is usually limited to the interdental papillae, and pyogenic granulomas may form. Geographic tongue (benign migratory glossitis), which may be confused with pathological forms of glossitis, presents as continuously changing areas of loss and regrowth of filiform papillae with thickened white borders surrounded by red patches, creating a map-like appearance of the tongue. Geographic tongue is considered to be a harmless, normal variant requiring no treatment.

Management

Most cases of stomatitis are effectively treated with outpatient care unless severe or resulting from an underlying disease requiring inpatient care (e.g., advanced syphilis). For example, if severe dehydration secondary to oral pain and dysphagia is present, parenteral fluids may be required.

- ▲ All behaviors or conditions contributing to lesion formation should be stopped or corrected (e.g., smoking, eating hot or spicy foods, or wearing ill-fitting dentures).
- ▲ Underlying causative infections should be treated appropriately but treatment specific to oral inflammation is primarily symptomatic and pharmacologic.
- ▲ Baking soda or salt water rinses three or more times a day (1/2 tsp. salt or sodium bicarbonate in 8 oz. water) may be sufficient to relieve mild discomfort. Alternatively, oral rinses of half strength 3 percenthydrogen peroxide solution (1:1 with water)
- ▲ Liquid antacids such as attapulgite (Kaopectate), aluminum hydroxide (Amphogel), or magnesium hydroxide (Maalox) may effectively relieve pain when taken qid.
- ▲ Equal amounts of anti-histaminic elixirs such as diphenhydramine (Benadryl) may be mixed with liquid antacids (1:1) to reduce inflammation.
- ▲ Nonprescription analgesics such as acetaminophen (Tylenol) 650 mg q4h to q6h may be used to relieve mouth pain.
- ▲ A viscous solution of 2 percent lidocaine may be applied to oral lesions q3h as a topical anesthetic or used as a gargle and swallow (15 mL) before meals and q3h prn.
- ▲ Severe attacks in adults may require topical gel-based 0.1 percent triamcinolone (Kenalog) or fluocinonide applied at bedtime and, if needed, tid after meals.
- ▲ Anti-inflammatory oral steroid "bursts" may be appropriate in severe cases of stomatitis and glossitis, but all oral medications should be monitored for toxicity because significantly more absorption than expected may result from open oral ulcers. In addition, steroids would not be indicated in immunosuppressed patients or those with viral infections, although antiviral medications like amantadine (Symmetrel) may be appropriate.

For cases of HSV, ice cubes applied locally for an hour to newly formed lesions may prove helpful; likewise, drinking cool liquids and sucking on frozen juice bars may reduce discomfort.

- ▲ Pharmacological prepartions for HSV may be helpful such as Valtrex 1 g bid for 2 days or Famvir 500 mg bid for 5 days.
- ▲ High fluid intake and antiseptic mouthwashes (without alcohol, which may be irritating and painful) may help prevent secondary bacterial infection.

In cases of candidiasis, antifungal agents should be used in conjunction with antibiotics and oral hygiene.

- ▲ Nystatin (Mycostatin, Nilstat), a polyene antibiotic, is formulated for use as a pastille (lozenge) or suspension 400,000 to 600,000 units PO (swish and swallow) qid. Because it is not absorbed across the gastrointestinal tract, the drug must remain in contact with the organism and must be reapplied several times a day.
- ▲ Clotrimazole (Lotrimin, Mycelex), an imidazole agent, is not well absorbed and must be administered at least qid as a 10-mg trouche.
- ▲ Ketoconazole (Nizoral) 200 to 400 mg PO qd × 7 to 14 days, another imidazole, is absorbed across the gastrointestinal tract and provides systemic therapy by the oral route. It should not be used routinely for routine oral candidiasis, however, because of possible drug interactions and potential liver toxicities. The triazole agent fluconazole (Diflucan) 200 mg PO on the first day then 100 mg qd for 7 to 14 days is well absorbed systemically and only rarely causes liver toxicity, although other drug interactions, as well as drug resistance, have been documented.
- ▲ Hydrocortisone-iodoquinol (Vytone) cream can be used to ease the discomfort of angular cheilitis. It combines the anti-inflammatory and antipruritic effects of hydrocortisone with the antifungal and antibacterial properties of iodoquinol.
- ▲ In terms of hygiene, toothbrushes should be changed frequently. A patient with candidiasis who wears dentures or partials must also treat the appliances to combat the infection.

Treatment of erythema multiforme requires eliminating exposure to the offending agent in the case of drug hypersensitivity or specific treatment to the underlying infectious agent (e.g., acyclovir for HSV infection). Specialist care by a dermatologist and close inpatient observation is required for severe cases that risk progression to Stevens-Johnson syndrome or toxic epidermal necrolysis. Vincent's stomatitis requires oral penicillin V potassium (Pen-Vee K; 250 to 500 mg q4h to q6h) to fight infection, as well as significant fluid intake of at least four to six glasses of nonacidic fruit juice or water per day. Severe gangrenous stomatitis requires IV antibiotic treatment and debridement of wounds.

Autoimmune disorders such as systemic lupus erythematosus, bullous pemphigoid, and pemphigus vulgarus are primary treated with systemic corticosteroids. The mucosal lesions of lupus may be treated with topical or intralesional steroids if located on the lips, while lesions of the oral cavity respond to antimalarials, provided no drug hypersensitivity manifests. However, for recalcitrant cases, increasingly potent immunosuppresive medications may be necessary. Treatment of any of these disorders typically require specialist care and rapid referral.

Dehydration and malnutrition can result from altered eating habits due to oral pain. Secondary bacterial infections may complicate any type of ulcerative oral lesion. Recent scarification of lesions may progress to facial space infection, tonsillar or cervical lymph gland infection, involvement of the vocal cords, bronchial tubes, rectum, vagina, and even sepsis. Thus, oral surgery may be needed to trim away rough, highly inflamed, infected gum tissue. Glossitis may become chronic if inadequately treated, and severe gangrenous or necrotizing stomatitis seen in severe HIV-infected cases may lead to death if untreated.

Patient Education

The importance of proper oral hygiene and healthful nutritional habits should be stressed to all patients. Patients should be instructed to brush their teeth with a soft-bristled toothbrush at least twice daily and to floss regularly (once a day, if possible). Patients should also wear protective headgear whenever bicycling, skating, or playing contact sports, to prevent cases of trauma-related tongue injury. Increased intake during treatment should be encouraged, as well as maintaining the recommended medication regimen while avoiding hot, spicy, salty, or acidic foods, and carbonated or alcoholic beverages. Patients may be instructed to drink through a straw if lesions are particularly painful. A liquid diet may be recommended during the first 2 to 3 days, if pain is severe. Milk, liquid gelatin, yogurt, ice cream, and custard are usually well tolerated. Severe cases of Vincent's stomatitis may even call for at-home rest during the first few days of treatment.

The contagious nature of pathogen-related forms of stomatitis or glossitis should be emphasized. The most effective means of avoiding secondary manifestations of reactivated HSV infection, for example, is to refrain from behaviors which put the individual at risk of HSV infection or reinfection—most notably, promiscuous, unprotected sex with multiple partners and physical contact with persons who have active herpetic lesions. Kissing and oral sex should be avoided if an individual is actively infected, and frequent handwashing during active flare-ups of herpetic lesions aids in preventing autoinfection and viral transmission. It is also helpful to inform patients of the high prevalence rate of HSV infection, to reduce the stigma commonly associated with herpes. Early treatment of primary or secondary HSV infection may also help to prevent stomatic or labial involvement. Wearing zinc oxide-containing sunscreens on the lips and face helps to prevent herpes labialis flare-ups when exposed to excessive sunlight.

Long-range, the most effective means of avoiding stomatitis is to refrain from risk behaviors such as smoking, eating hot or spicy foods, drinking alcohol, and practicing poor dental hygiene. Avoiding exposure to affected persons, especially in the case of HSV, as well as avoiding exposure to allergens, chemical irritants, or foods that seem to trigger attacks is also recommended. Care should be taken to fit all dentures and dental prostheses properly to prevent mechanical injury, and for cases related to bruxism (tooth grinding), a night-guard prosthesis with removable splints to reduce biting pressure on tooth surfaces may reduce damage to dentition, in turn, preventing related inflammation. Early treatment of viral, bacterial, and fungal infections may prevent stomatic and glossal involvement. Wearing protective headgear during bicycling, skating, and contact sports could prevent many means of trauma-related injury.

Temporomandibular Joint Disease

Temporomandibular joint (TMJ) *disease* is a collective term that refers to disorders affecting the masticatory musculature, the temporomandibular joint and associated structures, or both. The terms *craniomandibular disorders* (CMD) and *temporomandibular disorders* (TMD) are synonymous with the more familiar term temporomandibular joint disease (TMJ). Most current research favors the phrase *temporomandibular disorder* (TMD). Although TMD has been traditionally viewed as one syndrome, it is actually a cluster of related disorders in the masticatory system that has many features in common. The most common presenting symptom is pain in the muscles of mastication, the preauricular area, and/or the TMJ. Chewing, bruxism (clenching, grinding, or gnashing of the teeth during nonfunctional movements of the mandible), or other jaw functions tend to aggravate the pain. TMDs are considered to be a subclassification of musculoskeletal disorders.

Epidemiology and Causes

Symptoms of TMD in individuals are common, yet not every person with symptoms would be considered to have the disorder. Epidemiologic studies in specific populations show that about 75 percent have at least one sign of joint dysfunction (joint noise) and about 33 percent have at least one symptom (face or joint pain). It is estimated that only 5 percent of these individuals are in need of treatment for TMD. For many patients, TMD can be mild and self-limiting, while for others, it may progress to chronic pain and discomfort, which will require consultation with multiple professionals over many years.

Signs and symptoms of TMD generally increase in frequency and severity from the second through the fourth decade of life. The majority of patients are between age 15 and 45, with a mean age of onset of 35. The vast majority of patients with TMD (84 percent) are women, yet some data

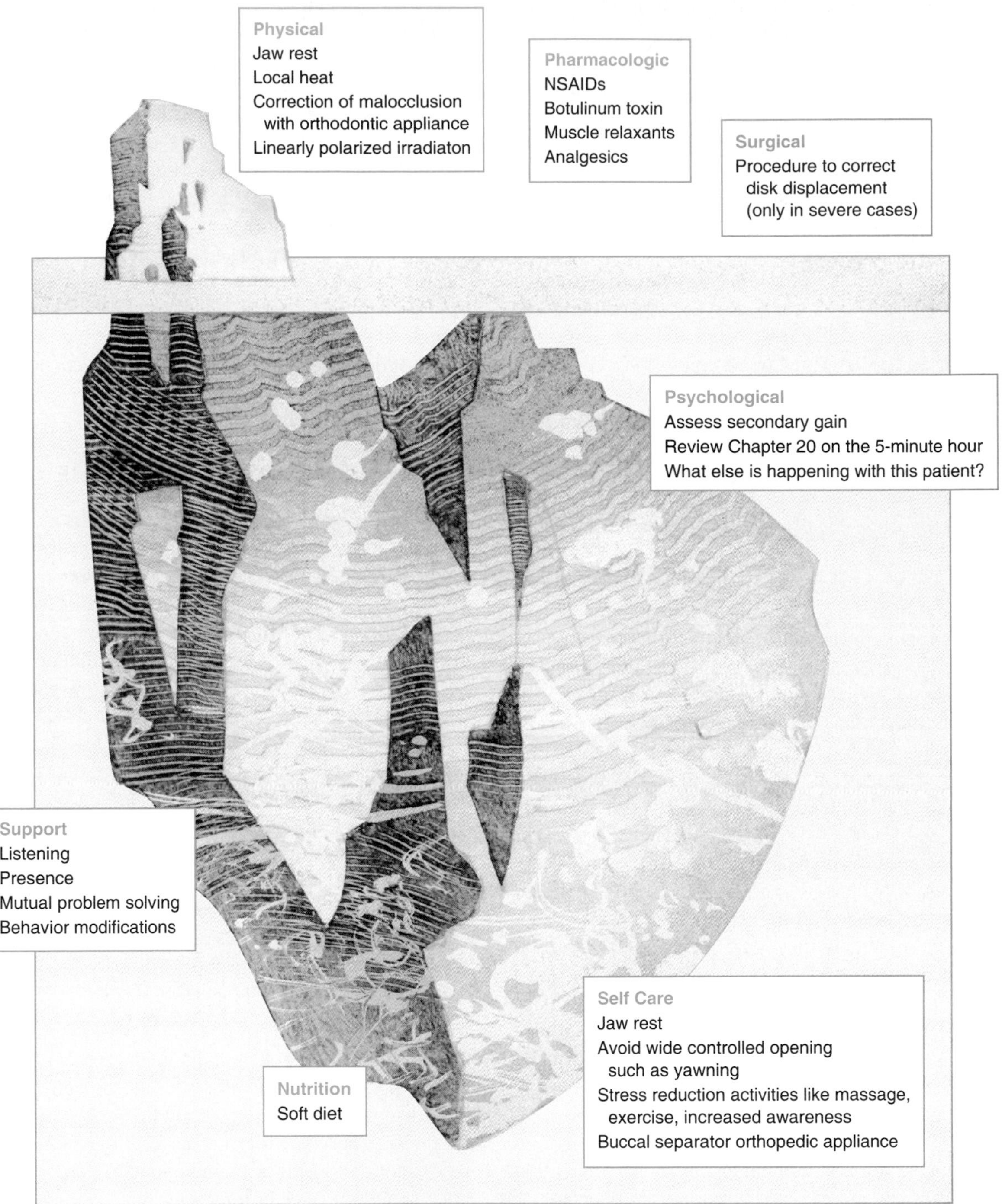

demonstrate that men have symptomatology but do not present for treatment. Symptoms may be self-limiting or may fluctuate over time, as suggested by the declining incidence with increasing age. The lack of a universally accepted classification scheme with diagnostic criteria makes it difficult to accurately determine the prevalence of TMD.

Because TMDs are diverse and multifactorial, a universal etiology does not exist. It may be more appropriate to differentiate contributing factors into predisposing, initiating, and perpetuating categories. *Predisposing factors* increase the risk of orofacial pain or TMD development. *Initiating factors* cause the onset of the disorder, and *per-*

petuating factors interfere with healing and complicate management. Contributing factors are not necessarily etiologic; they may be the result of the disorder instead.

Predisposing factors include biomechanical, genetic, or psychological factors that increase the chances of an individual developing TMD. Initiating or precipitating factors generally fall into two main categories—macrotrauma as a result of a single event, or microtrauma in the form of repetitive adverse loading of the masticatory system. Perpetuating factors include personality, social, emotional, and cognitive factors that are often related to the stresses of daily living. The dividing line between categories is not always clear cut. Some initiating factors (e.g., bruxism) may also act to maintain the disorder after onset. Table 7.6 presents contributing factors to TMD.

Pathophysiology

The TMJ is one of the most complex joints in the body. It is a synovial, encapsulated joint that is stress bearing. The TMJ differs from other joints in the body in that its articular surfaces are covered with fibrocartilaginous tissue rather than with the chondrocartilage found in other joints. The articular disc separates the upper and lower joint spaces. Pain from the TMJ arises from injury to the retrodiscal tissue or the capsular ligament. Locking of the joint may occur secondary to jaw malocclusion and, most commonly, anterior disc dislocation. However, several variations of articular disc displacement have been noted with the condition, as joint laxity from underlying connective tissue disorders and even asymetric body alignment from poor posture have been cited as risk factors. Dental manipulation of the jaw as well as degeneration of the TMJ from rheumatoid or osteoarthritis often underlie extracapsular joint dysfunction, as misalignment of the TMJ places pressure on nearby ear structures, resulting in otalgia (ear pain), tinnitus, vertigo, hearing loss, and tongue pain.

TMJ pain may also be intracapsular in origin and involve the masticatory musculature, known as TMJ myofascial pain syndome or simply TMJ syndrome. Similar to all skeletal muscles, the TMJ muscles are susceptible to muscle splinting, spasm, or inflammation. Pain that originates in the orofacial area may be referred to other areas, such as the neck, shoulders, and head, and TMJ syndrome often coexists with fibromyalgia. However, pain from the masticatory musculature is usually related to mandibular dysfunction. Abnormal chewing patterns, chronic tension of the jaw musculature, and facial trauma all predispose to muscle dysfunction. Stress-related jaw clenching as well as psychogenic nocturnal bruxism (unconscious nighttime teeth grinding) have also been strongly associated with TMJ syndrome. The importance of psychologic stress in the development of this disorder is further bolstered by the observation that a worse prognosis is associated with a diminished capacity for supportive interpersonal relationships.

Table 7.6 Factors Contributing to TMD

Biomechanical factors
Past injuries
Skeletal malformations
Postural imbalances
Occlusal factors (alteration in bite-controversial)
Cervical disorders
Macrotrauma
Contact sport
Motor vehicle accident
Whiplash
Psychological factors
Personality
Social
Emotional
Cognitive
Anxiety
Depression
Mental disorders
Substance abuse
Systemic medical conditions
Rheumatic
Hormonal
Infectious
Nutritional
Metabolic disorders
Microtrauma
Oral parafunctional
Habits
Bruxism
Nail biting
Gum chewing
Genetic factors

Clinical Presentation

Subjective

Patients may present with several complaints that lead to the suspicion of TMD or with only one symptom. The most common presenting symptom is pain (89 percent), followed by jaw noise (85 percent) and limited jaw movement (40 percent). Ear symptoms account for 28 percent of clinical presentations. Only 4 percent of patients present with obvious jaw dislocation.

Pain is usually localized in the muscles of mastication, the preauricular area, and/or the TMJ. Chewing or other jaw functions frequently aggravate the pain. Patients may complain of poorly localized pain in the face or head, which is dull, unilateral, centered in the temple, above and behind the eye, or in and around the ear. Other less obvious symptoms may include tinnitus, sinus symptoms, a foreign body sensation in the external ear canal, decreased hearing, neck or shoulder pain, visual disturbances, limited jaw opening, and popping or grating joint sounds. Patients may present with a history of trauma to the TMJ or cervical disc area (such as whiplash).

Several questionnaires have been developed to assist the health-care professional in screening for TMD.

Any patient who presents with symptomatology (complaints of orofacial pain, headaches, ear pain, or tinnitus) should be screened for TMD by asking questions such as: Do your jaw joints make noise? Does using your jaw—such as chewing, talking, and/or yawning—cause you pain or difficulty? Have you had jaw joint problems before, and were you tested? When moving your jaw, does it ever get "stuck," "lock," or "go out"? Is opening your mouth difficult or does it cause pain? Do you ever have pain in the head and neck area, such as the face, ears, temples, and/or forehead? Has your jaw, neck, or head ever been injured? If so, when? Do you clinch or grind your teeth at night or during the day? If you have tinnitus, does the ringing sound change in any way as you open and close your mouth while applying external pressure to the joint? Do you have frequent headaches, neckaches, or toothaches?

Objective

Because many of the presenting symptoms of TMD may be secondary to underlying medical conditions, a complete examination should be done in order to exclude metabolic, nutritional, neurologic, or hormonal etiologies. Visual acuity should be assessed. Special attention should be directed to observation of the patient's balance, gait problems, or unusual habits. The muscles of mastication and the TMJ should be palpated using a bimanual technique. Muscles to be palpated include the masseter, temporalis, medial pterygoid, digastric, and mylohyoid. Tenderness, enlargement, swelling, and unusual texture should be noted. Cervical muscle groups should also be palpated to differentiate craniocervical disorders. The oral exam may reveal ground-down teeth, which would indicate bruxism.

Next, the TMJ should be examined with the mouth in the closed position, which will allow palpation of the lateral aspect. On opening of the jaw, assessment of mandibular range of motion and TMJ sounds can assist with diagnosis. A mandibular opening of less than 40 mm is considered restrictive; the mandible may deviate to one side or the other when opened (asymmetrical opening). Joint sounds may be described as clicking, popping, or crepitus. Pain may also be elicited with mandibular movement and should be noted.

Diagnostic Reasoning

Diagnostic Tests

Initial testing for diagnosing TMD may first include ruling out other underlying medical conditions. Laboratory testing should include CBC with differential, platelets, chemistry panel, ESR, rheumatoid factor, and thyroid stimulating hormone. Radiographic imaging (x-ray films) may be helpful in confirming a clinical diagnosis of TMD. The clinician must remember that even if anatomical changes are found, imaging results rarely have any bearing on clinical outcome. Imaging testing is confirmatory at best, but the diagnosis may be made by history and clinical exam alone. Films are best reserved when dental anomalies are suspected or severe symptoms are refractory to conservative treatment. A transcranial view (lateral oblique projection) is the most common film taken of the TMJ. This view is useful for identification of gross osseous pathology and degenerative or traumatic changes of the joint; however, it is subject to distortion and shows only the lateral one-third of the condylar head and may not be sensitive enough to detect condylar displacement.

Subsequent testing should most likely be ordered by the dentist, otolaryngologist, or oral surgeon upon referral of the patient. This could include panoramic films, CT, or MRI. CT provides the clearest picture of the osseous structures, and with contrast, can help visualize the soft tissue of the head and neck, but it is not useful in the diagnosis of disk displacement of the TMJ. MRI visualizes the soft tissues of the joint without radiation and the injection of contrast dye. MRI can be used to determine disc position and morphology. MRI may also show arthritic changes in the TMJ. Moreover, disk displacement seen on MRI may also be observed in asymptomatic patients; so these findings should never guide therapy alone. Diagnostic injections with anesthesia, synovial fluid analysis, or biopsy of suspicious areas by the specialist may be useful for differentiating diagnosis.

Differential Diagnosis

Because of the extensive list of contributing factors and potential symptoms, it may be difficult to arrive at a diagnosis of TMD. Accurate diagnosis is essential, and has traditionally been the weak link in the chain of management of TMD. Disorders of the intracranial structures should be ruled out initially, because they may be life-threatening and require immediate attention. New or abrupt onset of pain, progressively more severe pain, interruption of sleep by pain, and systemic symptoms such as weight loss, ataxia, fever, and neurologic symptoms (e.g., seizures, paralysis, vertigo) are characteristic of intracranial disorders. Table 7.7 presents common differential diagnoses for TMD.

Management

Effective care of patients with TMD involves understanding and treating the whole patient via an individualized program. A multidisciplinary approach is frequently indicated. Contributing factors must be addressed rather than concentrating on eliminating signs and symptoms. The goals for management are similar to those of any musculoskeletal condition—reduction or elimination of pain and restoration of acceptable mandibular function. Complete resolution of TMD may not always be possible, however, as in the case of permanent damage to joint structures. In these cases, the term "cure" or "treatment" has been abandoned for the term "management."

Initial therapy should be reversible and is designed to be palliative and to promote healing. Acute disk displacement or active trigger points may require rapid treatment/

Table 7.7 Differential Diagnosis: TMD

Sinusitis
Atypical facial pain
Cervical disorders/arthritis
Glaucoma
Lyme disease
Otitis media and otitis externa
Temporal arteritis
Neuralgia
Foreign body or cerumen in the ear
Mastoiditis
Neoplasm
Dental pain/abscess
Headaches (cluster, migraine, tension, vascular)
Psychogenic pain
Anxiety disorders
Mood disturbances
Depression
Intracranial disorders (neoplasm, aneurysm, abscess, hemorrhage, hematoma, edema)

referral. In general, however, the practitioner can initiate management with conservative therapies such as self-help techniques and pharmacotherapy.

One of the most significant contributions toward management of TMD can be made by adjustment in diet consistency, education and alteration of oral parafunctional habits, and application of ice (for acute symptomatology) or moist heat (for chronic symptomatology). On occasion, self-treatment alone may control signs and symptoms; specific recommendations are listed in the section on Patient Education.

Physical therapy may be employed, primarily as an adjunct to other therapeutic modalities, in an attempt to relieve pain of musculoskeletal origin and restore normal masticatory function. Physical therapy for TMD may include electromodalities and therapeutic exercises as prescribed by a physical therapist. Behavioral therapy is indicated for patients with behavioral and emotional problems and/or noxious habits that accompany TMD. Stress relief and pain control methods such as counseling, hypnosis, biofeedback, and guided imagery are safe and noninvasive.

Pharmacotherapy can be beneficial in controlling pain and inflammation associated with TMD. Careful monitoring of the patient's tolerance to prescribed medications, as well as the effectiveness of the drug, is indicated. To avoid potential abuse of any drug that may produce dependence, dosing at regular intervals for a definite period of time is preferred, as opposed to prn dosing. Drugs Commonly Prescribed 7.2 presents the drugs that are commonly used to treat TMD. Injection of trigger points with anesthetic agents may be beneficial; however, it is most likely that this would be done by the specialist (dentist or oral maxillofacial surgeon) that the patient has been referred to.

For the majority of cases of TMD, any necessary subsequent management will be initiated and followed by

Drugs Commonly Prescribed 7.2: TMD

Drug	Indication	Dosage	Comments
Tricyclic Antidepressants			
Amtriptyline (Elavil)	TMD (Chronic)	25 mg tid to qid or 75 mg qhs	Begin with low nightly dose (10 mg) and increase. Orofacial pain, sleep disorders, muscle relaxation, and decreased bruxism
Benzodiazepenes			
Clonazepam (Klonopin)	TMD	0.05 mg tid	Short course of 1–2 weeks only Acute pain secondary to masticatory muscle spasm or TMJ pain
Diazepam (Valium)	TMD	2–10 mg bid to qid	Muscle relaxation, anti-anxiety, and sedative effects Usually ordered with NSAID
Nonopioid Analgesics			
Acetaminophen (Tylenol)	TMD	1000 mg tid to qid	Orofacial/TMJ
Ibuprofen (Motrin/Advil)	TMD	400–800 mg tid to qid	Inflammatory pain
Anticonvulsants			
Baclofen (Atrofen)	TMD	Initially 100 mg bid	Neuropathic pain
Skeletal Muscle Relaxants			
Cyclobenzaprine HCl (Flexeril)	TMD (Acute)	10 mg tid Max: 60 mg/day	Muscle relaxation Do not use for longer than 2–3 weeks. Brief trial only in conjunction with PT
Corticosteroids			
Methylprednisolone (Medrol/Solumedrol)	TMD (Acute and Severe)	Dose pack	Severe unremitting pain in the TMJ related to inflammatory conditions

the dentist, otolaryngologist, or oral surgeon that the patient has been referred to. Most of the therapies employed by these practitioners are not considered part of initial therapy for TMD because they are irreversible procedures. These therapies include orthodontics, prosthodontics, occlusal equilibration, or surgery. Wearing an intraoral appliance with an occlusal appliance or splint may be recommended, generally by a dentist. At the present time, this type of therapy is highly controversial and may not be considered an option by many practitioners, although it may be indicated for patients with gross structural changes in the alignment of the TMJ. Surgery, including arthroscopic surgery or arthrotomy, may be recommended by an oral maxillofacial surgeon. Surgery may be indicated in patients who do not respond to nonsurgical therapy and who have disabling pain or dysfunction related to TMD.

Follow-Up and Referral

The decision to refer a patient with TMD to a specialist should be made based upon the individual practitioner's knowledge level and comfort in treating TMD. Once other systemic conditions have been ruled out, the practitioner may choose to begin initial management of TMD symptoms. Follow-up should be early and repeated (e.g., in 1 to 2 weeks initially, and then monthly), especially if pharmacotherapy is ordered. If there is any uncertainty about the diagnosis, then referral should be made at this time to a dentist or otolaryngologist or to an oral maxillofacial surgeon who is knowledgeable in the treatment of TMD. If initial therapy is unsuccessful, or if advanced management is indicated, appropriate referrals should be undertaken.

Patient Education

Home care and patient education is an integral component to the management of TMD. The majority of patients achieve relief of symptoms with conservative therapy, including self-care techniques. Patient information for management of TMD includes the following recommendations:

- Limit jaw function by eating softer foods, taking smaller bites, and not opening wide when eating. Avoid foods like apples, corn on the cob, hard breads, raw vegetables, steak, and so on.
- To help reduce stress, strive for a nutritionally balanced diet and an active exercise program.
- Ice packs can be used for acute pain and muscle spasm. Place an ice pack over the temple area and side of face for 10 minutes, three or four times a day. For chronic pain, moist heat should be used following the same guidelines.
- Disengage your teeth—the rule is "lips together, teeth apart."
- Do not chew gum or ice.
- Sleep on your back with a pillow under your knees. Do not use firm, full pillows under your head. Orthopedic pillows can be helpful in reducing head and neck pain. Do not sleep on your stomach.
- When talking on the telephone, do not support the receiver with your shoulder.
- Prevent wide-opening when yawning. Do not sit with your chin resting on your hand.
- Practice good posture. If you must sit for long periods of time, try to stand and move around frequently in order to stretch your muscles.

Bibliography

General

Buchman, DD: Herbal Medicine. Wings Books, New York, 1996.

Buttaro, T, et al: Primary Care: A Collaborative Practice, ed 2. CV Mosby, St. Louis, Mo., 2003.

Dombro, M: Griffiths' 5-Minute Clinical Consult. Lippincott, Williams & Wilkins, Philadelphia, 2006.

Duke, JA: The Green Pharmacy. Rodale Press, Emmaus, Pa., 1997.

Epstein, O, et al: Clinical Examination, ed 2. Times Mirror International Publishing Limited, 1997.

Hagen, P: Mayo Clinic Guide to Self Care. Mayo Foundation for Medical Education and Research, Rochester, Minn., 1997.

Institute for clinical Systems Improvement (2005) National Guideline Clearinghouse: accessed at **http://www.guideline.gov/summary**

Leiberman, S, and Bruning, N: The Real Vitamin and Mineral Book, ed 2. Avery Publishing Group, New York, 1997.

Meredith, P, and Honsin, N: Adult Primary Care. WB Saunders, Philadelphia, 1999.

Murray, M, and Pizzorno, J: Encyclopedia of Natural Medicine, ed 2. Prima Publishing, Rocklin, Calif., 1998.

Noble, J (ed): Textbook of Primary Care Medicine, ed 3. CV Mosby, St. Louis, Mo., 2001.

Page, LR: Healthy Healing: A Guide to Self-healing for Everyone, ed 10. Healthy Healing Publications, Del Rey Oaks, Calif., 1997.

Rakel, R (ed): Conn's Current Therapy. WB Saunders, Philadelphia, 2006.

Robinson, D, et al: Primary Care Across the Lifespan. CV Mosby, St. Louis, Mo. 2000.

Seller, RH: Differential Diagnosis of Common Complaints, ed 5. WB Saunders, Philadelphia, 2004.

Uphold, C, and Graham, MV: Clinical Guidelines in Family Practice. Barmarrae Books, Gainesville, Fla., 2003.

Youngkin, E, et al: Pharmacotherapeutics: A Primary Care Clinical Guide, ed 2. Appleton & Lange, Stanford, Conn., 2003.

Hearing Impairment

Malmstrom, J: Gerontologic nurse practitioner care guidelines: Assessing and managing hearing deficits in the older adult. Geriatric Nursing 2691:57–59, 2005.

Spiro, SR: A cost-effectiveness analysis of earwax softeners. Nurse Pract 22(8):28, 30–31, 166, 1997.

Visual Disturbance

Congdon, NG, Friedman, DS, and Lietman, T: Important causes of visual impairment in the world today. JAMA 290(15):2057–2060, 2003.

Goldzweig, CL, Rowe, S, Wenger, NS, MacLean, CH, and Shekelle, PG: Preventing and managing visual disability in primary care: Clinical applications. JAMA 291(12):1497–1502, 2004.

Kennedy, MS: Growing older, seeing less: Blindness and visual impairment are on the rise in older Americans. AJN, Am J Nurs 104(7):21, 2004.

Rowe, S, MacLean, CH, and Shekelle, PG: Preventing visual loss from chronic eye disease in primary care: Scientific review. JAMA 291(12):1487–1495, 2004.

Trudo, EW, and Stark, WJ: Cataracts lifting the clouds on an age-old problem. Postgrad Med 103(5):114–126, 1998.

USPSTF Recommendations: A summary of recent health care findings from an independent panel of experts. AJN, Am J Nurs 105(2):88–89, 2005.

Watkinson, S: Visual impairment in older people: The nurse's role. Nurs Standard 19(17):42–55, 2005.

Glaucoma

Assaad, MH, et al: Glaucoma drainage devices: Pros and cons. Curr Opin Ophthalmol 10(2):147–153, 1999.

Craig, JE, and Mackey, DA: Glaucoma genetics: Where are we? Where will we go? Curr Opin Ophthalmol 10(2):126–134, 1999.

Glaucoma: Early detection can minimize vision loss. Mayo Clinic Health Letter 2005 Jul; 23(7): 1–3.

Medeiros, FA: Optic disc assessment: Five rules to guide clinicians. Ocular Surg News. 2005 Jun 15; Suppl:7–9.

Rahim, SA, Sahlas, DJ, and Shadowitz, S: Blinded by pressure and pain. Lancet 365(9478):2244, 2005.

Screening for glaucoma: Recommendation statement. Am J Nurse Pract 9(9):49–50, 52–55, 2005.

Stewart, WC: Perspectives in the medical treatment of glaucoma. Curr Opin Ophthalmol 10(2):99–108, 1999.

Sycha, T, Vass, C, Findl, O, Bauer, P, Groke, I, Schmetterer, L, and Eichler H: Interventions for normal tension glaucoma. Cochrane Library 2, 2004.

Wilensky, JT: The role of medical therapy in the rank order of glaucoma treatment. Curr Opin Ophthalmol 10(2):109–111, 2004.

Otitis Externa

Alper, BS: Evidence-based medicine. Choosing an antibiotic for otitis externa. Clin Advisor 7(3):126, 2004.

Beers, SL, and Abramo, TJ: Otitis externa review. Pediatr Emerg Care 20(4):250–256, 2004.

Blenkinsopp, A, Paxton, P, and Reid, S: Nurse prescribers. Otitis externa… latest in a series. Primary Health Care 13(9):33–34, 2003.

Felis, MJ: Protocol. Acute otitis externa. Lippincott's Primary Care Practice 4(5):529–533, 2000.

Hajioff, D: Clinical evidence concise. Otitis externa. Am Fam Phys 70(9):1741–1742, 1633–1636, 2004.

Hoskins, P: Advisor forum: Clinical pearls. Useful otitis externa treatment. Clin Advisor 7(6):[98], 2004.

Sander, R: Otitis externa: A practical guide to treatment and prevention. Am Fam Physician 63:927–941, 2001.

Simpson, KL, and Markham, A: Ofloxacin otic solution: A review of its use in the management of ear infections. Drugs 58(3):509–531, 1999.

van Balen, FAM, Smit, WM, Zuithoff, NPA, and Verjeij, TJM: Clinical efficacy of three common treatments in acute otitis externa in primary care: Randomised controlled trial. BMJ 327(7425):1201–1203, 2003.

Otitis Media

Alsarraf, R, et al: Measuring direct and indirect costs of acute otitis media. Arch Otolaryngol Head Neck Surg 125(1):12–18, 1999.

Brook, I, and Gober, AE: Resistance to antimicrobials used for therapy of otitis media and sinusitis: Effect of previous antimicrobial therapy and smoking. Ann Otol Rhinol Laryngol 108(7 Pt 1):645–647, 1999.

Dowell, S, et al, and the Drug-resistant *Streptococcus pneumoniae* Therapeutic Working Group: Acute otitis media: Management and surveillance in an era of pneumococcal resistance—A report from the Drug-resistant *Streptococcus pneumoniae* Therapeutic Working Group. Pediatr Infect Dis J 18:1–9, 1999.

Hoppe, HL, and Johnson, CE: Otitis media: Focus on antimicrobial resistance and new treatment options. Am J Health Syst Pharm 55(18):1881–1886; 1932–1933, 1998.

Jensen, PM, and Louis, J: Criteria, performance and diagnostic problems in diagnosing acute otitis media. Fam Pract 16(3):262–268, 1999.

Klugman, KP, and Feldman, C: Penicillin- and cephalosporin-resistant *Streptococcus pneumoniae*. Emerging treatment for an emerging problem. Drugs 58(1):1–4, 1999.

Kujdych, N: Acute otitis media, reining in resistant bacteria. Adv Nurse Pract 30–35, 1999.

McCracken, GH, Jr: Treatment of acute otitis media in an era of increasing microbial resistance. Pediatr Infect Dis J 17:576–579, 1998.

van Balen, FAM, Smit, WM, Zuithoff, NPA, and Verjeij, TJM: Clinical efficacy of three common treatments in acute otitis externa in primary care: Randomised controlled trial. BMJ 327(7425):1201–1203, 2003.

Ménière's Disease

Ervin, S. Meniere's disease: Identifying classic symtpoms and current treatments. J Am Assoc Occup Health Nurses 52(4):156–158, 2004.

Kim, HH, Wiet, RJ, and Battista, RA: Trends in the diagnosis and the management of Ménière's disease: Results of a survey. Otolaryngol Head Neck Surg 132(5):722–726, 2005.

Rhinitis

Berger, WE, et al: Double-blind trials of azelastine nasal spray monotherapy versus combination therapy with loratadine tablets and beclomethasone nasal spray in patients with seasonal allergic rhinitis. Rhinitis Study Groups. Ann Allergy Asthma Immunol 82(6):535–541, 1999.

Day, J: Pros and cons of the use of antihistamines in managing allergic rhinitis. J Allergy Clin Immunol 103(3 Pt 2):S935–S399, 1999.

Heyden, M.: Rhinitis. The Nurse Practitioner 29(12):27–39, 2004.

LaForce, C: Use of nasal steroids in managing allergic rhinitis. J Allergy Clin Immunol 103(3 Pt 2):S388–S394, 1999.

Mason, UG: Today's approach to managing rhinitis in women, hormonal forms of rhinitis pose unique clinical challenges. Womens Health Primary Care 2(8):661–669, 2004.

Settipane, RA: Complications of allergic rhinitis. Allergy Asthma Proc 20(4):209–213, 1999.

Sussman, GL, et al: The efficacy and safety of fexofenadine HCl and pseudoephedrine, alone and in combination, in seasonal allergic rhinitis. J Allergy Clin Immunol 104(1):100–106, 1999.

Terrien, MH, et al: Comparison of the effects of terfenadine with fexofenadine on nasal provocation tests with allergen. J Allergy Clin Immunol 103(6):1025–1030, 1999.

Terrye, M: Recognizing and treating non-infectious rhinitis. J Acad Nurse Pract 15(9):398–410, 2003.

Zagaria, M, and Buonanno, A: A patient-oriented approach to the management of allergic rhinitis. Clin Rev 15(9):59–69, 2005.

Sinusitis

Adelglass, J, et al: Comparison of the effectiveness of levofloxacin and amoxicillin-clavulanate for the treatment of acute sinusitis in adults. Otolaryngol Head Neck Surg 120(3):320–327, 1999.

Ah-see, K: Sinusitis (acute). [Journal Article, CEU, Exam Questions]. Am Fam Phys 69(11):2635–6, 2519–2521, 2004.

Alper, BS, and Hickner, JM: Stat consult. Acute sinusitis.Clinical Advisor. 8(3):86, 89–90, 2005.

Clifford, K, et al: Double-blind comparative trial of ciprofloxacin versus clarithromycin in the treatment of acute bacterial sinusitis. Sinusitis Infection Study Group. Ann Otol Rhinol Laryngol 108(4):360–367, 1999.

Evans, KL: Diagnosis and management of sinusitis. BMJ 309(26):1994.

Gooch, WM, III: Antibacterial management of acute and chronic sinusitis. Managed Care Interface 12(2):92–94, 1999.

Krouse, HJ, and Krouse, JH: Complementary therapeutic practices in patients with chronic sinusitis. Clin Excell Nurse Pract 3(6):346–351, 1999.

Leung, AKC, and Kellner, JD: Acute sinusitis in children: Diagnosis and management. J Pediatr Health Care 18(2):72–76, 2004.

Lindbaek, M: Acute sinusitis: Guide to selection of antibacterial therapy. Drugs 64(8):805–819, 2004.

New guidelines for sinusitis target prescribing practices. Disease Manage Advisor 10(3):27–30, 2004.

Piccirillo, JF. Clinical practice. Acute bacterial sinusitis. N Engl J Med 351(9):902–10, 945–948, 2004.

Poole, MD: A focus on acute sinusitis in adults: Changes in disease management. Am J Med 106(5A):38S–47S; discussion 48S–52S, 1999.

Ulualp, SO, et al: Possible relationship of gastroesophagopharyngeal acid reflux with pathogenesis of chronic sinusitis. Am J Rhinol 13(3):197–202, 1999.

Wong K. Heal thyself. Spotlight on sinusitis: We've nosed out the best natural remedies for keeping your passages clear. Altern Med (60):29–30, 32, 2003.

Temporomandibular Joint Disease

Birkner, KM: TMJ/temporomandibular joint syndrome. Consultant, May 2001.

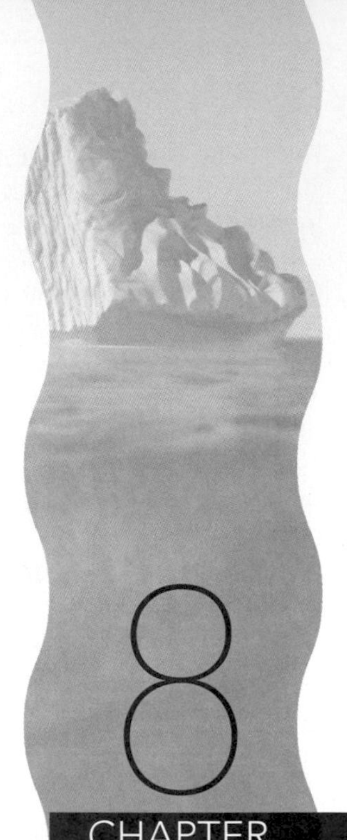

Respiratory Problems

Jill E. Winland-Brown, EdD, MSN, APRN, BC
Brian O. Porter, MD, PhD, MPH
Linda E. Moody, PhD, APRN, FAAN
Theresa Beckie, PhD, RN
Mary Webb, PhD, RN

Common Complaints

Cough

Each year more Americans seek medical treatment for a cough than for any other complaint. In the United States, the treatment costs for these visits exceed $1 billion annually. Cough is the body's natural protective mechanism for clearing the airways of secretions and irritants. Cough may be associated with a number of conditions, disorders, and diseases that alter pulmonary secretions (bronchitis, pulmonary edema), increase sensitivity of the cough receptors and airways (asthma), directly stimulate the receptors (aspiration), indirectly stimulate receptors (reflux), or affect psychological health. Cough may be associated with the following conditions: asthma, chronic obstructive pulmonary disease (COPD), bronchiectasis, cystic fibrosis, pneumonias, tuberculosis (TB), lung cancer, interstitial lung disease (ILD), cardiac tamponade, pharyngitis, and gastroesophageal reflux disease (GERD), to mention just a few.

In extreme cases of debilitation or in certain neuromuscular conditions, the cough mechanism may be impaired. There are times when the cough mechanism should be supported to clear the airways of unwanted irritants and times when it should be suppressed. These issues are discussed in relation to the underlying condition that initiates the cough mechanism.

Differential Diagnosis

The differential diagnosis of cough requires a comprehensive history and assessment to provide appropriate treatment and management. One patient may present with the complaint of a dry, hacking cough of sudden onset (*acute cough*); another may present with a cough of longer duration. A *chronic cough* is defined as one that lasts longer than 3 weeks. Many patients try over-the-counter (OTC) measures for a chronic, nagging cough and delay seeking treatment or seek treatment only when the cough becomes productive or when there is blood in the sputum.

A diagnosis can be made about 80 percent of the time via a thorough history by exploring with the patient the following details regarding the onset and nature of the cough:

- ▲ When did the cough first start? What factors may have prompted the cough (e.g., recent respiratory infection or exposure to noxious agents)? Is there a seasonal pattern? Is it related to work or hobbies?
- ▲ When does the cough occur—on arising, at bedtime, during exercise, or throughout the night?
- ▲ What factors seem to stimulate the cough or make it worse? Is the cough aggravated by exposure to certain chemicals, body position, exercise, or cold air?
- ▲ Has the patient identified any factors that seem to provide relief from the cough, such as sitting upright or avoiding exposure to certain agents? What measures have been tried to alleviate the cough?
- ▲ What is the quality of the cough—is it dry and hacking, wet, raspy, deep, or throaty?
- ▲ Is the cough productive or unproductive? If the patient produces sputum with the cough, ask the patient to describe the amount of sputum produced per day (e.g., 1 tsp, 1 tbsp, etc.), the color (e.g., yellow, gray, green, brown, clear, white, blood-tinged), and consistency (e.g., thick, ropy, frothy, or tenacious).

In addition, it is essential to find out if the patient has signs and symptoms associated with the cough, such as pedal edema, dizziness, chest pain, fatigue, dyspnea, hoarseness, fever, tachypnea, chills, heartburn, wheezing, and hemoptysis. The patient should be asked to describe in detail the onset of the associated signs and symptoms. Standard data regarding the patient's medical history should be recorded, including hospitalizations, surgeries, and major illnesses, particularly recent illnesses and respiratory allergies. The patient's lifestyle should be explored, such as occupation and work history; hobbies; exposures to noxious agents; and use of alcohol, tobacco, and other substances. The most common cause of chronic cough is cigarette smoking, which triggers the cough reflex by direct bronchial irritation. In general, a cough of acute onset occurs as a result of a lower respiratory tract infection, but it may be caused by other conditions that accompany a chronic cough.

The patient needs to be asked about the use of prescription and OTC drugs. Certain antihypertensive drugs such as angiotensin-converting enzyme (ACE) inhibitors and beta-blockers can cause hypersensitive airways and wheezing and cough. Other drugs such as nitrofurantoin (Macrobid, Macrodantin) may cause interstitial fibrosis and associated cough.

For the physical exam, focus on the following:

- ▲ Check the ears for cerumen or hairs impinging on the tympanic membrane, which may cause cough (Arnold's reflex).
- ▲ Examine the nose for discharge, edema, polyps, and sinus tenderness. In the throat, look for cobblestoning of the oropharynx, which suggests postnasal drip.
- ▲ Palpate the neck for enlarged lymph nodes or masses.

A complete assessment of the thorax and chest should be done to rule out cardiac or pulmonary problems. If the patient has not coughed during the visit, ask the patient to reproduce the cough and listen to its sound and character. The lungs should be auscultated, especially for crackles (formerly called rales) and rhonchi. The patient should be asked to produce a forced expiration while the practitioner checks for wheezes. Crackles will often clear after the patient is asked to cough and clear the airways. The presence of heart murmurs, gallops, and carotid bruits should also be assessed

Any of the following conditions may cause cough:

- ▲ Postnasal drip: This common problem is most often associated with allergic or vasomotor rhinitis and less often with sinusitis. Patients often describe a sensation of tickling or trickling in the back of the throat.
- ▲ Postinfection: Following a bout with the flu or viral illness involving the respiratory tract, patients may have a cough for 8 or more weeks because of bronchial hyperreactivity.
- ▲ COPD: *Chronic bronchitis*, the most common type of COPD, is defined as a chronic productive cough that persists for 3 months of the year or longer for 2 or more successive years. Most smokers eventually develop chronic bronchitis.
- ▲ Asthma: Asthma is a reversible obstructive pulmonary disease, a reactive airway disease, and is often accompanied by cough and wheezing. The cough may be productive or dry.
- ▲ GERD: In most cases, cough associated with GERD is thought to be caused by stimulation of the distal esophagus, but in a small percentage of cases it may be due to microaspiration.
- ▲ Drugs: Cough occurs in about 10 percent of patients who take ACE inhibitors such as captopril (Capoten) and enalapril (Vasotec). A complete history of prescribed and OTC drugs, including any herbal preparations, should be taken.
- ▲ Occupational and environmental factors: Exposure to air pollution, industrial dust and pollutants, second-hand smoke, and other pollutants may cause chronic cough.
- ▲ Other possible causes of cough: Tumors (bronchogenic or mediastinal), pulmonary embolism, aortic aneurysm, congestive heart failure (CHF), aspiration, bronchiectasis, TB, sarcoidosis, foreign body, diaphragmatic irritation (which may be seen in ascites), bronchiectasis, lung abscess, *Pneumocystis*, and psychogenic factors.

In most cases, the underlying cause can be determined from a history and physical exam, but it may be necessary to consider the judicious use of one or more of the following diagnostic aids in conjunction with the differential diagnosis process. For example, if one suspects TB, then a Mantoux purified protein derivative (PPD) (tuberculin intradermal skin test) should be done.

Spirometry is helpful to determine the presence of obstructive or restrictive lung disease. A chest x-ray film should be taken if there are signs and symptoms of pneumonia, TB, possible tumor, aspiration, foreign body, or ILD. Sinus films may be useful to rule out sinusitis when the patient presents with a history of chronic postnasal drip and chronic sinus infections.

Computerized tomography (CT) scanning can detect small peripheral nodules, evaluate coin lesions (solid, cystic, or calcified), and distinguish the chest wall from areas of pleural or parenchymal disease. Chest vessels can be separated from lymph nodes and other solid, nonvascular structures. The CT scan has replaced bronchography in diagnosing bronchiectasis. CT scan may help to better delineate endobronchial, parenchymal, or mediastinal masses. Pulmonary angiography is indicated when pulmonary thromboembolism is suspected.

A white blood cell count (WBC) and differential is helpful in diagnosing a bacterial infection. Fungal serology should be done to identify coccidiomycosis, histoplasmosis, and aspergillosis if the history of exposure is positive.

A Mantoux (PPD) intradermal skin test should be done when TB is suspected. A positive test result should be followed up with a chest x-ray film. For patients who are immunocompromised, the test may have to be repeated because of anergy.

Treatment

Because a cough is a symptom, treatment is always directed toward resolving the underlying cause(s) and removing any identified triggers. In patients with chronic cough who are weak and debilitated, the goal is to reduce complications from uncontrolled, forceful coughing, such as fractured ribs, pneumothorax, aspiration, exhaustion, sleep deprivation, and post-tussive syncope.

With severe, acute coughing that disrupts sleep and causes pain or extreme fatigue and weakness, it may be necessary to treat with antitussives, but these drugs have a limited role and should be used on a short-term basis. Nonnarcotic agents such as dextromethorphan (Benylin) or pseudoephedrine/brompheniramine/dextromethorphan (Dimetapp DM), q3 to 4h, are used. When sleep or eating is interrupted by persistent cough, the preferred choice is codeine, 8 to 30 mg q3 to 4h, but only on a short-term basis. (Patients with terminal lung cancer should receive codeine in sufficient doses to keep them comfortable.)

Decongestants and antihistamines, alone or in combination, are indicated in cases of allergic rhinitis and postnasal drip. Antihistamines are most useful for those who have allergic upper airways disease but are usually avoided in asthmatic individuals. Intranasal steroid sprays or aerosols such as beclomethasone (Vancenase, Beconase) or fluticasone (Flonase) may be useful also.

Expectorants are intended to decrease sputum viscosity and are used when the patient has a productive cough and needs help in clearing the airways. Suppression of a productive cough, however, may lead to complications such as pneumonia, as the patient may not be able to clear the airways and lungs of sputum. While expectorants may work for some, increasing the patient's water intake to 3 to 4 L/day is the most cost-effective means of helping to liquefy secretions.

Two herbal remedies are currently used but have not been thoroughly researched. Horehound has been suggested as a cough suppressant and licorice is supposed to calm a cough and have expectorant qualities.

Encouraging the patient to stop smoking should be a priority. A chronic cough may not disappear in ex-smokers for a year or more.

Patients with GERD usually respond to a course of antireflux therapy, which usually includes antacids, histamine$_2$ receptor blockers, and proton pump inhibitors. The benefits may not be noticed for several weeks, however.

Educating the patient and family about potential environmental and occupational factors that precipitate cough is essential. Explore ways to avoid exposure to irritants. If a family member smokes, the dangers of secondhand smoke should be explained to the patient and family. Adequate hydration (increasing fluids) and adequate room humidification may also help reduce coughing.

Dyspnea

Like pain, *dyspnea* is a perceived sensation. Patients with dyspnea usually describe a sense of difficult breathing or inability to get sufficient air into or out of the lungs. Dyspnea may also be described as a feeling of breathlessness, suffocation or smothering, air hunger, and labored breathing. In many cases of dyspnea, the respiratory rate is rapid and cough may be present, depending on the underlying disease or cause of the dyspnea. Dyspnea may be caused by a number of different health problems. In an older patient, dyspnea is the major atypical presentation for ischemic heart disease and myocardial infarction (MI). Dyspnea in aging patients may be difficult to evaluate when there are associated comorbidities.

Dyspnea is one of the most commonly occurring complaints for which patients seek help from health-care providers. Dyspnea, or shortness of breath, is estimated to be the third most frequent reason for seeking medical attention. Although dyspnea occurs primarily in patients with respiratory and cardiac disorders, it may also occur in other conditions such as lung neoplasms with metastasis, neuromuscular myopathies, neuropathies, spinal cord lesions, diaphragmatic disorders, and in panic disorders. In patients receiving hospice care, it is the second most common symptom, next to pain.

Differential Diagnosis

In the majority of cases, dyspnea is a result of cardiac or pulmonary decompensation. There are several symptoms associated with dyspnea, such as tachypnea (rapid breathing), orthopnea (dyspnea relieved in the sitting or upright position), and paroxysmal nocturnal dyspnea (sudden episodes of acute dyspnea at night). The causes of dyspnea are often complex. The common causes and precipitants of dyspnea follow:

- Pulmonary: COPD, asthma, pulmonary parenchymal disease ILD, pulmonary hypertension, severe kyphoscoliosis, exogenous mechanical factors (ascites, massive obesity, extensive pleural effusion)
- Cardiac: CHF, pulmonary venous congestion (mitral stenosis, mitral regurgitation)
- Hematologic: severe chronic anemia
- Psychogenic: anxiety and panic disorders

Dyspnea may be acute or chronic, and patients with COPD may have both acute and chronic dyspnea. It is important to do a complete workup to determine the underlying cause of the dyspnea so appropriate treatment can be initiated. Dyspnea caused by acute anxiety may mimic cardiopulmonary decompensation and patients with pulmonary hypertension may have episodes that resemble anxiety-related dyspnea. Onset of dyspnea at rest, accompanied by a sense of chest tightness, a feeling of suffocation, and an inability to "get air in," is a common presentation of anxiety-related dyspnea. In the absence of heart and lung disease, a history of multiple somatic complaints, emotional difficulties, no activity limitations (exercise intolerance), and dyspnea unrelated to activities provides evidence for psychogenic-related dyspnea.

About 75 percent of cases of dyspnea are caused by respiratory conditions that may be acute or chronic. The majority of other causes of dyspnea are cardiac in origin. It is important to explore with the patient the details of the onset and character of the dyspnea. The clinician should note whether the patient has dyspnea at rest or on exertion. Standard questions include: (1) How many flights of stairs did the patient climb before dyspnea occurred (e.g., one-flight dyspnea)? (2) How many blocks did the patient walk before dyspnea occurred (e.g., one-block dyspnea)? (3) How many feet did the patient walk before dyspnea occurred (e.g., 100-feet dyspnea)? The rate of the patient's speech during exercise can provide good clinical information.

Exploring when the dyspnea first occurred and what the patient was doing at the time is essential. Specific questions should be directed toward precipitating factors and factors that alleviate the dyspnea. Questions should explore potential environmental exposure (e.g., recent travel) or exposure to agents (e.g., through occupation or hobbies) that aggravate the dyspnea. Paying attention to other signs and symptoms that may be associated with the dyspnea, such as cough, peripheral edema, dizziness, wheeze, fever, chest pain, heartburn, leg pain, and paresthesias are also critical.

A complete physical examination should be done, with particular attention directed to the pulmonary and cardiovascular systems. The examiner should check for tachycardia, tachypnea, fever, and hypertension. The quality of breath sounds (increased, decreased, or absent) should be noted, along with the presence of crackles, rhonchi, wheezes, egophony, and fremitus. Assessment should include checking for third and fourth heart sounds, murmurs, friction rubs, jugular venous distension, pedal edema, and calf tenderness. A visual analog scale (0 to 100 mm) or the Borg graphical rating scale (0, for no dyspnea, to 10, for worst dyspnea ever had) is useful in assessing the degree of dyspnea. The scale can be used again on the patient's next visit to compare outcome effects of treatments.

Diagnostic tests are guided by data from the history and physical exam and the suspected causes of the dyspnea. Chest x-ray films are useful in ruling out tumors, TB, pneumonias, and other major pulmonary disorders. A complete blood count (CBC) should be done to rule out anemia and infection. A blood chemistry profile is done if a metabolic acidosis is suspected and to differentiate anion-gap acidosis from nonanion-gap acidosis. Oximetry to measure the saturation level of oxygen may be useful in assessing whether the patient may be dyspneic because of hypoxemia. If the O_2 saturation level is less than 90 percent, arterial blood gas (ABG) analysis should be done. Levels of dyspnea have not been found to correlate well with physiologic measures.

If there is suspicion of carbon monoxide (CO) exposure, a carboxyhemoglobin (COHb%) level should be obtained. COHb% levels of 4 to 15 percent may be found in heavy smokers. Levels above 20 percent may cause dyspnea and headache; levels greater than 40 percent may cause seizures and death.

Peak expiratory flow rate (PEFR) is a simple, inexpensive test that can be done with a hand-held flow meter in the office or at the bedside. This test determines the degree of expiratory airflow obstruction in asthma and COPD. Full spirometry is useful in determining whether the patient has obstructive, restrictive, or mixed (obstructive and restrictive) lung disease (see the section on Cough). Diffusion capacity should be checked if ILD is suspected.

Treatment

Initial treatment is directed at helping the patient find relief from the shortness of breath by removing the underlying cause and contributing factors. Subsequent management is directed at prevention and assisting the patient with management of chronic dyspnea in conditions such as COPD or ILD. In cases of dyspnea caused by hypoxemia, supplemental oxygen may be indicated if mismatching is present. In cases of shunting, the cause of the shunting must be corrected. For subsequent management, see the sections on Asthma, Chronic Bronchitis and Emphysema (COPD), and Interstitial Lung Disease.

For treatment of dyspnea related to cardiac disorders such as CHF, refer to the chapter on Cardiovascular Problems. Appropriate diuretics to relieve fluid overload may improve breathing, and supplemental oxygen may be necessary in some cases.

For anxiety-related dyspnea, psychiatric referral may be needed if other simple measures have been tried without good results. Dyspnea caused by rapid overbreathing during anxiety attacks can be corrected through patient education. Until the patient learns a rebreathing technique, it may be helpful to prescribe short-term use of anxiolytics such as buspirone HCl (BuSpar) 20 to 30 mg/day.

Hemoptysis

Hemoptysis is defined as expectoration of blood. The patient often reports coughing up blood or sputum that is streaked or tinged with blood. In addition, hemoptysis may be manifested as fresh (bright red) or old blood or, in the case of bleeding from an infected lung cavity, it may present as slow oozing or frank bleeding. In cases of profuse hemoptysis, blood clots may be expectorated.

Differential Diagnosis

About 80 percent of hemoptysis cases have inflammatory causes such as bronchitis, bronchiectasis, pneumonia, and TB. Other less common causes may include neoplasms that damage a pulmonary vessel and rupture a pulmonary artery. Use of pulmonary artery balloon catheters has increased the incidence of pulmonary artery rupture. Cardiovascular causes of hemoptysis include left ventricular failure, mitral stenosis, pulmonary embolism or infarct, primary pulmonary hypertension, and aortic aneurysm. Clotting defects may also cause hemoptysis. Bleeding may occur anywhere in the respiratory tract, including the nose, sinuses, and mouth.

About 95 percent of pulmonary blood circulation is supplied by the pulmonary artery and its branches, which is a low-pressure system. Bronchial circulation, a high-pressure system, originates from the aorta and usually provides about 5 percent of the blood to the lungs, mostly to the airways and supporting structures. When bleeding occurs, it usually arises from the bronchial circulation, unless trauma or erosion has affected a major pulmonary vessel. Pulmonary venous bleeding is modest and occurs in pulmonary venous hypertension, especially in conjunction with left heart failure.

The patient usually presents with a complaint of "coughing up" blood. To most people, the presence of blood in the sputum or coughing up blood is a frightening experience and most will seek immediate medical attention. As in differential diagnosis of dyspnea and cough, a similar line of questioning should be pursued regarding onset, amount, aggravating and alleviating factors, and the presence of other associated symptoms such as dyspnea, cough, dizziness, fatigue, and chest pain. Bronchopulmonary bleeding may present as hematemesis (vomiting of blood). The patient may swallow blood during the night and may vomit blood on arising.

The history and physical examination are focused along the same lines as for the complaints of cough and dyspnea. In addition, if the examiner suspects that the hemoptysis is due to a pulmonary neoplasm, the exam should focus on the pulmonary system and lymph node enlargement. If there is a history of epistaxis, the nasopharynx should be examined carefully.

Further diagnostic tests may be indicated, depending on the results of the history and physical examination. The common causes of hemoptysis will direct the laboratory tests. If hemoptysis occurs in patients age 45 or younger, it is likely caused by mitral stenosis, TB, bronchiectasis, or lung abscess. For patients older than age 45, common causes of hemoptysis include bronchogenic carcinoma, bronchitis, TB, and pulmonary embolus with infarction. In massive hemoptysis (loss of more than 600 mL of blood in 24 hours, which may occur in lung cancer, TB, bronchiectasis, and lung abscess), the condition is life threatening and constitutes a medical emergency. There may be time to do only chest radiographs and a CBC before emergency surgery or bronchoscopy.

For nonemergency cases, in which the sputum is tinged or streaked with blood, there is time to do the essential tests to identify the cause of hemoptysis. In addition to chest x-ray films and a CBC, sputum for acid-fast bacilli (AFB) should be done if TB is suspected. For suspected pneumonia or lung abscess, sputum for culture and sensitivity should be done. Patients who present with hematemesis may also have hemoptysis caused by aspiration; a chest x-ray film is indicated for these patients.

Patients with a history of thromboembolism may be taking anticoagulants. If so, clotting times should be checked, to rule this out as a cause of the hemoptysis.

Because of the exertion (forceful expiratory maneuvers) required by the patient during spirometry, measurement of lung volumes during periods of active hemoptysis is not recommended.

Treatment

Massive hemoptysis requires immediate treatment, surgery, or bronchoscopy. During this time, prevention of aspiration and keeping the airway open are of utmost importance. Endotracheal intubation may be necessary. Supplemental oxygen and replacement of blood loss may be necessary, depending on the ABG results and hemoglobin count.

Treatment of chronic hemoptysis is directed toward the underlying cause. When the cause is inflammation, as in chronic bronchitis, TB, and bronchiectasis, the patient must be educated to stop smoking, comply with use of prescribed medications (e.g., antibiotics, bronchodilators), perform pulmonary toilet (breathe deeply and clear the lungs) regularly, and avoid exposure to second-hand smoke and other noxious agents that might precipitate cough.

Education of the patient and family regarding the causes of the hemoptysis is essential. The patient needs to know what factors may precipitate the hemoptysis and how it can be prevented. The patient should be taught to note any change in the color, amount, and consistency of the blood expectorated. Any sudden increase should be reported to the health-care provider immediately for prompt medical attention.

Common Problems

Asthma

Asthma is a chronic, inflammatory, obstructive disease of the airways. It may occur at any age and may be characterized by wheezing (airways spasm), tightness in the chest, breathlessness (dyspnea), and cough. The signs and symptoms may remit spontaneously or exacerbate in response to intrinsic (stress) or extrinsic (environmental) triggers. The severity of asthma is highly unpredictable, ranging from mild attack to complete airway obstruction and death.

Epidemiology and Causes

Asthma affects more than an estimated 100 million people worldwide, and the numbers are increasing rapidly. In the United States, more than 31 million Americans have been diagnosed with asthma at some point in their lives. African Americans have asthma-related mortality rates that are higher than the rates for Caucasians. Despite newer anti-asthmatic drugs, asthma is responsible for more than 134 million days of restricted activity and about half a million hospitalizations annually. In the United States, 5500 deaths each year are attributable to asthma. Increases in the prevalence of and mortality associated with asthma in the last decade, despite pharmacologic advances, led to the formation in the early 1990s of the National Education and Prevention Program (NAEPP) by the NHLBI of the National Institutes of Health (NIH). Publication of the Expert Panel Report: Guidelines for the Diagnosis and Management of Asthma has led to an increased emphasis on patient education and self-management. The goals are to decrease the mortality and morbidity associated with asthma and to help patients with asthma to improve their quality of life.

Although the exact cause is unknown, three principal triggers for exacerbations of asthma have been identified:

- Allergens and environmental factors: Allergens may include inhaled substances, such as molds, pollens, dust, animal danders, cosmetics, and tobacco smoke; food additives with sulfite (preservative) agents; and medications, especially beta-blockers and aspirin or aspirin-containing drugs.
- Infections: Upper respiratory infections (URIs) are common precursors to an asthma attack. Viral infections commonly precede an asthma episode.
- Psychologic factors: Stressful events at work or home or a series of crises may precipitate an asthma attack. Many times the stressors may be overlooked or dismissed.

Inflammation of the airways contributes to bronchial hyperreactivity, airflow limitation, and the resultant characteristic signs and symptoms of asthma: wheezing, breathlessness, chest tightness, and cough. The stage is then set for acute bronchoconstriction, airway edema, mucus-plug formation, and airway narrowing and bronchial obstruction.

Pathophysiology

Asthma is a chronic inflammatory disease characterized by reversible, hyper-reactivity of the bronchi and bronchioles to a variety of stimuli. Genetic predisposition, allergy, environmental factors, stress, and infectious agents are factors that play a role in the etiology of asthma. Immunologically mediated inflammation, the major pathologic mechanism of this disease, involves mast cells, eosinophils, lymphocytes, neutrophils, and macrophages, which may directly infiltrate the airway at both smooth muscle and basement membrane layers. These cells release a variety of mediators that stimulate bronchoconstriction, vasodilation, edema formation, and increased mucus production, including histamine, interleukins, leukotrienes, tumor necrosis factor (TNF), bradykinin, thromboxanes, fibroblast growth factor, and prostaglandins.

In particular, CD4+ T helper (Th) cells bearing a Th2 phenotype (predominantly humorally mediated immunity) and resistant to apoptotic killing produce interleukin (IL)-3, IL-4, IL-5, and granulocyte-macrophage colony-stimulating factor (GM-CSF) after being stimulated by the offending allergen, which, in turn, upregulates the allergic response and airway hypersensitivity. Th1 T cells (predominantly cell-mediated immunity) have been implicated to a lesser extent. Eosinophils are a rich source of leukotrienes that directly cause contraction of bronchial smooth muscle and increase vascular permeability. Activated B lymphocytes transform into plasma cells, synthesizing large amounts of IgE antibody that binds and activates tissue mast cells and eosinophils. Mast cell-bound IgE molecules then become cross-linked by environmental allergen, which activates histamine release and further IL-4 and IL-5 production, thereby provoking bronchial smooth muscle contraction and vasodilation.

With each acute exacerbation of asthma, inflammatory mediators incite a structural remodeling of the airways. The alveoli remain largely unaffected, as this is not a parenchymal disease. Rather, airway remodeling entails thickening of the bronchial and bronchiolar mucosa, submucosa, and smooth muscle layers which contributes to the persistence of disease. Increased collagen is deposited below the basement membrane, while the loose areolar connective tissue found between epithelial and smooth muscle layers also hypertrophies. Therefore, prevention of acute episodes, which minimizes the amount of remodeling, is key to the proper treatment of asthma.

Asthma is an obstructive pulmonary disease with hypoxia as the universal finding during acute exacerbations. With acute bronchospasm, residual volume increases in the lungs, and peak expiratory flow rate diminishes. Inflammation and constriction of the bronchioles increase airway resistance, decrease inspiratory capacity and expiratory volumes, and lead to ventilation–perfusion mismatching and altered arterial blood gas concentrations. As a result of hyperventilation, respiratory alkalosis and hypocapnea are common findings with each episode. As an acute attack resolves, narrowing in the larger airways tends to reverse first, while the peripheral airways remain most constricted. If such an attack progresses, however, and fails to reverse, respiratory acidosis and an elevated arterial carbon dioxide concentration typically result, signaling impending respiratory failure. Indeed, severe irreversible bronchoconstriction and inflammation, termed *status asthmaticus*, can be fatal.

Clinical Presentation

The clinical presentation varies and depends on whether the patient is currently experiencing an acute attack or is seeking help to manage chronic asthma. It is importanat to note that not all people with asthma wheeze, and that not everyone who wheezes has asthma.

Subjective

During an acute attack, the patient may present with a complaint of breathlessness and may be unable to talk or may be able only to blurt out short sentences. There may be profuse sweating and a complaint of air hunger. In patients who are severely obstructed there may be no wheezing; only cough may be present.

The patient may present complaining of wheezing, persistent and recurrent cough, difficulty breathing, and/or tightness in the chest, particularly at night or in the early morning. Endurance problems during exercise may occur. Any single symptom or combination may occur and symptoms are usually worse at night. The disease spectrum varies from a few mild episodes in a lifetime to daily debilitating symptoms. Food additives, particularly metabisulfite, certain dairy products, and, for some individuals, monosodium glutamate, may also cause symptoms. An extreme emotional state such as excessive laughing and/or crying may precipitate or exacerbate an attack.

Objective

Reversible airflow limitation and diurnal variation as measured by peak flow meter are objective signs and symptoms of asthma. Variability between morning and evening peak expiratory flow (PEF) may reflect airway hyper-responsiveness and indicate asthma instability and severity. Nasal discharge, mucosal swelling, frontal tenderness, nasal polyps, and allergic "shiners"—dark discoloration beneath both eyes—should be noted. The clinician should also check for manifestations of allergic skin conditions such as eczema. Wheezing during forced exhalation is no longer considered a reliable indicator. It may be absent between attacks and may be obscured during acute attacks related to diminished breath sounds.

Audible inspiratory and expiratory wheezing may be heard. The patient may be using the accessory muscles of breathing (scalene and sternocleidomastoid) and sitting upright. Auscultation of the chest may reveal inspiratory and expiratory wheezes.

Diagnostic Reasoning

Expiratory airflow measurements are essential to the differential diagnosis of asthma. The essential elements to consider in making the diagnosis of asthma are listed in Table 8.1.

Differentiating asthma from other diseases is usually not difficult, particularly with the aid of pulmonary function tests (PFTs), a complete history, and laboratory test results. Spirometry is recommeded for the diagnosis of asthma. A very common feature of asthma is nocturnal awakening with one or more of the following symptoms: dyspnea, cough, and wheezing. Persistent wheezing localized to one area of the lung, with paroxysms of cough, is indicative of endobronchial disease such as foreign body aspiration, neoplasm, or bronchial stenosis. Acute left ventricular heart failure may initially present as asthma (wheezing), but the findings of moist, basilar crackles, gallop rhythms, and other signs of heart failure exclude the diagnosis of asthma.

Allergic rhinitis and eczema often accompany a diagnosis of asthma. Concurrent treatment for these conditions is critical. Effective treatment of allergic rhinnitis (discussed in Chapter 7) is critical as another mode to prevent triggering acute asthma attacks.

Table 8.1 Essential Elements to Consider When Diagnosing Asthma

History	• Cough (especially nocturnal) • Recurrent wheeze (absence does not rule out asthma) • Recurrent episodic dyspnea • Recurrent chest tightness
Symptoms worsen in relation to specific factors	• Airborne chemicals or dust • Animals with fur or feathers • Changes in weather • Exercise • Gastroesophageal reflux • Sensitivity to ASA, other NSAIDs & sulfites • Dust mites in house (mattresses, furniture, carpets) • Menses • Mold/pollen • Nighttime (patient awakens) • Nonselective beta blockers • Pollen • Smoke (tobacco, wood, etc.) • Strong emotional expression (laughing or crying hard) • Viral infection/rhinitis/sinusitis
Reversible (at least partially) airflow limitations with diurnal variability	• Variation in PEFR of at least 20% between first morning measurement (before taking an inhaled, short-acting beta-adrenergic agoinst) and early afternoon measurement (after using the inhaler)
Exclusion of alternate diagnosis	

Diagnostic Tests

To establish the diagnosis of asthma, episodic symtoms of airflow obstruction must be present, airflow obstruction must be at least partially reversible, and the provider attempts to rule out any alternative diagnoses. Spirometry measurements are helpful in diagnosing and then in evaluating the management of the disease. Forced vital capacity (FVC) and forced expiratory volume in 1 second (FEV_1) are helpful measurements. Pre- and postbronchodilator PFTs, including spirometry and diffusing capacitiy, to determine the response to bronchodilators are essential in the differential diagnosis and subsequent management of asthma. The diagnosis is made by demonstrating the reversibility of the airway obstruction from the pre- and post-PFTs. Reversibility is defined as a 15 percent or greater increase in the FEV_1 after two puffs of a beta-adrenergic agonist have been inhaled. When spirometry is nondiagnostic, bronchial provocation testing may be useful with histamine, methacholine, or exercise

A chest x-ray film may show only hyerinflation, but may incude thickening of the bronchial wall and diminished peripheral lung vascular shadows.

ABG analysis is included in the initial workup to establish a baseline and to determine the degree of hypoxemia and the need for supplemental oxygen. The results of the ABG analysis and spirometry, along with the clinical history and findings on exam, are triangulated to classify the severity of the asthma, as shown in Table 8.2.

A CBC, with special attention to the sedimentation rate and eosinophil count, is done. Levels of nasal

Table 8.2 Classification of Asthma Severity

Classification	Clinical Features Before Treatment	Daily Medication Required to Maintain Control
Mild intermittent	• Intermittent symptoms less than once a week, brief exacerbations (lasting from a few hours to a few days)* • Nighttime asthma symptoms less than twice a month • Asymptomatic and normal PEF between exacerbations • PEFR or FEV_1: >80% predicted • PFT variability >20%	• Intermittent reliever medication taken as needed only; inhaled short-acting beta-2 agonist or cromolyn before exercise or allergen exposure • Intensity of treatment depends on severity of exacerbation • No daily medication needed
Mild persistent	• Symptoms more than 2× per week but less than 1× per day, may be several times at night/month • Exacerbations may affect activity and sleep • Nighttime asthma symptoms more than twice a month • PEFR or FEV_1: >80% predicted • PFT variability 20%–30%	• One daily controller medication: low-dose inhaled corticosteroids (ICs); cromolyn/nedocromil; leukotriene modifiers • Inhaled beta-2 agonists as needed
Moderate persistent	• Symptoms daily, but not continual, >1 week, nighttime • Exacerbations affect activity and sleep • Daily use of inhaled short-acting beta-2 agonist • PEFR or FEV_1: 60%–80% predicted • PFT variability >30%	• Daily controller medications: combination inhaled medium-dose corticosteroid (ICs) and long-acting bronchodilator (especially for nighttime symptoms); cromolyn-nedocromil; leukotriene modifiers
Severe persistent	• Continuous daily symptoms, frequent nighttime symptoms • Frequent exacerbations • Physical activities limited by asthma • PEFR or FEV_1: ≤60% predicted • PFT variability >30%	• Inhaled beta-2 agonists as needed • Multiple daily controller medications: combination high-dose inhaled corticosteroid, and long-acting bronchodilator, cromolyn/nedocromil; leukotriene modifiers; may need long-term corticosteroids • Inhaled beta-2 agonist as needed

Source: National Asthma Education and Prevention Program (NAEPP): Expert panel report: Guidelines for the diagnosis and management of asthma update on selected topics. U.S. Department of Health and Human Services, Public Health Service, National Institutes of Health (NIH), National Heart, Lung, and Blood Institute (NHBLI), Bethesda, Md: NIH publication 02-5074, 2003.

*The presence of one of the features of severity is sufficient to place a patient in that category.

eosinophils, serum eosinophils, and IgE are assessed to determine the allergic status of the patient. Intradermal skin testing may be indicated if the allergic status is significant.

Infections often precede an asthma attack. If infection is suspected (because of a productive cough with colored sputum), a sputum test for culture and sensitivity should be done.

When persistent asthma is present, skin testing may be useful to determine sensitivity to environmental allergens.

Differential Diagnosis

Airflow obstruction may result from foreign body aspiration or viral infections, as well as a variety of underlying pulmonary infections, such as aspergillosis, TB, hypersensitivity pneumonitis, or habitual cough. Hyperventilation syndrome, mitral valve prolapse, recurrent pulmonary emboli, CHF, and chronic obstructive lung disease may mimic asthma. In addition, for some sensitive patients, cough may be secondary to use of certain drugs, such as ACE inhibitors, beta-blockers, aspirin, and nonsteroidal anti-inflammatory drugs (NSAIDs). One key feature to making the diagnosis of asthma is the reversibility of the phenomenon.

Management

An aggressive approach to asthma management is recommended to improve symptoms in the short term, prevent recurrence of symptoms, and/or manage a potentially chronic problem—all with the goal of improving the patient's quality of life by achieving and maintaining control of symptoms. The principles of management include:

1. Identification of factors that exacerbate the condition
2. Daily monitoring of peak expiratory flow with a symptom record (see Asthma Attack Trigger Diary)
3. Written instructions on managing an acute asthma attack
4. Intensive education and follow-up, emphasizing joint decision making

Initial and subsequent management of asthma is aimed at first removing the triggers or precipitants that can be identified. The step therapy approach is a guide to assist the provider in working with the patient to make the best treatment decisions. As a rule, the highest appropriate step should be used to gain early control. The therapy should be "stepped up" if control is not maintained. The clinicain should always review the patient's medication technique, adherence, and control of triggers at each visit. The stepwise approach, according to the severity of the asthma, is shown in the Treatment Flowchart 8.1.

Asthma management can require daily pharmacotherapeutics with inhaled steroids, long-acting beta-2 agonists, and/or leukotriene antagonists. Asthma may be present in the older adult. In patients with other comorbidities, management may be complicated. Daily medications for those with mildly persistent to severe asthma may significantly reduce and control symptoms, leading to improved quality of life.

In the management of chronic asthma, ABG analysis and PFTs are done periodically to measure how well the patient is responding to treatment. The patient can be taught to use a hand-held peak flow meter to measure the peak expiratory flow rate (PEFR) and gauge response to treatment. Several peak flow rate readings should be done when the patient is stable, to establish a baseline (or "personal best"). This baseline can be used as a benchmark for guiding the therapy. Once the patient's condition is stabilized, the daily PEFR monitoring can be done by the patient. If the PEFR reading is less than 80 percent of the patient's personal best, adjustments in medications or lifestyle may be necessary.

Inhaled corticosteroids are the treatment of choice, above other forms of inhaled meds and theophylline. Recent genetic and epidemiological studies appear to imply that certain individuals (especially of African American ethnicity) have a negative reaction to long-term beta-agonist bronchodilators, such as salmeterol. These individuals seem to do worse on long-term beta-agonist therapy. Salmeterol (Serevent) is no longer used as a single agent because of safety concerns regarding increased morbidity and mortality when used without an accompanying steroid. When used in combination with an inhaled corticosteroid (Advair Discus), it is extremely effective.

The step therapy approach is a guide to assist the provider in working with the patient to make the best treatment decisions. As a rule, the highest appropriate step should be used to gain early control. The therapy should be "stepped up" if control is not maintained. The clinician should always review the patient's medication technique, adherence, and control of triggers at each visit (Beclovent) to the lungs rather than the oropharynx (Drugs Commonly Prescribed 8.1).

Follow-Up and Referral

Step down therapy gradually if review of patient's status at 1- to 6-month intervals suggests reduction of treatment is warranted. Smoking cessation for patients with asthma is a must. (For more information on smoking cessation, see Smoking Addiction in this chapter.) The patient should avoid exposure to second-hand smoke. Family members also need to be educated about the hazards of second-hand smoke. Regular visits to their primary-care provider can be combined with appropriate referrals to specialists, as necessary.

The use of immunotherapy in asthma remains controversial and its effectiveness has not been well established. For most patients, avoidance of the allergens and triggers, along with the appropriate use of medications, is adequate therapy. If avoidance of certain allergens is impossible and medications fail, referral to an allergist for immunotherapy may be indicated. However, unless the patient's symptoms are exacerbated by exposure to an allergen and the allergen can be confirmed by skin-prick testing, it is unlikely that immunotherapy will be effective.

Treatment Flow Chart 8.1 Asthma

Step 1: Intermittent Asthma

Controller

Daily medications:

- None needed

Reliever

- Short-acting bronchodilator (inhaled beta-2 agonist as needed for symptoms), but less than once a week
- Intensity of treatment will depend on severity of exacerbation
- Inhaled beta-2 agonist or cromolyn before exercise or exposure to allergen

↓

Step 2: Mild Persistent Asthma

Controller

Daily medications:

- Either inhaled corticosteroid 200-500 μg, cromoglycate, nedocromil, or sustained-release theophylline
- Leukotriene receptor antagonist (Singulair)
- If needed, increase inhaled corticosteroids (up to 800 μg, if inhaled corticosteroids currently equal 500 μg), or add long-acting bronchodilator, especially for nighttime symptoms (long-acting inhaled beta-2 agonist, sustained-release theophylline, or long-acting oral beta-2 agonist)

Reliever

- Short-acting bronchodilator (inhaled beta-2 agonist as needed for symptoms), not to exceed three to four times a day

↓

Step 3: Moderate Persistent Asthma

Controller

Daily medications:

- Combination inhaled corticosteroid (Advair) and long-acting beta-2 agonist
- Inhaled corticosteroid 800-2000 μg, and
- Long-acting bronchodilator, especially for nighttime symptoms (long-acting inhaled beta-2 agonist, sustained-release theophylline, or long-acting oral beta-2 agonist)

Reliever

- Short-acting bronchodilator (inhaled beta-2 agonist as needed for symptoms), not to exceed three to four times in 1 day

↓

Step 4: Severe Persistent Asthma

Controller

Daily medications:

- Combination inhaled corticosteroid (Advair) and long-acting beta-2 agonist or
- Inhaled corticosteroid 800-2000 μg, and
- Long-acting bronchodilator (either beta-2 agonist, sustained-release theophylline, and/or long-acting oral beta-2 agonist), and
- Oral corticosteroid (long-term)

Reliever

- Short-acting bronchodilator (inhaled beta-2 agonist as needed for symptoms)

Step Up: If control is not achieved, consider step up, but first review patient medication technique, compliance, and environmental control (avoid all allergens or other trigger factors).

Step Down: Review treatment every 3 to 6 months. If control is sustained for at least 3 months, a gradual stepwise reduction in treatment may be viable.

Source: Adapted from the National Heart, Lung, and Blood Institute: Expert panel report 2: guidelines for the diagnosis and management of asthma. USDHHS, July 1997 (currrent as of summer 2005).

Drugs Commonly Prescribed 8.1: Asthma

Drug	Indication and Formulation	Dosage	Comments
Short-acting beta-2 agonists Provide smooth muscle relaxation	First-line defense for acute attack; may be used prophylactically prn before exercise. Increased need (usage) indicates need to change treatment regimen.		Adverse reactions: Tachycardia, palpitations, tremor, hypokalemia Use with caution in elderly patients.
Albuterol (Ventolin, Proventil)	Syrup: 2 mg/5 mL MDI (metered-dosage inhaler) 90 μg/puff DPI (dry powder inhaler) 200 μg/puff Nebulizer 5 mg/mL (0.5%)	2–4 mg PO 3–4 times daily (tid–qid). May increase dose gradually to maximum dose of 24 mg/day. 2 puffs q4–6h prn 2 puffs tid–qid prn, 2 puffs 5 min before exercise 1.25–5 mg (0.25–1 cc) in 2–3 cc of N/S q4–8h; may be mixed with cromolyn or ipratropium nebulizer solution	As above
Pirbuterol (Maxair)	Tablets, 2 mg, 4 mg MDI (metered-dosage inhaler)	2–4 mg PO q6–8h 200 μg/puff 2 puffs tid–qid prn	As above
Terbutaline (Brethine, tablets, SC)	Tablets Injectable—subcutaneous (SC)	2.5–5 mg tid at 6-hour intervals Inject 0.25 mg into lateral deltoid. May repeat after 15–30 min; maximum: 0.5 mg/q4h	Antagonized by beta-blockers For acute attack
Long-acting beta agonists	Appropriate for patients with moderate to severe asthma Use before sleep to prevent nocturnal attacks. May be used to prevent exercise-induced asthma.		Should not be used as a rescue inhaler. Should not be used in place of anti-inflammatory therapy.
Albuterol sulfate extended relief (Proventil Repetab)	Tablets	4-mg tabs q12h	
Anticholinergics	Used in conjunction with beta-2 agonist to increase overall effect		Not for primary treatment of acute attack.
Ipratropium bromide (Atrovent)	MDI (metered-dosage inhaler): 18 μg/puff Nebulizer: 0.02% (500 μg in 2.5 mL) for oral inhalation	2 puffs qid Maximum: 12 puffs/day 500 μg tid–qid	Do not give to patients with glaucoma or BPH. May precipitate HA, palpitations.
Combination beta-2 agonist and anticholinergic	May use when second aerosol bronchodilator needed		When used in combination, overall effect is increased.
Combivent	Ipratropium bromide 18 μg and albuterol (as sulfate) 90 μg MDI (metered-dosage inhaler)	2 puffs/qid Maximum: 12 puffs/day	Use with caution with other anticholinergics and sympathomimetics.

Drug	Indication and Formulation	Dosage	Comments
Leukotriene receptor antagonists	Long-term control. Prophylaxis and treatment of chronic asthma—NOT for acute attack.		NOT FOR ACUTE ATTACK
Montelukast (Singulair)	Prophylaxis and mild persistant cases 4- and 5-mg tablets Oral granules 4 mg/packet	Chewable tablets For both—10 mg/night	Monitor with potent CYP450 indices
Zafirlukast (Accolate)	Prophylaxis and chronic treatment of asthma 10-mg and 20-mg tablets	20 mg twice daily	Take at least 1 h before meals OR 2 h after meals
Inhaled nonsteroidal anti-inflammatories	Asthma prophylaxis; prevention of bronchoconstriction before known precipitant (e.g., exercise). Effect lasts for 1–2 h. Maintenance therapy		NOT FOR TREATMENT OF ACUTE ATTACK. AVOID ABRUPT CESSATION. MONITOR RENAL AND HEPATIC FUNCTION.
Cromolyn sodium (Intal)	MDI (metered-dosage inhaler): 0.8 mg/puff Nebulizer: 20 g/2 mL	2–4 puffs tid–qid 2 puffs 10–60 min before exposure to precipitants 20 mg administered by power-operated nebulizer qid	As above Adverse reactions: Bronchospasm, throat irritation, bad taste. Acts as a mast cell stabilizer.
Nedocromil sodium (Tilade)	MDI (metered-dosage inhaler): 1.75 mg/puff	2–4 puffs qid	As above
Inhaled corticosteroids	Maintenance treatment of asthma and prophylactic treatment in asthma		
Beclomethasone (Beclodisk)	Not for acute attack 40 or 80 μg/puff	2 puffs tid–qid or 4 puffs bid for severe asthma; maximum: 10 puffs/day	Rinse mouth after use. Avoid excessive use.
Budesonide (Pulmicort)	Dry powder delivery system 200 or 400 μg inhaler	1–2 puffs 1–2 times/day (800 μg max per day)	Monitor infections; susceptible to oral candidiasis. Rinse mouth after use. Avoid excessive use.
Fluticasone (Flovent)	MDI: 44, 110, 220 μg/puff DPI: 50-, 100-, 250-mcg dose	Dosage range from 88 μg bid to 440 μg bid Dosage range: from 2 to 6 inhalations (50 mg) up to 500 mcg twice daily	Monitor infections; susceptible to oral candidiasis. Rinse mouth after use. Avoid excessive use.
Flunisolide (AeroBid, Bronalide)	250 μg/puff (MDI)	Initially, 2 puffs bid; maximum: 8 puffs/day	Has mint flavor. Contains menthol.
Triamcinolone (Azmacort)	MDI 100 μg/inhalation	2 puffs bid–qid; maximum: 12 puffs/day	

(continued)

Drugs Commonly Prescribed 8.1: Asthma (continued)

Drug	Indication and Formulation	Dosage	Comments
Combination inhaled corticosteroid and long-acting beta-2 agonist			
Fluticasone and Salmeterol (Advair Diskus)	Moderate to severe persistent asthma	100, 250, or 500 μg fluticasone per dose plus 50 μg salmeterol per dose dry powder 1 puff twice daily	
Systemic corticosteroids	For long-term treatment of severe persistent asthma. Short courses or "bursts" effective for establishing control when initiating therapy or during a period of gradual deterioration.		
Methylprednisolone (Medrol) Prednisolone Prednisone (Deltasone)		Give 7.5–60.0 mg/day in a single dose or qid as needed for control. Short "burst" 40–60 mg/day as a single dose or in 2 divided doses over 3–10 days; tapering not necessary.	Use with caution in patients with TB, hypothyroidism, cirrhosis, ulcerative colitis, etc. MAY MASK INFECTION, HYPOKALEMIA, HYPERNATREMIA; GLUCOSE INTOLERANCE; BONE DEMINERALIZATION
Methylxanthine Theophylline (Bronkodyl, Theobid, Uniphyl), Aminophylline (Phyllocontin)	Long-acting bronchodilator for use in moderate and severe persistent asthma. Occasionally used as mild persistent asthma (step 2). Advantage is that bid level can be measured and theophylline may have some anti-inflammatory properties.	Loading dose: 6 mg/kg, then 2 mg/kg q8h for 2 doses, then 1–2 mg/kg q12h for maintenance dose To maintain steady state, keep serum concentration levels between 5 and 15 μg/mL	Not for use in acute attack. Many drug interactions; contraindicated in seizure disorders, arrhythmias, active peptic ulcer disease. **Adverse reactions:** Nausea, headaches, irritability, restlessness, convulsions, diuresis

Patient Education

A list of reasonable expectations (Table 8.3) for patients with asthma should be reviewed with the patient and family. If there are problems in certain areas, spend time exploring potential triggers that might be removed or problematic areas such as noncompliance or improper use of inhalants.

The patient and family should be educated about the following areas for self-care management:

1. Basic asthma facts
2. How to recognize early symptoms of an exacerbation and how to initiate a predetermined plan of action
3. Role of medications (long-acting and short-term)
4. Skills for inhaler (spacer) and daily peak flow-meter monitoring (for patients with moderate to severe persistent asthma). While some medications have "built-in" spacers, spacers are universally recommended for metered-dose inhalers (MDIs) to obtain maximum benefit.
5. Use of a nebulizer if necessary. Nebulizers may be necessary when patients cannot take in adequate breaths.
6. Environmental control
7. Avoidance measures
8. Importance of pneumococcal and annual influenza vaccination

Patient and family education is essential for control of triggers and recognition of warning signals. An Asthma

Table 8.3 **Reasonable Expectations for Patients with Asthma**

When entering into a treatment plan, the patient with asthma is entitled to expect to:
- Be able to participate fully in any activity.
- Be able to sleep through the night.
- Be free of severe symptoms day and night.
- Be satisfied with asthma care.
- Have the best possible pulmonary function.
- Need fewer or no emergency visits or hospitalizations due to asthma.
- Not miss work or school because of asthma.
- Use fewer medications with minimal adverse effects.

The provider is responsible for the following:
- Asking patients about their concerns and issues at each visit.
- Continually teaching and reinforcing key educational points.
- Ensuring ongoing and open communication with the patient and family.
- Reviewing short-term goals agreed on at the initial visit.
- Reviewing the asthma action plan for worsening symptoms and exacerbations.
- Reviewing the daily self-management plan and steps the patient needs to take.
- Supplying patients with appropriate educational materials for self-management and prevention.

Attack Trigger Diary, such as the one shown in Table 8.4, may be used. Reinforcement of medication use and proper use of the hand-held flow meter should be reviewed at each visit. It should be mentioned that rescue courses of systemic glucocorticoids may be needed at times to prevent acute attacks. Once patients have been followed for some time and have learned self-management, most patients with no cognitive impairment can be instructed on the proper use of glucocorticoids to prevent acute attacks.

The patient and family should be educated to the full extent possible to permit self-management and prevention of acute fatal attacks. Although asthma is a chronic dis-

Table 8.4 **Asthma Attack Trigger Diary**

Date, Time, and Location of the Attack	What Precipitated the Attack? (suspected trigger)	What Relieved the Attack? (medications, etc.)	Peak Flow Meter Reading

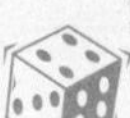

RISK FACTORS 8.1

Risk Factors for Fatal Asthma

- Comorbidity (cardiovascular or pulmonary disease such as COPD)
- Current use of or recent withdrawal from systemic glucocorticoids
- Difficulty perceiving airflow obstruction or its severity
- History of sudden severe exacerbations
- Hospitalization or emergency care for asthma within past month
- Illicit drug use
- Low socioeconomic status and urban residence
- Prior intubation for asthma
- Sensitivity to *Alternaria*
- Serious psychiatric disease or psychosocial problems
- Three or more emergency visits for asthma in the past year
- Two or more hospitalizations for asthma in the past year
- Use of three or more canisters of inhaled, short-acting beta-2-adrenergic agonists per month

ease, patients occasionally do die from an acute asthma episode. The risk factors for fatal asthma are included in Risk Factors 8.1.

Patients with any of the risk factors need some additional teaching time so they can learn self-management techniques to learn to reduce risk factors to the extent possible. An algorithm for self-management that is similar to the one shown in the Treatment Flowchart 8.2 should be reviewed the patient and family. It is extremely important that thc paticnt be trained to use the hand-held flow meter and learn to determine the predicted (personal best) PEFR. During exacerbations, the patient should compare a current reading to the baseline PEFR as a guide to determine how severe the attack is and to gauge medication use accordingly.

The value of the algorithm as a guide for the patient and family as to when to get emergency help should be emphasized. A family member should be educated as to how to handle an acute attack, in case the patient becomes severely hypoxic and cognitively impaired.

A caring relationship between the provider, the patient, and family may prove pivotal to effective disease management and improved quality of life. Self-care is an essential component of treatment.

Scant data exist on the prevalence of complementary therapy for asthma. One national survey study estimated that 59 percent of 4741 respondents in the United Kingdom had tried some form of complementary therapy. The three adjunct therapies most frequently used in the United Kingdom were breathing techniques, homeopathy, and herbal preparations. Even less research exists on the effectiveness of these therapies, so patients and families should be cautioned about their judicious use. The use of breathing exercises and devices such as the inspiratory pressure threshold device has been studied in COPD but not in asthma. More research is needed in this area.

Nutritional therapies have been used in the treatment of asthma. It is known that certain foods may precipitate an asthma flare. To treat this, Moses Maimonides, the noted thirteenth-century physician, prescribed a spicy, herbal mixture of chicken broth that contained herbs such as fennel, parsley, oregano, mint, and onion. Hydration from such a robust broth is also a helpful component in asthma treatment. Onions and garlic have been known to have some protective effect against allergic reactions.

Strong coffee was a widely used treatment for asthma in eighteenth-century Europe and continues to be used as an effective bronchodilator today. Although drinking teas has never been particularly favored as an asthma treatment, tea leaves were the original source of theophylline, whose name means "tea leaf."

Chronic Bronchitis and Emphysema (Chronic Obstructive Pulmonary Disease [COPD])

There are two primary forms of lung disease—obstructive and restrictive. *Obstructive lung diseases* are those in which the expiratory flow rate is impaired. *Restrictive lung diseases* are those in which the lung volumes are reduced due to musculoskeletal disorders, tumors, lung resection, or ILD. Obstructive lung diseases are further classified as reversible (such as asthma) and irreversible (such as chronic bronchitis and emphysema). The American Thoracic Society (ATS) has defined *chronic bronchitis* as a clinical disorder characterized by excessive mucus secretion in the bronchial tree. It is

TREATMENT FLOWCHART 8.2

SELF-MANAGEMENT OF ASTHMA EXACERBATIONS

Assess Severity:

- Measure PEFR: >50% personal best or predicted value suggests severe exacerbation
- Note signs and symptoms: cough, wheezes, chest tightness; accessory muscle use and suprasternal retractions suggest severe exacerbations

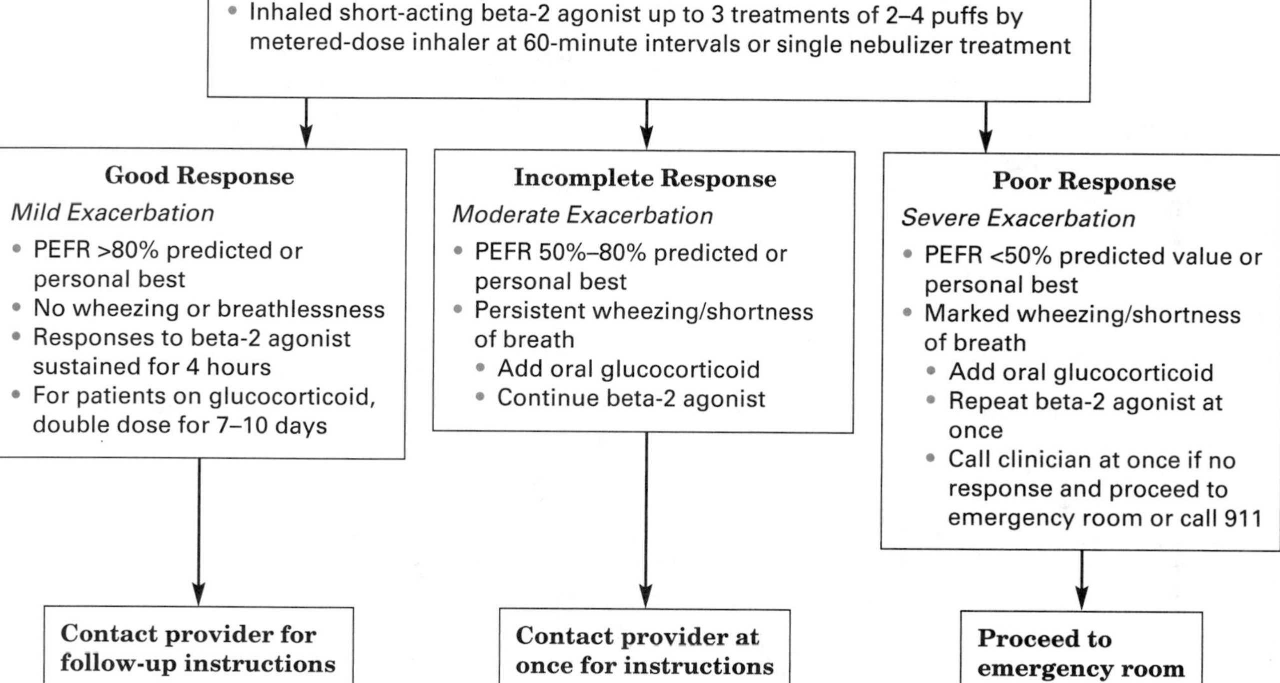

manifested by chronic or recurrent cough (with or without sputum production), present on most days for a minimum of 3 months of the year, for at least 2 successive years. In addition, dyspnea with or without wheezing is present. While over 14 million Americans have been diagnosed with COPD, an equal number are probably afflicted but not diagnosed.

Epidemiology and Causes

Chronic bronchitis and emphysema are grouped together as *chronic obstructive pulmonary diseases* (COPD). The ATS defines COPD as a disease state characterized by the presence of airflow obstruction due to chronic bronchitis or emphysema. Asthma is not classified as COPD, but is sometimes referred to as a reversible obstructive condition, whereas emphysema is irreversible. Chronic bronchitis is usually irreversible, but it may be partially reversible if there is a bronchospastic component and a significant response to bronchodilators. The prevalence and mortality rates for chronic bronchitis and emphysema increase with age. The COPD death rate for women almost tripled between 1980 and 2000. More women than men died of COPD in 2000. COPD is the fourth leading cause of death in the world and projected to be the third leading cause of death by 2020. There are almost 120,000 deaths due to COPD annually in the United States

Morbidity and mortality are higher in persons with low incomes and less education. It is difficult to estimate the prevalence of chronic bronchitis because there is considerable overlap of conditions: Some patients have all

RISK FACTORS 8.2

Risk Factors for COPD

Established risks:
- Age
- Male gender
- Cigarette smoking
- Reduced lung function
- Occupational exposures
- Air pollution
- $Alpha_1$-antitrypsin phenotypes

Probable or possible risks:
- Infections of the respiratory tract
- Allergic conditions
- Bronchial reactivity
- Climate
- Poor socioeconomic resources
- Alcohol intake
- Diet and nutrition
- ABO, ABH secretor, cell phenotypes
- Impaired immune function
- Familial factors

three (asthma, chronic bronchitis, and emphysema), and some have two of the three conditions.

Several studies have established certain predisposing and risk factors for morbidity and mortality from COPD. The established and probable risk factors for COPD are shown in Risk Factors 8.2.

Cigarette smoking is responsible for 80 to 90 percent of the cases of COPD, and is also the risk factor most amenable to modification for preventing or deterring the development of COPD. Educational intervention at an early age can help reduce smoking and some other risk factors, such as occupational exposure, exposure to air pollution and allergens, and respiratory infections. If certain genetic risk factors are present, the patient should be educated about periodic baseline testing for pulmonary function and about routine checks to prevent respiratory infections and reduce risks to the extent possible. The probability of a person developing COPD within 10 years can be calculated using the Tecumseh Index, in which points are allotted for the three major risk factors of age, number of cigarettes smoked per day, and FEV_1 as a percentage of the value predicted. Stopping smoking at any age has some beneficial effect for lung function even though there may be permanent damage to lung tissue.

Pathophysiology

COPD is a progressive disease characterized by airflow limitation that is not fully reversible. The disease process involves a combination of the pathologic mechanisms of emphysema and chronic bronchitis. In addition, hyperreactivity of the airways is a common feature. Thus, COPD is a disease of both the lung parenchyma and the small airways (bronchioles).

Emphysema is characterized by destruction of alveolar walls due to an imbalance of proteinase–antiproteinase enzymatic activity. In healthy lung tissue, protective antiproteinases counteract protein-degrading enzymes secreted by white blood cells. Chronic inflammation, caused by long-term cigarette smoking or chronic exposure to lung irritants, for example, repeatedly recruits white blood cells to the alveoli. In contrast to the atopic processes of asthma, the lymphocytic infiltration of COPD consists predominantly of CD8+ T cells, rather than CD4+ T helper cells. Neutrophil and monocyte-/macrophage-derived proteinases progressively degrade the alveolar walls overcoming antiproteinase defenses. Overdistended, hyperinflated, less elastic alveoli are the result of the recurring injury over time. Weak elastic recoil of alveoli leads to air trapping, increased

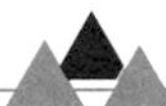

NURSING RESEARCH-BASED PRACTICE 8.1

Preparing Nurses for the Global Pandemic of Chronic Obstructive Pulmonary Disease

Kara, M: J Nurs Scholar 37:2, 127–133, 2005.

The purpose of this integrative review of the literature was to raise awareness of the global pandemic of chronic obstructive pulmonary disease (COPD), its multiple underlying causes, and how to fight it, with particular attention to needs in nursing education. The main underlying causes of COPD are both individual and environmental factors, and the disease usually results from an interaction between those two factors. The prevalence of COPD is highest in countries where cigarette smoking has been, or still is, very common, and it is lowest in countries where smoking is less common, or total tobacco consumption per person is low. COPD is to some extent a preventable disease especially by preventing exposure to tobacco smoke and to occupational dusts and chemicals including vapours, irritants, fumes, and indoor and outdoor air pollution. The main implication for nurses and nursing curricula is to expand the focus from the individual to include population-based intervention programs.

residual lung volume, reduced expiratory flow, and retained carbon dioxide. Individuals experience hypercapnea but can maintain adequate oxygenation early on in the disease process.

Desensitization of the central respiratory receptors to Pco_2 occurs with long-term hypercapnea. Pco_2 accumulation in the blood under normal circumstances, stimulates individuals to breath independently. However, persons who endure long-term states of hypercapnea lose this normal respiratory stimulus to breathe. Hypoxia becomes the stimulus for breathing instead of Pco_2. Hypoxia is sensed by peripheral chemoreceptors in the arteries, such as the carotid bodies. The individual who has endured hypercapnea for a prolonged period of time begins to rely on low oxygen levels to drive breathing. Consequently, supplemental oxygen must be used judiciously in these individuals because of their hypoxic drive to breathe. High levels of supplemental oxygen as well as respiratory depressants of any kind (e.g., sedatives, narcotics) can suppress the hypercapneic individual's hypoxic drive to breathe independently.

Cigarette smoking is the major environmental risk factor for development of COPD. Although smoking cessation slows progression of disease, reversal of pathologic changes does not occur. There is a proven causal relationship between cigarette smoking and COPD; however, there is marked variability in the pulmonary function of persons with similar smoking histories. This has led to investigation into genetic risk factors for COPD. One such genetic risk factor is alpha-1 antitrypsin deficiency. Alpha-1 antitrypsin is a major anti-proteinase enzyme that can counteract alveolar destruction. Individuals can inherit different genetic mutations that lead to variable degrees of deficiency of this enzyme. Individuals with complete absence of alpha-1 antitrypsin have an increased susceptibility to emphysema and develop the disease early in life.

Compared to emphysema, chronic bronchitis is the more common pathologic mechanism involved in COPD. Airflow obstruction in chronic bronchitis is caused by bronchiole edema, hyperplasia of mucus-producing goblet cells, and bronchiole smooth muscle hypertrophy. Clinically, chronic bronchitis, presents as a long-term cough or recurrent sputum production, primarily upon morning awakening, extending over 3 months for a period of at least 2 years. Individuals with hypoxia and cyanosis due to ventilatory obstruction and suboptimal oxygenation of the blood. In chronic bronchitis, long-term hypoxia leads to pulmonary vasoconstriction which can result in pulmonary hypertension. This increased pulmonary resistance against the right ventricle can lead to right ventricular failure or cor pulmonale. Chronic hypoxia also stimulates renal erythropoietin, which initiates and perpetuates red blood cell synthesis in the bone marrow, thereby increasing hemoglobin concentration and hematocrit.

Acute exacerbations of chronic bronchitis are highly characteristic of this disease. Increased purulent sputum production and worsened shortness of breath are the hallmark of such episodes, which may also be accompanied by fever and increased oxygen requirements for those patients on supplemental oxygen. While viral bronchitis requiring only supportive care is the most common etiology of such exacerbations, bacterial involvement must be considered with increased sputum production lasting over a week or new chest x-ray findings. *Streptococcus pneumoniae* is the most common agent, followed by *Haemophilus influenzae* and *Moraxella catarrhalis*, similar to the causative agents of sinusitis and community-acquired pneumonia. Antibacterial therapy is often instituted empirically, however, without the need for cultures or Gram stain evidence.

The respiratory symptoms of COPD logically follow patterns of pulmonary neuromuscular anatomy, as bronchiole smooth muscle is innervated by beta-2 adrenergic and cholinergic nerve receptors. The bronchiole constriction in COPD is largely cholinergically mediated. For this reason, blockade of cholinergic receptors by anticholinergic drugs enhances the ability of bronchioles to dilate in COPD. Increased mucous production is also counteracted by these agents. In contrast, beta-receptor activation mediates bronchodilation, as reflected in the therapeutic benefits of inhaled beta-agonist drugs. Inhaled and oral steroids, on the other hand, function by decreasing overall airway inflammation mediated largely by T cells.

There is a normal age-related decline in pulmonary function: The forced expiratory volume in 1 second (FEV_1) declines by 0.02 to 0.04 L per year. Cigarette smoking accelerates the decline by two- to threefold. Though smoking cessation slows the rate of decline, it will not reverse most pathologic changes. Pulmonary function patterns and physical findings for various pulmonary conditions are shown in Table 8.5. The PFT results reflect the underlying pathology of the condition.

It is common for patients to have mixed lung disease (both restrictive and obstructive). For example, patients with chronic bronchitis may also present with a restrictive ILD such as sarcoidosis. In cases like this, all lung volumes would be reduced, the diffusing capacity would be reduced, and the ABGs would be abnormal (showing hypoxemia and possibly carbon dioxide retention).

Age and FEV_1 are the strongest predictors for mortality in COPD (Table 8.6). High mortality rates occur when COPD is complicated by respiratory infection (acute bronchitis exacerbations) or cor pulmonale from chronic pulmonary hypertension. These conditions increase risk for ventilation–perfusion mismatch, hypoxemia, hypercapnea, respiratory acidosis, and respiratory failure.

Clinical Presentation

Subjective

The typical smoker who develops COPD may be asymptomatic for 10 to 20 years except for more frequent colds, persistent morning cough, and upper respiratory infections.

Table 8.5 Pulmonary Function and Physical Findings in Obstructive and Restrictive Lung Diseases

Parameters	Asthma	Chronic Bronchitis	Emphysema	Restrictive Disease
Forced vital capacity (FVC)	Normal	Normal to increased	Normal to increased	Decreased
Residual volume (RV)	Normal; increased during attacks	Increased	Increased	Decreased or normal
Total lung capacity (TLC)	Normal to increased	Normal	Normal to increased	Decreased
RV/TLC	Normal to increased	Increased	Increased	Normal
Expiratory flow rates	Normal to decreased	Normal to decreased	Normal to decreased	Normal to increased
FEV_1/FVC	Normal to decreased	Decreased	Decreased	Normal to increased
Bronchodilator response (% change)	>15%	0–15%	None	None
Diffusing capacity	Normal to increased	Normal to decreased	Decreased	Normal or decreased (depends on type of disease)
PaO_2	Normal; decreased during attack	Decreased	Normal in mild to moderate disease; decreased in severe disease	Normal or decreased
$PaCO_2$	First decreased, then increased during acute attack	Increased	Normal until advanced disease, then increased	Normal or decreased; increased in very advanced disease
Breath sounds	Marked decrease during acute attacks If FEV_1 = 0.5 L or less: absent	If FEV_1 = 1 L: barely audible		Normal or decreased in pneumonia, atelectasis
Crackles (rales)	Coarse crackles during infections	Coarse crackles during infections	No	Varies with type of restrictive disease
Wheezes (rhonchi)	High-pitched; continuous	Forced expiratory wheezes	No	No

Table 8.6 Severity of COPD Based on the Pulmonary Function Measures: Forced Expiratory Volume in One Second (FEV_1) and Forced Vital Capacity (FVC)

Stage 1: Mild COPD	$FEV_1 \geq 80\%$ predicted $FEV_1/FVC < 70\%$
Stage 2: Moderate COPD	$50\% \leq FEV_1 < 80\%$ $FEV_1/FVC < 70\%$
Stage 3: Severe COPD	$30\% \leq FEV_1 < 50\%$ $FEV_1/FVC < 70\%$
Stage 4: Very severe COPD	$FEV_1 < 30\%$ predicted or $FEV_1 < 50\%$ predicted with chronic respiratory failure* $FEV_1/FVC < 70\%$

*Respiratory failure is defined as $PaO_2 < 60$ mm Hg with or without $PaCO_2 > 50$ mm Hg while breathing room air.

Source: Adapted from Global Initiative for Chronic Obstructive Lung Disease (GOLD). Global strategy for the diagnosis, management, and prevention of chronic obstructive pulmonary disease, updated 2004. National Heart, Lung, and Blood Institute, World Health Organization.

Men, in particular, may wait until the dyspnea becomes severe before seeking medical help, or may seek help only when they need antibiotics for a chronic productive cough. They may ignore symptoms of fatigue, shortness of breath, and cough because of embarrassment. Older persons may attribute the shortness of breath and fatigue to functional decline related to aging. The onset of COPD is typically in the fifth decade or later with a 20-pack-year smoker (number of packs of cigarettes per day times number of years).

With advanced disease in which chronic bronchitis predominates, pulmonary hypertension may result from chronic alveolar hypoxia and cor pulmonale develops. Patients with these signs and symptoms are often called "blue bloaters" because of the edema and cyanosis that accompany their condition. A CBC may reveal polycythemia to compensate for the chronic hypoxemia.

Patients who primarily have emphysema ("pink puffers") have severe dyspnea but usually present with relatively normal ABGs that are maintained because of high minute ventilation. As the disease progresses, the dyspnea increases because the diffusing capacity is severely reduced. These patients often appear very thin and may have the typical "barrel chest" resulting from hyperinflation.

A patient with an acute exacerbation of chronic bronchitis may present with cough and increased sputum that is thick and colored (yellow, brown, gray, or green); fever may also be present. Sudden onset of cough with minimal sputum, chills, fever, and myalgia is more indicative of a viral infection. Remember that older adults often have blunted responses to infection.

Patients with COPD usually present with a complaint of chronic productive cough (chronic bronchitis) and increasing shortness of breath or dyspnea on exertion (emphysema). Associated symptoms may include fatigue, weakness, hemoptysis, loss of appetite, nausea, and dizziness. By the time there is dyspnea on exertion, the disease is usually well advanced. Patients may report having to sleep sitting up or with three or more pillows to relieve dyspnea. They may report awakening during the night with severe dyspnea (paroxysmal nocturnal dyspnea), which is relieved by sitting upright.

Objective

The physical findings will vary depending on the severity of the COPD. Physical findings are often not significant in mild to moderate COPD. In emphysema or mixed disease, the chest exam may indicate hyperinflation. There may be flattening of the diaphragm, tachypnea, and use of the accessory muscles of respiration (scalene, sternocleidomastoids). In hyperinflation, the predominant palpable or ausculatory cardiac contraction may be noted in the epigastrium rather than in the left intercostal space. On auscultation, breath sounds are distant and are not augmented much with deep breathing. End expiratory wheezes may be heard on forced expiration. Patients with a bronchospastic component may have inspiratory and expiratory wheezes. Measurement of forced expiratory time is useful to determine if airway obstruction is present. When auscultating the lungs, have the patient take a full inspiration, then listen while the patient exhales through the mouth until airflow stops. Normal duration is 3 seconds, but in COPD the time is prolonged because of airway obstruction.

Coarse crackles may be present during an acute exacerbation. Neck vein distension, especially during expiration, may occur as a result of increased intrathoracic pressure. The patient's feet and ankles should be examined for edema that may occur as the disease progresses and cor pulmonale develops. The nailbeds should be examined for clubbing (hypertrophic osteoarthopathy), which often occurs in patients with pulmonary pathology. Other causes of clubbing are atrioventricular (AV) shunt, subacute bacterial endocarditis, inflammatory bowel disease, and biliary cirrhosis.

During the physical exam, the patient's ability to follow commands and respond to questions should be documented. Changes in mental status may be caused by hypoxemia or hypercapnia rather than dementia. Fatigue is a common findng.

Diagnostic Reasoning

The diagnostic approach to the patient is directed at assessment of the type of obstructive disease (primarily bronchitis, emphysema, or mixed) and whether it is reversible or irreversible. The possibility of underlying restrictive disease must be eliminated. Patients who have chronic bronchitis and have smoked for 20 years or longer should be evaluated for lung cancer.

Diagnostic Tests

Initial Testing. The initial diagnostic evaluation should include PFTs (spirometry, diffusing capacity, and ABGs). The standard PFTs should include pre- and post-bronchodilator testing to determine if there is a significant response to bronchodilators. The diagnostic criterion for COPD is an FEV_1/FVC ratio that is less than 70 percent. The FEV_1 (percent of predicted value) is the most useful parameter to assess severity of obstruction (see Table 8.6).

Even though bronchitis and emphysema usually occur together in most patients, it is important to distinguish the severity of the bronchitis and the emphysema and to identify how much of a bronchospastic component is present in order to direct treatment appropriately. In chronic bronchitis and emphysema, narrowing of the airways is present that usually results in an increase in airway resistance and a decrease in maximal expiratory flow rates. In emphysema, the loss of elastic recoil accounts for a decrease in the caliber of the airwars (from loss of radial traction on the airways). The elastic recoil properties of the lung serve as a major determinant of the expiratory flow rates. Maximal expiratory flow rates represent a complex and dynamic interplay between airway caliber, elastic recoil pressures, and airway collapsibility. As a result of the altered pressure-airflow relations in COPD, the work of breathing is increased in bronchitis and emphysema. The maldistribution of inspired gas (through ventilation) and blood flow (through perfusion) is always present to a degree in COPD. When the mismatching is severe, it is reflected in the ABGs as hypoxemia or hypercarbia.

Chest radiography will appear normal in patients with early COPD. In patients with chronic bronchitis, chest x-ray films may reveal increased lung markings in the lower lobes and peribronchial thickening. In patients with emphysema, the radiograph may show hyperinflation (low flat diaphragm, enlarged retrosternal space), hypovascularity, areas of hyperlucency and bullae formation, and a small cardiac silhouette. Chest CT scans are used to evaluate the extent and distribution of emphysematous cysts for possible surgery. In recurrent bronchitis, CT scans may be used to rule out bronchiectasis.

Laboratory tests should include a CBC and differential. The hemoglobin, hematocrit (Hct), and red blood cell (RBC) count should be evaluated to rule out anemia or polycythemia. Serum $alpha_1$-antitrypsin levels should be done in patients who develop COPD at an early age (younger than 45), those with clinical emphysema who have not smoked, and those with a family history of young onset of COPD. A blood chemistry profile is done to assess the electrolyte (K, Na, Cl) and nutritional status (total protein, albumin) and to rule out renal or liver problems.

For an exacerbation of chronic bronchitis, sputum should be tested via Gram stain. Sputum culture and sensitivity is done to confirm the findings of the Gram stain. The Gram stain is the best clinical method for diagnosing an acute exacerbation because the bacteria can be seen and quantified. Patients with COPD often are colonized by low numbers of bacteria, including *Streptococcus pneumoniae, Haemophilus influenzae,* and *Moraxella catarrhalis,* which will grow in culture even though they are not present in sufficient numbers to be seen with Gram stain. If the Gram stain shows neutrophils but no bacteria in a patient with chronic bronchitis, the acute exacerbation is probably viral or chlamydial, even when the sputum culture yields *Haemophilus* or *Pneumococcus.* A negative Gram stain indicates that such culture results represent bacterial colonization rather than a true infection.

An electrocardiogram (ECG) should be done if the patient has not had a baseline test and especially if there are signs of cardiac disease or in advanced COPD. Atrial arrhythmias are common in older adults and in pulmonary patients of any age. ECG changes in pulmonary disease include peaked P waves in leads II, III, and aV_F, and changes associated with right ventricular hypertrophy. Cardiac abnormalities may have implications for the drugs selected to treat the COPD.

Assessing degree of functional status and quality of life of patients with COPD should be done initially to determine the potential for rehabilitation and to direct appropriate therapy. The SF-36 Health Survey is a valid, reliable tool used worldwide to assess the physical and emotional health and is recommended for patients with chronic illnesses such as COPD. The tool is widely available.

Subsequent Testing

Annual spirometry, CBC with differential, chemistry profile, and chest radiographs should be done to measure the patient's decline in pulmonary function and to screen for other lung diseases that may be related to smoking. Gram stain, culture, and sensitivity test of sputum and ABG analysis are done as needed during acute exacerbations. Pulse oximetry is a noninvasive test that can be done in the office to screen for hypoxemia. An oxygen saturation of 90 percent or less at rest warrants monitoring ABGs. The ATS recommends ABG monitoring for hypoxemia and hypercapnia in patients with advanced disease—those with an FEV_1 less than 50 percent of the predicted value.

Differential Diagnosis

Acute bronchitis, asthma, bronchiectasis, bronchogenic carcinoma, acute viral infection, normal aging of lungs, occupational asthma, sleep apnea, and chronic sinusitis are all conditions that need to be ruled out to make a diagnosis of COPD and emphysema. In young adults, cystic fibrosis needs to be ruled out. Patient history and PFT results (including decreased FEV_1 with concomitant reduction in FEV_1/FVC ratio) as well as poor or absent reversibility will all assist in making the diagnosis of COPD.

Management

It is essential to diagnose COPD early in patients, as the estimated direct medical costs of COPD in 2002 were 18 billion dollars. After the initial diagnosis is made, education of the patient and family is critical for therapy to be effective. The patient and family need to understand that although COPD is not a curable disease, with proper management and smoking cessation, the symptoms can be controlled and quality of life improved. For patients with severe symptoms who are not benefitting from maximal medical therapy, lung volume reduction surgery and transplantation may be an option.

Smoking cessation improves declining lung function. After 5 years without cigarettes, the lung function returns to almost that of a nonsmoker. Patients should be urged at each clinic visit to stop smoking; family members should also be encouraged to do the same if they smoke. For more information on smoking cessation, see Smoking Addiction in this chapter.

Pharmacologic Therapy

A stepwise approach to therapy, similar to that for asthma and hypertension, is used. Drugs most commonly used for management of COPD symptoms are beta-2 agonists, anticholinergics, combination short-acting beta-2 agonists plus anticholinergic in one inhaler, xanthines, inhaled glucocorticosteroids, and systemic glucocorticosteroids. Antibiotics are warranted in the presence of a prolonged illness, especially with purulent sputum.

Inhaled Beta-2 Agonist Bronchodilators. Inhaled short acting beta-2 agonists (beta-adrenergic agonists) are the first line of therapy in the GOLD (Global Initiative for Chronic Obstructive Lung Disease) Stage I. The major goals of therapy are to prevent bronchospasm with long-acting bronchodilators and use "rescue" medication to alleviate acute episodes of bronchospasm. Each episode of acute bronchospasm causes permanent remodeling of the bronchioles; therefore prevention of these episodes is critical. Inhaled short-acting beta-2 agonists (albuterol [Proventil, Ventolin], pirbuterol [Maxair Autohaler]) are prescribed as "rescue" medication for intermittent symptoms of acute shortness of breath. Patients may experience adverse reactions from beta-2 agonists that include tremors, nervousness, and dysrhythmias. Long-acting beta agonists are not first-line therapy but may be used for maintenance therapy to prevent acute bronchospastic episodes. They should not be used without inhaled steroids.

Inhaled Anticholinergic Bronchodilators. Inhaled anticholinergic bronchodilators such as ipratropium bromide (Atrovent) are recommended for maintenance therapy in COPD. Bronchospasm in COPD has been found to be mainly cholinergically mediated; therefore anticholinergic inhalers are effective. These drugs are well tolerated by older adults and are not systemically absorbed. Ipratropium is taken routinely, usually two puffs qid. A long acting anticholinergic agent in a dry powder form such as tiotropium (Spiriva) may be effective and is only inhaled once daily. As a scheduled bronchodilator, tiotropium offers significant advantages to patients whose symptoms are not controlled by albuterol. Tiotropium is the recommended therapy for GOLD Stage II along with albuterol as a rescue medication. Some inhaler medications for COPD contain a combination of anticholinergic and beta-2 agonist bronchodilator which act synergistically. Formoterol plus ipratropium, albuterol, or a combination may also be used in Stage II. These are also recommended in Stage III and IV along with the addition of an inhaled corticosteroid. A combination of inhaled corticosteroid and long-acting B_2 agonist is fluticasone and salmeterol (Advair Diskus). Patients seem to do better with one inhaler rather than two.

Corticosteroids. Inhaled corticosteroids are recommended as maintenance therapy for asthma. The dosing of inhaled steroids such as beclomethasone (Beclodisk), budesonide (Pulmicort), fluticasone (Flovent), and triamcinolone (Azmacort), among others, should be individualized. Good inhaler technique with a spacing device and frequent mouth rinsing are advised to avoid oral candidiasis. Combination corticosteroid and beta-2 adrenergic agonist inhalers are effective to counteract bronchoconstriction and inflammation.

Systemic steroids should be used in the management of an exacerbation for only 10 to 14 days. Some clinicians report that 15 to 20 percent of patients do respond both subjectively (perceived dyspnea) and objectively (FEV_1 and improved exercise performance) with low-dose long-term systemic steroids. Systemic steroids should be used only when the other drugs have failed and when there is an acute exacerbation and there is a bronchospastic component to the COPD. Patients who are likely to respond to steroids are those who have blood and sputum eosinophilia, positive skin test results, elevated levels of serum IgE, and a history of allergy and bronchodilator response. Before starting the oral steroids, baseline spirometry should be done; then the patient should start taking oral prednisone 30–60 mg qd for 2 weeks. Spirometry is repeated. An improvement in FEV_1 of 15 percent indicates a positive response. The dose should then be tapered to a low daily or alternate-day maintenance dose, 7.5 to 10 mg qd or 15 mg every other day. The adverse effects of systemic steroids are well known (e.g., gastric ulcer, osteoporosis, masked infections, secondary infections) and the patient should be monitored carefully for adverse reactions.

Beta-2 adrenergic agonists and anticholinergic, and corticosteroid medications are available in metered-dose inhalers (MDIs) and dry powder inhalers (DPIs). Use of these inhaler devices requires patient education. The clinician should observe a patient demonstration of proper inhaler technique because there are differences in the technique used with each type of dispenser. Many patients have difficulty mastering the proper inhaler technique to gain optimal pulmonary delivery of medication. Spacers can be used with some inhalers to enable better delivery of the drug. Nebulizers can also be used to facilitate delivery of some inhaler medications. Regardless of the method used, ongoing patient education is essential to ensure proper inhalation of the medication.

Xanthines. Aminophylline or theophylline may be used as a third-line drug if the beta-2 agonists and the anticholinergic drugs are not effective. These preparations have a very narrow therapeutic index and blood levels should be monitored closely for toxicity. The therapeutic levels are 5 to 15 mcg/mL. The therapeutic benefit may be the result of improved muscle contractility and decreased muscle fatigue. Therapy should be initiated with low doses, then increased gradually because of the narrow therapeutic range. Xanthines interact with other drugs commonly taken by patients with COPD: cimetidine (Tagamet), erythromycin, ciprofloxacin (Cipro), and beta-blockers, among others. If the patient is taking a xanthine, it is safer not to use these drugs, to avoid drug toxicity.

Antibiotics. Antibiotics are often needed for acute exacerbations of chronic bronchitis when purulent sputum is present. Most pulmonologists recommend the empiric use of antibiotics to treat acute episodes when the cough increases and the character and amount of the sputum changes (increase in amount, color, and consistency), even in the absence of fever, pulmonary infiltrates, and leukocytosis. For empiric therapy, the antibiotic should be effective against the three most common pathogens (*Streptococcus pneumoniae, Haemophilus influenzae,* and *Moraxella catarrhalis*), stable against the effects of beta-lactamase, and convenient to take with few adverse reactions. Patients with COPD who have had a fairly stable course (few hospitalizations) and have not been exposed to many antibiotics may respond well to tetracycline or trimethoprim-sulfamethoxazole (Bactrim). The penicillins and some of the first- and second-generation cephalosporins may be used, but amoxicillin (Amoxil) and erythromycin (E-mycin) require multiple dosing and can cause significant diarrhea and gastric upset. Cefuroxime (Ceftin, Zinacef), cefaclor (Ceclor), and cefprozil (Cefzil) are all second-generation cephalosporins, a good empiric choice that can be given twice daily. Macrolides such as clarithromycin (Biaxin) are effective but tend to be overused in COPD. They have been shown to be effective in uncomplicated acute bronchitis. The macrolide regimens include azithromycin dosing packs (Z packs or Tri-packs) taken as 500 mg the first day, then 250 mg daily for 4 days, or 3-day courses of 500 mg daily. Some clinicians continue to prescribe one full 7- or 10-day course of azithromycin. Third-generation oral cephalosporins, such as cefdinir (Omnicef), cefoperazone (Cefobid), and ceftibuten (Cedax) are very effective against common respiratory pathogens and have few adverse effects and interactions with other drugs. They have two advantages—once a day dosing for COPD and few adverse gastrointestinal (GI) effects. Immunocompromised patients with a turbulent course should be treated carefully with the right antibiotic, even if it is the most expensive, to prevent respiratory failure and admission to an intensive care unit. Persistent gram-negative infection may require prolonged IV antibiotic administration. While these therapies have all been shown to have benefits of decreased morbidity, hospitalization risk, and so forth in one form or another, it is only home supplemental oxygen that has been shown to have an actual mortality-reducing benefit.

Diuretics. Diuretics may be necessary when there is evidence of cor pulmonale (right heart failure). Often the triad of prerenal azotemia, hypernatremia, and low cardiac output develops in cor pulmonale and loop diuretics may be used. Small doses of furosemide (Lasix) and potassium chloride supplements are used in conjunction with a sodium-restricted diet.

Mucolytics and Expectorants. Inhaled aerosols of water, saline, steam, or other agents do not improve mucociliary clearance or expectoration. Oral expectorants such as guaifenesin (Humibid, Robitussin) are usually ineffective. Chest physiotherapy and keeping the patient well hydrated is the most cost-effective way to clear the lungs.

Home Oxygen. Because hypoxia leads to pulmonary hypertension and increases the work of the right ventricle, low-flow oxygen may help prevent or deter development of cor pulmonale. Requirements for home oxygen include (1) a Pao_2 of 55 mm Hg or less or an oxygen saturation (Sa) below 85 percent and (2) a Pao_2 of 55 to 59 mm Hg if any of the following is present: erythrocytosis (Hct of 56 percent or more), cor pulmonale (P wave more than 3 mm in leads II, III, and aV_F), edema, or CHF. The goal of therapy is a Pao_2 of 60 mm Hg or Sao_2 of 90 percent, which usually can be accomplished with 1 to 2 L of oxygen per minute for 15 hours per day. The patient should be reevaluated with ABGs or oximetry at 1, 3, and 6 months, then annually. In advanced disease, supplemental oxygen has been shown to reduce the number of hospitalizations and increase the quality of life in individuals.

Surgery

Although surgery will not cure COPD, some patients have benefitted from one of three surgical procedures with an improved quality of life. Because of the typically poor pulmonary state of the patient, any surgery is extremely risky and should be performed using an epidural or spinal anesthesia rather than general anesthesia. A bullectomy involves resection of a bulla which may be effective in reducing the patient's dyspnea. Lung volume reduction surgery (LVRS) involves resecting 20 to 30 percent of the lung to reduce hyperinflation. Exercise capacity may be improved but it is highly unlikely that life expectancy would be improved because of the advanced nature of the disease. A lung transplant has been shown to improve; the quality of life, functional capacity, and exercise performance. The 2-year survival rate for lung transplantation is 75 percent. The decision for surgery should be made with the specialist and involve the entire family.

Follow-Up and Referral

Patients who are unstable and those with severe disease should be seen monthly. If the patient is stable, an annual visit would be the minimum. If the patient is on theophylline, the blood levels should be monitored every 6 to 12 months once the patient is on the desired dose. If the patient is on home O_2, ABGs should be checked whenever there is any condition change, or at a minimum, semiannually. It is important to monitor oxygen saturation (pulse oximetry) more frequently.

Follow-up for the patient with COPD includes the development of a close and supportive relationship with the health-care provider. Because smoking cessation is the single most effective way to reduce the progression of COPD, at every visit the patient should be asked about this.

Patient Education

Patients with COPD should avoid extremes in temperature and humidity when possible and limit their exposure to areas that have high levels of air pollution. Smoking should not be allowed in the home, car, or other confined places. Occupational exposure to fumes, vapors, dusts, and irritants may aggravate symptoms of dyspnea and bronchospasm. High altitude and air travel can pose problems for hypoxemic patients. Arrangements can be made with the airlines in advance for patients requiring oxygen.

Most lung infections are viral, so avoiding contact with crowds during flu season and limiting exposure to people with colds may help. In the fall, patients with COPD should receive influenza immunizations with polyvalent vaccine from early October through mid-November.. Amantadine HCl (Symmetrel) is useful if started within 48 hours of exposure to influenza A and can protect susceptible individuals during the 2-week latency period before the vaccine is effective. Oseltamivir (Tamiflu) is another abortive antiviral which helps shorten the duration and decrease the severity of influenza symptoms if used within the first 48 hours of symptom onset. Polyvalent pneumococcal vaccine should be given. For people older than age 65, [illegible] atory [illegible] should be r[illegible] tion and sub-se[illegible]

[illegible] not only deter functional [illegible] patient and family to maintain a po[illegible] ften, the best exercise for patients with mild t[illegible] ate obstructive disease is an individualized walking program. Physical therapy may also be beneficial; the therapist should prescribe specific breathing exercises, arm exercises, and others that will promote general physical reconditioning. Walking aids have been shown to support the diaphragm and ease the difficulty of breathing while walking. During attacks, use of slow, pursed-lipped breathing may help to decrease respiratory rate, reduce bronchospasm, and relieve dyspnea. Effective cough techniques and chest physiotherapy are also recommended.

Many patients with COPD find support groups helpful for them and their spouses or caregivers. These support groups are usually sponsored by local chapters of the American Lung Association and they are usually listed in the phone book. Other patients have used forms of meditation or guided imagery to help relieve dyspnea and anxiety.

Patients with chronic illness such as COPD often are depressed. The Beck depression scale can be used to screen for depression. Use of the selective serotonin reuptake inhibitor (SSRI) antidepressants in patients with lung disease is considered safe and may improve sleep, quality of life, and functional status.

Providers should have a frank discussion with patients and their family regarding end of life care such as advanced directives and health-care surrogates. Copies of all documents should be kept in the chart as well as with patients' families and attorneys.

Upper Respiratory Infections

Upper respiratory infections (URIs) include some of the most common infectious diseases encountered and account for millions of visits to health-care providers annually. The majority of URIs are caused by a virus. Bacteria cause about 25 percent of the cases. For the average adult, they are a source of discomfort, disability, and loss of time. For young children and older adults, these infections may be a cause of morbidity and serious illnesses. In children and older adults as well as adults with underlying respiratory diseases, these viral infections are frequently complicated by bacterial superinfections.

Epidemiology and Causes

Influenza (the flu), the common cold (viral rhinitis or acute coryza), and acute laryngitis are some of the more frequently occurring URIs that the practitioner will need to manage. Infections such as acute epiglottitis and respiratory syncytial virus (RSV) infection occur predominantly in infants and younger children, but may occur as a life-threatening infection in adults. RSV infection can cause severe cases of pneumonia and lower respiratory tract disease in older, institutionalized adults and adults with suppressed immune status. Acute epiglottitis can result in complete or partial airway obstruction (Table 8.7).

Influenza epidemics occur every year in the United States, with typically 5000 to 250,000 cases annually. In some years with more severe outbreaks, as many as 40,000 deaths have occurred. Most of these deaths occur in older persons, particularly those with underlying pulmonary or cardiac disease. Although influenza and colds may occur at any time, most cases occur during the winter and spring months. Acute laryngitis is generally associated with a viral URI and often persists for a week or more after other symptoms have cleared. The incubation period for most URIs of a viral nature is 1 to 4 days.

Community-acquired respiratory tract infections caused by streptococcus account for more than 20 million primary care provider visits annually and are a major reason for work and school absenteeism.

Pathophysiology

The common cold (coryza) is caused by viruses spread through direct inhalation of airborne droplet sprays aerosolized by the infected person while speaking, coughing, or sneezing, as well as hand-to-face transmission after handling fomites serving as reservoirs of infection. Hand-to-hand transmission, however, is probably the most common mode of transmission in adults, underscoring the importance of frequent handwashing in the prevention of new cases. Numerous serotypes of rhino-, adeno-, corona-, coxsackie-, and parainfluenza viruses are associated with the common cold. The ability of the majority of these viruses to mutate readily ensures their ability to consistently evade host immune mechanisms. The number of rhinovirus serotypes, for instance, numbers more than a hundred. Following infection, individuals develop immunity to a specific viral strain but are susceptible to repeated infection by the same parent virus after only minor changes in surface proteins or polysaccharides.

Symptoms of congestion, rhinorrhea, and sneezing result directly from inflammation and edema of upper airway mucosal surfaces. The cough reflex may be triggered by this same mucosal inflammation in the posterior pharynx. Following acute infection, postviral cough may persist for as long as 6 to 8 weeks due to postnasal drip—the persistent drainage of thin mucous down the posterior pharynx resulting in direct pharyngeal irritation.

Classic flu is caused by the orthomyxovirus influenza type A and, to a lesser extent, influenza type B. In addition to the viral rhinitis symptoms of the common cold, influenza infection further leads to generalized muscle aches and pains, fatigue, significant fever, and rigors (chills).

The Iceberg of

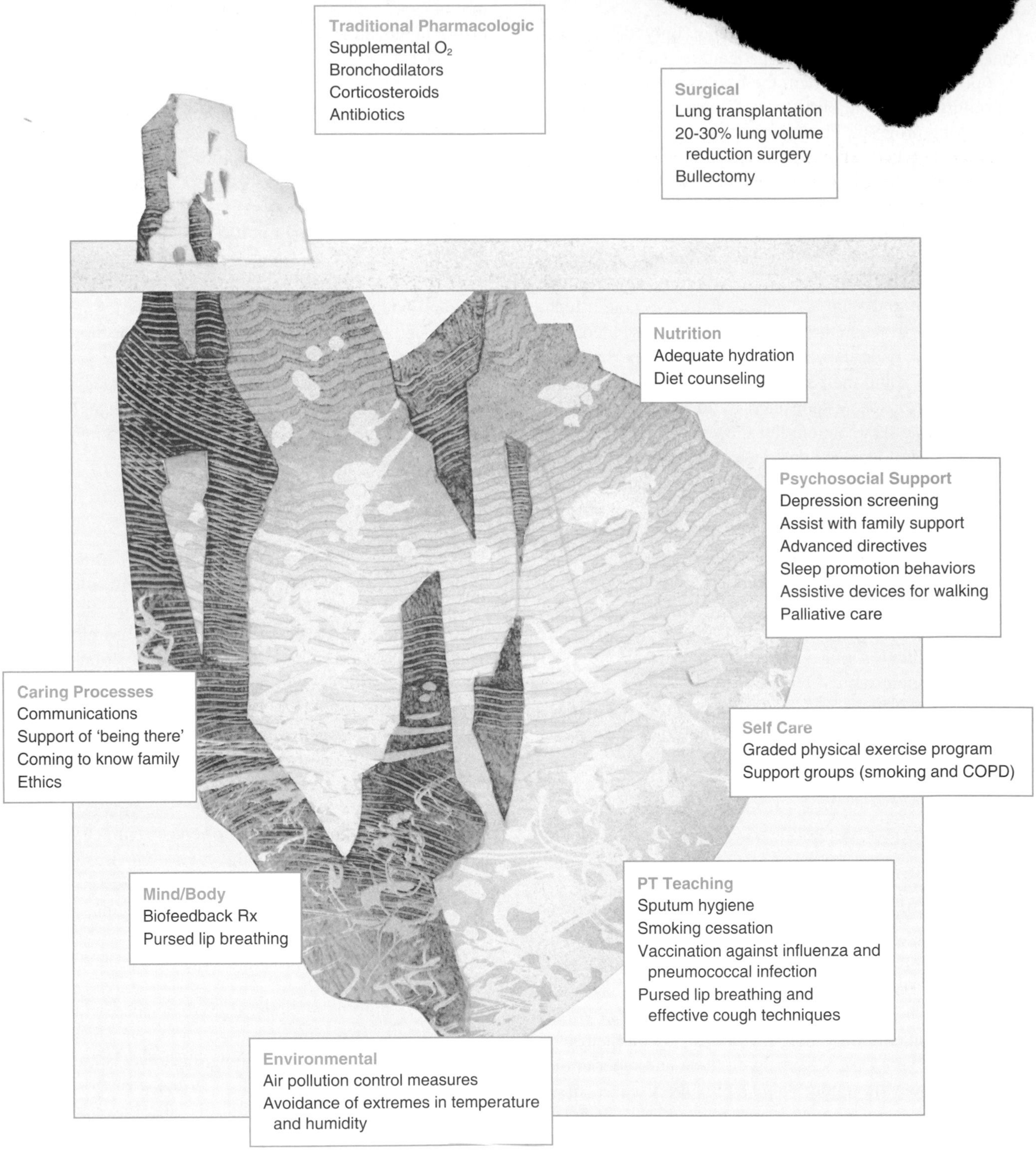

Traditional Pharmacologic
Supplemental O_2
Bronchodilators
Corticosteroids
Antibiotics

Surgical
Lung transplantation
20-30% lung volume reduction surgery
Bullectomy

Nutrition
Adequate hydration
Diet counseling

Psychosocial Support
Depression screening
Assist with family support
Advanced directives
Sleep promotion behaviors
Assistive devices for walking
Palliative care

Caring Processes
Communications
Support of 'being there'
Coming to know family
Ethics

Self Care
Graded physical exercise program
Support groups (smoking and COPD)

Mind/Body
Biofeedback Rx
Pursed lip breathing

PT Teaching
Sputum hygiene
Smoking cessation
Vaccination against influenza and pneumococcal infection
Pursed lip breathing and effective cough techniques

Environmental
Air pollution control measures
Avoidance of extremes in temperature and humidity

Table 8.7 Acute Epiglottitis

Acute epiglottitis is a life-threatening, rapidly progressing cellulitis of the epiglottis that may cause complete airway obstruction. Epiglottitis begins as a cellulitis between the tongue base and the epiglottis; the epiglottis is then pushed posteriorly. The epiglottis becomes swollen and threatens airway patency. Epiglottitis is more common and more severe in young children but it may occur in older children and adults.

Clinical Manifestations

Epiglottitis in adults should be suspected when odynophagia (pain upon swallowing) seems severe compared to pharyngeal findings. Other findings include dyspnea, drooling, and stridor.

Diagnostic Reasoning

Direct viewing of the epiglottis with a tongue blade and lighting should *never* be attempted because immediate laryngospasm and airway obstruction may result. It is recommended that children and adults be transported to the operating room while sitting up for visualization of the epiglottis with a fiberoptic laryngoscope, with preparations made for immediate airway control. The epiglottis will appear swollen and erythematous ("cherry red"), and an uncuffed endotracheal tube should be inserted.

Management

Acute epiglottitis requires emergency care for adequate airway control. No painful or stressful procedures should be performed on these patients unless preparations are in place for a planned intubation, such as in the O.R.

The patient with epiglottitis will require hospitalization for intravenous antibiotics such as cefuroxine (Ceftin), ceftriaxone (Rocephin), or ampicillin/sulbactam (Unasyn). Dexamethasone (Decadron) should also be administered IV and tapered as signs and symptoms resolve. Continuous pulse oximetry and careful monitoring of the patient's airway is critical. Patients who develop hypoxemia and respiratory distress will require intubation.

Influenza infection may also develop into frank viral pneumonia (lower airway infection), which may be further complicated by bacterial superinfection, particularly with *Staphylococcus aureus*. These additional manifestations and high potential for complicated disease underscore the importance of widespread yearly vaccination against influenza.

Repeated yearly vaccination is required because the influenza virus is capable of mutating its major surface proteins—hemagglutinin and neuraminidase—rendering protein-specific host antibody defenses ineffective and allowing for viral adherence and entry into host epithelial cells. Each year, a vaccine is developed using influenza proteins from the most likely serotype combination to lead to widespread infection for that year, as determined by complex disease modeling algorithms based on extensive Centers for Disease Control and Prevention (CDC) and World Health Organization (WHO) epidemiologic data. However, each vaccine is, in essence, a best guess, which may or may not provide adequate protection against the year's primary strain. In addition, other strains of the virus not covered by the vaccine may also cause numerous infections in any given year.

Most cases of laryngitis (inflammation of the vocal cords with extreme hoarseness and temporary voice loss) and croup (any combination of laryngotracheobronchitis with edema leading to airway obstruction with characteristic stridorous breathing) are caused by parainfluenza virus, respiratory syncytial virus (RSV), influenza virus, coxsackievirus, rhinovirus, and adenovirus. Laryngitis may also be caused by group A beta-hemolytic *Streptococcus pyogenes, Haemophilus influenzae,* and *Moraxella catarrhalis.* These same viral and bacterial agents, along with Neisseria gonorrhoeae and Epstein-Barr virus (EBV causing infectious mononucleosis) are also common causes of pharyngitis (see full discussion in Chapter 7).

RSV and influenza A (and less so influenza B) are the most common causes of bronchiolitis in children and adolescents, but adults tend to experience infection in the larger airways (i.e., acute bronchitis). Since the advent of widespread vaccination against *Haemophilus influenzae* type B (Hib vaccine) and Corynebacterium diphtheriae (DTaP vaccine), epiglottitis occurs only rarely in the United States (see Table 8.7). Bacterial tracheitis is a serious purulent infection of the subglottic trachea caused primarily by Staphylococcus aureus, with a toxic clinical presentation requiring hospitalization and IV antibiotic therapy

Clinical Presentation

The onset of influenza is usually abrupt, with fever, chills, malaise, myalgia, headache, nasal stuffiness, sore throat, and sometimes nausea. A nonproductive cough is usually present and occurs early in the course of illness. The fever may be as high as 103°F (39.4°C) in adults and typically lasts 3 to 5 days. Subjective findings in the person with the common cold include headache, myalgia, nasal congestion, watery rhinorrhea, sneezing, and a "scratchy throat." Laryngitis results in an inflammation of laryngeal mucosa and the vocal cords. Symptoms include hoarseness, aphonia, and, occasionally, pain on phonation, and deglutition. Physical findings in cases of URIs are usually minimal, with normal assessment findings on chest auscultation. Cervical lymphadenopathy may be present.

Diagnostic Reasoning

Diagnostic Tests

Diagnosis of influenza tends to be more accurate during epidemics. A successful presumptive diagnosis requires appropriate symptoms at the right time of the year and a knowledge of pattern of influenzal illnesses around the world. If necessary, the diagnosis can be confirmed by virology studies (e.g., nasal and pharyngeal cultures, cells from nasopharyngeal washings stained with monoclonal antibody fluorescence stains, and complement fixation studies on paired serum samples). Diagnosis of colds and laryngitis typically are based on the subjective presentation of the patient except when the etiologic agent in laryngitis is thought to be bacterial. In these situations, the practitioner should perform a throat culture to rule out group A beta-hemolytic streptococcal infection. Leukocytosis found on a CBC (complete blood count) may help to diagnose a bacterial infection.

Differential Diagnosis

Other conditions that need to be ruled out include allergic rhinitis, atypical *Mycoplasma* pneumonia, infectious mononucleosis, chlamydia, and possibly mumps, rubeola, and cytomegalovirus. Close attention to epidemiology (e.g., current outbreak in community) is important. Contact the Centers for Disease Control and Prevention (CDC) or the local health department to help determine the type of disease outbreak.

Management

Management of influenza and the common cold is generally symptomatic and is directed toward relief of symptoms and prevention of secondary infections. Antibiotics are not indicated for influenza or colds unless a secondary bacterial infection occurs. Mucopurulent rhinitis frequently accompanies the common cold and is not an indication for antimicrobial treatment. Although antibiotics are often viewed by the lay person as a viable treatment for a cold or the flu, these drugs have no effect on viruses and if taken injudiciously may produce resistant organisms.

Generally, most patients with influenza should rest at home until symptoms decrease in severity. The older patient or the patient with an underlying chronic illness may require hospitalization for influenza. In addition to rest, fluids, antipyretics, and analgesics are recommended. Cough suppressants with codeine may be necessary for adequate cough control. If the practitioner is reasonably confident that the virus in question is type A influenza, then the patient may benefit from amantadine (Symadine, Symmetrel). It is most effective if started early in the course of the disease. Relief from symptoms may still be produced if started 3 to 5 days into the disease process. Results of cultures or complement fixation do not provide information early enough for the practitioner to base the decision to use amantadine on those findings. A reduction in the dose of amantadine is required in the elderly who may develop CNS dysfunction. The use of Tamiflu in influenza may be initiated within 48 hours of symptom presentation to reduce the duration and severity of the course of the disease.

Rest, fluids, and antipyretics are also useful in controlling the discomfort associated with a cold. Decongestants such as pseudoephedrine (e.g., Sudafed) are widely used and may help control rhinorrhea and nasal congestion. These should be used only for 3 days and should not be used in the presence of hypertension. Nasal sprays such as phenylephrine (AK-Dilate, I-Phrine) or ocular decongestants such as oxymetazoline (e.g., OcuClear, Visine LR) are rapidly effective. Patients should be cautioned to use them only for a few days, because chronic use leads to a rebound congestion. Vitamin C and zinc lozenges with echinacea are currently popular "remedies" that are sold as OTC therapies. Despite numerous randomized trials, the evidence of effectiveness of zinc lozenges in reducing the duration of colds is lacking. The efficacy of vitamin C supplements to decrease the incidence of colds or to shorten the duration has also not been demonstrated. The only exception may be for the patient who has a possible vitamin C deficiency.

Treatment of laryngitis includes complete voice rest, steam inhalations, codeine or nonnarcotic cough suppressants for cough and pain, and a liquid or soft diet. If throat cultures are positive for group A beta-hemolytic *Streptococcus,* penicillin should be prescribed, if the patient is not allergic to penicillin. Erythromycin should be used for infections associated with *M. catarrhalis* or *H. influenzae.* Telithromycin (Ketek) is recommended for community-acquired respiratory tract infections caused by streptococcus. A dose of 800 mg once daily for 7 to 10 days is recommended for adults older than the age of 18. As a ketolide antibacterial, it has been shown to be effective against strains that are resistant to penicillin, erythromycin, and tetracycline. For particularly toxic bacterial infections such as bacterial tracheitis, blood cultures may be appropriate to rule out bacteremia.

For the management of croup, racemic epinephrine and dexamethasone are indicated and intubation is needed in only the most extreme cases. Bacterial tracheitis requires IV antibiotic therapy with nafcillin or an appropriate cephalosporin, or if methicillin-resistant *Staphylococcus aureus* (MRSA) is suspected, vancomycin or Linezolid. Because of impaired oral intake, all such infections, other than the common cold, may lead to dehydration requiring oral or IV rehydration therapy. In addition, hypoxemia based on pulse oximetry or blood gas analysis should be addressed with supplemental oxygen therapy. Bronchodilator therapy is often used as well, but randomized clinical trials do not consistently demonstrate its efficacy.

Follow-Up and Referral

The duration of an uncomplicated case of influenza is 1 to 7 days; the prognosis is excellent. Frequent complications do occur, however, including acute sinusitis, otitis media, purulent bronchitis, and pneumonia. Influenza causes necrosis of some respiratory epithelium, predisposing the infected person to secondary bacterial infections. The interaction between bacteria and influenza is bidirectional, with bacterial enzymes activating influenza viruses. If a fever persists for more than 4 days, if the WBC count rises to 12,000 or higher, or if the cough becomes productive, bacterial infection should be ruled out or verified and treated.

The most common complication of influenza is pneumonia; most fatalities result from bacterial pneumonia. The patient with bacterial pneumonia will experience gradual improvement of symptoms for 2 to 3 days and then develop cough and purulent sputum. Pneumococcal pneumonia is the most common bacterial pneumonia associated with influenza, but staphylococcal pneumonia is the most serious. Primary viral influenza pneumonia is the least common but has a high mortality rate among pregnant women and patients with rheumatic heart disease. The patient develops symptoms of influenza that become increasingly severe. Respiratory distress is often sufficient to require mechanical ventilation.

Most cases of the common cold and laryngitis are self-limiting. Complications of a cold may include pharyngitis, sinusitis, otitis media, tonsillitis, and chest infections. Unless symptoms of these complications are present, antibiotic therapy is not indicated. The patient with laryngitis needs to maintain voice rest until hoarseness and aphonia have resided. Any vigorous use of the voice such as shouting or singing may foster the formation of vocal cord nodules.

Patient Education

There currently is no immunization for the prevention of colds. Research has demonstrated that the best method of preventing transmission of infected droplets is through frequent hand washing, particularly in day-care facilities and congregate adult living facilities. During the cold and influenza seasons, the person with a chronic illness or a compromised immune status should be advised to avoid crowded, close situations and other persons who have obvious symptoms.

Trivalent influenza vaccine provides partial immunity (in approximately 86 percent of patients vaccinated) for a few months to 1 year. The vaccine's antigenic configuration changes yearly: It is based on the prevalent strains of the previous year, the viruses that are currently being seen in other parts of the world during the current year, and the estimated antibody response in persons previously infect with or vaccinated to these viruses. Vaccination in October or November of each year is recommended for all persons older than age 65; nursing home residents; adults and children with underlying conditions, including heart, pulmonary, malignant, and some metabolic diseases; and health-care workers. High-risk children have a particularly low influenza vaccination rate annually. Vaccination is also encouraged for members of any large groups who may be the principal vectors of influenza in their community such as schoolchildren, children in day care, college students, military personnel, and employees of large companies. Fewer than 20 percent of these populations are immunized each year. Low-income minority populations typically have lower vaccination rates than other populations. Medicare covers the cost of influenza and pneumococcal vaccination. Recent research has shown that obtaining yearly influenza vaccination can be influenced by the health-care provider's recommendations and phone calls offering encouragement and reminders. The practitioner may keep abreast of current epidemiological trends in influenza epidemics by accessing the Web site for the CDC at http://www.cdc.gov.

Pneumonia

Pneumonia is typically an acute inflammation of the lung parenchyma, usually infectious in origin. The lung tissue typically becomes consolidated as alveoli fill with exudate. Gas exchange may be impaired as blood is shunted around nonfunctional alveoli. The timely diagnosis and appropriate management of pneumonia in patients is critical because of the morbidity associated with bacterial etiologies as well as the increased mortality among older patients and those with underlying pulmonary disease. Community-acquired pneumonia occurs outside the hospital or is diagnosed within 2 days after hospitalization in a patient who has not resided in a long-term care facility for 2 weeks or more prior to the onset of the symptoms.

Epidemiology and Causes

It is estimated that in the United States almost 5 million people develop pneumonia annually. Of these, about 1.3 million persons with pneumonia are admitted to hospitals, and there are more than 64,000 deaths that occur per year. Approximately 70 to 80 percent of patients who develop community-acquired pneumonia (CAP) are age 60 and older or have a coexisting medical condition. CAP remains one of the 10 leading causes of mortality among elderly people in the United States today. This population is increasing, thus making adequate treatment of pneumonia a health-care priority. Nosocomial (hospital-acquired) pneumonias account for approximately 15 percent of all hospital-associated infections; pneumonia is second only to UTIs in terms of frequency among hospitalized patients. The most common pathogens associated with CAP and nosocomial pneumonia are shown in Table 8.8.

Pneumonia is frequently the terminal event in older adults and those debilitated by chronic diseases, particularly chronic respiratory disease. Oslev referred to pneumonia as "the special enemy of old age." *Pneumocystis carinii* pneumonia (PCP) affects more than half of all patients with acquired immunodeficiency syndrome (AIDS) and is one of the leading causes of death in this population. Other vulnerable populations include infants less than 6 months old, children younger than age 5, smokers, alcoholics, residents of nursing homes, young adults living in close quarters (e.g., college students and military recruits), and any patient with impaired swallowing capacity or cough reflex who is at risk for aspiration. Geographic location, the winter season,

Table 8.8 **Common Causes of Pneumonia**

Community-Acquired Pneumonia (CAP)	Nosocomial Pneumonia
Streptococcus pneumoniae (70% of all cases of bacterial pneumonia) Pneumococcal pneumonia (25%–35% of all CAP) *Staphylococcus aureus* *Klebsiella pneumoniae* *Moraxella catarrhalis* (less common) Atypical pneumonias: *Mycoplasma pneumoniae* (second most common cause of CAP) *Legionella pneumoniae* *Chlamydia pneumoniae* Fungi Oral anaerobes Viruses	Most are caused by gram-negative bacteria. Enteric aerobic gram-negative bacilli *Klebsiella pneumoniae* *Pseudomonas aeruginosa* *Staphylococcus aureus* (gram-positive) Oral anaerobes *Legionella pneumoniae* (which travel in cooling systems, condensers, and shower heads)

occupation, travel history, and pet or animal exposure are other factors associated with the development of pneumonia.

Pathophysiology

Pneumonia is an infection of the alveoli, distal airways, and interstitium of the lungs, and thus, predominantly a parenchymal disease. A pathogen, such as a bacterium, virus, fungus, or parasite, reaches the lower respiratory tract in sufficient number or with sufficient virulence to overwhelm the innate defenses of the respiratory tract. The inflammatory response is set in motion, which increases capillary permeability and attracts neutrophils, lymphocytes, platelets, and fibrinogen to the site of infection. Tissue fluid extravasates into the interstitial space from the pulmonary capillary bed, forming an exudate with a higher protein content than typical transudative fluid. As this exudate develops, an increasing amount of cellular debris accumulates, impeding optimal oxygen diffusion from the alveoli to capillaries with resultant hypoxemia. Vital capacity, lung compliance, residual capacity, and total lung capacity are diminished, while ventilation–perfusion mismatch occurs.

The spongy consistency of the lung tissue becomes fluid-filled and infiltrated by several lineages of white blood cells depending on the infective agent involved, including neutrophils, lymphocytes, and macrophages, as well as red blood cells and fibrin. Because of these changes, the area of pneumonia is often referred to as a consolidative focus which is typically dull to percussion on physical exam. Pneumonia may be classified as lobar, interstitial, miliary, or bronchopneumonia (Fig. 8.1). Lobar pneumonia involves an entire lobe of the lung, while interstitial pneumonia is a patchy or diffuse inflammatory process throughout regions of the interstitium. Miliary pneumonia consists of numerous discrete lesions resulting from hematogenous spread of infection, and bronchopneumonia is a patchy consolidation involving one or several lobes. Moreover, inflammation can also extend into the pleural space causing a parapneumonic effusion or inflammation of the pleural membranes, known as pleuritis or pleurisy.

Possible routes of infection include aspiration, aerosolization, hematogenous spread from a distant infected site, and direct spread from a contiguous infected site. Aspiration pneumonia occurs most often in postoperative, stroke, comatose, or otherwise mentally altered patients with an impaired swallowing reflex. Although *Streptococcus pneumoniae* remains the most common causative agent in aspiration pneumonia, anaerobic bacteria and gram-negative bacilli (i.e., gastrointestinal flora) must also be considered. Hematogenous spread to the lungs can take place in endocarditis, intravenous central catheter line infection, or from infection at other sites such as the urinary tract. Aerosolization, the most common means of infection, is the route by which most bacteria, *Mycobacterium tuberculosis*, fungi, and viruses reach the lungs.

In adults, the most common organisms involved in community-acquired pneumonia include viruses, *S. pneumoniae, Moraxella catarrhalis, Hemophilus influenzae, Legionella pneumophila,* and methicillin-sensitive *Staphylococcus aureus*, while nosocomial (hospital-acquired) pneumonia raises concerns for *Pseudomonas aeruginosa* and MRSA. Of note, increasing numbers of community-acquired MRSA infections are being reported, particularly among elderly nursing home residents, resulting in severe cases of necrotizing pneumonia. Extremely virulent strains of *S. aureus* expressing the Panton-Valentine leukocidin toxin are also surfacing in young adults with the same condition.

Streptococcus pneumoniae

The most common cause of CAP is the gram-positive bacteria *Streptococcus pneumoniae,* also referred to as pneumococcal pneumonia. *S. pneumoniae* is one of the leading causes of illness and death worldwide for young children, older adults, and persons with chronic, debilitating

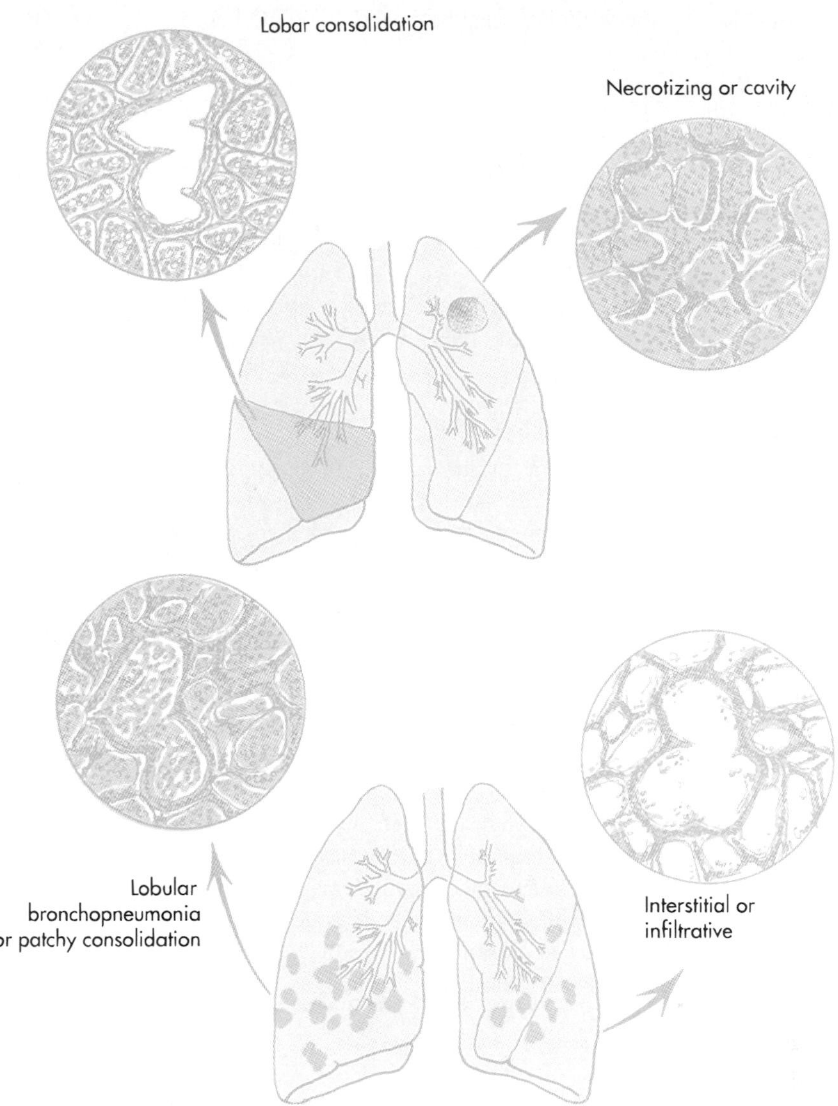

FIGURE 8.1 Forms of pneumonia. (Source: Price, SA, and Wilson, LM: Pathophysiology: Clinical Concepts of Disease Processess, ed 5. Mosby, St. Louis, 1996, p 565, with permission.)

pathology. The pathogenesis of pneumococcal pneumonia has been extensively studied and serves as a prototype for the management of other bacterial pneumonia.

Pneumococcal pneumonia occurs as a result of infected mucus or inhalation of organisms that have colonized in the nasopharynx. *S. pneumoniae* can be recovered from the nasopharynx of approximately 40 percent of healthy adults. In the normal host the bacteria is inactivated by opsonization with immunoglobulins and complement. Persons with defects in host-defense mechanisms (e.g., inadequate immunoglobulin production or deficiency, impaired phagocytic function, autoimmune disease, immunosuppression, or impaired mucociliary clearance) have a far greater susceptibility.

The lower lobes are most commonly infected because of the effects of gravity. On inhalation, the pneumococcus establishes itself in the alveoli, spreading rapidly through the pores of Kohn. Pneumococcal pneumonia typically includes four responsive stages of infection: engorgement, red hepatization, gray hepatization, and resolution. During engorgement, alveolar capillaries become congested, bacteria and exudate pours into alveoli from alveolar capillaries, and the bacteria multiply without inhibition. There is continued engorgement of the capillaries, with diapedesis of erythrocytes giving the lungs the gross appearance of liver (red hepatization). As the leukocyte count increases in the exudate, it compresses the capillaries and causes the lung tissue to assume a gray color (gray hepatization). At this point, phagocytosis is achieved by polymorphonuclear leukocytes. The presence of opsonizing antibody enhances the ingestion of the bacteria. The stage of resolution is reached when the pneumococci have been destroyed and macrophages are seen within the alveolar spaces where they lyse and absorb exudate. There often may be pleural involvement from contiguity to parenchymal lesions or by way of the lymphatics. As in the alveoli, there is an outpouring of fluid, followed by polymorphonuclear leukocytes and fibrin. The structure of the pleural space has fewer surfaces suitable for phagocytosis than do the alveoli. Control of the infection in the pleural area is more dependent on heat-stable (specific antibody) than heat-labile (complement opsins) antibodies.

Haemophilus influenzae

Haemophilus influenzae, a gram-negative bacteria, is the cause of the second most common CAP. It may occur in healthy individuals as well as in patients with chronic, debilitating diseases and chronic alcohol abuse. Development of *H. influenzae* pneumonia follows colonization of the upper respiratory tract. During viral infection epidemics, there is often an increase in the incidence of *H. influenzae* pneumonia.

Legionella pneumophila

Legionella pneumophila, a gram-negative bacteria, was identified in 1976 as a causative agent of pneumonia (Legionnaires' disease) during an American Legion convention in Philadelphia. The bacteria thrive in aquatic environments. The source of human infection has been associated with contaminated air-conditioning systems and showerheads. Within the hospital setting, contaminated respiratory tubing and equipment may serve as a source of *L. pneumophila.* The bacilli enter the lungs by aspiration, direct inhalation, and hematogenous dissemination. In the normal host, it is thought that the bacilli are cleared by the mucociliary process. This would explain the high incidence of the disease in patients with impaired mucociliary clearance (e.g., smokers, alcoholics, and older adults). Legionnaires' disease may occur in explosive outbreaks if large numbers of susceptible people are exposed to an infectious aerosol. Because of the low communicability of the disease, secondary cases should not occur.

Staphylococcus aureus

Staphylococcus aureus rarely causes pneumonia in healthy, young adults. Local pulmonary or systemic defense must be compromised before the organism can produce a pneumonia. *S. aureus* accounts for 2 to 9 percent of CAP in older adults or in patients with concomitant-conditions such as diabetes, chronic renal failure, bronchiectasis, or lung cancer, or risk factors such as residence in a chronic-care facility or IV substance abuse. Infections may also occur in previously healthy adults following a viral influenza with residual impaired bronchopulmonary mechanism.

Viral Pneumonia

Viral infections account for 5 to 15 percent of cases of adult CAP. Most viral infections are restricted to the upper respiratory system and tend to cause self-limiting symptoms. Some patients, particularly those with influenza infections, may develop pneumonia. Influenza may result in a primary viral pneumonia or, more commonly, a secondary bacterial pneumonia. Secondary pneumonia is most frequently caused by *S. pneumoniae* and *S. aureus.* Viral infections are transmitted by hand-to-hand contact or by aerosols (sneezing, coughing). The frequency of influenza as a cause of both CAP and nosocomial pneumonia increases in the winter months.

Mycoplasma Pneumonia

Mycoplasma pneumonia is also known as primary atypical pneumonia or "walking pneumonia" because of the predominance of constitutional symptoms. *Mycoplasma pneumoniae* is a class of bacterial L-forms, which are the smallest known free-living organisms. Children older than age 5 and young adults are at greatest risk for developing mycoplasmal pneumonia. Outbreaks can occur in populations living in close proximity, such as colleges, military bases, and prisons. Because of the long incubation phase of 2 to 3 weeks and the relatively low communicability, *Mycoplasma* pneumonia tends to move through the community slowly.

Chlamydia pneumoniae

Chlamydia pneumoniae has only recently been recognized as a pulmonary pathogen. *C. pneumoniae* is a gram-negative bacterium. Little is known about the mode of transmission and pathogenesis. The clinical features are similar to those caused by *M. pneumoniae.* Adult-onset asthma subsequent to infection with *Chlamydia* pneumonia has been documented. Recurrent infection is common.

Anaerobic Pneumonia

Anaerobic pneumonia may occur in the community and the hospital setting. *Prevotella melaninogenica,* anaerobic streptococci, and *Fusobacterium nucleatum* are commonly isolated anaerobic bacteria. Aspiration of oropharyngeal secretions normally occurs during sleep in healthy individuals but rarely causes disease. Individuals who are predisposed to aspiration of larger amounts of oropharyngeal secretions are at risk for anaerobic pneumonia. Alcoholism is the most frequent predisposing factor; others include dysphagia, cerebrovascular accidents (CVAs), seizures, and general anesthesia. Periodontal disease, which increases the number of anaerobic bacteria, is also associated with anaerobic infection. Pneumonia typically develops in dependent zones. Although body position at the time of aspiration determines which lung zones are dependent, anaerobic pneumonia most often develops in the posterior segments of the upper lobes and the superior and basilar segments of the lower lobes. The onset of symptoms is usually insidious. Empyema, lung abscess, or necrotizing pneumonia may be present by the time the patient seeks medical attention.

Nosocomial Bacterial Pneumonias

Nosocomial bacterial pneumonias are most frequently caused by gram-negative organisms such as *Pseudomonas aeruginosa, Klebsiella pneumoniae, Escherichia coli, Serratia, Proteus,* and *Enterobacter.* However, *Staphylococcus aureus* (especially methicillin-resistant *S. aureus, MRSA), S. pneumoniae,* and *H. influenzae* are frequently being reported among elderly nursing home residents. As in

CAPs, bacteria invade the lower respiratory tract by aspiration of oropharyngeal organisms, inhalation of aerosols containing bacteria, or by hematogenous spread from a distant body site. Patients at high risk for developing nosocomial bacterial pneumonia include postoperative patients, particularly those undergoing thoracoabdominal procedures, patients with endotracheal incubation and/or mechanically assisted ventilation, depressed level of consciousness, an episode of large-volume aspiration, underlying chronic lung disease, and patients age 70 and greater. Nosocomial pneumonia has a mortality rate of about 30 percent. Hospital-acquired pneumonia in patients on mechanical ventilation has mortality rates of about 48 percent. Patients who develop acute respiratory distress syndrome (ARDS) have a mortality rate greater than 68 percent.

Pneumocystis carinii Pneumonia

Pneumocystis carinii pneumonia (PCP) is the AIDS-defining opportunistic infection in 65 percent of HIV-infected individuals and is the major identifiable cause of death in 25 percent of patients with AIDS. Disease in adults represents reactivation of latent infection, because almost all people are infected with *P. carinii,* a protozoon, during the first decade of life. Most cases of PCP occur when the CD4-positive lymphocyte count has fallen below 200 to 250 cells. Pathologically, alveolar membranes become thickened, and mononuclear cell interstitial inflammation occurs as the disease progresses.

Cytomegalic Inclusion Virus

Cytomegalic inclusion virus (CMV) is a causative agent of pneumonia in immunocompromised patients. CMV is a type of herpes virus that results in latent infections and reactivation with shedding of the infected viruses. Pathologically, CMV produces an interstitial pneumonia that ranges from a mild disease to a fulminant course resulting in pulmonary insufficiency and death.

Clinical Presentation

While pneumonias may be classified as two different syndromes, typical and atypical, according to the clinical presentation, these two syndromes are very similar. The characteristics of the clinical manifestations do have some diagnostic value.

Subjective

The "typical" pneumonia syndrome is that which is seen in pneumococcal pneumonia as well as in pneumonia caused by *H. influenzae* and *S. aureus* (Table 8.9). The syndrome is characterized by a sudden onset of fever, cough, and chest pain. Generally, patients with a productive cough are more likely to have a bacterial infection. Patients with pneumococcal pneumonia produce sputum that has a characteristic rusty coloration; purulent sputum may also be evident. Fevers may run as high as 106°F (41.1°C), with peaks observed in the afternoon or evening. The chest pain tends to be pleuritic in nature and increases in intensity during coughing or upon inspiration. Patients often feel cold; about half experience teeth-chattering, shaking, and chills. Myalgia is a common complaint and may extend to tenderness in the calves and thighs. Severe myalgia, particularly when accompanied by vomiting, should strongly suggest the possibility of bacteremia. Respiratory and nonrespiratory symptoms are less commonly reported by older patients with pneumonia. The reduced prevalence of symptoms in older patients is most pronounced for the febrile response (chills and sweats) and for pain (myalgia, headache, and chest pain). Although the older adult may present with attenuated symptoms, this should not be misconstrued as an indication that such patients are less ill.

Table 8.9 Typical Pneumonia Syndrome Associated with Pneumococcal Pneumonia

Subjective Findings	Objective Findings
Sudden onset of fever (may be blunted in older adults)	Crackles
Productive cough	Dullness on percussion
Rust-colored or purulent sputum	Bronchophony, egophony, whispered pectoriloquy
Pleuritic-type pain	Pleural friction rub (severe consolidation)
Splinting	
Chills	Decreased or absent breath sounds
Myalgia	Dense, homogenous shadows in one or more lobes on x-ray

"Atypical" pneumonia is typically produced by *M. pneumoniae* but can also be caused by *L. pneumophila, C. pneumoniae, P. carinii,* and viruses. The atypical pneumonia syndrome is characterized by a more gradual onset, dry "hacking" cough, fever, and prominence of constitutional symptoms (e.g., pounding headaches, coryza, sore throat, shaking chills, and myalgia).

Pneumonias caused by anaerobic infections usually present with subacute or chronic constitutional and pulmonary symptoms. A chronic cough that produces purulent sputum is reported by the majority of patients. From 30 to 60 percent of patients report putrid sputum. This finding is considered to be virtually diagnostic of an aerobic infection and is associated with the development of tissue necrosis and cavitary lesions. Patients also present with chest pain that is dull or pleuritic in nature, hemoptysis, anemia, leukocytosis, and weight loss.

Patients with PCP present with fever, sweats, weight loss, nonproductive cough, decreasing exercise tolerance, and dyspnea on exertion. The median duration of symptoms is 1 month. Tachypnea is universal and is worsened by activity.

Objective

Physical examination of a person with typical pneumonia syndrome usually reveals an acutely ill patient who complains of chest pain and often splints on one side of the thorax. In some patients, crackles and dullness to percussion may be the only abnormality, particularly early in the disease. This finding may correlate with the period of outpouring of fluid into the alveoli. A second group of patients shows the classic signs of consolidation: egophony, bronchophony, whispered pectoriloquy, bronchial breath sounds, and dullness upon percussion. In patients with severe consolidation, crackles may be absent or minimal; a leathery pleural friction rub may be heard over the area of chest tenderness. Finally, a third group of patients has one or more areas of dullness, inspiratory crackles, and diminished breath sounds, a sign of mucus plugs in the smaller bronchioles. Objective findings in atypical pneumonia tend to be less pronounced. Fine to medium crackles may be heard early or at the very end of the inspiratory cycle. Dullness on percussion as well as crackles or wheezing are more likely to be observed later in the disease. Frank consolidation, pleural friction rubs, and pleural effusions are less common than in a typical pneumonia.

Although there is no "typical" syndrome of nosocomial pneumonia, one or more of the following clinical findings are present in most patients: fever, leukocytosis, purulent sputum, and a new pulmonary infiltrate on chest x-ray film. These findings must occur more than 48 hours after admission to the hospital to be considered suggestive of a nosocomial pneumonia.

Auscultation of the lungs is generally negative in patients with PCP, although fine crackles may occasionally be heard. Mucocutaneous lesions such as oral thrush, hairy leukoplakia, and Kaposi's sarcoma are common and suggest the presence of underlying HIV-related immunodeficiency in previously undiagnosed individuals. Physiologically, patients manifest arterial hypoxemia.

Diagnostic Reasoning

Diagnostic Tests

Initial Testing. Although a specific etiologic diagnosis is optimal in the management of CAP, limitations in diagnostic testing make this difficult. The responsible microbe is not identified in approximately 50 percent of patients, even when extensive diagnostic tests are performed. The three most helpful tests used in the initial establishment of a diagnosis of pneumonia include the chest radiograph, leukocyte count, and Gram stain of sputum specimens.

The chest x-ray study is important for three reasons. First, it may help distinguish whether a pneumonia is bacterial or viral in nature. Lobar infiltrates strongly suggest a bacterial infection. A bacterial pneumonia will show dense homogenous shadows involving one or more lobes. Diffuse interstitial infiltrates are suggestive of a viral, *Mycoplasma,* or *Chlamydia* infection. Lateral as well as anterior–posterior (AP) views are necessary to evaluate lesions lying directly behind the heart.

A second reason for a chest x-ray study is to rule out a pleural effusion, a complication occurring in approximately one-third of pneumococcal pneumonia patients. It is important to note that chest x-ray films may be normal in patients who are unable to mount an inflammatory response or early in an infiltrative process. Follow-up chest x-ray films are needed to see if the infiltrate clears completely. Younger patients and those with only single lobe involvement tend to have earlier resolutions.

Finally, cavities may be seen on chest x-ray films in patients with pneumonia caused by anaerobes, *S. aureus, S. pneumoniae* serotype III, *Mycobacterium tuberculosis,* aerobic gram-negative bacilli, and fungi. Cavities occur when necrotic material is discharged into airways, resulting in a necrotizing pneumonia (multiple small cavities, each less than 2 cm) or lung abscess (one or more cavities greater than 2 cm). Anaerobic abscesses are located in dependent segments, are most frequently seen in the right lung, and have air–fluid levels. Typical and atypical TB produce unilateral, well-drained, upper-lobe fibrocavitary disease. Cavities are rarely produced by *H. influenzae, M. pneumoniae,* viruses, and other serotypes of *S. pneumoniae.*

Although pulmonary infiltrates on x-ray films are considered suggestive of a nosocomial pneumonia, findings tend to be very nonspecific. Conditions such as an atelectasis, pleural effusion, pulmonary thromboembolism, and pulmonary edema may mimic nosocomial pneumonia on x-ray evaluation.

It may not always be practical or feasible to obtain a chest x-ray study, so good clinical judgment is essential. Factors that have been found to be predictive of pneumonia infiltrates on chest films include fever above 100°F (37.7°C), tachycardia, locally decreased breath sounds, and sputum production. Chest x-ray films may be normal when the patient is unable to mount an inflammatory response (e.g., in agranulocytosis), is in the early stages of an infiltrative process, or in PCP associated with AIDS.

To help identify those patients who need hospitalization, a WBC count should be done. The count may aid in differentiating between bacterial and viral pneumonia. Although there is no clear distinction, total WBC counts of more than 15,000 suggest a bacterial infection. A differential cell count is not a reliable indicator of causation. Leukopenia may be seen in severe infections, as well as in alcoholics, older adults, and in malnutrition. Blood cultures are indicated only for the patient who requires hospitalization or for cases of suspected nosocomial pneumonia.

A Gram stain of sputum remains the only diagnostic tool available to all practitioners at the onset of therapy. Caution needs to be exercised in the evaluation of a sputum specimen, because expectorated material is frequently contaminated by pathogenic bacteria that colonize the upper respiratory tract and the lower respiratory tract without causing disease. Large numbers of epithelial cells (more than 25 per low-power field) reflect contamination of the specimen with oral contents and mandate that another specimen be collected. If the sputum has been properly collected, polymorphonuclear leukocytes can be readily seen with a Gram's stain and the characteristic lancet-shaped, gram-positive diplococci associated with pneumococcal pneumonia are generally seen in abundance.

Gram stains are seldom useful in patients with atypical pneumonia because sputum is scant and most organisms that cause this syndrome cannot be detected by a Gram stain.

Acid-fast staining of sputum should be done when mycobacterial infection is suspected (Advanced Assessment 8.1).

A sputum culture is less valuable than a Gram stain for providing a casual diagnosis in bacterial pneumonia. Approximately 50 percent of patients with pneumococcal pneumonia have negative sputum cultures, even when large numbers of organisms are present on Gram's stain. Sputum cultures are also negative in 35 to 50 percent of cases of proven *H. influenzae* pneumonia. Isolation of the causative agent in atypical pneumonia is rare.

Sputum cultures may be valuable in the diagnosis of subacute and cavitary pneumonia. Mycobacteria grow well on culture media, and it has been estimated that sputum cultures can detect as few as 10 AFB per milliliter of concentrated sputum. For a more in-depth discussion of the use of sputum cultures for the isolation of mycobacteria, refer to the section on TB.

The usefulness of fungal cultures varies with the organism and the stage of the disease. Chronic forms of coccidiomycosis and blastomycosis may yield positive cultures in 70 to 100 percent of cases if multiple specimens are collected. Accurate positive cultures are not found in patients with histoplasmosis until the disease is in the chronic, cavitary stage. Fewer than 50 percent of patients with cryptococcosis have positive sputum cultures.

Expectorated sputum is usually collected in patients with a productive, vigorous cough, but may be scant in those with atypical pneumonia syndrome, in older adults, and in patients with altered mental status. If the patient is not producing sputum and can cooperate, respiratory secretions can be induced with ultrasonic nebulization of 3 percent saline solution. The use of more invasive procedures to induce sputum in the patient who is unable to produce a sputum specimen carries risks that must be weighed against the potential benefits. In patients who do not require hospitalization or in hospitalized patients who are not severely ill, the need to establish an accurate microbial diagnosis may not be crucial and empirical therapy can be started on the basis of clinical and epidemiological evidence alone. Patients who are hospitalized with CAP and are seriously ill or those who acquire a nosocomial pneumonia clearly need to have a specific causal diagnosis established. In these patients, it may be necessary to obtain specimens from the lower respiratory tract by fiberoptic bronchoscopy, transtracheal puncture, or percutaneous transthoracic lung puncture. Of these invasive procedures, fiberoptic bronchoscopy is currently the preferred technique for obtaining lower respiratory secretions. Specimens obtained by bronchoscopy should be tested with Gram and acid-fast stains, *Legionella* direct fluorescent antibody, and Gomori's methenamine silver stains and should be cultured for aerobic and anaerobic bacteria, *Legionella,* mycobacteria, and fungi.

Diagnostic testing for community-acquired pneumonia with *Streptococcus pneumoniae* may include a pneumococcal urinary antigen test which can detect a protein common to all pneumococcal serotypes. Within 15 minutes, this test can demonstrate the presence of pneumococcus in unconcentrated urine. This can facilitate more immediate decisions about antibiotic therapy. However, the sensitivity of this test varies and it is a complement to sputum and/or blood culture.

ADVANCED ASSESSMENT 8.1

Sputum Stains

Sputum Stain	Organism
Gram's stain	*S. pneumoniae* (gram-positive, lancet-shaped diplococci) *H. influenzae* (gram-positive coccobacilli) *S. aures* (gram-positive tetrads and grape-like clusters)
Acid-fast stain	Myobacterial infection
Fluorescent antibody: sensitivity diminished with concurrent use of inhaled pentamidine	*Legionella* infection
Giemsa stain: frequent false-positive and false-negative results	PCP
Gomori's methamine silver Periodic acid-Schiff stain	Fungal growth

Subsequent Testing. If the pneumonia is severe enough to require hospitalization, at least two blood samples should be obtained for culture as well as CBC and serologic analysis of sodium, urea, nitrogen, creatinine, and glucose. Liver and enzyme tests should be included if hepatic disease or malnutrition is suspected. Serologic studies are sometimes helpful in defining the etiology of certain types of pneumonia. An IgM titer, IgG titer, or IgG titer obtained by indirect immunofluorescence may be diagnostic of *M. pneumoniae* or *C. pneumoniae.* A *Legionella* titer or a urinary antigen test may help confirm Legionnaires' disease.

Pulse oximetry is indicated if the patient presents with respiratory distress, dyspnea at rest, or tachypnea or if the chest x-ray film shows multilobar pulmonary infiltrates. A blood gas analysis should be performed if the patient has known carbon dioxide (CO_2) retention, exacerbations of asthma, or COPD. Typically, a Pao_2 of less than 90 percent or a Pao_2 of less than 60 mm Hg indicates a need for supplemental oxygen. These threshold values must be modified if the patient is chronically hypoxemic.

Differential Diagnosis

Acute bacterial pneumonia should be differentiated from acute bacterial bronchitis. Both of these respiratory infections will cause fever and a productive cough. On auscultation, however, a patient with bronchitis will have clear lung sounds except for a few scattered rhonchi. In comparison, the patient with a bacterial pneumonia will likely have crackles, dullness to percussion, and abnormal breath sounds. Cavitary forms of pneumonia need to be differentiated from pulmonary TB and systemic mycoses, particularly coccidiomycosis and histoplasmosis. Likewise, the patient who presents with symptoms of PCP and a history of fever, weight loss, and pulmonary symptoms should be concurrently evaluated for TB, lymphomas, and brucellosis. Signs and symptoms secondary to central or endobronchial growth of a primary lung cancer will mimic those of a bacterial pneumonia (e.g., productive cough, fever, cough, dyspnea, hemoptysis). The practitioner needs to be aware of any occupational or environmental hazards to which the patient is exposed. For example, workers who develop berylliosis through exposure to beryllium (found in ceramics, high-technology electronics, and alloy manufacturing) may present with an acute pneumonia, or more commonly, with a chronic interstitial pneumonia. Exposure to moldy hay can result in symptoms of pneumonia (e.g., coughing, fever, chills, malaise, and dyspnea) within 4 to 8 hours following exposure. This disease (known as "farmer's lung") may become chronic.

Severe acute respiratory syndrome (SARS) should also be ruled out. Patients should be questioned about travel to an area with known transmission of SARS, as well as close contact with a person who has SARS. The causative agent is a coronavirus. Symptoms include a fever greater than 100.5°F (38°C), cough or respiratory distress. The diagnosis is by enzyme-linked immunosorbent assay (ELISA) or reverse transcriptase-polymerase chain reaction (RT-PCR) assays. Treatment is supportive care. The identification is critical from a public health standpoint rather than from the need of initiating SARS specific care which remains supportive

Management

The initial task in the management of patients with CAP is to determine whether the patient can be treated on an outpatient basis or whether hospitalization is required. The use of hospital services is costly and may further impair the patient's health because of the risk of nosocomial infections. The majority of patients with CAP with no comorbidity can be treated successfully as outpatients. Most patients, even those treated initially in a hospital, prefer outpatient treatment.

The decision to hospitalize a patient with CAP may be the single most important decision during the entire course of the illness. The Pneumonia Outcomes Research Team (PORT)—Pneumonia Severity Index (PSI) is a risk assessment tool used to determine the need for hospitalization of patients with pneumonia. The PSI uses calculations to categorize patients into five severity classes based on age, comorbidities, physical examination, and laboratory findings. Outpatient care can usually be recommended for patients in classes I, II, or III. However, patients suffering from substance abuse, severe psychosocial problems or those lacking social support may require hospitalization despite their PSI classification. This Community-Acquired Pneumonia Prognostic calculator may be found at www.ursa.kcom.edu/CAPcalc/default.htm.

Initial Management

Antimicrobial therapy represents the mainstay of treatment for patients with suspected or confirmed pneumonia. Additional management is supportive in nature and includes the use of analgesics for relief of chest pain and myalgia, antipyretics to control fever, increased fluid intake (at least 3 L over 24 hours), restricted activity or bed rest, a position of comfort (usually upright) to facilitate breathing, and humidified air to relieve irritated nares and pharynx. Expectorants may be indicated to decrease sputum viscosity and clear airways if a productive cough is present. While many promote the use of expectorants such as Guaifenesin (Robitussin, Benylin-E), the best and most cost-effective way to liquify secretions for ease of coughing and eliminating is hydration with water. Patients experiencing a dry, nonproductive cough may benefit from a cough suppressant with codeine

Patients requiring hospitalization need to have ongoing assessment for any indications of impaired respiratory status. Patients who manifest arterial hypoxemia will require supplemental oxygen therapy to maintain Po_2 above 80 mm Hg. In the past, chest physiotherapy had been widely used to mobilize secretions. However, percussion and postural drainage probably offer no added benefit to the patient who has an uncomplicated pneumonia without underlying pulmonary disease.

Treatment Standards/Guidelines 8.1 Empiric Antimicrobial Choices for Community-Acquired Pneumonia (CAP)

Patient Profile	Antimicrobial Agent
Uncomplicated CAP	
Without recent ATBX*	Macrolide Azithromycin (Zithromax) Clarithromycin (Biaxin) Erythromycin (Eryc) OR Doxycycline (Vibramycin)
With recent ATBX	Respiratory fluoroquinolone Gatifloxacin (Tequin) Gemifloxacin (Factive) Levofloxacin (Levaquin) Ciprofloxacin (Cipro) OR Azithromycin or clarithromycin PLUS High-dose amoxicillin (Amoxil) OR Azithromycin or clarithromycin PLUS High-dose amoxicillin–clavulanate (Augmentin)
Patient with CAP with a comorbidity	
Without recent ATBX	An advanced macrolide OR A respiratory fluoroquinolone
With recent ATBX	A respiratory fluoroquinolone alone OR An advanced macrolide PLUS A beta-lactam Amoxicillin–clavulanate (Augmentin) Cefpodoxime (Vantin) Cefprozil (Cefzil) Cefuroxime (Ceftin)
Patient with a suspected aspiration	Augmentin or clindamycin
Patient with CAP plus influenza	A beta-lactam OR A respiratory fluoroquinolone
Inpatient with CAP	
Without recent ATBX	An advanced macrolide OR A respiratory fluoroquinolone
With recent ATBX	As above but choose a different ATB than was recently used PLUS IV ceftriaxone (Rocephin)
Patient with community-acquired MRSA pneumonia†	Vancomycin (Vancocin) OR Linezolid (Zyvox)

*ATBX, antibiotic therapy.
†MRSA, methicillin-resistant *Staphylococcus aureus*

Source: Adapted from Guthrie, R, and Weis, MS: CAP and AECB: The need for a regimen that the bugs can't resist. Consultant 44 (Suppl, 7):S50–S52, 2004.

Community-Acquired Pneumonia (CAP). The Infectious Diseases Society of America (IDSA) has recommended specific therapy for CAP. The clinician must note whether the patient had recent antibiotic therapy or not, and determine what coexisting diseases are present, such as COPD and CHF. Treatment Standards/Guidelines 8.1 summarize the empirical treatment of the patient with CAP. Macrolides include azithromycin (Zithromax), clarithromycin (Biaxin), and erythromycin. Advanced macrolides refer to azithromycin and clarithromycin. Fluoroquinolones include gatifloxacin (Tequin), gemifloxacin (Factive), levofloxacin (Levaquin), and moxifloxacin (Avelox). Gemifloxacin is the only fluoroquinolone approved for multidrug-resistant *Streptococcus pneumoniae.* Beta-lactam agents refer to high-dose amoxicillin, high-dose amoxicillin–clavulanate (Augmentin), cefpodoxime (Vantin), cefprozil (Cefzil), cefuroxime (Ceftin), or ceftriaxone (Rocephin).

In an ICU setting, a third generation beta-lactam plus macrolide or a fluoroquinolone if *Pseudomonas* is not an issue should be prescribed. With beta-lactam or penicillin allergy, a fluoroquinolone with or without clindamycin may be used, depending on suspicion of anaerobes.

In the ICU, if *Pseudomonas* is a concern, an antipseudomonal penicillin should be ordered plus ciprofloxacin, because this is the fluoroquinolone with the best pseudomonal coverage. An aminoglycoside may also be added to this regimen, along with a fluoroquinolone or a macrolide. In this situation, if the patient has a beta-lactam allergy, aztreonam plus levofloxacin or aztreonam plus moxifloxacin or gatifloxacin with or without an aminoglycoside should be used.

Treatment regimens for community-acquired MRSA pneumonia, should typically start with vancomycin, until sensitivities are back, which may indicate susceptibility to Bactrim. Most recently, guidelines have established Linezolid (Zyvox) as an effective alternative therapy. Macrolides are used to effectively treat atypical pneumonias from mycoplasma or chlamydia.

Nosocomial Pneumonia. Antimicrobial therapy is the mainstay of therapy for nosocomial pneumonia as well as for anaerobic/cavitary pneumonia and PCP, but recommendations are less specific. Treatment for nosocomial pneumonia, like treatment of CAP, is usually empiric. Because of the high mortality rate associated with nosocomial pneumonia, treatment must be started as soon as pneumonia is suspected. Empiric therapy for nosocomial pneumonia in patients who are not in an ICU may consist of a beta-lactam antimicrobial agent against *P. aeruginosa* such as ceftazidime (Fortaz), piperacillin–tazobactam (Zosyn), ticarcillin–clavulanate (Timentin), or imipenem–cilastin (Primaxin). *S. aureus* has become increasingly methicillin-resistant. Such strains are resistant to all beta-lactam antibiotics and can be resistant to erythromycin, clindamycin, and the fluoroquinolones. Vancomycin should be prescribed when methicillin-resistant organisms are the possible cause of pneumonia, or linezolid as an alternative.

Empiric therapy for patients with ICU-associated or ventilator-associated pneumonia should be a combination of antibiotics directed against the most virulent organisms, such as *P. aeruginosa, Acinetobacter,* and *Enterobacter.* The most common regimen is a broad-spectrum beta-lactam (an antipseudomonal penicillin, a third-generation antipseudomonal cephalosporin, or imipenem/cilastin) plus an aminoglycoside. If the causative pathogen is isolated, it may be possible to switch to a regimen with a narrower spectrum.

The therapy for anaerobic/cavitary pneumonia depends on the pace of the illness and the degree of clinical toxicity. Clindamycin (Cleocin) is effective for most patients with anaerobic pulmonary infections and is the drug of choice. Anti-TB therapy should also be initiated if the clinical suspicion is high. Treatment of other causes of chronic cavitary pneumonia may be postponed until a diagnosis is established.

Nursing home residents should get a respiratory fluoroquinolone alone or Augmentin plus a macrolide. MRSA CAP has been seen in nursing home patients, as well as particularly sick young adults. In these patients, vancomycin is the intravenous treatment of choice, with Linezolid as the alternative for MRSA treatment. Sensitivities may reveal additional susceptibilities, though, allowing for narrowing of therapy.

Refer to Chapter 16 for the therapy of PCP.

Subsequent Management

The advent of antimicrobial therapy has greatly decreased complications that were commonly seen before the use of antibiotics. Pneumonia that is associated with bacteremia, leukopenia, or multiple lobe involvement increases the likelihood of complications and of death. The mortality rate for patients older than age 65 with bacteremia and involvement of more than three lobes is approximately 60 percent. Complications that do occur are more frequently found in patients with underlying chronic diseases.

The radiographic resolution of CAP is complete in half of patients after 2 weeks and in two-thirds of patients after 4 weeks. Follow-up x-ray studies should be done within 3 to 6 months for all patients who smoke or who are older than age 40. If an abnormality has not cleared on follow-up films, the patient should be evaluated for a possible cancer.

Pleural effusion represents the most common complication seen in patients with pneumonia. Fluid can be detected radiographically in the pleural space of more than 40 percent of patients hospitalized with pneumonia. In most cases, the amount is so small that needle aspiration is unsuccessful. If fluid is removed it typically is not purulent, nor can microbes be seen on a Gram stain.

Fluid that is purulent and has a gram-positive stain or has a pH less than 7.1 is indicative of an empyema. *Streptococcus pneumoniae, Streptococcus pyogenes,* and anaerobic pneumonias are associated with most cases of empyema. It is critical that the infected material be removed from the pleural space by means of a thoracentesis, needle aspiration, or thoracotomy. If this treatment is delayed, the patient is likely to require a prolonged hospital stay. Lung abscesses develop infrequently in *S. pneumoniae* but often occur as complications of pneumonias caused by gram-negative bacteria (e.g., *Klebsiella*), anaerobic bacteria, and *S. aureus.* Drainage of the abscess is essential to prevent further necrosis of the lung tissue. Prolonged antimicrobial therapy is critical for the successful treatment of this complication.

Delayed resolution results from persistent infection and is seen on x-ray studies as residual consolidation. Delayed resolution occurs most often in the patient who is older, malnourished, alcoholic, or has COPD. Progression of infiltrates in spite of antimicrobial therapy is a poor prognostic sign.

Metastatic infections that do occur tend to develop in the meninges, pericardium, heart valves, and skeletal system. Although these complications occur less frequently with antimicrobial therapy, persons with compromised health status remain at risk for the development of these infections. Possible metastatic infections include arthritis, pericarditis, endocarditis, and meningitis. Patients who develop arthritis will experience swollen, red, and painful joints. Purulent exudate may be aspirated from the joints. Meningitis caused by *S. pneumoniae* produces purulent cerebrospinal fluid (CSF). Patients with pneumococcal pneumonia who become disoriented, confused, or somnolent should have a lumbar puncture (LP).

Criteria for hospital discharge include the resolution of fever, an ability to take medications orally, no need for supplemental oxygen, no progression of an infiltrate seen on chest x-ray films, a decrease in the leukocyte count, and the presence of social and family support.

Follow-Up and Referral

Patients considered well enough for outpatient treatment do not need to be closely monitored unless symptoms worsen in spite of antibiotics. The patient should be contacted within 24 to 48 hours of starting therapy and should be scheduled for an office visit for 1 week and 4 to 6 weeks after the initial evaluation.

X-ray resolution of CAP is complete in 50 percent of patients after 2 weeks and in two-thirds of patients after 4 weeks. Examination at the second follow-up should include a chest x-ray film if clinical symptoms have not resolved. X-ray evaluations should be done for all patients who smoke. If an abnormality has not cleared on follow-up films, the patient should be evaluated for a possible cancer.

Smoking cessation is essential if respiratory health is to be maintained. Patients may be most receptive to antismoking counseling while they are still ill or recovering from pneumonia. The follow-up examination provides an opportune time for patient education. Pneumococcal and influenza vaccines should also be given at this time if indicated.

Patient Education

Influenza vaccine is strongly recommended for those older than age 65 and persons of any age who are at risk for adverse complication from influenza. A vaccine against the 23 most common serotypes of *S. pneumoniae* has been available since the early 1980s. The Advisory Committee on Immunization Practices recommends that it be administered to persons older than age 2 who have any of several underlying conditions (e.g., COPD, splenectomy, organ transplants) and to all persons age 65 or older. *Healthy People 2010* objectives target the vaccination of 60 percent of persons at risk for pneumococcal pneumonia by the year 2010. Despite the availability of the vaccine, it is underutilized. The increasing prevalence of multiantibiotic resistance of pneumococci makes immunization of high-risk individuals of utmost importance. For the very elderly patients and those who are institutionalized, revaccination every 5 years is indicated. Vaccine use tends to increase when efforts are made to raise awareness and promote the benefits of vaccination. The practitioner may obtain current and relevant data on pneumococcal vaccines, incidence rates of CAP and hospital-acquired pneumonia, drug therapy, and other pertinent information by contacting the CDC, the National Institute on Aging, and the National Foundation for Infectious Disease.

Tuberculosis

TB is one of the oldest human diseases. It is an infectious disease, most frequently caused by *Mycobacterium tuberculosis* in humans. In early writings, TB was called "consumption" because of its tendency to produce great wasting in its victims. During the 18th and 19th centuries it was known as the "white plague." TB is the leading cause of death worldwide from any single infectious agent. The pandemic of human immunodeficiency virus (HIV) infection and the emergence of drug-resistant TB have worsened the global problem of TB.

Epidemiology and Causes

TB had been considered to be under such good control that a possibility of eradication of the disease in the developing countries was considered to be an obtainable goal. Twenty years ago, this disease returned with a vengeance. It is estimated that 15 million persons in the United States are infected with *M. tuberculosis*. Worldwide, the majority of infected persons are living in developing countries; about 75 percent of these infected people are younger than age 50. Each year, 3 million people worldwide die from the disease. TB is the most common HIV-associated opportunistic infection in many developing countries. Currently the highest estimated case rates occur in Africa.

In the United States, TB is typically a disease of racial and ethnic minorities. The prevalence is three times higher in urban than in rural populations. Case rates are approximately 10 times higher in African American populations and about five times higher among Native Americans and Hispanics. TB among foreign-born residents of the United States accounts for approximately 40 percent of the national total. A factor in the increase of TB among foreign-born persons is the changing trends in countries of origin. Immigration has been increasing from Asia and Latin America, where TB rates are 5 to 20 times higher than those in the United States. Currently, the foreign-born population is concentrated largely in California, New York, Florida, Texas, and New Jersey.

Overall, approximately 10 percent of persons infected with M. tuberculosis will develop clinical TB sometime during their lives. About 5 percent of infected persons will manifest the disease within 1 year of infection. The remaining persons who develop the disease will have a delayed onset of TB, typically at a point of declined protective immunity, such as occurs in silicosis, diabetes mellitus, and diseases associated with immunosuppression, for example, HIV infection and immunosuppressive drugs. Susceptibility to TB is also greater during the first 2 years of life, at puberty, and during adolescence.

Geographically, the largest increases in reported TB cases have been in areas such as New York and Florida, which, in addition to having large foreign-born populations, also have a large number of AIDS cases. Outbreaks of drug-resistant (resistant to at least one anti-TB drug) and multidrug-resistant TB (resistant to isoniazid and rifampin) have occurred in hospitals, prisons, shelters for the homeless, nursing homes, and AIDS residential facilities.

The genus *Mycobacterium* includes the causative agents of TB and leprosy. Mycobacteria are aerobic, asporogenous, nonmotile, acid-fast rods. Of the 58 species of the genus *Mycobacterium,* the members of the TB complex (*M. tuberculosis, M. bovis, M. africanum,* and *M. microti*) are closely related, based on DNA homology studies. The TB complex does not occur in nature and depends on host transmission for its survival. *M. tuberculosis* is the major cause of human disease. Disease due to *M. bovis* is rare in the United States. *M. africanum* is a common cause of TB in Africa and *M. microti* is a pathogen for rodents.

Pathophysiology

Mycobacteria tuberculosis (TB) strains vary in virulence due to differences in the bacteria's genetic make-up. Similarly, persons display varying susceptibility to TB infection due to genetically conferred resistance, age, and comorbid conditions (e.g., chronic illness, immunosuppression). *M. tuberculosis* is most commonly transmitted from person to person by droplet nuclei which are aerosolized by coughing, sneezing, or speaking. Transmission from an infected individual to another is influenced by the intimacy and duration of contact, the degree of infectivity of the patient, and the shared contact environment. Patients with acid-fast staining organisms in their sputum are most infectious to others.

After *M. tuberculosis* organisms are inhaled, some are expelled by ciliated epithelium, and only a small fraction reaches the alveoli, leading to primary infection. There, alveolar macrophages attempt to phagocytose and contain the bacteria; however, virulent strains can multiply rapidly and overcome these macrophages, countering their oxidative bactericidal mechanisms. Nonetheless, activated macrophages react by releasing inflammatory mediators such as IL-12 and tumor necrosis factor-alpha (TNF-α), which contribute to fever, anorexia, and weight loss. Macrophages also stimulate the recruitment of T lymphocytes to the area of infection. Helper T (CD4+) and cytotoxic killer T (CD8+) lymphocytes are also integral in the effort to kill bacteria, as activated macrophages and T lymphocytes form granulomas or tubercles in an effort to confine bacterial growth by walling off the mycobacteria.

Within these tubercles, multiplication of the organisms is inhibited by low oxygen content and low pH. T lymphocytes release inflammatory mediators which neutralize the bacteria contained in the tubercle's central necrotic area known as the caseum because of its cheeselike appearance upon gross inspection. In a minority of cases, highly virulent strains of *Mycobacteria tuberculosis* may cause rapid infection, invading lung parenchyma, bronchioles, and blood vessels. Hemoptysis, a frequent clinical sign of active infection, may reflect the erosion of a granuloma into a pulmonary blood vessel. Old granulomas eventually calcify, identifiable as one or more Ghon complexes on chest x-ray film. Viable bacteria may remain dormant in these lesions for decades, only to be reactivated when the fine balance between host immunity and bacterial pathogenesis is tipped in favor of the mycobacteria. This results in secondary infection known as reactivation TB, seen typically in chronically ill or otherwise immunosuppressed individuals.

Mycobacteria can also spread via lymphatics or hematogenously, resulting in disseminated infection. Extrapulmonary sites of tuberculous infection include the lymph nodes, pleura, bones, meninges, peritoneum, pericardium, and genitourinary tract. Solid organs may be seeded at multiple tiny foci, taking on a millet seedlike appearance on gross inspection termed "miliary tuberculosis." Such pathologic findings have been noted as far back as the 1700s. Today, the term miliary TB has been extended to encompass all forms of progressive, disseminated TB infection but is still seen most often in children younger than 1 year of age.

When testing for TB, persons with previous exposure or infection develop a positive cell-mediated (type IV) delayed-type hypersensitivity skin reaction as a result of previously sensitized helper T lymphocytes (CD4+) which are attracted to the testing site when a small amount of mycobacterial antigen (purified protein derivative [PPD]) is injected intradermally. Reactions of this type typically require 48 to 72 hours to develop and are classified based on the degree of skin induration (rather than erythema) at the site of injection in relation to specific population norms.

Mycobacteria tuberculosis are aerobic and therefore particularly attracted to the apical segments of the upper lung lobes where high oxygen concentration favors their proliferation. While the upper lung zone is the most common site of accelerated growth of the bacilli, there may be a later progression at distant sites in the body. The kidneys, brain, and bones are the most common sites of distant progression.

Individuals may continue to discharge mycobacteria into the environment from pulmonary tubercles until multiple drug therapy is instituted to drive bacteria into a dormant state or eradicate infection completely. Although mycobacteria are almost always found in the bone marrow, liver, and spleen when disease occurs, uncontrolled multiplication of the bacilli in these organs is rare. Immunosuppressed individuals, particularly those with T-lymphocyte deficiencies and compromised cell-mediated immunity (e.g., persons living with HIV), are highly susceptible to tuberculous infection.

Clinical Presentation

Subjective

TB may mimic, or occur concurrently with pneumoconiosis, pneumonia, bronchiectasis, sarcoidosis, lung abscess, neoplasm, or fungal infections. It is very common for the onset to be insidious, with symptoms of anorexia, fatigue, digestive disturbances, a slow weight loss, irregular menses, and a lack of stamina. Persons may complain of being unable to complete a day's work. This pattern of onset will continue for several weeks or even months, when a low-grade elevation of temperature appears characteristically in the afternoon.

Pulmonary TB is characterized principally by a productive cough, purulent sputum, and repeated occurrences of coryza-like symptoms with rhinorrhea and nasal congestion. The cough progresses slowly over weeks or months to become more frequent and associated with the production of mucoid or mucopurulent sputum. The cough is usually due to sloughing of small caseous lesions within the presence of exudate in the bronchi. Sputum is characteristically yellow but is not tenacious or foul-smelling. Hemoptysis is a common symptom in patients with necrotizing or cavitary lesions. Blood usually appears as small streaks in the sputum. Dyspnea is uncommon in pulmonary TB and usually indicates extensive parenchymal involvement, massive pleural effusion, or other underlying cardiopulmonary disease.

A less frequently seen pattern of onset may be that of an acute febrile illness with an abrupt onset of high fever, chills, tachycardia, and weakness. A productive cough is seen, along with myalgia and sweating. Erythema nodosum may occur with the acute onset of symptoms. These patients may have paid no attention to milder symptoms that have preceded the acute episode. This is a common finding in the uneducated, alcoholics, or in persons debilitated by age or other disease.

Other less frequent modes of onset include pleuritic pain and hoarseness. Pleuritic pain, usually unilateral, tends to be accentuated by coughing or deep inspiration. Hoarseness is usually a result of involvement of the larynx and may be accompanied by severe pain. Constitutional symptoms tend to be general in nature and consist of night sweats, fatigue upon exertion, weight loss, and malaise.

In obtaining the health history, the clinician must keep in mind the chronicity of TB and the insidious nature of the onset of symptoms. Patients should be questioned about exposure to anyone with an open case of TB. Potential sources of exposure include the family as well as co-workers. Other significant disclosures obtained from a health history include a past diagnosis of pneumonia with recurrence, pleurisy, uncontrolled diabetes, alcoholism, malnutrition, and occupational exposures to quartz dust or silica. Other risk factors that should be taken into account are drug abuse, country of origin, corticosteroid use, and gastrectomy.

Objective

A complete examination of any patient suspected of having TB should always be performed. Although pulmonary TB is the most common form of TB, the clinician needs to be cognizant of any indications of extrapulmonary TB. Examination of the chest will usually provide the primary indications of pulmonary TB. Rhonchi, crackles, wheezing, and bronchial breath sounds may be heard upon auscultation but may have no radiographic counterparts. Dullness on percussion is commonly associated with pneumonic lesions. Persons with long-standing disease may manifest asymmetrical lung expansion, displacement of the trachea, and muscular atrophy. Although there are no specific changes related to pulmonary function, in patients with extensive parenchymal involvement, the vital capacity and other lung volumes may become decreased.

The patient should be examined for any evidence of present or past extrapulmonary TB in such structures as the genitourinary (GU) tract, lymph nodes, bones and joints, peritoneum, larynx, eye, abdominal organs, and the neurologic system (Table 8.10). Physical findings may include hepatomegaly, splenomegaly, and generalized lymphadenopathy. Abnormal behavior, headaches, and seizures may herald TB meningitis. Meningitis occurs frequently in infants and small children as a complication of early infection, but it may be seen in any age group. Bone and joint involvement, most often seen in older adults, may result in arthritis, osteomyelitis, fever, and localized pain. The lower spine and weightbearing joints are most often affected by skeletal TB. Genitourinary TB may present as recurrent UTIs with no growth of common pathogens, pyuria without bacteriuria, pelvic inflammatory disease (PID), amenorrhea, infertility, and perianal fistulas.

Diagnostic Reasoning

Diagnostic Tests

Initial Testing. The tuberculin skin test (TST) remains the standard test for determining infection with *Mycobacteria tuberculosis* but does not distinguish between active and latent infection. The TST tends to have a strong positive predictive value, but poorer negative predictive value. Skin testing on a patient suspected of being infected may easily be done in an office or clinic setting. It is useful as an

Table 8.10 Clinical Indicators of Extrapulmonary Tuberculosis

Extrapulmonary Sites	Clinical Manifestations
Genitourinary tract	Recurrent UTIs with no growth of common pathogens Pyuria without bacteriuria Unexplained hematuria Irregular menses, amenorrhea, PID, infertility Epididymitis Induration of the prostate
Bone and joints (lower spine and weight-bearing joints most common site)	Arthritis, osteomyelitis Fever and localized pain
Meninges	Headaches, convulsions Abnormal behavior
Peritoneum	Ascites, fever
Pericardium	Pericarditis
Lymph nodes	Hilar or mediastinal lymphadenitis Cervical and supraclavicular lymphadenopathy

epidemiologic tool to identify infected and especially recently infected people for preventive therapy and contact tracing. The ATS has developed criteria for tuberculin testing. Persons for whom tuberculin testing is routinely indicated are listed in the Screening Recommendations/Guidelines 8.1.

The most accurately and widely used method for skin testing is the Mantoux technique of injecting intermediate-strength PPD intradermally (TST). The reaction to intradermally injected tuberculin is the classic example of a delayed cellular hypersensitivity reaction. These reactions begin at 5 to 6 hours after injection and are maximal at 72 hours. In older adults or in persons who are being tested for the first time, the reaction may develop more slowly and may not peak until after 72 hours. A number of factors related to a decreased ability to respond to the tuberculin are included in Table 8.11. These factors do not negate testing in these situations because only a fraction of infected persons with these conditions may have falsely nonreactive results. If the lack of reaction to the testing is suspected to be a false response, then a repeat TST should be done. If generalized inability to respond is suspected, then it may be necessary to test delayed hypersensitivity using several other antigens to which the person has had a likely exposure. Anergy should be suspected if the person fails to respond to any of the antigens. Many infectious disease specialists think that anergy testing is no longer useful, as patients may have selective anergy to TB, but not to other antigens, so they are not helpful in ruling out TB.

It is possible to obtain an inaccurate interpretation of the patient's tuberculin response when the administration

SCREENING RECOMMENDATIONS/ GUIDELINES 8.1

Guidelines for Tuberculin Screening

- A person with signs and/or symptoms or current tuberculosis (TB)
- Recent contact with known TB cases
- A person at high risk of recent infection with *M. tuberculosis*
- Persons suspected of having TB
- A person with abnormal chest x-ray films compatible with past TB
- A person with medical conditions that increase the risk of TB
- Persons with HIV infection
  - Immigrant from Asia, Africa, Latin America
  - A person from a medically underserved or high-risk minority population
  - A resident or employee in a prison or long-term care facility
  - An employee in a health-care facility

SOURCE: American Thoracic Society. Diagnosis standards and classification of tuberculosis. Am Rev Respir Dis 145:525, 1990.

Table 8.11 Factors Contributing to a Decreased Response to Tuberculin Skin Testing

Infections:
- Viral: measles, mumps, chickenpox, HIV infection
- Bacterial: typhoid fever, brucellosis, typhus, leprosy, pertussis, recent or overwhelming *M. tuberculosis* infection
- Fungal: South American blastomycosis
- Live virus vaccinations: measles, mumps, polio

Nutritional factors: severe protein depletion

Diseases affecting lymphoid organs: Hodgkin's lymphoma, chronic lymphocytic leukemia

Drugs: corticosteroids and other immunosuppressive agents

Age: newborns, older adults

Stress: surgery, burns, mental illness, graft versus host reactions of the skin test is done incorrectly. Factors that may contribute to an inaccurate reading of the test include improper handling of the tuberculin, improper administration technique, and inaccurate reading of tuberculin test (e.g., by an inexperienced reader). To minimize reduction in potency by adsorption, tuberculin should never be transferred from one container to another and skin tests should be given soon after the syringe has been filled. Tuberculin should be kept refrigerated and stored in the dark as much as possible. The TST (0.1 mL) should be injected into the volar or the dorsal surface of the forearm, away from veins and into intact skin, free of lesions. The injection should be made just beneath the surface of the skin, with a one-quarter to one-half-inch 27-gauge needle and a tuberculin syringe. A discrete, pale elevation of the skin (a wheal) 6 to 10 mm in diameter should be produced when the injection has been done correctly. If the first test was improperly administered, another test dose can be given immediately, but in a site several centimeters from the original injection.

Tests should be read 72 hours after injection, using good lighting with the forearm slightly flexed at the elbow. The basis of reading the test is the presence or absence of induration, which is determined by inspection and palpation. The diameter of the induration is measured transversely to the long axis of the forearm and recorded in millimeters. The size of the TST reaction has nothing to do with erythema, but is based solely on induration, as it is a type IV T-cell–mediated immune response. History of BCG vaccination should be disregarded in interpreting the TST because immunity from BCG wanes over time.

Persons with sensitivity to tuberculin are known as reactors. The definition of a tuberculin reaction size that is indicative of an infection with *Mycobacteria tuberculosis* is influenced by the dose, dilution, and nature of the tuberculin preparation being used, immunologic factors, and the relative prevalence of tuberculin sensitivity resulting from infection with *Mycobacteria tuberculosis* and that resulting from other mycobacteria in the population being studied. Reactions caused by infections with mycobacteria other than *Mycobacteria tuberculosis* (cross-reactions) are common in many parts of the world. Generally, a reaction to *Mycobacteria tuberculosis* will be a larger reaction than would be seen in a cross-reaction. Guidelines for the classification of reactions to intradermal Mantoux tests have established three categories of positive reactions (5-mm, 10-mm, and 15-mm induration) based on the patient's immunosuppressive status, risk factors for exposure, and probability of cross-reaction (Table 8.12). A positive reaction in any patient represents only the presence of TB infection. In the United States, a positive TST without clinical TB infection (negative chest x-ray findings and no symptoms) should be treated to minimize the possibility of reactivation (secondary) TB. Standard regimens are INH for 9 months (least hepatotoxic regimen), rifampin for 4 months, or rifampin plus PZA for 2 months (but this is the most hepatotoxic regimen). LFT screening is needed while the patient is on therapy.

Table 8.12 Interpretation of Tuberculin Skin Testing

Diameter of Induration	Positive Results
>5 mm	• Persons with HIV infection or persons with risk factors for HIV infection and unknown HIV status • Persons who were recently exposed to clinically active TB, persons with organ transplants • Persons with chest films indicating healed TB
>10 mm	• Recent arrivals (<5 years) • Foreign-born persons from high-risk countries in Africa, Asia, Latin America • Medically underserved low-income populations and high-risk racial or ethnic minority populations • Intravenous drug abusers • Residents and employees of high-risk congregate settings: prisons and jails, nursing homes and other residential settings for elderly people, AIDS patients, homeless shelters • Mycobacteriology laboratory personnel. • Persons with medical conditions known to increase the risk for TB: diabetes, renal failure, silicosis, immunosuppressive therapy, hematological disorders (e.g., leukemia, lymphoma), gastrectomy, 10% or more below ideal body weight
>15 mm	• All other persons

Subsequent Testing. In patients in whom there is a clinical suspicion of TB, the first diagnostic step should be a combination of a standard AP and lateral chest x-ray film and a sputum examination for mycobacteria. The initial radiographic manifestation of an initial infection in the adult or a child is usually parenchymal infiltration accompanied by ipsilateral lymph node enlargement. The parenchymal lesions may be seen in any portion of the lung, but are seen most commonly in the apical and posterior segments of the upper lobes, or in the superior segments of the lower lobes. Lesions may be dense and homogenous, with lobar, segmental, or subsegmental distribution. Patients with HIV disease tend to have atypical radiographic findings. These patients tend not to have cavitations, and infiltrates are less likely to occur in the upper lobes. Cavitations are also seen infrequently in older patients and in those who may be immunosuppressed. Hematogenous TB is characterized by diffuse, finely nodular, uniformly distributed lesions on the chest x-ray film. The term "miliary" is applied to this appearance, because the nodules are about the size of a millet seed (approximately 2 mm in diameter).

Chest x-ray films that show no change in findings over a 3- to 4-month interval can generally be interpreted as showing a past TB or another disease. The use of a single chest x-ray film as a guide to the nature or the stability of the underlying disease is questionable. The terms "old" or "fibrotic" are not accurate terms to use when interpreting a single chest x-ray film. Any persistent infiltrate in an older person should be considered suggestive of TB. This form of TB is often missed in older adults, especially among patients residing in a nursing home.

In pulmonary TB, examination of sputum provides the most convenient method of identifying the presence of bacilli, in terms of low cost, widespread availability, ease of performance, and reliability. The patient must be instructed to produce material brought up from the chest by coughing. A series of at least three single specimens on different days should be collected from patients who have a productive cough. When a patient is unable to produce an adequate amount of sputum, it is possible to obtain by gastric lavage the bronchopulmonary secretions that the patient has unknowingly swallowed during the night. Gastric aspiration is done following a period of fasting for 8 to 10 hours; it should be performed before the patient arises. About 50 mL of gastric contents is required for this test, which is best performed in the hospitalized patient.

It is possible to induce sputum production by inhalation of hypertonic saline. These specimens will be thinner and more watery than sputum produced spontaneously. Sputum induced by this method may produce a violent and uncontrolled cough, so special methods of air control may be indicated. Occasionally, a pooled specimen, collected over a period of 10 to 24 hours, may be helpful if the methods previously described are not effec-tive or appropriate. This type of specimen is more subject to contamination and is best collected in an institutional setting.

Bronchial washings obtained with fiberoptic bronchoscopy may be indicated in patients who are unable to produce sputum or in those who are thought to have TB despite negative culture reports. When extrapulmonary TB is suspected, it is necessary to collect less common clinical specimens from sources such as urine, peritoneal, pericardial, and pleural fluids, bones and joints, and lymph nodes.

The detection of AFB in stained smears examined by direct microscopy provides the first evidence of the presence of mycobacteria in a clinical specimen. It is estimated that 50 to 80 percent of patients with pulmonary TB will have positive sputum smears. The sputum smear is the easiest and quickest procedure and provides the practitioner with a preliminary confirmation of the diagnosis. The smear also provides the practitioner with a quantitative estimate of the number of bacilli being excreted by the patient. These estimates should be described as rare, few, or numerous. The lowest concentration of organisms that can be detected by microscopic examination is 10 per milliliter of sputum. For direct microscopy of sputum, the most widely used method is the Ziehl-Neelsen staining method.

All clinical specimens suspected of containing mycobacteria must be inoculated onto culture media. Culture yield seems to be associated with the clinical presentation of the patient. One study reported that patients with cavitary disease tend to have a higher rate of positive cultures than do patients with focal infiltrates. The cultures should be incubated at 37°C and examined at weekly intervals. The time from the laboratory's receipt of the specimen to the report of the culture is usually 3 to 6 weeks. In rare situations, such as repeated contaminated specimens or patients with positive Gram stains and negative cultures, guinea pig inoculation may be necessary.

Susceptibility of tubercle bacilli to various anti-TB drugs may be determined by either the direct or the indirect test. The direct drug-susceptibility test is performed by using clinical specimens of AFB, which are inoculated directly onto drug-containing culture medium. Growth is then compared with growth on non–drug-containing medium. An indirect test is performed by using a subculture from the primary isolation as the inoculum. Although the direct test is preferred, because it is more representative of the bacterial population of the patient, the indirect test may be useful when the initial smear is negative but the culture is positive, when growth on the control medium is inadequate for a reliable test, or when a reference culture is submitted by another laboratory. In the past, the previously untreated patient with newly diagnosed TB was started on chemotherapy without prior drug-susceptibility testing. Recommendations for drug-susceptibility testing have been modified because of the emergence of drug-resistant bacilli and are discussed in the section on clinical management.

Differential Diagnosis

Difficulties in a differential diagnosis arise when the tubercle bacilli cannot be isolated by smear or culture and in situations in which other diseases such as carcinoma or pulmonary mycosis exist. Pulmonary lesions of small extent, particularly the solitary nodule or coin nodule, need to be differentiated from early carcinoma of the lung, pulmonary infarction, localized pulmonary fibrosis, and pneumonia of fungal, viral, mycoplasmal, or bacterial origin with delayed clearing or resolution. In extensive forms of pulmonary TB, bronchopneumonia and lobar pneumonia must be considered. The acute cavitary forms of TB must be differentiated from lung abscess. Other chronic pulmonary diseases that frequently are characterized by cavity formations include the systemic mycoses, particularly coccidiomycosis and histoplasmosis.

Pulmonary TB of hematogenous origin must be differentiated from other types of infection that may manifest in similar fashion: silicosis, berylliosis, asbestosis, sarcoidosis, diffuse interstitial fibrosis, scleroderma, metastatic neoplasms, or alveolar cell carcinoma. From the perspective of clinical manifestations, the APN must consider other conditions that may cause prolonged or obscure fevers, such as lymphoma, brucellosis, and HIV infection.

Management

The development of specific chemotherapeutic agents revolutionized the prognosis of TB and TB infection, making the disease truly curable and preventable. Drug treatment of TB should be viewed as both a personal health measure intended to cure the ill patient and as a public health measure intended to interrupt transmission of tubercle bacilli in the community.

Initial Management

In patients in whom the clinical and radiographic findings suggest a diagnosis of TB and the sputum examination reveals the presence of mycobacteria, a working diagnosis can be made and anti-TB chemotherapy can be started. For patients in whom TB is suspected but whose smear results are negative, an alternative is to begin therapy and wait for culture results. Initiating chemotherapy in the absence of a definitive diagnosis is a valid approach, but caution needs to be exercised in doing so in patients with HIV infection and multidrug resistance. X-ray findings in patients with AIDS are often atypical and may be indicative of a range of diagnostic possibilities. A presumptive diagnosis of TB in these patients may be more speculative.

The main goal of therapy is to eliminate all tubercle bacilli from the patient while avoiding the situation of clinically significant drug resistance. The treatment consists of administering multiple drugs that the organism is susceptible to, add new drugs to the regimen when it is suspected that treatment is not working; provide the maximum therapy in the shortest amount of time, and to insist on patient compliance. While curing the individual patient, the transmission of *Mycobacterium tuberculosis* to other persons needs to be minimized.

The current minimal acceptable duration of treatment for all children and adults with culture-positive TB is 6 months. The initial phase of a 6-month regimen should consist of a 2-month regimen of isoniazid (INH), rifampin (RIF), pyrazinamide (PZA) and ethambutol (EMB), or streptomycin in children who are too young to be monitored for visual acuity, should be included in the initial regimen until the results of the drug-susceptibility studies are available, unless there is little possibility of drug resistance (e.g., less than 4 percent primary resistance to INH in the community and the patient has had no previous treatment with anti-TB medication, is not from a country with a high prevalence of drug-resistant TB, or has no known exposure to a drug-resistant case). The second phase of therapy should consist of INH and RIF for a total of 4 months (daily treatment or 2 to 3 times per week). Therapy should be prolonged if the response is slow or otherwise suboptimal.

An alternative regimen for persons who cannot take PZA (e.g., pregnant women) consists of a 9-month regimen of INH and RIF. Ethambutol should also be included until the results of the susceptibility studies are available unless there is little possibility of drug resistance. Drug resistance is most common in HIV patients and immigrants. If INH resistance is confirmed, rifampin, plus PZA, plus ethambutol should be continued for a minimum of 6 months. For rifampin resistance, INH plus ethambutol should be used for 18 months or INH, PZA, and streptomycin for 9 months. In HIV patients, rifabutin should always be used because rifampin interacts with protease inhibitors and non-nucleoside retroviral inhibitors.

Recommended doses for the initial treatment of TB in adults are shown in Drugs Commonly Prescribed 8.2.

Directly observed therapy (DOT) should be considered for all patients because of the difficulty in predicting which patients will adhere to a prescribed regimen. When TB is initially diagnosed, the practitioner should explain to the patient about the disease, the treatment, and the necessity of completing the recommended therapy. If DOT is considered

Drugs Commonly Prescribed 8.2: Tuberculosis

Drug	Indication	Daily Dosage	Three Times Weekly Dosage
Isoniazid (INH)	Initial treatment of TB in adults	5 mg/kg max: 300 mg	15 mg/kg max: 900 mg
Rifampin (RIF)	Initial treatment of TB in adults	10 mg/kg max: 600 mg	10 mg/kg max: 600 mg
Pyrazinamide (PZA)	Initial treatment of TB in adults	15–30 mg/kg max: 2 g	50–70 mg/kg max: 4 g
Ethambutol (EMB)	Initial treatment of TB in adults	5–25 mg/kg max: 2.5 g	25–30 mg/kg max: 2.5 g
Streptomycin	Initial treatment of TB in adults	15 mg/kg max: 1 g	25–30 mg/kg max: 1.5 g

to be indicated, the patient and the practitioner should agree on a method that ensures the greatest rate of adherence and maintains confidentiality. DOT may require an outreach worker to go into the community and administer each dose of medication to the patient. Many patients can, however, receive the treatment at a center agreed on by the practitioner and the patient. Common community settings include TB clinics, community health centers, migrant clinics, homeless shelters, jails or prisons, nursing homes, schools, drug treatment centers, hospitals, HIV/AIDS clinics, or occupational health clinics. In some situations, a responsible person other than a health-care worker may be able to administer the chemotherapy. Possible resources in the community include correctional facility personnel, social and welfare caseworkers, clergy, teachers, and reliable volunteers.

HIV infection and other factors that compromise a patient's immune system are important considerations when practitioners select the most effective regimen. These factors are particularly important with drug-resistant TB because of the potential for rapid disease progression and death when patients receive inadequate treatment. See the recommendations for the treatment of TB among HIV-infected patients in Chapter 16.

DOT and experienced TB/HIV caregivers are considered to be critical to the effective treatment. Substituting rifabutin (Mycobutin) for rifampin (Rimactane, Rifadin) allows for the concurrent administration of anti-TB and antiviral drug therapies. Currently, recommendations indicate that HIV-infected patients should be treated for a total of 9 months and for at least 6 months following sputum conversion. Intermittent therapy has not been determined to be less effective than daily administration of chemotherapy.

Effective therapy for TB is essential for pregnant women. Untreated TB represents a greater hazard to a pregnant woman and her fetus than does treatment of the disease. Initial treatment should consist of INH and RIF. Ethambutol (Myambutol) should also be included unless primary INH resistance is unlikely. Streptomycin should not be prescribed for pregnant women because it may cause congenital deafness in the fetus. PZA is recommended by international TB organizations for use in pregnant women. In the United States, PZA is not currently recommended because it has not been determined if there is a risk of teratogenicity. Breast feeding does not need to be discouraged, because the small concentrations of anti-TB drugs in breast milk are not adequate to produce toxicity in the newborn. TB during pregnancy is not an indication for a therapeutic abortion.

Regimens that are adequate for treating adults with pulmonary TB should be effective in treating extrapulmonary disease. Bacteriologic evaluation of extrapulmonary TB may be limited by the relative inaccessibility of the disease site. Response to treatment often must be judged on the basis of clinical and radiographic findings. Surgery may be necessary to obtain specimens for diagnosis and to treat such processes as constrictive pericarditis. Corticosteroid therapy has been shown to be of benefit in preventing cardiac constriction from TB pericarditis and in decreasing the neurologic sequelae of TB meningitis.

Subsequent Management

Today, the majority of patients with TB may undergo treatment and remain in their own home setting. There may be specific patient situations that may mandate the need for hospitalization of the patient with TB. Some of the indications include very ill patients who have no responsible person at home to provide care, patients with advanced pulmonary disease with highly positive sputum smears or severe extrapulmonary disease, or the presence of associated medical problems that require hospitalization.

Adults should have measurements of serum bilirubin, hepatic enzymes, blood urea nitrogen (BUN), and creatinine and a CBC, including platelet count, before starting chemotherapy for TB. Visual acuity and red-green color perception tests are recommended before initiation of ethambutol, and a serum uric acid level should be measured before starting PZA. Patients should be advised to report symptoms suggestive of drug toxicity. For INH-containing regimens, symptoms of concern are anorexia, nausea, vomiting, fatigue or weakness, dark urine, icterus, rash, paresthesia of the hands and feet, fever, and abdominal tenderness. Routine monitoring of laboratory tests for evidence is not recommended, but monthly questioning for symptoms of drug toxicity is indicated. Patients with known liver disease or heavy drinkers may need to have periodic liver function tests (LFTs). Appropriate laboratory tests are mandatory if symptoms of drug toxicity should develop.

Periodic examination of the patient is necessary to observe for changes in symptoms, signs, body weight, and temperature. The single most important laboratory test is the bacteriologic examination of bronchopulmonary secretions. A progressive fall in the number of AFB in weekly or biweekly specimens is a good indicator of effective chemotherapy. Periodic laboratory checks of blood, urine, visual acuity, eighth-nerve function, renal function, and hepatic function are desirable based on the severity of the illness and the drugs being administered. Patients should be questioned closely for any symptoms of drug toxicity as well as the level of adherence.

It is not necessary to restrict physical activity and require bed rest for most patients. For patients who are experiencing fever, night sweats, anorexia, and bouts of coughing, bed rest may help make them more comfortable. Patients who present with a history of fever should have a normal temperature within 2 to 3 weeks following the initiation of chemotherapy. It may be necessary to suppress the cough reflex in patients who are experiencing severe coughing. Codeine and hydrocodone are the most useful for temporary treatment. If the patient is producing thick and tenacious secretions, suppression of the cough reflex is not desirable. These patients should be instructed in adequate hydration, air humidification, and prescribed an expectorant. Chest pain may manifest if the patient develops pleuritis.

Occasionally chest pain may be caused by a fractured rib resulting from hard coughing. An instillation of a local anesthetic about the rib fracture is preferred over the older method of strapping the chest. Coughing resulting in occasional episodes of streaked or bloody sputum requires no specific treatment other than managing the cough. There may be significant hemoptysis with bronchogenic spread of the TB; however, it tends to be self-limiting. In advanced chronic cavitary TB, fatal pulmonary hemorrhage or shock can occur if large pulmonary arteries or Rasmussen's aneurysm slough or ulcerate.

Follow-Up and Referral

The response to anti-TB chemotherapy in patients with positive bacteriology is best evaluated by repeated examinations of sputum. Sputum cultures should be done at least once monthly until sputum conversion is documented. After 2 months of treatment with regimens containing both INH and RIF, the majority of patients should convert to negative cultures. Patients whose sputum cultures have not become negative after 3 months of treatment should be carefully reevaluated. Drug-susceptibility tests should be repeated and treatment should be administered or continued under direct observation. If organisms are found to be resistant, the treatment regimen should be modified to include at least two drugs to which the organisms are susceptible and administered using DOT. Patients whose sputum no longer contains *M. tuberculosis* should have at least one further sputum smear and culture performed at the completion of therapy. X-ray evaluations during treatment are of less importance than sputum examination. A chest x-ray film at completion of treatment will provide a baseline comparison for any future films.

Shortness of breath in a patient without underlying pulmonary disease is suggestive of complications of pulmonary TB and requires further diagnostic inquiry. Sudden breathlessness may be a symptom of acute pleurisy with pleuritic pain, a pleural effusion, spontaneous pneumothorax, a massive extension of the TB, or an atelectasis. Patients who have coexisting emphysema or pulmonary disease may become dyspneic with only minimal involvement of the lungs.

Patients infected with *M. tuberculosis* who do not have the active disease still harbor small numbers of organisms. INH given for 6 to 12 months is effective in decreasing the risk of future TB in adults (300 mg per day) and children (10 to 14 mg/kg per day up to 300 mg per day) with TB infection demonstrated by a positive TB skin test reaction.

Preventive Therapy

The ATS has identified risk groups for whom preventive therapy is indicated (Table 8.13).

All persons with known HIV infection or suspected of having HIV who have positive skin tests should receive preventive therapy for TB. HIV-infected persons who are at high risk for TB but have negative skin tests should also be considered for preventive therapy.

Household members and other close contacts have a 2 to 4 percent risk of developing TB within the first year of exposure to the index case. The risk for very young children and adolescents may be twice the risk of the adult. People who do not develop TB disease within the first year will continue to be at risk for the disease throughout their life. Children should be treated even if their initial skin tests are negative. Skin testing should be repeated after 3 months of INH. If the skin test becomes positive, INH preventive therapy should be continued for a total of 9 months.

Persons with medical conditions such as diabetes, long-term use of adrenocorticosteroids, use of immunosuppressive therapy, IV drug use, hematologic disease, end-stage renal disease (ESRD), and conditions associated with rapid weight loss or chronic malnutrition are also at risk for TB. Other risk groups include foreign-born persons from high-prevalence countries (Asia, Africa, Latin America), medically underserved groups, especially high-risk racial or ethnic populations (African Americans, Native Americans, Hispanics), and residents of long-term care facilities (e.g., prisons, nursing homes, mental health facilities).

Bacille Calmette-Guérin (BCG) vaccination is an antimycobacterial vaccine developed from an attenuated strain of *Mycobacterium bovis*. Millions of persons worldwide have been vaccinated with BCG. It is not currently recommended because of multiple factors including its variable effectiveness against pulmonary TB. BCG vaccination in the United States should be used only after consultation with the local Health Department. The BCG vaccination should not be used in persons with impaired immune responses.

Because BCG vaccination has been widespread in the majority of countries outside the United States, the clinician will undoubtedly encounter patients who may be at risk for TB who have been vaccinated. Previous vaccination with BCG typically results in tuberculin test conversion, producing a reaction that may be difficult to distinguish from a natural mycobacterial infection. A large reaction to PPD tuberculin in BCG-vaccinated persons, especially among persons from countries with a high prevalence of TB, should be considered indicative of a possible TB infection and the patient should be evaluated appropriately. Reasons for not assuming that a large reaction to tuberculin testing is due to the BCG vaccination include (1) conversion rates after vaccination may be much less than 100 percent, (2) the mean reaction size among vaccines is often less than 10 mm, and (3) TB sensitivity tends to wane after vaccination.

To keep abreast of changes in treatment recommendations for TB, visit the Division of TB Elimination Web site at http://www.cdc.gov/nchstp/tb.

Patient Education

The necessity of educating the patient and the family about the disease, treatment, and importance of completing the

Table 8.13 **Groups for Whom Preventive TB Therapy Is Recommended**

Group	Comments
The following high-risk groups should be given treatment if their reaction to the Mantoux tuberculin skin test (PPD) is ≥ 5 mm:	
1. Persons with known HIV infection and those suspected of having HIV infection (persons with risk factors for HIV infection whose status is unknown)	HIV-infected persons who are at high risk for TB but have negative skin tests should be considered for preventive therapy.
2. Close contacts of persons with newly diagnosed infectious TB 3. Persons with fibrotic changes on chest x-ray exam consistent with old TB	Household members and other close contacts have a 2%–4% chance of developing TB within the first year of exposure to the index case. The risk for very young children and adolescents may be twice that of the adult. People who do not develop TB disease within the first year will continue to be at risk for the disease throughout their life. Children should be treated, even if their initial skin tests are negative. Skin testing should be repeated after 3 months of INH therapy. If the skin test becomes positive, INH preventive therapy should be continued for a total of 9 months.
4. Recent tuberculin skin test converters	A skin test conversion is defined as an increase in induration of 10 mm or more within 2 years for those younger than age 35 and 15 mm or more for those 35 or older.
5. Persons with medical conditions that increase the risk of TB:	
• Diabetes mellitus	The risk for this group may be 2 to 4 times that of the general population. Particularly at risk are poorly controlled insulin-dependent diabetics.
• Prolonged therapy with adrenocorticosteroids	TB that develops during corticosteroid therapy tends to be disseminated or presents in an obscure fashion. Prednisone (or equivalent) given daily at 15 mg or higher for 2–3 weeks markedly reduces tuberculin reactivity.
• Immunosuppressive therapy	Persons receiving other forms of immunosuppressive therapy are at an increased risk for TB.
• Hematological and reticuloendothelial diseases	Diseases such as leukemia and Hodgkin's disease may be associated with suppressed cellular immunity and an increased risk of TB.
• IV drug users known to be HIV-negative	Persons injecting illicit drugs may be at increased risk of TB even if not infected with HIV.
• End-stage renal disease (ESRD)	Persons with ESRD are predisposed to developing extrapulmonary TB with disseminated disease. As these patients may be anergic, a documented history or positive skin test is an indication for preventive INH therapy unless they have been treated previously.
• Clinical conditions associated with substantial rapid weight loss or chronic malnutrition	These conditions include intestinal bypass surgery for obesity (which carries an increased risk for disseminated TB), postgastrectomy, chronic peptic ulcer disease, chronic malabsorption syndromes, chronic alcoholism, and carcinomas of the oropharynx and upper GI tract that prevent adequate nutritional intake. The postgastrectomy state may increase the risk of developing TB even without weight loss.
Persons in the following groups who are under age 35 and have a positive tuberculin skin test (≥ 10 mm):	
• Foreign-born persons from high-prevalence countries	These countries include those in Latin America, Asia, and Africa that have a high prevalence of TB. Recent arrivals (<5 years)
• Medically underserved low-income groups, especially high-risk racial or ethnic minority populations	These groups include African Americans, Native Americans, and Hispanics.
• Residents of facilities for long-term care	These residents include those in correctional facilities, nursing homes, and mental health facilities. Staff of such facilities should also be considered for preventive therapy.
• Residents and staff of high-risk congregate settings (nursing homes, jails, homeless shelters)	

Group	Comments
• Mycobacteriology laboratory personnel	
• Persons with clinical conditions that make them high risk	HIV infection, substance abuse, recent infection with *M. tuberculosis* (within past 2 years), previous TB, PM, silicosis, prolonged immunosuppresive therapy, low body weight (<10% of normal), ESRD, chronic malabsorption
Persons with no known risk factors for TB may be considered for therapy if their reaction to the tuberculin test is ≥ 15 mm, This group should be given lower priority than the groups listed above.	

Sources: American Thoracic Society: Treatment of tuberculosis and tuberculosis infection in adults and children. ATS publication 99–6453. Am J Respir Crit Care Med 149:1359–1374, 1994.

Centers for Disease Control and Prevention: Prevention and treatment of tuberculosis among patients infected with human immunodeficiency virus: Principles of therapy and revised recommendations. CDC publication 99–5879. MMWR 47 (NORR-20), 1998.

recommended regimen is critical to the management of TB. The patient and family should understand the information and continue to be provided with reinforcement and encouragement throughout the course of therapy. Patients should be offered the option of participating in DOT. For patients who are administering their own medications, strategies that may be helpful for improving adherence include use of a weekly pill dispenser, marking off each day on a calendar as medicine is taken, taking pills at the same time every day (e.g., with breakfast or at coffee break), and asking a friend or family member to remind the patient to take pills.

Patients are typically considered to be infectious for about 2 to 3 weeks after initiation of drug therapy. If the patient is being cared for at home, he or she should not go to work or school. These patients should be instructed in controlling the spread of tubercle bacilli in microdroplets by using good hygienic measures, appropriate ventilation, and avoiding close contact with family and friends. Patients should sleep in a separate room until no longer considered infectious. Patients should be taught to always cover their mouths when they cough, sneeze, or laugh. Used tissues should be placed in a plastic or paper bag and discarded. If the weather is warm enough, patients should be instructed to place a fan in an open window to blow out air that may be contaminated with TB. Opening other windows in their room will help pull in fresh air.

Patients should be asked to identify any people who may need to be tested for TB infections, including coworkers, family members, and friends. All close contacts will need to undergo tuberculin skin testing and may require preventive INH therapy. Assurance should be provided to the patient and family by stressing that the majority of properly treated patients with TB are cured.

Some problems associated with TB among foreign-born patients stem from communication barriers, cultural and cognitive dissonance between practitioners and patients, and gaps in provider training. Education needs to be targeted to patients, providers, and community workers.

There are excellent TB control strategies available to the public from the CDC. Patients may access these guidelines via the Internet at http://www.cdc.gov and obtain guidelines written in an easily understood manner.

However, the problems of multidrug-resistant TB and issues of compliance with therapy among all populations remain a significant challenge for health-care providers. Practicing within a Circle of Caring enables the provider to approach these problems in a meaningful way.

Lung Cancer

Lung cancer arises from the epithelium of the respiratory tract. The four major histologic types are squamous-cell (epidermoid) carcinoma, small (oat)-cell carcinoma, large-cell carcinoma (including giant-cell and clear-cell), and adenocarcinoma. Squamous-cell carcinoma is named for the appearance of cells that resemble the epidermis of the skin. These cells usually contain the skin protein called keratin. Squamous-cell carcinomas arise most often from the bronchial lining and may grow to obstruct air passages. Adenocarcinoma, the most prevalent carcinoma of the lung of both sexes, resembles poorly formed glandular tissue. It may be difficult to determine whether an adenocarcinoma is a primary lung cancer or a metastatic tumor from elsewhere in the body. Fifty-five to 60 percent of adenocarcinomas are located in the periphery of the lung, not obviously related to any bronchus. Many organs in the body can develop adenocarcinoma that may metastasize to the lungs. Large-cell carcinomas, also called undifferentiated carcinoma, are characterized by a collection of poorly formed large cells that have abundant cytoplasm. These tumors may exhibit a glandlike structure and produce mucin.

Small-cell lung carcinomas (SCLCs) (oat-cell, intermediate, combined) are characterized by very small cells with scant cytoplasm. SCLC is a very rapidly growing tumor that usually metastasizes to distant tissue while

Table 8.14 Cellular Classification of Lung Cancer

Major Classification	Subclassification
SCLC	• Oat-cell carcinoma • Intermediate-cell carcinoma • Combined small-cell carcinoma (with squamous cell or adenocarcinoma)
NSCLC	• Squamous-cell (epidermoid) carcinoma Well-differentiated Moderately well-differentiated Poorly differentiated • Adenocarcinoma Well-differentiated Moderately well-differentiated Poorly differentiated Bronchoalveolar • Large-cell carcinoma Giant-cell Clear-cell

the tumor is quite small. The clinical effect of SCLC is much different from that of the other three forms of lung cancer, which is why lung cancers are usually classified in terms of small-cell and non–small-cell carcinomas (NSCLCs) (Table 8.14).

Epidemiology and Causes

Lung cancer is preventable, common, and lethal once it comes to clinical attention, and relatively resistant to current therapeutics. Lung cancer is the most frequent cause of cancer death in men and women in North America. There were an estimated 173,600 new cases of lung cancer in 2004; 93,000 in men and 80,600 in women. Eighty-six percent of patients die within 5 years. Lung cancer accounts for 32 percent of all cancer deaths in men and 25 percent in women. The death rate for women is now higher than of any other cancer because of increased cigarette smoking by women and because they may be more susceptible to the carcinogenic effects of tobacco smoke than are men. In every ethnic group men still have higher lung cancer incidence and mortality rates than women, although women are rapidly closing the gap. African American men have the highest lung cancer incidence and mortality rates. Lung cancer is the leading cause of cancer death in most racial and ethnic groups of women except Native American, Filipino, and Hispanic women. New lung cancers and lung cancer deaths peak in individuals 55 to 65 years of age.

Tobacco use, especially cigarettes, is the main cause of the progressive rise in mortality from lung cancer. Ninety percent of the lung cancer cases in men and 79 percent in women are attributed directly to cigarette smoking. The risk of lung cancer increases with the duration of smoking, with earlier age at onset of smoking, and for smoking unfiltered or high-tar cigarettes. Of continued note are the effects of environmental tobacco smoke (ETS), also called second-hand smoke, sidestream smoke, involuntary smoke, or passive cigarette smoke. Exposure to second-hand smoke is thought to increase the risk of dying from lung cancer by 30 percent.

Lung cancer also occurs in association with occupational and environmental exposure to carcinogenic agents from sources other than smoking. Environmental or occupational risk factors associated with lung cancer include benzpyrene and radon, mustard gas, and nickel and chromium particles associated with uranium mining, asbestos, arsenic fumes, radiation, and nuclear bombs. The combination of cigarette smoking and environmental exposure produces an additive effect such that smokers exposed to asbestos increase their risk of lung cancer 92 times.

Pathophysiology

The bronchial walls have three layers: an epithelial lining, a smooth muscle layer, and a connective tissue layer. The epithelial lining of the bronchi contains single-celled exocrine glands (the mucus-secreting goblet cells) and ciliated cells. High columnar pseudostratified epithelium lines the larger airways, changing to columnar cuboidal epithelium in the bronchioles. It is hypothesized that at sites of segmental bronchial bifurcations, air flow and mucus production are altered and bronchial epithelium becomes very susceptible to injury. Carcinogenic agents, such as tobacco smoke, are likely deposited and absorbed in these areas. Particle size in environmental tobacco smoke is smaller, and inhaled particles may travel to peripheral lung regions more readily than with mainstream smoke. This is thought to explain the excess of peripheral adenocarcinomas seen in passive smokers.

Cigarette smoke contains tumor initiators, promoters, and cocarcinogens. DNA-mutating agents in cigarettes produce alterations in both oncogenes (a class of genes that encodes proteins involved in normal cell-growth processes) and tumor-suppresser genes. Multiple genetic events occur, first resulting in dysregulated growth and eventually in a malignant cell. These alterations include bronchial epithelial changes progressing from squamous cell alteration or metaplasia to carcinoma in situ. Repeated carcinogenic irritation to the bronchial epithelium may cause increased rates of cellular replication. Healthy ciliated cells are replaced with a proliferation of basal cells, resulting in hyperplasia, dysplasia, carcinoma in situ, and invasive carcinoma.

Small-Cell Lung Cancer

SCLC, which accounts for 15 to 20 percent of lung cancers, invades the submucosa and is centrally located, developing around a main bronchus as a whitish gray growth that invades surrounding structures, eventually compressing the bronchi externally. The most striking difference between small-cell carcinoma and other forms of malignant lung neoplasms is the aggressiveness of this tumor, resulting in a more rapid growth, and early local and distant metastasis via the lymphatic and blood vessels. Oat-cell carcinoma, one of the three types of SCLC, is composed of cells with round to oval nuclei. The tumors are soft in consistency and have shiny gray cut surfaces. The more common intermediate cell type is characterized by cells with larger, more vesicular, fusiform or spindled nuclei. The third type is the combined type, in which small-cell carcinoma is combined with another cell type. The most important variant is the small-cell and large-cell, which is regarded as small-cell carcinoma for treatment purposes. It lacks sensitivity to radiation and chemotherapy but retains the aggressiveness of the "pure" small-cell carcinoma.

Non–Small-Cell Lung Cancer

NSCLC comprises approximately 85 percent of all primary lung carcinoma in the United States. The tumor suppressor gene *p53* has been reported to be associated with human cancer more commonly than any other gene. The gene is mutated in about 60 percent of all cases of NSCLC. It encodes for a protein with a central role in the regulation of transcriptional events in the cell nucleus, particularly in response to DNA-damaging agents, such as ionizing radiation and a variety of other carcinogens. The central role of normal p53 protein has led to its description as the "guardian of the genome." Although many efforts to improve survival have focused on expanding indications for both radiotherapy and surgery, little progress has been made.

Squamous-Cell Carcinoma. Squamous-cell carcinoma is the second most common lung cancer accounting for 25 to 35 percent of cases. It is more common in men than in women and occurs almost entirely in cigarette smokers.

These tumors arise from the basal cells of the bronchial epithelium and usually present as masses in the segmental, lobar, or mainstem bronchi. The tumors tend to be bulky and invade cartilage and the adjoining lymph nodes. Based on the degree of differentiation, these tumors are divided into three subtypes: well-differentiated, moderately well-differentiated, and poorly differentiated. Well-differentiated tumors may show epithelial pearl formation, whereas poorly differentiated tumors are characterized by keratinization. Because it is a relatively slow-growing tumor, several years may elapse between the development of a carcinoma in situ and clinical detection. Metastases of squamous-cell carcinomas are initially to hilar and mediastinal lymph nodes and then to the liver, adrenals, bones, and brain.

Adenocarcinoma. Adenocarcinoma, which represents 35 to 40 percent of all lung cancers, is the most prevalent carcinoma of the lung in both sexes and in nonsmokers. It forms acinar or glandular structures. Histologically, this tumor is divided broadly into well-differentiated, moderately well-differentiated, poorly differentiated, and bronchoalveolar types. They arise from the bronchial epithelium and may form in lung scars or fibrous tissue. Adenocarcinoma usually presents as a single peripheral nodule, usually in the periphery, although rapidly progressive multifocal disease may be present at diagnosis. Although adenocarcinomas are usually slow-growing tumors, they invade lymphatics and blood vessels early, and thus produce early metastases; nearly half are considered to be unresectable at the time of diagnosis. Grossly, central cavitation is uncommon. Areas of metastasis commonly include the brain, liver, bone, and adrenal glands. Patients with adenocarcinomas may have an associated history of chronic ILD such as scleroderma, rheumatoid arthritis (RA), recurrent pulmonary infections, and other necrotizing pulmonary disease.

The bronchoalveolar subtype of adenocarcinoma represents approximately 2 to 4 percent of all lung cancer. Often, it is associated with prior lung disease leading to fibrosis, including repeated pneumonias, idiopathic pulmonary fibrosis, asbestosis, scleroderma, and Hodgkin's disease. There is little correlation with this type of cancer and smoking. Bronchoalveolar carcinoma commonly arises in the periphery of the lung and it grows in a lepidic fashion along the alveolar septa. Grossly, these tumors may be categorized as solitary, multinodular, or diffuse. The solitary, well-differentiated bronchoalveolar cell carcinoma has a much better prognosis than the other forms; diffuse and multinodular forms usually are not amenable to therapy.

Large-Cell Carcinoma. Large-cell carcinoma, also called undifferentiated carcinoma, is the least common type of lung cancer, representing approximately 5 to 10 percent of cases. They are classified into two types: clear-cell and giant-cell. Large-cell carcinomas include all tumors that show no evidence of differentiation to small-cell, squamous-cell, or adenocarcinoma. These tumors tend to form large, bulky, somewhat circumscribed and necrotic masses, in the major or intermediate-sized bronchi or in the periphery, invade locally, and disseminate widely. The giant-cell variant of large-cell carcinoma is composed of huge, multinucleated, bizarre cells that are frequently associated with an extensive inflammatory cell infiltration. These tumors are usually large and peripheral and are very aggressive, highly malignant, and most often found at a late stage. These lesions show an ability to metastasize widely, with a predilection for the small intestine. Table 8.15 summarizes the characteristics of the types of lung cancer.

Clinical Presentation

Past history of a patient with suspected lung cancer must include any history of chronic respiratory problems as well as any prolonged exposure to environmental carcinogens. Habits must be assessed to determine the patient's risk of developing lung cancer. Smoking history includes the age when smoking started, the average number of packs smoked

Table 8.15 Characteristics of Lung Cancer

Lung Cancer Type	Tumor Type	Growth Rate	Metastasis	Manifestations	Treatment
SCLC	• 15%–20% • Neuroendocrine cells: Oat-cell carcinoma Combined small-cell (with squamous-cell carcinoma or adenocarcinoma)	Very rapid	Very early, via lymphatic and blood vessels	Obstruction of main bronchus; associated with paraneoplastic syndrome	• Not resectable • Treated with chemotherapy and radiation
NSCLC	• Squamous-cell (epidermoid) carcinoma • 25%–35% • Keratin-producing cells: Well-differentiated Moderately differentiated Poorly differentiated	Slow	Hilar and mediastinal lymph nodes, liver, adrenals, bone, brain	Most often in cigarette smokers; bulky mass in main stem bronchi	• Stage I and II: Resectable • Stage III: Chemotherapy and radiation • Stage IV: Chemotherapy (Refer to Table 8.17 for staging)
	• Adenocarcinoma • 35%–40% • Columnar cells: Well-differentiated Moderately well-differentiated Poorly differentiated Bronchoalveolar	Slow to moderate	Early and most frequently via lymphatic and blood vessels to brain, liver, bone, adrenal glands	Form glandular structures in scar or fibrous tissue; single distal pulmonary nodule	• Stage I and II: Resectable • Stage III: Chemotherapy and radiotherapy • Stage IV: Chemotherapy
	• Large-cell carcinoma • 5%–10% •Undifferentiated cells: Giant-cell Clear-cell	Rapid	Early and widespread to small intestine	Large, bulky necrotic masses in major or intermediate-sized bronchi or in periphery	• Stage I and II: Resectable • Stage III: Chemotherapy and radiotherapy • Stage IV: Chemotherapy

per day, and the number of years smoked. The type of tobacco (cigar, cigarette, snuff, or chewing tobacco) used by the patient must be determined. A positive family history of lung cancer may indicate that the patient is at a slightly higher risk to develop lung cancer. The genetic link, however, is not clear. A review of systems reexamines all pertinent present and past symptoms that relate to the chief complaint and usually completes the health history.

Clinical manifestations of lung cancer are dependent on the location of the tumor and the extent of spread. Ten to 25 percent of patients are asymptomatic at the time of diagnosis. Symptoms may be divided into four categories: intrathoracic or local–regional symptoms, symptoms resulting from extrathoracic involvement, nonspecific systemic symptoms, and paraneoplastic syndromes. Some cases of lung cancer are picked up during a routine chest x-ray study done for other reasons, for example, a preoperative physical for an unrelated surgery, or for a work physical, and so forth.

Intrathoracic or Local–Regional Symptoms

Subjective. The most common symptoms of local–regional disease are ambiguous and insidious; they include cough, sputum production, dyspnea, chest pain, hemoptysis, wheezing, postobstructive pneumonia, and pleural effusions. Cough resulting from bronchial irritation occurs in 60 percent of patients and often is attributed to a cold. The cough frequently goes away after a few days and returns intermittently. Cough may be produced by a small tumor acting as a foreign body, or by ulceration of the bronchial mucosa. Severe paroxysms of coughing may lead to cough fractures, rupture of an emphysematous bleb, or cough syncope. Cough and sputum production are not specific symptoms, because the majority of lung cancer patients also suffer from chronic bronchitis and emphysema due to cigarette smoking; however, a change in the character of the cough, a change in the quality and quantity of sputum, or unresponsiveness to previously effective therapy (e.g., bronchodilators, antibiotics, steroids) should raise the suspicion that a tumor is present.

Many patients with lung cancer experience dyspnea as a result of multiple disruptions in physiologic function of the respiratory system. Dyspnea has been reported in 26 to 60 percent of patients presenting with NSCLC and is often an ominous development, signifying intrathoracic extension or dissemination. Some patients may have dyspnea resulting from underlying pulmonary disorders such as pulmonary fibrosis or COPD. These patients may experience difficulties in airway clearance associated with excessive tracheobronchial secretions, thick tenacious secretions, muscle weakness, and chest pain. Central lung cancers cause dyspnea by means of obstruction, with or without postobstructive pneumonitis. Large pleural effusion or paralysis of a hemidiaphragm resulting from phrenic nerve involvement may also cause dyspnea. The assessment of dyspnea should include a description of the onset, duration, magnitude, and precipitating events. It is especially important to identify any interventions the patient has discovered that are helpful in relieving the dyspnea. Usually the chest radiograph in dyspneic patients demonstrates a sizable effusion, atelectasis of a lobe or entire lung, or clear evidence of intrapulmonary dissemination.

Chest pain with deep inspiration or coughing may be reported, as well as fatigue and anorexia. Chest pain in lung cancer may indicate local invasion of the pleura, ribs, and nerves. Pain may be dull, constant, and debilitating or intermittent and sharp, varying with the respiratory cycle. It may localize to the chest wall, or it may radiate to the midback, scapula, shoulder, or arm on the side of the tumor. The pain is usually a dull intermittent ache lasting from minutes to hours on the same side as the tumor and is not related to cough or respiration. Intercostal retractions, supraclavicular retractions, and/or use of accessory muscles on inspiration indicate obstruction to air inflow, whereas bulging interspaces on expiration are associated with outflow obstruction; either may be an indication of tumor. It is important to distinguish the chest pain that accompanies direct contiguous chest wall extension from painful rib metastases that are anatomically remote from the primary lesion.

Chest discomfort can be associated with atelectasis. Atelectasis develops in the patient with lung cancer secondary to mechanical obstruction of the airways, compression of lung tissue, and shallow breathing patterns. When the tumor obstructs the airway, it prevents or reduces alveolar ventilation to a region of the lung and produces atelectasis in that region. The size of the atelectic area depends on the size of the obstructed airway and the degree of obstruction. Localized compression of lung tissue occurs with large tumors and with large pleural effusions secondary to metastases.

Hemoptysis is seen in up to 30 percent of patients and occurs when the tumor erodes the epithelial layer or invades a blood vessel. It occurs more often in squamous-cell carcinoma and large-cell carcinoma than in SCLC. Typically, hemoptysis consists only of blood-streaked sputum, which is sometimes erroneously attributed to chronic bronchitis. The quantity of blood is usually small, but it can become massive and life-threatening. Hemoptysis usually prompts the patient to seek medical attention and is suggestive of endobronchial tumor. Inspection very seldom reveals any changes in the chest wall. Palpation may reveal lymph node enlargement.

Nonspecific Systemic Symptoms

Systemic symptoms of lung cancer include generalized weakness and fatigue, anorexia, cachexia, weight loss, and anemia. These nonspecific signs and symptoms are common in both SCLC and NSCLC. Weight loss, which usually (but not always) is accompanied by anorexia, occurs in more than one-half of the patients, and generalized weakness occurs in one-third. Fever and anemia occur in about 20 percent of patients. Fever generally is not considered to be paraneoplastic in patients with lung cancer; if present, it usually is associated with a documented infection or liver metastases.

Table 8.16 presents a summary of these clinical manifestations of lung cancer.

Table 8.16 Clinical Manifestations of Lung Cancer

Nonspecific systemic manifestations	Weakness Fatigue Fever Anorexia Cachexia Anemia Symptoms associated with paraneoplastic syndromes
Intrathoracic or local-regional manifestations	Cough Dyspnea Hemoptysis Wheezing Chest pain Stridor Hoarseness Vocal cord paralysis Hiccups Atelectasis Pneumonia Pancoast's syndrome Horner's syndrome Pleural effusion Pericardial effusion Superior vena cava syndrome
Manifestations resulting from extrathoracic involvement	Bone pain Headache Dizziness Lymphadenopathy CNS disturbances GI disturbances Jaundice Hepatomegaly Abdominal pain

Objective. Auscultation may reveal wheezing if an airway is partially obstructed. The wheezing is usually monophonic and localized, and does not disappear after a cough. Wheezing may be heard on both inhalation and exhalation. Absent or decreased breath sounds can be heard when normal lung tissue is replaced by tumor, or when the patient has a pleural effusion. Percussion reveals diminished resonance over lung tissue affected by a large tumor, pleural effusion, or pneumonia (consolidation). Decreased tactile fremitus may be associated with pleural effusion and tumors of the pleural cavity, whereas increased tactile fremitus may indicate a lung mass.

The most frequent peripheral sign of lung cancer is clubbing of the fingers, which at times is associated with generalized hypertrophic pulmonary osteoarthropathy (HPO), also known as Bamberger-Marie disease. HPO often resembles RA. The clinical syndrome consists of swelling of the soft tissues of the terminal phalanges, with curvature of the nails, pain and swelling of the joints, and periostitis of the long bones, with elevation of the periosteum and new bone formation. The incidence of HPO, most exclusively in patients with NSCLC, has been reported to be from 2 to 12 percent. It occurs only rarely, if ever, in small-cell tumors. Its occurrence is distributed equally among the other three major cell types of NSCLC. Removal of the pulmonary lesion may give dramatic remission of the arthralgia and peripheral edema.

Physical examination evidence for surgical nonresectability includes hoarseness, facial edema, arm pain, or changes in mental or emotional status. Hoarseness suggests vocal cord paralysis caused by recurrent laryngeal nerve compression by the tumor. Facial edema suggests compression of the superior vena cava by the tumor. Superior vena cava syndrome occurs when a lung tumor, usually SCLC, presses on the superior vena cava, partially or completely occluding it and impeding venous return from the head, neck, arms, and upper chest. Symptoms are related to venous obstruction, airway obstruction, and increased cerebral venous pressure. The most common symptoms include edema of the face, neck, arms, and upper torso. The conjunctiva may also be engorged. If the compression is untreated, neurologic symptoms related to increased intracranial pressure may ensue, including headache, dizziness, visual disturbances, and occasionally alterations in mental status. Associated upper airway obstruction or signs of cerebral edema are very poor prognostic signs.

Tumor compression of the cervical sympathetic nerve plexus causes Horner's syndrome, which consists of unilateral ptosis, miosis, and ipsilateral anhidrosis (lack of sweating due to extension of the tumor into the paravertebral sympathetic nerves). Horner's syndrome is often associated with radiographic evidence of destruction of the first and second ribs. Pancoast's syndrome, manifested as arm and shoulder pain, suggests invasion of the brachial nerve plexus by a superior sulcus tumor. In addition, there may be muscular atrophy and decreased range of motion (ROM) in the arm and shoulder; the patient may walk supporting the elbow of the affected arm.

Symptoms Due to Extrathoracic Involvement

Extrathoracic metastatic spread most often occurs in the lymph nodes, brain, bones, liver, and suprarenal glands. Bone pain caused by metastasis occurs in approximately 25 to 40 percent of patients, although pathological fractures are rare. Neurologic symptoms resulting from intracranial metastases are present in 3 to 6 percent of patients. These include hemiplegia, epilepsy, personality changes, confusion, speech defects, gait disturbances, or only nonspecific headache. Symptoms that relate to liver involvement (right upper quadrant pain) are less common or nonspecific (e.g., nausea, weight loss, anemia). Rarely, jaundice, ascites, or an abdominal mass is the major complaint. Neck, muscle, or subcutaneous tissue masses are present infrequently. Involvement of adrenal glands often is asymptomatic, and most adrenal metastases are discovered incidentally, either during staging evaluation or at autopsy. If symptomatic, it presents with unilateral pain in the flank, abdomen, or costovertebral angle. Although adrenal metastases are fairly common, signs of adrenal insufficiency are rarely seen.

Paraneoplastic Syndromes

Approximately 21 identified syndromes are associated with lung cancer that meet the usual definition of the term *paraneoplastic.* Approximately 2 percent of patients with lung cancer seek medical advice for systemic symptoms and signs not related to metastatic spread of the tumor, the so-called paraneoplastic syndromes shown in Table 8.17. The major categories of paraneoplastic syndromes include endocrine, neurologic, cardiovascular, skeletal, and cutaneous manifestation.

Paraneoplastic syndromes are often the first indication of the presence of tumor and may antedate the demonstrable tumor by a period ranging from months to years. SCLC is associated with paraneoplastic syndromes more frequently than the NSCLCs. The majority of metabolic manifestations are the result of secretion of endocrine or endocrine-like substances by the tumor.

Hyperadrenocorticism, in association with ectopic secretion of adrenocorticotropic hormone (ACTH), is a frequently observed hormonal syndrome in lung cancer, particularly with SCLC patients. It manifests as severe weakness, weight loss, edema, hypertension, hypokalemia, and hyperglycemia. The syndrome of inappropriate antidiuretic hormone secretion (SIADH), seen in 5 to 10 percent of all SCLCs, results from antidiuretic hormone (ADH) secretion by the tumor, and is associated with symptoms of water intoxication (anorexia, nausea, and vomiting). Symptoms include hyponatremia and low serum osmolality, characterized by mental status changes, lethargy, seizures, and confu-

Table 8.17 Paraneoplastic Syndromes Associated with Lung Cancer

Type of Cancer	Associated Paraneoplastic Syndrome
SCLC	• Ectopic ACTH (Cushing's syndrome) • Inappropriate antidiuretic hormone secretion (SIADH) • Lambert-Eaton myasthenic syndrome • Atrial natriuretic factor • Hyperpigmentation
NSCLC	• Humoral hypercalcemia • Hypertrophic pulmonary osteoarthropathy • Nephrotic syndrome • Hypoglycemia • Gynecomastia • Nonbacterial thrombotic endocarditis
All Lung Cancers	• Hypercoagulable state • Disseminated intravascular coagulation • Erythrocytosis • Granulocytosis • Neurologic and myopathic syndromes (dementia, limbic encephalitis, optic neuropathy, sensory neuropathy, sensorimotor peripheral neuropathy) • Dermatological syndromes (acanthosis nigricans, acquired ichthyosis, dermatomyositis)

sion. Hyponatremia resulting from the secretion of atrial natriuretic factor also can occur in some patients.

Hypercalcemia may be caused by bony metastases or excessive secretion by the tumor (usually squamous-cell) or parathyroid hormone (PTH)-related protein, so-called humoral hypercalcemia of malignancy. Although squamous-cell carcinoma is most commonly associated with hypercalcemia, other histologic types can cause the syndrome as well. An accompanying hypophosphatemia is also frequently found. Clinically, the hypercalcemic patient may have somnolence, irritability, confusion, or coma as well as anorexia, nausea, vomiting, constipation, and weight loss. The Eaton-Lambert myasthenic syndrome occurs in about 6 percent of patients with SCLC. This pseudomyasthenic syndrome is thought to be an autoimmune disorder in which the release of acetylcholine by the motor nerve terminals is impaired. Symptoms include proximal limb muscle weakness and fatigue, especially in the pelvis, thighs, arms, and shoulders, peripheral paresthesia, dry mouth, dysphagia, diplopia, ptosis, difficulty chewing, and double vision.

Diagnostic Reasoning

Early detection is the key to successful resection of the NSCLC tumors but mass screening programs have failed to affect mortality rates. The histological cell type and the stage of the disease are the major factors that influence choice of therapy for individuals. The currently accepted system for the staging of lung cancer is the Tumor–Node–Metastasis (TNM) classification presented in Table 8.18. This system is a code in which T denotes the extent of the primary tumor (ranging from T0 to T4), N indicates the nodal involvement (ranging from N0 to N3), and M describes the extent of metastasis (M0 or M1). The stage of disease (also in Table 8.18) is based on a combination of clinical (physical exam, radiologic, and laboratory studies) and pathological (biopsy of lymph nodes, bronchoscopy, mediastinoscopy, or parame-diansternotomy or other type of thoracotomy) staging.

The diagnostic approach for SCLC is the same as NSCLC, but the staging system is different. SCLC staging still focuses on disease extent but broadly classifies it as limited state (limited to one hemothorax with hilar and mediastinal nodes that can be included within a radiation therapy port) or extensive stage disease. The TNM staging system is not typically used for SCLC staging. The anatomic detail of the TNM classification system is unnecessary, as surgical resection is not a recommended treatment modality.

Diagnostic Tests

Initial Testing. A CBC should be ordered because anemia may be associated with lung cancer; along with a basic metabolic panel and hepatic panel checking for abnormalities in Na, K, Ca, and liver enzymes, and a prothrombin time (PT), partial thromboplastin time (PTT), and platelet count to assess for coagulopathies. An ECG should be done, as well as baseline PFTs. AP and lateral chest x-ray films remain the simplest method for identifying patients with lung cancer. The heart and other thoracic structures obscure large portions of the lung tissue, so it is important to evaluate both a frontal and a side view. The chest x-ray may demonstrate asymptomatic lung cancer and is almost always abnormal when the patient is symptomatic. A tumor nodule must be at least 2 to 3 mm before it is visible on the chest-radiograph. Associated atelectasis, postobstructive pneumonitis, abscess, bronchiolitis, rib erosion, pleural effusion, or bulky mediastinal lymphadenopathy may be identified

Table 8.18 Lung Cancer Staging

Tumor-Node-Metastasis (TNM) Stage Grouping for Lung Cancer	
Occult cancer	TX N0 M0
Stage 0	Tis N0 M0
Stage I	T1 N0 M0; T2 N0 M0
Stage II	T1 N1 M0; T2 N1 M0
Stage IIIA	T1 N2 M0; T2 N2 M0; T3 N0 M0; T3 N1 M0; T3 N2 M0
Stage IIIB	Any T N3 M0; T4 Any N M0
Stage IV	Any T Any N M1
TNM Definitions of Primary Tumor (T) Characteristics in Lung Cancer	
Primary (T)	
TX	Primary tumor cannot be assessed, or tumor proved by the presence of malignant cells in sputum or bronchial washings but not visualized by imaging or bronchoscopy.
T0	No evidence of primary tumor.
Tis	Carcinoma in situ.
T1	A tumor that is 3.0 cm or less in greatest diameter, surrounded by lung or visceral pleura and without evidence of invasion more proximal than the lobar bronchus (e.g., not in the main bronchus). (*Note:* The uncommon superficial tumor of any size with its invasive component limited to the bronchial wall, which may extend proximal to the main bronchus, is also classified as T1.)
T2	A tumor with any of the following features of size or extent: more than 3.0 cm in greatest dimension; involving the main bronchus, 2.0 cm or more distal to the carina; invading the visceral pleura; associated with atelectasis or obstructive pneumonitis that extends to the hilar region but does not involve the entire lung.
T3	A tumor of any size with direct extension to the chest wall (including superior sulcus tumors), diaphragm, mediastinal pleura, parietal pericardium; a tumor in the main bronchus less than 2.0 cm distal to the carina but without involvement of the carina; associated atelectasis or obstructive pneumonitis of the entire lung.
T4	A tumor of any size that invades any of the following: mediastinum, heart, great vessels, trachea, esophagus, vertebral body, carina; or tumor with a malignant pleural effusion.
Regional Lymph Nodes (N)	
NX	Regional lymph nodes cannot be assessed.
N0	No regional lymph node metastasis.
N1	Metastasis in ipsilateral peribronchial and/or ipsilateral hilar lymph nodes, including direct extension.
N2	Metastasis in ipsilateral mediastinal and/or subcarinal lymph node(s).
N3	Metastasis in contralateral mediastinal, contralateral hilar, ipsilateral or contralateral scalene, or supraclavicular lymph node(s).
Distant Metastasis (M)	
MX	Presence of distant metastasis cannot be assessed.
M0	No (known) distant metastasis.
M1	Distant metastases present; specify sites.

Note: Most pleural effusions associated with lung cancer are due to tumor; however, there are a few patients in whom multiple cytopathological examinations of pleural fluid are negative for tumor. In these cases, fluid is nonbloody and is not an exudate. When these elements and clinical judgment dictate that the effusion is not related to the tumor, the effusion should be excluded as a staging element and the patient should be staged as T1, T2, or T3.

on radiographs, thus raising a suspicion of primary lung malignancy. The four most common types of lung cancer usually present with slightly different chest radiographic patterns, but there is so much overlap that only biopsy and histological examination provide reliable evidence about the cell type. Mediastinal changes on radiograph may suggest lymphadenopathy or pleural effusions, and an elevated diaphragm may be seen with phrenic nerve involvement.

A chest CT scan with infusion of contrast material has become widely accepted as the primary cross-sectional modality for evaluation of the thorax and is recommended to stage NSCLC. The CT scan should extend inferiorly to include the liver and the adrenal glands. Because of its earlier metastases and unresectability, staging for SCLC is less useful for treatment and prognosis. A contrast-enhanced chest CT scan will: (1) characterize the size and location of the primary tumor and its relationship to other thoracic structures, (2) identify pathologically enlarged hilar and mediastinal lymph nodes, (3) identify satellite and other ipsilateral or contralateral pulmonary nodules, and (4) identify potential metastases to the liver and adrenal glands, both common metastatic sites.

Cytologic evaluation of sputum, bronchial washing, bronchial brushings, and fine-needle aspirations have a high diagnostic value, but the positive and negative predictive values of each, as well as their accuracy of diagnosis, depend on sampling error, tissue preservation, processing quality, and observer experience. Sputum cytology remains a simple test with a positive predictive value that can approach 100 percent, but it has a sensitivity rate of only 10 to 15 percent. If a diagnosis can be established through collective sputum cytology, invasive tests often can be averted. Automated sputum screening is currently being evaluated and may play an increasingly important role in early diagnosis. The highest yield occurs in patients with large, centrally located tumors. It is much less helpful in diagnosing peripheral lesions because relatively few cells are released from the lesion, and those that are released rarely get to the central airways. Early-morning sputum samples are collected for 3 to 5 days; deep coughing is recommended because coughing dislodges cancer cells into the sputum.

Flexible fiberoptic bronchoscopy (FFB) is an essential and standard technique for the evaluation of patients with pulmonary neoplasms. It remains the most important procedure for determining the endobronchial extent of disease. The extent and operability of the tumor are assessed by observing the site of the tumor and extent of airway involvement. When lesions are visible endobronchially, bronchial washings have a diagnostic yield of approximately 90 percent; bronchial brushings and bronchial mucosal forceps biopsy samples provide diagnosis of tissue in nearly 98 percent of visualized tumors. Under fluoroscopic control, transbronchial forceps biopsies, brushings, and washings can diagnose peripheral, parenchymal lesions up to 80 percent of the time. The visual assessment of the primary tumor can also provide a clinically useful estimate of the probability of tumor complications such as airway obstruction, postobstructive pneumonia, or hemoptysis.

Transthoracic percutaneous fine-needle aspiration (fine-needle aspiration biopsy [FNAB]) is used when lung lesions cannot be visualized by bronchoscopy but are accessible percutaneously. A needle guided by CT or fluoroscopy is inserted into the lesion for aspiration of cells. This procedure is most suitable for peripheral pulmonary nodules. Pneumothorax is the most common complication, with an increased risk in the patient with COPD. A positive pleural fluid cytology proves the spread of malignancy to the pleural space. Thoracentesis and pleural biopsy combined provide up to a 90 percent diagnostic yield in patients with malignancy.

Mediastinoscopy is an invasive procedure used for the diagnosis and staging of lung cancer. A biopsy is recommended if mediastinal lymph nodes found on chest CT scan that are greater than 1.0 cm for the patient with clinically operable NSCLC. The patient with lymphadenopathy on chest CT scan will most likely have positive nodes on biopsy. Anterior cervical mediastinoscopy allows direct visualization and biopsy of mediastinal nodes with less risk than an exploratory thoracotomy.

Video-assisted thoracoscopic surgery (VATS) is used for the staging and diagnosis of lung cancer when less invasive techniques fail to yield a diagnosis. Small thoracotomy incisions are made through which thoracoscopic instruments are inserted. Visualization of the chest and mediastinum and assessment of pleural effusions are superior to that achieved using older scopes, which may help improve diagnostic accuracy.

Thoracoscopy is useful for pleural evaluation but less useful for evaluating the lung. It is more than 90 percent sensitive for the diagnosis of pleural-based malignancies and peripheral lung nodules, with a specificity of 99 percent. With a thoracoscope, the mediastinum can be entered and nodes biopsied. Thoracoscopy affords the potential for more complete staging of patients with suspected mediastinal nodal spread and it has become a valuable adjunct to cervical mediastinoscopy and anterior mediastinotomy. There is a concern, however, about seeding the thoracoscope entrance site with tumor cells.

Subsequent Testing. A head CT scan or brain magnetic resonance imaging (MRI), with and without infusion of contrast material is recommended only in patients who have signs or symptoms of central nervous system (CNS) disease. The finding of an isolated adrenal mass on ultrasonographic or CT scan examination requires biopsy to rule out metastatic disease if the patient is considered to be potentially resectable. NSCLC metastasizes to the adrenal glands in 18 to 38 percent of cases. A bone scan should be performed only in patients who complain of bone pain or chest pain, or who have an elevated serum calcium level or an elevated serum alkaline phosphatase level. It is estimated that between 9 and 15 percent of patients with newly diagnosed NSCLC have bony metastases at presentation, with the vertebral bodies most commonly being affected. Finally, the finding of an isolated hepatic mass on ultrasonographic or CT exam requires a biopsy to rule out metastatic disease if the patient is otherwise considered to be potentially resectable.

Differential Diagnosis

The symptoms of lung cancer develop gradually in most cases and are often attributed by the patient to a smoker's cough or cold, and by the patient's health-care provider to tracheobronchitis, pneumonia, influenza, pulmonary infarction, or lung abcess. Thus, it is common for a patient to delay seeking medical attention for several months from the first recognizable onset of symptoms. Several additional months of symptomatic treatment and antibiotics frequently pass before the health-care provider establishes the correct diagnosis. Much of the initial diagnostic task is to differentiate if this is a primary tumor or a metastatic cancer. This is evaluated on biopsy. Other differential diagnoses include tuberculosis, lymphoma, mycobacterium avium complex, sarcoidosis, or a foreign body aspiration that has been retained.

Management

Active patient participation in decision-making respects the fundamental ethical and legal doctrine of autonomy and is especially important for the patient with unresectable NSCLC, because the prognosis is often poor and symptom palliation is a central concern. Fewer than half the patients with lung cancer are candidates for resection and only a small percentage of these are cured, so most patients with the disease require some form of palliation. Therapy should include efforts to slow the growth of the tumor and to treat complications as they arise, but above all, symptoms should be relieved.

Surgery

Surgical resection offers the best chance of cure for lung cancer. The patient with stage I or II NSCLC is routinely resected via a thoracotomy. Pneumonectomy (removal of a whole lung) and lobectomy (removal of a single lobe) are the most common of these surgical procedures. The nature of the tumor dictates the procedure, whereas pulmonary function determines if the patient can withstand the procedure. Pneumonectomy is required when the tumor or lymph nodes involve proximal structures such that a lung-conserving operation will not allow complete resection. Lobectomy is the most common resection performed for lung cancer. Such a resection allows removal of the primary tumor, associated disease, and lymph node-bearing areas while leaving a significant amount of residual functional parenchyma. Survival is equivalent for patients undergoing lobectomy or pneumonectomy for all stages of disease when a complete resection is performed. For lesions close to the lobar orifice, an adequate margin of resection often cannot be achieved. In such circumstances, a portion of the main bronchus must be included with the resection. This type of resection is termed *sleeve resection,* and it is performed as a parenchyma-sparing procedure avoiding pneumonectomy.

Very limited resection in the treatment of lung cancer has been reserved for patients with extremely poor pulmonary function who could tolerate no more than a very limited resection because of their underlying medical condition or low pulmonary reserve. Limited resections include segmentectomy, wedge resection, or lumpectomy. Segmental resection is the removal of a lung segment, and wedge resection is the removal of a small, V-shaped wedge of lung tissue. Lesions that reside more deeply within the pulmonary tissue often are not amenable to wedge resection and may require precise, local excision with laser or electrocautery assistance (e.g., lumpectomy). These techniques are used to preserve as much lung tissue as possible, and they are performed for the removal of small tumors located close to the surface of the lung. The guiding principle of surgical therapy in lung cancer is to remove the tumor completely, leaving as much functioning pulmonary tissue as possible. The aim of most operations is curative, and procedures that leave gross tumor are not warranted. Resection is abandoned if the tumor extends beyond the lung, when pleural seeding is evident, or when fixed mediastinal nodes are present.

Patients with stage I disease have a 50 to 80 percent 5-year survival and patients with stage II disease have a 25 to 50 percent survival at 5 years. However, 75 percent of patients present with advanced disease and significant comorbidities. Treatment decisions should consider symptom control, quality of life, the patient's value or meaning of life, and their perceptions and attitudes about a specific treatment.

Chemotherapy

Neoadjuvant chemotherapy involves giving antineoplastic drugs prior to surgery or radiation therapy. Adjuvant chemotherapy involves administering antineoplastic drugs after surgery or radiation therapy. Given that chemotherapy for advanced disease is marginally beneficial and noncurative, its use must be governed judiciously, with each decision evaluated individually for each patient.

Current chemotherapeutic approaches consist initially of defining new combinations of established chemotherapeutic agents that may act synergistically (Table 8.19). In addition, new drugs with novel mechanisms of action are also being investigated, both as single agents, and subsequently, as agents to be used in combination with established drugs.

Non–Small-Cell Lung Cancer Chemotherapy. Chemotherapy modestly improves median survival with distant metastatic NSCLC compared with best supportive care, but is not curative.

If a patient has stage I or II disease, there is no agreement on the role of neoadjuvant chemotherapy. It is more widely used with patients with stage IIIA and IIIB disease. Patients with stage I and N0 stage II disease treated with multidrug platinum-based chemotherapy show improved survival of 3 months at 5 years. Because of the toxicity, risks versus benefits must be discussed with the patient and family. Newer drugs with less toxicity are currently being studied. With patients in stage IIIB and IV, chemotherapy has shown to improve the patient's quality of life by decreasing bothersome symptoms.

Among the most widely used agents for the treatment of NSCLC, cisplatin has demonstrated a response rate of about 20 percent in most single-agent trials in previously untreated patients. Among the vinca alkaloids, vinblastine (Velban, VLB) and vindesine (Eldisine) are considered active in NSCLC, with single response rates ranging from 11 to 28 percent in most published studies. Of the newer agents, the taxanes, paclitaxel (Taxol) and docetaxel

Table 8.19 **Chemotherapeutic Agents Used to Treat Lung Cancer**

Small-Cell Lung Cancer	Non–Small-Cell Lung Cancer
Cisplatin* (Platinol)	**Localized disease**
plus	Cisplatin* (Platinol)
Etoposide* (VePesid, Etopophos)	or
Cyclophosphamide (Cytoxan, Neosar, Procytox)	Carboplatin* (Paraplatin)
Doxorubicin (Adriamycin, Doxil)	Docetaxel* (Taxotere)
Vincristine (Oncovin, Vincasar)	**Advanced disease**
	Cisplatin* (Platinol)
	or
	Carboplatin* (Paraplatin)
	Docetaxel* (Taxotere)
	Gemfitizib* (Gefitinib)
	Etoposide* (VePesid)
	Vinblastine* (Velban)
	Vinorelbine* (Navelbine)
	Doxorubicin (Adriamycin)
	Mitomycin (MitoExtra)
	Ifosfamide (Ifex)
	Paclitaxel (Onxol, Taxol)

*Current treatment of choice.

(Taxotere) have demonstrated significant activity against NSCLC. Vinorelbine (Navelbine), an analogue of vinblastine, is a semisynthetic vinca alkaloid that has had a positive effect on survival.

More recently, platinum-based combination regimens are recommended. The ASCO Practice Guidelines recommend cisplatin (Platinol, CDDP) combined with vinorelbine (Navelbine), paclitaxel (Taxol), or vinblastine as effective first-line regimens shown to produce improved survival in controlled trials. They further suggest that for the patient with unresectable stage III NSCLC, who is a candidate for combined chemotherapy and radiation, the duration of chemotherapy should be two to eight cycles, and for stage IV not more than eight cycles. Despite numerous efforts to produce efficacious treatments, the outcome of patients with advanced NSCLC remains poor. More than 15 years after cisplatin was introduced into the treatment of patients with advanced NSCLC, drug therapy remains controversial because therapy is toxic and the benefit small. The ASCO panel does not recommend second-line chemotherapy treatment except for a patient with good performance status or who responds to initial chemotherapy and then experiences a long progression-free interval off treatment.

Small-Cell Lung Cancer Chemotherapy. Combination chemotherapy is capable of effecting high objective response rates in SCLC. Furthermore, the simultaneous administration of multiple agents is superior to the sequential administration of the same drugs. Chemotherapy is most effective in SCLC with an 80 to 100 percent response in limited-stage disease (50 to 70 percent complete response), and 60 to 80 percent response in extensive stage disease (15 to 40 percent complete response). Remissions last a median of 6 to 8 months. If the cancer recurs, the median survival time is 3 to 4 months. Among the regimens, cisplatin plus etoposide (VePesid) is the current treatment of choice for many reasons. In the setting of relapsed SCLC, the combination of cisplatin and etoposide is capable of producing objective response rates of equal to or more than 50 percent in patients who have experienced a recurrence after cyclophosphamide-based therapy. No other drug combination has yielded response rates of this magnitude in a similar setting. Further, in previously untreated patients, cisplatin plus etoposide yields excellent overall response rates and survival results that are equivalent to cyclophosphamide- or doxorubicin-based regimens, albeit with less host-related toxicity. Cisplatin and etoposide is particularly well suited for the simultaneous administration of radiotherapy, given its lower incidence of toxicity and the putative radiation-sensitizing effect of both drugs. Thus, for many clinicians, cisplatin plus etoposide has become the de facto standard induction regimen for the patient with SCLC.

Radiation

The basic indication for radiation therapy is inoperability. This form of therapy can modify the natural course of the disease, relieve distressing symptoms, and produce an apparent cure in an occasional patient. Long-term results, however, have been generally disappointing. One-year and 5-year overall survival rates range from 25 to 55 percent and from 4 to 10 percent, respectively. It is used as adjunctive therapy after surgery to improve tumor control and it is used as palliative therapy to control symptoms in others.

Non–Small-Cell Lung Cancer Radiation. Radiation therapy is commonly offered to the patient with inoperable NSCLC when the cancer has not spread beyond the thorax. In this case, the asymptomatic patient or the patient who is still functioning at a high level is most likely to benefit. In addition, radiation therapy is used to shrink the tumor and control symptoms in the patient with inoperable lung cancer and to prevent brain metastasis. Treating the tumor with radiation therapy may relieve hemoptysis, shoulder and arm pain, chest pain, and dyspnea. It can be used in superior vena cava obstruction to reduce the tumor size and alleviate obstruction. Although there are currently no data that demonstrate a survival advantage for postoperative adjuvant therapy in patients with completely resected stage II disease, regardless of whether the patient receives radiation therapy alone or radiation therapy and chemotherapy, most of these patients are treated with postoperative radiation therapy to decrease local recurrence. Unfortunately, prevention of local recurrence has not been shown to translate into survival benefit. The patient with a malignant pleural effusion or with distant metastatic disease is not appropriate for definitive thoracic radiotherapy.

Small-Cell Lung Cancer Radiation. SCLC is quite sensitive to both radiation and chemotherapy. In limited stage SCLC the addition of both radiation and chemotherapy can increase the 5-year survival rate from about 11 to 20 percent. Most oncologists consider thoracic radiation therapy in combination with chemotherapy for limited-stage disease to be the standard of care. The major contribution of thoracic irradiation is local tumor control, and local control of the intrathoracic tumor is a sine qua non for cure. Thoracic radiation therapy does reduce the risk of dying of SCLC but at the price of increased toxicity. Concurrent or alternating treatment schedules appear to improve response rates over sequential chemotherapy and radiation therapy, although toxicity is more intense with concurrent therapy.

A summary of the treatment of NSCLC is shown in Treatment Flowchart 8.3.

Follow-Up and Referral

When lung cancer is first detected, the patient should be referred to a specialist for staging and treatment decisions. The patient who has been successfully treated for lung cancer needs to be followed routinely. The goal of monitoring patients with unresectable lung cancer in complete remission is to detect symptomatic progression of their disease that may benefit from therapeutic intervention or symptom management. However, the great majority of patients with unresectable, stage III and stage IV disease will not achieve a complete remission, or, if achieved, the duration of remission will be short.

A history and physical examination should be performed every 3 months during the first 2 years, every 6 months thereafter through year 5, and yearly thereafter. For the patient treated with curative intent, there is no clear role for routine x-ray evaluation in the asymptomatic patient and for those in whom no interventions are planned. A yearly chest x-ray film to evaluate for potentially curable second primary cancers may be reasonable. CT of the chest/abdomen, bronchoscopy, CBC and routine chemistries, including liver function tests, should be performed only as indicated by the patient's symptoms. These tests do not appear to detect asymptomatic recurrent disease with a high frequency.

Patient Education

Assessment of learning needs and provision of information is likely to be of paramount importance for the patient at the time of initial biopsy, between diagnosis and definitive treatment, and at discharge. These are highly stressful times for patients, and they may be easily overwhelmed by the information regarding treatment options. It is important to assess what level of participation in the decision-making process is desired by the patient, because that will help direct informational interventions and can reduce anxiety and psychological distress. This is particularly important for patients who have a choice between two treatment options or are deciding between participating in a clinical trial or receiving standard therapy.

Smoking cessation, never initiating smoking, and avoidance of occupational and environmental exposure to carcinogenic substances are recommended as effective interventions to reduce the risk of a second primary lung cancer in the curatively treated patient. For the patient with distant metastatic disease, the outlook is poor and smoking cessation has little effect on overall prognosis but may improve respiratory symptoms. A tapering nicotine patch or other delivery system has been proved to increase the odds of smoking cessation when combined with behavioral interventions.

Recommendations for lifestyle change are the same for the patient with a history of lung cancer as for those who have no previous history of lung cancer. Epidemiological studies also suggest that people who consume relatively large amounts of fruits and vegetables have a lower risk of both cancer and cardiovascular disease. Antioxidant vitamins contained in fruits and vegetables prevent carcinogenesis by interfering with oxidative damage to DNA and lipoproteins; however, the use of antioxidants and/or chemopreventive agents for lung cancer (retinoic acid, beta-carotene, and selenium) is investigational.

When medical care for the patient with lung cancer shifts from curative to palliative, the patient and family must choose a care setting. Home or hospice care can provide familiar surroundings, feelings of normalcy, involvement of family, and a more comforting situation as they participate in readiness for death activities. Although hospice has proved to be an extremely effective model for terminal care, referrals to a hospice often are not made until the final days of life. The difficulty lies in predicting when death will occur, because Medicare reimbursement requires that a hospice patient have a life expectancy of 6 months or less. Supportive resources for self-care should be provided as

TREATMENT FLOWCHART 8.3

TREATMENT OF NON–SMALL-CELL LUNG CANCER

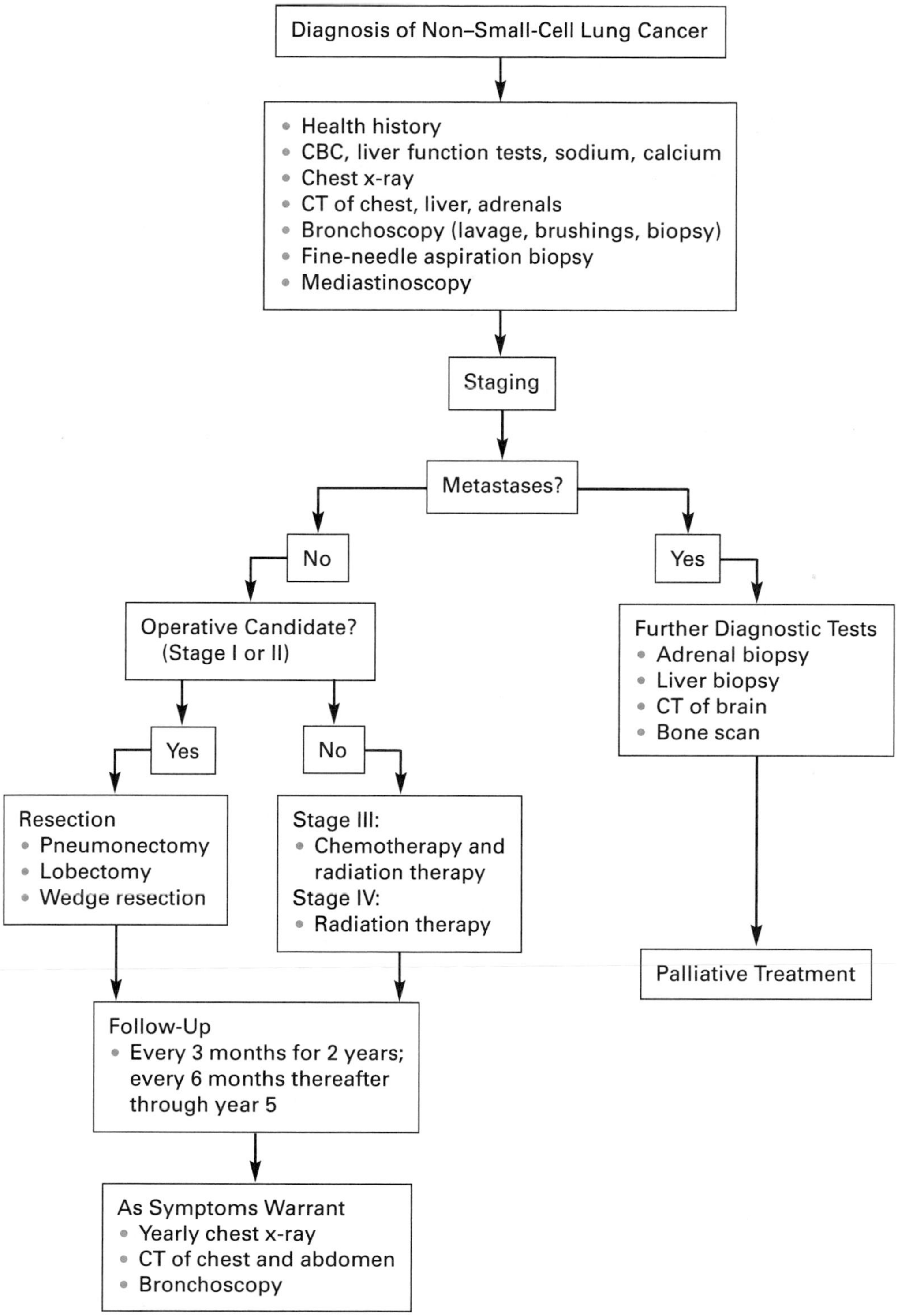

required by the individual situation. Patients will be able to manage less self-care as the disease progresses, and family members will require education with demonstration of care techniques and opportunities for questions and verbalization of feelings about caring for the one who is ill. Within the Circle of Caring model, collaborative planning is essential in helping the patient and family make informed choices and live in the moment.

Interstitial Lung Disease

ILD encompasses nearly 200 clinical disorders that affect the epithelium, the endothelium, or both cell surfaces of alveolar wall and satellite structures including terminal and respiratory bronchioles. ILD comprises a heterogeneous group of diseases that cause inflammation and fibrosis of the lower respiratory tract. The term *pulmonary fibrosis* is also applied to these diseases because fibrosis of the lung is the ultimate result of ILD. The term "interstitial" is misleading, in that most of these disorders have extensive alteration of alveolar and airway architecture as well. "Diffuse parenchymal lung disease" is, perhaps, a more appropriate descriptive term for this heterogeneous group of lung diseases, because the term *interstitium* usually refers to the microscopic anatomic space bounded by the basement membranes of epithelial and endothelial cells. The entire lung parenchyma is affected, however, in ILD.

The ILDs have many common features, including similarity of patient symptoms, comparable appearance of chest x-ray films, consistent derangements in pulmonary physiology, and typical histologic features. Four different infections may be associated with the cause or onset of most of the various diseases; disseminated fungus (coccidioidomycosis, blastomycosis, histoplasmosis); disseminated mycobacteria, *Pneumocystis* pneumonia, and certain viruses.

Although all the diffuse ILDs share the common morphologic characteristic of an abnormal lung interstitium, a satisfactory classification has been elusivebecause about 150 individual diseases have a component of interstitial lung involvement, either as primary disease or as a significant part of a multiorgan process, such as a collagen-vascular disease. Generally, ILDs are classified according to the type of agent that caused the lung injury. About one-third of patients with ILD have an identifiable agent responsible for inducing lung injury; however, the large majority of patients have disease attributable to no known cause. Therefore, ILDs are classified as those with a known cause and those with an unknown etiology; each of these groups are further subclassified according to the presence or absence of granuloma in interstitial or vascular areas.

Epidemiology and Causes

As many as 81 of every 100,000 Americans have some form of ILD. For patients with usual interstitial pneumonia (UIP), there is a slight male predominance with occurence between the ages of 55 and 60. There is a slightly younger age distribution associated with some of the other ILD's (age 40 to 45 for respiratory bronchiolitis-associated interstitial lung disease, and age 45 to 55 for nonspecific interstitial neumonitis). ILDs of known cause can be divided into several major subcategories. By far the largest group comprises occupational and environmental inhalant diseases; these include diseases resulting from inhalation of inorganic dusts, organic dusts, gases, fumes, vapors, and aerosols. Other categories include ILDs caused by drugs, irradiation, poisons, neoplasia, and chronic cardiac failure. The major subgroups within the category of unknown causes are idiopathic pulmonary fibrosis (IPF) and connective tissue (collagen vascular) disorders with ILD, including RA, systemic lupus erythematosus (SLE), progressive systemic sclerosis, polymyositis–dermatomyositis, and Sjögren's syndrome. Systemic vasculitides often have granulomas in tissue and include a variant of polyarteritis nodosa called allergic granulomatosis, lymphomatoid granulomatosis, and hypersensitivity vasculitis.

Seven major entities that are most frequently associated with diffuse ILD are (1) idiopathic pulmonary fibrosis, (2) bronchiolitis obliterans organizing pneumonia (BOOP), (3) connective tissue (collagen vascular) diseases (SLE, RA, progressive systemic sclerosis, and polymyositis–dermatomyositis), (4) systemic granulomatous vaculitides (Wegener's granulomatosis [WG], lymphomatoid granulomatosis, and allergic angiitis and granulomatosis), (5) drug-induced pulmonary disease, (6) sarcoidosis, and (7) hypersensitivity pneumonitis.

Pathophysiology

Interstitial lung disease (ILD) denotes a diverse group of conditions characterized by the common pathologic finding of pulmonary fibrosis and similar clinical presentation of restrictive lung findings (i.e., dyspnea on exertion and chronic nonproductive cough). The term "interstitial" used to describe this group of diseases is misleading because inflammation and fibrosis affects bronchioles, alveoli, and capillary endothelia, as well as the interstitium of the lower respiratory tract. Thus, a more illustrative term for this disease is pulmonary fibrosis. Sarcoidosis, hypersensitivity pneumonitis, pulmonary fibrosis in connective tissue disorders (e.g., systemic lupus erythematosus, rheumatoid arthritis, tuberous sclerosis, scleroderma), and occupational pulmonary diseases are all categorized as ILDs. Tissue injury and acute inflammation are believed to be the initial pathologic processes. In some conditions, such as sarcoidosis, the inciting antigen is unknown, whereas occupational pulmonary diseases are caused by repeated inhalation of environmental irritants, inorganic and organic dusts, fumes, or gases. For most ILDs, including idiopathic conditions, cigarette smoking is a primary risk factor.

In the majority of ILDs, there is a perpetuation of the inflammatory process with repeated tissue injury and aberrant wound healing with subsequent remodeling of the lung architecture. Infiltration of the lung parenchyma by various combinations of immune cells mediates this process, including neutrophils, lymphocytes, plasma cells, eosinophils, basophils, mast cells, and alveolar macrophages. Cytokine production (e.g., granulocyte-colony stimulating factor, transforming growth factor-β1, IL-1β, IL-8, TNF-α) drives these inflammatory and wound healing processes. Regions of chronic inflammation can develop granulomas consisting specifically of discrete masses of lymphocytes, macrophages, and fibroblasts. In turn, fibroblast proliferation and differentiation into myofibroblast forms (i.e., cells with both fibroblast and smooth muscle cell features) lead to fibrosis (collagen deposition) or scarring of the lungs and the development of cystic airspaces known as "honeycombing."

Such pathologic pulmonary tissue becomes less compliant and increasingly rigid, with consequential impedance of ventilation and gas exchange, characteristic of a progressive, minimally reversible restrictive lung disease. Diffusion capacity also worsens with increasing fibrosis of the lung parenchyma. In turn, ventilation–perfusion mismatch, hypoxemia, and pulmonary vasoconstriction develop, while increased resistance on the right ventricle may lead to *cor pulmonale* (right ventriculomegaly). Hypercarbia typically manifests only in end-stage disease. Total lung capacity, functional residual capacity, residual volume, and forced expiratory volumes (FEV and FEV_1) are all commonly decreased on pulmonary function testing; however, as fibrotic lung tissue is stiffer with greater elastic recoil, rapid exhalation of a major portion of the expiratory volume may be seen, as reflected in a normal or increased FEV_1/FVC ratio on PFTs – a key feature distinguishing restrictive from obstructive pulmonary disease.

Interestingly, recurrent dysregulated wound healing rather than neutrophilic or immune cell-mediated inflammation has been cited as the primary pathophysiologic mechanism in ILD, potentially explaining the ineffectiveness of anti-inflammatory and immunosuppressive treatments in many forms of ILD. Lung tissue biopsy is not required for the diagnosis of ILD, which may be made from a combination of clinical and radiographic findings including PFTs and certain serum markers of underlying connective tissue disease. However, the extent of lung fibrosis observed histopathologically is perhaps the most accurate prognostic indicator for this condition. In turn, much investigation has shifted toward antifibroblast therapies for ILD aimed at decreasing pulmonary collagen deposition.

Clinical Presentation

The typical patient with ILD presents with an insidious onset of dyspnea on exertion, often accompanied by fatigue and cough. This breathlessness has no other obvious cause such as asthma, obstructive airway disease, bronchitis, or heart failure. Although emphasis is usually given to this most common presentation of patients with ILD, the provider must recognize the variability of clinical presentations. Dyspnea is a virtually constant finding in patients with idiopathic pulmonary fibrosis (IPF), but it is by no means so consistent in other ILDs. Less common but important and sometimes misleading presentations include the following:

- Fatigue in the absence of dyspnea
- Dry cough without other respiratory symptoms
- Predominant systemic symptoms (e.g., fever, weight loss)
- Abnormal-appearing (90 percent) chest x-ray film in the absence of symptoms
- Incidental abnormalities of PFTs

Respiratory signs such as pleuritic chest pain, visceral chest pain, wheezing, or hemoptysis do not usually occur. Half of the patients have mucus hypersecretion and expectoration. This occurrence has been correlated with glandular hypertrophy in the airway mucosa and accumulated mucus in the airways. Clinical manifestations specific to the various types of ILD are discussed in Table 8.20.

Diagnostic Reasoning

Diagnostic Tests

Initial Testing. The symptoms of ILD are similar regardless of the underlying cause. In addition, the symptoms of lung involvement are nonspecific and could suggest many other causes, including obstructive lung disease, heart disease, or pulmonary vascular disease. The first symptom of ILD is usually progressive dyspnea on exertion or a nonproductive cough. The patient initially notices dyspnea only during heavy exertion but in very advanced stages of the disease, dyspnea occurs at rest.

The occupational and environmental history is the single most helpful tool to determine whether a respiratory problem may be related to an occupational or environmental exposure (Focusing the History 8.1). A careful history must include a detailed chronological account of the patient's employment activities, social activities, travel, immune status, pets, hobbies, and environment. A thorough review of the patient's past medical history, along with current and previous medications, is also important. The goal of these questions is to determine whether the patient has been exposed to agents known to cause ILD. Many patients have an occupational history that includes exposure to one or a variety of toxic inhalation products, and this may add uncertainty to the precise onset of symptoms and may suggest the contribution of several etiologic factors. The temporal relationship to the exposure may be obvious in some cases, but in others a low-grade exposure may provoke chronic illness without acute flares after exposure. The latency may be extremely long (e.g., more than 20 years for asbestosis) so that it is mandatory to take a detailed occupational history, including summer jobs and hobbies, in all patients with suspected ILD. Moreover, a history of smoking is associated with an increased risk for the development of IPF. Finally, the occurrence of familial cases of IPF suggests that genetic factors may modulate responses to causative agents.

Table 8.20 Interstitial Lung Diseases

Interstitial Pulmonary Fibrosis

A syndrome progressing from alveolitis to interstitial inflammation to fibrosis of the lungs.

Pulmonary Manifestations: Presents with dyspnea, cough, fatigue, adventitious crackles sounding like Velcro, tachypnea, finger clubbing, abnormal PFTs.

Management: No curative medical therapy. Nonspecific anti-inflammatory agents and immunosuppressive drugs are generally ineffective; other treatment options include cytotoxic agents and antifibrotic agents (colchicine or penicillamine).

Bronchiolitis Obliterans Organizing Pneumonia (BOOP)

A disease characterized by masses of granulation tissue in the lumens of small airways with patchy organizing pneumonia distal to these obstructions.

Pulmonary Manifestations: Presents with cough, flu-like illness, inspiratory crackles, expiratory squeaks, restrictive ventilatory defect and abnormal diffusing capacity; chest x-ray film shows patchy alveolar infiltrates often with a ground-glass appearance.

Management: Corticosteriod therapy.

Collagen Vascular Diseases

- **Systemic Lupus Erythematosus:** Chronic, multisystem inflammatory disease of connective tissue that involves the skin, joints, serous membranes (pleura, pericardium), kidneys, hematologic system, and CNS.
  Pulmonary Manifestations: May present with pleuritis with or without effusion, diaphragmatic dysfunction with reduced lung volume, acute lupus pneumonitis, diffuse alveolar hemorrhage, diffuse interstitial disease, pulmonary hypertension, and pulmonary thromboembolism.
  Management: NSAIDs, corticosteroids, immunosuppressive agents (cyclophosphamide [Cytoxan]), plasmapheresis (severe cases).
- **Rheumatoid Arthritis:** Chronic, systemic disease characterized by recurrent inflammation of the diarthroidal joints and related structures.
  Pulmonary Manifestations: Abnormal PFTs with reduced diffusing capacity and restrictive mechanics, pulmonary nodules, BOOP, pleuritis with or without effusion, ILD.
  Management: Rheumatoid lung disease responds very poorly to drug therapy; a trial of prednisone is usually given but fewer than 10% of patients have a measurable response.
- **Progressive Systemic Sclerosis (Scleroderma):** A disorder of connective tissue characterized by fibrotic, degenerative and occasionally inflammatory changes in the skin, blood vessels, synovium, skeletal muscle, and internal organs.
  Pulmonary Manifestations: Presents with dyspnea, bibasilar crackles, reduced lung compliance, pleural thickening and pulmonary fibrosis on x-ray, abnormal PFTs, pulmonary hypertension, recurrent aspiration pneumonia.
  Management: No specific drugs or combination of drugs have been proved effective; in general, corticosteroids are not beneficial and only a few patients respond to penicillamine (Cuprimine) therapy.
- **Polymyositis-Dermatomyositis:** Diffuse inflammatory myopathies of striated muscle, producing symmetrical weakness, usually most severe in the proximal muscles.
  Pulmonary Manifestations: The three types of lung disease classically described are interstitial pneumonitis, aspiration pneumonia due to esophageal dysmotility, and pneumonia secondary to hypoventilation as a result of respiratory muscle involvement.
  Management: Corticosteroids; cyclophosphamide (Cytoxan).

Systemic Granulomatous Vasculitis

- **Wegener's Granulomatosis:** Characterized by a triad of (1) necrotizing granulomatous vasculitis of the upper and lower respiratory tracts, (2) glomerulonephritis, and (3) variable degrees of vasculitis of small arteries and veins.
  Pulmonary Manifestations: Upper respiratory tract lesions include sinusitis, otitis media, nasal septal ulceration. Pulmonary manifestations vary from focal granulomatous vasculitis to diffuse alveolitis and capillaritis that may present as alveolar hemorrhage. Pulmonary function tests reveal a restrictive pattern.
  Management: Cyclophosphamide (Cytoxan) and prednisone; azathioprine (Imuran) and methotrexate (Folex, Rheumatrex) are alternative agents.
- **Lymphomatoid Granulomatosis:** A systemic disease consisting of angiocentric lymphoid granulomatous vasculitis, primarily of the lungs, with frequent involvement of the kidneys and skin.
  Pulmonary Manifestations: Presenting symptoms are usually cough, dyspnea; chest x-ray reveals multiple, bilateral, ill-defined or nodular densities that may cavitate.
  Management: Cyclophosphamide (Cytoxan) and corticosteroids; chemotherapy regimen if recurrence with malignant lymphoma.
- **Allergic Angiitis and Granulomatosis (Churg-Strauss Syndrome):** Rare disorder characterized by necrotizing angiitis of the lungs, heart, skin, and CNS with involved organs containing infiltration with eosinophils.
  Pulmonary Manifestations: Presents with an allergic history, often with asthma; chest x-ray abnormalities may range from patchy densities to large bilateral nodular infiltrates; cavitation is rare.
  Management: Corticosteriods, prednisone, azathioprine (Imuran), cyclophosphamide (Cytoxan), plasma exchange.
- **Drug-Induced Pulmonary Disease:** Iatrogenic and adverse complications of various drugs (cytotoxic agents, antibiotics immunosuppressives).
  Pulmonary Manifestations: Hypersensitivity pulmonary disease with dyspnea, nonproductive cough, lung crackles, tachypnea, diffuse linear streaks and densities in lower lung zones on x-ray.
  Management: Discontinuation of the drug or reduction in drug dosage in conjunction with corticosteroid therapy.
- **Sarcoidosis:** A multisystem syndrome of unknown etiology, involving complex cellular immune pathways; it most frequently affects the lung.
  Pulmonary Manifestations: Lung most common organ affected; PFTs reveal a restrictive pattern and small lung volumes; tissue biology demonstrates characteristic granulomas.
  Management: Corticosteroids, and other drugs such as hydroxychloroquine (Plaquenil), methotrexate (Folex).

- **Hypersensitivity Pneumonitis (Allergic Alveolitis):** Caused by inhalation of a variety of organic dusts. Dusts can be derived from animal dander and proteins; from fungi that contaminate vegetables, wood bark, or water-reservoir vaporizers; and from dairy and grain products. Colorful, descriptive names for the diseases underscore the frequent occupational nature of exposure.
  Pulmonary Manifestations: In acute form of disease, respiratory and systemic symptoms develop explosively within 4–6 hours after dust is inhaled and consists of dyspnea, cough, chills, fever, and malaise. Symptoms abate in 12 hours. With each reexposure the acute episode occurs again. The acutely ill patient is dyspneic with inspiratory crackles in lower lung zones. Chest x-ray film shows fine, diffuse alveolar filling and variable interstitial streaks; PFTs are abnormal.
  Management: Avoidance of inhaled substance, corticosteroids (prednisone).

Dyspnea in the patient with ILD is the result of increased work of breathing caused primarily by the stiffness of the lungs and by excessive minute ventilation. Hypoxemia, often aggravated by exercise, may amplify the sensation of dyspnea by carotid body stimulation. Unfortunately, patients do not always know what toxins they were exposed to and exposures to toxins may be easily overlooked, so that considerable investigation may be required.

FOCUS ON HISTORY 8.1

Taking an Occupational and Environmental History

General health history	• Does the patient think symptom/problem is related to anything at work? • When was the onset of symptoms, and how are they related to work? • Has the patient missed a day of work, and why? • Prior pulmonary problems • Medications • Cigarette use
Current or most relevant employment	• Job or process: title and description • Type of industry and specific work • Name of employer • Years employed
Exposure information	• General description of job process and overall hygiene • Materials used by worker and others • Ventilation/exhaust system • Use of respiratory protection • Are other workers affected? • Industrial hygiene samples and OSHA data
Environmental nonoccupational factors	• Cigarettes • Diet • Hobbies • Pets
Specific workplace exposures	• Fumes/dust/fibers • Gases • Metals • Solvent • Other chemicals: plastics, pesticides, corrosive agents • Infectious agents • Organic dusts: cotton, wood • Physical factors: noise, repetitive trauma • Radiation • Emotional factors, stress
Past employment	• List jobs in chronological order • Job titles • Exposures • Military service

For example, fungi in cooling systems or birds in the home may be a source of allergens that can elicit hypersensitivity pneumonitis. History of medication use is also critical to diagnosing ILD. Patients who have been using drugs (e.g., nitrofurantoin) for years may not report them as medications on routine questioning. Mineral oil taken as a laxative or nose drops also may not be considered medications.

Diseases in other organs may present as ILD, so a detailed review of systems is important. With occupational lung diseases, the physical exam is generally unrevealing about specific cause. It is most helpful in ruling out nonoccupational causes of respiratory symptoms or diseases such as cardiac problems or connective-tissue diseases. Chronic heart disease may present as ILD with dyspnea, cough, crackles, and interstitial-type abnormalities on the chest x-ray film. Malignancies of virtually any organ system may spread to the lungs and present as ILD. The manifestations of the collagen-vascular diseases (e.g., rashes, Raynaud's phenomenon, fevers, arthralgias, muscle weakness) may give important clues on history taking. Dysphagia or regurgitation may relate to either recurrent aspiration or collagen-vascular disease, especially scleroderma. The connective-tissue diseases may be difficult to rule out because the pulmonary manifestations occasionally precede the more typical systemic manifestations by months or years. Patients with AIDS complicated by pneumocystosis or lymphocytic interstitial pneumonia may first present with an insidious onset of dyspnea and fatigue, as do patients with other ILDs. Therefore, sexual preference and other possible risk factors for AIDS should be identified.

Abnormalities on the chest x-ray film may be the first clue to the presence of ILD; however, the patient with ILD may be asymptomatic, with normal or abnormal chest x-ray results, or may be symptomatic, with normal or abnormal chest x-ray results. The initial abnormality on the chest x-ray film is usually described as ground glass or a hazy appearance of the lungs. As disease progresses, diffuse abnormalities are found bilaterally. Pulmonary opacities (infiltrates) are usually described as small nodules (nodular), lines (reticular), or both (reticulonodular). Nodules are most commonly found in granulomatous diseases and hypersensitivity pneumonitis. The development of reticular densities is thought to be the result of edema, infiltration, or fibrosis of the septa in the periphery of the lung. A common characteristic of ILD is a progressively worsening in the opacities, with the development of honeycomb lung. The honeycomb-like appearance is created by the cystlike spaces that characterize the pathology of advanced ILD. Many ILDs have unique radiographic presentations. For example, WG is associated with lower lobe cavities and nodules, whereas sarcoidosis is associated with swelling of the lymph nodes of the hilum of the lung (hilar lymphadenopathy). The hila are composed of the pulmonary arteries and their main branches, the upper lobe pulmonary veins, the major bronchi, and the lymph nodes.

High-resolution computed tomography (HRCT) has become widely used for evaluating ILDs. In addition, HRCT is unsurpassed in the detection and localization of pericardial and pleural fluid collections. HRCT examines only 1 mm of lung at each level, thus revealing some of the lung parenchyma's delicate architecture. Several signs of ILDs may be noted on HRCT. The most common are interface signs—the thickened and irregular appearance of the normally smooth interface of lung parenchyma with bronchi, blood vessels, and visceral pleura. Although HRCT is an exceptional tool for evaluation of parenchymal lung disease, it is important to note its limitations. It cannot be used to study the entire thorax; conventional CT must be used to avoid missing abnormalities between images. Some HRCT findings may be difficult to interpret without a conventional CT image to use for reference.

Serologic tests for antinuclear antibodies and rheumatoid factor are positive in 20 to 40 percent, although rarely diagnostic, while antineutrophil cytoplasmic antibodies (ANCAs) may be diagnostic in some settings.

A transbronchial biopsy has become the leading invasive tool for evaluating and treating patients with a wide spectrum of pulmonary disorders. In addition, the technique of bronchoalveolar lavage (BAL) through the fiberoptic bronchoscope into a segmental or smaller bronchus provides a means to sample the cellular and soluble components of the lower respiratory tract. The area beyond the bronchoscope is washed with saline. The saline that is then aspirated back through the bronchoscope contains a small number of cells. The cells that are recovered include many from the alveoli and are representative of the cells associated with the inflammatory process. This procedure has aided in the diagnosis, pathogenesis, and assessment of activity of ILDs.

PFTs measure lung volumes and airflow with a spirometer. Whether the patient is symptomatic or not, PFTs should be performed to establish that disease is present, to determine its severity, and to monitor response to treatment. The sensitivity and specificity of these tests to diagnose the various ILDs is low, however. Routine spirometry values and lung volumes are often initially normal, as are resting blood gas measurements; only after exercise are gas-exchange abnormalities evident. The evaluation of the patient during exercise, although not constituting a direct measurement of respiration, gives more information than static measurements of lung volume or diffusing capacity regarding ventilation, blood flow, gas exchange, and control of breathing. PFTs usually show a purely restrictive defect in most patients with ILD. Obstructive lung disease develops gradually in some patients and more commonly in some diseases (sarcoidosis, hypersensitivity pneumonitis).

The compliance of the lungs decreases as lung involvement progresses. This is caused, in part, by fibrosis of the pulmonary parenchyma and the formation of cystic airspace. Diffusion capacity of the lung (DLCO) is a good reflection of alveolar capillary surface area. Destruction of lung parenchyma results in a reduction in DLCO as ILD progresses. An abnormal DLCO may be the earliest evidence of ILD found on standard PFTs.

Subsequent Testing. The use of the thoracoscope in combination with standard surgical instruments has led to the designation video-assisted thoracic surgery or video-assisted thoracoscopy (VATS). VATS provides the same access to the hemithorax as both thoracoscopy and thoracotomy. VATS procedures are particularly useful for obtaining lung biopsies in patients with diffuse ILD. With VATS, the visualization of the lung is better than it is with a limited thoracotomy and more areas of the lung can be sampled.

Transbronchial lung biopsy involves passing a forceps or needle through the bronchoscope. A specimen is obtained with forceps or aspirated through a needle. Pleural biopsy is useful in diagnosing granulomatous disease or malignancy of the pleura and should be performed only if these two diseases are suspected. If a specific diagnosis is not made by transbronchial biopsy, then an open lung biopsy is indicated. Open lung biopsy is the most definitive way to diagnose and stage the disease so that appropriate prognostic and therapeutic decisions can be made. Because of the age of the patient and the potential risks of the sur-gery in a compromised patient, empirical therapy may be initiated.

Differential Diagnosis

When confronted with a patient with unexplained dyspnea and fatigue, the list of Differential Diagnoses is immense. Pulmonary, cardiac, hematologic, renal, neuromuscular, and even endocrine diseases may present with exercise intolerance of dyspnea. A complete workup of these systems is required to determine the correct diagnosis. Some of the conditions that give rise to dyspnea, diffuse pulmonary infiltration, and granulomatous reaction include the following: extrinsic allergic alveolitis, asbestosis, silicosis, berylliosis, lymphoid granulomatosis, connective-tissue diseases, certain drugs, miliary TB, lymphoma, leukemias, PCP, and coccidiomycosis.

Management

Management of most ILDs is difficult, and different approaches are taken depending on the specific entity. Regardless of etiology, end-stage fibrosis is irreversible and untreatable. An extensive and aggressive diagnostic evaluation early on, even in the patient with relatively few symptoms is recommended. Early clinical intervention in patients who are more likely to develop lung disease could be of considerable benefit for the patient. A good example is the identification and assessment of disease progression in diffuse lung disease found in systemic sclerosis. The first course of action when faced with a patient with ILD is to determine whether exposure to environmental agents or drugs is the cause, and to discontinue the exposure. Therapeutic dilemmas arise because discontinuation of such drugs as tocainide or amiodarone may result in life-threatening dysrhythmias. Second, the best chance for therapeutic success begins with the correct diagnosis. Finally, in cases in which specific medication is employed, such as prednisone or cytotoxic agents, there is usually suppression rather than cure of the primary process. Many patients with ILD are older adults, so the decision to treat them with immunosuppressive drugs should not be taken lightly, because the toxicity and adverse effects of these medications can be substantial. In addition, anti-inflammatory and immunosuppressive treatments may be ineffective because of recurrent dysregulated wound healing rather than neutrophilic or immune cell-mediated inflammation. Investigational studies are looking at a shift toward antifibroblast therapies for ILD aimed at decreasing pulmonary collagen deposition.

Initial Management

Corticosteroids may be initiated in the therapy for ILD. A trial with them is reasonable, even for the patient who is in an advanced stage of the disease with relatively acellular and fibrotic changes in lung tissue. The best predictor of ultimate steroid responsiveness and a better prognosis is early benefit following the initial 1 to 2 months of steroid therapy. The dosage and duration of corticosteroid therapy depends on the specific disorder, but in general relatively high doses are used for the first 6 weeks (1 to 2 mg/kg per day, or 60 to 100 mg per day) over the ensuing 3 months. A period of 3 to 6 months is often required to determine the steroid responsiveness of fibrosing alveolitis, although patients with sarcoidosis and cryptogenic organizing pneumonia may respond much more quickly with lower dosages. Certain processes, such as idiopathic pulmonary fibrosis, commonly require therapy for 12 months or longer.

Subsequent Management

For the patient who is not well controlled with or responsive to corticosteroids, additional immunosuppressive therapy may be considered. Cyclophosphamide (Cytoxan), an alkylating drug, is a potent immunosuppressant and seems to be effective in patients with ILD who are not helped with corticosteroids. If improvement in the lung disease is documented after 3 months of this therapy, it should be continued for a 12-month interval. Azathioprine (Azasan, Imuran) has been used as an alternative to cyclophosphamide. Penicillamine (Cuprimine, Depen) has been used in some patients, with the rationale that it might prevent the cross-linking of abnormal collagen being synthesized in the interstitium and prevent or retard fibrosis. Exercise tolerance may be significantly improved with supplemental oxygen.

As the pulmonary vascular bed is impaired by progressive fibrosis, pulmonary hypertension and cor pulmonale can develop; right-sided CHF can be difficult to control.

Judicious use of diuretics is advised, for a significant decrease in intravascular volume may be deleterious for lung perfusion. Digitalis or antidysrhythmic drugs may be required, although adequate oxygenation is probably the best treatment for heart failure in this situation. Some patients may also develop obstruction to air flow and be troubled with wheezing and coughing that may respond to bronchodilators. Because infection may occur during immunosuppressive therapy, it is important to maintain a high index of suspicion and to treat infection aggressively. Prophylactic use of pneumococcal and influenza vaccines is encouraged. Finally, lung transplantation may be an option for patients with refractory disease limited to the chest.

Follow-Up and Referral

Reassessment of disease activity is generally performed at 3, 6, 12, and 24 months and more often if needed. Respon-siveness is defined as a decrease in symptoms: radiographic improvement, physiologic improvement, or no further decline in clinical, radiographic, or physiologic parameters. The patient should be followed for signs of infection that are masked by immunosuppressive drugs, pneumothorax, or development of lung cancer, which occurs in 5 to 10 percent of patients. The patient on steroids must be monitored closely during times of illness or stress and during steroid tapering or withdrawal. The patient should be encouraged to wear a medical identification bracelet. In view of exercise-related hypoxia, the patient should be assessed for benefit of supplemental oxygen during exercise. Patients with a collagen vascular disorder must be regularly assessed for progression or exacerbations of their chronic illnesses. For example, patients with RA require rest, joint protection, daily heat and exercise, and psychological support. Community resources such as a home care nurse, homemaker services, and vocational rehabilitation may be considered. Self-help groups may be beneficial for the patient. These diseases require the collaborative and integrated approach as emphasized in the Circle of Caring Model.

Specialized testing should be undertaken and the patient referred to a pulmonologist if no specific cause of dyspnea or cough can be found; if the symptoms exceed the physiologic or radiographic abnormalities identified; if empiric management (with bronchodilators, diuretics, smoking cessation) resulted in an atypical or unsatisfactory clinical outcome; if the patient needs an impairment or disability evaluation for workers' compensation or any reason; if specialized cardiopulmonary testing (e.g., lung biopsy) is needed; or if a therapeutic immunosuppressive or cytotoxic drug trial is contemplated.

Patient Education

Patients with ILD must be educated about the nature of their illness, the related diagnostic tests, and the treatment regimen for their particular type of lung disease (Table 8.21). For example, avoidance of exposure to antigens is paramount for those with hypersensitivity pneumonitis. All patients must be advised and assisted to stop cigarette smoking to prevent further lung damage. In many cases, the most comprehensive patient education occurs within the context of a pulmonary rehabilitation program.

Table 8.21 Educational Content for the Patient with Interstitial Lung Disease

- Respiratory anatomy and physiology
- Pathophysiology of interstitial lung disease
- Respiratory diagnostic tests:
  Chest x-ray
  PFTs
  Exercise tests
  Bronchoscopy
  HRCT
- Self-care measures:
  Pulmonary medications
  Diet
  Fluid intake
  Smoking cessation
  Environmental control
  Signs of infections
- Chest therapy:
  Relaxation and guided imagery
  Breathing retraining
  Controlling dyspneic episodes
  Postural drainage
- Progressive exercise conditioning:
  Walking programs
  Treadmill or bicycle exercise training
  Arm or leg ROM exercises
- Respiratory equipment:
  Oxygen therapy
  Hand-held nebulizer

The need to reduce repeated admissions into expensive ICUs brought about the proliferation of formal inpatient and outpatient pulmonary rehabilitation programs in the United States for patients with chronic lung disease. The target population for these programs has been severely disabled patients with COPD or ILD, who require a broad range of comprehensive services to keep them clinically stable and out of the hospital for long periods of time. Appropriate patients with all levels of respiratory impairment, not only the severely disabled, should be referred to such programs.

Each program has criteria for referral that generally include the following patient characteristics: dyspnea on exertion, inability to carry out selected activities of daily living (ADLs), repeated hospitalizations or need for home care services, time lost from work or school, and desire for educational update of self-care techniques. Moreover, the following laboratory features are inclusion criteria for pulmonary rehabilitation: reduced vital capacity in restrictive disease, reduced expiratory flow rates, hypercapnia, and hypoxemia at rest or during exercise.

The team teaches self-care educational content and implements a program of bronchial hygiene and physical conditioning, based on needs identified during the initial assessment. Group and individual instruction and counseling are provided by a variety of personnel. Patient progress is evaluated utilizing respiratory assessment parameters and teaching–learning tools. A final evaluation with recommendations for long-range treatment is forwarded to the referring clinician.

Sleep Apnea

Sleep apnea is defined as a temporary pause in breathing during sleep that lasts at least 10 seconds to as long as 90 seconds. The three patterns of apnea are central, obstructive, and mixed. Central apnea occurs when both airflow and respiratory efforts are absent. *Central apneas* occur as a result of an absence of neural output from the brainstem's respiratory centers, which leads to a lack of inspiratory effort. The respiratory center in the brain fails to respond to elevated carbon dioxide concentrations. In contrast, during *obstructive sleep apnea* (OSA), respiratory efforts persist, although airflow is absent at the nose and mouth. Airflow obstruction occurs when the tongue and the soft palate fall backward and partially or completely obstruct the pharynx. Finally, many adult patients exhibit mixed apneas in which both central and obstructive patterns occur.

Each apnea results in progressive asphyxiation until an arousal from sleep occurs, with a subsequent restoration of upper airway patency and airflow. A patient then usually returns to sleep quickly, resulting in another occlusion of the upper airway. Apnea and arousal cycles occur repeatedly, as many as 200 to 400 times during 6 to 8 hours of sleep. Sleep hypopnea is a period of hypoventilation or decreased airflow defined as a 50 percent reduction in thoracoabdominal movements, with a 4 percent fall in oxygen saturation lasting at least ten seconds during sleep. OSA/hypopnea is present when the respiratory drive is intact but the upper airway intermittently becomes obstructed during sleep. The *respiratory disturbance index* (RDI) (also called the apnea/hypopnea index)—the number of apneas plus hypopneas per hour of sleep—may be used to define and quantify the severity of OSA. The RDI is obtained by dividing the total number of events throughout the entire night by the total sleep time in hours. An index greater than 5 is abnormal, although it probably does not become clinically significant until it reaches 20. In general, as the RDI increases, so does the severity of symptoms.

Patients with OSA may experience a number of potentially adverse physiologic and neurobehavioral problems. Consequences of OSA are the result of daily exposure to abnormalities in breathing during sleep and result in long-term morbidity in the neurobehavioral and cardiovascular domains. Sleep-disordered breathing is an independent risk factor for the development of hypertension and, subsequently, left ventricular dysfunction. The patient with combined coronary artery disease (CAD) and OSA may have an increased cardiac risk because of worsening of the relationship between myocardial oxygen demand and supply as a result of apnea-associated hypoxemia and activation of the autonomic nervous system (Table 8.22). Moreover, cardiac dysrhythmias, usually occurring during apneic episodes, have been reported to be a significant complication of OSA. In addition, sleep quality may be influenced by apnea-associated activation of the CNS (arousals) and ischemia-associated arousals. Timely diagnosis and treatment of CAD as well as sleep apnea is necessary for these patients.

Table 8.22 Possible Consequences of Sleep Apnea

Pulmonary hypertension
Systemic hypertension
Cardiac dysrhythmias
Right or left ventricular failure
Right ventricular hypertrophy
MI (increased risk of)
Stroke (increased risk of)
Nocturnal angina
COPD (exacerbation of)
Insulin resistance
Endothelial cell dysfunction

OSA can cause mild pulmonary hypertension, even in the absence of pulmonary disease. Sustained pulmonary hypertension, often associated with clinical evidence of right ventricular failure, has been observed in about 20 percent of OSA patients. It is hypothesized that repetitive hypoxemia during sleep may lead to vascular remodeling in susceptible patients and thus cause pulmonary hypertension during the day. Further, because the patient with OSA is often obese or has pathological lung function resulting in abnormalities of daytime ABG values, pulmonary vasoconstriction is another mechanism inducing pulmonary hypertension.

Epidemiology and Causes

Sleep apnea is an extremely common clinical disorder; as such, it has major public health implications. Unrecognized and untreated OSA in the general adult population, most of whom are in the most productive period of their lives, contributes to significant and disabling psychomotor deficits. An estimated 40 million Americans are chronically ill with various sleep disorders and 38,000 cardiovascular deaths annually are directly attributable to OSA; yet, the vast majority of Americans with sleep disorders remain undiagnosed and untreated. This, in turn, costs billions of dollars in accidents in the home, at the workplace, and in traffic.

Approximately 4 percent of women and 9 percent of men have significant OSA. OSA is most prevalent in men older than the age of 50 and in postmenopausal women probably related to hormonal changes. Normal men have a significantly higher pharyngeal and supraglottic resistance than normal women, which makes them more susceptible to pharyngeal collapse and OSA, and may contribute to the male predominance of the syndrome. Pharyngeal resistance increases with age in normal men, possibly related to greater body weight, and it is widely believed that the risk of developing OSA increases with age in men. This assumption, however, is far from conclusive. Moreover, once a disorder is labeled as predominantly a male condition, clinicians may be less likely to think about it in women and, hence, less likely to refer women to sleep disorder centers. Compared to OSA, central sleep apnea syndrome is uncommon. In most sleep laboratories, patients with central sleep apnea syndrome constitute less than 10 percent of patients tested. The division between central and obstructive sleep apnea is not as clear-cut as it might appear, because many patients with central sleep apnea present with clinical features more suggestive of OSA; it is possible that in some patients, upper airway occlusion triggers a central, rather than an obstructive apnea. Support for this notion comes from the finding that some patients with central sleep apnea can be successfully treated with nasal continuous positive airway pressure (CPAP).

The cause of OSA is poorly defined but appears to be multifactorial; upper airway tract malformation, oropharyngeal muscle dysfunction, and abnormal respiratory drive each play a greater or lesser part (Risk Factors 8.3). A number of recognized anatomic abnormalities are associated with narrowing of the upper airway and predispose patients to OSA. Conditions associated with facial dysmorphism or mandibular abnormalities show a predisposition to OSA and include adenotonsillar hypertrophy, choanal atresia, micrognathia (small mandible), retrognathia, macroglossia, nasal septal deviation, and craniofacial dyostosis. Micrognathia is particularly associated with OSA, because a small or retropositioned mandible places the base of the tongue closer to the posterior pharyngeal wall and interferes with the efficiency of the genioglossus muscle in keeping the tongue out of the narrowed pharynx.

There is increasing evidence that sleep apnea has a familial distribution. Relatives of a person with sleep apnea have approximately twice the normal risk of having sleep apnea. Most adult patients with OSA, however, have no specific skeletal or soft tissue lesion obstructing the upper airway, but they often have a small, congested oropharyngeal airway. Symptoms of sleep apnea are present two to six times more frequently in family members of affected patients than in a control population.

Obesity and alcohol consumption are well recognized as aggravating factors. One possible explanation for the relationship between obesity and OSA is that the upper airway is narrowed in the obese patient as a result of increased fat deposition in the pharyngeal walls. Fat in the neck plays the largest role. Neck (or collar) size is the best indicator of the presence of sleep apnea. Approximately 30 percent of snoring males with a collar size larger than 17 inches will have OSA. Neck size in women is less well investigated, but when it is over 15 inches, it increases the risk for sleep apnea. Another possible explanation for this relationship is the fact that the obese patient often has smaller lung volumes, particularly functional residual capacity, than the nonobese patient; this, in turn, can indirectly influence upper airway size and contribute to upper airway narrowing. Any factor that interferes with the arousal mechanism, such as alcohol consumption, could lead to more profound and prolonged apneas. Alcohol, which reduces upper-airway muscle tone, and sedatives or hypnotics, which reduce the arousal mechanism, exacerbate OSA. There is considerable evidence that OSA carries a substantial morbidity and mortality, particularly from cardiovascular complications.

RISK FACTORS 8.3

Risk Factors for Mortality or Complications from Community-Acquired Pneumonia

Age: Over age 65

Presence of coexisting illness:
- Chronic pulmonary disease
- Diabetes mellitus
- Chronic renal failure
- CHF
- Chronic liver disease of any etiology
- Previous hospitalization within 1 year of the onset of pneumonia
- Suspicion of aspiration
- Altered mental status
- Postsplenectomy state
- Chronic alcohol abuse or malnutrition

Abnormal physical findings:
- Respiratory rate above 30/min
- Diastolic BP 60 mm Hg or below and/or systolic BP 90 mm Hg or below
- Temperature above 101°F
- Evidence of extrapulmonary sites of disease (e.g., septic arthritis, meningitis)
- Decreased level of consciousness or confusion

Abnormal laboratory findings:
- WBC count $<4 \times 10^6$/L or $>30 \times 10^6$/L
- $Pao_2 < 60$ mm Hg or $Paco_2 > 50$ mm Hg on room air
- Hemoglobin <9 g/dL
- X-ray showing more than one lobe involvement, pleural effusion, evidence or rapid spreading
- Severe electrolyte or renal abnormality not known to be chronic (e.g., BUN > 50 mg/dL, creatinine > 1.2 mg/dL, sodium <130 mEq/L)

Pathophysiology

Sleep is divided into two states—rapid eye movement (REM) sleep and non–rapid eye movement (NREM) sleep. NREM sleep is further divided into four stages, based on changes in the electroencephalogram (EEG) pattern. Normal sleep begins with stage I, which is characterized by slow eye movements, usually preceding sleep onset. Stage II involves further slowing of the EEG, with the presence of sleep spindles and slow eye movements. Stage III is manifested by low-frequency delta waves with occasional sleep spindles but no slow eye movements. Finally, stage IV is characterized by high-voltage delta waves. REM sleep is characterized by desynchronized, low-voltage, fast activity that occurs about every 90 minutes beginning after 1 to 2 hours of NREM sleep. The normal adult sleeper alternates between NREM sleep and REM sleep approximately every 90 minutes through the night.

Typically, during the lighter stages of NREM sleep, the breathing pattern is irregular because of the decrease in respiratory drive associated with the stimulatory effect of wakefulness and decreased metabolic rate associated with sleep. In the deeper stages of NREM sleep, breathing is typically very regular; however, overall ventilation is reduced compared to that during wakefulness. During REM sleep, the respiratory drive is irregular because of the transient decrease in ventilatory response to chemical and mechanical stimuli. The influence of sleep on the upper airway is similar to its effects on other skeletal muscles, resulting in a general loss of muscle tone, and a reduction in tidal volume and minute volume. The sleep structure of the patient with OSA is characterized by the loss of physiologic REM/NREM alternation as well as by a deficit of REM and slow-wave sleep. This can be caused by sleep fragmentation as a result of the high amount of arousals related to respiratory events.

Central Sleep Apnea

Etiological factors of central sleep apnea are found mainly in disturbances in the respiratory control system in the brainstem. The cause of such disturbances of the breathing control system remains unclear in most cases, however. Central apneas are commonly seen in altitudes where hypoxemia induces hyperventilation with associated alkalosis. Cheyne-Stokes respiration with central apneas may also occur in the patient with CHF. Neurologic diseases affecting the brainstem may cause breathing pattern disorders in sleep. Well-known neurologic diseases such as arteriosclerosis in the older adult, infarctions, tumors, hemorrhage, trauma with damage of this region, encephalitis, poliomyelitis, or other infectious diseases may cause central apnea during sleep, even though no abnormalities of breathing patterns are present during wakefulness. If the neural pathways from medullary respiratory groups to motor neurons of the ventilatory muscles are interrupted, the metabolic control of breathing may be disturbed. This may occur after cervical cordotomy.

Obstructive Sleep Apnea

The underlying pathophysiology of sleep apnea is complex and not fully understood. However, it is generally accepted that patency of the upper airway is dependent upon the action of oropharyngeal dilator and abductor muscles, which are normally activated in a rhythmic fashion during inspiration. The available evidence indicates that in OSA, the site of upper airway obstruction is the pharynx and that obstruction of the pharynx during sleep is a result of an imbalance between the forces that serve to dilate the pharynx and those that promote pharyngeal closure. The upper airway is subjected to collapse when the force produced by these muscles, for a given cross-sectional area (CSA) of the upper airway, is exceeded by the negative airway pressure generated by inspiratory activity of the diaphragm and intercostal muscles. Upper airway obstruction can occur if the suction pressure is too high, or the counteracting forces of the dilating muscles are too weak, for any given suction pressure.

The subsequent obstructive apnea results in progressive and sometimes profound hypoxia and hypercapnia. These apnea-associated changes in Po_2 and Pco_2 stimulate ventilation, resulting in increasing inspiratory efforts. Eventually the progressive hypoxemia and hypercapnia and/or the associated increase in inspiratory effort result in arousal of the patient. With this usually transient arousal occurs augmentation of upper airway dilator muscle activity to an extent proportionately greater than the simultaneous augmentation of diaphragm activity. This leads to deocclusion of the pharynx and restoration of airflow. During the subsequent brief period of ventilation, Po_2 rises and Pco_2 falls. The rapid resumption of sleep, however, results in reocclusion of the upper airway. This cycle of events may therefore recur hundreds of times each night, triggering recurrent arousals that may contribute to many of the clinical features of OSA (Fig. 8.2).

Clinical Presentation

Subjective

The diagnosis of OSA is not difficult to make: the symptoms are typical and the major risk factor is relatively obvious. Patients with sleep apnea have both nighttime and daytime symptoms (Table 8.23). Hypersomnolence is the single most important presenting symptom of sleep apnea and frequently identifies which patient will require and accept specific therapy.

Hypersomnolence is not tiredness, fatigue, or lassitude, but rather, clear-cut, uncontrollable sleepiness. It develops over a long period and is first experienced by a patient as sleep onset when attention is not demanded (e.g., when watching television, sitting in a college lecture, or waiting at a traffic light). Eventually more alerting situations are affected such as long-distance driving or quiet conversation. Daytime symptoms include a morning headache (from hypercapnia) and neuropsychologic disturbances, including falling asleep while performing purposeful activities. These episodes can occur during work or social functions and can lead to embarrassment, domestic discord, decreased work

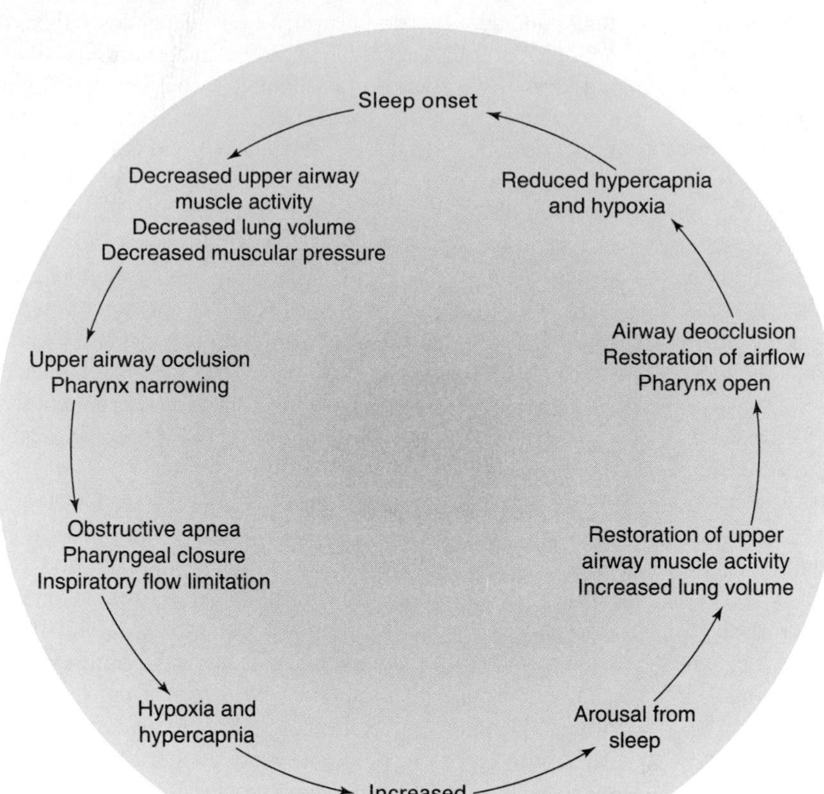

FIGURE 8.2 Pathogenesis of obstructive sleep apnea.

productivity, loss of employment, and an increased incidence of accidents. The patient may complain of nocturnal restlessness, frequent urination or enuresis, and choking.

The patient usually reports impaired intellectual performance, such as decreased concentration, ambition, and memory loss. Patients with sleep apnea also report limiting social contact because of their fear of sleepiness and falling asleep. Personality changes such as irritability and moodiness are seen in about 50 percent of patients and more severe psychiatric disturbances such as major depression and psychosis have been reported. Sexual dysfunction is common (e.g., diminished libido, even though men with apnea can obtain an erection). Persons with sleep apnea may note nocturnal palpitations or skipped heartbeats. OSA is characterized by loud snoring that is repeatedly interrupted by episodes of complete upper airway obstruction and resolves with temporary arousal. The snoring of OSA is both loud (it can be heard in an adjacent room) and habitual (it occurs nightly). Hypoxemia and hypercarbia of varying degrees frequently accompany apnea or hypopnea. It is not uncommon for some patients to regularly desaturate to oxygen saturation levels below 70 percent and, occasionally, below 60 percent. Apneas and hypopneas often result in arousal from sleep, which then terminates the breathing disturbance and a surge in blood pressure (BP). Once aroused, the CNS can respond appropriately to the partial or complete closure of the pharynx with a brief contraction of the pharyngeal dilating muscles. This restores upper airway patency and permits resumption of airflow, with subsequent reversal of the hypoxemia and hypercarbia. Arousals often last for only 1 to 3 seconds and are not recognized by the patient. Occasionally, during the arousal that terminates the apneic event, the bed partner may witness arm flailing or other gross movements.

On awakening in the morning, the patient is often completely unaware that he or she aroused several hundred

Table 8.23 Conditions Presenting with Excessive Daytime Sleepiness

- Sleep apnea syndromes
- Narcolepsy
- Idiopathic hypersomnia
- Periodic limb movements in sleep
- Psychiatric disorders
- Drug and alcohol dependency
- Insufficient sleep syndrome
- Circadian disorders (jet lag, shift work)
- Obesity-hypoventilation syndrome (Pickwickian syndrome)
- Hypothyroidism
- Seizure disorder
- Depression

times during the night. It is believed that recurrent arousals and the consequent sleep disruption are the causes of many of the daytime symptoms and effects of sleep apnea. Automobile accidents have been reported to occur 2.0 to 2.6 times more frequently among patients with OSA than among other individuals, a consequence that contributes to many unnecessary and costly days in the hospital.

Clinically, patients with central sleep apnea usually shows less daytime sleepiness than do patients with other types of apnea. Sleep disruption, frequent awakening, shortness of breath after awakening, and signs of right heart failure such as peripheral edema are observed quite often. The patient with central sleep apnea tends to have a normal body weight. Psychiatric symptoms such as depression may occur as well. As in obstructive apnea, oxygen desaturation and consequent hemodynamic disorders may be observed.

Objective

The predominant clinical manifestations of OSA reflect the risk factors: obesity (particularly of the upper body), increased neck size, crowded oropharynx (tonsillar hypertrophy and enlargement of soft palate (uvula) and tongue, as well as lateral peritonsillar narrowing), retrognathia, and micrognathia.

Diagnostic Reasoning

Diagnostic Tests

OSA should be suspected whenever hypersomnia and snoring coexist. The recording of specific historical details from the patient and his or her spouse is crucial to the diagnosis, particularly since the patient sometimes does not realize the severity of the sleepiness. This is perhaps because he or she finds it socially unacceptable or has slipped into it so gradually. Initial testing may take the form of determining how easy it is for a patient to fall asleep, or alternatively, how difficult it is for the person to remain awake. This type of testing may include both subjective and objective assessments. Two common subjective assessments of sleepiness are the Stanford Sleepiness Score (SSS) and the Epworth Sleepiness Scale (ESS). The SSS is used to record the degree of sleepiness experienced by a patient at a given time and does not necessarily relate to his or her overall propensity to fall asleep (Advanced Assessment 8.2). The ESS measures sleepiness as a reflection of a patient's tendency to fall asleep during specific nonstimulating situations, as assessed over an interval of time. A value of 10 is considered abnormal.

The definitive test for sleep apnea is an overnight polysomnogram. This all-night recording of the patient's sleep, performed in a sleep center, is the "gold standard" for identifying the presence, type, and severity of sleep apnea. The standard raises two major problems, however: first, the test is not accessible to many patients, because it is limited to specialized sleep centers; second, it is expensive. The polysomnograph is a multichannel recorder that records the patient's eye movements, airflow, respiratory movements, leg movements, EEG readings, pulse oximetry, ECG readings, and snoring. From such records, apneas, hypopneas, and snoring-related arousals are scored. The RDI is calculated from the number of apneas plus hypopneas per hour. Recently, multichannel devices that record a limited number of parameters (e.g., respiratory movements, airflow, snoring, pulse oximetry, and ECG) have been introduced for home studies, which may be comparable to a full polysomnogram.

The development of large numbers of limited diagnostic systems in recent years represents a recognition of the logistic problems involved in access to large sleep centers. Unfortunately, there is no uniformity among these devices,

ADVANCED ASSESSMENT 8.2

Epworth Sleepiness Scale

In contrast to just feeling tired, how likely are you to doze off or fall asleep in the following situations? (This refers to your usual life in recent times. Even if you have not done some of these things recently, try to work out how they would have affected you.)

Use the following scale to choose the most appropriate number of each situation:

0 = would never doze
1 = slight chance of dozing
2 = moderate chance of dozing
3 = high chance of dozing

Situation	Chance of Dozing
Sitting and reading	
Watching TV	
Sitting inactive in a public place (theatre or at a meeting)	
As a passenger in a car for an hour without a break	
Lying down to rest in the afternoon when circumstances permit	
Sitting quietly after lunch without alcohol	
In a car, while stopping for a few minutes in traffic	

and the only consistent variable common to all such systems is the oxygen saturation level. Most offer some measure of respiration, based either on nasal flow or chest bands. In the patient with OSA, the polysomnogram demonstrates frequent episodes of apnea with corresponding periods of oxygen desaturation as demonstrated by pulse oximetry. The effort to breathe remains intact during the periods of OSA, as evidenced by the movement of the lower chest and abdomen.

If the polysomnogram is negative for OSA in the patient with significant daytime sleepiness, a multiple sleep latency test (MSLT) should be performed in a sleep center to rule out narcolepsy. The MSLT is performed the day after the polysomnogram. The patient is instructed not to take any medications such as sedatives and certain antidepressants for 2 weeks before the test. The patient is allowed to take four or five 15- to 20-minute naps 2 hours apart. Healthy subjects have a sleep latency of 10 to 20 minutes in the MSLT. A test is considered consistent with excessive daytime sleepiness if sleep onset occurs within 5 minutes. The presence of two sleep-onset REM episodes in the appropriate clinical setting is diagnostic of narcolepsy.

The syndrome of periodic limb movements (PLMs) (also known as nocturnal myoclonus or periodic leg movements) consists of stereotypic periodic leg (or arm) movements during sleep that may or may not be associated with arousals. If enough arousals occur, sleep may be so fragmented that daytime sleepiness results. Because patients with narcolepsy frequently have PLMs, any patient with excessive daytime sleepiness and PLMs on a polysomnogram should be questioned carefully concerning narcoleptic manifestations.

An otolaryngologic exam should be performed. In addition, screening with a home nocturnal pulse oximetry has a high negative predictive value if no desaturations are seen. Erythrocytosis is common. A hemoglobin level and thyroid function tests should also be performed.

Differential Diagnosis

A number of disorders present with excessive daytime sleepiness (Table 8.23). Drug addiction and depression can masquerade as sleep apnea, especially in the older adult patient, in whom a number of apneas during sleep may be considered normal. Certain diagnostic tests, such as ABGs, thyroid function testing, PFTs, the ECG, and chest x-ray exam, are routinely indicated to determine the potential cause, presence, or severity of signs of hypoxic exposure occurring as the result of repetitive apneas during sleep. A recording of the patient's usual amount and pattern of sleep may be instructive.

Management

Obstructive Sleep Apnea

Currently, the first line of treatment for OSA is medical management. The treatments for OSA include:

- ▲ General measures: avoidance of alcohol, sedatives, and hypnotics; weight loss; and other (less effective) measures, including pharmacologic agents, oxygen therapy, and nasal dilators
- ▲ Specific measures: position therapy, positive airway pressure (CPAP, bilevel systems, auto-CPAP), and oral appliances

As with the most modern diseases, OSA and its treatment are highly dependent on patient behavior. Clinicians have both an opportunity and a responsibility to advise patients of the profound influence that their behavior can have on disease severity and outcome. For patients who cannot tolerate medical treatment or who do not desire long-term medical therapy, surgical treatment of sleep apnea should be considered.

Elimination of Risk Factors. A reasonable first step in the management of the patient with sleep-disordered breathing is to identify and subsequently eliminate, or avoid, the risk factors. The adverse effects of alcohol on upper airway stability during sleep and the arousal response to chemical stimuli mandate that the patient with OSA be instructed to abstain from alcohol. Although not invariably associated with OSA, obesity is usually present in this patient population. Weight reduction may result in significant improvement in OSA and sleep quality, and may obviate the need for further therapeutic interventions. Efforts in this regard represent a major, lifelong therapeutic challenge, best approached by utilizing the multidisciplinary resources of the physician, nutritionist, psychologist, and a peer support system. It is difficult to accomplish and maintain weight loss, but it is very beneficial to patients with sleep apnea when they do so. Benefits of weight loss in obese patients with sleep apnea include reduced respiratory disturbance index, BP, and optimal CPAP pressure; improved pulmonary function, daytime ABGs, polycythemia, sleep structure, and oxygen saturation; elimination of snoring; and prevention of relapse after surgical treatment.

The relationship between sleep in the supine position and augmentation of snoring and sleep apnea in some patients is apparent. It has been hypothesized that the effects of gravity in promoting posterior movement of the tongue with apposition against the posterior pharyngeal wall are magnified in the supine position. Although manipulation of the sleeping position is not an effective therapy for the majority of patients with sleep-disordered breathing, it may be all that is needed in selected patients. It has been suggested that there may be a decreased incidence of sleep-disordered breathing events during sleep in the lateral decubitus position. Position therapy can be accomplished by sewing pockets for one or two tennis balls in the back of patients' nightshirts in an attempt to prevent them from assuming the supine position. Devices to train people to sleep in the lateral position have been described.

Devices that Maintain Upper Airway Patency. CPAP administered through a nasal mask has become the most common treatment for OSA. Nasal CPAP also effectively reduces or eliminates mixed apneas, including both the central and obstructive components. A continuous flow of air is delivered from a blower unit to a tightly fitting nasal mask held in place by head straps. Nasal CPAP acts as a pneumatic splint preventing collapse of the upper airway in all phases of respiration. The device is used for the entire sleep period every night. The optimal CPAP pressure is determined by technologists during polysomnography. Typically, 5 to 20 cm H_2O is the pressure needed to abolish apneas, snoring, and oxyhemoglobin desaturations in all positions and during REM sleep. Although CPAP use is associated with few serious complications, it does elicit a number of complaints. Minor adverse effects of CPAP include feelings of suffocation, nasal drying or rhinitis, ear pain, difficulty in exhaling, mask and mouth leaks, chest and back pain, and conjunctivitis. Most of these can be alleviated.

Newer automatic CPAP devices continuously adjust the positive pressure to the required levels. In the automatic CPAP mode, the positive pressure is maintained as long as ventilation remains stable; however, any respiratory disorder results in a progressive increase in the pressure. If a breathing disturbance has not occurred for more than 4 minutes, the positive pressure decreases again. For many patients who use it at home regularly, CPAP quite dramatically eliminates apneas and hypopneas, improves sleep architecture, and reduces daytime sleepiness, even for those with mild sleep apnea. The effectiveness of CPAP is limited, however, by incomplete patient compliance.

Oral Appliances. Oral appliances are an effective noninvasive alternative to CPAP in patients with mild to moderate sleep apnea. Although oral appliances are effective in some patients with OSA, they are not universally effective. There are major design differences in the numerous oral appliances that are now available, and this may have an impact on their success and compliance rates. A novel anterior mandibular positioner has been developed with an adjustable hinge that allows progressive advancement of the mandible. This appliance may be an effective first-line treatment for the patient with mild to moderate OSA and may be associated with greater patient satisfaction than CPAP. For these devices to treat sleep apnea effectively, the mandible should be advanced to 50 to 75 percent of the maximal forward protrusion of the jaw. In most patients, dental appliances lessen but do not abolish OSA and snoring. In many patients treated with an oral appliance, the RDI still remains high, with more than 20 events per hour after treatment. The side effects of oral appliances include excessive salivation, dental misalignment, and pain in, or damage to, the temporomandibular joint (TMJ).

Surgical Management

Surgery for OSA is designed either to bypass the obstructing region of the upper airway or to modify the upper airway in such a fashion that it is less likely to lose patency. The obstruction may result either from a wide variety of structural aberrations, such as nasal deformity, nasal polyps, hypertrophic tonsils and/or adenoids, craniofacial disproportion, neoplasms, or, as in most cases, no detectable anatomic abnormalities. Accordingly, a variety of surgical procedures have been applied to the management of these patients.

Extensive excision of soft tissue in the oropharynx, termed uvulopalatopharyngoplasty (UPPP), was developed to improve pharyngeal function during sleep. The procedure involves a bilateral tonsillectomy and a submucosal resection of redundant tissue. A variable portion of the posterior margin of the soft palate and the uvula is also removed and the palatopharyngeus muscle may also be resected. In the absence of weight gain or other confounding factors, a success rate of 50 percent has been sustained for at least 1 year postoperatively. However, even OSA patients who are UPPP failures often have substantial reduction in snoring following surgery, despite persistent apnea. A repeat polysomnogram is necessary to assess the therapeutic outcome of surgery. The success rate in patients undergoing UPPP appears to be partly related to the location of the obstructing tissue: Patients with retropalatal obstruction removal experience better results than those with retroglossal obstruction removal. The preoperative presence of tonsils has been associated with improved success of UPPP.

The patient undergoing surgical reconstruction of the airway for OSA, such as UPPP, often has coexisting medical problems, especially cardiovascular disease, which can complicate treatment. The uncertainty regarding the proper predictive parameters for surgical success greatly limits optimal patient selection. Further, a significant number of patients have difficulty at induction and intubation for general anesthesia. Men with increased neck circumference and associated skeletal deformities should be evaluated carefully and considered for fiberoptic intubation.

Laser-assisted uvulopalatoplasty (LAUP) is a procedure to treat snoring in the outpatient setting. The procedure entails reshaping the palate and tonsillar pillars in one to seven serial sessions under local anesthesia. Each session lasts approximately 15 minutes and is generally well tolerated; the incidence of complications is low. The procedure is successful in reducing snoring in 90 percent of patients. However, the success rate in patients with OSA is not yet clear.

A variety of maxillofacial and nasal surgical procedures may be performed to normalize the bony relationships of the maxilla and mandible to minimize the likelihood of airway collapse during sleep. Many of these procedures are preceded by UPPP and, if the results are unsatisfactory, a second stage involving mandibular advancement is undertaken. These procedures require a great deal of surgical and orthodontic expertise, along with careful consultation with anesthesia services and pulmonary medicine.

Nasal surgery has been performed on patients with OSA in an effort to reduce the predisposition to collapse during sleep. A nasal septoplasty is performed if gross nasal septal deformity is present. The definitive therapy is a tracheostomy. Because of the drastic nature of this procedure, it is limited to patients with life-threatening arrhythmias or severe disability who have not responded to conservative therapy.

Central Sleep Apnea

Medical treatment is ineffective in the patient with central sleep apnea. Implantation of a diaphragm-pacing device is an aggressive measure, the efficiency of which has not been proven by long-term clinical trials. Diaphragm pacing may precipitate upper airway occlusion during sleep due to dysynchrony between activation of the diaphragm and the upper airway and laryngeal dilators. Thus, tracheostomy is often performed concomitantly with diaphragm pacing. These difficulties, in conjunction with the resource-intensive nature of the procedure and subsequent care have made this technique one that is infrequently employed in the clinical setting of central sleep apnea.

The use of a timed bilevel system (BiPAP) device is able to normalize blood gases during sleep. The BiPAP prevents development of severe pulmonary artery hypertension during sleep. BiPAP delivers a higher airway pressure during inspiration (when the airway is most likely to be occluded) and a lower airway pressure during expiration (patient exhales against less resistance). Cardiac dysrhythmias decrease significantly. Improvement of the respiratory situation and of the hemodynamics using a timed BiPAP device may reduce mortality rate in these patients. Bilevel systems are more expensive than conventional CPAP systems, however, and the algorithms to adjust the inspiratory and expiratory pressures are essentially empiric. Consequently, bilevel systems are now reserved for patients who cannot tolerate CPAP, especially for those who experience difficulties with exhalation or chest pain as a result of the hyperinflation produced by the applied positive pressure.

Follow-Up and Referral

In recent years, COPD and sleep apnea syndrome have been found to coexist in many patients, who are at increased risk of respiratory insufficiency. The detection of small airway disease may be difficult in OSA patients, because this syndrome is associated with various pulmonary function abnormalities resulting from obesity and upper airway obstruction. Both of these factors can be responsible for airway obstruction. Patients with both disorders frequently have marked hypoxemia, hypercapnia, and pulmonary hypertension, so they should be referred for investigation of both COPD and sleep apnea. The patient with this so-called "overlap syndrome" is at a higher risk of developing respiratory insufficiency and pulmonary hypertension than the patient with "pure" OSA. Finally, a hypoxemic stress is placed on the coronary circulation during sleep that may contribute to nocturnal mortality in the patient with COPD.

Patient Education

Because CPAP is a safe and effective treatment of OSA, it is important to improve patient compliance with regular CPAP use. Only 75 percent of patients continue to use CPAP after 1 year, citing the noise, interferance with positioning, and complaints of bed-partners. Systematically collected data on family members' learning needs and descriptions of the psychosocial impact of CPAP technology treatments on family function and quality of life are essential to developing a comprehensive protocol for teaching and counseling for CPAP therapy. The effect of group patient education sessions on compliance with CPAP therapy has proved to be a simple and effective means of improving treatment of OSA. Nasal discomfort and lack of perceived benefit are possible characteristics of patients with poor compliance; these patients might benefit from education sessions and emotional support. The personal contact and teaching, along with interaction with other OSA patients, may provide an atmosphere of encouragement and support.

Counseling may be needed concerning the potential loss of employment because of poor performance or poor decision making related to profound fatigue from sleep deprivation. Problems of depression, extreme sleepiness, and the effects of hypoxia on cognition pose special difficulties for teaching these patients; their family members must be educated. Family problem-solving skills for managing equipment, overcoming psychosocial barriers to regular nightly use, and eliminating the physiologic side effects of CPAP such as oral dryness are important skills and knowledge for this patient population. Home follow-up programs could help patients to eliminate reported physiologic adverse effects of CPAP treatments, monitor cardiac stability, and provide ongoing education and family function assessment as evidenced in other follow-up programs. A follow-up program would be cost-effective when quality of life is considered or when compared with hospital admissions for traffic accidents or the severe cardiovascular sequelae associated with OSA.

Teaching must include nutrition counseling. Weight loss may be curative, but as 10 to 20 percent of body weight loss is required, many patients give up. Strict avoidance of alcohol and hypnotic medications must also be stressed. One of the developmental objectives from *Healthy People 2010* is to reduce the proportion of vehicular crashes caused by persons with excessive sleepiness. Educating patients to be aware of this and to take corrective action is an important role of the health care provider.

Smoking Addiction

A pack-a-day smoker takes more than 70,000 puffs per year. Each puff delivers a rich assortment of chemicals into the lungs and blood. Each puff also reinforces the habit a little more and augments the establishment of secondary reinforcers, such as the sight and smell of cigarettes, the lighting procedure, and the milieu and context of a meal with a cup of coffee or a cocktail. Nicotine fulfills all the criteria of a drug addiction: compulsive use, psychoactive effects, withdrawal symptoms, and drug-reinforcing behavior. Tolerance and physical dependence, manifested by an abstinence-mediated withdrawal syndrome, contribute to the strong control exerted by nicotine on smoking behavior. Although nicotine is the most popular suspect for the reinforcing agent in tobacco, there are other possibilities. Tar and carbon monoxide are the two most likely contenders. Tobacco use is the leading preventable cause of illness, particularly cardiovascular disease, cancer, and lung disease, in the United States. Cigarettes are responsible for one in every five deaths in the United States. Besides the loss of life and the reduction in the quality of life, billions of medical expenses a year can be directly attributed to cigarette smoking.

There are hazards for nonsmokers who breathe the smoke of others' cigarettes (passive smoking or environmental tobacco smoke). *Environmental tobacco smoke* (ETS) is defined as a combination of the smoke emitted by a burning cigarette, cigar, or pipe, and the smoke exhaled by smokers. Passive smoking is associated with a modestly increased risk of lung cancers and possibly other cancers and has been classified by the Environmental Protection Agency (EPA) as a known human carcinogen. Exposure to ETS causes about 3000 deaths from lung cancer per year in nonsmoking U.S. adults and damaging the respiratory health of hundreds of thousands of children who live in homes with a parent who smokes cigarettes. It has been estimated that between 150,000 and 300,000 cases of respiratory illness occurring in infants and children up to 18 months of age may stem from exposure to ETS, which increases the risk of lower respiratory tract infections.

Epidemiology and Causes

Substantial gains have been made in reducing smoking prevalence in the United States, although still almost 1 in 4 Americans smoke. More than 430,000 deaths per year in the United States are attributed to tobacco use. At the current rate, an estimated 5 million persons younger than the age of 18 will die prematurely from a disease related to smoking. At the cost of 50 billion dollars per year for medical expenses, this problem is epidemic in proportion. The initiation of smoking by adolescents is now of great concern, but smoking also has become an important issue of women's health. Despite the publicizing of health risks, women continue to start smoking and to persist at high rates.

Although the reduction in overall smoking prevalence represents a major victory for public health, there are many groups within the population that have not experienced these gains. For example, low socioeconomic status (SES) and low educational attainment are now the primary predictors of smoking status in the United States and Canada. Although there have been some important strides made in the reduction of smoking among the U.S. population, there are important target groups that continue to smoke at disproportionately high rates. These groups have been less likely to experience the benefits of tobacco control efforts.

Recently, the use of forms of smokeless tobacco (plug, leaf, and snuff) has increased. "Dipping snuff," the placing of a coarse, moist powder between the cheek and gum, which results in the direct absorption of nicotine and other carcinogens through the oral tissue, has caused the greatest concern. Oral cancer occurs more frequently among snuff dippers as well as among pipe and cigar smokers compared with nonusers of tobacco.

The use of tobacco products is a complex, learned behavior that is woven into the fiber of daily life and is linked to how the smoker deals with the world. Numerous daily activities, thoughts, and emotions serve as powerful cues to smoke. Such conditioned ties become paired with positive neuroregulatory effects of nicotine to reinforce the addictive process. Personal characteristics such as education level, belief in one's ability to change, and coping skills are determinants of tobacco use. Similarly, environmental factors such as the level of acceptance of smoking in the home, peer group, workplace, and community norms influence smoking behavior.

The tobacco industry's drive for profits is the root cause of why cigarette smoking continues to thrive in the United States despite towering and irrefutable evidence that it is a health hazard and a form of drug addiction. Legislative initiatives to control cigarette smoking in the United States are appreciated but not as stringent as they should be. Millions of dollars are spent every day on tobacco advertising. The estimated 3000 children and youths who become regular smokers each year suffice to ensure an enduring supply of adult smokers. Bans on smoking in the workplace and in some restaurants have done little to discourage smokers from smoking.

Pathophysiology

When cigarettes are smoked, approximately 4000 chemicals and gases are inhaled into the lungs. Many carcinogens have been isolated from cigarette smoke; 3,4-benzpyrene is the most dangerous. At least 43 other components have been identified as carcinogens, cocarcinogens, tumor promoters, tumor initiators, and mutagens. The primary active (and addictive) ingredient in tobacco is nicotine. In its purest state, nicotine is an extremely toxic, clear, oily liquid with a characteristic odor. At low doses it acts as a stimulant; at high doses it depresses the central nervous system (CNS).

Nicotine enters the body through a variety of routes. Inhalation of smoke from a cigar, cigarette, or pipe is perhaps the most common route. During smoking, some absorption of nicotine occurs through the membranes of the mouth, throat, and bronchi as well as the alveoli of the lungs. In the case of snuff and chewing tobacco, nicotine reaches the bloodstream by absorption through the mucous linings of the mouth, nose, and throat.

Inhalation is the quickest and most effective delivery method. It is estimated that 90 percent of the nicotine that reaches the alveoli of the lungs in each breath is absorbed into the blood. Although an average cigarette contains from 15 to 20 mg of nicotine, only 1 to 2 mg from each cigarette smoked is actually delivered to the mouth. About 25 percent of the nicotine is immediately carried to the brain, where it easily crosses the blood–brain barrier and interferes with normal brain biochemistry. In humans, 60 mg of nicotine is a lethal dose.

Acute Effects of Nicotine Use

Outside the CNS, nicotine affects the transmission of nerve signals by mimicking acetylcholine. It occupies receptor sites at the synapses and prevents the transmission of nerve impulses from neuron to neuron and from neuron to muscle cells. Smoking exerts its deleterious effects primarily on the cardiovascular and pulmonary systems (Table 8.24). Nicotine, a direct adrenergic agonist, causes the release of epinephrine, which increases heart rate, systemic vascular resistance, and blood pressure. Smoking directly increases coronary vascular resistance, especially at sites of atherosclerotic plaques and stenosis. Inhaled cigarette smoke also exerts a negative inotropic effect on the myocardium, possibly due to the binding of carbon monoxide (CO) to cytochrome oxidase and myoglobin, resulting in increased myocardial oxygen consumption and decreased oxygen delivery. These changes are accompanied by the constriction of the blood vessels beneath the skin, a reduction in the motility in the bowel, and a loss of appetite.

CO, a component of tobacco smoke, is present in cigarette smoke in similar concentrations as in automobile exhaust. CO has a binding affinity for the hemoglobin molecule 250 times greater than that of oxygen, thereby reducing the smoker's oxygen-carrying capacity. In heavy smokers, as much as 15 percent of circulating hemoglobin may be bound to CO, reducing the oxygen-carrying capacity of the blood. In addition, CO shifts the oxyhemoglobin dissociation curve to the left, inhibiting the release of oxygen. The half-life of the COHb complex is 4 hours when the individual is breathing room air. The heart's need for oxygen is increased because of the sympathetic stimulatory effect of nicotine. Because the blood's oxygen-carrying capacity is reduced, the heart must pump more rapidly to adequately supply tissues with oxygen.

The effects of smoking on the respiratory system are diverse. The irritating effect of the smoke causes hyperplasia of cells, including goblet cells, which subsequently results in increased mucus production. Hyperplasia reduces airway diameter and increases the difficulty in clearing secretions. Smoking is known to disrupt mucociliary function and its ability to clear particles from the peripheral airways before any abnormality in pulmonary function is measured; smoking may cause actual loss of ciliated cells. Smoking also produces abnormal dilation of the distal air space, with destruction of alveolar walls. Many cells develop large, atypical nuclei, which is considered a precancerous condition. Smoking also alters pulmonary immune defense mechanisms by depressing neutrophil chemotaxis, decreasing immunoglobulin levels, reducing natural killer lymphocyte activity, decreasing macrophage adherence, and altering immunoregulatory T-lymphocyte activity.

In the CNS, nicotine activates receptors within the brain. Stimulation of the brain is seen by changes in EEG patterns, reflecting an increase in the frequency of electrical activity. This is part of a general arousal pattern signaled by the release of the neurotransmitters norepinephrine, dopamine, acetylcholine, and serotonin. Heavy tobacco use, resulting in high levels of nicotine in the bloodstream, eventually produces a blocking effect, as more and more receptor sites are filled. The result is a generalized depression of the CNS. When the blood levels of nicotine reach a critical point, the brain's vomiting center may be activated.

Chronic Effects of Nicotine Use

The chronic effects of nicotine include the development of tolerance and chemical dependence. These phenomena cause the user to consume greater quantities of nicotine for longer periods than the user had originally planned and thus endanger the user's health. Dependence on nicotine is

Table 8.24 **Effects of Tobacco Smoke**

Cardiovascular Effects	Respiratory Effects
Increased myocardial oxygen consumption	Decreased mucociliary clearance
Increased heart rate	Bronchospasm
Increased systemic vascular resistance	Cough
Decreased myocardial inotropic activity	Sputum accumulation
Decreased myocardial oxygen supply	Decreased circulating immunoglobulin levels
Carboxyhemoglobin (reduced available hemoglobin)	Decreased neutrophil chemotaxis
Coronary artery vasospasm	Decreased pulmonary macrophage count and adherence
Oxyhemoglobin dissociation curve shifted to the left	Altered T-lymphocyte immunoregulatory activity
	Decreased natural killer lymphocyte activity
	Decreased function of alpha$_1$-antitrypsin

quickly established in the majority of those who use it. Although psychological dependence may occur as well, the development of physical dependence, the establishment of tolerance, and the presence of withdrawal symptoms have all been demonstrated. Nicotine withdrawal symptoms include dysphoric or depressed mood, insomnia, irritability, frustration, anger, anxiety, poor concentration, restlessness, decreased heart rate, and increased appetite.

To understand better the neuropsychopharmacologic basis of why people smoke, researchers performed positron emission tomography (PET) scans on smokers and abstainers and found that smokers had 40 percent less of a brain enzyme known as monoamine oxidase B (MAO B). The mechanisms of MAO inhibition by cigarette smoke are not known. The enzyme breaks down dopamine, a neurotransmitter associated with feelings of pleasure. Given that nicotine stimulates dopamine release and that dopamine produces pleasurable effects, it is virtually significant in reinforcing and motivating smoking behavior. Therefore, smoking seems to create a self-perpetuating cycle: less MAO B leads to more dopamine, which leads to more pleasure, which leads to more smoking, which leads to less MAO B and so on. The researchers proposed that reduction of MAO B activity may synergize with nicotine to produce the diverse behavioral and epidemiological effects of smoking.

Clinical Presentation

Subjective

Demographic, anthropometric, physiologic, and laboratory features that distinguish cigarette smokers from nonsmokers reflect both baseline differences between these groups and the effects of smoking. Smokers drink more alcohol, coffee, and tea than do nonsmokers. Their weight and BP are slightly lower and their heart rate (HR) is slightly faster than those of nonsmokers. Women who smoke are at increased risk for early menopause, decreased bone density, and osteoporosis. Smoking has also been shown to decrease fertility in those attempting pregnancy and to impair uteroplacental function, which adversely effects the fetus during pregnancy. Further, sudden infant death syndrome is two to four times more common in infants whose mothers smoke during pregnancy. Smokers have impaired maximum exercise performance and impaired immune systems compared to nonsmokers. A markedly increased number of pulmonary alveolar macrophages is present in smokers, and the function and metabolism of these cells are abnormal. In smokers, the ratio of high-density lipoprotein (HDL) cholesterol to low-density lipoprotein (LDL) cholesterol is reduced.

A causal association is present between smoking and coronary heart disease, atherosclerotic peripheral vascular disease, cerebrovascular disease, lung and laryngeal cancer, oral cancer, esophageal cancer, COPD, intrauterine growth retardation, and low-birth-weight babies. In addition, smoking is considered by many to be the probable cause or a contributing cause for other conditions such as unsuccessful pregnancies, increased infant mortality, peptic ulcer disease, and cancers of the bladder, breast, pancreas, uterus, and kidney (Table 8.25). Smokers are at risk for increased fractures, premature wrinkling, gingival recession, dental caries, periodontal disease, cataracts, and glaucoma. Depression is twice as common among those who smoke than in people who have never smoked and has been linked to increased smoking initiation and to failures in smoking cessation efforts. A strong association also exists between smoking and other substance abuse disorders, especially alcohol. Clinical manifestations of these specific diseases, though beyond the scope of this chapter, are all clinical manifestations, directly or indirectly, of cigarette smoking.

Objective

The smoker usually demonstrates many observable signs of tobacco addiction. The smell of tobacco smoke lingers on the individual's clothing, and on his or her skin and hair. The breath and sputum often smell of stale tobacco and the fingers and nails are often stained from tobacco use. Use of smokeless tobacco may manifest in periodontal disease, a gum disease that may result in the loss of teeth, abrasive damage to the enamel of the teeth caused by the tobacco during processing, and oral cancer. The patient may also have lumps in the jaw or neck area; color change in lumps inside the lips; or white, smooth or scaly patches in the mouth or throat or on the lips or tongue. A patient who smokes may present with a red spot or sore on the lips or gums or inside the mouth that does not heal or difficulty or abnormality in speaking or swallowing.

Signs of cardiopulmonary disease often accompany tobacco addiction. A productive cough, dyspnea, wheezing, and fatigue should alert the clinician to respiratory problems related to smoking. Frequent bouts of pneumonia, influenza, and bronchitis as well as chronic diseases such as emphysema, ILD, or chronic airway obstruction often result from cigarette smoking. Cardiovascular signs of smoking including tachycardia, cardiac dysrhythmias, increased blood pressure, decreased peripheral blood flow, and angina must all be assessed to determine the risk for and extent of cardiovascular disease.

Nicotine dependence is related to the amount and duration of smoking and manifests as withdrawal symptoms. These signs and symptoms begin within a few hours of the last cigarette, peak 48 to 72 hours later, and return to baseline within 3 to 4 weeks of quitting. Criteria for nicotine dependence disorder are published in the *Diagnostic and Statistical Manual of Mental Disorders*. They include dysphoric or depressed mood, insomnia, irritability or anger, frustration, anxiety, concentration difficulties, decreased heart rate, and increased appetite or weight gain.

Diagnostic Reasoning

Asking the patient about smoking status and recording this information in the medical record takes only an additional 15 seconds and serves as a reminder to the practitioner to discuss the problem with each smoker. In spite of this, only

Table 8.25 **Diseases Associated with Cigarette Smoking**

Cardiovascular	• Atherosclerotic cardiovascular disease (CAD; carotid vascular disease; mesenteric, renal, iliac disease; abdominal aortic aneurysm) • Coronary artery spasm • Arrhythmias • Peripheral vascular diseases (thromboangiitis obliterans, deep vein thrombosis, pulmonary embolus)
Endocrine	• Altered hormone secretion • Graves' disease • Antidiuresis • Goiter
Gastrointestinal	• Peptic ulcer disease (gastric, duodenal) • Gastroesophageal reflux disease • Chronic pancreatitis • Crohn's disease • Colic adenomas
Genitourinary	• Glomerulonephritis • Benign prostatic hypertrophy
Immune/musculoskeletal	• RA • Osteoporosis
Infectious	• TB • Pneumococcal infection • Meningococcal infection
Integumentary	• Skin wrinkling • Psoriasis
Malignancies	• Respiratory tract malignancies • Lung cancer (squamous-cell, adenocarcinoma, large-cell, small-cell) • Laryngeal cancer • Oral cancer • Others (esophagus, pancreas, bladder, uterine, cervical, breast, kidney, anus, penis, stomach, liver, leukemia)
Pediatric	• Effects on children of parental smoking (asthma, rhinitis, otitis, pneumonia, increased risk for child to begin smoking)
Psychiatric	• Depression • Schizophrenia
Reproductive	• Ovarian failure • Decreased sperm quality • Pregnancy-related diseases (prematurity, premature rupture of membranes, spontaneous abortion) • Fetal/infant-related diseases (low-birth weight, impaired lung growth, sudden infant death syndrome, febrile seizures, reduced intelligence, behavioral disorders, atopic disease or asthma)
Respiratory	• COPD • Asthma • Eosinophilic granuloma of the lung • Respiratory bronchiolitis • Goodpasture's syndrome • Sleep apnea • Pneumothorax
Sensory and head and neck	• Loss of olfaction • Loss of taste • Cataracts • Periodontal disease

20 percent of smokers receive any medical quitting advice during visits to healthcare providers. All patients should be asked if they use tobacco and should have their tobacco-use status documented on a regular basis as a new vital sign. Several questionnaires measuring self-reported tobacco dependence have been used. The six-question Fagerstrom Test for Nicotine Dependence (FTND) predicts the level of nicotine dependence and may help predict smoking cessation success as well as influencing nicotine replacement dosages (Advanced Assessment 8.3).

Diagnostic Tests

Laboratory assays of smoking-related biochemical compounds such as thiocyanate, cotinine, nicotine, and COHb can be performed to verify smokers' reports of smoking sta-

ADVANCED ASSESSMENT 8.3

The Fagerstrom Test for Nicotine Dependence

Question	Score
1. How soon after you wake do you smoke your first cigarette? 3 = within 5 minutes 2 = 6–30 minutes 1 = within 30 minutes 0 = after 30 minutes	
2. Do you find it difficult to refrain from smoking in places where it is forbidden (e.g., church, library, cinemas, etc.)? 1 = yes 2 = no	
3. Which cigarette would you most hate to give up? 1 = the first one in the morning 0 = any other	
4. How many cigarettes a day do you smoke? 3 = 31 or more 2 = 21–30 1 = 11–20 0 = 10 or fewer	
5. Do you smoke more frequently during the early morning than the rest of the day? 1 = yes 0 = no	
6. Do you smoke if you are so ill that you are in bed most of the day 1 = yes 0 = no	
TOTAL SCORE	

SOURCE: Heatherton, TF, Kozlowski, LT, Frecker, RC, Gaferstorm, KO: The Fagerstrom test for nicotine dependence: A revision of the Fagerstrom Tolerance Questionnaire. Br J Addiction 86:1119-1127, 1991.
NOTE: the higher the score, the more severe the addiction. A total of 7 or greater may indicate more severe withdrawal symptoms, greater difficulty quitting, and possibly the need for higher-dose nicotine supplements.

tus or abstinence. There are four potential sources of objective information to determine whether or not a person has smoked: urine, blood, breath, and saliva.

A urine sample can be assayed for the constituents of the cigarette smoke itself or for excretion products that are associated with the physiologic effects of smoking. Nicotine excretion in smokers correlates well with the number of cigarettes smoked and inversely with pH of the urine. Urine metabolites of epinephrine can also be measured; however, a potential for false-positives related to severe anxiety exists.

Carbon monoxide (CO) is found in the blood of those who smoke and combines to form carboxyhemoglobin (COHb). A value of 2 percent is used as a suggestion that smoking has occurred. However, one must take environmental and occupational sources of CO into account. Although COHb increases proportionately with number of cigarettes and varies with nicotine content, discretion is necessary in interpreting the data.

The determination of mean alveolar CO partial pressure makes it possible to determine the COHb levels of the blood with a high degree of correlation. Also, by subtracting expired CO from inspired CO, it is possible to determine if a smoker is an inhaler. Smokers have higher levels of both expired CO and thiocyanate. To measure CO, the patient is instructed to inhale deeply and to hold his or her breath for 10 to 15 seconds before expiring with full force through the inflow valve of the monitor (EC_{50} monitor, Bedfont, Technical Instruments, Sittingbourne, UK). Levels of 9 parts per million (ppm) or lower are considered to indicate a nonsmoking status.

Cotinine is a major metabolite of nicotine and is a useful marker. A sample of at least 3 mL of unstimulated saliva is collected in a plastic cup. The presence of nicotine in saliva can be determined by gas chromatography and an alkali flame ionization detector but it is difficult to distinguish a pattern of smoking. Moreover, nonsmokers who have ingested cigarette smoke passively may also have nicotine in their saliva.

Differential Diagnosis

The best way to rule out differential diagnoses is to ensure that for every patient at every clinic visit, tobacco-use status is queried and documented. The cause of a smoker's cough and dyspnea must be explored to rule out other explanatory causes such as lung cancer, ILD, allergies, and infections. Unfortunately, many patients with symptoms of cough, dyspnea, sputum production, and changes in pulmonary function testing not only are smokers but also suffer from some form of lung disease or disorder. Smokers tend to have unique laboratory findings such as increases in Hct, total WBC count and platelet count. They may also have decreases in leukocytes, vitamin C levels, serum uric acid, and albumin.

Management

The changing face of health-care delivery in the United States indicates the need to incorporate smoking cessation as a regular part of clinical care, particularly in the current managed care environment. The Agency for Health Care Policy and Research (AHCPR) has an extensive review and synthesis of the outcome of smoking cessation strategies, as well as recommendations for the delivery of smoking interventions in clinical practice. The Practice Guideline's key findings emphasize the importance of offering cessation treatment to every smoker at every office visit. Patients who are counseled to quit are 1.6 times as likely to attempt quitting. The Guideline proposed a series of recommendations for primary care clinicians, smoking cessation specialists, and health-care administrators and purchasers of health insurance, as well as specific strategies for carrying out each of the recommendations (Table 8.26). Clinicians aiding patients in smoking cessation should remember the four As: Ask, Advise, Assist, and Arrange. The following discussion is based on these guidelines.

The goal of every practitioner ought to be to change clinical culture and practice patterns to ensure that every patient who smokes is offered treatment. It is essential to provide a brief but effective smoking cessation intervention for all tobacco users at each clinical visit.

Initial Management

Smoking Cessation Programs. Once the patient has been identified as a smoker, it is important to advise the patient of

Table 8.26 Strategies to Help Your Patient to Quit Smoking

Goal	Intervention	Strategy
Ask: Systematically identify all tobacco users at every visit.	Implement an office-wide system that ensures that, for *every* patient at *every* visit, tobacco-use status is queried and documented.	Expand the vital signs to include tobacco use • Data collected by health-care team • Implemented using preprinted progress note paper that includes the expanded vital signs, a vital signs stamp, or, for computerized records, includes an item assessing tobacco-use status
Advise: Strongly urge all smokers to quit.	In a clear, strong, and personalized manner, urge every smoker to quit.	Advice should be • Clear: "I think it is important for you to quit smoking now and I will help you." "Cutting down while you are ill is not enough." • Strong: "As your health-care provider, I need you to know that quitting smoking is the most important thing you can do to protect your current and future health." • Personalized: Tie smoking to current health/illness, and/or the social and economic costs of tobacco use, motivation level/readiness to quit, and/or the impact of smoking on children and others in the household.
Ask: Identify smokers willing to make an attempt to quit.	Ask every smoker if he or she is willing to make an attempt to quit at this time.	Encourage staff to reinforce the cessation message and support the patient's quit attempt. • If the patient is willing to make a quit attempt at this time, provide assistance. • If the patient prefers a more intensive treatment or the clinician believes intensive treatment is appropriate, refer to interventions administered by a smoking cessation specialist and follow up with the patient regarding quitting. • If the patient clearly states he or she is not willing to make a quit attempt at this time, provide a motivational intervention.

Goal	Intervention	Strategy
Assist: Aid the patient in quitting.	Help the patient with a quit plan.	Set a quit date. Ideally, the quit date should be within 2 weeks, taking patient preference into account. In preparation for quitting, the patient should • Inform family, friends, and coworkers of quitting and request understanding and support. • Remove cigarettes from his or her environment. Before the patient quits, recommend that he or she avoid smoking in places where he or she spends a lot of time. • Review previous quit attempts. Ask: What helped you? What led to relapse? • Anticipate challenges to planned quit attempt, particularly during the critical first few weeks. • These include nicotine withdrawal symptoms.
	Encourage nicotine replacement therapy except in special circumstances.	Encourage the use of nicotene patch, gum, lozenges, inhaler or nasal spray. Consider the initiation of x bupropion medication therapy for smoking cessation.
	Give key advice on successful quitting.	• Abstinence: Total abstinence is essential. "Not even a single puff after the quit date." • Alcohol: Drinking alcohol is highly associated with relapse. Those who stop smoking should review their alcohol use and consider limiting or abstaining from alcohol during the quit process. • Other smokers in household: The presence of other smokers in the household, particularly a spouse, is associated with lower success rates. Patients should consider quitting with their significant others or developing specific plans to stay quit in a household where others still smoke.
	Provide supplementary material.	• Sources: Federal agencies, including AHCRP; nonprofit agencies (American Cancer Society, American Lung Association, American Hospice Association); private local and state health departments. • Type: Culturally, racially, educationally, and age-appropriate for the patient. • Location: Readily available in every office.
Arrange: Schedule follow-up contact.	Schedule follow-up contact, either in person or via telephone.	• Timing: Follow-up contact should occur soon after the quit date, preferably during the first week. A second follow-up contact is recommended within the first month. Schedule further follow-up contact as indicated. • Actions during follow-up visit: Congratulate success. If the patient is still smoking, review circumstances and elicit a recommitment to total abstinence. Remind the patient that a lapse can be used as a learning experience. Identify problems already encountered and anticipate challenges in the immediate future. Assess nicotine replacement therapy use and problems. Consider referral to a more intense or specialized program.

Source: Adapted from Fiore, MC, Baily, WC, Cohen, SJ, et al: Smoking Cessation. Clinical Practice Guideline No. 18. US Department of Health and Human Services, Public Health Service, Agency for Health Care Policy and Research. USDHHS, Rockville, MD, 1996, AHCPR publication 96–0692.

the need to quit. This should be done after the patient's chief complaint has been addressed. The patient's response will determine the proper strategy to pursue. The patient must be informed of how unhealthy smoking is. Pregnant smokers should be strongly encouraged to quit throughout pregnancy. Because of the serious risk of smoking to the pregnant smoker and fetus, pregnant smokers should be offered intensive counseling treatment. Patients should choose a quit date, usually within a month. This will provide a chance to develop effective alternative behaviors to smoking. Periods of extreme stress or depression are not optimal times to attempt smoking cessation.

Before initiating a smoking cessation program, the clinician must know in which state of smoking cessation the client is in at that time. This is the first step of the provider-initiated smoking cessation program. Most smokers transition through five stages of behavioral change in their attempts at cessation—precontemplation, contemplation, preparation, action, and maintenance. By understanding the smoker's stage of behavior and readiness to change, the clinician can better assist him or her to achieve a successful cessation.

Smokers in the *precontemplation stage* have no desire to quit in the next 6 to 12 months. These individuals usually benefit from motivational interventions that increase awareness of the adverse affects of smoking. Smokers who are giving serious thought to and are interested in quitting but are not yet ready to do so are in the *contemplation stage.* These smokers also will benefit from motivational counseling emphasizing the negative effects of smoking. Smokers who are serious about quitting and have taken the initial steps toward cessation are in the *preparation phase.* Individuals in this stage benefit from interventions that assist them in quitting. These interventions include providing information about nicotine replacement and developing behavior modification skills.

During the *action stage,* the smoker quits smoking. The action stage lasts from several weeks to 6 months after cessation, which is a common time of relapse. Because of the likelihood of relapse during this stage, interventions should address relapse prevention, including congratulating successes and rewarding positive behavioral changes with more frequent contacts by the clinician. When a smoker has abstained from cigarettes for 6 months, the *maintenance stage* begins. Most successful quitters relapse and recycle through these stages three or four times before attaining long-term abstinence; some may take several years to move through these stages until abstinence can be maintained.

Effective smoking cessation requires behavior modification. The behavior of smoking is usually linked to a variety of triggers (e.g., stress, foods or beverages, driving). When a patient is able to recognize the triggers, healthy alternative behaviors can be substituted. It is crucial to develop alternative coping strategies to overcome the urge to smoke. Such strategies include deep breathing and relaxation exercises, chewing gum, exercise, drinking water, sucking on a piece of sugarless candy, and eating carrot or celery sticks.

Patients with any chronic health problem need support from their clinician, their families and other persons. The clinician can help the patient handle particularly difficult triggers and can treat any underlying behavior problems, such as anxiety or depression. The family can provide invaluable positive reinforcement to the patient during this time. If there are other smokers in the patient's household, the clinician should encourage them to quit smoking at the same time as the patient. It is very difficult for a person to refrain from smoking in the long term when a spouse or a family member continues to smoke. Many patients benefit from the support of groups such as Nicotine Anonymous, the American Lung Association's Freedom from Smoking program, and the American Cancer Society's Freshstart program.

Hypnosis. The goal of hypnosis in smoking cessation is to enable the smoker to achieve an altered state of consciousness that enhances the ability to quit. However, the hypnotic trance is generally not measurably different from deep muscle relaxation. The effects of hypnosis are often short-lived. Controlled trials of hypnosis have generally not documented long-term efficacy for smoking cessation. Hypnosis is of low reliability, with published quit rates ranging between 0 and 88 percent. Although it is of uncertain value, hypnosis remains a commercially popular stop-smoking method. The primary advantage of hypnosis is that it may be an attractive alternative for people who have failed to quit with other methods.

Aversion Conditioning. Aversion conditioning is based on the premise that smoking is a learned response that can be extinguished by creation of an association between smoking and a negative sensation. Among the aversion techniques utilized for smoking cessation are electric shock; nausea-inducing drugs; hot, smoky air treatments; and rapid smoking. High quit rates were reported in some of the early smoking cessation trials using aversion conditioning; however, these high rates may be attributed, in part, to factors related to patient selection, because arguably only the most highly motivated persons are willing to undergo therapies such as electric shock or the breathing of hot, smoky air. Additionally, aversion conditioning techniques may represent a health hazard.

Subsequent Management

Pharmacologic Approaches. Although some smokers may need antidepressants or anxiolytics, it is difficult to predict who will benefit from these adjunctive therapies. Bupropion (Zyban) is an antidepressant and smoking deterrent. Bupropion is a weak inhibitor of the neuronal uptake of norepinephrine and dopamine but has no effect on serotonin. Its dopaminergic and noradrenergic activities are responsible for its efficacy in smoking cessation, with the dopaminergic activity affecting areas of the brain having to do with the reinforcement activity affecting nicotine withdrawal. Bupropion appears to have no effect on patient depression scores, so it is unlikely that the mechanism for the efficacy of bupropion is through its antidepressant effects. Bupropion is well tolerated, with the most frequent adverse effects being headache, insomnia, and dry mouth. Antidepressants are associated with a small risk of seizure. Moreover, patients with a history of severe head trauma, eating disorders, recent MI, unstable heart disease, or active alcoholism should not take bupropion.

The dosage of 300 mg per day (150 mg per day for 3 days followed by 150 mg bid) is begun 1 to 2 weeks before smoking cessation. It is important for the steady-state plasma levels of bupropion to be reached (usually within 8 days) before smoking cessation is begun. This dosing schedule has been found to lead to less weight gain during the medication phase. The duration of treatment is usually 7 to

12 weeks. For maintenance therapy, bupropion SR 150 mg bid for up to 6 months should be considered. As with the nicotine replacement products, behavioral modification therapy should coexist. For heavily addicted smokers, nicotine replacement therapy and bupropion can be coadministered concurrently.

Health-care providers need to be aware of the nuances of smoking cessation. For example, individuals often experience constipation during cessation, as the gastrointestinal (GI) system adjusts to withdrawal from the stimulating effects of nicotine. The use of a bulk-forming agent such as Metamucil, increased dietary fiber, and increased fluids will alleviate the problem. A form of exercise, such as walking, is an excellent, affordable stress reliever. A walking program also assists with reducing the expected mean weight gain of 5 to 7 pounds that occurs with smoking cessation. Nicotine is an appetite depressant, and once its effects have cleared from the body, food tastes better.

Nicotine Replacement Therapies (NRT). Nicotine is the drug of choice to assist smoking cessation. The nicotine patch, gum, and lozenges are available over-the-counter, and nicotine nasal spray and inhalers are available by prescription (Drugs Commonly Prescribed 8.3).

Increased access through OTC availability has substantially increased the number of quitters in the United States. Evaluations of the efficacy of nicotine gum through

Drugs Commonly Prescribed 8.3: Nicotine Replacement Therapies

Drug	Dosage	Advantages	Disadvantages
Transdermal patch		*Continuous delivery*	*Expensive*
Habitrol (worn 24 h/day)	21 mg/day for 4–6 weeks, then 14 mg/day for 2–4 weeks, then 7 mg/day for 2–4 weeks	Fewer compliance problems than gum	Risk of skin irritation
Nicoderm CQ (worn 24 h/day)	21 mg/day for 4–6 weeks, then 14 mg/day for 2–4 weeks, then 7 mg/day for 2–4 weeks, then 7 mg/day for 2–4 weeks	Less instruction required than gum	Risk of insomnia or nightmares
Nicotrol (worn 16 h/day)	15 mg/day for 4–12 weeks, then 10 mg/day for 2 weeks, then 5 mg/day for 2 weeks	Once daily dosing	Nausea, vertigo
Gum (nicotine polacrilex)		*Useful on "as needed" basis*	*Requires good dentition*
Nicorette	2 mg/piece; max 30 pieces/day 4 mg/piece; max 24 pieces/day	Provides oral gratification Patient control Delayed weight gain	Risk of mouth irritation Dyspnea, nausea Risk of developing dependence
Nasal spray		*Useful on "as needed" basis*	
Nicotrol (10-mL bottle)	0.5 mg/spray; 2 sprays; daily range 8–40 mg/day for 3 months	Rapid delivery	Risk of nasal and throat irritation Runny nose Watery eyes
Inhaler			
Nicotrol inhaler	13 µg/puff; 6–16 cartridges/day for 3 months	Mimics smoking behavior	Risk of cough, irritation of mouth and throat
Lozenge			
Commit	2 mg 4 mg; max 20 lozenges/day		May cause hiccoughs, heartburn
Other			
Bupropion hydrochloride (Zyban)	150 mg/day for 3 days, then 150 mg bid for 7–12 weeks	Non-nicotine, less weight gain	Risk of seizures, headache, dry mouth, insomnia

12-month follow-up suggest that the gum improves smoking cessation rates by approximately 40 to 60 percent as compared with control interventions. Efficacy is increased when nicotine gum use is combined with an intensive psychosocial intervention. The efficacy of the nicotine patch overall appears to be somewhat stronger than that for the gum. The patch has been found to double the 6- to 12-month abstinence rates over those yielded by placebo interventions.

The cost of the patch remains relatively high, however, which places this cessation strategy out of the reach of some smokers. Although the manufacturer of nicotine gum has developed a series of strategies for increasing access to NRT among underserved populations, it is not clear if the penetration of such programs can match the need for an effective strategy among lower-income and other underserved groups.

The gum must be correctly chewed to a softened state and then placed in the buccal mucosa. Clients should not eat for 15 minutes before or during use of the nicotine gum. A piece of gum should be chewed intermittently over a 30-minute period. Initially, one piece is chewed every 1 to 2 hours over 6 weeks with a maximum of 24 pieces in 24 hours. Time intervals for gum use are gradually increased to 2 to 4 hours for 3 weeks, then every 4 to 8 hours for 3 weeks. Fewer than 10 percent of patients will become dependent on the gum, although many will require long-term use (1 to 2 years) to maintain abstinence. Nicotine absorption is decreased by acidic foods and beverages, which should be avoided during use. Irritation and trauma to the oral mucosa, teeth, and dental work can occur. Many patients experience jaw ache, GI discomfort, hiccups, and cardiostimulation.

The doses delivered by the 16- and 24-hour nicotine patches range from 5 to 22 mg of nicotine. Nicotine patches are applied every morning and worn for 16 to 24 hours per day. Patches are usually indicated for 6 to 8 weeks to promote long-term abstinence. Patients should be instructed to change the application site daily to minimize skin irritation. The highest-dose patch should be considered if the patient smokes more than 20 cigarettes per day and has no active cardiovascular disease. Because a dose-response effect has been found, researchers recommend that a higher nicotine dose is more effective for smoking cessation. The adverse effects of the patches include skin reactions, insomnia, vivid dreams, and myalgias. If vivid dreams or insomnia occur, the patient should be instructed to remove the patch before going to bed and then to apply a new patch upon arising.

The nicotine nasal spray (Nicotrol nasal spray) delivers nicotine in a more rapid manner and thereby serves as a better substitute than nicotine gum or a nicotine patch. The device is similar to nasal antihistamine sprays. The nasal spray delivers 0.5 mg of nicotine per spray. Smokers are instructed to use 1 to 2 doses per hour for 3 months. The nasal spray delivers nicotine more rapidly than gum, patch, or inhaler but less rapidly than cigarettes. Peak levels occur within 4 to 15 minutes and are about two-thirds of those associated with cigarettes. Patients initially experience nasal and throat irritation, rhinitis, sneezing, coughing, and watering eyes. Tolerance to these effects develops in the first week. The spray may cause serious dysrhythmias, elevated blood pressure, and angina in post–myocardial infarction patients. Use of the spray is not recommended in patients with several other chronic diseases, including asthma, peptic ulcer disease, chronic nasal disorders, severe renal impairment, liver disease, diabetes, and hyperthyroidism.

Researchers have found that the use of a nicotine patch with a nicotine nasal spray is significantly more effective for long-term smoking cessation than with either alone. The results suggest an increased efficacy in prevention of relapse with more intake of nicotine or by combining different types of NRT. The combination of a nicotine patch and nicotine nasal spray may be successful not only because of the high level of substitution but also because of the opportunity to respond quickly to the smoker's need. Researchers have suggested that using a patch for 5 months with a nicotine nasal spray for 1 year provides a more effective means of stopping smoking than using a patch alone.

The nicotine inhaler (Nicotrol inhaler) is a plastic rod with a nicotine plug that provides a nicotine vapor when puffed on. Each active cartridge contains approximately 10 mg of nicotine and 1 mg of 1-menthol. The menthol is added to decrease the throat irritation caused by the nicotine. Although the device is designed as an inhaler, this label is a misnomer because the device does not deliver a significant amount of nicotine to the lungs; rather, the device delivers nicotine bucally. This occurs whether smokers use deep or shallow puffs. One puff from the inhaler provides about 13 mg of nicotine at room temperature. Because each active cartridge contains about 10 mg of nicotine, 80 puffs from the nicotine inhaler would approximate the amount of nicotine delivered by one cigarette. This level of nicotine delivery can only be achieved by puffing intensively (2 to 4 puffs per min) over 20 to 30 minutes. Consequently, users of the nicotine inhaler must work harder to get nicotine compared to individuals who smoke cigarettes. Patients use 6 to 16 cartridges per day for 3 months, then taper for 6 to 12 weeks as needed. The most common adverse effects are cough and irritation in the mouth and throat. The inhaler has the potential to assist in the smoking cessation process not only by providing nicotine replacement but also by mimicking the behavioral aspects of smoking. Such a device clearly blurs the line between cigarette and nicotine-delivery device, however. In effect, the patient is brand switching (i.e., switching from their usual brand of cigarette to a smoke-free nicotine-delivery device) even though the effort required to obtain nicotine from the inhaler is greater than that required from a cigarette. Combining the nicotine inhaler with nicotine patch may increase the efficacy over using the patch alone, because the inhaler would serve to supplement the nicotine provided by the patch and not be the sole provider of nicotine.

A summary of smoking cessation strategies is presented in Treatment Flowchart 8.4.

TREATMENT FLOWCHART 8.4

SMOKING CESSATION STRATEGIES

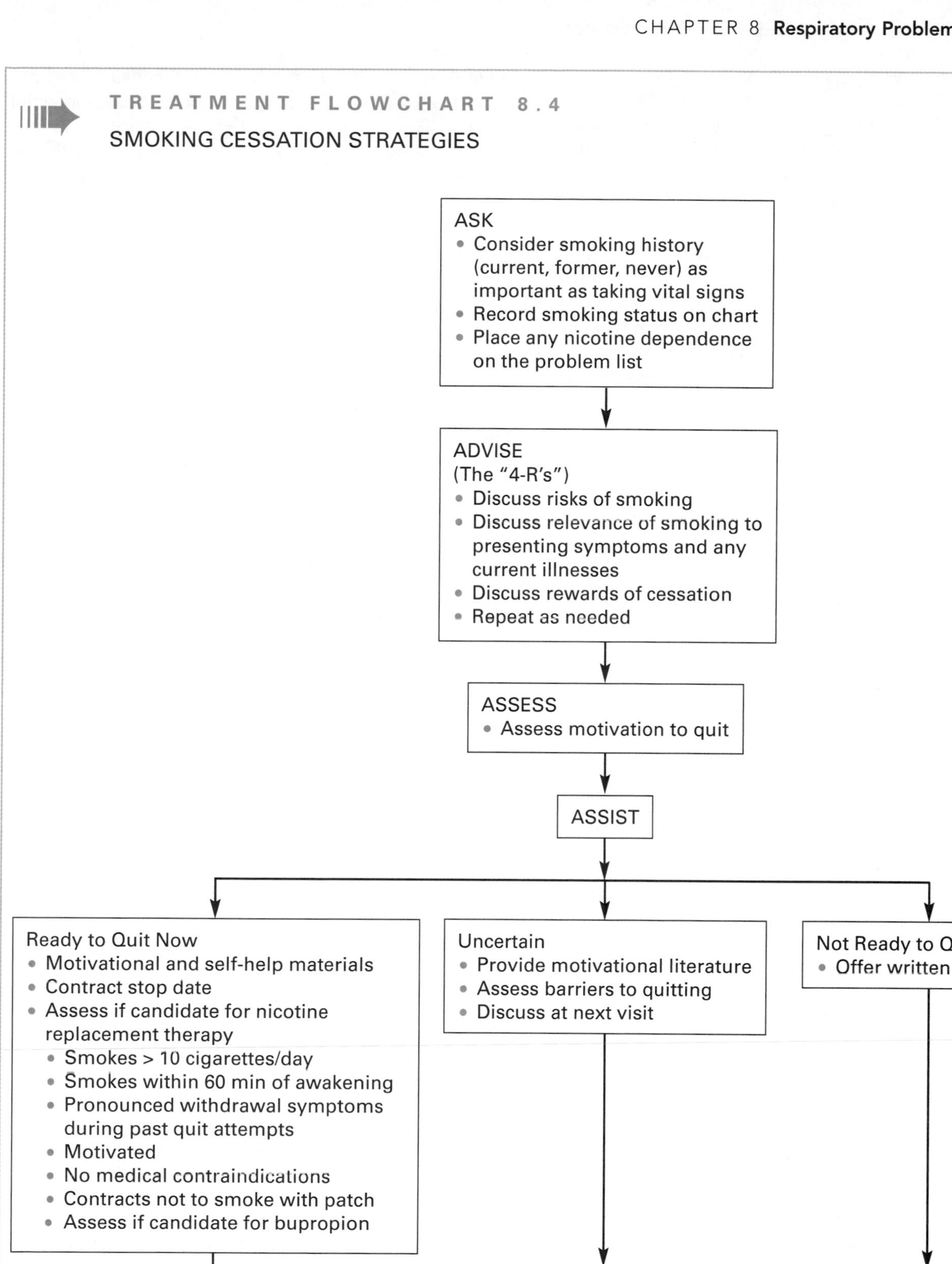

Follow-Up and Referral

As with any serious medical problem, follow-up is essential after the initial intervention. A supportive phone call the week after the quit date can be made by a health-care worker with the reinforcement of the self-help materials that have been provided. Office follow-up by the clinician at 1 and 3 months after the quit date can help the patient who has quit smoking to cope with persistently difficult triggers or situations; this support can help the patient who may have relapsed get back on the right track. In the case of relapse, the client should be assisted to set another quit date, revisit the reasons for quitting, and begin the process again. Assure patients that stable abstinence is commonly achieved only after five or six attempts.

Patient Education

For years, cigarette smoking was viewed as largely a social or psychological habit. As such, the ability to quit was considered a measure of personal motivation and willpower. Motivation to stop smoking, combined with sufficient psychological resources, was seen as a driving force behind successful cigarette abstinence. Thus, if smokers could be educated about the health risks of cigarette smoking, they could theoretically become sufficiently motivated and psychologically empowered to quit. Unfortunately, the anticipated benefits of achieving smoking cessation through education were overoptimistic and simplistic. More than 80 percent of current smokers indicate they would like to quit but cannot. Educational programs to aid smoking cessation have produced disappointing results and high long-term failure rates. Only about 4 percent of smokers are able to quit each year. Nonetheless, it is helpful to give the patient some age-specific smoking cessation literature.

It is important to understand the meaning of smoking to the individual patient, to hear the "patient's voice." Assisting the patient in ceasing smoking involves an empowerment process that enhances the patient's motivation and self-esteem. The provider can facilitate this process by providing available cessation information to both the patient and the family. There must be a family-focused emphasis, with shared commitment and participation. Providers can encourage patients to identify daily stressors and assist them to reframe situations and develop alternative coping strategies. Equally important is developing an enhanced self-efficacy, which includes accepting and believing in the ability to succeed. Providers need to ask how the patient usually deals with stress and give simple, usable

THE PATIENT'S VOICE 8.1

Battleground

"What is it with you and your cigarettes, anyway?" I angrily thought to myself after yet another heated debate with my father about smoking. As usual, he had been defending cigarettes as a source of pleasure, saying he always enjoyed smoking. He was against federal attempts to regulate levels of nicotine or restrict access. After smoking for 60 years, he quit last year, when the severity of his lung disease nearly took his life. Why couldn't I make him understand that cigarettes were killing people?

He must have sensed my frustration or read my mind, because as his O_2 concentrator clicked off and on, the looked at me and said softly, "You know, Snicklefritz, it was cigarettes that saved my life many times during the war." My father rarely talks about THE WAR. He was a combat infantryman, a machine gunner, part of the Fifth Division known as 'Roosevelt's Red Devils." He started slowly...

"At night we were the point. Machine gunners never got relieved. The cold was the worst. You couldn't imagine the cold. Raining—below freezing. We would take turns sleeping. You couldn't sleep for more than an hour. You had to rely on your buddies to wake you up. You had to keep moving to keep from freezing. Many only lasted one night and had to be sent back because their feet were frozen. I think we lost more men to cold that winter than from enemy fire.

"I remember standing up one night with tracers going by my head, yelling 'Go ahead and shoot me—put me out of my misery!' My buddy had to pull me down. He said. 'Have a cigarette—calm yourself!' We had to cover our heads with raingear to keep anyone from seeing to light up and give away our positions. You can't imagine the warmth and comfort in one cigarette. We were worried about living through the night.

"There were times warmth of a cigarette was the only thing that kept us alive. We were short of supplies that winter, but they always kept us in cigarettes. Even our K-rations came with a pack—I'll give them that."

As he talked, I tired to imagine, to understand, the inhuman conditions he was describing and the meaning cigarettes held for him. As I listened to my father's story and watched him pull his arms to his chest and cup his hands to his face, as if he were holding something as precious as life itself, I finally heard what he had been saying for years. I began to feel my anger slipping away—anger with my father for smoking all those years and for nearly dying before my 3-year-old son had a chance to come to know him.

I felt my eyes fill with tears, not for the suffering my father had experienced during the war, but for the suffering he experienced because his daughter, the nurse, never understood.

—Shirley Countryman Gordon from "Nightingale Songs" Publication of Florida Atlantic University College of Nursing

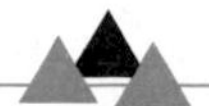

NURSING RESEARCH-BASED PRACTICE 8.2

Bialous, SA, Sarna, L, Wewers, ME, Froelicher, ES, and Danao, L: Nurses' Perspectives of Smoking Initiation, Addiction, & Cessation. Nurs Res 53(6):387–395, 2004.

While one of the goals of *Healthy People 2010* is to reduce the overall smoking prevalence of all Americans to 12%, it is estimated that 18% of registered nurses smoke. RNs are the largest group of health professionals and recognize the need for smoking cessation. This qualitative study utilized eight focus groups in four states and through content analysis identified four major theses:

- Initiation of smoking and addiction
- Myths and misconceptions about quitting
- Overcoming addictions
- Strategies for enhancing successful cessation

Nurses felt guilty about their smoking and cited non-supportive colleagues as contributing to their shame affecting their public image of nurses. To be sucessful, nurses wished for several strategies in addition to smoking cessartion interventions currently available. They wanted confidentiality from the general public about their smoking, and support/counseling regarding their feelings of guilt and shame.

The end result was the development of the Tobacco Free Nurses Initiative, a national program to support nurses' smoking cessation efforts. (http://www.tobacco-freenurses.org).

alternative coping strategies. A telephone hotline with recorded messages that empower and encourage can be an effective way to manage and overcome the desire to smoke. Information about the rewards of smoking cessation, such as improved health with lower blood pressure and improved circulation and lung functioning, should be provided. Individuals who cease smoking report more energy, enhanced taste and smell, money saved, freedom from addiction, feeling better about oneself, and better performance in sexual and sports activities. Smokers over age 55 should be informed that despite many years of smoking, smoking cessation will improve their health. They will enjoy a better quality of life as an ex-smoker and their risk for lung and other smoking-associated cancers will be reduced. Smokers die 5 to 8 years earlier than persons who have never smoked. Additional rewards for older adults can be the satisfaction of being a positive role model for other family members and making a contribution to the improved health of their grandchildren. To enhance recovery from nicotine addiction and prevent relapse, both individual and group cessation counseling and education must include a family focus.

Bibiography

General

American Psychiatric Association: Diagnostic and Statistical Manual of Mental Disorders, ed 4 (DSM-IV-TR). Author, Washington, D.C., 2000.

Cavanaugh, BM: Nurse's Manual of Laboratory and Diagnostic Tests. FA Davis, Philadelphia, 2003.

Cotran, RS, Kumar, V, and Collins, T: Robbins Pathologic Basis of Disease, ed 6. WB Saunders, Philadelphia, 1999.

Guyton, AC, and Hall, JC: Textbook of Medical Physiology, ed 10. WB Sunders, Philadelphia, 2000.

Kasper, DL, Fauci, AS, Longo, DL, Braunwald, E, Hauser, SL, and Jameson, JL (eds): Harrison's Principles of Internal Medicine. McGraw- Hill, New York, 2005.

Papadakis, MA, and McPhee, SJ: Current Consult Medicine. Appleton-Lange/McGrawHill, New York, 2005.

Prendergast, TJ, and Ruoss, SJ: Pulmonary Disease . In McPhee, SJ, Lingappa, VR, Ganong, WF, and Lange, JD: Pathophysiology of Disease: An Introduction to Clinical Medicine. Appleton-Lange/McGraw-Hill, New York, 2000.

Tierney, LM, McPhee, SJ, and Papadakis, MA: Current Medical Diagnosis and Treatment, ed 44. Appleton & Lange, Stamford, Conn., 2005.

Youngkin, EQ, Sain, KJ, Kissinger, JF, and Israel, DS (eds): Pharmacotherapeutics: A Primary Care Guide, ed 2.Pearson/Prentice Hall, Upper Saddle River, NJ, 2005.

Asthma

Asch-Goodkin, J: Eliminating disparities in asthma management. Patient Care Nurse Practit 5:68–83, 2000.

Busse, WW, and Lemanske, RF: Advances in immunology: Asthma. N Engl J Med 344(5):350–362, 2001.

Institute for Clinical Systems Improvement (ICSI): Diagnosis and management of asthma. Bloomington (MN); Institute for Clinical Systems Improvement, National Guideline Clearinghouse. http://www.guideline.gov, March 2005 (Accessed July 14, 2006).

McFadden, ER: Asthma. In Kasper, DL, Fauci, AS, Longo, DL, Braunwald, E, Hauser, SL, and Jameson, JL (eds). Harrison's Principles of Internal Medicine. McGraw-Hill, New York, 2005.

Murphy, KR, Cecil, B, and Sarver, NL: Helping patients breathe easier. Nurse Pract 49(10):39–55, 2004.

National Asthma Education and Prevention Program (NAEPP). (2003). Expert panel report: Guidelines for the diagnosis and management of asthma update on selected topics—2002. U.S. Department of Health and Human Services, Public Health Service, National Institutes of Health (NIH) / National Heart, Lung, and Blood Institute (NHBLI). Bethesda, MD: NIH publication no. 02-5074.

http://www.nhlbi.nih.gov/guidelines/asthma

http://www.healthypeople.gov/Document/HTML/Volume 2/24Respiratory.htm

Chronic Bronchitis and Emphysema (COPD)

Buch, K, Bensadoun, E, and Doherty, DE: Anticholinergics for maintenance therapy in patients with COPD.J COPD Manage 5(1):9–14, 2004.

Cambach, W, et al: The long-term effects of pulmonary rehabilitation in patients with asthma and chronic obstructive pulmonary disease: a research synthesis. Arch Phys Med Rehabil 80:103–111, 1999.

Campbell, SC: Pharmacolocy of inhaled bronchodilators in COPD. J COPD Manag 3(2):10–15, 2002.

Cooper, CB, and Zagaria, MAE: New advances in COPD management—long-acting anticholinergic agent for maintenance therapy. Clin Rev Ther Spotlight Self-Study Suppl, Jan, 2005.

Doherty, DE: COPD: A contemporary overview. In a supplement to The Clinical Advisor, Jan. 2005—Breathing Easier: New concepts in COPD Management, 3–9, 2005.

Global Initiative for Chronic Obstructive Lung Disease (GOLD). (2004). Global strategy for the diagnosis, management, and prevention of chronic obstructive pulmonary disease, 2004. National Heart, Lung, and Blood Institute, World Health Organization. Bethesda, Md.

Lareau, SC, et al: Dyspnea in patients with chronic obstructive pulmonary disease: Does dyspnea worsen longitudinally in the presence of declining lung function? Heart Lung 28:65–73, 1999.

National Heart, Lung, and Blood Institute and National Institutes of Health: For selected NHLBI Clinical Trials go to http://apps.nhlbi.nih.gov/clinicaltrials/Advsearch.ASP (Accessed July 14, 2006).

O'Brien, GM, et al: Improvements in lung function, exercise, and quality of life in hypercapnic COPD patients after lung volume reduction surgery. Chest 11:75–84, 1999.

Prendergast, TJ, and Ruoss, SJ: Pulmonary disease . In McPhee, SJ, Lingappa, VR, Ganong, WF, and Lange, JD: Pathophysiology of Disease: An Introduction to Clinical Medicine. Appleton-Lange Medical Books/McGraw-Hill, New York, 2000.

Reilly, JJ; Silverman, EK, and Shapiro, SD: Chronic obstructive pulmonary disease. In Kasper, DL, Fauci, AS, Longo, DL, Braunwald, E, Hauser, SL, and Jameson, JL (eds): Harrison's Principles of Internal Medicine. McGraw-Hill, New York, 2005.

Skrepneck, GH, and Skrepneck, SV: Epidemiology, clinical and economic burden, and natural history of chronic obstructive pulmonary disease and asthma. Am J Managed Care 10(5 Suppl):S129–137, 2004.

Lung Cancer

Litzky, L: The pathology of non–small cell lung carcinoma. In Alfred Fishman (ed): Fishman's Pulmonary Diseases and Disorders. McGraw-Hill, New York, 1998, pp 1739–1758.

Roth, J: Gene replacement strategies for lung cancer. Curr Opin Oncol 10:127–132, 1998.

Sone, S, et al: Mass screening for lung cancer with mobile spiral computered tomography scanner. Lancet 351:1242–1245, 1998.

Sorensen, M, et al: Current therapy for small cell lung cancer. Curr Opin Oncol 10:133–138, 1998.

Zumsteg, M, and Casperson, D: Paraneoplastic syndromes in metastatic disease. Semin Oncol Nurs 14:220–229, 1998.

Pneumonia

Aujesky, D, Auble, TE, Yealy, DM, et al: Prospective comparison of three validated prediction rules for prognosis in community-acquired pneumonia. Am J Med 118:384–392, 2005.

Guthrie, R, and Weis, M: Strategies for improving management of community-acquired pneumonia and acute exacerbations of chronic bronchitis Consultant 44(7):S3–S4, June 2004 (Suppl).

Guthrie, R, and Weis, M: CAP and AECB: The need for a regimen that the bugs can't resist. Consultant 44(7):S50–S52 June 2004 (Suppl).

Levison, ME: Pneumonia, including necrotizing pulmonary infections. In Fauci, AS, et al (eds): Harrison's Principles of Internal Medicine, ed 14. McGraw-Hill, New York, 1998, p 1437.

Regueiro, CR: The latest approaches to managing pneumonia. Clin Advisor Nov. 25–31, 2004.

Regueiro, CR: The latest approaches to community-acquired pneumonia. Cortlandt Forum, Sept. 31–40, 2004.

Stauffer, JL: Lung. In Tierney, LM, et al (eds): Current Medical Diagnosis and Treatment, ed 25. Appleton & Lange, Stamford, Conn., 1998, p 215.

Sleep Apnea

Chediak, A: Pathogenesis of obstructive sleep apnea. Respir Care 43:265–272, 1998.

Flemons, W, and Tsai, W: Quality of life consequences of sleep-disordered breathing. J Allergy Clin Immunol 99:S750–S756, 1997.

Gil, D: Sleep apnea. In Wilkins, RL, and Dexter, JR (eds): Respiratory Disease: A Case Study Approach. FA Davis, Philadelphia, 1998, pp 394–409.

Guilleminault, C, and Robinson, A: Sleep-disordered breathing and hypertension: Past lessons, future directions. Sleep 20(9):806–811, 1997.

Johns, M: A new method of measuring daytime sleepiness: The Epworth Sleepiness Scale. Sleep 14:540–546, 1991.

Kim, H, et al: Sleep-disordered breathing and neurophysiologic deficits. Am J Respir Crit Care Med 156:1813–1819, 1997.

Kramer, N, et al: Enuresis and obstructive sleep apnea in adults. Chest 114:634–637, 1998.

Merritt, SL, Gyllenhaal, C, Peterson, SD, Block, K, and Gochenour, T: Herbal Remedies: Efficacy in controlling sleepiness and promoting sleep. Nurse Pract Forum 11(2) June, 87–100, 2000.

Narkiewicz, K, et al: Sympathetic activity in obese subjects with and without obstructive sleep apnea. Circulation 98:772–776, 1998.

Phillips, B: Clinical diagnosis of sleep apnea. Respir Care 43:288–291, 1998.

Schwab, R, et al: Sleep apnea syndromes. In Fishman, AP (ed): Fishman's Pulmonary Diseases and Disorders. McGraw-Hill: New York, 1998, pp 1617–1637.

Smith, CE, et al: Continuous positive airway pressure: Patients' and caregivers' learning needs and barriers to use. Heart Lung 27:99–108, 1998.

Strohl, KP: Consequences of sleep-disordered breathing. Respir Care 43:277–283, 1998.

Tami, TA, et al: Identification of obstructive sleep apnea in patients who snore. Laryngoscope 108:508–513, 1998.

Smoking Addiction

Andrews, J: Optimizing smoking cessation strategies. Nurse Pract 23:47, 48, 51, 52, 57, 61, 64, 67, 1998.

Blondal, T, et al: Nicotine nasal spray with nicotine patch for smoking cessation: Randomized trial with six year follow up. BMJ 318:285–288, 1999.

Hughs, J, et al: Recent advances in the pharmacotherapy of smoking. JAMA 281:72–76, 1999.

Hurt, R, et al: A comparison of sustained-release bupropion and placebo for smoking cessation. N Engl J Med 337:1195–1202, 1999.

Pohl, J, and Caplan, D: Smoking cessation: Using group intervention methods to treat low-income women. Nurse Pract 23:13–37, 1998.

Rennard, S, and Daughton, D: Cigarette smoking and disease. In Fishman, AP (ed): Fishman's Pulmonary Diseases and Disorders. McGraw-Hill, New York, 1998, pp 697–708.

Sheahan, S, and Wilson, S: Smoking cessation tips: Family system and addiction perspectives. J Am Acad Nurse Pract 10:393–401, 1998.

Tobacco Use, Chap. 27 Healthy People 2010—Centers for Disease Control and Prevention.

http://www.healthypeople.gov/Document/HTML/Volume2/27Tobacco.htm (Accessed July 14, 2006).

Tonnesen, P, et al: Higher dosage nicotine patches increase one-year smoking cessation rates: Results from the European CEASE trial. Eur Respir J 13:238–246, 1999.

Tuberculosis

http://www.cdc.gov/nchstp/tb—Division of TB elimination Web site

ATS/CDC: Targeted tuberculin testing and treatment of latent tuberculosis infection. Pub 99-6422. MMWR 49 (No RR-6), 2000.

American Thoracic Society: Diagnostic standards and classification of tuberculosis in adults and children. Pub 99-6423. Am J Resp Crit Care Med 161:1376–1395, 2000.

Hinthorn, D, and Bader, MS: Tuberculin skin testing: Indication, interpretation, and management. Adv Stud Med 4(10):534–542, 2004.

Jerant, AF, Bannon, M, and Rittenhouse, S: Identification and management of tuberculosis. Am Fam Phys 61(9):2667–2678, 2000.

Mitchell, AE, and Parish, TG: Using combination therapy for smoking cessation. Clin Rev 15(5):40–45, 2005.

Neff, M. ATS, CDC, and IDSA update recommendations on the treatment of tuberculosis. Am Fam Phys 68(9):1854, 1857–1858, 1861–1862, 2003.

Raviglione, MC, and O'Brien, RU: Tuberculosis, In Kasper, DL, Fauci, AS, Longo, DL, Braunwald, E, Hauser, SL, and Jameson, JL (eds):

Harrison's Principles of Internal Medicine. ed 16. McGraw-Hill, 2005, pp 953–966.

Upper Respiratory Infections

Durand, M, et al: Infections of the upper respiratory tract. In Fauci, AS, et al (eds): Harrison's Principles of Internal Medicine, ed 14. McGraw-Hill, New York, 1998, p 179.

Snow,V, Mottur-Pilson, C, and Gonzales, R: Principles of appro priate antibiotic use for treatment of nonspecific upper respiratory tract infections in adults. Ann Intern Med 134(6):487–489, 2001.

Wimett, L, and Laustsen, G: Telithromycin (Ketek) for community-acquired respiratory tract infections. Nurse Pract 29(9):56–60, 2004.

Resources

American Cancer Society, Inc.
http://www.cancer.org
American Sleep Apnea Association
http://www.sleepapnea.org
American Sleep Association
http://www.americansleepassociation.org
National Sleep Foundation
http://sleepfoundation.org
Asthma and COPD (selected Web sites)
Allergy, Asthma, and Immunology Online
http://allergy,mcg.edu/physicians/manual/manual:html
wwwnhbi.nih.gov/guidelines/asthma
American Lung Association
http://www.lungusa.org
National Institute of Allergy and Infectious Disease
http://www.niaid.nih.gov
Cancer Care, Inc.
http://www.cancercare.org
http://rex.nci.nih.gov and http://cancernet.nci.nih.gov
National Institutes of Health
National Heart, Lung, and Blood Institute
http://www.nhlbi.nih.gov/nhlbi/nhlbi.htm
National Library of Medicine
http://www.nlm.nih.gov
CDC's SARS website
http://www.cdc.gov/ncidod/sars/infectioncontrol.htm
Patient Education (selected Websites):
http://www.betterhealth.com
http://www.cdc.gov
http://www.medscape.com
Smoking Cessation
American Lung Association
http://www.lungusa.org
http://www.meds.com/pdq/small_cellpro.html
Smoking Cessation Behavior Modification
http://www.clc.gov/tobacco/how2quit.htm

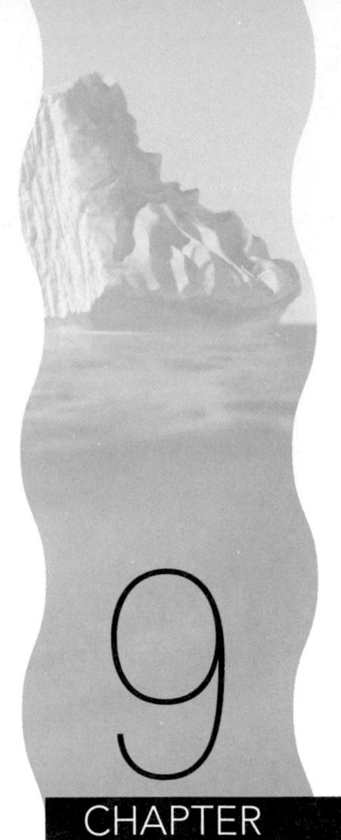

Cardiovascular Problems

Jill E. Winland-Brown, EdD, MSN, APRN, BC
Brian O. Porter, MD, PhD, MPH
Margaret A. Fitzgerald, DNP, APRN, BC, NP-C, FAANP, CSP

Common Complaints

Chest Pain

Chest pain is a discomforting sensation in the chest area. Although chest pain is often associated with cardiovascular problems, it may also have pulmonary, gastrointestinal (GI), musculoskeletal, neurologic, psychogenic, or idiopathic causes. If the chest pain is related to coronary artery disease (CAD), the incidence increases after age 35 in men and in postmenopausal women. In individuals up to 50 years of age, it occurs more frequently in men, then occurs equally in men and women, with a higher incidence in black men.

Differential Diagnosis

Obtaining a focused health history and physical exam is essential for accurate assessment and appropriate treatment for a patient with chest pain. Critical components of the history include appraisal of the major symptoms of heart disease, including chest pain, dyspnea, syncope, and congestive heart failure (CHF). The clinician should ask patients in all age groups about tolerance of exercise, especially whether exercise provokes any of the aforementioned complaints. The history of the present illness (HPI) of the person with chest pain should focus on personal risk factors for cardiovascular disease.

The clinician should obtain a complete chest pain symptom analysis including location, quality, duration, aggravating or relieving factors, and associated symptoms or signs. In particular, localized, fleeting, and moving pain is rarely indicative of serious cardiac pathology. Anxiety and bereavement can cause diffuse pain lasting for hours and chest tenderness, often associated with sighing. Costochondritis is often described as localized, and it can be replicated with arm movement or pressing on the area of tenderness.

In contrast, the discomfort of angina pectoris is classically described as a diffuse, retrosternal sensation, often with radiation, and a heavy, burning sensation, usually lasting more than 1 minute but less than 10 minutes. Exertional symptoms are usually more common in individuals with fixed atherosclerotic lesions. In assessing the person with known angina pectoris, it is critical to ascertain if there has been a change in the symptom pattern, because this may indicate an alteration in vessel patency such as that found in accelerated atherosclerosis or vessel spasm. The word "pain" should be used with caution in taking the history of a person with suspected myocardial ischemia, because the patient may deny that pain is present but may agree that tightness, burning, fullness, or other sensations more aptly describe the complaint.

The terms "unstable angina," "preinfarct angina," and "crescendo angina" are synonymous, used to describe the condition in which there is a new onset of cardiac ischemic chest pain at rest, but without evidence of acute myocardial infarction (MI). Reports of symptoms at rest are more likely to be associated with coronary artery vasospasm, a condition usually seen in patients with coronary atherosclerosis. The combination of two mechanisms of lumen narrowing leaves the patient at considerable risk for an acute coronary syndrome—in these cases rapid and accurate assessment is vital to ensure appropriate disposition and treatment.

About one-third of patients with angina pectoris will have simultaneous dyspnea, caused by transient increase in pulmonary venous pressures that accompany ventricular stiffening during an episode of myocardial

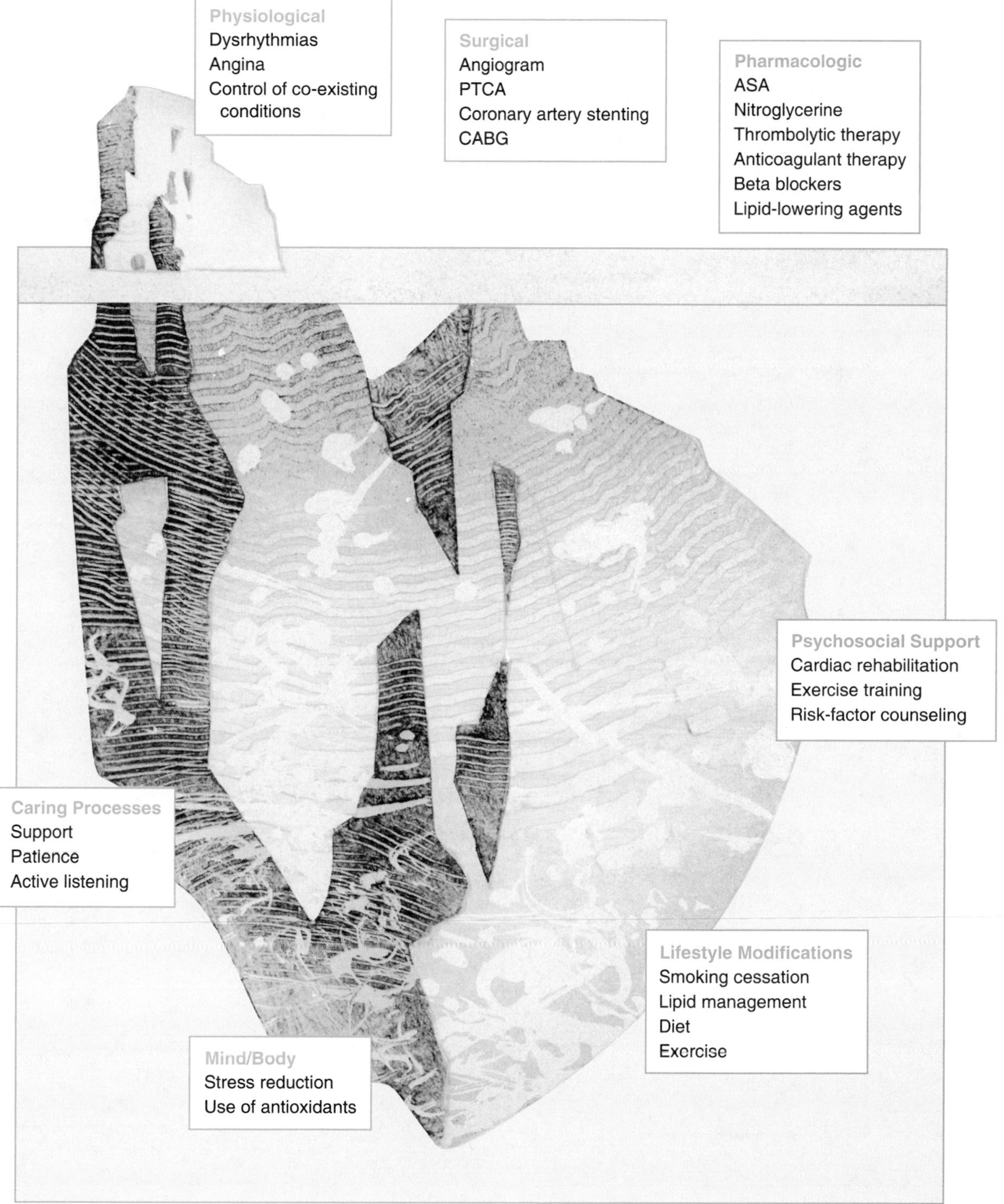

ischemia. The presence of diaphoresis with chest pain is particularly worrisome, often indicating a significant drop in cardiac output during the episode of pain and subsequent decreased perfusion of the skin. In contrast to the patient who complains of anginal pain, the patient who is experiencing an acute MI often complains of anginal-like chest pain that lasts in excess of 20 minutes but occasionally waxes and wanes during that period. The pain is frequently accompanied by dyspnea, diaphoresis, nausea, and dizziness. The pain may radiate to the neck, jaw, shoulder, or arm

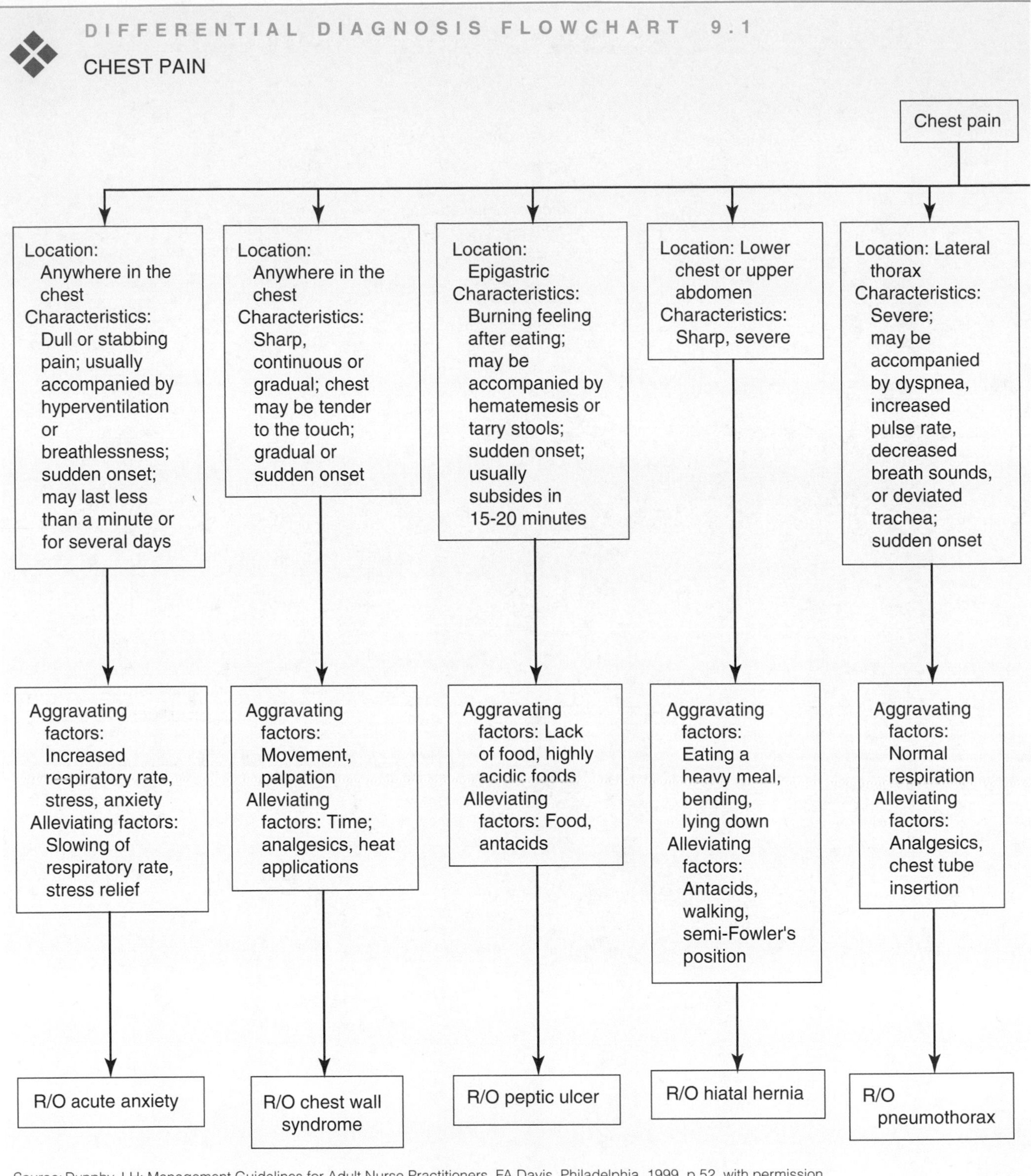

Source: Dunphy, LH: Management Guidelines for Adult Nurse Practitioners. FA Davis, Philadelphia, 1999, p 52, with permission.

(left side more than right). Patients show extreme variation in the amount of pain experienced with an MI, from the patient who complains of a "vise around the heart" to someone who is apologetic for seeking assistance with "just a bit of indigestion that will not clear up." In particular, women, older adults, and people with diabetes mellitus are likely to have minimal or atypical symptoms with an acute MI. A more detailed discussion of the pain of angina and MI is provided in the sections on treatment of those conditions later in the chapter (Differential Diagnosis Flowchart 9.1).

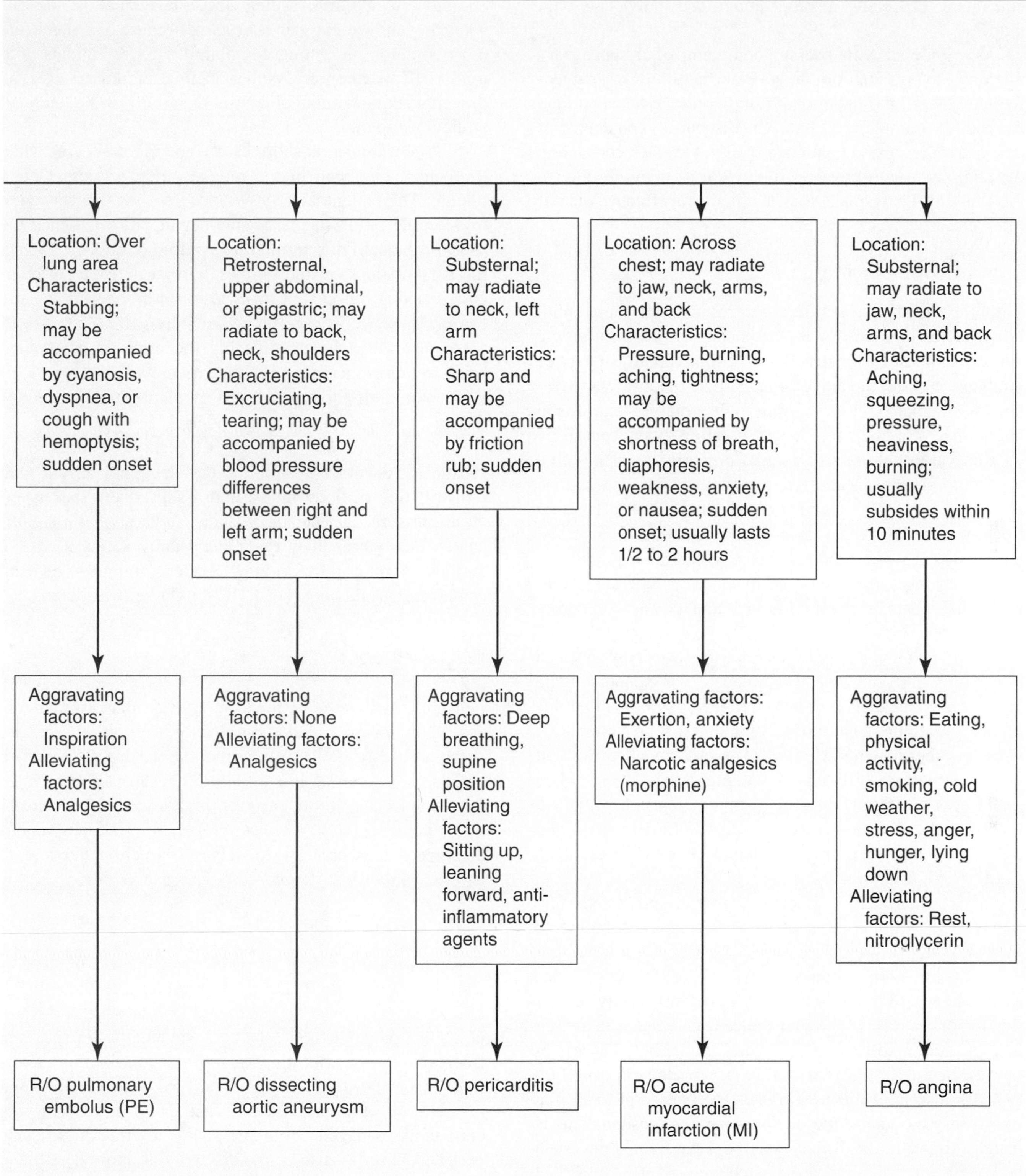

Dyspnea: Shortness of Breath

Dyspnea, or shortness of breath, is a highly subjective complaint, yet it is one of the most common cardiac symptoms. The challenge to the clinician is to determine its etiology. As with any complaint, the patient with dyspnea should be asked about precipitating factors, quality, duration, alleviating factors, and the length of time needed to relieve the symptom after discontinuing the precipitating event. In addition, dyspnea may be an anginal equivalent, especially in older adults and individuals with diabetes.

Patients with a chief complaint of dyspnea vary markedly in presentation; however, because this is a subjective complaint, the patient's report should be taken as fact. As with the complaint of pain, the discomfort and degree of dyspnea represents the patient's reality; however, correlating the complaint with physical findings may help to establish the cause of the dyspnea, thus leading to an effective plan of intervention.

Differential Diagnosis

The origin of dyspnea differs according to the cause. With left-sided cardiac outflow tract blockage, such as in severe aortic stenosis or obstructive cardiomyopathy, dyspnea likely arises from the decrease in cardiac output. When dyspnea is associated with recurrent myocardial ischemia, as in angina pectoris, the shortness of breath is likely caused by an increase in pulmonary vascular pressure, coupled with a transient decrease in cardiac output. In right-sided cardiac problems, such as tricuspid and pulmonic valvular dysfunction, the complaint of dyspnea usually arises from increased pulmonary pressures and resistance to cardiac emptying.

Noncardiac causes of dyspnea include anxiety or emotional distress, pneumothorax, and physical deconditioning.

The patient's assessment of the severity of dyspnea may differ from the objective findings. For example, some patients who have been observed to have rather marked difficulty breathing have little complaint of breathlessness, whereas other patients who have few objective findings will describe marked difficulty breathing. In addition, when asked about difficulty breathing, one patient may admit to feelings of suffocation, in that getting sufficient air in and out of the lungs is a problem, whereas others will describe a need to take deep breaths.

Dyspnea is a poorly sensitive and nonspecific marker for cardiovascular disease. Factors contributing to the complaint of breathlessness in the absence of heart disease include poor conditioning and exercise intolerance related to inactivity and obesity. The patient usually reports that the onset of this type of dyspnea accompanies increased activity, and resolves rapidly when the activity ceases. In any event, in cardiovascular disease, dyspnea is usually a result of increased stiffness in the lungs caused by increased pulmonary blood volume or pulmonary congestion. This is usually found in conditions with poor cardiac output, such as CHF, recurrent myocardial ischemia, poorly controlled hypertension, and valvular dysfunction and heart disease.

When dyspnea is the complaint, it is essential for the clinician to assess the change in the patient's ability to perform average daily activities. In particular, dyspnea often is first detected by the patient as the inability to talk during exertional activities. Pinpointing the onset of the symptoms and concurrent events may be helpful in determining its etiology. In addition, asking about cosymptoms such as wheezing and weight gain is crucial, because dyspnea is the most common presenting complaint in CHF. Patients with mild CHF may report dyspnea in this circumstance, even though walking without objects in the arms may be tolerated without symptoms.

Orthopnea is shortness of breath that begins when the patient has been in a supine position for less than 1 minute. The patient usually compensates for this sensation by sleeping on an increased number of pillows, hence the use of the qualifying term "three-pillow orthopnea." When the person slides off the pillows, shortness of breath reoccurs, causing the person to awaken. Orthopnea is usually caused by CHF, as a result of increased right-sided heart pressures, which happens during the night as right-sided heart pressures increase after the patient has been supine for a few hours, mobilizing fluid that pooled in the extremities during the waking, more active hours.

Paroxysmal nocturnal dyspnea is shortness of breath that occurs 2 to 4 hours into sleep, concurrent with redistribution of body fluids, and a subsequent rise in left atrial pressure. The person awakens suddenly, with significant difficulty breathing. He or she usually stands or sits up, getting symptom relief in about 10 to 30 minutes. As with orthopnea, the diagnosis of CHF should be considered.

Leg Aches

Leg aches associated with peripheral vascular disorders are caused by impaired blood flow to the extremities. Peripheral vascular disease (PVD) affects the arteries and veins. When the disease is arterial, it is usually the result of accumulated fatty streaks and fibrous plaques (high levels of low-density lipoproteins [LDL]). Venous problems relate to venous incompetence secondary to valve obstruction, leading to chronic venous insufficiency and varicose veins.

Differential Diagnosis

Patients presenting with leg aches may have a number of disorders other than PVD, so a thorough history and physical examination must be performed to rule out thrombosis, phlebitis, polycythemia, anemia, Raynaud's disease, and Buerger's disease. Because some of the contributing factors to PVD may be smoking, high blood pressure (BP), and diabetes, these problems must be addressed and underlying conditions managed. Both peripheral arterial disease and peripheral venous disease are discussed in more detail later in the chapter.

Palpitations

In addition to the major symptoms of cardiac disease, palpitations are commonly reported by the individual who has or is at risk for heart disease. *Palpitations* are defined as the awareness of the beating of one's heart and may be benign or pathologic in nature. When questioning the patient with palpitations, the clinician should obtain a detailed description of the sensation. If the patient reports a sensation of a strong but regular rhythmic beating of the heart after stress or exertion, this likely indicates a normal physiologic response to the increased catecholamine production. If there is a report of skipped or missed beats, particularly with the sensation that the heart "stopped" momentarily after the extrasystole, this may indicate the presence of an atrial or ventricular ectopic beat.

Differential Diagnosis

Atrial ectopias are most often benign, occurring with excessive coffee, alcohol, or tobacco use. On occasion, atrial ectopias occur with cardiac pathology, sometimes as a precursor to a supraventricular rhythm such as multifocal atrial tachycardia or atrial fibrillation. This is most likely in the patient with chronic obstructive pulmonary disease (COPD) or rheumatic heart disease.

Ventricular ectopias are somewhat more likely to indicate cardiac pathology than atrial ectopias; however, these beats are more common in older adults. If the patient is at high risk for or has known heart disease, the clinician must carefully assess the complaint of palpitations, because ventricular extrasystoles may indicate increased risk for sudden cardiac death.

Another variation on the presentation of palpitations is the patient who complains of a sudden onset of a very rapid heartbeat or fluttering of the heart. The etiology may be a supraventricular or ventricular tachycardia, often with equally rapid and unpredictable cessation of the rhythm, or a rhythmic paroxysm. Although this type of rhythmic sensation is usually regular, such as in paroxysmal supraventricular tachycardia or ventricular tachycardia, it may also be irregular, such as in intermittent atrial fibrillation. In any case, the clinician should query the patient carefully about cosymptoms such as chest pain related to decreased coronary artery filling and increased myocardial oxygen demands, as well as about symptoms associated with low cardiac output.

Diagnostic testing should be directed by information obtained in the health history and physical exam. As with cardiac-related syncope, blood chemistries, hemoglobin, and hematocrit (Hct) should be evaluated to help rule out electrolyte imbalance or anemia as a possible, though less common, cause of palpitations. Ambulatory cardiac monitoring, whether for a short period of time, such as 24 hours, or longer, until at least one event is recorded, is most helpful in ascertaining the presence of a potentially lethal cardiac rhythm disturbance. Echocardiography may be necessary to assess cardiac outflow tract patency and to help rule out valvular stenosis or hypertrophic cardiomyopathy.

Intervention should be directed at the underlying cause of the palpitations. For example, if a rhythm disturbance such as recurrent supraventricular or ventricular tachycardia is the cause, treatment directed at eliminating this is warranted. In any event, the clinician should consult with a clinician who has expertise in this area to ensure patient safety and optimal outcome.

Differential diagnoses of palpitations are presented in Differential Diagnosis Flowchart 9.2.

Peripheral Edema

Peripheral edema is the accumulation of fluid within the interstitial spaces of the extremities. When the edema involves the lower extremities, it is a symptom of an underlying disorder; it may be caused by cardiac conditions (e.g., heart failure, chronic venous insufficiency, or thrombophlebitis), renal and hepatic disease, or by trauma, tumors, or inflammation. Peripheral edema occurs equally among men and women.

Differential Diagnosis

Peripheral edema is usually diagnosed via the history and physical exam, although laboratory findings assist in determining the cause of the edema. Specific diagnostic tests the clinician should order include complete blood count (CBC), urinalysis, serum chemistries, and a thyroid profile. X-ray studies may be ordered if trauma or osteomyelitis is suspected, and a chest x-ray film should be ordered to assess the heart and lungs. A computed tomography (CT) scan may help to assess the edema distribution and pinpoint the extent of venous and lymphatic obstructions. An electrocardiogram (ECG) is essential for assessing cardiac function, and Doppler studies may be ordered to evaluate for deep vein thrombosis. It is essential that the underlying cause be identified and treated, or the peripheral edema will remain, possibly causing tissue ischemia from compressed and diminished arterial circulation. Differential diagnoses of peripheral edema are presented in Differential Diagnosis Flowchart 9.3.

Syncope

Syncope is loss of consciousness that occurs abruptly as a discrete episode and usually lasts for a short period of only a few minutes. The implied pathology is decreased cerebral blood flow caused by marked cardiac output. Cardiac-related syncope is an ominous sign associated with high rates of mortality. One of the most common cardiac causes of syncope is a ventricular rhythm disturbance such as a ventricular tachycardia. A less common reason for cardiac syncope is profound bradycardia, usually with a heart rate (HR) below 40 beats per minute. The patient regains consciousness with the resumption of a rhythm capable of producing adequate cardiac output for cerebral perfusion.

DIFFERENTIAL DIAGNOSIS FLOWCHART 9.2

PALPITATIONS

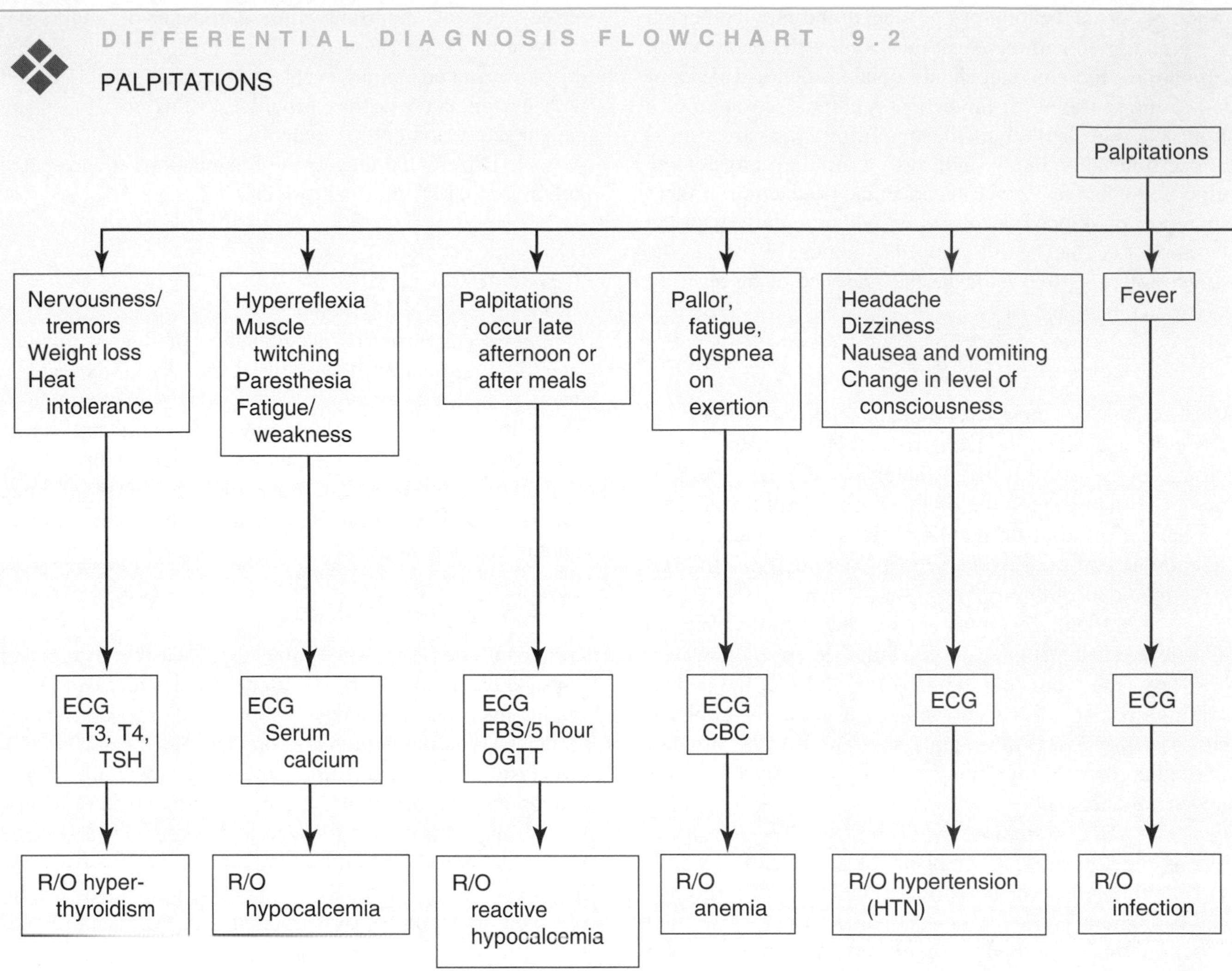

Source: Dunphy, LH: Management Guidelines for Adult Nurse Practitioners. FA Davis, Philadelphia, 1999, p 89, with permission.

Differential Diagnosis

Cardiac outflow tract blockage, such as the obstruction that may occur in hypertrophic cardiomyopathy and aortic valve stenosis, can also produce syncope. This is most often seen in response to increased activity or stress, when the outflow tract blockage impedes the increase in cardiac output needed to meet the increased demands for oxygen. This leads to syncope that typically lasts for a few seconds and ends when the "rest" of the syncopal episode helps balance supply and demand.

Presyncope is a momentary "blackout" or "gray-out" that would lead to syncope if the causative cardiac condition continued. The etiology is usually the same as for syncope. In contrast, in vertigo, the person has the sensation of staggering or veering in a certain direction or spinning. The sensation can often be reproduced by a change in head position. In vertigo, the cause is usually something other than decreased cerebral blood flow, often an inner ear disturbance, for example.

Diagnostic testing for cardiac-related syncope should be directed by the information obtained in the health history and physical exam. Blood chemistries, hemoglobin, and Hct should be checked to help rule out electrolyte imbalance or anemia as a possible, though less common, cause of syncope. Ambulatory cardiac monitoring, whether for a short period of time such as 24 hours or longer, until at least one event is recorded, is most helpful in ascertaining the presence of a potentially lethal cardiac rhythm disturbance. Echocardiography may be necessary to assess cardiac outflow tract patency and to rule out valvular stenosis or hypertrophic cardiomyopathy.

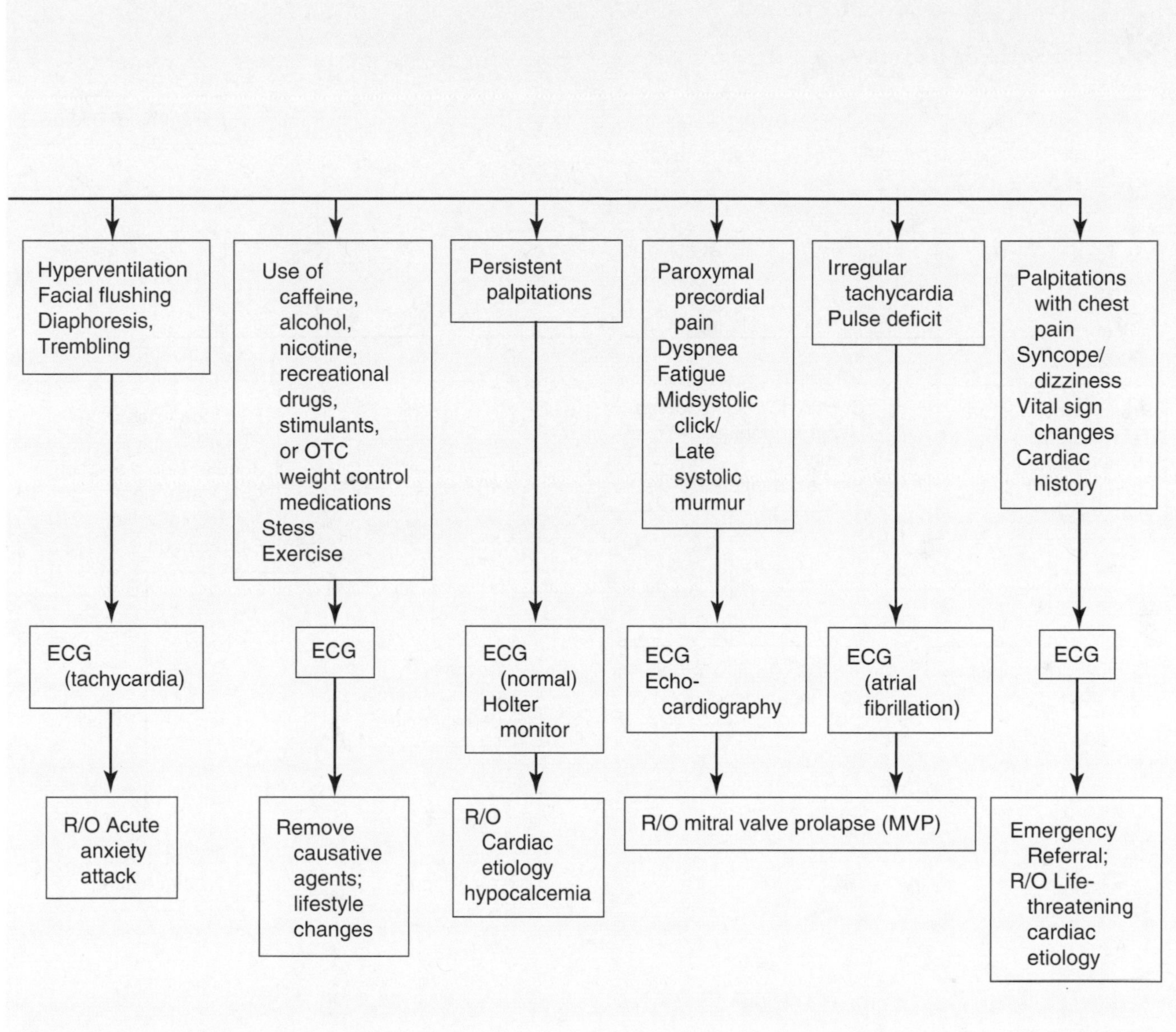

Intervention in cardiac-related syncope should be directed at the underlying cause. If a rhythm disturbance such as recurrent ventricular tachycardia is the cause, treatment directed at eliminating it is warranted. A pacemaker may be needed if recurrent bradycardia is found. In any event, the clinician should consult with a clinician who has expertise in this area to ensure patient safety and an optimal outcome.

Common Problems

Hypertension

Hypertension (HTN) is one of the most common chronic health problems seen in the primary-care setting. *Hypertension* in adults age 18 and older is defined as a systolic blood pressure (SBP) greater than 140 mm Hg and/or a diastolic blood pressure (DBP) of greater than 90 mm Hg, based on the average of two or more properly measured seated BP readings on each of two or more office visits. The Seventh Report of the Joint National Committee on Prevention, Detection, Evaluation, and Treatment of High Blood Pressure cite the following three categories for adults age 18 and older (Table 9.1):

- ▲ Prehypertension (SBP 120 to 139 mm Hg/DBP 80 to 89 mm Hg)
- ▲ Stage 1 hypertension (SBP 140 to 159 mm Hg/DBP 90 to 99 mm Hg)
- ▲ Stage 2 hypertension (SBP ≥160 mm Hg/DBP ≥100 mm Hg)

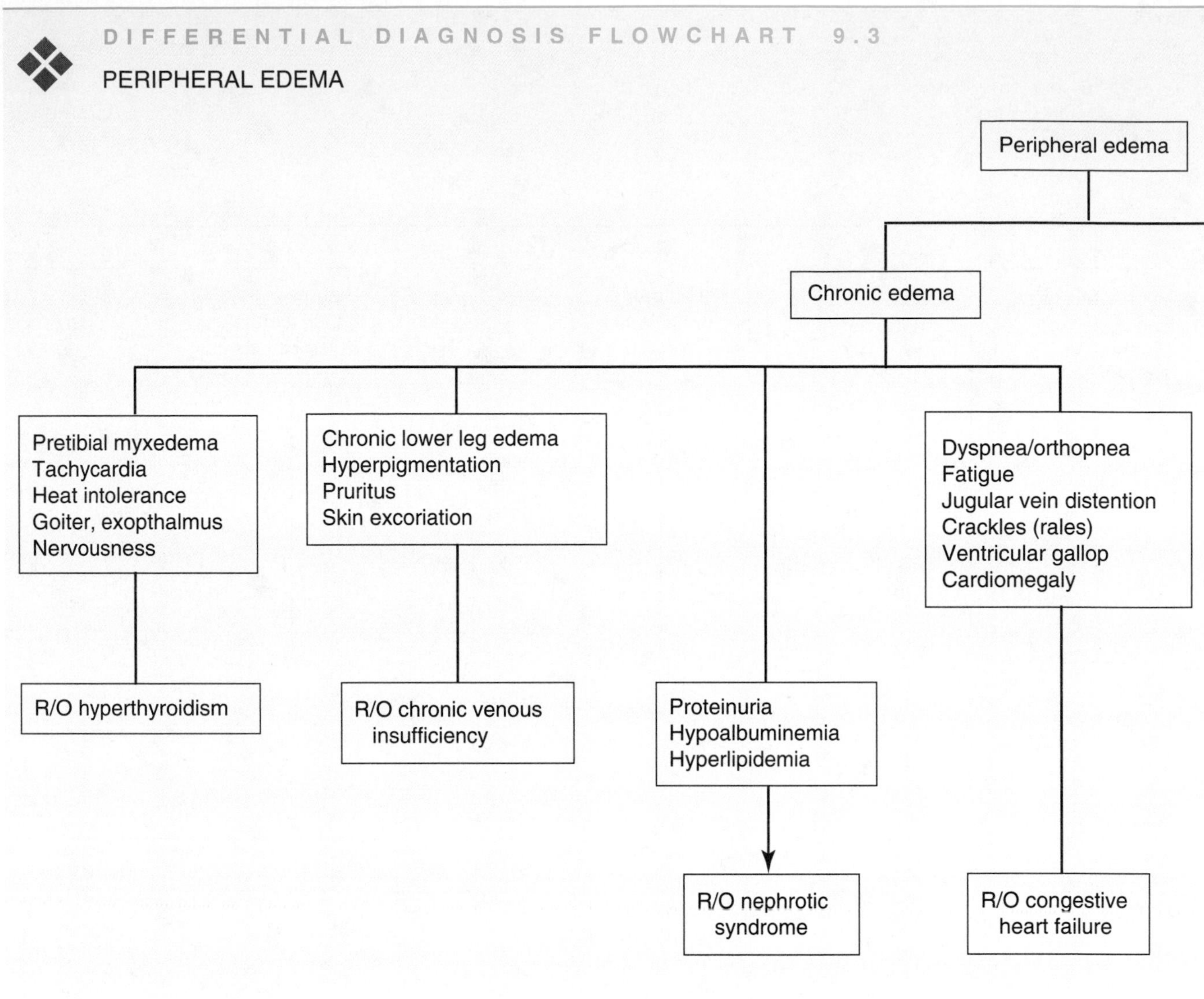

Source: Dunphy, LH: Management Guidelines for Adult Nurse Practitioners. FA Davis, Philadelphia, 1999, p 92, with permission.

More than 95 percent of patients with elevated BP have primary or essential HTN, with no single identifiable cause; this type of HTN results from the interplay of multiple genetic and environmental factors, including lifestyle influences. Fewer than 5 percent of patients, therefore, have secondary HTN; or a specific, possibly reversible, cause of elevated BP such as certain cardiac, renal, and endocrinologic problems or the use of vasoconstricting medications.

After decades of a steady reduction in rates of HTN-related diseases, researchers have reported a recent leveling of coronary heart disease rates, coupled with a slight increase in end-stage renal failure and age-adjusted stroke rates. These changes are likely caused by a number of factors including a growing aging population; however, the role of undetected untreated and inadequately controlled HTN contributes significantly. Considering this, the clinician should be committed not only to the detection and treatment of HTN but also to its prevention. When a patient develops HTN, primary prevention measures have not been successful. The clinician must aggressively monitor the patient and encourage his or her participation in the management of the disease.

There is a specific listing for Heart Disease and Stroke in the *Healthy People 2010* objectives as cardiovas-

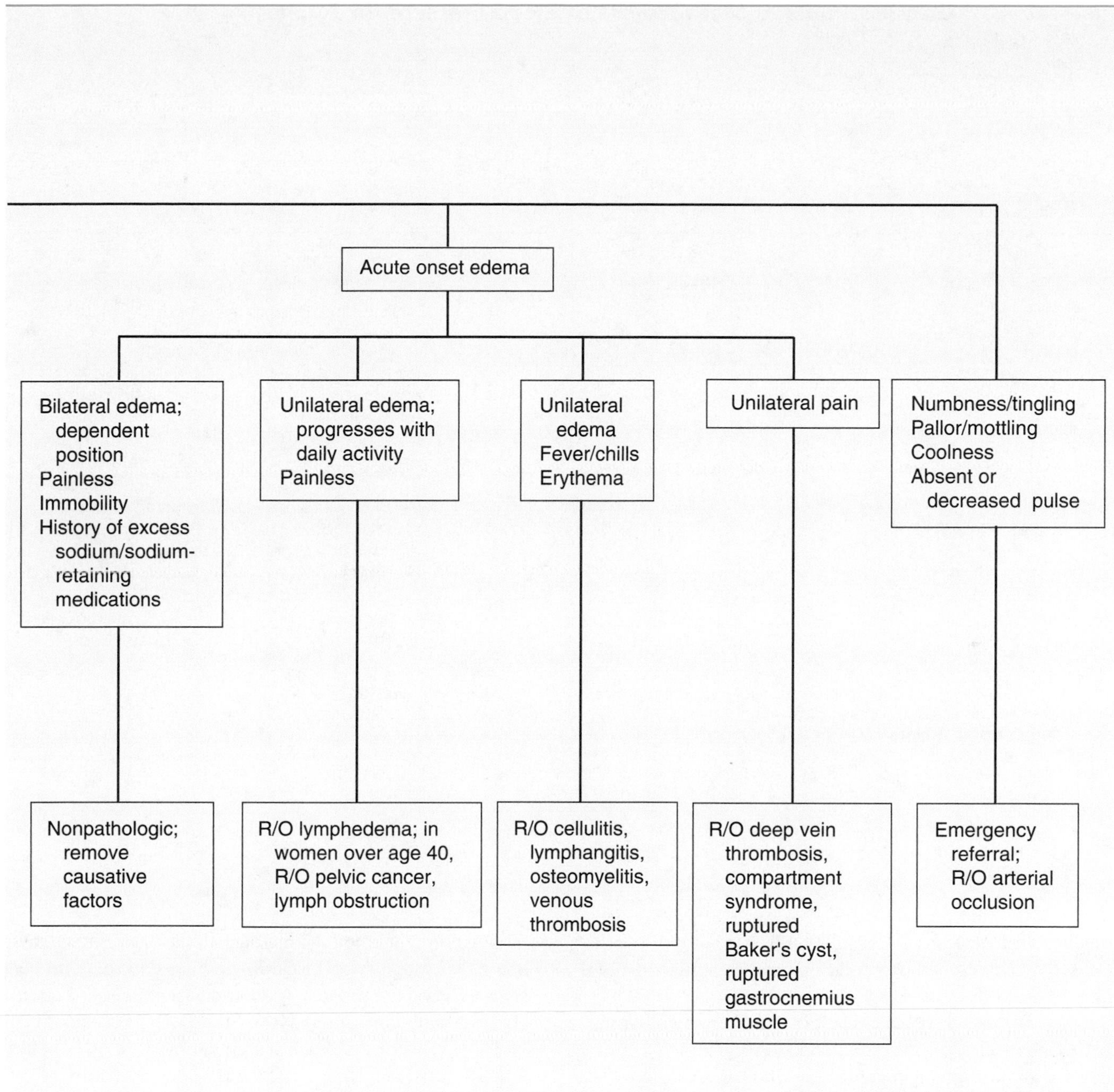

cular disease is so prevalent in our population. The goal is to improve cardiovascular health and quality of life through the prevention, detection, and treatment of risk factors; early identification and treatment of heart attacks and strokes; and prevention of recurrent cardiovascular events. There are 16 objectives, with 4 relating to blood pressure.

Epidemiology and Causes

HTN occurs in about 20 percent of the population of the United States (about 50 million persons). It occurs more often in men than in women and is more common in black men. The usual age at onset is by 30 years; however, it is usually not often detected until later in life. The prevalence increases with age. HTN can lead to ischemic heart disease, heart failure, diabetic hypertension, chronic kidney disease, and cerebrovascular disease. An increase in body mass index (BMI >30 kg/m^2), referred to as the metabolic syndrome, contributes to high blood pressure and cardiovascular disease. Today, 122 million Americans are considered overweight or obese, a situation that is reaching epidemic proportions

The onset of diastolic HTN, with or without systolic elevation, after age 60 is unusual. If this is found, the

Table 9.1 Classification and Management of Blood Pressure for Adults Aged 18 Years or Older

				Management*		
					Initial Drug Therapy	
BP Classification	Systolic BP, mm Hg*		Diastolic BP, mm Hg*	Lifestyle Modification	Without Compelling Indication	With Compelling Indications**
Normal	<120	and	<80	Encourage		
Prehypertension	120–139	or	80–89	Yes	No antihypertensive drug indicated	Drug(s) for the compelling indications[†]
Stage 1 hypertension	140–159	or	90–99	Yes	Thiazide-type diuretics for most; may consider ACE inhibitor, ARB, beta-blocker, CCB, or combination	Drug(s) for the compelling indications Other antihypertensive drugs (diuretics, ACE inhibitor, ARB, beta-blocker, CCB) as needed
Stage 2 hypertension	≥160	or	≥100	Yes	Two-drug combination for most (usually thiazide-type diuretic and ACE inhibitor or ARB or beta-blocker or CCB)[‡]	Drug(s) for the compelling indications Other antihypertensive drugs (diuretics, ACE inhibitor, ARB, beta-blocker, CCB) as needed

ACE, angiotensin-converting enzyme; ARB, angiotensin-receptor blocker, BP, blood pressure; CCB, calcium channel blocker.
*Treatment determined by highest BP category.
**See Table 9.1
†Treat patients with chronic kidney disease or diabetes to BP goal or less than 130/80 mm Hg.
‡Initial combined therapy should be used cautiously in those at risk for orthostatic hypotension.

Source: Chobanian AV, et al: Seventh report of the Joint National Committee on Prevention, Detection, Evaluation, and Treatment of High Blood Pressure. Hypertension 42(6): 1206–1252, 2003.

diagnosis of new-onset secondary HTN should be considered. In particular, renovascular disease is a common cause of new-onset diastolic HTN.

Primary HTN is a result of the interplay of a number of genetic, environmental, and lifestyle issues. HTN is more common among individuals whose parents or other close family members have HTN. In these individuals, diminished ability to excrete excessive sodium, coupled with long-term high dietary sodium intake, appears to be a predisposing factor to increased peripheral vascular resistance (PVR) and rise in BP.

Pathophysiology

Pathophysiology of Essential Hypertension

Arterial blood pressure measurements of less than 120 mm Hg systolic and less than 80 mm Hg diastolic are considered ideal values. HTN is consistent elevation of arterial blood pressure: a systolic value of greater than or equal to 140 mm Hg or a diastolic value of greater than or equal to 90 mm Hg. HTN is diagnosed when *either* systolic or diastolic pressure falls within this range. Numerous studies have shown there is a linear progression of cardiovascular damage with consistent BP values above a systolic measurement of 120 mm Hg or diastolic measurement of 80 mm Hg. For individuals 40 to 70 years of age, each increment of 20 mm Hg in systolic BP or 10 mm Hg in diastolic BP doubles the risk of cardiovascular disease (CVD), across the entire BP range from 115/75 mm Hg to 185/115 mm Hg. The precursor stage of hypertension has been designated as *prehypertension*: a systolic BP greater than or equal to 121 to 139 mm Hg or diastolic BP greater than or equal to 81 to 89 mm Hg. Persons with prehypertension have a higher risk for cardiovascular disease than do normotensive individuals.

The term "essential hypertension" describes high BP that has no identifiable etiology after thorough clinical examination excludes possible secondary causes. Although etiology is unknown, endothelial dysfunction is the key pathophysiological process involved in essential HTN. The arterial endothelium is an important regulator of vascular tone, vascular structure, thrombosis, and inflammation. Endothelial dysfunction is central to a wide array of cardiovascular disorders, including HTN, atherosclerosis, and myocardial ischemia. Vascular tone is maintained by endothelium-derived mediators such as nitric oxide, endothelin-1, and angiotensin II. Nitric oxide, a major vasodilator, counteracts the potent vasoconstrictors endothelin-1 and angiotensin II, which regulate normal vascular tone. In essential hypertension, there is an imbalance in the vasodilator and vasoconstrictive substances secreted by the endothelium. Plasma levels of nitric oxide are diminished whereas levels of endothelin-1 and angiotensin II are elevated. Reasons for this imbalance have not been elucidated, and it is not clear whether endothelial dysfunction precedes or is the result of HTN.

Other investigations have found that renin levels are markedly abnormal in some hypertensive individuals, despite normal renal function. Renin oversecretors experience constant cycling of the renin–angiotensin–aldosterone cascade, which raises blood volume and blood pressure. Low renin secretors, in general, are salt-sensitive hypertensive individuals. Ingestion of sodium increases water reabsorption into the bloodstream, which raises blood volume and blood pressure. The cause of renin imbalance in some persons with essential hypertension is unknown. Measuring plasma renin levels may assist in clinical diagnosis and treatment.

HTN is a common disorder that occurs with aging in industrialized societies. Data from the Framingham Heart Study suggest that individuals who are normotensive at 55 years of age have a 90 percent lifetime risk of developing HTN. There is a particular rise in systolic BP that progresses throughout life, with a difference of 20 to 30 mm Hg between early and late adulthood. Worldwide epidemiologic evidence demonstrates that age-related HTN is uncommon in societies where individuals maintain lower body weight, lower consumption of sodium, higher intake of potassium, and greater levels of physical activity. These findings indicate that high BP is influenced by environmental and lifestyle factors and is not an inevitable consequence of aging. Smoking, obesity, and stress are examples of modifiable lifestyle factors that raise BP.

Genetic and ethnic influences also play a role in the development of HTN. Persons with a family history of HTN are four times more likely to suffer HTN than those with no family history of the condition. Studies show that the genetic contribution to essential HTN is complex, and multiple genes are likely involved. Most genetic effects involve gene–gene interactions and gene–environment interactions. Genes that encode components of the renin–angiotensin–aldosterone system are being extensively studied. Results of this line of investigation have implicated mutations in the angiotensinogen gene and angiotensin-converting enzyme (ACE) gene.

Studies of hypertension in African Americans demonstrate that ethnicity is related to hypertension susceptibility and plays a role in the efficacy of specific types of drugs. Morbidity and mortality due to HTN and HTN-related disorders are more common in African Americans than in Caucasian, non-Hispanic Americans. HTN also seems to follow a more malignant course in African Americans. Compared to Caucasian Americans with HTN, African Americans have an increased risk of left ventricular hypertrophy, heart failure, and renal failure.

HTN has localized and systemic adverse effects. Locally, high blood pressure creates a shearing force against the arterial walls, which injures the endothelium and accelerates development of atherosclerosis. Endothelial injury initiates a detrimental localized reaction of vasoconstriction, inflammation, platelet aggregation, fibrin and lipid deposition—the rudiments of arteriosclerotic plaque formation. Target organs that are damaged by HTN include the heart (left ventricular hypertrophy and CAD resulting in angina or acute myocardial infarction), the kidneys (chronic renal insufficiency), the brain (transient ischemic attacks and cerebrovascular accidents), the eyes (retinal hemorrhages and hypertensive retinopathy), and the peripheral arteries (peripheral vascular disease).

In summary, the etiology and pathophysiology of essential HTN is incompletely understood. It is a complex, multifactorial disorder that involves genetic and environmental factors, diet and lifestyle practices, imbalances in vasoactive substances, and dysfunction of the arterial endothelium.

Pathophysiology of Secondary Hypertension

Secondary HTN is elevated blood pressure due to an identifiable, underlying condition. Detection of secondary HTN is critical in order to reverse the source of the pathologic process and prevent hypertensive target organ damage. Less common than essential HTN, secondary HTN has an overall frequency of 5 to 10 percent in primary care practices. Secondary HTN is often distinguished from essential HTN by certain assessment findings, such as age at onset younger than 30 years or older than 50 years, BP higher than 180/110 mm Hg at diagnosis, significant target organ damage at diagnosis, hemorrhages and exudates on funduscopic examination, renal insufficiency, left ventricular hypertrophy, accelerated or malignant hypertension, and poor response to therapy. Resistant HTN is often due to unexplored, reversible secondary causes.

Reversible causes of HTN include obesity, obstructive sleep apnea, renovascular disease, chronic steroid therapy, Cushing's syndrome, primary hyperaldosteronism, pheochromocytoma, coarctation of the aorta, thyroid disease, parathyroid disease, and excess alcohol intake. Secondary HTN can also be drug-induced, and a thorough history of the patient's medications, including herbal supplements, over-the-counter (OTC) agents, and any illicit drug use is essential. Common drugs that can cause HTN include non-steroidal anti-inflammatory drugs (NSAIDs), cyclooxygenase-2 inhibitors (Cox-2 inhibitors), sympathomimetics such as decongestants and anorectics (diet pills), oral contraceptives, erythropoietin, cocaine, amphetamines, steroids, tacrolimus, cyclosporine, and herbal ephedra supplements. Licorice, smoking, and chewing tobacco also raise blood pressure.

"White Coat" Hypertension

"White coat" HTN is a transient rise in blood pressure experienced by a patient when in the clinical or hospital setting, most likely due to anxiety. This condition of "pseudohypertension" is common in primary care practice. The "white coat" effect can lead to overestimation of blood pressure and prescribing of unnecessary antihypertensive treatment. In addition, the patient's transiently high BP can be misinterpreted as ineffectiveness of antihypertensive therapy. Patients with "white coat" HTN are more accurately assessed through the use of ambulatory blood pressure monitoring, which provides an automated 24-hour recording of the patient's BP during normal daily activities that can be reviewed by the clinician. Alternatively, the patient may be instructed to measure and record intermittent BP readings over several weeks with reliable, consistent equipment for later review.

Pathophysiology of Malignant Hypertension (Hypertensive Emergency)

Malignant HTN is diagnosed when a patient presents with severely elevated blood pressure in the range of ≥ 180 mm Hg/110 mm Hg and evidence of acute target organ damage. Although the terms are often used interchangeably, hypertensive emergency or hypertensive crisis denotes this process occurring acutely. If not treated with immediate parenteral antihypertensive therapy in an acute care setting, a hypertensive emergency may prove fatal. In contrast, a significantly elevated BP alone with *no evidence* of target organ damage *does not* constitute an emergency. In turn, an isolated finding of severely elevated BP can be reduced over the course of hours with oral medications in an outpatient setting. In hypertensive emergency, acute target organ damage most commonly involves the neurologic, cardiac, or renal systems. Acute cerebrovascular events, papilledema, acute myocardial ischemia or infarction, pulmonary edema, aortic dissection, acute renal failure, Tepistaxis, states of catecholamine excess, and preeclampsia/eclampsia are conditions associated with severely elevated BP. A patient presenting with acutely severe BP elevation requires a thorough clinical examination which includes funduscopy, electrocardiogram, urinalysis, serum creatinine measurements, and chest x-ray study. A CT scan of the head to rule out stroke may be necessary. Evidence of target organ damage includes the following:

- papilledema, hemorrhages, or exudates on funduscopic examination
- change in mental status or neurologic deficits on physical examination
- ECG consistent with myocardial ischemia or infarction
- chest x-ray film showing heart failure or aortic dissection
- renal dysfunction evidenced by hematuria, proteinuria and elevated serum creatinine

The primary care provider should refer patients with hypertensive emergency to an acute care setting for appropriate diagnostic testing, monitoring, and treatment.

Clinical Presentation

Subjective

Typically the diagnosis of HTN is made after several routine office visits with the patient complaining of no symptoms. Occasionally, if the BP is extremely elevated, the patient may present with a headache that occurs on awakening and is located in the occipital area.

Objective

A systematic approach should be used when assessing the person with or at risk for HTN. The assessment should include two measurements of BP in both arms, with the patient preferably seated, and after standing for at least 2 minutes. The higher readings should be recorded.

When a person has been diagnosed with or is suspected to have HTN, assessment should include a focused health history and physical examination, staging of BP elevation, and investigation for evidence of hypertensive target organ damage (TOD).

This exam should include funduscopic examination, palpation of the chest for PMI, auscultation of the heart, abdominal assessment for bruits or widened aortic diameter and enlarged kidneys, examination of the carotid arteries for bruits, palpation of peripheral pulses, and a neurologic examination. Evidence of target organ damage (TOD) includes retinopathy which may appear as arteriolar narrowing, arteriovenous nicking, hemorrhages, or exudates. A bruit may be auscultated over either carotid artery, indicating stenosis. The chest may demonstrate a displaced PMI and/or an S4 heart sound indicating left ventricular hypertrophy (LVH). Auscultation of an S4 heart sound is associated with decreased elasticity of the LV that occurs in LVH. The patient should also be evaluated for the presence of heart failure, a known sequela of long-standing hypertension. An S3 gallop, pulmonary crackles, jugular venous distension, and peripheral edema are signs of heart failure. A bruit heard in the abdomen may indicate an aneurysm or renal artery stenosis. Palpation of a widened aortic pulsation is associated with abdominal aortic aneurysm (AAA). Diminished peripheral pulses and sensation in the lower extremities can indicate peripheral arterial disease. Neurologic examination can reveal deficits associated with transient ischemic attacks (TIAs) or a cerebrovascular accident (CVA) (Advanced Assessment 9.1).

The history should include a thorough investigation of cardiovascular risk factors such as age, gender, postmenopausal status, diet, activity level, alcohol and caffeine use, smoking, dyslipidemia, diabetes, family history of heart disease, and current medications. Some medications, such

ADVANCED ASSESSMENT 9.1

Hypertension

Assessment	*Common Hypertension-Associated Findings*
Blood Pressure Measurement	
Proper technique:	SBP >140 mm Hg
Cuff size at least 80% of upper arm	DBP >90 mm Hg
Rest for 5 minutes before measurement	
Arm resting at level of the heart	
Average 2 readings at least 2 minutes apart (if >5 mm Hg difference, obtain additional readings)	
Physical Examination	
Height, weight, BMI	Obesity (BMI >27), especially with central or truncal pattern
Waist measurement	Men: >39 inches
	Women: >34 inches
Funduscope	Hypertensive retinopathy (arteriolar narrowing, arteriovenous nicking, hemorrhages, exudates, papilledema)
Carotid arteries	Bruits
Neck veins	Distension
Thyroid	Enlargement
	Nodules
Cardiac	PMI and apex displaced laterally; greater than one intercostal space
	S3, S4 heart sounds
	Murmur or mitral regurgitation
Lungs	Crackles
	Bronchospasm
Abdomen	Bruits, masses, abnormal aortic pulsations
	Enlarged kidneys
Extremities	Absence of peripheral arterial pulsations
	Bruits
	Edema
Diagnostic Tests	
Urinalysis	Proteinuria
BUN	Increased
CBC	May show anemia
Potassium	Increased or decreased
Blood glucose	May be increased
Triglycerides, HDL, LDL	Increased
12-lead ECG	May show target organ damage

as NSAIDs or OTC cold remedies, may exacerbate BP elevation. Excess use of alcohol is often the source of refractory HTN. Culture and ethnicity should be assessed within the history as well. Compared to Caucasians, African Americans have a higher risk of hypertension, diabetes mellitus, and renal impairment which requires aggressive management of blood pressure and specific drug therapy.

Particular care must be taken when assessing an older patient with HTN. If severe vessel rigidity is present in the brachial artery, the BP cuff may be unable to compress the calcified vessel well, leading to a falsely high pressure. This phenomenon is known as *pseudohypertension.* Although it may raise the BP by 30 mm Hg or more, it does not by itself represent a disease state.

Diagnostic Reasoning

Diagnostic Tests

Diagnostic testing of a patient who has or is suspected of having HTN should focus on the evaluation of target organs and concurrent conditions as well as on excluding certain causes of secondary HTN. Additional testing may be indicated, particularly when concurrent diseases such as diabetes mellitus or hyperlipidemia are present (Advanced Assessment 9.1).

The ECG is an important screening tool to assess for cardiac target organ damage in the hypertensive patient. It can be used to assess the presence of left atrial enlargement, left ventricular hypertrophy, myocardial ischemia or infarction, premature ventricular contractions, and atrial fibrillation. Left atrial enlargement is one of the earliest ECG findings associated with hypertension. An echocardiogram is most useful to detect the presence of increased left ventricular wall thickness and hypertrophy.

Differential Diagnosis

The key to differential diagnosis is to determine the underlying etiology of the HTN, whether it is essential or secondary, for instance, and to assess the degree of hypertension (prehypertension, hypertension, malignant or benign, etc.). A presumptive diagnosis is made if the average of at least two seated BP measurements on at least two or more visits exceeds either 90 mm Hg DBP or 140 mm Hg SBP in adults older than age 18.

Management

The key to hypertension management is not only the reversal of HTN-related disease trends, but also the prevention of target organ damage. The following are Public Health approaches to achieve a downward shift in the distribution of a population's BP, thus potentially reducing morbidity, mortality, and the lifetime risk of an individual becoming hypertensive.

- Develop community health programs to stress reducing calories, saturated fat, and salt in processed foods.
- Encourage food manufacturers and restaurants to reduce the sodium in the food supply by 50 percent over the next decade.
- Increase community/school opportunities for physical activity.
- Address the diversity of racial, ethnic, cultural, linguistic, religious, and social factors in the delivery of community services to increase the community's receptiveness to use of public health services.
- Improve opportunities for treatment and control of HTN. Health-care providers can help break down barriers to the diagnosis and treatment of HTN. Examples include nursing and work-site clinics and offering health services on evenings and weekends, which increases the likelihood of those who work during the weekday hours having access to care.

Patient-specific goals include:

- An awareness regarding the risks involved in prehypertension. Prehypertension (SBP of 120 to 139 mm Hg and/or DBP of 80 to 89 mm Hg) imparts an increased risk of developing HTN. In addition, teens and young adults with high normal BP are at markedly increased risk of developing HTN in their fourth and fifth decades of life. Behavioral therapies such as a program of regular aerobic exercise and a diet that is lower in fat and sodium and higher in potassium should be initiated to help avoid HTN.
- Knowing one's own body mass index (BMI). This should serve as a guide to weight loss rather than just looking at ideal body weight.
- Improving HTN control in persons already diagnosed. Many with HTN have a BP greater than 140/90 mm Hg, demonstrating inadequate control.
- Reducing cardiovascular risks. Many patients with HTN will have additional modifiable cardiovascular disease risk factors such as diabetes mellitus, hyperlipidemia, tobacco use, and inactivity; therefore, a comprehensive plan to treat HTN must also address these issues.

The use of lifestyle modifications (Table 9.2) should be a part of every patient's regimen to prevent or treat elevated blood pressure. In addition, Nursing Research-Based Practice 9.1 cites research using a nursing intervention as a possible BP lowering action. The fear of a rise in mortality with excessive BP reduction has not been supported with large-scale studies. When caring for the person with HTN, the clinician should bear in mind that cardiovascular mortality is considerably reduced if the SBP is less than 120 mm Hg and the DBP less than 80 mm Hg. The clinician should work with the patient on a plan of lifestyle modification and medications as needed to lower the BP as much as is tolerated without symptoms. In particular, the presence of diabetes mellitus and/or renal impairment should compel the clinician and patient to work together to maintain meticulous BP control at SBP levels less than 120 mm Hg and DBP less than 80 mm Hg to minimize the development of

Table 9.2 Lifestyle Modifications to Manage Hypertension*

- Weight reduction: Maintain normal body weight (BMI, 18.5–24.9 kg/m^2)

Approximate SBP reduction, range: 5–20 mm Hg/10 kg weight loss

- Adopt DASH (Dietary Approaches to Stop Hypertension) eating plan: Consume a diet rich in fruits, vegetables, and low-fat dairy products with a reduced content of saturated and total fat.

Approximate SBP reduction, range: 8–14 mm Hg

- Dietary sodium reduction: Reduce dietary sodium intake to no more than 100 mmol per day (2.4 g sodium or 6 g sodium chloride)

Approximate SBP reduction, range: 2–8 mm Hg

- Physical activity: Engage in regular aerobic physical activity such as brisk walking (at least 30 minutes per day, most days of the week).

Approximate SBP reduction, range: 4–9 mm Hg

- Moderation of alcohol: Limit consumption to no more than 2 drinks (1 oz or 30 mL ethanol [e.g., 24 oz beer, 10 oz wine, or 3 oz 80-proof whiskey]) per day in most men and to no more than 1 drink per day in women and lighter weight persons.

Approximate SBP reduction, range: 2–4 mm Hg

*For overall cardiovascular risk reduction, stop smoking. The effects of implementing these modifications are dose and time dependent, and could be greater for some individuals.

Source: Chobanian AV, et al: Seventh report of the Joint National Committee on Prevention, Detection, Evaluation, and Treatment of High Blood Pressure. Hypertension 42(6):1206–1252, 2003.

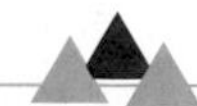

NURSING RESEARCH-BASED PRACTICE 9.1

Adding story-centered care to standard lifestyle intervention for people with stage one hypertension.

Liehr P, Meininger JC, Vogler R, Chan W, Frazier L, Smalling S, Fuentes, F: Adding story-centered care to standard lifestyle intervention for people with Stage one hypertension. Appl Nurs Res 19:16-21, 2006.

This study examined the blood pressure (BP) lowering effect of adding story-centered care (carefully attending to another's narrative) to standard lifestyle intervention (exercise training, nutrition counseling) for people with Stage 1 hypertension. Subjects ($N = 24$), who were university and hospital employees, were unmedicated and received standard lifestyle intervention; half were randomly assigned to story-centered care. Twenty-four hour BP was measured four times at 8-week intervals, twice before and twice after the intervention. Subjects who received story-centered care had greater decreases ($p < .05$) in awake systolic BP over the 6-month study period. Neither systolic nor diastolic sleep BP was significantly affected. Story-centered care showed promise for contributing to the BP-lowering effect of lifestyle intervention. Approaches for integrating story-centered care into the treatment of people with hypertension is challenging but warrants further attention.

nephropathy. In addition to public health programs, community-affiliated programs, including parish-based programs and neighborhood and work-site health promotion events, should be utilized to assist patients.

Special Considerations for Older Adults

Nearly one-half of all adults age 65 and older develop isolated systolic hypertension (ISH), defined as a SBP above 160 mm Hg with a normal DBP (86 or below), as a consequence of atherosclerotic thickening of the vessels. More than two-thirds of persons older than age 65 develop HTN in general. Given its frequency, the development of ISH is often viewed as an unavoidable part of aging, but clinicians should be aware that behavior-based therapies used to avoid and treat HTN can also help minimize age-associated increases in BP. Older adults benefit greatly from the treatment of ISH, yielding significant reduction in CHF and cardiovascular and cerebrovascular disease.

Even in persons older than 50 years of age, SBP greater than 140 mm Hg is a much more important cardiovascular disease risk factor than diastolic blood pressure. Patients with a normal BP at age 55 have a 90 percent lifetime risk for developing HTN. In a patient with a BP of 115/75 mm Hg, the risk of CVD doubles with each increment of 20/10 mm Hg.

Pharmacologic Therapy

Lifestyle modifications should be used for patients with prehypertension. No antihypertensive drug therapy is indicated if there is no other compelling indication other than the prehypertension. For most patients with stage 1 hypertension, in addition to lifestyle modifications, thiazide-type diuretics should be ordered. Thiazide diuretics continue to be recommended as first-line, proven antihypertensive drugs. These agents are useful in the presence of ISH as well as being inexpensive and an efficacious agent. They are also helpful with patients with osteoporosis as they help preserve bone density. Thiazide diuretics are well documented for reducing stroke and cardiovascular-related mortality and morbidity; however, the clinician should choose antihypertensive therapy with concurrent disease or comorbid conditions in mind. Examples of antihypertensive drugs that can be used in patients with concurrent disease include choices from the following groups:

- Angiotensin-converting enzyme inhibitors (ACEIs—drugs with generic names ending in -pril, such as captopril and enalapril) and perhaps angiotensin receptor blockers (ARBs) in the presence of heart failure, and MI with systolic dysfunction to help limit myocardial remodeling. These should be ordered when certain comorbid conditions including renal insufficiency and diabetes mellitus are present, and may assist in preserving or enhancing renal function.
- Angiotensin II receptor blocking agents (ARBs) are helpful in antihypertensive individuals with comorbid conditions such as heart failure and type 2 diabetes. Because they have a higher cost than ACEIs, and long-term research is lacking, ARBs should be reserved for patients who develop a cough when taking ACEIs.
- Beta-blockers (BBs—drugs with generic names ending in -lol, such as atenolol, nadolol, or propanolol) should be used in the presence of angina, post-MI (ability to reduce cardiac workload and enhance rhythm stability), atrial tachycardia (blunt tachycardia response), migraine headache (nonselective for reduction in frequency and severity of headache), and essential tumor (nonselective). These drugs may help to reduce the tremor resulting from blockage of beta-2 receptor sites.
- Long-acting dihydropyridine (DHP) calcium channel blockers (CCBs) are used in patients with ISH as well as in patients with hypertension and stable angina pectoris.
- Alpha-adrenergic antagonists (alpha-blockers) are usually effective in patients with benign prostatic hyperplasia as

they facilitate bladder emptying by decreasing prostate size.

- Additional drugs may include combination drugs, such as ACEIs and CCBs, ACEIs and diuretics, ARBs and diuretics, BBs and diuretics, drugs with central sympatholytic actions and diuretics, and combinations of diuretics. (See Drugs Commonly Prescribed 9.1.)

Initial therapy should consist of a low dose of the agent chosen. If the agent is well tolerated but BP control has not been achieved, the dose should be increased. If the BP continues to be elevated, and the patient is in stage 2 hypertension, a second antihypertensive agent should be added, preferably a low-dose diuretic. Because renal sodium retention increases as the BP drops, the addition of a low-dose thiazide diuretic to enhance sodium excretion may provide the added antihypertensive effect needed.

Small doses of two agents from different classes may have a synergistic effect in lowering BP while avoiding the problems of higher doses of either agent given alone and may possibly give additive therapeutic benefit (Table 9.1). These combination products may be appropriate for first-line antihypertensive therapy. In particular, a very low dose (12.5 mg) of hydrochlorothiazide (HCTZ) has the ability to potentiate the effect of other agents without producing negative metabolic effects.

If treatment continues to be ineffective, substitute another drug from a different class or add a second agent from a different class. If the desired effect has still not been achieved, continue to add drugs from other classes. A cardiologist should be consulted if the HTN remains uncontrolled.

Choosing the Best Drug. Most patients with HTN require two or more antihypertensive medications to achieve the goal blood pressure of less than 140/90 mm Hg, or less than 130/80 mm Hg for patients with diabetes or chronic kidney disease. If the blood pressure is greater than 20/10 mm Hg above the goal blood pressure, the clinician should consider prescribing two agents, one of which usually should be a thiazide-type diuretic.

Certain patient characteristics, including ethnicity, may influence the choice and efficacy of an antihypertensive agent. A common perception is that the best antihypertensive effect for African Americans and older adults with HTN can be achieved by using a combination of diuretics and calcium channel blockers. This should not be viewed, however, as a contraindication to using beta-blockers, ACEIs, or ARBs. Indeed, these drugs may offer significant benefit when concomitant disease is present or poses significant risk. Beta-blockers, ACEIs, and ARBs may be used in all groups; however, when these drugs are used in older adults and African Americans, higher doses may be needed and a longer period of time may elapse before the onset of action is seen.

An agent with once daily dosing (24-hour activity with at least 50 percent of action in the last 12 hours) is recommended. (See Drugs Commonly Prescribed 9.1.) The clinician should prescribe a once-daily dose, especially if patient adherence is a problem. This provides the patient with persistent, smooth control of HTN, and adherence to drug therapy is improved. In addition, with longer-acting formulas, there is less risk of hypertensive rebound resulting from a missed dose, providing protection against risk of stroke, MI, or sudden death from cardiac arrest induced by a dramatic increase in BP.

In certain clinical situations, some medications should be used with caution or are contraindicated because they may have unfavorable effects on comorbid conditions (Table 9.3).

Age-Related Concerns. Certain age-related physical changes predispose older adults to difficulty with HTN drug therapy. Because this group benefits significantly from control of HTN, the appropriate drug should be chosen with care and with consideration of particular factors including loss of baroreceptors, which increases the risk for postural HTN. As a result, BP should be measured with the patient in both standing and sitting positions. In addition, older adults should be instructed to change position slowly while on antihypertensive medication.

The force of myocardial contractility decreases with age, leaving older adults more sensitive to hypertensive medications with negative inotropic effects, such as beta-blockers. Because of lower circulating volume, diuretics, particularly effective antihypertensive agents for this age group, should be used in lower doses (12.5 mg HCTZ or its equivalent). Older adults usually have decreased renal excretory capacity; therefore, smaller doses of medications are required. The adage “start low and go slow” should be followed. The dose titration of antihypertensive drugs should be monitored closely with every dose adjustment.

Concurrent Use of Select Medications

Through their sodium-retaining effect, NSAID use can negate the BP-lowering effects of select antihypertensive medications such as ACEIs and diuretics. In addition, use of vasoconstricting medications such as decongestants (e.g., pseudoephedrine [Advil Cold and Sinus, Benadryl Allergy], phenylpropanolamine [Tavist D]), caffeine, and drugs of abuse (e.g., cocaine, amphetamines) can cause persistently elevated BP readings in spite of intervention. Excessive alcohol use may also prevent many antihypertensive medications from achieving full therapeutic effect. In addition, one of the first manifestations of alcohol withdrawal is BP elevation. Nicotine and many of the chemically active, vasoconstricting substances ingested with cigarette smoke can also contribute to inadequate BP control.

On occasion, a given clinical condition necessitates the use of a drug such as cyclosporine, erythropoietin, or certain antidepressants known to cause BP elevations. In this case, the antihypertensive therapeutic agent must be chosen with care and an adequate dose prescribed.

(Text continued on page 414)

Drugs Commonly Prescribed 9.1: Hypertension

Drug	Initial Dose	Dosage Range	Effective with Comorbid Conditions	Conditions Exacerbated by this Drug	Comments
Diuretics					
Thiazide diuretics					
Hydrochlorothiazide (HCTZ) (Hydro-Diuril)†	12.5 mg daily	25–50 mg once daily	Heart failure, diabetes type 2 (low dose only), osteoporosis	Gout, renal failure, hepatic impairment	Inexpensive, generally well tolerated; enhances efficacy of other HTN agents; avoid in pregnancy
Loop diuretics					
Furosemide (Lasix)	20 mg bid	40–320 mg in 2 or 3 doses		Renal stones, electrolyte imbalances, increases calcium excretion	Try HCTZ first if possible. Loop diuretics are poor antihypertensives by themselves.
Bumetanide (Bumex)	0.25 mg bid	0.5–10 mg in 2 or 3 doses			
Aldosterone receptor blockers					
Spironolactone (Aldactone)†	12.5 or 25 mg daily	12.5–100 mg once daily		Hyperkalemia, metabolic acidosis, gynecomastia	Useful in patients with refractory hypertension
Combination hydrochlorothiazide and triamterene Dyazide (25/50 mg)* and Maxzide (25/37.5 mg)†	1 tablet	1–2 tablets daily		Gout, renal and hepatic impairment, GI disturbances, hyperkalemia	Use in patients with need for potassium-sparing diuretic.
Beta-adrenergic blockers (BBs)			In general, most BBs effective with stable angina pectoris, post-MI, acute coronary syndromes, heart failure, hyperthyroidism, migraine headaches, arrhythmias, essential tremor, preoperative hypertension	Depression, impotence	Use cautiously in patients with pulmonary disease. May have adverse effects on lipid levels. May worsen hyperglycemia in diabetics. Use with caution with peripheral vascular disease.
Acebutolol (Sectral)	200 mg once daily	200–1200 mg in 1–2 doses			
Atenolol (Tenormin)†	25 mg	25–200 mg daily			
Bisoprolol (Ziac)*,†	5 mg/6.25 mg	2.5–10 mg plus 6.25 mg			
Carvedilol (Coreg)	6.25 mg	12.5–100 mg in 2 doses			
Metoprolol (Lopressor,	50 mg in 1–2 doses	50–200 mg in 1–2 doses			
Toprol-XL)†	50 mg	50–200 mg once daily			
Nadolol (Corgard)†	20 mg	20–160 mg once daily			
Propranolol (Inderal)	20 mg bid	40–320 mg in 2 doses			

(continued)

Drugs Commonly Prescribed 9.1: Hypertension (continued)

Drug	Initial Dose	Dosage Range	Effective with Comorbid Conditions	Conditions Exacerbated by this Drug	Comments
Angiotensin-converting enzyme inhibitors (ACEIs)				Hyperkalemia	Works well with African American patients, although may increase the risk of angioedema.
Benazepril (Lotensin)	10 mg once daily	5–40 mg in 1–2 doses	Diabetes, heart failure		
Captopril (Capoten)	25 mg bid	50–300 mg in 2–3 doses			
Enalapril (Vasotec)	5 mg once daily	5–40 mg in 1–2 doses	MI with systolic dysfunction		Avoid use in pregnancy. May cause chronic cough.
Fosinopril (Monopril)	10 mg once daily	10–80 mg in 1–2 doses	Chronic kidney disease		Effective for prevention of recurrent stroke.
Lisinopril (Prinivil, Zestril)†	5–10 mg once daily	5–40 mg once daily			
Angiotensin II receptor blockers (ARBs)				Hyperkalemia, angioedema, renal impairment	Avoid use in pregnancy.
Irbesartan (Avapro)†	150 mg once daily	150–300 mg once daily	Heart failure, MI with systolic dysfunction		
Irbesartan and HCTZ (Avalide)†	150 mg/12.5 mg once daily	150–300 mg/12.5 mg once daily			
Losartan (Cozaar)	50 mg once daily	25–100 mg in 1–2 doses	Diabetes, chronic kidney disease		
Losartan and HCTZ* (Hyzaar)†	50 mg/12.5 mg once daily	1–2 tablets once daily			
Valsartan (Diovan)†	80 mg once daily	80–320 mg once daily			
Valsartan and HCTZ* (Diovan HCT)†	80 mg/12.5 mg once daily	80–320/12.5–25 mg once daily			
Calcium channel blockers (CCBs)				Heart failure	All CCBs potentiated with grapefruit juice
Benzothiazepines					
Diltiazem (Cardizem LA)†	180–240 mg daily	180–540 mg daily	Stroke (CCBs have a protective effect)		CCBs may cause lower extremity edema.
(Cardizem SR)	90 mg bid	180–360 mg in 2 doses	Stable angina pectoris		Avoid in patients with recent MI or pulmonary congestion
(Dilacor XR)†	180 or 240 mg daily	180–480 mg daily			

(continued)

Drug	Initial Dose	Dosage Range	Effective with Comorbid Conditions	Conditions Exacerbated by this Drug	Comments
Dihydropyridines					
Amlodipine (Norvasc)†	5 mg daily	5–20 mg daily	Atrial tachycardia or fibrillation		Combination meds not for initial treatment.
(Lotrel-amlodipine plus benazepril)*	2.5 mg/10 mg daily	2.5 mg/10 mg, 5 mg/10 mg daily, 5 mg/20 mg, 10 mg/20 mg daily	Diabetes mellitus type 1 and 2		Amlodipine is the only CCB with established safety in patients with severe heart failure.
Felodipine					
(Plendil)†	5 mg daily	5–20 mg daily			
(Lexxel*-felodipine plus enalapril)	5 mg/2.5 mg	5/2.5 mg, 5/5 mg 1–2 doses daily			
Nifedipine					
(Adalat CC)†	30 mg daily	30–120 mg daily			
(Procardia XL)†	30–60 mg daily	30–120 mg daily			
Diphenylalkylamines					
Verapamil					
(Calan)	80 mg three times daily	80–360 mg in divided doses			
(Calan SR)	180 mg daily	180–480 mg in 1–2 doses			
(Verelan)†	120 mg daily	120–480 mg daily			
(Tarka-verapamil plus trandolapril)*,†	2/180 mg 1/240 mg daily	2/180 mg, 1/240 mg, 2/240 mg, 4/240 mg once daily			
Alpha-adrenoceptor blockers					
Prazosin (Minipress)	1 mg HS	2–20 mg in 2 or 3 doses	BPH	Orthostatic hypotension	Caution: Syncope common with first dose.
Terazosin (Hytrin)	1 mg HS	1–20 mg in 1 or 2 doses	Dyslipidemia	Sexual dysfunction	May positively affect lipid levels.
Doxazosin (Cardura)†	1 mg HS	1–16 mg daily			Provides short-term relief of BPH. Avoid use in pregnancy.

*Combination drugs.
†Once daily dosing.

Table 9.3 Antihypertensive Medications that are Contraindicated or to be Used with Caution

Drug	Contraindicated or Use with Caution	Comments
Beta-blockers	In asthma and obstructive pulmonary disease	Use with caution because of the risk or worsening bronchospasm.
Beta-blockers	In peripheral vascular disease (PVD)	Use with caution because of the risk of worsening claudication symptoms.
Beta-blockers (except carvedilol [Coreq])	In heart failure	Use with caution because of negative inotropic effects.
Calcium channel blockers (except amiodipine, felopine)		
Calcium channel blockers (shorter to intermediate acting; including SL nifedipine)	In heart failure, 2nd- and 3rd-degree block (unless pacemaker in place)	Use with caution because of possible risk of increased mortality.
ACE inhibitors and ARB	In pregnancy	Use with caution because of the risk of fetal hypotension and intrauterine fetal demise.
Diuretics (high dose)	In diabetes mellitus	Use with caution because of risk of increasing insulin resistance and negatively affecting glucose control.

Concurrent health problems that are inadequately treated may also affect the BP. The normal pain response includes vasoconstriction; therefore, inadequate control of both acute and chronic pain can cause a rise in BP.

Follow-Up and Referral

For the patient on lifestyle modification, a follow-up visit should be scheduled every 3 to 6 months to determine effectiveness and adherence to the regimen. If ineffective, pharmacologic therapy should be initiated. HTN can be controlled only if the patient is motivated. Using the Circle of Caring model and involving the patient in his or her own care may assist to increase motivation.

After initiation of antihypertensive therapy, a follow-up visit should be scheduled in 2 to 3 weeks for a BP check or even in 1 to 2 weeks for an electrolyte or side effect check. Once the BP goal is reached, visits can be scheduled every several months. More frequent visits may be needed if comorbid conditions exist. Serum potassium and creatinine levels should be monitored several times per year. Lifestyle modifications need to be stressed at each visit, particularly with vigorous promotion of tobacco avoidance. Low-dose aspirin therapy should be initiated when BP control is achieved. If aspirin therapy is started when the patient is still hypertensive there is a potential risk of hemorrhagic stroke.

Patient Education

A patient-directed interdisciplinary team approach is critical to successful HTN care. This team should include representatives from nursing, pharmacy, medicine, and nutrition for the continued education of the patient and family and therapeutic monitoring during antihypertensive therapy. This is stressed to improve patient adherence to behavioral and pharmacologic therapy.

The Framingham Scoring System (Box 9.1) is helpful to the clinician to evaluate the risk of patients for having an acute coronary event in the next 10 years. At a patient's annual visit, this risk assessment may be done by the clinician as a teaching tool to encourage patients to change behaviors such as smoking, exercise, and diet. A clinical example of using the Framingham Scoring System to evaluate the risk of a specific patient having an acute coronary event is provided in Box 9.1.

As this patient has a greater than 20 percent risk of having an acute coronary event in the next 10 years (Box 9.1), patient teaching is extremely important. Using the Circle of Caring, the patient will be involved with the clinician in addressing diet, exercise, smoking, and every modifiable risk factor that may be positively changed.

Numerous factors influence the efficacy of HTN therapy. Certain issues should be considered when HTN persists. Nonadherence to therapy is the most common reason for persistent HTN. The most common reasons for nonadherence are lack of perceived benefit of the intervention, difficulty with provider follow-up, and adverse effects of medication. The clinician must work with the patient to develop a plan of care that will meet therapeutic goals and fit with the patient's needs. Choosing well-tolerated drugs for intervention and continually acting as the patient's advocate and coach for lifestyle changes are critical.

Oral contraceptives may increase the blood pressure and the risk of HTN increases with the length of use. BP should be monitored regularly in women taking oral contraceptives. If a woman becomes hypertensive while taking oral contraceptives, the clinician should advise the patient to consider other forms of birth control.

The frequency of erectile dysfunction (ED) is significantly higher in men who are hypertensive than in men who are normotensive. If ED occurs, the antihypertensive

Box 9.1 Framingham Scoring System

An asymptomatic, overweight, 60-year-old man with untreated prehypertension, dyslipidemia, and smoking history presents for a yearly physical examination. He has no history of diabetes or CAD. The patient has a BMI (body mass index) of 27, BP of 138/83 mm Hg, and smoking status of one pack per day. What is his risk of an acute coronary event in the next 10 years?

Lipid Profile

Total cholesterol	271 mg/dL
Triglycerides	238 mg/dL
LDL	186 mg/dL
HDL	35 mg/dL

Framingham Point Score (male)

Risk Factors	Points	Risk Category Explanation
Age 60 (male)	10	
Total cholesterol	2	
HDL	2	
BP	1	
Smoking	1	
TOTAL POINTS	16 pts.	(see chart for meaning of score)
10 year risk = 25%		High risk; multiple risk factors; and greater than 20% risk of acute coronary event in next 10 years

Source: 2001 Third Report of the NCEP Expert Panel on Detection, Evaluation, and Treatment of High Blood Cholesterol in Adults. JAMA 285:2486–2497, 2001.

medication should be discontinued and treatment restarted with another agent. Hypertensive men should be advised that there is a lower risk of ED in men who are physically active, not obese, and nonsmokers. Therefore these lifestyle modifications should be encouraged for all men to forestall ED.

Because some older adults develop postural hypotension with hypertensive drug therapy, the clinician must insist that these patients change position slowly while on HTN medication, and that they sit on the edge of the bed for several minutes before standing. In addition, patients with postural hypotension should be urged to avoid volume depletion by drinking adequate quantities of water. Lifestyle modifications cannot be stressed enough. Teaching at every visit should reinforce the suggestions listed in Table 9.2.

Dyslipidemia

Dyslipidemia, also referred to as *hyperlipidemia*, is a general term for elevated concentrations of any or all of the lipids in the plasma. A major risk factor for CVD, increasing lipid levels positively correlate with a growing risk of ACS.

Epidemiology and Causes

The correlation between dyslipidemia and coronary events is well documented. Elevated lipid levels present the greatest risk factor for the development of CAD. In the United States CAD claims the lives of approximately 700,000 men and women each year. The Framingham Heart Study (the largest ongoing cohort study of heart disease in the United States) has documented that 40 percent of participants who developed an MI had a total cholesterol (TC) level between 200 and 250 mg/dL. A patient with a TC level greater than 259 mg/dL is three times more likely to develop CAD than a patient with a level less than 200 mg/dL. It is important to recognize that dyslipidemia is only one of the many factors that increases the risk of developing CAD. The greater the number of risk factors present, the greater the probability of developing clinically significant CAD.

Pathophysiology

Dyslipidemia is a heterogeneous metabolic disorder that involves levels of lipids and lipoproteins that increase risk of atherosclerosis. Lipoproteins are molecules that carry cholesterol in the bloodstream. Lipoproteins differ in size, density, atherogenicity, and are divided into several classes—very low density lipoprotein (VLDL), intermediate density lipoprotein (IDL), low-density lipoprotein (LDL), lipoprotein (a) (Lp[a]), and high-density lipoprotein (HDL). Atherogenesis is mediated by the lower density lipoproteins: Lp(a), VLDL, IDL, and LDL. These small LDL particles migrate into the inflamed region of the blood vessel wall, where they are oxidized and phagocytosed by macrophages to form foam cells, ultimately leading to the formation of fatty streaks and atherosclerotic plaques. LDL cholesterol (LDL-C) is the specific type of cholesterol that constitutes the lipid core of arteriosclerotic plaque deposits. In clinical analyses, Lp(a), LDL, IDL, and VLDL are combined into the single fraction of LDL. Desirable levels of LDL are dependent on the existence of other CVD risk factors (see Tables 9.4 and 9.5). Triglycerides (TGs) are large lipid molecules formed from dietary fats that also contribute to atherogenesis. To prevent cardiovascular disease, the desirable level of TG is less than 150 mg/dL (see Table 9.6).

Atherogenic forms of cholesterol–lipoprotein complexes include all types of non-HDL cholesterol- and triglyceride-transporting proteins: LDL, IDL, Lp(a), and VLDL. Total cholesterol in the blood arises both from ingested fats and liver synthesis. The measurement of total blood cholesterol is based on LDL-C, TG, and HDL-C. The following equation is used to calculate total cholesterol = LDL-C + TG/5 + HDL-C. The desirable level of total cholesterol in the blood is less than 200 mg/dL (see Table 9.7).

Table 9.4 LDL Classifications

LDL Cholesterol (mg/dL)	Classification of Level
<100	Optimal
100–129	Near optimal/above optimal
130–159	Borderline high
160–189	High
>190	Very high

Table 9.5 Classification of Serum Triglycerides

Normal	<150 mg/dL
Borderline high	150–199 mg/dL
High	200–499 mg/dL
Very high	>500 mg/dL

HDL cholesterol (HDL-C) is excreted and not deposited on the arterial wall. HDL removes excess cholesterol from blood vessels and delivers it back to the liver through reverse cholesterol transport. Once in the liver, cholesterol is excreted into the intestine as bile. HDL also plays a protective role by blocking the oxidation of LDL, which, in turn, inhibits atherogenesis. A low HDL level (less than or equal to 40 mg/dL) is considered a cardiovascular risk factor, whereas a high level of HDL-C (greater than or equal to 60 mg/dL) is considered cardioprotective (see Table 9.7). An HDL-C level less than or equal to 60 mg/dL is a negative cardiovascular risk factor, subtracting one factor from the total number of CVD risk factors.

Primary goals of treatment of dyslipidemia are lowering elevated LDL, lowering elevated TG, and raising suboptimal levels of HDL, which seek to prevent CVD development. Tables 9.4 to 9.7 show lipid values and classifications according to the Guidelines of the National Cholesterol Education Program, National Institutes of Health, National Heart, Lung and Blood Institute.

Dyslipidemia can also arise as a result of a genetic disorder such as familial hypercholesterolemia. Behavioral factors such as dietary consumption of fats and a lack of physical activity also play a role. This lipid disorder can be part of a constellation of abnormalities known as metabolic syndrome. Metabolic syndrome is characterized by abdominal obesity, glucose intolerance, insulin resistance, hyperinsulinemia, dyslipidemia, and HTN.

It is important to assess patients for secondary causes of dyslipidemia before instituting lipid-lowering treatment. Treatment of the primary disorder can correct the dyslipidemia. Secondary causes of dyslipidemia include obesity, diabetes mellitus, hypothyroidism, nephrotic syndrome, end-stage renal disease, hepatic disorders, excessive alcohol consumption, estrogen administration, Cushing's

Table 9.6 Total Blood Cholesterol Classifications

Total Blood Cholesterol (mg/dL)	Classification of Level
<200	Desirable
200–239	Borderline high
>240	High

Table 9.7 HDL Classifications

HDL Cholesterol (mg/dL)	Classification of Level
<40	Low
>60	High (optimal; cardio-protective)

syndrome, and glycogen storage disease. Certain drugs can cause lipid abnormalities such as thiazide diuretics, steroids, beta-blockers, HIV protease inhibitors, isotretinoin, and growth hormone.

In summary, dyslipidemia is a major risk factor for atherogenesis and cardiovascular disease. Elevated TG, low levels of HDL-C, and high levels of LDL particles characterize this disorder. The pathophysiology of metabolic syndrome is discussed here because dyslipidemia is a significant part of that syndrome. For more information on the metabolic syndrome, see Chapter 15.

Metabolic Syndrome

Metabolic syndrome is a common disease characterized by a combination of atherogenic and diabetogenic factors. Increased BMI, elevated systolic BP, hypertriglyceridemia, hyperglycemia, and low levels of protective HDL-C are found in affected persons. Any three of the above conditions occurring together can establish the diagnosis (Table 9.8). Etiology is unknown; however, environmental, genetic, and behavioral factors contribute to the development of metabolic syndrome, particularly physical inactivity and excess body fat. Elevated BMI is apparent as central obesity, with the affected individual demonstrating an "apple shape" or high waist circumference. Metabolic syndrome is also

Table 9.8 Components of the Metabolic Syndrome

Risk Factor (three required for diagnosis)	Defining Level
Abdominal obesity	Waist circumference
Men	>40 inches
Women	>35 inches
Triglycerides	>150 mg/dL
HDL-C	
Men	< 40 mg/dL
Women	< 50 mg/dL
Blood pressure	≥ 130 / ≥ 85 mm Hg
Fasting glucose	> 110 mg/dL

Source: From the Expert Panel on Detection, Evaluation, and Treatment of High Blood Cholesterol in Adults. Executive Summary of the Third Report of the National Cholesterol Education Program (NCEP). JAMA 285;2486–2497, 2001.

a proinflammatory and prothrombotic disorder causing endothelial injury, as evidenced by elevations of C-reactive protein (CRP), increased platelet aggregation, and increased fibrinogen levels. In addition to hyperglycemia and deranged lipid metabolism, peripheral tissues are resistant to insulin. The pancreas oversecretes insulin to overcome tissue resistance, which results in hyperinsulinemia. Obesity enhances insulin resistance and predisposes the individual to type 2 diabetes mellitus.

Obesity is believed to significantly contribute to the development of metabolic syndrome. The National Cholesterol Education Program (NCEP) recommends obesity as the primary target for intervention. Abdominal obesity is defined as a high waist-to-hip ratio. Weight loss improves serum lipid profiles, reduces blood pressure, decreases insulin resistance, and ameliorates glucose intolerance.

Clinical Presentation

Subjective

Typically, the patient may present without symptoms when diagnosed with dyslipidemia. Often, however, concurrent problems exist, such as HTN or CAD.

Objective

The clinician, on noting an abnormal lipid profile, may be the first to diagnose dyslipidemia in the unsuspecting patient. Physical examination may reveal a carotid bruit and corneal arcus. In some forms of dyslipidemia, yellowish skin deposits of cholesterol called xanthomas may occur. These deposits commonly occur around the eyelids (xanthelasma) and extensor tendons. Interestingly, even with effective lipid-lowering therapy, these deposits tend not to regress.

Diagnostic Reasoning

Diagnostic Tests

The third Adult Treatment Panel guidelines from the National Cholesterol Education Program (ATP III NCEP) of the National Heart, Lung, and Blood Institute (NHLBI) recommends that beginning at age 20, adults have a fasting lipid profile that includes TC, LDL, HDL, and TG level every 5 years. Determination of cardiovascular risk is based on the Framingham scoring system, which calculates the 10-year risk of coronary events. Points are allocated based on age, gender, total cholesterol level, smoking status, HDL cholesterol level, and systolic BP. (An example is shown in the HTN section.) Patients are classified at highest risk if they have any of the following disorders: known CAD, diabetes, mellitus, peripheral vascular disease, abdominal aortic aneurysm, carotid artery disease, or a 10 year risk of a coronary event of more than 20 percent as determined by the Framingham scoring system. The scoring system can be found at http://www.nhlbi.nih.gov/guidelines/cholesterol/-profmats.htm.

Even if a patient exhibits only some of the risk factors, more frequent analyses should be considered. Once dyslipidemia is diagnosed, frequent analyses must be done to monitor the progress of treatment.

A TC level gives only a slanted view of the overall health of the artery. It is essential to obtain a lipid profile to evaluate the relationship between the LDL and HDL. If the set of laboratory findings seems inconsistent with what the clinician suspects, a second determination should be done. If the first two LDL tests differ by more than 30 mg/dL, a third test should be obtained within 1 to 8 weeks and the average value of the three tests should be used.

Differential Diagnosis

Some potential causes of secondary dyslipidemia are listed in Table 9.9. Elevated TC levels may be present in CAD, type II familial hypercholesterolemia, idiopathic hypercholesterolemia, obstructive jaundice, biliary cirrhosis, hypothyroidism, von Gierke's disease, pregnancy, uncontrolled diabetes mellitus, other pancreatic disease, chronic nephritis, glomerulosclerosis, and obesity. Decreased TC levels may be present in malabsorption, starvation, liver disease, severe cell damage, HTN, chronic anemia, Tangier disease, and drug therapy with agents such as adrenal corticotrophic hormones and antibiotics.

Elevated TG levels may be present in liver disease, alcoholism, nephrotic syndrome, renal disease, hypothyroidism, uncontrolled diabetes mellitus, pancreatitis, gout, glycogen storage disease, MI (increased levels may last for 1 year), metabolic diseases related to endocrinopathies, von Gierke's disease, stress, high carbohydrate diet, and HTN. Decreased triglyceride levels may be present in malnutrition, hyperthyroidism, exercise, and malabsorption syndrome.

An elevated HDL level may be associated with chronic liver disease or chronic intoxication, long-term aerobic exercise or vigorous exercise, and estrogen and birth control pills. A decreased HDL level may be caused by hypertriglyceridemia, hypothyroidism, end-stage liver disease, diabetes mellitus, obesity, chronic inactivity, uremia, and homozygous Tangier disease.

An increased LDL level may be the result of familial hypercholesteremia and secondary causes such as diet high in cholesterol and saturated fat, nephrotic syndrome,

Table 9.9 Potential Causes of Secondary Hyperlipidemia

Causes	Lipid Abnormality
Inactivity	HDL ↓
Alcohol abuse	TG ↑, HDL ↑, LDL ↑
Diabetes mellitus	TG ↑, HDL ↓, TC ↑
Hypothyroidism	TG ↑, TC ↑
Thiazide diuretic use (high dose)	TC ↑, LDL ↑, TG ↑
Beta-blocker use (high dose)	LDL ↑, HDL ↓
Chronic renal insufficiency	TC ↑, TG ↑

chronic renal failure, pregnancy, porphyria, diabetes mellitus, multiple myeloma, steroids, and estrogens. A decreased LDL level may be the result of malnutrition and malabsorption syndromes.

An increased VLDL level may be caused by familial hyperlipidemia and secondarily by alcoholism, obesity, diabetes mellitus, chronic renal disease, pancreatitis, pregnancy, estrogen, birth control pills, and progestins. A decreased VLDL level may be the result of malnutrition and malabsorption syndromes.

Management

The principal goal of treatment is to decrease lipid levels to normal or below normal, depending on the number of risk factors for CAD present, and to prevent the sequelae of CAD, angina, and MI. Table 9.10 lists the lipid goals and treatment guidelines from the NCEP ATP III.

Diet

Initially, if the patient has borderline dyslipidemia, a cholesterol-lowering diet is recommended. Diets very low in total fat or in saturated fat, however, may lower HDL cholesterol as much as LDL cholesterol. A sensible nutritional approach is the best recommendation. Most nutritionists advocate reducing total fat to 25 to 30 percent and saturated fat to less than 7 percent of calories. Dietary cholesterol should be limited to less than 200 mg/day. This will replace fat, particularly saturated fat, with carbohydrate, usually result in fewer total calories consumed, and facilitate weight loss in overweight patients. The Mediterranean diet as well as omega-3 fatty acids found in certain fish have been shown to decrease cholesterol levels in some patients.

The current recommendation for patients with evidence of CAD is to keep the LDL cholesterol level less than 100 mg/dL. In the past, patients with no risk of CAD and LDL cholesterol above 130 mg/dL were candidates for lipid-lowering management. Recent research has suggested that even patients with moderate degrees of LDL cholesterol elevation (100 to 130 mg/dL) can benefit from aggressive treatment aimed at achieving levels of LDL less than 100 mg/dL. NCEP guidelines with each renewal keep recommending lower LDL goals. At present driving LDL levels down to or below 70 is not recommended. Desirable serum HDL levels should be more than 40 mg/dL, and the LDL-to-HDL ratio should be less than 3.5.

If the patient is trying diet therapy alone, a 3- to 6-month trial period should be sufficient to determine if this therapy will be effective in reducing lipid levels. If the patient is unable to achieve the desired effect, pharmacologic therapy should be initiated. Many authorities recommend aggressive management with drug therapy to ward off the sequelae of CAD.

Pharmacologic Therapy

For years, diet has been the cornerstone of treatment for hyperlipidemia; however, recent studies have demonstrated that diet alone is often insufficient in lowering cholesterol. To achieve LDL levels less than 100 mg/dL, pharmacologic therapy is often required. One risk factor for CAD is hyperhomocysteinemia, which is estimated to occur in 30 percent or more individuals with CAD. Folic acid (400 mg qd) and vitamin B_6 (pyridoxine) supplementation (200 mg qd) reduce homocysteine levels and may prove to be a beneficial and cost-effective treatment for patients with premature atherosclerosis. The Federal Drug Administration

Table 9.10 Lipid Goals and Treatment Guidelines from the NCEP ATP III

Risk Category	LDL Cholesterol Goal	Recommended Treatment
Very high risk: CVD plus diabetes, high blood pressure, and cigarette smoking, or metabolic syndrome	<70 mg/dL	If LDL cholesterol is ≥ 100 mg/dL, initiate lifestyle modification and drug therapy
High risk: CVD, diabetes, or multiple risk factors with a 20% chance or MI in 10 years	<100 mg/dL	If LDL, cholesterol is ≥ 100 mg/dL, initiate lifestyle modification and drug therapy
Moderately high risk: Two or more risk factors with a 10%–20% chance of MI in 10 years	<130 mg/dL (<100 mg/dL = ideal)	If LDL cholesterol is ≥ 100–129 mg/dL, treat with lifestyle modification and drug therapy
Moderate risk: Two or more risk factors with a chance or MI in 10 years of less than 10%	<130 mg/dL	If LDL cholesterol is ≥ 160 mg/dL, treat with lifestyle modification and drug therapy
Low risk: Zero or one risk factor	<160 mg/dL	If LDL cholesterol is ≥ 190 mg/dL, treat with lifestyle modification and drug therapy

Source: Grundy, SM, et al: Implications of recent clinical trials for the National Cholesterol Education Program Adult Treatment Panel III Guidelines. Circulation 110:227–239, 2004.

(FDA) mandates that grains be fortified with folic acid to reduce neural tube defects in infants may also have a positive impact on the incidence of premature vascular disease in the United States.

The 3-hydroxy-3 methylglutaryl coenzyme A (HMG-CoA) reductase inhibitors (medications with generic names ending in -statin) are the first-line drugs of choice in the majority of patients. The most commonly used statins include fluvastatin (Lescol), lovastatin (Mevacor), pravastatin (Pravachol), simvastatin (Zocor), and atorvastatin (Lipitor). Most statins reduce LDL levels by 30 to 40 percent; however, atorvastatin (Lipitor) reduces LDL levels by 40 to 60 percent and has been shown to have the greatest effect on lowering of TGs. There is no effect on homocystine, and the liver is the major route for excretion.

Adverse effects of the statins include elevations of liver enzymes to levels more than three times normal, which warrants discontinuation of the statin; however, patients may be restarted at lower doses after the liver enzyme levels return to normal. Monitoring should be done at 6 to 12 weeks, then every 6 months. The clinician should caution patients about use of statins with other hepatoxic drugs and alcohol consumption. Other adverse effects include muscle weakness and, in extreme cases, rhabdomyolysis with significant elevations in serum creatine phosphokinase (CPK, creatine kinase) levels. Gastrointestinal complaints include dyspepsia and abdominal pain.

Once the initial dose of statin medication has been prescribed, the clinician must consider whether to increase the dose or add another agent. The addition of oral niacin (1 to 2 g per day) or a low dose of a bile-acid sequestrant (e.g., cholestyramine, colestipol) may produce a greater reduction in LDL than simply increasing the dosage of the statin medication. The antibiotic neomycin (2 g per day) may also be used to bind bile acids, thus lowering LDL levels via a mechanism similar to the bile acid sequestrants. Niacin, however, is associated with significant flushing, hot flashes, and pruritus, although this may be countered by pretreatment with NSAIDs, such as aspirin or ibuprofen 30 to 60 min before each dose. In addition, bile acid sequestrants may be complicated by gastrointestinal side effects such as nausea, bloating, and elevations in serum liver enzymes. However, a low-dose combination regimen may reduce adverse effects of any single agent. Low-dose regimens may also increase compliance because of reduced medication cost.

The fibric acid derivatives fenofibrate (200 mg PO qd with food) and gemfibrozil (600 mg PO bid) are currently approved in the United States for lipid-lowering therapy, with their most profound effects being decreases in triglyceride levels by 35 to 50 percent and increases in HDL by 15 to 25. Clofibrate, an additional drug from this class, is now avoided because of its association with cholangiocarcinoma. The fibrates' main side effect are myopathies, which are enhanced in the presence of concurrent statin therapy. CPK levels should be checked if a patient complains of myalgias to help determine whether these agents should be stopped.

Ezetimibe (Zetia; 10 mg PO qd) reduces dietary as well as biliary cholesterol absorption directly at the intestinal surface, likely via effects on cholesterol transport proteins within the intestinal brush border. However, absorption of TGs and the fat-soluble vitamins A, D, E, and K is not affected. Ezetimibe is often used in combination with a first-line statin drug. However, warnings have been issued citing adverse effects of ezetimibe similar to those of the statins, including musculoskeletal pains, rhabdomyolysis, and liver enzyme elevation (drug-induced hepatitis).

Drugs Commonly Prescribed 9.2 presents commonly used cholesterol-lowering drugs.

Follow-Up and Referral

The clinician should be very well equipped to treat the patient with hyperlipidemia. Consultation with a nutritionist may be recommended if the patient cannot follow or understand a cholesterol-lowering diet. The patient on diet therapy alone should be seen at monthly intervals to monitor weight and encourage the patient to reach the desired goal. Patients who have been started on statins must return in 6 to 12 weeks for liver function tests (LFTs), dosage adjustment, or commencement of combination therapy. Once LFTs have been verified to be within a normal range, the patient may then return at 6-month intervals for several visits, then yearly, to monitor the progress with lipid profiles.

Patient Education

It is important for the clinician to provide ongoing support and reinforcement to patients undertaking both dietary and pharmacologic therapy for dyslipidemia. Many patients do not like to take medications and feel that diet alone is sufficient to keep them "under control." Sometimes, showing the patient the lab results and having a discussion about what the numbers mean, especially the ratio of HDL to TC, in terms of the risk of having an MI, is an effective way to get the patient to take a hard look at potential benefits of combined therapy. In addition, discussing the patient's Framingham Heart Score to predict the risk of having an acute coronary event might help to motivate a patient in adhering to a diet, exercise, and drug treatment program. Using the Circle of Caring Model, patients can be encouraged through the highs and lows that typically occur when initiating long-term changes.

Coronary Heart Disease (Atherosclerotic Coronary Artery Disease)

Coronary heart disease (CHD), also referred to as coronary artery disease (CAD), is the leading cause of death in the United States, responsible more than one in five or approximately 700,000 deaths per year. Mortality from CAD has declined over the years because of patient education regard-

Drugs Commonly Prescribed 9.2: Hyperlipidemia

Drug	Dosage: Initial Daily Dose	Dosage: Maximum Daily Dose	Effect on Lipids	Comments
HMG-CoA reductase inhibitors (statins)				
Atorvastatin (Lipitor)	10 mg daily	80 mg daily	LDL: –25 to –40% HDL: +5% to +10% TG: ↓	Monitor liver function tests before initiating therapy and 12 weeks after.
Fluvastatin (Lescol)	20 mg daily	40 mg daily	LDL: –20% to –30% HDL: +5% to +10% TG: ↓	Do not use with gemfibrozil. Take in evening.
Lovastatin (Mevacor)	10 mg daily	80 mg divided	LDL: –25% to –40% HDL: +5% to +10% TG: ↓	Side effects: myositis (especially in patients taking fibrates or niacin)
Pravastatin (Pravachol)	20 mg daily	40 mg daily	LDL: –25% to –40% HDL: +5% to +10% TG: ↓	
Simvastatin (Zocor)	5 mg daily	80 mg daily	LDL: –25% to –40% HDL: +5% to +10% TG: ↓	
Nicotinic acid Niacin (Niaspan)	100 mg daily	3–4.5 g divided	LDL: –15% to –25% HDL: +25% to +35% TG: ↓	Flushing or pruritus common. Flushing may be decreased with ASA 81–325 mg or another NSAID 30 min prior to dose. Take with food. Avoid alcohol and hot drinks at dosing. May potentiate effects of antihypertensives. Use with caution with anticoagulants (monitor PT and platelet counts).
Bile acid sequestrants				
Cholestyramine (Questran)	4 g bid	24 g divided doses	LDL: –15% to –25% HDL: +5% TG: same or ↑	Mix with liquids.
Colesevelam (WelChol)	625 mg, 6–7 tablets at once	Same	LDL: –10% to –20% HDL: +10% TG: same or ↑	GI symptoms common, with constipation and gas. Use psyllium to prevent.
Colestipol (Colestid)	5 g bid	30 g divided doses	LDL: –15% to –25% HDL: +5% TG: same or ↑	
Folic acid derivatives Fenofibrate (Tricor)	160 mg daily	Same	LDL: –10% to –15% HDL: +15% to +20% TG: ↓	Take with food. Side effects greater when taking other lipid lowering agents. Side effects: cholelithiasis, hepatitis, and myositis. When taken with a statin, increased risk of myopathies.
Gemfibrozil (Lopid)	600 mg daily	1200 mg divided doses		
Cholesterol absorption inhibitor Ezetimibe (Zetia)	10 mg daily	10 mg daily	LDL: –15% to –20% HDL: < +5% TG: same or ↑	Long-term effects not yet established.

ing risk factors and early recognition and treatment of symptoms; management of existing problems such as HTN, dyslipidemia, and diabetes; and because of improved technologies such as thrombolytic drugs.

Epidemiology and Causes

Risk factors for CAD are classified as nonmodifiable, modifiable, or contributing and are listed in Risk Factors 9.1. Nearly 13 million Americans have CAD, and the incidence increases with age. More than 10 times the number of women die from CVD each year than from breast cancer.

The narrowing of the coronary arteries as a result of atherosclerosis causes angina. A thrombus, coronary artery vasospasm, aortic stenosis, aortic insufficiency, severe HTN, or idiopathic subaortic hypertrophic stenosis may also cause angina. Angina is the number one symptom of CAD. Angina is the presenting symptom in CAD in 38 percent of men and 61 percent of women. Middle-aged and older men and postmenopausal women are most prone to developing angina. Variant angina may occur in patients with normal coronary arteries who have cyclically recurring angina at rest that is unrelated to effort. Unstable angina tends to last longer and have greater intensity than the pain of stable angina.

RISK FACTORS 9.1

Coronary Artery Disease (CAD)

Category	*Risk Factors*
Nonmodifiable	Male gender Increasing age Family history or CAD African-American race
Modifiable	Hypertension (>140 mm Hg SBP and/or ≥90 mm Hg DBP) Smoking Sedentary lifestyle Hyperlipidemia (total cholesterol [TC] >200 mg/dL, high-density lipoprotein [HDL] <40 mg/dL, with optimal levels ≥60 mg/dL, low-density lipoprotein [LDL] >130 mg/dL, with optimal levels at ≤ 100 mg /dL, TC to HDL ratio >7.5) For women: natural or surgical menopause without estrogen replacement therapy; oral contraceptive use combined with cigarette smoking
Contributing	Diabetes mellitus Obesity Stress

Pathophysiology of Arteriosclerosis and Coronary Artery Disease

The coronary arteries perfuse the dynamic cardiac muscle with oxygenated blood as needed for energy. The coronary arteries must be capable of dilation to deliver sufficient blood flow to the myocardium with the changing energy needs of the heart pump. In addition, the lumen of each coronary artery needs to be patent to transport blood flow without impediment. In CAD, arteriosclerotic plaque hinders optimal blood flow and dilation of the coronary arteries. Coronary arteries become obstructed and incapable of vasodilation which severely impedes perfusion of the myocardium. During physical exertion, when the myocardium requires increased blood flow, the limitations of the coronary arteries become most apparent. Coronary artery blood flow becomes insufficient for the oxygen demands of the myocardium.

This coronary insufficiency, in turn, leads to ischemia of heart muscle. Ischemia creates anaerobic conditions for the myocardium, particularly if acute occlusion results. Anaerobic metabolism yields inadequate energy (approximately 5 percent of normal) for myocardial demand, allowing for less than a 20-minute period of tissue viability post-occlusion. Lactic acid is created as a waste product, leading to localized tissue acidosis. Irritating to muscle tissue, lactic acid build-up is the source of chest pain in ischemic heart disease. The term *angina pectoris* means *chest pain* due to ischemia of the heart muscle. If myocardial ischemia is prolonged, MI ensues. Thus, if untreated, CAD progresses to ischemia of the heart muscle or angina pectoris, which can then lead to MI.

Atherosclerosis (arteriosclerosis) is a systemic disease affecting all arteries of the body. If CAD is diagnosed, it is likely that arteriosclerosis is present throughout all arterial systems. Likewise, if vascular disease is identified in target end-organs, CAD is likely to already be present. The process of arteriosclerosis begins with endothelial injury which can be incited by a number of etiologic agents. Free radicals, HTN, hyperglycemia of diabetes, and hyperlipidemia have been found to be agents of injury to arterial endothelial cells. Endothelial injury provokes an inflammatory reaction that attracts T cells, macrophages, monocytes, and platelets to the site. White blood cells secrete mediators, such as interleukins (ILs), tumor necrosis factor-alpha (TNF-α), and C-reactive protein (CRP) which perpetuate the inflammatory reaction. Platelets aggregate and form microthrombi. Inflammation is now thought to be the major force that drives atherosclerosis. This is supported by elevated levels of *high sensitivity C-reactive protein (hs-CRP),* an inflammatory marker, in individuals with coronary arteriosclerosis.

Inflammation of the endothelium depletes nitric oxide, a major vasorelaxant of the arterial muscle wall. This depletion results in a net vasoconstrictive effect. Other pro-inflammatory mediators stimulate proliferation of vascular smooth muscle within the arterial wall which intensifies the vasoconstrictive effect further. Concurrently, macrophages within the vessel wall engulf and ingest LDLs, forming "foam cells." The disruption of the arterial endothelium by inflammation, lipid-laden macrophages, platelets, and vasoconstricting mediators are the initiating events of arteriosclerosis or atherogenesis.

In the process of atherogenesis, an initial fatty streak on the arterial wall evolves over time, serving as a nidus for fibrin deposition to become a fibrous, calcified plaque. "*Arteriosclerosis*" means "*hardened arteries,*" which is an apt term for the rigid arteries resulting from long-term plaque formation. Arteries lose significant vasodilation capacity and are lined by calcified arteriosclerotic plaque. The lipid-rich, calcified plaque becomes brittle, unstable, and easily ruptures with mechanical stress. When disruption of the plaque occurs, this induces platelet aggregation and activation of the coagulation cascade. A thrombus forms at the site that can embolize, lodge, and obstruct the lumen of narrowed arteries. In patients who die of unstable angina or MI, pathologic studies find that death occurs as a result of ruptured plaque with associated thrombosis. Obstruction due to thrombosis is the most common cause of ischemia in *any* arterially supplied region of the body. Common sites of arteriosclerosis are the coronary arteries, cerebral arteries, and peripheral arteries of the lower extremities. Consequently, ischemia-prone regions of the body are the myocardium, brain, and lower extremities. Prolonged, severe episodes of ischemia can lead to MI, ischemic stroke, and peripheral arterial insufficiency.

Clinical Presentation

Subjective

In most patients, CAD develops many years before the patient is aware of its existence. Because collateral circulation develops, the patient is usually unaware that anything is wrong unless other concomitant conditions are present, such as dyslipidemia or HTN. Typically, symptoms of CAD are not reported until 75 percent of the coronary artery is narrowed. Eventually, if CAD is uncorrected, the patient will usually present with exertional angina, which should lead the clinician to suspect CAD. Associated symptoms may include radiation of the discomfort to the left arm and jaw, nausea, shortness of breath, and light-headedness (syncopal episodes).

Objective

The clinician should note all the peripheral pulses; auscultate for carotid bruits; note jugular venous distension (JVD); take the BP sitting, lying, and standing; and examine the skin condition for evidence of decreased perfusion. The history should include a detailed description of other risk factors that are present, which will guide further assessment for resultant problems such as angina. (Pertinent questions related to angina are covered later in this chapter.) Because atherosclerosis is a widespread problem, patients with CAD also have a much higher incidence of PVD and cerebrovascular disease than other individuals. The clinician should assess for other symptoms that suggest vascular insufficiency such as intermittent claudication or TIAs.

Diagnostic Reasoning

Diagnostic Tests

An ECG, stress test, nuclear scanning, and angiography may be ordered to determine the extent of the CAD and which vessels are affected. ECGs are discussed in detail in the section on Myocardial Infarction.

An exercise ECG, or a stress test, may be ordered to detect and evaluate CAD. Carefully controlled and supervised exercise increases the myocardial oxygen demands, which assists in evaluating the coronary arteries' ability to meet the increased demands successfully. When the patient is unable to achieve a vigorous level of exercise, a dipyridamole thallium-201 test may be used. It may produce false-positive readings, especially in women, and in cases of certain drugs and electrolyte imbalances. A stress test is contraindicated in acute CVD (e.g., MI, unstable angina, or heart failure) because the heart cannot respond to an increased demand for oxygen.

Nuclear scanning (technetium-99m ventriculography) studies the motion of the left ventricular wall and measures the ventricle's ability to eject blood, referred to as the ejection fraction (normally 55 to 75 percent). When ischemia is present because of a narrowed coronary artery, the segment of the myocardium it serves exhibits diminished wall motion (hypokinesis) or contractility that is represented as pooled blood within the ventricular and atrial chambers.

Contrast-enhanced CT scan imaging is a noninvasive imaging method of assessing overall "plaque burden." The extent to which atheromatous plaque undermines the integrity of an artery wall is termed "plaque burden." Estimating "plaque burden" can assess the risk of atheromatous plaque to rupture and cause ischemia. This CT scan, also termed CT calcium scoring, can evaluate the overall burden of calcified atherosclerotic plaque.

A cardiac catheterization with angiography for coronary artery visualization is performed, commonly after the patient is stabilized in acute coronary syndrome (ACS) or if there is high suspicion of ACS. Visualization of the coronary arteries confirms diagnosis of CAD and can evaluate the extent of stenosis of coronary arteries.

Ultrasonography can be used with cardiac catheterization to add diagnostic information. Intravascular ultrasonography (IVUS) used during cardiac catheterization measures "plaque burden" through real-time intraluminal imaging of vessel walls. IVUS can also be used to assess plaque regression when the patient is on antilipemic drug therapy.

Because arteriosclerosis is a chronic inflammatory condition, the biomarker CRP is commonly elevated in individuals with CAD. CRP is an acute phase inflammatory protein produced by the liver and by the smooth muscle cells within arteriosclerotic coronary arteries. An elevated level of CRP found on the laboratory test, hs-CRP (high-sensitivity C-reactive protein), has been shown to be an independent predictor of risk of MI, stroke, peripheral arterial disease, and sudden cardiac death. Measurement of hs-CRP adds to the total cardiac risk assessment of the patient and should not be solely relied on as a confirmatory test.

Epidemiologic studies show that an elevated level of the amino acid homocysteine is an independent risk factor for arteriosclerosis and CAD. Homocysteine requires folic acid, vitamin B_6, and vitamin B_{12} for its metabolism. The amino acid accumulates in the blood and injures the endothelium when there are inadequate levels of the B vitamins and folate for its proper metabolism. Therefore, elevated serum homocysteine levels add to the cardiac risk assessment of a patient.

Differential Diagnosis

Differential diagnoses for CAD include GI, pulmonary, or cardiac problems that are not related to ischemia. Gastroesophageal reflux disease (GERD), esophageal spasm, or biliary colic can present with symptoms similar to MI or angina. Patients with CAD or MI often present with epigastric pain that is misinterpreted as "heartburn" or related pain. This misinterpretation is often the reason for a patient's delay in obtaining prompt medical evaluation.

Patients with anxiety or panic attacks often present to the emergency department with symptoms which mimic angina or MI. Extreme stress can precipitate chest pain, dizziness, dyspnea, and hyperventilation which mimic the symptoms of angina or MI. Costochondritis, a musculoskeletal problem, can also present as chest pain that may be misinterpreted as CAD by patients. The pain of costochondritis can usually be reproduced by pressing on the sternum and costochondral regions of the chest.

Persons with diabetes may experience angina or silent MI with minor symptoms or no symptoms at all. Patients with CAD may experience nausea and vomitng, dyspnea, epigastric pain, diaphoresis, or dizziness with no complaint of chest pain. These symptoms are referred to as "anginal equivalents." Women experiencing angina or MI commonly present with "anginal equivalents" rather than with chest pain. Historically, clinicians have underestimated the risk of CVD in women. Atypical presentation of ACS in women contributes to lack of early recognition of cardiac symptoms by both patients and clinicians. Women classically delay seeking medical care for ischemic symptoms, which contributes to their overall higher morbidity and mortality with cardiac events.

Pneumothorax, pneumonia, pericarditis, pulmonary embolism, mitral valve prolapse, and aortic dissection are other less common causes of chest pain. The diverse causes of pain and that of ischemic chest pain (angina) must be determined. Because chest pain is so often the impetus to the diagnosis of CAD, the pain characteristics that drive the differential diagnoses need to be carefully assessed. In a young otherwise healthy adult, reproducible point tenderness is likely musculoskeletal chest wall pain and not ischemic. Pleuritic pain worsens on inspiration and is likely from lung pathology such as pneumonia, especially if accompanied by fever and productive cough. Clinicians need to have a high level of suspicion and complete a thorough cardiac risk assessment to rule out MI in all patients complaining of chest pain or symptoms known as "anginal equivalents."

Management

The principles of management include establishing the diagnosis, controlling the symptoms, and preventing the disease progression that may lead to MI or sudden death. During a cardiac catheterization, fibrinolytic agents may be infused directly into an occluded coronary artery in an attempt to restore coronary blood flow. Other therapeutic approaches may include balloon angioplasty, stent placement, and coronary artery bypass graft (CABG). A stent-like prosthesis requires the use of anticoagulants after 4 to 8 weeks.

Risk-Factor Modification

Risk-factor modification is essential to stop the progression of CAD. This involves aggressive lowering of lipid levels (which is discussed in the Dyslipidemia section), strict glycemic control in patients with diabetes (see Chapter 15), aggressive antihypertensive therapy (discussed in the Hypertension section), smoking cessation (see Chapter 8), and modifying the lifestyle to include regular exercise, stress reduction, and a heart-healthy diet (less than 300 mg cholesterol and 7 percent or less of total calories from saturated fatty acids).

Complementary Therapies 9.1 presents suggested vitamin, mineral, and herbal supplementation for various cardiovascular disorders.

Pharmacologic Therapy

Pharmacologic agents are used to control the symptoms of angina and to prevent subsequent events (see discussion in the Angina Pectoris section). Most clinicians recommend low-dose daily aspirin (81 to 325 mg) to decrease the incidence of a first MI in middle-aged men and women. Coated aspirin is recommended for individuals with gastric problems. The dose should be decreased if there is a tendency to bruise. There is still controversy regarding dosage and concomitant use if patients are on other anticoagulants.

Follow-Up and Referral

Patients need to understand the chronicity of this disease and be committed to frequent follow-ups for control of risk factors. The clinician should refer the patient to a cardiologist for a stress test and for any further cardiac workup indicated by the results.

COMPLEMENTARY THERAPIES 9.1

Cardiovascular Disorder	Supplement	Dosage	Comments
Angina	Hawthorn: active ingredient is vitexin-2′-rhamnoside	100–250 mg tid	May potentiate the effects of antihypertensives, ACE inhibitors, digitalis drugs, and nitrates.
	Magnesium	200 mg qd	Prevents coronary artery spasm
Arteriosclerosis/ Atherosclerosis/ Hyperlipidemia	Beta-glucans	2 tablespoons oat bran, or 3 tablespoons of dry oatmeal	Soluble fiber that decreases cholesterol
	Selenium	200 mcg qd	Selenium is an antioxidant that helps limit the oxidation of LDL cholesterol. Found in nuts, meat, seafood, sunflower seeds.
	Vitamin B complex	B-50 (B12 50 mcg; Folic acid 400 mcg; 50 mg all other B vitamins) 1 tablet bid with food.	Decreases homocysteine
	Vitamin B_3—Niacin	500 mg inositol hexaniacinate tid	This form of niacin not only lowers LDL, and triglycerides, but also raises HDL cholesterol.
	Vitamin C	800–1000 mg qd	Vitamin C is an antioxidant that may help prevent the oxidation of LDL cholesterol.
	Vitamin E	400 IU qd	Prevents oxidation of LDL cholesterol—research on heart disease prevention continuing. Doses over 800 IU may inhibit absorption of other vitamins and may interfere with blood clotting.
	Flaxseed oil	1 tablespoon of oil in the morning (2.5 g)	High in alpha-linolenic acid (Omega-3 fatty acids) and linoleic acid (Omega-6 fatty acids); also has some anti-inflammatory properties.
	Garlic	400–600 mg qd	Active ingredient is allicin. May decrease blood clotting
	Lycopene	10 or more servings of tomato products per week	Antioxidant—may prevent oxidative damage of free radicals.
Congestive Heart Failure	Coenzyme Q_{10}	100 mg/bid	Antioxidant—prevents cell damage by free radicals. Strengthens heart muscle
Hypertension	Calcium	1000–1500 mg qd	
	Magnesium	400 mg qd	Relaxes vascular smooth muscle thereby decreasing BP
	Flaxseed oil	1 tablespoon of oil in the morning (2.5 g)	High in alpha-linolenic acid (Omega-3 fatty acids) and linoleic acid (Omega-6 fatty acids); also has some anti-inflammatory properties
	Hawthorn	100–250 mg tid	May potentiate the effects of antihypertensives, ACE inhibitors, digitalis drugs, and nitrates.

Sources: Bascom, A: Incorporating herbal medicine into clinical practice. FA Davis, Philadelphia, 2002. http://www.wholehealthmd.com

Blumenthal, M, Goldberg, A, and Brinckmann, J (eds): Herbal medicine expanded Commission E Monographs. Newton, Mass. American Botanical Council, Austin, Tex; Integrative Medicine Communications, 2000.

Table 9.11 Types of Angina

Type of Angina	Characteristics
Stable	Chest pain: Transient episodes related to activities that increase myocardial oxygen demand. Duration: Typically lasts 3–15 min. Associated signs and symptoms: Nausea, vomiting, shortness of breath. Relief: rest and/or nitroglycerin tablets.
Unstable	Chest pain: Similar to stable angina but more severe and brought on with less exertion; may occur at rest. Duration: Prolonged. Associated signs and symptoms: Nausea, vomiting, shortness of breath, diaphoresis. Relief: Not relieved by rest and/or nitroglycerin tablets; relieved by morphine.
Variant (Prinzmetal's)	Chest pain: Episodes unrelated to activities that increase myocardial oxygen demand. Duration: Cyclic; often occurs during sleep (most common in early morning hours); pain intensifies quickly and lasts longer than that of stable angina. Associated signs and symptoms: Palpitation, syncope, bradycardia. Relief: May subside with exercise.

Source: Adapted from Sommers, MS, and Johnson, SA: Davis's Manual of Nursing Therapeutics for Diseases and Disorders. FA Davis, Philadelphia, 1997, with permission.

Patient Teaching

On each visit, the clinician should stress risk-factor modification. The lifestyle modifications listed in Table 9.2 for managing hypertension are good activities for overall cardiovascular health.

Acute Coronary Syndromes

Acute coronary syndrome (ACS) is a term used for the disorders of myocardial ischemia—stable angina, unstable angina, variant angina (Prinzmetal's), or MI. While ACS really refers to acute conditions, stable angina is covered in this section. While angina pectoris (chest pain related to ischemia of the myocardium) is described as chest discomfort, the pain may radiate elsewhere. S*table angina* (chronic exertional) is a diagnosed condition of myocardial ischemia that is predictable in pattern and frequency and controlled with medication.

Unstable angina is myocardial ischemia that is newly diagnosed or previously diagnosed angina that has changed in pattern, frequency, or severity. Unstable angina is commonly a forerunner of acute MI. Table 9.11 presents the types of angina and their characteristics.

A *myocardial infarction* (MI) is necrosis or death of part of the myocardium as a result of prolonged ischemia (an insufficient supply of oxygenated blood). The location and extent of the infarction determines the prognosis in addition to the speed with which reperfusion is supplied to "cut-off" areas. Because the use of early reperfusion therapy increases the likelihood of survival and improves left ventricular function, the patient with a suspected MI should be assessed rapidly and prompt, appropriate care provided.

Epidemiology and Causes

About 1.5 million MIs occur annually in the United States. The mortality rate is approximately 30 percent for a severe MI. More men than women experience MIs, and the majority (55 percent) occur in individuals who are older than 65 years of age. Eighty percent of patients who die from an MI are older than age 65. Men have about a 20 percent chance of having an MI or CAD. MIs are more common in Western societies. African Americans have a higher incidence of MI, which is probably related to the fact that African Americans have a higher incidence of HTN, a major contributing factor to an MI.

The contributing factors for an MI include the same risk factors as for CAD (see Risk Factors 9.1), as well as tachycardia, left ventricular hypertrophy (LVH), anemia, increased platelet aggregation, and abuse of illegal substances.

Pathophysiology of Acute Coronary Syndromes

Acute coronary syndrome (ACS) is a broad term to describe a continuum of disorders that arise from coronary artery occlusion. ACS is either an episode of angina pectoris or a MI. In both angina and MI, decreased myocardial perfusion occurs because of coronary artery narrowing caused by thrombus formation subsequent to rupture of atherosclerotic plaque. In stable angina, coronary occlusion causes brief ischemia which is treatable. In unstable angina, coronary occlusion leads to ischemia with high risk for MI. When ischemia is prolonged, MI occurs. The two types of MI are classified according their electrographic changes—NSTEMI (non-ST-segment elevation myocardial infarction) and STEMI (ST-segment elevation MI). NSTEMI indicates an infarction caused by a *nonocclusive* thrombus which *partially* interrupts perfusion of the myocardium. NSTEMI indicates an infarction affecting only part of the myocardial wall, rather than full thickness. STEMI, an ST-segment elevation MI, is caused by an *occlusive* thrombus that leads to complete *transmural* MI—an infarction of the full thickness of the myocardial wall. The majority of MIs are due to nonocclusive thrombi that cause partial wall infarctions.

After myocardial ischemia occurs, anaerobic metabolism becomes the predominate form of energy production in the affected cardiac tissue. Anaerobic metabolism yields low energy that can sustain the heart tissue only for a maximum of 20 minutes. Death of myocardial tissue (infarction) occurs as energy requirements are not met by anaerobic metabolism, thus underscoring the importance of acute beta-blocker therapy in the management of MI to decrease cardiac workload and myocardial oxygen demand. Moreover, lactic acid, a waste product of anaerobic metabolism, is noxious to surrounding cells, further disrupting cell function.

The pharmaceutical treatment of ACS is directed primarily at dissolution of the intracoronary thrombus by antiplatelet (e.g., aspirin, glycoprotein IIb/IIIa receptor antagonists), anticoagulant therapy (e.g., heparin), and relief of symptoms by anti-anginal (e.g., nitroglycerin, beta-blockers, supplemental oxygen therapy) and analgesic (morphine sulfate) medications. After MI is confirmed, urgent evaluation for salvage of viable myocardial tissue is initiated through reperfusion treatments based on coronary angiographic studies.

An infarcted region of the myocardial wall is an area of necrosis that disrupts the conduction system and decreases the strength of the heart muscle as a mechanical pump. *Dysrhythmias* and *heart failure* are common sequelae of MI. The more damage to the heart muscle, the greater the risk of heart failure. *Papillary muscle rupture* is also a common complication that results from MI. Heart valve leaflets are attached to papillary muscles via stringlike membranous attachments called chordae tendineae. Disrupted papillary muscles and ruptured chordae tendineae cause valvular dysfunction that may manifest as a heart murmur due to turbulent blood flow. MI of the LV with papillary muscle rupture can cause dysfunction of the mitral valve, and mitral regurgitation is a common complication of left ventricular MI.

Clinical Presentation

Subjective

With angina the patient will complain of chest discomfort that may be described as pressure, tightness, burning, or heaviness. The pain may radiate to the arms, chest, back, neck, jaw, or teeth. Patients frequently describe the discomfort as indigestion because it may be accompanied by nausea or vomiting. Shortness of breath and diaphoresis may also be present, either at rest or with physical activity. The patient may also be anxious, light-headed, and tachycardic. The pain may frequently occur after meals because of increased oxygen consumption during the meal, or it may be brought on by psychological stress. Rest and nitroglycerin, either sublingual (SL) or spray, may relieve the symptoms of stable angina. The patient may be in denial and will often rationalize that the symptoms are caused by indigestion or overexertion.

In acute MI, the patient often complains of angina-like chest pain lasting more than 20 minutes but occasionally waxing and waning during that period. Often, dyspnea, diaphoresis, nausea, and dizziness are also reported. Radiation of the pain to the neck, jaw, shoulder, or arm (left more often than right) is usually described. The degree of distress with these symptoms varies greatly, however, from the patient who complains of an "elephant standing on my chest" to the patient who is apologetic for seeking assistance with "just a bit of indigestion that will not clear up." In particular, women, older adults, and persons with diabetes mellitus are likely to have minimal or atypical symptoms with an acute MI.

About 15 percent of patients suffer a painless MI that may either be detected on a future ECG or on autopsy or if the patient presents with other symptoms that prompt the clinician to question the possibility of an MI. This occurs more often in an older patient or a patient with diabetes or HTN. In this instance, the patient may complain of dyspnea, general upper abdominal pain, exacerbation of heart failure, or acute confusion.

Objective

In a patient with angina, the clinician may auscultate a transient third (S3) or fourth (S4) heart sound, a transient mitral regurgitant murmur, and/or a carotid arterial bruit. The patient should be asked to describe the pain in terms of its quality, location, radiation, precipitating factors, alleviating factors, and associated signs and symptoms during the attack. In addition, the patient may appear dyspneic and be diaphoretic.

In a patient with a MI, the clinician may observe pallor, cool, diaphoretic skin, crackles on auscultation, a third (S3) or fourth (S4) heart sound, murmurs, edema of the extremities, and possibly neck vein distension. In addition, the patient may have a low-grade fever. The presence of diaphoresis with chest pain is particularly worrisome, often indicating a significant drop in cardiac output during the episode of pain and subsequent decreased perfusion of the skin.

The cardiac examination should include inspection, palpation, and auscultation. As with any physical examination, the cardiac exam should begin with the general survey, in which the clinician begins to develop a picture of the overall health status of the patient and continues to gather diagnostic clues.

Diagnostic Reasoning

Diagnostic Tests

The best laboratory tests to rule out MI are cardiac-specific troponin I and T (cTnI and cTnT). Cardiac troponins are cardiac proteins released from dead heart muscle and they are not detected in the blood of healthy individuals. Troponin levels rise within the first 2 to 4 hours after MI and remain elevated for 7 to 10 days.

Serum cardiac enzymes, which include the specific MB isoenzyme of CPK, are also released from necrotic heart muscle after MI. The CPKmb isoenzyme level rises within 4 to 8 hours after MI and generally returns to normal by 48 to 72 hours. The other cardiac enzymes are serum glutamic oxaloacetic transaminase (SGOT) and lactate dehydrogenase (LDH). These become elevated much later in the course of MI and are not indicators of acute MI.

A blood level of the CPKmb fraction remains elevated in the blood more briefly than cardiac troponin. Therefore, episodes of recurrent ischemic discomfort and recurrent MI are more readily diagnosed with a rise in CPKmb fraction. The prolonged elevation of cardiac troponins does not allow recognition of repeat episodes of acute MI within the first few days after the initial insult. The rise in CPKmb fraction correlates better with infarct size than does troponin level. If the diagnosis of MI remains uncertain, serum cardiac biomarkers should be measured on admission, at 6 to 9 hours post-admission, and again after 12 to 14 hours.

Myoglobin is a muscle protein that rises in the blood within only a few hours after MI. It is one of the earliest serum cardiac markers to rise after MI, however, it is nonspecific for cardiac muscle death and can rise with skeletal muscle injury. Blood levels return to normal within 24 hours of infarction and cannot be relied on for diagnosis of MI.

Other laboratory tests which include complete blood count (CBC), erythrocyte sedimentation rate (ESR), serum electrolytes, blood urea nitrogen (BUN), and serum creatinine should be drawn. Leukocytosis is a nonspecific indicator of myocardial injury. White blood cell counts often reach levels of 12,000 to 15,000/μL. ESR, a general indicator of inflammation, also rises after MI and remains elevated for several days.

After the patient is stabilized, cardiac catheterization with angiography is a procedure that gives clinicians significant prognostic information. When the patient is assessed angiographically, coronary artery occlusion can be estimated along a scale called the Thrombolysis in Myocardial Infarction (TIMI) grading system. The TIMI scale grades coronary artery occlusion from grade 0, indicating complete occlusion, to grade 3, indicating full perfusion of the coronary artery within full normal flow.

In addition, radionuclide imaging can detect reversible ischemic regions or fixed infarcted areas. Radionuclide substances are distributed in proportion to myocardial blood flow. This type of myocardial perfusion imaging reveals a "cold spot" during the first few hours after MI. However, it cannot distinguish acute MI from the scarring of the myocardium from an MI suffered in the past.

Also, echocardiography can be done to detect wall motion abnormalities, right and left ventricular function, valvular or septal defects, and LV ejection fraction. Echocardiography is a noninvasive procedure that is easily performed, however, it is not recommended as a relaible diagnostic test of MI.

12-Lead Electrocardiogram (ECG). Although chest pain can be caused by a number of conditions, assessing for life-threatening cardiac conditions such as angina and acute MI is critical. In the emergency clinical setting, a 12-lead ECG can reveal either myocardial ischemia, ST-segment elevation MI (STEMI), non-ST segment elevation MI (NSTEMI), or dysrhythmias.

An ECG should be performed promptly: The presence of an ST-segment elevation greater than 1 mm in contiguous leads usually indicates acute coronary artery occlusion, usually from thrombosis. In addition, clinically significant ST-segment elevation largely dictates reperfusion therapy. The ECG will further delineate the location of the MI and its corresponding coronary artery.

Ischemic and injured cells have an altered action potential and altered patterns of depolarization and repolarization. Infarcted cells have no action potential, which leads to changes in the ECG.

Myocardial ischemia is demonstrated by enlargement and inversion of the T wave caused by altered late repolarization. The ischemic area remains depolarized when adjacent areas have returned to the resting state. Myocardial injury is demonstrated by ST-segment changes. With epicardial injury, injured cells depolarize normally but repolarize more rapidly than do normal cells. This causes an elevation in the leads facing the areas of injury. In endocardial injury, the ST segment is more likely to be depressed (usually 1 mm or more) in the leads facing the injury. The decision to proceed with thrombolytic therapy is based in large part on the presence of ST-segment elevation in two or more ECG leads. Because of the absence of depolarization of the cells in the area of an acute MI, Q waves show up about 1 to 3 days following the infarction. An abnormal Q wave is usually 0.04 seconds wide and 25 percent or greater in depth than the R wave is tall. Figure 9.1 presents the typical serial ECG changes seen with an acute MI.

At times, myocardial perfusion halts temporarily, then is reestablished in a relatively short period of time. This may be the result of vessel spasm or sudden drop in BP, such as with severe blood or fluid loss. In this situation, a small portion of subendocardial tissue is damaged, yet adjoining myocardial tissue remains viable. As a result, ECG changes are present but differ significantly from those in a classic transmural MI. Q waves do not form because electrically active tissue backs up the area of infarction. Because tissue injury, ischemia, and infarction are subendocardial rather than oriented toward the epicardium, as in transmural MI, injury pattern is reflected in ST-segment depression. The ECG changes are transient—present only during the acute event and during tissue healing. Thus, if not found during the acute presentation, a non–Q wave MI may never be diagnosed. There may be a temptation to think of a non–Q wave MI as a "small heart attack" with limited long-term

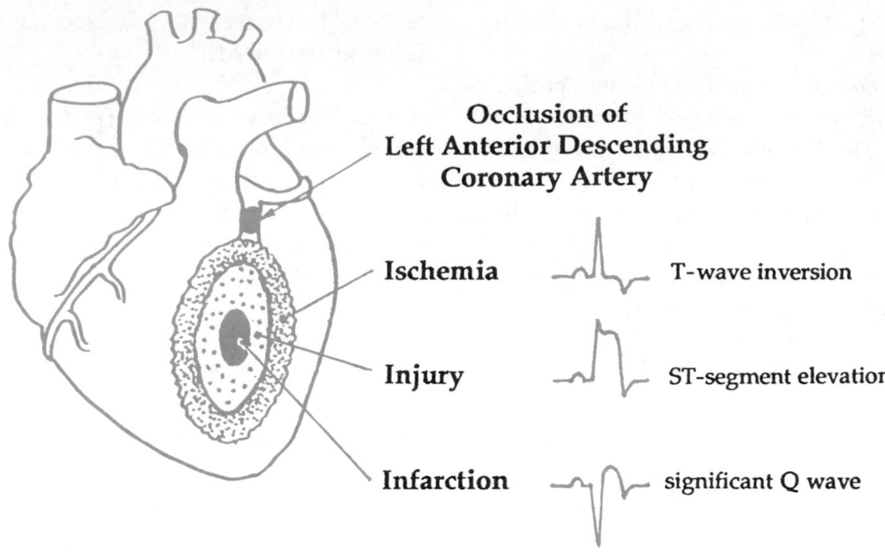

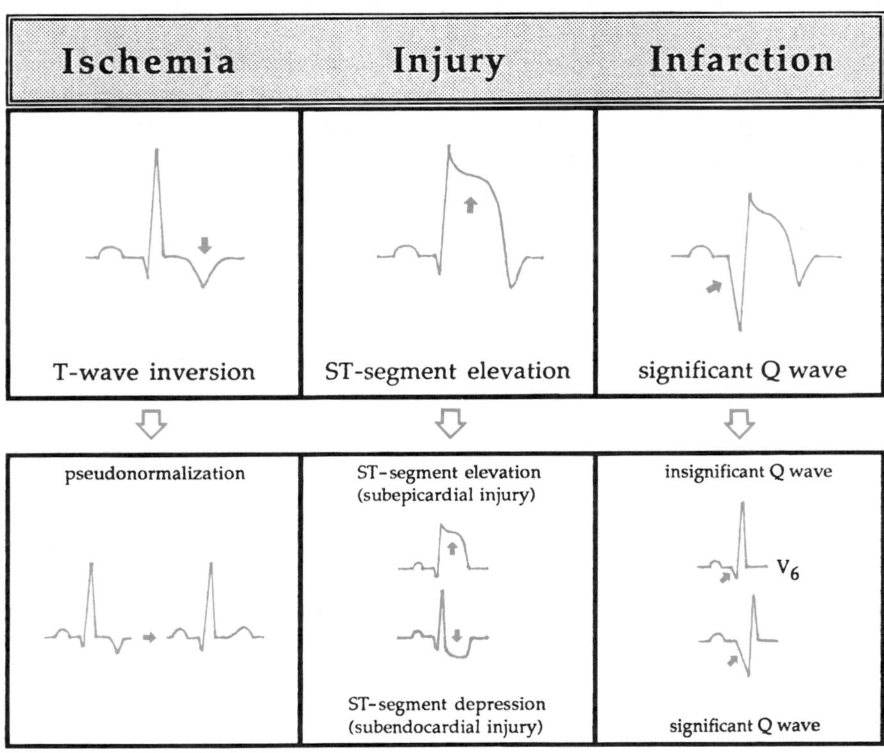

FIGURE 9.1 Typical ECG changes seen with an acute myocardial infarction. (Source: Lipman, B, and Cascio, T: ECG Assessment and Intervention. FA Davis, Philadelphia, 1994, with permission.)

sequelae. These patients have well-demonstrated risk for future MI and other cardiac events, particularly during the next 3 to 6 months. The majority of patients with non–Q wave MIs are older adults (age 70 or more) with a history of prior MI and CHF. Figure 9.2 illustrates the difference between Q wave and non–Q wave MIs.

The 12-lead ECG presents 12 leads, or "views," of the heart, to detect myocardial damage. Leads I, II, and III are the three standard (bipolar) leads. Leads aV_R, aV_L, and aV_F are augmented or unipolar leads; the chest or precordial leads (V_1 to V_6) view the heart in a horizontal plane. Figure 9.3 shows the normal ECG wave configuration of a normal 12-lead ECG.

By identifying the leads that contain the ECG changes, the location of the myocardial damage and its corresponding coronary artery can be determined (Table 9.12).

The 12-lead ECG can also provide information about axis deviation. Electrical axis is, for all practical pur-

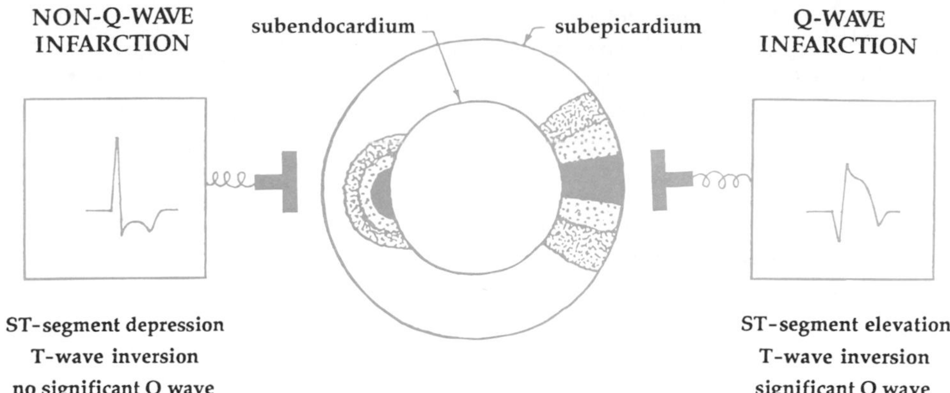

FIGURE 9.2 Q wave versus non-Q wave myocardial infarction. (Source: Lipman, B, and Cascio, T: ECG Assessment and Intervention. FA Davis, Philadelphia, 1994, with permission.)

poses, synonymous with the wave of myocardial depolarization. Healthy myocardial tissue depolarizes in a predictable pattern; therefore recording in the ECG a predictable electrical axis. The normal wave of depolarization travels down the heart and to the left. This normal axis shows as a positive QRS complex in lead I and lead aV_F. This is because the net ventricular forces travel toward the pole of lead I and down toward the pole of lead aV_F.

With cardiac disease, the wave of depolarization swings away from areas of damage or necrosis, creating axis deviation, or a change from the norm. When the axis is shifted to the left, the QRS complex is positive in lead I and negative in lead aV_F. Left axis deviation is subdivided into normal left axis deviation (NLAD) and abnormal left axis deviation (ALAD). NLAD is often seen in the presence of LVH. ALAD is seen in a block of the anteriosuperior division of the left bundle branch, often referred to as a left anterior fascicular block (LAFB). ALAD is also seen in Q wave inferior-wall MI and a right apical pacemaker. Right axis deviation (RAD) is seen in a block of the posterior inferior division of the left bundle block, often referred to as a left posterior fascicular block (LPFB). RAD is also caused by an extensive Q wave lateral-wall MI and may be seen in right ventricular hypertrophy (RVH).

Axis deviation is occasionally present in the absence of cardiac disease. In pregnancy, the heart is shifted in the cavity because of the height of the diaphragm. This may cause a left axis deviation. In addition, adults with abdominal obesity may demonstrate left axis deviation. In infants and children and tall, thin adults right axis deviation is normal. Advanced Assessment 9.2 presents a quick quadrant method for determining axis deviation.

The 12-lead ECG may also provide information about heart chamber enlargement. Chamber enlargement or hypertrophy is usually a consequence of obstruction of blood flow out of the affected area of the heart. For example, left atrial hypertrophy is a common consequence of mitral valve stenosis because the atrium must generate excessive

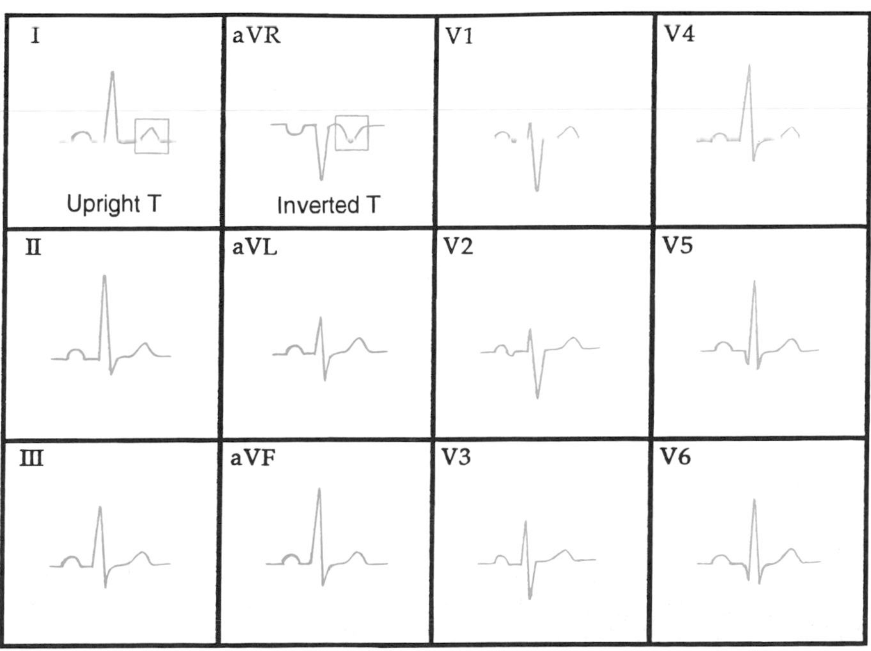

FIGURE 9.3 The normal 12-lead ECG. (Source: Lipman, B, and Cascio, T: ECG Assessment and Intervention. FA Davis, Philadelphia, 1994, with permission.)

pressure, thereby becoming enlarged, as a result of forcing open a stiff, diseased valve. The following are the typical ECG findings:

- Right atrial hypertrophy (RAH), also known as P pulmonale
  - Peaked P wave in leads II, III, aV_F, V_1
  - P wave more than 2.5 mm in leads II, III, aV_F
- Left atrial hypertrophy (LAH), also known as P mitrale
  - Notched P wave more than 0.10 seconds in leads II, III, aV_f
  - Prominent negative P terminale in V_1 (more than 1:1)
- Right ventricular hypertrophy (RVH)
  - Reversal of R wave progression in the precordial leads
  - Although not routinely seen, RVH may be seen in patients with COPD.
- Left ventricular hypertrophy (LVH), which uses the Estes Scoring System:
  - 3 points for any or all of the following: voltage of 25 mm or more (S wave in V_1 or V_2; R wave in V_5 or V_6 and/or voltage of 20 mm or more (R or S wave in leads I, II, III, aV_F, aV_L)
  - 1 point for secondary ST-segment T-wave changes if the patient is taking digitalis
  - 3 points for secondary ST-segment T-wave changes if the patient is not taking digitalis
  - 3 points for an abnormal P terminal in V_1
  - 2 points for left axis deviation
  - 1 point for an RS interval of more than 0.09 seconds
  - 1 point for ventricular activating time in V_5; 0.05 seconds or more in V_6.

If the patient has 4 points, there is the probability of LVH; 5 points is a strong indication of LVH.

Differential Diagnosis

Differential diagnoses for angina may include an acute MI, esophagitis, esophageal spasm, peptic ulcer, gastritis, cholecystitis, costochondritis, pericarditis, aortic dissection, pulmonary embolus (PE), pulmonary HTN, pneumothorax, anxiety, and panic disorders.

Differential diagnoses for MI include pericarditis, myocarditis, acute aortic dissection, pneumothorax, PE, acute cholecystitis, esophageal spasm, unstable angina, biliary tract disease, and panic attack.

Management

In ACS, the goal is to promptly diagnose and treat the underlying condition appropriately. In the primary care setting, the clinician can attempt to stabilize the patient with ASA and nitroglycerin. However, the patient experiencing ACS needs to be transferred to a hospital emergency medical setting, preferably one with access to a cardiac catheterization lab.

Stable Angina

If a patient presents with ischemic chest pain and nitroglycerin and rest relieve the chest pain, the result implies stable angina. Chronic anginal pain is typically of short duration, usually 3 to 5 minutes, but may last up to 30 minutes or longer. For a patient with chronic stable angina who is currently having an attack, rest and nitroglycerin should be ordered. Nitroglycerin may be given as a tablet SL (Nitrostat 0.3, 0.4, or 0.6 mg) or spray SL (Nitrolingual 0.4 mg). One tablet or one spray should be used under the tongue every 5 minutes for three doses. If the pain has not been relieved after three doses, the local emergency medical services system should be called and the patient transported immediately to the ED.

After the patient's chest pain has been relieved, a beta-blocker and/or long-acting nitrate may be prescribed. Beta-blockers decrease myocardial oxygen demand by interfering with the effects of the sympathetic nervous system on the beta-1 receptors in the heart. Long-acting nitrates, topical or oral, may be added to the beta-blocker regimen to decrease myocardial oxygen supply by coronary artery vasodilation. Many beta-blockers may be used such as atenolol (Tenormin) 50 mg qd; nadolol (Corgard) 40 mg qd initially with a maintenance dose of 80 mg qd; or propranolol (Inderal) 80 mg qd initially in two divided doses, with a maintenance dose of 120 to 240 mg in two doses daily.

Table 9.12 Location of Myocardial Infarction

Location of MI	Leads	Reciprocal Changes	Coronary Artery Affected
Anterior	V_2–V_4	II, III, aV_F	Left anterior descending (LAD)
Anteroseptal	V_1–V_3	None	LAD
Anterolateral	I, aV_L, V_4–V_6	II, III, aV_F	LAD, left circumflex
Inferior	II, III, aV_F	I, aV_L	Right coronary artery (RCA) in 80%–90% left coronary artery (LCA) in 10%–20%
Posterior	V_1–V_3	R wave greater than S wave, depressed ST segment, elevated T wave	RCA, left circumflex
Lateral	I, aV_L, V_5–V_6	V_1–V_2	Left circumflex

> ## ADVANCED ASSESSMENT 9.2
> ### Assessing Axis Deviation
> The quadrant method is a rapid, accurate way of assessing electrocardiogram (ECG) electrical axis. Although it does not yield an exact degree measurement, such as obtained when using an ECG ruler, this method can be done without the use of special equipment. When using the quadrant method, do the following:
> - Examine leads I and aV_F for the presence of a positive or negative QRS complex
> - Determine the results as:
>
>   Normal axis: positive complex (tall R wave) in leads I and aV_F
>
>   Left axis deviation: positive complex (tall R wave) in lead I; negative complex in aV_L
>
>   Right axis deviation: negative complex in lead I, R in aV_F
>
>   Extreme right axis deviation: negative complex in lead I and aV_F

Long-acting nitrates, topical or oral, may include the nitroglycerin transdermal patch (Transderm), supplying 0.1, 0.2, 0.4, 0.6, or 0.8 mg/hour. The patch should be in place for 12 hours and removed for 12 hours. Isosorbide dinitrate (Isordil Titradose) is another good long-acting nitrate that is taken orally. The initial dosage should be 5 to 20 mg q4 to 6h PO. Maintenance dosage is 10 to 40 mg q6h. There should be a daily dose-free interval of at least 14 hours. All of the aforementioned doses may be taken daily as prophylaxis to prevent recurrent angina.

All patients with diagnosed angina should be placed on daily aspirin therapy to help prevent coronary thrombosis. Aspirin (ASA) 81 to 325 mg qd may be taken (use coated ASA if gastric problems exist). Ticlopidine (Ticlid) 250 mg bid with food may be ordered for patients who are allergic to aspirin or those with a history of GI bleeding.

Unstable Angina

With unstable angina, the goal is to diagnose the underlying condition and treat appropriately. If rest and nitroglycerin do not relieve the chest discomfort, the patient must be immediately transported by ambulance to the ED for further evaluation. Treatment Flowchart 9.1 presents the management of unstable angina.

Variant (Prinzmetal's) Angina

Prinzmetal's angina is an atypical form of angina pectoris that occurs as a result of vasospasm of otherwise normal coronary arteries. Pain is experienced at rest, and an ECG, when taken during the attack, will indicate ST-segment elevation rather than depression. This ECG change will abate when the patient is treated with nitroglycerin (see previous section) and drugs that influence calcium metabolism. A calcium channel blocker such as verapamil HCl (Calan) 80 to 120 mg tid (40 mg in older adults or lightweight patients). Increase daily or weekly if needed to a maximum of 480 mg daily.

Myocardial Infarction

The goal of management is to salvage the ischemic myocardium before it becomes necrotic by reperfusing the area as soon as possible. After that, the goal becomes directed at preventing future attacks.

If an MI is suspected at the time of a clinical visit, a 12-lead ECG should be done promptly. Immediate interventions of rest, aspirin, and nitroglycerin administration should be implemented. Nitroglycerin can be administered sublingually as a tablet or spray. If relief is not achieved within 2 to 3 minutes after the initial dose of nitroglycerin, a second or third dose can be given at 5-minute intervals for a total of three doses. A 162- to 325-mg aspirin tablet can also be administered in the ambulatory clinical setting. Aspirin exerts an antiplatelet effect, and nitroglycerin decreases preload and coronary spasm, thus contributing to the overall beneficial effect in an acute MI. The patient should initially chew one aspirin and then take one by mouth. This initiation of thrombolytic therapy given at the time of onset (within 70 minutes) of the symptoms, before hospitalization, has lowered the mortality rate of patients.

The patient should then be transferred to an emergency medical setting. The clinician should begin an IV, provide oxygen, and monitor the patient until the emergency medical system (EMS) can be activated. Once the patient is stabilized, emergency care clinicians can determine if the patient is a candidate for reperfusion treatment with thrombolytic agents or primary percutaneous coronary intervention (PCI). They should be used only for patients with acute MI associated with ST-segment elevation (STEMI) or with left bundle branch block (LBBB). Thrombolytic agents, such as alteplase (recombinant tissue plasminogen activator [tPA]), reteplase (rPA), or tenecteplase (TNK), are most effective when administered early in the course of an MI. The first thrombolytic agent, streptokinase, is not commonly used as it is non-fibrin-specific. For the BEST therapeutic effect, thrombolytics should be administered within the first 3 hours (ideally 30 minutes) of presentation of symptoms of MI. Studies have shown that thrombolytic therapy can be of benefit up to 12 hours after initial presentation of symptoms of MI. Alternatively, thrombolytic therapy can be combined with antiplatelet agents known as glycoprotein IIb/IIIa inhibitors.

Cardiac catheterization with angiography can decipher whether or not the patient is a candidate for reperfusion therapy, percutaneous translumninal coronary angioplasty (PTCA), coronary artery stenting, or coronary artery bypass grafting (CABG). Immediate coronary angiography and primary PCI which includes stenting, of the infarct-related

TREATMENT FLOWCHART 9.1

UNSTABLE ANGINA

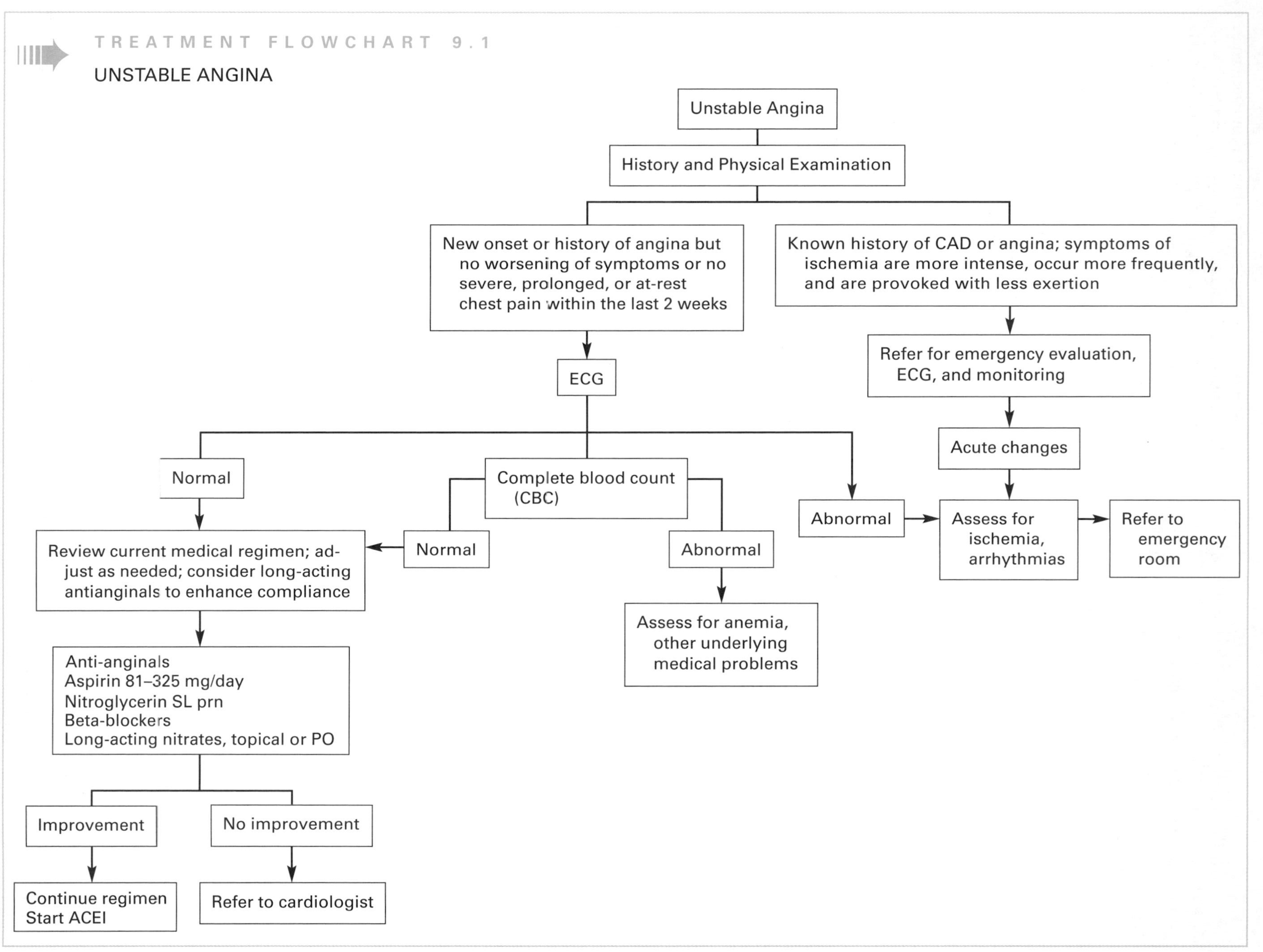

artery have been shown to be MORE effective than thrombolysis if done within 90 minutes for STEMI. This is referred to as "door to balloon" time. It is done only in specialized centers. Stenting may be done in conjunction with the platelet glycoprotein IIb/IIIa antagonist abciximab in patients with acute MI.

The American Heart Association (AHA) has published Guidelines for the Management of Patients with Acute Myocardial Infarction. Developed from consensus of nursing and medical experts and evidence-based health care, the AHA recommends the following for a person with suspected MI:

- ▲ Community systems, including primary-care providers, should work together to ensure prompt initial care of the patient with suspected MI. Once the patient enters care in the emergency department (ED), initial evaluation should occur within 10 minutes.
- ▲ The following care should be provided immediately: Administration of oxygen via nasal prongs; sublingual nitroglycerin unless SBP is less than 90 mm Hg and heart rate is less than 50 or more than 100 beats per minute; adequate analgesia with morphine sulfate or meperidine; and aspirin (ASA) 162 to 325 mg PO. The ASA should be administered regardless of whether or not thrombolytic therapy is being considered. Chewable ASA has a more rapid effect and is preferred.
- ▲ Clinically significant ST-segment elevation largely dictates reperfusion therapy by use of thrombolytic therapy or primary PTCA. When thrombolysis is used, heparin is usually given for 48 hours to ensure continued vessel patency. A viable alternataive to unfractionated heparin if renal insufficiency is not present is a low molecular weight heparin such as enoxaparin sodium (Lovenox).
- ▲ If LBBB is present on ECG and the clinical scenario is consistent with acute MI, the same level of care should be offered. Patients with presentations suggestive of MI but without ST-segment changes should not receive thrombolysis, as it may cause more harm.
- ▲ The patient should be hospitalized and placed on continuous ECG monitoring for rhythm disturbances. Serial 12-lead ECGs should be obtained and results correlated with clinical measures of myocardial necrosis such as creatine kinase (CK) or (CPK) isoenzymes and troponin T or I.
- ▲ Aspirin therapy should be continued; the use of heparin should also be considered in the presence of a large anterior MI or LV mural thrombus because of increased risk of embolic stroke. Initially, the dosage for aspirin should be 325 mg/day, with anywhere from 81 mg to 325 mg given once per day after discharge ad infinitum.
- ▲ If no contraindications are present, beta-blocker therapy and ACE inhibitor therapy should be initiated promptly because the use of these products is associated with reduced mortality and morbidity post-MI. Beta-blocker therapy should be continued indefinitely, with ACE inhibitor use being most appropriate for patients with LV dysfunction characterized by systolic ejection fraction less than 40 percent or in the presence of CHF. Beta-blockers exert their beneficial effect in patients with an MI by reducing myocardial oxygen demand, reducing myocardial wall stress, and antagonizing the arrhythmogenic effects of catecholamines. ACE inhibitors reduce the progressive ventricular dilatation and remodeling after an MI, and in some studies have been shown to reduce myocardial reinfarction (for an unknown reason). ACE inhibitors also reduce the incidence of CHF, thus reducing mortality in patients with large myocardial infarcts and in patients with left ventricular dysfunction.
- ▲ Before hospital discharge, the patient should undergo standard exercise testing to assess functional capacity and the efficacy of the current medical regimen, as well as to assess the risk for a subsequent cardiac event.
- ▲ Ongoing care includes a goal of reducing LDL cholesterol to less than 100 mg/dL using diet, exercise, and, if necessary, drug therapy. This is in keeping with an overall plan to reduce or eliminate all cardiac risk factors, including inactivity, smoking, and obesity.
- ▲ Coronary artery bypass surgery is not usually done during an evolving MI unless the patient has a serious complication such as acute severe mitral regurgitation with or without papillary muscle rupture, acute septal rupture, or a free wall rupture that might be associated with a pseudoaneurysm, refractory cardiogenic shock, or recurrent severe ischemia postinfarction that cannot be managed with drugs and PTCA.

Follow-Up and Referral

As previously stated, patients with unstable angina should be referred to the ED and a cardiologist for a complete evaluation. Patients with stable angina may be managed by the clinician with either beta-blockers and/or long-acting nitrates with nitrolingual tabs or spray prn for emergency and prophylactic use. Patients should be followed every 3 months to determine their adherence to risk factor modification strategies. From the instant the clinician suspects a patient is experiencing an acute MI, the patient must be immediately transported to the ED and be evaluated by a cardiologist. The clinician may follow the patient posthospitalization. When the cardiologist discharges the patient from his or her care, the clinician may become involved in the follow-up care. The cardiologist should have already referred the patient to a cardiac rehabilitation program before discharge. The clinician should take an active role in encouraging the patient to adhere to the prescribed program.

On discharge, the patient should be prescribed nitroglycerin (SL or spray) and a beta-blocker with instructions when to take it. In addition, the patient should be taking a daily enteric-coated aspirin of at least 81 mg, as well as a statin cholesterol-lowering drug. For patients with residual myocardial ischemia or with significant left ventricular dysfunction, a longer-acting nitrate such as isosorbide (Isordil) should also be considered. Research has shown that with the addition of a diuretic, there has been a decrease in mortality.

Patient Education

Patients should be taught about their medications, usage, adverse effects, and how to take nitroglycerin prophylactically. In addition, the clinician should stress that nitroglycerin tablets should remain in the light-resistant bottle in which they are packaged and not be put in another pill box or remain in areas that are or could become warm and humid. Once opened, the bottle must be dated and discarded after 6 months.

The clinician should assist the patient to reduce CAD risk factors and factors that exacerbate angina. The patient should be placed on a low-fat diet, with minimal calories if weight reduction is necessary. Coexisting conditions such as HTN, anemia, hyperthyrodism, and CHF should be aggressively managed. The clinician should encourage the patient to enter a cardiac rehabilitation program of safe exercise and risk-factor modification. The clinician should also encourage the patient to adhere to activity limitations determined by exercise tolerance testing and to stop smoking. Patients may be taught to use nitroglycerin prophylactically before any stressful exercise such as sexual intercourse. Anxiety and fear often accompany anginal attacks because the patient may fear the onset of an MI. Patients and their families should be allowed to express their fears and concerns and should be collaborative partners in necessary lifestyle changes. As with all cardiac conditions, family members should learn cardiopulmonary resuscitation (CPR).

Patient teaching after the patient has experienced an acute MI involves aggressive risk factor modification to prevent a recurrence. Lifestyle modifications should be stressed as stated in Table 9.2. Patients should be referred for cardiac rehabilitation to improve exercise tolerance, cardiac symptoms, blood lipid levels, and psychosocial well-being. Exercise training through cardiac rehabilitation increases the arterial oxygen saturation and improves the oxygen uptake by the peripheral tissues, thereby improving the efficiency of oxygen transport and use by the peripheral tissues, resulting in a decrease in the cardiac output required to perform exercises.

There are three phases of cardiac rehabilitation: Phase I begins in the early in-hospital postinfarct phase with range-of-motion exercises progressing to an increase in the activities of daily living (ADLs). Phase II is a structured outpatient program of exercise training and risk-factor counseling and education. Phase III establishes a lifelong pattern of regular aerobic exercise and further modification of risk factors; it is usually undertaken in a community wellness center (The Patient's Voice 9.1).

THE PATIENT'S VOICE 9.1

Myocardial Infarction

It was 4:30 A.M.... Damn, what a case of indigestion.... Have to get to the golf course....It's the first day of the senior's tournament, and employees will be there early. Driving to work, the indigestion seemed to be subsiding. Arrived at work and started getting things organized for the day's events. Started pulling kegs of beer to be placed around the course when the pain started coming back and I got nauseated. Pain getting worse now. Now it's starting to feel like someone is sitting on my chest. Someone called the paramedics. I'm in the ambulance now. I'm sweating, feeling clammy, ... chest pain continues. We get to the hospital. The people there ask if I'm allergic to anything. Pain is getting worse. They're sticking tubes and needles in me. A doctor tells me I'm having a heart attack . . . and not to worry, they have it all under control. Not worry—what does he think! Then he tells me he's going to give me a clot-busting drug. I'm trying to listen, but I really don't understand what's going on. The chest pain is starting to go away. I'm only 40 ... I can't be having a heart attack! This isn't happening to me!

At every visit to the office, the patient should be educated about risk-factor modification, such as smoking cessation, lipid management, control of coexisting conditions such as diabetes mellitus and HTN, stress reduction, and the use of antioxidants. Several studies have shown the beneficial effects of vitamin E (alpha-tocopherol) 400 to 800 IU qd to be the inhibition of the oxidation of LDL, which helps prevent atherosclerosis.

Heart Failure

Heart failure is a condition in which cardiac output is insufficient to meet the body's demands. Each patient presents differently, because there are various causes and stages of heart failure. The patient with left ventricular failure (LVF) presents with symptoms of pulmonary origin due to a back up of hydrostatic pressure into the pulmonary arterial system. Right ventricular failure symptoms occur as a result of hydrostatic pressure build up in the venous system. Clinical manifestations of systemic edema occur with right ventricular failure. Biventricular heart failure can cause a combination of these clinical manifestations. Clinicians use the term "heart failure" to describe all types of conditions in which cardiac supply is less than metabolic demand. Previously patients with heart failure were generally hospitalized, but many now may be managed at home. Early identification of patients at risk for heart failure and patient education is key, not only for the prevention of the disease but also for the quality of life of these patients.

Epidemiology and Causes

Heart failure, unlike other cardiac disorders, has been increasing in incidence and prevalence, especially in the older adult population. This disease afflicts approximately 4 million Americans, with 400,000 new cases being diagnosed each year. The incidence is increasing because of the use of newer medications and technologies that have increased survival at the expense of increased morbidity. Heart failure is the most common discharge diagnosis in patients older than age 65; it is diagnosed in 10 percent of the population by the time they reach age 75 years. The annual mortality rate is as high as 60 percent, and the 5-year survival rate for patients with severe heart failure is about 50 percent. Approximately 200,000 patients each year die of heart failure. The cost for care and evaluation of patients with heart failure exceeds $10 billion in resources each year.

Heart failure occurs after a cardiac abnormality has been present for years, when an increased demand is placed on a heart in an already compensated state and there is further deterioration. It is critical for the APN to identify not only the underlying cause of heart disease but also the precipitating cause of the heart failure. Prompt treatment and elimination of precipitating causes may save the patient's life. Table 9.13 presents causes of heart failure and their effects on the heart.

Ongoing research is being conducted to explore the neurohormonal hypothesis of heart failure. This research began with the discovery that ACE inhibitors and possibly beta-blockers were better in reducing mortality than potent afterload-reducing drugs (Nursing Research–Based Practice 9.2). In the neurohormonal model, active molecules that are released in heart failure are toxic to the myocardium. Currently, noradrenaline, angiotensin, vasopressin, endothelin, and tumor necrosis factor-alpha (TNF-α) are being studied for their relationship to heart failure. Clearly, heart failure involves a number of complex physiologic changes that are progressive. Because of the increasing incidence of heart failure, new theories are being generated to explain the elusiveness of this disease process to intervention and cure.

Pathophysiology

Heart failure is a constellation of clinical manifestations that result from the heart's inability to pump adequate amounts of blood to meet the demands of peripheral body tissues. It can result from a dysfunctional ventricle that is unable to eject an adequate amount of blood (*systolic dysfunction*) or from the inability of the ventricle to fill with a sufficient amount of blood (*diastolic dysfunction*). There are numerous etiologies of heart failure; however, ischemic heart disease and long-standing HTN are common underlying causes. Ischemic heart disease causes diminished coronary supply of the myocardium which weakens strength of contractility of the ventricles. HTN creates excess mechanical stress on the ventricles, resulting in the structural change of hypertrophy and eventual dilatation. Factors that increase risk of heart failure include obesity, valvular disorders, CAD, anemia, diabetes mellitus, chronic renal insufficiency, myocarditis, dysrhythmias, thyrotoxicosis, PE, and sleep apnea. There are also differences in susceptibility to heart failure associated with gender, race, and genetic background.

Table 9.13 Precipitating Causes of Heart Failure

Precipitating Causes	Effect on the Heart
Infection	Increases demand on the heart secondary to fever, tachycardia, hypoxemia, and increased metabolic demands.
Anemia	Increased cardiac rate to meet peripheral oxygen demands leads to increased cardiac demand.
PE	Increased pulmonary arterial pressure leads to increased right ventricular afterload.
Pregnancy, thyrotoxicosis	Adequate tissue perfusion in these conditions requires increased cardiac output.
Arrhythmias	Tachyarrhythmias decrease diastole and lead to cardiac ischemia. Loss of "atrial kick" leads to increased atrial pressures. Abnormal intraventricular conduction can lead to decreased cardiac output, which will lead to further attempts to compensate. Any arrhythmia that alters the formula: cardiac output = HR × SV has the potential to increase demands on an already decompensated heart.
Rheumatic heart disease and other forms of myocarditis	Alterations in cardiac output increase cardiac demand secondary to infectious or inflammatory processes.
Infective endocarditis	Valvular damage, fever, and inflammatory processes increase cardiac demand.
Physical, dietary, environmental, and emotional excesses	Electrolyte disturbances, alteration in medication regimen, excessive heat or humidity, physical overexertion.
Systemic HTN	Sudden elevation of arterial pressure leads to increased systemic vascular resistance (SVR) and increased cardiac workload.
MI	May lead to impaired ventricular function.

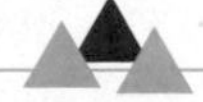

NURSING RESEARCH-BASED PRACTICE 9.2

Factors Affecting the Symptom Burden in Chronic Heart Failure

Gusick, GM: Factors affecting the symptom burden in chronic heart failure. J Card Fail, 11 (6, Suppl):179, 2005.

Background: Heart failure (HF) is a health problem of epidemic proportions and a clinical syndrome that leads to progressively severe symptoms, which contribute significantly to the burden of the disease. Several factors may affect the symptom burden of patients with HF, including physiological, psychological, and spiritual factors. This study was designed to examine the inter-relationship of physiological, psychological, and spiritual factors affecting symptoms for patients with HF.

Objectives: The aims of this study were to examine symptom burden of heart failure patients related to: (1) the physiological factor of brain natriuretic peptide (BNP); (2) the psychological factor of depression; (3) the spiritual factors of self transcendence and purpose in life; and (4) combined effects of physiological, psychological and spiritual factors. One additional aim was to describe symptom intensity related to symptom burden.

Methods: A cross-sectional nonexpermental correlational design was used to examine factors affecting symptom burden in 105 patients with HF from a southwestern medical center outpatient heart failure clinic. Both men and women were included; average age was 56.6 (SD = 16.86). All measures except BNP were obtained by patient self-report

Results: The mean number of symptoms present was 8.17 (SD = 3.34) with the three most common symptoms being shortness of breath on exertion, fatigue, and weakness. The mean symptom intensity was 365.66 (SD = 199.50) on a summative scale of visual analogue reports for 13 symptoms. The mean BNP level was 292.64 pg/mL (SD = 571.11). The prevalence rate for depression was 43.6% with a mean score of 3.48 (SD = 2.75) on the Center for Epidemiological Studies–Depression scale (CES-D 10) scale. In a multivariate analysis, depression was the only significant predictor of symptom burden ($r = .474$; $p < .001$), accounting for 18% of the varience. Spirituality had an interaction effect with depression ($p \leq .001$), serving as a moderator between depression and symptom burden.

Conclusion: HF is a chronic and progressive syndrome characterized by severe symptoms, hospitalizations and disability. Depression is significantly related to symptom burden and this relationship is moderated by spirituality.

Regardless of etiology, heart failure provokes hemodynamic changes, neurohormonal stimulation, vasoactive substance secretion, and cardiac structural alterations (myocardial remodeling)—all of which have systemic consequences. Heart failure may be described as *systolic* versus *diastolic* dysfunction, *right-sided heart failure* versus *left-sided heart failure, right ventricular* versus *left ventricular failure,* or *forward* versus *backward failure.* These contrasting terms are descriptions that illustrate the different pathophysiologic mechanisms of heart failure for academic purposes. However, clinically, most patients with heart failure exhibit a combined clinical presentation of the preceding descriptions.

The terms *systolic dysfunction* and *forward failure* describe the same process in heart failure. In both *systolic dysfunction* and *forward failure*, the diminished ejection of blood from a weakened ventricle sets off a detrimental cascade of events. The weakened ventricle cannot pump sufficient blood volume forward into the arterial system, which results in decreased cardiac output and hypoperfusion of organs. Hypoperfusion of the arteries and kidney stimulate a *neurohormonal response*, which attempts to increase circulation. BP drops in the hypoperfused arteries and this drop is sensed by baroreceptors, pressure sensors within arterial walls. Baroreceptors stimulate the *sympathetic nervous system* to constrict the arteries in efforts to raise BP. Hypoperfusion of the kidneys stimulates renin, which provokes the *renin–angiotensin–aldosterone cascade*. Renin circulates in the bloodstream and when it reaches the liver, angiotensinogen is released. Angiotensinogen circulates and when it reaches the lungs, this proenzyme is converted to angiotensin I. Within the lungs, a key reaction occurs; angiotensin I is converted to angiotensin II by angiotensin converting enzyme (ACE).

Angiotensin II acts in various ways to further raise BP and increase blood volume. Angiotensin II is a potent vasoconstrictor that directly incites peripheral arterial vasoconstriction. It also stimulates the adrenal gland to secrete aldosterone, a hormone that acts at the nephron to increase sodium and water reabsorption into the bloodstream and to excrete potassium. Angiotensin II also directly provokes genetic changes within cardiac myocytes to promote hypertrophic remodeling. Increased BP and blood volume, increased peripheral vascular resistance, and myocardial hypertrophy are the net results of sympathetic stimulation and activation of the renin–angiotensin–aldosterone cascade. These effects, although compensatory mechanisms, raise blood volume and peripheral resistance which increase workload on the weakened heart pump. As the ventricle endures greater workload, further systolic dysfunction occurs, and the neurohormonal mechanism is cyclically activated. This cycle increases blood volume and leads to fluid overload and further deterioration of systolic function.

Diastolic dysfunction or *backward failure* describes an abnormality of filling, distensibility, or relaxation of the ventricles. There is elevated filling pressure in the left and/or right ventricle, which causes backward buildup of hydrostatic pressure into the atria. In left ventricular diastolic dysfunction or backward failure, there is a backup of hydrostatic pressure into the left atrium and, in turn, the pulmonary venous system, which results in the extravasation of fluid into the pulmonary interstitium. If hydrostatic pressure builds to high levels, pulmonary capillary wedge pressure increases; high amounts of fluid build in the pulmonary interstitial spaces, which is called *pulmonary edema*. Clinical manifestations of fluid in the pulmonary interstitium are dyspnea, cough, orthopnea, paroxysmal nocturnal dyspnea, and crackles heard on auscultation of the lungs. The classic sign of pulmonary edema is *pink, frothy sputum*. *Orthopnea* is a term that describes the inability of the patient to breathe comfortably while lying supine. As a patient endures diastolic dysfunction or backward failure, the backup of pulmonary fluid in the interstitial spaces creates breathing difficulty. Patients breathe easier with the head of the bed elevated because this position disperses fluid downward into the lung bases. Patients often report needing two or three pillows to breathe comfortably, termed two-or-three-pillow orthopnea. Frequently patients report awakening in the middle of the night feeling breathless or awakening due to a "nightmare." This nighttime hypoxia due to fluid accumulation in the pulmonary tissues is *paroxysmal nocturnal dyspnea (PND)*.

Left-sided heart failure or *left ventricular failure* (LVF) is the most common type of heart failure. Most often the LV becomes dysfunctional due to long-standing hypertension. Systemic hypertension increases resistance against the LV, thereby increasing workload. This leads to left ventricular hypertrophy and eventually the LV decompensates into failure. In addition, the LV is vulnerable to ischemic insults due to coronary artery disease and may endure MI. One of the most common sites of arteriosclerosis is the left anterior descending (LAD) artery, a branch of the left main coronary artery, a major supplier of the LV. Repeated ischemic episodes can lead to weakening of the LV with eventual failure. LVF can occur as systolic dysfunction (forward failure) and/or diastolic dysfunction (backward failure) as described previously. The classic clinical presentation of LVF involves the pulmonary signs and symptoms of exertional dyspnea, cough, orthopnea, PND, crackles heard on auscultation, and the hemodynamic finding of elevated pulmonary capillary wedge pressure. These symptoms are a result of the buildup of hydrostatic pressure backward into the pulmonary vasculature due to a failing LV. Ejection fraction (EF) is decreased in LV systolic dysfunction to less than 50 percent of total ventricular volume (normal EF ranging from 55 to 70 percent). In contrast, in diastolic dysfunction, EF may be normal or even increased to greater than 70 percent, representing the need for the LV to eject a larger proportion of its total blood volume during systole to compensate for reduced diastolic filling.

Right-sided heart failure or *right ventricular failure* (RVF) most commonly occurs as a result of LV failure. The same cardiac muscle comprises both right and left ventricles, which endure biochemical and hemodynamic stresses during heart failure. Therefore, in the clinical setting, often manifestations of right- and left-sided heart failure appear together. The RV can undergo systolic dysfunction (forward failure) and/or diastolic failure (backward failure) in the same manner as the LV. In right-sided heart failure, the classic signs and symptoms are due to backup of hydrostatic pressure into the venous system. Venous congestion of the superior vena cava is reflected in the classic sign of jugular venous distension. Venous congestion of the inferior vena cava is reflected in the GI system as hepatomegaly, splenomegaly, and peritoneal edema (*ascites*). Depending on the position of the patient, peripheral edema is apparent as either sacral edema or ankle edema.

Isolated right ventricular failure can also occur due to pulmonary disease. The term *cor pulmonale* is used to describe right-sided heart failure, which is a result of a pathologic pulmonary process, such as pulmonary fibrosis, recurrent pulmonary emboli, or other phenomena leading to pulmonary hypertension due to arterial vasoconstriction in the pulmonary vascular bed. Chronic hypoxia is a common cause of pulmonary arterial vasoconstriction. The high pulmonary arterial pressure leads to increased resistance against the RV. The RV hypertrophies in response to the increased workload initially. However, eventually the hypertrophic RV decompensates from the excess workload, leading to right ventricular failure. This syndrome is then called *cor pulmonale*.

The most common cause of right-sided heart failure, however, is initial left-sided heart failure. In this case, right-sided heart failure does not occur in isolation, but rather results from a failure of forward cardiac output. This leads to vascular congestion in the pulmonary arterial bed with increased capillary wedge pressure, which is eventually transmitted to the RV, thus compromising its function as it attempts to pump against this increased resistance.

Heart failure evokes the secretion of vasoactive substances and cytokines which initially help the body adapt to changes from reduced cardiac output. However, in chronic heart failure, these substances cause further myocardial damage and impairment of cardiac function. When cardiac muscle contraction is weakened, *endothelin,* a potent vasoconstrictor, is secreted by the arterial endothelium in response to a drop in blood pressure. Although endothelin helps the body compensate by raising blood pressure, chronic secretion increases afterload and resistance against the heart pump. Another substance, *tumor necrosis factor–alpha (TNF-α)*, is found in the circulation and heart muscle during heart failure. TNF-α is an anorexigenic cytokine that also increases wasting of lean body mass. Two important vasodilator peptides are released with dilation of the atria and ventricles in heart failure: *atrial natriuretic peptide (ANP)* and *brain natriuretic peptide (BNP)*. These are natural diuretic substances that counteract the excess water reabsorption and fluid overload caused by activation of the renin–angiotensin–aldosterone cascade in response to decreased cardiac output, by stimulating the excretion of sodium and water. Circulating serum BNP level is a useful indicator of the degree of heart failure, when compared to a baseline value obtained in the absence of acute cardiac decompensation.

There are four stages of heart failure classified as A to D that describe the evolution and progression of disease. Patients in stage A of heart failure are at high risk but do not have structural abnormalities or symptoms. This group includes patients with HTN, diabetes, CAD, previous exposure to cardiotoxic drugs, or a family history of cardiomyopathy. Patients in stage B of heart failure have structural abnormalities but no symptoms. This group includes patients with left ventricular hypertrophy, previous MI, left ventricular systolic dysfunction, or valvular heart disease. Patients with stage C have structural abnormalities and current or previous symptoms of heart failure. Patients with stage D have refractory symptoms of heart failure at rest despite medical therapy, are hospitalized, or require specialized interventions or hospice care.

Clinical Presentation

Subjective

The patient with heart failure will present complaining of symptoms related to the pulmonary system, central nervous system (CNS), and generalized systemic and organ systems.

Complaints related to the pulmonary system are cough, orthopnea, dyspnea, and paroxysmal nocturnal dyspnea. Orthopnea refers to dyspnea that is positional. The patient feels more dyspneic in a recumbent position but relief when sitting or standing. The number of pillows that the patient sleeps on can grade the severity of orthopnea. Two related symptoms are dry nocturnal cough, seen early in heart failure, and dyspnea in the left lateral decubitus position. As heart failure progresses, the degree of dyspnea increases. If the progression is gradual, the patient may not be aware of the dyspnea. Assessment of the patient during activity may be necessary to elicit this symptom. Paroxysmal nocturnal dyspnea occurs as a result of hypoxia from the accumulation of fluid in the pulmonary interstitium. The patient is usually not aware that he or she is hypoxic and may describe paroxysmal nocturnal dyspnea as awakening during sleep because of a "nightmare" or extreme shortness of breath. The clinician must have a high level of suspicion because the description of paroxysmal nocturnal dyspnea varies from patient to patient. Slight relief may be noted with sitting, standing, or inspiration of fresh outdoor air. When severe coughing and wheezing are associated with this symptom, the condition is sometimes referred to as *cardiac asthma*. Patient symptoms related to the CNS range from delirium, insomnia, anxiety, and headache all the way to hallucinations and unresponsiveness.

Patient complaints of systemic and organ symptoms are many. Patients may complain of fatigue and generalized weakness, which are associated with low cardiac output and may occur at rest or with increased activity. These symptoms may also be caused by blood volume depletion and electrolyte imbalance secondary to overdiuresis. Patients may also notice a decreased urine output during the day as well as nocturia that is the result of enhanced renal filtration secondary to recumbency. During the waking hours, renal filtration of sodium and water is decreased in the heart failure patient. Nocturia may not be present if concurrent renal failure is present. The patient may also complain of peripheral and dependent edema. Patients may present with ascites, fullness, nausea, vomiting, constipation, upper abdominal pain, or anorexia, conditions related to liver, spleen, and intestinal congestion. They may also report light-headedness, near-syncope, or syncope. In addition, the patient may be confused or have difficulty concentrating, an impaired memory, headache, insomnia, or anxiety. Some patients may present with chest pain.

Objective

A complete physical examination is necessary to diagnose the condition and determine the etiology of heart failure and provide the clinician with enough information to optimize intervention techniques. On general inspection, the clinician may note breathlessness, dyspnea on exertion, peripheral cyanosis (as a result of low cardiac output), pallor in extremities, and distended peripheral veins. There may be jugular venous distension (JVD) along with abnormal pulsations. A skeletal deformity (as seen in Marfan's syndrome) may be noted. In addition, the patient may have dependent edema, jaundice (suggesting hepatic congestion), ascites, or anasarca.

Vital signs may show tachycardia; pulsus alternans (a weak pulse alternating with a strong pulse); atrial fibrillation, which may contribute to heart failure; rapid, shallow respirations at rest or with minimal exertion; and possibly Cheyne–Stokes respirations. Cheyne–Stokes respirations are crescendo–decrescendo patterns of respiratory swings terminating in apnea. Cheyne–Stokes respirations are caused by the prolonged circulation time from the heart to the brain.

On cardiac assessment, the clinician may note lateral and downward shift in the point of maximal impulse (PMI) secondary to cardiac enlargement, the presence of a third heart sound (S3) in adults older than age 40, and the sudden development of the murmurs of mitral or tricuspid regurgitation.

When performing a lung assessment, the clinician may note crackles (rales), generally heard bilaterally in the bases or in the most dependent regions of the lungs on inspiration. Wheezing may also be present, as well as pleural effusion (stony dullness, or shifting of dullness with position changes is characteristic of percussion with pleural effusion). In evaluating these symptoms, the clinician should also consider arterial embolism, which is present in 4 percent of the patients with primary dilated cardiomyopathy.

Diagnostic Reasoning

Diagnostic Tests

The clinician should initially order laboratory tests to assist in the diagnosis. Cardiac myocytes and endothelial tissue manufacture and secrete a family of structurally related peptide hormones termed natriuretic peptides. Atrial natriuretic peptides (ANPs) are secreted in response to the atrial stretch that occurs in heart failure due to increased hydrostatic pressure within the atria. These peptides have diuretic, vasodilating, and kaliuretic (potassium-wasting) effects. B-type natriuretic peptide (BNP) is abundant in the heart and rapidly rises in the bloodstream in the presence of heart failure. A blood test can show elevated BNP within 15 minutes. In patients with the symptom of dyspnea, which can be either cardiac or pulmonary in origin, the BNP blood test can be used to rule out heart failure. BNP is a cardiac marker that can be used in combination with other more definitive tests and is not solely relied on to diagnose heart failure. BNP can be elevated in pulmonary edema, COPD, pulmonary embolism, renal disease, and other conditions. However, a BNP level which is greater than 500 pg/mL is highly indicative of heart failure. After instituting treatment for heart failure, the clinician can rely on BNP levels to monitor therapeutic effectiveness. In addition, there is a pharmacologic form of BOP, nesiritide, which is used to treat heart failure.

An echocardiogram is the diagnostic test utilized after demonstrable elevation of BNP. Echocardiography is the single best test to confirm a diagnosis of heart failure. Abnormalities of systolic and diastolic function are easily visualized and ejection fraction can be estimated. An echocardiogram can also visualize different etiologies of heart failure, diseases of the pericardium, myocardium, and heart valves.

A CBC may show severe anemia associated with high-output heart failure. A urinalysis that shows proteinuria may indicate nephrotic syndrome and red blood cells (RBCs) or cellular casts may indicate glomerulonephritis. A serum albumin elevation may indicate volume overload caused by renal failure. An ESR should be ordered because the ESR is typically decreased secondary to impaired fibrinogen synthesis and decreased fibrinogen concentration in patients with heart failure. Electrolytes may show hyponatremia, which may be either genuine (secondary to prolonged sodium restriction and diuretic therapy) or dilutional (secondary to expansion of extracellular volume). Hyponatremia may also signal pronounced activation of the renin–angiotensin system. Hypokalemia may be secondary to diuretic therapy or activation of the renin-–angiotensin–aldosterone axis. Hyperkalemia may be secondary to renal failure as a result of the heart failure, especially if ACE inhibitors have been used. The blood urea nitrogen (BUN) and creatinine may be elevated secondary to decreased renal blood flow. LFTs may show abnormalities as a result of hepatic congestion. There is also a decreased hepatic blood flow; therefore, drugs metabolized by the liver should be appropriately dosed. An arterial blood gas (ABG) study may also be ordered. Finally, the thyroxine (T_4) and thyroid-stimulating hormone (TSH) levels may indicate that the heart failure is aggravated by hypo- or hyperthyroidism.

The clinician may also order the following diagnostic procedures to gather information in the diagnosis of CHF. Although there is no specific ECG pattern for CHF, an ECG may help diagnose the underlying cause, such as an MI. A chest x-ray film will show an alteration in cardiac silhouette as evidenced by a change in cardiac size and shape, a change in cardiothoracic ratio (cardiothoracic ratio more than 0.50 is considered cardiomegaly), and specific chamber enlargement. A chest x-ray film may also show pulmonary venous congestion as evidenced by distension of the pulmonary veins upward from the hila. Normally in the upright position, larger vessels are seen in the bases; however, with increasing capillary pressures, there is compression of the vessels to the lower lobes and dilation of upper lobe vessels. This might present on x-ray studies as an equalization of upper and lower lobe vessel size; loss of definition of pulmonary vascular markings, which is usually caused by perivascular edema; haziness of hilar shadows; and thickness of interlobular septa (Kerley B lines). Kerley B lines usually result from distended lymphatic vessels. As PCWP exceeds 25 mm Hg, alveolar edema is indicated by diffuse haziness, usually extending downward toward both lung fields (butterfly pattern). An echocardiogram can be used to identify underlying structural defects such as valvular defects, systolic dysfunction, and abnormal cardiac wall thickness. A radionuclide angiocardiography uses Technetium-99m (multigated acquisition [MUGA] scan). This multigated blood pool imaging technique, is useful in measuring the ejection fraction (EF) and wall-motion abnormalities; and right-heart catheterization is useful for determining response to therapy; it can be used in a monitored intensive care unit.

Left-heart catheterization is not usually indicated in heart failure; however, once the condition is stabilized, catheterization can be useful in identifying the underlying causes of the failure. Left-heart catheterization may be performed by the cardiologist if sudden murmurs are auscultated, including severe mitral regurgitation that may be caused by ruptured chordae tendineae, severe aortic regurgitation that may be caused by bacterial endocarditis, or perforation of the interventricular septum or papillary muscle rupture.

Heart failure severity has traditionally been described with the symptom-based New York Heart Association (NYHA) classification system. The newer American College of Cardiology/American Heart Association (ACC/AHA) supplements this with a staging system

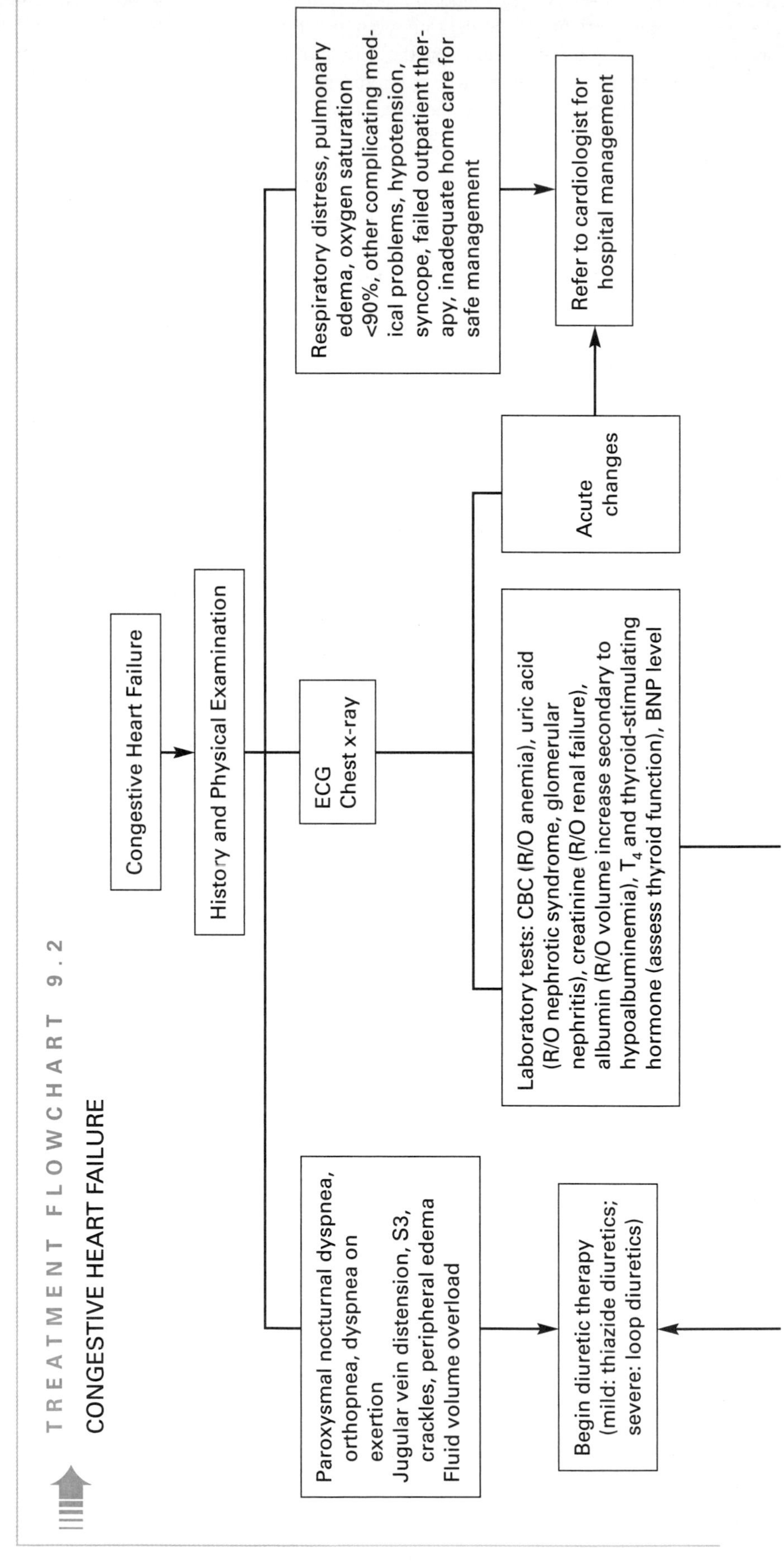
TREATMENT FLOWCHART 9.2
CONGESTIVE HEART FAILURE
Congestive Heart Failure
History and Physical Examination
Paroxysmal nocturnal dyspnea, orthopnea, dyspnea on exertion
Jugular vein distension, S3, crackles, peripheral edema
Fluid volume overload
Begin diuretic therapy (mild: thiazide diuretics; severe: loop diuretics)
ECG
Chest x-ray
Laboratory tests: CBC (R/O anemia), uric acid (R/O nephrotic syndrome, glomerular nephritis), creatinine (R/O renal failure), albumin (R/O volume increase secondary to hypoalbuminemia), T4 and thyroid-stimulating hormone (assess thyroid function), BNP level
Acute changes
Respiratory distress, pulmonary edema, oxygen saturation <90%, other complicating medical problems, hypotension, syncope, failed outpatient therapy, inadequate home care for safe management
Refer to cardiologist for hospital management

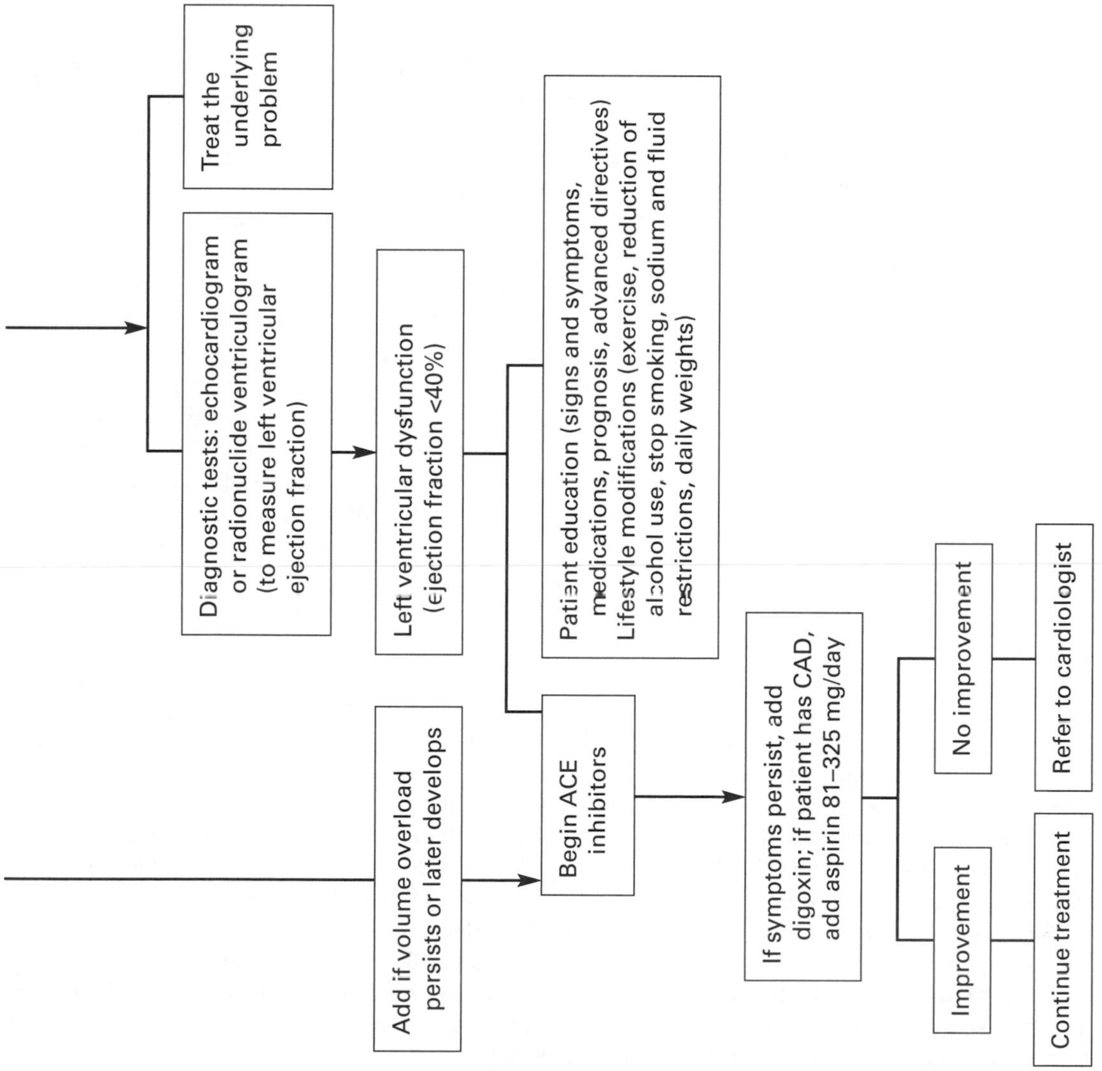

Diagnostic tests: echocardiogram or radionuclide ventriculogram (to measure left ventricular ejection fraction)

Treat the underlying problem

Left ventricular dysfunction (ejection fraction <40%)

Add if volume overload persists or later develops

Begin ACE inhibitors

Patient education (signs and symptoms, medications, prognosis, advanced directives)
Lifestyle modifications (exercise, reduction of alcohol use, stop smoking, sodium and fluid restrictions, daily weights)

If symptoms persist, add digoxin; if patient has CAD, add aspirin 81–325 mg/day

Improvement

Continue treatment

No improvement

Refer to cardiologist

describing the progressive phases of heart failure. The two systems are complementary with the NYHA system describing sysmptom severity and the ACC/AHA system providing a framework for a stage-based therapeutic approach.

NYHA Classification of Heart Failure Severity

I. Patients with asymptomatic heart failure
II. Patients with heart failure symptoms with significant exertion
III. Patients with heart failure symptoms with minor exertion
IV. Patients with heart failure symptoms at rest

ACC/AHA Staging Criteria of Heart Failure

A. Patients at risk for developing left ventricular dysfunction
B. Patients with left ventricular dysfunction who have not developed symptoms
C. Patients with left ventricular dysfunction with symptoms
D. Patients with refractory end-stage heart failure

Differential Diagnosis

The symptoms of heart failure can be vague and progress slowly, or they can be sudden and overwhelming. In either event, the symptoms and findings of what appears to be heart failure may have other causes such as anxiety neurosis, lung disease, venous insufficiency, nephrotic syndrome, hepatic cirrhosis, superior vena cava syndrome, constrictive pericarditis, or pericardial effusion.

Management

The principles of management include identifying and treating precipitating or aggravating conditions, recognizing and treating underlying cardiac disease, and managing the cardiac failure.

When managing heart failure, the clinician must consider treatments that will decrease the cardiac workload, decrease the clinical volume overload, optimize LV function, reduce mortality, and control atrial fibrillation. Treatment Flowchart 9.2 presents an algorithm for the treatment of CHF.

To decrease the cardiac workload, the clinician must order rest until the patient's "dry weight" (non-CHF weight) is achieved, order vasodilators, encourage weight loss if appropriate, and control HTN. Analysis of data acquired from the Systolic Hypertension in the Elderly Program indicates a marked effect in preventing development of heart failure in older patients with isolated systolic hypertension when diuretic therapy was instituted.

To decrease clinical volume overload, diuretics should be initiated at the first signs of volume overload (e.g., orthopnea, paroxysmal nocturnal dyspnea); however, the clinician should avoid overdiuresis, which will lead to hypotension or renal insufficiency and may interfere with other medications. For mild heart failure, thiazide diuretics are used, and for severe failure, loop diuretics, such as furosemide (Lasix) or bumetanide (Bumex) should be ordered. Doses of these agents can be increased during acute CHF exacerbations to counteract fluid overload. All patients should be on a sodium-restricted diet.

For severe heart failure, IV nesitiride, a synthetic B-type natriuretic peptide, can be added to the regimen to stimulate diuresis. Spironolactone, an aldosterone antagonist, has been shown to be of benefit because it is a potassium-sparing diuretic. As a compensatory mechanism in heart failure, the sympathetic nervous system is stimulated. Sympathetic stimulation causes arterial vasoconstriction and increased heart rate which have detrimental effects on the weakened heart. For this reason, beta-2 adrenergic blockers, such as carvedilol, have been recommended as part of the drug treatment regimen. Beta-2 adrenergic blockade slows heart rate, decreasing the work of the heart, and limits peripheral arterial vasoconstriction, decreasing afterload against the ventricles.

To optimize left-ventricular function, digoxin (Lanoxin) or other inotropic agents should be ordered. Digoxin increases the force of contraction in patients with left-ventricular dysfunction but has no known effect on mortality. Digoxin should be used in conjunction with other medications in patients with severe heart failure. It may not be necessary in patients who become asymptomatic following treatment with angiotensin-converting enzyme inhibitors (ACEIs) and diuretics. Inotropic agents that may be ordered include dopamine (Intropin), dobutamine (Dobutrex), and amrinone (Inocor).

To reduce mortality, the health-care provider should order ACEIs, which are indicated for all patients with LV systolic dysfunction unless there are specific contraindications, such as history of intolerance or adverse reactions to these agents, serum potassium more than 5.5 mEq, or symptomatic hypotension. ACEIs may be the sole therapy for a patient with fatigue and mild dyspnea on exertion.They are referred to as the "cornerstone of heart failure therapy." Diuretics should be added to this therapy if symptoms persist or volume overload becomes obvious. ACEIs have been demonstrated to counteract many of the neurohumoral changes in heart failure and, therefore, decrease mortality. For patients who cannot tolerate ACEIs, angiotensin receptor blockers (ARBs) can be used. Vasodilators and nitrates can also be used in those who cannot tolerate ACEIs.

Controlling atrial fibrillation is essential in treating CHF. Atrial fibrillation in patients with asymptomatic or symptomatic left ventricular systolic dysfunction is associated with an increased risk of progression of the dysfunction and mortality. Because of this, anticoagulation treatment is instituted in heart failure to decrease the formation of thrombi in the dysfunctional heart chambers. Long-term oral anticoagulation with warfarin (coumadin) is usually recommended.

When heart failure is first diagnosed, the collaborating physician should be consulted regarding digitalization and/or appropriate pharmacologic therapy. Once drug therapy is initiated, the clinician may manage the patient. Increasingly around the country, heart failure clinics are becoming popular referral resources.

Other treatments include the following:

- Regular exercise should be encouraged for all patients with stable heart failure, as it improves functional status and decreases symptoms.
- Cardiac rehabilitation programs, although not specifically indicated for patients with heart failure, might benefit patients who are anxious about exercising on their own or those who have low cardiac output.
- Dietary sodium restriction to 2 g/day or lower.
- Limitation of fluid intake should be advised for each patient based on his or her status.
- Alcohol consumption should be discouraged. A patient should drink no more than one glass of beer or wine or a mixed drink with no more than 1 ounce of alcohol per day.
- The patient should record his or her weight daily and notify the clinician if a weight gain of 3 to 5 pounds or more occurs within 1 week.
- Immunization with influenza and pneumoccocal vaccines may reduce the risk of a respiratory infection.
- All barriers to adherence must be removed to assist the patient with management of the disease. Some barriers include the cost of medications, adverse effects, and the complexity of the medical regimen.
- The patient must be counseled concerning the prognosis, so that he or she may have the benefit of understanding the rationale for decisions made about care. This must be done while maintaining hope. The clinician should explain that good quality of life is still possible with cooperation in the treatment regimen. The patient must be given information regarding the prognosis so that plans can be made for the future.
- The patient should be encouraged to complete advanced directives.

A cardiac catheterization should be performed as many patients may benefit from various reperfusion treatments such as percutaneous cardiac transluminal angioplasty (PCTA), coronary artery bypass grafting (CABG), or stenting. Heart failure often causes ventricular remodeling and dysrhythmias such as left bundle branch block (LBBB). These conditions lead to unsynchronized ventricular contractions. Cardiac resynchronization therapy (CRT) has been shown to improve cardiac mechanics by inducing concordant contraction of the two ventricles. CRT involves implantation of a biventricular pacing device and if necessary, an implantable cardioverter defibrillator (ICD). Implantation of an internal cardiac automated defibrillator may be considered for primary prevention in chronic CHF patients (NYHA functional class II or III) with ischemic or nonischemic cardiomyopathy, or with a patient with an EF less than or equal to 35 percent, given the patient's increased risk of sudden cardiac death due to an increased risk of sustained ventricular tachycardia and ventricular fibrillation. CRT may also be used for patients with NYHA class III or IV heart failure with persistent symptoms who are already receiving optimal medical therapy. Heart transplantation may be considered for patients who have exhausted all other treatment recommendations with poor effect. Psychological support is essential; patient support groups have been shown to be very effective in helping patients cope with their conditions and follow the prescribed regimens.

Follow-Up and Referral

Referral to a cardiologist is recommended on onset of symptoms of heart failure; however, initial treatment should begin immediately in the clinician's office, with a phone referral made directly to the cardiologist. Patients in acute failure may be hospitalized. The clinician and the cardiologist will establish a plan of care with the patient and will decide who will manage the patient on an ongoing basis. It must be clear to all involved what the plan of care is to be.

Patients in chronic cardiac failure may be treated on an outpatient basis. After a complete and detailed baseline history and physical examination, subsequent visits for the patient in chronic failure should assess the patient's cardiac status thoroughly. Questions regarding the patient's health-related quality of life (e.g., sleep, sexual function, mental health, or outlook on life, appetite, and social activities) should also be asked. After the patient, family, and caregiver have been educated on the condition, they should be encouraged to communicate all signs, symptoms, fears, and concerns with the clinician. Patients are likely to experience changes in symptoms before there is evidence of deterioration on physical examination.

Frequency of follow-up should depend on the underlying cause of heart failure. Generally, the patient is seen by the clinician at least every 3 months. Intensive home-care surveillance has been shown to decrease the need for hospitalization and improve the functional status of older adult patients with CHF.

Patient Education

Successful management of patients with heart failure requires an active partnership between the patient and all health-care providers. One of the most critical points in decreasing the possibility of the patient becoming "crippled" by the disease process is a thorough education regarding the condition and encouragement to take responsibility for personal care. The clinician should encourage and assist the patient to:

- Keep a record of daily weights and notify the clinician of a 3- to 5-pound or more weight gain in 1 week or less.
- Advise the clinician of symptoms or concerns.
- Exercise regularly.
- Rest with elevation of lower extremities.
- Use elastic stockings to reduce the risk of venous thrombosis and PE.
- Ensure emotional rest.

- Maintain an optimum body weight.
- Discuss with the clinician changes made in self-care. The clinician should explain to the patient that some things can be changed, and that by discussing what he or she wants to change with the clinician, before making changes, an "informed" change can be made.

In working closely with the patient and possibly the family to plan the patient's care, the clinician should never lose sight of the high esteem with which his or her opinions and directions are taken. In discussing the plan of care with the patient and family, the clinician should keep in mind that the family, who fears losing their loved one, will attempt to ensure that the plan is followed to the letter; therefore, the clinician should remember to "build in," and teach the patient and family how to "build in," some humane adaptations to the plan of care. For instance, as the clinician stresses that the diuretic must be taken every morning, he or she must realize that if the patient has an important family function one morning and chooses to take the diuretic later in the day, the mandate may cause needless stress and guilt. The patient may be frightened of getting into distress if he or she does not follow the orders. The family may "harass" the patient for deliberately not following the plan of care, or the patient may feel that participation in events that take place in the morning is forbidden. Any or all of these perceived restrictions compromise the quality of the patient's life and are unnecessary. It is critical that the clinician ensure that the patient understands the rationale for decisions about his or her care.

With the increasing incidence of heart failure, researchers have begun to look at areas of patient involvement in self-care and the impact on outcome. Exercise training is now being recommended for most individuals with moderate-to-severe heart failure. Activity intolerance associated with chronic heart failure has been studied from the perspective of physiologic variables; however, very little research has been conducted on the outcomes of exercise training based on subjective data. A research study examined the perception of vigor as a subjective measure of personal health. In this study of person–environment interaction in patients with heart failure, the researcher found that an astute evaluation of the patient's environment, including his or her physical and social milieu, is warranted when assessment of energy level is undertaken. Purposeful activity and exercise should be encouraged and supported. During interviews with patients with heart failure, the researcher noted the hopeful and life-loving attitudes of the participants involved in exercise training in her study, which suggested coping strategies not often attributed to a population experiencing terminal illness. She concluded that reinforcement of these attitudes may be a key intervention in reversing the energy-draining sequelae of illness patterns experienced by the individual with a failing heart.

Coaching and encouraging a terminally ill patient in self-care is time consuming and can be draining. The clinician will need to have authentic presence and respond to calls for care that are often not timed with the patient's regularly scheduled appointment; however, the time invested in each patient cannot be charged appropriately on a ledger or justified to other patients who may be late for their visit with the clinician. Nonetheless, to patients with lifelong terminal illness, the importance of life and the significance of the effects of their illness are directly related to their perceptions of the attention and care they perceive being given.

Dysrhythmias

Dysrhythmias the clinician may encounter in primary-care practice include the atrial arrhythmias of atrial fibrillation, premature atrial contractions (PACs), atrial tachycardia, atrial flutter, and supraventricular tachycardia (SVT). Ventricular arrhythmias encountered include premature ventricular contractions (PVCs) and ventricular tachycardia (VT). First-, second-, and third-degree heart blocks and arrhythmias associated with digitalis toxicity are other arrhythmias commonly encountered.

Atrial Arrhythmias

Atrial Fibrillation. Atrial fibrillation is one of the most common arrhythmias that clinicians will encounter in clinical practice. In most cases, atrial fibrillation will be associated with a rapid ventricular response and most patients will have some type of underlying heart disease. In these patients, the loss of atrial contribution to left ventricular blood volume (atrial "kick"), along with a rapid ventricular rate, can have serious hemodynamic effects caused by diminished cardiac output. These effects may be seen in the form of hypotension, diaphoresis, dizziness, and syncopal episodes.

The loss of mechanically effective atrial contractions in atrial fibrillation leads to stasis of blood in the left atrium which predisposes to formation of embolic atrial thrombi. Thrombi that form in the left atrium then have a propensity to travel into the LV and into the aorta where they are propelled into the arterial circulation. A common route for the thrombus from the aorta is to the brachiocephalic artery, carotid artery, and then into the cerebral circulation. This pathway makes atrial fibrillation a risk factor for ischemic stroke because a thrombus often lodges in a branch of the middle cerebral artery. Compared to persons in sinus rhythm, those in atrial fibrillation have a 6-fold increased risk of stroke. For those with rheumatic heart disease, the risk of stroke is 18-fold.

Premature Atrial Contractions. PACs are very common, yet in most cases have no clinical significance. PACs are usually a benign arrhythmia that does not require pharmacologic intervention unless there are underlying causes that can be corrected. This arrhythmia is commonly seen in young healthy individuals. Cardiac stimulants such as caffeine, nicotine, alcohol, or over-the-counter (OTC) medications sometimes induce PACs. They are rarely, if ever, symptomatic and are frequently seen in patients with obstructive lung disease and CHF.

Supraventricular Tachycardia. Supraventricular tachycardia (SVT) is often described as a "catch-all" term that encompasses rapid arrhythmias above the ventricles. There continues to be confusion over specific terminology of these SVTs. Some experts feel that the confusion arises from failure to understand the mechanism and inability to differentiate true atrial tachycardias or atrial flutters from paroxysmal supraventricular tachycardias (PSVTs) that use reentry circuits. The use of the term *paroxysmal atrial tachycardia* (PAT) further confounds the terminology issue. This term is often incorrectly used for all SVTs (whether paroxysmal or not) that are not atrial flutter or atrial fibrillation.

Research has shown that the two most common forms of PSVT are atrioventricular node reentry tachycardia (AVNRT) and orthodromic circus movement tachycardia (CMT). For purposes of this discussion, the condition SVT is subdivided into PSVT, which includes AVNRT and CMT, and non-PSVT, which includes atrial tachycardia of nonreentry origin and atrial flutter. Although atrial fibrillation can also be classified as an SVT, this rhythm is discussed separately. Current Advanced Cardiac Life Support (ACLS) treatment standards require that the APN be able to differentiate the aforementioned atrial tachycardias that are included under the term "SVT."

The atrial rate differentiates atrial tachycardia from atrial flutter. This rate difference is particularly pertinent when the clinician is attempting to discern if the arrhythmia is an atrial tachycardia with block (seen in digitalis toxicity) or an atrial flutter. Both rhythms can present with more than one observable P wave before the QRS. An atrial tachycardia rate is slower than an atrial flutter rate. Atrial flutter is less common than atrial fibrillation and most commonly occurs in older adults. These patients typically have some form of organic heart disease.

Ventricular Arrhythmias

Premature Ventricular Contractions. PVCs are usually a benign arrhythmia that does not require pharmacologic intervention unless the rhythm progresses to VT. VT may be associated with any form of heart disease. It may be sustained or nonsustained. In patients who have had an MI, nonsustained VT is a risk factor for sudden cardiac death.

Heart Blocks

Atrioventricular (AV) blocks are classified as to the degree of severity of the disturbance of the impulse going through the electrical conduction system between the atria and ventricles. Heart blocks may be permanent or transient and are classified as first, second, or third degree. A *first-degree AV block* is the mildest form, with a regular rhythm and only a prolonged PR interval. *Second-degree AV block* may further be classified as type I (Mobitz I or Wenckebach) and type II (Mobitz II). For purposes of this discussion, the terms "type" and "Mobitz" are combined as Mobitz type I and Mobitz type II. Mobitz type I occurs in the AV nodal area with progressive lengthening of the PR interval until a QRS complex (ventricular contraction) is dropped. Mobitz type II occurs within or below the bundle of His, with a normal or lengthened PR interval and a periodic drop of a QRS complex in a set ratio of atrial to ventricular contractions. A *third-degree AV block* occurs when the atria beat regularly and at a normal rate but no excitation is transmitted from the atria to the ventricles. In turn, the atria and ventricles contract independently at their own intrinsic rates. This complete lack of coordination between the chambers of the heart severely compromises cardiac output and can prove fatal.

Third-degree heart block is classified as third degree at the junctional level or third degree at the ventricular level. A second-degree Mobitz type I block does not progress to Mobitz type II; rather, a Mobitz type I block typically progresses to a third-degree block with an idiojunctional response. In contrast, a second-degree Mobitz type II block progresses to third-degree heart block with an idioventricular response that carries a more ominous prognosis. If a rhythm presents with two P waves with a normal rate to every 2 R waves (referred to as 2:1 conduction), the origin of nodal or subnodal pathology must be determined. This rhythm is often referred to as second-degree AV block undifferentiated.

Dysrhythmias Associated with Digitalis

One of the most common agents used in the treatment of CHF and supraventricular tachyarrhythmias is digitalis. It is the second most common cause of various degrees of AV block. There is a narrow therapeutic range for this drug; signs of toxicity can occur before acute symptoms are recognized. Digitalis toxicity can produce virtually any arrhythmia. Those arrhythmias most commonly seen in digitalis toxicity are atrial tachycardia with AV nodal block, accelerated junctional rhythms, atrial fibrillation with a slow or regular ventricular response, second-degree heart block or Mobitz type I (Wenckebach), and ventricular dysrhythmias. The serum digitalis levels may not reflect the amount of digitalis bound to the myocardial membrane, where it cannot be measured. A finding of a normal digitalis level should not be the determining factor in assessing digitalis toxicity. The onset of atrial tachydysrhythmias, noncardiac subjective symptoms, and pertinent medication history should make the APN highly suspicious of digitalis toxicity. ECGs representing these rhythms are presented in Figure 9.4.

Epidemiology and Causes

Atrial Arrhythmias

Most patients with atrial fibrillation have some form of heart disease. The most common form is CAD associated with CHF, followed by HTN and rheumatic heart disease.

ATRIAL ARRHYTHMIAS

Atrial fibrillation

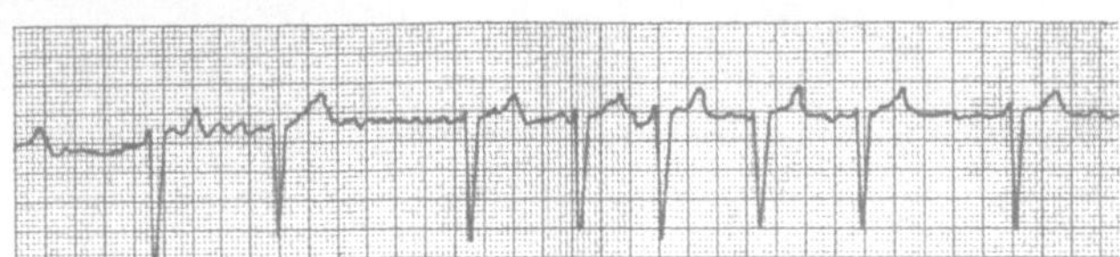

Fibrillatory waves distort the baseline, and the R-R interval is characteristically irregular. The ventricular rate is approximately 70 bpm. (*Source:* Textbook of Advanced Cardiac Life Support. American Heart Association, 1987, p 73.)

Atrial premature complexes (APCs) or premature atrial contractions (PACs)

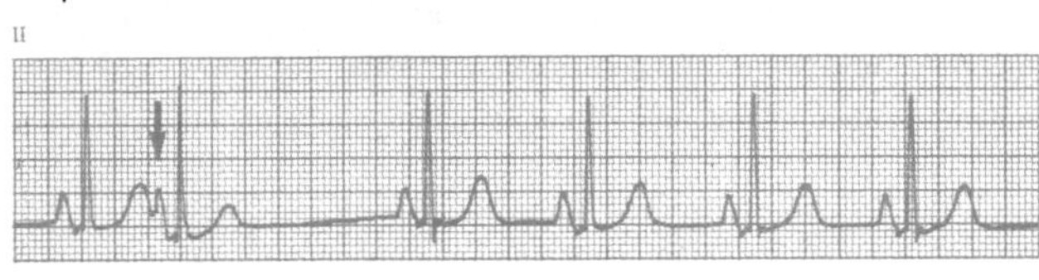

A

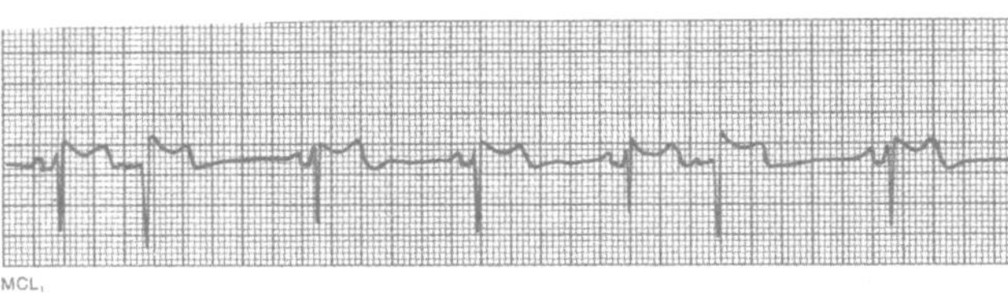

B

(A) Sinus rhythm with one APC. An ectopic P wave (*arrow*) is clearly visible before the early QRS complex. The QRS is narrow because conduction in the ventricles is undisturbed. (*Source:* Conover, MB: Understanding Electrocardiography: Arrhythmias and the 12-lead ECG, ed 5. CV Mosby, St. Louis, 1988, p 103.) *(B)* Sinus bradycardia with two APCs. (*Source:* Brown, KR, and Jacobson, S: Mastering Dysrhythmias: A Problem-Solving Guide. FA Davis, Philadelphia, 1988, p 44.)

Atrial tachycardia

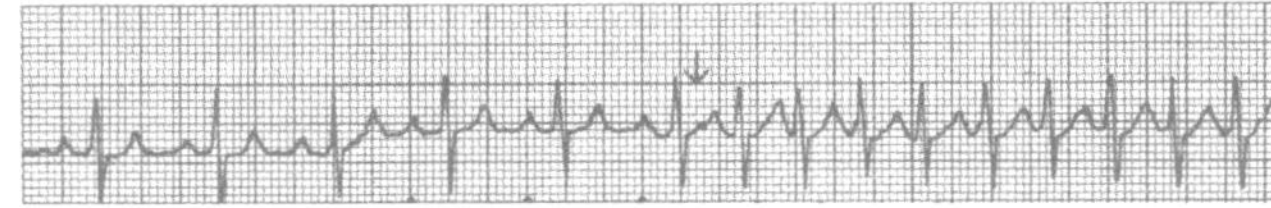

Sinus tachycardia with an episode of atrial tachycardia initiated by an APC (*arrow*). There is a 1:1 conduction at a rate of 185 bpm. (*Source:* Textbook of Advanced Cardiac Life Support. American Heart Association, 1987, p 70.)

Atrial flutter

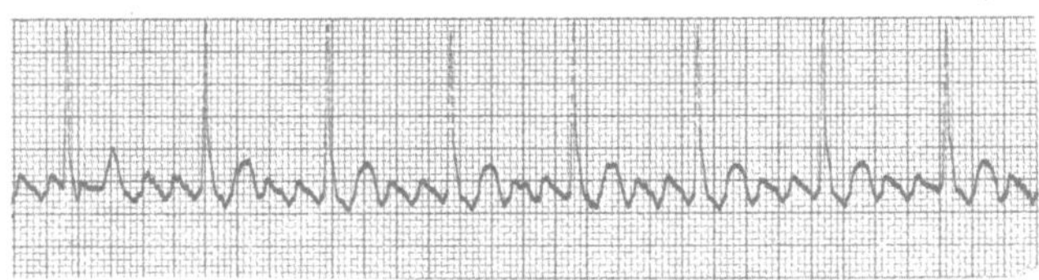

A

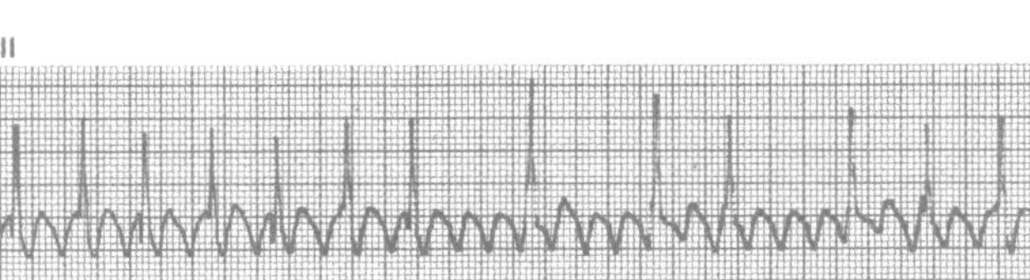

B

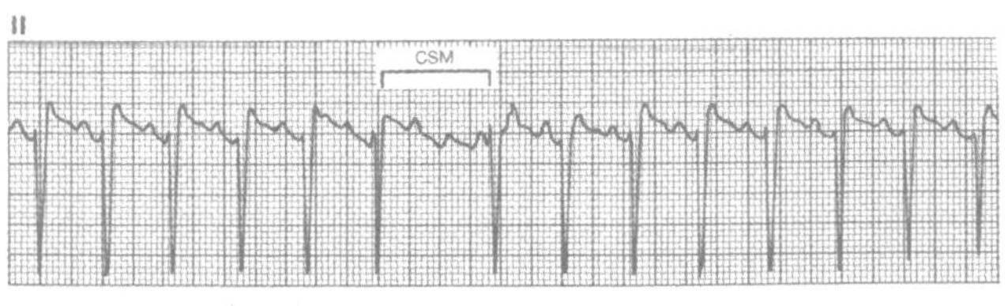

C

A characteristic sawtooth pattern to the baseline. *(A)* Atrial flutter with a 4:1 conduction. The R-R interval is regular. (*Source:* Brown, KR, and Jacobson, S: Mastering Dysrhythmias: A Problem-Solving Guide. FA Davis, Philadelphia, 1988, p 221.) *(B)* Atrial flutter with variable conduction. The R-R interval is irregular. (*Source:* Conover, MB: Understanding Electrocardiography: Arrhythmias and the 12-lead ECG, ed 5. CV Mosby, St. Louis, 1988, p 117.) *(C)* Atrial flutter with a 2:1 conduction. Initiation of carotid sinus massage temporarily slows the ventricular rate enough to unmask the flutter waves. (*Source:* Brown, KR, and Jacobson, S: Mastering Dysrhythmias: A Problem-Solving Guide. FA Davis, Philadelphia, 1988, p 244.)

FIGURE 9.4 Common arrhythmias.

VENTRICULAR ARRHYTHMIAS
Ventricular premature contractions (VPCs) or premature ventricular contractions (PVCs)

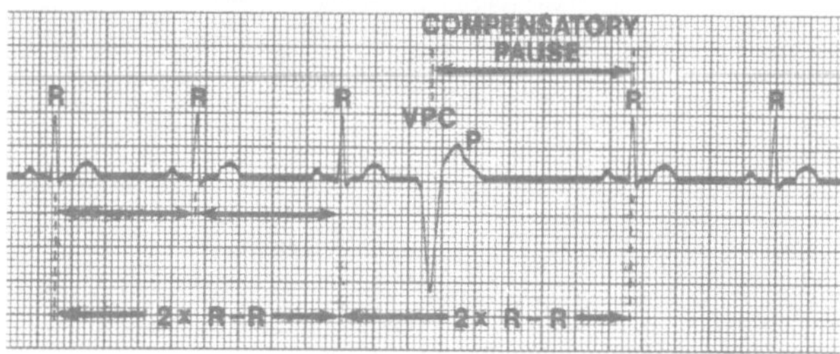

A

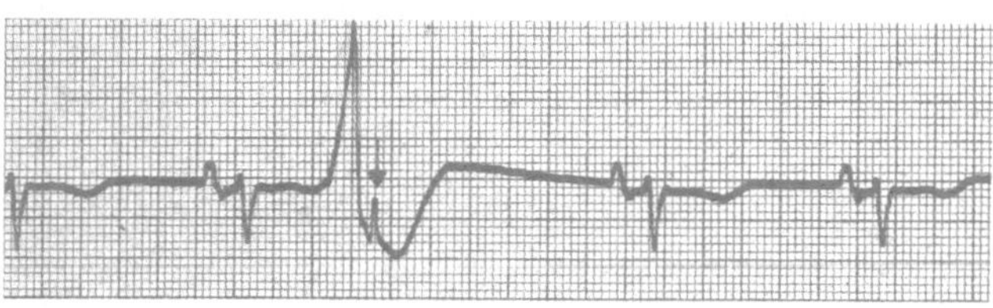

B

(A) The ectopic QRS complex (the VPC) is wide, abnormally shaped, and appears earlier than expected. The length of the compensatory pause following a VPC indicates that sinus node discharge was undisturbed. A nonconducted sinus P wave distorts the T wave (the P wave appears on time). (*Source:* Lipman, BC, and Lipman, BS: ECG Pocket Guide. Year Book Medical Publishers, Chicago, 1987, p 62.) *(B)* The P wave immediately following the VPC (*arrow*) indicates that the ectopic impulse was conducted retrogradely into the atria. (*Source:* Conover, MB: Understanding Electrocardiography: Arrhythmias and the 12-lead ECG, ed 5. CV Mosby, St. Louis, 1988, p 187.)

VPC couplets

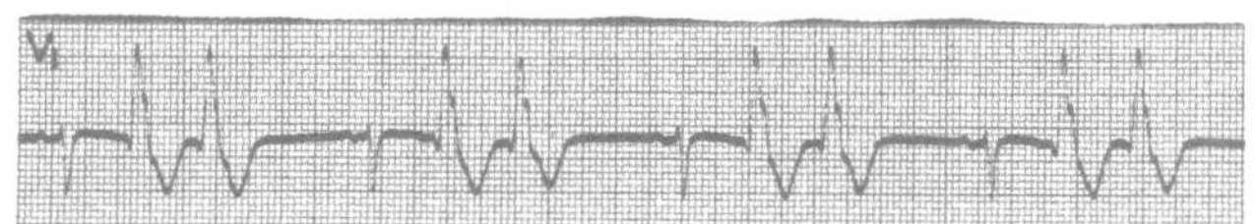

Pairs of uniform VPCs originating from the same ectopic site. (*Source:* Marriott, HJL: Practical Electrocardiography, ed 7. Williams and Wilkins, Baltimore, 1983, p 432.)

VPC triplets

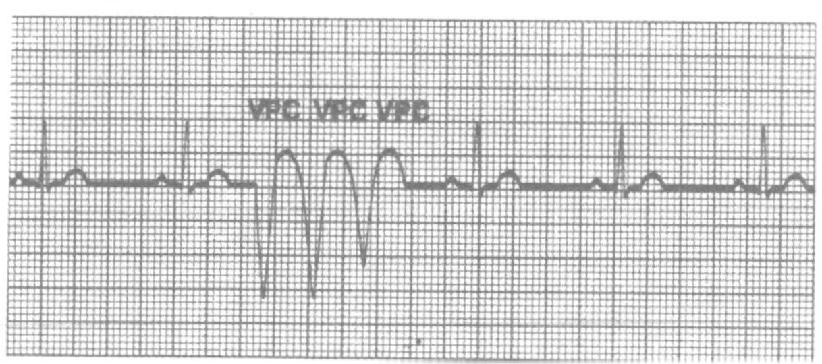

Three uniform VPCs in a row, originating from the same ectopic site. Generally, three VPCs in a row is considered to be ventricular tachycardia. (*Source:* Lipman, BC, and Lipman, BS: ECG Pocket Guide. Year Book Medical Publishers, Chicago, 1987, p 65.)

VPC bigeminy

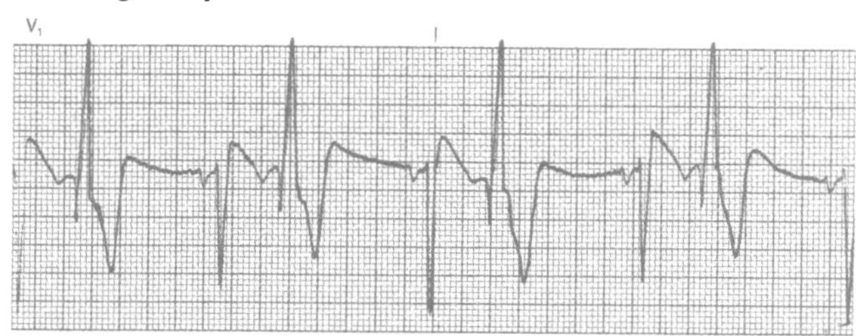

A uniform VPC, occurring from the same ectopic site, occurs every other beat. (*Source:* Lounsbury, P, and Frey, SJ: Cardiac Rhythm Disorders: A Nursing Process Approach, ed 2. Mosby-Year Book, St. Louis, 1992.)

FIGURE 9.4 (continued)

VPC trigeminy

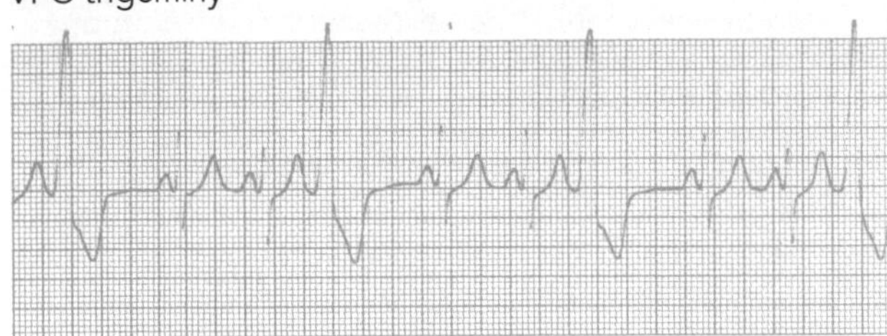

A uniform VPC, occurring from the same ectopic site, occurs every third beat. (*Source:* Walraven, G: Basic Arrhythmias, ed 2. Brady, Englewood Cliffs, N.J., 1986, p 350.)

VPC quadrigeminy

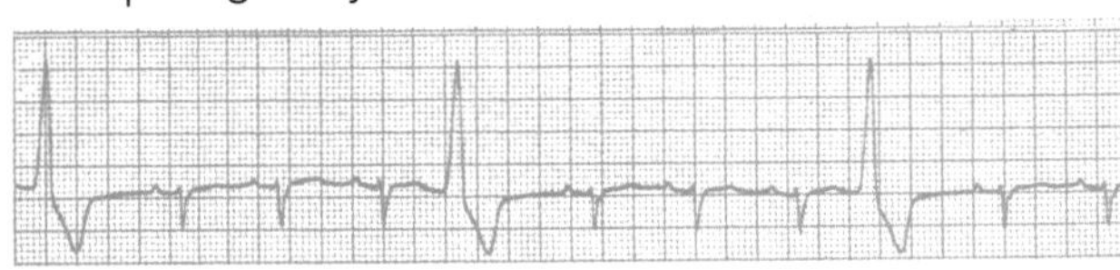

A uniform VPC, occurring from the same ectopic site, occurs every fourth beat. (*Source:* Chung, EK: Electrocardiography: Practical Applications with Vectorial Principles, ed 3. Appleton & Lange, Norwalk, Conn., 1985, p 248.)

Ventricular tachycardia (VT)

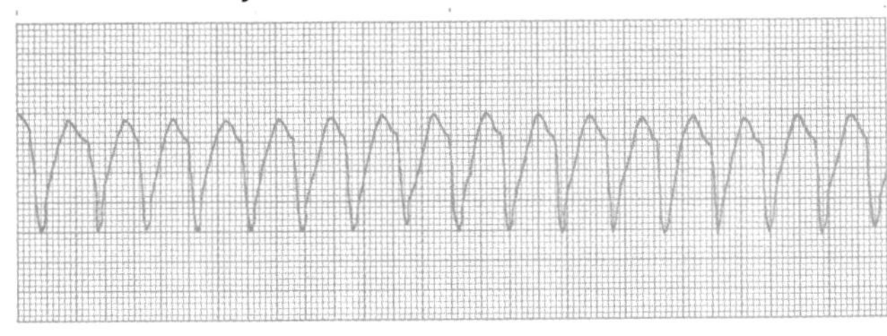

A

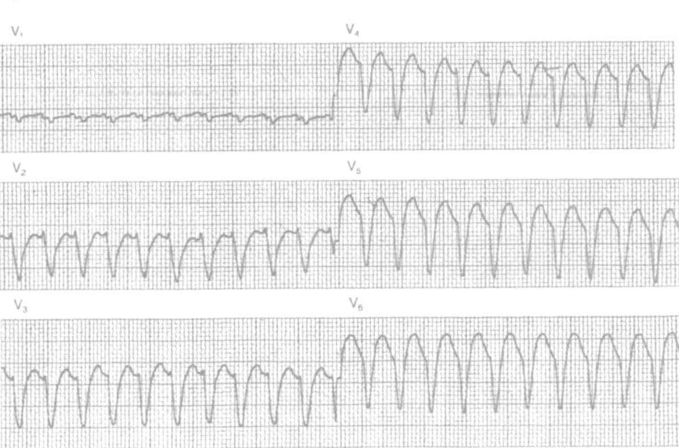

B

(A) The ventricular rate is approximately 167 bpm. The QRS complexes are wide, they look alike, and the R-R interval is regular. (*Source:* Walraven, G: Basic Arrhythmias, ed 2. Brady, Englewood Cliffs, N.J., 1986, p 282.) *(B)* The QRS complexes are negative in all six precordial leads. (*Source:* Lounsbury, P, and Frey, SJ: Cardiac Rhythm Disorders: A Nursing Process Approach, ed 2. Mosby-Year Book, St. Louis, 1992.)

ATRIOVENTRICULAR (AV) BLOCKS

First-degree AV block

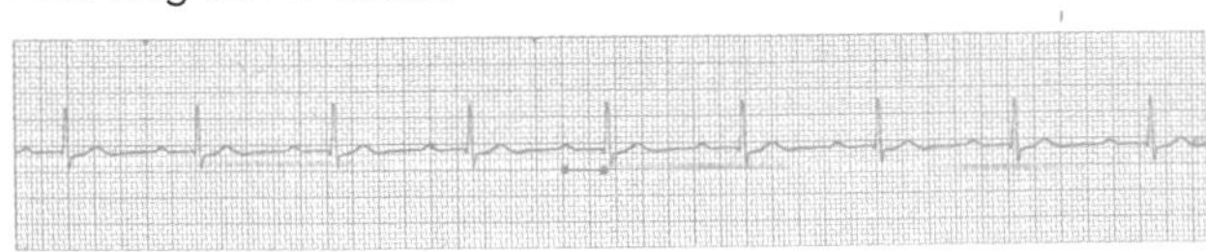

The PR interval is consistently prolonged at 0.20 seconds or longer. The underlying rhythm is sinus. (*Source:* Brown, KR, and Jacobson, S: Mastering Dysrhythmias: A Problem-Solving Guide. FA Davis, Philadelphia, 1988, p 223.)

FIGURE 9.4 (continued)

Second-degree AV block, type I

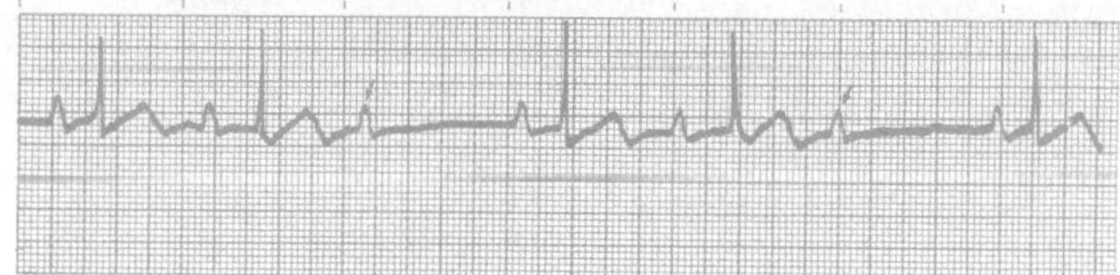

A

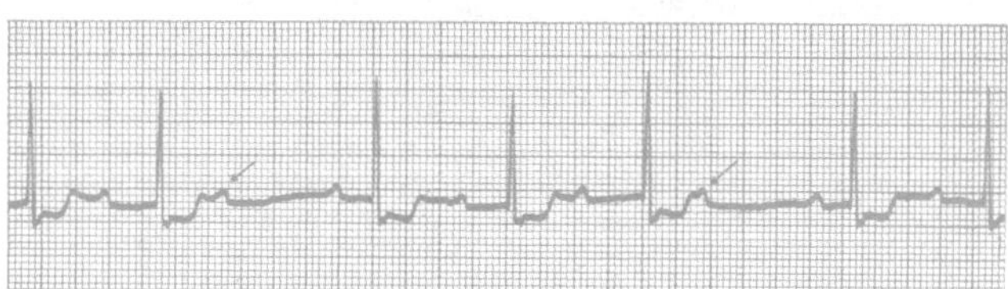

B

Group beating is present. The PR interval lengthens until a beat is dropped (*arrows*). The QRS complexes are narrow. *(A)* The nonconducted P waves (*arrows*) are easily visible. (*Source:* Brown, KR, and Jacobson, S: Mastering Dysrhythmias: A Problem-Solving Guide. FA Davis: Philadelphia, 1988, p 18.) *(B)* The nonconducted P wave distorts the T wave of the preceding QRS complex. (*Source:* Textbook of Advanced Cardiac Life Support. American Heart Association, 1987, p 81.)

Second-degree AV block, type II

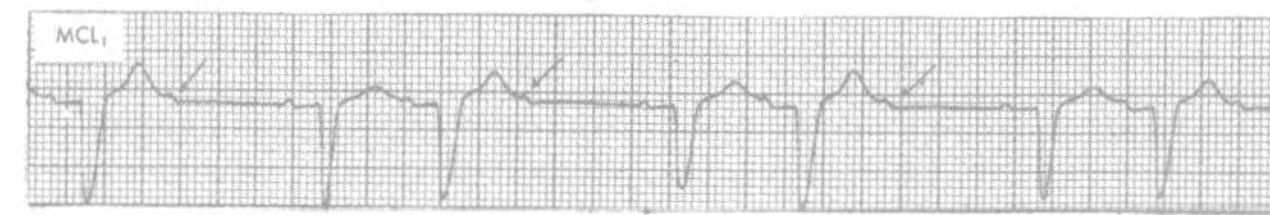

A

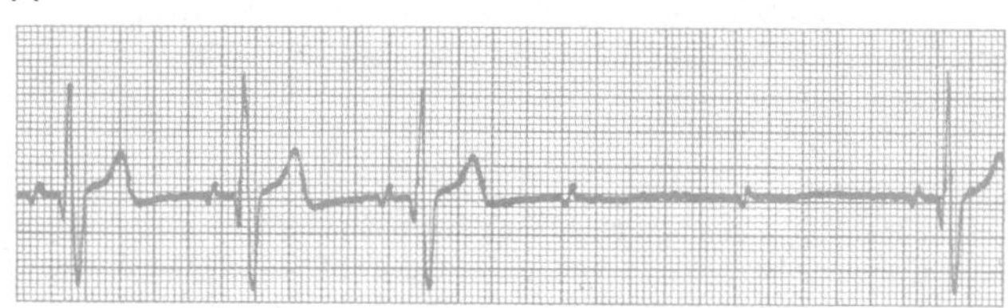

B

The PR interval remains fixed. The QRS complexes are wider than normal. *(A)* The nonconducted P waves are visible in the terminal portion of the T wave. (*Source:* Marriott, HJL, and Conover, MB: Advanced Concepts in Arrhythmias, ed 2. CV Mosby, St. Louis, 1989, p 249.) *(B)* The ventricular rate slows when all conduction pathways into the ventricles are blocked. Conduction resumes after a pause of just over 3 seconds. (*Source:* Textbook of Advanced Cardiac Life Support. American Heart Association, 1987, p 82.)

Third-degree AV block

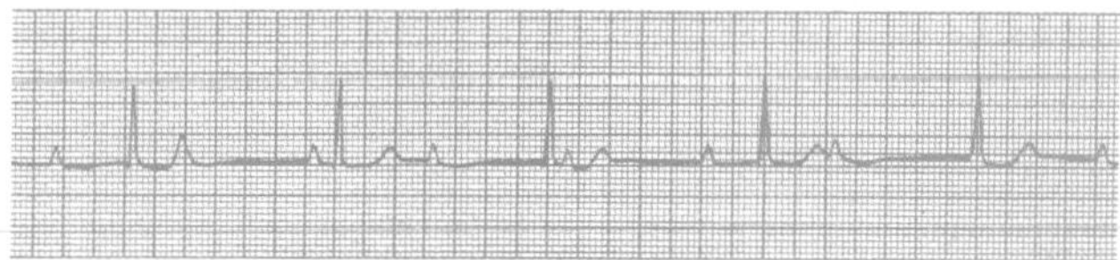

A

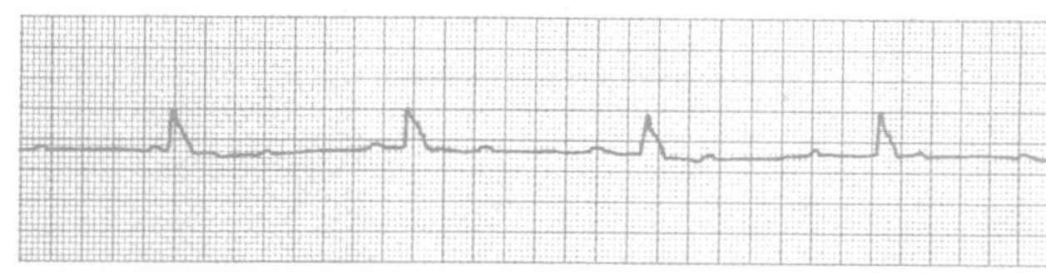

B

The P-P and P-R intervals are nearly regular, but the atrial and ventricular rates are different. There is no relationship between the P wave and the QRS complex. *(A)* Third-degree AV block with a junctional escape pacemaker. The QRS complexes are narrow, and the ventricular rate is 44 bpm. *(B)* Third-degree AV block with a ventricular escape pacemaker. The QRS complexes are wide, and the ventricular rate is 37 bpm. (*Source:* Textbook of Advanced Cardiac Life Support. American Heart Association, 1987, p 83.)

FIGURE 9.4 (continued)

DIGITALIS TOXICITY
The digoxin effect

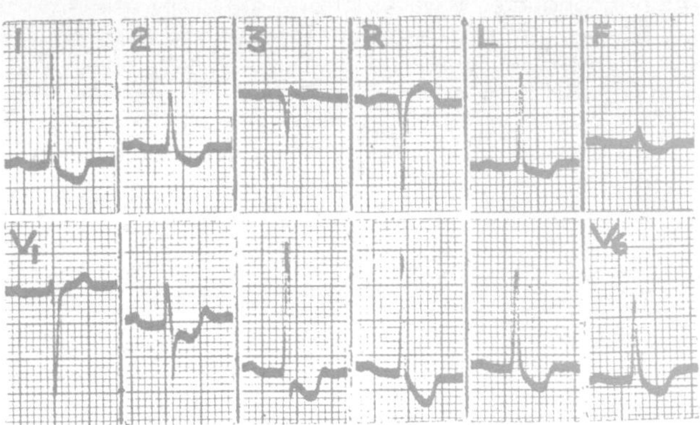

The ST segments are depressed, with a "scooped-out" look in several leads. (*Source:* Marriott, HJL: Practical Electrocardiography, ed 7. Williams and Wilkins, Baltimore, 1983, p 425.)

Digitalis toxicity

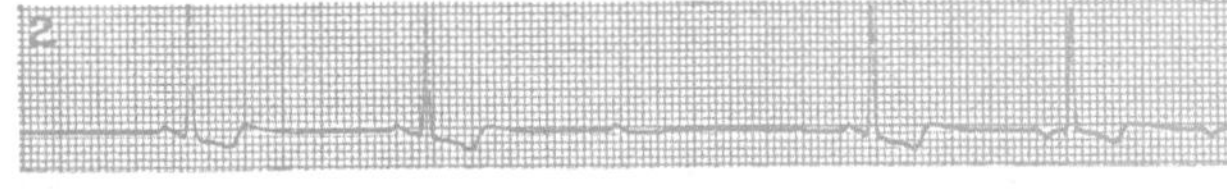

A

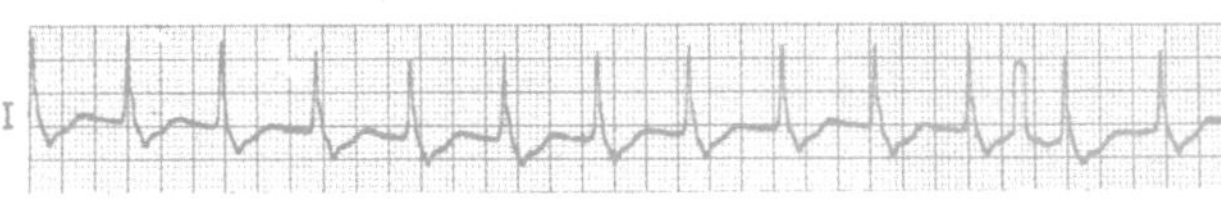

B

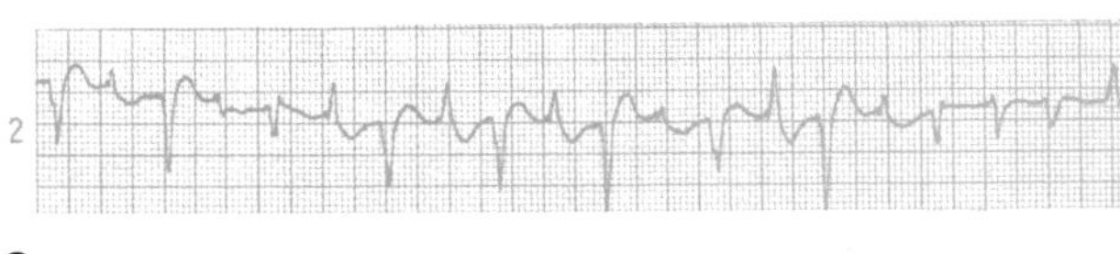

C

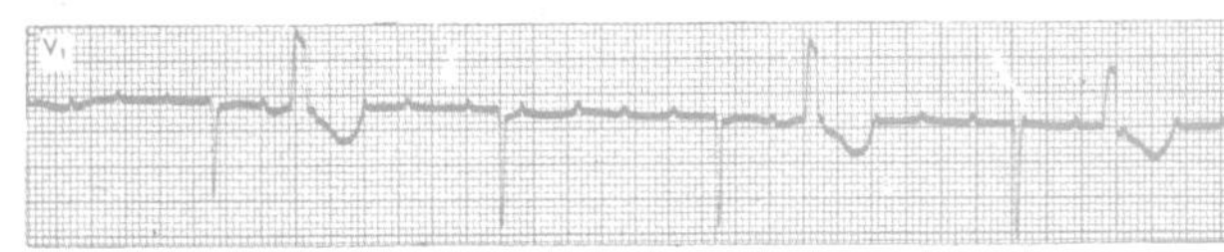

D

A wide variety of dysrhythmias and heart blocks may accompany digitalis toxicity. *(A)* The initial portion of this rhythm is sinus bradycardia. Toward the end of the strip an ectopic junctional pacemaker takes over; note the inverted P preceding the last QRS complex. (*Source:* Marriott, HJL: Practical Electrocardiography, ed 7. Williams and Wilkins, Baltimore, 1983, p 432.) *(B)* Junctional tachycardia at approximately 100 bpm. Note the inverted P wave in the terminal portion of the QRS complex. (*Source:* Chung, EK: Electrocardiography: Practical Applications with Vectorial Principles, ed 3. Appleton & Lange, Norwalk, Conn., 1985, p 517.) *(C)* Atrial fibrillation with bidirectional ventricular tachycardia. There is alternating polarity of the QRS complexes. Bidirectional VT is associated with advanced digitalis toxicity and a poor prognosis. (*Source:* Chung, EK: Electrocardiography: Practical Applications with Vectorial Principles, ed 3. Appleton & Lange, Norwalk, Conn., 1985, p 514.) *(D)* Atrial tachycardia with a 4:1 block and VPCs. (*Source:* Marriott, HJL, and Conover, MB: Advanced Concepts in Arrhythmias, ed 2. CV Mosby, St. Louis, 1989, p 66.)

FIGURE 9.4 (continued)

Frequently, the precipitating event is an acute illness, electrolyte imbalance, or major cardiac surgery. Atrial fibrillation is seen in 60 percent of patients after valvular surgery and in 33 to 42 percent of patients with mitral stenosis. Other causes of atrial fibrillation include abrupt discontinuation of beta-blockers, alcohol ingestion (sometimes called "holiday heart"), hyperthyroidism, acute MI, and cor pulmonale. A danger of untreated atrial fibrillation, with or without rapid ventricular response, is the significant increased risk of embolic stroke. The risk of stroke is increased in untreated atrial fibrillation after 48 to 72 hours; therefore, it is important to diagnose and treat this arrhythmia in an expeditious manner.

PACs typically have no clinical significance. In a normal patient, tobacco, caffeine, alcohol, or emotional stress may cause PACs. PACs may also result from stretch of the myocardium as a warning of developing CHF. In patients with organic heart disease, common causes of PACs are mitral stenosis and cor pulmonale secondary to atrial enlargement. Occasionally in patients with organic heart disease, PACs may precipitate PSVT, atrial flutter, and atrial fibrillation.

Ventricular Arrhythmias

Frequent PVCs are seen in patients with cardiomyopathies of differing etiologies and arteriosclerotic heart disease (ASHD). These patients are rarely symptomatic and in general do not need to be treated. In patients with frequent PVCs it is worthwhile to rule out acute underlying causes of ventricular ectopy such as hypokalemia, hypomagnesemia, hypoxia, myocardial ischemia, or digitalis toxicity. Other common causes are stress and stimulants such as alcohol and nicotine. Sustained ventricular tachycardia is associated with a prior MI or CAD, electrolyte disturbances, and digitalis toxicity.

Heart Blocks

A first-degree heart block is the mildest form and may be seen in patients with CAD and digoxin toxicity. A transient second-degree AV block type I may be associated with an acute inferior MI. It may also be associated with CHF or digitalis toxicity. A Mobitz type II AV block is a less common second-degree heart block; it is marked by an intermittent blocked impulse that can occur at the bundle of His or the right or left bundle branches. This type of block may occur as the result of an anterior wall MI. As this block progresses, complete heart block with an idioventricular response may follow. Insertion of a temporary pacemaker as soon as a Mobitz type II block is discovered is the standard of care. Other causes of AV block at this level are acute infections, valvular heart disease, and digitalis toxicity. This is not commonly a transient arrhythmia and can progress to third-degree AV block at the ventricular level; therefore, it must be monitored and treated appropriately.

Arrhythmias Associated with Digitalis

The epidemiology and cause of this arrhythmia are discussed under this heading in the previous section.

Pathophysiology

The mechanism of atrial fibrillation remains controversial. Cardiac disease associated with atrial enlargement is the primary cause of the rapid firing (400 to 700 beats per minute) of the ectopic foci throughout the atrium. Although electrical atrial activity is very rapid, only a small islet of myocardium is depolarized rather than the entire atrium. Because the atrium does not contract as a whole, there is no P wave. The chaotic atrial activity is seen as a wavy line between the QRS complex and is referred to as fibrillatory waves. These impulses are transmitted in variable fashion from the atria to the ventricles. The ventricular response rate to atrial fibrillation may be fast or slow, depending on the refractory nature of the AV node and the degree of AV nodal heart block or conduction delay within the AV node. In turn, therapy may be geared toward rate control with AV nodal slowing agents, rather than toward complete resolution of the dysrhythmia with anti-arrhythmic medications.

Normally, electrical impulses from the sino–atrial node within the atria are conducted down the AV node to the His–Purkinje conduction system, disseminating throughout the two ventricles, thereby leading to subsequent contraction. However, in addition to the AV node, in some individuals a fast conducting accessory pathway exists between the atria and ventricles that bypasses the AV node. The tissue in these pathways depolarizes at a faster rate owing to the presence of faster inward sodium transport channels. One of the most common and well-characterized examples of these bypass tracts is the bundle of Kent accessory tract, which is seen in individuals with Wolff–Parkinson–White (WPW) syndrome. Because conduction down this bypass pathway directly transmits a depolarizing impulse to the ventricles faster than impulses sent down the AV node, this has been termed a "preexcitation" syndrome. EKG patterns in these patients demonstrate QRS fusion beats with a characteristic shape produced by the overlap of QRS complexes transmitted via each pathway in temporal proximity, hence creating a fusion complex. The first portion of the upswing in the R wave in this complex has a characteristic slanted appearance with a less steep angle than the remainder of the upward deflection, termed a "delta wave." Figure 9.5 shows a delta wave present in WPW syndrome.

The most common mechanisms of PSVT observed in symptomatic patients are CMT (40 percent of cases) and AVNRT (50 percent of cases). CMT is distinguished by the dependence of the circular, reentrant impulse on an accessory conduction pathway, separate from the AV node itself. Thus, the fast bypass tract found in WPW syndrome is a perfect setup for CMT. Normal physiology dictates that cardiac conducting tissue becomes refractory (i.e., resistant to depolarization and electrical conduction) for a brief period of time following transmission of an electrical impulse. Bypass pathways such as that seen in WPW syndrome typically have shorter refractory periods than the AV node. Once depolarizing impulses are transmitted down the AV node to the ventricles, the refractory nature of the AV node prevents retrograde conduction back up this pathway. However, the same impulse may be conducted in retrograde fashion from the ventricles back up the accessory bypass tract to the atria. In turn, this impulse may then be conducted back down the AV node, which will have recovered from its refractory state by this time, only to circle back around once again to the atria via the fast accessory pathway. This type of circular, orthodromic conduction accounts for 90 percent of CMT cases, with a P wave occuring immediately after the QRS complex, rather than before it. The remaining 10 percent of CMT cases are considered antidromic, with the depolarizing impulse intially conducted down the fast accessory tract, only to circle back up the slower AV nodal pathway to the atria to complete the circular movement.

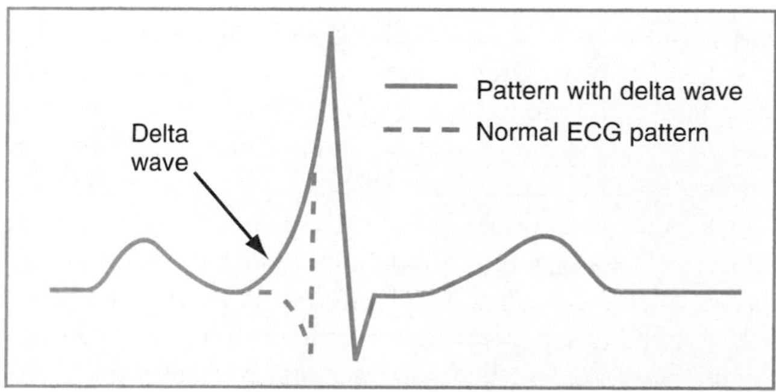

FIGURE 9.5 Delta wave present in Wolff–Parkinson–White syndrome.

In AVNRT, PSVT typically results from an interplay of two conducting pathways within the AV node itself—one fast and one slow. The key aspect of this type of PSVT is that reentry of the impulse is dependent on an AV nodal pathway, as opposed to an accessory bypass pathway. In AVNRT, the fast AV nodal conducting pathway has a refractory period that lasts longer than that of the slow AV nodal pathway. Thus, if an electrical impulse enters both pathways of the AV node simultaneously, the fast pathway will remain refractory longer. In turn, if an early PAC then enters the AV node while the fast accessory pathway is still refractory, it can only depolarize the ventricles via transmission down the slower AV nodal pathway. By the time the impulse has traveled down this open slow pathway, the fast pathway is no longer refractory, and the impulse may travel in retrograde fashion back up to the atria via the fast pathway, and then back down again to the ventricles via the slow pathway. This mechanism activates the atria and the ventricles nearly simultaneously, which places the P wave within the QRS complex, distorting its terminal portion.

PVCs and VT may be the results of enhanced normal automaticity from catecholamines within the His–Purkinje system or abnormal automaticity anywhere in the ventricles from ischemia, injury, or electrolyte imbalances. Another mechanism for these arrhythmias is reentry through slowly conducting tissue within the His–Purkinje system or the ventricular myocardium related to catecholamines or digitalis excess.

Digitalis toxicity may cause delayed after-depolarizations that are oscillations in transmembrane potential that follow full repolarization of the membrane. These oscillations are caused by interference of the sodium–potassium pump by digitalis. Digitalis competes with potassium for a binding site on the cellular membrane wall, which disables the sodium–potassium adenosine triphosphatase (ATPase) pump. Triggered activity is also another important mechanism in the pathophysiology of digitalis toxicity.

The mechanism of AV block is delayed conduction or nonconduction of an atrial impulse when the AV junction is not physiologically refractory. In first-degree AV block, there is not an actual block but rather a prolongation of conduction. In second-degree block, there is non-conduction of some of the atrial impulses. The pathology is either in the AV node itself or within or below the bundle of His. The QRS complex duration assists the APN in localizing the level of block. A narrow QRS complex is seen if the ventricular response is initiated at the level of AV node and conducted down both bundle branches simultaneously, as seen in Mobitz type I block. A wider QRS complex indicates that the block is located further down the conduction system at the bundle of His or within the bundle branches, resulting in a broader QRS complex. These criteria may not be helpful if the patient has a preexisting right or left bundle branch block, however. Such a patient could present with a prolonged PR interval with a broad QRS complex, and the pathology could be either in the AV node or within or below the Bundle of His. The clinician would then need to carefully assess the PR interval for varying lengths and Wenckebach conduction patterns. If the patient is in a 2 P wave for every wide QRS complex (2:1 conduction) pattern, the origin of pathology is difficult to determine from the ECG.

Clinical Presentation

Subjective

A patient presenting with atrial fibrillation may complain of shortness of breath, palpitations, angina, changing level of consciousness, and syncope. If the patient is aware of palpitations, the clinician should have him or her "tap" out the rhythm in the palm of the hand. The irregular tapping at irregular intervals can differentiate this rhythm from the regular patterns of other arrhythmias.

A patient experiencing SVT will complain of dizziness, shortness of breath, and chest pain. As part of taking the patient's history, the clinician should ask about polyuria that is associated with SVT. Polyuria is present in 20 to 50 percent of patients with PSVT or atrial fibrillation. It is thought to be related to the cardiac secretion of atrial natriuretic factor released by changes in rhythm and atrial pressure.

A patient presenting with nonsustained VT may complain of palpitations, or may present with symptoms similar to those of patients with sustained VT. Usually patients with sustained VT will have complaints compatible with a loss of cardiac output, such as decreased levels of mentation and hypotension.

If the patient is taking digitalis, the clinician should question him or her about anorexia, nausea, and vomiting. In addition, the patient should be asked about changes in the quality of color vision, especially red and green color distortions. These changes may be subtle; patients often do not volunteer them unless asked. Scotomas and flickering halos, although advanced signs, may also be present. Neurologic symptoms such as headache, malaise, memory lapses, and insomnia may also be reported.

A patient experiencing first-degree heart block will be asymptomatic. With a third-degree AV block, the patient may exhibit signs of symptomatic bradycardia. The origin of the block may determine the degree of symptomatology. Patients with second-degree AV Mobitz type I that progresses into a third-degree block with an idiojunctional response may or may not exhibit overt signs or report symptoms of a bradycardia. The hemodynamic symptom present will depend on the rate of the junctional response (anywhere from 40 to 60 beats per minute), the status of the patient's left ventricular ejection fraction, and the loss of atrial kick (up to 20 to 30 percent of the cardiac output). A patient whose Mobitz type II heart block progresses to third-degree with a ventricular response of 20 to 40 beats per minute will almost always exhibit signs and symptoms of a severe bradycardia such as profound changes in level of consciousness and hypotension, which will prohibit reports of subjective data.

Objective

Atrial Fibrillation. Physical examination of the patient with atrial fibrillation will yield an irregularly irregular heart rhythm. In most cases the rate is rapid (100 to 180 beats per minute). Some patients with a diseased AV node present with a slow or normal ventricular rate. Patients can be asymptomatic, although most cases present with some symptoms such as palpitations, dizziness, a decrease in BP, or are mildly symptomatic with new-onset activity intolerance. In a few cases, a CVA can be the presenting manifestation of atrial fibrillation. *Cannon waves,* which are unpredictable expansions of the jugular pulse caused when the atria contract against closed AV valves, causing a reflux of blood into the jugular vein, may be seen. When present, Cannon waves signify AV dissociation as a result of the atrial fibrillation. The ECG strip will show fibrillatory waves representing an atrial rate of 350 to 600 beats per minute, with a ventricular rate of 100 to 180 beats per minute. The rhythm is irregular. There are no discernible P waves, and a coarse or fine fibrillatory wave (f wave) is present. It is the hallmark of this arrhythmia and represents chaotic atrial activity. The PR interval cannot be measured and the QRS wave is usually normal.

Premature Atrial Contractions. PACs may be found on a routine ECG. The rate is usually 60 to 100 beats per minute with a regular rhythm except when the premature beats are present. The premature beats have different P wave configuration because of origination outside the sinus node. The PAC PR interval may be different from the sinus PR interval and the QRS complex may be normal, aberrant (wide, different QRS complex), or absent.

The most common cause of a pause on an ECG rhythm strip is a blocked or nonconducted PAC. This occurs when the PAC comes so early that it falls in the T wave. If the AV node is still refractory, the early P wave does not conduct and a pause is seen on the rhythm strip. If the clinician looks closely at the T wave and compares it to the patient's other T waves, the early nonconducted P wave can be seen distorting that specific T wave. If the nonconducted PACs present in a bigeminal pattern, the rhythm may be mistaken for profound sinus bradycardia or sinoatrial (SA) block. The clinician should always assess for nonconducted P waves within preceding T waves in any pauses observed on the ECG.

Observation of the neck veins may help the clinician rapidly distinguish between PSVT and VT. During PSVT, the atria contract against closed AV valves, resulting in a rapid, regular expansion of the neck veins (the same mechanism as Cannon waves). This physical finding has been called the "frog sign" because the rapid, regular expansion of the neck veins resembles the puffing motion of a frog. The patient's family may have noticed the frog sign of PSVT.

Supraventricular Tachycardia. The ECG of a patient in SVT will show a regular rhythm with a rate of 150 to 250 beats per minute. The P waves are ectopic and distorted and may be initiated by a PAC. The PR interval is shortened, and the QRS complex may be normal or distorted. If the patient is in atrial flutter, the atrial rate will be regular, at 250 to 350 beats per minute, and the ventricular rate may be regular or irregular. The P waves are discernible and "march out" (can be mapped out with a caliper) consistently throughout the strip. The PR interval cannot be calculated and the QRS complex has a variable conduction.

Premature Ventricular Contractions. The ECG of a patient with PVCs will usually show a rate of 60 to 100 beats per minute. The rhythm will be irregular secondary to the premature ventricular beat. The PVC usually obscures the P waves; however, P waves may be visible if the PVC is late in diastole. These P waves are not related to the ectopic beat and occur at the same regular rate of the preceding sinus P waves. The PR interval is not measurable on the PVC. The QRS complex for the PVC is wide and bizarre. It may be observed in patterns of ventricular bigeminy, trigeminy, or couplets. In the setting of an acute ischemic event, PVCs that occur close to the preceding T wave (R on T phenomena) may precipitate ventricular fibrillation.

Ventricular Tachycardia. The ECG of a patient with VT will show a rate over 100 beats per minute, with a regular rhythm; the P waves will be buried in the QRS complex or discernible after the QRS complex because of retrograde conduction. The PR interval is not measurable and the QRS complex is wide and bizarre.

Heart Blocks

In first-degree AV block, the pulse will usually be 60 to 100 beats per minute. The ECG rhythm is usually regular, with a P wave preceding each QRS complex and a prolonged PR interval longer than 0.20 milliseconds. QRS complexes follow every P wave and are usually a normal width.

A patient with second-degree AV block Mobitz type I will have a ventricular rate of 50 to 70 beats per minute, although it may vary. The atrial rate is regular, whereas the ventricular rate is irregular. P waves precede each QRS complex and the PR interval progressively lengthens. The QRS complex is usually normal in width, unless a preexisting bundle branch block is present. As the PR interval progresses, eventually the QRS comples disappears for a beat. In contrast, in a Mobitz type II AV block, the PR interval may be prolonged or normal, but it remains constant, unlike the progressively lengthening PR of a type I. The blocked P wave may occur in patterns of 2 to 1, 3 to 1, or 4 to 1 that can be regular or irregular. The width of the QRS complex indicates indicates where the block is located. The wider the complex, the lower the block is located below the AV node. The P wave is regular and the PR interval constant, with a wide QRS following every P wave until the QRS complex is not conducted.

With a third-degree block, the ABV node (if the block is of a Mobitz I origin) or the ventricles (if the block is a Mobitz II in origin) set up an autonomous rhythm with a ventricular rate of 25 to 60 beats per minute. The atrial rate is 60 to 100 beats per minute. P waves are present and regular, but there is no relationship to the QRS complex. The PR interval cannot be calculated, and the QRS complex is wider and longer than 0.12 ms if the block is at the ventricles; it is normal if the block is at the junctional level.

Arrhythmias Associated with Digitalis. The digitalis effect on the ECG of a patient on digitalis therapy may be a scooping deformity of the ST segment. The other characteristic effect that may be observed is ST-segment depression and asymmetric T-wave inversion. This characteristic may be difficult to differentiate from left ventricular strain. Not all patients exhibiting digitalis effect are toxic; moreover, not all patients on digitalis exhibit a digitalis effect. In patients with sinus rhythm, a slightly prolonged PR duration is considered a therapeutic effect; however, an alarming prolonged duration may signify digitalis toxicity. The clinician must monitor the trends of PR intervals on patients taking digitalis.

Diagnostic Reasoning

Diagnostic Tests

An ECG is the routine diagnostic test to determine the type of dysrhythmia. so as to appropriately direct treatment. The most definitive diagnostics are confirmed by electrical physiology studies (EPS). Electrophysiologic testing using intracardiac electrocardiographic recordings and programmed atrial and/or ventricular stimulation is used in the diagnosis and management of complex dysrhythmias. Electrophysiologic testing can evaluate recurrent syncope of possible cardiac origin and differentiate supraventricular from ventricular dysrhythmias.

Tilt-table testing, or autonomic testing, is useful in patients with dysrhythmias when syncope may be due to a vasovagal response. The patient is tilted to approximately 70 degrees in conjunction with isoproterenol infusion. Syncope due to bradycardia and/or hypotension, will occur in about one-third of patients with recurrent syncope.

Transesophageal echocardiography (TEE) is a diagnostic procedure used to visualize and rule out the presence of thrombi in the left atrium prior to cardioversion in atrial fibrillation. The presence of clots in the left atrium are contraindications to cardioversion.

Differential Diagnosis

The differential diagnoses should consider conditions that could mimic the symptoms of dysrhythmia, such as panic attack, anxiety, valvular disorders, and syncopal episodes either neurogenic or cardiac in origin.

Management

Management of these patients by a clinician depends upon the expertise of the clinician. If the clinician is at all unsure of the management of an arrhythmia, he or she should consult with the collaborating physician or cardiovascular specialist.

Atrial Fibrillation

The goal of treatment in atrial fibrillation is to slow down the heart rate and then convert the patient back to normal sinus rhythm (NSR) by using medications or electrical synchronized cardioversion. Recent evidence has shown, however, that ventricular rate control should be the primary goal of treatment.

Many patients with atrial fibrillation after cardioversion return to atrial fibrillation within a short period of time. This is seen particularly in patients with long-standing atrial fibrillation or in patients with advanced heart disease and a very large left atrium. Patients with new-onset atrial fibrillation or chronic atrial fibrillation with a very rapid ventricular response should be admitted to a unit where telemetry is available, so that the response to treatment can be carefully monitored. Drugs that convert atrial fibrillation to sinus rhythm are amiodarone (Cordarone), disopyramide (Norpace), flecainide (Tambocor), propafenone (Rythmol), and ibutilide. Digoxin is effective only for rate control at rest and should be used only as a second-line agent. Elective synchronized cardioversion is recommended if acute ischemic heart disease is present along with a rapid ventricular rate (120 to 200 beats per minute) or if the patient is in clinical distress.

For the patient in atrial fibrillation, rapid digitalization is recommended with 0.75 mg to 1.25 mg digitalis (Lanoxin) PO or IV over 24 hours in three or more divided doses q6 to 8h. The maintenance dose is 0.125 mg to 0.5 mg daily.

Sccessful cardioversion and prevention of recurrence of atrial fibrillation depends on atrial size and the length of time in atrial fibrillation. Before electrical or pharmacologic cardioversion is attempted, anticoagulants should be considered. Anticoagulation therapy should be initiated in all patients who remain in atrial fibrillation greater than 48 hours or experience atrial fibrillation of unknown duration. Patients may be placed on IV heparin for rapid anticoagulation or started on warfarin (Coumadin), which takes approximately 5 days to achieve its full anticoagulant effect. A prothrombin time (PT) with international normalized ratio (INR) is drawn and the patient started at 5 mg/day, with the dose adjusted according to the patient's INR. The target INR is between 2 and 3, and most patients require a maintenance dose of 2 to 7.5 mg/day. The PT should be checked at regular intervals to make sure the INR remains within the appropriate range. If the patient is hospitalized, these levels are usually monitored daily, but typically take 2 to 3 days to equilibrate in response to dosing changes. Once the patient is discharged, levels should be checked every week with the dosage adjusted accordingly, until the clinician has established the patient's individual response and optimal dose. Once a constant appropriate INR range has been established, PTs should be monitored monthly. The clinician should try to maintain patients in chronic atrial fibrillation who are difficult to convert with a controlled ventricular rate and keep them on anticoagulant therapy indefinitely.

Premature Atrial Contractions

Treatment of PACs is not indicated unless patients are symptomatic or there are underlying causes that can be corrected. Simple measures such as stopping smoking, reducing caffeine intake, and improving electrolyte imbalance may reduce the incidence of PACs. If symptoms persist, Holter monitoring may be indicated and the patient should be instructed to maintain a diary of activities. The patient should be monitored for the first 3 months to establish whether this is an acute or chronic condition. A cardiologist should follow the patient.

Supraventricular Tachycardia

The initial treatment for stable SVT consists of vagal maneuvers, such as carotid sinus pressure. Vagal maneuvers increase parasympathetic tone and slow the conduction through the AV node. These techniques include coughing, lying on the floor while elevating legs against the wall, or squatting. If the clinician has the experience and knowledge of carotid sinus massage, this maneuver is usually effective. The vagal maneuver of carotid sinus massage is contraindicated in patients with carotid artery stenosis, bruits, or a history of transient ischemic attacks, or in patients older than age 65 years who may have an exacerbated parasympathetic response to carotid pressure. Facial immersion in cold water (dive reflex) is another method used. The clinician must never use eyeball pressure as a vagal maneuver because it may cause retinal detachment and is unpleasant for the patient.

In the case of PSVT, adenosine (Adenocard) is the treatment of choice; 6 mg in a peripheral IV is given rapidly. If treatment is unsuccessful, the dosage is increased to 12 mg and may be repeated once. Adenosine blocks the AV node and has an extremely short half-life of less than 10 seconds. Because of this short half-life, it is critical that this drug be delivered to the heart by a rapid IV push followed by a rapid saline flush. Adenosine does not usually cause a drop in BP and has replaced verapamil in the emergency treatment of PSVT. Verapamil hydrochlorate (verapamil HCl) may be used to treat tachyatrial arrhythmias and is given as a 2.5 to 5 mg IV bolus over 1 to 2 minutes; a second dose of 5 to 10 mg may be given IV 15 to 30 minutes after the first dose.

Pharmacologic intervention to prevent irritability may include beta-blockers and calcium channel blockers. If the patient is symptomatic with atrial flutter, is hypotensive, has ischemic pain, or has severe CHF, synchronized cardioversion is usually recommended. Pharmacologic intervention may involve beta-blockers and calcium channel blockers along with digitalis.

Patients who have recurrent symptomatic and refractory PSVT will need to see an electrophysiologist for possible radiofrequency ablation of the accessory pathway. Ablation therapy is often chosen over a lifetime course of prophylactic drugs.

Premature Ventricular Contractions

Treatment for PVCs is not usually needed in healthy adults because many adults experience PVCs with no untoward effects. If the patient is having PVCs related to an MI, however, it must be determined whether the PVCs are caused by a problem with oxygenation, hypotension, electrolyte or acid–base imbalance, other medications, or by an increased catecholamine state from unrelieved ischemic pain or anxiety. Typically, therapy in this case involves treating the underlying cause, such as the hypoxia, pain relief, electrolyte imbalance, or the alteration in hemodynamics with nitroglycerin, oxygen, pain medications, and beta-blockers.

Heart Blocks

Treatment for a first-degree AV block is not advised because it is an asymptomatic arrhythmia. For a Mobitz type I AV block, treatment is observational. If symptomatic bradycardia develops, a temporary or transcutaneous pacemaker may be needed, whereas a permanent pacemaker may be required for a Mobitz type II AV block. For third-degree heart block, the underlying pathologic sites must be determined to prevent complications. The ability to determine whether this block has an idiojunctional response versus an idioventricular response is necessary for determining appropriate interventions. Third-degree heart block is considered an emergent and potentially life-threatening condition.

Dysrhythmias Associated with Digitalis

Management for digitalis toxicity depends upon the degree of symptomatology. If the patient exhibits common manifestations such as marked prolongation of the PR interval or a slow ventricular response in atrial fibrillation, temporary withdrawal of the digitalis may be sufficient. Once the patient's condition has stabilized, the dosage is adjusted to prevent recurrence. Early recognition and intervention by the clinician are important. The mortality rate is extremely high for unrecognized digitalis toxicity. The clinician providing care for patients taking digitalis is obligated to closely evaluate for signs of digitalis toxicity.

If the patient presents with severe arrhythmias or hemodynamic compromise because of digitalis, emergency IV administration of Fab fragments, digoxin-specific antibodies, may be initiated. These antibodies reverse the cellular effects of digoxin. Digoxin immune Fab ovine (Digibind) is an example of a Fab fragment. It is a digoxin antagonist. The IV dose is based on the amount of digoxin or digitoxin to be neutralized. The contents of one vial neutralize 0.5 mg of digoxin. Electrolyte disturbances must be corrected. If the patient is severely hemodynamically unstable, a temporary ventricular pacemaker must be inserted until the patient is stabilized. Digitalis toxicity is diagnosed by subjective and ECG symptoms and digitalis levels. The concurrent use of quinidine sulfate, amiodarone, verapamil, and erythromycin all have the potential to increase digitalis levels. The digitalis dose should be tailored to the patient's weight and renal status because digitalis is excreted by the kidneys.

Premature Ventricular Contractions and Ventricular Tachycardia

Implantable cardioverter defibrillator (ICD) devices are multiprogrammable anti-arrhythmic devices capable of treating bradydysrhythmias, ventricular fibrillation, and ventricular tachycardia. These devices offer anti-tachycardia pacing as well as low- and high-energy shocks in multiple ranges of tachycardia rates. Placed under the skin in the left chest, these pacemakers last 6 hours or longer. Patients need close follow-up with a cardiologist and extensive patient education. Patients should carry a device identification card at all times. The American College of Cardiology/American Heart Association/North American Society of Pacing and Electrophysiology (ACC/AHA/NASPE) guidelines delineate indications for ICD thearpy.

Follow-Up and Referral

A cardiologist should be consulted to establish the plan of care. The cardiologist may order a Holter monitor to establish if there is a routine pattern to the rhythm. Electrophysiologic studies may be indicated to evaluate the patient for ablation therapy for PSVTs, such as WPW syndrome.

Patient Education

The education of a patient for atrial fibrillation should include a list of foods and prescription and OTC drugs that interfere with warfarin (Table 9.14). The patient on warfarin is at risk for bleeding; therefore, the clinician should provide literature on medical alert identification jewelry and instruct the patient how to assess for signs of bleeding, such as bruising and dark stools and how to use electric razors and night lights. Patients should be taught to check their pulse rate. If the pulse rate is decreased (below 60 beats per minute) or the patient notices bursts in the rate, it should be reported to the clinician.

Valvular Disorders and Murmurs

Mitral and aortic valve disorders are the most common of the heart valve disorders. These disorders may be congenital or acquired and may be symptomatic or asymptomatic.

Table 9.14 Drugs and Foods that Interact with Warfarin

Increased Anticoagulant Effect	Decreased Anticoagulant Effect
Drugs	Drugs
Acetaminophen (Tylenol)	Carbamazepine (Tegretol)
Allopurinol (Zyloprim)	Cholecystyramine (Questran)
Amiodarone (Cordarone)	Griseofulvin (Grifulvin)
Cisapride (Propulsid)	Oral contraceptives (Ortho TriCyclen, Loestrin)
Cephalosporins (Keflex)	Rifampin (Rifadin)
Disulfiram (Antabuse)	Spironolactone (Aldactone)
Erythromycin (E-Mycin)	Sucralfate (Carafate)
Fluoroquinolones (Cipro, Levaquin)	Foods
Gemfibrozil (Lopid)	Chronic alcohol abuse
H_2-blockers (Pepcid, Zantac)	
Fluconazole (Diflucan)	
Metronidazole (Flagyl)	
NSAIDs (Advil, Motrin)	
Penicillins (Pen VK)	
Propranolol (Inderal)	
Quinidine (Quinaglute)	
Selective serotonin re-uptake inhibitors (SSRIs: sertraline [Zoloft], fluoxetine [Prozac])	
Sulfonylureas (Glucotrol, Amaryl)	
Tetracycline (Achromycin)	
Trimethoprim-sulfamethoxazole (Bactrim)	
Valproate (Depakene)	
Foods	
Excessive alcohol	
Vitamins A, C, E	

Many are detected during heart auscultation when alterations in the normal heart rhythm, presence of extrasystoles, murmurs, and abnormal heart sounds are heard.

Heart murmurs are the sound of turbulent blood flow. Blood traveling through the chambers and great vessels is normally a silent event. When the flow is sufficient to generate turbulence in the wall of the heart or great vessel, a murmur occurs.

Murmurs may be benign, in that the clinician simply hears the blood flowing through the heart but no cardiac structural abnormality exists. Certain cardiac structural problems, however, such as valvular and myocardial disorders, can contribute to the development of a murmur.

Benign systolic ejection murmurs such as physiologic murmurs are found in the absence of cardiac pathology. The term implies that the reason for the murmur is something other than obstruction to flow and is present with a normal gradient across the valve. This murmur may be heard in up to 80 percent of thin adults or children if the cardiac exam is performed in a soundproof booth; it is best heard at the left sternal border. It occurs in early to midsystole, leaving the two heart sounds intact. In addition, the patient with a benign systolic ejection murmur denies cardiac symptomatology and has an otherwise normal cardiac exam, including an appropriately located PMI and full pulses. No cardiac pathology is present with a physiologic murmur, so no endocarditis prophylaxis is needed.

A *hemic murmur* is heard in hyperkinetic or high-volume states such as anemia, fever, or response to exercise. The murmur is crescendo–decrescendo and harsh, and both heart sounds are preserved. Because there is no cardiac pathology associated with this condition, it resolves when its underlying cause is gone. As with a physiologic murmur, no structural cardiac abnormality is present and no endocarditis prophylaxis is needed.

An *aortic sclerosis murmur* is also called the 50/50 murmur, as it is present in about 50 percent of adults older than age 50. Its etiology is likely fibrotic and/or calcific changes in the aortic valve. The valve can open enough to prevent a significant gradient but is restricted enough to cause the murmur. It differs from an aortic stenosis murmur in having an early peak and resolution as well as lack of hemodynamic significance.

Types of Valvular Disorders

Aortic stenosis is the inability of the aortic valves to open to optimum orifice. The aortic valve normally opens to 3 cm^2; aortic stenosis usually does not cause significant symptoms until the valvular orifice is limited to 0.8 cm^2. The disease is characterized by a long symptom-free period, with rapid clinical deterioration at the onset of symptoms, including dyspnea, syncope, chest pain, and CHF. The clinician should look for a small pulse pressure on BP, a characteristic of severe aortic stenosis.

The murmur of *mitral regurgitation* arises from mitral valve incompetency or the inability of the mitral valve to close properly. This allows a retrograde flow from a high-pressure area (ILV) to an area of lower pressure (left atrium). Mitral regurgitation is most often caused by the degeneration of the mitral valve, most commonly by rheumatic fever, endocarditis, calcific annulus, rheumatic heart disease, ruptured chordae, or papillary muscle dysfunction. In mitral regurgitation from rheumatic heart disease, there is usually also some stenosis. Once the person is symptomatic, the disease progresses in a downhill course of CHF over the next 10 years.

Mitral valve prolapse (MVP) is the most common valvular heart problem with an incidence of 2.4 percent in the general population based on two-dimensional echocardiographic criteria. In most cases, MVP is a benign condition. However, MVP with mitral regurgitation may predispose the individual to thrombi and endocarditis. In the past, the prevalence of MVP was overestimated owing to lack of the availability of specific diagnostic procedures. Patients given this diagnosis more than 10 years ago may not have the disorder at all and should be reevaluated with two-dimensional echocardiography (Table 9.15 presents the common valvular disorders.)

Epidemiology and Causes

Bacterial endocarditis, rheumatic heart disease, and aortic calcification are common etiologies of valvular disorders that cause heart murmurs. Bacterial endocarditis is most often due to septicemia caused by *Staphylococcus aureus* or *Streptococcus* viridans (alpha-hemolytic) infection. Valvular deformities are among a spectrum of abnormalities associated with endocarditis. Intravenous drug abusers and patients with indwelling intravenous catheters are at risk for bacterial septicemia which can lead to endocarditis. Patients with prosthetic heart valves, heart murmurs, or valvular damage require prophylactic antibiotics to prevent endocarditis prior to any invasive procedures such as dental or surgical interventions.

Rheumatic heart disease is another cause of heart valve injury. Rheumatic heart disease is a result of rheumatic fever, an infection caused by group A beta-hemolytic *Streptococcus* infection. The pathologic mechanism involves antibodies developed by the body against the bacteria. Antistreptococcal antibodies are thought to cross-react with the body's own tissues and "mistakenly" attack the heart valves in susceptible individuals. Because of the wide availability of antibiotics, rheumatic fever has become a less common etiology of valvular disease.

Calcification of the aortic valve is a common finding in elderly patients who present with an aortic heart murmur. A calcified aortic valve is often a result of long-standing arteriosclerosis. This calcification causes narrowing of the aortic valve resulting in an audible disturbance in blood flow through the valve.

In childhood and younger adults, aortic stenosis may be present; it is usually caused by a congenital bicuspid (rather than tricuspid) valve or by a three-cusp valve with

Table 9.15 **Common Valvular Disorders**

Disorder	Murmur Characteristics	Physical Examination	Diagnostic Findings
Aortic stenosis	Grade: 1–4/6, harsh systolic usually crescendo-decrescendo pattern. Heard best: Second right intercostal space (RICS), apex. Radiation: To carotids. Other: Softens with standing.	Cardiac: May have diminished S2, slow-filling carotid pulse, narrow pulse pressure, loud S4, heaving PMI. Other: Anxiety, difficulty breathing, compromised mental status, cyanosis, peripheral edema, hair loss, shiny skin over shins, cool extremities, decreased SBP, pulmonary edema.	Chest x-ray: Aortic valve calcification, left ventricle (LV) enlargement, prominent ascending aorta. ECG: LVH, sinus tachycardia, atrial fibrillation, AV conduction delay, left or right bundle branch block (LBBB, RBBB). Echocardiogram: Limited aortic valve movement, thickened left ventricular wall. Cardiac catheterization: Increased pressure gradient in systole across aortic valve, decreased size or aortic orifice, increased left ventricular end-diastolic pressure.
Aortic regurgitation	Grade: 1–3/4 high-pitched blowing diastolic murmur. Heard best: Third left intercostal space (LICS). Radiation: Other: May be enhanced by forced expiration, leaning forward.	Cardiac: Usually with S3 wide pulse pressure, sustained thrusting apical impulse, palpitations, dyspnea, orthopnea, PND, syncope, signs of LV failure, peripheral edema, flushed skin, cardiomegaly. Other: More common in men, usually from rheumatic heart disease; occasionally caused by third-degree syphilis, fatigue, weakness, anxiety, compromised mental state.	Chest x-ray: Aortic valve calcification, LV enlargement, dilation of ascending aorta. ECG: LVH, sinus tachycardia, PVCs. Echocardiogram: Dilated and hyperdynamic LV, enlargement of aortic root and LA, early closure of mitral valve, diastolic fluttering of aortic valve. Cardiac catheterization: Decreased aortic diastolic pressure, increased LVEDP, decreased regurgitant flow, reflux through aortic valve.
Aortic sclerosis	Grade: 2–3/6 systolic ejection murmur. Heard best: Second RIC. Radiation: Other: "50 over 50" murmur (found in 50% of those over age 50).	Cardiac: Full carotid upstroke, no S4.	Echocardiogram: Benign thickening and/or calcification of aortic valve leaflets. Cardiac catheterization: No change in valve pressure gradient.
Mitral stenosis	Grade: 1–3/4 low-pitched late diastolic murmur. Heard best: Apex. Radiation: Localized. Other: Short crescendo-decrescendo rumble, often with opening snap; enhanced by left lateral decubitus position, squat, cough; also immediately post–Valsalva maneuver.	Cardiac: Accentuated S1 in mitral area, atrial fibrillation, dyspnea, orthopnea, PND. Other: History or rheumatic fever; protracted latency period, then gradual decrease in exercise tolerance, fatigue, hoarseness, ruddy cheeks, peripheral edema, anorexia, enlarged liver, crackles, bloody productive cough.	Chest x-ray: LA and RV enlargement, pulmonary venous congestion ECG: LAH, RVH, P-mitrale, prolonged notched P waves, atrial fibrillation. Echocardiogram: Thickened mitral valve with diminished movement of leaflets, left atrium (LA) and right ventricle (RV) enlargement.

Disorder	Murmur Characteristics	Physical Examination	Diagnostic Findings
			Cardiac catheterization: Increased pressure gradient across mitral valve, increased left atrium pressure (LAP) and pulmonary vascular resistance, increased LVEDP, increased PAWP, decreased CO.
Mitral regurgitation	Grade: 1–4/6 high-pitched blowing systolic murmur, often extending beyond S2. Heard best: Right lower sternal border (RLSB). Radiation: Radiates to axilla, often with laterally displaced PMI. Other: Sounds like a loon—"haa," "hoo." Decreased with standing Valsalva maneuver; increased by squat, hand grip.	Cardiac: History of ischemic heart disease, endocarditis, RHD, other valve abnormalities, dyspnea, orthopnea, paroxysmal nocturnal dyspnea (PND), diaphoresis, cyanosis, JVD, peripheral edema. Other: Weakness, fatigue, anxiety, abdominal respirations, enlarged liver, crackles.	ECG: Atrial fibrillation, P mitrale (if patient is in sinus rhythm). Doppler echocardiogram: Detects and quantifies mitral regurgitation.
Mitral valve prolapse	Grade: 1–3/6 late systolic crescendo murmur with honking quality. Heard best: Apex. Other: Follows midsystolic click; with Valsalva or standing, click moves forward into earlier systole resulting in a longer sounding murmur; with hand grasp, squat, click moves back further into systole, resulting in a shorter murmur.	Cardiac: Recurrent chest pain in the precordium and substernal areas, dyspnea, syncope. Other: Often seen with minor thoracic deformities (e.g., pectus excavatum, strait back, shallow AP diameter) or high arched palate, fatigue, lightheadedness, migraine headache, exercise intolerance, anxiety, panic attacks; arm span often greater than height.	Chest x-ray: Normal. ECG: Normal. Two-dimensional echocardiogram: Demonstrates MVP.
Atrial septal defect (uncorrected)	Grade: 1–3/6 ejection murmur. Heard best: Pulmonic area.	Cardiac: Widely split S2 RV heave. Other: CHF, exertional dyspnea.	Auscultation: A split S2 may be heard.

leaflet fusion. This defect is most often found in males and is commonly accompanied by a long-standing history of becoming excessively short of breath with increased activity such as running. The physical examination is usually normal except for the associated cardiac findings.

Mitral valve prolapse occurs in about 2 to 4 percent of the population and is usually detected in young adulthood. It is more common in women younger than age 20; the incidence is equal in men and women after age 20.

Pathophysiology

Normal heart valves allow one-way, unimpeded forward blood flow through the heart. The entire stroke output is able to pass freely during one phase of the cardiac cycle, and there is no backflow of blood. When a heart valve fails to open to its normal orifice, it is stenotic. When it fails to close appropriately, the valve is incompetent, causing regurgitation of blood to the previous chamber or vessel. Both of these events place the patient at significant risk for embolic disease.

Treatment for a first-degree AV block is not advised because it is an asymptomatic arrhythmia. For a Mobitz type I AV block, treatment is observational. If symptomatic bradycardia develops, a temporary or transcutaneous pacemaker may be needed, whereas a permanent pacemaker may be required for a Mobitz type II AV block. For third-degree heart block, the underlying pathologic sites must be determined to prevent complications. The ability to determine whether this block has an idiojunctional response versus an idioventricular response is necessary for determining appropriate interventions. Third-degree heart block is considered an emergent and potentially life-threatening condition.

Clinical Presentation

Subjective

The patient may be asymptomatic or, depending on the specific problem, may complain of dyspnea, orthopnea, paroxysmal nocturnal dyspnea, fatigue, hoarseness, palpitations, weakness, chest pain, heart failure, vertigo, syncope, and peripheral edema. The patient may or may not know whether or not he or she has a heart murmur. (Table 9.16 lists the signs and symptoms of specific valvular disorders.)

Objective

When evaluating an adult with a cardiac murmur, the clinician should ask about major symptoms of heart disease, including chest pain, CHF symptoms, palpitations, syncope, and activity intolerance. The bell of the stethoscope is most helpful for auscultating lower-pitched sounds, whereas the diaphragm is best used for hearing higher-pitched sounds. Systolic murmurs are graded on a 1 to 6 scale, from barely audible to audible with stethoscope off the chest (grades IV to VI must have a palpable thrill). Diastolic murmurs are usually graded on the same scale but are graded from 1 to 4, because these murmurs are not loud enough to reach grades 5 and 6. Advanced Assessment 9.3 gives more information about the cardiac examination, including assessing heart murmurs.

Diagnostic Reasoning

Diagnostic Tests

Initially, the clinician may discover a murmur on physical exam. Depending on the associated symptoms, the clinician may refer the patient for subsequent testing or may refer the patient directly to a cardiologist for more invasive testing. Two-dimensional echocardiography is the definitive procedure to diagnose heart valve disorders.

Various diagnostic tests used to detect valvular lesions or structural heart changes include an echocardiography, ECG, chest x-ray film, and cardiac catheterization. The clinician usually should order an echocardiogram, ECG, and chest x-ray film to confirm a definitive diagnosis of a murmur and then refer the patient to a cardiologist unless the clinician and patient agree on an initial course of therapy as a trial, such as in MVP. The ECG can reveal LVH. The chest x-ray film may show an enlarged cardiac silhouette, left ventricular prominence, calcification of the aortic valve, and dilation and calcification of the ascending aorta. An echocardiogram is useful in demonstrating the underlying pathologic process, whether the lesion involves the aortic root, or if valvular disease is present. Cardiac catheterizations can provide an accurate assessment of regurgitation and stenosis, along with left ventricular function and pulmonary artery pressures. Coronary angiography is often indicated to determine the presence of CAD before valve surgery.

Differential Diagnosis

The differential diagnosis for MVP include hypertrophic cardiomyopathies, papillary dysfunction, coronary artery spasm and/or disease, anxiety disorders, and congenital cardiac anomalies.

The differential diagnoses for mitral stenosis include atrial myxoma or vegetation caused by endocarditis, anemia, and thyrotoxicosis. For mitral regurgitation, the differential diagnoses include rheumatic or ischemic heart disease, MVP, infective endocarditis, mitral annular dilation or calcification, congenital valve deformities, cardiac trauma, and prosthetic mitral valve malfunction.

Management

The principle of management is to help the patient maintain a normal cardiac output, thus preventing manifestations of heart failure, venous congestion, and inadequate tissue perfusion. For an asymptomatic patient, no treatment is indicated, except for possibly prophylactic antibiotic therapy discussed in the section on Aortic Valve Disorders.

Mitral Valve Disorders

Mitral Valve Prolapse. There is no medical treatment to correct MVP. Symptomatic management includes lifestyle changes, such as beginning a mild exercise program to reduce plasma catecholamines, lower the HR, decrease stress, and increase the cardiac output and blood volume. Beta-blockers may be prescribed for patients with MVP to help control palpitations; however, because fatigue is a problem with this disorder, it may be exacerbated by beta-blockers.

Antibiotic prophylaxis to prevent infective bacterial endocarditis may be prescribed to some persons with MVP, not all. Antibiotic prophylaxis is considered if certain high-risk echocardiographic characteristics are present such as leaflet redundancy, leaflet thickening, or left atrial or ventricular enlargement. Anticoagulation with aspirin (81 to 325 mg/day) is prescribed for some individuals with MVP who also have had a history of TIA, ischemic stroke, or atrial fibrillation.

Persons with MVP and severe mitral regurgitation should be followed with stress echocardiography periodically. Surgical intervention is indicated for MVP with severe mitral valve regurgitation.

Mitral Stenosis. For symptomatic mitral stenosis, cardiac glycosides (digitalis) may be used to control ventricular response or cardioversion, followed by quinidine to maintain the sinus rhythm if the patient has atrial fibrillation. Diuretics and sodium restriction should be initiated to reduce the blood volume and pulmonary and systemic venous pressures, along with anticoagulation therapy with warfarin (coumadin) if there is a history of systemic embolism, atrial fibrillation, or a large left atrium. Surgical intervention may be required for some patients; it may

ADVANCED ASSESSMENT 9.3

The Cardiac Examination and Assessment of Heart Murmurs

Area of Examination	*Assess*	*Possible Clinical Correlation*
Skin temperature	Variations from normal	Cool, moist skin may indicate a decrease in cardiac output Cool, dry skin may reflect environmental temperature or use of vasoconstricting substances such as sympathomimetics (caffeine, nicotine)
Skin color	Central cyanosis	Poor blood oxygenation
	Peripheral cyanosis	Excessive removal of oxygen from the blood
	Palmar erythema	Suggests liver impairment
	Pallor	May be present in severe anemia (hemoglobin [Hgb] <8 g)
Pulse	Rate	Note presence of bradycardia, tachycardia
	Rhythm	Regular, irregular, regularly irregular (extrasystoles), irregularly irregular (likely atrial fibrillation)
	Character and volume	Normally full and rapidly filling
Blood pressure (BP)	Pulse pressure	Narrow pulse pressure may be found in volume depletion, aortic stenosis Wide pulse pressure may be found in aortic regurgitation
Point of Maximum Impulse (PMI)	Location	Normally located at fifth ICS at midclavicular line With hypertrophy, PMI shifts laterally and may cover more than one ICS
Apical impulse	Sensation	Normally a gentle tapping sensation Forceful, thrusting seen with ventricular overload Diffuse, weak seen in cardiac hypertrophy Sustained in poorly controlled hypertension, aortic stenosis Double apex impulse in ventricular aneurysm
Heart sounds	S1 (normal heart sound)	Marks onset of systole, heard just before palpation of carotid artery High-pitched, click-like sound
	Variations from normal S1	Unusually loud: mitral stenosis Unusually soft: In mitral stenosis, S1 becomes softer as the valve calcifies and becomes more rigid and less mobile. (mitral stenosis, mitral regurgitation) Abnormally wide split: delay in closure of tricuspid valve (RBBB)
	S2 (normal heart sound)	Marks end of systole; vibration of aortic and pulmonic valve after closure
	Physiologic split S2	Occurs at end of systole Widest split at peak inspiration; may disappear with sitting, standing Normal finding in younger adult; usually disappears by middle-age
	Fixed split S2	Occurs at end of systole No closure of split with position change; does not increase with inspiration Occurs with atrial septal defect, pulmonary stenosis
	Paradoxical split S2	Occurs with coarctation of the aorta
	S3 (third heart sound, ventricular gallop, protodiastolic gallop)	Likely produced by the rapidly filling ventricles at a point where ventricular filling slows or by a recoil of the heart as it is pushed against the chest Occurs in early diastole Heard best by the diaphragm; no change with respiration, although occasionally inspiration or expiration will increase its sound Found in disorders of systolic emptying, CHF, valvular heart disease, ischemic heart disease, hypertrophic cardiomyopathy
	S4 (fourth heart sound, atrial gallop, presystolic gallop, S4 gallop)	May be caused by the tug of the chordae and papillary muscles in the state of poor ventricular compliance Found in disorders of diastolic filling; poorly controlled hypertension, angina, ischemic heart disease

include mitral commissurotomy, balloon valvuloplasty, or mitral valve replacement.

Mitral Regurgitation. For an symptomatic patient with mitral regurgitation, vasodilators should be initiated to reduce ventricular filling volume and to decrease systemic vascular resistance. Digitalis and anticoagulants should be prescribed to control the ventricular rate and decrease the embolic complications if the patient has atrial fibrillation. Sodium restriction and diuretics will relieve symptoms of CHF if they are present in patients with mitral regurgitation. A mitral valve replacement may be required.

Aortic Valve Disorders

Aortic Stenosis. Aortic valve replacement or aortic commissurotomy may be required for aortic stenosis.

Aortic Regurgitation. For the patient with symptomatic aortic regurgitation, digitalis and diuretics can be used to treat the symptoms of heart failure; arterial vasodilators will reduce the left ventricular afterload. Aortic valve replacement may be required.

Follow-Up and Referral

The clinician should follow the patient at regular intervals for close monitoring as well as whenever a new drug has been added or a dosage changed. The patient should be referred to the collaborating physician or cardiologist when the diagnosis is unconfirmed, or when the symptoms are not well managed with medical therapy.

Patient Education

Valvular heart disorders require lifelong management. Patients may benefit from maintaining a diary to monitor the effectiveness of lifestyle changes and compliance with drug therapy in controlling symptoms of the disorder. Patients with MVP should be instructed to begin a gradual program of exercise and to avoid caffeine, decongestants, and products containing ephedrine, alcohol, chocolate, and cheeses. They should be encouraged to drink at least eight glasses of water a day to prevent dehydration. Patients with aortic stenosis often require activity restrictions. The patient should understand how to pace activity, note an improvement in fatigue, and accept the activity restrictions.

A critical part of the evaluation of a person with a heart murmur is the decision to offer antimicrobial prophylaxis. No prophylaxis is needed with benign murmurs. Treatment Standards/Guidelines 9.1 presents the treatment guidelines for bacterial endocarditis prophylaxis. Patients with beta-hemolytic streptococcal infections (the precursor to rheumatic heart disease) must be identified and treated promptly.

Treatment Standards/Guidelines 9.1 Bacterial Endocarditis Prophylaxis

The following are the American Heart Association's guidelines for bacterial endocarditis prophylaxis when undergoing dental, oral, respiratory tract, or esophageal procedures:

Recommended for:

High-risk patients:

- Prosthetic heart valves
- Previous bacterial endocarditis
- Complex cyanotic congenital heart disease
- Surgically constructed systemic pulmonary shunts or conduits

Moderate risk patients:

- Most other congenital cardiac deformities, including ventricular septal defect (VSD)
- Rheumatic heart disease and other acquired cardiac defects, including after successful surgical repair
- Hypertrophic cardiomyopathy
- Mitral valve prolapse (with valvular regurgitation and/or thickened valves)

Not recommended for:

Risk no greater than the general population:

- Isolated ostium secundum atrial septal defect
- Surgical repair of atrial septal defect, ventricular septal defect, patent ductus arteriosus with residua beyond 6 months
- Mitral valve prolapse without significant mitral regurgitation or notation of redundant or thickened tissue around the valve
- Physiologic, functional, or innocent heart murmurs either currently present or diagnosed in the past
- Previous Kawasaki disease without valvular dysfunction
- Previous rheumatic fever without valvular dysfunction
- Cardiac pacemakers (intravascular and epicardial)

Endocarditis prophylaxis:

No penicillin allergy:

- Amoxicillin: adults 2 g 1 hour before procedure; children 50 mg/kg 1 hour before procedure

If penicillin allergic:

- Clindamycin: adults 600 mg; children 20 mg/kg OR
- Cephalexin or cefadroxil: adults 2 g; children 50 mg/kg OR
- Azithromycin or clarithromycin: adults 500 mg; children 50 mg/kg

Source: Adapted from Dajani, AS, et al: Prevention of bacterial endocarditis: Recommendations of the American Heart Association. JAMA 277:1794–1801, 1997.

Peripheral Vascular Disease/ Deep Venous Thrombophlebitis/ Thromboembolism

Peripheral vascular disease (PVD) consists of two distinct types of disorders—arterial and venous disease. Because of the nature of blood flow and vessel structure, the mechanisms of PVD are completely different for arteries and veins. Both types of PVD involve the blood vessels of the lower extremities. Chronic venous insufficiency is a common problem found in primary care settings.

Most PVD disorders of the arteries are a consequence of arteriosclerosis which impedes circulation from the heart to the lower extremities. Arterial blood flow is obstructed, causing ischemia of the muscles in the lower extremity in arterial insufficiency (also called peripheral arterial disease [PAD]). Other types of arterial PVD include aneurysms and arteritis (inflammation of the arteries).

The major types of venous PVD involve valve weakening, venous stasis, and venous clot formation. Valves within the veins assist in maintaining blood flow upward from the lower extremities to the heart. Weakened valves within the veins allow venous blood to pool in the lower extremities which enhances the potential for clot formation. Major types of venous PVD include chronic venous insufficiency and deep venous thromboembolism. Thrombophlebitis usually occurs in the lower extremities. When involving the deep veins of the pelvis or extremities, it is referred to as *deep venous thrombosis* (DVT). A thrombus begins by attaching itself to the vessel wall or valve cusp in the venous system. Then it lyses spontaneously, propagates, or embolizes. Unfortunately, which of these three events will occur cannot be predicted. If a clot breaks away from the vessel wall, it becomes an embolism, which may travel through the venous system and lodge in the lungs, causing a life-threatening pulmonary embolism (PE).

Epidemiology and Causes

Peripheral artery disease is caused by atherosclerosis, blood clots, trauma, spasms of smooth muscles in the arterial walls, and congenital structural defects in the arteries. Approximately 8 million people have PAD, and its most common symptom is intermittent claudication. In patients older than age 70, 20 percent suffer from PAD. The 5-year mortality rate for PAD approaches 30 percent as patients die from comorbid conditions of CAD and cerebrovascular disease. PAD is more common in men than women and nine times more common in smokers.

Chronic venous insufficiency and varicose veins usually result from venous incompetence gsecondary to valve obstruction. More than 20 percent of the population are affected with chronic venous insufficiency; the incidence increases with age. There are no significant ethnic predispositions. Chronic venous insufficiency is more common in women than men. Risk Factors 9.2 presents a comparison of the arterial and venous risk factors. DVT and PE are complications encountered during the treatment of medical and surgical patients. Risk Factors 9.3 presents risk factors for DVT. Approximately 300,000 to 600,000 hospitalizations can be associated with DVT and PE each year. Up to 50,000 deaths occur annually because of PE. It is estimated that there are more than 2 million cases per year of DVT. The actual number of cases is underdiagnosed because of the silent nature of the problem.

RISK FACTORS 9.2

Peripheral Vascular Disease

Arterial Risk Factors (Peripheral Arterial Disease)	Smoking: Vasoconstriction/spasm-decreased circulation Obesity: Increased cardiac workload Inactivity: Decreased circulation Hypertension: Increased fibrous tissue, which decreases stretch of arterial walls, which increases peripheral vascular resistance High cholesterol: Atherosclerotic plaque, which increases hyperlipidemia Diabetes: Increase in atherosclerosis of smaller vessels
Venous Risk Factors	Coagulation abnormalities Abdominal/pelvic surgery: Venous pooling/stasis Estrogen/oral contraceptives Pregnancy: Venous congestion Obesity: Increased in cardiac workload, venous pooling Heart disease: Venous stasis Advanced neoplasm: Coagulation abnormalities; interference with venous blood flow

Patients undergoing various types of surgical procedures, such as orthopedic, gynecologic-obstetric, urologic, neurosurgical, and general surgical procedures are at high risk for developing DVT and PE. Of these groups, orthopedic patients appear to be especially prone to thrombosis, particularly patients with hip fracture. All elective orthopedic surgical patients undergoing lower extremity surgery are at risk for DVT. The risk is greatest for patients undergoing hip surgery and knee reconstruction, for which DVT rates range from 45 to 70 percent.

Patients with various types of medical diseases, usually chronic, are also at a high risk for venous thrombotic events. The risk of DVT in pregnancy has been reported to be five times higher than in nonpregnant patients in the same age group and may be increased postpartum. A silent DVT may cause a postphlebitic syndrome. Up to 800,000 Americans have or have had venous ulceration. The postphlebitic syndrome can result in significant loss of workdays for these patients. A frequent complication of DVT is PE, which can obstruct blood flow to the lungs and cause sudden death without signs or symptoms. It is often not possible to recognize DVT until it is too late. More than 80 percent of patients who died from a pulmonary embolism showed DVT on autopsy.

Pathophysiology

Atherosclerosis is the most common cause of arterial insufficiency of the lower extremity, also referred to as PAD. Arteriosclerotic plaque obstructs optimal arterial blood flow to the muscles of the lower extremity. With increased muscle activity there is an increased need for arterial blood flow. For this reason, during ambulation or exercise, limitations of arterial blood flow cause muscle pain due to ischemia. This cramping muscle pain is referred to as *intermittent claudication* since in the initial stages of PAD, ischemia occurs periodically. Muscle activity of the lower extremity requires increased circulation and arterial vasodilation. PAD causes lack of arterial vasodilatory ability. Thus, as PAD worsens, arterial circulation diminishes and less muscle activity causes pain due to worsening ischemia. Eventually pain at rest occurs which is a sign of severe PAD. In general, the clinical manifestations of PAD are extremity pain (claudication), weak pulse, pallor, paresthesias, and palpable coolness of the lower extremity. Longstanding PAD causes muscle atrophy, diminished hair growth, and discolored, hardened toenails of the extremity. All of these signs and symptoms are due to lack of arterial blood supply to the lower extremities. Early recognition of the signs of PAD and treatment are critical because severe ischemia can lead to the need for amputation.

Arteriosclerotic plaque formation within the lower extremities is accelerated by the presence of diabetes mellitus; therefore, PAD is more common in persons with diabetes. Hyperglycemia in diabetes causes endothelial injury, damaging arterial vessels. Clinical manifestations of arterial insufficiency are apparent in the lower extremities of individuals with diabetes. Many suffer the complications of diminished circulation of the legs which include poor wound healing and peripheral neuropathy. The smaller caliber arterial vessels of the most distal regions of the lower extremity are initially affected. Therefore, careful periodic physical assessment of the feet and lower extremities is recommended in persons with diabetes, inspecting for poor wound healing and diminished peripheral pulses.

Aneurysms, another manifestation of arterial PVD, result from weakening in arterial walls, which renders them susceptible to rupture. The most common cause of this weakening is arteriosclerosis. Aneurysms appear as bulges in the arterial wall and are classified according to location. The aorta and cerebral arteries are the most common sites of aneurysms. In the aorta, a dissecting aneurysm, which is an incomplete tear in the vascular wall, may occur when elevated BP leads to separation of the layers of aortic tissue.

Arteritis, a form of vasculitis, involves inflammation of arterial blood vessels. Inflammation decreases the vasodilatory capacity of arteries and may cause spasm of the arteries. This condition is often associated with autoimmune disease. *Raynaud's phenomenon* is a result of cold-induced vasospasm of the small blood vessels in the fingers and toes, causing a characteristic blanching that sometimes extends to the hands or feet. A tricolor change may also be stimulated, which appears first as blanching of the finger tips and toes, followed by cyanosis and rubor (redness).

Clots can originate anywhere in the venous system, but the majority begin in the deep veins of the pelvis and lower extremities, with a significant number at or above the popliteal vein. Clots that originate in the proximal veins are potentially more dangerous because they are larger in size and result in more clinically significant thromboembolic events.

The causative factors in the formation of blood clots are referred to as *Virchow's triad* (see Risk Factors 9.3). Clots are likely to form when two of the three factors in the triad—stasis, vessel wall damage, and coagulation changes—are altered. Stasis of blood may result from immobility, edema, or anesthesia; blood tends to coagulate in and around the valve cusps of the veins, thus increasing the likelihood of clot formation. Vessel wall damage may result from trauma, surgical incision, laceration, venous wall distension from immobility or anesthesia, or a previous DVT. Coagulation changes leading to activated coagulation factors as a result of damaged endothelium may be the result of surgery, trauma, injury, disease states (such as sepsis, infection, or cancer), pregnancy, or foreign substance invasion via IV lines or catheters. The damaged endothelium causes the local activation of coagulation factors as platelets come in contact with the exposed collagen found in connective tissue, including skin, bone, ligaments, and cartilage. The platelets release substances, which cause vasoconstriction and accelerate clotting.

RISK FACTORS 9.3

Risk Factors for DVT

Virchow's Triad	*Clinical Risk Factors for DVT*
Venous Stasis	Immobility Venous insufficiency Prolonged sedentary position Post-stroke Post-myocardial infarction Heart failure
Vessel Injury	Trauma Surgery (especially orthopedic) Indwelling intravenous catheters (lower extremity)
Hypercoagulability	High estrogen states (oral contraceptives or hormone replacement therapy) Pregnancy/postpartum period Cancer Inherited coagulation abnormalities

Source: Teri Capriotti, DO, MSN, CRNP.

Once formed, a DVT can propagate, embolize, or lyse. When the clot propagates, it extends proximally and becomes larger and thus more dangerous, by obstructing blood flow, which causes the vein to dilate and the vessel wall to be damaged. When a clot embolizes, it travels; it may lodge itself in the arteries of the lungs, resulting in PE. When a clot lyses, it breaks down. Even if a clot lyses, it can still cause irreversible valve damage by allowing blood to reflux in the veins. The damage sets up a cycle of pooling and HTN known as the postphlebitic syndrome. Patients with this syndrome experience chronic pain, swelling, and venous ulcers.

Chronic venous insufficiency is a disorder of the valves within the deep veins of the lower extremities. Valves within veins assist venous blood to flow upward toward the heart, regulating unidirectional flow by preventing retrograde flow of venous blood away from the heart. Weakened venous valves do not form tight closures, failing to prevent retrograde blood flow. The appearance of superficial varicose veins may be associated with chronic venous insufficiency. However, superficial varicose veins are benign in most cases and are treatable with conservative measures. However, under more severe circumstances, venous stasis results, as excess pressure builds up in the legs, causing distension of the veins, thinning and scaling of the skin with dusky discoloration (stasis dermatitis), and eventually large venous ulcers. In addition, dependent edema and poor wound healing result.

Deep venous thrombophlebitis/thromboembolism (DVT) is a critical disorder of the veins of the lower extremity. The presence of a thrombus within a deep vein with an accompanying inflammatory response is termed *deep venous thrombophlebitis or deep venous thrombosis.* A venous thrombus can dissolve, propagate, or embolize. If the thrombus breaks away from the wall of the vein and travels upward toward the heart, it is termed a *venous thromboembolism*. The factors that predispose to deep venous thrombosis are known as *Virchow's Triad*: hypercoagulability of the blood, venous stasis, and vascular injury. Common causes of hypercoagulability are estrogen use, pregnancy, and neoplasms. Venous stasis occurs most often as a result of immobility. Vascular injury can be due to surgery or trauma. Orthopedic surgery is a major risk factor for DVT, and there is a high incidence of concurrent DVT in persons with cancer of the pancreas, lungs, breast, genitourinary tract, and stomach.

The signs of DVT may be subtle. Overt signs of DVT include tenderness and ropiness along the course of a vein, warmth, erythema and edema over a localized region of the leg, and distension of venous collaterals. Findings are typically unilateral, as well. The most common complaint is calf pain. A positive "*Homan's sign*" (pain on dorsiflexion of the foot) may be indicative of DVT; however, this is an unreliable diagnostic indicator.

Pulmonary embolism (PE) is a potential complication of deep venous thromboembolism. The venous thrombus may break free from the venous wall and travel from the lower extremity to the inferior vena cava and up to the right atrium, RV, and into the pulmonary arterial circulation. This may cut off blood flow to an entire lung segment, resulting in potentially fatal perfusion–ventilation (V:Q) mismatch. In addition, any abnormal communication between the right and left chambers of the heart (e.g., atrial septal defect, patent foramen ovale, ventricular septal defect) creates the potential for cerebral thromboembolism (i.e., cerebrovascular accident or stroke).

It is critical to diagnose DVT early because the complication of pulmonary embolism can be life-threatening. A pulmonary embolism is a thrombus that obstructs circulation within the lungs causing lack of oxygenation of blood. Signs of pulmonary embolism can be subtle or severe depending on the size of the embolus. Sudden death can result from pulmonary embolism and may not be heralded by clearly, observable signs of DVT.

Clinical Presentation

Subjective

The patient with peripheral artery disease will usually present with intermittent leg pain (intermittent claudication) in both calves that increases in severity until the patient stops walking. The pain is described as severe, "grabbing," and cramplike. There is usually no complaint of pain at times of rest or in any other area but the calves. The pain lasts minutes (at most) and is relieved by rest and does not reoccur until the patient walks the same distance again. The patient usually denies swelling, pain at night, or color or temperature changes. The patient may also complain of thick toenails with cornlike material under the nails. Eventually, the lower legs and ankles may assume a purple-black color characteristic of cyanosis and gangrene.

The patient with chronic venous insufficiency will complain of dependent edema, venous engorgement (varicose veins), and localized pain. The patient may complain of a darkened color in the lower extremities, along with dryness and scaling of the skin.

Although many calf thrombi are silent, if the patient is aware of a problem, the presenting complaint will be pain in the calf muscle, slight swelling, or muscle tenderness.

Objective

Taking a thorough history distinguishes the cause of leg pain in more than 90 percent of patients. Assessing the risk factors assists in the diagnosis. The next step should be to determine the rapidity of onset of symptoms. PVD must be differentiated from a limb-threatened state that may need immediate treatment. If the onset of claudication has been gradual, this is more consistent with the progressive obliteration of the lower extremity vessels and the formation of collateral circulation, as seen with PVD, rather than an acute event such as an embolus from the heart or a proximal abdominal aortic aneurysm (AAA).

The clinician should evaluate the cervical, radial, ulnar, brachial, femoral, popliteal, dorsalis pedis, and posterior tibial pulses bilaterally. A consistent grading system should be used. Usually 0 refers to an absent pulse, 1+ a diminished pulse, 2+ normal, and 3+ bounding. The clinician should keep in mind that about 10 percent of the population has absent pedal pulses. Because a bruit indicates turbulence and possible artherosclerotic narrowing, the following pulse sites should be assessed using the diaphragm of a stethoscope: cervical, supraclavicular, abdominal, flank, and inguinal areas.

To differentiate chronic venous insufficiency from PAD, the clinician should raise the patient's legs for several minutes. When the legs are dependent again, the patient with PAD will have pale, dusky red (rubor) extremities and the patient with chronic venous insufficiency will have improved color in the extremities. Aneurysms may be palpated in the abdomen at the level of the umbilicus, and in the popliteal fossae. Circulatory checks should be done to assess for acute arterial ischemia. The 6 P's of PAD include pain, pulselessness, paresthesia, paralysis, poikilothermia (coolness), and pallor. The clinician should do a sensory examination to rule out peripheral neuropathy associated with ischemia in patients with diabetes.

With PAD, the clinician may observe decreased or absent peripheral extremity pulses. The affected leg may be smaller in size as a result of muscular atrophy. The clinician will note thinning of the skin, loss of hair over the affected area, and possible leg ulcers. The extremity may be cool and pale, and the toenails will be thickened. The patient will have a history of delayed wound healing. When the extremity is dependent, it will appear reddish blue in color.

In patients with chronic venous insufficiency, the clinician may note a brownish hyperpigmentation of the extremities, edema, subcutaneous fibrosis, and possibly leg ulcers. When the clinician elevates the extremity, the sharp, deep muscle pain may be lessened. The peripheral pulses may be normal or diminished. There may be superficial ulcers around the medial malleolus.

With thrombophlebitis, the clinician may note slight swelling, muscle tenderness, and pain in the calf muscle while eliciting a Homan's sign. The clinician may assess for warmth or heat of the affected extremity and note distension of the superficial veins. A slight fever and tachycardia may also be present. An acute DVT in the femoral or iliac veins may show symptoms of tenderness over the veins, swelling, and a slightly bluish skin color.

Diagnostic Reasoning

Diagnostic Tests

If arterial insufficiency is suspect and the pulses are absent, a Doppler flow study should be performed, which can quantify the degree of the ischemia. Part of the Doppler flow study includes calculating an ankle–brachial index (ABI), which involves a comparison of arm BP to the ankle pressures, using a BP cuff and a Doppler. The normal ratio of ankle to brachial pressure is more than 0.9. An ABI reading of 0.6 to 0.9 indicates claudication, and levels less than 0.5 indicate severe ischemia. Although an arteriogram is not usually ordered as a diagnostic tool, it should be obtained preoperatively, after the patient has been assessed by a vascular surgeon.

To confirm venous insufficiency, if the history and physical examination are inconclusive, a venogram may be performed. This is a radiologic test in which the vein is injected with a radiopaque dye. Sequential films will show the engorged and tortuous veins. In addition, a plethysmography may be done to determine the changes in the fluid volume of the extremities. The air-cuff plethysmography measures the changes in the circumference of a limb by recording the changes in pressure in a air-filled cuff surrounding the extremity. This test is rarely done because the history, physical examination, and other tests are usually adequate to confirm the diagnosis.

Additional assessment tools and diagnostic procedures for peripheral artery disease also include a walking impairment questionnaire (WIQ), treadmill exercise testing, lipid profile, and magnetic resonance angiogram. The WIQ is used to assess the ability of patients to walk defined distances, speeds, and climb stairs.

If a diagnosis of DVT is suspected, the clinician should order an ultrasound. The diagnosis is established when there is lack of compressibility of the vein. Occasionally, the thrombus is actually imaged, but this is not necessary to confirm the diagnosis.

If the results of the ultrasound are inconclusive, a vascular surgeon may order an ascending venogram. The ascending venogram has long been considered the "gold standard" for diagnosis of venous thromboembolism, although if an ultrasound confirms the diagnosis, usually no further testing is done. An ascending venogram is performed by injecting a contrast material into a vein in the foot. Sequential x-ray films are taken that may show abnormalities such as vein-filling defect, formation of collateral veins, or abrupt termination of the contrast material along the vein. One risk of the ascending venogram, however, is an actual DVT, because the invasive nature of the procedure may actually cause the thrombus to release.

Magnetic resonance imaging (MRI) is an alternative to a venogram. MRI is expensive and should be reserved for those who cannot tolerate the intravenous dye needed for a venogram. Venous ultrasound and venogram are more cost effective.

The D-dimer assay can be helpful in the diagnosis of DVT. D-dimer is a breakdown product of fibrin and is positive in venous thrombosis and pulmonary embolism. However, the D-dimer assay has low specificity and sensitivity and cannot be solely relied on for diagnosis.

Differential Diagnosis

Differential diagnoses for peripheral artery disease and chronic venous insufficiency may include thrombosis, phlebitis, polycythemia, anemia, Raynaud's disease, Buerger's disease, aneurysms, and peripheral neuropathy.

Patients with chronic venous insufficiency may exhibit some of the symptoms of DVT. Patients who suffer from chronic venous insufficiency have swelling and dilated superficial veins. They may also complain of aching or fatigue in the legs while standing or walking. Other differential diagnoses for DVT include cellulitis, lymphedema, and a strained muscle.

Management

Treatment for peripheral vascular disease is aimed at improving blood flow by removing or lessening the cause of impaired circulation. Because the condition is usually chronic and irreversible, treatment involves education and lifestyle changes. Treatment Flowchart 9.3 presents the assessment and management of PVD.

It is essential to diagnosis deep venous thrombosis early, so as to prevent PE. Certainly, prevention of DVT is superior to treatment. To prevent DVT, prophylactic modalities fall into three categories—pharmacologic, physical or mechanical, or the combined use of both types of modalities.

Peripheral Artery Disease

Patients with PAD should be counseled about modification of risk factors, and HTN and diabetes should be aggressively managed. The clinician should encourage the patient to walk at least 30 minutes three to four times per week. Any ulcers or traumatic lesions to the extremities will need immediate care. The patient should be encouraged to keep the legs dependent (below the level of the heart) to improve blood flow and, therefore, oxygenation in the extremities. Tight bandages and stockings should be avoided.

Although drug therapy is not a substitute for exercise, some medications have been helpful in extending ambulation distances for more than 25 percent of patients.

Previously, pentoxifylline (Trental) (400 mg tid with food) was prescribed as it was thought to decrease the blood viscosity and increase RBC flexibility. This drug recently has been taken off more and more formularies because many authorities consider it ineffective for leg pain. Aspirin may also be prescribed to decrease platelet aggregation. Clopidogrel (Plavix) (75 mg qd) is a platelet inhibitor and is used to prevent atherosclerotic ischemic events in patients with PAD. Cilostazol (Pletal) (100 mg bid without food) may be ordered specifically to treat leg pain and cramping due to the blockages from atherosclerosis in the leg arteries. It lengthens the pain-free walking distance for patients with claudication. Cilostazol is a phosphodiesterase-3 inhibitor that causes vasodilation and in addition inhibits platelet aggregation. Cilostazol should not be prescribed in the presence of any degree of CHF, as this is a contraindication to its use. Surgical intervention and angioplasty are used selectively in patients with severe PAD.

Chronic Venous Insufficiency

For the patient with chronic venous insufficiency, conservative treatment is effective in alleviating symptoms in 85 percent of patients. The dependent edema can be a guide to the effectiveness of therapy. The clincian should order light exercise, support or compression stockings, and weight loss

TREATMENT FLOWCHART 9.3

PERIPHERAL VASCULAR DISEASE

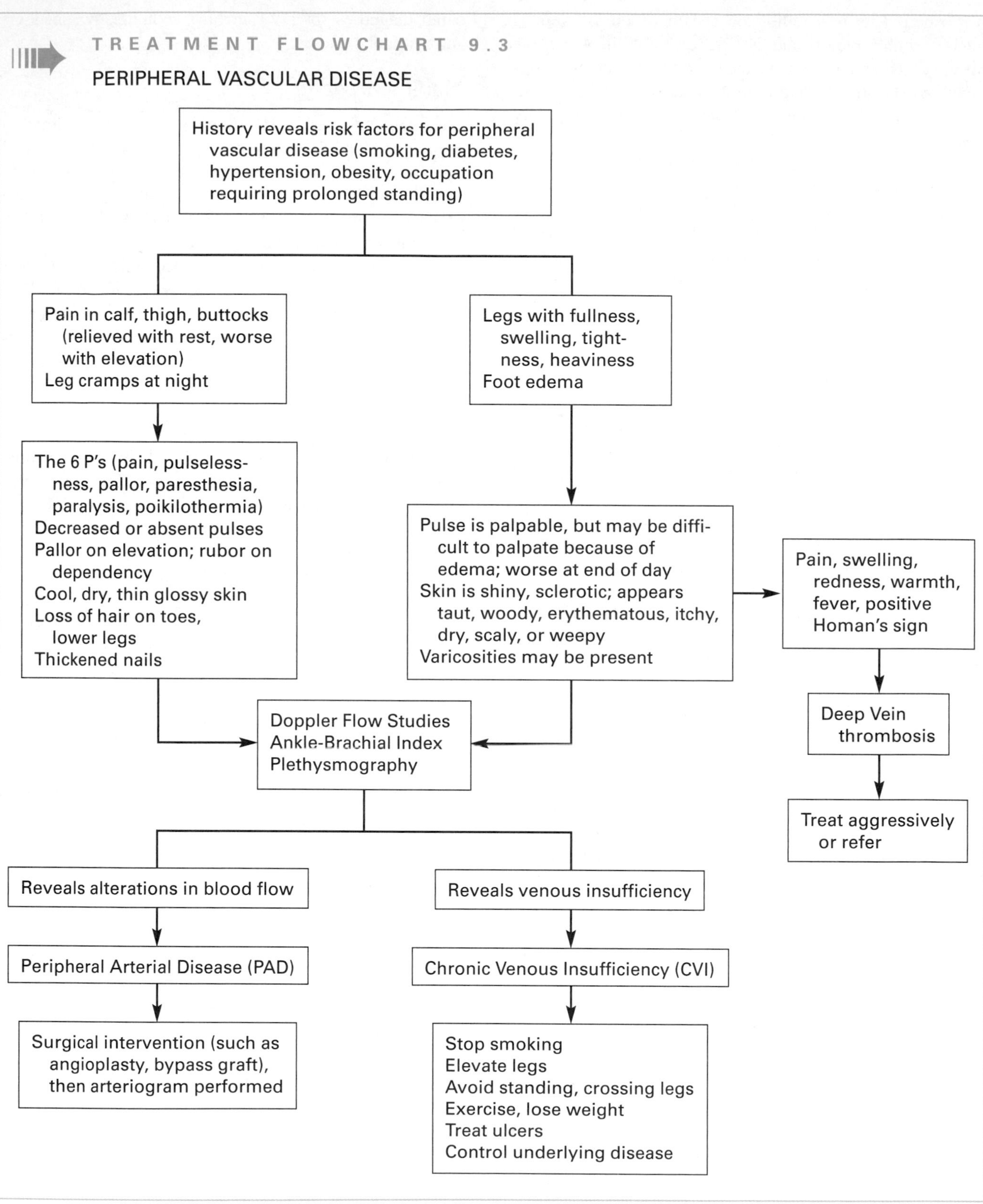

and should stress the need to elevate the legs several times each day for approximately 30 minutes. Subsequent management involves aggressively treating any ulcers and reducing factors that cause atherosclerosis.

Deep Vein Thrombosis

Patients with deep venous thrombosis can be treated in an inpatient or outpatient setting. In the hospital, patients are treated aggressively with anticoagulant therapy with IV unfractionated heparin and monitored for signs of further thrombosis or iatrogenic bleeding. An initial IV bolus of heparin (5000 to 10,000 units IV) should be followed by a continuous infusion at 1000 units per hour. The dosage of heparin should be adjusted according to the partial thromboplastin time (PTT). The goal is to achieve a PTT of two times the control value. Alternatively, low molecular weight heparin (LMWH) can be used as outpatient management of DVT until warfarin is at therapeutic level. Candidates for outpatient therapy must have a supportive environment, be hemodynamically stable, without renal failure, and not at high risk for bleeding. Enoxaparin (Lovenox), dalteparin (Fragmin), and tinzaparin (Innohep), are examples of types of LMWH. LMWH can be administered subcutaneously once or twice daily. Lovenox may be used at 1 mg/kg injected SC q12h. In this case, PTT need not be followed, although Factor Xa levels may be measured to assess for therapeutic response to comfirm the appropriateness of the dose. The side effect of thrombocytopenia is less likely and less laboratory testing is required. Simultaneous initiation of warfarin and LMWH has not shown any adverse effects.

Only unfractionated heparin is readily reversible after several hours, once the IV drip is turned off. Subcutaneously injected low molecular weight heparins, on the other hand, will exert its effect for at least 12 hours after each dose. Warfarin therapy should be initiated after the patient has been on heparin for 1 to 5 days. Warfarin should be started at 5 to 10 mg PO qd, with the dose adjusted to the PT and INR, as stated previously.

If anticoagulant therapy is contraindicated, filtering devices such as an umbrella may be used to trap emboli before they reach the lungs and cause a PE. Inferior vena caval filters are mechanical barriers that are inserted in the large vena cava under percutaneous radiologic guidance. Although they do not prevent clot formation, they prevent clot migration from the legs to the lungs.

Patients should also elevate the affected limb, apply heat, and limit activity. Graded elastic compression stockings are also recommended.

Thrombolysis is not indicated for DVT except in cases of massive ileofemoral thrombus. Thrombolytic agents are indicated for patients with massive pulmonary embolism and associated hemodynamic instability. The role of thrombolysis in patients with lesser size pulmonary emboli is controversial.

Follow-Up and Referral

All patients with peripheral artery disease should be followed at least every 3 months to assess the effectiveness of lifestyle changes, skin care, and management of ulcers. If ulcers are present, the patient may need to be seen on a weekly basis. Patients with peripheral artery disease may be referred to a vascular surgeon for evaluation and potential surgery, including a balloon angioplasty in the distal extremity or an arterial graft using a section of the great saphenous vein or a synthetic graft.

If the clinician is following a patient with superficial thrombophlebitis as an outpatient, the patient should be seen in the office at 48 hours following diagnosis and initiation of treatment. If the patient is hospitalized, the patient will be under the care of a vascular surgeon; most patients with acute DVT are hospitalized for about 1 week. Follow-up therapy for these patients includes anticoagulant therapy for 6 months after an initial episode of DVT and for 1 year after each subsequent episode. The clinician will follow the patient after he or she is released from the hospital. The patient on warfarin must be seen daily until the target PT range is achieved (usually in the hospital), then on a monthly basis thereafter.

Patient Education

Patients who have been diagnosed with PAD or chronic venous insufficiency should be counseled about the modification of risk factors. They should totally abstain from nicotine. It is essential to control HTN and diabetes if present. Dietary control must include limitation of fat and salt intake. Patients must be taught to do meticulous daily foot care that includes inspecting feet daily for sores, ulcers, and abrasions, including the use of a mirror to check the soles of the feet. Patients should not walk barefoot and should wear well-fitting support shoes. They should not soak their feet and should be careful trimming their nails. All patients should be taught to watch for the signs and symptoms that might indicate progressive ischemia, such as increased pain, increased pallor or cyanosis, and rest pain.

Patients with chronic venous insufficiency must be encouraged to wear their stockings during the day and to elevate their legs several times during the day. Patients with PAD should be encouraged to perform Buerger–Allen exercises three to four times per day. The clinician should teach the patient to raise and lower the extremities, with each of five repetitions taking about 2 minutes. The legs should be raised to a 45-degree angle, then lowered again to the supine position. The changes in position cause the veins of the legs to refill by gravity.

Exercise therapy is recommended for peripheral artery disease because it stimulates collateral vessel growth in the lower extremities. Patients should be encouraged to walk distances until moderate pain occurs, stop until pain subsides, and then resume walking. A supervised treadmill walking program three times a week over a 6-month period is part of cardiovascular rehabilitiation. Treadmill grade and speed are gradually increased over time as the patient improves.

Patients should be educated about deep venous thrombosis and treated prophylactically, depending on the number of risk factors exhibited and the resulting need for hospitalization or surgery. To prevent DVT, prophylactic modalities should be used for all patients at risk, including those pharmacologic, physical or mechanical, or a combination of the two.

Pharmaceutical modalities prevent coagulation changes in the blood that result in clot formation or prevent extension of the clot. Low-dose heparin, administered SC, is considered the mainstay of therapy for DVT, although this agent has proved to be relatively ineffective in orthopedic procedures. Some potential complications of low-dose heparin therapy include bleeding, wound hematoma, and thrombocytopenia. Low-dose heparin therapy is contraindicated for neurosurgical procedures, especially intracranial procedures.

If low-dose heparin is used prophylactically, 5000 IU of heparin SC q8 to 12h should be administered preoperatively for surgical patients and at the time of confinement to bed for medical patients and then continued. Warfarin may be used instead and is effective for orthopedic procedures and general surgical procedures. However, because warfarin does not provide adequate anticoagulation for 3 to 5 days after its initiation, high-risk patients should also have nonpharmacolog prophylaxis with intermittent pneumatic compression (IPC) for at least the first 5 days of therapy. External pneumatic compression and gradient compression stockings are effective alternatives for decreasing lower leg thrombosis if lower extremity trauma does not preclude their use.

Dextran, originally introduced as a plasma expander, is effective in very high-risk orthopedic and gynecologic surgery patients. Dextran inhibits platelet adhesiveness and aggregation; it is used in patients who are at risk for DVT but are also at high risk for bleeding with anticoagulants. The usual dose of dextran for perioperative prophylaxis is 500 mL IV, administered as a continuous infusion over 6 hours, once daily. This is usually followed by infusions of 500 to 1000 mL IV on the day of surgery and of 100 to 500 mL IV for several days postoperatively, depending on the type of surgery.

Physical modalities that prevent DVT by reducing stasis include leg elevation, massage, passive leg exercises, and early ambulation. Although these techniques are somewhat effective, each has some drawbacks and should be combined with other physical measures such as graduated elastic compression or external pneumatic compression devices. Graduated compression stockings provide safe, simple, and inexpensive prophylaxis. Besides preventing stasis, they also prevent venous distension, which potentially initiates vessel wall damage. Pneumatic compression devices are more effective at emptying the veins, sustaining femoral blood flow velocity, and expelling the blood from behind the valve cusps in the femoral vein, thus stimulating fibrinolysis.

Education for patients recovering from DVT includes teaching about the need to avoid trauma to the affected veins. The clinician should be educated regarding potential adverse effects of the anticoagulant medication, including signs and symptoms of bleeding, and when to seek medical care. The patient must avoid food fads and crash diets and should not drink alcohol or take vitamin E, cold medicines, antibiotics, aspirin, cimetidine (Tagamet), thyroid hormones, or NSAIDs without first consulting the clinician. Immobility should be discouraged. Patients must know when to return for a follow-up PT if they are on warfarin.

Superficial Thrombophlebitis

For a very mild, superficial case of thrombophlebitis, the application of heat, combined with elevation of the extremity, may suffice. Anticoagulation therapy consists of warfarin (Coumadin), although this does not provide adequate anticoagulation for 3 to 5 days after its initiation. Frequent laboratory monitoring of PT is necessary. The dose of warfarin should be adjusted to maintain a therapeutic PT, which is 1.5 to 2 times the control, or about 15 to 17 seconds. This may also be reported as an international normalized ratio (INR): A target INR of 2.0 to 3.0 is utilized. Frequent monitoring is required to ensure the dose of warfarin is safe and effective. NSAIDs may be used for pain. Patients should not smoke and bed rest should be maintained for 3 to 5 days.

Deep Vein Thrombosis

Patients with DVT must be hospitalized initially to begin aggressive anticoagulant therapy with heparin intravenously and to monitor for signs of further thrombosis, or bleeding. An initial IV bolus of heparin (5000 to 10,000 units IV) should be followed by a continuous infusion at 1000 units per hour. The dosage of heparin should be adjusted according to the partial thromboplastin time (PTT). The goal is to achieve a PTT of two times the control value. Warfarin therapy should be initiated after the patient has been on heparin for 1 to 5 days. Warfarin should be started at 5 to 10 mg PO qd, with the dose adjusted to the PT and INR, as stated previously.

If anticoagulant therapy is contraindicated, filtering devices such as an umbrella may be used to trap emboli before they reach the lungs and cause a PE. Inferior vena caval filters are mechanical barriers that are inserted in the large vena cava under percutaneous radiologic guidance. Although they do not prevent clot formation, they prevent clot migration from the legs to the lungs.

Bibliography

General

Dunphy, LH: Management Guidelines for Nurse Practitioners: Working with Adults, ed 2. FA Davis, Philadelphia, 1999.

Tierney, L, McPhee, S, and Papadakis, M: Current Medical Diagnosis and Treatment, ed 44. Appleton & Lange, Norwalk, Conn., 2005.

Kasper, OL, Fauci, AS, Longo, DL, Braunwald, E, Hauser, SL, Jameson, JL (eds): Harison's Principles of Internal Medicine. McGraw-Hill, New York, 2005.

Papadakis, MA, and McPhee, SJ: Current Consult Medicine. Lange Medical Books/McGraw-Hill, New York, 2005.

Dyslipidemia

Brewer, HB: Rising to the challenge of the new NCEP ATP III guidelines: Exceeding current therapeutic limitations. Am J Manage Care 8(2): S23–S32, 2002.

Chilton, RJ: Pathophysiology of coronary heart disease: A brief review. J Am Osteopath Assoc 104(9 Suppl 7):S5–S13, 2004.

Cleeman, JI, Davidson, MH, and Pasternak, R: Implementing the new ATP III cholesterol guidelines. Patient Care Nov: 19–46, 2002.

Cui, Y, Blumenthal, RS, Flaws, JA, Whiteman, MK, Langenberg, P, Bachorik, PS, and Bush, T: Non-high density lipoprotein cholesterol level as predictor of cardiovascular disease mortality. Arch Intern Med 161:1413–1419, 2001.

Deen, D: Metabolic syndrome: Time for action. Am Fam Phys 69(12):2875–2882, 2004.

Expert Panel on Detection, Evaluation, and Treatment of High Blood Cholesterol in Adults. Executive Summary of the Third Report of the National Cholesterol Education Program (NCEP): JAMA 285; 2486–2497, 2001.

Galbut, BH, and Davidson, MH: Practical applications of the NCEP ATP III updates. Patient Care 39(3):31–38, 2005.

Grundy, SM, et al: Definition of metabolic syndrome: Report of the National Heart, Lung, and Blood Institute/American Heart Association. Circulation 109(3):433–438, 2004.

Grundy, SM: Non-high density lipoprotein cholesterol level as potential risk predictor and therapy target. Arch Intern Med 161:1379–1380, 2001.

Grundy, SM, Cleeman, JI, Merz, CN, et al: Implications of recent trials for the National Cholesterol Education Program Adult Treatment Panel III Guidelines. Circulation 110:227–239, 2004.

Krantz, MJ, and Garcia, JA: Dyslipidemia in high risk patients: A rational approach to therapy. Consultant Sept 1:1321–1328, 2004.

Lakka, HM, Laaksonen, DE, Lakka, T, Niskanen, LK, et al: The metabolic syndrome and total and cardiovascular disease mortality in middle aged men. JAMA 288(21):2709–2716, 2002.

LaRosa, JC, Grundy, SM, Waters, DD, Shear, C, Barter, P, Fruchart, J-C, Gotto, AM, Greten, H, Kastelein, JJP, Shepherd, J, Wenger, NK, for the Treating to New Targets (TNT) Investigators: Intensive lipid lowering with atorvastatin in patients with stable coronary disease. N Engl J Med 352(14):1425–1435, 2005.

Morgan, JM, Carey, CM, Lincoff, A, and Capuzzi, DM: The effects of niacin on lipoprotein subclass distribution. Prevent Cardiol 7:182–189, 2004.

Nambi, V, Hoogwerf, BJ, and Sprecher, DL: A truly deadly quartet: Obesity, hypertension, hypertriglyceridemia, and hyperinsulinemia. Cleve Clin J Med 69(12):985–994, 2002.

Nash, DT: The metabolic syndrome: Early clues, effective management. Consultant May: 859–863, 2004.

National Institutes of Health (NIH): National Heart, Lung, and Blood Institute (NHLBI). National Cholesterol Education Program (NCEP). ATP III guidelines at-a-glance quick desk reference. U.S. Department of Health and Human Services. NIH publication no. 01-3305, 2001.

Pitt, B: Low density lipoprotein cholesterol in patients with stable coronary disease—Is it time to shift our goals? N Engl J Med 352(14): 1483–1484, 2005.

Spratt, KA: Reducing the risk of coronary heart disease via lipid reduction. J Am Osteopath Assoc 104(9 Suppl 7):S9–S13, 2004.

Dysrhythmias

Lipman, B, and Cascio, T: ECG Assessment and Interpretation. FA Davis, Philadelphia, 1994.

Coronary Artery Disease, Angina Pectoris, Myocardial Infarction

ACA/AHA 2002 guideline update for the management of patients with unstable angina and non-ST segment elevation myocardial infarction. A report of the American College of Cardiology/American Heart Association Task Force on Practice Guidelines (Committee on the Management of Patients with Unstable Angina). Accessed online May 2004 at http://www.americanheartorg/

Ambrose, JA, and Dangas, G: Unstable angina: Current concepts of pathogenesis and treatment. Arch Intern Med 160:25–37, 2000.

Braunwald, E: Unstable angina: Diagnosis and management. Rockville, Md.: U.S. Dept of Health and Human Services, Public Health Service, Agency for Health Care Policy and Research, National Heart, Lung, and Blood Institute. Clinical practice guideline no.10; AHCPR publication no. 94–0602, 1994.

Chilton, RJ: Recent discoveries in assessment of coronary artery disease: Impact of vascular mechanisms on development of atherosclerosis. J Am Osteopath Assoc 101(9 Suppl):S1–S5, 2001.

Coudrey, L: The troponins. Arch Intern Med 158:1173–1180, 1998.

Dayspring, TD: Prevention of first myocardial infarction. J Clin Pharmacol 41:1–9, 2001.

Keely, EC, and Grines, CL: Primary coronary intervention for acute myocardial infarction. JAMA 291(6):736–739, 2004.

Krantz, MJ, and Garcia, JA: Dyslipidemia in high-risk patients: A rational approach to therapy. Consultant Sept 1:1321–1328, 2004.

Kushner, I, and Sehgal, AR: Is high sensitivity C-reactive protein an effective screening test for cardiovascular risk? Arch Intern Med 162:867–869, 2002.

Monaco, C, Mathur, A, and Martin, JF: What causes acute coronary syndromes? Applying Koch's postulates. Atherosclerosis 179(1):1–15, 2005.

Patel, VB, and Topol, EJ: The pathogenesis and spectrum of acute coronary syndromes: From plaque to thrombosis. Cleve Clin J Med 66(9):561–570, 1999.

Perers, E, Caidahl, K, Herlitz, J, Sjolin, M, Karlson, BW, Karlsson, T, and Hartford, M: Spectrum of acute coronary syndromes: History and clinical presentation in relation to sex and age. Cardiology 102(2):67–76, 2004.

Plutzky, J: The vascular biology of atherosclerosis. Am J Med 115(8A): 55S–61S, 2003.

Reeder, GS: Contemporary diagnosis and management of unstable angina. Mayo Clin Proc 75:953–957, 2000.

Scirica, BM, and Morrow, DA: Troponins in acute coronary syndrome. Prog Cardiovasc Dis 47(3):177–188, 2004.

Wiviott, SD, and Braunwald, E: Unstable angina and Non-ST segment elevation myocardial infarction: Part I. Initial evaluation and management, and hospital care. Am Fam Phys 70(3):525–538, 2004.

Heart Failure

American Heart Association, Aurigemma, GP, and Gaasch, WH: Diastolic heart failure. N Engl J Med 351(11):1097–1105, 2004.

Aurigemma, GP, and Gaasch, WH: Diastolic heart failure. N Engl J Med 351(11):1097–1105, 2004.

Braunwald, E: Heart failure and cor pulmonale. In Kasper, D, Fauci, A, Longo, D, Braunwald, E, Hauser, SL, and Jameson, JL: Harrison's Principles of Internal Medicine, ed 16. McGraw Hill, New York, 2005.

Hunt, SA, et al: ACC/AHA 2005 guidelines update for the diagnosis and management of chronic heart failure in the adult: A report of the American College of Cardiology/American Heart Association Task Force on Practice Guidelines (Writing Committee to Update the 2001 Guidelines for the Evaluation and Management of Heart Failure). Available at http://www.acc.org/clinical/guidelines/failure/index.pdf

Jessup, M, and Brozena, S: Medical progress: Heart failure. N Engl J Med 348(20):2007–2018, 2003.

Redfield, MM: Understanding "diastolic" heart failure. N Engl J Med 350(19):1930–1931, 2004.

Schrier, RW, and Abraham, WT: Mechanisms of disease: Hormones and hemodynamics in heart failure. N Engl J Med 341(8):577–585, 1999.

Vasan, RS, and Benjamin, EJ: Diastolic heart failure—No time to relax. N Engl J Med 344(1):56–58, 2001.

Zile, MR, Baciu, CF, and Gaasch, WH: Diastolic heart failure—Abnormalities in active relaxation and passive stiffness of the left ventricle. N Engl J Med 350(19):1953–1959, 2004.

Hypertension

August, P: Physiology of the renin-angiotensin-aldosterone system and its pathophysiologic role in some forms of hypertension. J Clin Hypertens 7(1):36–37, 2005.

Chobanian, AV, et al: Seventh report of the Joint National Committee on Prevention, Detection, Evaluation, and Treatment of High Blood Pressure. Hypertension 42(6):1206–1252.

Elliot, WJ: Clinical features and management of selected hypertensive emergencies. J Clin Hypertens 6(10):587–592, 2004.

Gibbons, GH: Physiology, genetics, and cardiovascular disease: Focus on African Americans. J Clin Hypertens 6(4 Suppl 1):11–18, 2004.

Greenlund, KJ, Croft, JB, and Mensah, GA: Prevalence of heart disease and stroke risk factors in persons with prehypertension in the United States, 1999–2000. Arch Intern Med 164:2113–2118, 2004.

Mathew, RG, and Reyes, IM: Hypertensive emergencies and urgencies: Update on management. Consultant March: 341–345, 2004.

National Institutes of Health, National Heart, Lung and Blood Institute. The Seventh Report of the Joint National Committee on Prevention, Detection, Evaluation, and Treatment of High Blood Pressure (The JNC 7 Report). JAMA 289(19):2560–2572, 2003.

Parati, G, Bilo, G, and Mancia, G: White coat effect and white coat hypertension: What do they mean? Cardiovasc Rev Rep 24:477–484, 2003.

Perez del Villar, C, Garcia-Alonso, CJ, Feldstein, CA, Juncos, LA, and Romero, JC: Role of endothelin in the pathogenesis of hypertension. Mayo Clin Proc 80(1):84–96, 2005.

Pickering, TG: Measurement of blood pressure in and out of the office. J Clin Hypertension 7(2):123–129, 2005.

Pickering, TG: Treatment of hypertension in the elderly. J Clin Hypertens 6(10 Suppl 2):18–23, 2004.

Saunders, E: Managing hypertension in African-American patients. J Clin Hypertens 6(4 Suppl 1):19–25, 2004.

Schwartz, GL, and Sheps, SG: Hypertension: Etiology and genetics. ACP Medicine, 2004. Retrieved on 3/10/05 from http://www.medscape.com

Touyz, RM, and Schiffrin, EL: Role of endothelin in human hypertension. Can J Physiol Pharmacol 81(96):533–541, 2003.

Weber, MA: Endothelial dysfunction: Linking hypertension to systemic and local disease. Cardiovasc Rev Rep June: 42–54, 1998.

Whelton, PK: Epidemiology and the prevention of hypertension. J Clin Hypertens 6(11):636–642, 2004.

Williams, B: Angiotensin II and the pathophysiology of cardiovascular remodeling. Am J Cardiol 87(8A):10C–17C, 2001.

Metabolic Syndrome

Deen, D: Metabolic syndrome: Time for action. Am Fam Phys 69(12): 2875–2882, 2004.

Expert Panel on Detection, Evaluation, and Treatment of High Blood Cholesterol in Adults. Executive Summary of the Third Report of the National Cholesterol Education Program (NCEP): JAMA 285; 2486–2497, 2001.

Grundy, SM, et al: Definition of metabolic syndrome: Report of the National Heart, Lung, and Blood Institute/American Heart Association. Circulation 109(3):433–438, 2004.

Lakka, HM, Laaksonen, DE, Lakka, T, Niskanen, LK, et al: The metabolic syndrome and total and cardiovascular disease mortality in middle aged men. JAMA 288(21):2709–2716, 2002.

Nambi, V, Hoogwerf, BJ, and Sprecher, DL: A truly deadly quartet: Obesity, hypertension, hypertriglyceridemia, and hyperinsulinemia. Cleve Clin J Med 69(12):985–994, 2002.

Nash, DT: The metabolic syndrome: Early clues, effective management. Consultant May:859–863, 2004.

Thrombosis

Braunwald, E: Chapter 219: Valvular heart disease. In Kasper, DL, Fauci, AS, Longo, DL, Braunwald, E, Hauser, SL, and Jameson, JL: Harrison's Principles of Internal Medicine, ed 16. McGraw-Hill, New York, 2005.

Creager, MA, and Dzau, VJ: Chapter 232: Vascular diseases of the extremities. In Kasper, DL, Fauci, AS, Longo, DL, Braunwald, E, Hauser, SL, and Jameson, JL: Harrison's Principles of Internal Medicine, ed 16. McGraw-Hill, New York, 2005.

Resources

American College of Cardiology
http://www.acc.org

American Heart Association
http://www.americanheart.org
(Contact AHA for local state affiliate)

American Medical Association (AMA)
http://www.ama-assn.org
(Contact AMA online for specific topics as well as to register for online access to *JAMA* and *Archives* journals)

Nova Online Cardiac Resources
http://www.pbs.org/wgbh/eheart/resources.html

Abdominal Problems

Debera J. Thomas, DNS, APRN, BC

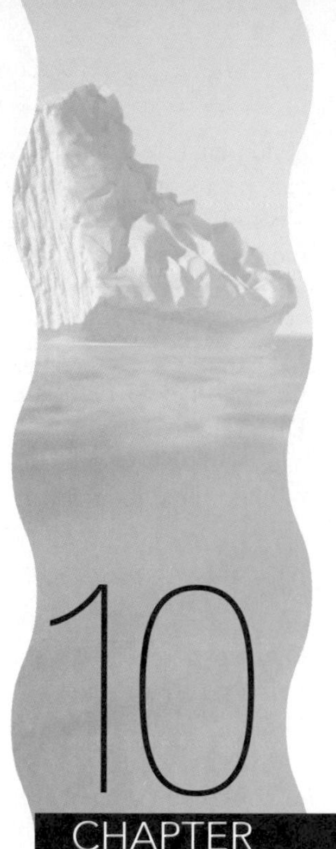

10

CHAPTER

Common Complaints

Abdominal Pain

Abdominal pain is one of the most common complaints for which people seek medical attention. Up to 90 percent of all visits to the emergency room involve some form of abdominal pain, ranging from that associated with typical influenza to the intense pain of appendicitis, peptic ulcer disease, or bowel obstruction. The causes of abdominal pain are numerous; a few are serious enough to require surgical intervention. Conditions associated with an acute abdomen can be inflammatory, metabolic, or structural; therefore, any acute abdominal pain must be evaluated quickly and precisely. Abdominal pain that occurs without any other signs or symptoms is rarely a serious problem.

Differential Diagnosis

Total patient presentation must be considered when evaluating abdominal pain. A careful history is key to determining the severity of the condition. The onset, timing, and characteristics of the pain are useful in the diagnostic reasoning. The presence or absence of bowel sounds is also an important diagnostic factor. Tachycardia, tachypnea, and hypertension often indicate the intensity of the pain. Many nonsurgical conditions can present with classic acute surgical abdomen symptoms such as intense pain, rebound tenderness, and guarding. All patients with abdominal pain should undergo rectal, genital, and pelvic evaluations. Blood found in the stool or intense pain upon exam may indicate more serious conditions.

The mechanism responsible for the abdominal pain is what gives certain characteristics to the pain. For example, pain that originates from pain receptors located in the viscera (organs) produces pain that is poorly localized and is described as dull. This is known as *visceral pain* and is caused by distension or spasm of a hollow viscus. Distension of an organ capsule, such as Glisson's capsule around the liver; vascular compromise; and mucosal irritations cause pain that is visceral in nature. Conversely, *parietal pain,* described as sharp and is well localized, is caused by irritation of the peritoneum. Appendicitis often causes this type of pain as the peritoneum becomes involved. *Abdominal pain* described as colicky, which simply means that it comes and goes, may result from gallstones or renal stones. *Burning pain,* caused by irritation of the gastric mucosa by gastric contents, is associated with peptic ulcers and esophagitis.

A thorough history and physical examination are essential to narrow the list of differential diagnoses of patients with abdominal pain, First, the nature of the pain should be elicited in order to provide clues to the mechanism of the pain. Location of the pain is valuable information, but it is important to remember that abdominal pain can be referred from areas outside of the abdomen. Timing of the pain (onset, duration, frequency, and relationship to associated symptoms) can help eliminate some causes. The palliative and provocative aspects of the pain can give clues about the cause of the pain. For example, does moving, eating certain foods, assuming different positions, or taking medications make the pain better or worse? Associated symptoms will further narrow the list of diagnostic possibilities. Some causes of abdominal pain will necessitate a surgical referral. Any time the pain is very severe and associated with a rigid abdomen, referral to a physician is essential. Abdominal pain can be the presenting symptom of many different pathophysiologic processes, ranging from very mild gastritis to more serious forms of abdominal pain associated with bowel obstruction or appendicitis.

A complete blood count (CBC), serum chemistries, liver function tests (LFTs), urinalysis (UA), and abdominal films will help determine the acuity of the problem. The Differential Diagnosis Flowchart 10.1 presents selected causes of abdominal pain and their characteristics. Treatment of abdominal pain depends on the cause.

Constipation

Constipation is a very common symptom in Western society. It is the most common gastrointestinal (GI) disorder in the United States, particularly in older adults and sedentary individuals. There is no single definition of constipation, although it is often defined as a change in a person's normal bowel pattern, either a decrease in frequency or more difficult defecation. The APN and the patient must have a similar operational definition of constipation and what a normal bowel pattern is for that patient.

The most common cause of constipation in the United States is a lack of dietary fiber. Experts recommend a diet that contains 30 grams of fiber for optimal bowel health. The average American consumes only about 10 grams per day. Other common causes of constipation are habitual use of laxatives, irritable bowel syndrome (IBS), decreased physical activity, a change in environment or travel, use of medications with constipating potential, suppression of the urge to defecate, and painful defecation caused by anorectal problems. Other less common but serious causes of constipation include bowel tumors, metabolic disorders such as hypothyroidism, diabetes, hypercalcemia, and pregnancy.

Generally, there are three categories of constipation: simple constipation, disordered motility, and secondary constipation. *Simple constipation* results from a diet that is low in fiber and high in simple carbohydrates and meat. Some people have difficulty defecating in an environment other than their own home; they frequently suppress the urge to defecate, thereby promoting simple constipation. The next most common category of constipation is *disordered motility,* which is seen most often in older adults and is caused by slowed transit time. Megacolon and megarectum are also common disorders of motility, but they most frequently occur in children. Other conditions that cause disordered motility and constipation include IBS and diverticular disease. *Secondary constipation* often is a result of medications such as codeine, morphine, analgesics, calcium channel blockers, antidepressants, antiparkinsonian drugs, cough medicine, and aluminum antacids. Table 10.1 presents a list of constipating drugs. Other common causes of secondary constipation are chronic laxative use, prolonged immobilization, and organic diseases of the lower GI system.

Table 10.1 Medications that Commonly Cause Constipation

Aluminum-containing antacids
Anticholinergics
Anticonvulsants
- Phenobarbital
- Phenytoin
- Carbamazepine

Antidepressants
- Amitriptyline
- Doxepin
- Imipramine
- Nortriptyline
- Protriptyline

Antihistamines
Antihypertensives
- Calcium channel blockers
- Clonidine

Antiparkinsonian drugs
Antipsychotics
Bismuth-containing products bismuth subsalicylate (Pepto-Bismol)
Iron preparations
Nonsteroidal anti-inflammatory drugs
Opiates
- Codeine
- Morphine
- Heroin
- Fentanyl
- Methadone
- Propxyphene

Sympathomimetics

Chronic constipation rarely results from a serious condition and the patient can usually be treated symptomatically and by increasing the fiber in the diet. Those whose constipation developed with a recent disability, a change in diet, recent depressive illness, or with the ingestion of constipating medication can also be treated symptomatically. It is in patients who develop constipation that cannot be explained, have abdominal pain, report blood or mucus in their stool, or require a substantial increase in their laxative use that a more serious cause of constipation should be investigated. Constipation occurs in fewer than 30 percent of patients with colon cancer.

Differential Diagnosis

An accurate description of the feces can give clues to the cause of the constipation. For example, ribbonlike stools often indicate a motility disorder but can also be caused by an organic narrowing of the distal or sigmoid colon. If the patient complains of a progressive decrease in the diameter of the stools, this suggests an organic lesion. If steatorrhea and greenish-yellow stools are associated with the constipation, the practitioner should look for a small bowel or pancreatic lesion. Constipation alternating with diarrhea is often a result of IBS.

The cause of constipation is multifactorial, which can make the differential diagnosis difficult. Differential Diagnosis Flowchart 10.2 presents various causes of constipation.

Treatment

The management of simple constipation is straightforward. Most patients respond well to education about bowel habits, activity, and dietary intervention. Some patients may require pharmacologic intervention as well. Patients should be instructed to slowly increase the amount of dietary fiber to 20 to 30 grams per day, with at least 12 to 15 grams at breakfast. Mild exercise after the morning meal is often helpful in stimulating peristalsis and promoting defecation. Uninterrupted toilet time in the morning is also helpful. Adequate hydration is essential in the prevention of constipation; patients should be encouraged to drink at least 64 ounces of fluids daily.

Treatment with a pharmacologic agent may be needed for patients who do not respond to increases in fiber, fluids, and exercise. Most drugs should be used for a short time only, and most are available without a prescription. Because these agents are available without a prescription, patients may have self-medicated for some time and by the time they seek medical attention, they may either have overused laxatives or may have a more serious underlying pathology. The only agents that are appropriate for long-term use are the bulking agents. The different agents used in the treatment of constipation are listed in Table 10.2.

Diarrhea

Just as with constipation, there is no single definition of diarrhea, but it is generally defined as an increase in the frequency, volume, or fluid content of bowel movements over what is normal for the individual. Because dietary intake of fiber in the United States is low, the average daily stool for each individual weighs about 200 grams. For most individuals, if the daily stool is more than 200 grams or the frequency of bowel movements is more than three times a day, the patient's condition can be considered diarrhea. Diarrhea is one of the most common presenting complaints in primary-care practice.

There are several types of diarrhea. The first is *osmotic diarrhea,* which is seen in patients with injury to the small intestine that results in malabsorption or maldigestion of nutrients, as in patients with short bowel syndrome. Lactase deficiency or disaccharidase deficiency can also cause osmotic diarrhea, as can ingestion of poorly absorbed solutes such as magnesium sulfate, laxatives, and sorbitol. Osmotic diarrhea usually responds to fasting.

Another type is *secretory diarrhea,* which produces voluminous watery stools but is unresponsive to fasting. Secretory diarrhea is primarily the result of bacterial enterotoxins (most notably from cholera and strains of *Escherichia coli*), but it can also be caused by laxative abuse, bile salt malabsorption which stimulates colonic secretion, and by endocrine tumors that stimulate pancreatic or intestinal secretion.

Diarrhea is associated with *morphological changes* within the mucosa of the intestinal wall that occur with inflammatory conditions of the intestines, and these changes can result in acute or chronic diarrhea. Both Crohn's disease (CD) and ulcerative colitis (UC) cause inflammation of the mucosa of the intestinal lumen, resulting in diarrhea.

Diarrhea can also result from *altered intestinal motility* secondary to diabetic neuropathy, dumping syndrome, or IBS. Some medications, such as antibiotics, can induce diarrhea by disrupting the normal balance of bacteria. Pathogenic bacteria also cause increases in the GI motility and intestinal secretions.

Differential Diagnosis

Differential diagnosis of diarrhea is aided by separating acute diarrhea from chronic diarrhea. *Acute diarrhea* usually has an abrupt onset and lasts for less than 1 week. Nausea, vomiting, or fever may be associated with acute types of diarrhea. On the other hand, *chronic diarrhea* lasts for more than 2 weeks or recurs over months or years. When diarrhea occurs suddenly in an otherwise healthy patient without signs or symptoms of other organ involvement, the most likely cause is an infectious agent, most often viral. The most frequent causes of chronic diarrhea are IBS, medications, dietary factors, inflammatory bowel disease, and colon cancer.

A thorough history and comprehensive review of systems can elicit information that the patient may not think is important but can facilitate diagnosis. For example, recent travel is particularly important because viral, bacterial, and protozoan causes are endemic in many areas. Hikers and campers in the United States who drink unfiltered water are at a high risk for giardiasis. Focusing the History 10.1 presents important information to obtain from the patient's history.

Acute viral gastroenteritis is the most common cause of diarrhea. (Gastroenteritis is discussed in detail later in this chapter.) Other common causes of diarrhea the practitioner should consider are IBS, inflammatory bowel disease (IBD), ingestion of magnesium-containing antacids, lactose intolerance, antibiotic therapy, laxative abuse, and acquired immunodeficiency syndrome (AIDS). Differential Diagnosis Flowchart 10.3 presents the differential diagnosis of diarrhea.

Dyspepsia and Heartburn

The frequency with which patients present with dyspepsia and heartburn as their chief complaint has been diminishing probably because of the availability of over-the-counter

(Text continued on page 482)

DIFFERENTIAL DIAGNOSIS FLOWCHART 10.1

ABDOMINAL PAIN

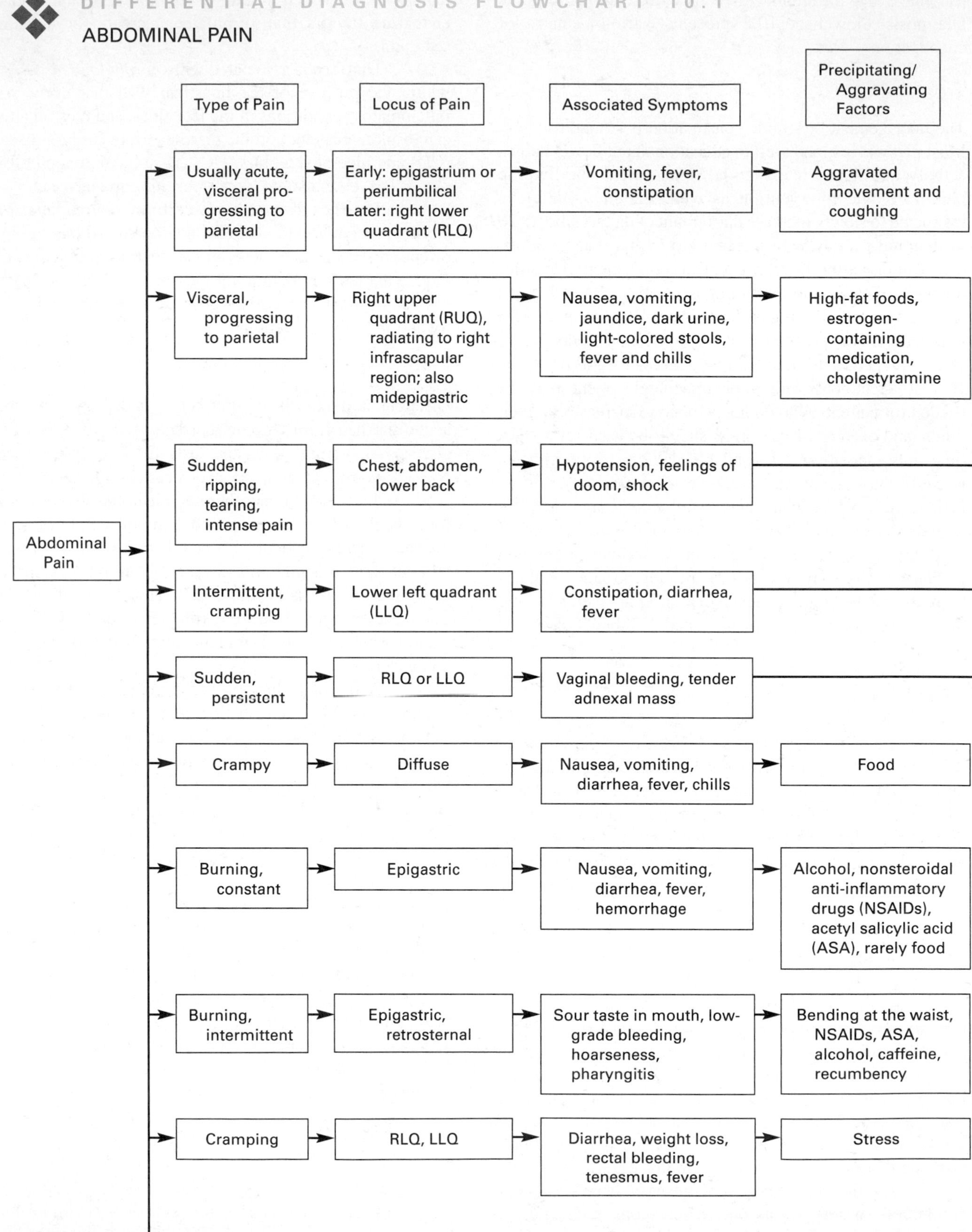

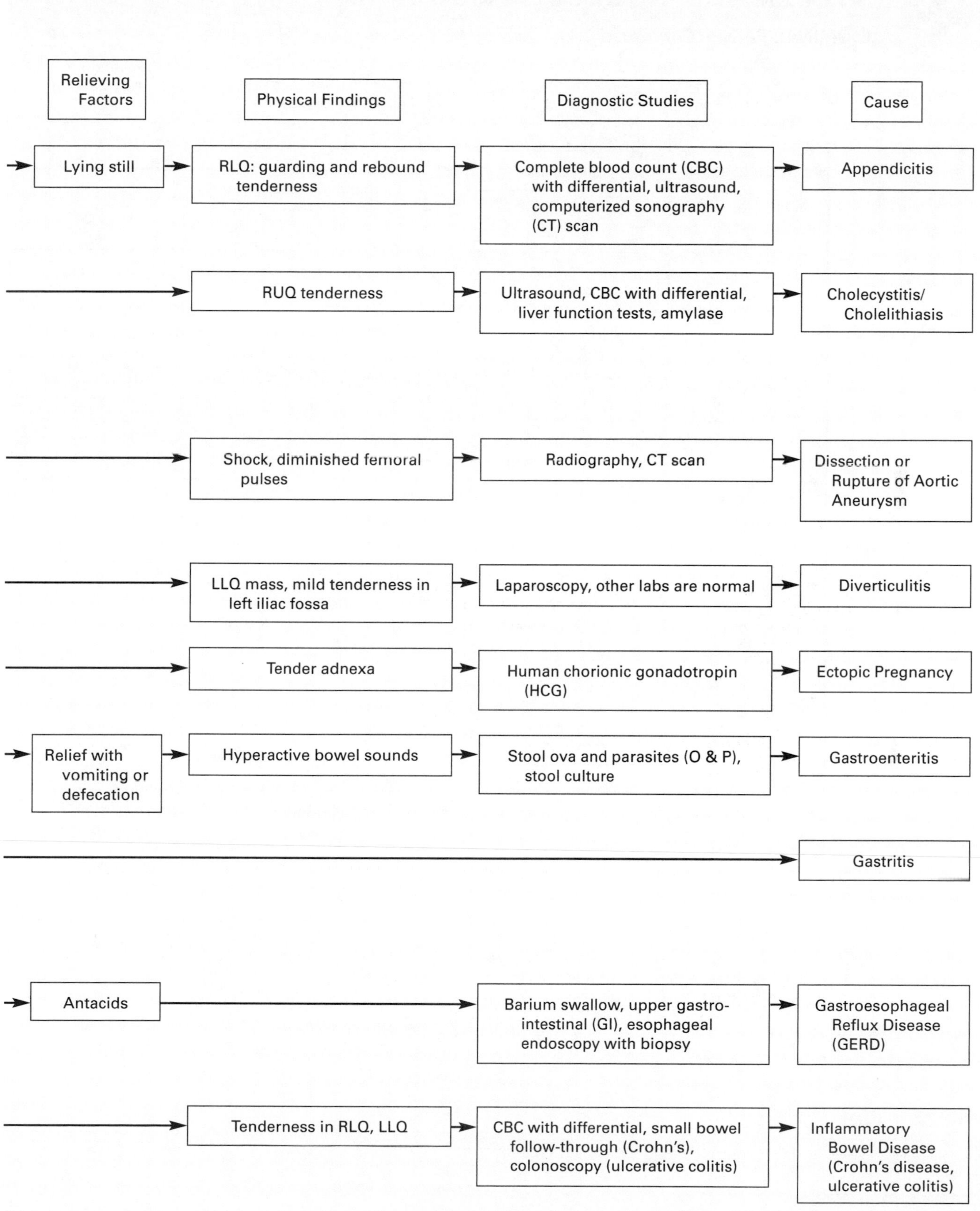

Relieving Factors
Physical Findings
Diagnostic Studies
Cause
Lying still
RLQ: guarding and rebound tenderness
Complete blood count (CBC) with differential, ultrasound, computerized sonography (CT) scan
Appendicitis
RUQ tenderness
Ultrasound, CBC with differential, liver function tests, amylase
Cholecystitis/ Cholelithiasis
Shock, diminished femoral pulses
Radiography, CT scan
Dissection or Rupture of Aortic Aneurysm
LLQ mass, mild tenderness in left iliac fossa
Laparoscopy, other labs are normal
Diverticulitis
Tender adnexa
Human chorionic gonadotropin (HCG)
Ectopic Pregnancy
Relief with vomiting or defecation
Hyperactive bowel sounds
Stool ova and parasites (O & P), stool culture
Gastroenteritis
Gastritis
Antacids
Barium swallow, upper gastro-intestinal (GI), esophageal endoscopy with biopsy
Gastroesophageal Reflux Disease (GERD)
Tenderness in RLQ, LLQ
CBC with differential, small bowel follow-through (Crohn's), colonoscopy (ulcerative colitis)
Inflammatory Bowel Disease (Crohn's disease, ulcerative colitis)

DIFFERENTIAL DIAGNOSIS FLOWCHART 10.1

ABDOMINAL PAIN (*Continued*)

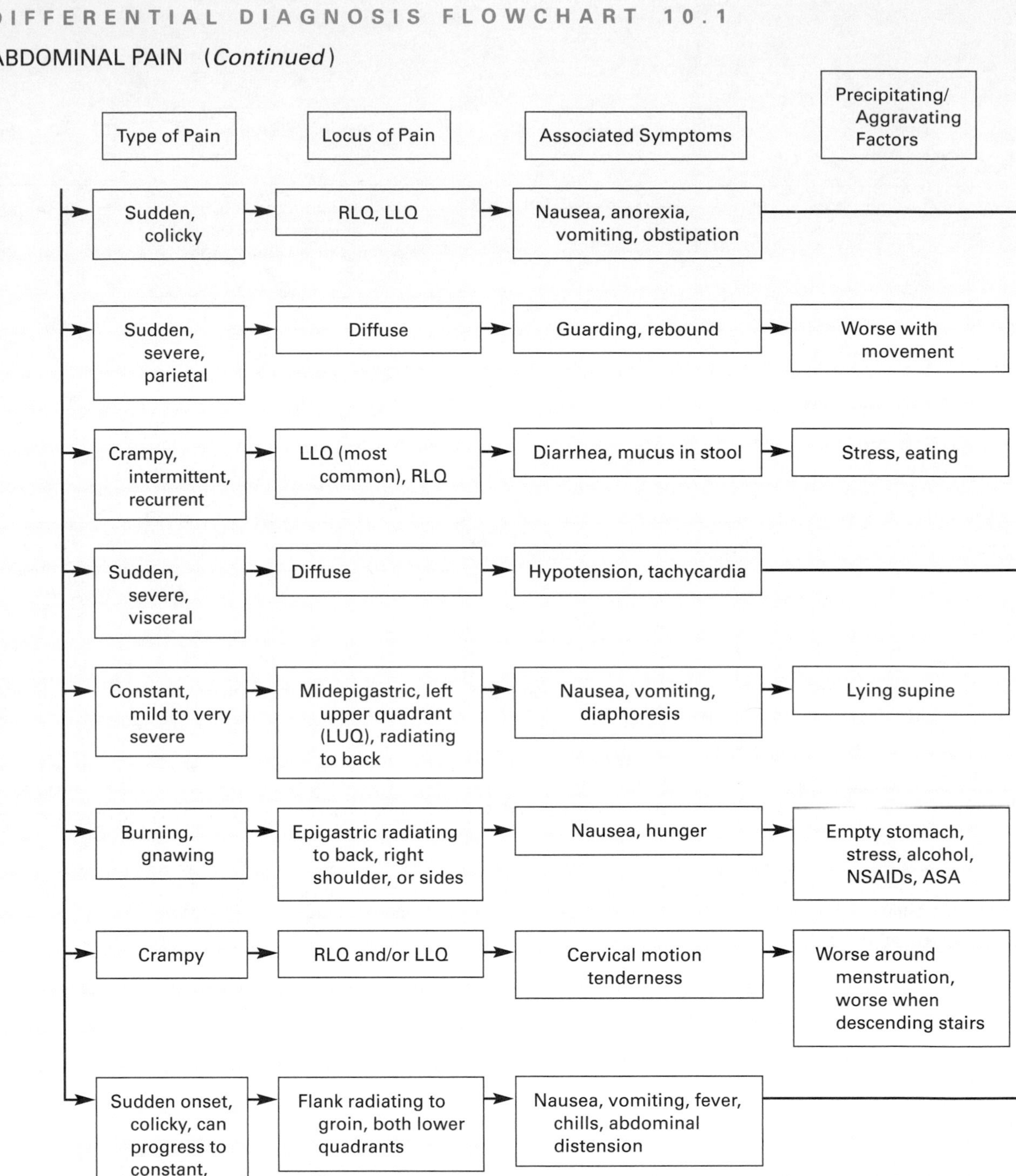

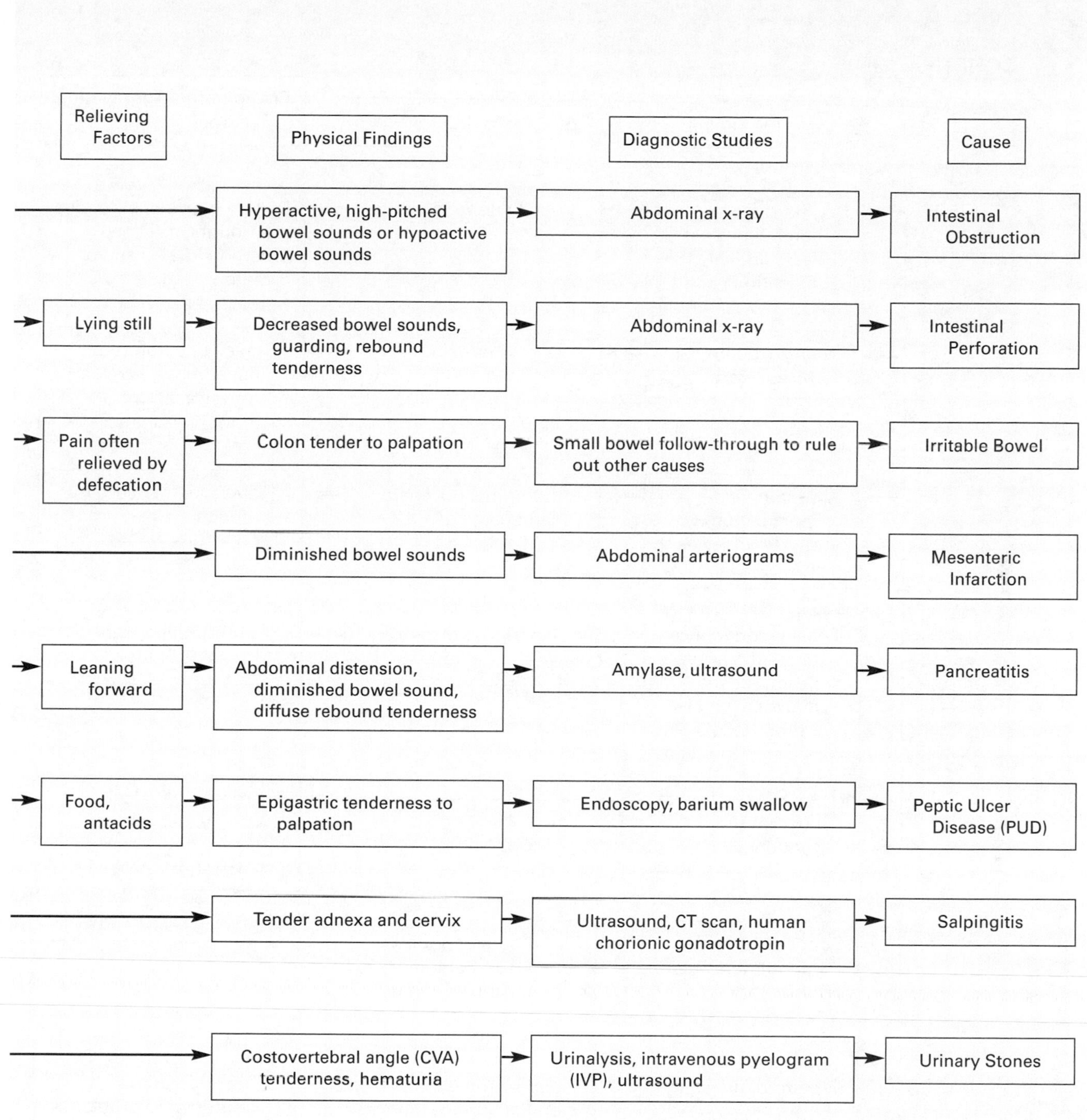
Relieving Factors
Physical Findings
Diagnostic Studies
Cause
Hyperactive, high-pitched bowel sounds or hypoactive bowel sounds
Abdominal x-ray
Intestinal Obstruction
Lying still
Decreased bowel sounds, guarding, rebound tenderness
Abdominal x-ray
Intestinal Perforation
Pain often relieved by defecation
Colon tender to palpation
Small bowel follow-through to rule out other causes
Irritable Bowel
Diminished bowel sounds
Abdominal arteriograms
Mesenteric Infarction
Leaning forward
Abdominal distension, diminished bowel sound, diffuse rebound tenderness
Amylase, ultrasound
Pancreatitis
Food, antacids
Epigastric tenderness to palpation
Endoscopy, barium swallow
Peptic Ulcer Disease (PUD)
Tender adnexa and cervix
Ultrasound, CT scan, human chorionic gonadotropin
Salpingitis
Costovertebral angle (CVA) tenderness, hematuria
Urinalysis, intravenous pyelogram (IVP), ultrasound
Urinary Stones

DIFFERENTIAL DIAGNOSIS FLOWCHART 10.2

CONSTIPATION

Constipation →

Symptoms	Associated Symptoms	Precipitating/Aggravating Factors
Dry, hard stools less than 5 times per week; difficult defecation	Usually none in adults	Dietary intake of excessive amounts of refined carbohydrates and/or meat
Vague abdominal discomfort	Anorexia	Travel, uncomfortable lavatories, decreased physical activity, immobilization
Alternating constipation with diarrhea, mucus in stool	Abdominal distension and pain	Stress, eating certain foods
Fecal incontinence or soiling often described as diarrhea, small-caliber stools	Abdominal pain	Immobility, age, dehydration
Dry, hard stools with a decreased frequency		Decreased physical activity, decreased dietary fiber, decreased fluid intake
Suppression of painful defecation, hard stools	Blood noted on toilet paper, in the toilet, or on the surface of feces	
Suppression of painful defecation	Blood noted on toilet paper, in the toilet, or on the surface of feces	Pregnancy, cirrhosis of the liver, prior hemorrhoid problems
Dry, hard stools	Anorexia	Ingestion of medications listed in Table 10.1
Early morning rushes, decreased effectiveness of laxatives, blood, pus, or mucus in stool.	Abdominal pain, distension. Late signs: weight loss, anorexia, anemia	

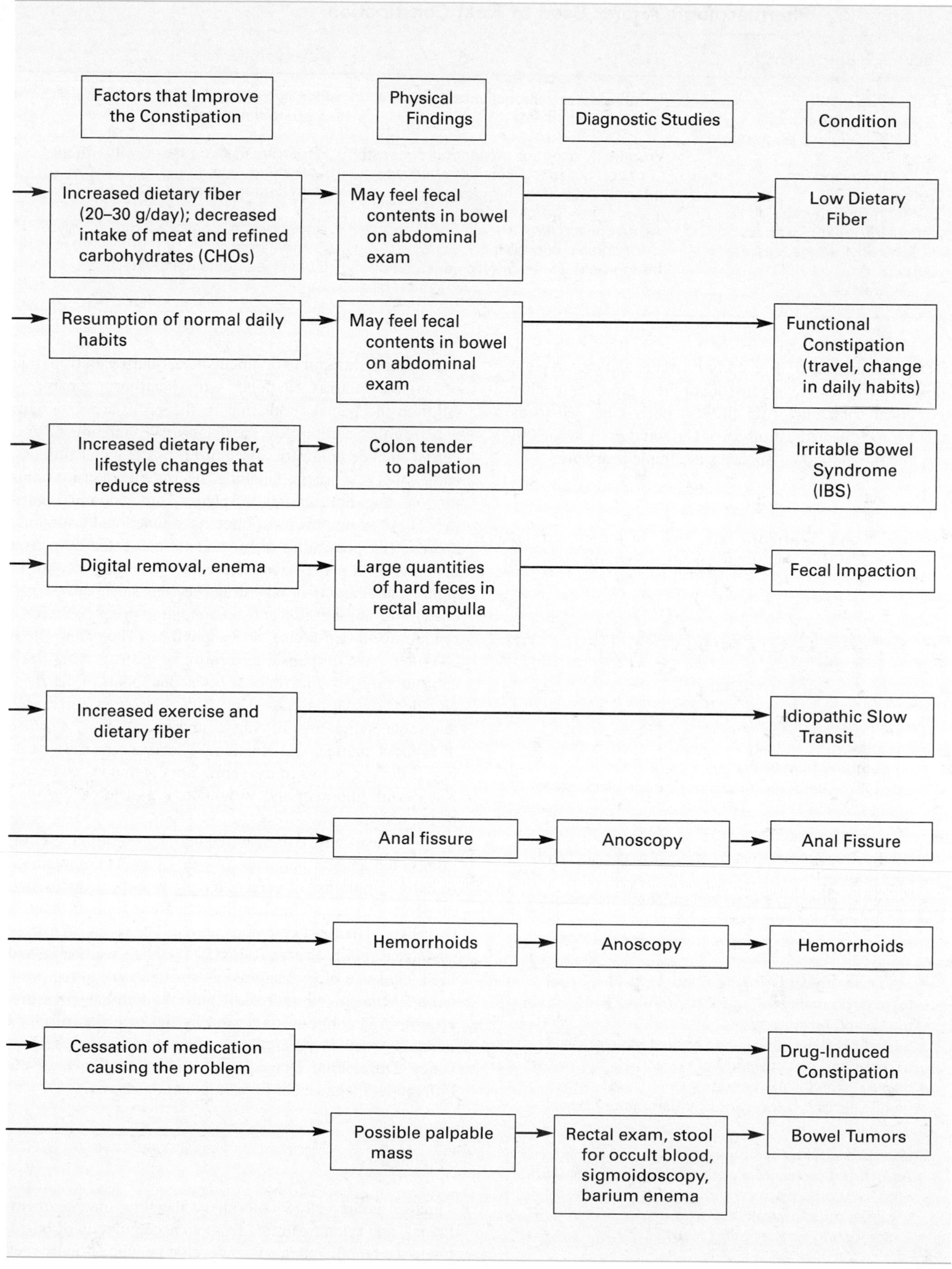
Factors that Improve the Constipation
Physical Findings
Diagnostic Studies
Condition
Increased dietary fiber (20–30 g/day); decreased intake of meat and refined carbohydrates (CHOs)
May feel fecal contents in bowel on abdominal exam
Low Dietary Fiber
Resumption of normal daily habits
May feel fecal contents in bowel on abdominal exam
Functional Constipation (travel, change in daily habits)
Increased dietary fiber, lifestyle changes that reduce stress
Colon tender to palpation
Irritable Bowel Syndrome (IBS)
Digital removal, enema
Large quantities of hard feces in rectal ampulla
Fecal Impaction
Increased exercise and dietary fiber
Idiopathic Slow Transit
Anal fissure
Anoscopy
Anal Fissure
Hemorrhoids
Anoscopy
Hemorrhoids
Cessation of medication causing the problem
Drug-Induced Constipation
Possible palpable mass
Rectal exam, stool for occult blood, sigmoidoscopy, barium enema
Bowel Tumors

Table 10.2 Pharmacologic Agents Used to Treat Constipation

Pharmacologic Agent	Use	Adverse Effects
Bulking agents Psyllium preparations Methylcellulose preparations	Irritable bowel, chronic constipation, diverticulitis	Flatulence, bloating; requires adequate fluid intake
Stool softeners Docusate sodium	Frequently used for prevention of constipation but most likely not effective	Hepatotoxic if combined with irritant laxatives
Saline laxatives Magnesium hydroxide	Intermittent use in chronic constipation and bowel preparation	Dehydration, electrolyte imbalance
Stimulant/irritant laxatives Bisacodyl, senna, cascara	Acute constipation; should not be used for chronic constipation	Dependence, dehydration, electrolyte imbalance
Lubricants Mineral oil	Intermittent use in chronic constipation	Lipid pneumonia if aspirated

(OTC) histamine-2 (H_2)-receptor blockers and proton pump inhibitors. Aggressive advertising of these products by pharmaceutical companies over the last decade has led to the increase in self-medication for what could be a serious illness that the individual mistakes as simple heartburn.

Differential Diagnosis

Dyspepsia and heartburn are two different entities. *Heartburn* is occasionally described as extreme pain, and this makes it difficult to distinguish heartburn pain from that of angina pectoris. Patients with heartburn sometimes describe the pain as radiating to the back, arms, or jaw, which further complicates the diagnosis. Symptoms of *dyspepsia* include epigastric discomfort, postprandial fullness, early satiety, anorexia, belching, nausea, heartburn, vomiting, bloating, borborygmi, dysphagia, and abdominal burning. These symptoms most often have functional or organic causes. The possibility of an organic cause for dyspepsia increases as a person ages. Patients who ingest alcohol in significant amounts or take drugs such as salicylates, corticosteroids, nonsteroidal anti-inflammatory drugs (NSAIDs), erythromycin (E-Mycin), or theophylline (Theo-Dur, Theo-24) often have dyspepsia as a result of gastritis. Giardiasis can cause dyspepsia with only occasional bouts of diarrhea. Nonulcer dyspepsia caused by *Helicobacter pylori* causes the same symptoms of vague abdominal pain, a sense of fullness, nausea, and bloating, which are worse after eating. If the symptoms of dyspepsia are continuous and associated with anorexia and weight loss, gastric cancer may be the cause.

Heartburn, a retrosternal burning sensation, is common in the general population, with 7 percent complaining of daily symptoms, 14 percent having weekly episodes, and 36 percent experiencing heartburn at some time or other in their lives. The most common cause of heartburn is gastroesophageal reflux disease (GERD). Pregnant women have a high incidence of esophagitis, most often later in the pregnancy because of increased intra-abdominal pressure. Heartburn is commonly relieved by the ingestion of alkali (antacids) and is precipitated and aggravated by recumbency. Differential Diagnosis Flowchart 10.4 reviews the differential diagnosis of heartburn and dyspepsia.

FOCUS ON HISTORY 10.1

Diarrhea

Characteristics of Feces

- Frequency
- Amount and fluidity
- Color and characteristics: blood, tarry, black, steatorrhea, mucus

Other History

- Diet history: intolerance to lactose or certain foods
- Recent travel
- Source of drinking water: well or city water supply
- Medication use: magnesium-containing antacids, antibiotics, chemotherapy, immunosuppressive agents
- Medical/surgical history: diabetes mellitus, hyperthyroid, human immunodeficiency virus (HIV), organ transplant, GI surgery
- Sexual practices: frequency of anal intercourse, number and sex of partners
- Social history: living conditions
- Family history: colon cancer, inflammatory bowel disease

Dimensions of the Problem

- Associated symptoms: abdominal pain, fever, vomiting, neurologic symptoms, headache, malaise, myalgia, muscle weakness
- Exacerbating or alleviating factors

Jaundice

Jaundice is the yellow coloring of the skin, mucous membranes, and sclera resulting from an accumulation of bilirubin in the blood. Patients who develop jaundice usually seek medical attention promptly because it is so dramatic, frightening, and difficult to ignore.

The hyperbilirubinemia that causes the jaundice can be a result of increased production, decreased uptake, decreased conjugation, or decreased excretion of bilirubin. The etiology of hyperbilirubinemia is shown in Table 10.3. Hyperbilirubinemia and jaundice in most patients result from cholestasis, either because of impaired bile formation and/or bile flow, which can be the result of extrahepatic biliary tract obstruction, or hepatic parenchymal disease.

Differential Diagnosis

Understanding the laboratory values is essential to determine the type of problem causing the hyperbilirubinemia and establish a differential diagnosis. Icterus is not usually evident until the serum bilirubin level exceeds 2 to 3 mg/dL. The normal serum bilirubin level is 0.3 to 1.0 mg/dL. Most bilirubin is formed from the heme portion of the breakdown of red blood cells. This initial bilirubin is unconjugated and therefore not soluble in water. When measured in the serum, it is reported as indirect bilirubin. This form of bilirubin is reversibly bound to albumin and transported to the liver, where it is taken up by the hepatocyte and conjugated with glucuronic acid. Conjugated bilirubin, which is water soluble, is transported from the hepatocyte into the bile. It is measured in the serum as the direct fraction of bilirubin. Only conjugated bilirubin, by nature of its water solubility, is found in the urine of patients with hyperbilirubinemia. Problems in the metabolism of bilirubin can occur at any point of the cycle.

Serum levels of the transaminases—aspartate aminotransferase (AST) and alanine aminotransferase (ALT)—are good indicators of hepatocyte damage from a variety of causes. Elevated transaminase levels reflect the activity of the disease process, but the actual serum levels do not necessarily correlate with the overall severity of the liver disease, nor with the prognosis. AST is found in hepatocyte mitochondria and cytoplasm and in nonhepatic tissues such as skeletal muscle, the heart, and brain. ALT is found primarily in hepatocyte cytoplasm, making it a much more specific marker for hepatocyte damage. Levels of AST and ALT that are below 300 U/L are nonspecific; however, some extreme elevations can be quite diagnostic. For example, it is very uncommon for the AST to be elevated 15 times the normal value in biliary obstruction except when it occurs suddenly or is associated with cholangitis. Striking elevations of ALT and AST (greater than 1000 U/L) occur in patients with acute viral hepatitis, toxin- or drug-induced hepatitis, and ischemic liver injury. If the ratio of AST to ALT is high, it generally indicates severe hepatic necrosis, most often caused by alcoholic hepatitis.

Alkaline phosphatase is found in the biliary canalicular membranes and is useful in assessing cholestasis. Cholestasis is also characteristically accompanied by an increase in the serum gamma-glutamyl transpeptidase (GGT) and 5′-nucleotidase. Extreme elevations in alkaline phosphatase (greater than three times normal) in conjunction with elevation of the GGT indicate a mechanical obstruction of the biliary system by a tumor, stricture, or stone. Because alkaline phosphatase is also found in bone, an isolated elevation of that enzyme without elevation of the GGT is indicative of a bone disorder rather than a cholestatic process.

A patient who presents with jaundice often has complaints of pruritis, anorexia, nausea, vomiting, fever, light-colored stools, weight loss, and fatigue. Examination may reveal right upper quadrant (RUQ) pain and tenderness, dark urine, and abdominal distension. Pruritus, dark urine, and light-colored stools in conjunction with the jaundice are indicative of cholestasis, either intrahepatic or extrahepatic, such as cholelithiasis, cirrhosis, or other biliary obstruction.

Melena

Melena is defined as black, tarry stools that test positive for occult blood. The most common cause of melena is upper GI bleeding, but bleeding in the small bowel or the right colon can also produce melena. It is the action of gastric acid and intestinal secretions that reduces bright red blood to black, tarry stools. To produce melena, about 100 to 200 mL of blood must be present. Because of GI transit time, it is possible for melena to continue for several days after the acute bleeding has stopped.

Differential Diagnosis

Some patients may present with black, tarry stools that do not test positive for blood. The most common causes for this are iron supplements, bismuth subsalicylate (Pepto-Bismol), and a variety of foods. Table 10.4 lists common causes of GI bleeding. Signs and symptoms associated with GI bleeding depend on the source, rate of bleeding, and coexistent diseases. A CBC can give clues to the severity and duration of the bleeding. Endoscopy is useful in diagnosing the upper GI tract as the source of the bleeding.

Nausea and Vomiting

Nausea is an unpleasant sensation in the stomach that is difficult to define because it is a sensory experience. It is often accompanied by diaphoresis, increased salivation, and the vasovagal signs of hypotension and bradycardia. Nausea can occur alone or precede vomiting. Vomiting is the forceful expulsion of gastric contents; it is a reflex response to stimulation of receptor sites in the mucosa of the upper GI tract, the labyrinthine apparatus in the inner ear, higher cortical centers in response to emotional stimuli, or the chemoreceptor trigger zone (CTZ) of the medulla oblongata. Afferent nerve fibers carry these impulses to the vomiting center,

(Text continued on page 488)

DIFFERENTIAL DIAGNOSIS FLOWCHART 10.3

DIARRHEA

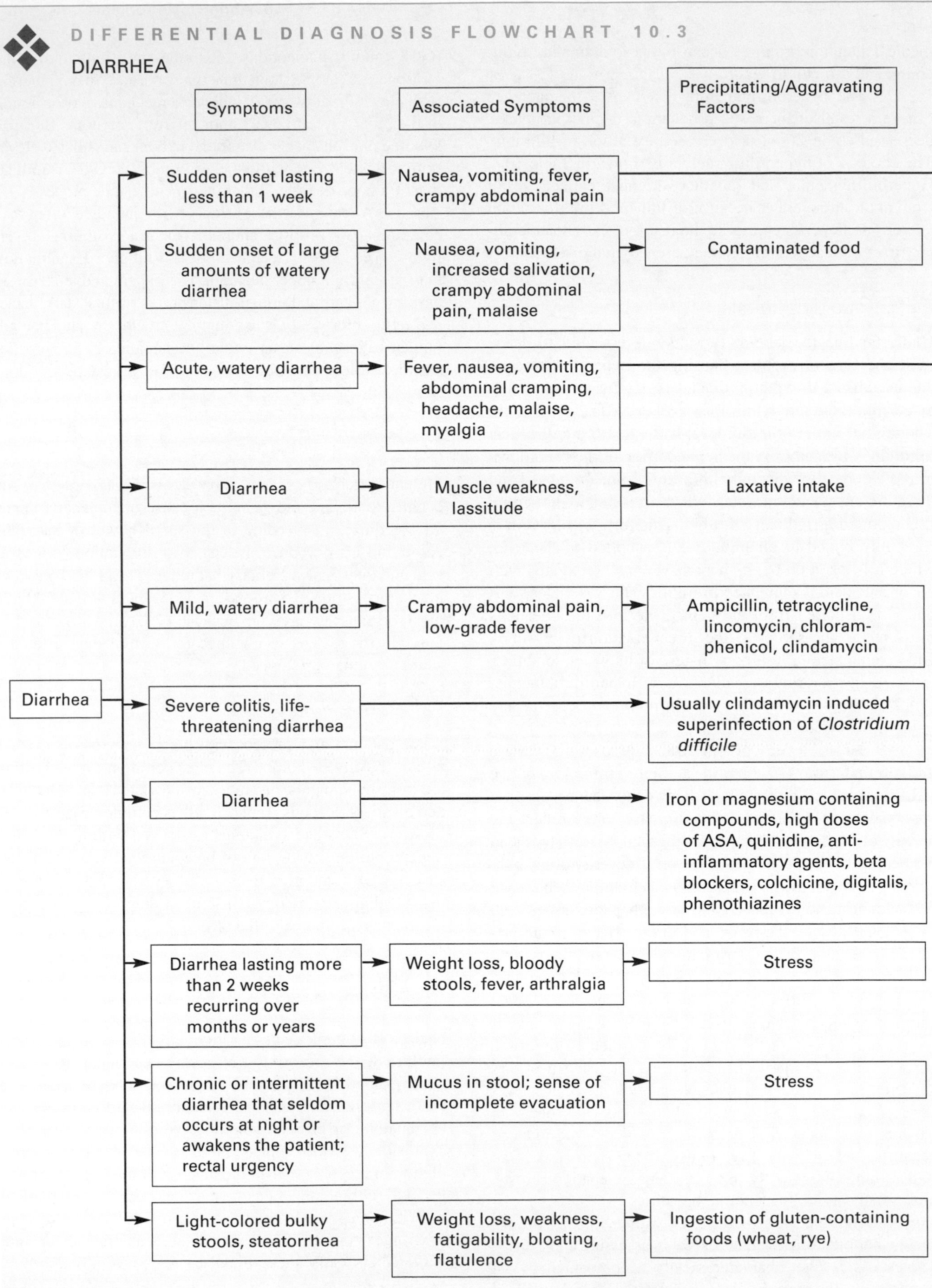

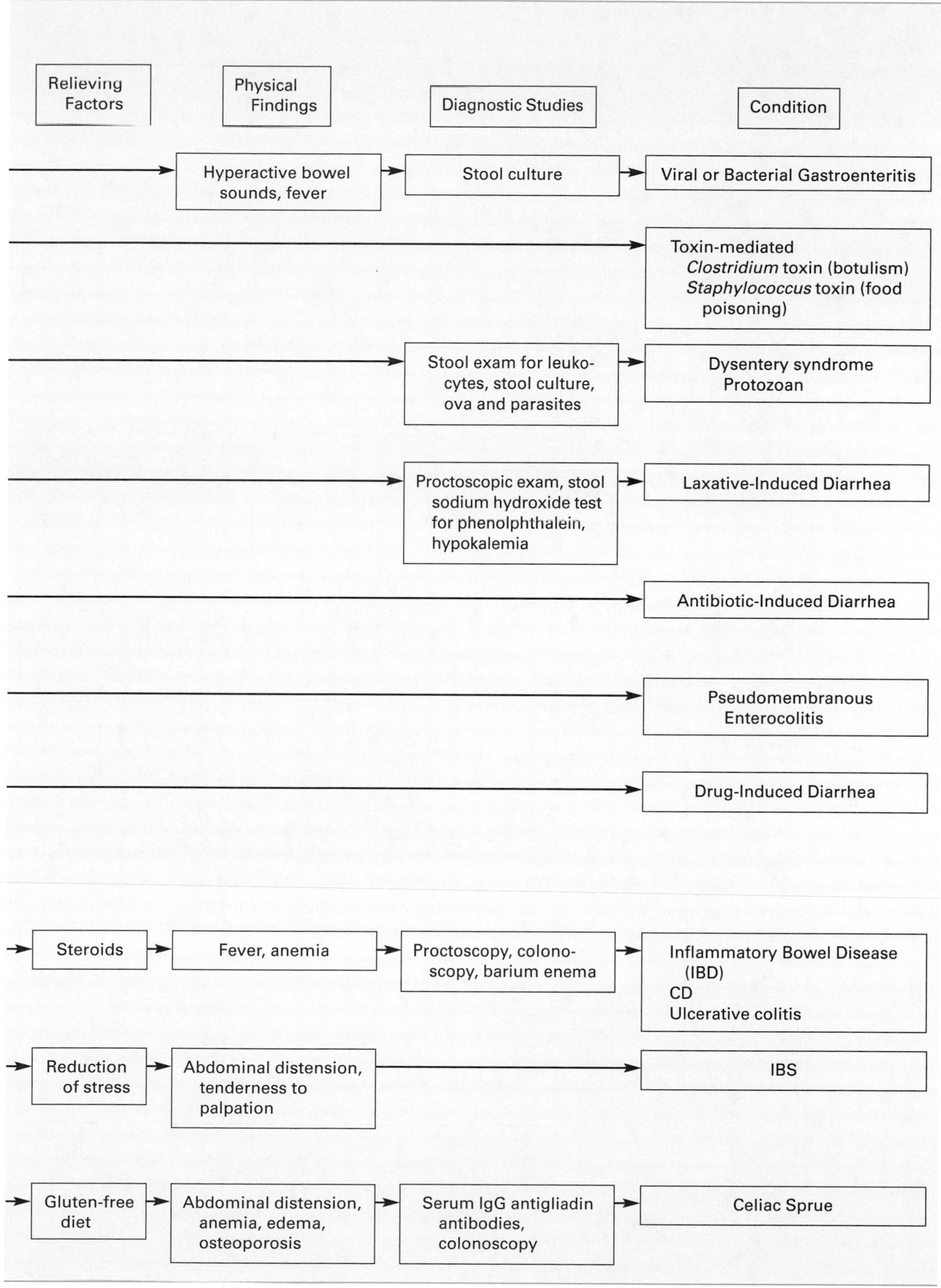

Relieving Factors
Physical Findings
Diagnostic Studies
Condition
Hyperactive bowel sounds, fever
Stool culture
Viral or Bacterial Gastroenteritis
Toxin-mediated
Clostridium toxin (botulism)
Staphylococcus toxin (food poisoning)
Stool exam for leukocytes, stool culture, ova and parasites
Dysentery syndrome
Protozoan
Proctoscopic exam, stool sodium hydroxide test for phenolphthalein, hypokalemia
Laxative-Induced Diarrhea
Antibiotic-Induced Diarrhea
Pseudomembranous Enterocolitis
Drug-Induced Diarrhea
Steroids
Fever, anemia
Proctoscopy, colonoscopy, barium enema
Inflammatory Bowel Disease (IBD)
CD
Ulcerative colitis
Reduction of stress
Abdominal distension, tenderness to palpation
IBS
Gluten-free diet
Abdominal distension, anemia, edema, osteoporosis
Serum IgG antigliadin antibodies, colonoscopy
Celiac Sprue

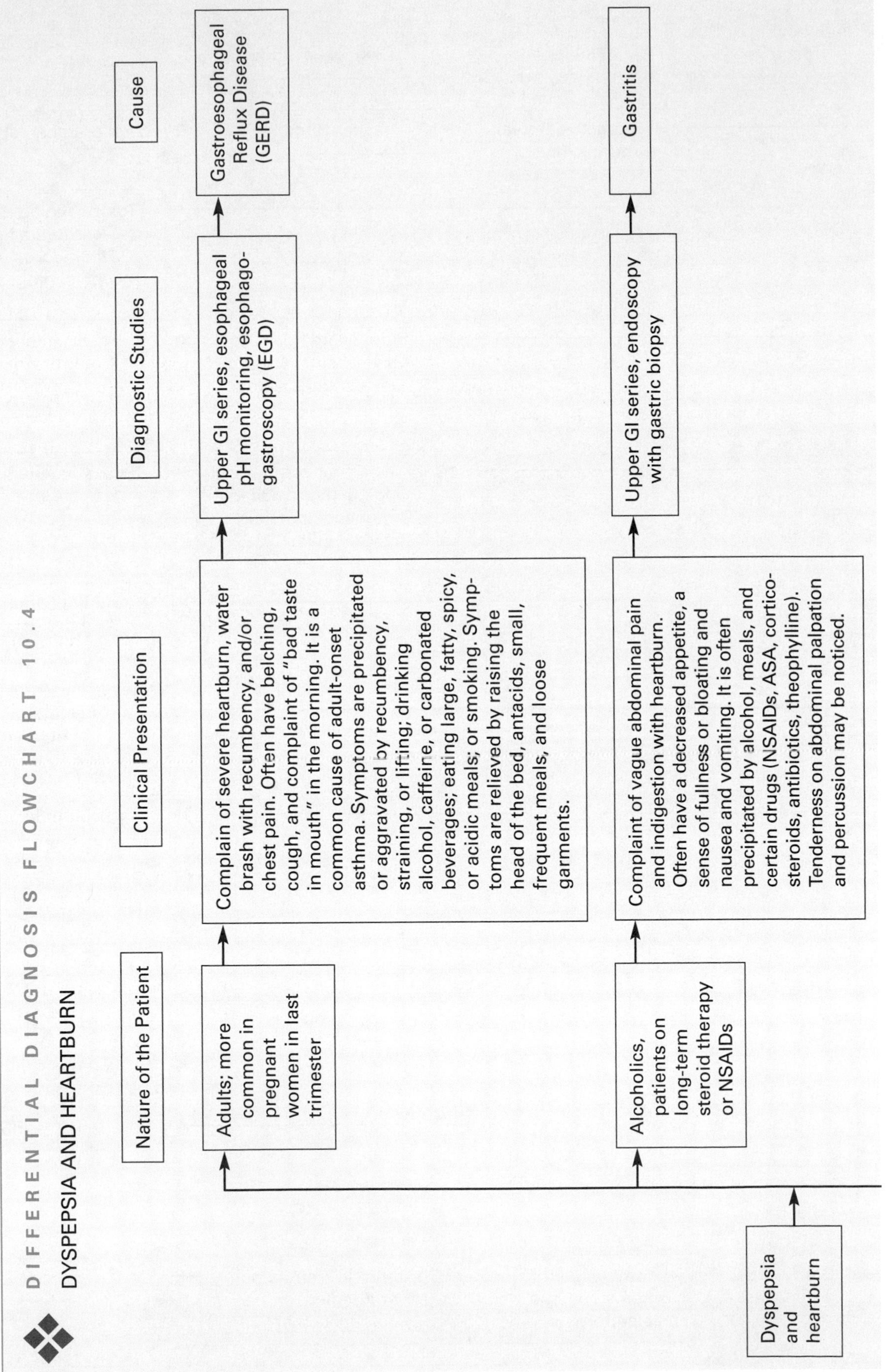
DIFFERENTIAL DIAGNOSIS FLOWCHART 10.4
DYSPEPSIA AND HEARTBURN
Nature of the Patient
Clinical Presentation
Diagnostic Studies
Cause
Dyspepsia and heartburn
Adults; more common in pregnant women in last trimester
Complain of severe heartburn, water brash with recumbency, and/or chest pain. Often have belching, cough, and complaint of "bad taste in mouth" in the morning. It is a common cause of adult-onset asthma. Symptoms are precipitated or aggravated by recumbency, straining, or lifting; drinking alcohol, caffeine, or carbonated beverages; eating large, fatty, spicy, or acidic meals; or smoking. Symptoms are relieved by raising the head of the bed, antacids, small, frequent meals, and loose garments.
Upper GI series, esophageal pH monitoring, esophago-gastroscopy (EGD)
Gastroesophageal Reflux Disease (GERD)
Alcoholics, patients on long-term steroid therapy or NSAIDs
Complaint of vague abdominal pain and indigestion with heartburn. Often have a decreased appetite, a sense of fullness or bloating and nausea and vomiting. It is often precipitated by alcohol, meals, and certain drugs (NSAIDs, ASA, cortico-steroids, antibiotics, theophylline). Tenderness on abdominal palpation and percussion may be noticed.
Upper GI series, endoscopy with gastric biopsy
Gastritis

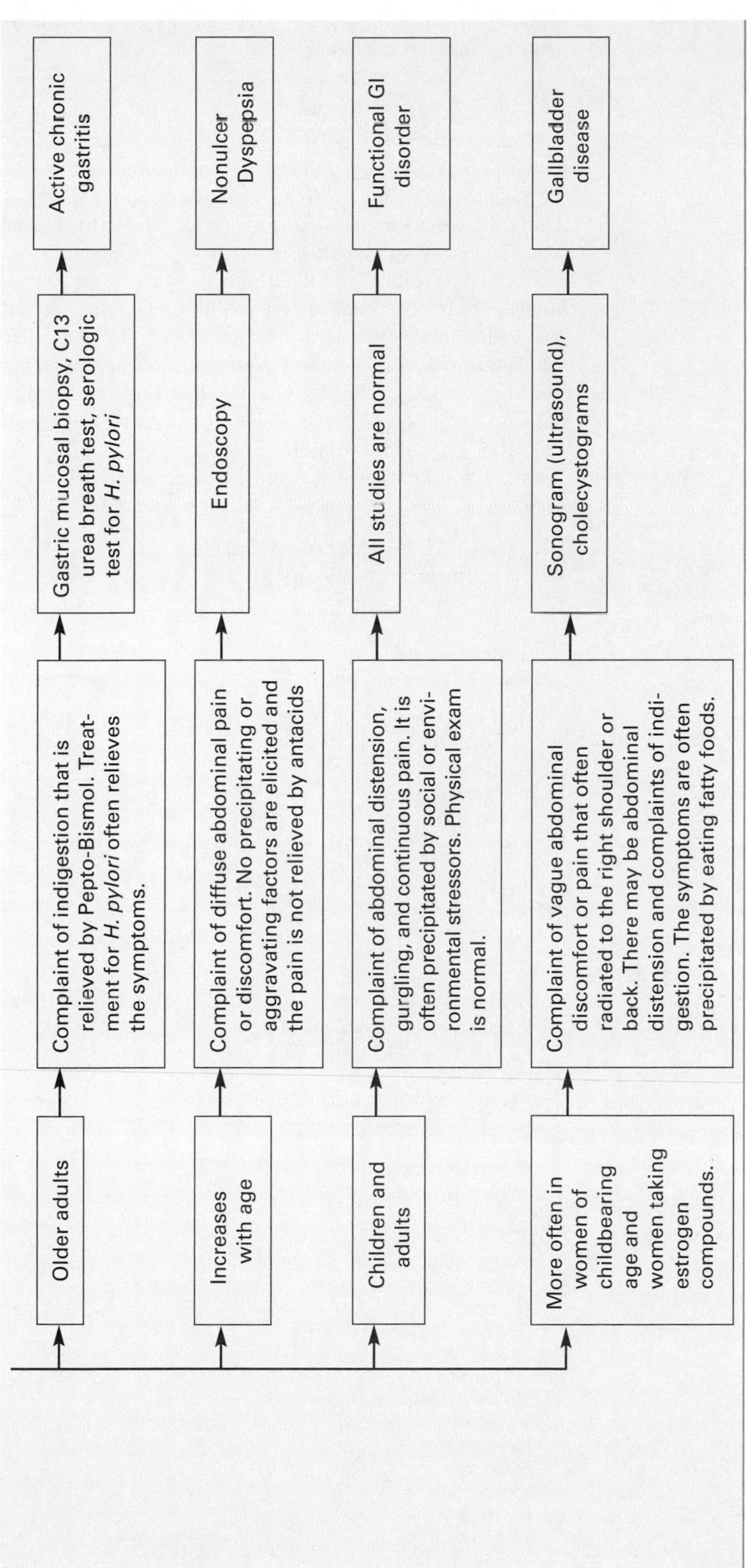
Older adults
Complaint of indigestion that is relieved by Pepto-Bismol. Treatment for H. pylori often relieves the symptoms.
Gastric mucosal biopsy, C13 urea breath test, serologic test for H. pylori
Active chronic gastritis
Increases with age
Complaint of diffuse abdominal pain or discomfort. No precipitating or aggravating factors are elicited and the pain is not relieved by antacids
Endoscopy
Nonulcer Dyspepsia
Children and adults
Complaint of abdominal distension, gurgling, and continuous pain. It is often precipitated by social or environmental stressors. Physical exam is normal.
All studies are normal
Functional GI disorder
More often in women of childbearing age and women taking estrogen compounds.
Complaint of vague abdominal discomfort or pain that often radiated to the right shoulder or back. There may be abdominal distension and complaints of indigestion. The symptoms are often precipitated by eating fatty foods.
Sonogram (ultrasound), cholecystograms
Gallbladder disease

Table 10.3 Etiology: Hyperbilirubinemia

Increased Production
Hemolysis, resorption of hematomas, ineffective erythropoiesis
- Megaloblastic anemia, iron deficiency anemia, sideroblastic anemia
- Thalassemia minor
- Polycythemia vera
- Lead poisoning

Decreased Clearance
Inherited disorder of bilirubin metabolism
- Gilbert's syndrome, Crigler-Najjar syndrome, Dubin-Johnson syndrome, Rotor's syndrome

Cholestasis
- Hepatocellular disease
  Viral, drug-induced or alcoholic hepatitis
- Biliary tract obstruction
  Choledocholithiasis, tumor, sclerosing cholangitis, chronic pancreatitis, pancreatic cancer, primary biliary cirrhosis
- Drugs
  Antibiotics (erythromycin, trimethoprim/sulfamethoxazole, amoxicillin/clavulanic acid, nitrofurantoin, griseofulvin)
  Analgesics (propoxyphene, sulindac, diflunisal)
  Allopurinol
  Warfarin
  Steroids (contraceptive and anabolic)
  Phenytoin
  Thiazide diuretics
  Phenothiazines
  Tricyclic antidepressants
  Haloperidol
  Parenteral gold
  Oral hypoglycemics (chlorpropamide, tolbutamide)

where efferent fibers then send impulses to relax the gastric fundus and the gastroesophageal sphincter, to contract the pylorus, and to cause reverse peristalsis in the esophagus. The abdominal muscles and diaphragm contract, increasing the intra-abdominal pressure, which forces the gastric contents out through the mouth.

Table 10.4 Common Causes of Gastrointestinal Bleeding

Upper GI Tract
Peptic ulcer
  Gastric ulcer
  Duodenal ulcer
Gastric erosions
Erosive esophagitis
Esophageal varices
Lower GI Tract
Diverticular disease
Colon cancer
Intestinal polyps
IBD
  Ulcerative colitis (UC)
  CD
  Infectious colitis
Meckel's diverticulum
Small bowel neoplasm

Differential Diagnosis

Gastroenteritis is the most common cause of nausea and vomiting in adults and children. Contaminated food should be considered in cases of acute nausea and vomiting, especially when more than one person is affected. Gastritis, usually associated with alcohol consumption or drugs (aspirin, NSAIDs, antibiotics, and illicit drugs), is also a very common cause of acute nausea and vomiting in adults. Nausea and vomiting are listed as adverse effects of a large number of medications; they are also common presenting symptoms for many disease entities such as hepatitis, myocardial infarction, and peptic ulcer. Table 10.5 provides common causes of nausea and vomiting.

A bit of detective work is necessary to determine

Table 10.5 Common Causes of Nausea and Vomiting

GI Disorders and Problems
Gastroenteritis
Acute GI infections
Food poisoning
Gastritis, including alcoholic
Peptic ulcer disease
Hepatitis
Food intolerance
Celiac sprue
Lactase deficiency
Ingestion of fatty foods
Intestinal obstruction
Appendicitis
Cholecystitis
Peritonitis
Diabetic gastric atony
CNS Disorders and Problems
Increased intracranial pressure
Migraine headache
Meningitis
Acute labyrinthitis
Ménière's disease
Altitude sickness
Other Disorders and Problems
Motion sickness
Uremia
Bulimia nervosa
Diabetic ketoacidosis
Adrenal insufficiency
Acute myocardial infarction
Congestive heart failure
Acute Systemic Infections Accompanied by Fever
Pregnancy
Adverse Effect of Drugs and Chemicals
Antibiotics (erythromycin, metronidazole)
Opiates
Estrogen
Ipecac
Digitalis
Chemotherapy
Theophylline

the cause of the nausea and vomiting. The circumstances surrounding the episode or episodes give clues to the cause. Vomiting following a meal can occur with gastritis and in digitalis toxicity. If the vomiting occurs 1 to 2 hours after eating, then diseases of the biliary tract or pancreas should be suspected. Projectile vomiting without nausea is classically a sign of a neurologic source, such as increased intracranial pressure. If the nausea and vomiting occur in the early morning, the cause may be uremia, pregnancy, or chronic alcohol ingestion. The duration of the nausea and vomiting depends on the cause. Infectious agents in the GI tract usually cause nausea and vomiting only for 24 hours or less. On the other hand, nausea as a result of pregnancy can last for weeks.

The characteristics of the vomitus are important in determining the cause. For example, repeated vomiting without bile staining is indicative of pyloric obstruction, which can be caused by scars from an ulcer or a tumor, whereas vomiting of undigested food could indicate an esophageal obstruction. The odor of the vomitus is important information to elicit from the patient in determining the cause. Odorless vomitus indicates a lack of gastric acid, possibly from esophageal stricture or achalasia. Fecal odor, on the other hand, indicates a bowel obstruction or gastrocolic fistula.

In the continued search for the cause of nausea and vomiting, associated symptoms can further narrow the field of possibilities. Ménière's disease or middle ear disturbances should be suspected if the patient complains of vertigo, tinnitus, or hearing loss. Nausea and vomiting often accompany migraine headaches, which are usually unilateral. Nausea and vomiting with diarrhea and abdominal pain are often caused by gastroenteritis. Differential Diagnosis Flowchart 10.5 delineates the differential diagnosis of nausea and vomiting.

Treatment

Management of nausea and vomiting is aimed at the underlying cause, which is covered in detail under the specific diagnoses in this chapter and in other chapters of this book. Symptomatic relief, however, is useful for the comfort of the patient and in preventing complications such as dehydration and electrolyte imbalance. Table 10.6 presents a list of medications commonly used for the control of nausea and vomiting. Complementary Therapies 10.1 lists the uses of vitamins, minerals, and herbs for GI problems.

Common Problems

Gastroesophageal Reflux Disease

Esophageal reflux is the backward flow of stomach or duodenal contents into the esophagus without associated retching or vomiting. It can occur in otherwise healthy people. If symptoms become severe or frequent or are associated with esophageal mucosal damage, the potential for serious clinical consequences becomes more likely and the esophageal reflux is considered a disease. Gastroesophageal reflux disease (GERD) is a syndrome that results from esophageal reflux; the characteristic symptoms are caused by repeated exposure of the esophageal mucosa to the deleterious effects of GI contents and the gradual breakdown of the mucosal barrier.

Epidemiology and Causes

Although GERD can occur at any age, the incidence increases after age 50. The prevalence of GERD is equal across gender, ethnic, and cultural groups and is a very common condition. Thirty-five to 45 percent of the adult population complain of heartburn at least once a month, and 10 percent of the adult population complain of symptoms daily. The figures may be significantly underestimated, because many people with mild symptoms use OTC H_2-receptor blockers or antacids. Many individuals also believe that it is normal to have symptoms from time to time and attribute their symptoms to stress or dietary indiscretion.

The primary cause of GERD is the inappropriate, spontaneous, transient relaxation of the lower esophageal sphincter (LES) to an unknown stimulus. In most patients, the resting or baseline LES pressure is normal (10 to 30 mm Hg). In patients who have more severe disease, the LES is incompetent, with a resting pressure of less than 10 mm Hg. The incompetent LES results in free reflux during abdominal straining, lifting, bending, and recumbency. Gastric contents are acidic, and it is this low pH (less than 3.9) that causes the injury to the esophageal mucosa in the majority of patients with GERD. Normally, refluxate is cleared and neutralized by swallowing salivary bicarbonate and esophageal peristalsis. Decreased swallowing (by two-thirds) during sleep, coupled with recumbency, significantly increase the duration of exposure of the mucosa to acid at night.

Historically, the presence of a hiatal hernia, which displaces the LES into the thorax, was believed to be the major cause of GERD. This is now disputed because, although most patients with hiatal hernias do experience reflux, not all patients who have reflux have hiatal hernias. The two conditions are related but separate. Delayed gastric emptying, which often worsens as people age, causes increased intra-abdominal pressure and may contribute to reflux. Obesity is also a risk factor for GERD. A number of foods and pharmacologic agents are known to lower LES pressure. Table 10.7 lists the common substances that reduce LES pressure or cause direct gastric mucosal irritation.

Pathophysiology

Physiologically, gastric acid is prevented from refluxing into the esophagus by the presence of two areas of high pressure in the distal esophagus. The upper esophageal sphincter is a 3-cm segment at the proximal end of the esophagus. The

(Text continued on page 493)

DIFFERENTIAL DIAGNOSIS FLOWCHART 10.5

NAUSEA AND VOMITING

Nausea and Vomiting

Clinical Presentation	Diagnostic Studies	Cause
Acute onset of nausea and vomiting usually accompanied by diarrhea, fever, and abdominal pain. Physical exam reveals hyperactive bowel sounds.	None unless infectious cause is suspected, such as *Salmonella,* etc., then stool culture and ova and parasites	Gastroenteritis
Acute or chronic nausea and vomiting usually occurs soon after a meal and frequently accompanied by abdominal pain. History may reveal alcohol or drug ingestion or contact with other persons who have similar symptoms (suggesting viral infection).	Endoscopy	Gastritis
Acute or chronic nausea and vomiting. History reveal medication use. Some medications cause gastritis as mentioned above, others may stimulate the chemoreceptor trigger zone or vomiting center directly. Examples of drugs that commonly cause nausea and vomiting are cytotoxic drugs, codeine, digitalis (cardiac glycosides), quinidine, salicylates, theophylline, antihypertensives, antibiotics, iron preparations, NSAIDs, nicotine, and Nicorette gum.	Serum drug levels	Drug-induced nausea and vomiting

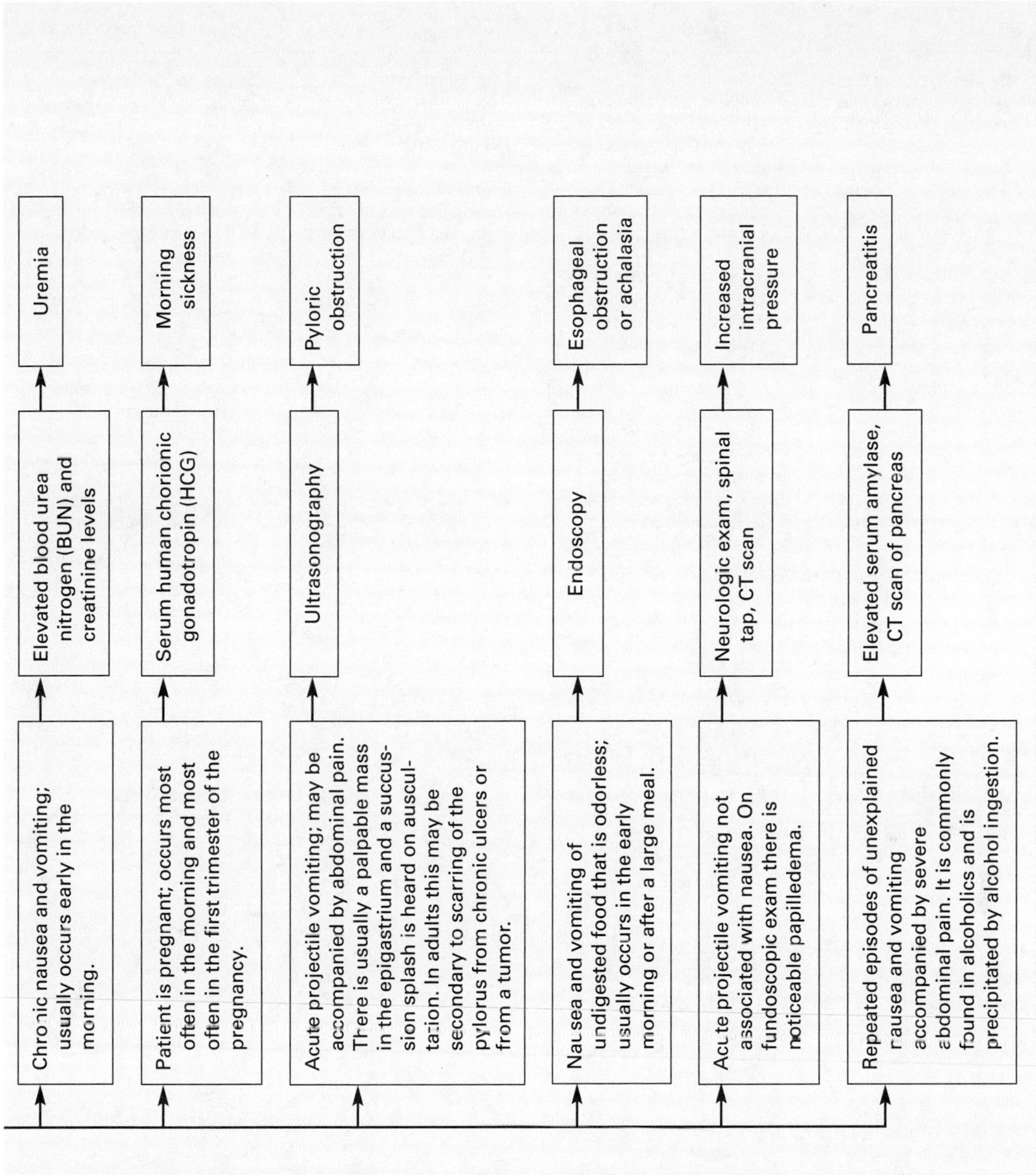
Chronic nausea and vomiting; usually occurs early in the morning.
Elevated blood urea nitrogen (BUN) and creatinine levels
Uremia
Patient is pregnant; occurs most often in the morning and most often in the first trimester of the pregnancy.
Serum human chorionic gonadotropin (HCG)
Morning sickness
Acute projectile vomiting; may be accompanied by abdominal pain. There is usually a palpable mass in the epigastrium and a succussion splash is heard on auscultation. In adults this may be secondary to scarring of the pylorus from chronic ulcers or from a tumor.
Ultrasonography
Pyloric obstruction
Nausea and vomiting of undigested food that is odorless; usually occurs in the early morning or after a large meal.
Endoscopy
Esophageal obstruction or achalasia
Acute projectile vomiting not associated with nausea. On fundoscopic exam there is noticeable papilledema.
Neurologic exam, spinal tap, CT scan
Increased intracranial pressure
Repeated episodes of unexplained nausea and vomiting accompanied by severe abdominal pain. It is commonly found in alcoholics and is precipitated by alcohol ingestion.
Elevated serum amylase, CT scan of pancreas
Pancreatitis

Table 10.6 **Medications for the Control of Nausea and Vomiting**

Medications	Mechanism and Site of Action	Indications	Adverse Effects
Antihistamines (e.g., dimenhydrinate, promethazine, hydroxyzine, meclizine)	Mechanism of action unclear; site of action is labyrinth efferents causing central venous system (CNS) depression	Motion sickness Drug-induced nausea Postoperative During labor	Sedation, dry mouth, blurred vision, headache
Antidopaminergics (phenothiazine derivatives, e.g., prochlorperazine)	Blocks D_2-dopaminergic receptors in the chemoreceptor trigger zone	Chemotherapy- and radiation-induced nausea and vomiting Postoperative	Sedation, dry mouth, urinary retention, constipation, extra-pyramidal effects
Antidopaminergics and cholinergics (e.g., metoclopramide)	Blocks D_2 receptors in the chemoreceptor trigger zone and stimulates upper GI motility	Postoperative Diabetic gastroparesis	Restlessness, drowsiness, fatigue, extrapyramidal effects
Cholinergic antagonists (antimuscarinics, e.g., scopolamine)	Blocks muscarinic receptors in the labyrinth, chemoreceptor trigger zone, and vomiting center, causing inhibition of parasympathetic functions	Motion sickness	Dry mouth, blurred vision, tachycardia, constipation, sedation
Serotonin receptor antagonists (e.g., ondansetron, granisetron)	Block serotonin stimulation and subsequent vagal afferent discharge	Chemotherapy- and radiation-induced nausea and vomiting	Anxiety, euphoria, depression, headache, insomnia, restlessness, weakness

COMPLEMENTARY THERAPIES 10.1

Complementary Therapies for Gastrointestinal Problems

Gastrointestinal Problem	Treatment or Agent	Dosage or no. of treatments
Appetite, poor	Vitamin A	25,000 IU qd
	Calcium	1500 mg qd
	Magnesium	750 mg qd
	Vitamin B complex	100 mg qd before meals
	Zinc	80 mg qd
	Copper	3 mg qd
Celiac disease	Vitamin A	15,000 IU qd
	Beta-carotene	10,000 IU qd
	Vitamin E	400 IU qd
	Vitamin B complex	100 mg tid
	Vitamin B_{12}	As directed on label
	Folic acid	As directed on label
	Vitamin K	As directed on label
	Zinc lozenges	1–15 mg 5 times a day
	Copper	3 mg qd
Constipation	Vitamin C	1000–4000 five times a day
	Senna (*Cassia senna*)	1–2 tsp dried leaves per 8 oz water taken as a tea (not to be taken for longer than a few days)
Diarrhea	Potassium	200 mg qd
Diverticulitis	Vitamin B complex	100 mg tid
	Vitamin K	100 μg qd
Food poisoning	Potassium	200 mg qd
	Vitamin C	2000 mg qid
	Vitamin E	600 IU qd
	Selenium	200 μg qd

Gastrointestinal Problem	Treatment or Agent	Dosage or no. of treatments
Heartburn/GERD	Vitamin B complex	50 mg tid with food
	Vitamin B_{12}	200 μg tid
	Chamomile	350–500 mg tid–qid as a tea or tincture
Hepatitis	Milk thistle (*Silybum marianum*)	140 mg tid (oral)
Indigestion/dyspepsia	Vitamin B complex	100 mg tid with food or meals
	Vitamin B_1	50 mg tid
	Vitamin B_{12}	1000 μg bid
IBD	Acupuncture	8–12 treatments
	Acidophilus	1 tab tid
	Vitamin B complex	100 mg tid
	Vitamin B_{12}	200 μg qd
	Folic acid	200 μg qd
	Vitamin C	1000 mg tid
	Vitamin K	As directed on label
	Vitamin A	25,000 IU qd
	Vitamin E	Up to 800 IU qd
	Zinc	50 mg qd
IBS	Vitamin B complex	50–100 mg tid with food or meals
	Vitamin B_{12}	200 μg bid
	Acupuncture	8–12 treatments
Malabsorption syndrome	Vitamin C	1000–4000 mg bid with juice
Nausea	Ginger	250 mg qid
Peptic ulcer disease (PUD)	Vitamin E	400–800 IU qd
	Licorice root	5–15 mg tid

LES is a 2- to 4-cm segment of the esophagus just proximal to the gastroesophageal junction that prevents the reflux of gastric contents. These areas of the esophagus are under muscular, hormonal, and neural control. The anatomic placement of the LES within the abdomen supports its function, as does the acute angle (angle of His) that is formed as the esophagus enters the stomach.

Esophageal reflux occurs when the gastric volume (e.g., a large meal) or the intra-abdominal pressure is elevated (e.g., in pregnancy). It can also occur when the sphincter tone of the LES is decreased (e.g., by caffeine) or when the LES undergoes inappropriate relaxation. Gravity, saliva, and peristalsis combine to return refluxed contents to the stomach. As the esophagus becomes inflamed with repeated exposure to gastric acid, it cannot eliminate the refluxed material as quickly or efficiently, prolonging the duration of the contact with each subsequent exposure.

Because gastric contents are so irritating to the esophageal mucosa, an inflammatory response is established. With repeated exposure, the inflammation becomes chronic. In response to chronic inflammation, there is increased blood flow to the area and erosion occurs. Frank bleeding is unusual, but minor capillary bleeding is common. As the erosion heals, the body replaces the normal squamous epithelium with metaplastic columnar epithelium (Barrett's epithelium) containing goblet and columnar cells. This new

Table 10.7 Substances that Reduce Lower Esophageal Sphincter Pressure or Irritate the Gastric Mucosa

Food Substances	*Nonfood Substances*
Alcohol	Anticholinergic drugs
Caffeinated beverages (cola, tea, coffee)	Beta-adrenergic blocking agents
Chocolate	Calcium channel blockers
Citrus fruits	Diazepam
Decaffeinated coffee	Estrogen and progesterone
Fatty foods, fats (butter, margarine, shortening), and oils	Nicotine, including second-hand smoke
Onions	Theophylline
Peppermint and spearmint	
Tomatoes and tomato-based products (ketchup, cocktail sauce, tomato sauce, tomato paste)	

epithelium is more resistant to acid and, therefore, supports esophageal healing. Barrett's epithelium is a premalignant tissue, however, and presents a 40-fold risk for the development of esophageal adenocarcinoma. Fibrosis and scarring also accompany the healing process, leading to esophageal strictures.

Clinical Presentation

Subjective

The most typical symptom of GERD is heartburn, ranging in degree from mild to severe. It is usually associated with other symptoms, including regurgitation, water brash (reflex salivation), dysphagia, sour taste in the mouth in the morning, odynophagia, belching, coughing, hoarseness, or wheezing, usually at night. Substernal or retrosternal chest pain may also be present, but additional questioning can determine if the pain is activity induced, leading to the conclusion that the pain may be cardiac in origin. Factors that precipitate or make the symptoms worse, such as reclining after eating; eating a large meal; ingesting alcohol, chocolate, caffeine, fatty or spicy foods, or nicotine; wearing constrictive clothing; or working in an occupation in which heavy lifting, straining, or working in a bent over position is involved also help establish the diagnosis of GERD. It is equally important to ask what the patient does that makes the symptoms better, such as taking antacids, sitting upright after a meal, or eating small meals.

Patients with chronic GERD may present with dysphagia as their chief complaint. The dysphagia is usually present only with the first swallow of every meal and is not progressive. Should the patient complain of progressive or persistent dysphagia, adenocarcinoma or the development of a stricture should be suspected.

Objective

The physical exam of the patient with GERD is usually normal. The only physical sign may be a stool positive for occult blood on rectal exam resulting from microhemorrhages in the irritated esophageal epithelium.

Diagnostic Reasoning

Diagnostic Tests

Diagnosis of GERD is usually made by history alone and has a sensitivity of 80 percent. The severity of the symptoms does not correlate well with the severity of the disease; some patients with the most severe disease have virtually no symptoms. GERD may also manifest with atypical symptoms such as adult onset asthma, chronic cough, or sore throat.

When the diagnosis of GERD is unclear or when the patient fails to respond to 4 weeks of empiric therapy, the most accurate method of diagnosing the disease is by ambulatory esophageal pH monitoring, which involves placing pH probes 5 cm above the LES. If the pH is less than 4 above the LES and correlates with the occurrence of symptoms, the test is definitive for GERD. Esophageal manometry is indicated to determine the location of the LES before placement of the pH-monitoring probe. Upper endoscopy with a biopsy is the test of choice to document the type and extent of tissue damage (e.g., Barrett's esophagus) in the esophagus. Endoscopy is normal in 50 percent of symptomatic patients, however.

Differential Diagnosis

The symptoms of GERD are similar to those of PUD and the two conditions often coexist. Unlike GERD, however, PUD usually produces epigastric pain and tenderness on palpation. One pattern that can help differentiate GERD from PUD is that heartburn from PUD is usually relieved by food. This is not the case in GERD; instead, the symptoms are worse shortly after eating. Another possible differential diagnosis is gallbladder disease, which usually presents with epigastric or right subcostal pain. Nausea and possibly vomiting are usually associated with cholelithiasis and cholecystis; this is not the case in gastric reflux. There may be a strong association between the ingestion of a high fat meal and the development of the symptoms of cholelithiasis. Occasionally, GERD may present with chest pain. In these patients, the practitioner must differentiate between symptoms of cardiac origin and those of GERD. If the pain is of cardiac origin (e.g., angina), the patient's history usually reveals that the pain is associated with exercise and is relieved by rest and nitrates. Patients with angina are often treated with medications (calcium channel blockers, beta-adrenergic blockers, nitrates) that decrease the LES pressure and produce a coexistent esophageal reflux, which complicates the differential diagnosis further.

Management

The principal aim of the management of GERD is to eliminate or reduce symptoms and to prevent the complications of esophageal stricture, esophageal ulcer, Barrett's esophagus, pulmonary aspiration, and esophageal hemorrhage. The focus of management is patient education, coupled with pharmacologic intervention in a stepped care approach. In addition to the stepped care approach, other medications that the patient may be taking for other conditions may need to be modified because many of them decrease LES pressure.

Step 1

Step 1 involves lifestyle modifications, including dietary modifications (a weight loss plan) if the patient is overweight; eating small frequent meals; avoiding foods that are known to cause heartburn, with the emphasis placed on the main meal of the day at midday; avoiding bedtime snacks; and eating no meal less than 4 hours before bedtime. The patient should be instructed to reduce caffeine intake slowly (to prevent withdrawal symptoms) and to eventually eliminate the intake of all caffeinated beverages, as well as eliminating any foods that reduce LES pressure or cause direct mucosal irritation. Other lifestyle changes include smoking cessation, avoiding tight belts or garments, and sleeping with the head of the bed elevated. These lifestyle modifications may be sufficient to control symptoms.

Step 1 also includes the use of antacids or OTC histamine-2-(H_2)-receptor blockers such as cimetidine (Tagamet), ranitidine (Zantac), or nizatidine (Axid) for the rapid relief of occasional symptoms when they occur. Gaviscon, an alginate-antacid combination, appears to be superior to plain antacids in the reduction of upright reflux. The measures in step 1 should be stressed to all patients regardless of the severity of the disease.

Step 2

Step 2 is prescribed for patients with more frequent, mild-to-moderate symptoms that do not respond well to step 1 treatment. It includes a trial of prescription H_2-receptor blockers or a proton pump inhibitor. These agents should not be used in combination, especially with older adults. The H_2-receptor antagonists (ranitidine, nizatidine, famotidine) should be taken at least twice a day, or cimetidine four times a day. H_2-receptor blockers are considerably less expensive than proton pump inhibitors and are effective in 66 percent of patients when used in conjunction with lifestyle modifications. Step 2 therapy should be continued for 8 to 12 weeks. For symptoms that persist, long-term continuous or intermittent therapy may be needed.

Step 3

Patients that have severe symptoms and have endoscopically documented erosive esophagitis or Barrett's esophagus are treated with proton pump inhibitors once a day such as omeprazole, rabeprazol, pantoprazole, or lansoprazole. An 8-week course of once a day treatment usually heals 80 percent of the cases, while twice a day dosing heals 95 percent of cases. Chronic maintenance therapy with proton pump inhibitors may be necessary for severe erosive esophagitis.

Step 4

Step 4 is reserved for the 5 to 20 percent of patients who do not respond to any of the above treatments; these patients are referred for surgical fundoplication (Nissen or Belsey fundoplication). Advances in technology have led to successful interventions using laproscopic techniques. Before surgical intervention, other causes of refractory GERD, such as gastrinoma, proton pump resistance, pill-induced esophagitis or patient noncompliance are investigated.

Treatment Standards/Guidelines 10.1 outlines the stepped approach to the treatment of GERD and includes medications, dose, and dosing schedule.

Follow-Up and Referral

GERD is a lifelong condition, and patients must be reevaluated on a regular basis to minimize the development of severe complications. Patients with mild-to-moderate symptoms should be instructed in the appropriate lifestyle modifications and treated with antacids or OTC H_2-receptor blockers for a period of about 4 weeks. If on the 4-week follow-up visit there is no improvement in the symptoms, then the patient can be advanced to step 2 treatment for 8 to 12 weeks. If this regimen is ineffective, the patient should be referred to a gastroenterologist. Patients who have self-medicated for a length of time may have developed erosive esophagitis or Barrett's esophagus and need aggressive treatment.

Treatment Standards/Guidelines 10.1
Stepped Treatment for GERD

Step 1	Trial for 4 weeks; if symptoms persist, move to Step 2 Dietary and Lifestyle Modifications Pharmacologic therapy: Antacids prn (Maalox TC or Mylanta-II 10–15 mL or 2–4 tablets, Gaviscon 2–4 tablets) OTC H_2-receptor antagonists prn (cimetidine 200 mg, ranitidine 75 mg, nizatidine 75 mg, famotidine 10 mg)
Step 2	Trial for 8–12 weeks; if symptoms persist, may refer to gastroenterologist or move to Step 3 Dietary and Lifestyle Modifications Pharmacologic therapy: H_2-receptor antagonists (cimetidine 400–800 mg bid, ranitidine 150 mg bid, nizatidine 150 mg bid, famotidine 20 mg bid) OR Proton Pump Inhibitors (omeprazole 20 mg, rabeprazole 20 mg, lansoprazole 30 mg, esomeprazole 20 mg, or pantoprazole 40 mg qd)
Step 3	Trial for 8–12 weeks; if symptoms persist, may choose Step 4. Dietary and Lifestyle Modifications Pharmacologic therapy: Proton pump/inhibitors (omeprazole 20–40 mg daily, lansoprazole 30 mg daily)
Step 4	Dietary and Lifestyle Modifications Surgical Intervention (Nissen fundoplication)

Patient Education

Education for patients with GERD includes instructing them on appropriate lifestyle modifications. Patients who are obese should be referred to a dietitian for counseling about weight loss. Dietary modifications are the keystone for lifestyle change; they include reducing the ingestion of foods that are irritating to the gastric mucosa and those that reduce LES pressure. Factors that increase intra-abdominal pressure should be avoided, such as large meals, tight or restrictive clothing, and bending or straining. It is most helpful for patients to eat small, frequent meals, with the main meal at midday. Eating less than 4 hours before bedtime, including snacks, should be avoided because this increases the chance of reflux. Patients should be instructed to sleep with the head of the bed elevated, which can be accomplished by placing blocks or bricks under the legs of the head of the bed.

Sleeping with more pillows does not have the same effect as raising the head of the bed. With the head elevated, gravity helps in preventing reflux at night, when the swallowing reflex is reduced. Patients should be given assistance in smoking cessation, but the use of supplemental nicotine should be avoided because it reduces LES pressure. Programs for stress management have not been found to be helpful in reducing the symptoms of GERD.

Gastroenteritis

Gastroenteritis, also known as enteritis or gastroenterocolitis, is defined as an inflammation of the stomach and intestine that manifests as anorexia, nausea, vomiting, and diarrhea. Gastroenteritis can be acute or chronic and can be caused by bacteria, viruses, parasites, injury to the bowel mucosa, inorganic poisons (sodium nitrate), organic poisons (mushrooms or shellfish), and drugs. Chronic causes include food allergies and intolerance, stress, and lactase deficiency. Gastroenteritis caused by bacterial toxins in food is often referred to as food poisoning; it should be suspected when groups of individuals present with the same symptoms.

The symptoms and subsequent electrolyte imbalances are usually self-limiting in the healthy adult but can have serious consequences for older adults and immunocompromised or pediatric patients. The severity of the illness is indicated by the presence of dehydration secondary to profuse watery diarrhea, fever greater than 101°F (38.3°C), vomiting, or dysentery (frequent small stools containing blood and mucus). A careful history and physical exam provides clues about the causative agent and the suspected vector of transmission. Travel, dining, and antibiotic history should be included as part of the assessment.

Epidemiology and Causes

Acute gastroenteritis results most often from an infectious agent. Although it is one of the most frequent diagnoses in primary-care practice (about 30 percent of patients seen each year), the exact number of individuals affected is not known, because acute gastroenteritis presents with a group of nonspecific symptoms that often go unreported or the etiology cannot be determined. Estimates are that the annual rate for gastroenteritis is approximately one episode per adult per year in the United States and Western Europe. Food- and water-borne outbreaks are of particular importance and gain the attention of the news media in an effort to identify and treat all the individuals who may have been exposed to the potentially harmful pathogen.

The most common mode of transmission for acute infectious gastroenteritis is the fecal–oral route from contaminated food or water. Person-to-person transfer of the disease is more common within the hospital setting and within daycare centers where there are larger groups of people capable of transmitting the disease. Groups considered at high risk for developing gastroenteritis include anyone traveling to a developing country, immunocompromised patients, anyone engaging in anal intercourse, residents of institutions or nursing homes, infants and children attending daycare centers, and individuals consuming raw shellfish and seafood.

Bacterial pathogens account for 30 to 80 percent of acute gastroenteritis cases and are an important cause of morbidity in tropical areas and in travelers to areas of high risk for the pathogens (traveler's diarrhea). Areas considered high risk for developing traveler's diarrhea include Mexico, Africa, Southeast Asia, and developing countries in the Middle East or Latin America. Table 10.8 presents the most common bacterial, viral, and parasitic causes of gastroenteritis.

Gastroenteritis can also be caused by dietary factors such as coffee, tea, and sodas containing caffeine, medications (primarily antacids and antibiotics), and metabolic factors, including diabetes mellitus, hyperthyroidism, and adrenal insufficiency.

Pathophysiology

Pathophysiological causes of gastroenteritis are numerous; however, bacterial, viral, and parasitic infections are among the most common. Almost all forms of enteric infection manifest with diarrhea. Diarrheal diseases cause an increase in the frequency of stools, less well formed feces, and an increase in the fecal water content. The definition of diarrhea is dependent on each patient's normal bowel habits. Diarrhea is not considered a medical emergency unless it affects children or older adults who are less able to regulate their fluid intake. Diarrhea is a major cause of infant mortality in developing nations.

The GI tract has several defenses against the development of infection. When bacterial or viral pathogens can overcome these barriers, they proliferate, causing varying degrees of gastroenteritis. The acidity of the stomach is normally maintained at a pH of 2, which creates a hostile environment for most microorganisms. This acidic barrier protects the small bowel and colon from ingested pathogens. If the organism is resistant to the acid environment or the patient has taken medications that alter the pH, the organism may thrive and cause illness.

Another host defense mechanism is the constant peristalsis of the small bowel, which prevents the colonization of pathogens within the lumen. Patients who have small bowel stasis as a result of obstruction, diverticuli, or blind loop syndrome frequently develop an overgrowth of bacteria within the stagnant segment, causing gastroenteritis resulting from the increased number of bacteria in the small bowel. In contrast, the colon is relatively stagnant; it typically harbors about 1 billion bacteria per gram of intestinal contents. The normal stool is primarily composed of water

(text continued on page 504)

Table 10.8 Organisms Causing Gastroenteritis

Pathogen	Pathogenesis	Duration/Onset	Clinical Findings	Diagnosis and Treatment
Bacterial Pathogens:				
Bacillus cereus	Type of food poisoning from formation of enterotoxins within food or gut; two forms, differing in duration of illness	Duration is normally less than 24 h. Onset is within 1–8 h after exposure.	Illness begins with vomiting and proceeds to diarrhea; no fever. Commonly occurs in rice dishes; the spores are heat resistant and not affected by cooking.	No antibiotic treatment is required; oral hydration and supportive care
Campylobacter jejuni	Primarily found in eggs and poultry but may be found in domestic animals. Organism invades the intestinal mucosa and produces a cholera-like toxin. Organism grows within ileum and jejunum.	Duration of illness is from 2–6 days. Onset of symptoms approximately 48 h after ingestion of pathogen.	Common cause of traveler's diarrhea from ingestion of contaminated water. Symptoms include fever, bloody diarrhea, and abdominal pain. Stool is positive for polymorphonuclear neutophil (PMNs).	Normally self-limiting. Erythromycin ethylsuccinate (EES) can be used in severe cases. Rapid antibiotic resistance is common. Stool culture requires special media. Quinoline antibiotics have been effective in increasing recovery.
Clostridium botulinum	Anaerobic gram-positive bacillus that produces seven distinct toxins. In the food-borne type the toxin is ingested with contaminated food. Once absorbed, the toxin blocks the release of acetylcholine from peripheral nerve endings. Canned foods are the primary source.	Duration of illness depends on diagnosis and treatment. Mortality is high. Onset is abrupt, although incubation can be as long as 4–8 days.	GI symptoms often precede neurological findings, which are bilateral, symmetrical, and occur in a descending fashion. Initial neurological symptoms include dry mouth, diplopia, and loss of pupillary reflex. Dysphagia and dysarthria can lead to aspiration pneumonia. Progression of neurological insult leads to paralysis of the diaphragm and death if mechanical ventilation is not employed.	Diagnosis is made by isolation of organism in suspected food, the serum, or feces. Symptoms are often confused with Guillain-Barré. Treatment is to first eliminate any unabsorbed food (toxin) by inducing vomiting or by gastric lavage, then administration of trivalent antitoxin (A, B, or E) from the Center for Disease Control and Prevention (CDC). The antitoxin does not reverse the existing neurological symptoms but prevents progression. Little benefit if given after 72 h. Toxin may cause serum sickness or anaphylaxis. Mechanical ventilation must be considered in an emergency.

(continued)

Table 10.8 **Organisms Causing Gastroenteritis** (continued)

Pathogen	Pathogenesis	Duration/Onset	Clinical Findings	Diagnosis and Treatment
Clostridium difficile	Gram-positive anaerobe maintained in spore from. It colonizes bowel when normal bowel flora are suppressed by antibiotics. It produces two toxins; toxin A, an enterotoxin, and toxin B, a cytotoxin causing pseudomembranous colitis and necrosis.	Duration and intensity of disease varies. Onset normally is in a hospitalized patient who has had recent antibiotic treatment.	Symptoms range from none to acute abdomen secondary to toxic megacolon with perforation; symptoms usually begin after initiation of antibiotics. Profuse, watery, or mucoid diarrhea, which may be blood tinged, accompanied by fever, abdominal cramping and distension, WBCs greater than 20,000, and ascites. Metabolic acidosis indicates severe colitis or toxic megacolon. Common cause of nosocomial infections in hospitals.	Diagnosis is confirmed with isolation of toxin A or B in the stool. Culture alone is no longer diagnostic because of the number of patients who are asymptomatic carriers. Flexible sigmoidoscopy may reveal pseudomembranous colitis. It is associated with recent abdominal surgery. It is treated with oral metronidazole (Flagyl) 250 mg qid for 10 days, vancomycin (Vancocin) 125 mg qid for 10 days. Relapse (20%) is treated with second course of above. Patients with multiple relapses may require 30 days of antibotic treatment. Avoid antimotility agents.
Clostridium perfringes	Found in soil, feces, air, water. Outbreaks caused most often by contaminated meat. Type A enterotoxin causes mild to moderate gastroenteritis. Type C enterotoxin can be fatal.	Duration of illness is similar to mild gastritis lasting 1–4 days without medical intervention. Fatal cases are less common. Onset is usually within 12 h of ingestion of contaminated food.	Abrupt onset of diarrhea without fever. If fatal, cases have severe diarrhea with abdominal pain and distension.	Diagnosis is made by isolating organism in food or feces. Cultures usually show many clostridia in food or feces. No treatment is necessary for mild forms other than supportive care. Penicillin may be useful in severe cases.
Escherichia coli (E. coli)	Five identified strains classified by pathogenesis of diarrhea. All are gram-negative rods.	Dependent on strain; epidemics are due to ingestion of contaminated meat or dairy products.		

Pathogen	Pathogenesis	Duration/Onset	Clinical Findings	Diagnosis and Treatment
(*E. coli*) *(Continued)*	Enterohemorrhagic *E. coli* (EHEC). Most serious; produces a hemorrhagic infection; 0157:H7 strain produces two toxins, which inhibit protein synthesis in intestinal cells.	Duration typically 1–8 days. Onset is 24 h after ingestion of contaminated food.	Acute onset of dysentery with 12–24 h of abdominal cramps, watery diarrhea, and fever is followed by bloody stools. Can cause hemorrhagic infection of colon and can be fatal. Complications include hemolytic-uremic syndrome (HUS) or thrombolytic thrombocytopenic purpura (TTP). WBCs are greater than 20,000; azotemia; dehydration. Infants and older adults are most prone to adverse effects.	Diagnosis is by isolation of *E. coli* 0157:H7 in stools. Look for the source of undercooked meat. It can be transmitted in feces and dirty diapers. Treatment is supportive. Antibiotics have not proved effective.
	Enterotoxigenic *E. coli* (ETEC). Adheres to the mucosa of small bowel releasing toxins, which cause diarrhea.	Duration 2–4 days. Incubation period is 24–36 h.	Most common cause of traveler's diarrhea from contaminated food or water. Mild fever, abdominal cramps, watery stool, nausea, and vomiting are common.	Usually self-limiting, requiring no treatment other than supportive care. It is common in developing countries.
	Enteropathogenic *E. coli* (EPEC)	Duration is 1–3 days; 12–36 hour incubation period.	Profuse, watery, foul-smelling diarrhea. It is of special concern to infants and older adults who are prone to dehydration.	Usually self-limiting. Infants and older adults may require hospitalization. It is rare in the United States.
	Enteroinvasive *E. coli* (EIEC) causes invasion and proliferation within enterocytes, much like *Shigella* infection.	Duration is 4–10 days; 12– to 72-hour incubation period.	It is an uncommon cause of food-borne dysentery in the United States. Patients have fever, anorexia, cramps, and watery diarrhea. Stools may be mucoid or bloody. Clinical presentation is much like that of *Shigella* infection.	May isolate leukocytes in stool. Diarrhea is self-limiting. Food poisoning of this kind is rare in the United States.
	Enteroadherent *E. coli* (EAEC) is rare and adheres to liver cells.		Mild, nonbloody diarrhea; strain is uncommon.	No leukocytes in stool.

(continued)

Table 10.8 **Organisms Causing Gastroenteritis** (continued)

Pathogen	Pathogenesis	Duration/Onset	Clinical Findings	Diagnosis and Treatment
Vibrio cholerae	Commonly found in areas with poor sanitation; food and water contaminated with feces. Enterotoxin causes hypersecretion in small intestine. Rarely found in the United States but may be endemic along the Gulf Coast.	Incubation is 1–3 days. Duration is 1–2 weeks.	Most cases in the United States are hemolytic and are transported here from contaminated foods. Diarrhea can be severe, causing septicemia, especially in immunocompromised patients, children, or older adults. Diarrhea is profuse, "rice water" and can be life threatening. There is no abdominal cramping or fever. Patients may stool at the rate of 1 L/h.	To diagnose *V. cholerae* a special *Vibrio*-selective medium must be used in the stool culture. Diarrhea requires prompt replacement of fluids and electrolytes. Antibiotic: tetracycline 500 mg PO q6h for 2 days or Bactrim DS q12h for 2 days.
Vibrio parahaemolyticus	Pathogen found in seafood. Produces toxins in the gut or invades intestinal mucosa. Outbreaks frequent in summer; usually associated with improperly cooked seafood.	Incubation period 8–24 h. Duration is 1–3 days.	Patient presents with abdominal cramping, headache, fever. Usually associated with explosive, noninflammatory, watery diarrhea, which may be bloody depending on the degree of mucosal destruction.	Stool is positive for *Vibrio*. Often diagnosed when a group of people become sick after consuming seafood. Food cultures are positive.
Yersinia enterocolitica	Primarily transmitted via fecal-oral route; food borne. It is rare in the United States; more common in northern Europe and Canada. Organism forms an enterotoxin and invades the intestinal epithelium.	Onset and incubation are unknown. Duration usually resolves in 1–3 weeks.	Symptoms include fever, abdominal pain, and bloody diarrhea. Older children may develop mesenteric adenitis, which presents with fever, right lower quadrant pain, and leukocytosis; similar to symptoms of appendicitis. Adults may present with polyarthritis, Reiter's syndrome, and erythema nodosum. *Yersinia* can cause bacteremia.	Diagnosis is made by isolation of organism in the stool. Stool also tests positive for fecal leukocytes. Treatment for severe cases is tetracycline 250–500 mg q6h for 7–10 days; ciprofloxin 500 mg PO bid; Tobramycin 3–5 mg/kg/day q8h.

Pathogen	Pathogenesis	Duration/Onset	Clinical Findings	Diagnosis and Treatment
Salmonella	One of the major causes of diarrhea worldwide. 3 species: *S. typhi, S. choleraesuis, and S. enteritidis.* Primarily found in chicken, eggs, and livestock, causing 85% of community-acquired *Salmonella* outbreaks. Individuals must ingest 10,000–1 million organisms to become infected.	Duration is 2–5 days; onset is 8–48 hours after ingestion. Patients may become "chronic carriers," defined as individuals with positive stool cultures 1 year after initial disease.	Peak incidence is in summer and fall. Symptoms begin with nausea and vomiting, followed by colicky abdominal pain and bloody or mucoid diarrhea. Enteric fever results from organisms entering the bloodstream via the bowel lymphatics, causing bacteremia, headache, and myalgias. Tissue abscesses may develop. Stools may be foul smelling.	Diagnosis is made by isolation of organism in stool. No treatment is necessary unless associated with fever and systemic disease. Treatment includes trimethoprim-sulfamethoxazole (Bactrim DS) or a quinoline, Norfloxin 400 mg or Ofloxin 400 mg PO bid for 7–10 days. Stress proper handling of food, thorough cooking, and good hand washing.
Shigella	One of the most common causes of bacillary dysentery. Several species: *S. sonnei* is isolated in 75% or cases in United States. Because of poor hygiene and overcrowding, it is spread via fecal-oral route and requires only a small number of organisms to produce disease. Organism causes epithelial invasion of intestinal mucosa.	Duration usually 4–7 days and is self-limiting. Incubation period of 1–2 days after exposure or ingestion of pathogen.	Initially patients present with watery diarrhea and high fever. Later colitis-type symptoms develop: abdominal cramps, tenesmus, urgency, frequent small stools with blood and mucus. Low-grade fever may persist for 2–20 days. Complications can include hemolytic-uremic syndrome (HUS) and colitis.	Diagnosis is made by isolation of organism in stool or rectal swab. In severe cases sigmoidoscopy shows mucosal hyperemia, friability, and ulceration. Treat with Bactrim DS bid for 3 days if infection was acquired in the United States.
Staphylococcus	Common cause of food poisoning. Caused by ingestion of enterotoxin found in improperly handled or stored foods. Enterotoxins produced by *Staphylococcus* act on receptors in the gut, which then transmit impulses to medullary centers.	Abrupt onset 1–8 h after ingestion of contaminated food. Duration is usually less than 24 hours.	Abrupt onset of nausea, vomiting, colicky abdominal cramps, profuse watery diarrhea.	Definitive diagnosis is made only if contaminated food source is tested; otherwise, diagnosis is made based on short incubation and duration of symptoms.

(continued)

Table 10.8 **Organisms Causing Gastroenteritis** (continued)

Pathogen	Pathogenesis	Duration/Onset	Clinical Findings	Diagnosis and Treatment
Entamoeba histolytica (amebiasis)	Transmitted via contaminated food and water, primarily in tropical areas with poor sanitation. Common in Mexican migrant workers and military personnel returning from the Far East. Human host becomes a reservoir after ingesting cysts from source and can transmit disease via fecal-oral route. Venereal transmission is common in the male homosexual population.	Most common clinical variant is the asymptomatic cyst carrier who can be a reservoir for an undertermined length of time. Duration can be weeks to months.	Symptoms include abdominal cramps, abdominal pain and weight loss. Diarrhea contains blood and mucus. Patients may have hepatomegaly and pain over the cecum and ascending colon. Some patients may have fever, tenesmus, and acute dysentery illness. Complications can include peritonitis, toxic megacolon, and hepatic abscess. The encysted ameba is passed into the environment, where it can survive for up to 10 days.	Diagnosis is important to distinguish amebiasis from ulcerative colitis because treatment with glucocorticoids can accelerate amebic colitis and enhance systemic invasion. Sigmoidoscopy reveals discrete rectosigmoid ulcers with normal intervening mucosa. Indirect hemagglutination test is effective in detecting invasive amebic disease but remains positive long after treatment. Treat with metronidazole (Flagyl) 750 mg tid for 7–10 days.
Cryptosporidium	Enteric protozoan parasite that invades the small bowel located just below the basement membrane. Causes two distinct syndromes—one in immunocompetent and one in immunosuppressed individuals. Common cause of water-borne outbreaks from inadequate filtration. Parasite products an exotoxin.	Incubation is 1–3 weeks. Usually self-limiting but can last 1–2 weeks in immunocompromised patients.	Outbreaks can occur after ingestion of water contaminated with livestock waste. Also common in day-care centers and patients with AIDS. Immunocompromised patients develop severe cholera-like diarrhea, which can last for months and cause daily fluid losses of 5–10 L/day.	Diagnosis by isolation of parasite in stool. Commercially available immunofluorescent antibody test can also assist diagnosis. Leukocytes not present in stool. Intestinal mucosa not inflamed but with ulcerations. Suggested treatment includes paromomycin (Humatin) 500 mg PO qid with food for 14–28 days, then 500 mg bid indefinitely. If treatment fails, then azithromycin (Zithromax) 2.4 g PO on day 1, 1.2 g PO for 27 days, and then 600 mg/day for maintenance indefinitely.

Pathogen	Pathogenesis	Duration/Onset	Clinical Findings	Diagnosis and Treatment
Viral Pathogens:				
Rotavirus	Very common cause of gastroenteritis in industrialized areas. Organism most often implicated in deaths from diarrhea. Frequently involves small bowel. A disaccharidase deficiency is common after rotavirus infections. Rotavirus is an RNA virus with four antigenic serotypes.	Incubation period 24–36 h. Duration is 4–6 days.	Common in children under age 3. Peak incidence at age 6–24 months. Uncommon in adults because most have developed immunity. Symptoms include low-grade fever and copious watery diarrhea. Outbreaks are more common in winter months.	Diagnosis is made by electron microscopy. Serologic enzyme-linked immunosorbent assays (ELISA) tests are available. No leukocytes found in stool.
Norwalk virus	Cube-shaped virus with seven known antigenic variants. It can cause large epidemics spread by contaminated water. It is transmitted by the fecal-oral route. It is a common cause of absenteeism due to "viral gastroenteritis."	Incubation is 18–48 h. Duration is 48–72 h	Illness can be very debilitating to some patients. Symptoms are mild and brief and include vomiting, frequent watery diarrhea, diffuse myalgias, chills, and sometimes fever. Often causes family outbreaks.	No known antiviral therapy is available. Fluid and electrolyte replacement is the treatment of choice. Virus can be isolated with electron microscopy but is costly and the disease is self-limiting.
Protozoal Pathogens:				
Giardia lamblia	Approximately 4% of healthy United States citizens harbor *G. lamblia* in their intestines and are asymptomatic. *G. lamblia* is a protozoa that attaches to the mucosa of the small bowel. Patients with hypogammaglobulinemia and achlorhydria are predisposed to giardiasis. It is transmitted via oral-anal intercourse and is a common cause of traveler's diarrhea and diarrhea in children who attend day-care centers.	Incubation is 1–4 weeks. Duration usually 1–6 weeks.	Symptoms range from nonspecific complaints of bloating, flatulence, nausea, and watery, noninflammatory diarrhea to chronic diarrhea with weight loss, anorexia, and malabsorption.	Diagnosis can be made by examination of stool but is most often made by duodenal aspirate or small bowel biopsy. Stool exam is positive for trophozoites in about 50% of confirmed cases. Treatment with quinacrine hydrochloride (Atabrine) 100 mg tid after meals for 5–7 days or metronidazole (Flagyl) 250 mg tid for 5–7 days.

and bacteria. These beneficial bacteria protect against potential pathogens by consuming available nutrients and by producing by-products that create a hostile environment to the invading pathogens.

The GI tract also produces specific immunoglobulins that protect against invading organisms. Following exposure to certain organisms, immunoglobulins may even protect against future invasions by the same organism, much like an antigen–antibody response. IgA, a secretory immunoglobulin, may help defend against many of the bacteria that cause gastroenteritis by invading the intestinal mucosa.

Ingestion of contaminated food can result in clinical symptoms of gastroenteritis, but this depends on the number and virulence of the organisms in the food. Almost all bacteria are capable of producing mild diarrhea if ingested in large enough quantities. Other organisms (e.g., *Shigella, Salmonella, Campylobacter, Cryptosporidium*) have such a high virulence that only a small inoculum can produce symptoms.

Often, the incubation time of the pathogen, coupled with the presenting symptoms, will give specific clues for establishing a diagnosis. Infectious processes of the small intestine often result in watery, secretory, or a malabsorptive type of diarrhea; whereas infections of the large intestine tend to produce bloody diarrhea and abdominal pain. Gastroenteritis with an onset of nausea and vomiting within 6 hours after exposure to the pathogen suggests food poisoning resulting from the ingestion of a preformed toxin such as that of *Bacillus cereus.* Incubation periods greater than 14 hours and the initial symptom of vomiting are highly suggestive of viral infections.

Clinical Presentation

Subjective

Patients with gastroenteritis present with varying degrees of nausea, vomiting, diarrhea, fever, and abdominal pain and cramping. Symptoms depend on the underlying cause, but can also include fatigue, malaise, anorexia, tenesmus, and borborygmus. Individuals with profuse diarrhea may complain of rectal burning and hematochezia from rectal abrasion and bleeding. Patients may complain of symptoms that suggest dysentery, including passage of numerous small-volume stools containing blood and mucus. Reports of voluminous stools are suggestive of a source in the small bowel or proximal colon, whereas small stools accompanied by a sense of urgency suggest a source in the left colon or rectum. Bloody stools suggest mucosal damage and an inflammatory process secondary to invasive pathogens. Frothy stools and flatus suggest a malabsorption problem.

Objective

The physical exam is usually normal except for the aforementioned GI problems. Depending on the degree of dehydration, the skin turgor may be poor and mucous membranes may be dry. Vital signs may reflect dehydration, such as a fever with an increase in temperature and heart rate. Older and very young patients with gastroenteritis may show signs of severe dehydration such as orthostatic hypotension and dizziness. Patients who have had prolonged illness and are malnourished may present with edema resulting from hypoalbuminemia.

Diagnostic Reasoning

Diagnostic Tests

Evaluation of the history is of vital importance to the appropriate diagnosis and management of the patient with gastroenteritis. The patient must be questioned thoroughly about the temporal association of symptoms with the suspected pathogen. Patient history should include a thorough drug history, including OTC drugs, antibiotics, antacids, laxatives, alcohol, and sugar substitutes. It is important to know the patient's travel history, surgical history, and sexual orientation and practices. The duration of the illness is important in the differential diagnosis, because acute diarrhea is usually caused by infectious agents or toxins, whereas chronic diarrhea usually has a noninfectious etiology.

Laboratory diagnosis of acute gastroenteritis is not always necessary in patients with nonbloody diarrhea and no evidence of systemic toxicity. In the average, otherwise healthy adult, the disease will normally run its course without incident and there is no need for costly evaluation. Selection of the most appropriate tests is based on information received from the history and physical exam. Patients with severe diarrhea and dehydration should have stool examination for consistency, blood, and fecal leukocytes. Numerous fecal leukocytes in patients with acute diarrhea is indicative of diffuse colonic inflammation and is highly suggestive of an invasive pathogen such as *Shigella, Salmonella,* or *Campylobacter.* Other causes of leukocyte-positive stools include *Clostridium difficile, Yersinia, Vibrio parahaemolyticus,* and *Escherichia coli.* In patients with chronic diarrhea, fecal leukocytes suggest IBD or ischemia.

A stool culture should be done on any patient that has severe diarrhea, a fever of 101.3°F (38.5°C) or higher, the presence of bloody stools, or stools that test positive for leukocytes, lactoferrin, or occult blood, because these findings are indications of a bacterial pathogen. Routine stool culture will identify the presence of *Shigella, Salmonella, Campylobacter, Aeromonas,* and *Yersinia.* In diarrheal illnesses that are suspected to be caused by eating contaminated hamburger meat, stools can be cultured for *E. coli.*

Blood cultures should be obtained from patients who show clinical signs of typhoid or enteric fever or from any hospitalized patient who has an intestinal illness with high fever. It is essential that the blood cultures be obtained before initiation of antibiotic therapy.

Stools should be examined for ova and parasites in cases of persistent diarrhea, especially if the symptoms began after travel to Russia, Nepal, the Rocky Mountains, or other mountainous regions, or after exposure to infants in a daycare center. Parasites should also be considered in homosexual males or any patient with AIDS who presents with diarrhea, as well as in a patient with diarrhea who lives in a community where a water-borne outbreak has occurred. If a patient has diarrhea that has lasted longer than 2 weeks and the stool is negative for fecal leukocytes, a stool exam for parasites should be considered. Patients with intestinal amebiasis usually have no leukocytes in their stool, because of the noninflamed areas of intestinal mucosa between the areas of ulceration as well as the lytic effects of the exotoxins produced by the parasite. If parasitic infection is highly suspected but the stool culture is negative, a small bowel biopsy is indicated to identify the causative agent. Immunofluorescent antibody tests and diagnostic enzyme-linked immunosorbent assay (ELISA) tests are more sensitive than microscopic studies for identifying *Giardia* and *Cryptosporidium.*

In patients with epidemiological evidence, stool samples should be sent to the laboratory for specific enteropathogen studies that are not normally detected with routine stool culture, such as enterohemorrhagic colitis (*E. coli* 0157:H7), *Vibrio cholerae,* other noncholera vibrios and other Shigatoxin-producing *E. coli.* Routine stool culture identifies certain strains of *Yersinia* and *E. coli* 0157:H7; however, some strains can be detected only by research laboratories. Any patient who develops diarrhea after initiation or completion of antibiotic therapy should have tissue culture assay or an ELISA test for *C. difficile* toxin.

Viral gastroenteritis should be suspected in patients who present with vomiting as the major symptom and in cases where food- or water-borne contamination is suspected and the incubation period is greater than 12 hours. Although there are commercially available test kits that identify rotaviruses, their application is limited because there is no known treatment for viral causes of illness.

Flexible sigmoidoscopy is usually reserved for patients with colitis that is unresponsive to antibiotic therapy and for patients with persistent diarrhea undiagnosed by lab oratory evaluation. Tissue biopsy can help identify the offending pathogen as well as differentiate infection from chronic inflammatory changes consistent with inflammatory bowel diseases or celiac disease.

Differential Diagnosis

The differential diagnosis of gastroenteritis, particularly in patients with persistent or chronic diarrhea and severe abdominal pain, should include IBS, IBD, ischemic bowel disease (especially in patients with peripheral vascular disease), partial bowel obstruction, and pelvic abscess. Other considerations for diagnosis should include ruling out complications from diabetes mellitus, small bowel diverticulosis, Whipple's disease, chronic pancreatitis, and any surgical alteration of the GI tract that might interfere with normal absorption.

Management

All patients who present with diarrhea require fluid and electrolyte management, particularly children, older adults, and immunosuppressed patients. Patients who are dehydrated and able to tolerate oral fluid replacement should be instructed to drink fluids with a sodium content of 45 to 75 mEq/L (Pedialyte or Gatorade) or be provided with oral rehydration salts. In patients who are severely dehydrated, or those who have chronic diseases and are hypotensive, hospitalization for intravenous hydration may be indicated. In otherwise healthy adult patients who are not dehydrated, sports drinks, diluted fruit juices, and broths or soups are usually adequate for fluid and sodium replacement.

Patients with diarrhea require a diet that includes calories that come from boiled starches and cereals (potatoes, pasta, rice, wheat, and oats), which will facilitate enterocyte renewal, with the addition of salt for the duration of illness. Once stools have started to become formed, the diet can be advanced as tolerated. Some authors advise avoiding dairy products; however, this is not necessary unless there is clinical evidence of lactose intolerance.

Nonspecific symptomatic treatment of acute diarrhea can decrease the occurrence by 50 percent and is most effective against secretory diarrhea. Antimotility drugs are the most frequently prescribed and most effective drugs for the treatment of symptomatic gastroenteritis. These agents work by slowing intraluminal peristalsis, thereby slowing the passage of fluids through the lumen, which facilitates absorption. Patients with febrile dysentery should not receive antimotility medications because slowing the intraluminal time may prolong the duration of the disease. Drugs Commonly Prescribed 10.1 lists medications commonly recommended for the symptomatic treatment of acute diarrhea.

Empirical antimicrobial therapy is recommended for patients with severe diarrhea, especially those with fever or stool positive for leukocytes. Traveler's diarrhea is treated empirically with trimethoprim-sulfamethoxazole (Bactrim DS), one double-strength tablet bid for 3 days. Other antibiotics that are effective for milder forms of illness include a single dose of ciprofloxacin (Cipro) 500 mg, norfloxacin (Noroxin) 400 mg, or ofloxacin (Floxin) 300 mg. Antibiotic prophylaxis, which has a 90 percent effectiveness rate, for people traveling in high-risk areas, includes the antibiotics mentioned above in daily doses continuing for 2 days after returning home. Nonantibiotic preventive therapy includes bismuth subsalicylate (Pepto-Bismol), two tablets before each meal and at bedtime for a total of eight tablets/day for the entire trip. This remedy has an approximate 60 percent effectiveness rate.

Follow-Up and Referral

Follow-up is not usually required except in those patients suffering from the chronic forms of infectious diarrhea such as from *C. difficile.* Often, patients with serious infectious diarrhea will require home administration of intravenous

Drugs Commonly Prescribed 10.1: Symptomatic Treatment of Acute Diarrhea

Drug	Indication	Dosage	Comments
Bismuth subsalicylate (Pepto-Bismol)	Acute diarrhea	30 ml or two tablets every 30 minutes for eight doses May repeat same regimen on day 2.	Not as effective as loperamide in acute diarrhea. Do not use with antibiotics in patients with HIV infection.
Loperamide (Imodium)	Acute diarrhea	Initial dose (OTC) 4 mg (2 tablets), then 2 mg after each loose stool, not to exceed 8 mg/day. Prescription dose should not exceed 16 mg/day for a 2-day limit.	Drug of choice for afebrile, nondysenteric cases of acute diarrhea. Minimal central opiate effect.
Diphenoxylate with atropine (Lomotil)	Acute diarrhea	Two tablets (4 mg) qid for 2 days	Prescription only. For use in afebrile, nondysentery cases of acute diarrhea. Has central opiate effects. Overdose possible. Atropine has adverse effects that may limit its use.

antibiotics. Patients who require sigmoidoscopy for biopsy of intestinal mucosa for identification of the pathogen should be referred to a gastroenterologist.

Patient Education

The aim of patient education is prevention of the spread of disease from patients with infectious diarrhea to other individuals. Teaching includes good hand washing and safe disposal of waste products. Any infant or child with infectious diarrhea should not attend daycare until the diarrhea has stopped or the child has completed the prescribed course of antibiotics. Good hand-washing technique is imperative to prevent household outbreaks of the disease.

Patients traveling in high-risk areas should be instructed to consume only safe foods and beverages there and on the airplane leaving the area. "Safe" foods include acidic foods such as unpeeled citrus fruits; dry foods such as breads and cereals; steamed foods and beverages such as coffee, tea, and vegetables; foods containing high amounts of sugar such as syrups, jellies, and jams; and bottled carbonated drinks such as soda and beer. It is generally not considered safe to drink bottled water (unless bottled from a safe source) or to eat raw uncooked vegetables, including salad. Patients with known HIV infection and any other individual with a known debilitating illness who may not tolerate any degree of gastroenteritis should be encouraged to take antibiotic prophylaxis.

Peptic Ulcer Disease

Peptic ulcer disease (PUD) is a generic name for both gastric ulcers and duodenal ulcers. A peptic ulcer is a break in the surface mucosa of the stomach or duodenum, which results when there is disruption of the normal mucosal defenses and the tissue is exposed to the damaging effects of acid and pepsin. By definition, a peptic ulcer penetrates the muscularis mucosa and is usually larger than 5 mm in diameter. The initial damage to the mucosa is usually a result of infection by *H. pylori* or medications, particularly NSAIDs.

Epidemiology and Causes

A person's lifetime risk of developing a peptic ulcer is from 5 to 10 percent. Approximately 500,000 new cases are diagnosed each year in the United States. Men and women are almost equally affected by peptic ulcers, with the incidence in men slightly more. Most duodenal ulcers occur in patients between age 30 and 55, but gastric ulcers are more prevalent between age 55 and 70.

A variety of conditions are considered to be risk factors for the development of PUD, but the three major causes are infection with *H. pylori,* chronic ingestion of aspirin and other NSAIDs, and acid hypersecretion such as in Zollinger-Ellison syndrome. Genetics, blood type, personality type, and cigarette smoking may also play a role in the development of PUD. Patients with chronic obstructive pulmonary disease (COPD), cirrhosis, renal failure, and renal transplant have a higher incidence of PUD than the general public, but the mechanism is not known. Dietary factors such as caffeine, alcohol, and spicy foods are no longer considered to be ulcerogenic.

Pathophysiology

Almost all patients with gastric ulcers have normal or subnormal amounts of gastric acid secretion. Only about 35 percent of patients with duodenal ulcers have demonstrated above-average rates of acid secretion, usually as a result of gastrin hypersecretion with hypergastrinemia, elevated histamine production, and increased neuronal release of acetylcholine from vagal hyperfunction. The breakdown of the local mucosal defenses appears to play a larger role in the pathogenesis of ulcer formation. Mucosal defense is supported by surface mucus and bicarbonate, which form a thin alkaline gel coating mucosal cells, and by prostaglandin-enhanced mucosal blood flow and cell renewal.

A variety of factors can affect the development of ulcers. Cigarette smoking increases ulcer formation, which is proportional to the amount smoked. The mechanism by which cigarette smoking causes ulcer formation is unclear. Aspirin and other NSAIDs decrease the mucosal defense mechanisms by inhibiting prostaglandin synthesis, leaving the area vulnerable to the effects of gastric hydrochloric acid and pepsin. Many infectious agents have been detected in patients with ulcer disease, but *H. pylori* is the most important. As many as 75 percent of patients with duodenal ulcers are infected with *H. pylori,* and the bacterium is present in the majority of gastric ulcer patients, although the association with gastric ulcers is less. Not everyone with *H. pylori* infection, however, develops PUD.

Clinical Presentation

Subjective

The hallmark of PUD is a complaint of a burning or gnawing (hunger) sensation or pain (dyspepsia) in the epigastrium, which is often relieved by food or antacids. These complaints, however, are not specific or sensitive enough to be diagnostic of ulcer disease. Patients with PUD usually describe an episodic pattern of complaints in which the pain tends to cluster and last for minutes, with the episodes separated by periods of no symptoms. It is this alternating pattern that is more predictive of ulcer disease than the nature of the symptoms themselves. Almost half the patients with NSAID-induced ulcers are asymptomatic, however, and 60 percent of patients with complications have no history of prior symptoms.

Nocturnal pain is present in two-thirds of patients with duodenal ulcers and one-third of those with gastric ulcers. Nausea and anorexia sometimes occur in patients with gastric ulcer, whereas vomiting and weight loss are indications of more serious complications such as gastric malignancy or pyloric obstruction. Patients with duodenal ulcers may report a reduction in pain after eating; patients with gastric ulcers tend to experience more intense pain after eating, which is a result of secretion of gastric acids.

Objective

The physical examination is not useful in differentiating PUD from other types of upper GI disorders. Patients with duodenal ulcers often demonstrate an epigastric tenderness 2.5 cm to the right of the midline, but this may also be present with cholecystitis, pancreatitis, nonulcer dyspepsia, and other GI disorders. Reports of melena or coffee-ground-like emesis usually indicate a bleeding ulcer, and a perforated ulcer may present with abdominal rigidity.

Diagnostic Reasoning

Diagnostic Tests

Most routine laboratory tests are normal in patients with ulcer disease unless there is significant bleeding or vomiting, wherein the results show anemia, fluid, and electrolyte disturbances. The diagnostic standard for PUD is upper GI endoscopy. It is much more accurate in diagnosing ulcer disease than the previously used upper GI radiographic series. Endoscopy also does not involve exposure to radiation, which is a concern, particularly in pregnant patients.

Research has implicated *H. pylori* gastritis in 90 to 95 percent of both duodenal and gastric ulcers that are not associated with NSAIDs. A simple serology test for *H. pylori* can be done. *H. pylori* can also be diagnosed by direct bacteriologic analysis by an esophagogastroduodenoscopy (EGD) biopsy. EGD is an expensive, invasive procedure with possible complications; therefore, it is ordered for examination of individuals who have failed the standard triple drug therapy for *H. pylori* (see p 509) or for those who require direct visualization of the gastric mucosa for acute bleeding. There are a number of other ways to diagnose *H. pylori.* A serologic antibody (ELISA) test can be used to detect infection with *H. pylori,* but the test does not distinguish between active or past (treated) infection, and is expensive. Urease is plentiful in patients with *H. pylori* infection. Breath tests for *H. pylori* are based on the production of ammonia from the metabolism of urea by urase. These breath tests indicate active infection and are a noninvasive way of diagnosing *H. pylori* infection, although negative tests have a poor predictive value because false-negative results are more likely than truly negative findings.

In patients for whom an increase in gastric acid secretion is suspected, a fasting serum gastrin level should be drawn. Levels higher than 200 pg/mL should be confirmed on repeat testing and followed by basal and peak acid-output measurements. Zollinger-Ellison syndrome should be suspected in patients whose fasting serum gastrin level is above 600 pg/mL and who have a basal acid output of more than 15 mmol/h.

Differential Diagnosis

PUD must be distinguished from other causes of epigastric distress, which can be problematic because a variety of thoracic and upper abdominal disorders can cause similar pain. Diseases to be considered in the differential diagnosis should include nonulcer dyspepsia, cholecystitis, pancreatitis, IBS, GERD, gastric cancer, myocardial ischemia, gastritis, and gastroenteritis. If the pain does not respond to food or antacids and there is severe pain and rebound tenderness, the cause is not likely to be an uncomplicated peptic ulcer. If the patient presents with weight loss, anemia, or exacerbation of the pain when eating, gastric cancer should be suspected.

Management

The principal aim of management for patients with PUD is to relieve pain, heal the ulcer, and prevent complications or recurrences. Pharmacologic therapy is the foundation of management for PUD, but nonpharmacologic measures, such as smoking cessation should be used as well. Cigarette smoking increases the risk for PUD, and, in patients with documented ulcers, smoking impairs healing, promotes recurrence, and increases the morbidity and mortality. Dietary measures are used on an individual basis. If spicy foods cause discomfort for a particular patient, they should be avoided, but they themselves are not ulcerogenic and do not inhibit healing, as was once thought. Pharmacologic intervention for PUD consists of H_2-receptor antagonists, proton pump inhibitors, and agents that enhance the mucosal defenses, such as antacids, sucralfate (Carafate), bismuth subsalicylate (Pepto-Bismol), and prostaglandin analogs (misoprostol), and antibiotics.

Proton Pump Inhibitors

The proton pump inhibitors (PPI) are now the drugs of choice for treating PUD because they are more effective and are easier to use. The duration of action of the PPIs is more than 24 hours, whereas H_2-receptor blockers inhibit only 65 percent of acid secretion over 24 hours. Another advantage of PPIs over H_2-receptor blockers is that the PPIs are given on a once a day dosage schedule while H_2-receptor blockers require at least BID dosing. The usual dosage is either omeprazole 20 mg, rabeprazole 20 mg, lansoprazole 30 mg, esomeprazole or pantoprazole 40 mg. All of the PPIs inhibit parietal cell hydrogen-potassium adenosine triphosphatase (ATPase), which mediates hydrogen ion secretion. Proton pump inhibitors heal 90 percent of duodenal ulcers in 4 weeks of therapy and 90 percent of gastric ulcers after 8 weeks. Long-term use of these drugs is associated with slightly decreased absorption of vitamin B_{12} and iron.

H_2-Receptor Blockers

If a patient has mild symptoms and no indicators of complications or a more serious disease, then empiric therapy with H_2-receptor blockers should be instituted for 2 weeks. After the initial treatment period, if symptoms persist or are worse, then upper endoscopy should be considered for a more definitive diagnosis. When H_2-receptor blockers are used for peptic ulcer treatment, the standard treatment is to administer an H_2-receptor blocker once a day at bedtime or half the daily dose twice a day for 8 weeks. Over 80 percent of ulcers are healed by the completion of this regimen. H_2-blockers effectively reduce basal and food-stimulated secretion of gastric acid and thue facilitate healing; they are generally well tolerated. Cimetidine (Tagamet), however, inhibits the hepatic cytochrome P-450 system and can increase levels of other medications that are metabolized by these enzymes, including warfarin (Coumadin), theophylline (Theo-Dur), and phenytoin (Dilantin). The other H_2-blockers have fewer adverse effects.

Other Pharmacologic Agents

Antacids were traditionally the mainstay of ulcer treatment for decades and are still useful today. They neutralize acid rapidly, are generally well tolerated, and are inexpensive. One of the major disadvantages is that they require frequent (1- to 3-hour) dosing, which can contribute patient nonadherence. They should be used with caution in patients with renal failure because of the risk of aluminum and magnesium toxicity. Antacids that contain calcium should not be used in patients with PUD because calcium causes rebound acid secretion.

Sucralfate is an aluminum hydroxide salt of sucrose that enhances the mucosal defenses and is used in healing duodenal ulcers and in the long-term treatment to prevent recurrence. Sucralfate works by forming a protective barrier to the action of acid and pepsin in the ulcer base. It also stimulates mucus, bicarbonate secretion, and prostaglandin production, and binds fibroblast growth factor. Studies have shown that sucralfate 1 g qid heals duodenal ulcers as well as H_2-blockers do.

Bismuth preparations promote ulcer healing by stimulating mucosal bicarbonate and prostaglandin production. Bismuth also has antimicrobial action against *H. pylori* and has been shown to eradicate the organism in up to 33 percent of the cases. The two types of bismuth preparation available in the United States are bismuth subsalicylate and ranitidine bismuth citrate. Bismuth causes feces to darken or turn black. Patients should be warned of this effect to lessen their anxiety when it happens.

Misoprostol (Cytotec), a prostaglandin analog, stimulates ulcer healing by promoting mucus and bicarbonate secretion. It is indicated for use only as a prophylactic measure to prevent ulcer formation in patients who require treatment with NSAIDs for other conditions.

There are a number of regimens used to eradicate *H. pylori,* enhance ulcer healing, and prevent ulcer recurrence. Comparatively speaking, it is more cost effective to employ a regimen to eradicate *H. pylori* than it is to maintain a patient on long-term therapy. Most regimens use a combination of several drugs, including bismuth, amoxicillin (Amoxil), tetracycline (Tetracap), clarithromycin (Biaxin), metronidazole (Flagyl), H_2-antagonists, and proton pump inhibitors for a period of 2 weeks. Triple drug therapy combining two antibiotics, clarithromycin and either amoxicillin or metronidazole, with a proton pump inhibitor has been shown to be very effective in the eradication of *H. pylori.* The use of amoxicillin is preferred over metronidazole because there are resistant strains of *H. pylori* and the adverse effects of metronidazole hamper patient adherence. Eradication of *H. pylori* has also been demonstrated by combining bismuth subsalicylate and two antibi-

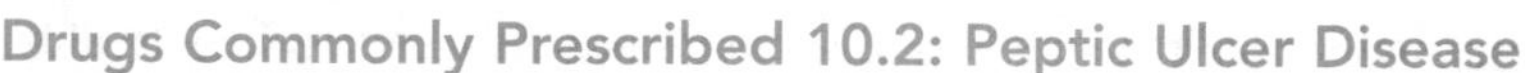

Drugs Commonly Prescribed 10.2: Peptic Ulcer Disease

Drug	Indication	Dosage
Single-Drug Therapy		
Antacids		
Mylanta II	PUD	30 mL qh + 3 h pc + hs
Sucralfate	PUD	1 g qid or 2 g bid
H_2 blockers		
Cimetidine	PUD	400 mg bid or 800 mg qhs
Ranitidine	PUD	150 mg bid or 300 mg qhs
Famotidine	PUD	20 mg bid or 40 mg qhs
Nizatidine	PUD	150 mg bid or 300 mg qhs
Proton pump inhibitors		
Omeprazole	PUD	20 mg qam
Lansoprazole	PUD	15 mg qd
Combination Therapy		
Omeprazole OR	Active *H. pylori*-associated PUD	20 mg bid for 2 weeks
lansoprazole		30 mg bid for 2 weeks
AND		
Metronidazole PLUS clarithromycin		500 mg bid for 2 weeks
		500 mg bid for 2 weeks
Amoxicillin PLUS clarithromycin	Active *H. pylori*-associated PUD	1 mg bid for 2 weeks
		500 mg bid for 2 weeks
Bismuth subsalicylate PLUS	Active *H. pylori*-associated PUD	2 tablets qid for 2 weeks
tetracycline PLUS metronidazole		500 mg qid for 2 weeks
		250 mg qid for 2 weeks

otics, but the dosing schedule is qid and has a higher incidence of adverse effects. Drugs Commonly Prescribed 10.2 presents the drugs used for PUD.

Follow-Up and Referral

In patients empirically treated for ulcers, follow-up is necessary only if symptoms recur. If after 2 weeks the patient has seen no improvement or symptoms have progressed, referral to a gastroenterologist for upper endoscopy is indicated. Any time a gastric ulcer is suspected rather than a duodenal ulcer, the patient should be referred to a gastroen terologist because the incidence of gastric cancer in these patients is increased. In patients treated with an *H. pylori* eradication regimen, retesting for *H. pylori* is necessary only if symptoms recur. Follow-up is necessary for any patient who does not respond to therapy or who experiences worsening symptoms.

Patient Education

The most important aspect of patient education is to stress the importance of following the treatment regimen prescribed. The patient's anxiety can be eased by informing him or her of possible bothersome side effects of any medications, such as a change in fecal color when taking bismuth preparations. If the patient is taking sucralfate in conjunction with an antacid, proton pump inhibitor, or H_2 blocker, it should stressed that the sucralfate cannot be taken at the same time as the other medications or at the same time as digoxin, ciprofloxacin, or phenytoin because sucralfate binds to all of these medications. Dispelling myths about ulcers is also an important part of patient education.

Cholecystitis

Cholecystitis is an acute inflammation of the gallbladder wall, which is usually the result of an impacted calculus within the cystic duct, causing inflammation proximal to the obstruction. Cholelithiasis is found in 90 to 95 percent of patients presenting with cholecystitis. Cholecystitis without gallstones, acalculous cholecystitis, is a very serious disease. It usually occurs in patients who are already critically ill because of trauma, burns, surgery, or sepsis, and have had no oral intake or have been supplemented with hyperalimentation. Patients present with severe pain and tenderness in the epigastrium or RUQ of the abdomen accompanied by nausea, vomiting, fever, and leukocytosis.

Epidemiology and Causes

Cholecystitis/cholelithiasis is much more prevalent in Western societies. Researchers estimate that the disease affects approximately 20 million Americans, the majority of whom are not aware they have cholelithiasis. About 50 percent of these asymptomatic patients never require treatment. Gallstones form in people as early as their 30s. In fact, 75 percent of American Indian women over the age of 25 have gallstones. The risk of requiring a cholecystectomy increases with age as a consequence of complications secondary to the lithiasis. By age 65, about 20 percent of women and 10 percent of men have symptoms related to gallstones that require medical attention. As many as 5000 to 6000 deaths each year are attributed to gallstone-related disease.

Cholesterol stones are the most common form and account for 75 percent of all gallstones. The remaining 25 percent are pigmented stones, which are categorized as black or brown depending on their chemical composition. Cholesterol stones contain between 50 and 90 percent cholesterol; the remainder of the stone is made of calcium salts from bilirubin pigment, carbonate, bile acids, phospholipids, fatty acids, and proteins. Risk Factors 10.1 describes the risk factors associated with cholelithiasis.

The well-known mnemonic regarding the typical cholelithiasis patient is the "six Fs": fat, female, forty, flatulent, fertile, and fat intolerant. After age 50, the gender distribution is equal. Pregnancy also predisposes women to cholelithiasis, presumably because of the increased abdominal pressure as well as increased cholesterol levels during the third trimester. Any condition that increases the development of cholelithiasis increases the chance of developing cholecystitis.

Pathophysiology

Ninety-five percent of cholecystitis cases are associated with cholelithiasis. Cholesterol stones are the most common form of gallstones. Cholesterol is insoluble in water; it is therefore made soluble though interaction with bile salts and phospholipids, allowing it to be carried within the bile. There are two known transport systems for cholesterol within the bile, vesicular and micellar, both of which exist in the bile to maintain equilibrium. When this equilibrium is disturbed and the bile contains more cholesterol than can be maintained, crystallization of the cholesterol, referred to as nucleation, occurs. Gradual deposition of cholesterol on these crystals leads to the development of a cholesterol gallstone. Although this process seems to contribute to the formation of gallstones, not all people with cholesterol-saturated bile form stones. Thus, there is more to the process of lithogenesis than is known.

The gallbladder is of primary importance in the development of gallstones because it provides an arena for bile stasis and allows time for the slow crystallization of cholesterol, which may also be enhanced by yet unknown proteins or other materials within the bile. Biliary cholesterol is increased by ingestion of estrogen and oral contraceptives, multiparity, and inflammatory terminal ileal disease, which decreases the bile acid pool. Bile stasis, which can contribute to gallstone formation, is increased by strictures within the ductal system, parenteral hyperalimentation, fasting, and mechanical obstruction secondary to tumor or cyst formation.

The pathogenesis of pigmented stones is less well understood but seems to be directly related to elevation in levels of unconjugated bilirubin. Any disease state that increases the amount of bilirubin increases the risk for pigmented lithogenesis. Black pigmented stones are formed within the gallbladder and are commonly associated with hemolytic diseases and in patients with cirrhosis and those who require long-term parenteral hyperalimentation. Black pigmented stones are more fragile and seem to crush more easily than cholesterol stones.

Brown pigmented stones are composed of alternating layers of calcium bilirubinate and calcium fatty acids. Chronic bacterial infections are believed to be partly responsible for the formation of brown pigmented stones because the enzymes the bacteria produce predispose stone formation. Brown stones are typically found within the intrahepatic ducts and are rarely found within the gallbladder.

The pathophysiological changes occurring within the gallbladder before the diagnosis of acute cholecystitis are directly related to the amount of time the duct has been obstructed and the degree of inflammation that has taken place. The earliest pathological findings are erythema, edema, and a fibrosuppurative exudate. Tissue examination reveals inflammatory infiltration, hemorrhage, and edema resulting in ulceration of the mucosa within a short period of time. The result is the development of gangrene, with abscess formation. As the acute process resolves, collagen deposits develop, usually within 1 to 2 weeks. The gallbladder eventually contracts and becomes scarred, causing thickening of the wall. Often the gallbladder becomes filled with pus preceding the development of gangrene. Perforation may occur, most often at the fundus, but it can occur anywhere there is erosion of an impacted stone. Perforation of the gallbladder allows bile to spill into the peritoneal cavity, causing bile peritonitis and abscess and fistula formation.

RISK FACTORS 10.1

Risk Factors Associated with Cholelithiasis

Cholesterol Stones	Pigmented Stones
Female gender	Hemolytic diseases
Obesity	Increasing age
Pregnancy	Hyperalimentation
Increased age	Cirrhosis
Drug-induced (oral contraceptives, clofibrates)	Biliary stasis
Cystic fibrosis	Chronic biliary infections
Rapid weight loss	
Spinal cord injury	
Ileal disease with extensive resection	
Diabetes mellitus	
Sickle cell anemia	

Clinical Presentation

Subjective

Acute cholecystitis causes various symptoms, ranging from generalized GI complaints to intractable pain. Most patients complain of indigestion, nausea, and vomiting, especially after consuming a meal high in fat. Acute cholecystitis usually begins with acute, colicky-type pain. About 80 percent of patients report that they have experienced this type of pain before. However, the pain associated with acute cholecystitis persists, and as the inflammation progresses the pain localizes over the RUQ. Patients may complain of referred pain that radiates to the middle of the back, to the infrascapular area, or to the right shoulder. The pain is increased by any movement including respiration. If the inflammation extends to the peritoneal area, the pain worsens and the abdominal muscles become rigid and a fever is usually evident.

Objective

Physical findings are dependent on the degree of inflammation present. As the pain over the RUQ becomes severe, there is often involuntary guarding of the abdominal muscles over the right side. A positive Murphy's sign is elicited when the right subcostal region is so tender that there is painful splinting with deep inspiration or when palpation over the RUQ area causes transient inspiratory arrest. The gallbladder is palpable in fewer than 50 percent of the patients. Fever is usually low grade, 99 to 101°F (38.3°C); high fever suggests sepsis. Patients may develop mild jaundice from edema of the common bile duct. Hyperbilirubinemia should raise the suspicion of choledocholelithiasis. Bowel sounds may be diminished.

In most cases, acute cholecystitis subsides spontaneously, with improvement in the first few days and no symptoms after about 4 days. If symptoms persist or become more severe, the potential for perforation, gangrene, empyema, and septic shock increases. Rebound tenderness, shaking chills, or increased fever should raise suspicion that perforation has occurred. Surgical referral is indicated early in the disease process.

Diagnostic Reasoning

Diagnostic Testing

During the acute presentation of cholecystitis, there is usually mild elevation of the white blood cell (WBC) count, to 15,000/mL. Serum transaminases can be elevated up to four times the normal amount; aspartate aminotransferase (AST) and alanine aminotransferase (ALT) can be elevated to 300 U/L. Alkaline phosphatase is elevated two to four times above normal levels and the bilirubin can be as high as 4 mg/dL. Profound elevation of the alkaline phosphatase and bilirubin is highly suggestive of choledocholithiasis. An elevation in amylase can be the result of passage of a stone through the common bile duct but may also indicate gallstone pancreatitis.

Abdominal x-ray films may reveal gallstones, enlarged gallbladder, or air within the biliary system or peritoneal cavity. The gold standard for diagnosis of acute cholecystitis is ultrasound; it is a quick, noninvasive, reliable, and cost-effective means of identifying the presence of cholelithiasis. Radionuclide scanning following administration of technetium-99m (99m-Tc) is the most accurate means of confirming the clinical diagnosis of cholecystitis with cystic duct obstruction. If the gallbladder fills with the isotope, the diagnosis of cholecystitis is highly unlikely; however, if the bile duct is visualized and the gallbladder is not, this is highly suggestive of cholecystitis. Oral cholangiograms are of no benefit in the acutely ill patient.

Differential Diagnosis

The differential diagnosis of acute cholecystitis in the presence of RUQ pain, nausea, vomiting, and fever includes pancreatitis, myocardial infarction, appendicitis, peptic ulcer, pneumonia, and hepatitis. Most of these potential diagnoses can be effectively ruled out via standard laboratory tests and ultrasound. Electrocardiogram (ECG) can rule out myocardial infarction and is necessary as part of preoperative studies.

Management

Treatment of cholelithiasis depends on many variables, including age, presenting symptoms, past medical history, and size, type and number of gallstones involved. Patients with symptomatic cholelithiasis can often be safely managed on an outpatient basis. Patients must be advised to avoid foods high in fat, which can provoke an attack. Nonsurgical options for the treatment of gallstones include dissolution of the stone by oral ingestion of ursodeoxycholic acid (ursodiol) or direct dissolution by percutaneous instillation of methyl-tertiary-butyl ether. Both types of dissolution therapies are of limited value and can be used only with cholesterol stones. It should be stressed that with these treatments recurrence is almost 100 percent and the length of treatment may be as long as 2 years.

Patients who are deemed poor surgical risks can also undergo extracorporeal shock wave lithotripsy along with chemical dissolution in an attempt to reduce the size of the stone. Patients who continue to have biliary colic or have developed other complications should be hospitalized for further treatment, with prompt referral to a gastroenterologist and or a surgeon.

Initial Management

Initial treatment begins with definitive diagnosis. For many, the diagnosis of gallstones is made as an incidental finding during medical treatment for another problem. These patients are often asymptomatic and require no further treatment except an awareness of the signs and symptoms of a "gallbladder attack." Patients who are considered a poor surgical risk can be treated nonsurgically with dissolution therapy or lithotripsy. Those who remain symptomatic despite treatment or have developed other complications should be hospitalized in an attempt to reduce the risk of a life-threatening event such as perforation or septic shock.

Management of acute cholecystitis includes rehydration with intravenous fluids and replenishing electrolytes as indicated by laboratory results. Patients are not allowed anything by mouth, and if vomiting is persistent, a nasogastric (NG) tube is inserted. Pain is managed with intramuscular analgesic agents. A third-generation cephalosporin is started once the diagnosis is made. If sepsis is suspected, an aminoglycoside is added to the antibiotic coverage.

The treatment of choice for acute cholecystitis is early surgical intervention. Patients in the acute phase of the disease are usually stabilized before a cholecystectomy is scheduled. Patients who are considered a poor surgical risk may benefit from cholecystotomy, either operatively or percutaneously. Emergency decompression with cholecystotomy may be necessary to remove stones and purulent material before a cholecystectomy, which should be deferred for 6 to 8 weeks.

The mortality associated with acute cholecystitis is 5 to 10 percent and is usually associated with patients older than age 60 with comorbid conditions and those with septic complications. Approximately 50 percent of patients who do not choose to undergo cholecystectomy have a reoccurrence within 5 years, and complications are common.

Subsequent Management

The most common complications of acute cholecystitis are empyema and perforation. Perforation into the abdominal cavity can occur early in the disease process and is associated with a 30 percent mortality rate. Perforation may also occur into another hollow viscus or into the colon, causing draining fistulas, which may relieve the symptoms associated with cholecystitis. Surgical removal of the gallbladder with fistula repair is indicated when the patient is medically stable for surgery.

Follow-Up and Referral

Patients with acute cholecystitis require referral to a general surgeon for removal of the gallbladder. Referral should be made after diagnosis of acute cholecystitis. Follow-up includes routine postoperative visits according to the surgeon. Patients who have persistent symptoms after the removal of the gallbladder (postcholecystectomy syndrome) may have a mistaken diagnosis, a functional bowel disorder, retained or recurrent common bile duct stones, or spasm of the sphincter of Oddi. Patients with incidental findings of asymptomatic gallstones should be referred to a surgeon and given the option for elective surgery, medical dissolution therapy, lithotripsy, or contact solvent dissolution.

Patient Education

Patient education for individuals declining surgical intervention should include the risks and benefits of each therapy. Dietary counseling should include weight loss for those patients who are obese and the avoidance of fatty foods that provoke attacks. Patients taking oral contraceptives should be given information about alternative forms of birth control, and menopausal women taking estrogen should be counseled about alternative sources of phytoestrogens, such as soy products.

Acute Pancreatitis

Acute pancreatitis is defined as an acute inflammation of the pancreas and the surrounding tissues resulting from the release of pancreatic enzymes into these tissues. These enzymes cause a chemical burn in the retroperitoneal spaces, which leads to systemic toxicity. The degree to which the microcirculation within the pancreas is preserved determines the histological classification of pancreatitis. If the microcirculation remains intact, the process is defined as acute interstitial pancreatitis, but if the microcirculation is disrupted, necrotizing pancreatitis results. Acute pancreatitis normally resolves both clinically and histologically.

Epidemiology and Causes

Although there are many causes of acute pancreatitis, approximately 80 percent of all hospital admissions for acute pancreatitis are caused by biliary tract disease (passing of a gallstone) and alcoholism. The remaining 20 percent are caused by infection (mumps), hyperlipidemia (particularly types I, IV, and V), metabolic disorders (hyperparathyroidism, hypercalcemia), drugs (furosemide, valproic acid, sulfonamides, thiazides), endoscopic retrograde cholangiopancreatography (ERCP), structural abnormalities of the pancreatic duct (stricture, carcinoma, pancreatic divisum), structural abnormalities of the common bile duct and ampullary region, surgery (particularly of the stomach and biliary tract), vascular disease (atherosclerosis, severe hypotension), or trauma.

Acute pancreatitis is usually the result of some other process, such as passing of a gallstone, excessive alcohol intake, or some other biliary tract disease. Clinical pancreatitis is seen in up to 9.5 percent of alcoholic patients and histologic evidence is found in 17 to 45 percent of this group. Cholelithiasis is present in 60 percent of nonalcoholic patients with pancreatitis.

Pathophysiology

Pathologic changes associated with pancreatitis range from acute edema and cellular infiltration to necrosis and hemorrhage. Although the exact pathogenesis is not known, temporary impaction of the sphincter of Oddi by a gallstone before its passage into the duodenum may cause edema or obstruction of the ampulla of Vater, with subsequent reflux of bile into the pancreatic ducts and injury to the acinar cells. This cascade of events causes an autodigestive process within the pancreas that can progress to shock and death without appropriate intervention. Inflammation is confined to the pancreas in edematous pancreatitis and the mortality rate is less than 5 percent.

When inflammation and tissue necrosis extends beyond the pancreas, the associated mortality is 10 to 50 percent. Pancreatic exudate containing toxins and activated enzymes permeates the retroperitoneum and causes a chemical burn that increases the permeability of the blood vessels within the peritoneal cavity. As a result, large amounts of protein-rich fluid from the circulation is sequestered in these third spaces producing hypovolemia and shock. As these toxins and enzymes enter the systemic circulation they can further reduce vascular tone, and, thus, the ability to correct the hypotension and shock.

Acute pancreatitis can be classified as either mild or severe. Mild acute pancreatitis normally improves within 48 to 72 hours and does not involve other organ systems. There is minimal interstitial edema, with only occasional microscopic acinar cell necrosis. Severe, acute pancreatitis is often associated with complications and multisystem organ failure. It can be a life-threatening condition and the patient may require monitoring in the intensive care unit (ICU).

Complications during the first few days of diagnosis are associated with hemodynamic instability; shock, renal failure, and respiratory compromise secondary to adult respiratory distress syndrome (ARDS) and hypoxemia. Pancreatic necrosis with secondary gram-negative sepsis has an associated 100 percent mortality rate unless there is extensive surgical debridement of the infected tissue. Up to 25 percent of patients diagnosed with acute pancreatitis develop some degree of fluid collection within a few days of diagnosis that resolves spontaneously half of the time and the rest form pseudocysts, abscesses, and other necrotic collections.

Pancreatic pseudocysts take at least 4 weeks to form and resolve spontaneously after about 6 weeks in 40 percent of the cases. If the pseudocyst does not resolve within 12 weeks after acute pancreatitis, the risk of complications in symptomatic patients (infection, bleeding, rupture) are reported as high as 60 percent, but there is little associated risk in asymptomatic patients. The decision for invasive intervention will depend on the progression of symptoms and cyst size.

Clinical Presentation

Subjective

The patient with acute pancreatitis usually presents with abrupt onset of deep epigastric pain that persists for hours to days and may radiate straight through to the back. The pain is intense and often refractory to large doses of parenteral narcotics. It is aggravated by any vigorous activity such as coughing and by lying supine; it improves when the patient is seated and leaning forward. The patient appears acutely ill, often with intractable nausea and vomiting. In some cases, depending on the severity, the patient may experience sweating, weakness, and anxiety. The patient may report a history of ingestion of alcohol or a big meal before onset of symptoms or mild biliary colic preceding the episode.

Objective

On physical exam, there is severe abdominal tenderness, particularly over the epigastric area, which may be accompanied by guarding but without rigidity or rebound tenderness, and there may be milder pain in the lower abdomen without guarding or rigidity. Abdominal distension is present in approximately 20 percent of the patients. Bowel sounds can be hypoactive or absent if associated with paralytic ileus. The rectal exam is normal, and the stool is usually negative for occult blood.

The patient is tachycardic (100 to 140 beats/min) with rapid, shallow respiration. Inspiratory effort is poor because deep inspiration causes pain. Blood pressure may be high secondary to pain or low if shock is imminent. The patient's temperature may initially be normal or subnormal but increases to 100.4 to 102.2°F (38° to 39°C) within a few hours. Mild jaundice and scleral icterus may be present. The patient's skin may be pale, cool, and clammy if shock is present.

Uncommon findings that can result from the pancreatic inflammatory process include left-sided pleural effusion, bluish discoloration over the flanks (Grey Turner's sign) or around the umbilicus (Cullen's sign), jaundice caused by impingement upon the common bile duct, and epigastric mass secondary to pseudocyst development.

Diagnostic Reasoning

Diagnostic Tests

The diagnosis of pancreatitis is strongly suggested through the history and physical exam; however, because many other diseases present with similar symptoms, further testing is necessary. The gold standard for diagnosis is an elevated serum amylase (up to three times the normal level); however, in one-third of patients with alcoholic pancreatitis, the serum amylase level may be normal. The diagnosis of pancreatitis is supported by a concurrent elevation of the serum lipase. Serum amylase and lipase levels are increased on the first day of acute symptoms and return to normal in 3 to 7 days. These levels remain normal if there has been repeated prior damage to the acinar cells, rendering them incapable of further enzyme secretion. The level of elevation of amylase and lipase is not indicative of the severity of the disease.

The WBC count is usually between 12,000 and 20,000 cells/mL. The hematocrit can be as high as 50 to 55 percent because of hemoconcentration resulting from sequestered fluids in the third spaces.

A decrease in serum calcium may indicate saponification and is indicative of the severity of the pancreatitis. Calcium levels below 7 mg/dL (with normal serum albumin) can cause tetany and are associated with poor prognosis. Elevated C-reactive protein is correlated with pancreatic necrosis. The risk of infection is positively correlated with pancreatic necrosis and accounts for most of the deaths. Pancreatic necrosis requires surgical intervention and CT-guided aspiration of the necrotic tissue for Gram stain and culture is indicated.

Patients presenting with biliary pancreatitis have an elevation of the liver enzymes. When ALT is up to three times the normal limit, the positive predictive value is 95 percent that the pancreatitis is caused by biliary disease (gallstones). Concomitant rises in the AST, alkaline phosphatase, and bilirubin suggest gallbladder disease.

Diagnostic imaging, especially CT of the abdomen, can provide fast and accurate information for the definitive diagnosis of acute pancreatitis. Although the CT scan can be normal in 15 to 30 percent of patients with mild acute pancreatitis, it is the most efficient means of discerning acute pancreatitis from other potentially fatal intra-abdominal processes. CT is also helpful in monitoring the progression or resolution of pancreatic pseudocysts.

Ultrasonography (US) is the gold standard for identification and location of gallstones and is considered mandatory because studies have shown that the morbidity associated with gallstone pancreatitis is dramatically reduced once the stone is removed. US can also detect dilatation of the common bile duct (CBD), indicating obstruction. ERCP with sphincterotomy and stone extraction can be performed and has been proved to decrease morbidity and mortality.

If there is evidence that the pancreatitis is severe, additional testing with intravenous (IV) contrast is recommended; the necrotic pancreas has damage to its microcirculation and, thus, is not enhanced with IV contrast. If the microcirculation remains intact, there is uniform enhancement of the pancreas. Pancreatic necrosis is associated with a much higher morbidity, mortality, and infection rate.

Pancreatic infection is a complication that requires immediate diagnosis and intervention. Infection should be suspected when the patient has persistently elevated WBCs and fever. The patient normally looks toxic. Positive blood cultures and visualization of gas bubbles within the retroperitoneum on CT support the diagnosis.

Ranson's criteria are the most widely accepted and utilized system for assessing the severity of acute pancreatitis. Identification of early prognostic signs may provide the best indication of a serious outcome and can alert the practitioner that the patient may require transfer to the ICU. Listed within Table 10.9 are the 11 objective signs used to classify the severity of pancreatitis. Mortality rates correlate directly with the number of diagnostic criteria present. Pancreatitis is classified as severe when three or more of Ranson's criteria are met.

Differential Diagnosis

Differential diagnosis of acute pancreatitis is made by history and physical exam and supported by laboratory data and imaging studies. The gold standard for diagnosis is serum amylase; however, in cases in which the level is normal or mildly elevated, diagnosis can be confirmed by CT scan. CT scan is useful in differentiating other intraabdominal processes from acute pancreatitis. Laboratory data are helpful in differentiating other causes of acute abdominal pain with associated hyperamylasemia. Table 10.10 differentiates hyperamylasemia resulting from pancreatic and nonpancreatic causes.

Table 10.9 Ranson's Criteria for Assessing the Severity of Pancreatitis

At admission or at time of diagnosis
1. Age older than 55 years
2. White blood cell (WBC) count greater than 16,000/μL
3. Blood glucose greater than 200 mg/dL
4. Base deficit greater than 4 mEq/L
5. Serum lactate dehydrogenase (LDH) greater than 350 IU/L
6. AST greater than 250 U/L

During the initial 48 hours
1. Hematocrit (Hct) drop of more than 10 percentage points
2. Blood urea nitrogen (BUN) rise of greater than 5 mg/dL
3. Arterial Po_2 of less than 60
4. Serum calcium (Ca) of less than 8 mg/dL
5. Estimated fluid sequestration of greater than 6 L

Number of Diagnostic Criteria	Mortality Rate (%)
0–2	1
3–4	16
5–6	40
7–8	100

Management

Treatment of acute pancreatitis is aimed at limiting the severity of pancreatic inflammation, preventing further complications by interrupting the pathological processes, and managing the symptoms as they arise. Mild acute pancreati-

Table 10.10 Hyperamylasemia: Pancreatic and Nonpancreatic Causes

Pancreatic Hyperamylasemia	Nonpancreatic Hyperamylasemia
Pancreatic pseudocyst	Salivary adenitis (secondary to mumps)
Perforated duodenal ulcer	Ruptured ectopic pregnancy
Small bowel perforation	Post–abdominal surgery
Mesenteric infarction	Lactic acidosis
Mesenteric vascular thrombus	Diabetic ketoacidosis
Opiate administration	Leaking aortic aneurysm
Post ERCP	Renal insufficiency

tis usually resolves spontaneously in a few days, so these patients can be managed conservatively as outpatients. Fasting is necessary until the symptoms of acute inflammation have subsided.

Treatment includes maintaining fluid status with parenteral fluids to prevent hypovolemia and hypotension. Pain is controlled with meperidine (Demerol) rather than with other opiates, to prevent increased pressure within the sphincter of Oddi although research indicates that morphine causes no more spasms in the sphincter of Oddi than meperidine. The patient is allowed NPO, and NG tube insertion should be considered when there is persistent nausea, vomiting, or evidence of ileus. The use of empiric antibiotics, H_2-receptor antagonists, and pancreatic enzyme inhibitors have not been proven effective and are not recommended.

Judicious introduction of clear liquids can be instituted once the patient is pain free, the amylase and lipase have returned to normal range, and bowel sounds have returned. The diet may be advanced to regular low fat as the patient tolerates.

Patients with more severe pancreatitis tend to have sequestered larger amounts of fluid as a result of the "chemical burn" sustained by the tissues within the retroperitoneal space. These patients are usually transferred to the ICU under the care of a gastroenterologist or surgeon. Aggressive volume replacement is necessary and may require invasive hemodynamic monitoring to maintain appropriate fluid balance. Fluid resuscitation is an important part of therapy and 6 to 8 L/day may be required. Some patients may require infusion of fresh frozen plasma or serum albumin or blood transfusions, which can increase the risk of the development of ARDS. Cardiac function and fluid status can be monitored with a central line or pulmonary artery catheter. Measurement of hourly urine output is also necessary. If hemodynamic stability is not achieved through volume replacement, vasopressors may be necessary.

Daily monitoring of serum calcium, magnesium, glucose, electrolytes, total protein, albumin, amylase, lipase, and CBC with subsequent correction of abnormalities is required. In febrile patients, cultures of blood, urine, and sputum should be obtained, as well as CT-guided needle aspiration of necrotic areas of the pancreas with initiation of appropriate broad-spectrum antibiotic coverage as necessary to prevent increased morbidity and mortality. Arterial blood gas (ABG) readings should be obtained daily and hypoxemia treated accordingly. The patient may require assisted ventilation if hypoxemia persists or ARDS develops.

Correction of serum glucose is done with caution and should not begin until levels are greater than 250 mg/dL. Hypocalcemia is often corrected with the administration of albumin-containing fluids. Neuromuscular irritability, if present, can be corrected with 10 percent solution of calcium gluconate. If there is a coexisting hypomagnesemia, correction of the magnesium level will often restore the calcium to its normal level. In patients with renal impairment, magnesium must be replaced cautiously.

Patients with severe pancreatitis must be maintained in a fasting state for prolonged periods of time, often for 2 to 4 weeks. Administration of antacids through an NG tube can help to prevent stress ulceration. The nutritional needs of the patient can be maintained with total parenteral nutrition (TPN) until the gut becomes functional and then enteral feedings can be started, using the distal jejunum to reduce pancreatic stimulation. Oral feedings should not be started until any and all complications have been treated and the patient is free from nausea and vomiting and amylase and lipase levels have returned to normal.

Surgical intervention is normally reserved for a pancreatic pseudocyst that has persisted for more than 6 weeks with ongoing symptomatology, necrotizing pancreatitis, pancreatic abscess, or severe hemorrhagic pancreatitis. Despite surgical intervention, the mortality rate for necrotizing pancreatitis remains high.

For pancreatitis caused by cholelithiasis, surgical intervention is determined by the presenting course of events. If biliary decompression is necessary, it can often be accomplished with ERCP. If the pancreatitis is mild, a cholecystectomy can be performed at a later time.

Follow-Up and Referral

Patients presenting with mild pancreatitis can usually be managed by the practitioner as previously mentioned. Patients with more severe acute pancreatitis or those who do not respond to conservative treatment must be referred to a gastroenterologist for management because the patient often requires intensive care. Surgical referral should be made once the diagnosis of pancreatitis is made. The patient who develops a pseudocyst requires long-term follow-up with serial CT scans to observe the resolution or growth of the cyst, which may require surgical intervention. The patient who has gallstone disease should have a cholecystectomy.

The prognosis of the patient with pancreatitis correlates directly with the severity of the inflammatory process. Patients with interstitial or edematous pancreatitis even with systemic complications have a mortality rate of 1 to 2 percent; however, patients with necrotizing pancreatitis have a mortality rate of 10 percent with sterile necrosis and up to 30 percent with infected necrosis.

In patients for whom no cause has been found, studies have suggested that half of these patients have occult gallstone disease (biliary sludge) or sphincter of Oddi dysfunction. These patients require repeated abdominal US exams to detect the development of biliary sludge. Patients with hereditary hypercholesterolemia are often missed because serum triglycerides are not obtained until after several days of fasting, at which time the triglyceride level may have fallen to within normal limits.

Patient Education

Patients with biliary disease as the cause of the pancreatitis should be informed of the need for a cholecystectomy as well as the benefit of reducing their dietary intake of fat. If the etiology of pancreatitis is alcohol abuse, the patient must be encouraged to abstain. Patients with genetic hyperlipidemia require diet instruction and information on avoidance of precipitating factors such as alcohol, estrogens, and certain drugs. These patients may benefit from lipid-lowering medications and must be taught to control their diabetes if present. If a drug is the suspected cause of the pancreatitis, it should not be restarted.

Chronic Pancreatitis

Chronic pancreatitis is defined as a slowly progressive inflammatory process that results in irreversible fibrosis of the pancreas with destruction and atrophy of the exocrine and endocrine glandular tissue. There are varying degrees of ductal dilatation and fibrosis. There can be intraductal formation of protein plugs, which calcify and cause further dilatation and obstruction. Chronic relapsing pancreatitis is defined as acute attacks that occur in the setting of chronic pancreatitis and are usually precipitated by a specific event such as binge drinking or the passage of a stone.

Epidemiology and Causes

There is little reliable information on the prevalence or incidence of chronic pancreatitis. Alcoholism accounts for between 70 and 80 percent of the cases in industrialized countries. These patients, on average, have consumed 120 grams of alcohol (eight 12-ounce beers, 8 ounces of 100 proof whiskey, or 30 ounces of wine) per day for 10 years. Although there is no threshold for alcohol consumption and the development of chronic pancreatitis, there is a statistically significant increase in those individuals who consume 120 grams per day. Diets high in protein in combination with either high or low fat can further predispose patients to pancreatic injury from alcohol.

Other causes of chronic pancreatitis include untreated hyperparathyroidism, severe malnutrition (especially protein calorie deficiency in developing countries), hereditary pancreatitis, and obstruction of the main pancreatic duct caused by stenosis, stones, tumor, or cystic fibrosis. In 10 to 30 percent of those with chronic pancreatitis, the cause is unknown, but patients are divided into two groups: (1) those who present with abdominal pain (usually between ages 15 and 30) and (2) older individuals (ages 50 to 70) who present, often without pain, with pancreatic calcifications, glandular insufficiency, and diabetes.

The tropical or nutritional form of chronic pancreatitis is most often found in India, Indonesia, and Africa. In these countries, the disease begins in early childhood and results in death in early adulthood because of complications. Malnutrition has a significant role, but it is not the sole cause because many areas with comparable malnutrition do not have equal prevalence of the disease.

Pathophysiology

The pathogenesis of chronic pancreatitis is not known but is the result of irreversible structural damage with permanent functional impairment of the pancreatic gland. For individuals who have alcohol-related disease, ductal obstruction is thought to be caused by changes in the chemical composition of the pancreatic juice, leading to protein plugging, calcification, and subsequent pancreatic damage. Another theory postulates that continuous injury to the acinar cells causes inflammation, necrosis, and fibrosis. Analysis of pancreatic juice obtained from alcoholic patients revealed protein plugs but not always chronic pancreatitis. Proponents of the theory favoring repeated damage to the pancreatic acinar cells believe that ductal obstruction is a result of changes in the pancreatic juice that cause increased viscosity and damage to the gland itself. These changes in the enzymatic properties result in chronic inflammation and fibrosis of the gland. Biliary disease has not been identified as a causative factor in the development of chronic pancreatitis.

With the progressive inflammatory changes occurring with chronic pancreatitis, it is not uncommon to find a fibrotic common bile duct and jaundice secondary to the obstructed CBD. Upper GI bleeding can result from the formation of gastric varices or the development of a pseudoaneurysm in an artery within the pancreatic area. Steatorrhea and diabetes mellitus result from destruction of the pancreatic gland with subsequent endocrine and exocrine insufficiency. Steatorrhea develops as lipase and protease secretion drops below 10 percent of normal. Islet cell destruction reduces insulin secretion, causing glucose intolerance and diabetes.

Clinical Presentation

Subjective

The most frequent presenting symptoms are intractable abdominal pain, weight loss, and diarrhea, but symptoms can be as mild as dyspepsia, nausea, and vomiting. Abdominal pain is usually epigastric or in the LUQ, may radiate to the back or left lumbar region, and is described as dull and constant. Pain may be absent in 5 to 10 percent of the cases or may represent an exacerbation of acute or relapsing pancreatitis. Pain may precede the development of other symptoms of chronic pancreatitis by years. The pain is often precipitated or aggravated by food or alcohol intake. In some patients, the pain diminishes over time (5 to 15 years) and is associated with burnout or calcification of the gland. Between 10 and 20 percent of older adults with idiopathic chronic pancreatitis have no pain with the disease.

Weight loss may result from anorexia caused by pain and nausea, malabsorption secondary to pancreatic exocrine insufficiency, or poorly controlled diabetes mellitus. Diabetes mellitus is present in approximately 50 percent of patients and is often the presenting sign in those individuals who have no pain associated with pancreatitis. Steatorrhea develops after the pancreas loses the ability to secrete digestive enzymes, which results in bulky, foul-smelling, fatty stools. Patients often complain of "oil leakage" from the rectum or an "oil slick" in the toilet bowl, which is indicative of pancreatic insufficiency.

Objective

Abdominal assessment in patients presenting with pain reveals mild to moderate epigastric tenderness with no rebound tenderness or guarding. A palpable abdominal mass is suggestive of a pancreatic pseudocyst. Bowel sounds may be absent in patients with paralytic ileus. Lung sounds may be diminished in the bases, which is indicative of pleural effusion.

Diagnostic Reasoning

Diagnostic Tests

Diagnosis of chronic pancreatitis is normally made through evaluation of pancreatic function and radiographic visualization of structural abnormalities such as pancreatic calcification or abnormalities in the size or consistency of the pancreatic tissue. The patient usually presents with chronic abdominal pain, weight loss, exocrine insufficiency (malabsorption), and diabetes mellitus.

Tests for pancreatic function include assessment of endocrine and exocrine function. A 2-hour postprandial blood sugar level greater than 200 mg/dL or fasting glucose greater than 120 mg/dL on two occasions is diagnostic for diabetes mellitus. Glucosuria may also be present. Serum amylase level may remain within normal limits because the pancreas has lost the ability to mount a response due to the chronicity of the disease. Malabsorption is documented by a 72-hour stool analysis for fecal fat content. Although helpful for diagnosis of exocrine function, steatorrhea is not diagnostic of chronic pancreatitis because patients do not develop steatorrhea until lipase falls below 10 percent of normal.

Pancreatic insufficiency can be confirmed by the Bentiromide (NBT [Nitroblue Tetrazolium]-PABA [para-aminobenzoic acid]) test, which measures urinary excretion of pancreatic chymotrypsin, or a secretin stimulation test, which is more sensitive but is unavailable in many places. The test involves placing a tube within the duodenum and collecting pancreatic secretions after IV stimulation with secretin. Collections that are of normal volume and low in bicarbonate (HCO_3–) suggest chronic pancreatitis; collections low in volume and normal HCO_3– suggest pancreatic cancer. The detection of decreased fecal chymotrypsin or elastase help to diagnose pancreatic insufficiency, but these tests do not have widespread availability.

Imaging studies include plain films of the abdomen, which may show intraductal stones or a calcified pancreas caused by pancreaticolithiasis and mild ileus. CT scan and/or ultrasound of the abdomen may show an abnormal size or consistency of the pancreas, a pancreatic pseudocyst, or dilated pancreatic ducts. ERCP may also show abnormality of the main pancreatic duct or its secondary branches. Although not available everywhere, magnetic resonance cholangiopancreatography (MRCP) is an excellent alternative to ERCP.

Differential Diagnosis

Differential diagnosis includes diseases that present with persistent abdominal pain such as PUD or mesenteric ischemia, and diseases that result in weight loss and abdominal pain, including abdominal malignancies, especially cancer of the pancreas, and intestinal disorders that may present with steatorrhea. The diagnosis of chronic pancreatitis can be confirmed by visualization of the calcified pancreas on x-ray films, which will also rule out most other disease processes.

Management

The treatment of chronic pancreatitis is aimed at preventing further pancreatic damage, managing pain, and supplementing exocrine and endocrine function. The major cause of chronic pancreatitis is alcohol abuse. Patients must abstain from alcohol completely because it frequently precipitates attacks. Narcotics are necessary to manage pain, and addiction is not uncommon. Recent studies have investigated the use of pancreatic enzymes in the treatment of chronic pain. A trial of high doses of a non–enteric-coated pancreatic enzyme supplement (pancrelipase, e.g., Viokase 8) with meals and at bedtime in conjunction with a gastric acid-secretion inhibitor (proton pump inhibitor or H_2-receptor blocker) can be attempted in an effort to quell the pain by enhancing the inhibition of pancreatic enzyme by the feedback loop. Patients whose pain is not managed by analgesics or pancreatic enzyme therapy should be considered for operative treatment.

Malabsorption is managed with a low-fat diet (less than 50 g/day) and oral pancreatic-enzyme supplementation. Oral supplementation should be administered 20 to 30 minutes before meals and snacks. The usual dose is 30,000 units of lipase. Non–enteric-coated pancrelipase formulations (pancrelipase, e.g., Viokase or Cotazym) should be given with H_2-receptor antagonists to prevent degradation by gastric acids. Enteric-coated preparations (pancrelipase, e.g., Pancrease or Creon, or pancreatin, e.g., Donnazyme) are stable at an acid pH and should not be given with acid neutralizers because this will promote enzyme release within the stomach. Fat-soluble vitamin (A, D, E, and K) replacement may be required. Favorable outcomes are weight gain, decreased number of stools per day, decrease in oil seepage from the rectum, and subjective improvement in well being.

Endocrine insufficiency is controlled with insulin supplementation. Extreme caution must be used with insulin supplementation as there is a deficiency of glucagon secretion, which can lead to prolonged hypoglycemia. Serum glucose levels of 200 to 250 mg/dL are considered acceptable and do not require treatment. The principal step in the management of diabetes associated with chronic pancreatitis is the correction of poor nutritional habits, malabsorption and malnutrition, and the elimination of alcohol. Normal insulin requirements range from 5 to 15 units per day but may fluctuate up to 40 units per day. It is best to maintain these patients at a higher than normal glucose level to avoid hypoglycemia while avoiding significant glucosuria.

Surgical intervention may be required to drain unresolving pseudocysts, for relief of pain, or to treat other complications associated with chronic pancreatitis. The goal of surgical intervention is to alleviate biliary tract disease, establish the free flow of bile into the duodenum, and remove obstruction of the pancreatic duct. Distal pancreatectomy may be necessary if the disease is located at the tail of the pancreas, and Whipple procedure is performed when disease is most extensive at the head of the pancreas. These procedures relieve the pain for 60 to 80 percent of the patients.

In patients with alcoholic pancreatitis, ERCP examination often reveals alternating stricture and dilatation ("chain of lakes") of the pancreatic duct. Treatment for this is a modified Puestow procedure (lateral pancreaticojejunostomy), which is 70 to 80 percent effective for pain relief.

Follow-Up and Referral

Follow-up of the patient with chronic pancreatitis will depend on the complications resulting from the disease and the medical and surgical interventions employed to remedy the disease. The patient undergoing surgical or other invasive treatment is under the care of the surgeon or the gastroenterologist, and follow-up will initially be prescribed by them. Once the patient has been released from the referring provider, follow-up should be directed by any complications.

Patients who have developed pseudocysts that have not resolved spontaneously will require periodic CT scans to monitor resolution or evolution of the cysts. Cysts that are consistently larger than 6 cm and are expanding should be referred for invasive treatment.

A nutritionist may be helpful in managing any protein calorie malnutrition. The pancreas is very nutrition sensitive and an improper diet can lead to atrophy and fibrosis. Follow-up with the nutritionist is often necessary for control of diabetes mellitus as well.

Patient Education

Patients should be taught about the natural history of this chronic disease, the common complications, and what to expect in the long term. Patients with chronic pancreatitis can expect that after 5 to 10 years, the episodes of pancreatic pain diminish in frequency and may in fact disappear. Patients should fully understand their medicine regime, including appropriate time of medication and adverse effects. Patients have a tendency to be more compliant when they understand that the goal of treatment is to control diarrhea and gain body weight. Patients can be provided with written instructions to assist with adherence.

Patients should be cautioned against long-term narcotic analgesic use because it can result in drug dependence. If long-term narcotic use is necessary, patients may benefit from referral to a pain control clinic to learn how to relieve pain using nonpharmacotherapeutic measures.

Hepatitis

Hepatitis is a common problem throughout the world and has many causes, including infectious, drug, vascular, and metabolic etiologies. Many cases of hepatitis are subclinical. Symptoms may be "flu-like" and go unreported, so that the true incidence of the disease may be underestimated. Table 10.11 lists some of the causes of acute hepatitis.

Acute viral hepatitis is a systemic infection that predominantly affects the liver and can lead to liver inflammation and necrosis. There are many viral agents that cause hepatitis, but the most common, and the ones that have public health concerns are hepatitis A (HAV), hepatitis B (HBV), hepatitis C (HCV), hepatitis D (HDV), and hepatitis E (HEV). All are endemic to the United States except HEV which is common in Southeast Asia, India, parts of Africa and Mexico. The prevalence of acute hepatitis has been slowly rising for the past few years.

Epidemiology and Causes

Hepatitis A

HAV is a small, single-stranded RNA virus of the picornavirus family. There are an estimated 138,000 infections and 75,000 cases of clinical illness resulting from HAV annually in the United States. HAV is endemic in the United States, with period outbreaks occurring in certain populations: Native-Americans, Alaskan natives, and some Hispanic populations. Because the symptoms of HAV are

Table 10.11 Causes of Acute Hepatitis

Viral	Cytomegalovirus; Epstein-Barr virus; hepatitis A, B, C, D, and E viruses; herpes virus; rubella; varicella-zoster virus; yellow-fever virus
Nonviral	Amebic abscess, bacterial abscess, Lyme disease, syphilis
Metabolic disorders	Alpha-1-antitrypsin deficiency, Wilson's disease
Vascular disorders	Budd-Chiari syndrome, congestive heart failure, ischemia (hypotension, shock)
Drugs	Acetaminophen, allopurinol, ASA (high doses), captopril, carbamazepine, isoniazid, ketoconazole, methyldopa, NSAIDs, procainamide, sulfonamides
Toxins	Alcohol (ethanol), carbon tetrachloride, herbs, mushrooms

often mild and nonspecific, many cases are undetected. Many other cases are asymptomatic, making it almost impossible to quantify the number of infections annually. Risk factors include crowded conditions, such as prisons, nursing homes, and day-care centers, and poor sanitation. Contaminated food or water are common sources of HAV.

Transmission is by the oral–fecal route, but has been detected in blood. People contract HAV by consuming contaminated water or ice, raw shellfish harvested from sewage-contaminated water, and fruits, vegetables, or other foods eaten uncooked that may have become contaminated while handling, but also through transfusion of infected blood. The virus is killed by heating at 185°F for 1 minute. Adequate chlorination of water also kills the virus. According to the CDC Viral Hepatitis Surveillance Program, household or sexual contact with a person who has HAV is the most frequently reported source of infection, accounting for 24 percent of the cases. The incubation period is 4 to 6 weeks. Excretion of HAV in feces occurs up to 2 weeks before clinical illness. It is rarely found in feces after the first week of illness. Blood and stools are infectious throughout the incubation period and early illness until the aminotransferase levels peak. A person is most infectious about 2 weeks before and during the first week that symptoms appear.

Chronic HAV does not occur. There is no carrier state, and HAV causes no long-term damage. HAV may persist for up to 1 year with relapses before full recovery. The mortality rate is less than 0.2 percent.

Hepatitis B

HBV is a DNA hepadnavirus with 7 different genotypes. It replicates in the liver and accounts for about 34 percent of all cases of hepatitis and for 5 to 10 percent of cases of chronic hepatitis and cirrhosis. However, the risk of chronic HBV is as high as 90 percent for infected infants. The frequency of infection and the mode of transmission vary in different parts of the world. According to the CDC, in the United States, Canada, Western Europe, Australia, and South Africa, the infection is of low endemicity and occurs primarily in adolescents and adults; 5 to 8 percent of the total population have been infected, and 0.2 to 0.9 percent have chronic infection. More than 1 million people in the United States have chronic HBV infection, and, although the overall prevalence of HBV in the United States is only 2 to 3 percent, the prevalence in the native Alaskan population is 6.4 percent and 14 percent among African-Americans. Despite these figures, the incidence of HBV has decreased by almost 50 percent in the last decade.

High-risk groups include male homosexuals, IV drug abusers, first-generation immigrants from endemic regions (Southeast Asia, China, and the Middle East), and people with multiple sex partners. Increased numbers of cases have been reported resulting from heterosexual transmission. Other high-risk groups include nurses, physicians, dentists, and personnel working in clinical and pathology labs and blood banks where direct needle-stick contamination may occur. The risk of infection from a contaminated needle is 10 to 30 percent. Patients and staff at hemodialysis centers are also at high risk. The risk of contracting HBV from a blood transfusion is now one in 600,000 units transfused in the United States.

Transmission is usually by direct contact with infected blood or blood products or by sexual contact. The highest concentrations of HBV are found in the blood; however, other body fluids such as semen, cervical secretions, saliva, and wound exudates contain lower concentrations of hepatitis B surface antigen (HBsAg). Parenteral exposure is the most efficient route of transmission, most often occurring in IV drug abusers sharing or using nonsterilized contaminated needles and health-care workers by accidental needle sticks. HBV can be transmitted from contact with contaminated inanimate objects because the virus is capable of living in the open environment for approximately 1 week. HBV is not transmitted via the fecal–oral route. The vast majority (90 percent) of acute HBV infections occurs in young adults, especially men. HBsAg-positive mothers may transmit HBV to their babies during childbirth. HBV is not spread through food, water, or casual contact. The average incubation period for HBV is 12 to 14 weeks but can be anywhere from 6 weeks to 6 months.

The mortality rate for acute HBV infection is 0.4 to 1 percent but is higher for superimposed hepatitis D. About 10 percent of patients infected with HBV develop chronic hepatitis. The risk of chronic infection with HBV is inversely proportional to the age when infection occurred. These patients are at an increased risk for cirrhosis and hepatocellular cancer. Infection with HBV is also associated with arthritis, glomerulonephritis, and polyarteritis nodosa.

Hepatitis C

HCV is a single-stranded RNA virus with at least 6 genotypes and an incubation period of 6 to 7 weeks. Transmission is similar to the routes for HBV, and before 1990, HCV was responsible for 90 percent of cases of post-transfusion hepatitis, but now only 4 percent of the cases of HCV infection are attributable to blood transfusion. IV drug use accounts for about 50 percent of HCV today. There is a small risk of sexual and maternal-neonate transmission but tends to be in patients with high circulating levels of HCV RNA. For many patients infected with HCV, the source is never determined. Most acute cases are undetected. Seventy to 90 percent of patients develop chronic hepatitis. Of this group, 20 percent progress to chronic liver disease, liver failure, or hepatocellular carcinoma.

Hepatitis D

HDV is a defective RNA virus that requires HBsAg for its replication. Only individuals with HBV are at risk for HDV. The major risk factor for HDV is IV drug use. Transmission is by the parenteral route and should be suspected in any HBsAg-positive person with acute or chronic hepatitis. New cases of HDV are uncommon in the United States today, probably because of widespread vaccination for HBV. Incubation is 1 to 6 months, and the mortality rate is 3 percent.

Hepatitis E

HEV, formerly called enterically transmitted non-A non-B hepatitis, is an RNA virus. HEV is responsible for water-borne hepatitis outbreaks and seen in endemic form in Southeast Asia, India, North Africa, and Mexico. There have been relatively few cases in the United States; however, with global travel, this will change. The illness is self-limiting and there is no carrier state. The incubation period is from 2 weeks to 2 months. The mortality rate is low except in pregnant women, in whom the mortality rate is 10 to 20 percent. Table 10.12 lists the features of hepatitis A, B, C, D, and E.

Hepatitis G

Hepatitis G is a flavivirus that is transmitted percutaneously. It is associated with a chronic viremic state that can last at least 10 years. It appears that coinfection with HGV improves the survival in patients with HIV infection. The virus has been detected in a small percentage of blood donors (1.5%), 50 percent of IV drug users, 30 percent of hemodialysis patients, and 20 percent of hemophiliacs. There is no evidence at this point that HGV causes liver damage.

Chronic Hepatitis

Chronic hepatitis, characterized by elevated aminotransferase (ALT, AST) levels for more than 6 months, occurs in 1 to 2 percent of immunocompromised adults with HBV and as many as 90 percent of neonates and infants with HBV. Chronic hepatitis occurs in up to 90 percent of the people infected with HCV. Cirrhosis develops in 40 percent of patients with chronic HBV, and 20 percent of those with chronic HCV are at high risk for developing hepatocellular carcinoma as well.

Pathophysiology

Hepatitis is an inflammation of the liver. It can result from a variety of causes. Viral hepatitis usually presents in one of three clinical manifestations; anicteric, icteric, or cholestatic. Despite the presentation, the progression of the disease follows the same pattern differing only in severity, enzymatic abnormality and possible outcomes. The pathologic lesions of hepatitis are similar to those caused by other viral infections. Regardless of the type of hepatitis causing the infection, all the liver acini cells are affected by patchy cell dropout, acidophilic hepatocellular necrosis, scarring, Kupffer cell hyperplasia, and mononuclear inflammatory infiltrate. The degree of cellular change is proportionate to the severity of infection. Hepatocellular injury is mediated by cell-mediated immune response. Cytotoxic T cells and natural killer cells play an important part by killing the infected cells and releasing inflammatory cytokines. An intense immune response can decrease the chance of chronic infection; however, it does foster development of hepatocellular necrosis. Histologic examination of tissue from livers infected with hepatitis demonstrate that even early on in the disease process regeneration has already started.

Normally, in patients infected with hepatitis the underlying reticulin network is preserved allowing for complete histologic recovery. If extensive necrosis of the bridging acini occurs, however, the inflammatory process can damage and obstruct the bile caniculi, causing cholestasis and obstructive jaundice. In most mild cases of hepatitis the liver parenchyma is not damaged; HBV and HCV tend to be the more severe forms of hepatitis, with histologic evidence of parenchymal inflammation and necrosis. Although the histological changes in the liver tissue are the same for each type of hepatitis, occasionally HBV can be diagnosed from the presence of "ground glass" hepatocytes caused by HBsAg-infiltrated cytoplasm and by using special staining techniques that detect certain viral components. These findings are most often associated with chronic HBV infection. The long-term, asymptomatic chronic-carrier state is thought to result from an immunologic tolerance to the hepatitis virus. The virus is not totally cleared by the immune system and the hepatocellular injury is minimal, leading to a lifelong asymptomatic carrier state. This carrier state is most common in infants, whose immune system is immature and may be unable to overcome the virus. This chronic-carrier state is associated with a 10- to 100-fold risk of hepatocellular carcinoma.

HCV causes hepatocellular injury through direct cytopathic invasion by the virus. The viral load is directly proportionate to the histologic inflammation seen on liver biopsy. HCV is capable of rapid mutation, which allows it to elude immunity by development of resistant strains to the existing antibodies. Autoimmune hepatitis is most commonly associated with HCV, lending itself to the multiple extrahepatic manifestations of the disease. These patients develop autoimmune responses leading to membranous glomerulonephritis, vasculitis, dermatitis, pulmonary fibrosis, and rheumatoid arthritis. Chronic HCV occurs in approximately 50 percent of the cases, with inflammatory changes leading to cirrhosis within 20 years.

Different drugs can cause different histopathologic abnormalities in the liver. For example, acetaminophen damages hepatocytes by producing toxic metabolites that damage the cellular and subcellular structures of the liver. Hepatic injury resulting from sepsis is caused by direct bacterial invasion of the parenchyma, circulating endotoxins, and hypoxia. Cytotoxic lymphocytes attack hepatocyte membrane antigens in autoimmune chronic active hepatitis. All of these agents result in varying degrees of hepatocyte injury.

Clinical Presentation

Subjective

The clinical presentation of viral hepatitis is extremely variable. It can vary from asymptomatic infection without jaundice to a sudden severe infection and death in a few days.

Table 10.12 **Key Features of Hepatitis A, B, C, D, and E**

Features	Hepatitis A (HAV)	Hepatitis B (HBV)	Hepatitis C (HCV)	Hepatitis D (HDV)	Hepatitis E (HEV)
Transmission	Fecal–oral, sewage, contaminated water, and shellfish and possibly blood	Percutaneous, permucosal through infected blood and body fluids, sexual	Percutaneous, community, a large percentage have no known risk factors	Percutaneous, but must have coinfection with HBV	Fecal-oral
Incubation period (days)	15–50 (average 20–37)	25–160 (average 60–110)	42–49	Same as for HBV	10–56
Laboratory tests	Anti-HAV IgM (acute); anti-HAV IgG (resolving)	HBsAg (confirms), IgM anti-HBs (acute phase), IgG anti-HBs (resolving/immunity), HBeAg, anti-HBe, anti-HBc (persists in carriers)	Anti-HCV appears in 6–37 weeks	Anti-HDV appears late	Anti-HEV IgM detected within 26 days of jaundice; IgG antibody persists
Immunity/immunization	45% of United States population has antibodies against HAV; HAV vaccine available	5%–15% of U.S. population has anti-HBs; HBV vaccine available	Unknown; no vaccine available	People immune to HBV are also protected against HDV	Unknown
Prevalence	Increasing in adults	Decreasing in the United States	4% of posttransfusion hepatitis; 50% IV drug users	Common in IV drug abusers	Rare in United States; endemic in Southeast Asia, India, North Africa, Mexico
Course/mortality	Does not progress to chronic state; mortality is 0–0.2% with fulminant hepatitis	Chronic liver disease occurs in 1%–5% of adults and 80%–90% in children; mortality is 0.3%–1.5%.	Chronic active hepatitis develops in 70%–90% of cases; 20% develop chronic liver disease; mortality is the same as for HBV	Chronic liver disease develops if present in chronic HBV; mortality is 2%–20% for acute icteric hepatitis	Does not progress to chronic liver disease; mortality is 1%–2% but as high as 10%–15% in pregnant women

Table 10.13 displays the clinical findings and corresponding laboratory values for the different phases of viral hepatitis.

Prodromal Phase. During the prodromal phase, the onset may be abrupt or insidious with anorexia, nausea, vomiting, malaise, upper respiratory infection, or flu-like symptoms. The patient may also complain of myalgia, arthralgia, and easy fatigability. Many patients report a distaste for smoking if they are smokers. Nausea and vomiting occur frequently. Diarrhea or constipation may be reported. In the early stage of acute HBV, skin rashes and arthritis may be seen.

Fever is usually present but rarely exceeds 103°F (39.4°C) except in HAV, in which it may go higher. Chills may mark an acute onset. A decrease in fever often coincides with the onset of jaundice.

Abdominal pain is usually mild and constant in the RUQ or epigastrium. The pain can be aggravated by jarring or exertion. It is occasionally severe enough to simulate cholecystitis or cholelithiasis.

Icteric Phase. During the icteric phase, jaundice and dark urine appear, usually 5 to 10 days after the initial symptoms, although some patients do not experience jaundice. With the onset of jaundice, the prodromal symptoms worsen and are followed by progressive clinical improvement.

Convalescent Phase. The convalescent phase is marked by an increased sense of well-being. The jaundice, abdominal pain and tenderness, and fatigability disappear and the appetite returns. Chronic HBV begins at this point in the case of chronic disease.

The acute illness usually subsides over 2 to 3 weeks. Complete clinical and laboratory recovery happens by the ninth week in HAV and after 16 weeks in HBV. Five to 10 percent of the cases may last longer, and less than 1 percent have an acute fulminant course. Hepatitis B and C may become chronic.

Hepatomegaly is present in 50 percent of the patients with viral hepatitis and splenomegaly is seen in 15 percent of the cases. Lymphadenopathy, especially in the cervical and epitrochlear areas, is commonly present. Signs of general toxemia may vary from minimal to severe. The clinical features of all the types of viral hepatitis are similar with the exception of onset. Hepatitis A and E usually have an abrupt onset, whereas hepatitis B, C, and D have a more insidious onset and the liver enzyme levels are higher. HVC is often asymptomatic.

Diagnostic Reasoning

Diagnostic Tests

Laboratory tests are used to diagnose, identify the serologic type, and determine the current status of the disease.

Hepatitis A. Two types of antibodies to HAV can be detected by radioimmunoassay (RIA) and ELISA. The first type of antibody to HAV is the IgM antibody (IgM anti-HAV), which appears about 4 weeks after exposure or just before hepatocellular enzyme elevation occurs and disappears in 3 to 6 months. Detection of IgM is the diagnostic test for acute hepatitis A. The second type of antibody, IgG anti-HAV, appears about 2 weeks after the IgM anti-HAV begins to increase and peaks after about 1 month of disease. The IgG antibody persists for more than 10 years and provides immunity. If the IgM is elevated in the absence of IgG, acute hepatitis is suspected. If IgG is elevated in the absence of IgM, this indicates previous exposure to HAV, noninfectivity, and immunity to recurring HAV infection.

Table 10.13 Clinical Findings: Viral Hepatitis

Stage	Subjective and Objective Complaints	Laboratory Tests
Incubation	None	HBsAg late in the stage HBeAg
Prodromal	Onset abrupt or insidious Anorexia, nausea, vomiting, malaise, upper respiratory infection (nasal discharge, pharyngitis), myalgia, arthralgia, easy fatigability, fever (HAV), abdominal pain	HBsAg in HBV
Icteric	Jaundice, dark urine, light-colored stools Continued prodromal complaints with gradual improvement	Anti-HBc Anti-HAV (IgG and IgM) Anti-HCV HBsAg becomes negative High urine bilirubin Markedly elevated ALT and AST Elevated LDH, bilirubin, alkaline phosphatase Marked increased PT indicates increased mortality
Convalescent	Increased sense of well-being Appetite returns Jaundice, abdominal pain, and fatigability abate	Anti-HAV IgG Anti-HBs Decreased liver enzymes

Hepatitis B. Acute and chronic HBV can be differentiated from other forms of viral hepatitis by serologic markers representing the body's immunologic response. The HBV is made up of an inner core surrounded by an outer capsule. The outer capsule contains HBsAg (hepatitis B surface antigen). The inner core contains the HBV core antigen (HBcAg). The hepatitis Be-antigen (HBeAg) is also found within the core. Antibodies to these antigens are called anti-HBs, anti-HBc, and anti-HBe.

Detection of HBsAg is diagnostic for HBV and is the first test to order when HBV is suspected; it will remain positive throughout the acute phase of the illness and if it persists longer, may indicate chronic hepatitis. HBsAg rises before the onset of clinical symptoms, peaks during the first week of symptoms, and returns to normal by the time the jaundice subsides. HBsAg indicates acute infection and infectivity. Anti-HBs appears about 4 weeks after the disappearance of the surface antigen and signifies recovery from the infection and noninfectivity as well as immunity.

There are no tests available to detect the HBV core antigen (HBcAg), but the IgM anti-HBc appears shortly after HBsAg is detected and can persist for 3 to 6 months. The anti-HBc level is elevated during the time lag between the disappearance of HBsAg and the appearance of anti-HBs; this interval is called the *core window.* During this window, anti-HBc is the only detectable marker of a recent hepatitis infection. Anti-HBs is composed of IgG and IgM antibodies. The IgM titer is diagnostic for acute hepatitis, whereas the IgG antibody is usually positive for life after infection.

HBeAg is generally not used for diagnostic purposes but rather as an index of viral replication and infectivity. The presence of HBeAg correlates with early and active disease and with high infectivity in patients with acute HBV infection. HBeAg appears during the incubation period shortly after the detection of HBsAg. The continued presence of HBeAg predicts the development of chronic HBV infection. Table 10.14 displays the serology testing and results for HBV infection.

Hepatitis C. The diagnosis of HCV is based on enzyme immunoassays (EJA or RIBA [recombinant immunoblot assay]) that detect antibodies to HCV (anti-HCV). Limitations of the enzyme immunoassay include moderate sensitivity for the diagnosis of acute HCV (false-negative) and low specificity (50 percent) in healthy blood donors and some people with elevated gamma-globulin levels (false-positive). In these particular cases, a diagnosis of HCV may be confirmed by use of a polymerase chain reaction (PCR) to detect HCV RNA. The risk of transfusion-associated HCV has decreased from 10 percent in the early 1990s to less than 0.1 percent today as a result of the testing of donated blood for HCV.

Hepatitis D. Diagnosis of HDV is by detection of anti-HDV or HDV RNA in the presence of hepatitis B markers. Rising titers of anti-HDV indicate acute infection and are detectable early in the disease.

Hepatitis E. HEV is diagnosed by history and exclusion of other causes. There is no antigen or antibody test currently available for the accurate serologic identification of HEV.

Additional Testing. In any patient in whom hepatitis is suspected, liver enzyme levels should be checked for signs of injury. Elevated aminotransferases are the hallmark of all forms of acute hepatitis. AST is usually markedly elevated early in hepatitis. ALT is often very elevated early in hepatitis, as is LDH. All of these hepatocellular enzymes are elevated during the acute and chronic active phase of hepatitis. AST and ALT levels fluctuate during the course of the disease for unknown reasons. Bilirubin and the alkaline phosphatase are usually elevated and may remain elevated after the AST and ALT have normalized.

The WBC count is normal or low, especially in the preicteric phase. Large atypical lymphocytes may occasionally be seen and are similar to those found in infectious mononucleosis. Mild proteinuria is common, and there is bilirubinuria just preceding and during the icteric phase. The prothrombin time may be prolonged in severe hepatitis and signifies increased mortality. Liver biopsy is rarely indicated unless there is evidence of liver damage from a chronic state of hepatitis.

Table 10.14 **Serologic Testing for Hepatitis B**

Interpretation	HBsAg	Anti-HBs	HBeAg	Anti-HBe	Anti-HBc
Acute hepatitis (confirms diagnosis)	+	−	+	−	IgM
Acute hepatitis	−	−	+ or −	−	IgM
Recovery from hepatitis (immunity)	−	+	−	+ or −	IgG
Vaccination (immunity)	−	+	−	−	−
Chronic HBV with active viral replication	+	−	+	−	IgG
Chronic HBV with low viral replication	+	−	−	+	IgG

Differential Diagnosis

Differential diagnosis for hepatitis includes other viral diseases that affect the liver, such as infectious mononucleosis, cytomegalovirus infection, and herpes simplex virus. Drug- or toxin-induced liver damage should be included in the differential diagnosis list as well. Conditions that cause jaundice must also be included in the differential diagnosis of hepatitis.

Management

The principle of the management of hepatitis includes prevention of transmission and symptomatic relief. Vaccinations are available to prevent HAV and HBV. Vaccination against HAV is recommended for people living or traveling to endemic areas and prevents infection for at least 20 years. Immune globulin is recommended for close contacts of people with HAV within 2 weeks of exposure because it may prevent or lessen the severity of the disease.

HBV vaccine is recommended for people with high-risk factors, such as health-care workers, day-care workers, IV drug users, male homosexuals, household contacts of HBsAg carriers, heterosexual contacts of HBsAg carriers, people with anticipated multiple transfusions, and patients undergoing dialysis.

Treatment for hepatitis, no matter what the cause, is largely supportive. Patients rarely require hospitalization. Balanced nutrition with adequate calories and fluids is recommended, and avoidance of alcohol is stressed. Activity is generally restricted during the acute phase and during a relapse with gradual resumption of activity.

Treatment of chronic HBV is currently intramuscular interferon alfa-2b in a dose of 5 million units per day or 10 million units 3 times a week. Candidates include patients with compensated liver disease, persistent elevated ALT, detectable HBsAg and HBeAg, low concentrations of HBV DNA, and fibrosis seen on liver biopsy. The response rate after this expensive therapy, however, is about 40 percent.

HCV causes chronic hepatitis and liver damage. Treatment with peginterferon and ribavirin in the acute phase decreases the risk of chronic hepatitis. This treatment has a high sustained viral response rate (SVR) for those infected with genotype 2 or 3 and a liver biopsy is not necessary. However, SVR is not as good in persons with genotypes 1a, 1b, and 4. Pegylated interferon is a slow release, long acting drug that is given once a week in a dose of 180 mg for 48 weeks has been shown an SVR in 38 percent of patients that already have chronic hepatitis C. SVR in patients that have genotype 2 or 3 is about 80 percent. The goals of treatment include clearing the viremia, improving symptoms, slowing the progression to cirrhosis, and decreasing the risk of primary hepatocellular carcinoma.

Response to therapy is judged by an ALT returning to normal by 12 weeks and negative viral markers (HCV RNA). After the ALT has returned to normal, treatment is slowly discontinued. Consuming alcohol increases the risk of these patients progressing to cirrhosis and liver failure, so abstinence from all forms of alcohol (including in medications) is especially important.

Hepatic transplantation is indicated for patients with advanced liver disease as a result of chronic HCV and in fact, it is the most common reason for liver transplantation in the United States.

Follow-Up and Referral

Any patient diagnosed with HCV should be referred to a hepatologist for follow-up because the chance of developing chronicity is great with this type of hepatitis. Patients with HAV usually do not require follow-up. Patients with HBV should be seen in 1 month and should have blood drawn for HBsAg after 6 months. Persistent elevation of HBsAg indicates a chronic state, and these patients should be referred to a hepatologist.

Patient Education

Patients and their intimate contacts should be given careful instructions about the cause of hepatitis, the mode of transmission, and measures to prevent the transmission. It is recommended that household contacts and sexual contacts be given passive immunity (immunoglobulin) for HAV and HBV as well as active immunization. Hand washing and personal hygiene can help prevent the spread of the disease. Patients should also be taught not to share personal items such as toothbrushes, razors, and eating utensils during the period of infectivity. Patients with chronic hepatitis or a carrier state should be instructed to practice safe sex.

Patients who develop chronic liver disease as a result of hepatitis can contact the American Liver Foundation at www.liverfoundation.org.

Cirrhosis and Liver Failure

Cirrhosis is the end result of hepatocellular injury involving the entire liver, resulting in fibrosis and nodular regeneration, and represents permanent and irreversible damage. Fibrous bands are formed during nodular regeneration in an attempt by the liver to repair itself and give the liver a hobknobbed appearance. The fibrotic changes that occur within the liver parenchyma cause disruption and compression of the vascular, biliary, and lymphatic vessels and result in many of the characteristic findings common to liver failure. Cirrhosis and fibrosis are not synonymous terms; fibrotic changes are characteristic findings of cirrhosis.

Epidemiology and Causes

In the Western Hemisphere, cirrhosis is a leading cause of death in individuals older than age 40. Although there are many causes of cirrhosis (Table 10.15), chronic alcohol abuse remains the leading pathological insult in the United States.

Table 10.15 Causes of Cirrhosis

Alcohol
Direct hepatotoxins
- Carbon tetrachloride
- Phosphorus

Indirect hepatotoxins
- Tetracycline
- Methotrexate

Acetaminophen
- Mushroom toxin-*Amanita phalloides*
- Alkylated anabolic steroids
- 6-Mercaptopurine

HBV and HCV
Autoimmune chronic active hepatitis
Diabetes mellitus and insipidus
Thyroiditis
Ulcerative colitis
Glomerulonephritis
Biliary cirrhosis
Primary biliary cirrhosis
Primary sclerosing cholangitis
Chronic pancreatitis
Sclerosing cholangitis
Vasculitis
Cholelithiasis
Cystic fibrosis
Genetic diseases
- Wilson's disease
- Hemochromatosis
- Galactosemia

Vascular/congestive disorders of the liver
- Budd-Chiari syndrome
- Ischemic hepatitis/shock liver
- Right-sided heart failure (chronic)

Alcoholic cirrhosis, also known as Laennec's, portal, fatty, or micronodular cirrhosis, is the most common type of cirrhosis in the United States. An estimated 18 million people in the United States abuse alcohol, but only 25 percent of alcoholics develop cirrhosis. It is estimated that more than 30,000 people in the United States alone die from liver disease caused by alcohol abuse each year. Men are affected three times more often than women.

Alcoholic cirrhosis is often associated with nutritional and vitamin deficiencies but occurs in well-nourished individuals as well as alcoholics. Studies have found no safe amount of alcohol that can be ingested daily without causing cirrhosis, which supports the theory that there are additional factors (genetic, environmental, nutritional) that may influence the development of alcoholic liver disease. Women tend to develop cirrhosis more quickly with less alcohol intake than men, which suggests that a smaller, leaner body mass and enhanced absorption are both factors in the development of alcoholic cirrhosis.

There are three consequences of alcohol abuse: fatty liver, alcoholic hepatitis, and alcoholic cirrhosis. Alcoholic hepatitis results from moderate to severe alcoholic abuse for years and can lead to alcoholic cirrhosis quickly even with abstinence, but it is not an obligatory phase in the development of cirrhosis.

Primary biliary cirrhosis (PBC) is a disease that almost exclusively affects women between the ages of 40 and 60. It is an autoimmune disease that causes destruction of the intrahepatic bile ducts resulting in cholestasis. Autoimmune disorders such as scleroderma, Raynaud's syndrome, autoimmune thyroid disease, celiac disease and Sjögren's syndrome have been linked to the development of PBC.

Primary sclerosing cholangitis (PSC) is most common men between the ages of 20 and 40 and is associated with IBD as well as with the histocompatible antigen HLA-B8, -DR3 and –DR4, suggesting a genetic link. It is characterized by diffuse inflammation and fibrosis throughout the biliary tree. Factors contributing to the development of PSC are anything that obstructs or inhibits the flow of bile through both the extrahepatic and intrahepatic bile ducts. Smoking is associated with a *decreased* risk of PSC.

Budd–Chiari syndrome (BCS) is a disorder resulting from hepatic vein thrombosis and outflow obstruction, which can occur anywhere from the hepatic veins to the inferior vena cava (IVC) or the right atrium. Other disease processes associated with this form of cirrhosis are coagualopathies, lymphoreticular malignancies, ischemic hepatitis resulting from profound hypotension associated with shock, and liver arteriovenous malformations (AVMs) characteristic of hemorrhagic telangiectasia. There are numerous causes for BCS, and definitive diagnosis is found in only approximately 65 to 75 percent of cases. In the Western Hemisphere, thrombosis of the hepatic veins is most often associated with myeloproliferative and coagulation disorders as well as oral contraceptive use. Venous thrombosis is also an associated risk factor in the third trimester of pregnancy. Malignant tumors arising from within the liver or metastatic renal carcinoma can result in mechanical obstruction of the inferior vena cava (IVC), causing thrombosis within the hepatic veins and resulting in cirrhosis.

Wilson's disease and hemochromatosis are both autosomal recessive metabolic disorders that often present with hepatocellular dysfunction and can lead to cirrhosis if left untreated. The liver is the primary organ involved in the metabolism of both iron (hemochromatosis) and copper (Wilson's disease); overload of either metal can cause cirrhosis. Hemochromatosis is diagnosed primarily in middle-aged whites, whereas Wilson's disease is a disease of adolescents and young adults.

Pathophysiology

Cirrhosis is the irreversible, end stage of liver injury caused by a variety of insults. Fibrotic scarring and hepatocellular changes result from chronic inflammation, obstruction, toxic, metabolic, and congestive injuries. The morphologic changes resulting from the injury are often classified according to the size of the regenerative nodules: Patients may have micronodular, macronodular, and mixed forms of cirrhosis. The liver can develop cirrhosis as a result of severe acute injury, as is seen with hepatitis; or subsequent to moderate damage sustained over months, as seen with obstructive biliary diseases; or from chronic continuous abuse as seen in alcoholic cirrhosis.

With cirrhosis, the normal lobular liver architecture is replaced by diffuse disorganization, resulting in proliferation of bands of fibrous tissue and nodular regeneration of the surviving hepatocytes. The extent to which this occurs depends on the degree of injury, the length of exposure to the injury, and the liver's reaction to the insult. The end result is a decrease in the total liver cell mass because of the collagen formation or fibrosis. During the repair process, there is distortion of the microcirculation, resulting in an increased resistance to blood flow and thereby causing portal venous hypertension. As the liver attempts to repair itself, it develops a series of collateral vessels from the newly regenerated nodules to the existing portal vein and hepatic artery. These vessels, which are much less efficient than those of the normal circulation, cause portal hypertension.

Histologic classification of cirrhosis is useful for describing the major anatomic changes that result from the various insults. This type of classification gives no etiologic information other than narrowing the scope to those injurious agents resulting in this specific histologic category of injury. Moreover, it is important to remember that at any point in the disease process, a patient may exhibit varying degrees of histologic change.

Micronodular (Laennec's) cirrhosis is characterized by regenerative nodules that are 1 cm in diameter or less, no bigger than normal liver lobules. Histologic examination fails to identify portal tracts and hepatic venules. Alcohol abuse often results in this type of cirrhosis; the theory being that there is continuous damage being done to the liver, preventing it from regenerating. Initially the liver becomes enlarged and fatty as changes in lipid metabolism lead to fatty infiltrates. As the disease progresses, the liver atrophies and hardens. Fibrous tissue forms in thin, regularly spaced bands throughout the liver, which in time result in a decreased liver mass.

Macronodular cirrhosis is characterized by larger nodules (diameters of 5 cm), which may be multinodular with varying size nodules and may contain central veins. These nodules are surrounded by broad fibrous bands of varying thickness, which correspond to postnecrotic types of cirrhosis as seen following hepatitis. As the normal liver architecture collapses, the portal tracts converge between the fibrous scars, which is a key histological finding. *Mixed cirrhosis* has characteristics of both micro- and macronodular cirrhosis.

Drug-induced liver disease can be the result of the drug's metabolism itself or a combination of several drugs together. The resultant liver toxicity may be caused by metabolism that is enhanced, altered, or the result of idiosyncratic processes such as hypersensitivity or certain genetic makeups. Intrinsic hepatic injury is drug-dose dependent, whereas idiosyncratic drug reactions are more frequent and are not dose dependent. Patients who have hypersensitivity reactions to a drug develop hepatotoxicity secondary to the formation of drug metabolites, which are harmful to the liver.

PBS and PSC are both chronic cholestatic liver diseases that affect adults. There is a immunologic component to both diseases that causes inflammation and fibrosis, which ultimately results in bile duct destruction. Liver biopsy in patients with PBC is of limited value because the disease varies from portal tract to portal tract; biopsy is, however, helpful to validate cirrhotic changes. The beginning stages of PSC are characterized by portal infiltration of lymphocytes, plasma cells, macrophages, and eosinophils. These inflammatory changes are followed by "ductular proliferation," which is characterized by the replacement of mature bile ducts with small, ineffective ones. The inflammatory changes lead to fibrosis and as fibrotic changes ensue, increased signs of cholestasis appear. The end result of these changes is cirrhosis.

Primary sclerosing cholangitis can involve any part of the biliary tract from the ampulla of Vater to the small bile ducts within the liver. The lumens of these ductal systems can be narrowed or completely obstructed by fibrous scar tissue resulting in the key functional abnormality, which is cholestasis. The biopsy results show fibrosis with inflammatory changes as described for PSC. Bacterial infections that often occur in the area above the strictures and in the presence of longstanding disease lead to biliary cirrhosis.

The pathophysiology of liver disease caused by hereditary factors is essentially the same for both Wilson's disease and hereditary hemochromatosis. Wilson's disease results from decreased hepatic excretion of copper and excessive absorption of copper from the small intestine. There is a gradual accumulation of copper within the tissues, resulting in hepatotoxicity. Initial presentation of Wilson's disease may vary from acute hepatitis or chronic hepatitis, neuropsychiatric disease, cirrhosis, or fulminant hepatic failure in young adults. Histological examination of the initial lesions reveal hepatic steatosis, with increased glycogen deposits. These lesions eventually progress to fibrosis and finally cirrhosis.

Hereditary hemochromatosis is characterized by increased intestinal absorption of iron. Liver biopsy reveals increased iron deposition, predominantly within the hepatocytes. When levels of iron exceed 20,000 μg/g of liver tissue, fibrosis and cirrhosis usually ensue.

Vascular causes of liver disease, which include BCS and congestive hepatopathology, cause cirrhosis as the end result of necrosis. Liver biopsies show centrilobular congestion, hemorrhage, necrosis, and dilatation. The resultant disruption of the hepatic circulation causes portal hypertension, fibrosis of the surrounding tissues, and ultimately cirrhosis.

Clinical Presentation

Cirrhosis is often an incidental finding on an annual exam, revealed either by an asymptomatically enlarged liver or an elevation of the liver enzymes. The clinical manifestations of cirrhosis are the result of hepatocellular damage and portal hypertension. The cumulative effect of these signs and symptoms is often referred to as "the stigmata of liver disease." The onset of symptoms is usually gradual, and patients with cirrhosis may appear well and remain asymptomatic for years.

Subjective

Initial complaints generally include weakness, anorexia, weight loss, and fatigue. Malnutrition is usually evident and can be the result of anorexia or the effect of reduced bile salt excretion, resulting in fat malabsorption and deficiency of fat-soluble vitamins.

As cirrhosis advances, patients may present with upper GI bleeding from esophageal varices, which develop secondary to portal hypertension. As the liver continues to fail, patients may present with ascites and/or encephalopathy. Patients with cirrhosis may complain of abdominal pain that is caused by the enlargement of the liver and stretching of Glisson's capsule or by the ascites itself.

Menstrual abnormalities, loss of libido, impotence, sterility, and gynecomastia are manifestations of increased levels of estrogen that result from the liver's inability to inactivate hormones. These symptoms may prompt individuals to seek medical attention. Previously undiagnosed cirrhosis is often the underlying cause of symptoms in patients presenting with one of the aforementioned complaints.

Objective

The physical exam findings depend on the stage and severity of the disease process. Initial exam findings may reveal an enlarged firm liver edge (which is the left lobe) palpable below the right costal margin; however, in patients with advanced disease the liver may be small and difficult to palpate. Often, a firm smooth mass is palpable over the epigastric area, which is the right lobe of the liver (Reidel's lobe). Occasionally nodular deformities may be palpable along the liver edge. These areas of liver enlargement are dull to percussion and can aid in measuring the expanse of the liver.

Manifestations of cirrhosis that are nonspecific but suggestive of chronic liver disease include spider nevi, which are normally found over the anterior chest; pectoral alopecia; generalized muscle wasting; Dupuytren's (palmar) contractions; parotid gland enlargement; palmar erythema; hair loss; and testicular atrophy. Patients may have dilated cutaneous veins called caput medusae radiating out from around the umbilical area. These varicose veins are a result of the shunting of blood to the paraumbilical veins and are a manifestation of portal hypertension. Signs of vitamin and mineral disturbances are glossitis, cheilosis, and peripheral neuropathies. Fever may indicate complications such as peritonitis, cholangitis, or hepatitis.

Jaundiced sclera, skin, and mucous membranes usually develop in the later stages of cirrhosis. The hyperbilirubinemia is a consequence of the liver's inability to conjugate and excrete bilirubin. Patients with hereditary hemochromatosis may have slate-colored skin from increased levels of iron stored in the tissue. Pruritus, although nonspecific, is often the presenting symptom in several forms of cirrhosis and can develop as a result of bile salts accumulating in the skin. Disruption in the liver's ability to synthesize clotting factors may manifest with bruising and complaints of a tendency to bleed. Peripheral edema results because of the decreased plasma osmotic pressure caused by hypoalbuminemia.

Ascites is a direct result of portal hypertension, which is a consequence of increased portal vein pressure. As liver function fails and healthy hepatic cells are replaced with fibrous nodules, the blood flow through the liver is impaired, causing increased resistance and back pressure that result in the accumulation of serous fluid within the abdomen. An abdominal exam reveals a positive fluid wave as well as shifting dullness on percussion. Splenomegaly results from splenic vein congestion. Esophageal varices, another consequence of portal hypertension, may be discovered after bleeding causes hematemesis, hematochezia, and/or melena. Hemorrhoids, which result from portal hypertension, are also present and cause bright red bleeding from the rectum.

Hepatic encephalopathy can range from mild confusion to coma and is the result of increasing blood ammonia, which is toxic to the brain. Characteristics of encephalopathy include asterixis (liver flap), reversal of sleep–wake patterns, tremors, hyperactive deep-tendon reflexes, dysarthria, delirium, and drowsiness.

Patients who present with Wilson's disease may have golden brown rings of color—called Kayser–Fleischer rings—located within Descemet's membrane of the cornea. These rings are usually found in patients with CNS involvement and are seen with a slit lamp.

Diagnostic Reasoning

Diagnostic Tests

Results of initial laboratory testing varies depending on the stage of the disease process. If cirrhosis is in the early stages, laboratory results may be normal; however, in other patients, elevation of liver enzymes may be the only indicator of liver disease. Laboratory testing may reveal abnormalities but these are nonspecific unless correlated with the history and physical examination.

Alcoholic cirrhosis may manifest in different ways depending on other coexisting processes such as malnutrition or hepatitis. The CBC commonly shows a macrocytic anemia and, depending on the severity of the disease, pancytopenia from the overall suppression of the bone marrow.

The mean corpuscular volume does not correct quickly with abstinence from alcohol and may be the only key to occult alcohol use. Anemia can represent suppression of erythropoiesis from folic acid deficiency, occult losses from the GI tract, or a combination of the two. The white cell and platelet counts can vary depending on whether there is infection or splenic sequestration. As the liver continues to fail and liver cell mass decreases, the prothrombin time (PT) increases as the liver loses the ability to synthesize the proteins necessary to produce clotting factors.

The blood chemistry may show mild to moderate increases in ALT and AST levels; if, however, the patient has a superimposed alcoholic hepatitis, the classic enzyme elevation of ALT/AST may be reversed, with an AST/ALT ratio ranging from 2:1 to 3:1. The levels of AST/ALT do not reflect the severity of the disease process. The GGT level is a good measurement of recent alcohol ingestion and declines rapidly with abstinence. Alkaline phosphatase levels may be markedly elevated when there is biliary obstruction. Serum bilirubin levels can be as high as 30 mg/dL. Hypoalbuminemia is common and contributes to the development of edema.

The diagnosis of alcoholic cirrhosis may be difficult to differentiate from alcoholic hepatitis, which is a reversible process, unless a liver biopsy is obtained. Histological examination reveals hepatocellular necrosis and evidence of Mallory bodies within the damaged cells. Depending on the stage of the disease, there is fatty infiltration and fibrosis. In early disease, there are micronodular changes, which over time develop into macronodular cirrhosis.

Abdominal ultrasound is helpful in determining the size of the liver and any ascites or nodule formation. Doppler studies, in combination with US, are used to evaluate patency of the venous system, which, if disrupted, can lead to portal hypertension. Any nodular findings that are suspicious for malignancy should be biopsied. If a patient presents with melena or hematemesis, an esophagogastroscopy should be performed to assess for esophageal varices or ulcerative processes.

Diagnosis of cholestatic liver disease, specifically PBC and PSC, may be made in conjunction with various autoimmune disease processes. The initial hepatic blood workup usually shows an alkaline phosphatase level that is three to four times normal, with mild to moderate increases in the transaminases. The cholecystatic nature of both processes leads to prolonged PT.

Patients with PBC may also present with mild elevation of serum bilirubin and more often hypercholesterolemia. Serum IgM levels are elevated in 50 percent of cases. Antimitochondrial antibodies (AMAs) are found in 95 percent of the patients with PBC; titers can exceed 1:500. Definitive diagnosis is made via liver biopsy, which reveals granulomatous bile duct destruction and accumulation of inflammatory cells within the portal tracts with resultant segmental necrosis of the interlobular and septal bile ducts (chronic nonsuppurative destructive cholangitis). Ultrasonic evaluation of the biliary tree is negative for biliary obstruction.

Laboratory studies of patients with PSC show the typical cholestatic profile; however, unlike with patients with PBC, the AMA is negative. Total cholesterol levels increase as the disease progresses. Endoscopic or transhepatic cholangiography reveals characteristic beading and stricturing of the intra- and extrahepatic bile ducts. Liver biopsy is diagnostic for fibrous obliterative cholangitis, with the hepatic ductal system being replaced with fibrous cords of connective tissue. The end result for both PBC and PSC is biliary cirrhosis.

Diagnosis of cirrhosis caused by vascular disorders such as BCS and other veno-occlusive diseases is normally made through imaging studies because laboratory findings are nonspecific. Serum bilirubin, transaminases, and alkaline phosphatase can be elevated as much as four times normal. A CT scan demonstrates failure of the hepatic veins to opacify, indicating an occlusive process. Pulsed Doppler studies illustrate absent hepatic flow; a normal pulsed Doppler effectively rules out BCS. Venographic studies also demonstrate narrowing and obstruction of the hepatic venous system. Histologic examination reveals centrilobular congestion with associated hemorrhage and necrosis.

Wilson's disease and hemochromatosis are inherited metabolic liver diseases that result in cirrhosis if diagnosis and treatment are not made early. Diagnosis of Wilson's disease is suggested by elevated serum copper levels in conjunction with low serum ceruloplasmin levels. Once an abnormal ceruloplasmin level has been documented, a 24-hour urine check for copper should be completed. Definitive diagnosis is made through quantitative copper levels in the liver on biopsy. The majority of patients with Wilson's disease have histologic findings consistent with hepatic steatosis, which in time progresses to fibrosis and cirrhosis.

Iron metabolism studies are used to diagnose hereditary hemochromatosis and should be collected with the patient in the fasting state. The presence of an elevated transferrin saturation level in combination with an elevated ferritin level is suggestive of hereditary hemochromatosis. Liver biopsy is necessary for definitive diagnosis. Histologic studies with quantitative iron levels greater than 20,000 μg/g are consistent with advanced disease and cirrhosis.

Differential Diagnosis

The patient who presents with cirrhosis can be a diagnostic challenge. The differential diagnosis of cirrhosis varies little between the different etiologies, so the challenge is determining the cause in an attempt to prevent further liver damage. The differential diagnosis of alcohol-induced liver disease includes biliary tract disease, idiopathic hemochromatosis, nonalcoholic fatty liver disease, drug toxicity, and/or viral hepatitis. Ultrasonic examination of the liver can often rule out obstructive process. Alcoholics with chronic pancreatitis frequently develop jaundice secondary to stricturing of the common bile duct, which is differentiated through ERCP. A liver biopsy is often the only definitive test for differentiating many of the hepatobiliary diseases from each other. Thorough history and physical examination can suggest a diagnosis, but histologic study is necessary to distinguish one process from another.

Alcoholic patients also have a high incidence of coinfection with hepatitis, the cause of which is often unclear; this can alter the typical serological findings. A hepatitis panel will reveal active or prior infection. Drug toxicity, specifically with acetaminophen, even in low doses, can alter transaminase levels and necessitates obtaining a careful drug history from each patient. Because of the preexisting liver injury, alcoholics who present with acetaminophen toxicity have significantly higher morbidity and mortality with relatively low doses of acetaminophen.

The differential diagnosis of cholestatic liver disease must include all other causes of chronic cholestasis, such as tumors, strictures, or obstructions resulting from stone formation. Autoimmune chronic active hepatitis can mimic the signs and symptoms of PBC; however, laboratory studies will show a low or negative titer for AMA. Ultrasonic examination may reveal biliary duct dilatation, a process consistent with both PBS and PSC, thus making cholangiography the diagnostic test of choice.

Management

Treatment of cirrhosis is aimed at identifying and removing the causative agent and treating the symptoms.

Alcohol-Induced Liver Disease

In a patient with alcohol-induced liver disease, the most effective treatment remains abstinence. Patients who continue to ingest alcohol and present with ascites can increase their 2-year survival rate to 95 percent if they can completely abstain from alcohol. Those who continue to drink have a 2-year survival rate of less than 25 percent. The liver has a remarkable regenerative potential, and despite slow progress the patient can become functional if he or she is motivated to remain abstinent. Nutritional assessment with dietary supplementation to ensure adequate caloric intake (25 to 35 kcal/kg body weight/day) is imperative because many patients with alcohol-induced liver disease are also malnourished. Protein intake should be increased to 1 to 1.5 gram per kilogram of body weight per day unless there is evidence of hepatic encephalopathy, which necessitates a reduction in protein intake. Daily vitamin and mineral supplementation is also indicated: Specifically, patients should receive a multivitamin, B_{12}, folate, thiamine, magnesium, and zinc supplementation. Patients who continue to show clinical deterioration despite abstinence can be considered for liver transplantation, provided they have remained alcohol-free for more than 6 months.

Treatment of Complications

Many of the complications of alcohol-induced liver disease are the direct result of the development of portal hypertension and include ascites, hepatic encephalopathy, anemia, hemorrhage, spontaneous bacterial peritonitis, hepatorenal syndrome, hepatopulmonary syndrome, and hepatocellular carcinoma. Table 10.16 presents the treatment of these complications. Portal hypertension is the result of disruption of the hepatocellular circulation causing an increase in portal venous pressure. As the liver becomes progressively more cirrhotic, there is development of collateral venous circulation to overcome the increased resistance to blood flow. The collateral circulation that develops between the portal and systemic circulation, specifically the azygos vein, is a much weaker system and results in dilated, tortuous vessels commonly known as varices. Development of varices within the esophagus and submucosa of the gastric fundus predispose patients to hemorrhage when the portal pressure gradient is greater than 12 mm Hg.

Irreversible, Chronic Liver Disease

Liver transplantation is the treatment of choice for irreversible chronic liver disease. Patients with cirrhosis, hepatitis C, primary biliary cirrhosis, primary sclerosing cholangitis, alcoholic liver disease, autoimmune hepatitis, and genetic disorders of the liver are diseases for which transplantation has been successful. Five-year survival rates are documented as high as 80 percent with the advancement in surgical techniques and immunosuppressive agents such as cyclosporine and tacrolimus (FK506). Contraindications to transplantation include malignant hepatobiliary processes, sepsis and advanced cardiopulmonary disease. In cases of hepatitis B and C, the virus can infect the new liver.

Primary Biliary Cirrhosis

Treatment of primary biliary cirrhosis (PBC) is symptomatic. Pruritus is often the most aggravating manifestation of PBC. Cholestyramine (Questran) or colestipol relieves itching in patients with cholestasis by lowering serum bile acids and increasing the intestinal secretion of bile by preventing its resorption. The usual dose is 4 g or 5 g respectively in water or juice tid until the pruritus has been controlled, and then the dosage is decreased to that which maintains control of the symptom. Rifampin (Rifadin), 150 to 300 mg bid has been beneficial in relieving pruritus in some cases, and ondansetron, a 5-HT3 serotonin receptor antagonist, shows promise as well.

Fat-soluble vitamin deficiency occurs with the onset of steatorrhea and can be enhanced with the administration of cholestyramine. Vitamins A, D, E, and K can be replaced orally. Laboratory studies will reveal vitamin K deficiency as a prolonged PT. The deficiency can be treated with 5 to 10 mg of vitamin K PO; subsequent monitoring of the PT will indicate whether therapy is adequate. Overdosage of vitamin A can cause hepatotoxicity, so

(Text continued on page 532)

Table 10.16 Complications of Alcohol-Induced Liver Disease

Portal Hypertension and Variceal Hemorrhage

Portal hypertension is the result of disruption of the hepatocellular circulation causing an increase in portal venous pressure. As the liver becomes progressively more cirrhotic, there is development of collateral venous circulation to overcome the increased resistance to blood flow. The collateral circulation that develops between the portal and systemic circulation, specifically the azygos vein, is a much weaker system and results in dilated, tortuous vessels commonly known as varices. Development of varices within the esophagus and submucosa of the gastric fundus predisposes patients to hemorrhage when the portal pressure gradient is greater than 12 mm Hg.

The most common site of variceal hemorrhage is from within the esophagus and can be life threatening, with a mortality rate of approximately 50%. Patients with a massive acute hemorrhage require immediate attention to prevent hemodynamic instability and shock. Endoscopic examination can help identify the site of the bleeding and allows for banding or sclerotherapy, the treatments of choice for acute variceal bleeding. Pharmacologic intervention includes intravenous infusion of vasoconstricting agents that assist in decreasing portal pressures. Octreotide causes reduced splanchnic and hepatic blood flow and is effective in reducing portal pressures. Octreotide (Sandostatin) can be infused at 50 to 250 μg/h. A combination of band ligation or slerotherapy and octreotide is the most effective treatment for bleeding varices. Patients who have failed both endoscopic and pharmacologic intervention require emergent insertion of a Sengstaken-Blakemore tube for balloon tamponade of the bleeding variceal site. The risk for aspiration, esophageal rupture, or rebleed is great, and patients normally require inten-sive care monitoring.

Some patients may benefit from surgical placement of a portacaval shunt or more recently placement of a transjugular intrahepatic portosystemic shunt (TIPS). Both procedures are performed to decrease portal hypertension but are associated with a high operative mortality rate especially if performed on an urgent basis. Portacaval shunts are effective in reducing esophageal bleeding but carry an associated risk of developing postshunt encephalopathy and hepatic failure of about 50% and eliminates the possibility for future hepatic transplantation.

The risk of rebleeding from esophageal varices is about 70%, so patients should be placed on preventative therapy. The most well-known pharmacologic intervention is the initiation of a nonselective beta-blocker such as propranolol (Inderal) or nadolol (Corgard) to reduce portal pressure. Dosages of propranolol can range from a starting dose of 40 mg bid up to a total daily dose of 200 mg. The goal of treatment is to reduce the resting heart rate by 25% but not below 60 beats/min. The usual contraindications to beta-blocker therapy must be considered before initiation of therapy. Also, any patient with known alcohol-induced cirrhosis should have beta-blocker therapy as tolerated to decrease the risk of initial variceal bleed.

Prevention of recurrent bleeding can also be accomplished using sclerotherapy or variceal banding. Although both procedures are equally effective, endoscopic banding is associated with lower complications from ulcers or strictures than sclerotherapy. Surgical decompression of the portal system by shunt insertion or TIPS procedure can also be performed to reduce the risk of future variceal bleeding. Complications resulting from these procedures include hepatic encephalopathy, infection, shunt stenosis, and shunt occlusion.

Ascites

Ascites, the excess accumulation of serous fluid within the peritoneal cavity, is associated with unfavorable outcomes. Abdominal paracentesis should be performed and the ascitic fluid analyzed for cell count, culture, and albumin level. The serum albumin level minus the ascitic albumin level equals the serum-ascites albumin gradient (SAAG). A SAAG level greater than 1.1 g/dL is highly suggestive of portal hypertension but offers no information regarding the cause of the ascites. Ascites results from a combination of increased hydrostatic pressure (portal hypertension), decreased oncotic pressure (hypoalbuminemia), peripheral vasodilatation probably mediated by nitric oxide released from the splanchnic vasculature, volume expansion resulting from a disturbance in the renin-angiotensin system with subsequent sodium and water retention, and impaired activation of aldosterone by the liver.

Ascites can be clinically observed on physical examination when 1000 mL or more of fluid has accumulated within the abdominal/peritoneal cavities; smaller amounts are detectable with the use of ultrasound. Shifting dullness to percussion and a positive fluid wave are two findings consistent with the diagnosis of ascites.

Treatment of ascites begins with sodium restriction of 400-800 mg/day. The goal of treatment for the patient with ascites and peripheral edema is a daily weight loss of approximately 1 pound; if fluid is mobilized too quickly it can further impair renal function by causing a prerenal azotemia. Treatment of ascites includes daily monitoring of weight, serum electrolytes, and renal function. Patients who present with ascites and have hyponatremia (serum levels less than 125 mEq/L) need fluids restricted to 800-1000 mL/day. Although some patients respond with sodium and water restriction, diuretic therapy is usually required. Spironolactone (Aldactone), a potassium-sparing, aldosterone antagonist, is started at 100 mg/day and increased by 100 mg/week until diuresis is achieved or a maximum dose of 400 mg/day is reached. Adverse effects include painful gynecomastia and hyperkalemia. If effective diuresis has not been achieved, then a loop diuretic is added. Furosemide (Lasix) is started at 40 mg/day and is titrated up to 240 mg/day as necessary.

Approximately 10% of patients with cirrhosis are resistant to diuretic therapy despite spironolactone 400 mg/day and furosemide 160 mg/day. These patients have persistent tense ascites and may also develop azotemia with creatinine levels greater than 2.0 mL/dL as a result of the intense diuretic regime. The treatment for this "intractable" ascites is a large-volume paracentesis, but the practitioner must first determine whether the patient is adhering to the medical regime, especially sodium restriction. If a large-volume paracentesis is necessary, up to 4 to 6 L of fluid can be removed per procedure. Intravascular volume expanders can be infused simultaneously to prevent hemodynamic instability secondary to removal of large volumes of ascitic fluid. Large-volume paracentesis is often the treatment of choice, because it requires a shorter hospital stay and has fewer complications in comparison to diuretic therapy with regard to electrolyte imbalance and renal insufficiency.

The procedure can be performed daily until ascites is resolved, and then the patient can be maintained on diuretic therapy. The two major complications of paracentesis are spontaneous bacterial peritonitis (SBP) and hepatorenal syndrome.

Spontaneous Bacterial Peritonitis

Spontaneous bacterial peritonitis is a common complication of cirrhosis that can be fatal. Patients may present with abdominal pain, increasing ascites, fever, and progressive encephalopathy. Definitive diagnosis is made by paracentesis. The gold standard for the diagnosis of SBP is a total white cell count of greater than 300 cell/μL with a polymorphonuclear neutrophil (PMN) cell count of greater than 250/μL. The protein concentration is usually less than 1 g/dL. Gram-negative bacilli are the causative pathogen in 70% of SBP, with *Escherichia coli* being isolated in 50% of the cases. Gram-positive organisms are isolated in approximately 25% of the cases, and infection with anaerobic organisms is rare due to the high oxygen content of the ascitic fluid. Because the mortality rate for untreated SBP is 50%, initiation of treatment is suggested before culture results are obtained. Cefotaxime (Claforan) is a broad-spectrum, third-generation cephalosporin and is considered the treatment of choice for SBP. The usual dose is 2 g IV q8h for 5 days. Post-SBP prophylaxis can be accomplished with norfloxacin 400 mg/day.

Hepatorenal Syndrome

Hepatorenal syndrome is a terminal complication frequently associated with advanced liver damage and is almost always found in patients with advanced ascites. The syndrome is characterized by oliguria, hyponatremia, azotemia, low urine sodium (less than 10 mEq/L), and hypotension. The hallmark to diagnosis is a disproportionate rise in creatinine with respect to the blood urea nitrogen (BUN). Histologically, the kidneys are normal, and diagnosis is often one of exclusion. Individuals with decompensated cirrhosis and ascites can precipitate hepatorenal syndrome after large-volume paracentesis, aggressive diuresis aimed at decreasing ascites, or sepsis. Patients are often misdiagnosed with prerenal failure and the only way to differentiate between the two is through insertion of a central venous catheter and assessment of venous pressures. Treatment includes restoring the intravascular volume and avoiding any procedures that will dramatically disturb the patient's volume status, such as large-volume paracentesis and aggressive diuresis. The definitive treatment of patients with hepatorenal syndrome is liver transplantation.

Hepatic Encephalopathy

Hepatic encephalopathy, also known as portosystemic encephalopathy, is a complex process involving a change in mental status resulting from the failure of the liver to detoxify elements of gut origin and shunting of this blood from the portal to the systemic circulation and then to the brain. Nitrogenous agents such as ammonia are believed to enter into the CNS by way of shunted blood resulting in disturbances in neurological function. Although ammonia is thought to be the sole toxin responsible for hepatic encephalopathy, the serum levels do not correlate with the degree or presence of encephalopathy.

The diagnosis of hepatic encephalopathy is made clinically and often follows an event such as increased dietary protein, GI bleeding, constipation, infection, deterioration in hepatic function, hypokalemia, azotemia, alkalosis, and hypovolemia. Physical exam findings include an altered mental status such as personality (mood) changes, decreased reaction time, and intellectual deterioration as well as neuromuscular dysfunctions such as asterixis or metabolic flap, absence of fixed sensory or motor deficits, and hyperreflexia. Other findings include fetor hepaticus (garlic odor of the breath caused by exhalation of sulfur-containing mercaptans), hyperthermia, and hyperventilation. Obtaining a fasting arterial blood ammonia level or a spinal fluid glutamine level can be helpful in confirming the diagnosis of hepatic encephalopathy although they are not necessary.

Treatment of hepatic encephalopathy begins with identification and treatment of factors that precipitate encephalopathy in patients with liver disease.

- GI Bleeding. Increases production of ammonia and other nitrogenous toxins.
- Increasing Dietary Intake of Protein. Provides building substrate for formation of nitrogenous toxins in the intestine.
- Diuretic-Induced Problems. Overdiuresis causes in creased circulation of urea and ammonia production. Hypovolemia resulting in hypokalemia and alkalosis enhances the transfer of ammonia across the blood-brain barrier.
- Constipation. Decreases transit time within the intestine, which enhances contact time with ammonia-forming bacteria in the colon.
- Drugs Causing CNS Depression. Impaired liver function causes alteration in degradation and may accumulate, causing further depressant effects.
- Infection. Increases catabolism and production of nitrogenous toxins.

For instance, GI bleeding and diets high in protein provide the basic elements for formation of ammonia and other nitrogenous compounds from the action of bacteria in the gut, which can induce or aggravate the symptoms of encephalopathy. Colonic bacteria responsible for the formation of ammonia and other nitrogenous compounds can be reduced by administering oral neomycin (Mycifradin Sulfate Oral, Neo-Tabs Oral) 0.5 to 1.0 g q4-6h for 5 to 7 days. Lactulose (Cephulac, Heptalac) is a non-absorbable synthetic disaccharide, which, when digested by intestinal bacteria, is fermented and causes acidification of the colon contents. The lower stool pH binds the ammonia in the colon, rendering it nonabsorbable. Lactulose also changes the bowel flora so that there are fewer ammonia-forming bacteria. The initial dose of lactulose is 30 mL three to four times daily and is titrated until the patient has two or three softly formed stools daily.

Iron Deficiency Anemia

Iron deficiency anemia is a common finding in alcoholics. It can be treated with ferrous sulfate taken tid after meals. To avoid the constipating effect of iron, a stool softener can be given as well. If there is evidence of a macrocytic anemia, the patient may benefit from 1 mg of folic acid daily.

Hepatopulmonary Syndrome

Hepatopulmonary syndrome is a recently recognized pulmonary complication of cirrhosis and portal hypertension, which manifests through abnormal arterial oxygenation. The diagnosis is made when there is intrapulmonary dilatation in the absence of other morphological pathology. The results are reversible with liver transplantation.

dosage must be individualized based on serum levels and response to treatment.

Patients with PBC often have associated osteoporosis, which has no known treatment. If patients have been diagnosed with PBC and have osteomalacia, calcium supplementation with 500 mg tid and vitamin D replacement once weekly is indicated.

Several immunosuppressive agents including corticosteroids, methotrexate, and azathioprine and the antifibrinogenic colchicine have been effective in reducing elevated serum alkaline phosphatase and bilirubin levels. Ursodeoxycholic acid (ursodiol), a choleretic, acts by stimulating excretion of bile by the liver, is much less toxic, and has been effective in reducing symptoms and improving long-term survival.

Surgical reconstruction of the biliary tract, choledochoduodenostomy, and choledochojejunostomy are palliative treatments that alleviate the symptoms of PBC. If there is notable stricturing within the biliary tree, patients often do well with stenting. Liver transplantation for advanced PBC is the treatment of choice.

Hemochromatosis and Wilson's Disease

Two important but treatable inherited metabolic causes of cirrhosis are hemochromatosis and Wilson's disease. Early diagnosis and treatment is key to the management of hereditary hemochromatosis (HHC) and begins with liver biopsy for definitive diagnosis. If treatment is initiated in the precirrhotic phase, the disease can be controlled with weekly phlebotomies of 1 unit (500 mL) of blood, which contains approximately 250 mg of iron. This process is continued until there is depletion of the iron stores (which can be 2 years or more). Every 2 to 3 months iron metabolism studies monitor the patient's progress. Once the iron stores are depleted, when serum ferritin levels fall below 50 ng/mL and transferrin saturation is less than 50 percent, patients can be maintained with periodic phlebotomies. Patients who are exhibiting cardiac symptoms may require the use of iron-chelating agents such as deferoxamine. Administered intramuscularly, it increases the urinary excretion of iron up to 5 to 18 g annually. Phlebotomy decreases the cardiac conduction defects and lowers insulin requirements. Patients should be instructed to consume a low-iron diet that eliminates foods such as red meat, and they should avoid alcohol, vitamin C, raw shellfish, and any supplement containing iron. Patients may require specific treatment of diabetes mellitus, heart disease, arthropathy, hypopituitarism, and portal hypertension, all complications due to HHC. Patients whose disease has progressed to cirrhosis must be monitored for hepatocellular carcinoma either by liver ultrasound or measurement of α-fetoprotein levels. Because the disease is inherited, screening of all first-degree relatives is necessary.

Wilson's disease is also an inherited disease that, if diagnosed and treated early, can prevent the development of neurologic or hepatic damage. Treatment includes both dietary and medicinal components. Limiting dietary intake of copper (legumes, animal organs, and shellfish) should become a lifelong habit. The administration of oral penicillamine (Depen) 0.75 to 2 g/day in divided doses induces the urinary excretion of chelated copper. If GI upset or hypersensitivity prohibits the use of penicillamine, trientine (Syprine) 250 to 500 mg tid can be substituted. Oral administration of zinc 50 mg tid as maintenance therapy also promotes excretion of copper in the feces. Patients who are receiving penicillamine, an antimetabolite of vitamin B_6, should receive pyridoxine (supplemental vitamin B_6) 50 mg/week. Liver transplant is the treatment of choice for patients with cirrhosis or fulminant hepatitis. Siblings and family members should be screened for the disease.

Vascular or Congestive Liver Disorders

Management of patients who present with vascular or congestive liver disorders, such as those with BCS and other hepatic occlusive diseases, is essential. Because of the many causes of BCS, initial treatment must begin with finding and treating the cause of the hepatic congestion. Hepatic vein thrombus is difficult to manage and requires a multidisciplinary approach including a hematologist, surgeon, hepatologist, and gastroenterologist. Ascites is initially managed with sodium restriction and diuretics; however, over time this is usually ineffective and most patients will require large-volume paracentesis or shunting for symptomatic relief.

If diagnosis of acute thrombus is made early, thrombolytic therapy can be instituted and long-term anticoagulation with Coumadin can help prevent further thrombus formation. Surgical decompression shunting for refractive ascites can delay development of hepatic failure or cirrhosis but often results in graft thrombus. Patients with associated myeloproliferative diseases and hypercoagulopathies may benefit from low-dose aspirin therapy and chemotherapy as directed by a hematologist.

Follow-Up and Referral

Any patient with advanced liver disease should be referred to a hepatologist or gastroenterologist trained to treat the disease and the subsequent complications. All patients require referral for liver biopsy to establish a definitive diagnosis. It is the responsibility of the practitioner to recognize the onset of the disease process and obtain all the necessary testing in order to provide the most complete information to the accepting consultant. Patients with end-stage liver disease should be referred to a liver transplant facility. Patient follow-up can be shared between the primary-care practitioner and the consulting physician. Patients with chronic or advanced liver disease will require indefinite monitoring of their liver function tests as well as their fluid and electrolyte status. Maintaining good nutrition is an important component of treatment of any disease process. Patients with advanced liver disease may benefit from consultation with a registered dietitian, who can review dietary restrictions and help patients understand how to achieve a balanced diet.

Patient Education

Patients with hepatic failure should be taught to check their weight daily as a way to monitor increasing fluid retention and ascites, which may indicate a developing complication. Patients with cirrhosis have a life-threatening terminal disease; therefore, attention must be given to promoting psychological well-being. Patients should be provided with education regarding medications to avoid to prevent further hepatotoxicity, such as acetaminophen (Tylenol), vitamin A, cocaine, tetracycline (Sumycin), phenytoin (Dilantin), and ethyl alcohol. Patients with liver failure should always ask their health-care provider about the potential liver toxicity of each of their medications. Patients with hepatic encephalopathy should avoid CNS depressants, which might intensify their lethargy or fatigue. These patients may also require education about the need for self-administering enemas if they become constipated, in order to decrease the time for bowel absorption of nitrogen-based compounds. All patients with ascites must be informed of the signs and symptoms of infection, which may indicate developing spontaneous bacterial peritonitis.

Abdominal Hernias

An abdominal hernia is the protrusion of a peritoneally lined sac through some defect or weakened area in the abdominal wall. There are several different types of hernias, which are usually classified by the anatomical location of the protrusion.

Epidemiology and Causes

It is estimated that up to 10 percent of the population has some form of hernia. *Groin hernias* are the most common type and are classified as *indirect inguinal hernias,* which are responsible for 50 percent of hernias treated; *direct inguinal hernias,* which represent 25 percent of hernias seen; and *femoral hernias,* which represent 10 percent of hernias. Hernias occurring through the anterior abdominal wall are called *ventral hernias;* these account for only 15 percent of all hernias. Ventral hernias are further broken down into epigastric hernias (5 percent), incisional hernias (5 percent), and umbilical hernias (3 percent).

Groin hernias are by far the most common type of hernia and occur in both men and women. Indirect inguinal hernias are the most common and occur in both genders, although they are frequently seen in young men. Direct inguinal hernias are more common in men older than age 40 and are caused by a congenital abnormality. Femoral hernias occur more often in women than men and are rare in children.

The recurrence rate of hernias in general is about 10 percent, with direct and indirect hernias having a recurrence rate that is approximately equal. The subsequent recurrence rate of recurrent hernias is much higher, at 35 percent.

Ventral hernias include all other hernias of the anterior abdominal wall. Epigastric hernias are much more common in men than in women and are multiple in 25 percent of the cases. The peak age of incidence is age 20 to 50. Umbilical hernias are considered a normal occurrence in newborn infants, with about 20 percent of infants being affected. These hernias are more common in males of all ages and in African Americans of either gender. The presence of an umbilical hernia is considered normal until the child reaches the age of 2. Incisional hernias are considered the only iatrogenic type of herniation. Approximately 2 to 11 percent of all patients undergoing abdominal surgery develop incisional hernias. Women are affected twice as often as are men.

Hernias occur because there is sufficient pressure to force tissue out through a defect in the abdominal wall as well as a potential space for that protrusion. The etiology of hernias is multifactorial, with biological, congenital, and environmental influences contributing to their development.

Pathophysiology

In general, for any type of groin hernia to occur, two of the body's protective mechanisms must be overcome. The first of which is called the *shutter mechanism,* whereby the internal oblique muscle and the transversus abdominis muscles contract to overlap, strengthening the posterior wall of the inguinal canal. Second, a *closure* or *sphincter-type mechanism* causes contraction of the musculature, displacing the transversalis fascia, which in effect decreases the diameter of the deep inguinal ring.

Indirect Inguinal Hernias

Indirect inguinal hernias result when tissue herniates through the internal inguinal ring, which extends the length of the spermatic cord. With continued pressure, the sac can actually reach the scrotum, where it is then palpable just proximal to Hesselbach's triangle. The pathophysiology of indirect inguinal hernias in most cases begins with the herniation of tissue through a still-patent vaginal process that remains after the descent of the testes. In women, the vaginal process exists within the canal of Nuck. Indirect inguinal herniation is caused by a combination of this congenital defect and a disruption in the functioning of the sphincter mechanism as a result of a variety of environmental conditions, including increased abdominal pressure and trauma to the area.

Direct Inguinal Hernias

Direct inguinal hernias occur when the transversus abdominis and internal oblique muscles are attached, forming a high arch on the inferior border that results in a faulty shutter mechanism. Any environmental factors that increase abdominal pressure enhance the chance of herniation. As with indirect inguinal hernias, the presence of this congenital defect does not explain why herniation is more common later in life.

Femoral Hernias

Femoral herniation occurs at the fossa ovalis where the femoral artery exits from the abdomen. It is presumed to be caused because women have a larger femoral canal and smaller iliopsoas muscles. Other factors that contribute to femoral herniation are femoral engorgement during pregnancy and the size of the female pelvis.

Epigastric Hernias

Epigastric hernias occur along the midline between the xiphoid process and the umbilicus. The fibers along the linea alba are brought together in a patch-work type closure; the defect exists within this decussation. As these fibers weaken, the contents can herniate through the abdomen. Epigastric hernias are three times more likely to occur in men than in women. Peritoneal fat, bowel, and omentum are the most common abdominal contents to protrude through the wall.

Umbilical Hernias

Umbilical hernias that develop in adulthood occur through a weakening in the abdominal wall around the umbilical ring. The herniation of abdominal contents through this defect is also dependent on environmental factors that increase intra-abdominal pressure. Of particular importance when diagnosing an umbilical hernia is to look for underlying ascites secondary to liver disease.

Incisional Hernias

Incisional hernias can occur anywhere along a surgical incision into the abdomen. They are classified into those that cannot be controlled by surgical technique and those that can be controlled by surgical technique. Controllable factors include the type of incision chosen and choice of suture and surgical techniques. Factors that are considered uncontrollable include the prior medical history of the patient, age, steroid use, nutritional status, obesity, and surgical complications of the surgery, especially wound sepsis.

Clinical Presentation

Subjective

In any patient presenting with an abdominal hernia, the provider must determine whether there is an abnormal increase in intra-abdominal pressure that has contributed to the herniation. A thorough history and physical exam, with special attention to the genitourinary, respiratory, and GI systems, will provide clues. All male patients who present with an abdominal hernia, regardless of age, require a prostate examination to determine if there is any obstructive process inhibiting urinary output, which in effect increases intra-abdominal pressure. Patients should be evaluated for ascites, which also increases intra-abdominal pressure.

Patients who have respiratory difficulty, such as obstructive pulmonary disease processes, have an increased risk of hernia because of the increased abdominal pressure associated with coughing and the downward expansion of the diaphragm found with hyperinflated lungs.

Objective

The presentation of inguinal hernias is not always obvious and is quite often an incidental finding on routine exam. Patients may present with complaints of pain while straining or lifting heavy objects or a swelling in the groin area. In general, the physical examination for all groin hernias begins with visual inspection of both groins as well as the genitalia. With the patient standing, the spermatic cord is located on both sides and is palpated for any swelling into the scrotum. Once the inguinal canal has been palpated, three additional areas must be examined. After invaginating the scrotal sac, the examining finger follows the spermatic cord up to the external inguinal ring and the fascia of the external oblique muscle. The posterior wall is inspected for weakness or bulging and the inguinal ring is also palpated for structural soundness. Once these areas have been examined, the provider then withdraws the finger slightly and the patient is asked to cough, which increases the intra-abdominal pressure. If the provider feels the presence of a tissuelike sac tapping against the finger, then hernia is present. Other findings indicative of herniation are feeling a rush of fluid (peritoneal) under the examining finger or a patient's report of pain. In a female patient, the femoral areas are palpated while the patient increases intra-abdominal pressure by performing the Valsalva maneuver. Any bulging in the area is considered a positive finding.

Once a groin hernia has been diagnosed, the practitioner must determine whether the hernia is incarcerated or strangulated, both of which require immediate surgical attention, or whether a more chronic situation is present, which can be cared for electively. Most often this can be determined by patient history as well as the physical ability to reduce the hernia on examination. A strangulated hernia is a nonreducible herniation in which the blood supply to the herniated tissue is compromised. An incarcerated hernia is a hernia that has caused a bowel obstruction as a result of the protrusion.

An indirect inguinal hernia presents as a soft swelling within the internal ring, when either provoked or unprovoked, and often descends into the scrotum. A direct inguinal hernia presents as a bulge in the area of Hesselbach's triangle (Fig. 10.1). Direct inguinal hernias are usually painless and easily reducible. The hernia bulges anteriorly, pushing against the side of the examining finger. Femoral hernias are more common on the right side and may be accompanied by severe pain. There is a palpable bulge through the femoral ring and the inguinal canal is empty. Normally, it is the intestine that has herniated through the abdominal wall.

Epigastric hernias are normally asymptomatic and present as a small bump or bulge along the midline above the umbilicus. There may be variation in size with increasing

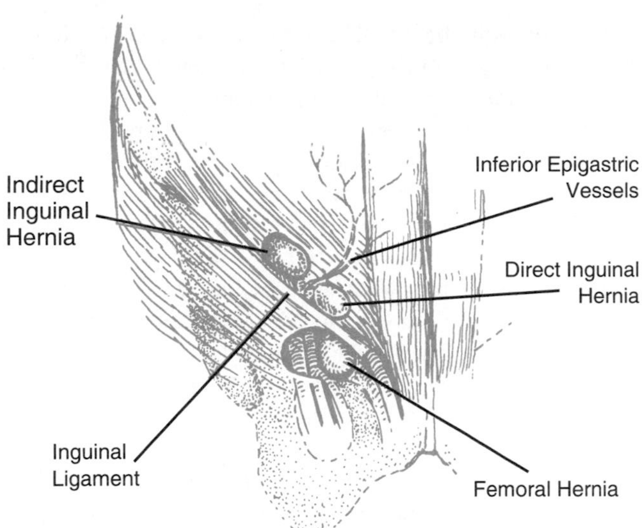

FIGURE 10.1 Locations of indirect and direct inguinal and femoral hernias. Anterior view of the groin, showing locations of indirect inguinal hernia, direct inguinal hernia, and femoral hernia, based on anatomic landmarks. (Source: Kozol, AK, et al: When to Call the Surgeon: Decision Making for Primary Care Providers. FA Davis, Philadelphia, p 170, with permission.)

intra-abdominal pressure. Peritoneal fat, omentum, and bowel are usually the tissues that herniate through the abdomen. The smaller hernias tend to be more painful because they involve the herniation of the preperitoneal fat, which is irritating. Larger hernias must be examined for incarceration and obstruction.

Incisional hernias manifest along the incision line of a previous abdominal operation and can be painful. Patients with incisional hernias may also have signs and symptoms of bowel obstruction, which are discussed in the Bowel Obstruction section of this chapter.

Diagnostic Reasoning

Diagnostic Tests

Hernias are diagnosed almost exclusively by physical examination findings, as described in the preceding text. On occasion, a radiographic study is necessary to determine if an obstructive process is taking place. Other studies, such as pulmonary function testing or evaluation of a mass or lesion within the abdomen, may be indicated to assess the cause and/or extent of increased intra-abdominal pressure.

Differential Diagnosis

The differential diagnosis list for hernia is limited. It includes hydrocele, psoas abscess, femoral adenopathy or inguinal adenopathy, and ectopic testis.

Management

When a hernia is detected, the patient should be referred to a surgeon. Despite the evolution of hernia repair over the century, the underlying principles remain the same: reinforce the two natural defense mechanisms discussed previously; decrease the size of the inguinal ring; and strengthen the posterior wall of the canal. Repair of femoral hernias is accomplished by reducing the size of the canal, whereas repair of indirect hernia is accomplished by dissecting the hernial sac and reduction of the repaired tissue. Frequently, there is not sufficient tissue to reconstruct and strengthen the posterior wall of the canal and synthetic mesh materials are used. Laparoscopic surgery has decreased the recovery time and allowed for a single intervention for bilateral hernia repair. All ventral hernias should be repaired to decrease the possibility for incarceration.

Postoperatively, the patient may experience incisional pain, which is relieved by oral analgesics. Pain that persists for more than a few days suggests impending wound infection. Normally, there is slight postoperative swelling, ecchymosis, and erythema of the skin, up to the scrotal area in male patients. Hernia repair with significant scrotal involvement may result in increased scrotal edema, which can be relieved with ice packs, elevation, and wearing a scrotal support. In female patients, swelling is usually limited to the surgical site but may extend to the labia and vulva.

Follow-Up and Referral

All patients with abdominal hernias require surgical consultation, whether emergently or electively, and appropriate referral should be made. The patient is usually seen in the surgeon's office 3 to 7 days after surgery.

Patient Education

Following typical groin surgery, the patient is allowed to return to normal activities, including work, after about 1 week but is instructed to avoid heavy lifting or contact sports for at least 4 to 6 weeks. Patients who have undergone laparoscopic repair of groin hernias are allowed to resume regular activities, including heavy lifting, as soon as 2 days postprocedure. Patients who have had a ventral hernia repair should follow routine postoperative instruction as directed by the surgeon.

Appendicitis

The appendix is a fingerlike projection located at the apex of the cecum just below the ileocecal valve. It has no known function in humans; however, it is thought to have some immunologic function, based on the amount of lymphoid tissue it contains. The appendix fills with food, just as the cecum does, but, because the lumen of the appendix is smaller, it has a tendency to become obstructed. Appendicitis is the inflammation of the variform appendix caused by an obstruction and/or infection. It is the most common cause of acute RLQ abdominal pain requiring surgical intervention. Acute appendicitis results in more than 200,000 appendectomies annually.

Epidemiology and Causes

Appendicitis can occur at any age; however, it is most common between ages 10 and 30. It is rare in infants and in older adults and is often associated with higher morbidity within these age groups because of delayed diagnosis and intervention. During the peak incident years, men are twice as likely to be diagnosed with appendicitis as are women, but the occurrence in both genders tends to equalize over the life span. It is estimated that appendicitis will affect 10 in 100,000 people in the United States, with a lifetime risk for individuals projected at 7 to 10 percent.

Appendicitis is more common in Western countries, where people have diets that are low in fiber, high in fat, and high in refined sugars and other carbohydrates. Obstruction of the appendix by a variety of pathological processes is the cause of the majority of appendicitis. Other contributing factors include intra-abdominal tumors and positive family history. Recent roundworm infestation or viral infection of the GI tract have also been implicated.

Pathophysiology

Appendicitis typically begins with dilatation of the appendix, followed by obstruction and subsequent bacterial infection. When the lumen of the appendix is obstructed by hardened feces (fecalith), inflammatory processes (including parasites, viruses, or bacteria), strictures, neoplasms, or foreign bodies (including vegetable or fruit seeds or barium), the mucosa of the appendix continues to secrete fluid, which further distends the lumen, impairing the venous blood flow and leading to tissue necrosis. Left untreated, this increased distension impedes arterial inflow. Bacteria continue to proliferate and, in the absence of treatment, perforation of the appendix occurs. The incidence of perforation in patients with appendicitis is between 17 and 40 percent, with rates as high as 60 to 70 percent in older adults because of the nonspecific presenting symptoms.

Clinical Presentation

Subjective

The diagnosis of acute appendicitis is made clinically and is based primarily on the patient's history and physical examination. The historical presentation of signs and symptoms are important keys to prompt diagnosis and treatment; therefore, it is important to obtain a thorough and accurate account of the events. The classic presentation of appendicitis begins with the acute onset of mild to severe colicky, epigastric, or periumbilical pain. The pain is often vague at first, but within 24 hours usually it shifts and localizes over the RLQ and is exacerbated by walking or coughing. In male patients the pain may radiate into the testicles; pain (rigidity) also may be associated with abdominal muscle spasm in male or female patients. Most patients complain of nausea and anorexia after the onset of pain, which may or may not be associated with vomiting. If vomiting is present, the patient usually reports that abdominal pain was present before vomiting began. The sensation of constipation is typical, although diarrhea is present in some patients.

A mildly elevated temperature of 99 to 100°F is common. If the patient with RLQ pain presents with shaking chills (rigors), perforation of the appendix should be suspected. An important point to remember is that the very young and older adults may have an atypical presentation, which can mimic other less acute disease processes. For example, older adults with appendicitis may present with weakness, anorexia, abdominal distension, and mild complaints of pain. A delay in the diagnosis in this age group has led to an associated increase in morbidity and mortality.

Objective

On physical examination, the patient may or may not look toxic, depending on the degree of pain and other symptoms. The patient may have hypertension and tachycardia proportionate to the degree of fever and pain. When the patient is lying recumbent, the client may flex up the right knee in order to relieve the tension on the iliopsoas muscle, which overlies the appendix. Palpation of the abdomen early in the process may reveal diffuse tenderness over the umbilicus and midepigastric areas. As the process progresses, the tenderness localizes over the RLQ and may be accompanied by guarding. Guarding is defined as the voluntary contraction of the abdominal muscles in anticipation of examination, as opposed to rigidity, which is caused by the involuntary reflexive spasm of the muscles of the abdominal wall. Rebound tenderness is tested by placing the palmar aspect of the hand on the abdomen and pressing hard enough to depress the peritoneum. This may cause the patient pain, but the clinician should keep the abdomen depressed with constant pressure until the patient becomes accustomed to the pressure and the pain decreases. Then, without warning, the clinician should remove the hand suddenly, preferably when the patient's attention is directed elsewhere. If positive for rebound tenderness, the patient will grimace in pain, which is a more reliable sign than a subjective complaint of pain. Asking the patient to cough helps to localize exactly from where the pain is coming. Advanced Assessment 10.1 outlines exam maneuvers that aid in the diagnosis of appendicitis.

A rectal examination can be performed, but it is open to greater subjective interpretation. Patients with appendicitis will normally perceive greater tenderness and fullness on the right than on the left during the rectal exam. The provider must keep in mind that both the bowel as well as the appendix are mobile organs; they can shift posteriorly or suprapubically, causing altered exam findings. Bowel sounds are a nonspecific finding—they may be present, absent, or decreased in patients with appendicitis.

Other physical exam findings can include alterations in vital signs consistent with increased pain, such as tachycardia or elevated blood pressure. Patients may be reluctant to take a deep breath for fear they will cause themselves pain.

ADVANCED ASSESSMENT 10.1

Physical Examination Maneuvers for Diagnosing Appendicitis

Maneuver	Examination	Comments
Rovsing's sign	Deep palpation over the LLQ with sudden, unexpected release of pressure.	This causes tenderness over the RLQ and is considered a positive finding.
Psoas sign	The patient is instructed to try to lift the right leg against gentle pressure applied by the examiner or by placing the patient in the left lateral decubitus position and extending the patient's right leg at the hip.	An increase in pain is considered positive and is an indication of the inflamed appendix irritating the psoas muscle.
Obturator sign	With the right hip and knee flexed, the examiner slowly rotates the right leg internally, which stretches the obturator muscle.	Pain over the RLQ is considered a positive sign and indicates irritation of the muscle by the inflamed appendix.
McBurney's sign	Pressure is applied to McBurney's point, which is located halfway between the umbilicus and the anterior spine of the ilium.	Pain when pressure is applied to this area is considered a positive response.

If there is perforation of the appendix, there may be a sudden cessation of the pain, which is considered an emergency. Findings consistent with peritonitis include diffuse abdominal tenderness with rigidity. The patient may exhibit signs of septic shock, with marked leukocytosis, fever, and hemodynamic instability.

Diagnostic Reasoning

Diagnostic Tests

Laboratory findings are not diagnostic and are nonspecific, so they must be used in combination with data from the history and physical exam. The CBC usually reveals a mild to moderate leukocytosis (WBC 10 to 20,000 μg/L) with a left shift. Urinalysis show microscopic hematuria or pyuria in 25 percent of patients. Women should have a urine human chorionic gonadotrophin (hCG) test completed to rule out (ectopic) pregnancy. The lack of laboratory findings should not preclude the diagnosis of appendicitis.

No radiologic exam is of diagnostic importance early in appendicitis, but x-ray studies become more important as appendicitis progresses. A chest x-ray film rules out pneumonia as a source of abdominal pain and is necessary as part of the preoperative procedure in most hospitals. Plain x-ray films of the abdomen may show evidence of a fecalith, a gas-filled appendix, small bowel ileus, a deviation in the bowel gas pattern, or a loss of the right iliopsoas shadow. Any of these findings are suggestive of appendicitis when combined with a suspect history and physical exam.

A CT of the abdomen is helpful in ruling out other diagnostic possibilities, as well as determining if there has been perforation of the appendix or development of a periappendiceal abscess. An abdominal US helps to visualize the inflamed appendix and is also useful in ruling out other potential diagnoses. Diagnostic laparoscopy may be considered in female patients to rule out ectopic pregnancy, tuboovarian processes, or pelvic inflammatory disease (PID).

Differential Diagnosis

The differential diagnoses of appendicitis include a host of problems, which include, but are not limited to, urinary tract infection (UTI), ectopic pregnancy, ovarian cyst, pneumonia, gastroenteritis, Crohn's disease, diverticulitis, mesenteric adenitis, pancreatitis, PID, and cholelithiasis. If the diagnosis of appendicitis remains questionable after the history and physical examination have been completed and initial lab work has been obtained, then radiographic studies are helpful in ruling out many of the processes found within the differential diagnoses. For women of childbearing age, the clinician should always obtain a pregnancy test before ordering any radiographic studies. In some cases, laparotomy or laparoscopy may be required to assist in definitive diagnosis.

Careful attention must be given to the sexual and menstrual history of all female patients because of the myr iad of potential gynecological problems that present with the same signs and symptoms as appendicitis. A pelvic exam and a diagnostic laparotomy are often necessary for differential diagnosis.

Many GI disorders have symptoms that mimic those of appendicitis, and watchful waiting may be indicated in some cases. If appendicitis is at all a suspicion, however, the prudent practitioner will follow these patients closely until a diagnosis has been reached.

Management

The treatment of appendicitis is surgical; therefore, once a definitive diagnosis is made, prompt referral to a surgeon should be made. The high percentage of unnecessary appendectomies is still considered acceptable in lieu of the morbidity and mortality associated with perforation. The incidence of appendiceal perforation ranges from 17 to 40 percent in patients with appendicitis; it is as high as 60 to 70 percent in older adults. With effective treatment the mortality is less than 1 percent; however, in the older adult population, mortality remains at 5 to 15 percent.

Preoperative management includes correction of fluid and electrolyte imbalances; bed rest; NPO, with placement of a NG tube if indicated; and IV antibiotics. Narcotics should be avoided if possible because they mask any developing symptoms that might indicate a complication such as perforation. Laxatives are contraindicated in patients with appendicitis because they may cause the appendix to rupture. Stool softeners may be given if the patient is complaining about constipation and diarrhea is not present.

Third-generation cephalosporins are the antibiotics of choice. If there has been perforation and peritonitis is suspected, antibiotic coverage for both gram-negative aerobic and anaerobic organisms is recommended. Some of the choices include ampicillin, gentamicin, clindamycin, metronidazole (Flagyl), ampicillin-sulbactam (Unasyn), and ticarcillin/clavulanate (Timentin).

Patients are normally discharged the same day as surgery unless there are complications. Early ambulation is encouraged, with progression to full activity as soon as possible. Diet is advanced when bowel sounds return. The patient is given standard postoperative guidelines for individuals who have had abdominal surgery.

Follow-Up and Referral

The patient is normally followed by the surgeon, who will see the patient 5 to 7 days postoperatively to remove the sutures. If there was perforation of the appendix and the patient must remain hospitalized, the surgeon will follow the patient until discharge.

Patient Education

The patient will be given standard postoperative instructions from the surgeon, which should include a return to the hospital if anorexia, nausea, vomiting, abdominal pain, fever, or chills develop. Patients should understand that they are not to do any heavy lifting for at least 2 weeks.

Inflammatory Bowel Disease

Inflammatory bowel disease (IBD) is the term used to describe a chronic immunologic disease that manifests in intestinal inflammation. The disease is characterized by exacerbations and remissions that are experienced throughout an individual's lifetime and therefore result in significant disruption in the quality of life. The Patient's Voice 10.1 describes the impact of CD on a 39-year-old woman with a 20-year history of the disease.

Ulcerative colitis (UC) and Crohn's disease (CD) are both inflammatory bowel diseases that share similar characteristic and causes, but are considered two separate diseases. UC involves only the mucosal surface of the colon, which ultimately results in friability, erosions, and bleeding. It is also known as regional enteritis because of the characteristic segmental presentation of the diseased bowel, which is clearly separated by normal areas (skipped areas) of bowel mainly in the rectosigmoid area but can involve the entire colon. CD can involve all or any layer of the bowel wall as well as any portion of the GI tract from the mouth to the anus. Disease of the terminal ileus is present in about 80 percent of patients with CD, and in 20 percent of the cases only the colon is involved.

THE PATIENT'S VOICE 10.1

Crohn's Disease

As a 39-year-old woman with a 20-year history of severe CD, I remain undecided as to which has been most difficult to deal with: the symptoms of the disease—uncontrolled diarrhea, bowel incontinence, malnutrition, pain, bloating, and flatulence, to name a few; the results of the symptoms—fatigue, malaise, anemia, anorexia, anxiety, embarrassment, guilt, fear, and shame; or the constant discipline necessary to incorporate lifestyle changes instrumental to the adaptation and management of this debilitating disorder—diet, stress elimination, exercise, rest, vitamin supplementation, and prescription compliance. Experience with CD has taught me that health and wellness is a personal choice and that whatever intestinal ailments or conditions one struggles with, incorporating the dietary changes necessary to promote wellness through nutrition, particularly raw, fresh fruit and vegetable juices, should be part of a comprehensive approach to achieving optimal health.

SOURCE: Cynthia Tagliaferri

Epidemiology and Causes

The incidence and prevalence of these diseases varies widely, which supports a multifactorial theory in the development of the disease. Research supports a genetic predisposition for IBD even though less than 15 percent of cases are familial. A gene on chromosome 16 that encodes the protein, nucleotide-binding oligomerization domain 2 (*NOD2*) has variants that are found in about 62 percent of patients with CD. Genes associated with IBD have also been found on chromosomes 10 and 7 that encode for proteins that mediate epithelial cell–cell interactions and the transport of molecules in and out of cells. Another factor is the ability of bacteria in the gut to cause inflammation. Researchers believe that there is an exaggerated cell-mediated immune response to the bacteria. The intestinal epithelium plays an important role in the immune response, interacting with microbes and antigens and communicating with immune cells triggering the production and secretion of cytokines and chemokines.

The incidence of IBD is about equal in men and women. The highest prevalence for the disease is in Scandinavian and Northern European countries. The overall incidence and prevalence for both of these diseases is about equal worldwide, with incidence rates between 3 and 10 per 100,000 and prevalence rate between 30 and 50 per 100,000. The age at onset is frequently in early adulthood, but can be anywhere from age 10 to 40. Table 10.17 compares UC and CD.

Pathophysiology

Ulcerative Colitis

The inflammatory process of UC is confined to the mucosa of the colon and rectum and begins with neutrophil infiltration at the base of the crypt of Lieberkühn. The disease most often occurs in the rectum and sigmoid colon. The mucosa in this area is thinner, and has a dark red and velvety appearance in susceptible individuals. The cytokines released from the macrophages and neutrophils during the inflammatory response are responsible for tissue damage. Ulcers form in the eroded tissue and abscesses form in the crypts. These abscesses become necrotic and ulcerate. The muscularis mucosae becomes edematous and thickened, narrowing the lumen of the colon. Bleeding, cramping pain, and the urge to defecate result from the mucosal destruction. The characteristic stool is diarrhea that contains blood and purulent mucus. There is also a loss of the absorptive surface leading to large volumes of watery diarrhea. Fecal leukocytes are always present with active colitis. Absence of these inflammatory changes within the deeper layers of the intestinal mucosa helps to differentiate UC from other inflammatory processes. Patients diagnosed with severe UC are at risk for a perforated colon. They require close observation and should have consultation with a surgeon.

Crohn's Disease

CD is an inflammatory process that begins in the submucosa of the intestine and gradually spreads to involve the mucosa and serosa. Any portion of the GI tract can be affected, but the terminal ileum is the most common site. There are abnormalities in the intestinal immune response where proinflammatory cytokines, interleukins, and tissue necrosis factor produce areas of tissue damage. Typically, some haustral segments are affected while others are not, creating a pattern called skip lesions. The ulcerations form longitudinal and transverse fissures, extending inflammation into Peyer's patches and the lymphoid tissue. The typical lesion is granulomatous with projections of inflamed tissue that is surrounded by scar tissue. It is described as a "cobblestone" appearance. With progression of the disease, fibrosis thickens the bowel wall, narrowing the lumen. Serosal inflammation causes bowel loops to adhere to one another, contributing to transmural inflammation, ulceration, and fibrosis, which can lead to obstruction, fistulas, and shortening of the bowel.

Table 10.17 Comparison of Ulcerative Colitis and Crohn's Disease

Feature	Ulcerative Colitis	Crohn's Disease
History		
Age of onset	Age 10–40	Age 15–25; age 50–80
Etiology	Unknown	Unknown
Genetic tendency	Familial tendency	Familial tendency
Nicotine use	Nonsmoker	Smoker
Assessment Findings		
Serologic	+ (positive) for antineutrophil cytoplasmic antibodies (pANCA)	− pANCA
Fever/malaise	With severe disease	Common
Weight loss	Uncommon	Common
Rectal bleeding	Common	Dependent on location of lesion; occurs in about 50% of cases
Abdominal pain	Usually mild	Can be moderate to severe
Abdominal mass	Negative	May be present
Perianal lesions	Absent	May develop fissures, abscess
Fistulas	Absent	Common
Strictures	Uncommon	Common
Histologic/Endoscopic Findings		
Rectal involvement	Always	50% of the cases
Distribution	Confined to colon; continuous	Any portion of GI tract; discontinuous, skipped lesions
Mucosa	Friable, granular	Cobblestone appearance
Ulceration	Crypt abscess development	Aphthous or linear ulcers
Inflammation	Surface involvement	Transmural involvement

Individuals with IBD are at greater risk for developing colorectal cancer than the general population. Clinical findings suggest that carcinoma is less common in patients with CD than with UC and is attributed to the treatment of CD with colectomy.

Clinical Presentation

Subjective

Individuals with mild forms of UC commonly report four or fewer loose bowel movements per day associated with abdominal cramps that are relieved with defecation, small amounts of blood and mucus in the stool, and sometimes tenesmus. Usually there are no associated systemic symptoms. With moderate disease, patients have four to six loose stools a day containing more blood and mucus. They also have systemic symptoms such as tachycardia, mild fever, weight loss, and may have mild edema depending on the serum albumin level. Severe disease manifests with more frequent bloody bowel movements (6 to 10) per day; abdominal pain and tenderness; and symptoms of anemia, hypovolemia, and impaired nutrition.

The most common presenting symptoms of CD are abdominal cramping and tenderness, fever, anorexia, weight loss, spasm, flatulence, and RLQ pain or mass. Individuals may report an increase in symptomatology during periods of stress or emotional upset or after meals consisting of poorly tolerated foods such as fatty or spicy foods or milk. Stools are soft or semiliquid. Observable blood is found in the stool intermittently; when present, it occurs in larger amount than with UC. Because of the loss of healthy bowel mucosa, there may be insufficient resorption of bile salts, causing steatorrhea (foul-smelling, fatty stools). CD can involve the entire thickness of the bowel wall, causing microperforations and symptoms of acute localized peritonitis, which can mimic appendicitis or diverticulitis. If there is fistula formation, these symptoms may dominate the clinical picture.

Several patterns of symptom onset have been manifested—gradual, with vague abdominal discomfort, malaise, cramping, and bloody, mucopurulent stools; abrupt, with frequent periods of bloody diarrhea, anorexia, fever, and weight loss; and abrupt and fulminating, with sudden, violent diarrhea occurring nocturnally, high fever, intense abdominal cramping, signs of peritonitis, weight loss, and anorexia. Stools may contain blood, mucus, and/or pus. Typically, CD has a more insidious and gradual onset. Individuals often experience intermittent symptoms long before presenting for medical attention. The disease is characterized by periods of acute exacerbation alternating with complete remission.

If the UC is confined to the rectal or sigmoid area the stools can be normal or hard and dry; however, the rectum will continue to dispel mucus containing both red and white blood cells. As the disease process moves proximally, the stools become looser. Patients may report eating less to decrease the frequency of bowel movements, which leads to more pronounced nutritional deficiencies.

Objective

On physical exam, there may be tenderness in the LLQ or across the entire abdomen, often accompanied by guarding and abdominal distension. A digital rectal exam should be performed to assess for anal and perianal inflammation, rectal tenderness, and blood in the stool. Depending on the severity of the disease and the extent of potential complications, signs and symptoms of ileus and peritonitis may be found. Perirectal abscesses and fistulas are not associated with UC.

The physical exam may reveal abdominal tenderness with a tubular, tender mass in the RLQ. Fifty percent of individuals with CD have perianal involvement, including anal fissures, perianal fissures, and edematous, pale skin tags, which are often misdiagnosed as prolapsed hemorrhoids. Extraintestinal findings include episcleritis, erythema nodosum, nondeforming peripheral arthritis, and axial arthropathy, which may be more apparent than bowel symptoms and should prompt the practitioner to look for a diagnosis of CD.

CD tends to present in one of four patterns: (1) inflammation, RLQ abdominal pain, and tenderness, often presenting as appendicitis; (2) obstruction, fibrosis, and stenotic changes within the bowel, causing recurrent obstruction associated with severe colic, abdominal distension, constipation, and vomiting; (3) diffuse jejunoileitis involving the jejunum and ileum and characterized by both inflammation and obstruction, which can result in malnutrition and chronic debility; and (4) abdominal fistulas and abscesses, normally occurring late in the disease process and causing fever, generalized wasting, and abdominal masses. Although CD is uncommon among children, those with CD often present with extraintestinal symptoms, especially growth retardation, fever of unknown origin, and anemia.

Diagnostic Reasoning

Diagnostic Tests

Definitive diagnosis is made by correlating the symptoms with the history and physical exam. The results of diagnostic testing help to differentiate UC from CD. Stool analysis and cultures are obtained to rule out bacterial, fungal, or parasitic infection as the cause for diarrhea. The stool is also examined for mucus and blood, which are normally present with UC.

Patients with CD who have small intestine involvement may also require evaluation for malabsorption, which manifests as anemia secondary to bleeding and iron deficiency; for macrocytic anemia from inflammation of the terminal ileum and poor absorption of folate; and for hypocalcemia and vitamin D deficiency, hypoalbuminemia, and steatorrhea resulting from bile salt deficiency. Liver function tests may be helpful in screening for primary sclerosing cholangitis and other liver problems associated with

IBD. Fluid and electrolyte disturbances are common in both diseases because of the extracellular fluid loss. CD may also present with an elevated WBC and sedimentation rate as well as a prolonged PT.

Imaging studies are necessary to confirm the diagnosis of IBD. Contrast radiography and endoscopy are the primary diagnostic tools. The diagnosis of UC should be supported with sigmoidoscopy, which defines the actual extent of the mucosal inflammation. Early in the disease the mucous membrane is granular, friable, and edematous, with loss of the normal vascular pattern. In many patients, there may be scattered areas of hemorrhage that bleed with minor trauma. The resulting ulcerations develop after the mucosa breaks down, leaving the mucous membranes dotted with numerous bleeding and pus-oozing ulcers. Severe disease is characterized by copious amounts of purulent exudate. Colonoscopy should be avoided in individuals with severe colitis or deep ulcerations because of the risk of perforation or the development of toxic megacolon. Although there are periods of remission, sigmoidoscopy always shows some degree of friability and granulation in patients with UC. Biopsy results reveal chronic inflammation.

Plain films of the abdomen can help estimate the severity and proximal extent of the disease by demonstrating loss of haustration and the absence of formed stool within the diseased sections of bowel.

Every patient with UC requires a colonoscopy to determine the extent of the disease, but in order to avoid perforation, this is normally reserved for patients who have already begun treatment. Colonoscopy is preferred over BE as it allows direct assessment of the colon and permits histologic examination through biopsy. Ulcers suggestive of UC are shallow and confluent; they are erythematous, edematous, and friable, causing them to bleed easily. Individuals with UC usually have disease that begins in the rectum and extends proximally, without "skipped areas." Although BE is informative, it is contraindicated in individuals with moderate or severe disease because it can precipitate toxic megacolon.

Definitive diagnosis of CD is normally made via x-ray studies. The earliest manifestations of CD are aphthous and linear ulcers, which are best visualized with air contrast BE or small bowel follow-through depending on the location of the lesions. BE may show reflux of barium into the terminal ileum. The ileum is stiff and nodular, and the lumen shows signs of thickening and narrowing. In advanced disease, the upper GI tract with small bowel follow-through may show the characteristic "string sign"—ileal strictures and evidence of bowel loop separation resulting from marked circumferential inflammation and fibrosis.

Colonoscopy reveals ulcers that are either minor erosions or deep longitudinal fissures. Segmental transverse fissuring creates the characteristic cobblestone appearance and is usually found above the rectum and rectosigmoid areas. Biopsies may be obtained to rule out pseudopolyposis, adenomatosis, or cancer. CT is often used in the evaluation of CD to identify bowel wall thickening or abscess formation. If an abscess is found, CT may be useful for guided drainage of the abscess.

Differential Diagnosis

Differential diagnosis of UC must begin with the exclusion of an infectious cause for the colitis before treatment is initiated. Enteric infection is ruled out through fresh stool culture for ova and parasites. Infectious colitis caused by *Entamoeba histolytica*, *Campylobacter enteritidis* and *Shigella* species and *Chlamydia* species can cause acute colitis, which is difficult to differentiate from UC both clinically and endoscopically. The distinction must be made because treatment with corticosteroids can be catastrophic. Obtaining a thorough travel, sexual, and antibiotic history is imperative. If the individual has had antibiotic exposure within the last 30 days, a stool for *Clostridium difficile* should be obtained. Homosexual men practicing anal intercourse should be screened for infectious proctitis as a cause of colitis. Individuals with HIV are susceptible to many opportunistic infections, which must also be considered as part of the differential diagnosis and treatment.

Older adults, patients with a history of coagulation disorders, and young women using oral contraceptives should be examined for ischemic colitis. Radiographic findings of "thumbprinting" and segmental distribution of lesions are typical of ischemic colitis. Although colon cancer rarely presents with fever and purulent diarrhea, it should be ruled out as a cause for bloody diarrhea.

As with UC, evaluation of CD must begin with ruling out infectious enteritis as the source of colitis. Enteric tuberculosis and fungal disease must also be considered in the differential diagnosis of CD. *Yersinia enterocolitica* enteritis, although a self-limiting infection, may require a 3-month follow-up examination because the initial clinical presentation is so similar to CD.

Although only 20 percent of patients with CD have disease that is limited to the colon, differentiation from UC must be made. CD is the more likely diagnosis when there is evidence of perianal disease and rectal bleeding. RLQ pain without a history of chronic bowel symptomatology may mimic appendicitis, PID, ectopic pregnancy, ovarian cysts, or tumors; all of these must be ruled out in the differential diagnosis of CD. Both diverticular disease and ischemic colitis can present with the segmental involvement and luminal stricturing characteristic of CD.

Many drugs have been implicated in drug-induced colitis, the most common being NSAIDs and antibiotics. Many individuals who routinely take NSAIDs suffer damage to the GI tract characterized by bloody diarrhea and weight loss. Some antibiotics alter the bowel flora, allowing overgrowth of pathogens such as *Clostridium difficile,* which produces a toxin that is damaging to the bowel mucosa and can cause bloody diarrhea, abdominal pain, and weight loss. Although initial radiographic studies may be similar to those for CD, endoscopic examination reveals a more segmental distribution of lesions, and biopsy results are not supportive of inflammatory disease.

Colon cancers can cause bloody diarrhea; however, they usually do not have the associated fevers, leukocytosis, and purulent discharge. Diverticulitis can cause abdominal pain, fever, leukocytosis, obstruction, and diarrhea; however, endoscopic evaluation reveals the characteristic mucosal herniations in the bowel wall.

Management

There is no cure or definitive treatment for IBD. The initial therapy should depend on the severity of the presenting symptoms and must be individualized. Medical therapy is directed at reducing inflammation, correcting or maintaining fluid and electrolyte balance, and relieving the signs and symptoms of the disease.

Ulcerative Colitis

Initial treatment of UC includes nutrition counseling. Patients should avoid caffeine, raw fruits, vegetables, and other foods high in fiber, which can cause trauma to the already inflamed mucosal surface. Some patients may benefit from a lactose-free diet, but that is not recommended unless a trial produces symptomatic relief. A bland diet that is high in calories and protein yet low in fat can help to control diarrhea and flatulence and maintain nutrition and weight. Parenteral nutrition may be necessary in individuals with severe anorexia or uncontrollable diarrhea.

Antidiarrheal medications should be avoided in the acute phase, but can be helpful for patients with mild symptoms. Patients with mild to moderate diarrhea may benefit from diphenoxylate with atropine (Lomotil) 2.5 to 5.0 mg PO bid up to qid, loperamide (Imodium) 2 mg after each bowel movement, or codeine 15 to 30 mg PO q4 to 6 h.

Disease that is limited to the rectosigmoid area can often be successfully treated with topical steroids or mesalamine (Drugs Commonly Prescribed 10.3). Steroid enemas and foams (e.g., hydrocortisone [Cortifoam] 100 mg) should be administered nightly for 2 weeks. If effective, this treatment will bring about remission in 70 percent of initial episodes of idiopathic UC. Patients may then taper the dose over the next week to prevent the side effects associated with rapid steroid withdrawal. Mesalamine (Rowasa), a form of 5-aminosalicylate (5-ASA), is more expensive; it is sometimes more effective than hydrocortisone for patients with refractory or left-sided colitis and is available in enema and suppository form. Oral preparations of 5-ASA medications (e.g., Asacol) help to maintain remission after the enemas have been discontinued. 5-ASA preparations lack the sulfapyridine moiety (a byproduct of the metabolism of sulfasalazine and responsible for most of the drug's toxicity), have fewer adverse effects, and are better tolerated for prolonged courses of treatment. Subsequent exacerbations of UC tend to show increasing resistance to therapy, requiring longer treatment regimens.

More advanced disease usually requires the addition of a systemic glucocorticoid in combination with sulfasalazine or 5-ASA therapy. Glucocorticoids are especially helpful in controlling the extracolonic manifestations of UC, which include peripheral arthritis, ankylosing spondylitis, erythema nodosum, anterior uveitis, and pyoderma gangrenosum. Peripheral arthritis and the skin lesions often parallel the course of the disease. Oral prednisone (Prelone), up to 40 to 60 mg in single or divided doses, must be tapered and not discontinued abruptly.

Drugs Commonly Prescribed 10.3: 5-Aminosalicylic Acid Medications

Drug	Indication	Dosage	Comments
Mesalamine preparations			
Enemas	Distal colitis	4 g/60 mL retained for 8 h; 1 enema qhs for 3–6 weeks	Topical, rectosigmoid preparation: may require tapering to discontinue.
Asacol	IBD in the small intestine and colon	400–800 mg PO tid; maximum of 1600 mg tid	Enteric pH-sensitive coating; may be effective in treating terminal ileitis, Crohn's colitis.
Pentasa	IBD in the small intestine and colon	1 g PO qid	Agent released slowly through stomach, small and large bowel
Olsalazine	UC	500–1000 mg PO bid	Bacterial hydrolysis; can cause diarrhea, which is reduced with dose reduction and administration with meals.
Sulfasalazine	Initial treatment of UC and CD	500 mg PO bid; increase over 1 week to 1–1.5 g qid	Many adverse effects; may be given with folic acid 1 mg qd

Severe or fulminant UC is manifested by 10 or more bloody stools per day, abdominal tenderness, fever, colon dilatation, fever, and tachycardia. Patients often require hospitalization for these symptoms. Patients with severe disease must be monitored closely for the development of toxic megacolon and colonic perforation. Any patient who does not show improvement after 7 to 10 days of maximized therapy should be considered for surgical intervention. Subtotal or total colectomy is often required to prevent perforation of the bowel and its complications. Some individuals may require restoration of their fluid volume and electrolytes as well as blood transfusions, depending on the severity of the diarrhea and bleeding.

Immunosuppressive agents, azathioprine (Imuran), cyclosporine, and metabolite 6-mercaptopurine (6MP), are used in cases of UC that are unresponsive to other medical treatment and in patients who are not surgical candidates. The long-term use of immunosuppressive agents for relapse prevention must be balanced with the increased risk of developing a malignancy. Most commonly, these agents are used to allow patients to reduce the maintenance dosage of glucocorticoids.

Individuals who progress to fulminant disease are at risk for developing toxic megacolon—an atonic and distended, thin-walled colon. Approximately 1 to 2 percent of patients with UC develop this complication, which is characterized by fever, sepsis, electrolyte imbalances, hypoalbuminemia, and dehydration. Definitive diagnosis is made when the radiographic measurement of the midtransverse colon is dilated to greater than 6 cm. The patient is at risk for perforation until the dilatation is reduced. If medical reversal is not accomplished within 48 hours, surgical intervention is indicated and consultation should be made early.

Patients with toxic megacolon should receive nothing PO, an NG tube should be placed for intermittent suction, and all antidiarrheal medications should be discontinued. Fluid and electrolyte disturbances, particularly hypokalemia, should be corrected, and total parenteral nutrition may be required until the patient is able to tolerate oral food and fluids. Broad-spectrum antibiotics for peritonitis prophylaxis and parenteral administration of glucocorticoids are indicated. Patients must be monitored closely for signs and symptoms of perforation, which may be blunted because of the large doses of glucocorticoids. Loss of hepatic dullness on percussion may be the first sign of perforation. Daily abdominal x-ray films are necessary to assess colon distension and the presence of free air within the abdomen.

Emergent total colectomy is indicated for patients who do not respond to intensive medical therapy within 48 hours or who have massive hemorrhage or perforation. Surgical intervention is sometimes done in stages for patients who are severely ill. The most common procedure is the proctocolectomy with a Brooke ileostomy; it is a curative and functional procedure. Surgical intervention is also considered in patients who require large maintenance doses of glucocorticoids, are experiencing quality of life issues caused by severe diarrhea, or in children who are manifesting signs of growth retardation.

Crohn's Disease

Treatment of CD parallels that of UC including sulfasalazine (Azulfidine), 5-ASA medications, and glucocorticoids. There is no curative therapy for CD; therefore, treatment is aimed at suppressing the inflammatory process and symptomatic relief of complications. The patient with CD has a much greater incidence of relapse once medications are discontinued; 70 percent of patients started on steroid therapy must remain on the therapy to prevent relapse. The use of 5-ASA medications concomitantly with steroids has been helpful in successful weaning of the steroids. Oral prednisone 40 to 60 mg/day is used as initial outpatient treatment. Once maximal response has been achieved, the dose can be tapered over 2 to 4 months. Some patients may require a daily maintenance dose of 5 to 10 mg/day. As with UC, steroids are often helpful in managing the extraintestinal manifestations of the disease. Patients with disease within the rectum may benefit from enema preparations as well.

Sulfasalazine (Azulfidine) remains the treatment of choice for CD but is limited by the high incidence of intolerance, including nausea, anorexia, rash, and headache. The initial dose of sulfasalazine for treatment of mild to moderate disease of the colon or ileocolon is 500 mg bid; the dose can be increased to 3 to 4 g/day. Clinical improvement is usually noted in 3 to 4 weeks, at which time the medication can be tapered to 2 to 3 g/day for 3 to 6 months. Sulfasalazine interferes with folic acid absorption, so patients should receive folic acid 1 mg/day while taking this medication. Patients with disease that is confined to the small intestine or those who do not tolerate sulfasalazine may benefit from other 5-ASA preparations.

The use of immunosuppressive medications has been shown to be effective in patients with CD that is unresponsive to other treatments and in individuals dependent on high-dose steroids, or in those with nonhealing fistulas. The clinical benefit of 6MP (the active metabolite of Imuran and azathioprine) can take up to 3 months before being realized. These drugs can cause bone marrow suppression and pancreatitis; therefore, patients must be monitored frequently for leukopenia. The risk for developing malignancy is low but still must be considered. Patients remain on treatment for up to 2 years; in extremely refractory cases, treatment is continued indefinitely. Cyclosporine (Neoral, Sandimmune), an immunosuppressant drug typically used to prevent organ transplant rejection, is helpful in patients with steroid-resistant CD. Its use remains experimental and it should be administered by practitioners who are experienced in caring for patients with complicated CD.

Infliximab is an IgG anti-TNF antibody that is proving helpful in patients with moderate to severe CD as an immunomodulatory agent. Rapid improvement is seen when infliximab is used initially. The regimen includes an initial dose of 5 mg/kg and then again at 2 weeks and 6 weeks with maximal response seen in the first 2 weeks. The side effects include infusion-related reactions and hypersensitivity reactions as a result of the development of antinuclear antibodies. This can be reduced by concomitant administration of other immunosuppressive medications. Serious infections may develop while patients are being treated with this medication.

The use of metronidazole has been effective in patients who are intolerant of sulfasalazine, although its use is also limited by adverse effects, including nausea, anorexia, metallic taste, furry tongue, and paresthesias. Although the mechanism of action is not clear, metronidazole has been effective in the treatment of perianal disease and in controlling Crohn's colitis. There is a high rate of relapse, however, once the drug has been discontinued. Other antibiotics such as ciprofloxacin, ampicillin, and tetracycline have been effective in controlling Crohn's ileitis and ileocolitis.

Surgical intervention for CD is normally not indicated except for complications including intestinal obstruction, fistulas and abscess drainage, or perforation. Patients with fistula formation (which may be enterocutaneous, enterovaginal, or enterovesicular) should be managed with bowel rest, parenteral nutrition, and antibiotic therapy before surgery is considered. Surgery is not curative and must be reserved for complications that are resistant to medical therapy. Intestinal obstruction caused by stricture formation is often successfully treated with strictureplasty, thus avoiding multiple surgeries and the risk of short bowel syndrome. Patients with symptoms of obstruction should avoid foods that contain nuts or seeds.

As with UC, the use of anticholinergic and antidiarrheal medications should be avoided in patients with severe disease because the drugs may precipitate toxic megacolon or ileus. Loperamide (Imodium), diphenoxylate (Lomotil), and codeine may be helpful in controlling chronic diarrhea in patients with mild Crohn's colitis.

Follow-Up and Referral

UC and CD are both complex illnesses with periods of exacerbation and remission requiring lifelong intervention and follow-up. Adjustment of therapy is based on symptom analysis and examination. Confirmation of the diagnosis and uncontrolled exacerbations should be referred to the physician. Referral to a gastroenterologist is often necessary for endoscopic evaluation and tissue biopsy. Long-term use of steroids and immunosuppressive drugs dictates ongoing patient follow-up. Repeat evaluation may be indicated if symptoms of a major complication have developed. Routine colonoscopy for colon cancer surveillance is necessary in any patient with long-standing disease. Stool analysis for occult blood is not an effective means of surveillance. Individuals whose disease is not controlled with established medical therapy of low-dose prednisone and sulfasalazine or other 5-ASA medications should be referred to a gastroenterologist who is knowledgeable in the treatment of these chronic disease processes.

Patient Education

All patients need to be informed about the disease process, the treatment options, and the expected outcome of the treatment regimens. Patients must be a part of the treatment plan and must have the knowledge necessary to make informed decisions. Education about the disease, diagnostic and laboratory tests, and diet and lifestyle changes should be included in the education. Open, honest information is important in helping patients to develop realistic expectations with regard to treatment and outcomes.

The importance of adequate rest and stress reduction in an attempt to decrease bowel motility and promote healing is essential. Stress management techniques, such as guided imagery should be taught, and patients can be referred for counseling if necessary. Patients should be provided with the information and addresses for national organizations such as the Crohn's and Colitis Foundation of America, Inc. that have up-to-date information and local support groups.

Dietary concerns for patients with CD include a low-residue diet when obstructive symptoms are present. Patients on a low-residue diet should avoid all foods high in fiber, including whole grain breads and cereals, all fresh fruits and vegetables, and seeds and nuts. Patients are allowed to have canned fruits and vegetables and should have only white breads. If the patient is unresponsive to medical treatment or is exhibiting signs of growth retardation, oral elemental or parenteral nutrition may be necessary. Patients who are intolerant of lactose should be taught to avoid dairy foods. When patients are not in the middle of an acute attack, they can eat whatever they can tolerate.

Dietary instruction for patients with UC is the same as that for CD. If they are not having symptoms of an acute attack, patients may eat whatever they can tolerate. During an acute exacerbation, parenteral nutrition or oral supplementation for malnutrition may be necessary. Some patients will ask questions about the use of diet as a treatment. Studies to date show that diet is ineffective as a treatment or therapy for UC. Foods that can cause diarrhea and gas-producing foods should be avoided during acute attacks.

Female patients with IBD require special guidance and counseling before pregnancy.

Irritable Bowel Syndrome

Irritable bowel syndrome (IBS) is a functional GI disorder that is characterized by abdominal pain or discomfort. To be considered IBS, the patient must also have two of these features: abdominal pain or discomfort that is relieved by defecation; change in frequency in stool; and a change in the appearance of the stool. Patients usually have other symptoms such as frequent stools (more than three per day), or fewer stools (less than three per week), passing mucous, feelings of straining, urgency or incomplete evacuation, flatulence, and abdominal distension. IBS is a common GI problem encountered in primary care. When patients present for medical attention, they have usually had the complex of symptoms for several weeks to several months.

Epidemiology

Traditionally, women have been affected more often than were men, at a rate of 3:1. Recent epidemiological studies, however, suggest that men and women are affected equally, but that men are underdiagnosed based on the current IBS diagnostic criteria. It is estimated that 9 to 20 percent of the general population is affected by symptoms that can be classified within the diagnosis of IBS but fewer than one-third of those individuals seek medical attention. Typically, the symptoms first present in late adolescence and early adulthood but rarely in patients older than age 50.

Pathophysiology

The exact cause of IBS is unknown. IBS was once considered to have no organic cause, but several mechanisms have been identified. Normal bowel function is regulated by segmental contractions that limit the movement of bowel contents through the colon. An increase in these contractions causes constipation, and a decrease in the contractions results in frequent stooling or diarrhea. Myoelectric studies of colonic movement in individuals with IBS were inconclusive for diagnostic criteria, but the studies did demonstrate patterns of hypermotility, including high-amplitude pressure waves in patients, with pain as the predominant symptom during an acute IBS attack. Likewise, patients with diarrhea-predominant IBS had decreased and lower amplitude pressure waves. Studies have confirmed alterations in colonic activity during periods of emotional stress, in which motility is decreased or inhibited with depression and increased with feelings of hostility and anger.

Another major investigative focus of IBS has centered on visceral hypersensitivity. Approximately 50 percent of the patients with IBS have perceptual abnormalities including heightened gut sensitivity, leading to a lower tolerance for abdominal pain and distension of the colon with gas and feces. Studies in which the rectums of IBS patients were distended by balloon dilatation resulted in spastic contractions, leading to the characteristic symptoms seen with IBS. Patients with IBS are acutely aware of the intraluminal activities occurring with the digestive process. Sensations range from mild discomfort and tugging to frank pain. In summary, IBS patients do show evidence of abnormal colonic smooth muscle activity; however, the level at which the lesion originates is yet unknown.

Up to one-third of patients with IBS develop the disorder after bacterial gastroenteritis. It appears that patients with increased life stressors are more prone to developing IBS postinfection. Although the importance is unknown at this time, increased inflammatory cells have been found in all layers of the bowel in some patients with IBS.

The correlation between the symptoms of IBS and food intolerance is high. Careful diet history is necessary to distinguish between the two. The most common dietary triggers are lactose, fructose, sorbitol, and glutens. There is also a correlation between depression, anxiety, and somatization in patients who seek medical attention for their IBS symptoms.

Clinical Presentation

Subjective

Individuals with IBS typically present with symptoms that fall into two broad categories—those with abdominal pain and altered bowel habits, consisting of both diarrhea and constipation, and those with painless diarrhea.

Most patients with abdominal pain describe their pain as originating over some area of the colon, with the LLQ being most often affected. The pain can be sharp and burning with cramping or a diffuse dull ache. The description of the pain usually remains constant for the individual but can vary greatly among the patient population. Pain is often precipitated by eating or stress and can be relieved with a bowel movement or passing of flatus. The pain associated with IBS is usually not significant enough to interfere with sleeping nor is it great enough to wake the patient from sleep.

More than 50 percent of patients with IBS describe an overly acute sensory ability with regard to the GI tract and the digestive process. This visceral hypersensitivity is manifested by frequent complaints of abdominal distension, gas, and belching. Many of these symptoms occur 2 hours after having a meal and are often thought to be food intolerances. Patients typically complain of urgency to defecate, abdominal pain, bloating, and gas. Some patients with IBS have upper GI complaints, including dyspepsia, pyrosis, nausea, and vomiting.

Patients who present with painless diarrhea usually report an urgent need to defecate immediately on awakening or after eating. Although diarrhea rarely occurs nocturnally, urgency is so great that it may cause incontinence.

Alteration in bowel habits is the most consistently reported symptom. The typical presentation is diarrhea alternating with constipation. Patients report that constipation that was once responsive to laxatives has become continuous and that the stool has become harder and is decreased in caliber. Many patients complain of a sense of incomplete evacuation and thus repeated attempts at defecation are necessary within a short period of time. Periods of predominant constipation can last for months, interrupted by periods of diarrhea and then back to constipation. Patients who have diarrhea as their predominant symptom complain of frequent, low-volume (less than 200 mL), loose stools. Diarrhea does not normally occur at night; however, it can be exacerbated by eating or stress. Many patients report the passage of large volumes of mucus within the stool. This differs from the mucus occurring with colitis because there is no associated inflammatory process nor is there any blood in the stool, other than if there is an incidental finding of hemorrhoids.

Patients diagnosed with IBS frequently have an associated psychiatric diagnosis, which presents in the form of anxiety, depression, and somatoform disorders. IBS symptoms are often precipitated by a recent stressful life event such as marital discord, death, or abuse.

Objective

As with any illness, a thorough and detailed patient history is the key to definitive diagnosis. The physical examination is usually normal except for tenderness in some area of the colon, most often the LLQ and over the umbilicus or epigastric area in those with small bowel involvement. Digital rectal exam is normal but may reveal tenderness and exacerbate symptoms in some individuals.

There is usually no associated weight loss or deterioration in health. History of psychosocial stressor can often be correlated with the onset of symptoms. Key to diagnosis is the lack of other systemic symptoms such as fever, leukocytosis, or bloody stools, which might suggest an organic cause for symptoms.

Diagnostic Reasoning

Diagnostic Tests

IBS is diagnosed based on a careful history and physical that reveals the characteristic increase in bowel symptoms with the onset of pain, relief of pain with defecation, heightened sensation of bowel activity, or sense of incomplete defecation. The criteria used for diagnosing irritable bowel syndrome are provided in Advanced Assessment 10.2.

Initial laboratory testing should include CBC, erythrocyte sedimentation rate (ESR), chemistry panel including electrolytes and serum amylase, urinalysis, and stools for occult blood, ova and parasites, and cultures. Any abnormal lab value should prompt further investigation in the direction of the abnormal finding, because most laboratory studies in the patient with IBS are normal and any diagnostic clue as to the cause is helpful. If WBCs are found in the stool, it suggests an infectious or inflammatory process and not IBS.

Flexible proctosigmoidoscopy enables the provider to see up to 60 cm of the colon. No abnormalities are seen with IBS except for maybe an increased volume of mucus; however, increased tenderness and spasm may inhibit passage of the scope beyond 15 cm. Patients who present for initial treatment at age 40 or older should also be given an air contrast BE or colonoscopy.

Food intolerances should be ruled out, especially in patients who present with diarrhea and gas as predominant symptoms. Lactase deficiency can be identified with a hydrogen breath test or lactose tolerance test. Other intolerances are identified by removing the most common causative agents from the diet for 3 weeks and then slowly reintroducing them to the diet one at a time.

ADVANCED ASSESSMENT 10.2

Criteria for Diagnosing Irritable Bowel Syndrome

Abdominal pain or discomfort that is consistently relieved by defecation or has been associated with a change in the frequency or a change in the consistency of the stool for a period of 3 months either continuously or recurrently within that time frame.

AND

Defecation with varying patterns of constipation and diarrhea 25% of the time

AND

Two or more of the following:

Altered stool frequency

- Altered stool form including hard, loose, watery, mucoid
- Altered sensory act of defecation including straining, urgency, tenesmus

Passage of mucus

- Varied degrees of bloating and abdominal distension

IBS is no longer a diagnosis of exclusion; thus, the practitioner must direct diagnostic testing as information is received and lends itself toward an organic cause of the symptoms. Patients should not be subjected to endless batteries of expensive and uncomfortable tests in search of an organic disease. Laboratory findings that support a cause other than IBS include elevated ESR, anemia, leukocytosis, blood or WBCs in the stool, or stool volumes greater than 300 mL.

Differential Diagnosis

The differential diagnosis of IBS can include any of the processes in Table 10.18, with emphasis on the organic GI disorders. Most of the disease processes can be ruled out with careful history and physical exam. Patients presenting with diarrhea as the dominant symptom should have thyroid function tests, 24-hour stool check for fecal fat, and stool weight and stool testing for laxative content. Patients who present with constipation as their predominant symptom may require referral to a specialist who can measure colonic transit time. A careful medication history is necessary for either presentation.

Patients with epigastric pain must have the pain differentiated from that produced by biliary tract pain, ulcerative disease, or malignancies of the stomach and pancreas.

Management

The initial step to successful management of IBS is making the diagnosis and then identifying the symptom pattern for each individual patient. The therapy includes diet, education, and pharmacologic and supportive interventions. The

Table 10.18 Differential Diagnosis of Irritable Bowel Syndrome

- Food intolerance
  - Lactase deficiencies
  - Caffeine
  - Fermentable carbohydrates
  - Artificial sweeteners
- Fat or bile acid intolerances
- Pathogen-recipitated processes
  - Intestinal parasites
  - Bacterial overgrowth
- Medication-induced alterations in bowel motility
  - Laxative abuse
  - Magnesium-based antacids
  - Antibiotics
  - Opiate analgesics
- Functional upper GI disorders
  - Dyspepsia
  - Pyrosis
  - GERD
  - Peptic ulcer disease
  - Cholelithiasis
  - Biliary pain
  - GI malignancy
- Functional lower GI disorders
  - Inflammatory bowel disease
    - Crohn's disease
    - Ulcerative colitis
  - Diverticulitis
  - Intestinal obstruction
  - Hemorrhoids
  - Lower GI malignancy
  - Ascites
- Endocrine disorders
  - Hypothyroidism
  - Hyperthyroidism
  - Autonomic diabetic neuropathy
- Psychological disorders
  - Depression
  - Anxiety

patient with IBS requires reassurance and guidance throughout the course of the disease. Patients must understand that there is no proven treatment and the therapy is often symptomatic. Much of the recent literature suggests that there is a high degree of placebo effect with varying treatments.

A careful diet history is important in identifying foods that may precipitate symptoms. IBS is often confused with lactose intolerance and can be evaluated by removing lactose from the diet for 2 weeks and monitoring the symptoms. Other foods that are frequently identified in producing IBS syndromes include caffeine, legumes (and other fermentable carbohydrates), and artificial sweeteners. If any foods are identified that provoke symptoms, they should be eliminated from the diet. Patients who seem to suffer from postprandial discomfort may alleviate symptoms by eating a lower-fat diet that contains more protein. Dietary consultation can be helpful in assisting patients in developing a diet program that is palatable to them.

Diets high in fiber are beneficial regardless of predominant bowel habit. Patients are encouraged to increase their fiber intake to 20 to 30 grams per day. The hydrophilic properties of fiber or bulk-producing agents help to prevent excessive hydration or dehydration of stool and are thus indicated for both diarrhea and constipation symptom presentations. Foods high in fiber include whole grains, cereals, fruits, and vegetables; however, they must be introduced slowly for IBS patients in order to avoid the sensation of bloating. Bulk-producing agents can be substituted for individuals who choose not to change their diet. Commercially prepared bulk-producing agents are started once a day and increased gradually to three to four times daily. Patients are encouraged to continue treatment for at least 2 months before termination in order to allow the bowel to adjust to the bulking agents. All patients should try to drink at least eight 8-ounce glasses of water per day. Those individuals with constipation as their predominant symptom should be aware that fiber-bulking agents are not overnight laxatives and they should not abandon this therapy because they did not get overnight results.

Pharmacologic treatment is reserved for patients with moderate to severe symptoms and is directed at specific symptoms. Antidiarrheal medications are used only as a temporary measure. When the diarrhea is severe, episodic use of loperamide (Imodium) 2 mg or diphenoxylate (Lomotil) 2.5 to 5.0 mg q6h can be used as needed. The use of codeine, tincture of opium, and paregoric should be avoided because of their addictive nature. Patients who anticipate stressful situations can use antidiarrheals prophylactically.

Patients with constipation who have not responded to a high-fiber diet, hydration, exercise, and bulking agents may benefit from intermittent use of stimulant laxatives such as lactulose or magnesium hydroxide. Long-term use of laxatives is discouraged.

Antispasmodic agents have been used successfully in controlling abdominal pain caused by intestinal spasm. Patients who suffer with postprandial pain not responsive to diet therapy can benefit from dicyclomine 10 to 20 mg three to four times a day by mouth or hyoscyamine 0.125 to 0.75 mg twice a day. Anticholinergics should be avoided in patients with glaucoma and benign prostatic hypertrophy (BPH) because of the adverse effects and used with caution in the elderly.

Patients that have an associated psychological component to their IBS can obtain relief with serotonin receptor agonists (tegaserod) or antagonist (alosetron). Tegaserod is used for patients with predominantly constipation while alosetron is used when the patients has severe IBS with diarrhea predominant. Both of these medications have only been tested in women, so their efficacy and side effect profile may differ with male patients. Individuals with IBS need reassurance and understanding that their disease is chronic. They often benefit from support groups and counseling. Psychiatric interventions that teach behavior modification and biofeedback or can provide psychotherapy or hypnosis are helpful alternative measures for patients with refractory IBS.

Follow-Up and Referral

The emotional support provided by regular follow-up appointments is important in the management of patients with IBS. A strong, honest relationship with the patient is necessary to allay fears and prevent unrealistic expectations of the patient regarding their disease. Follow-up is important to encourage preventive behaviors including high-fiber diet, regular exercise, and avoiding foods that precipitate symptoms. Patients who are not responding to treatment should be referred to a gastroenterologist.

Patients who have IBS are often dissatisfied with treatment because no organic cause of their symptoms can be found. A second opinion is helpful in the management of these individuals; however, they must also be discouraged from continuing to search for organic causes for their symptoms. Referral for psychological intervention tends to be more helpful in patients with intermittent symptoms; those with chronic pain or intractable symptoms usually respond poorly.

Patient Education

Care of patients with IBS requires a positive and honest practitioner–patient relationship. Education is important in reducing the number of return visits for symptoms common to patients with IBS. The patients should understand that they have a real intestinal disorder, which is characterized by hypersensitivity to certain foods, hormonal changes, and stressors. Patients should be taught how to recognize these triggers and how to avoid or diminish their effects. Patients should understand the chronicity of their disease, but that they do not have a shorter life expectancy because of it. A thorough understanding of the treatment regime and setting realistic goals regarding treatment is the key to building a positive relationship with the patient. Patients must understand that the goal of treatment is to improve their symptoms, not cure the disease, and that improvement in symptoms can be a time-consuming process.

Dietary education is paramount to relief of the symptoms. Increasing fiber and water intake is an important component of the treatment. Teaching patients how to read nutrition labels will help them to quantify the amount of fiber they are consuming daily. Patients must be encouraged to take an active role in their treatment program and understand that elimination of foods that trigger symptoms can be time consuming and requires their careful attention.

Establishing good bowel habits is also important in the treatment of IBS. A high-fiber diet and increasing water intake to eight 8-ounce glasses per day can help in maintaining a regular bowel program. Patients who suffer with constipation should avoid laxatives and instead practice bowel training. Allowing adequate time after breakfast to sit on the toilet without straining can help establish a daily schedule.

Helping patients recognize and understand environmental stressors that trigger symptoms should be included in patient education. Involving the patient's family is important in establishing a support system. A resource available to patients for both education and support is the International Foundation for Bowel Dysfunction (IFBD).

Bowel Obstruction

Bowel obstruction is the consequence of any condition that inhibits the normal flow of chyme through the intestinal lumen. It can be complete or partial and can involve any segment of the large or small bowel. Bowel obstruction is considered simple when it results from a mechanical blockage or functional (paralytic ileus) when there is a disruption in motility.

Epidemiology and Causes

Intestinal obstruction can be classified according to the onset. Acute obstruction is sudden and can be caused by torsion, herniation, or intussusception (the slipping of a proximal piece of intestine into the part below it). Chronic obstruction usually indicates a slow gradual process often from tumor growth or strictures. Obstructions are also classed according to the degree of obstruction, either complete or partial and the location of the obstructing lesion. Obstructions can develop within the lumen, as in the case of foreign bodies, tumors or intraluminal fibrosis. This type of obstruction is considered intrinsic. Conversely, they can be extrinsic or from obstruction that arise outside the intestine. For example, intussusception, torsion (volvulus), fibrosis, and hernia can all cause intestinal obstructions from outside the bowel. Another aspect in the classification of intestinal obstruction is the effect it has on the intestinal wall. A simple obstruction indicates that there is no impairment of the blood supply to that portion of the intestine. A strangulated obstruction means that the lumen is obstructed and the blood supply is compromised. Bowel obstruction can be a complication of adhesions that are fibrous bands of tissue that develop after a surgical procedure.

Pathophysiology

There are numerous physiological alterations resulting from an intestinal obstruction related to the onset, location of the obstruction, and the amount of intestine proximal to the obstruction. Immediately after the obstruction begins there is distention of the intestine with sequestration of fluid and gas proximal to the obstruction. The gas is a result of bacterial fermentation and swallowed air. When the intestine begins to distend, its ability to absorb water and electrolytes decreases and more is left in the lumen adding to the distention. Sources of water and electrolytes include saliva, gastric juice, bile, pancreatic juice as well as intestinal secretion. Within 24 hours as much as 8 liters can accumulate in the intestinal lumen, leading to vomiting. Because of the vomiting and sequestration of fluid and electrolytes in the intestinal lumen, profound fluid and electrolyte imbalances result leading to dehydration, hemoconcentration, and ultimately hypovolemic shock. The increasing distention causes pressure on the diaphragm, thereby reducing the respiratory volume leading to atelectasis and pneumonia.

Depending on the location and stage of the intestinal obstruction, alkalosis or acidosis is possible. Alkalosis occurs early in intestinal obstruction or if the obstruction is in the proximal portion of the small bowel. This occurs because gastric juice which is high in hydrogen ions, does not get absorbed through the intestinal lumen, resulting in loss of the ion. However, later in the course of obstruction, or if the obstruction is more distal, acidosis occurs because alkaline pancreatic secretions and bile cannot be reabsorbed. Potassium is sequestered in the intraluminal fluid causing hypokalemia which promotes acidosis and atony of the intestinal wall.

As pressure within the intestinal lumen increases, arterial blood flow may be compromised leading to ischemia, necrosis, perforation, and peritonitis. Metabolic acidosis is compounded by the buildup of lactic acid that results from the decreased arterial blood flow. Venous return is reduced leading to edema within the bowel wall. As the edema progresses, there is an increase in capillary permeability causing fluid to be lost into the peritoneum, contributing to the hypovolemia already present.

Clinical Presentation

Subjective

In general, patients with obstruction generally complain of a sudden onset of colicky abdominal pain accompanied by nausea and vomiting. The pain is usually intermittent and corresponds to peristaltic waves. Patients with obstruction at the jejunum or below may have emesis that has changed to a brownish, feculent type material. They may complain of initial bouts of diarrhea, but this is soon followed by constipation.

In the later stages of obstruction, patients may have constipation and lack of flatulence. It is important to obtain information regarding previous abdominal operations, which may help in the diagnosis of intestinal obstruction. The abdominal pain of small bowel obstruction is usually centered about the umbilicus or in the epigastric area, and vomiting usually occurs early in the disease process. If the arterial circulation to the bowel is compromised, the pain becomes more constant and severe. Perforation produces severe generalized abdominal pain as well as the classic signs of peritonitis.

Objective

The physical examination should include careful inspection for abdominal scars and the presence of hernias. The patient may show signs of dehydration including poor skin turgor, dry mucous membranes, sunken eyeballs, and tachycardia. Blood pressure may be elevated depending on the degree of pain and if there is evidence of strangulation and subsequent ischemia. The degree of abdominal distension depends on the level of obstruction. The more distal the obstruction, the greater the length of proximal intestine producing greater distention. Also, if the obstruction is in the distal portion of the intestine, vomiting may only occur late in the course of the disease. The abdomen may be tender to palpation if there is strangulation present. Bowel sounds are high pitched and hyperactive; they may be accompanied by rushes, which coincide with the colicky abdominal pain. Patients with strangulation tend to have increased distension, abdominal tenderness, tympany to percussion, and hypoactive or absent bowel sounds. Sometimes a mass is palpable. If perforation has occurred, there may be a short period of pain relief, which is soon followed by increased pain, rebound tenderness, and fever, all suggestive of peritonitis.

Patients presenting with large bowel obstruction usually have a more gradual onset of symptoms, beginning with increasing constipation and abdominal distension. Large bowel obstruction is rare in patients younger than age 50. Lower abdominal cramps are unproductive of feces and are painful. Patients report a several-day history of no stools or flatus production. Vomiting occurs if there is an incompetent ileocecal valve or if there is a resultant superimposed, small bowel obstruction. The most common cause of large bowel obstruction is carcinoma of the sigmoid colon or diverticulosis.

Physical examination findings include a distended abdomen, particularly over the transverse and descending colon, with the presence of borborygmi. Patients are normally afebrile unless diverticulitis is suspected. There is usually no abdominal tenderness or guarding unless there are areas of ischemic bowel or associated small bowel obstruction with impending cecal perforation. A mass may be palpable over the area of obstruction. Rectal examination reveals an empty vault without tenderness unless there are obstructing rectal carcinomas. The systemic manifestations of large bowel obstructions are much less serious than those caused by small bowel obstruction.

Diagnostic Reasoning

Diagnostic Tests

Before diagnostic testing, patients must be thoroughly examined for any type of hernia that may be precipitating the obstruction. Diagnosis of small bowel obstruction is usually confirmed by supine and upright abdominal x-ray films that reveal a ladderlike distension of the small bowel. Upright films show multiple air-fluid levels within the loops of small bowel, which are the hallmark of small bowel obstruction. Findings indicative of other causes of small bowel obstruction are evidence of foreign body or actual mass suggestive of infarcted bowel. Oral contrast with small bowel follow-through can identify areas of partial obstruction. Oral barium studies are contraindicated and must be avoided unless large bowel obstruction has definitely been ruled out.

Laboratory studies include CBC and chemistry profile but are rarely useful for the diagnosis. Leukocytosis can indicate impending ischemia or strangulation of the bowel but is not diagnostic of such. Chemistry evaluation can help with proper fluid and electrolyte replacement. Serum amylase may be elevated and can lead to the erroneous diagnosis of pancreatitis. A finding of metabolic acidosis or an elevated lactic acid are highly suggestive of intestinal infarction.

Abdominal x-ray films of patients with large bowel obstruction usually show distension of the intestine down to the level of the obstruction. It is important to note the size of the cecum because, as the diameter approaches 14 cm, the danger of perforation is imminent. If air is noted under the diaphragm, it is likely that perforation of the cecum or sigmoid colon has occurred.

Differential Diagnosis

Volvulus, a twisting of the bowel upon itself, can happen suddenly, with loss of blood supply to the area and subsequent ischemia. Cecal volvulus presents as a large gas bubble within the midabdomen or LUQ on abdominal x-ray film. A volvulus of the sigmoid colon usually only occurs in older adults. It typically appears as a "coffee bean" dilatation arising from the pelvis. For both cecal and sigmoidal volvulus, a BE is done to reveal the precise location of the obstruction.

Colonoscopy and endoscopy are contraindicated in patients suspected of mechanical bowel obstruction because, in order to visualize the intestine, air must be introduced into the colon and can increase the chance of perforation. The differential diagnosis of small and large bowel obstruction is presented in Table 10.19.

Table 10.19 Differential Diagnosis of Bowel Obstruction

- Pseudo-obstruction
- Toximegacolon
- Twisting of a loop of bowel
  - Cecal volvulus
  - Sigmoid volvulus
- Incarcerated or strangulated hernias
  - Abdominal
  - Femoral
  - Inguinal
- Kinking of a loop of bowel
  - Adhesions secondary to previous abdominal surgery
- Concentric narrowing of the lumen of the intestine
  - Neoplasms
  - Diverticulitis
  - CD
- Foreign body
  - Gallstones
  - Ingested objects
- Intussusception
- Paralytic ileus

Management

All patients with suspected intestinal obstruction should be hospitalized and immediately referred to a surgeon. Therapy must be administered as definitive diagnosis is being obtained. Most patients with a bowel obstruction will require placement of an NG tube to decrease passage of secretions, aid in decompression, and ameliorate vomiting if present. Rehydration with IV fluids and replacement of electrolytes should be done as indicated by laboratory studies. Placement of an indwelling urinary catheter is necessary to accurately monitor urine output, which is recorded on a daily intake and output sheet.

Treatment of small bowel obstruction proceeds after the aforementioned therapies have been instituted and the patient is medically stabilized. Patients with upper small bowel obstruction are prone to alkalosis and hypokalemia caused by emesis; they must be monitored carefully, with IV fluid and electrolyte replacement as necessary. All medications that can decrease intestinal motility, including anticholinergics, narcotics, and calcium channel blockers, should be discontinued. If strangulation is suspected, the patient should be started on broad-spectrum antibiotic therapy, which provides coverage for anaerobic and gram-negative organisms. Laparotomy is indicated for all patients with complete bowel obstruction.

Patients with a large bowel obstruction are rehydrated and stabilized as previously described. If the patient has evidence suggestive of sigmoidal volvulus, an initial attempt to reduce the volvulus can be made with sigmoidoscopy, but surgery is required if unsuccessful. Patients with CD, intestinal lymphoma, or diverticulitis with subsequent concentric narrowing of the intestinal lumen may be given a trial of medical therapy specific to the disease process in an attempt to relieve the obstruction before surgical intervention.

Obstructing carcinomas can be treated with surgical resection and anastomosis. (Colon cancer is discussed later in this chapter.) If fecal impaction has been identified as the cause, it can often be removed digitally. If the impaction is barium and is located within the sigmoid colon, open laparotomy is required for removal. Adhesions can be relieved by surgical intervention; however, the chances are great that they will reoccur. Hernia reduction is indicated if this is the determined cause of obstruction. All patients who have undergone surgical intervention as definitive therapy must be monitored for paralytic ileus postoperatively.

Follow-Up and Referral

All patients with suspected bowel obstruction must be referred to a surgeon, who will manage the patient's hospitalization and postoperative care. The prognosis of appropriately treated simple intestinal obstruction is good, with a mortality rate of less than 2 percent. If strangulation is suspected and intervention is delayed, the mortality can be as high as 25 percent.

Because patients are usually acutely ill, postoperative teaching should be delayed until the patient is more receptive to instruction. Initial follow-up visits should be with the consulting surgeon, who will direct the patients' care until they are released to their primary-care provider.

Patient Education

Follow-up of patients with bowel obstruction will be guided by the surgeon. Care of the incision including dressing changes and signs and symptoms of infection are provided before discharge from the hospital. Once the patient has been cleared by the collaborating surgeon, the patient will return to the primary care setting. Patients should be instructed to report any recurrent abdominal pain with or without vomiting, fever, or problems regarding bowel function. Laxatives should not be taken without consulting the primary-care provider first. Stool softeners are prescribed as needed and patients are encouraged to avoid foods that cause constipation. Patients should refrain from strenuous activity for at least 6 to 8 weeks.

Diverticular Disease

Diverticular disease is the term used to describe the inflammatory changes that occur within the diverticular mucosa of the intestine (diverticulitis) as well as the asymptomatic, uninflamed outpouchings called diverticulosis. Diverticula are pouchlike protrusions of the intestinal mucosa that occur most often within the descending and sigmoid segments of the colon. They decrease in frequency in the cecum and rarely are found in the rectum. Diverticula tend to form at weakened areas of the intestinal wall, usually where arterial vessels perforate the colon. The inner layer of these pouch like protrusions form a narrow neck, which is continuous with the inner layer of the colon, and the sac herniates through the muscle wall. Most diverticula are asymptomatic and pose a problem only when they become inflamed or bleed. Most diverticula are found incidentally with endoscopy or BE. Diverticula vary in size from 3 mm to 3 cm in diameter.

Epidemiology and Causes

Diverticula are uncommon in individuals younger than age 40, with the prevalence increasing steadily after that. Over one-third of the United States population is affected by age 60. Diverticular disease is more common in developed nations than in less developed countries, with estimates as high as 40 to 50 percent in Western populations. The incidence is 2200 to 3000 per 100,000 people, occurring equally among men and woman. Diverticula are a rare finding in pediatric patients. Although they are common in older adults, it may be difficult to diagnose diverticular disease in these patients because of their blunted immune response.

Although there is no known cause for diverticular disease, a low-fiber diet has been implicated, because it causes increased intraluminal pressures within the colon, which lead to mucosal herniation through the weaker areas in the bowel wall. Other factors believed to contribute to the formation of diverticula include hypertrophy of the segments of the circular muscle of the colon, chronic constipation and straining, irregular and uncoordinated bowel contractions, obesity, and weakness of the bowel muscle brought on by aging. Risk factors are directly related to the suspected causes of the disease: older than age 40, low-fiber diet, previous diverticulitis, and the number of diverticula present within the colon. Diverticula occur most often in the LLQ; a RLQ presentation is a rare condition, with a higher incidence in Asian populations.

Pathophysiology

The exact cause of diverticulosis is unknown; therefore, the pathophysiology is based on the speculative findings already mentioned. As a consequence of increased ingestion of refined foods and decreased fiber intake, the stool bulk is decreased and the colon transit time is increased leading to the development of diverticula. Diverticula are thought to result from the increased pressure produced with the segmental contraction of the muscular portion of the wall of the colon. This increased pressure causes the herniation of the bowel wall through the weaker points in the muscle layer of the colon, normally occurring along the teniae at the penetration site of colonic vasculature. Inflammation occurring around the diverticular sac is often caused by the retention of undigested food and bacteria, which when formed into a hardened mass is called a *fecalith.* This mass in turn can disrupt the blood flow and lead to abscess formation. When the opening of this saclike projection becomes occluded and inflammation ensues, it can progress to the point of rupture. Acute diverticulitis is the result of this localized inflammation within the wall of the colon or peritoneum, causing the characteristic LLQ abdominal pain and tenderness. If the perforation is not localized, the patient can develop acute peritonitis and septic shock.

Fistula formation following acute diverticulitis is the result of a tract forming between the colon and other structures within the abdomen. These fistulas include colovesicular fistulas (urinary bladder), colovaginal fistulas (vagina), enteroenteric fistulas (loop of bowel), and colocutaneous fistulas (peritoneal tissue). Pericolitis is inflammation around the colon, which can result in fibrous strictures and obstruction.

Bleeding is a common complication of diverticulosis and is the most common cause of substantial lower GI bleeding. Postbleeding examinations have discovered that most bleeding occurs from uninflamed rather than inflamed diverticuli.

Clinical Presentation

Subjective

Approximately 25 percent of patients with diverticular disease develop symptoms. Patients with diverticulosis characteristically present with pain in the LLQ of the abdomen. Some patients report that the pain is worse after eating, which may be a result of colonic distension, and that the pain is sometimes relieved with a bowel movement or passing flatus. Elimination patterns may alternate between diarrhea and constipation, and there may be associated abdominal distension and tenderness. Diverticulitis may present with bleeding, which can be massive and is not associated with pain or discomfort.

When the diverticula have become inflamed, there are the usual signs and symptoms of infection—fever, chills, and tachycardia. Patients typically present with localized pain and tenderness in the LLQ of the abdomen with associated anorexia, nausea, and vomiting. If there is fistula formation, there are symptoms associated with the particular organ involved. Patients may complain of dysuria, pneumaturia (passage of air in the urine), and or fecaluria (passage of fecal matter in the urine) if there is fistula formation involving the bladder. Patients may be concerned about the development of hematochezia or frank bleeding from the rectum.

Objective

A physical exam reveals tenderness in the LLQ of the abdomen, and—if the patient can tolerate more vigorous examination—a firm, fixed mass may be identified in the area of the diverticuli. Patients may have rebound tenderness with involuntary guarding and rigidity. Bowel sounds may initially be hypoactive or can be hyperactive if an obstructive process has developed. Examination of the rectum may reveal tenderness, and the stool is usually positive for occult blood.

Diagnostic Reasoning

Diagnostic Tests

Initial laboratory testing can show mild to moderate leukocytosis, depending on whether the patient presents with diverticulitis or with a more advanced inflammatory process such as peritoneal abscess. The WBC is usually normal in patients with diverticulosis. Hemoglobin and hematocrit may be low if there is associated rectal bleeding. If there is fistula formation between the diverticula and the bladder, urinalysis may show elevated levels of both WBCs and RBCs and urine culture may be positive. Patients with signs suggestive of peritonitis should have a blood culture to assess for bacteremia.

Abdominal x-ray films should be obtained on all patients with suspected diverticulitis, especially if there are signs of perforation or peritonitis. Plain films of the abdomen can reveal free air (indicating perforation), ileus, or obstruction (small or large bowel). A BE outlines the lumen of the bowel clearly defining diverticula and is thus most helpful in the diagnosis of the disease process. If perforation is suspected, the study can be preformed with Gastrographin, a water-soluble contrast medium. Barium studies help to identify sinus tracts, fistula formation, or obstructive processes. Diverticula are often an incidental finding on colonoscopy; however, colonoscopy is much less sensitive for the diagnosis of diverticular disease than BE. Colonoscopy may be helpful in ruling out cancer as the source of the symptomatology, as is cystoscopy in evaluation of colovesicular fistula.

Although diverticulitis can often be diagnosed clinically, a CT scan with oral contrast is a much more sensitive and accurate test for cases in which confirmatory testing is necessary. CT scan can also determine if there is clinical deterioration by measuring the thickness of the bowel wall and assessing for the development of phlegmon over time using serial exams.

Patients who present with lower GI bleeding may require radioisotope scanning to locate the site of bleeding. Angiography is often nondiagnostic because the rate of bleeding is too slow or has stopped.

Differential Diagnosis

The differential diagnosis of diverticular disease includes IBS, carcinoma of the colon, IBD, lactose intolerance, PID, ovarian cyst, colitis (infectious or ischemic), appendicitis, and pyelonephritis. Most often the diagnosis can be made using the clinical findings and initial noninvasive ultrasonography. BE or colonoscopy are most helpful for definitive diagnosis of diverticulitis and colon surveillance for other colonic disease processes.

Management

With early detection and treatment of diverticulitis and the associated complications, the prognosis is good. An incidental finding of uncomplicated diverticulosis requires no further intervention and can be managed with a high-fiber diet or daily fiber supplementation with psyllium. Treatment of a patient presenting with mild symptoms can often be managed on an outpatient basis with rest, oral antibiotics, and a clear liquid diet. Initial antibiotic therapy varies with the extent of the inflammatory process and can include metronidazole (Flagyl) 500 mg PO tid with ciprofloxacin (Cipro) 500 mg PO bid, or trimethoprim/sulfamethoxazole (Bactrim DS) 160/800 mg PO bid for 7 to 10 days. The symptoms usually subside quickly; then the diet can be advanced to soft, low roughage and next to high fiber as tolerated. Pain due to spasms can be managed with antispasmodics such as hyoscyamine (Levsin) 0.125 mg q4h, dicyclomine (Bentyl) 20 to 40 mg qid, buspirone (BuSpar) 15 to 30 mg/day, and/or meperidine (Demerol) 100 to 150 mg/day in divided doses.

Patients with more acute illness require hospitalization for intravenous antibiotics and hydration, analgesia, bowel rest, and possible NG tube placement. If the patient requires analgesia, morphine sulfate should be avoided because it increases intraluminal pressures within the colon and causes or exacerbates the presenting symptoms or perforation. An NG tube should be placed if there is evidence of ileus or if there is intractable nausea and vomiting.

The choice of antibiotics will depend on the severity of the disease process and should cover both gram-negative bacteria and anaerobic organisms. If cultures are obtained from the diverticular abscess, antibiotic coverage can be altered according to the results of the culture. Use and dosage of aminoglycosides should depend on renal function as indicated by the creatine clearance. Patients who are immunocompromised will require broader antibiotic coverage, including an anti-*Pseudomonas* agent. IV antibiotic therapy is normally continued for 7 to 10 days and may be continued orally for an additional 7 to 10 days after discharge, depending on the severity of the illness.

Patients will usually experience relief in symptoms after 3 to 5 days of antibiotic therapy and may resume oral intake as tolerated. Once patients are able to maintain adequate nutrition and hydration, they can be discharged. A BE should be scheduled for 2 weeks after discharge to evaluate treatment.

Patients whose case is complicated by bleeding that does not subside will require angiography to locate the site of bleeding; they may also require infusion of vasopressin (Pitressin) 0.2 to 0.3 U/min via an intraarterial catheter placed during the radiographic procedure. If the patient shows signs and symptoms of acute blood loss, transfusion may be indicated. Twenty percent of patients who have experienced diverticular bleeding bleed again within a year.

If there is no improvement or if there is clinical deterioration after 72 hours of medical treatment, surgical intervention may be indicated. Approximately 20 to 30 percent of patients with the diagnosis of diverticulitis require surgical management. Surgery is usually required for patients who have had several episodes of diverticulosis within 2 years or for those who have had a single episode of diverticulitis with complications. Findings including free peritonitis and large abscesses, which do not respond to medical treatment, are indications for emergent surgical intervention. The surgical procedure of choice is colon resection with a temporary colostomy. Once the inflammation and infection have resolved, the patient can undergo elective reanastomosis of the colon. Patients who have undergone the surgical procedure will require routine postoperative care, with emphasis on pain management, pulmonary hygiene, hydration, nutrition, and wound assessment.

Localized abscesses can be drained percutaneously with the assistance of the interventional radiologist. Once the inflammation and infection have resolved, the patient may require an elective single-stage colon anastomosis in which the affected portion of the colon is removed. Despite medical treatment, it is estimated that up to 40 percent of patients with diverticulitis continue to experience symptoms, and approximately half of these patients will need surgical intervention.

Follow-Up and Referral

To evaluate or diagnose diverticular disease, all patients will require colonoscopy at some point during their disease process; therefore, referral to a gastroenterologist is indicated for symptoms that do not respond to treatment after 6 months. Early in the disease process patients with diverticulitis should consult with a surgeon who can follow them and determine the necessity for emergent surgical intervention if complications should develop. If patients respond well to antibiotic therapy but suffer subsequent attacks of diverticulitis, they should be referred to a surgeon for elective removal of the affected portion of the bowel. Any patient who has had an acute attack of diverticulitis before the age of 40 will usually require surgical intervention and should be referred accordingly. Follow-up BEs can be repeated every 3 years if symptoms persist or after corrective surgery has been completed.

Patient Education

Patients diagnosed with diverticular disease will need to make modifications in their diets with an emphasis on increasing the amount of dietary fiber. Diet changes should be made slowly to avoid bloating, gas, and other GI problems that may discourage compliance. Fiber can be increased by eating bran, fresh fruits, vegetables, and whole grains. The goal of diet therapy is to avoid constipation and straining during bowel movements, which can further increase intraluminal pressures and cause complications. Patients must be cautioned to avoid undigestible roughage, which can become lodged within the diverticula and exacerbate symptoms.

Patients should also be instructed to drink at least ten 8-ounce glasses of water a day to have regular, soft bowel movements. If patients continue to have constipation despite increasing their fiber and fluid intake, a bulk-forming laxative such as psyllium (FiberCon, Metamucil) can be added.

Patients who have had a colostomy will need instruction regarding follow-up care, including how to assess the stoma and the skin (for skin breakdown) and how to clean, empty, reclose, and change the colostomy pouch. Diet instruction as previously discussed is important for patients with a colostomy to prevent constipation and promote bowel regularity.

Symptoms will recur in approximately one-third of all patients with diverticulitis who were initially treated with medical management. All patients with diverticular disease, therefore, should be instructed to return for follow-up if they develop signs and symptoms of infection or other associated complications of diverticulitis. Patients who present with another episode of diverticulitis warrant elective surgical resection. Patients should understand that despite adherence to diet and medication, they may have another attack.

Colorectal Cancer

Colorectal tumors are both curable and preventable; however, the systematic screening of such cancers is in its infancy. Their presentation can be either symptomatic or asymptomatic and is dependent on the location of the tumor. Polyps, the most benign form of tumors, are classified as hyperplastic (nonneoplastic), adenomatous (neoplastic), or submucosal (lipomas). Adenomatous polyps are believed to be the precursors to the malignant adenocarcinomas, which comprise over 95 percent of all malignant tumors of the colon. Over the past 20 years, there has been a decline in the mortality associated with colorectal carcinoma, which has been attributed to improvement in screening, diagnosis, and treatment. Cure rates of colorectal carcinoma are estimated to be as high as 50 percent. Improvement in diagnosis and screening techniques have been attributed to advances in genetics and microbiology. .

Epidemiology and Causes

Colorectal cancer is second only to lung cancer in the number of cancer deaths in the United States. Over a lifetime, colorectal cancer will affect 1 in 17 Americans. Approximately 6 percent of Americans, or 134,000 individuals, will develop colorectal cancer every year, with 40 percent (55,000) of these cases being fatal. Of these 134,000 new cases of colorectal cancer, half will occur in the rectosigmoid area, and 25 percent are fund in the cecum and ascending colon. The higher incidence of colorectal cancer found within the rectum may be due in part to easier accessibility for examination and diagnosis.

Age is the most important risk factor for developing colorectal cancer in the United States. The risk increases steadily with age, especially after age 45, and is rare in individuals under age 35 unless they are predisposed to rare genetic diseases. The older adult population is at the greatest risk of developing colorectal carcinoma, with the median age at the time of diagnosis being 71 years. Colon cancer affects men and women equally; however, rectal cancers are more common in men. The overall survival rate of patients with colorectal cancer is approximately 50 to 55 percent and is attributed to early detection and treatment. African American males and low-income minorities have, for unknown reasons, lower survival rates in comparison to national data for other groups. It is presumed—though not proved—that the lower survival rates among minorities are in part a result of decreased accessibility to or underutilization of health care.

Seventh-Day Adventists and Mormons are two religious groups that subscribe to a vegetarian diet and have a lower incidence of colorectal cancer. In the past, studies have shown that the Japanese have had a lower incidence of colorectal cancer; however, Japanese Americans who have adopted a diet high in fat and refined carbohydrates have a higher incidence of this type of cancer. In general, groups that migrate from areas of low to high incidence of colorectal experience a change in cancer incidence that parallels that of the new region.

Other risk factors for developing colorectal carcinoma include a family history and a personal history of adenomatous polyps (multiple polyps or individual polyps greater than 1 cm in size) or colon cancer. Twenty-five percent of patients diagnosed with colon cancer have a family history of colon cancer. The risk of developing colon cancer is directly proportional to the number of first-degree relatives affected: For patients who have one first-degree relative with colon cancer, the risk increases two- to threefold. Disorders involving increased colon mucosal cell turnover (such as IBD and UC) have been implicated in greater risk for colon cancer. Familial adenomatous polyposis is an autosomal dominant condition that results in the development of thousands of adenomas within the colon but accounts for less than 1 percent of colon cancers. Other hereditary conditions that increase the chance of developing colorectal cancer include Peutz-Jeghers syndrome, Gardner's syndrome, and Turcot syndrome. Patients with a family history or personal history of gynecological (breast, ovarian, endometrial) cancers and individuals diagnosed with Barrett esophagus also have an increased risk of developing colon carcinoma.

Although the etiology of colorectal cancer (adenomas) is unknown, both environmental and genetic factors have been implicated. Geographic variances and a positive correlation in the incidence of disease among migrant workers both suggest that environmental factors play a role. Diets high in fat, red meat, and refined carbohydrates and low in plant fiber have been correlated with the areas of highest incidence of colorectal cancer, whereas areas with the lowest incidence of colorectal cancer have diets high in fiber and rich in vegetables and fruits. It has been theorized that the excess fat interacts with colonic bacteria to form deconjugated bile acids, which have been associated with tumor-producing activity, increased deposition of fatty acids within the cell membranes, and increased synthesis of prostaglandins, which further stimulates cell proliferation. Ketosteroids are thought to be metabolic byproducts of cholesterol that induce genetic damage and have been found in higher concentrations among high-risk populations. Products of pyrolysis—decomposition of organic matter secondary to increases in temperature such as those resulting from char-broiling and frying—have also been implicated in carcinoma of the colon. Geographical areas with low levels of selenium also have higher incidence of colorectal cancer.

Conversely, diets high in fiber tend to reduce the transit time within the colon, thus decreasing exposure to potentially carcinogenic substances and altering the gut flora and decreasing fecal pH. (Populations with the highest incidence of colorectal cancer have an associated higher fecal pH.) When fecal contents take longer to transit the bowel, the deionized bile acids and free fatty acids stay in contact with the intestinal mucosa, which has been associated with development of colorectal cancer.

Pathophysiology

Adenocarcinomas account for more than 95 percent of colorectal malignancies. The evolution from adenoma to invasive carcinoma can take up to 10 years. *Adenomas* are benign neoplasms composed of granular epithelium that are not capable of metastasis or invasion of the muscularis mucosa. They are either sessile (attached by a broad base) or pedunculated (attached by a stalk). Most smaller adenomas (less than 1 cm in diameter) are of the tubular type, and less than 1 percent contain carcinoma. As the polyps increase in size (greater than 2 cm in diameter), they begin to show villous changes with increasing dysplasia; the chance of one of these polyps containing cancer is about 50 percent.

Most adenocarcinomas of the colon form hard, nodular areas that grow irregularly. Colon cancers are staged or classified according to histological changes in the infiltrative character of the tumor. The most common classifications used today are the Joint Committee Classification, Duke's staging system and the tumor, node, and metastasis (TNM) system (Table 10.20). Histologically, colon cancers vary from well-differentiated cells that appear normal (grade 1) to highly anaplastic, poorly differentiated cells (grade 4). The accuracy of specimen collection is crucial. The most accurate method of evaluating a polyp is by removing the entire lesion for cytologic examination. If the polyp is less than 7 mm in diameter, tissue for biopsy can be obtained while the polyp is destroyed through "hot" (fulguration) biopsy.

Metastatic progression of colon cancer usually involves spread by local invasion, lymphatic extension with spread to the mesenteric lymph nodes first and then hematogenous spread through the portal system to the liver. In some patients, the cancer metastasizes throughout the peritoneal cavity and to the lungs. Rectal carcinoma spreads by direct extension through the perirectal fat to the lymph nodes and less often to the lung and distant organs through hemorrhoidal circulation. Prognosis of colorectal carcinoma is a function of several factors, including poorly differentiated tissue histology, mucin production, aneuploidy (DNA abnormalities), tumor invasion to other organs, perforation, and venous involvement. The prognosis is not influenced by tumor size.

Colon cancers can develop as polyps within the lumen of the intestine or as a mass on the wall of the colon. Bulky polypoid tumors are more common within the right colon, whereas tumors that encircle the bowel, causing obstruction, are more common on the left side of the colon. Tumor growth is normally slow and, in most cases, is asymptomatic until the tumor becomes large. Diagnosis is usually made late in the course of the disease, often after metastasis, thereby making a surgical cure difficult. Colon cancers that produce intracellular mucin are called "signet ring"-type carcinomas; these tumors have a tendency to be more aggressive in their spread.

Several types of colon cancers have been linked to specific genetic defects. Hereditary nonpolyposis colorectal cancers (HNPCCs) include two autosomal dominant conditions that have been associated with a markedly increased risk for developing colon cancer. Although these patients have few or no adenomatous polyps, individuals diagnosed with Lynch syndrome I are at increased risk of developing colon cancer at an early age. This cancer has a propensity for the right side of the colon. Lynch syndrome II includes the features of Lynch syndrome I as well as an increased risk of developing tumors within the ovary, uterus, urinary tract, and stomach.

Clinical Presentation

Subjective

Signs and symptoms in patients with colorectal cancer will vary, depending on the tumor size, anatomic location, and associated complications, if any. There are very few early

Table 10.20 Staging Classifications of Colorectal Cancer

Duke's Stage	TNM Class*	Description	Five-Year Survival Rate
A	T1	Tumor invades submucosa	Greater than 80%
	T2	Tumor invades muscularis	
B_1	T3	Tumor penetrates through bowel wall	60%–80%
B_2	T4	Tumor invades adjacent organs	
C_1	Any T	Any bowel wall perforation with lymph node involvement	20%–50%
	N1	1–3 pericolic or perirectal lymph nodes	
C_2	N2	4 or more pericolic or perirectal lymph nodes	
	N3	Metastasis to lymph nodes along a vascular trunk	
D	Any T Any N M1	Presence of distant metastasis	3%–25%

Source: Adapted from Tierney, L, et al: Current Medical Diagnosis of Treatment, ed 44. A Lange Medical Books/McGraw Hill, New York, 2005.
*American Joint Committee on Cancer

warning signs of colorectal carcinoma; in fact, most individuals are totally asymptomatic. Frequently, the cancer is found incidentally during abdominal surgery or during screening sigmoidoscopy.

Patients may present with melena or bright red bleeding from the rectum, depending on the location of the tumor. A change in bowel habits, including constipation alternating with diarrhea or a change in stool caliber (described as narrowed or ribbonlike), can be signs of colon cancer. Stools streaked with blood may be mistakenly dismissed as a sign of hemorrhoidal irritation. Abdominal pain is a rare presenting symptom but may indicate obstruction resulting from tumors on the left side of the colon, which has a smaller diameter lumen, or from invasion of the bowel wall by a tumor. Patients rarely report colicky pain as a result of a right-sided colon cancer because of the larger diameter of the colon and the liquid consistency of the stool. Patients with rectal cancer may complain of tenesmus (spasm of the anal sphincter), urgency, and/or hematochezia. Patients with chronic occult blood loss from an undiagnosed tumor may experience weakness and fatigue caused by iron-deficiency anemia. Weight loss and anorexia are common with any malignant process but are usually manifested late in the disease process.

Objective

Physical examination may reveal a mass within the abdomen or an enlarged liver, which may be suggestive of metastasis. A digital rectal examination should be done even though most tumors are not palpable. The stool should be tested for occult blood, which, if positive, is pathognomonic for right-sided colon cancer. Approximately 50 percent of patients with a positive fecal occult blood test have either an adenoma (38 percent) or a neoplasm (12 percent). Conversely, fecal occult blood testing is positive in only 60 to 70 percent of patients with known large intestinal cancers; however, annual screening can reduce colorectal mortality by 33 percent.

Diagnostic Reasoning

Diagnostic Tests

Although there are no definitive laboratory tests for diagnosis of colorectal cancer, a CBC should be obtained to assess for iron deficiency anemia or anemia of chronic blood loss, either of which can be common findings in patients with colorectal cancer. Liver function tests (LFTs) may reveal an elevation of the liver enzymes, especially of alkaline phosphatase if there has been metastasis to the liver and/or bone. Usually, when there is liver metastasis, the bilirubin level tends to remain normal until late in the disease process.

The serum immune assay for carcinoembryonic antigen (CEA) was developed with the intent of providing an early means of detection for colon cancer; however, the test is too insensitive and nonspecific for screening. CEA levels have been poorly correlated with the stage of cancer; however, this test is useful for monitoring a patient's response to therapy, whether surgical or chemotherapeutic. CEA levels usually normalize after colon resection, and levels that remain elevated are associated with poor prognosis. A secondary spike in the CEA level after surgery is highly suggestive of reoccurrence and must be evaluated.

Colonoscopy with a biopsy and BE are used to establish definitive diagnosis of colorectal cancer. Air contrast BE enables the radiologist to detect small defects or lesions within the intestinal mucosa. Colonoscopy is a more specific and sensitive test that can be used as follow-up to the findings of the BE; colonoscopy can also be used by itself to provide more definitive data through the biopsy of the suspect lesions. Colonoscopy establishes the diagnosis of colon cancer with almost 100-percent accuracy and is thus the diagnostic procedure of choice. Flexible sigmoidoscopy can be used for confirming lesions within the rectosigmoid area; however, full colon examination with colonoscopy is preferred. CT scan is used for evaluation of distant metastasis. Endoscopic US has been used to stage regional rectal cancers and is more accurate than CT scan in this particular area.

Patients with colonic polyps will require histologic examination of the polyp. Polyps larger than 7 mm should be totally removed by snare cautery. Polyps that are less than 7 mm in size are usually not malignant and can be removed by "hot" biopsy, which destroys the polyp while obtaining the necessary tissue for cytologic exam.

Differential Diagnosis

The symptoms of colorectal cancer are nonspecific; therefore, many disease processes can mimic the presenting symptoms of colon carcinoma and must be differentiated from it. Most of the inflammatory and irritable bowel disease processes can be confused with colon carcinoma. Ischemic colitis, diverticular disease, IBS, IBD, or infectious colitis can form strictures within the bowel that are indistinguishable from colon carcinoma. Colonoscopy with biopsy of the lesion is the diagnostic procedure of choice. Any patient over age 50 who presents with iron deficiency anemia, stool positive for occult blood, change in bowel habits, or hematochezia should have a thorough evaluation to rule out the possibility of neoplasm.

Management

The first step in the treatment of colon cancer is the staging of the disease. The staging of the cancer is of critical importance not only for the determination of the patient's long-term survival but also for determining which patients should receive adjuvant therapy. Staging of a neoplasm first involves understanding the characteristics used to describe the histological findings: tissue of origin (adenocarcinoma, sarcoma), origin of specimen (colon, breast), and the degree of tissue differentiation. Staging of the carcinoma includes both the primary site as well as the metastatic sites and allows for the development of the most optimal treatment plan based on those findings. More than half of all cancers are not curable using approved treatments available today. Many of the treatment regimens involve some form of experimental drugs or procedures; therefore, accurate staging is necessary to determine the efficacy of the treatment.

The only known cure for colon cancer is surgical resection. This is the treatment of choice for all patients who can tolerate the surgery. Even patients who have known metastasis can benefit from surgical intervention to reduce the chance of developing an intestinal obstruction or rectal hemorrhage later in the disease process. Most patients with colorectal cancer present with penetration of the mass through the bowel wall and with associated lymph node involvement. The surgeon will decide, based on the staging, what type of surgical resection is appropriate. The anatomic location of the tumor—left or right side of the colon—will dictate whether left or right hemicolectomy is performed. A wide margin of intestine (with careful ligation of the total arterial blood supply) will be resected to ensure mesenteric and associated lymph node drainage is removed.

Lesions located within the rectosigmoid area are usually treated with anterior resection, which protects the rectal sphincter. (The rectum is the distal 8 to 11 cm of large bowel.) If the rectal lesions are small and are discovered early, they can sometimes be treated by local incision, laser photoablation, or cryosurgery. Larger lesions located within this lower portion of the large bowel usually require a combination of abdominal-perineal resection with a colostomy. Unresectable rectal cancers can be palliated with a diverting colostomy, or, if the patient is a poor surgical candidate, laser fulguration of the tumor mass can minimize the bleeding and maintain the patency of the rectum.

Adjuvant chemotherapy for colon cancer is based on the stage of the disease (see Table 10.20). From 6 months to 1 year of chemotherapy with 5-fluorouracil (5-FU) and levamisole continues to be the treatment of choice for carcinomas classified as stage III (node-positive) and, although it is not curative, it enhances the survival rate. Evaluation of the treatment is based on the initial response of the tumor to the therapy (e.g., shrinkage) as well as improvement in the 5-year survival rate.

Rectal carcinomas are typically treated with chemotherapy as well as radiation therapy. Radiation therapy for rectal cancer may involve both pre- and postoperative radiation therapy. Depending on the size of the tumor, preoperative radiation therapy can help shrink the tumor, making it more amenable to resection. Postoperative combination therapy with 5-FU and radiation therapy has been effective in reducing both local and metastatic node occurrences.

Twenty percent of patients with colorectal cancer have known metastases at the time of diagnosis. Patients with known metastases to the liver may have improved survival rates with resection. Some patients with liver metastases have opted for infusions of 5-FU into the hepatic artery or portal vein, which has proved superior in the treatment of hepatic disease; however, this treatment has little effect on the overall survival rate for colorectal cancer and can be extremely toxic to the patient. Radiation therapy is often employed as a palliative measure for patients whose pain has been unresponsive to chemotherapy or other treatment modalities.

Although the oncologist will manage the patient's chemotherapy, the primary care practitioner will continue to work closely with the patient to treat any of the numerous adverse effects caused by the chemotherapy and/or the radiation therapy. The potential toxic effects of adjuvant therapy for colorectal cancer are numerous and can range from nausea, vomiting, and weight loss to cystitis and radiation proctitis. Radiation therapy to the pelvic area can cause severe GI disorders, including intractable diarrhea and even malabsorption syndromes.

Follow-Up and Referral

Initial assessment and screening for colorectal carcinoma is the responsibility of every primary-care provider. Patients who are known to be at higher risk for the development of colorectal cancer, such as those who have a first-degree relative with the disease, a family history of adenomas, a personal history of adenomas or colorectal cancer, or a longstanding history of IBD will require a more in-depth screening by a practitioner who is well trained in this area. Screening for high-risk patients should include colonoscopy, which is best done by an experienced gastroenterologist. The recommended screening for average- and high-risk individuals is provided in Screening Recommendations/Guidelines 10.1.

Follow-up is vitally important in the treatment of colorectal cancer. In an effort to prevent occurrence or reoccurrence, scheduled colon surveillance is required. Early detection and removal of adenomas can improve survival rates. Close surveillance is necessary for patients who have undergone "curative resection" surgery. Recommendations include office visits every 3 months, which should include a CEA level, annual CT of the abdomen and pelvis, and chest x-ray film for the first 3 years postoperatively. Colonoscopy should be completed postoperatively; but, if the exam was not completed at that time, a colonoscopy should be scheduled for 3 months postoperatively and then again at 1 year, with special attention to anastomotic recurrences. If the results of the exam are within normal limits, patients may continue with follow-up exams every 3 years. Patients whose CEA levels normalize or stabilize after surgery and then spike suddenly require a thorough examination.

Patients who have undergone surgical resection of a colon cancer and have a temporary or permanent colostomy may benefit from assistance from a enterostomal therapist. Consultation with a urologist for urologic or sexual dysfunction resulting from surgical or radiation therapy may provide medical and social support. Patients suffering

SCREENING RECOMMENDATIONS / GUIDELINES 10.1

Colon Cancer Screening Recommended by the American Cancer Society

Risk	Screening Recommendations
Average risk	Annual fecal occult blood (FOB) test Flexible sigmoidoscopy every 5 years beginning at age 50 or colonoscopy every 10 years
High risk (general)	Annual FOB testing Double contrast barium enema OR Colonoscopy every 3–5 years starting at age 40
Specific High-Risk Groups	
Prior colorectal cancer	Colonoscopy 1 year postfinding, then every 3 years
HNPCC	Colonoscopy screening must begin 10 years before the age of onset of the earliest affected family member OR Colonoscopy every 1–2 years beginning at age 20–25 and continuing until age 35 and then yearly
IBD	Annual colonoscopy beginning 8 years after onset of disease
First-degree family history	Colonoscopy every 3–5 years beginning 5 years before the age of onset of the youngest affected relative

from metastatic disease can be referred to hospice service personnel who are trained in providing comfort and support to both the family and the patient. They can give guidance regarding home and hospital care and are specially trained in providing appropriate analgesia for patients. Criteria for admission to the hospice program differs from one area to another; most require a physician statement that the patient has less than 6 months to live and is receiving only palliative or supportive treatments. Some hospice services require patients to have a "do not resuscitate" (DNR) order in place as a condition for admission.

Patient Education

Patient education should focus first on the prevention of colon cancer, stressing a diet that is low in fat and refined carbohydrates and high in fiber, fruits, vegetables, and complex carbohydrates. Some studies have shown favorable statistics when individuals supplement their diets with vitamins E and C and beta carotene as well as pursue a lifestyle that includes exercise. The risk/benefit/cost ratio makes these preventative measures worth suggesting.

Hemorrhoids

Hemorrhoids are defined as a mass of dilated and tortuous veins that represent prolapsed submucosal tissue. Hemorrhoids are classified as either internal or external, depending on their location. The primary cause of hemorrhoids is believed to be straining during defecation, which is further complicated by constipation, prolonged sitting, pregnancy, and anal infection. Some hemorrhoids are asymptomatic and require no treatment; others can result in profuse bleeding, requiring emergency ligation.

Epidemiology and Causes

Every year approximately 1 million people, or 5 percent of the American population, visit their medical provider for symptoms of hemorrhoids. Although hemorrhoids can occur at any age, their incidence increases with age.

Although the cause of hemorrhoids is not completely known or understood, there has been an increase in the development of countries where there is a known deficiency of dietary fiber. Thus, increased straining during defecation has been recognized as an important predisposing factor in the development of hemorrhoids. Heredity may also be a factor because 10 percent of the patients with hemorrhoids have a family history of the disease. Patients suffering from illnesses characterized by chronic diarrhea, such as IBD, are also more likely to develop hemorrhoids.

Pathophysiology

External hemorrhoids are dilated, varicose veins originating from the inferior hemorrhoidal plexus and are located below the anal rectal line. Internal hemorrhoids are a dilatation of the veins within the superior hemorrhoidal plexus and are located within the distal rectum and the anal canal.

The inferior hemorrhoidal plexus is prone to increased distension during defecation, which can result in rupture of a vessel and subsequent development of a perianal hematoma or thrombus within one of the vessels of the plexus. Patients who have a thrombosed hemorrhoid may present with a painful perianal lump.

Internal hemorrhoids are further classified by the degree of prolapse present. Table 10.21 describes the difference between each degree of prolapse.

Clinical Presentation

Subjective

External hemorrhoids may present with an abrupt onset of pain that is associated with the development of a perianal lump. Many patients complain of more intense pain after defecation or other straining maneuvers, which result in further inflammation and engorgement. Mucus discharge from the anus can lead to poor hygiene and complaints of pruritus. The natural history of a resolved hemorrhoid is the formation of external skin tags, which are asymptomatic but may be irritating and interfere with daily hygiene.

Objective

On physical examination, external hemorrhoids may not be visible at rest but usually protrude on standing or with the Valsalva maneuver. Thrombosed hemorrhoids may appear as shiny, blue masses located at the anus. Evidence of hemorrhoidal skin tags may appear at the site of resolved hemorrhoids; these skin tags are fibrotic and painless.

Internal hemorrhoids most often present with rectal bleeding described as bright red streaks on the toilet paper. Patients may report that blood actually drips into the toilet after a bowel movement. Occasionally the bleeding is sufficient enough to cause anemia, which in any case merits further investigation.

Diagnostic Reasoning

Diagnostic Tests

Initial diagnosis is made by visual inspection of the anal area. Digital rectal examination is not considered an accurate means of diagnosis because most internal hemorrhoids are soft swellings that usually are not palpable, nor are they painful unless they have thrombosed, become infected, or a fissure has developed. External hemorrhoids can usually be diagnosed at physical exam, whereas internal hemorrhoids are visible on physical examination only if they have prolapsed.

Definitive diagnosis of internal hemorrhoids requires anoscopy for a proper inspection of the anal canal. With the anoscope in place, the patient is asked to strain as he or she would while having a bowel movement so that the degree of prolapse can be assessed. Patients may undergo proctosigmoidoscopy in order to effectively rule out any precipitating or coexisting diseases of the colon or rectum.

Table 10.21 Classification of Internal Hemorrhoids

Severity	Description of the Process
First degree	Protrude into the lumen of the anal canal, usually without the sensation of protrusion.
Second degree	Protrude beyond the anal canal during defecation but spontaneously reduce when defecation is completed.
Third degree	Protrude beyond the anal canal during defecation but must be manually reduced after the completion of the bowel movement.
Fourth degree	Protrude beyond the anal canal and are permanently prolapsed despite attempts at manual reduction.

Differential Diagnosis

The differential diagnosis of hemorrhoids includes polyps, carcinoma of the anus, anorectal fistula, cryptitis, papillitis, or rectal prolapse. Proctosigmoidoscopy is an effective means of establishing the appropriate diagnosis.

Management

Initial treatment for symptomatic external hemorrhoids is focused on adequate pain relief with oral analgesia and sitz baths. If the hemorrhoids do not spontaneously regress, care is directed at decreasing straining with defecation and modification of toilet habits. Patients are encouraged to avoid sitting on the toilet for long periods of time, to use some form of bulk-forming laxative, and to increase their daily fiber intake slowly to 25 to 35 grams to establish regular, formed stools. Patients who suffer from diarrhea should be treated accordingly to control frequent loose stools. Individuals who suffer from pruritis should be instructed to maintain anal hygiene. Sitz baths, witch hazel, and application of topical hydrocortisone creams are all effective in controlling pruritus. If the external hemorrhoids continue to be painful or bothersome despite treatment, referral for surgical excision should be made.

Medical treatment of internal hemorrhoids follows the same principles previously outlined, with attention toward avoiding straining during defecation, modification of diet with the addition of fiber, increasing fluids, and the addition of bulking agents. If medical treatment is not effective, there are a number of nonsurgical treatments that may be employed. First-degree hemorrhoids can be treated by injection sclerotherapy or infrared coagulation. Infrared coagulation, much like electrocoagulation, uses high-intensity light to shrink the swelling. Second- and third-degree hemorrhoids are normally treated with rubber band ligation, in which a rubber-banded ring is placed around the base of the hemorrhoid. This band acts a tourniquet, strangulating the tissue while fixing the mucosa proximal to the ligation into the muscularis. All of the nonsurgical techniques used to treat internal hemorrhoids are associated with some degree of pain and bleeding.

Large, advanced-degree hemorrhoids will most often require referral to a surgeon for a formal hemorrhoidectomy. Again, proper anal hygiene and correction of chronic constipation and diarrhea are essential to prevent the recurrence of hemorrhoids.

Follow-Up and Referral

Excision of a single external hemorrhoid, evacuation of a thrombosed external hemorrhoid, and injection sclerotherapy of simple internal hemorrhoids can all be performed in the office by a trained provider. Band ligation and other specialized treatment of hemorrhoids will require referral to a gastroenterologist more familiar with these procedures. Follow-up will be based on the patient's postprocedure course. Most patients will require no further care except for instruction on proper anal hygiene and diet. The addition of a nonirritating laxative postprocedure will usually prevent the development of constipation and the associated fear of defecation.

Patient Education

Patient education for hemorrhoids is aimed at preventing the problem through increasing fiber in the diet. Fiber should be increased to 25 to 35 g/day, but this should be done slowly to prevent bloating and gas formation. Teaching patients to read the labels of their food can help them gain control over their nutrition. Often, patients associate salad and cereal with very high levels of fiber. This is not accurate information in many cases, for example, most breakfast cereals have only 1 to 3 g of fiber per serving, and iceberg lettuce has very little fiber as well. OTC bulking agents, such as psyllium (Metamucil), can be suggested to help eliminate constipation. It is important to teach patients the necessity of drinking no less than 64 ounces of water a day.

Bibliography

General

Barker, LR, Burton, JR, and Zieve, PD: Principles of Ambulatory Medicine, ed 6. Lippincott Williams & Wilkins, Philadelphia, 2003.

Bascom, A: Incorporating Herbal Medicine into Clinical Practice. FA Davis, Philadelphia, 2002.

Dambro, MR. Griffith's 5-Minute Clinical Consult. Lippincott Williams & Wilkins, Philadelphia, 2003.

Hayes, A, Buffum, M, Lanier, E, Rodahl, E, and Sasso, C: A music intervention to reduce anxiety prior to gastrointestinal procedures. Gastroenterol Nurs 26(4):145–149, 2003.

Huether, SE: Alterations in digestive function. In McCance, KL, and Huether, SE (eds): Pathophysiology: The Biologic Basis for Disease in Adults Children, ed 4. CV Mosby, St. Louis, Mo., 2002, pp 1261–1313.

Kee, JL: Laboratory and Diagnostic Tests with Nursing Implications, ed 6. Prentice-Hall, Upper Saddle River, N.J., 2002.

McQuaid, KR: Alimentary tract. In Tierney, LM, et al (eds): Current Medical Diagnosis and Treatment, ed 44. Lange/McGraw-Hill, New York, 2005, pp 518–628.

Thompson, DL: Complementary healthcare practices: East meets west: the use of traditional Chinese medicine for gastrointestinal disorders. Gastroenterol Nurs 26(6):266–268, 2003

Tierney, LM, McPhee, SJ, and Papadakis, MA: Current Medical Diagnosis & Treatment, Lange/McGraw-Hill, New York, 2005.

Wagner, D: Complementary healthcare practices: Thought on complementary approaches to intestinal disease. Gastroenterol Nurs 26(1):41–44, 2003.

Liver, Biliary, and Pancreatic Diseases

Brown, VK: Hepatitis C: Risk factors, prevention, and management. Clin Excell Nurse Pract 5(6):35–39, 2002.

Buckley, K: The cleansing diet. Hepatitis 4(6):19–22, 2002

CDC: (2003). Hepatitis C epidemiology. Available at: http://www.cdc.gov/ncidod/diseases/hepatitis/c_training/edu/1/epidem-trans-2.htm. Accessed March 10, 2003.

CDC: Notifiable diseases/deaths in selected cities weekly information. MMWR Morbid Mortal Weekly Rep 53(52):1213–1221, 2005.

Friedman, LS: Liver, biliary tract, & pancreas. In Tierney, LM, et al (eds): Current Medical Diagnosis and Treatment, ed 44. Lange/McGraw-Hill, New York, 2005, pp 629–678.

Losue, K: Chronic hepatitis C: Latest treatment options. Nurse Pract 27(4):32–49, 2002

Plec, CE: Milking it. Hepatitis 5(3):15–17, 2003.

Deutsch, KF: Hepatitis C: The silent epidemic. Clin Advisor May, 10–18, 2003.

Shapira, SC, and Yoshida, EM: Hepatitis B: Latest treatment guidelines. Consultant 45:605–610, 2005.

Swaroop, VS, Chari, ST, and Clain, JE: Severe acute pancreatitis. JAMA 291(23):2865–2868, 2004.

Tokita, H, et al: Risk factors for the development of hepatocellular carcinoma among patients with chronic hepatitis C who achieved a sustained virological response to interferon therapy. J Gastroenterol Hepatol 20:752–758, 2005.

Wilson, TR: The ABCs of hepatitis. Nurse Pract 30(6):12–21, 2005.

Upper GI Diseases

Biddle, W: Gastroesophageal reflux disease: Current treatment approaches. Gastroenterol Nurs 26(6):228–236, 2003.

Der, G: An overview of proton pump inhibitors. Gastroenterol Nurs 26(5):182–190, 2003.

Hemminger, LL, and Wolfsen, HC: Photodynamic therapy for Barrett's esophagus and high grade dysplasia: results of a patient satisfaction survey. Gastroenterol Nurs 25(4):139–141, 2002.

Huether, SE: Alterations in digestive function. In McCance, KL, and Huether, SE (eds): Pathophysiology: The Biologic Basis for Disease in Adults & Children, ed 4. CV Mosby, St. Louis, Mo., 2002, pp 1261–1313.

O'Malley, P: Gastric ulcers and GERD: the new "plagues" of the 21st century. Clin Nurse Spec 17(6):286–289, 2003.

Ours, TM, Fackler, WK, Richter, JE, and Vaezi, MF: Nocturnal acid breakthrough: Clinical significance and correlation with esophageal acid exposure. Am J Gastroenterol 98(3):545–550, 2003.

Rockey, AD: What you need to know about Barrett's esophagus. Gastroenterol Nurs 25(6):237–240, 2002.

Saddler, D: Gastroesophageal reflux disease. Gastroenterol Nurs 26(3):125–126, 2003.

Williams, JL: Gastroesophageal reflux disease: Clinical manifestations. Gastroenterol Nurs 26(5):195–200, 2003.

Wollner, T: Eradicate *H. pylori* with effective treatment regimens. Nurse Pract 29(6):40–44, 2004.

Lower GI Diseases

Erlinger, TP, Platz, EA, Rifai, N, and Helzlsouer, KJ: C-reative protein and the risk of incident colorectal cancer. JAMA 291(5):585–590, 2004.

Fasano, A, et al: Prevalence of celiac disease in at-risk and not-at-risk groups in the United States: A large multicenter study. Arch Intern Med 163(3):359–361, 2004.

Gisbert, JP, Gomollon, F, Mate, J, and Pajares, JM: Role of 5-aminosalicylic acid (5-ASA) in treatment of inflammatory bowel disease: A systematic review. Digest Dis Sci 47(3):471–488, 2002.

Hampton, T: Scientists explore pathogenesis of IBD. JAMA 292(22): 2708–2713, 2004.

Hilsden, RJ, Verhoef, MJ, Best, A, and Pocobelli, G: Complementary and alternative medicien use by Canadian patients with inflammatory bowel disease: Results from a national survey. Am J Gastroenterol 98(7):1563–1568, 2003

Manthey, MW, Ross, AB, and Soergel, KH: Cryptosporidiosis and inflammatory bowel disease: Experience from the Milwaukee outbreak. Digest Dis Sci 42(8):1580–1586, 1997.

Mow, WS, et al: High-level serum antibodies to bacterial antigens are associated with antibiotic-induced clinical remission in Crohn's disease: A pilot study. Digest Dis Sci 49(7/8):1280–1286, 2004.

Nandakumar, G, Morgan, JA, Silverberg, D, and Steinhagen, RM: Familial polyposis coli: clinical manifestations, evealuation, management and treatment. Mt Sinai J Med 71(6):384–391, 2004.

Paraskeva, PA, Axix, O, and Darzi, A: Laparoscopic surgery for colon cancer. Surg Clin North Am 85(1):49–60, 2005.

Pasch, B, and Serhan, CN: Is C-reactive protein an inflammation opsonin that signals colon cancer risk? JAMA 291(5):623–624, 2004.

Smith, MM, and Bryant, JL: Mind-body and mind-gut connection in inflammatory bowel disease. Gastroenterol Nurs 25(5):213–217, 2002.

Stein, P: Ulcerative colitis-diagnosis and surgical treatment. AORN 80(2).242–262, 2004.

Su, LJ, and Arab, L: Report: alcohol consumption and risk of colon cancer: Evidence from the national health and nutrition examination survey I epidemiologic follow-up study. Nutr Cancer 50(2):111–119, 2004.

Young, LS, and Thomas, DJ: Celiac sprue treatment in primary care. Nurse Pract 29(7):42–45, 2004.

Zimmerman, J: Extraintestinal symptoms in irritable bowel syndrome and inflammatory bowel diseases. Digest Dis Sci 48(4):743–749, 2003.

Resources

American Liver Foundation
(800)223-0179
http://www.liverfoundation.org

Crohn's and Colitis Foundation of America
386 Park Avenue, South, 17th Floor
New York, NY, 10016-8804
(800)932-2423 ext. 12
http://www.ccfa.org

International Foundation for Bowel Disfunction (IFBD)
Box 17864
Milwaukee, WI 53217
(414)241-9479

Renal Problems

Debera J. Thomas, DNS, APRN, BC
Brian O. Porter, MD, PhD, MPH

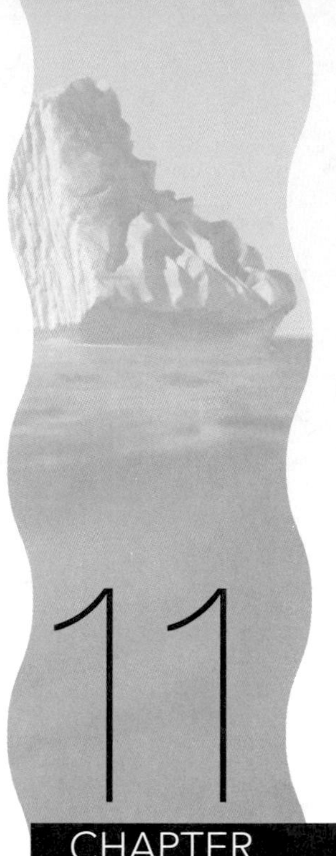

Common Complaints

Dysuria

Dysuria is the subjective experience of pain or a burning sensation on urination, and can include frequency, hesitancy, urgency, and strangury (slow, painful urination). Symptoms of dysuria can be secondary to several different medical conditions or certain medications; for example, a light burning sensation or discomfort can be normal when associated with concentrated acidic urine. Dysuria is most commonly associated with lower urinary system infection.

Differential Diagnosis

Dysuria is most often associated with a bladder problem and rarely with renal disease Inflammatory lesions of the prostate, bladder, and urethra—including prostatitis in men, urethrotrigonitis in women, and bladder and urethral infections in men and women—are the most common causes of dysuria. When caused by bladder problems, frequency of urination usually occurs secondary to diminished bladder capacity or with pain when the bladder becomes distended. Urinary frequency may be a manifestation of urinary incontinence and can occur with prostatic hypertrophy or neurogenic bladder disorders.

Other conditions associated with dysuria are bladder tumors, chronic renal failure, nephrolithiasis, and occasionally diseases of the upper urinary system. Dysuria may also be associated with diseases outside the renal system such as sexually transmitted diseases (STDs), vaginitis, or prostatitis. For example, female patients may present with symptoms of dysuria or external irritation from the urine passing over the irritated labia. The dysuria may or may not be accompanied by vaginal discharge. Any woman who presents with dysuria should be questioned about an associated vaginal discharge or irritation. The symptoms of dysuria may lead to other diagnoses, including urethral strictures, prolapsed uterus, pelvic peritonitis, cancer of the cervix or prostate, dysmenorrhea, and conditions of the prostate. Prescribed medications such as opiates and those used to prevent motion sickness can also cause dysuria.

Urinalysis is the easiest, most noninvasive, and most economical way to identify urinary tract infections (UTIs) and other renal problems (Advanced Assessment 11.1). Once the underlying problem has been identified, appropriate treatment can be instituted.

Conditions associated with dysuria, such as bladder tumors, chronic renal failure, nephrolithiasis, and infections of the upper and lower urinary system, are discussed in the Common Problems section of this chapter. Problems associated with conditions of the prostate are discussed in Chapter 12 and those associated with dysmenorrhea in Chapter 13.

Hematuria

Hematuria is defined as blood in the urine and can be visible (gross) or occult (microscopic). It is characterized by more than three red blood cells (RBCs) per high-power microscopic field (hpf). Normal urinary excretion of RBCs is 2,000,000 per day, which corresponds to two or three RBCs per hpf. It actually takes very little blood to make the urine look very red. Urine starts to "pink up" at between 20 and 30 RBCs per hpf and becomes red at about 100 RBCs per hpf. There is a direct relationship between the quantity of blood found in the urine and the likelihood of pathology.

ADVANCED ASSESSMENT 11.1

URINALYSIS

Name	Abnormal Value	Common Differential Diagnosis
Appearance	Colorless	Diabetes insipidus, diuretic agents, fluid overload
	Dark	Hematuria, malignancy, stones, acidic urine
	Cloudy	UTI, hematuria, bilirubin, mucous
	Pink/red	Hematuria, hemoglobin, myoglobin, beets, food coloring
	Orange/yellow	Phenazopyridin, rifampin, bile pigments
	Brown/black	Myoglobin, bile pigments, melanin, cascara, iron preparation
	Green	Bile pigments, methylene blue, indigo carmine
	Foamy	Proteinuria, bile salts
Specific Gravity	Increased	Dehydration, congestive heart failure, adrenal insufficiency, diabetes mellitus, nephrosis, ADH
	Decreased	Diabetes insipidus, pyelonephritis, glomerulonephritis (GN), excess fluid intake
pH	Acidic	Diet, medications, acidosis, ketoacidosis, chronic obstructive pulmonary disease (COPD)
	Alkaline	Diet, sodium bicarbonate, vomiting, metabolic alkalosis, UTI
Bilirubin	Positive	Jaundice, hepatitis
Blood	Positive	Kidney stones, tumors, kidney disease, trauma, infection, injury from instrumentation, coagulation problems, menses
Glucose	Positive	Diabetes mellitus, pancreatitis, Cushing's disease, shock, burns, steroids, renal disease, hyperthyroidism, cancer
Ketones	Positive	Starvation, diet, ketoacidosis, vomiting, diarrhea, pregnancy
Nitrate	Positive	Infection
Protein	Positive	Kidney disease, pregnancy, CHF, diabetes mellitus, cancer, benign cause
Leukocyte esterase	Positive	Infection
Reducing substance	Positive	Medications, glucose, fructose, galactose
		Liver disease, hyperthyroidism

Transient hematuria occurs on one occasion while *persistent hematuria* occurs on two or more consecutive occasions. Both transient and persistent hematuria can be a sign of serious underlying disease. Urine color can vary widely from light pink to dark red, and is sometimes characterized as "smoky." The color of urine is dependent on the amount of blood present, as well as on dietary intake, use of medications, the dilution, and the pH of the urine. For example, the ingestion of beets can color the urine red to pink, while medications such as rifampin and phenazopyridine (Pyridium) can give urine a reddish-orange color. The presence of porphyrins, hemoglobin, or myoglobin can color the urine reddish-brown. Pus in the urine is indicative of bacterial infection, such as cystitis, urethritis, or prostatitis.

Rates of hematuria can be as high as 15 percent in the general population but are usually less than 1 percent. The age, gender, and activity level of the patient with hematuria should be considered on assessment. For example, long-distance runners and other athletes can have rates of hematuria as high as 18 percent. However, even transient hematuria in men older than age 50 may be an indication of serious disease, with up to 2.4 percent of this population having urinary tract malignancies, typically a transitional cell carcinoma. In men older than age 60, this incidence of urinary tract malignancy increases to 9 percent. In older men with gross hematuria, the rate of associated malignancy is as high as 20 percent. In general, there is a higher correlation between underlying malignancy and gross hematuria as opposed to microscopic hematuria, especially in patients with a history of cigarette smoking.

Differential Diagnosis

A drug history is important because many drugs can cause hematuria. In addition, dietary substances such as caffeine, spices, tomatoes, chocolate, alcohol, citrus fruits, and soy sauce may act as bladder irritants. The patient's drug and food intake history should be assessed to rule out these substances as the causative agent. The drugs involved may be prescribed, over-the-counter (OTC), herbal, supplemental vitamins, or recreational in nature.

Some medications, beta-lactam antibiotics, sulfonamides, nonsteroidal anti-inflammatory drugs (NSAIDs), rifampin, ciprofloxacin (Cipro), allopurinol (Zyloprim), cimetidine (Tagamet), and phenytoin (Dilantin) can cause *nephritis,* which can result in destruction nephrons and subsequently can lead to impaired renal function and hematuria. Other conditions such as anticoagulation and papillary necrosis can result from the use of anticoagulants such as warfarin (Coumadin), heparin, aspirin, and NSAIDs. Glomerulonephritis can be caused from the use of hydralazine, hydrocarbons (including glue and paint sniffing), gold, penicillamine, amphetamines, NSAIDs, allopurinol, and paraquat. Urolithiasis (discussed later in this chapter) can occur from the use of carbonic anhydrase inhibitors, triamterene, sulfonamides, and vitamin D metabolites and often presents with hematuria.

Menstrual history is always important in a female patient, as well as history of recent strenuous exercise, streptococcal infection (especially poststreptococcal glomerulonephritis), or nephrolithiasis; family history (e.g., of polycystic kidney disease); and recent travel (potential exposure to parasitic infections). Gross painless hematuria is a cardinal symptom of certain malignancies such as bladder cancer.

The physical examination may reveal costovertebral angle tenderness, which could indicate pyelonephritis, tumor, or glomerulonephritis. An abdominal mass may indicate a neoplasm (renal cell cancer) or polycystic kidney disease. Suprapubic tenderness is indicative of a bladder etiology, whereas urethral discharge indicates a urethritis. An enlarged prostate could indicate benign prostate hypertrophy (BPH), whereas a tender prostate would more likely be suggestive of prostatitis; a prostate nodule may indicate a neoplasm. Skin lesions (e.g., ecchymosis) may indicate an underlying coagulopathy or vasculitis.

The most important diagnostic test in cases of hematuria is urinalysis. One major drawback of doing a urine dipstick test is that it detects the presence of heme (an iron-containing nonprotein portion of the hemoglobin molecule) in the urine but not RBCs. If the dipstick is positive for heme, but the number of RBCs on the microscopic exam is within normal limits then myoglobinuria and hemoglobinuria should be suspected. When hematuria of renal origin is suspected, laboratory test should include antinuclear antibodies (ANAs); immunoglobulins; cryoglobulins; antiglomerular basement membrane antibodies; a full chemistry panel, including creatinine clearance and blood urea nitrogen (BUN); complete blood count (CBC) and platelets; antistreptolysin O (ASO) titer; serum protein electrophoresis; and a Venereal Disease Research Laboratory (VDRL) test (to rule out syphilis). If these studies indicate a renal problem then the patient should be referred to a nephrologist, who will probably do a renal biopsy. A urine culture and sensitivity should be done on all patients with hematuria, and if bacterial infection is found, treatment with appropriate antibiotics should be instituted with reevaluation for a persistent hematuria 2 weeks after completion of treatment.

Isolated asymptomatic hematuria is often found on a routine screening urinalysis with no apparent source determined by history and physical exam. The possibility of occult malignancy or other potentially serious etiology increases with age and if the patient is older than age 40, he or she should be evaluated for urologic tumor. Patients younger than age 40 should be monitored at least monthly for 3 months and if the hematuria persists then a more aggressive workup is indicated.

Examination of the morphology of RBCs present in the urine using phase-contrast microscopy can provide clues as to the etiology of hematuria. Dysmorphic RBCs may indicate glomerular disease. A fresh urine sample is essential, since the changes in morphology occur if the urine is allowed to sit. If the hematuria persists without evidence of infection, an IVP (intravenous pyelogram) or renal ultrasound should be done to assess kidney structure. A computed tomography (CT) scan is the preferred imaging method for follow-up if a possible solid renal mass is found. Other tests that should be done include a prothrombin time (PT) and partial thromboplastin (PTT), a purified protein derivative (PPD) test, erythrocyte sedimentation rate (ESR), an ANA test and complement level, antistreptococcal enzyme titers (ASO, anti-DNase B), cryoglobulin screen, and a urinalysis for cytology.

Cystoscopy is done to evaluate the upper urinary tract, while cytology can be done to evaluate the lower urinary tract. If the findings of these studies are negative and the patient continues to have gross hematuria, further investigation should include a CT scan, arteriogram, and/or ureteroscopy. The outcome of these studies will determine whether a referral for urologist or nephrologist follow-up is necessary.

The causes of hematuria are grouped according to anatomic site of the blood source. For example, *isolated hematuria* (no other abnormal urine components) may be from bleeding anywhere from the renal pelvis to the urethra, but is rarely caused by systemic disease. RBC casts usually indicate injury to the nephron and are diagnostic of hematuria of a renal origin. However, intact uniform RBCs with no casts suggests hematuria originating in the lower urinary tract. The presence of bacteria in the urine is diagnostic of a bacterial origin, as is fever. Acute cystitis and urethritis produce gross hematuria and are more common in women. The presence of both proteinuria and hematuria is suggestive of glomerular or interstitial nephritis. Hematuria accompanied by colicky flank pain suggests a ureteral stone. When bleeding occurs only at the beginning or end of urination then a prostatic or urethral source is likely. Hematuria accompanied by hypertension, edema, and a sore throat or a skin infection may be indicative of glomerulonephritis. Thirty percent of patients with gross hematuria are diagnosed with a malignancy of the prostate, urethra, bladder, kidney, or ureter. Table 11.1 lists possible differential diagnoses of hematuria.

Table 11.1 Differential Diagnosis: Hematuria

Problem	Differential Diagnoses
Urethra	Urethritis (gonococcal, non-gonococcal) Stricture Calculus Trauma
Prostate/male genitourinary tract	Infection (prostatitis, epididymitis) Benign prostatic hypertrophy (BPH) Tumor
Kidney	Infection (pyelonephritis) Nephrolithiasis Cancer (renal cell) Trauma Glomerular disease (vesculitis, idiopathic) Ischemia (embolism, thrombosis, papillary necrosis) Allergic interstitial nephritis (drug induced)
Ureters	Nephrolithiasis Tumor Endometriosis
Bladder	Infection (bacterial, parasitic) Calculus Tumor Endometriosis Drugs (hemorrhagic cystitis)
Pseudohematuria	Menstrual contamination Phenothiazines Red food dye Quinine Rifampin Hemoglobinuria
Systemic Illness	Intense exercise Coagulopathies (thrombocytopenia, hemoglobinopathy, sickle cell)

Proteinuria

The primary proteins found in urine are globulin and albumin. *Proteinuria* is usually indicative of a renal pathology, most often glomerular in origin. Proteinuria can be functional as a result of acute illness, emotional stress, or excessive exercise and is a benign process. It can also develop from overproduction of filterable plasma proteins, especially Bence Jones proteins associated with multiple myeloma. Abnormalities in the glomerular basement membrane produce glomerular proteinuria. Damage to the proximal tubule where filterable proteins are reabsorbed can result in tubular proteinuria.

Intermittent proteinuria is most often asymptomatic and discovered incidentally through urine dipstick testing and is associated with functional disorders. Continuous proteinuria is associated with renal pathology. The dipstick test does not detect Bence Jones proteins or light chain immunoglobulins and is most sensitive to albumin. A false-negative reading can occur because of a diluted urine sample, alkaline pH (normal 4.5 to 8 [usually 5.5 to 6.5]), or Bence Jones proteinuria. The most accurate way to quantify the amount of protein in the urine is a 24-hour urine collection; however, a spot urine albumin to urine creatinine ratio can be measured and is a close approximation of the 24-hour urine measurement. A 24-hour urine with more than 165 mg of protein is considered abnormal and a specimen with more than 3.5 grams is indicative of a nephrotic problem. A urine albumin to urine creatinine ration of less than 0.2 is normal and corresponds to an excretion of less than 200 mg/dL of protein.

Differential Diagnosis

Proteinuria may occur from "benign" causes. Causes of benign, or functional, proteinuria include orthostatic proteinuria, exercise, environmental conditions, fever, and acute illnesses. Orthostatic proteinuria occurs when the protein level is elevated only when the patient has been standing but not while he or she has been reclining. Exercise-induced proteinuria may occur in athletes such as runners or boxers; it may be accompanied by elevated catecholamines, hemoglobinuria, or hematuria. Proteinuria caused by environmental conditions such as emotional stress, exposure to cold, prolonged lordotic posture, and excess in the body's norepinephrine level will resolve spontaneously when the precipitating element is eliminated or removed. A mild, transient proteinuria may result from an albumin infusion or acute illnesses such as fever, congestive heart failure (CHF), acute pulmonary edema, head injury, or cerebral vascular accident; this type of proteinuria typically resolves as the medical condition improves.

When proteinuria is identified in a low-risk (nondiabetic or nonpregnant) patient, the urine should be tested for Bence Jones protein, the presence of which suggests multiple myeloma. In addition, a full chemistry panel should be done, including a fasting blood sugar (FBS), a lipid profile, urine culture and sensitivity, and a CBC with differential. If the patient's urine is positive for Bence Jones proteins, a serum protein electrophoresis should be done. Proteinuria associated with multiple myeloma, lymphosarcoma, Hodgkin's disease, and leukemia is called Bence Jones proteinuria. Bence Jones proteinuria is characterized as a free monoclonal light chain of protein.

Any persistent proteinuria that is not classified as functional proteinuria requires further workup, beginning with a 24-hour measurement of urine protein and creatinine levels. If the excretion rate is above 3.0 to 3.5 g/day, the patient, by definition, has nephrotic syndrome and must be referred to a nephrologist. Nephrotic syndrome can lead to acute renal failure (ARF), hypertension, and end-stage renal failure.

If the excretion rate of protein is more than 2 grams in 24 hours a glomerular cause is most likely and further evaluation is warranted. If renal function is normal in a patient with an elevated urine protein, the patient should then be evaluated for orthostatic proteinuria. This involves having the patient collect a urine specimen on awakening but before assuming an upright position for longer than 1 minute. After the patient has been standing or walking for 2 hours, a second specimen is collected. If the patient has orthostatic proteinuria the first specimen will be free of protein and the second will be positive for protein, and referral to a nephrologist is necessary. Although this condition is largely benign and self-limiting, orthostatic proteinuria is not well understood. Patients with nonorthostatic proteinuria and normal renal function in whom no Bence Jones proteins have been detected should also be referred to a renal specialist for renal biopsy. Proteinuria associated with a specific disease process involving the renal system is presented in Table 11.2.

Management of proteinuria depends on the underlying cause. Angiotensin-converting enzyme (ACE) agents have been found to reduce proteinuria by decreasing interglomerular pressure. If hyperlipidemia and/or hypertension are present, they should be aggressively treated. Patients found to have chronic renal failure (CRF) should also be aggressively managed to prevent or delay the onset of end-stage renal disease (ESRD).

Common Problems

Urinary Incontinence

Urinary incontinence (UI) is the involuntary loss of urine from the bladder. Incontinence is so frequent in women that many consider it normal. Incontinence is also common in older men as a result of an enlarging prostate. Incontinence can affect a person's quality of life and may be psychologically devastating. Ignoring the incontinence, or inadequate treatment of this condition, can lead to social isolation, body image problems, anxiety, or depression, therefore, prompt treatment is essential.

Epidemiology and Causes

Urinary incontinence costs more than $16 billion per year and affects more than 13 million Americans. One study estimates that more than 40 percent of American women are affected, and researchers have found a strong association between urinary incontinence and major depression. The prevalence of urinary incontinence in the community population varies from 5 percent to 15 percent depending on age and gender, and more than 50 percent of the patients in long-term care facilities have incontinence. Women are more likely than men to have incontinence and the incidence increases with age; in fact, the risk of urinary incontinence increases 14 percent with each decade of life.

Transient UI is characterized by a sudden onset and can have several causes including delirium, infection, pharmacologic agents, or underlying systemic illnesses such as diabetes, fecal impaction, and restricted mobility. Table 11.3 presents popular mnemonics (memory aids) for the causes of urinary incontinence. Most new-onset incontinence that occurs in the hospital resolves with appropriate treatment, but this acute transient phase can become a chronic problem if left untreated.

The basic types of persistent UI are categorized as stress, urge, overflow, and functional urinary incontinence. A patient may present with mixed symptoms of urge and stress incontinence. Table 11.4 provides an overview of the types of urinary incontinence.

Pathophysiology

An understanding of incontinence requires knowledge of the physiology of micturition. Three major components are involved in urine storage and release: the central nervous system (CNS), the bladder, and the bladder outlet (urethral sphincters). Within the CNS, micturition is controlled by both the cortical (central) and brainstem (pontine) micturition centers. The cortical micturition center coordinates inhibitory stimuli from the frontal lobes and basal ganglia, permitting bladder relaxation and filling, as well as urethral

Table 11.2 Proteinuria

Type of Proteinuria	Major Mechanism	Disease Process
Bence Jones proteinuria	Elevated plasma concentration	Multiple myeloma (lymphosarcoma, leukemia, Hodgkin's disease)
Tamm-Horsfall proteinuria	Increased tubular cell secretion	Normal mucoprotein in urine
Tubulointerstitial area involvement	Decreased tubular reabsorption of normal filtered protein	Pyelonephritis
Altered glomerular capillary permeability	Increase of filtered proteins	Glomerulonephritis, nephrotic syndrome
pH >8.0	High-alkaline urines	False-positive

Table 11.3 Urinary Incontinence

DIAPERS
D Delirium
I Infection, inflammation
A Atrophic vaginitis, atrophic urethritis, atonic bladder
P Psychologic problems (e.g., depression), prostatism, pharmacologic agents
E Endocrine abnormalities (e.g., diabetes, hypercalcemia, hypothyroidism)
R Restricted mobility (e.g., severe arthritis, orthostatic hypotension, restraints), retention
S Stool impaction
DRIP
D Delirium
R Restricted mobility, retention
I Infection, inflammation
P Polyuria (e.g., endocrine abnormalities), psychologic problems, prostatism, pharmacologic agents

sphincter closure to prevent urinary leakage, as the bladder increases in size. These efferent signals emanate from spinal levels T11 to L2 and are mediated by alpha-adrenergic receptors and cholinergic somatic stimulation. This maintains urethral pressure along the bladder outlet by both internal and external sphincters. Alpha-adrenergic stimulation causes muscle contraction of the internal sphincter, while the external sphincter is under voluntary control of striated muscle tissue (allowing patients to "hold their urine" for purposes of social appropriateness).

In contrast, bladder emptying is mediated by the parietal lobes and thalamus, which modulate afferent proprioceptive stimuli from the distended bladder wall detrusor muscle, sensing an increase in bladder pressure that is interpreted as bladder fullness. Once the patient has the urge to void, inhibition by the cortical micturition center ceases. In turn, the brainstem micturition center sends impulses from the pons down the spinal cord to the sacral micturition center at S2 to S4, subsequently triggering the bladder detrusor muscle to contract via cholinergic stimulation of parasympathetic M2 and M3 type muscarinic receptors found within the smooth muscle of the bladder walls. This latter action is simulated by the pharmacologic agent bethanechol (Urecholine), which is used to treat urinary retention from an atonic or poorly responsive bladder. In addition, preganglionic sympathetic inhibition relaxes the urethral sphincter, allowing for the egress of urine.

Age-related changes that may affect urologic functioning are decreased bladder capacity, increased post-void residual urine volume (greater than 50 mL), increased disinhibition of bladder contractions (i.e., overactive bladder), increased nocturnal sodium and fluid excretion (nocturia), urinary overflow phenomena resulting from increased urethral resistance in men related to benign prostatic hypertrophy (BPH), and weakness of the pelvic muscle walls in women. Postmenopausal estrogen deficiency can result in decreased competence of the internal and external sphincters via atrophy of the urethral mucosal epithelium. This results in atrophic urethritis, loss of compliance, and a diminished urethral mucosal seal, which may all contribute to various types of urinary incontinence, for example, stress and urge incontinence. It is important to note, however, that normal aging in and of itself does not cause urinary incontinence.

Clinical Presentation

Subjective

All assessments of the urinary system should begin with a detailed medical and surgical history, including the patient's voiding history. A voiding history includes the date of onset; number of times per day or night the patient voids; amount of urine voided each time; fluid-intake history, with types of fluids consumed; and the characteristics of the urinary incontinence, such as "occurs when sneezing," nocturia, frequency, urgency, or dysuria. Information regarding underlying medical conditions such as diabetes, cancer, acute illness, and neurologic disease should be elicited.

Objective

Physical examination of the patient is aimed at identifying the underlying pathophysiologic causes of incontinence, which can be multiple. The neurologic assessment is important in differentiating diagnoses such as cerebrovascular accident (CVA) and Parkinson's disease and should include an assessment of the functional and cognitive ability. This provides information about limitations in mobility, self-care ability, mental status, and communication barriers, such as aphasia or language.

An abdominal exam should be done to rule out constipation, fecal impaction, masses, distended bladder, or cystitis, which can lead to incontinence. A pelvic examination will reveal the pelvic muscle strength, conditions such as uterine prolapse, and any problems associated with perineal structures. Inspection of the skin around the pelvic area is important. For example, in women, there may be atrophic vaginitis and in men there may be abnormalities of the foreskin, penis, or perineum. A rectal exam should be done to determine the sphincter tone and the presence or absence of feces, to support causative complications such as fecal impaction. In men, a prostate examination is crucial in evaluating urinary tract complaints. The skin condition should be evaluated for breakdown or pressure areas during the pelvic examination because incontinence can lead to skin breakdown in the perineal area and buttocks which then can lead to decubitus ulcers. In female patients, particularly post-menopausal women, the perineum should be assessed for dryness and atrophy from decreased estrogenization of the vaginal mucosa.

During the physical exam, signs of CHF should be assessed; a cough stress test (which will allow direct observation of urine loss with a full bladder), as well as catheterization to determine postvoid residual volume should be

Table 11.4 Types of Urinary Incontinence

Type	Cause	Assessment	Management
Stress	Failure to store due to hypermobility of bladder neck, intrinsic sphincter deficiency, neurogenic sphincter deficiency Medications: sedatives, hypnotics, antispasmodics	History of vaginal deliveries, urine leakage with cough or sneeze Evidence of urine loss Pelvic exam, pad test, stress test, urinalysis culture and sensitivity, video-urodynamics, cystometrogram	Pelvic floor re-education with biofeedback (Kegel exercises) Weight loss if obese Electrical stimulation Hormone replacement therapy (estrogen) Alpha-adrenergic agonist Surgical correction of hypermobile bladder neck Periurethral bulking injections
Urge	Failure to store due to urinary tract infection; vaginitis; bladder stones and tumors; cortical, subcortical, and suprasacral lesions; cerebrovascular accident; dementia; multiple sclerosis; Parkinson's disease; spinal cord transection Medications: diuretics, narcotics	History of dysuria, frequency, urgency, hematuria, nocturia Evidence of a large amount of urine loss, evidence of unstable detrusor with decreased capacity Assess perineal hygiene Pelvic exam, smear, neurologic exam, urinalysis, culture and sensitivity, cystometrogram, video-urodynamics	Antimicrobial agents, antiseptics, topical estrogen, anticholinergics, smooth muscle relaxers, tricyclic antidepressants, impramine Pelvic floor re-education with biofeedback (Kegal exercises) Prompted voiding and scheduled voiding Fluid intake management Removal of bladder stones, resection and/or tumor treatment
Overflow	Failure to empty due to underactive detrusor, outlet obstruction, diabetes mellitus Medications: anticholinergics, disopyramide, antihistamines, calcium channel blockers	History of hesitancy, dribbling, decreased, stream, feeling of not emptying, constipation Neurologic exam, prostate exam (for males), prostate-specific antigen (for males), urinalysis, culture and sensitivity, serum creatinine, voiding cystometrogram, video-urodynamics	Scheduled toileting (Credé's maneuver) Treatment of underlying conditions Collection devices (intermittent or suprapubic) Alpha-blockers Resection of prostate, balloon dilation
Functional	Delirium, fecal impaction, manual dexterity and immobility Medications: diuretics, hypnotics, alcohol, narcotics, decongestants	Fecal impaction Assess sleep patterns, mental state, hearing, vision, functional ability, intake and output, accessibility, infection, neurologic function	Remove barriers Provide barrier-free environment Bowel and bladder program Collection devices Physical therapy Habit training

done as well. The patient or caretaker should be instructed to keep a voiding record for 3 to 7 days (Table 11.5). For patients with a questionable history of UI, a "pad test" can be done. This involves having the patient take oral Pyridium, which will color the urine orange, then wear a sanitary pad that can be checked at intervals for staining.

Diagnostic Reasoning

Diagnostic Tests

A urinalysis and urine culture and sensitivity should be done, as well as measurements of serum electrolytes, blood urea nitrogen (BUN), creatinine, calcium (for polyuria in the absence of diuretics), and glucose. Catheterization to assess postvoiding residual volume is important even on initial evaluation of the patient. Further testing will also depend on whether the onset of incontinence is acute, in which case testing related to other concurrent conditions may be warranted. The urinalysis is often normal but may show glycosuria (in patients with diabetes), proteinuria (in patients with glomerular disease), white blood cells (WBCs—in patients with a bacterial infection), RBCs (which may indicate the presence of a tumor), or bacteria (another sign of infection). A urine culture that is positive for bacteria also indicates infection; specific findings can be used to guide antibiotic therapy.

Other diagnostic options include urodynamic testing and cystometry, cystometrogram, video-urodynamics,

Table 11.5 Voiding Record

Time (record actual time if possible)	Urge to Void (yes or no)	Leaking Episode (large or small)	Activity at Time of Leakage	Did You Void (urinate) in the Toilet?	Fluid Intake (include amount and time)
12 midnight					
1 AM					
2 AM					
3 AM					
4 AM					
5 AM					
6 AM					
7 AM					
8 AM					
9 AM					
10 AM					
11 AM					
12 noon					
1 PM					
2 PM					
3 PM					
4 PM					
5 PM					
6 PM					
7 PM					
8 PM					
9 PM					
10 PM					
11 PM					

and a post-void residual catheterization to indicate the amount of retained urine. Reviewing the patient's use of medications for possible drug interaction, obtaining an accurate record of intake and output, and evaluating for other risk factors contributing to UI are also important. Patients who have indwelling catheters should be urodynamically evaluated for possible bladder retraining. Renal ultrasound may show renal pathology; a transrectal ultrasound can provide evidence of prostate disease; and a pelvic ultrasound may demonstrate pelvic pathology. A cystogram may show abnormal sphincter pressure or bladder pathology.

Differential Diagnosis

Many older patients may be described as "compensated incontinents." Any alteration—either physiologically or psychologically—such as a hospitalization, may precipitate an acute onset of incontinence. The administration of IV hydration in an acutely ill or older adult may be sufficient to precipitate incontinence. While the end-point is the same for all types of incontinence (involuntary bladder emptying), the context in which this occurs may vary markedly. Thus, the primary goal of differential diagnosis is for the clinician to correctly identify the type and etiology of incontinence, which in turn drives management and treatment decisions.

In persistent UI, a number of factors must be evaluated. Normal micturition requires the coordination of both the central and peripheral nervous systems. The cerebral cortex exerts an overall inhibitory influence on the sacral spinal cord reflex. Delirium, dementia, parkinsonism, and stroke may all lead to urge incontinence without awareness. The brainstem, on the other hand, and the suprasacral spinal cord exert a predominantly facilitating and coordinating influence that may be overcome in disorders such as stroke and multiple sclerosis, leading to overflow incontinence without awareness. This is referred to as neurogenic or detrusor–sphincter dysynergy. Local irritation and bladder or outflow obstructions may also lead to urge incontinence without awareness. Injuries to the sacral cord, which controls reflex bladder filling and emptying, persistent outlet obstruction, and diabetes mellitus may all lead to an acontractile bladder and overflow incontinence without awareness. Likewise, the bladder and lower genitourinary tract must perform their storage and emptying function properly for normal micturition. Failure to store urine may be a result of a hyperactive or poorly compliant bladder (e.g., secondary to cystitis, stones, tumor, or diverticuli), leading to urge incontinence. Laxity of pelvic floor muscles, bladder outlet, or sphincter weakness all may cause diminished outflow tract resistance, leading to stress incontinence. The bladder may fail to empty completely if it is poorly contractile as a result of diabetes mellitus, thus resulting in overflow incontinence. Increased outflow obstruction may be caused by anatomic obstruction by the prostate, stricture, or cystocele, resulting in chronic urinary retention and overflow incontinence.

Mixed types of incontinence are the norm rather than the exception; many patients have an overlap of pathologies. Just as multiple etiologic factors must be considered, a broad variety of interventions must be made available and are best approached through the Circle of Caring.

Management

Stress Incontinence

Stress incontinence is the involuntary loss of urine resulting from increased intra-abdominal pressure such as coughing, sneezing, and laughing. In this condition, the bladder is unable to retain urine because of hypermobility of the bladder neck, intrinsic sphincter deficiency, neurogenic sphincter deficiency, or use of medications such as sedatives, hypnotics, alpha-blockers, and/or antispasmodics. Patients who present with stress incontinence report urine leakage with coughing or sneezing, and typically have a history of vaginal deliveries, and/or hysterectomy, as well as evidence of urine loss. A detailed history guides the diagnostic workup which will then include a pelvic exam, pad test to determine the amount and frequency of leakage, cough stress test, urinalysis with culture and sensitivity, video-urodynamics, and/or cystometrogram.

Once the diagnosis of stress incontinence has been made, treatment should be individualized and instituted to meet the patient's needs. Noninvasive treatments include pelvic floor reeducation (Kegel exercises) with biofeedback, weight loss (if the patient is obese), electrical stimulation, and medications such as alpha-adrenergic agonists, which improve the muscle tone of the urinary tract. Eliminating diuretics will also improve symptoms. Surgical options include correction of hypermobile bladder neck and periurethral bulking injections. See Drugs Commonly Prescribed 11.1 for a list of medications used for UI.

Urge Incontinence

Urge incontinence, also known as detrusor instability, is the involuntary leakage of urine resulting from inability to delay voiding. The patient has the sensation of a full bladder but is not able to store the urine long enough to reach the toilet. This failure can be caused by urinary tract infection; vaginitis; bladder stones; bladder tumors; cortical, subcortical, and suprasacral lesions; CVA; dementia; multiple sclerosis; Parkinson's disease; prostate problems; spinal cord transection; and medications such as diuretics and narcotics. The patient's history and physical examination may reveal evidence of dysuria, increased frequency or urgency, hematuria, large amounts of urine loss, and unstable detrusor muscle with decreased capacity, or nocturia. Assessment should include perineal hygiene, pelvic exam and a vaginal discharge smear, neurologic exam including an assessment of mental status, and a urinalysis with a culture and sensitivity should be ordered. Invasive procedures that may be needed include the cystometrogram and video-urodynamics.

Treatment begins conservatively, with pelvic floor reeducation and biofeedback, if the patient is capable. A prompted and/or scheduled voiding by a caregiver, with management of the patient's fluid intake, may be useful for patients who have cognitive impairments or are forgetful. Medications such as antimicrobial agents may be necessary to treat underlying conditions. Other medications may include topical estrogen, anticholinergics, smooth muscle relaxers, and tricyclic antidepressants to improve the neuromuscular function of the bladder and sphincter (Drugs Commonly Prescribed 11.1). Surgical treatment may be indicated for the removal of bladder stones or tumors.

Overactive Bladder

The term overactive bladder (OAB) is often used interchangably with urge incontinence; however, they are different conditions. OAB is a syndrome of symptoms that include urgency, frequency, and nocturia all of which are associated with involuntary contractions of the detrusor muscle. Urge incontinence may or may not be a feature of this syndrome; about one-third have urge incontinence. OAB may occur as a component of other types of urinary incontinence, such as with stress incontinence. The cause of OAB is multifactorial in that it can include disorders of the lower urinary tract, ingestion of alcohol and caffeine, use of a variety of prescribed drugs, or neurologic conditions. This condition is most common in women and often results in anxiety and depression because of the restricted daily functioning. Sexual dysfunction can occur because of the fear of urine loss during sexual intercourse.

Treatment for OAB first begins with identifying women with the problem. It is estimated that only about 6 to 27 percent of women with this condition seek treatment. Nonpharmacologic methods mentioned earlier are used to manage OAB as well, but pharmacotherapy plays an important role. Antimuscarinic agents are the most commonly used drugs and are affective because they block the parasympathetic stimulation of the detrusor muscle by blocking acetylcholine. See Drugs Commonly Prescribed 11.1 for a complete list of medications used for OAB.

Drugs Commonly Prescribed 11.1: Urinary Incontinence

Drug	Indication	Dosage	Comments
Anticholinergic/antispasmotic agents			
Oxybutynin Ditropan	Urge incontinence OAB Stress incontinence	2.5 mg PO up to qid (immediate-release form)	*Contraindications* Closed angle glaucoma Myasthenia gravis Partial or complete gastric obstruction Severe colitis
Ditropan XL		5–30 mg PO qd (extended release)	*Side Effects* Dry mouth Drowsiness Blurred vision Urinary hesitance
Transdermal system		3.9 mg for 3–4 days (apply twice weekly)	Urinary retention Decreased GI motility
Muscarinic receptor antagonist agents			
Tolterodine Detrol	Urge incontinence OAB		*Contraindications* Urinary retention Gastric retention Closed angle glaucoma *Side Effects*
Detrol LA (extended release)			Dry mouth Headache Constipation Vertigo/dizziness Abdominal pain
Topical estrogen			
Premarin cream (conjugates estrogen)	Stress incontinence Urge incontinece associated with atrophic vaginitis	0.5–2 g daily—3 weeks on 1 week off (0.625 mg conj estrogens/g)	*Contraindications* Hypersensitivity Breast cancer Thromboembolic disorders
Estrace cream		1 g 1–3 times per week	Estrogen-dependent neoplasia Abnormal genital bleeding
Estring		Insert ring deeply into the upper third of vagina and leave in place for 3 months then replace.	Pregnance *Side Effects* PMS-like syndrome Amenorrhea Nausea/vomiting Headache Dizziness Depression Changes in libido Dysmenorrhea Breakthrough bleeding Breast tenderness Photosensitivity Endometrial cystic hyperplasia
Alpha-1-adrenergic blocking agents (men)			
Tamsulosin hydrochloride Flomax	BPH and related urinary symptoms	0.4–0.8 mg qd	*Contraindications* Hypersensitivity to tamsulosin
Terazosin hydrochloride Hytrin		1–5 mg q hs	Hypersensitivity to prazosin, terazosin or doxazosin
Doxazosin mesylate Cardura		1–8 mg q hs	*Side Effects* Orthostatic hypotension Palpitations Dizziness Impotence GI upset Headache

(continued)

Drugs Commonly Prescribed 11.1: Urinary Incontinence (continued)

Drug	Indication	Dosage	Comments
Tricyclic antidepressants Imipramine Tofranil Janimine Generics	OAB Urge incontinence	10–25 mg PO qd up to tid	*Contraindications* Hypersensitivity to tricyclic antidepressants Use of MAO inhibitors *Side Effects* Dry mouth urinary retention Blurred vision Orthostatic hypotension Sedation Confusion in the elderly Tachycardia Anxiety and nervousness Sexual dysfunction Constipation

Overflow Incontinence

Overflow incontinence is the involuntary leakage of small amounts of urine. This is caused by an overdistended bladder in a patient who does not feel the need to void because of an atonic detrusor muscle, outlet obstruction, BPH, diabetes mellitus, or use of medications such as anticholinergics, disopyramide (Norpace), antihistamines, diuretics, or calcium channel blockers. The history and physical examination may indicate hesitancy, dribbling, nocturia, decreased stream, feeling of not emptying the bladder, and/or constipation. A neurologic exam, prostate exam, urinalysis with culture and sensitivity, serum creatinine, voiding cystometrogram, and/or video-urodynamics should be done.

The treatment consists of treating the underlying condition, teaching scheduled toileting, Credé's maneuver, and the prescribing of medications such as alpha-blockers (Drugs Commonly Prescribed 11.1). It may be necessary to discontinue certain medications or to alter dosages to reduce the adverse effects causing overflow incontinence. Teaching scheduled toileting and Credé's maneuver to force the urine from the bladder may be helpful. The Credé maneuver involves applying pressure over the symphysis pubis and slowly pressing down. This is particularly helpful in patients who have a spinal cord injury or other neurologic problems. Alternative collection devices may be indicated, including the use of external catheters; pads; and indwelling, intermittent, or suprapubic catheterization. In the case of outlet obstruction, a resection of the prostate may be necessary.

Functional Urinary Incontinence

Functional UI is incontinence that occurs in a normal functioning urinary system. The leakage of urine is caused by factors outside the lower urinary tract and can be transient in nature. The causes of functional incontinence may vary from delirium or fecal impaction to lack of manual dexterity and immobility problems. Medications such as diuretics, hypnotics, narcotics, and decongestants as well as alcohol may also play a role. Assessment for fecal impaction, sleep pattern disturbances, mental status, hearing and vision, functional ability, fluid intake, accessibility, infection, and neurologic function is essential.

Treatment for functional incontinence consists of removing barriers, education regarding a scheduled bowel and bladder program, use of collection devices, physical or occupational therapy, and habit training. Barriers to elimination may be identified when the patient cannot remove clothing or reach the toilet in sufficient time to avoid leakage. By identifying the barrier(s), interventions to resolve the problem can be developed. Some solutions include the use of Velcro closures (which are easily managed by arthritic hands and fingers) instead of buttons and zippers, bedside commodes for night-time use to eliminate the amount of time needed to get to the bathroom, or monitors for obtaining immediate assistance in getting out of bed and to the toilet.

A caregiver may be necessary to assist the patient in toileting; therefore, it is imperative to assess the caregiver's ability to provide care and determine his or her level of competency. Nursing research shows that caregivers want to give "good" care; however, the caregiver must be physically capable of providing the care through manual dexterity, strength, and cognition. Further, the caregiver must be able to comprehend and follow through with instructions that may be complex and require problem-solving ability.

Identifying patients who need physical or occupational therapy to improve their functional skills may be required. Initiation of a bowel and bladder program can decrease the incidence of constipation and fecal impaction; patients should also be encouraged to retrain the bladder to empty completely on a regular basis. For patients who cannot avoid urinary incontinence, alternatives are available to keep them clean and dry. Condom catheters are effective in keeping male patients dry, and pads of various types are available for both males and females. Indwelling catheters, suprapubic catheters, and intermittent catheterization are options for urine collection in patients who cannot maintain bladder function or have frequent or regular urinary incontinence.

Medications used to treat incontinence are effective for patients who suffer from the inability to store urine. Pharmacologic agents should be used in conjunction with other treatment modalities such as toileting and behavioral modification. Scheduled toileting along with regulation of fluid intake can have a positive effect on bladder control. Behavioral modification treatment such as pelvic floor reeducation is designed to increase pelvic floor muscular strength and endurance. Reeducation is accomplished through Kegel exercises of the targeted muscle group using biofeedback for a period of 4 to 6 weeks. Kegel exercises are the tightening and releasing of the pubococcygeal and levator ani muscles. This is accomplished by tightening the muscle group used to avoid defecation or urination. The patient may experience results within 2 weeks to several months of initiating the program. This treatment is noninvasive and, when appropriate, should be attempted before surgical intervention (Table 11.6).

Vaginal cones or rings may be used to retain the uterus in a more normal position. Cones can reduce the pressure on the bladder of the prolapsed uterine musculature.

Surgical intervention may be appropriate if all other measures have failed or in conjunction with the previous conservative approaches. Surgery may be indicated to correct anatomic abnormalities such as prolapsed uterus, hypermobile bladder neck, or obstructions such as enlarged prostate or tumors. Surgery should be used as the last treatment option unless the causative agent is diagnosed as a tumor or severe obstruction.

Obviously, a multidimensional approach is necessary to deal with this multicausal problem. Advanced Practice Nursing Interventions illustrates the management of urinary incontinence.

Follow-Up and Referral

Close follow-up of patients is essential for patients with incontinence. This may be biweekly at first, while the patient is being taught the exercises and the medication dosage is being adjusted. Quarterly follow-up visits may be sufficient once incontinence is under control and medication dose has been stabilized. The patient should be monitored for adverse effects of medication and orthostatic hypotension. Periodic urinalysis should be done to detect any urinary tract infections early. Women should have regular pelvic exams to detect pelvic abnormalities early, and men should have regular rectal exams to pick up prostatic abnormalities.

Table 11.6 Kegel Exercises

Instructions for the patient

- Locate the correct muscle. To do so, try stopping your urine flow by contracting the muscle. When the urine slows or stops, you are using the pubococcygeus (PC) muscle.
- Squeeze the muscle for 2 seconds. (Do not hold your breath or contract your abdomen, buttocks, or thighs.) Then relax for 10 seconds. This is one repetition. Do 10 repetitions twice a day.
- After you have mastered the technique, begin to lengthen the time you contract the muscle. Increase the time by 1 second every few days until you are able to contract the muscle for 10 seconds at a time (and relax for 10 seconds). Continue to do 10 repetitions twice a day.

Patient Education

Patient and family education is crucial in the treatment of urinary incontinence. Environmental assessment should include recommendations about proximity of toilet facilities. An individualized toileting schedule should be geared to each patient's pattern of incontinence. Bladder training in the form of timed voiding, working up to 3-hour intervals, is an important intervention. Good general nutritional and exercise practices are important to the upkeep of overall health. Support and encouragement are essential. Interventions geared toward preventing social isolation, setting up support services necessary, and optimism in dealing with the problem are important interventions in the primary care setting.

Lower Urinary Tract Infections

A lower UTI occurs when the normal sterile condition of the urinary tract system is invaded by pathogenic bacteria. Infections of the lower urinary tract can occur in the urethra, bladder, and prostate. Infection of the urethra (*urethritis*) and infection of the urinary bladder (*cystitis*) usually occur together. Women may be diagnosed with chronic inflammation of the bladder wall (*interstitial cystitis*). *Prostatitis* is infection of the prostate gland.

Infections are classified as acute, chronic, recurrent, complicated, or uncomplicated. The *acute infection* is characterized by an onset of UTI in a previously symptom-free individual. The infection becomes *chronic* when it is unresolved after the usual treatment is rendered. UTIs become chronic because of obstructions, antibiotic-resistant bacteria, or the presence of multiple strains of bacteria that are not susceptible to the antibiotic therapy prescribed. A UTI is considered *recurrent* when it recurs within 2 weeks of the original infection. A *complicated* UTI is either an acute or chronic infection that is accompanied by factors that complicate the infection, such as catheters (e.g., indwelling, suprapubic, or intermittent), underlying chronic disease, or pregnancy. An *uncomplicated* UTI is one that can be resolved without addressing such complicating factors.

Epidemiology and Causes

Lower UTI is a common problem that affects approximately 20 percent of women and 1 percent of men each year. UTI rarely occurs in men younger than age 50 and is usually

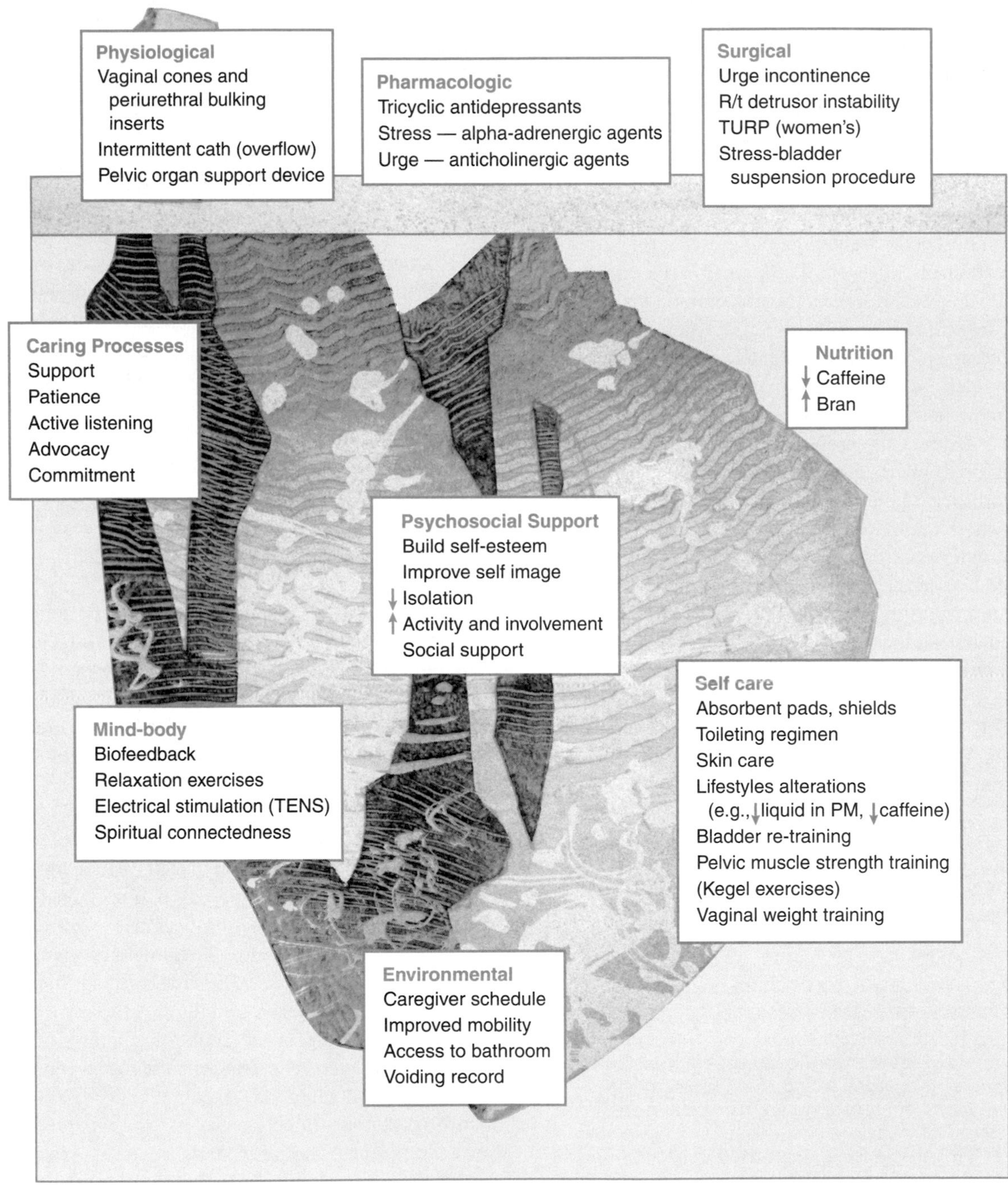
The Iceberg of Incontinence
Advanced Nursing Practice
Management of Urinary Incontinence
Traditional Medicine
Physiological
Vaginal cones and periurethral bulking inserts
Intermittent cath (overflow)
Pelvic organ support device
Pharmacologic
Tricyclic antidepressants
Stress — alpha-adrenergic agents
Urge — anticholinergic agents
Surgical
Urge incontinence
R/t detrusor instability
TURP (women's)
Stress-bladder suspension procedure
Caring Processes
Support
Patience
Active listening
Advocacy
Commitment
Nutrition
↓ Caffeine
↑ Bran
Psychosocial Support
Build self-esteem
Improve self image
↓ Isolation
↑ Activity and involvement
Social support
Mind-body
Biofeedback
Relaxation exercises
Electrical stimulation (TENS)
Spiritual connectedness
Self care
Absorbent pads, shields
Toileting regimen
Skin care
Lifestyles alterations (e.g., ↓ liquid in PM, ↓ caffeine)
Bladder re-training
Pelvic muscle strength training (Kegel exercises)
Vaginal weight training
Environmental
Caregiver schedule
Improved mobility
Access to bathroom
Voiding record

caused by urinary catheters, anatomic abnormalities of the urinary tract, unprotected anal intercourse, or vaginal intercourse with a woman who has a bacterial infection. UTI may occur at all ages but is more prevalent in sexually active adults, very young children, or frail older adults. Other populations at risk include individuals with predisposing conditions such as a suppressed immune system, pregnancy, urinary obstruction, catheter dependency, neurogenic bladder, or diabetes mellitus. UTIs account for more than 7 million visits to primary-care providers each year.

Lower UTI may be the result of other conditions within the renal system. A urethral obstruction can create stasis of urine, providing a medium for bacterial growth. Other conditions that can contribute to UTI are a descending infection from the kidney, an anatomically short urethra (in female patients), and acute infections elsewhere in the body. UTI may also occur as a result of poor or nonsterile catheterization technique or re-use of disposable catheters, poor hygiene, unprotected anal intercourse, or simply from an indwelling catheter which, as a foreign body, serves as a nidus of infection.

Interstitial cystitis is found primarily in women. Statistically, one in every 350 persons seeking treatment for bladder pain is diagnosed with interstitial cystitis, also known as painful bladder disease. The cause of this condition is unknown at this time but some researchers theorize that there is an abnormality in the bladder surface that allows potassium and urea to leak and absorb into the bladder interstitium. Other factors being investigated are lymphatic, infectious, neurologic, psychologic, autoimmune, and vasculitic. Interstitial cystitis does not respond to antibiotics.

Pathophysiology

Lower UTIs usually occur as a result of contamination from the patient's own gastrointestinal tract. Bacteria may be introduced into the urinary tract from fecal contamination secondary to poor perineal hygiene, unprotected sexual intercourse, and/or an anatomically shortened urethra in women. The use of a spermicide during intercourse (especially with diaphragm forms of contraception) alters the vaginal microenvironment, predisposing to bacterial colonization. Immunosuppressed or medically compromised patients may have difficulty in suppressing bacterial growth as bacteria ascend the urethra. Patients who are dependent on catheters are at risk for introduction of bacteria into the urinary tract through contamination of the catheter. Alkaline urine is a common complication of diabetes mellitus. The elevated pH of the urine creates a medium in which bacteria can grow and proliferate. Renal stones can also create an environment that promotes bacterial growth, as the blockage causes stasis of urine or reflux. In turn, contamination can occur in the kidney when urine "backs up" in the kidney due to vesicoureteral reflux, in which the urine back-flows freely into one or both ureters, leading to urinary stasis.

In women, approximately 80 to 90 percent of cases of uncomplicated UTI are a result of the gram-negative rod bacteria *Escherichia coli.* The second most common cause (5 to 20 percent of cases) of uncomplicated bacterial infection is the gram-positive coccus *Staphylococcus saprophyticus*, although this agent is rare in complicated UTI. Other gram-negative rods identified as causative pathogens in a smaller number of cases, but particularly in complicated UTI, are *Proteus mirabilis, Klebsiella, Enterobacter, Serratia,* and *Pseudomonas*. In addition, the gram-positive coccus *Enterococcus* has been identified. *Staphylococcus aureus* is a gram-positive coccus that can be introduced into the urinary tract system through instrumentation or as a complication of renal stones. Fungi, particularly *Candida* species, may also be causative agents in complicated UTI that fails to respond to antibiotic therapy, especially in the presence of an indwelling catheter. Candiduria may be asymptomatic, and fungal structures should be sought on urine microscopy, as fungal colonies may be more difficult to elaborate on standard urine culture, in turn leading to delays in treatment.

In up to 50 percent of all bacterial species associated with cystitis, genetic virulence determinants may be identified that contribute to the uropathogenicity of these organisms, such as adherence factors that allow for greater binding to the uroepithelium. Another is the urease gene, expressed by certain gram-negative bacteria such as *Proteus, Klebsiella, Ureaplasma, Providencia,* and *Pseudomonas* species. This enzyme splits urea molecules within the urinary tract, creating ammonium and hydroxyl ions that produce an alkaline microenvironment. This higher pH facilitates survival of these bacteria, particularly when housed within triple phosphate (magnesium ammonium phosphate) stones, also known as struvite stones.

Cystitis is rare in men, as the increased length and drier environment around the urethra contribute to less frequent bacterial colonization. In addition, prostatic fluid has inherent anti-bacterial properties. When UTI does occur in men, it is often associated with abnormal urethral anatomy, or it may be the result of inadequate treatment of prostatitis. Most antibiotic agents do not penetrate the prostatic tissue and, therefore, do not eliminate the infection. As a result, the bladder is reinfected from contaminated prostatic fluid.

Two well-documented phenomena related to classic UTI are asymptomatic bacteruria and the dysuria–pyuria syndrome. As the name implies, in asymptomatic bacteruria patients experience no obvious clinical symptoms or signs of UTI (including altered mental status in the elderly), yet urinalysis and culture consistently yield findings consistent with bacteruria. In contrast, the dysuria-pyuria syndrome (also called "acute urethral syndrome") is characterized by painful urination with white blood cells on microscopic urinalysis in the absence of a positive bacterial culture. Such a condition may be due to organisms such as *Chlamydia* that do not grow well on standard urinary culture. This condition may be difficult to distinguish clinically from vaginitis due to sexually transmitted infection, however.

Clinical Presentation

Subjective

The presenting signs and symptoms of UTIs vary widely in intensity and occurrence. Women may present with urethritis and cystitis simultaneously. The most frequently reported symptoms in both males and females are dysuria, urinary frequency or urgency, nocturia, hematuria, low back or suprapubic pain, urinary incontinence, or cloudy, foul-smelling urine. These symptoms can occur in any combination. In elderly patients, altered mental status may be the sole manifestation of UTI and should create a high level of suspicion.

Urethritis in men is rare; if left untreated or treated inadequately, it can lead to complications such as urethral strictures, periurethral abscess, urethral diverticuli, and fissures. Vaginal discharge in women and urethral discharge in men may suggest STDs. Purulent urethral discharge (*Neisseria gonorrhoeae*) or whitish-mucoid discharge (*Chlamydia trachomatis*) should be treated aggressively, with the appropriate antibiotic therapy.

Objective

The physical examination should include a clean-catch, midstream urine sample for urinalysis. The urinalysis will reveal an infectious process in the urinary tract system and may exhibit any of the following: cloudy appearance, alkaline pH, hematuria, elevated levels of nitrites, leukocyte esterase (detecting pyuria of greater than 10 leukocytes per hpf), and urine sediments of RBCs, WBCs, mucus, and bacterial overgrowth. Of note, the Enterobacteriaceae convert urinary nitrates to nitrites, producing positive results on urine dipstick analysis if present in adequate numbers (greater than 100,000 organisms/mL). In contrast, however, staphylococci do not convert this substrate and are not detectable by this test. Moreover, false-positive urinary nitrite tests may result in the presence of the urinary tract analgesic phenazopyridine. A urine culture and sensitivity may be ordered to speciate and determine the sensitivity of the causative organism to specific antibiotic therapy.

Patients with interstitial cystitis may present with the need to urinate frequently because of reduced bladder capacity. This may occur up to 60 times per day in extreme cases. Other symptoms include pain or discomfort in the abdominal area that holds the bladder.

Diagnostic Reasoning

Diagnostic Tests

Diagnosis of lower UTI is made based on the subjective complaints of the patient and a clean-catch midstream urine sample showing the presence of bacteria, especially if more than 100,000 organisms/mL of the same morphology are present in a sample from a female patient. Traditionally, this concentration of bacteria (i.e., 100,000 cfu/mL on urine culture) has been used to define UTI, but in light of increasing evidence that UTI may result from far lower bacterial loads, UTI is currently defined as a urine sample with greater than 100 organisms/mL in the presence of characteristic clinical symptoms. The method of urine collection also influences interpretation of the urine culture, as the sterility of commonly performed "clean catch" techniques is heavily dependent on the patient's ability to self-clean around the urethra prior to voiding. Sterile wipes containing iodine, chlorhexidine, or other acceptable cleaning agent must be used to wipe the urethral opening at least 2 to 3 times consecutively in a direction away from the perineum to minimize contamination by anorectal flora. Alcohol swabs are unacceptable cleaning agents. Straight catheterization samples obtained with sterile technique are the most reliable, while samples obtained from receptacles connected to indwelling catheters may prove unreliable owing to repeated manipulation of the collecting bag.

While urine culture is considered the gold standard with the greatest sensitivity for laboratory confirmation of UTI, urinalysis with microscopy is also helpful and provides rapid results. Urinalysis also typically indicates pyuria (greater than 10 neutrophils per hpf on microscopic exam) and often the presence of RBCs. Hematuria is common in UTI but not with urethritis or vaginitis; however, blood in the urine is not marker of complicated infection. UTIs may be treated with empiric antibiotic therapy based on knowledge of the most common bacterial etiologies. However, a urine culture and sensitivity testing will definitively identify the infecting microorganism and the appropriate antibiotic therapy. Although the diagnosis of UTI is made both clinically and by urinalysis, it is generally agreed that urine culture and sensitivities are indicated if complicated infection is suspected, if atypical symptoms are present, or if symptoms persist or recur within 1 month of the patient's receiving an empiric course of antibiotic therapy and a new regimen is desired.

Interstitial cystitis has been a diagnosis of exclusion; however, a helpful diagnostic tool for this condition is the Potassium Sensitivity Test (PST). This test involves slow instillation of 40 mL of sterile water into the bladder and the patient is asked to grade the discomfort on a 0 to 5 scale, with 5 being the most severe. This establishes a baseline. Then the water is emptied and potassium chloride solution is instilled into the bladder and the discomfort graded as in the instillation of water. Interstitial cystitis is suggested when there is a 2-point increase in the pain or urgency, indicating abnormal epithelial dysfunction.

Differential Diagnosis

The differential diagnosis of tumors, upper UTI (pyelonephritis), vaginitis, and STDs must be explored. Tumors of the renal system and upper UTI are discussed in this chapter. Vaginitis and STDs are discussed in Chapters 12 and 13. Patients with lower UTI differ from those with upper UTI in that they do not exhibit signs of sepsis such as fever and chills, have WBC casts in the urine (reflecting the passage of neutrophils through the renal tubules), or experience flank and costovertebral angle tenderness on exam.

Management

Pharmacologic antimicrobial management is the mainstay of treatment. Drugs Commonly Prescribed 11.2 presents the oral agents typically used for the treatment of lower UTI. Epidemiologic surveillance has revealed increasing rates of resistance in *Escherichia coli* isolates to ampicillin and sulfonamides (including trimethoprim-sulfamethoxazole or Bactrim), but only a small percentage of these isolates were resistant to nitrofurantoin (Macrodantin, Macrobid), which is known to concentrate in the urine. Nitrofurantoin is also effective against many gram-positive cocci such as *Enterococcus faecalis*, while other key uropathogens such as *Proteus*, *Enterobacter*, and *Klebsiella* may be highly resistant. Thus, both trimethoprim-sulfamethoxazole and nitrofurantoin may be used as empiric therapy for uncomplicated UTI only and, in fact, may prove to be inadequate. Indeed, one of the strongest risk factors predicting microbial resistance to trimethoprim-sulfamethoxazole is the previous use of this or any other antimicrobial agent for any type of infection within the past 3 months.

The fluoroquinolones (e.g., ofloxacin, ciprofloxacin, gatifloxacin, levofloxacin), on the other hand, have widespread efficacy against most uropathogens, although their increasing use as first-line empiric therapy has clearly been associated with steadily rising rates of resistance, as well. Thus, for uncomplicated UTI, a 3-day regimen of trimethoprim-sulfamethoxazole should be used empirically in patients with no history of sulfa drug allergy, previous hospitalization, or antibiotic use for any reason within the past 3 months, in geographic areas where *Escherichia coli* resistance to this agent is known to be less than 20 percent (e.g., the Northeastern United States, as opposed to the Western United States). A 7-day course of nitrofurantoin should be used as an alternative in patients with documented sulfa allergies or in those with previous antibiotic use within the last 3 months.

The cost-effective 3-day treatment regimen for uncomplicated lower UTI reduces the risk of nonadherence and the development of *Candida* vaginitis due to clearance of normal urogenital flora. It is recommended for trimethoprim-sulfamethoxazole or the fluoroquinolones, but not nitrofurantoin which requires a longer course of therapy for maximum efficacy. Complicated UTI, on the other hand, requires at least 10 to 14 days of antibiotic therapy. The antimicrobial effects of these medications persist for several days after the final dose is administered. In particularly severe cases of UTI (especially in high-risk groups such as elderly or bed-bound patients) or in cases involving urinary tract instrumentation, hospitalization and broad-spectrum IV antibiotic coverage (e.g., ceftriaxone, piperacillin-tazobactam, or ampicillin plus gentamicin) may be required until symptoms wane and urine culture and antibiotic sensitivities confirm the most appropriate antibiotic choice. The same approach may be required for upper UTI (i.e., pyelonephritis).

Empiric treatment of UTI in men (by definition, a complicated UTI) should be extended to at least 7 days. Nitrofurantoin and beta-lactams should be avoided, while fluoroquinolones are generally the antibiotics of choice, given their effectiveness in treating occult prostatic infection.

Treatment of UTI during pregnancy is especially important, as an established link exists between premature delivery and UTI (especially pyelonephritis). Empiric therapy may include amoxicillin (Amoxil) 500 mg PO bid or 250 mg PO tid, nitrofurantoin (Macrobid, Macrodantin) 100 mg PO bid, or cephalexin (Keflex) 500 mg PO bid to qid. Broader spectrum regimens may include amoxicillin-clavulanate (Augmentin) 500 mg/125 mg PO bid or cefpodoxime (Vantin) 100 mg PO bid. Most clinicians will choose to treat UTI during pregnancy for one full week. Fluoroquinolones should be avoided, given concern for their effects on bone and cartilage formation in the developing fetus, and trimethoprim-sulfamethoxazole should be avoided in the first and third trimesters of pregnancy. In women with a prior history of recurrent UTI, postcoital prophylaxis with a single oral dose of nitrofurantoin 50 mg or cephalexin 250 mg has been shown to be highly effective.

Fungal UTI due to *Candida* infection is typically associated with an indwelling urinary catheter and nearly half of all cases resolve simply with removal of the catheter. However, re-insertion of a new catheter is associated with a high rate of relapse. Antifungal treatment is typically not required for asymptomatic colonization, but if indicated in the presence of dysuria, an appropriate regimen would be fluconazole (Diflucan) 200 mg PO (or IV for hospitalized patients) qd for 7 to 14 days.

The management of asymptomatic bacteruria deserves special mention. This condition should be treated with antibiotics in pregnant women, as it increases the risk of premature delivery. Although some studies suggest treatment in girls beyond pre-school age is not warranted owing to the high rate of recurrent asymptomatic infection without obvious sequelae, general practice also calls for treating asymptomatic bacteruria in young children. Treatment is also indicated in patients before they undergo a urologic procedure to avoid operating on a contaminated field, after removal of a bladder catheter in place for less than 1 week, and in any patient with an underlying structural abnormality of the urinary tract, vesicoureteral reflux, or struvite stones. In contrast, treatment of this condition in adult men, nonpregnant women, the elderly, diabetic persons, and spinal cord patients with indwelling urinary catheters is not warranted. Although asymptomatic bacteruria may be a harbinger of future UTI, antibiotic therapy has not been shown to persistently eradicate bacteruria or urinary tract colonization in these populations.

After completion of antibiotic treatment, follow-up cultures may be obtained to ensure complete eradication of the pathogen in patients with a history of recurrent infection, during pregnancy, or in those prone to complicated UTI. Chronic or recurrent UTI may be prevented through prophylactic treatment either on a daily basis or after sexual intercourse, but this should be done only after all options to

Drugs Commonly Prescribed 11.2: Urinary Tract Infections

Drug	Indication and Dosage	Comments
Trimethoprim and sulfamethoxazole (TMP-SMX) Bactrim, Septra (80 mg TMP/400 mg SMZ) Bactrim DS (160 mg TMP/800 mg SMZ) [double strength]	*Pre- or postcoital prophylaxis* • Bactrim or Septra $^1/_2$ tab PO ×1 *Acute uncomplicated UTI* • Bactrim DS 1 tab PO q 12 h × 3 days *Complicated UTI or pyelonephritis* • Bactrim DS 1 tab PO q 12 h × 10–14 days	*Contraindications* Hypersensitivity to trimethoprim or sulfonamides Allergy to sulfa Folate deficiency megaloblastic anemia Pregnancy at term and lactation *Side Effects* Abdominal distress Nausea Rash Neutropena *Special Instructions* Take with a full glass of water Complete full course of therapy
Fluoroquinolones Ciprofloxacin (Cipro) (Cipro XR) [extended release] Levofloxacin (Levaquin) Gatifloxacin (Tequin) Ofloxacin (Floxin) Norfloxacin (Noroxin)	*Uncomplicated UTI or reinfection* • Cipro 250 mg PO bid × 3 days • Cipro XR 500 mg PO qd × 3 days *Uncomplicated UTI* • 250 mg PO qd × 3 days *Complicated UTI/acute pyelonephritis* • 250 mg PO qd × 10 days *Uncomplicated UTI* • 400 mg PO × 1 dose or 200 mg PO × 3 days *Complicated UTI/acute pyelonephritis* • 400 mg PO qd × 7–14 days *Uncomplicated UTI* • 200 mg PO q 12 h × 3 days *Complicated UTI* • 200 mg PO q 12 h × 10 days *Uncomplicated UTI (E. coli, Klebsiella pneumonia, or Proteus mirabilis)* • 400 mg PO q 12 h × 3 days • 400 mg PO q 12 h × 7–10 days for other gram-negative bacteria	*Contraindications* Hypersensitivity to fluoroquinolones Tequin may prolong the QT interval in the ECG of some patients with hypokalemia and patients taking quinidine, procainamide, amiodarone or sotalol. *Side Effects* Nausea Abdominal discomfort Diarrhea Photosensitivity Dizziness Superinfections Tequin may cause headache and vaginitis in addition to the above mentioned side effects. *Special Instructions* Complete the full course of therapy. Do not take at the same time as antacids, calcium, iron or zinc preparations • Norfloxacin, ofloxacin cannot be taken with food or milk
Aminopenicillins Amoxicillin (Amoxil) Amoxicillin and potassium clavulanate (Augmentin)	*Uncomplicated pyelonephritis* • 500 mg PO tid × 10–14 days *Uncomplicated UTI (mild)* • 500 mg/125 mg PO bid × 10–14 days *Uncomplicated UTI (severe)* • 875 mg/125 mg PO × 10–14 days *Complicated UTI/pyelonephritis* • 875 mg/125 mg PO bid × 10–14 days • 500 mg/125 mg PO tid × 10–14 days	*Contraindications* Penicillin allergy *Side Effects* Hypersensitivity reactions Urticarial rash Nausea Diarrhea Superinfections *Special Instructions* Complete full course of therapy May decrease effectiveness of oral contraceptives Augumentin should be given with food to decrease nausea

Drug	Indication and Dosage	Comments
Anti-infective Nitrofurantoin (Macrodantin, Furadantin)	UTI 50–100 mg PO qid × 7–10 days	*Contraindications* Hypersensitivity to nitrofurantoin Renal function impairment Anuria or oliguria Pregnancy in third trimester, labor, or delivery *Side Effects* Nausea Vomiting Anorexia Abdominal discomfort *Special Instructions* Take with food May cause urine to darken
Urinary analgesic Phenazopyridine (Pyridium)	Relief of pain, burning, urgency and frequency from UTI 200 mg PO tid after meals	*Contraindications* Hypersensitivity to phenazopyridine *Side Effects* Headache Rash Itching *Special Instructions* Take after meals May turn urine reddish-orange color and stain fabric
Antispasmodic Flavoxate (Urispas)	Relief of dysuria, urgency, frequency and incontinence 100–200 mg PO tid–qid	*Contraindications* Use with caution in patients with glaucoma and older adults *Side Effects* Nausea Vomiting Dry mouth Headache Drowsiness Blurred vision Vertigo

eliminate the causative factors of UTI have been explored. Strategies should be emphasized to decrease the incidence of infection through the guidelines outlined in the Patient Education section.

Although appropriate antibiotic treatment is often adequate to relieve dysuria, certain medications may also be prescribed for the first few days to decrease the pain and discomfort of UTI. Use of these agents should not be prolonged, however, given their significant side effect profile. Effective treatment may involve anticholinergics, which produce an antispasmodic effect, including atropine (Donnatal), hyoscyamine (Levsin, Cystospaz), propantheline (Pro-Banthine), or oxybutynin (Ditropan). However, anticholinergics may also contribute to urinary retention (especially in the elderly), which is a clear risk factor for UTI, and should thus be used with caution. Analgesics may be prescribed such as phenazopyridine (Pyridium), but this alters the color of urine to orange and may cause urinary leakage secondary to anesthetization of the urethra and sphincter.

Interstitial cystitis does not respond to antibiotics. However, this condition may be treated with pentosan polysulfate sodium (Elmiron), which tends to reduce the bladder wall inflammation. This drug has been shown to improve symptoms in 38 percent of the patients with interstitial cystitis. Complementary therapies used for lower UTI are presented in Complementary Therapies 11.1.

Follow-Up and Referral

Patients should follow up with a midstream, clean-catch urine sample for urinalysis to evaluate for the presence of WBCs or a culture and sensitivity for all recurrent infections. UTI that is secondary to other pathologic conditions will not resolve until the primary causative factor is

COMPLEMENTARY THERAPIES 11.1

Lower Urinary Tract Infections

Therapy	Dosage	Comments
Vitamins		
Vitamin A	10,000 IU qd	Pregnant women: no more than 10,000 units/day
Vitamin C	1000 mg qd	Take in divided doses for better absorption and to avoid diarrhea
Vitamin E	600 IU qd	Can interfere with anticoagulation therapy
Beta-carotene	15,000 IU qd	Larger doses can turn skin orange
Minerals		
Calcium	1500 mg qd	Should be taken with optimal daily allowance of vitamin D (400 IU qd) for better absorption
Magnesium	750–1000 mg qd	Use with caution in patients with renal disease
Herbs		
Cranberry	300–400 mg PO bid standardized cranberry extract capsules	Prevents the adherence of bacteria to the bladder wall (proanthocyanidins, active ingredient, inhibits adhesion of *E. coli* to uroepithelial cells)

addressed. Indwelling urinary catheters should be changed every 4 to 6 weeks with new equipment using sterile technique. It is important to maintain adequate hydration and to monitor the urine output for signs of obstruction or renal failure. Urinary tract obstructions must be identified and removed to reduce the chances of chronic infection and renal damage leading to renal insufficiency and failure. It may be necessary to prescribe analgesics for the patient to reduce the pain associated with the UTI. Pain-relieving medications such as phenazopyridine (Pyridium) can be effective but should be prescribed for no more than 3 days.

Self-medication is usually adequate for female patients who have relatively few recurrences of UTI. If a diagnosis of recurrent bacterial UTI is confirmed, the patient should be given a supply of an antibiotic (preferably trimethoprim-sulfamethoxazole or nitrofurantoin) and instructed to take it for 3 to 7 days whenever the symptoms recur. The patient should keep a diary of her infections and response to treatment and review it annually with a health professional so as to track medication-associated problems. The patient should also be advised to notify the clinician if symptoms such as flank pain, fever, hematuria, or lack of response to treatment occurs.

If UTI recurs frequently (e.g., monthly), prophylactic therapy should be prescribed. After a course of 10 to 14 days of a suitable antibiotic (e.g., a fluoroquinolone), the patient should begin low-dose antimicrobial prophylaxis every other day at bedtime over a 4- to 6-month period. This regimen has proved as effective as daily dosing. Night-time therapy is recommended because the patient generally does not void for a prolonged period, thus giving the bacteria the opportunity to adhere to the bladder wall. If this period of prophylaxis has been effective, the patient may switch to self-medication. If the frequency of recurrence increases at this point, however, prophylaxis should be extended to every other night indefinitely. However, all lifestyle issues should be investigated first.

Patient Education

Patient education should focus on teaching the patient to prevent recurrence of UTI. This is accomplished by advising the patient to follow these guidelines:

- Complete the full course of antibiotic therapy even if all symptoms subside (treatment may be anywhere from 3 to 14 days in duration).
- Perform proper hygiene for toileting by wiping front to back after urinating or defecating.
- Increase fluid intake to eight 8-ounce glasses of water per day; this is most important to continue flushing out bacteria.
- Take vitamin C to acidify the urine, which will help to decrease the bacteria's ability to proliferate.
- Self-medicate if indicated.
- Wear cotton underclothes rather than nylon to avoid moisture buildup and avoid wearing "thong" underpants.
- Avoid the use of harsh soaps or feminine hygiene products that can irritate the urethra.
- Drink water before sexual intercourse and empty the bladder before and after intercourse activities.
- Use condoms to provide a barrier to infection from intercourse.
- Use proper techniques for self-catheterization to reduce the incidence of introducing bacteria.
- Empty the bladder frequently to avoid stasis of urine.
- Take showers instead of tub baths or bubble baths to avoid chemical irritation of the urethra.

- ▲ Keep a diary of urinary symptoms and review it annually if recurrent infections are a problem.
- ▲ Avoid tampons, especially if there is a pattern of becoming infected during the menstrual cycle, which may be related to the type of sanitary protection.
- ▲ Empty the bladder completely, possibly by double-voiding (i.e., completely emptying the bladder two times in 5 minutes), especially if recurrent infections are a problem.

The patient should also be educated regarding any potential adverse effects of medication, including urinary leakage associated with phenazopyridine (Pyridium) treatment or the subsequent development of vaginal yeast infections.

Upper Urinary Tract Infection: Pyelonephritis

Pyelonephritis is an infection of the kidney that is characterized by infection within the renal pelvis, tubules, or interstitial tissue that may be unilateral or bilateral. The condition may be classified as either acute or chronic. The chronic condition leads to changes in the kidney that create atrophy and scarring of the kidney and calyceal deformity that may eventually lead to renal failure.

Epidemiology and Causes

Pyelonephritis occurs in both men and women, but it is more common in women. The occurrence is higher in older adults (especially if institutionalized or hospitalized), children, and in immunocompromised patients. Community-acquired pyelonephritis is estimated to occur in approximately 15.7 persons per 100,000 per year, whereas hospital-acquired pyelonephritis occurs in approximately 7.3 persons per 10,000 hospitalized persons. The incidence and risk of developing this disease is increased in patients with predisposing factors including anatomic abnormalities such as ureterovesical reflux, urinary obstruction, stress incontinence, multiple or recurrent UTIs, renal disease, kidney trauma, pregnancy, and metabolic disorders such as diabetes mellitus. Having an indwelling urinary catheter is always a prominent risk factor for pyelonephritis, especially in hospitalized elderly women. An episode of acute pyelonephritis within the prior year also puts the patient at increased risk, as does frequent receptive vaginal intercourse (more than 3 times per week) and recent spermicide use. Most of these risk factors alter the vaginal microenvironment and predispose individuals to lower UTI, as well.

In acute pyelonephritis, the actual insult to the kidney may be hematogenous seeding or urinary tract reflex, but most commonly it is an ascending infection from the bladder. It can often be attributed to untreated lower UTI that spreads to the upper urinary system or is introduced through instrumentation. Chronic pyelonephritis usually has no specific pathologic explanation if anatomic abnormalities have been ruled out.

Pathophysiology

Pyelonephritis is typically caused by fecal flora that colonize the vaginal introitus and subsequently ascend along the urinary tract to the kidneys. It is unclear whether lower UTI always precedes pyelonephritis, as many patients present without clinical evidence of prior cystitis. However, bacteria are believed to enter through the urethral meatus and ascend upward from the lower urinary tract (urethra and bladder) to one or both kidneys via the ureters, the bloodstream (i.e., hematogenous spread), or the lymphatic system.

Escherichia coli (70 to 95 percent of cases), *Proteus mirabilis, Klebsiella,* and *Pseudomonas* are the most common gram-negative causative agents. Five to 10 percent of cases are caused by gram-positive organisms, including *Enterococcus, Staphylococcus saprophyticus,* and *Staphylococcus aureus* (particularly in severe infection). *Ureaplasma urealyticum* and *Mycoplasma hominis* are rarer causative agents. In patients with normal urogenital systems, nearly all bacterial agents of pyelonephritis express virulence factors that contribute to their uropathogenicity (e.g., the *pap* and *sfa* operons and pathogenicity islands found in virulent *Escherichia coli* strains).

In acute pyelonephritis, swelling of the renal parenchyma occurs as a result of the patchy distribution of the acute infectious process throughout the kidney. In rare instances, scarring of the renal parenchyma leading to kidney atrophy, renal hypertension, and renal failure may occur if left untreated. When the infection is severe, abscesses may develop in the renal medulla leading to necrosis of the renal papillae. This infection can be potentially life threatening in the elderly, in children, or in immunocompromised patients. In addition, diagnosis and treatment in pregnant women is particularly critical, as upper UTI has a clear association with premature delivery.

Chronic pyelonephritis is usually caused by a recurrent or chronic bacterial infection of the kidney, often related to the presence of instrumentation such as an indwelling catheter that serves as a nidus of infection. Patients often have other urological problems such as vesicoureteral reflux, neurogenic bladder, or urinary obstruction caused by renal tumors, stones, or prostatic hypertrophy. The persistent unresolved infection and inflammation cause fibrosis (scarring) of the tubulointerstitium, which may lead to hypertension as the body senses decreased renal blood flow or eventually chronic renal insufficiency.

Clinical Presentation

Subjective

The patient with acute pyelonephritis may present with a sudden onset of fever, persisting over a few hours or days and ranging up to 103°F (39.5°C). The patient may present with shaking, chills, nausea, and vomiting as well as unilateral flank or localized back pain over the affected kidney (i.e., costovertebral angle tenderness), fatigue, diarrhea, or other symptoms resembling those of a gram-negative sepsis.

Signs of urinary urgency or frequency and suprapubic discomfort may be present. Otherwise, the patient may be largely asymptomatic and then progress to full-blown sepsis (i.e., urosepsis). In the elderly patient, altered mental status may be the initial manifestation of pyelonephritis.

Chronic pyelonephritis may present with the patient complaining of fatigue, nausea, decreased appetite with weight loss, nocturia, and/or polyuria. Patients may present with symptoms of renal failure resulting from asymptomatic chronic pyelonephritis that has persisted for several years. Symptoms of renal failure are discussed in detail later in this chapter.

Objective

The physical examination will elicit marked tenderness on deep abdominal palpation and/or percussion of the affected flank and back overlying the affected kidney (i.e., costovertebral angle tenderness). Patients may be hypertensive and with severe pyelonephritis may remain symptomatic for several days, even if appropriate antibiotic therapy is administered.

Patients with chronic pyelonephritis may show minimal symptoms or symptoms similar to those of acute pyelonephritis. The early signs and symptoms may be vague; chronic pyelonephritis usually is first diagnosed when the patient presents with impaired renal function caused by damage to the kidneys.

Diagnostic Reasoning

Diagnostic Tests

The diagnosis of pyelonephritis is confirmed through urinalysis, which is positive for bacteria, proteinuria, leukocyte esterase, urinary nitrites, hematuria, pyuria, and specifically WBC casts (reflecting the passage of neutrophils through the renal tubules), as well as urine culture, which typically demonstrates greater than 100,000 cfu/mL, allowing for identification of the causative organism. Any of these findings may be altered, however, if the patient is already on antibiotic therapy, and colony counts may be as low as 10,000 cfu/mL in some cases. Blood cultures may also be positive in 10 to 20 percent of mild to moderate pyelonephritis, reflecting urosepsis.

Cystoscopy with ureteral catheterization, renal ultrasound (to reveal hydroureter and/or hydronephrosis), or intravenous pyelogram (IVP) may be indicated. However, the nuclear medicine-based dimercaptosuccinic acid (DMSA) scan is most sensitive for detecting pyelonephritis and renal scarring. Although rarely used, renal biopsy in acute pyelonephritis may reveal abscess formation with neutrophilic invasion. The area of the infection is wedge-shaped, pointing toward the medulla, while the glomeruli are spared. Findings in chronic pyelonephritis will include fibrosis, scarring, and reduction of renal tissue, with calyceal clubbing, dilation, and distortion. A voiding cystourethrogram (VCUG) may reveal vesicoureteral reflux, which predisposes to both lower and upper UTI.

Differential Diagnosis

It can be difficult to differentiate pyelonephritis from cystitis; however, the presence of WBC casts is diagnostic for pyelonephritis. Hematuria is also often present in lower and upper UTI, but not in vaginitis or urethritis. Chronic pyelonephritis can sometimes be diagnosed through IVP, DMSA scan, and ultrasound, which may identify atrophied kidneys with "clubbing" of the affected calyces. A definitive diagnosis of chronic disease is made by identifying persistent pyuria and by positive urine cultures. Sometimes, chronic pyelonephritis is diagnosed only via kidney biopsy.

Management

Aggressive therapy is necessary to prevent permanent damage to the kidneys, a potential complication of upper versus lower UTI. Tissue penetration of antibiotics into the renal medulla appears more important that serum or urine levels. Oral antibiotics may be prescribed in mild cases of acute pyelonephritis, characterized by the absence of nausea and vomiting or signs of sepsis. Trimethoprim-sulfamethoxazole taken orally for 14 days may be as effective as oral amoxicillin or amoxicillin-clavulanate for 6 weeks in young women with their first pyelonephritis and without anatomic abnormalities. However, given the prevalence of sulfonamide and ampicillin resistance among common uropathogens, trimethoprim-sulfamethoxazole and amoxicillin are likely to be ineffective in cases of recurrent or moderate to severe pyelonephritis (except in cases of *Enterococcus* infection, which calls for the addition of amoxicillin [Amoxil] 500 mg PO tid). Nitrofurantoin should be avoided, as it does not achieve adequate tissue levels. Other effective choices are third-generation cephalosporins (e.g., cefixime, cefpodoxime, ceftriaxone), aminoglycosides (e.g., gentamicin, tobramycin), or aztreonam, with fluoroquinolones reserved for antibiotic-resistant organisms, hence the critical need for early urine culture to guide pharmacotherapy. Drugs Commonly Prescribed 11.2 presents the oral agents commonly prescribed for lower UTI and mild to moderate pyelonephritis (not requiring hospitalization or IV therapy).

Hospitalization may be indicated, depending on the patient's ability to maintain adequate fluid intake and to tolerate oral antibiotics, along with the severity of the symptoms and evidence of bacteremia. Hospitalization of patients who are pregnant, vomiting, or dehydrated should be strongly considered. Likewise, the patient's degree of systemic illness (bacteremia or urosepsis), age, history of chronic disease, or of nonadherence to therapy may lead to the assessment that hospitalization is necessary. Ninety-five percent of patients demonstrate a good response within 48 hours to IV antibiotic treatment and may be discharged on appropriate oral medication, once urine culture and antibiotic sensitivity results are available and subsequent antimicrobial therapy may be narrowed in spectrum. Treatment courses should typically last for 7 to 10 days for mild to moderate cases, 14 days for severe cases, or 21 days in particularly slow responders. Ample evidence has demonstrated that once common 6-week regimens lead to increased adverse effects without improved treatment effectiveness.

Common choices for non-*Enterococcal* infection include ceftriaxone 1 gram IV qd, gentamicin 3 to 5 mg/kg IV qd, or tobramycin 3 to 5 mg/kg IV qd. Fluoroquinolones are also appropriate choices, except in pregnant women, given concerns over their effects on bone and cartilage formation in the developing fetus. This class of antibiotics has virtually equivalent absorption when administered orally or intravenously at the same dose (see Drugs Commonly Prescribed 11.2). Thus, IV fluoroquinolone preparations should only be used for patients with active nausea and vomiting. When enterococcal infection is suspected, ampicillin 1 to 2 grams IV q6h should be combined with either gentamicin or tobramycin at 1 mg/kg IV q8h added for synergy. Another option for empiric therapy is the broad-spectrum antibiotic piperacillin-tazobactam (Zosyn) 3.375 g IV q6h given over 30 minutes. If the creatinine clearance is between 20 and 40 mL/min then the dose should be 2.25 g q6h. If the creatinine clearance is less than 20 mL/min, the dose should be 2.25 g q8h.

If the patient does not respond adequately within 48 hours, he or she should be reevaluated, the cultures reviewed, and an ultrasound, IVP, or DMSA scan performed. IV antibiotics may need to be administered for up to 7 to 10 days in severe cases. During treatment the patient must increase fluid intake and an accurate intake and output record must be maintained for appropriate fluid management. Surgery may be indicated to remove or correct secondary causes of UTI such as urinary obstruction or anatomic abnormalities and neuropathic genitourinary tract lesions. Diagnostic studies requiring insertion of instruments should be delayed until the urine is sterile or free of bacteria and/or pus, to avoid the complications of bacteremia or septic shock. A urological anatomic evaluation should be performed for all men with pyelonephritis and women with recurrent pyelonephritis to elicit structural abnormalities that may be contributing to or causing the condition.

Follow-Up and Referral

If undergoing outpatient treatment, the patient should be seen 48 hours later to assess responsiveness to therapy. Similarly, patients in the hospital should be evaluated in 48 hours for response to therapy and consideration of discharge. Follow-up urine cultures are not routinely recommended in aysmptomatic patients. However, in those with recurrent pyelonephritis, reculturing at 2, 6, and 12 weeks after antibiotic therapy is initiated may be done to ensure complete and lasting eradication of infection. Further treatment decisions are based on clinical findings such as fever, pain, and culture of bacteria. When a diagnosis of chronic pyelonephritis is determined, the patient should be referred to a nephrologist because of the severe damage that can occur to the kidney. As discussed previously, a renal ultrasound, renal colic CT scan, or voiding cystourethrogram may detect structural abnormalities, renal stones, or vesicoureteral reflux—all of which predispose to infection. Patients should also be monitored and treated for other conditions secondary to the pyelonephritis such as hypertension, chronic infection, renal insufficiency, or renal failure.

Patient Education

The focus should be on teaching the patient to prevent recurrence of lower UTI and of pyelonephritis by following these instructions:

- Complete the antibiotic therapy even if symptoms subside.
- Prevent or reduce the incidence of lower UTIs by following the guidelines under Patient Education in the next section.
- Increase fluid intake to eight 8-ounce glasses of water per day.
- Report any recurrence of UTI symptoms immediately.
- Take vitamin C to acidify the urine, which will help to decrease the bacteria's ability to proliferate.
- Control hypertension with medications, dietary regimen, and lifestyle changes as detailed in Chapter 9.

Nephrolithiasis

Nephrolithiasis is a condition in which stones (renal calculi) that originate in the kidney. The calculi form from calcium salts (approximately 75 to 85 percent), struvite (approximately 10 to 15 percent), uric acid (approximately 7 percent), and cystine (1 to 2 percent). These stone formations often cause acute episodes of urinary tract obstruction, infection, and abdominal pain in adults.

Epidemiology and Causes

This disease peaks in people between the ages of 20 and 30 with a range of 20 to 60 years. It affects approximately 2 to 5 percent of individuals at some time during their lifetime, or about 70 to 210 per 100,000 of the population. Some stones such as calcium oxalate occur more often in men, whereas struvite stones are more common in women. Formation of renal calculi is more prevalent in the Southeast, West, and Midwest. The patient may report a sedentary lifestyle or occupation that exposes him or her to high environmental temperatures. Renal stones can occur because of obstruction, urinary stasis, infection, dehydration and urine concentration, increased consumption of calcium or vitamin D, excessive excretion of uric acid, or vitamin A deficiency; Hereditary factors can also predispose the patient to kidney stone formation.

Calcium oxalate and calcium phosphate stones account for 65 to 85 percent of all cases of kidney stones. These types of stones are found predominantly in men and in individuals whose diet is high in salt, animal fat, animal protein, and oxalate from green leafy vegetables. Interestingly, a low-calcium diet is also a risk factor, as it leads to increased oxaluria, since less oxalate is complexed with calcium within the GI tract. Vasectomy is a risk factor as well, while hypertension doubles the risk of stone formation for reasons that are as yet unclear. Patients with calcium oxalate or calcium phosphate stones typically are not characterized by hypercalcemia except with certain disorders such as hyperparathyroidism, sarcoidosis, and hyperuricemia, which may lead to hypercalciuria or hyperuricosuria. Loop diuretics such as furosemide (Lasix) also promote calciuria, while hypocitriuria and hyperoxaluria similarly predispose to calcium stone formation, as an increased amount of calcium is available for complexing with oxalate or phosphate within the urinary tract. Inflammatory bowel disease is associated with marked hyperoxaluria, while medullary sponge kidney disease is found in 10-30 percent of persons with calcium stones.

Struvite stones are found predominantly in women; these stones are associated with UTIs. They occur when the urine pH is high (alkaline; greater than 7.0) and a urea-splitting organism such as *Proteus* or *Klebsiella* is present. Uric acid stones are formed from an increase in uric acid production or ineffective elimination of uric acid, as found in gout. This may result from dietary intake of foods high in uric acid, acidic urinary pH (e.g., type I renal tubular acidosis, significant bicarbonate loss associated with severe diarrhea), regional enteritis, hereditary factors (including a predisposition to gout), or ulcerative colitis. Uric acid stones account for approximately 15 to 20 percent of all cases of nephrolithiasis. Cystine stones are created because of a rare autosomal recessive disorder called cystinuria. These stones are formed when there is a metabolic error that causes a decrease in tubular reabsorption in the kidney, leading to urinary cystine concentrations greater than 250 mg/L. Cystine stones account for approximately 1 to 3 percent of all cases of renal stones.

Pathophysiology

Renal stone formation occurs when normally soluble mineral substances supersaturate the urine and deposit out of solution as crystals, which serve as nuclei for stone-forming substance such as calcium oxalate, calcium phosphate, triple-phosphate struvite (magnesium ammonium phosphate), uric acid, or cystine. Stone formation may also be facilitated by extremes in the urinary pH (alkaline or acid). This crystal combination becomes trapped within the renal system, where it continues to attract other crystals, causing the stone to increase in size. Stones are typically anchored at the ends of collecting ducts at sites of epithelial injury. The calculi vary in size and composition and typically grow within the renal tubules, calyces, renal pelvis, ureters, or bladder. Large stones are called staghorn calculi if they span more than one of the renal calyces. Although over the span of years their presence in the kidneys may lead to chronic renal failure, unless they fragment and pass through the urinary system, they are generally asymptomatic.

The four major types of stones, their characteristics, causes, etiology, diagnosis, and treatment are listed in Table 11.7. These forms are not mutually exclusive and share certain risk factors. Thus, many patients have renal stones of a mixed etiology. Calcium stones are light in color; their crystals characteristically resemble RBCs in shape and size or may be a larger "dumbbell" form. Formation of these stones may be secondary to hypercalcemia or idiopathic. Hyperoxaluria and hyperuricosuria are more associated with calcium oxalate stones, while calcium phosphate stones are more associated with primary hyperparathyroidism. Struvite stones are flat and consist of hexagon-shaped crystals that are radiopaque. They often form secondary to UTI caused by *Proteus mirabilis*. Staghorn calculi are more likely to be stru-

Table 11.7 Renal Calculi

Type of Stone (percentage of all stones)	Characteristics	Causes	Management
Calcium (75%–80%)	Resembles RBCs in shape and size or large dumbbell form Light color	Idiopathic, hypercalcemia, or increased levels of uric acid	Thiazide diuretics Diet Cholestyramine or oral calcium Surgery
Struvite (15%)	Flat, hexagon shape Radiopaque	Alkaline urine, infection with urea-splitting organisms such as *Pseudomonas*	Antibiotic therapy Surgery
Uric acid (7%)	Teardrop-shaped or flat square plates Red-orange color	Increased uric acid production, high intake of uric acid, acidic urine, regional enteritis, ulcerative colitis, or idiopathic	Allopurinol Fluid replacement Diet Surgery
Cystine (<1%)	Lemon yellow and sparkle	Hereditary	Force fluids D-Penicillamine Tiopronin

vite stones. Uric acid stones are radiolucent and red-orange, with a teardrop or flat square shape. Formation of these stones may be associated with a hereditary etiology of gout or with idiopathic causes. Uric acid crystals may also serve as a nidus for calcium stone formation. Cystine stone crystals are lemon yellow, hexagonal, and sparkle under light microscopy. They have a hereditary etiology. Finally, certain medications strongly promote crystalluria and predispose to renal stones, including topiramate, triamterene, and sulfadiazine. The protease inhibitor indinavir (Crixivan) used to treat HIV-positive patients may actually precipitate within the renal collecting system, causing direct stone formation.

The incidence of recurrence of certain stones is approximately 40 to 50 percent within 5 years, with an estimated one-third of patients eventually losing a kidney if the condition is left untreated or inadequately treated. Complications can occur when the stone obstructs the flow of urine. This can lead to urinary retention, accumulation of uremic wastes, end-stage renal failure, and/or electrolyte imbalances. Stones can further compromise the patient, by predisposing to UTI and hematuria.

Clinical Presentation

Subjective

The patient with an acute episode of nephrolithiasis may present with a variety of signs and symptoms, depending on the location, size, and type of stone. Onset is usually sudden, with renal colic, which is a type of flank pain that is not relieved by changes in position or other measures. The pain may present with a referral pattern that originates in the flank or kidney area and radiates across the abdomen down into the groin, perineal area, and inner thigh. This colicky pain occasionally progresses to constant pain at a level that can be excruciating and intractable. Other symptoms of renal calculi may include nausea, urinary frequency, vomiting, diaphoresis, dysuria, hematuria, and weakness. The patient may report a history of a recent or chronic UTI, previous diagnosis with nephrolithiasis, a dietary history consistent with stone formation, or alterations in voiding patterns.

Objective

The patient may present with abdominal distension and guarding on palpation, flank tenderness on percussion, and decreased or absent bowel sounds on auscultation. Fever may be present if there is acute infection related to obstruction. Blood pressure (as well as pulse rate and respiratory rate) may be elevated because of pain.

Diagnostic Reasoning

Diagnostic Tests

The diagnostic workup should begin with a routine urinalysis, CBC, and blood chemistry profile. The urinalysis may be normal or it may show RBCs, WBCs, crystals, cast minerals, bacteria, pus, and an alkaline or acidic pH. Table 11.8 identifies the tests and the expected results that would lead to the suspicion of renal calculi. Either gross or microscopic hematuria is observed in the majority of cases but may be absent in up to 30 percent of cases, depending on the time of presentation. Identification of the type of stone formation is important for the appropriate treatment to be instituted. The results of these tests should lead the clinician to continue the diagnostic workup with noninvasive tests to identify obstructions, masses, or anatomic abnormalities. Further diagnostic tests include the kidney, ureters, and bladder (KUB) x-ray studies, abdominal or transvaginal ultrasonography (used for pregnant women and those of child-bearing age in whom radiation must be avoided), or noncontrast helical computed tomography (CT) scan (contrast is avoided due to potential renal toxicity). Invasive procedures may be necessary to visualize or assist in removing the stone through IVP, cystourethroscopy, or other surgical procedures.

Differential Diagnosis

The differential diagnosis for renal calculi may include a variety of diseases, including appendicitis, diverticulitis, mesenteric adenitis, pancreatitis, ileus, peptic ulcer disease, abnormalities of the fallopian tubes and ovaries including ovarian cysts, ectopic pregnancy, gall bladder disease, and abdominal aneurysms. A tentative diagnosis of renal

Table 11.8 Tests for Renal Calculi

Test	Rationale
Urinalysis	Shows RBCs, WBCs, crystals, casts, minerals, bacteria, pus, abnormal pH
24-hour urine	May show increased levels of creatinine, uric acid, calcium, phosphorus, oxylate, or cystine
Serum chemistry	May show increased levels of magnesium, calcium, uric acid, phosphorus, protein, and electrolytes
Serum BUN and creatinine	Shows BUN elevated secondary to urinary tract obstruction; creatinine elevated secondary to damage to the kidney
CBC	May show infection or septicemia
Kidney and upper bladder	Shows calculi and/or anatomic changes
IVP	Shows calculi and any abnormality in anatomic structures
Cystourecteroscopy	May show calculi and/or abnormal structural defects
CT scan	Identifies calculi and other masses in the renal system

calculi is made from the history and the findings of the physical examination showing increased intensity of colic with flank pain or a pattern of referred pain, coupled with flank tenderness. As hematuria may be the only presenting sign of stone formation, malignancy (renal cell carcinoma), which is typically painless, must also be considered. Diagnosis of renal stones is confirmed by urinalysis that is positive for blood and visualization by radiography or ultrasound.

Management

Treatment goals are to decrease the symptoms and complications arising from existing stones and prevent subsequent recurrence. It is important, therefore, to decrease the concentration of stone-forming substances in the urine. An intake of six to eight 8-ounce glasses of water a day is essential; this high fluid intake must continue indefinitely. Most stones smaller than 5 mm pass spontaneously; rates of spontaneous passage steadily decrease for stones larger than this and is highly unlikely for stones larger than 10 mm.

Initially, pain management is the priority. Oral NSAIDs in doses of 600 to 800 g tid or oral narcotics such as hydrocodone-acetaminophen (Vicodin, Lortab), acetaminophen-codeine (Tylenol #3), or oxycodone-acetaminophen (Percocet) are often necessary. In some cases, intramuscular or intravenous narcotic analgesics may be necessary, but most studies have demonstrated NSAIDs are as effective as oral opiates, albeit slower-acting. In addition, they have also been shown to relax ureteral smooth muscle, which may facilitate stone passage. Antispasmodics such as flavoxate or oxybutynin may also provide temporary relief, but the anticholinergic effects of these medications must be taken into account as they may lead to urinary retention. Warm compresses to the lower back, focused breathing, imagery, and diversional activities may provide minimal relief.

Certain drugs help to reduce urinary excretion of stone-forming substances. Most notably, thiazide diuretics (e.g., hydrochlorothiazide) reduce calcium excretion; allopurinol reduces uric acid production by inhibiting xanthine oxidase; and D-penicillamine affects the excretion of cystine. Importantly, loop diuretics such as furosemide (Lasix) and triamterene increase calciuria and typically worsen renal stone formation.

Noninvasive or invasive surgical interventions may be necessary if the stone does not pass spontaneously; these are presented in Table 11.9. Noninvasive procedures to treat renal calculi are aggressive and have many of the same risks that occur with surgery. Extracorporeal shock wave lithotripsy (ESWL) sends shock waves throughout the outside of the body to disrupt proximal and mid-ureteral calculi and is preferred for stones smaller than 10 mm. NSAIDs should be avoided at least 3 days prior to this therapy to minimize the risk of bleeding. The percutaneous ultrasonic lithotriptor (PUL) applies therapeutic ultrasound waves to the outside of the body to achieve the same results. A lithotriptic agent may also be used to dissolve the calculi stones.

Invasive procedures may be necessary to remove the stone because of the location of the stone or the failure of noninvasive procedures to destroy the stone. The procedure chosen is dependent on the location, size, and type of stone (e.g., struvite stones typically require ESWL or surgical intervention). First- and second-generation lithotriptors originally visualized stones via fluoroscopy or ultrasonography. However, advances in urethroscopy with flexible fiber optic systems now allow for the direct visualization of stones virtually anywhere along the urinary tract from the urethra to the renal pelvis. Stones may be crushed via electrohydraulic or laser lithotripsy in conjunction with these visualization techniques. Flexible ureteroscopy combined with laser lithotripsy is now the preferred treatment for

Table 11.9 Surgical Procedures for Renal Calculi Management

Procedure	Type of Procedure	Location of Calculi	Description
Lithotripsy	Invasive	Bladder or urethra	Crushing of the calculi under direct visualization using a lithotriptoscope
Lithotony	Invasive	Renal system	Arthroscopic removal of the calculi
Lithonephrotomy	Invasive	Kidney	Incision of the kidney to remove the calculi
Lithotomy	Invasive	Bladder or urethra	Incision of the bladder or ureter to remove the calculi
Ureteral stent	Invasive	Kidney or ureter	Stent is placed in front of the calculi to facilitate elimination
Lithotropic	Noninvasive	Renal system	Agent used to dissolve calculi
Percutaneous ultrasonic lithotriptor (PUL)	Noninvasive	Renal system	Ultrasound waves are applied to the outside of the body to crush the calculi
Extracorporeal shock wave lithotripsy (ESWL)	Noninvasive	Renal system	Shock waves are applied to the outside of the body to crush the calculi

proximal ureteral stones larger than 10 mm. The patient is then able to eliminate the stones naturally after they are crushed into smaller pieces. *Lithotomy* is an incision into the bladder or ureter to remove calculi or place a ureteral stent, while lithotony specifically denotes arthroscopic extraction of a renal stone from the bladder. Ureteral stents may be placed within the ureters to facilitate the passage of stones through natural elimination. *Lithonephrotomy* is an incision into the kidney to remove a stone.

Preventative measures may be taken to reduce the incidence of recurrence. The incidence of calcium-based stones may be reduced by increasing fluid intake (greater than 2 L/day) and taking thiazide diuretics or allopurinol. In addition, an acidic diet higher in meat content actually promotes calcium excretion. Hypocitruria and hyperuricosuria may both be treated with potassium citrate supplementation. However, this may alkalinize the urine, creating another risk factor for stone formation, and care must be taken to stop this drug if urine pH is greater than 6.0. In similar fashion, appropriate treatment of UTI must be initiated to avoid recurrence of struvite stones, while the urease inhibitor acetohydroxamic acid (Lithostat) 250 mg PO tid to qid may be given as adjunctive therapy to prevent urinary alkalinization, if infection with urease-producing organisms is confirmed.

Oxalate-containing stones should be prevented with a low-oxalate diet (see Patient Education). Struvite stone production may be decreased by preventing UTIs through patient education and self-care as previously discussed, maintenance of antibiotic therapy, or acidifying the urine with methenamine mandelate. Uric acid stones may be decreased through diet modification (see Patient Education) or medications that facilitate uric acid excretion, such as allopurinol. Recurrence of cystine stones may be reduced through maintenance doses of D-penicillamine, tiopronin, or captopril which binds cystine via sulfhydryl moieties.

Follow-Up and Referral

Most patients with renal calculi are treated and followed on an outpatient basis. The patient may need hospitalization for secondary complications that can occur, such as severe nausea and vomiting leading to dehydration, urinary obstruction, decreased renal function, severe bleeding, intractable pain, and significant infection. The patient should be referred to a urologist and/or nephrologist for stone removal under these circumstances or if stone formation is thought to be secondary to a metabolic abnormality.

Patient Education

The patient should be instructed to increase fluid intake to six to eight 8-ounce glasses per day unless prevented by cardiac complications, such as congestive heart failure. Increasing fluids will assist in the elimination of the stones. The patient should monitor intake and output and strain the urine for passed stones. The OTC drugs that contain phosphorus or calcium, such as many antacids (e.g., Tums), and most vitamin supplements, especially vitamin D_3 should be avoided. The role of vitamin C supplementation is controversial. While some promote high-dose vitamin C supplementation to acidify the urine and facilitate stone dissolution (especially the calcium phosphate type), excess vitamin C (1 g/day) is known to undergo chemical conversion to oxalate, which may promote oxaluria and calcium oxalate stone formation. In contrast, vitamin B_6 and magnesium are both known to decrease oxaluria by facilitating oxalate metabolism. Magnesium further competes with calcium, reducing calcium-containing stone formation. In turn, supplementation of vitamin B_6 and magnesium has been shown to reduce the incidence of oxalate stones, although the ideal doses have not been established.

The patient should be encouraged to increase his or her activity level as tolerated, because inactivity contributes to stone formation secondary to calcium shifts and urinary stasis. Dietary modification is also key. In general, caffeine should be avoided, and beer and wine consumption must be only in moderation. A low-oxalate diet is appropriate for calcium oxalate stones, which avoids oxalate-rich foods including beets, black tea, chocolate and cocoa, lamb, nuts, rhubarb, and spinach. A low-phosphorus diet for calcium phosphate or struvite stones avoids milk products and cola drinks. A low-purine diet is often effective in reducing stones formed from excess uric acid. This diet is achieved by limiting intake of purine-rich foods, such as organ meats, red meats, seafood (especially sardines, anchovies, and scallops), poultry, legumes, whole grains, and alcohol (which decreases uric acid clearance).

Renal Tumors

Renal tumors (*neoplasms*) are characterized by abnormal tissue formations on or around the kidney that may cause or contribute to renal disease. They may be primary or secondary (resulting from malignant spread), although the latter are rarely clinically relevant and are typically found during postmortem examination. *Renal adenomas* (benign tumors) and adenocarcinomas are rare; these tumors usually create complications requiring surgical removal.

Epidemiology and Causes

Renal cell carcinomas originating in the renal cortex are the most common (85 percent) malignant renal tumors. These tumors occur most often in the parenchyma of the kidney, with ureteral and urethral tumors occurring rarely. Histologically, they are classified as clear cell (75-85 percent), chromophilic or papillary (15 percent), chromophobic (5 percent), and the uncommon forms of oncocytic and collecting duct tumors. Transitional cell carcinomas are the next most common, comprising 5-8 percent of all tumors; these typically affect the bladder and are discussed extensively in the next section.

Renal tumors are responsible for approximately 3 percent of all adult malignancies. The incidence is higher in men (although the difference in incidence has been decreasing over time), with onset between ages of 55 and 70 years and rarely occurring in people younger than 35 years of age. These cancers are curable in more than 90 percent of patients if they are superficial and/or localized in the renal pelvis or ureter. Tumors that are invasive have a 10 to 15 percent chance of being cured. In children, nephroblastoma (Wilms' tumor) is common, comprising 5 percent of primary tumors, while sickle cell disease has a known, albeit rare, association with carcinoma of the renal medulla.

Obesity, exposure to asbestos, cadmium, and/or gasoline, the use of phenacetin- and aspirin-containing analgesics, and chronic hemodialysis for acquired polycystic kidney disease are all risk factors for renal cell carcinoma. Cigarette smoking has a 25 to 30 percent correlation with the development of renal cell carcinoma.

Pathophysiology

The urinary system is lined with transitional cell epithelium where tumors may form. The tumors often are asymptomatic and grow undetected until complications from the tumor present. The tumors are usually encapsulated and located near the cortex unilaterally. Renal neoplasms may be diagnosed as benign or malignant; they may be identified as either primary (originating in the kidney) or secondary (originating or spread from another source). Primary malignancies usually spread through the lymph nodes and blood vessels to the lungs, liver, and bone. Metastatic disease that spreads to the kidney, usually from the lung, is more common than primary renal neoplasms. Metastatic lesions to the ureter typically originate via hematogenous spread from breast or colorectal primary lesions. Direct extension into the ureter may also occur from cervical or colonic neoplasms, as well as pelvic retroperitoneal lymphoma. Benign renal neoplasms are rare but should be removed because of complications that may occur such as pain, bleeding, and obstruction.

Carcinogen exposure has been associated with specific gene mutations which appear to underlie the development of various forms of hereditary renal cell carcinoma, for example, the von Hippel-Lindau tumor suppressor gene on chromosome 3p25 to 26 (associated with both sporadic and hereditary clear cell carcinoma, i.e., von Hippel-Lindau disease), the fumarate hydratase gene, the Birt-Hogg-Dube tumor suppressor gene on chromosome 17p, and the c-met oncogene on chromosome 7 which codes the hepatocyte growth factor receptor (associated with hereditary papillary renal cell carcinoma), the *ras* gene family, and *p53* overexpression (implicated in cellular division). However, definitive causal relationships between these various mutational hot spots and renal cancer have not been proven.

Clear cell carcinomas consistent display mutations spanning the 3p14 to 3p26 chromosomal region. In contrast, chromophilic carcinomas lack these mutations but have been associated with various trisomies, including chromosomes 12, 16, and 20. Chromophobic carcinomas, which arise from the intercalated cells of the collecting duct system, typically display hypodiploidy with a wide variety of whole chromosomal deletions. The much less common oncocytic carcinomas have been associated with deletions in chromosome 11q13, but as with collecting duct tumors, no consistent chromosomal abnormalities have been identified.

Clinical Presentation

Subjective

Signs and symptoms vary depending upon the size of the tumor. Early signs of tumor growth are silent: approximately 40 percent of the time patients present with gross hematuria as the only symptom. The patient may at times complain of a dull, achy flank pain or abdominal mass.

Objective

Examination of the patient may reveal other symptoms that may present alone or in combination with hematuria. General signs of advanced disease include weight loss and fatigue; more specific signs and symptoms of renal tumors include intermittent fever (not associated with infection), palpable abdominal mass, and nephralgia. Metastasis of renal cancer indicates a poor prognosis; it typically involves the lungs, lymph nodes, liver, bones, and contralateral kidney.

Diagnostic Reasoning

Diagnostic Tests

The diagnosis of renal mass is initially confirmed by IVP with nephrotomography; however, it is often impossible to determine if the mass is solid or cystic with this test. Generally speaking, a cancerous tumor splays, distorts, or occludes the visualization of the collecting system and prevents normal filling and draining of the renal system. Although hematuria is common, urine cytology is not consistently reliable for diagnosing these tumors. Ureteroscopy or ultrasonography with IVP can be used to differentiate a potentially neoplastic tissue from a cyst formation by direct or indirect visualization of the entire renal system. Once tissue biopsy samples are obtained, flow cytometric analysis is used to determine the ploidy (DNA content) of the tumor, while histologic analysis determines morphology and tumor grade (degree of cellular differentiation). Urine cytology samples often provide inadequate tissue for such analyses, however, and the mass must be biopsied directly. Figure 11.1 presents a flowchart for the appropriate diagnostic evaluation of a renal mass.

Magnetic resonance imaging (MRI) and CT scan are useful in preoperative workup and staging of the metastatic lesion. It is necessary to stage the advancement of the tumor to initiate appropriate treatment. Staging of the neoplasm is confirmed through surgical intervention. Staging identifies the tumor advancement and potential for survival.

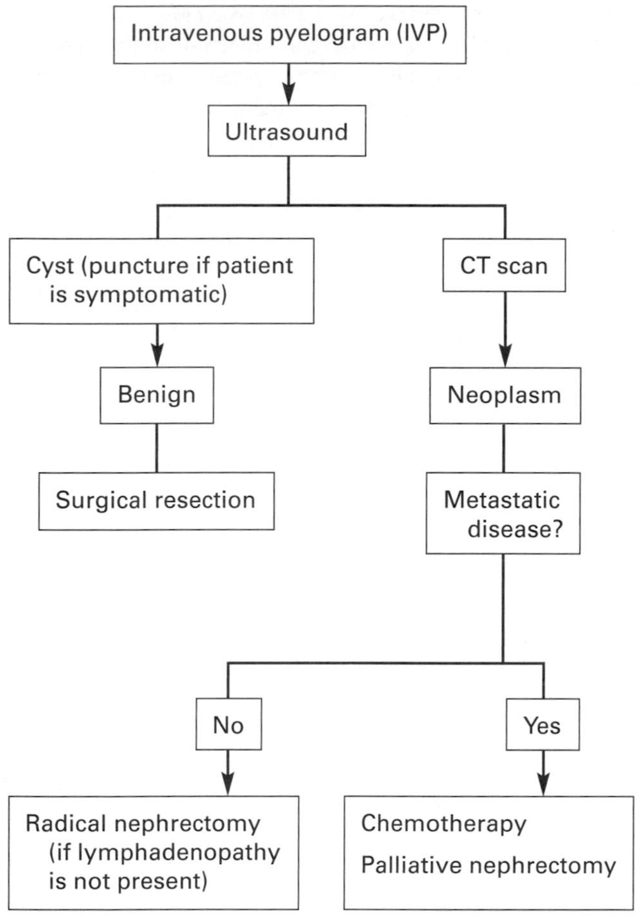

FIGURE 11.1 Renal mass workup.

- ▲ Stage I is defined as a tumor confined within the kidney capsule; it is treated by nephrectomy. The 5-year survival rate is 60 to 75 percent.
- ▲ Stage II is defined as the invasion of the renal capsule that is confined within the Gerota's fascia; it is treated by nephrectomy. The 5-year survival rate is 47 to 65 percent.
- ▲ Stage III is defined as involvement of the regional lymph nodes ipsilateral, renal vein, or vena cava. The 5-year survival rate is 5 to 15 percent.
- ▲ Stage IV is defined as distant metastasis, with a 5-year survival rate of less than 5 percent.

Approximately 30 percent of patients with renal tumors have metastatic disease when the diagnosis is established. The most common sites of metastasis are the lung (50 to 60 percent), bone (30 to 40 percent), regional nodes (15 to 30 percent), brain (10 percent), and adjacent organs.

Differential Diagnosis

Differentiation of a renal cyst from a renal tumor is done by biopsy. Renal calculi and renal infarction must be ruled out, as well as (rarely) renal tuberculosis. In addition, polycystic kidney disease and hydronephrosis must be considered and may be ruled out on biopsy.

Management

As with any cancer, treatment of renal tumors requires immediate specialist referral to a urologist or surgical oncologist, often with additional consultation by a medical oncologist or nephrologist, depending on the patient's renal function. Treatment for a renal neoplasm is primarily surgical with a partial or total nephrectomy, with or without regional lymphadenectomy if no metastatic disease is present. Less radical surgical interventions have been suggested by a vocal minority of urologists, who stress the poor prognosis of advanced renal tumors, regardless of surgical intervention, as well as increased morbidity and mortality associated with radical surgery.

No universal standards have been accepted for the treatment after nephrectomy. Chemotherapy is not effective with this type of cancer; however, immunotherapy using lymphokine-activated killer (LAK) cells with or without interleukin 2 (IL-2) may be helpful for selected patients. Radiation therapy is controversial but may be used in combination with nephrectomy or for palliative effects in patients with bone metastasis.

Follow-Up and Referral

For follow-up of patients with a total nephrectomy, a CT scan of the abdomen and renal fossa should be done in 3 to 6 months; then the patient may be followed with renal ultrasound every 6 months for 3 years, then annually, unless symptoms occur. Chest x-ray studies are done quarterly for a year to monitor for pulmonary metastasis.

At the time of the neoplasm diagnosis, the patient should be referred to a urologist for a surgical evaluation and to an oncologist for cancer treatment. The patient should be seen by the primary-care provider as needed for problems not related to the cancer and to assist the patient with counseling regarding grief, death and dying, body image changes, and quality of life.

Patient Education

The patient needs preparation for the surgical intervention. Postoperatively, the focus is on pain management and promoting comfort, through the use of moist heat, analgesic/narcotics, or positioning on the side with pillows and back support. Additional interventions include preventing pneumonia and atelectasis by encouraging the patient to do coughing and deep breathing exercises, incision care, and monitoring bowel and bladder function.

Bladder Tumors

Bladder tumors are abnormal tissue masses that occur in the bladder wall lining, which is composed of transitional cell epithelium, or "urothelium." These tumors commonly recur in spite of aggressive treatment.

Epidemiology and Causes

Bladder tumors are the most common cancer of the urinary system; they represent approximately 2 percent of all malignant tumors and result in 3 percent of cancer deaths per year. Bladder cancer is the fifth most common neoplasm in the United States; it occurs in men three times more often than women, most often in adults between ages 60 and 70. It is also more common among non-Hispanic white men than in other ethnic and racial groups.

There is a significant correlation between bladder tumors and risk factors including cigarette smoking, presence of renal tumors, exposure to aromatic amine dyes known as arylamines (e.g., beta-naphthylamines, xenylamine, 4-nitrobiphenyl, and benzidine), arsenic, chronic use of phenacetin-containing analgesics, saccharin (in rodent studies), chronic lower UTI, schistosomiasis, and recurrent nephrolithiasis. Other predisposing factors include previous radiation treatment for cervical, ovarian, or prostate cancer, and prior cyclophosphamide chemotherapy.

Pathophysiology

The second most common form of renal carcinomas arise from the transitional cell uroepithelium (urothelium), which lines the mucosal surfaces of the collecting tubules, renal calyces, renal pelvis, ureters, bladder, and urethra. Transitional cell carcinomas account for 90 percent of all tumors of renal pelvic or ureteral origin. Bladder tumors are primarily transitional cell carcinoma, which have the most favorable prognosis, but may also include squamous cell carcinoma and adenocarcinoma. Bladder tumors are described as papillary (90 percent) or nonpapillary (10 percent). Papillary bladder lesions form as a small protuberance attached to a stalk. Nonpapillary lesions are more invasive and have a poorer prognosis. Primary bladder cancer tends to metastasize to the lymph nodes, liver, bones, and lungs. Bladder cancer may be secondary to local extension and/or metastatic disease from adjacent organs such as the cervix in women and the prostate in men.

Genetic analyses of transitional cell carcinomas demonstrate a loss of heterozygosity at any one of multiple chromosomal locations, including 9q (most common), 5p, 8p, 10q, 11p, and 17p—all of which may represent sites of tumor suppressor genes. Genetic predispositions also appear to exist, based on allelic variants of the p450 cytochrome enzyme complex. For instance, smokers afflicted with bladder cancer express p450 enzyme variants which lead to increased activation of arylamine metabolites, a required step for their role in bladder carcinogenesis. Along this same line, allelic variants exist for the *N*-acetyltransferase gene *NAT2*, which (along with *NAT1*) serves as the primary pathway for the metabolism and detoxification of arylamines via *N*-acetylation. Individuals with *NAT2* variants conferring a "slow-acetylation" phenotype are up to 17 times more likely to develop bladder cancer than those with a "fast-acetylation" phenotype. A similar phenomenon exists regarding the glutathione-*S*-transferase M1 gene (*GSTM1*), which contributes to detoxification of carcinogenic compounds via conjugation to glutathione and the facilitation of excretion. In the United States, nearly 50 percent of white men display deletions in both alleles of this gene, effectively eliminating any enzymatic activity from the *GSTM1* gene product.

Transitional cell carcinomas often present multifocally along the urinary tract, spreading via intraluminal seeding or intraepithelial migration in a process known as "field cancerization." However, these multifocal tumors still display monoclonality along their entire distribution. Squamous cell carcinoma, a less common form of bladder cancer that also accounts for 7 percent of renal pelvis tumors, is typically associated with inflammatory processes, including chronic UTI and renal calculi. These tumors tend to be deeply invasive and carry a poor prognosis.

Clinical Presentation

Subjective

The patient with a bladder tumor frequently is asymptomatic until he or she has an episode of hematuria that varies in severity from microscopic to gross amounts and may be intermittent or continuous. Other presenting symptoms may include dysuria, frequency, chills, low-grade fever, weight loss, and urinary urgency. Patients with advanced disease may complain of pelvic pain and symptoms associated with urethral obstruction.

Objective

The physical examination may be positive for a palpable mass and/or metastatic manifestations. The urinalysis shows trace to gross hematuria, possibly with abnormalities in protein level, RBCs, or WBCs. The serum CBC may indicate that anemia is present.

Diagnostic Reasoning

Diagnostic Tests

The diagnosis of bladder tumor is confirmed by visualization of the lesion through cystoscopy and biopsy. A urine cytology positive for transitional cell cancer can confirm the diagnosis; however, negative results do not rule out the possibility of bladder cancer. Cystoscopic evaluation can be used to confirm the suspected diagnosis, to determine the location of the tumor, and to aid in the staging of the tumor. The cystoscopy should include a bladder washing for cytology and a mucosal biopsy. An abdominal or pelvic CT scan, with or without IVP, may be useful for determining the metastatic progress of the disease.

In general, transitional cell carcinomas are staged from A to D, according to level of invasion: stage 0 tumors are confined to the mucosa; stage A tumors invade the lamina propria; stage B tumors invade the muscular layer; stage C tumors extend to the peripelvic fat or renal parenchyma; while stage D indicates metastatic disease. The T (tumor) N (node) M (metastasis) system of the American Joint

Committee on Cancer may also be used, with nodal metastases reflecting stage IV cancer. When transitional cell carcinomas are looked at as a whole, in situ disease has a 5-year survival rate of 95 percent, localized disease nearly 90 percent, regional disease at just over 60 percent, and distant disease only 17 percent.

Urine tumor marker tests can detect recurrent tumors. The *N*-benzoyl-L-tyrosyl-*p*-aminobenzoic acid (BTA) and nucleoside 5′-monophosphate (NMP22) tests are more sensitive for recurrent tumors than urine cytology.

Differential Diagnosis

Because this disease most often presents as painless hematuria, differential diagnoses associated with this condition must be ruled out, such as stones, infections, trauma, other tumors such as renal cell carcinoma, atriovenous malformations, and glomerulonephropathies. Differential diagnosis for bladder irritability includes inflammation, stones, neurologic dysfunction, and foreign bodies. Biopsy is necessary for definitive diagnosis.

Management

Treatment is dependent upon the type, size, and degree of invasion of the bladder tumor, which is classified as superficial, invasive, or metastatic. *Superficial tumors* involve the bladder mucosa and submucosa; they are treated by endoscopic resection or laser resection. These tumors tend to recur and the patient must be reexamined every 6 months. *Invasive tumors* involve the muscle and/or perivesical fat around the bladder. These tumors are treated with radical cystectomy or with radiation and chemotherapy. The 5-year survival rate is 65 to 75 percent with treatment. *Metastatic tumors* involve the lymph nodes, bone, or viscera and are treated with radiation and/or chemotherapy. This stage of the disease has a 5-year survival rate of 10 to 15 percent.

For the majority of bladder tumors, surgical resection is the treatment of choice. Immediate referral to a urologist or surgical oncologist is critical, as well as follow-up with a medical oncologist and/or nephrologist, depending on functional renal status. Intravesical chemotherapy may prevent recurrence, but radiation therapy for bladder tumors is less effective than the other interventions. Treatment options are presented in Treatment Standards/Guidelines 11.1.

Follow-Up and Referral

All patients diagnosed with bladder cancer should be referred to a urologist for evaluation and treatment. Obtain a urinalysis and cystoscopy every 3 to 6 months because of the increased risk of recurrence of bladder tumors. Patients who have been diagnosed with advanced metastatic disease should be referred to an oncologist. Home health or hospice care may be appropriate for patients who need skilled care and ongoing patient teaching; an ostomy nurse may be necessary for patients who have undergone an ileostomy or urostomy.

Patient Education

Teach the importance of ongoing follow-up care. For terminal patients, many issues must be addressed and discussed in order to give patients and their caretakers an improved quality of life. Some of these are fear and anxiety, grieving, anticipation, self-image issues (including loss of hair), nausea and vomiting, weight loss, anorexia, impotence, sterility, pain, fatigue, loss of job, loss of family member, and potential for infection. Ileostomy/urostomy teaching is indicated for patients whose bladders have been surgically removed. Preventive measures include not smoking and avoidance of other chemical carcinogens.

Acute Renal Failure

Acute renal failure (ARF) is the sudden and rapid deterioration of renal function, resulting in an accumulation of nitrogenous wastes. The terms acute renal failure and acute renal insufficiency are most often used interchangeably; however, some authorities believe acute renal failure should be reserved to describe only those cases requiring hemodialysis during acute treatment. The time course of ARF reflects

Treatment Standards/Guidelines 11.1 Bladder Tumors

Type	Stage	Treatment Options	Characteristics
Superficial	**Stage I** Mucosal (O) Submucosal (A) Careinoma in situ (OIS)	Endoscopic or laser resection intravesical immunotherapy OR intravesical chemotherapy	Recurrence is common; follow up every 6 months
Invasive	**Stage II** Bladder muscularis (B)	Simple or radical cystectomy, radiation, chemotherapy	Survival rate 65 to 75% after 5 years
	Stage III Periovesical fat (C)	Same as stage II	Survival rate 30 to 65% after 5 years
Metastatic	**Stage IV** Lymph node (D1) Bone or viscera (D2)	Treatment is palliative only Systemic chemotherapy and/or radical cystectomy or external beam radiation therapy	Survival rate 10 to 15% after 5 years

a process that has developed over days to weeks that is often completely reversible, while chronic renal failure (see next section) typically develops over months to years and is almost never fully reversible.

The most common causes of ARF are associated with intrarenal injury caused by renal hypoperfusion or nephrotoxins. The signs and symptoms vary with each patient and can range from mild azotemia to uremia. Persons with ARF usually do not experience the profound neurologic and musculoskeletal disorders seen in patients with chronic renal failure (CRF). Although recovery from ARF may be rapid and complete, this disorder nonetheless has a high mortality rate, estimated at anywhere between 5 and 80 percent, depending on the patient's age, the cause of ARF, and the extent of multiorgan involvement.

Epidemiology and Causes

It is estimated that 5 percent of all hospitalized patients develop ARF; for patients in intensive care units (ICUs), the rate is as high as 15 percent. Two to 7 percent of all post–open heart surgery patients are estimated to develop ARF. Fifty percent of ARF that develops in hospitalized patients is considered iatrogenic. ARF affects all ages and both sexes.

Risk factors for ARF include surgery, especially for older patients or patients of any age with elevated creatinine levels. Community-based ARF occurs more frequently among vulnerable populations such as individuals with underlying renal disease, multiple myeloma, or diabetes. ARF is also one of the potential risks related to open-heart surgery and other cardiac procedures (e.g., cardiac catheterization) and use of IV contrast dyes. Any problem that causes decreased blood flow to the kidneys can lead to ARF: anaphylactic shock caused by drug or transfusion reactions, ingestion of nephrotoxic substances (aminoglycosides, angiotensin-converting enzyme [ACE] inhibitors in renal artery stenosis), malignancy, sepsis, cardiac problems, aneurysm, liver cirrhosis, trauma, dehydration, or shock.

The etiologies of ARF are classified into three major groups based on the anatomic nature of the lesion, which may be prerenal, intrarenal (or intrinsic renal), or postrenal. *Prerenal* is the name given to any condition that leads to an overall decrease in renal perfusion; etiologies in this group include hypovolemia, renovascular disease, decreased cardiac output, systemic vasodilation, renal vasoconstriction, and impairment of renal autoregulation of blood flow, which is often associated with drugs such as ACE inhibitors or NSAIDs. *Intrarenal* refers to disorders that affect the renal parenchyma itself, such as glomerulonephritis, acute tubular necrosis (often caused by ischemic insult or nephrotoxic drugs such as aminoglycosides), interstitial nephritis (often an allergic type of reaction to various drugs or transfusion reactions), and tubular obstruction. Immune-mediated phenomena may lead to ARF following acute bacterial infection, for example, thrombotic thrombocytopenic purpura (TTP), hemolytic uremic syndrome (HUS) following *Escherichia coli* gastroenteritis. *Postrenal* refers to any etiology that might lead to an obstruction of flow of urine from the kidneys, including ureteral obstruction, bladder neck obstruction, or urethral obstruction. Major causes include benign prostatic hyperplasia/hypertrophy (BPH), prostate or bladder cancer, and metastatic disease affecting the urinary tract. An important consideration in the male patient with preexisting BPH is the use of OTC sympathomimetic decongestants and other cold remedies, the alpha-agonist properties of which may lead to acute worsening of prostatic hypertrophy with resultant anuria.

Table 11.10 presents the major causes of ARF. Complications commonly seen as a result of ARF include intravascular volume overload, metabolic acidosis, anemia, hyperkalemia, and uremic syndrome which is characterized by nausea, vomiting, anorexia, pericarditis, and both central and peripheral nervous system abnormalities including altered mental status, seizures, or coma. *Prerenal*, *intrarenal*, and *postrenal* mechanisms of ARF are not mutually exclusive, however, and many patients present with a combination of these pathologies.

Pathophysiology

Prerenal Azotemia

Prerenal azotemia is caused by decreased blood flow to the kidneys, usually associated with poor systemic perfusion. Etiologies includes hypovolemia, altered peripheral vascular

Table 11.10 Major Causes of Acute Renal Failure

Prerenal Acute Renal Failure
Fluid and electrolyte depletion
Hemorrhage
Septicemia
Cardiac failure
Liver failure
Heat stroke
Burns
Intrarenal Acute Renal Failure
Ischemia
Toxins
Radiocontrast agents
Hemoglobinuria
Myoglobinuria
Acute GN
Arterial or venous obstruction
Tubulointerstitial nephritis
Pyelonephritis
Papillary necrosis
Precipitation from hypercalcemia
Urates
Myeloma protein
Postrenal Acute Renal Failure
Prostatism
Bladder tumor
Pelvic tumor
Retroperitoneal tumor
Renal calculi

resistance, diminished cardiac output, CHF, renal artery disorders such as vasculitis and to a lesser extent thromboembolic disease as well as chronic liver diseases such as cirrhosis and the hepatorenal syndrome.

The kidney's compensatory mechanisms to hypoperfusion are autoregulation and activation of the renin–angiotensin–aldosterone axis via the release of renin. In the face of damage to select renal tissue, these mechanisms attempt to shunt blood to undamaged nephrons in a process called adaptive hyperfiltration. Autoregulation depends on the body's ability to control afferent arteriole dilation and efferent arteriole constriction in order to maintain normal glomerular filtration rate (GFR), creatinine clearance. The release of renin activates the proenzyme angiotensinogen to the biologically inactive angiotensin I. In turn, angiotensin converting enzyme (ACE) converts angiotensin I into angiotensin II, one of the most potent vasoconstricting agents in the body. Its production results in peripheral vasoconstriction and increased sodium reabsorption via increased aldosterone production. Antidiuretic hormone (ADH) is released in response to the increased plasma sodium concentration. ADH further enhances vasoconstriction and increases water reabsorption, thereby decreasing urinary output and increasing blood volume.

These mechanisms attempt to maintain systemic and renal perfusion. However, if the adaptive mechanisms of the kidneys fail, ARF develops because of hypoperfusion. As a result, glomerular filtration and the excretion of urea decrease, along with increased sodium and water reabsorption, resulting in an overall increase in BUN. Thus, while adaptive hyperfiltration is initially beneficial, allowing normal serum creatinine to be maintained in the face of mild renal insufficiency, prolonged activation of this compensatory mechanism leads to progressive renal failure.

Intrarenal (Parenchymal) Azotemia

Intrarenal azotemia results from injury to renal tissue; it is usually associated with intrarenal ischemia, toxins, or both. This condition, called *acute tubular necrosis* (ATN), is the most common cause of intrarenal azotemia and acute renal failure in general.

In ischemic ATN, the ischemic event refers to prolonged hypoperfusion and ischemia of the kidneys, with a sustained mean arterial pressure (MAP) in adults of less than 75 mm Hg. When renal autoregulation fails, the sympathetic nervous system (SNS) responds by initiating the renin–angiotensin system as the kidney attempts to redirect blood flow to the remaining healthy neurons in a process called adaptive hyperfiltration, as explained above. Again, however, this initially compensatory mechanism can eventually lead to progressive renal failure, as the SNS response and possibly endothelin production may lead to severe afferent renal arteriole constriction. As a result, overall glomerular hydrostatic pressure, glomerular blood flow, and GFR are decreased.

The length of the ischemic episode determines the amount and degree of renal cellular damage, which may continue after MAP and renal reperfusion are restored. Studies in animal models have demonstrated a number of immunologic mechanisms contribute to renal tubular injury, most notably early complement activation, intracellular adhesion molecule-1 (ICAM-1) expression, which may promote neutrophilic damage to the endothelium, T-cell-mediated cytotoxicity, macrophage activation, and pro-inflammatory cytokine expression (e.g., tumor necrosis factor-α [TNF-α], IL-6, IL-7, various chemokines).

Renal blood flow can be reduced by 50 percent after an ischemic episode; this is termed *no-reflow phenomenon.* The kidneys are unable to synthesize vasodilating prostaglandins, which usually exacerbates the ischemic injury. Blood flow is redistributed from the cortex to the medulla as a result of SNS stimulation and angiotensin II production. This further decreases glomerular capillary flow and worsens tubular ischemia, because these structures are located primarily in the cortex.

With renal ischemia, the availability of nutrients and oxygen for basic cellular metabolism and the tubular transport system is diminished. There is a significant decrease in the production of adenosine triphosphate (ATP) by the mitochondria, and, with insufficient oxygen and ATP, metabolism shifts from aerobic to anaerobic. This shift corresponds with extracellular and intracellular acidosis that alters kidney function. Ischemia also causes a decrease in renal cellular potassium, magnesium, and inorganic phosphates, and an increase in intracellular sodium, chloride, calcium, and reactive oxygen species. Sodium and calcium exchange is abnormal because of low ATP, altered Ca-ATPase activity, and increased intracellular sodium. This results in an increase in cellular calcium, which seems to increase cell injury. The formation of oxygen-free radicals further exacerbates cellular damage and apoptosis (programmed cell death) during reperfusion after a prolonged renal ischemic event, an event termed "reperfusion injury."

The basement membrane is altered by tubular cellular edema and becomes necrotic because of prolonged tubular ischemia. Tubular obstruction occurs from sloughed necrotic cells and cast formation, which seems to be facilitated by a translocation of basement membrane cellular adhesions proteins called integrins to the luminal membrane. Tubular hydrostatic pressure and Bowman's capsule hydrostatic pressure, which opposes the glomerular hydrostatic pressure, increase as a result of tubular obstruction. This decreases GFR. Injury to the basement membrane increases tubular permeability, allowing tubular filtrate to leak back into the interstitium and peritubular capillaries, further decreasing tubular filtration.

Ischemic ATN is usually associated with oliguria (less than 500 mL/day in adults) because of extensive nephronal injury. Other clinical indications of ATN include decreased urea excretion and elevated BUN, decreased creatinine clearance and elevated serum creatinine, abnormal renal handling of sodium, and an inability to concentrate urine. Urinary osmolality may approximate plasma osmolality of 300 to 350 mOsm/L, a condition called *isosthenuria.*

Toxic ATN involves exposure to toxic by-products of microorganisms or to nephrotoxic agents. Renal toxic drugs often cause allergic interstitial nephritis, characterized by eosinophilic damage. Toxic ATN begins with an event that causes injury to tubular cells. Subsequent pathophysiology is similar to that of ischemic ATN because there is tubular cell necrosis, cast formation, tubular obstruction, and altered GFR. Unlike in ischemic ATN, the basement membrane is usually intact, however, and the injured necrotic areas are more localized. Other differences are nonoliguria, which occurs more often with toxic ATN than with ischemic ATN, as well as the extent of injury with toxic ATN, which may be less than with ischemic ATN. The healing process, therefore, can be more rapid in patients with toxic ATN.

There are several reasons why the kidney is so susceptible to toxic damage. Blood continuously circulates through the kidney, repeatedly exposing the kidney to all components in the blood. Also, the kidney is the major excretory organ for toxic substances, and, as these substances await transport within renal cells, they disrupt cellular function. If liver disease is present, substances that are usually detoxified by the liver can overload the kidney. The kidney also transforms many substances into metabolites that can be toxic to the kidney, while the countercurrent mechanism concentrates bodily substances as well as other substances that, in increased concentrations, can be toxic to the kidney.

Postrenal Azotemia

Bilateral (ureteral) or distal (bladder outlet or urethral) postrenal obstruction impedes urine flow and results in oliguria or frank anuria. Urine congestion increases pressure retrograde through the collecting system and nephron and slows the tubular fluid flow rate and GFR. There is increased reabsorption of sodium, water, and urea, which results in decreased urine sodium, increased urine osmolality, and increased BUN. The decreased GFR results in a decreased creatinine clearance and, therefore, in an increased serum creatinine level. If the postrenal obstruction is prolonged, the collecting system dilates and compresses parenchymal tissue. The nephron is injured, which results in dysfunction of the concentrating and diluting mechanism, causing the urine osmolality and sodium level to be similar to those of plasma. If the postrenal obstruction is temporary, there is little dilation of the collecting system and loss of renal tissue.

Clinical Presentation

Subjective

Symptoms of ARF are not usually present until the GFR falls to approximately 10 to 15 percent of normal. The symptoms reported are usually secondary to the accumulation of toxic metabolites such as urea, including fatigue, malaise, nausea, vomiting, pruritus, and mental status changes. Of note, the development of uremic syndrome symptoms bears no direct correlation to increases in BUN or serum creatinine, despite the critical role of hemodialysis in clearing the body of as yet unidentified uremic toxins. Oliguria or even anuria may also be a presenting symptom of ARF but is not present in every case; urine output depends largely on the stage of ARF as well as the precipitating cause. In some cases, fluid overload may be present, resulting in dyspnea and orthopnea.

A detailed history can give clues to the etiology of ATP. The patient should be questioned about history of drug use, surgery, trauma, or infection, as possible sources of renal insult. However, the actual diagnosis of ARF is often made by routine laboratory assessment.

There are multiple signs and symptoms of ARF and four identified stages: initiating, oliguric, diuretic, and recovery. The *initiating stage* begins when the kidney is injured; this stage is variable in length, from minutes to several days (e.g., damage caused by contrast dye is done within 2 minutes). Decreased urine volume and other signs and symptoms of renal impairment may then become evident. These may include anorexia, lethargy, nausea, headache, muscle cramps, and fatigue. The cause of ARF must be determined and the plan of treatment should be established, in consultation with a nephrologist.

The *oliguric stage* usually lasts from 5 to 15 days but can persist for weeks, depending on the nature of renal damage. Renal repair begins as tubular cells regenerate. Destroyed basement membrane is replaced with fibrous scar tissue, and nephrons become obstructed with inflammatory products. Decreases in glomerular filtration, tubular transport of substances, urine formation, and renal clearance occur. When ARF persists for weeks or longer, renal endocrine functions are altered such as a decrease in the secretion of erythropoietin. The longer this stage persists, the poorer the prognosis.

The next phase is the *diuretic stage*, defined as beginning when urine output is greater than 400 mL per day, and when the BUN begins to fall. It is considered to last until the BUN is stabilized or is in the normal stage.

The fourth and final stage, referred to as the *convalescent phase*, extends from the time the BUN is stable and the urine output normal to the day the patient returns to normal activity. The entire process may take 10 months and some patients never recover but instead progress to CRF.

Objective

The objective manifestations of ARF depend on the stage of the disorder and may be extremely variable; however, these signs can provide an assessment of the degree of renal failure and provide clues as to the underlying etiology. Orthostatic vital signs, skin turgor, and distension of jugular veins should be assessed to obtain information on the patient's fluid balance. Signs of fluid depletion can point to a prerenal etiology, whereas signs of fluid overload suggest a greater degree of renal impairment. Severe proteinuria may lead to generalized edema (anasarca) due to the lack of intravascular oncotic pressure from hypoalbuminemia. Abdominal bruits can suggest renovascular disease. In cases of polycystic kidney disease or hydronephrosis, the kidneys may be palpable. A pelvic or renal exam may reveal causes of outflow obstruction such as an enlarged prostate or pelvic mass.

Diagnostic Reasoning

Diagnostic Tests

Elevated BUN and serum creatinine levels assist in establishing the diagnosis of ARF. GFR is difficult to measure directly, and is most commonly estimated using a simplified formula for creatinine clearance (see Diagnostic Tests section under Chronic Renal Failure for complete discussion). However, as acute trends are most important in the diagnosis and follow-up of ARF, direct serum creatinine levels are often used as an estimate of renal function. However, it is critical to remember that these absolute values are heavily influenced by a patient's muscle mass, age, gender, as well as the presence of any underlying renal disease. As such, serum creatinine levels may over- or underestimate renal function in certain populations (e.g., elderly or obese patients).

Serum electrolyte levels (sodium, potassium, chloride, bicarbonate, calcium, phosphate) should also be monitored for potentially life-threatening abnormalities that may develop secondary to impaired renal function. The presence of RBCs, either alone or as casts, may suggest a vascular or glomerular lesion, whereas WBCs and white cell casts are seen in interstitial nephritis and cases associated with infection. Eosinophiluria, in particular, is characteristic of allergic interstitial nephritis (AIN) due to renal toxic drugs. "Muddy-brown" granular casts and epithelial cell casts are strongly associated with ATN but are not considered very specific. Moreover, their absence does not exclude intrinsic renal disease.

Urinary sodium tends to be less than 20 mEq/L in prerenal disease, whereas the kidneys "leak" or "spill" sodium by failing to reabsorb this electrolyte in ATN, resulting in urinary sodium values typically greater than 40 mEq/L. However, variations in water reabsorption also affect urinary sodium concentration. Thus, the fractional excretion of sodium (FENA), which is defined as 100 percent times (urine sodium/serum sodium) divided by (urine creatinine/serum creatinine), is more helpful in distinguishing prerenal azotemia from ATN. The FENA is generally less than 1 percent in prerenal disease related to hypoperfusion, because the kidneys try to preserve intravascular volume by maximally conserving sodium. A FENA of greater than 2 percent reflects acute tubular necrosis, but values between 1 and 2 percent are considered inconclusive. Of note, FENA has little or no predictive value in the presence of diuretic therapy, as natriuresis is a mechanistic outcome of both thiazide and loop diuretics. Thus, increased urinary sodium may not exclude a prerenal etiology nor implicate ATN. In addition, FENA is less helpful when ATN is superimposed upon a chronic intravascularly depleted state, such as in hypoalbuminemic cirrhotic liver disease.

ATN is also characterized by an inability to concentrate urine; thus, urine osmolality is typically lower than 450 mOsm/L and in many cases lower than 350 mOsm/L. In contrast, the urine is highly concentrated in prerenal azotemia due to the secretion of ADH and intensified water reabsorption, producing urine osmolalities greater than 500 mOsm/L. As renal tubular function worsens under prerenal conditions, however, this distinction tends to blur, and concentrating ability may wane as ischemic damage sets in.

If a glomerular process is suspected, measurement of anti-nuclear antibody (ANA), anti-neutrophil cytoplasmic antibody (ANCA—seen in Wegener's granulomatosis), antiglomerular basement membrane (anti-GBM) antibodies, complement levels, and cryoglobulins can help the clinician determine whether immune-mediated disease is present.

A 24-hour urine test is the best way to measure proteinuria. A protein loss of more than 3.0 to 3.5 grams every 24 hours indicates a glomerular lesion, whereas lesser amounts in the urine are more indicative of an interstitial disorder.

Renal ultrasound is commonly used to assess kidney size and rule out hydronephrosis. Ultrasound is used instead of IVP to avoid the risk of radiocontrast nephrotoxicity. If hydronephrosis indicative of obstruction is detected, the patient should be referred to a urologist. CT scan, retrograde pyelogram, and cystoscopy may all be useful in determining the exact location of the obstruction. Renal scan may be helpful in detecting unilateral renal artery stenosis but is less sensitive in detecting bilateral renal artery disease. Renal artery stenosis is better diagnosed via CT scan or MRI/MRA, although direct renal angiography is still considered the, albeit invasive, gold standard for diagnosis.

If the noninvasive workup proves inconclusive, renal biopsy may be indicated in some cases. Most notably, biopsy is performed in cases of isolated glomerular hematuria with proteinuria to confirm acute nephritic syndrome, to better characterize nephrotic syndrome or suspected vasculitis, and to aid in the diagnosis of acute or subacute renal failure of unknown etiology. Percutaneous versus open biopsy techniques are chosen based on the propensity for bleeding diatheses and the difficulty in reaching the affected kidney as determined by renal imaging.

Differential Diagnosis

The main diagnostic challenge in ARF is to determine the underlying cause. This is often complicated by fluid and electrolyte alterations. A thorough assessment of the patient involves taking a thorough history, physically assessing the patient, and ordering appropriate laboratory studies. When determining whether or not prerenal azotemia exists, the patient's history can provide information indicating poor renal and/or systemic perfusion. This information may include surgery, high fever, alterations in diet or fluid status such as a patient made NPO and given bowel preparation repeatedly for diagnostic tests, or a low-sodium diet with fluid restriction, use of diuretics and antihypertensives, anaphylactic drug or transfusion reaction, penetrating or nonpenetrating abdominal trauma, hemorrhage, burns, shock, excessive sweating and dehydration, peritonitis, malignancies, sepsis, neurogenic shock, drug overdose, acute myocardial infarction, CHF, cardiac tamponade, cardiac dysrhythmias, cardiac arrest survival, renal artery emboli, thrombi, stenosis, aneurysm, occlusion, trauma, and liver cirrhosis.

Physical assessment findings may vary depending on the etiology of ARF and need to be correlated with the patient's history and laboratory findings, such as fluid volume depletion or oliguria. Findings on physical exam consistent with a prerenal etiology may include dry mucous membranes, poor skin turgor, reduced jugular venous pressure, hypotension, oliguria, or weight loss. Significant laboratory findings are increased urine osmolality and specific gravity, decreased urine sodium and urea, increased BUN, increased BUN to plasma creatinine ratio (a ratio greater than 20:1 because plasma creatinine is usually normal), normal urinary sediment (in most cases), and oliguria.

Prolonged azotemia caused by prerenal condition often leads to intrarenal failure. Nephrotoxic agents that may cause damage to the kidneys are drugs such as antineoplastics, anesthetics, antimicrobials, and anti-inflammatory agents; x-ray contrast media; biologic substances (e.g., toxins, tumor products, and heme pigments from hemoglobin or myoglobin); environmental agents (e.g., pesticides and organic solvents); heavy metals (e.g., lead, mercury, and gold); and plant and animal substances (e.g., toxic mushrooms and snake venoms).

Other factors that may injure renal (parenchymal) tissue include inflammatory processes related to bacterial or viral infection and toxemia of pregnancy; immune processes, such as autoimmunity, hypersensitivity, and tissue or organ transplant rejection; trauma or radiation to the kidney; and obstruction (e.g., neoplasm, stones, and scar tissue). Intravascular hemolysis related to transfusion reaction and microangiopathic hemolytic anemia as seen in TTP and HUS also causes damage to renal tissue. In addition, systemic and vascular disorders, such as renal vein thrombosis, nephrotic syndrome, Wilson's disease, malaria, multiple myeloma (direct proteinaceous deposition of immunoglobulin light chains into the renal parenchyma), sickle cell disease, malignant hypertension, diabetes mellitus, and systemic lupus erythematosus, and all cause intrarenal injury. Pregnancy-related disorders, such as septic abortion, preeclampsia, abruptio placentae, intrauterine fetal death, and idiopathic postpartum renal failure can also cause damage to the kidneys.

Data that identify an event, a series of events, an agent, or agents that may have caused renal injury, especially those related to ischemia or exposure to toxins should be collected during the history. These may include nephrotoxins; radiologic tests that require administration of a dye; hypersensitivity reaction to a drug or dye; recent infections, trauma, or sepsis; antineoplastics, with or without radiation therapy; multiple myeloma or pregnancy; and a history of cardiac, renal, or liver disease.

There is no one specific finding that pinpoints intrarenal azotemia during physical assessment. Findings on exam must be correlated with history and laboratory findings. Differentiating prerenal problems and actual ATN is a challenge. Because prerenal problems often correspond with the onset phase of ATN and because this is a reversible phase, it is essential for diagnosis and aggressive management to begin early. Laboratory plasma values, urinalysis, and microscopic examination of the urine provide important data that can help to differentiate prerenal azotemia from ATN.

Prerenal problems are indicated by high urinary specific gravity and osmolality, low urinary sodium caused by decreased renal blood flow, avid tubular sodium reabsorption, and decreased GFR. The kidneys interpret this as a state of dehydration and respond with aldosterone and ADH to maximize sodium and water reabsorption from the distal tubule and collecting duct into the peritubular capillary plasma. This results in a small amount of very concentrated urine with high specific gravity and high osmolality. Despite maximal sodium reabsorption, urine is concentrated because of urea or other solutes. Urinary and plasma creatinine levels often show wide variation in prerenal problems, with a slower rate of rise than in ATN and periodic decreases in serum creatinine.

ATN is characterized by altered renal ability to conserve sodium; clinically, ATN is seen as a urinary sodium level greater than 20 mEq/L. Laboratory serum sodium levels vary in ATN, depending on the state of hydration. Oliguria is usually associated with postischemic ATN, whereas either oliguria or nonoliguria may be associated with nephrotoxic ATN. Creatinine clearance is severely decreased and plasma creatinine rises about 0.5 to 1 mg/dL per day in ATN. BUN to serum creatinine ratio does not typically exceed 10 to 15 to 1 in ATN.

Response to therapy is another factor that distinguishes ATN from prerenal problems. The kidneys typically respond very quickly to therapy aimed at correcting an underlying prerenal problem in which no actual nephron damage has occurred; however, in ATN, response to treatment of the underlying cause may be minimal depending on the degree of *nephron damage*. Additional therapy for ATN should be aimed at correcting alterations related to inability of the kidneys to maintain their functions.

Postrenal azotemia results from interference with the flow of urine from the kidneys and is associated with obstruction or disruption of the urinary tract. Ureteral, bladder, bladder neck, or urethral obstruction may be the result of calculi, urinary tract or bladder neoplasms, or sloughed papillary tissue; strictures, trauma, or blood clots; congenital or developmental abnormalities; foreign objects or surgical ligation; prostatic hypertrophy; retroperitoneal fibrosis; abdominal and pelvic neoplasms; pregnancy; neurogenic bladder; bladder rupture; or use of drugs such as antihistamines and ganglionic blocking agents. History should focus on collecting data that indicate obstruction or disruption of the urinary tract. Significant findings include change in urine volume, history of prostatic disease or abdominal neoplasms, history of urinary tract stones or nephralgia, pregnancy, recent abdominal surgery, and paralysis (e.g., quadriplegia).

Postrenal azotemia physical assessment findings also vary with etiology and need to be correlated with laboratory and history findings (e.g., nephralgia associated with moving urinary tract stones or rapidly developing hydronephrosis; or bladder distension associated with prostate, bladder neck, or urethral disorders). Laboratory findings include urine volume variations such as oliguria, polyuria, or abrupt anuria; urine osmolality variations (may be increased or similar to plasma osmolality); urine specific gravity variations; a decrease in urine sodium and urine urea; and a BUN to serum creatinine ratio that is normal to slightly increased. Microscopy of the urinary sediment is usually normal unless UTI is present.

Management

Approximately 50 percent of patients with ARF are nonoliguric and have less severe signs and symptoms than oliguric patients. Because frequent causes of death are cardiac arrest resulting from hyperkalemia, gastrointestinal bleeding, and infection, the patient should be monitored very closely and treated appropriately on a day-to-day basis. The main goal is to keep the patient alive and to determine the underlying cause of the renal failure. The etiology of ARF will determine long-term management strategies.

In many cases of ATN, which is often caused by nephrotoxic agents, the removal of the offending agent will allow renal function to return gradually to normal. In the meantime, supportive measures should be provided, often in the form of peritoneal or hemodialysis. Prerenal azotemia secondary to absolute hypovolemia necessitates the restoration of intravascular volume. Replacement of fluids depends on the mechanism of loss. Gastrointestinal fluid loss is generally hypotonic and should be replaced accordingly; fluid loss as a result of hemorrhage usually indicates the need for administration of both saline and RBCs. In addition, fluid and electrolytes must be managed. Hyperkalemia in ARF can be life-threatening; emergent management is required in patients with extreme elevation of potassium levels (more than 6.5 mmol/L) or in any patient with electrocardiogram abnormalities.

Certain diseases, such as glomerulonephritis or Wegener's granulomatosis, require immunosuppressive treatment with prednisone and cyclophosphamide to prevent irreversible renal damage. Postrenal azotemia involves identification of the level of obstruction followed by treatment to relieve the obstruction. If the obstruction is high, at the vesicoureteral junction or in the ureter or renal pelvis, percutaneous nephrotomy or ureteral stent placement by a urologist is necessary. For urethral obstruction, bladder catheterization or placement of a suprapubic tube may be sufficient to relieve the obstruction. Intermittent bladder catheterization 4 to 5 times a day poses less risk of UTI than an indwelling urinary catheter and is the preferred method for urinary outflow in cases of bladder atony and neuromuscular compromise such as with spinal cord injury. However, the presence of a bladder outlet or urethral obstruction, which is more likely to cause ARF, may necessitate placement of a long-term catheterization device until surgical intervention is possible.

In cases of intrarenal (intrinsic) failure, supportive methods are necessary while waiting for the kidneys to respond to reversal of the underlying problem. Several indications exist for temporary hemodialysis including, but not limited to, fluid overload unresponsive to diuretic therapy; hyperkalemia with symptoms or EKG changes; uremic encephalopathy; severe metabolic acidosis; cardiorespiratory failure; pleuritis, pericarditis, and other forms of inflammatory serositis. Forms of dialysis include traditional intermittent hemodialysis via large-bore venous and arterial catheters, peritoneal dialysis which operates by osmotic diffusion via an indwelling dialysate within the peritoneal cavity, and continuous renal replacement (CRRT), which is a prolonged form of low-flow arteriovenous or venovenous hemofiltration appropriate for hemodynamically unstable patients.

Follow-Up and Referral

After hospitalization, patient follow-up is necessary in about 1 week, then 1 month, 3 months, 6 months, and annually thereafter, providing there are no further complications. Blood chemistries, such as a basic metabolic profile as well as a CBC, should be checked at each follow-up visit. The patient should be assessed for signs and symptoms of fluid overload, such as crackles upon lung auscultation, elevated blood pressure (BP), shortness of breath, weight gain, jugular vein distension, and/or edema.

Patient Education

During the recovery stage there is no special form of treatment other than general healthy living. Lack of knowledge is a major problem with regard to acute episodes of renal failure. Patients require continual education throughout their clinical pathway and their treatment of ARF. Follow-up care, support, and prevention of another episode should be the teaching focus.

Chronic Renal Failure

Chronic renal failure (CRF) is characterized by a progressive loss of functioning nephrons, eventually leading to end-stage renal disease (ESRD). As the functional reserve of the kidneys is lost, signs and symptoms of renal failure appear. These signs may arise as sequelae of ARF, but most often CRF arises as a complication of chronic systemic disease, such as diabetes or hypertension. The time frame for the development of CRF is typically thought of as ranging from months to years, while ARF typically sets in over days to weeks (see previous section).

Epidemiology and Causes

According to the Third National Health and Nutrition Examination Survey (NHANES), a population-based representative study of the entire country, approximately 11 percent of the United States population suffers from CRF. The number of people with a chronic elevation of creatinine greater than 2.0 mg/dL is estimated to be 2.8 per 100,000. There are approximately 160,000 patients with ESRD on chronic dialysis in the United States, with about 42,000 new patients placed on dialysis each year. Older adults represent 33.8 percent of new patients. Diabetes mellitus and hypertension cause about 70 percent of ESRD. Compared to the general population, African Americans are 3.9 times more likely to have ESRD and 6.7 times more likely to have hypertensive ESRD. It is estimated that HIV-associated nephropathy may soon be the third leading cause of ESRD (after diabetes mellitus and hypertension) in African Americans ages 20 to 64. Men are 1.3 to 1.4 times more likely than women to have ESRD. The peak age for onset of ESRD is between ages 65 and 75. Geriatric patients have the highest incidence and morbidity and mortality rates, because renal disease can result from many age-related illnesses. Some older patients do tolerate dialysis quite well, however.

The major underlying conditions leading to ESRD are diabetes mellitus and primary hypertension (approximately 70 percent), glomerulonephritis, cystic diseases, and other urologic diseases (approximately 15 percent), and assorted other causes (approximately 15 percent). Renal artery stenosis and chronic ischemic renovascular disease may cause up to 20 percent of CRF cases in persons older than 50 years. Analgesic abuse (e.g., NSAIDs), cigarette smoking, collagen vascular disease, AIDS-related nephropathies (on the rise), cirrhosis, and multiple myeloma are examples of other risk factors for the development of CRF. Several hereditary renal diseases (e.g., polycystic kidney disease and Alport syndrome, which also causes congenital deafness) can lead to CRF in children and some adults.

Hypertension is present in at least 85 percent of patients with CRF. Hypertensive- and diabetic-related CRF is a form of microvascular end-organ damage caused by these cardiovascular risk factors. Thus, these patients must also be evaluated for other forms of end-organ damage related to atherosclerotic disease, as a significant correlation exists between microvascular CRF, peripheral vascular disease, coronary artery disease, and cerebrovascular disease.

Pathophysiology

The pathophysiology of renal failure is manifested somewhat differently depending on the underlying cause, although the end result is the same—a nonfunctional kidney. Diabetic nephropathy is the most common cause of ESRD and involves several mechanisms, including hyperglycemia, hormonal imbalances, and renal hemodynamic changes. Hyperglycemia leads to alterations in tubuloglomerular feedback, abnormalities in polyol (e.g., sorbitol) metabolism, and the formation of advanced glycosylation end products (AGEs) in tissues. Increase in circulating AGE peptides parallel the severity of renal dysfunction in diabetic nephropathy. Ultimately, defects in glomerular cellular metabolism lead to hemodynamic changes in the kidney.

Hormonal imbalances associated with diabetes and ESRD include decreased insulin, increased growth hormone and glucagon, and altered concentrations of or responsiveness to vasoactive hormones (angiotensin II, catecholamines, prostaglandins). Growth hormones and glucagons (both elevated in poorly controlled diabetes) have been shown to produce glomerular hyperfiltration in the laboratory in recent studies.

Renal hemodynamic changes implicated in diabetes and ESRD involve glomerular hypertension and glomerular hyperfiltration. Changes in circulating levels of vasoactive hormones, or altered responsiveness to them, can result in hyperfiltration. Regardless of the inciting event, factors such as hyperglycemia-induced increases in extracellular fluid volume, renal hypertrophy, and/or altered glycoregulatory or vasoregulatory hormone action, contribute to increased pressure and flow across the glomerular membrane, resulting in glomerular hypertension. This, in turn, along with associated renal vasodilation and hyperfiltration, increases transglomerular protein filtration. This leads to proteinuria and mesangial deposition of circulating proteins. As a result, mesangial expansion and glomerulosclerosis cause destruction of nephrons and the glomerulus becomes a fibrinous scar that can no longer function. In addition, a positive feedback stimulus for compensatory hyperfiltration is initiated, with further increase in GFR and progressive renal injury. Ultimately, it is glomerular hypertension that mediates the progressive nephron destruction. Based on this glomerular hypertension–hyperfiltration hypothesis, therapies directed at lowering glomerular hypertension would protect the kidney from further progression of nephropathy.

Hypertensive nephropathy is the second most commonly occurring cause of renal failure. The kidney is one of the major organs injured by hypertension. The resultant disease is termed *nephrosclerosis.* Benign nephrosclerosis is associated with chronic, mild, or moderate hypertension in which renal insufficiency develops slowly. The renal arterial vessels become thickened while the lumens become narrowed, resulting in decreased renal flow and autoregulation. Renal tubular changes correlate with the degree of reduction in renal blood flow. Signs and symptoms vary with the severity of renal injury; they include proteinuria, nocturia, casts, and azotemia. Patients with benign nephrosclerosis are very susceptible to ARF when a situation occurs that decreases blood flow to the kidney. Treatment is focused on control of hypertension.

Malignant nephrosclerosis is associated with marked hypertension, headache, CHF, and blurred vision. Unlike the progression of benign nephrosclerosis, renal failure develops rapidly. Renal arterioles and glomerular capillaries become thickened and necrotic and tubules atrophy. Signs and symptoms are hematuria with red cell casts, proteinuria, and azotemia. Treatment includes immediate reduction of BP, which is necessary to prevent permanent renal loss and damage to other organs.

Renal artery stenosis occurs when the renal artery and the branches become thickened, stiff, and narrow because of atheromatous plaques (two-thirds of cases) or fibromuscular dysplasia (one-third of cases). As the body perceives the decreased blood flow (i.e., hypoperfusion) via the stenotic renal arteries as hypovolemia, the renin–angiotensin–aldosterone axis is activated, and mild to severe hypertension results from the retention of sodium and water. This condition becomes critical if both renal arteries are affected or if blood flow is compromised in patients with only a single solitary kidney, either congenitally or following live organ donation of the other kidney. Other signs include a bruit auscultated in the flank or mid-abdominal region over the affected renal artery and an elevated blood renin level from the ipsilateral renal vein. The incidence of fibromuscular dysplasia is higher in women than in men, especially from 20 to 40 years of age. The treatment required is angioplasty or surgical repair to stent or reconstruct the stenotic vessels, along with medical therapy consisting of antihypertensives and diuretics.

Glomerulonephritis (GN) is the third most common cause of renal failure. GN is an inflammatory process that primarily affects the glomerular capillaries. It is also a major cause of ESRD. Approximately 25 percent of GN cases result from non-immune mechanisms, whereas 60 to 75 percent stem from autoimmune mechanisms. Glomerular injury can be divided into two major categories based on pathology: *nephritis,* which is characterized by glomerular inflammation and/or necrosis, and *nephrosis,* which is characterized by abnormal permeability of the glomerular membrane. This allows macromolecules such as albumin to pass. These two forms of injury are not mutually exclusive. A single etiology can produce both forms of injury.

The immunologic injury that characterizes glomerulonephritis functions in several different ways. Antiglomerular basement membrane (anti-GBM) disease is a result of direct glomerular injury occurring as a result of inflammation triggered by antibodies directed against components of the glomerular basement membrane. Linear deposits of immunoglobulin are seen via immunofluorescence (IF) microscopy of renal tissue. IF also reveals granular immunoglobulin deposits. Part of the inflammatory response that occurs is secondary to the glomerular deposition of immune complexes, composed of antibody bound to a variety of circulating antigens. This is referred to as *immune complex disease.* Finally, pauci-immune ANCA disease is characterized by the presence of serum antibodies against the neutrophil cytoplasm that are associated with the multisystem disease. Minimal or no immunoglobulin is seen by IF, hence the name "pauci-immune." Nonetheless, the glomerular injury is still believed to be immune in nature.

The hallmark of nephrosis is increased permeability of the glomerular capillary wall to macromolecules, including serum proteins. Inflammatory changes are generally not seen but may be present. In classic forms of glomerulonephrosis, nephrotic syndrome develops, and various degrees of proteinuria may be present. In addition to hypertension, other characteristic findings include hypercholesterolemia with lipiduria and central edema from hypoalbuminemia due to albuminuria. In more than two-thirds of cases of glomerulonephrosis in adults, the cause is idiopathic; in the remainder, nephrosis is secondary to systemic disease such as diabetes, lupus, or amyloidosis.

Clinical Presentation

Subjective

Because of the significant functional reserve of the kidneys, symptoms do not generally appear until renal function (as measured by the GFR) declines to 10 to 15 percent of normal. At about 30 to 40 percent of normal GFR, biochemical evidence of renal failure may be apparent, but patients typically remain asymptomatic. Early prominent symptoms in renal failure include anorexia, lassitude, fatigability, and weakness.

The inability of the kidneys to perform their normal excretory, metabolic, and endocrine functions results in *uremia,* a complex syndrome that includes a variety of physiologic and clinical abnormalities. Dermatologic abnormalities may result in the patient complaining of pruritus and dry skin; gastrointestinal alterations may manifest themselves as complaints of anorexia, nausea, vomiting, and hiccupping. Neurologic complaints may include emotional lability or depression, insomnia, fatigue (especially on exertion), confusion, headache, seizures, and coma. There may be a urine odor to the breath and perspiration, complaints of shortness of breath, a metallic taste in the mouth, impotence, nocturia, and muscle cramps. The patient may present with foot drop, infection, bleeding, or gout. Often the patient is being treated for a major systemic disease such as diabetes. It is, therefore important to be alert to the potential for the onset of CRF.

Objective

The patient may appear pale, with a characteristic uremic frost appearance to the skin, or, conversely, hyperpigmentation may be apparent. There may be bruising and asterixis (i.e., hand-flapping upon hyperextension of the wrists with complete forward extension of the upper extremities). Peripheral neuropathy and altered mental status may be present, along with peripheral edema and ascites from severe proteinuria and the resulting hypoalbuminemia, as well as auscultatory crackles and a pericardial rub. There may be an elevated BP and a hard, rapid pulse. Some abnormalities are the result of the accumulation of toxic metabolites; others are caused by underproduction (e.g., of vitamin D and erythropoietin) or overproduction (e.g., renin) of biochemically active substances produced by the kidney.

Diagnostic Reasoning

Diagnostic Tests

If a patient has a condition known to predispose the individual to the development of CRF, especially if that patient is in a high-risk population, biochemical monitoring (BUN, creatinine, and creatinine clearance) should be done to detect renal failure before it becomes clinically apparent. Serum creatinine can track the progression of CRF; however, the GFR (normally about 140 to 180 L/day) can fall to 40 to 50 percent of normal with only small changes in serum creatinine levels. Accurate measurement of the GFR itself is based on experimental calculations of renal inulin clearance. Inulin is a polymer of fructose secreted from the blood exclusively via the renal glomeruli and displaying no tubular reabsorption. Measurement of inulin clearance, however, requires a complex assay too cumbersome for daily clinical use and tends to be reserved solely for research purposes.

Alternatively, GFR can be estimated using the Cockcroft-Gault formula for creatinine clearance: (140 minus age × lean body weight in kilograms) divided by (72 stable serum creatinine in mg/dL). This value is multiplied by 0.85 (i.e., reduced by 15 percent) for women. It is important to realize that trends in GFR (as estimated by creatinine clearance or serum creatinine levels) are far more important in assessing renal function and stability of CRF than are the absolute values of these indices. This is especially true of direct serum creatinine measurements, whose interpretation must take into account a patient's muscle mass, age, and gender. Thus, creatinine clearance is a far more informative diagnostic tool as a measure of renal function.

Although no universally agreed upon definition of chronic kidney disease exists, GFR and proteinuria are often used to stratify CRF patients by disease severity. The Third National Health and Nutrition Examination Survey defined stage 1 disease as persistent albuminuria with a normal GFR greater than 90 mL/min/1.73 m^2 of body surface area (BSA); stage 2 disease has persistent albuminuria with a GFR between 60 and 89 mL/min/1.73 m^2 of BSA; stage 3 disease is defined as a GFR between 30 and 59 mL/min/1.73 m^2 of BSA; stage 4 disease is defined as a GFR between 15 and 29 mL/min/1.73 m^2 of BSA; and stage 5 disease is ESRD, defined as a GFR less than 15 mL/min/1.73 m^2 of BSA. According to this study, the distribution of CRF in the United States is as follows: stage 1 = 3.3 percent, stage 2 = 3 percent, stage 3 = 4.3 percent, stage 4 = 0.2 percent, and stage 5 = 0.2 percent.

Routine monitoring of the CBC can detect anemia secondary to erythropoietin deficiency. Monitoring of urinalysis can detect increasing proteinuria. When renal function declines further, closer monitoring of routine laboratory tests to detect dangerous electrolyte imbalances (e.g., hyperkalemia) and acidosis is required.

Numerous laboratory alterations occur in patients who have developed ESRD. A CBC will usually reveal a normochromic, normocytic anemia; decreased hematocrit; increased bleeding time; capillary fragility; thrombocytopenia; and a decreased immune responsiveness. Blood chemistries typically reveal some of the following abnormalities: decreased active vitamin D; elevated ammonia, BUN and serum creatinine, uric acid, sulfate, potassium, phosphate, parathyroid hormone, and glucose levels, along with insulin resistance and a type IV hyperlipidemia. Urinalysis may reveal proteinuria (the greater the proteinuria, the quicker the progression of CRF) and coarse granular casts. Ketosis may artificially raise creatinine levels, and certain drugs (cimetidine, trimethoprim, cefazolin) may also alter diagnostic test results.

Twenty-four-hour urine studies (protein, creatinine clearance) may be done, although samples often are difficult to obtain in ambulatory patients and have been largely replaced by spot urine checks. Complement levels, ANA, serum and urine protein electrophoresis may all provide data as to the underlying pathophysiology of CRF

Renal ultrasound performed at least at baseline is indicated in all cases of CRF. Among other pathology, sonography may reveal decreased kidney size (less than 11 cm), polycystic kidney disease, or an obstructed ureter or bladder outlet with hydroureter and/or hydronephrosis. Renal CT scan/CT angiography or MRI/MRA may detect and localize harder to visualize structural abnormalities, renal parenchymal disease, or renal artery stenosis. Duplex Doppler ultrasonography to assess renal vascular flow has a high sensitivity and specificity for arterial stenosis if conducted by an experienced ultrasonographer, but renal angiography remains the diagnostic gold standard for this condition. However, unilaterally decreased kidney size on renal imaging is highly suggestive of vascular occlusive disease and may be quite helpful as a screening method. Renal biopsy is not utilized for CRF as much as for ARF, unless noninvasive modes of testing are unable to suggest a likely etiology.

Differential Diagnosis

The differential diagnosis of CRF is aimed at identifying the underlying etiology or etiologies of renal failure, as discussed earlier. Although the terms *chronic renal failure* and *chronic renal insufficiency* are often used interchangeably, some authorities reserve the use of CRF to imply a dialysis-dependent state, while CRI denotes an earlier form of the condition not yet requiring dialysis or kidney transplantation, but which may clearly progress to CRF. The signs and symptoms and diagnostic test results commonly seen in the three stages of CRF (decreased renal reserve, renal insufficiency, and ESRD) are presented in Table 11.11.

Table 11.11 Differentiating the Stages of Chronic Renal Failure

Stage	Renal Function	Signs and Symptoms
I. Decreased renal reserve	40%–75% of normal kidney function remains	Asymptomatic (normal BUN and serum creatinine)
II. Renal insufficiency	20%–49% of normal kidney function remains	Decreased: GFR, solute clearances, urine concentration, hormone secretion Increased: BUN, serum creatinine Mild azotemia polyuria Nocturia Anemia
III. End-stage renal disease	Less than 15% of normal kidney function remains	Markedly increased: BUN, serum creatinine Increased: serum phosphorus, serum potassium Decreased: serum calcium Anemia Metabolic acidosis Hyperuricemia Fluid overload Oliguria with urine osmolality similar to plasma osmolality Uremic syndrome

Management

General principles of CRF management include (1) the determination and control of underlying etiology, (2) monitoring changes in renal function, (3) conservative treatment of the physiologic effects of CRF, and (4) instituting more aggressive treatment (dialysis and/or renal transplantation) when appropriate in later stages of treatment-refractory disease. Glucose levels and hypertension must be strictly controlled in diabetic patients. For any patient with proteinuria of more than 1 g/day, the target BP is 125/75 mm Hg; for a patient with proteinuria of less than 1 g/day, the goal is a BP of 130/80 mm Hg. Given the importance of maintaining renal perfusion, systolic blood pressures lower than 110 mm Hg should be avoided. ACE inhibitors or the newer class of angiotensin II receptor blockers (ARBs) should be used for BP control in patients with diabetes mellitus given their renoprotective effects. If monotherapy with one of these agents is insufficient to control BP, a diuretic should be added, followed by a calcium channel blocker (diltiazem or verapamil) or a beta-blocker, as needed. If combination therapy using agents from these additional classes proves ineffective, an ACE inhibitor or ARB should be added (whichever class was not used initially).

Pharmacologic BP management is equally as important for the medical treatment of renal artery stenosis. However, ACE inhibitors and ARBs are usually avoided in patients with bilateral renal artery stenosis, as their vasodilatory effects on the efferent renal arterioles effectively decrease GFR in the presence of reduced afferent blood flow from stenotic renal arteries. In turn, this may precipitate potentially devastating acute on chronic renal failure. Percutaneous angioplasty or surgical revascularization with arterial stenting should be considered for patients with severe hypertension refractory to pharmacotherapy, recurrent episodes of flash pulmonary edema due to CRF-related fluid overload, and progressive renal insufficiency which fails to improve despite effective blood pressure control. Individuals with particularly severe CRF (serum creatinine greater than 4 mg/dL) or chronically atrophied kidneys (less than 7 cm) are unlikely to respond to such interventions, however. Revascularization is more likely to be effective in patients whose renal function rapidly declines, particularly after beginning ACE inhibitor or ARB therapy.

Dietary therapy is a cornerstone of conservative management of CRF. Restriction of fluid (limited to maintain a serum sodium concentration of 135 to 145 mEq/L) and sodium (especially if volume expanded) may decrease secondary hypertension or CHF, although volume depletion must be avoided given the potential for acute worsening due to renal hypoperfusion. Restricted protein intake is recommended (0.6 to 1.0 g/kg/day), although an adequate caloric intake (40 to 50 cal/kg/day) should be maintained, as malnutrition is a common complication of CRF. Consultation by a skilled nutritionist is recommended at the time of diagnosis and periodically as the disease progresses and the patient's nutritional needs change. Foods rich in essential amino acids are the most effectively utilized source of nitrogen. Restriction of dietary phosphate (800 mg/day) and potassium may be necessary because of reduced excretion and the potential for hyperphosphatemia and hyperkalemia. Strict dietary restrictions may be unnecessary in older patients because they often have low protein and sodium intake, but treatment regimens must be individualized.

Low-dose Kayexalate (sodium polystyrene sulfonate) 5 mg PO qd to tid with meals may be used as a potassium binder for hyperkalemia. Oral phosphate binders such as calcium carbonate (2.5 to 20 g/day), calcium acetate

(Phos-Lo; 1334 mg tid), or sevelamer (Renagel; 800 mg tid) are typically taken with meals when GFR falls below 30 mL/min. Sevelamer is used when CRF is complicated by iatrogenic hypercalcemia. Aluminum- and magnesium-containing salts should be avoided, owing to cumulative toxicity.

Given the kidneys' reduced ability to synthesize activated vitamin D in CRF and the propensity for subsequent hypocalcemia and renal osteodystrophy, oral 1,25-dihydroxyvitamin D (calcitriol 0.25 mg qd) and calcium carbonate (600 mg bid) supplements should be given, along with a renal-specific multivitamin (Nephrocaps). Importantly, however, this chronic treatment may result in hypercalcemia and worsen coronary artery calcification. Thus, close monitoring of serum calcium levels is critical. Vitamin E may also be helpful in treating muscle cramps.

Anemia should be treated with erythropoietin (80 to 120 U/kg SC per week), taking care not to induce polycythemia (goal Hgb = 11 to 12 g/dL) with its attendant risk of stroke. Dosing usually begins around 10,000 U per week but may be adjusted upward in frequency or dose, as needed. Darbepoetin alfa is an alternative erythropoietic agent with a longer half-life, allowing for less frequent dosing (0.45 μg/kg SC per week). Patients with iron deficiency anemia should take ferrous sulfate 325 mg PO qd to tid with meals, with lower doses in elderly patients being less likely to induce constipation. Gentle transfusion with packed red blood cells may be required in cases of extreme or acutely worsened anemia, but care must be taken not to induce high-output heart failure or fluid overload, as the heart typically adapts to the chronic anemia of CRF. In relation to this, bleeding diatheses due to uremic platelet dysfunction are not uncommon in both ARF and CRF. Active bleeding in these patients should be treated with desmopressin (dDAVP), cryoprecipitate, estrogen, or dialysis to remove uremic toxins believed to be qualitatively inhibiting platelet function.

Hypercholesterolemia should be treated with a statin drug to an LDL goal of less than 100, as CRF is considered a coronary artery disease equivalent. Recent evidence suggests this goal should be even lower to minimize the rate of disease progression due to atherosclerotic renovascular disease. Dietary modification to restrict cholesterol and saturated fats is also critical to adequately address hyperlipidemia, especially hypertriglyceridemia.

Both hypovolemia (renal hypoperfusion) and renal toxic drugs may exacerbate CRF and must always be considered when acute on chronic renal failure is observed. A judicious trial of isotonic fluid repletion may be appropriate in patients displaying the physical stigmata of dehydration, while careful attention must be paid to the dosing of all chronic and newly started medications. All nephrotoxic agents (e.g., NSAIDs, radiocontrast dye) should be avoided.

Other measures to relieve symptoms include skin moisturizers for dry skin, while menthol or phenol lotion, a trial of capsaicin cream, or diphenhydramine (Benadryl) may all be useful in treating pruritus. It may be necessary to give diuretics for edema, but dehydration must be avoided. Thiazide diuretics may be tried first, but they are far less effective at a GFR less than 20 to 30 mL/min (approximated by serum creatinine levels of greater than 2.5 mg/dL); however, they do provide an additive effect when used with a loop diuretic initiated for refractory edema. Potassium-sparing diuretics should be avoided, owing to the kidneys' reduced ability to excrete potassium.

As CRF progresses, the patient will have increased difficulties with fluid balance and may experience episodes of hyperkalemia, hypertension, acidosis, and severe uremia with altered mental status and qualitative platelet dysfunction with a tendency for bleeding diatheses. Metabolic acidosis should be treated with sodium bicarbonate 600 mg bid initially to titrate serum bicarbonate to the 16 to 20 mEq/L range. However, patients must display adequate respiratory function to avoid the accumulation of metabolized carbon dioxide and respiratory acidosis. The potassium and calcium levels should be monitored during treatment of acidosis, because both might fall. Hospitalization may be required for control of fluid overload, hypertension, hyperkalemia, or infection.

A GFR less than 10 mL/min/1.73 m^2 of BSA, a serum creatinine level approaching 12 mg/dL, or BUN greater than 100 mg/dL all typically require more aggressive therapies to avoid life-threatening sequelae, including peritoneal or hemodialysis. Continuous venovenous or arteriovenous hemofiltration may be used in hemodynamically unstable patients, as an alternative to classic hemodialysis. Such therapies must be done only under the supervision of a nephrologist, however. Life-threatening indications for dialysis include pericarditis, diuretic-refractory fluid overload (e.g., pulmonary edema), medication-resistant or rapidly worsening hypertension, uremic syndrome with an attendant bleeding diathesis or neurologic symptomatology, and persistent nausea and vomiting. In addition, protein malnutrition in the face of a creatinine clearance of less than 20 mL/min is considered an indication for early dialysis.

Follow-Up and Referral

Patients with CRF should be referred to a nephrologist. The course of CRF is typically punctuated by periods of rapid deterioration, often precipitated by dehydration or infection. The rate of progression to kidney failure will depend in part on the underlying renal disease: It is usually more rapid in patients with diabetic nephropathy or severe hypertension and slower in patients with polycystic kidneys. In patients with advanced renal failure (creatinine levels greater than 10 mg/dL), however, mean survival time without intervention (e.g., dialysis or transplantation) is 100 to 150 days. Vascular access for hemodialysis (arteriovenous grafts or fistulae) must be obtained 2 to 3 months in advance to permit maturation of the fistulae and allow for potential revisions. Decisions regarding dialysis and transplantation

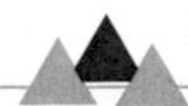

NURSING SITUATION 11.1

Giving Up Hope

Hope began her life as a juvenile diabetic. She became sick early in life, but did not let that stop her from having a rewarding career as a teacher. Her favorite hobby was painting—a talent that proved to strengthen her throughout her illnesses.

When I met Hope, she was 47 years old, her kidneys were no longer functioning, and she had lost one leg below the knee. She also had recently been diagnosed with breast cancer and had chosen to undergo chemotherapy. No longer able to work, she began to paint and continued to fight her illness. Each complication drained her body more. She endured peritoneal dialysis and then hemodialysis after a bout with peritonitis. Finally, her breast cancer metastisized to the peritoneal cavity.

Hope returned from hemodialysis early one day. It would be for the last time. Her sixth dialysis shunt was no longer patent. I then realized why I had been drawn to Hope. She no longer needed medicine or therapy; she needed someone to help her die.

I'll never forget that day. Hope looked at me through her tears and said, "I don't want to die." Not knowing exactly what to say, I looked in her eyes and told her it was time. Her life was in someone else's hands now, not hers. She didn't have any more decisions to make and she could try to find peace. Although her soul was strong, her body was not. By letting go, she wasn't giving up; she was saving herself.

I feel that we, as clinicians, touch life in the most profound way by giving certain patients permission to die. The true challenge lies in knowing when medicine is no longer what the patient needs.

SOURCE: Lisa Astalos Chism, L: An unforgettable case. The Clinical Advisor, February 1998, p 12.

require a team approach with the primary-care provider, nephrologist, patient, and family. Comprehensive evaluation of the patient's medical, psychological, and social situation is necessary for successful planning.

The patient may need to be hospitalized to control fluid overload, hypertension, hyperkalemia, or infection. In general, the multiplicity of metabolic demands on the patient with CRF will require careful and close follow-up and constant adjustments in treatment. The most important cornerstone of care is the monitoring and treatment of all underlying disorders known to lead to chronic renal failure. Successful therapy depends in good part on the maintenance of a strong relationship between the health-care provider and the patient and family. Nowhere is a Circle of Caring approach more important than in a chronic, progressive disorder such as CRF. Interventions should be geared toward minimizing the patient's dependence and social isolation. (See Nursing Situation 11.1.)

Patient Education

For care to be effective, the patient and family must have a good understanding of the chronic and progressive nature of CRF, of the importance of treating all underlying systemic diseases such as diabetes and hypertension, and of the specifics of the treatment plan. Avoidance of infection is important, as is maintaining a healthy diet as recommended. Patients should know when and how to report bleeding, fever, decreases in urine output, or episodes of nausea and vomiting.

Bibliography

General

Bagnis, CI, et al: Herbs and the kidney. Am J Kidney Dis 44(1):1–11, 2004.

Barker, LR, Burton, JR, and Zieve, PD: Principles of Ambulatory Medicine, ed 6. Lippincott Williams & Wilkins, Philadelphia, 2003.

Bascom, A: Incorporating Herbal Medicine into Clinical Practice. FA Davis, Philadelphia, 2002.

Brown, WW, et al: Early detection of kidney disease in community settings: The Kidney Early Evaluation Program (KEEP). Am J Kidney Dis 42(1):22–35, 2003.

Carcio, H: Urodynamic testing. Adv Nurse Pract 13(10):45–54, 2005.

Dambro, MR: Griffith's 5-Minute Clinical Consult. Lippincott Williams & Wilkins, Philaelphia, 2003.

Howell, AB, Vorsa, N, Der Marderosian, A, and Foo LY: Inhibition of the adherence of p-fimbriated *Escherichia coli* to uroepithelial-cell surfaces by proanthocyanidin extracts from cranberries. N Engl J Med 339(15): 1085–1086, 1998.

Kee, JL: Laboratory and Diagnostic Tests with Nursing Implications, ed 6. Prentice-Hall, Upper Saddle River, N.J., 2002.

Kontiokari, T, et al: Reandomised trial of cranberry-lingonberry juice and lactobacillus GG drink for the prevention of urinary tract infections in women. BMJ 322(7302):1571, 2001.

Lakkis, J, and Weir, MR: Pharmacological strategies for kidney function preservation: are there differences by ethnicity? Adv Renal Replace Ther 11(1):24–40, 2004.

Sampselle, C: Teaching women to use a voiding diary. AJN 103(11): 62–64, 2003.

Simmerville, JA, Maxted, WC, and Pahira, JJ: Urinalysis: a comprehensive review. Am Fam Phys 71(6):1153–1162, 2005.

Stoller, ML, and Carroll, PR: Urology. In Tierney, LM, et al (eds):

Current Medical Diagnosis and Treatment, ed 44. Lange/McGraw-Hill, New York, 2005, pp 629–678.
Tierney, LM, McPhee, SJ, and Papadakis, MA: Current Medical Diagnosis & Treatment. Lange/McGraw-Hill, New York, 2005.
Wallace, M, and Sadovsky, R: What clinicians should know about urinalysis. Clin Advisor 8(4):39–47, 2005.
Watnick, S, and Morrison, G: Kidney. In Tierney, LM, et al (eds): Current Medical Diagnosis and Treatment, ed 44. Lange/McGraw-Hill, New York, 2005, pp 867–901.
Braunwald, E, et al (eds): Harrison's Principles of Internal Medicine, ed 16. McGraw-Hill, New York, 2005.
Youngkin, E, et al: Pharmacotherapeutics: A Primary Care Guide, ed 2. Pearson/Prentice Hall, Upper Saddle River, N.J., 2005.

Acute Renal Failure

Cox, CD, and Tsilouris JP: Preventing contrast nephropathy: What is the best strategy? A review of the literature. J Clin Pharmacol 44(4):327–337, 2004.
Druml, W: Nutritional management of acute renal failure. J Renal Nutr 15(1):63–70, 2005.
du Cheyron, D: Atrial natriuretic peptide to prevent acute renal failure: Old concept with new promise. Crit Care Med 32(6):1421–1422, 2004.
Herget-Rosenthal, S: One step forward in the early detection of acute renal failure. Lancet 365(9466):1205–1206, 2005.
Kodner, CM, and Judrimoti, A: Diagnosis and management of acute interstitial nephritis. Am Fam Phys 67(12):2527–34, 2539, 2461–3 passim, 2003.
Liu, KD: Molecular mechanisms of recovery from acute renal failure. Crit Care Med 31(8) (Suppl):572–581, 2003.
Noble, DW: Acute renal failure and diuretics: Propensity, equipoise, and the need for a clinical trial. Crit Care Med 32(8):1794–1795, 2004.
Parikh, CR, et al: Urinary interleukin-18 is a marker of human acute tubular necrosis. Am J Kidney Dis 43(3):405–414, 2004.
Rabb, H: Novel urinary markers for early diagnosis of ARF. Am J Kidney Dis 42(3):599–600, 2003.
Schrier, RW, and Wang, W: Mechanisms of disease: Acute renal failure and sepsis. N Engl J Med 351(2):159–169, 2004.
Singri, N, Ahya, SN, and Levin, ML: Contemporary updates: Linking evidence and experience. Acute renal failure. JAMA 289(6):747–751, 2003.
Slawson, D: Are diuretics helpful for acute renal failure in critically ill patients? Evidence-Based Practice 6(3):7–8, 2003.
Uchino, S, et al: Diuretics and mortality in acute renal failure. Crit Care Med 32(8):1669–1677, 2004.
Weinmann, ME: Acute renal failure. Emerg Med Serv 32(12):7172, 2003.

Bladder Tumors

Beitz, JM, and Zuzelo, PR: The lived experience of having a neobladder. West J Nurs Res 25(3):294–321, 2003.
Cope, D: Vitamin E may reduce bladder cancer mortality. Clin J Oncol Nurs 75(5 Part 1):506, 2003.
Felknor, SA, et al: Bladder cancer screening program for a petrochemical cohort with potential exposure to beta-mapthylamine. J Occup Environ Med 45(3):289–294, 2003.
Gray, M, and Simms, TW: NMP-22 for bladder cancer screening and surveillance. Urol Nurs 24(3):171–172, 177–179, 186, 2004.
Harvard Health Watch: Bladder cancer in women: no time to wait. Havard Womens Health Watch 11(7):3–5, 2004.
MacVicar, GR, and Pienta, KJ: Current chemotherapy options: Valuating therapy for locally advanced or high-risk bladder cancer. Contemp Urol 16(11):14–21, 2004.
Moyer, P: Study: Absence of hematuria does not rule out bladder cancer. Oncol Times 26(19):62, 64, 2004.
Pashos, CL, et al: Bladder cancer: Epidemiology, diagnosis, and management. Cancer Pract 10(6):311–322, 2002.
Richard, E: Links: Dietary folate, genetic instability and bladder cancer risk. Positive Health June(89):8, 2003.
Schellhammer, PF, et al: Superficial bladder cancer: Insight and expertise. Contemp Urol May: (Suppl):3–24, 2004.
Schoenberg, M, and Grossman, HB: Point and counterpoint. Bladder cancer follow-up: Can urine biomarkers replace cystoscopy? Contemp Urol 17(2):21–22, 25–26, 28, 2005.
Sengupta, N, Siddiqui, E, and Mumtaz, FH: Cancers of the bladder. J Roy Soc Promot Health 124(5):228–229, 2004.
Stein, JP, and Resnick, MI: Contemporary issues and management of bladder cancer. Urol Clin North Am 32(2):121–246, 2005.
Williams-Cox, D: A mixed-method study into quality of life for bladder cancer patients. Prof Nurse 19(6):343–347, 2004.
Zietman, A, and Skinner, E: Quality of life after radical treatment for invasive bladder cancer. Semin Radiat Oncol 15(1):55–59, 2005.

Chronic Kidney Disease

Bernardi, A, et al: Factors affecting nutritional status, response to exercise, and progression of chronic rejection in kidney transplant recipients. J Renal Nutr 15(1):54–57, 2005.
Brewster, UC, and Perazella, MA: Early renal disease: Tips on recognition and prevention. Consultant 44(13):1613–1620, 2004.
Burrows-Hudson, S: Chronic kidney disease: An overview. AJN 105(2): 40–50, 2005.
Chen, J, et al: The metabolic syndrome and chronic kidney disease in U.S. adults. Ann Intern Med 140(3):167–174, 2004.
Coulston, AM: New name, old problem: Chronic kidney disease, formerly known as chronic renal failure. Nutr Today 39(3):139–142, 2004.
Cowley, BD Jr: Recent advances in understanding the pathogenesis of polycystic kidney disease: Therapeutic implications. Drugs 64(12): 1285–1294, 2004.
Eknoyan, G, et al: Proteinuria and other markers of chronic kidney disease: A position statement of the National Kidney Foundation (NKF) and the National Institute of Diabetes and Digestive and Kidney Diseases (NIDDK). Am J Kidney Dis 42(4):617–622, 2003.
Feest, T: Epidemiology and causes of chronic renal failure. Medicine (UK) 31(6):49–52, 85–86, 2003.
Holcomb, SS: Evaluating chronic kidney disease risk. Nurse Pract 30(4): 12–27, 2005.
Ideura, T, et al: Effect of nonsupplemented low-protein diet on very late stage CRF. Am J Kidney Dis 41(3) (Suppl 1):S31–34, 2003.
Iseki, K, et al: Significance of hyperuricemia as a risk factor for developing ESRD in a screened cohort. Am J Kidney Dis 44(4):642–650, 2004.
Jablonski, A: The illness trajectory of end-stage renal disease dialysis patients. Res Theory Nurs Pract 18(1):51–72, 2004.
Jaffery, JB, and Becker, BN: Evaluation of eHealth Web sites for patients with chronic kidney disease. Am J Kidney Dis 44(1):71–76, 2004.
Johnson, CA, et al: Clinical practice guidelines for chronic kidney disease in adults: Part II. Am Fam Phys 70(6):1091–1097, 2004.
Kasinskas, C, and Piazza, D: Chronic renal failure—a clinical pathway. Acute Care Perspect 13(3):1, 3–4, 2004.
Loghman-Adham, M: Medication noncompliance in patients with chronic disease: Issues in dialysis and renal transplantation. Am J Manage Care 9(2):155–171, 2003.
Loos, C, et al: Effect of end-stage renal disease on the quality of life of older patients. J Am Geriatr Soc 51(2):229–233, 2003.
Luk,WS: The HRQoL of renal transplant patient. J Clin Nurs 13(2):201–209, 2004.
Mitch, WE: Treating diabetic nephropathy—are there only economic issues? N Engl J Med 351(19):1934–1936, 2004.
Russell, CL, et al: Medication-taking beliefs of adult renal transplant recipients. Clin Nurse Specialist 17(4):200–210, 2003.
Singh, RB, et al: Randomized, double-blind, placebo-controlled trial of coenzyme Q10 in patients with end-stage renal failure. J Nutr Enviorn Med 13(1):13–22, 2003.
Snively, CS, and Gutierrez, C: Chronic kidney disease: Prevention and treatment of common complications. Am Fam Phys 70(10):1921–1928, 2004.
Tarver-Carr, ME, and Powe, NR: Chronic kidney disease: Principles for prevention and management in African Americans. Consultant 43(13): 1513–1524, 2003.
Vora, J: Diabetic nephropathy: Detection and treatment of renal disease in patients with diabetes. Adv Studies Med 4(10G):S1022–1029, S1032–1034, 2004.
Wasen, E, et al: Renal impairment associated with diabetes in the elderly. Diabetes Care 27(11):2648–2653, 2004.
Yu, HT: Progression of chronic renal failure. Arch Intern Med 163(12): 1417–1429, 2003.

Hematuria

American Academy of Family Physicians. Information from your family doctor: Microscopic hematuria. Am Fam Phys 71(1):135–136, 2005.

Baum, NH: Curbside consults: Hematuria from bicycling or running? Postgrad Med 114(2):62, 2003.

Baum, NH: Curbside consults: How to work up hematuria of unknown origin? Postgrad Med 118(1):4, 2005.

Bloom, TL, and Kolon, TF: Clinical challenge: Gross hematuria in a healthy adolescent: cystourethroscopy was key in diagnosing our young patient's multiple episodes of the painless, yet uncommon, condition. Clin Advisor 8(1):99–100, 2005.

Ruewster, UC, and Perazella, MA: Hematuria: Review questions. Hosp Phys 39(7):17–18, 2003.

Butler, M, and Noyes, DT: Advisor forum: Evaluating persistent hematuria. Clin Advisor 7(6):76, 2004.

Cohen, RA, and Brown, RS: Microscopic hematuria. N Engl J Med 348(23):2330–2338, 2371–2372, 2003.

Gleich, P: Hematuria: Is it from UTI or something more serious? Consultant 44(6):749–754, 2004.

Jones, W, and Murdock, CB: Hematuria: is it benign or cause for concern? Emerg Med 34(12):35–40, 2002.

Jonkers, IJ, Bruijn, JA, and Vleming, L: A case of minimal change disease evoling into steroid-dependent nephrotic syndrome with hematuria. Am J Kidney Dis 44(4):773–777, 2004.

Novak, K, and McLaughlin, K: 4 steps: Getting to the bottom of hematuria. Can J Diagn 21(9):101–107, 2004.

Slawson, D: Is computed tomography or urography preferred for evaluating microhematuria? Evidence-Based Pract 6(2):10–11, 2003.

Nephroliathiasis

Bennett S, Hoffman, N, and Monga, M: Ephedrine-and guaifenesin-induced nephrolithiasis. J Altern Comp Med 10(6):967–969, 2004.

Bhandari, A, and Menon, M: Nephrolithiasis: Reducing the risk of recurrence. Contemp Urol 15(2):36, 39–40, 42, 2003.

Daudon, M, and Jungers, P: Drug-induced renal calculi: Epidemiology, prevention and management. Drugs 64(3):245–275, 2004.

Moyad, MA: Complementary and preventive medicine. Calcium oxalate kidney stones: another reason to encourage moderate calcium intakes and other dietary changes. Urol Nurs 23(4):310–313, 2003.

Pathophysiology, diagnosis, and medical management of nephrolithiasis. Patient Care Nurse Pract Apr (2 p), 2004.

Ramey, SL, Franke, WD, and Shelly, MC II: Relationship among risk factors for nephrolithiasis, cardiovascular disease, and ethnicity: Focus on a law enforcement cohort. AAOHN J 52(3):116–121, 2004.

Safriel, Y, Malhotra, A, and Sclafani, SJ: Hematuria as an indicator for the presence of absence of urinary calculi. Am J Emerg Med 21(6):492–493, 2003.

Zarychta, WA: Case of the month...nephrolithiasis. J Am Acad Phys Assist 17(9):52, 2004.

Proteinuria

Boulware, LE, et al: Screening for proteinuria in US adults: A cost-effectiveness analysis. JAMA 290:3101–3114, 2003.

Daly, H: A campaign to raise awareness of microalbuminuria screening. Prof Nurse 19(5):275, 2004.

Donnelly, R, and Rea, R: Microalbuminuria: How informative and reliable are individual measurements? J Hypertens 21(7):1229 1233, 2003.

Eknoyan, G, et al: Proteinuria and other markers of chronic kidney disease: A position statement of the National Kidney Foundation (NKF) and the National Institute of Diabetes and Diagestive and Kidney Diseases (NIDDK). Am J Kidney Dis 42(4):617–622, 2003.

Harwell, TS, et al: Testing for microalbuminuria in 2002: Barriers to implementing current guidelines. Am J Kidney Dis 42(2):245–248, 2003.

Levene, LS, et al: What characteristics are associated with screening positive for microalbuminuria in patients with diabetes in the community? Pract Diabetes Int 21(8):287–292, 2004.

Matsui, J, et al: LDL particle size and lipid composition are risk factors for microalbuminuria in normotensive and normocholesterolemic patients with type 2 diabetes. Diabetes Res Clin Pract 66(3):229–236, 2004.

Segura, J, Ruilope, LM, and Zanchetti, A: On the importance of estimating renal function for cardiovascular risk assessment. J Hypertens 22(9):1635–1639, 2004.

Staples, B, et al: Land contamination and urinary abnormalities: Cause for concern? Occup Environ Med 60(7):463–467, 2003.

Wallace, M, and Sadovsky, R: What clinicians should know about urinalysis. Clin Advisor 8(4):39–47, 2005.

Renal Tumors

American Cancer Society: Cancer Facts and Figures, 1999. Author, Atlanta, Ga., 1999.

Coppin, C, et al: Immunotherapy for advanced renal cell cancer. The Cochrane Library no. 3, 2005.

Dale, DC, Federman, DD, and Levinson, W. What's new in medicine. Imaging studies for renal cancer. Clin Advisor 6(5):107–109, 2003.

Jazieh, AR, Kyasa, MJ, and Hutchins, L: Phase I clinical trial of tamoxifen and interferon alpha in the treatment of solid tumors. J Appl Res 4(3):464–469, 2004.

Middelton, L, and Lessick, M: Inherited urological malignant disorders: Nursing implications. Urol Nursing 23(1):15–30, 2003.

Quinn, DL: Clinical challenge: no relief from recurrent right flank pain. Clin Advisor 6(11):37–38, 2003.

Strauss, W, and Zimmerman, RW: Advisor forum: The latest on renal cancer. Clin Advisor 7(1):57, 2004.

Urinary Incontinence

Appell, RA: Overactive bladder: refining treatment strategies for different patient populations. Clin Advisor (Suppl) Nov:3–13, 2004

Bushnell, DM, et al: Quality of life of women with urinary incontinence: Cross-cultural performance of 15 language versions of the I-QOL. Qual Life Res 14:1901–1913, 2005.

Eslami, MS, and Friedman, JL: Urinary incontinence: Is there effective therapy? Consultant 44(7):905–915, 2004.

Gibbons, L, and Choe, JM: Helping women quell urinary incontinence. Clin Advisor 7(5):21–28, 2004.

Gray, ML: Gender, race, and culture in research on UI. AJN 3(Suppl):20–25, 2003.

Gray, ML: Stress urinary incontinence: Myths, misconceptions, and other impediments to the diagnosis and treatment of stress urinary incotinence. Am J Nurse Pract (Special Suppl):15–22, May 2004.

Holroyd-Leduc, JM, and Straus, SE: Management of urinary incontinence in women: Clinical applications. JAMA 291(8):996–999, 2004.

Jumadilova, Z, et al: Urinary incontinence in the nursing home: Resident characteristics and prevalence of drug treatment. Am J Manage Care 11:S112–S120, 2005.

Miller, KL: Stress urinary incontinence in women: Review and update on neurological control. J Womens Health 14(7):595–608, 2005.

Newman, DK: Stress urinary incontinence: Therapeutic strategies for managing stress urinary incontinence in women. Am J Nurse Pract (Special Suppl):23–32, May 2004.

Newman, DK, and Giovannini, D: The overactive bladder: A nursing perspective. AJN 102(6):36–45, 2002.

Ouslander, JG: Management of overactive bladder. N Engl J Med 350(8):786–799, 2004.

Palmer, MH: Stress urinary incontinence: Prevalence, etiology, and risk factors in women at 3 life stages. Am J Nurse Pract (Special Suppl):5–14, May 2004.

Rosenberg, MT, and Hazzard, MA:. Pharmacologic management of overactive bladder in women. Womens Health Primary Care 8(3):140–148, 2005.

Sampselle, CM: State of the science on urinary incontinence: Behavioral interventions in young and middle-age women. AJN 3(Suppl):9–19, 2003.

Williams, KS, et al: Clinical and cost-effectiveness of a new nurse-led continence service: A randomised controlled trial. Br J Gen Pract 55(518):696–703, 2005.

Wyman, JF: Treatment of urinary incontinence in men and older women. AJN 3(Suppl):26–35, 2003.

Urinary Tract Infections

Alcaide, M, and Lichtstein, DM: How best to treat urinary tract infections in adults: A rational approach. Consultant 44(8):1145–1151, 2004.

Dell, JR: Understanding chronic pelvic pain in women: Diagnosing and managing women with interstitial cystitis. Female Patient 29(Sept):13–18, 2004.

Hooton, TM: Optimizing treatment for acute uncomplicated cystitis. Clin Rev 13(9):109–116, 2003.

Mehnert-Kay, SA: Diagnosis and management of uncomplicated urinary tract infections. Am Fam Phys 72(3):451–456, 2005.

Rosenberg, MT, Moldwin, RM, and Stanford, EJ: Early diagnosis and management of interstitial cystitis: What primary care clinicians should know. Womens Health Primary Care 7(9):456–463, 2004.

References

Nursing Research–Based Practice: 14.1

Beitz JM, Zuzelo PR: The lived experience of having a neobladder. West J Nurs Res 25(3): 294–321, 2003.

Resources

American Cancer Society
http://www.cancer.org
American Urological Association
http://www.auanet.org
Mayo Clinic
http://www.mayohealth.org
National Association for Continence
http://www.nafc.org
National Bladder Foundation
http://www.bladder.org
National Kidney Foundation
http://www.kidney.org
University of Pennsylvania Cancer Center
http://www.oncolink.upenn.edu

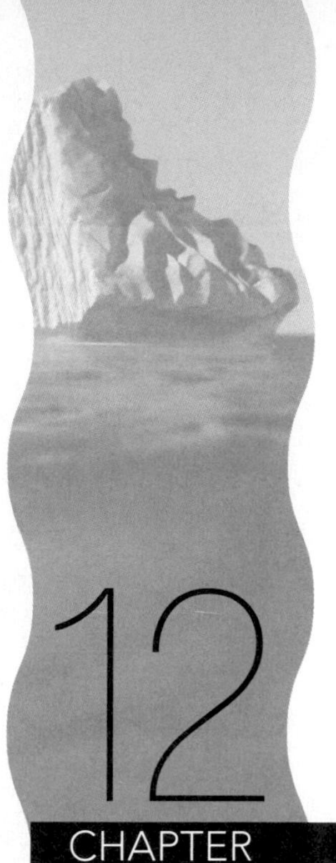

Men's Health Problems

Debera J. Thomas, DNS, APRN, BC
Brian O. Porter, MD, PhD, MPH

Common Complaints

Erectile Dysfunction

Erectile dysfunction (ED), sometimes referred to as impotence, is the failure to consistently maintain a sufficiently rigid erect penis to allow for sexual intercourse and is considered a facet of male sexual dysfunction. ED can also manifest as a lack of sexual desire or inability to ejaculate. ED can result from many causes including physiologic, endocrine, vascular, and neurologic.

ED is classified as mild if the patient fails to achieve a satisfactory erection in 2 out of 10 attempts. If all attempts at satisfactory erection fail then the ED is classed as severe. Moderate ED is somewhere in between mild and severe. It is difficult to estimate the number of men with ED because the definition is broad and some men may be reluctant to seek medical attention for the problem. In the United States, between 10 and 30 million men are believed to suffer from ED at some time in their lives. Aging affects sexual functioning, and more than 25 percent of men older than 65 years of age have ED. Most cases of ED have an identifiable organic as opposed to a psychogenic cause. Episodes of impotence occur in about half of all adult men at one time or another in their lives and are not pathological.

Normal sexual function in men has five phases: libido, erection, ejaculation, orgasm, and detumescence. For an erection to occur, there must be an intact autonomic and somatic nerve supply to the penis and the pudendal arteries. Erection begins with neurologic and vascular stimulation and is maintained by increased arterial blood flow, increased venous resistance, and relaxation of the smooth muscle of the sinusoids in the corporal bodies of the penis. Additional rigidity of the penis is accomplished by contraction of the bulbocavernosus and ischiocavernosus muscles. The process is initiated by neurotransmitters, possibly nitric oxide, vasoactive intestinal peptide, acetylcholine, and prostaglandins, although the exact mechanism is unknown at this time.

In addition to the increase in arterial flow, the efflux of blood is reduced. As the erectile tissue expands, the peripheral veins are compressed against the enveloping tunica albuginea, which effectively impedes drainage of blood from the cavernous sinuses. The less turgid corpus spongiosum allows the urethra to dilate during ejaculation.

With continued sexual stimulation, the urethral meatus dilates and sperm move to the ejaculatory duct. Seminal fluid is added to the sperm cells by the seminal vesicles and prostate gland. At the time of vaginal penetration, the male secretions produced by the bulbourethral glands and the glands of the penile urethra combine with the female cervical secretions. The sperm cells move by emission into the prostatic urethra, where they become activated by seminal fluid and are motile. In the male, orgasm is concomitant with ejaculation, which is brought about by sympathetic activity transmitted along the hypogastric nerve and lateral pelvic plexus, and then through the prostatic and cavernous plexuses. Ejaculation is the strong rhythmic contraction of the vas deferens, seminal vesicles, epididymis, prostate, urethra, and penis. Retrograde ejaculation is prevented by partial bladder-neck closure, mediated by sympathetic nerves. Orgasm is a sensory phenomenon in which the rhythmic contractions of the muscle are perceived as pleasurable.

Postcoital resolution or detumescence results from the sympathetic outflow to the genital areas; the periarterial

The Iceberg of Erectile Dysfunction

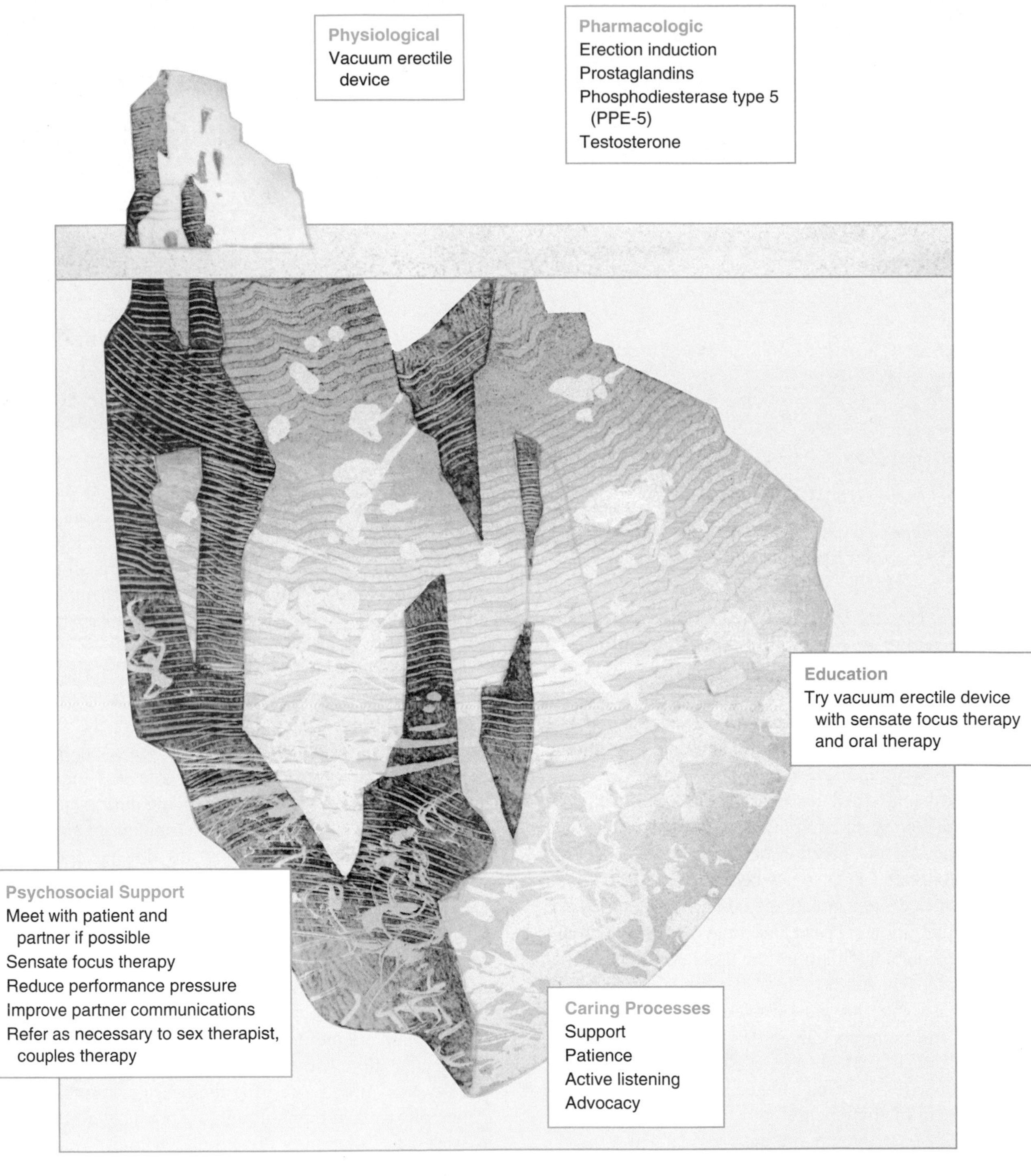

muscle increases its tone, thereby reducing the flow to the erectile tissues of the penis. A refractory period of variable duration follows.

Differential Diagnosis

Since male sexual dysfunction can manifest in many ways and because the causes are numerous, a careful history is essential for the correct diagnosis and subsequent treatment. As impotence is a very personal complaint, discussion requires a trusting relationship between patient and clinician and sufficient time during the visit for the patient to voice his concerns. He may complain of a loss of desire, inability to obtain or maintain erection, premature ejaculation, or an absence of emission or inability to achieve orgasm. Frequently, the patient has a combination of these symptoms. It is essential to determine whether or not the patient has normal erections, most likely during sleep or early in the morning. If an erection does occur, then an organic cause is most likely not the cause of the erectile dysfunction.

A physical exam, including a thorough genital examination to rule out any abnormalities of the penis itself, is done. The testes should be palpated for size or abnormal masses. If the length is less than 4 cm, hypogonadism should be considered. Evidence of feminization such as gynecomastia and abnormal body hair distribution should be assessed. All pulses should be palpated, including the penile pulse, which can be felt by pressing both corpora between the thumb and forefinger and palpating to either side of the midline. If there is an indication of a vascular etiology from either the patient's history or physical exam, an aortogram may be indicated.

A neurologic exam to evaluate the erectile reflex, including anal sphincter tone, perineal sensation, and the bulbocavernosus reflex, should be part of the physical exam. The reflex can be evaluated by squeezing the glans penis and noting the degree of anal sphincter constriction. An examination for signs of peripheral neuropathy, including distal muscle weakness and loss of tendon reflexes in the legs, is important, along with tests that will reveal any impairment of vibratory, position, tactile, and pain sensation.

Three categories of ED should be considered when determining the cause of the problem. First, there may be a failure to generate the nerve impulse that is required to initiate an erection. This can be caused by a number of endocrinologic or neurologic conditions as well as be psychogenic in origin. ED can be a result of a failure to fill, most often arteriogenic in origin. Another category is the failure to store, which is usually veno-occlusive in origin.

A loss of libido may indicate androgen deficiency arising from either pituitary or testicular disease and results in a failure to initiate the nerve impulse needed to initiate an erection. Plasma levels of testosterone and gonadotropins are measured to rule out this possibility. Endocrine factors are unlikely if the patient has normal semen volume. Some of the organic causes of erectile dysfunction are listed in Table 12.1.

Medications are a common cause of erectile dysfunction, either directly or by adverse effects. Loss of erection can be caused by central sympatholytics such as methyldopa, clonidine, and reserpine, whereas alpha-blockers cause few problems with erection. However, beta-adrenergic blocking agents and spironolactone can cause a loss of libido. Certain drugs, such as calcium channel blockers, can increase prolactin secretion and thereby cause erectile dysfunction. Some of the drugs of addiction can lower testosterone levels and lead to erectile dysfunction.

An understanding of vascular disease as a cause of ED is essential, because continual high blood flow into the vascular system of the penis is necessary to maintain an erect state. Atherosclerosis can cause failure to fill; therefore risk factors for this type of ED are heart disease, cigarette smoking, diabetes mellitus, aging, dyslipidemia, and hypertension. Trauma can also damage the pudendal and cavernous arteries, for example, from prolonged bicycling, and cause failure to fill. Leriche's syndrome, with impedance of

Table 12.1 Organic Causes of Erectile Dysfunction

Neurologic Diseases
Anterior temporal lobe lesions
Disease of the spinal cord
Loss of sensory input (secondary to diabetes mellitus, polyneuropathies), tabes dorsales (disease of dorsal root ganglia)
Disease of nervi ergentes (secondary to complete prostatectomy, retrosigmoid operations, aortic bypass)
Vascular Disease
Leriche syndrome
Endocrine Disorders
Testicular failure (primary or secondary)
Hyperprolactinemia
Penile Disorders
Failure of detumescence
Priapism
Penile trauma
Peyronie's disease
Medications
Phenothiazines
Thioridazine
Imipramine
Methyldopa
Guanethidine
Reserpine
Spironolactone
Alcohol
Heroin
Methadone
Estrogen
Beta-blockers
Antihypertensives
Thiazide diuretics

the blood flow into the penis, occurs as the result of obstruction of the distal aorta at the bifurcation of the common iliac arteries. Presenting symptoms of this syndrome are claudication and ED, either separately or in combination.

Because resistance to the efflux of blood from the penis is necessary to maintain an erection, anything that impairs this ability is considered as a failure-to-store defect. It can result from insufficient relaxation or fibrosis of the corporeal smooth muscle. Adrenergic agonists and/or psychological stress can cause insufficient relaxation of the corporeal smooth muscle while atherosclerosis and penile trauma can result in fibrosis. *Priapism,* persistent painful erection, is usually idiopathic, but can be associated with sickle cell anemia, chronic granulocytic leukemia, or spinal cord injury. The persistent erection disrupts this vascular network and can lead to fibrosis and subsequent failure to store.

Premature ejaculation seldom has an organic cause. It is usually related to anxiety about the sexual situation, performance-related fears, or an emotional disorder. Psychological disorders can preclude organic causes of ED. Depression, bipolar disorder, anxiety disorders, and relationship dysfunction may all cause ED.

The absence of emission may be produced by three organic disorders: retrograde ejaculation, sympathetic denervation, or androgen deficiency. Retrograde ejaculation may occur following surgery on the bladder neck or it may develop spontaneously in a male patient with diabetes. A postcoital urine sample can be analyzed to confirm the diagnosis. Smooth muscle contractions may not occur at the time of ejaculation as a result of the loss of the autonomic innervation of the prostate and seminal vesicles following sympathectomy. An androgen deficiency may lead to absence of secretions from the prostate and seminal vesicles. If libido and erectile function are normal, the absence of orgasm is almost always due to psychiatric disorder.

Penile diseases can cause ED. Structural causes of erectile dysfunction include microphallus, Peyronie's disease, scarring of the cavernosa, phimosis, hypospadias, and postsurgical sequelae. Peyronie's disease results from localized fibrotic thickening of the tissue around the corpora cavernosa. Plaque may be palpated along the penile shaft, usually on the dorsum, but plaque is sometimes present on any part of the corpora cavernosa. Inelasticity produces or curvature of the penile shaft on erection that may be very painful. There is a high correlation between Peyronie's disease and Dupuytren's contracture of the palmar fascia. Differential diagnosis of ED requires consideration of fibrosis secondary to trauma, severe urethritis, late-stage syphilitic lesions, penile infiltration with lymphogranuloma venereum, benign and malignant tumors, and congenital curvature. Urethral strictures produce an indurated area that may be identified by careful palpation along the penile urethra. A stricture can be identified more easily by the passage of a small urethral probe or catheter (urethral sound). Occasionally, strictures may be recognized by the presence of an indolent, firm, tender mass that may even involve the skin over the penile shaft. Restricted erections may cause ventral curvature of the penis, periurethral inflammations, and, at times, a purulent urethrocutaneous fistula. Zinc deficiency may also cause ED.

Initially, laboratory tests that rule out causes of ED should be done. These tests include a fasting blood sugar to rule out diabetes mellitus; lipid profile to rule out dyslipidemia; thyroid stimulating hormone (TSH); and a testosterone level. If the testosterone level is below 300 ng/dL, then a serum prolactin level is warranted. Laboratory tests for patients with established ED should include a complete blood count (CBC), a blood chemistry profile (including fasting glucose or glycosylated hemoglobin levels), a TSH level, and a prostate-specific-antigen (PSA) in men as young as 40 years if they have a family history of prostate cancer. Most men older than age 55 will have some abnormal laboratory findings or risk factors, but these may not necessarily be the cause of the ED. Several specialized tests can be done, but usually only if the cause of the ED is not apparent from the more standard tests. The most useful of these tests is the nocturnal penile tumescence and rigidity (NPTR) test and color Doppler sonography of the penis.

NPTR testing is useful to assess the patient's physical ability to achieve an erection. Sensors are placed at the base and tip of the penis and record the circumference and rigidity of the penis during sleep. Typically, the test is done from one to three nights. Men usually have erections during rapid eye movement (REM) sleep. A physiologic cause of ED is indicated if there is an absence or impairment of erections during sleep. This test is self-administered in the patient's home; however, it can be used in the clinical setting to determine erectile response to sexual stimuli.

There are, however, two medical conditions that cause ED in sexual situations, yet still allow normal erectile activity during NPTR. The first is disruption of the afferent nerves that amplify the erectile response to external sexual stimuli but are bypassed in the nocturnal erectile activity. The second is called *pelvic steal syndrome,* which may occur in physiologic states when the patient is awake, but not when he is asleep. This condition involves partial blockage of the iliac vessels and causes all erections to occur when the patient is at rest. Loss of erection ensues, however, with the gluteal muscle activity during thrusting.

Color Doppler sonography is being used to assess vascular causes of ED. It measures the integrity of arterial influx in the cavernous artery during erection by measuring the peak systolic velocity in this artery.

Treatment

A number of options are available for the treatment of ED. If an organic cause cannot be found, these men will most likely benefit from behaviorally based sex therapy. Treatments for ED are presented in Table 12.2 and include hormone replacement, vacuum constriction devices, vasoactive therapy, penile prostheses, and penile revascularization.

Table 12.2 Treatment for Erectile Dysfunction

Treatment	Usual Dosage	Adverse Effects	Contraindications	Instructions
Hormone replacement				
Parenteral agents				
• Testoterone cypionate (Depo-Testosterone) • Testosterone enanthate (Delatestryl)	50–400 mg q2–4 weeks 50–400 mg q2–4 weeks	Sodium retention with dependent edema, increased risk of bleeding, pain at injection site, mild gynecomastia, mood swings, lipid abnormalities	Serious liver, kidney, or cardiac disease, hypersensitivity. Do not use in men with cancer of the breast or prostate, allergy to mercury	Instruct the patient of the peak and trough effects that may lead to aggression, feelings of well-being, energy, and increased libido within 72 hours of injection. As the peak level falls, the patient may experience depressed mood and loss of libido.
Oral agents				
• Fluoxymesterone (Halostestin) • Methyltestosterone (Metandren)	2.5–20 mg qd 10–50 mg qd	Same as for parenteral agents Not used much as transdermal or parenteral agents because of the difficulty in achieving adequate blood levels due to high first-pass loss in the liver.	Same as above	
Transdermal				
• Testoderm patch	4–6 mg/24 hours	Same as for parenteral agents with the addition of skin irritation at the application site.	Same as above	Must be applied directly to scrotum.
• Testoderm TTS (Transdermal Testosterone System)	5 mg/24 hours			Testoderm TTS and Androderm can be applied anywhere on clean dry skin of the abdomen, back, upper arms, or thighs.
• Androderm	2.5 mg/24 hours	Same as above with less skin irritation		
• AndroGel (2.5- to 5-g packets) • Testim (5- to 10-g packets)	2–5 g applied once daily			Gel is applied directly to the skin of shoulders, upper arms, or abdomen. Wash hands following application and cover area with T-shirt to prevent absorption by partner. Avoid swimming or showering for 6 hours after application.
Vacuum constriction devices		Pain, ecchymosis	Priapism, sickle cell anemia, other blood disorders, lack of manual dexterity and hand strength.	If using ring, remove ring from base of penis after 30 minutes.

(continued)

Table 12.2 **Treatment for Erectile Dysfunction** (continued)

Treatment	Usual Dosage	Adverse Effects	Contraindications	Instructions
Vasoactive therapy				
Oral agents				
• Sildenafil (Viagra)	50 mg PO 1 hour before sexual activity (25–100 mg)	Headache, flushing, dyspepsia, nasal congestion, visual color changes, back, lower limb pain for all phosphodiesterase-5 inhibitors	Current use of nitrates or alpha-blockers.	Erections lasting more than 4 hours require immediate medical attention. Cannot be taken more than once a day.
• Vardenafil (Levitra)	10 mg PO once daily 1 hour before sexual activity (5–20 mg)			
• Tadalafil (Cialis)	10 mg once daily before sexual activity (5–20 mg)			
Injectables				
• Alprostadil (Caverject)	5–40 μg	Penile pain, prolonged erection, penile fibrosis, injection site hematoma, numbness, yeast infection, priapism. May also cause upper respiratory infection, headache, dizziness, hypotension.	Sickle cell anemia, penile fibrosis, coagulopathy, severe cardiovascular disease, myeloma, leukemia, penis deformity, morbid obesity, penile implant.	Patient should be instructed not to reuse needles and syringes, choose injection site along side of proximal third of the penis, alternate injection sites, avoid visible veins, and cleanse injection site with alcohol. Use only once every 24 hours, up to 3 times a week.
Transurethral suppositories				
• Alprostadil (Muse)	125–1000 μg		As above with the addition: do not use if partner is pregnant unless a condom is used.	After urinating, the patient slowly stretches the penis upward to its full length and inserts the applicator about 1 inch into the urethra. The patient then pushes the button on top of the applicator to release the suppository. A gentle rocking motion will separate the suppository from the applicator. After the applicator is removed, the patient massages the penis firmly between his hands for about 10 seconds while standing. An erection begins in about 5–10 minutes.

Common psychogenic causes of erectile dysfunction include performance anxiety and relationship problems. Referrals to sex therapy and/or marriage counseling may help some patients, especially in combination with other therapies.

Hormone Replacement

For men with documented testosterone deficiency who do not have prostate cancer, testosterone replacement is the treatment of choice. Testosterone replacement can be accomplished by several delivery methods which include injections, oral medication, topical patches, or topical gels.

Vacuum Constriction Devices

Most vacuum devices work in similar ways, using a process that takes about 2 minutes. The patient inserts his penis into the cylinder, then uses the pump to create a partial vacuum. This causes venous blood to enter the corpora cavernosa, initiating tumescence and rigidity. Once a sufficient erection is achieved, a latex constriction ring is placed around the base of the penis to help maintain the erection. This is a noninvasive procedure and complications are rare. Vacuum constrciton devices are now available over the counter and cost between $300 and $500.

Vasoactive Therapy

The development of drugs that decrease the breakdown of 5-cyclic guanosine monophosphate (cGMP) have revolutionized ED treament. cGMP is the intracellular second messenger of nitric oxide which is the primary vasodilator and neurotransmitter involved in the erectile response. The first of these drugs was sildenafil citrate (Viagra). Sildenafil is an orally active cGMP-specific phosphodiesterase inhibitor. It results in an increased blood flow necessary for successful penile erection. The standard dose is sildenafil 50 mg taken orally at least 1 hour before sexual activity. Contraindications that can cause severe hypotensive effects are listed in Table 12.2. Other, newer medications in this class are vardenafil (Levitra) and tadalafil (Cialis). Phosphodiesterase-5 inhibitors do not affect libido and do not initiate an erection without sexual stimulation.

Vasoactive prostaglandins have been shown to be an effective treatment for ED. Alprostadil (Caverject) 5 to 40 μg is injected directly into the base and lateral aspect of the penis using a tuberculin syringe. Erection occurs within 20 minutes and lasts for approximately 30 to 60 minutes. Prolonged erection (priapism) occurs rarely, but the patient should be instructed to seek medical attention if this does occur. Alprostadil is also available in a transurethral suppository in dosages of 125, 250, 500, or 1000 μg. Results have been good, with the suppositories producing an erection in about 5 to 10 minutes (see Table 12.2 for instructions for use).

Penile Prostheses

Several prosthetic devices are available, in a variety of sizes and diameters, that can be surgically implanted into the penis. They are placed directly in the corporal bodies. Penile prostheses may be rigid, semifirm, hinged, or inflatable. The inflatable devices are more natural appearing, however, there is more opportunity for mechanical failure. Implantation of a prosthesis, which is a highly reliable but invasive form of therapy, may help men who have failed therapy with other methods, but it is very expensive, ranging in cost from $9000 to $20,000. Implantation may be covered by some insurance plans. Most patients desiring implants prefer spontaneity and therefore choose this invasive treatment. Significant problems associated with implants are infection, erosion, and occasional mechanical failure (in fewer than 5 percent of patients). The most common types of implants are nonhydraulic (using semirigid rods) and hydraulic (using inflatables). Both types of implants involve surgical placement of two cylinders inside the corpus cavernosum. Healing takes 4 to 6 weeks, after which the patient may have intercourse.

Penile Revascularization

The experience with penile revascularization is limited and some patients fail to have a sufficient erection even after the procedure. Patients with arterial disorders may be candidates for the various procedures which include endarterectomy and balloon dilation, or arterial bypass. For patients with venous disorders, ligation of the deep dorsal vein or emissary vein or ligation of the crura of the corpora cavernosus may be somewhat effective.

In younger men, several conditions may warrant penile revascularization surgery. Men younger than age 45 whose impotence is caused by severe pelvic trauma are the best candidates for this surgery. In patients with impotence of sudden onset, the possibility that trauma to the peritoneum or pelvis may have led to vascular injury should be considered. A congenital shunt should be ruled out in any patient who reports that he has never had a full erection.

Nocturia and Incontinence

Nocturia is described as frequency of urination at night and disrupts the normal sleep cycle. Recording the number of times a patient urinates at night and making a reasonable estimate of the amount voided is extremely important. The frequency of urination may vary from large volumes of urine (polyuria) to small quantities passed at frequent intervals. Adult males normally void five to six times during the day and once or not at all during the night. As men age, nocturia is usually a sign of benign prostatic hypertrophy (BPH). Typically, 50 percent of men older than age 50 years have BPH, and the rate increases by 10 percent for every 10 years of age (e.g., to 60 percent of men older than age 60 years, to 70 percent of men older than age 70 years, and so on). BPH is discussed in more detail later in this chapter.

The occurrence of nocturia without discomfort may be due to diminished bladder capacity, overflow incontinence, or habit. In men with a normal bladder, the absence of nocturia while suffering from increased frequency of urination during the day suggests psychogenic origin. A rare finding might be a polyp or irritative lesion in the posterior urethra that is relieved by recumbence, so nocturia is not present.

Detrusor muscle instability may cause urinary incontinence as well as nocturia. Fifty percent of male patients in nursing homes are incontinent, whereas 15 to 30 percent of elderly men in the community have urinary incontinence, which may be caused by decreased bladder capacity, increased residual urine (from inability to empty the bladder), or involuntary bladder contractions. Moderate dribbling of urine may indicate overflow from a partially incompetent outlet and can be congenital or an acquired anomaly. Less common causes of incontinence are spinal cord disease, multiple sclerosis, tumors, trauma, syphilis, and diabetic neuropathy. Microorganisms can cause nocturia as well as incontinence and include *Klebsiella pneumoniae, Proteus mirabilis, Enterobacter, Staphylococcus,* enterococci (*Streptococcus* bacteria associated with the intestines), or *Pseudomonas.*

Medications, such as methyldopa, phenothiazides, diazepam, and diuretics, may also cause nocturia as well as precipitate or aggravate incontinence. Drugs that cause urinary retention include alpha-adrenergic agents, androgens, and sympathomimetic agents such as ephedrine and pseudoephedrine. Urinary retention can cause nocturia and incontinence.

Differential Diagnosis

Increased frequency may occur as a result of primary disease of the urinary tract, or may result from metabolic disease such as diabetes mellitus or diabetes insipidus; it may also be associated with emotional tension. Documentation of the pattern of urination during a 24-hour period is vital to a diagnosis of nocturia. Although a patient may complain if he awakens frequently to urinate, the precipitating events and activities of the day may also give a hint to the cause and effect. For example, alcohol intake prior to sleep may increase the number of times the patient urinates at night, and may also increase urine volume.

Urgency can be constant or intermittent and is a desire to urinate. Urgency and frequency of urination often occur together. Urgency is frequently the result of prostatic disease or bladder infection. Hesitancy refers to difficulty in initiating a urine stream. *Oliguria* is a decrease in urinary output and can be caused by a decrease in production of urine secondary to acute glomerulonephritis or other renal disease, as well as conditions that drastically decrease cardiac output. Dribbling can be symptomatic of disease; it may occur at night as well as during the day and usually indicates the presence of a urethral stricture or prostatic obstruction, but it may be caused by a neurologic disorder.

Treatment

Treatment of nocturia depends on identifying the cause. A simple urinalysis is performed to rule out urinary tract infection. A prostatic-specific antigen (PSA) blood test and a digital rectal exam (DRE) are done to rule out BPH. The results may indicate a need for further testing, as explained under Common Problems.

Testicular Pain

Testicular pain is probably the most urgent of patient complaints. Testicular pain as a single symptom is a fullness or heaviness of the scrotum, ranging from a dull ache to a sticking pain and may occur in a wide variety of patients with no differentiation based on culture, race, or socioeconomic status.

The tunica vaginalis is a remnant of the processus vaginalis; a painful hernia can occur when an evagination of the peritoneal cavity is occluded by the adult spermatic cord. A patent processus vaginalis predisposes the patient to indirect or congenital hernias. Partial occlusion of the processus vaginalis can result in fluid accumulation, or hydrocele, which cannot be distinguished from a hernia or an incompletely descended testicle until surgery is performed. Anterior and lateral to the testes, the processus vaginalis remains patent, forming the tunica vaginalis, which represents the detached portion of the peritoneal cavity within the scrotum.

Differential Diagnoses

A sign of testicular pain may be swelling of the testis, the epididymis, or the spermatic cord, or torsion of the testicle (the testicle may become twisted around the spermatic cord, causing acute pain; this condition is a urological emergency). Differential diagnoses for testicular pain include hydrocele, varicocele, epididymitis, and prostatitis. Pain from prostatitis usually occurs in the lower back and radiates to the testicles and is typically accompanied by fever. Cultures usually show *E. coli,* with or without fistula formation. Hernias, hydroceles, and hematomas all must be excluded. A detailed history and physical exam will direct the assessment to the exclusion of other diagnoses. A spermatocele may also cause testicular pain, although most spermatoceles are painless. A syphilitic gumma is a part of the differential diagnosis, as is a varicocele; however, these are usually not painful.

Because of the multiple possible diagnoses, specialized tests are performed. A scrotal ultrasound can clearly identify any mass originating in the testicles and is the simplest test. An echo-texture pattern reveals the presence of a hypoechoic mass that is distinct from surrounding normal testicular tissue, spermatoceles, hydroceles, or varicoceles.

Treatment

Treatment of testicular pain is dependent on finding the underlying cause for the pain and treating it appropriately.

Common Problems

Benign Prostatic Hyperplasia

Benign prostatic hyperplasia or hypertrophy (BPH) is one of the most common conditions affecting men older than age 40 years. The prostate gland is a walnut-size gland positioned at the base of the bladder and in front of the rectum. The prostate gland starts enlarging in puberty and stops growing at around age 20 years. It begins to enlarge again after age 50 years. The prostate has three distinct zones: the central zone, the peripheral zone, and the transition zone which lies adjacent to the urethra (see section on Prostate Cancer for a more detailed description of prostatic anatomy). BPH develops primarily in the transition zone, whereas carcinoma of the prostate usually develops in the peripheral zone.

Epidemiology and Causes

Aging is the predominant risk factor for BPH. Histologically, BPH is found in more than 50 percent of men older than age 50 years, in 70 percent of men older than age 70 years, and in 80 percent of men older than 80 years. Of these, 20 percent of men older than age 60 years have obstructive and irritative symptoms that are severe enough to require treatment. Genetic susceptibility of the disorder is also underscored by twin concordance and family history studies, with inherited forms predominating in men younger than 60 years of age.

Epidemiologic studies of BPH have been hampered by inconsistencies in the definition and clinical criteria of this disorder. Most authorities consider not only prostate size (greater than 30 mL) but also decreased urinary flow rates (less than 15 mL/sec) and significant postvoid residual bladder volumes (greater than 50 mL).

Evidence suggests that BPH arises from a systemic hormonal alteration, which may or may not act in combination with growth factors that stimulate stromal or glandular hyperplasia. One risk factor for BPH are intact testes—more specifically, functioning Leydig cells. Thus, BPH is rare in castrated men or in those who experience untreated hypogonadism before the age of 40 years. There has been no concrete evidence that dietary, environmental, or sexual practices are implicated in BPH.

Pathophysiology

Prostatic secretions form part of the seminal fluid during ejaculation. The ejaculatory ducts from the seminal vesicles pass through the prostate gland and enter the urethra. The prostate consists of two main sections. The inner section of the gland produces secretions needed to keep the lining of the urethra moist. The outer section contributes to seminal secretions.

The importance of dihydrotestosterone as a key androgenic hormone in the pathogenesis of BPH has been well supported. Although concentrations of this prohormone (which is subsequently converted into testosterone) do not differ in men with or without BPH, prostatic receptors for this hormone have a much more heterogeneous distribution in men with BPH, while in normal controls; these receptors predominate within the epithelia. Thus, while necessary to the pathogenesis of BPH, androgen exposure alone is not sufficient to cause the disorder. Similar, estrogen has been implicated as a necessary factor to maintain BPH in older men, but not sufficient to cause its pathogenesis alone. The data are conflicting, however. For instance, the concentration of estrogen receptors is actually lower in hyperplastic prostatic tissue, which the concentration of progesterone receptors does not differ in BPH versus the normal prostate.

The earliest histologic signs of BPH usually appear in men in their 30s and 40s. The development of pathologic BPH is similar in most cases. BPH usually presents as a predominance of stromal nodules (up to a fourfold increase), consisting primarily of smooth muscle and connective tissue, in the periurethral area of the transition zone. This may be followed by glandular hyperplasia (up to a twofold increase) with an increase in epithelial cells. Key growth factors including fibroblast growth factor, insulin-like growth factor-2 (IGF-2), and transforming growth factor (TGF)-β. In vitro data demonstrate even a wider array of growth factors that stimulate prostatic epithelial cell growth. Anti-apoptotic factors such as bcl-2 are also upregulated in BPH tissue, while animal studies have implicated higher numbers of stem cells in hyperplastic prostatic tissue.

There are two documented mechanisms of obstruction—static and dynamic. *Static constriction* is caused by the buildup of prostatic tissue, with direct obstruction of the bladder neck. *Dynamic constriction* is an increase in prostatic muscle tone through adrenergic stimulation, leading to constriction of the bladder neck. A predominance of alpha-adrenergic receptors in the sympathetic nervous system controls stromal hyperplasia. If middle-lobe enlargement of the prostate predominates, the symptoms produced are similar to those of a ball-valve obstruction at the bladder neck.

Obstruction of the bladder outlet forces the bladder to generate higher pressures than normal to achieve micturition. Increased muscle mass in the bladder leads to reduced bladder elasticity and compliance, which manifests as a reduction in bladder capacity. If the bladder-neck obstruction is not relieved, the bladder's smooth muscle begins to be replaced by connective tissue, leading to bladder failure.

Clinical Presentation

Subjective

Use of a standardized questionnaire such as the one from the American Urologic Association (AUA), the AUA Symptom Score Index (shown in Focusing the History 12.1), or the International Prostatic Symptom Score (I-PSA) is important in assessing the impact of BPH upon the patient. These questionnaires are designed to uncover the degree of symptomology in each patient. Total symptom scores may range from 0 to 35. Obstructive voiding symptoms can be mild, with a score of 0 to 8. A score of 9 to 19 is considered moderate; 20 or more indicates severe symptoms. Symptom scores are helpful to quantify the patient's symptoms. A score of 7 or higher on the AUA Symptom Score Index, for example, can reinforce the need for further investigation of the cause of the symptoms. Although the scores alone are not diagnostic, they help to support the diagnosis, as well as being useful in following a patient after initiating therapy to track the decrease in symptoms.

The symptoms of BPH vary, and are dependent upon the type of obstruction, but usually include a combination of obstructive and irritative voiding symptoms. Because the symptoms are not specific to BPH and may have other causes, a complete workup is necessary. BPH is non–life-threatening, but it is a lifestyle-changing diagnosis.

Symptoms of obstructive BPH include decreased force of stream, hesitancy, postvoid dribbling, sensation of

FOCUS ON HISTORY 12.1

AUA Symptom Score Index

Directions: Circle one number on each line.

Questions to be Answered	Not at all	Less than 1 time in 5	Less than half the time	About half the time	More than half the time	Almost always
1. Over the past month, how often have you had a sensation of not emptying your bladder completely after you finished urinating?	0	1	2	3	4	5
2. Over the past month, how often have you had to urinate again less than 2 hours after you finished urinating?	0	1	2	3	4	5
3. Over the past month, how often have you found you stopped and started again several times when you urinated?	0	1	2	3	4	5
4. Over the past month, how often have you found it difficult to postpone urination?	0	1	2	3	4	5
5. Over the past month, how often have you had a weak urinary stream?	0	1	2	3	4	5
6. Over the past month, how often have you had to push or strain to begin urination?	0	1	2	3	4	5
7. Over the past month, how many times did you most typically get up to urinate from the time you went to bed at night until the time you got up in the morning?	0	1 time	2 times	3 times	4 times	5 times

Total sum of the 7 circled numbers (AUA Symptom Score): ____________

SOURCE: Barry, MJ, et al: The American Urological Association symptom index for benign prostatic hyperplasia. J Urol 148:1549–1557, 1992.

incomplete bladder emptying, overflow incontinence, inability to voluntarily stop the urinary stream, urinary retention, double-voiding (voiding a second time within 2 hours), and straining. Irritative symptoms of BPH include nocturia, urinary frequency, urgency, dysuria, and urge incontinence.

Objective

A DRE is done to determine enlargement of the prostate gland. The prostate in BPH is usually a smooth, firm, elastic enlargement. If the prostate is not smooth, prostate cancer may be present. The size of the prostate does not correlate with the severity of the symptoms in men with BPH. Some men simply have large prostate glands. Many men with palpably enlarged prostates are not symptomatic, whereas some patients with small prostates have irritative or obstructive symptoms.

Objective findings may also include gross hematuria (in men older than 60 years of age), observation of a weak stream, distended bladder (to greater than 150 cc, detected by percussion), increased postvoid residual volume (more than 100 mL), and prostate enlargement (to more than the normal "walnut" size, weighing 20 g or less).

Diagnostic Reasoning

Diagnostic Tests

Laboratory tests include a urinalysis and PSA. Urinalysis is done to exclude infection or hematuria. Renal function should be assessed with a serum creatinine because 10 percent of patients with prostatism have renal insufficiency and are at high risk of postoperative complications after surgery for BPH. PSA is done to assess for prostate cancer. There may be an elevation of the PSA in either prostate cancer or BPH; therefore, the PSA value alone is not diagnostic of cancer or BPH. Acute lower urinary retention or prostatitis will also elevate the PSA. The PSA in BPH is usually less than 10 ng/mL. PSA is a glycoprotein that aids in the liquefaction of the seminal coagulum. Although it is prostate specific, it should not be touted as a prostate cancer–specific enzyme. An elevated pH results from the chronic residual urine. If an obstructive uropathy is present, the serum creatinine level will be elevated. Urine cultures are sometimes positive for bacteria because of the chronic residual urine. Urine cytology should be done to rule out carcinoma, particularly when hematuria has been identified. An intravenous pyelogram (IVP) will show an increased postvoid residual (PVR) volume of urine, a large prostatic impression on the bladder, trabeculated bladder, bladder diverticula, upper tract dilation, and/or bladder stones.

Subsequent testing should be done by a urologist if initial treatment does not relieve symptoms, or if prostatic carcinoma is suspected. Uroflow, for example, measures the amount of urine voided per unit of time. Flow of less than 10 mL/sec is indicative of obstruction. This test is accurate when the voided volume is greater than 200 mL. A cystometrogram (CMG) measures bladder compliance and is usually reserved for patients with suspected neurologic disease or whose prostate surgery was unsuccessful in relieving symptoms. A cystoscopy is usually done only to determine the best surgical approach for BPH.

Differential Diagnosis

The differential diagnoses that must be considered when evaluating a patient with suspected BPH are numerous and fall into three distinct categories: bladder outlet obstruction, nonobstructive etiologies, and irritative symptoms. Table 12.3 presents the differential diagnosis for BPH.

When BPH is the presumptive diagnosis, other obstructive etiologies of the lower urinary tract (bladder calculi, bladder-neck contracture, urethral stricture and prostate cancer) should be explored. Careful history may reveal previous urethral instrumentation, urethritis, or trauma as the source of the obstruction. Bladder calculi may present with pain and hematuria. Irritative etiologies (bladder cancer, lower urinary tract infection, prostatitis, or urethritis) may present with hematuria, urgency, and frequency. A history of diabetes mellitus, stroke, neurologic diseases, or spinal cord injury can contribute to a neurogenic bladder, which has many of the same symptoms as BPH. Cancer of the prostate and BPH have many of the same symptoms. A PSA and DRE can help differentiate between these two disorders.

Table 12.3 Differential Diagnoses: Benign Prostatic Hyperplasia

Bladder-Outlet Obstruction
Bladder-outlet obstruction
Prostate cancer
Urethral stricture
Bladder-neck contracture (acquired or congenital)
Anterior or posterior urethral valve failure
Müllerian duct cysts
Inability of bladder neck or external sphincter to relax during voiding
Nonobstructive Etiologies
Neurogenic bladder (detrusor denervation)
Myogenic cause (detrusor muscle failure)
Diabetes mellitus
Parkinson's disease
Cerebrovascular accident (CVA)
Medications (parasympatholytics, sympathomimetics)
Psychogenic stress-induced performance anxiety
Irritative Symptoms
Neurogenic bladder (detrusor denervation)
Neoplasm
Bladder cancer
Bladder calculi
Prostatitis
UTI
Urethritis

Management

Medical Management

Most patients with BPH can be treated as outpatients; the goal is to relieve the symptoms, specifically nocturia. The Patient's Voice 12.1 illustrates the patient's need for symptom relief. Inpatient treatment is required to manage fluid and electrolyte abnormalities of obstructive uropathy.

Most urologists and primary-care providers have adopted a "watchful waiting" technique for BPH that has only mild symptoms. A patient with mild to moderate symptoms, minimal PVR, and no objective changes in the urinary tract may require just monitoring. The "watchful waiting" medical treatment is usually considered the most conservative and the most effective treatment for BPH as long as more serious conditions have been ruled out. Watchful waiting is also the prescribed treatment when BPH has little or no impact on the quality of life. As lifestyle changes do occur, however, or as the AUA score increases, several options may be offered to the patient. Avoidance of caffeine and alcohol, both known to be bladder irritants, is recommended. A patient with a high AUA symptom score, urinary retention, or complications of BPH, including a high PVR, renal insufficiency, hematuria, bladder stones, or anatomic or urinary tract abnormalities, should not be treated with medical management and watchful waiting. These conditions require more vigorous treatment.

Once prostatic cancer has been ruled out, medications may be tried initially to treat the BPH symptoms. Medications are used when no strong indication for surgery exists or when a patient refuses surgery or is a poor surgical risk. Because the prostate and bladder contain $alpha_1$-adrenergic receptors that cause the prostate and bladder neck to contract when bound, alpha-blockade decreases this affect and results in objective and subjective improvement in the manifestations of BPH. Most of the alpha-blockers used in the treatment of BPH are selective $alpha_1$-adrenergic agonists. These include the short-acting prazosin (Minipress) 1 to 5 mg bid or the longer-acting terazosin (Hytrin) 1 to 10 mg qd, and doxazosin (Cardura) 1 to 8 mg qd. The subtype $alpha_{1a}$-adrenergic receptors have recently been identified in the bladder neck and prostate with subsequent development of medications that target these receptors which include tamsulosin (Flomax) 0.4 or 0.8 mg qd and alfuzosin (UroXatral) 10 to 15 mg qd (immediately after the same meal each day).

The dosage of prazosin must be titrated, starting with 1 mg at bedtime for three nights and then adding another 1-mg dose in the morning. The dose can be increased to more than 2 mg bid, but the improvement in symptoms is minimal and the side effects increase and include orthostatic hypotension, dizziness, tiredness, retrograde ejaculation, rhinitis, and headache. The long-acting $alpha_1$-blockers have the advantage of once-a-day dosing, but still require a gradual dose titration. For example, doxazosin is usually started at 1 mg qd for 7 days then increased to 2 mg qd for another week, and finally increased to 4 mg qd. Terazosin is started at 1 mg qd for 3 days then 2 mg qd for 11 days, then increased to 5 mg qd. The $alpha_{1a}$-adrenergic blockers (tamsulosin and alfuzosin) do not need to be titrated, but should be started at the lowest dose and increased if necessary.

Another class of medications used to treat BPH is the 5-alpha-reductase inhibitors including finasteride (Proscar) and the newest one, dutasteride (Avodart). These medications block the conversion of testosterone to dihydrotestosterone (DHT) by inhibiting the enzyme 5-alpha-reductase. DHT is primarily responsible for the enlargement of the prostate gland. The maximum reduction in prostate size (20 percent reduction) may not be seen until after 6 months of therapy. However, improvement in symptoms is seen only in men with very enlarged prostates (greater than 40 mL). Finasteride is well tolerated in most patients, but adverse effects include decreased ejaculate volume, reduced libido, and erectile dysfunction, in 3 to 5 percent of all patients. The adverse effects may decrease with time, however, and are reversible with the cessation of treatment. Finasteride also decreases the PSA concentration by almost 50 percent, which can complicate prostate cancer detection. Dutasteride (second-generation 5-alpha-reductase inhibitor) produces a more rapid reduction in DHT. For example, dutasteride 0.5 mg qd for 2 weeks reduced serum DHT concentrations by 90 percent and significant improvement in symptoms after 3 to 12 months of treatment. The side effects of dutasteride were similar to those of finasteride, but decreased over time and were only slightly higher than in the men receiving placebo.

Some research indicates that combination therapy of terazosin and finasteride is superior to single-medication

THE PATIENT'S VOICE 12.1

Nocturia

I had gradually been increasing the times I got up to go to the bathroom at night to urinate. It was getting to be a nuisance. I couldn't see going to the doctor's for just this, so I waited for my annual exam.

The doctor said that my exam only showed mild BPH and that my PSA was normal, so if I was able to go back to sleep right away, to live with getting up in the night to go to the bathroom. I didn't really like this answer, but didn't know what to do. Sure, I could go back to sleep, but after getting up three to four times during the night, it was becoming a nuisance. I made another appointment, since this was bothering me so much. This time, the nurse practitioner saw me. She said that if getting up several times a night was bothering me, that there were some medications I could try. I thought it was worth it, so I gave it a try. What relief! A simple pill and now I can sleep all night and wake up refreshed. I feel great...and I feel great that the nurse practitioner took the time to really listen to me and my concerns.

COMPLEMENTARY THERAPIES 12.1

Men's Health Problems

Problem	Therapy	Dosage	Comments
Benign Prostatic Hyperplasia (BPH)	Herbal: Saw palmetto	320 mg of a lipophilic fruit extract (two 80-mg caps bid)	Rare; stomach problems
	Herbal: Nettle	4–6 g daily as tea; 4 g (3–4 tsp) in 150 mg in 1 cup of hot water tid or qid	Local rash and irritation, mild GI upset
	Herbal: Pygeum	100–200 mg daily of lipid extract of the bark	No adverse effects noted
	Beta-carotene	15,000 IU daily	
	Magnesium	400 mg daily	
	Selenium	200/μg daily	Only exceed 100 μg if under medical care
	Vitamin A	10,000 IU daily	
	Vitamin B_6 (pyridoxine)	100 mg daily	
	Vitamin C	1000–4000 mg (1–4 g) daily	May cause diarrhea
	Vitamin E	Up to 1000 IU daily	Do not take with anticoagulants
	Zinc	160 mg (Vicon-C) in 2 divided doses daily	
Prostatitis	Vitamin B complex	50 mg tid	
	Vitamin B_6	50 mg bid	
	Zinc	80 mg daily	
	Vitamin A	5000–10,000 IU daily	
	Vitamin E	600 IU daily	
Impotence (erectile dysfunction, sexual anxiety)	Vitamin E	Up to 1000 IU daily	Do not take with anticoagulants
	Vitamin B_6	300 mg daily	
	Vitamin B_{12} (cyanocobalamin)	500 mg daily	
	Folic acid	1200 mg daily	
	Zinc	50 mg daily	May cause GI upset
	Aromatherapy: Ylang ylang	Via bath or vaporizer	Do not overuse
Urinary Infection (cystitis, urethritis)	Herbal: Cranberry	360–960 mL daily; 6 capsules = 90 mL	GI disturbances (diarrhea) with large dosage
	Aromatherapy: Bergamot essential oil	Via vaporizer, cold compress, or bath	Sensitivity with sunlight

therapy (either alpha-blockers or 5-alpha-reductase inhibitors) in long-term but not in short-term treatment. If a patient has reached the maximum dose of the alpha-blockers and symptoms continue to progress, finasteride can be added at that point to improve prostate size and symptoms.

Complementary therapies may also be used to treat BPH. Complementary Therapies 12.1 presents herbal therapies, along with vitamin and mineral therapies that may be used in the treatment of the symptoms of BPH as well as other men's health problems.

Invasive and Surgical Management

Urologic surgery is another treatment option for BPH and in fact is the second most common surgery in men (cataract surgery is the first). Prostate surgery is indicated when there is urinary retention or when other symptoms are intractable because of the prostatic obstruction, as gauged by the AUA index (that is, in patients with a score of greater than 8). Obstructive uropathy, recurrent and persistent UTIs resulting from the prostatic obstruction, or recurrent gross hematuria caused by the enlarged prostate also are indications for surgical resection.

Transurethral resection of the prostate (TURP) continues to be the surgical treatment of choice for a patient with BPH. Candidates for surgical intervention include patients with severe symptoms, high PVRs, complications, upper urinary tract changes, and those who fail medical therapy. TURP is performed through a cystoscope, using a diathermy loop for resection of prostatic tissue. It usually is performed under spinal or general anesthesia, with a urethral catheter maintained in place for 36 to 48 hours postoperatively. Some patients may also need to be discharged from the hospital with a urinary catheter in place for up to 2 weeks after surgery. Symptomatic improvement following a TURP occurs in 90 percent of the patients. Flow-stream rates are increased as much as 15 mL/sec. Unfortunately, a complication of TURP can be retrograde ejaculation, occurring in 65 percent of patients; another potential complication is erectile dysfunction, which occurs in up to 15 percent of patients. Less frequent problems include bleeding, UTI, and urethral stricture.

A transurethral incision of the prostate (TUIP) is limited to patients with moderate to severe symptoms and a small prostate who have an elevated bladder neck or posterior commissure hyperplasia. In this procedure, an instrument is passed through the urethra to make one or two cuts in the prostate and the prostate capsule, reducing urethral stricture. This procedure can be performed on an outpatient basis or during a 24-hour stay; TUIP has a lower complication rate than TURP.

Open prostatectomy is a surgical option reserved for prostate glands weighing more than 40 to 100 g. An open prostatectomy is the surgical removal of the inner portion of the prostate via a suprapubic or retropubic incision in the abdominal area. This procedure requires longer hospitalizations than the other two options, and has far more complications. Nonetheless, this may be the only alternative for a patient who has failed medical treatment, or when a carcinoma of the prostate is suspected.

There are several minimally invasive procedures for BPH. Transurethral laser-induced prostatectomy (TULIP) is a type of coagulation necrosis and is done under transrectal ultrasound guidance. Other types of laser surgery (coagulation necrosis) are performed under direct visualization. In laser procedures, the ablated tissue sloughed in 3 weeks to 3 months. The main advantage of laser surgery is that it is minimally invasive and can be done in the outpatient setting. There is also minimal blood loss and the occurrence of retrograde ejaculation and ED is reduced. Also, this procedure can be performed in patients who are taking anticoagulants.

Another minimally invasive procedure is transurethral electrovaporization of the prostate. This seems to provide results equivalent to those of laser ablation. In transurethral electrovaporization of the prostate, a grooved roller-blade electrode administers diathermic energy to the prostate, vaporizing the prostatic tissue. The procedure provides a patient with improved urinary flow through the urethra. Because this is a recent innovation, long-term studies are not yet available.

Transurethral microwave thermotherapy (TUMT) is another procedure that results in the ablation of prostatic tissue. In TUMT, microwave energy is applied to the prostate through a microwave antenna in a urethral catheter; temperature monitoring of the rectum and urethra is essential. Prostate tissue is heated to 55°C, resulting in necrosis of the tissue causing obstruction. Urethral cooling prevents urethral necrosis and limits postoperative irritative symptoms. One of the adverse effects of TUMT postoperatively is urinary retention, requiring catheterization. Although symptom score and urine flow rates are improved, long-term studies are needed to assess the efficacy.

In transurethral needle ablation (TUNA), two radiofrequency energy waves are administered to prostatic tissue via needle electrodes applied through a cystoscope. Temperatures up to 120°F (48.9°C) destroy the prostatic tissue that had caused the urinary retention or obstruction, while preserving prostatic urethral mucosa.

Another means of thermal tissue ablation in the high-intensity focused ultrasound (HIFU). A rectal probe delivers a short burst of high-intensity focused ultrasound energy that heats the prostate tissue resulting in coagulative necrosis. Clinical trials are ongoing and demonstrate symptom improvement, but long-term efficacy is not known yet.

Stents have been placed cystoscopically and may be effective in relieving severe urinary obstruction or retention without further surgical intervention. Within 4 to 6 weeks after placement, the stents become covered in urothelium. Stent placement is reserved for patients who are poor surgical risks or who have a limited life expectancy. Stent placement is being used less since the development of minimally invasive procedures such as the TUNA and TULIP.

Transurethral (balloon) dilatation of prostate (TUDP) involves the insertion of a catheter with a balloon at the end through the urethra and into the prostatic urethra. The balloon is then inflated to stretch the urethra at the stricture where it has been narrowed. Although this treatment has been associated with fewer complications, dilatation is less effective than other methods. It may provide only a temporary solution, with symptoms recurring within 2 years, and is rarely used today.

Follow-Up and Referral

Patient monitoring includes the use of the AUA symptom index, which should be monitored every 1 to 6 months; urodynamic testing, which should be done every 3 to 6 months; and DRE and PSA, which should be done yearly. In addition to the yearly PSA, urodynamic studies should be done every 3 to 6 months to evaluate flow rates and voiding pressures. Any patient with BPH who is suspected to have prostatic carcinoma should be referred to a urologist.

Patient Education

It is extremely important to stress to the patient with BPH that taking over-the-counter medications containing alpha-agonists or anticholinergic agents can cause acute urinary retention which can result in acute renal failure. These patients may require an indwelling urinary catheter until the acute urinary retention is resolved. The most common offending medications are various cold and flu preparations.

Patients should also be advised to avoid bladder irritants such as coffee, spicy foods, and alcohol. Patients should be instructed to void at least every 2 hours to help reduce the possibility of UTI.

Prostatitis

Prostatitis is one of several inflammatory and/or painful conditions affecting the prostate gland. Prostatitis accounts for about 25 percent of all office visits by men. The classification of the type of prostatitis is important for both diagnostic and treatment purposes. Patients may present with acute bacterial prostatitis, chronic bacterial prostatitis, nonbacterial prostatitis, or prostatodynia. Chronic nonbacterial prostatitis is the most common type; it is eight times more frequent than bacterial prostatitis.

In an effort to standardize this classification schema, the National Institutes of Health (NIH) suggested nonbacterial prostatitis and prostatodynia be grouped together as chronic prostatitis/chronic pelvic pain syndrome, which may be inflammatory or noninflammatory in nature. In addition, a final category of asymptomatic inflammatory prostatitis is used to denote persons with a significant inflammatory infiltrate in prostatic secretions but without overt pain or difficulty with urination.

Epidemiology and Causes

Acute bacterial prostatitis is always associated with a urinary tract infection (UTI) and has a characteristically abrupt onset. Chronic bacterial prostatitis is a major cause of recurrent bacteriuria. Nonbacterial prostatitis has findings similar to those associated with chronic bacterial prostatitis, but no evidence of bacterial infection will be present in a urine culture. Prostatodynia presents with signs and symptoms of prostatitis but without evidence of inflammation. Prostatitis occurs predominantly in sexually active men between ages 30 and 50 years. Chronic bacterial prostatitis is more common in patients older than 50 years old. Athletes who run long distances—including cross-country runners and athletes who have vigorous exercise regimens—may be predisposed to prostatitis, although the etiology is not well documented at present.

Acute and chronic bacterial prostatitis are both caused by an infection that originates from the ascending urethral flexion or from the reflux of urine into the prostatic ducts. Infection may also spread directly to the prostatic ducts from the rectum. Infection may spread via the lymphatic system or bloodstream, with prostatic calculi serving as a nidus for infection. The most common aerobic gram-negative bacteria involved in prostatitis include *Klebsiella, Pseudomonas, Enterobacter, Escherichia coli, Proteus mirabilis,* and *Neisseria gonorrhoeae.* The causative gram-positive bacteria are *Streptococcus faecalis* and *Staphylococcus aureus.* Some organisms suspected but as yet unproven are *Staphylococcus epidermidis, Micrococcus,* non–group D *Streptococcus,* and diphtheroids. Rarely, fungi and *Mycobacteria tuberculosis* have been implicated in chronic prostatitis. The cause of nonbacterial prostatitis is currently under scrutiny; however, *Ureaplasma, Trichomonas vaginalis,* and *Chlamydia trachomatis* may be involved. Risk factors for prostatitis are age (older than age 50 years), history of prostatic calculi, and history of a previously diagnosed UTI. Chronic prostatitis, in particular, is associated with a history of recurrent UTI, presumably due to repeated seeding of the urinary tract by the infected prostate.

Pathophysiology

The infectious processes resulting in acute or chronic bacterial prostatitis are a result of the organisms mentioned previously. Purulent prostatic discharge may or may not be evident in the absence of prostatic massage. Among patients who fall into the chronic prostatitis/chronic pelvic pain category, prostatic massage will effectively double the number of cases that are considered inflammatory, due to the presence of WBC in postmassage urine or seminal fluid.

The pathophysiology of nonbacterial prostatitis is less clear, but it may be related to a voiding dysfunction such as spasm of the bladder neck or urethra. The cause of prostatodynia is unclear, although it may be related to internal urethral sphincter problems or to abnormal tension of the pelvic floor musculature. Prostatodynia is also related to stress, anxiety, and depression.

Clinical Presentation

Subjective

The patient may present complaining of *tenesmus* (a spasmodic contraction of the anal sphincter), with pain and a persistent desire to empty the bowel or bladder accompanied by involuntary, ineffective straining efforts. Focusing the History 12.2 presents common signs and symptoms of the different types of prostatitis. Obstructive symptoms, including weak urine stream, incomplete bladder emptying, and terminal dribbling, are common in both acute bacterial prostatitis and prostatodynia. Irritative symptoms are present in all of the classifications but are more common in chronic bacterial prostatitis and prostatodynia. In addition, the patient with prostatodynia typically does not have a history of recurrent UTIs.

Objective

The practitioner should assess the patient for the signs and symptoms listed in Focusing the History 12.2. A rectal examination should be performed with care since vigorous manipulation of the prostate can result in septicemia.

Diagnostic Reasoning

Diagnostic Tests

A CBC will show leukocytosis and a shift to the left if the patient has acute bacterial prostatis. A urinalysis is done to

FOCUS ON HISTORY 12.2

Signs and Symptoms of Prostatitis

Type of Prostatitis	Common Signs and Symptoms
Acute bacterial prostatitis	General complaints: fever, chills, low back pain; malaise, arthralgia, myalgia Urinary complaints: frequency, urgency, dysuria, nocturia, bladder-outlet obstruction Physical exam: warm, tense, boggy, very tender prostate
Chronic bacterial prostatitis	General complaints: symptoms often absent, perineal pain, low back pain, lower abdominal pain, scrotal pain, penile pain, pain on ejaculation Urinary complaints: dysuria, irritative voiding Physical exam: normal, boggy, or focally indurated prostate
Nonbacterial prostatitis	Similar to chronic bacterial prostatitis Physical exam: prostate tender on palpation
Prostatodynia	General complaints: pelvic pain Urinary complaints: irritative voiding, abnormal flow

check for bacteriuria and if found then a fractional urine examination is indicated. In this test, the first 10 mL of urine in a void (VB_1), 10 mL from midstream (VB_2), expressed prostatic secretions (EPS) obtained by prostate massage, and 10 mL of urine following massage (VB_3) are obtained, cultured, and microscopically examined. If VB_1 shows the highest number of WBCs and colonies on culture, urethritis is diagnosed. If VB_2 is highest, cystitis is probable. If EPS and/or VB_3 are highest, chronic bacterial prostatitis is confirmed. Some clinicians feel that vigorous prostatic massage can lead to bacteremia; therefore, this is left up to the individual clinician's discretion. Because this test is cumbersome to perform and studies have shown that prescribing patterns do not differ substantially between clincians who do or do not perform this test, it is not necessarily done. A urine sample from a patient with nonbacterial prostatitis will show the presence of white blood cells (WBCs), but the urine culture will be negative. There are no abnormal laboratory findings associated with prostatodynia.

If a malignancy or abscess is suspected, computed tomography (CT) scanning or transrectal ultrasonography is indicated. A needle biopsy of the mass or aspiration of the abscess for culture may be done by the urologist.

Differential Diagnosis

The differential diagnosis for prostatitis includes cystitis, urethritis, pyelonephritis, epididymitis, prostatic abscess, malignancy, obstructive calculi, foreign bodies, and acute urinary retention. In the case of abscess, this is more common in men who are HIV positive. The manifestations of acute prostatitis can mimic those in acute diverticulitis, but history and laboratory tests usually differentiate between the two conditions. In the case of nonbacterial chronic prostatitis or chronic pelvic pain syndrome, the diagnosis is one of exclusion and other sources of perineal pain (hernias, testicular masses, and hemorrhoids) should be ruled out first. Asymptomatic inflammatory prostatis is not yet fully understood, and guidelines as to its natural history and need for treatment are not yet established.

Management

The main principle of management for prostatitis is to treat the patient on an outpatient basis if he does not have a fever. Hospitalization may be necessary if the patient is toxic, immunocompromised, has a proven or suspected abscess, or has signs of urosepsis.

An extremely ill patient with bacterial prostatitis should be treated in the hospital with ciprofloxacin (Cipro), 200 to 400 mg IV q12h until he has been afebrile for 24 to 48 hours, then oral ciprofloxacin 500 mg PO q12h or norfloxacin (Noroxin) 400 mg PO q12h is used to complete 4 to 6 total weeks of treatment.

Men with bacterial prostatitis may be treated on an outpatient basis for 4 to 6 weeks with antibiotics such as ofloxacin (Floxin), 400 mg PO bid q12h, ciprofloxacin 500 mg PO q12h, or norfloxacin 400 mg PO q12h. Alternatives to the quinolones are trimethoprim and sulfamethoxazole (TMP-SMX [160 mg/800 mg] Bactrim, Septra, Cotrim) one double-strength (DS) tablet q12h, or doxycycline (AK-Ramycin, AK-Ratabs, Doryx, Doxy-Caps, Doxychel Hyclate, Doxy-Lemmon, Vibramycin, Vibra-Tabs, doxycycline) 100 mg q12h.

It is extremely important that the patient with acute bacterial prostatitis be kept well hydrated. IV fluids must be given if the patient is hospitalized and is unable to consume liquids orally. Urethral catheterization is contraindicated in patients with acute bacterial prostatitis and percutaneous suprapubic catheterization is required if urinary retention develops.

The best cure rates in chronic bacterial prostatitis are associated with treatment with TMP-SMX, although other antibiotics such as carbenicillin, erythromycin, cephalexin, and the quinolones are effective as well. The patient with chronic infection is usually treated for 6 to 12 weeks.

The etiology of nonbacterial prostatitis in uncertain, but the patient may benefit from erythromycin 250 mg qid, TMP-SMX DS one tablet qd, or in combination with a fluoroquinolone. Other patients with nonbacterial prostatitis have responded to treatment with nitrofurantoin (Furadantin, Furalan, Furanite, Macrodantin, Nitrofan, Nitrofurantoin), 100 mg qd.

The irritative voiding symptoms associated with nonbacterial prostatitis may be treated with nonsteroidal, anti-inflammatory drugs (NSAIDs), muscle relaxants, anticholinergics, hot sitz pads, normal sexual activity, and regular mild exercise. Avoidance of spicy foods, caffeine, and alcohol may help some patients alleviate the irritative voiding symptoms. For patients with severe urinary retention, insertion of a suprapubic catheter may be necessary. Surgical resection for intractable chronic disease or to drain an abscess may also be performed.

Follow-Up and Referral

Depending on the acute nature of the illness and the patient's response to treatment, referral to a urologist may be warranted. The patient with hematuria or significantly elevated PSA should prompt immediate urologic referral. Patient monitoring for acute bacterial prostatitis should include a follow-up urinalysis and culture 30 days after beginning treatment. Chronic bacterial prostatitis requires urinalysis and culture every 30 days. Monitoring should continue until the patient no longer shows signs of infection. Suppression therapy with prophylactic antibiotics has also been tried if recurrent symptomatic infections occur.

Patient Education

The patient should be told that the prognosis for recovery from prostatitis is good, with a 55 to 97 percent cure rate. The cure rate depends on the population and the medications used. Prostatitis can, however, be difficult to cure and can last for a prolonged time. The National Kidney and Urologic Diseases Information Clearinghouse has printed information available for patient education.

Prostatodynia

Prostatodynia is often mistaken for prostatitis. It affects mostly young and middle-aged men and is a noninflammatory disorder that has many causes. Some of the causes include voiding dysfunction and pelvic floor dysfunction, but the prostate is normal.

Clinical Presentation

The reason that prostatodynia is mistaken for chronic prostatitis is that many of the symptoms are the same. The patient with prostatodynia may present with low back and perineal pain, hesitancy, and interruption of flow. Unlike in chronic prostatitis, there is no history of urinary tract infections with prostatodynia. On physical examination, the prostate is normal, but there may be increased anal sphincter tone and periprostatic tenderness.

Diagnostic Reasoning

Diagnostic Tests

Essentially, there are no tests that specifically diagnose prostatodynia. The urinalysis is normal, as are expressed prostatic secretions. There may be detrusor contraction without urethral relaxation, high urethral pressures, and spasms of the urinary sphincter on urodynamic tests. However, these tests are not performed unless the patient has no response after a trial of alpha-blockers or anticholinergic medication.

Differential Diagnosis

The differential diagnoses for prostatodynia include acute and chronic prostatitis and nonbacterial prostatitis. Because the urinalysis is normal, acute infection can be ruled out. The normal expressed prostatic secretions distinguish prostatodynia from nonbacterial prostatitis.

Management

The patient with prostatodynia is usually treated with alpha-blockers to reduce bladder-neck and urethral spasms. The most commonly used drugs are terazosin 1 to 10 mg PO qd or doxazosin 1 to 8 mg PO qd. Some patients benefit from warm sitz baths, while others need diazepam and biofeedback to relieve the pelvic floor muscle dysfunction. Psychotherapy is appropriate if sexual dysfunction accompanies prostatodynia.

Epididymitis

Epididymitis is an inflammation of the epididymis, the coiled structure connecting the sperm-producing rete testis to the vas deferens, allowing for maturation and immunosurveillance of the sperm. This results in scrotal pain, swelling, and induration of the posterior-lying epididymis, with eventual scrotal wall edema and involvement of the adjacent testicle, possibly with reactive hydrocele formation. The inflammation of the testicle results in a unilateral painful testicle known as *epididymo-orchitis*.

Epidemiology and Causes

There is a predisposition to epididymitis when the patient has a history of unprotected intercourse, a new sexual partner, a history of UTI with dysuria, or urethral discharge. Symptoms may also occur following heavy lifting or straining. Younger sexually active men or older men with UTI are the patients who most commonly present with epididymitis.

It may also (but rarely) occur in prepubertal boys, which likely heralds a structural abnormality in the genitourinary tract.

The causes of epididymitis in males younger than 35 years are usually sexually transmitted diseases (STDs) such as *Chlamydia* or *Neisseria gonorrhea* infections. There is usually a difference in the type of discharge. *Chlamydia* infection produces a serous urethral discharge, whereas gonorrhea produces a purulent discharge.

Causes of epididymitis in men 35 years of age and older include coliform bacteria (such as *Escherichia coli,* which is most common) and sometimes *Pseudomonas aeruginosa* or *Staphylococcus aureus.* Epididymitis is often associated with a distal urinary tract obstruction in men older than 35 years or with coliform infections in men engaging in insertive anal intercourse. Tuberculous epididymitis will present with sterile pyuria and nodularity of the vas deferens, as well as pain. Another cause of epididymitis is sterile urinary reflux following transurethral prostatectomy (TURP). A granulomatous reaction following bacille Calmette-Guérin (BCG) intravesical therapy for superficial bladder cancer may also cause epididymitis.

Rare causes of epididymitis include syphilis, brucellosis, blastomycosis, coccidioidomycosis, and cryptococcosis. When nonbacterial epididymitis and epididymo-orchitis occur, the cause is not clear, but may be secondary to retrograde extravasation of urine.

Pathophysiology

UTI, particularly prostatitis, predispose a patient to the development of epididymitis. Other risk factors include transmission of pathogens via indwelling urethral catheters or urinary instrumentation, or as a consequence of transurethral prostate surgery. A urethral stricture of any type may also be a risk factor. Epididymitis caused by STDs is transmitted through the urethra and may be accompanied by symptomatic or asymptomatic urethritis.

Other causes include immunosuppression, trauma, or reflux of urine from the urethra through the vas deferens, causing chemical inflammation and edema within the epididymis which leads to ductal obstruction. Predisposing factors for subacute presentations of epididymitis in otherwise healthy postpubertal male patients include heavy physical activity, prolonged bicycle or motorcycle riding, and sexual activity. These patients may have negative urinalyses and often do not experience dysuria.

Clinical Presentation

Subjective

The major complaint of patients with epididymitis is scrotal pain that often radiates along the spermatic cord or to the flank. The pain may appear relatively acute over several hours. Many experience pain at the tip of the penis and complain of urethral discharge or other symptoms of UTI, such as frequency of urination, dysuria, cloudy urine, or hematuria. Initially, only the lowermost tail section of the posterior-lying epididymis will be painful, tender, and indurated. Elevation of the testes and the epididymis will relieve the discomfort. Fever and chills occur with a severe infection and an abscess formation.

Objective

Physical exam reveals scrotal swelling, and the testis may be indistinguishable from the epididymis. The scrotum wall will be thick and indurated, and a reactive hydrocele may occur. In addition to nodularity of the vas deferens and tenderness of the epididymis, patients with the nonsexually transmitted variety of epididymitis will have pyuria. Rectal exam reveals a tender prostate.

Diagnostic Reasoning

Diagnostic Tests

Initially, a urinalysis will show pyuria and leukocytosis. A Gram stain of the urethral discharge may reveal gram-negative intracellular diplococci which are diagnostic of *Neisseria gonorrhoeae*. Culture of the penile discharge may be consistent with *Chlamydia* or gonorrhea infection. If no organisms are visible on the urethral smear, but WBCs are evident, the diagnosis is usually nongonococcal urethritis and *Chlamydia* is the most likely pathogen. A CBC shows increased WBCs with a left shift. Interstitial congestion and fibrotic scarring may be present. An ultrasound of the scrotum can confirm the diagnosis of epididymitis.

Differential Diagnosis

The differential diagnoses for epididymitis include epididymal congestion following a vasectomy, testicular torsion, torsion of the appendix testis, mumps, orchitis, testicular tumor, and testicular trauma. An epididymal cyst, spermatocele, hydrocele, or varicocele should also be ruled out as part of the differential diagnosis. In epididymitis, the pain often improves when the scrotum is elevated above the level of the pubic symphysis (Prehn's sign).

Management

Initial treatment includes bed rest with scrotal elevation and ice packs, along with appropriate antibiotics; in severe cases, a spermatic cord block with local anesthetics may be necessary to relieve the pain. In men younger than age 35 with sexually transmitted epididymitis, treatment is a one-time dose of ceftriaxone 250 mg IM in addition to doxycycline (Vibramycin), 100 mg bid for 10 days. If the patient is allergic to cephalosporins or tetracyclines, then a fluoroquinolone such as ofloxacin 300 mg PO bid or levofloxacin 500 mg PO qd can be given for 10 days. It is important to treat the sexual partner as well. For patients with nonsexually transmitted forms of epididymitis may be treated with ciprofloxacin 750 mg PO bid, ofloxacin 200 to 300 mg PO bid, or TMP-SMX (Bactrim, Septra), one DS tablet PO bid for 2 to 3 weeks. For patients with noninfectious epididymitis treatment is with NSAIDs, rest, and scrotal support. Antibiotic therapy is for patients who are refractory to conservative treatment. Tylenol with codeine may be used for moderate to severe pain. For the septic or toxic hospitalized patient, ceftriaxone (Rocephin), 1 to 2 g given IV or IM q24h, is the preferred treatment. An aminoglycoside (gentamicin) 1 mg/kg IV or IM q8h (adjusted to the patient's renal function after a loading dose of 2 mg/kg) may also be administered.

Surgical procedures may be needed, depending on the severity of the case. An aspiration of the hydrocele may assist in examination of the scrotal contents and relieve discomfort. A vasostomy to drain the infected material may be done as well. Scrotal exploration should be done if there is uncertainty in differentiating epididymitis from testicular torsion. Drainage of abscesses, epididymectomy, or orchiectomy may be considered in severe cases that do not respond to antibiotics. The activity of the patient following these procedures is limited to bed rest for a minimum of 1 to 2 days.

Follow-Up and Referral

Patient monitoring with office visits should continue until there are no signs of infection. Early treatment of prostatitis may prevent the development of epididymitis. Vigorous rectal examination of patients experiencing acute prostatitis should be avoided because this can lead to epididymitis. Prognosis is good if epididymitis is treated promptly. Pain improves in 1 to 3 days, but induration may last several weeks and take several months to resolve completely.

Complications of epididymitis include infertility or decreased fertility, recurrent epididymitis, abscess formation, or Fournier's gangrene (necrotizing synergistic infection), all possible when treatment is delayed or inadequate. Patients with sensory neuropathy as a result of diabetes may have little pain despite severe infections or abscesses; older adult patients may also present without significant pain.

Patient Education

The patient is instructed to limit activity and immobilize the scrotal contents which will relieve the pain and aid in treating the infection. The patient will need to wear an athletic supporter and avoid sexual contact and physical activity as long as pain persists. Patient education includes stressing the need to complete the full course of all antibiotics, even after the patient becomes asymptomatic.

Testicular Torsion

Testicular torsion is the twisting or rotation of the testes, resulting in acute ischemia. It is a urologic emergency. The torsion may vary from 90 degrees to 360 degrees about the spermatic cord. An even more common phenomenon is torsion of the testicular appendix or appendiceal torsion, in which a small vestigial remnant of the Müllerian duct located on the anterosuperior portion of the testis twists about its base.

The testis is approximately 4.5 cm × 3 cm × 2.7 cm. Within the scrotum, each testis is surrounded by the tunica albuginea, a tough layer of connective tissue, as well as the tunica vaginalis, which is a potential space formed by a membranous sac covering the anterior two-thirds of the testicle. A cryptorchid testis that fails to descend into the scrotal sac is most prone to undergoing torsion.

Epidemiology and Causes

Testicular torsion can occur at any age, from the newborn to age 80 years; however, two-thirds of the cases occur between 10 and 20 years with the peak at age 14 years. Testicular torsion is possible, but rarely occurs in older men. Torsion of the appendix testis is more common in children aged 7 to 14 years.

The contributing factors of testicular torsion are usually idiopathic and spontaneous. There is a history of trauma in 20 percent of the cases, with one-third of the patients having had prior episodic testicular pain. One initiating factor of torsion appears to be the contraction of the cremaster muscle, which may occur during sleep in approximately 50 percent of patients. The contraction of the cremaster muscle may also be stimulated by trauma, exercise (most frequently in runners), extreme cold (torsion is more common in winter months), and sexual stimulation. Paraplegics are also at high risk for developing testicular torsion, probably as a result of constant pressure while sitting. Other factors contributing to testicular torsion are possible alterations in testosterone levels and cremasteric contractions during the nocturnal sex response cycle, or a congenital abnormality of the tunica vaginalis or the spermatic cord.

Pathophysiology

If the base of the testis is inadequately fixed to the tunica vaginalis via the gubernaculum, the testis may twist around the spermatic cord under several of the conditions listed above. Arterial inflow becomes compromised and venous outflow is obstructed, resulting in ischemia of the testis. This is exquisitely painful and may lead to necrosis if it is not treated on an emergency basis. Irreversible cellular damage may result in as little as 6 to 12 hours. Even if the testis is salvaged, fertility may be permanently compromised owing to a disruption of the blood–testis immunologic barrier. This exposes germ cell antigens to the systemic circulation, resulting in sperm-specific antibodies which lead to permanent destruction of spermatozoa.

Clinical Presentation

Subjective

The most common symptom of testicular torsion is acute onset pain accompanied by swelling. Torsion of the appendices of the testis also presents with pain but it may be more gradual in onset. The patient may have pain for several days before seeking medical attention.

Objective

The most common clinical sign of testicular torsion is the absence of the cremasteric reflex. The testicle may also be high in the scrotum, with a transverse, rather than longitudinal, lie known as a "bell-clapper" deformity. Elevation of the testis does not relieve testicular pain, as is sometimes observed in epididymitis (Prehn's sign). However, this physical finding is insufficiently specific to distinguish between these two disorders. Occasionally with torsion of the appendices of the testis there may be a small lump that is palpable on the superior pole of the testis. If the skin is pulled tautly over it, the lump may appear blue ("blue dot sign"). This "blue dot" results from infarction and necrosis of the appendix testis and is present in about one fifth of cases.

Diagnostic Reasoning

Diagnostic Tests

Testicular torsion is diagnosed by the history and presenting manifestations. The only initial assessment required is a physical exam. Color Doppler ultrasonography or radionuclide scanning can be used to diagnose both testicular torsion and appendiceal torsion. Doppler ultrasound can detect an absent or reduced pulse with torsion, and an increased flow with an inflammatory process (Doppler ultrasound is reliable only in the first 12 hours following torsion). A radionuclide testicular scintigraphy with technetium 99-m (99m-Tc) pertechnetate will show absent or decreased vascularity in patients with torsion; increased vascularity will be evident in patients with inflammatory processes, including torsion of appendix testes.

Differential Diagnosis

Differential diagnoses for testicular torsion include epididymo-orchitis, an incarcerated or strangulated inguinal hernia, an acute hydrocele, a traumatic hematoma, an idiopathic scrotal edema, a torsion appendix testis, an acute varicocele, a testicular tumor, or Henoch-Schönlein purpura. Scrotal abscesses and leukemic infiltrates are also important considerations in the differential diagnosis and must be ruled out.

Some pathologic findings associated with testicular torsion include venous thrombosis, tissue edema, necrosis, and arterial thrombosis.

Management

Compression of the testicular vessels leads to ischemic necrosis of the testes within 6 hours. Failure to recognize the torsion and intervene immediately results in the loss of the testicle in 80 percent of the cases, with subsequent atrophy of the testis in 10 percent or more. Fertile resolution occurs in only 10 percent of patients.

On diagnosis, immediate referral of the patient to the emergency room is indicated. Testicular torsion is a urologic emergency. In the emergency room, manual reduction may be successful. Manual reduction of the testis is classically done with gentle external rotation of the testis toward the thigh, since most cases of torsion occur with medial rotation away from the thigh. However, retrospective studies have demonstrated lateral testicular torsion in up to one-third of cases. Relief of pain, resolution of the "bell-clapper" deformity, and a restoration of arterial blood flow are used as the primary indications of effective reduction of testicular torsion. Reduction is followed by surgical exploration. Any testis that is not clearly viable (and obvious) is removed. Surgical exploration via scrotal approach—with detorsion, evaluation of testicular viability, orchidopexy of the viable testicle, and orchidodectomy of the nonviable testicle—is the preferred surgical intervention.

For a patient with torsion of the appendix testis surgery may also be performed, but recovery is quicker, just several days. Conservative medical treatment may be initiated with rest, ice, and NSAIDs, but recovery is much slower and pain may persist from weeks to months. The dead appendiceal tissue is usually reabsorbed, though, and fertility is preserved.

Follow-Up and Referral

Testicular salvage is directly related to the duration of torsion; the salvage rate is 85 to 90 percent if torsion has persisted for less than 6 hours. The salvage rate becomes less than 10 percent if the duration of the torsion is greater than 24 hours. Depressed spermatogenesis occurs in 80 to 94 percent of individuals and may be related to the duration of ischemic injury.

Patient Education

As many as two-thirds of testes salvaged may atrophy in the first 2 to 3 years posttorsion. The possibility of testicular atrophy in a salvaged testis, with depressed sperm counts, necessitates patient education and understanding. Patients should be taught to seek immediate care when experiencing testicular pain, to prevent permanent sequelae.

Hydrocele

A *hydrocele* is a collection of peritoneal fluid within the scrotum around the testes, between the parietal and visceral (adjacent to the testis) layers of the tunica vaginalis—the two-layered sac that surrounds the testis and spermatic cord. A hydrocele forms when secretion of fluid into this potential space outweighs its reabsorption. These collections may range from only a few milliliters of fluid to enormous volumes measured in liters.

Epidemiology and Causes

The incidence rate of hydrocele is about 1 percent in adult males. Most hydroceles occur in men older than age 40 years. Causes of an acute hydrocele include nonspecific acute epididymitis, tuberculous epididymitis, trauma to the testes, tumor of the testes, or sequelae as complications of radiation therapy. Exstrophy of the bladder may increase the risk for hydrocele formation. Patients with Ehlers-Danlos syndrome have an increased risk for hydrocele, as are patients with a ventricular peritoneal shunt for dialysis or peritoneal dialysis.

Pathophysiology

A basic knowledge of scrotal anatomy is required to understand the pathogenesis of a hydrocele. The processes vaginalis originates as a diverticulum of the peritoneal sac that lines the abdomen, just inferior to the testis. During development, as the testis descends into the scrotum, it brings this diverticulum down with it, eventually becoming engulfed by it. The sac surrounding the testis (now called the tunica vaginalis) remains connected to the peritoneal sac via the processus vaginalis. Typically, throughout infancy and childhood, the connecting portion of the sac between the tunica vaginalis and the processus vaginalis gradually closes, breaking communication with the peritoneal sac.

Hydroceles in infants typically result from a patent processus vaginalis that fails to close during in utero development, allowing for the free flow of fluid between the peritoneal sac and the tunica vaginalis. These hydroceles have been directly correlated with the risk of indirect inguinal herniation in which gut contents bulge through the patent processus vaginalis. A noncommunicating hydrocele results from complete closure of the processus vaginalis, trapping peritoneal fluid within the tunica vaginalis. This type of hydrocele may be self-limited in adults. A hydrocele of the spermatic cord forms when the distal processus vaginalis closes but the midportion surrounding the cord remains patent and filled with fluid. The proximal portion may be opened or closed.

Rapidly forming hydroceles may result from reactive inflammatory processes within the scrotum such as testicular or appendiceal torsion, epididymitis, and even testicular cancer. A chronic hydrocele may result from gradual fluid accumulation within the tunica vaginalis in young boys or men, caused by an imbalance in fluid secretion, conduction, and reabsorption.

Clinical Presentation

Subjective

Patients with hydrocele typically present with swelling in the scrotum or inguinal canal. If the size of the scrotum fluctuates, a communicating hydrocele could exist. Hydroceles are usually painless, although patients report a sense of heaviness in the scrotum. If pain is present, it may radiate to the lower back.

Objective

The scrotum is transillumination with a penlight in a darkened room during the physical exam. The trapped fluid appears light pink, yellow, or red. The hydrocele can be illuminated to show the full size and shape, which assists in the diagnosis. The testes themselves do not transilluminate, nor do hematomas. Swelling may be noted in the groin or in the upper scrotum.

Diagnostic Reasoning

Diagnostic Tests

A detailed description of the events that precipitated finding the hydrocele should be obtained. Details of any trauma incurred will assist in the evaluation. If a hydrocele cannot be confirmed, the patient should be referred for an inguinoscrotal ultrasound, which can distinguish the presence or absence of bowel within the inguinal ring. A testicular nuclear scan is used to distinguish testicular torsion. Abdominal x-ray studies may be useful in distinguishing an incarcerated hernia from a hydrocele but are rarely needed.

Differential Diagnosis

The differential diagnoses for hydrocele includes indirect inguinal hernias (because of the location of the hydrocele), orchitis (inflammation or infection of the testes), or epididymitis, an inflammatory process that can produce symptoms that mimic those of a hydrocele, or varicocele. Pain is more likely to be present with epididymitis. Traumatic injury to the testes must be ruled out by history and physical exam. Torsion of the testicle, or torsion of the appendix of the testes must also be ruled out. Exploratory surgery is indicated for definitive diagnosis of a patent processus vaginalis in a communicating hydrocele. A mass of any type requires further evaluation for testicular or scrotal cancer.

Management

For adults, no treatment of a hydrocele is required unless complications are present or the clinician suspects a significant underlying cause, such as a tumor. If the hydrocele is painful, large, unsightly, or uncomfortable; however, several treatments are available. For example, a variety of outpatient surgical procedures are used to treat hydrocele. The Jaboulay-Winkelmann surgical procedure is for thick hydrocele sacs that form when the hydrocele has wrapped itself posteriorly around the cord structures. The Lord procedure is used for a thin hydrocele sac; the radial suture is used to gather the hydrocele sac posterior to the testis and the epididymis. The hydrocele can be surgically drained and the tunica vaginalis resected. Sclerotherapy (injection of a sclerotic irritant into the tunica vaginalis to induce scarring and adhesions between the adjacent layer of the tunica) and endoscopic procedures can also be performed to alleviate hydroceles. Aspiration of hydroceles is usually not done because the fluid rapidly reaccumulates; however, it may be done for a postoperative hydrocele.

Follow-Up and Referral

Patient monitoring for a hydrocele should be at 3-month intervals until the decision is made for or against surgery. Postoperatively, patient monitoring should be in 2- to 3-week intervals, followed by 2- to 3-month intervals until there is resolution.

Postoperative traumatic hydroceles are common and usually resolve spontaneously. Other possible complications may be injury to the vas deferens spermatic vessels, suture granuloma, hematoma secondary to the surgery, or a wound infection.

Patient Education

For patients with a hydrocele, no education beyond an explanation of the disease process is necessary, other than reassurance.

Varicocele

A *varicocele* is an abnormal degree of venous dilatation of the pampiniform plexus above the testes, which usually results in pain and engorgement of the testis.

Epidemiology and Causes

There is no ethnic predisposition or age differentiation among patients with varicoceles. The overall rate of incidence is 8 to 20 percent. In men evaluated for infertility, however, the rate of varicocele increases to 25 to 40 percent. A weak wall in the spermatic vein or excessive pressure are the leading causes of varicoceles.

Pathophysiology

The pathophysiology of a varicocele results from vascular engorgement of the internal spermatic vein. A varicocele almost always appears on the left or bilaterally, because the left spermatic (gonadal) vein empties into the left renal vein, whereas the right spermatic vein empties into the inferior vena cava. One of the longest veins in the body, the left spermatic vein, empties into the renal vein at a perpendicular angle. Compared to the right renal vein, the left renal vein has a higher intravascular pressure owing to its anatomic positioning between the aorta inferiorly and the superior mesenteric artery. In turn, if the valves of the left renal vein become incompetent because of this increased pressure, retrograde blood flow causes back-pressure to be transmitted to the pampiniform venous plexus which overlies the testis. In contrast, a unilateral right-sided varicocele may result from serious pathology causing increased pressure within the inferior vena cava, such as a tumor or thrombus.

Clinical Presentation

Subjective

The patient may present with pain and engorgement of the testes. The recognition of a varicocele is usually secondary to a problem with fertility, however. A patient with a varicocele often describes the sensation as feeling like a "bag of worms."

Objective

On physical exam, with the patient in an upright position, tortuous veins located posterior to and above the testis can be assessed. The engorged veins may extend up into the external inguinal ring, depending on development. Venous dilatation can be increased by having the patient perform the Valsalva maneuver in a recumbent position. The reverse is also true: In the recumbent position, the venous distension will abate. Testicular atrophy with impaired circulation may be present.

Diagnostic Reasoning

Diagnostic Tests

A system of grading has been established to better define varicocele. A *grade 1* varicocele is one that is palpable only when the patient performs the Valsalva maneuver. A *grade 2* varicocele is palpable when the patient is standing. A *grade 3* varicocele may be assessed with light palpation and visual inspection.

Sperm counts and motility of the sperm are significantly decreased in patients with a varicocele approximately 65 to 75 percent of the time. There is evidence of a progressive decline in fertility in men with varicocele. Scrotal ultrasound, venography (shows testicular venous reflux from a varicocele), and thermography (shows increase in temperature at the varicocele) all help to confirm the diagnosis.

Differential Diagnosis

A differential diagnosis for varicocele must include a hydrocele, a spermatocele, testicular tumor, epididymal cyst, and a renal tumor. A diagnostic priority is questioning the patient. It is essential to note whether the onset of the varicocele has been rapid or has resulted from a gradual increase in the varices of the testicles. In an elderly patient, the development of a varicocele may be a late sign of a renal tumor.

Management

After a varicocele has been diagnosed, referral to a surgeon is indicated although most patients do not require surgery because most varicoceles are minor. Surgical treatment of a varicocele involves ligation of the internal spermatic vein, which usually results in decompression of the varicocele and improvement of the quality of semen as well as decrease in the pain. The surgery can be either laparoscopic, anteriorly via an inguinal or subinguinal approach, or posteriorly via a lumbar approach, or even microsurgical. Embolization with coils is a second-line approach, but appears to have a higher complication rate owing to migration of the coils. Testicular atrophy is a definite indication for treatment. Conservative treatment in older men with only minor pain or for whom fertility is no longer an issue or for men with normal fertility may consist of NSAIDs and scrotal support. Treatment has not consistently improved sperm count or fertility in controlled trials.

Follow-Up and Referral

Complications of a varicocele (if not corrected) include infertility and testicular atrophy. A referral to a urologist is indicated and recommended for affirmation of the diagnosis and further explanation of treatment options. Any patient with a recent onset of varicocele, infertility, pain, or testicular atrophy should have a urology consult.

Patient Education

Education for the patient should include an explanation of the disease process, signs, symptoms, and implications. The patient should be taught how to monitor growth and symptoms of the varicocele, especially if it is right sided. To relieve pain, the patient should be encouraged to wear a scrotal support; for some patients, wearing jockey shorts (briefs) rather than loose boxer shorts is sufficient to relieve discomfort.

Prostate Cancer

To properly understand the pathophysiology, diagnosis, and treatment of carcinoma of the prostate, a brief review of prostatic anatomy is warranted. The prostate is composed of acinar glands and their ducts, which are arranged in a radial fashion with the stroma containing blood vessels, lymph vessels, and nerves. Ninety-five percent of all prostate cancers are acinar adenocarcinomas. The prostate gland secretes 0.5 to 2 mL of fluid a day, and this constitutes 10 to 20 percent of the seminal fluid of the ejaculate. The prostatic fluid contains citric acid, prostaglandins, and fibrinogen. The epithelial cells of the prostate gland are the only source of the glycoprotein prostate-specific antigen (PSA).

The prostate lies between the base of the urinary bladder and the upper surface of the levator ani and deep transverse peritoneal muscles. The anterior surface is adjacent to the retropubic space; the posterior surface lies adjacent to the seminal vesicles and recto-vesicular (rectum–bladder) septum.

The prostate is palpable per rectum. The prostate gland is 2 to 3 cm across and its midpoint is twice the breadth of the examining finger. A 20-g size is normal. A slightly enlarged gland is documented as +1, and is considered three finger-breadths across, with +2 being twice the normal breadth. Occasionally a +3 or +4 classification will present, which involves the anterior pelvic outlet with marked encroachment of the posterior lobe on the rectal wall, reducing the caliber of the rectal passage. A normal prostate posterior area can be palpated without moving the hand, but the clinician may need to move the hand side to side in order to palpate an enlarged prostate or nodular area.

The prostate gland is subdivided into five lobes, which include the left and right lateral lobes (which are extensive and make up what was formerly termed the anterior lobe), the left and right posterior lobes (which also include the apex of the gland), and the median lobe. Prostatic cancer is known to have a propensity for the gland's posterior and apical peripheral zone (thus palpable through the rectal wall), while benign prostatic hypertrophy tends to affect the transition zone that surrounds the urethra.

Epidemiology and Causes

Prostate cancer is the most common cancer found in American men and ranks second in the number of cancer deaths (lung cancer is number one). In fact, more than 40 percent of men older than 50 years of age have been found to have prostate cancer on autopsy and the prevalence increases with age. Clinical incidence of prostatic carcinoma is highest in North America and Europe and lowest in the Far East, suggesting that there may be environmental or dietary factors that increase prostate growth. In American men, those at highest risk for prostate cancer are African Americans, men with a family history of prostate cancer, and men with a diet high in fat, particularly animal fat.

Recently a major susceptibility focus for prostate cancer was found on chromosome one and is still under investigation. A man with a first-degree relative (a father or a brother) with prostate cancer is twice as likely to develop the disease and to do so at an earlier age. Occupational and environmental risks for development of prostate cancer include exposure to cadmium nitrates and heavy metals. As an occupational group, farmers are at the highest risk for development of prostate cancer. Further investigation continues on the subject of occupations as a risk factor.

Smoking has also been identified as a risk factor for prostate cancer; the risk appears to be proportional to the amount of smoking the patient does and may be related to the cadmium content of cigarettes. A patient's endogenous hormonal influences, characterized by increased levels of testosterone, have been shown to contribute to increased risk.

Pathophysiology

Prostate cancer is believed to result from a sequential accumulation of genetic abnormalities affecting the androgen receptors on prostatic tissue. These defects have been characterized as either genetic predispositions to disease which are seen to run in families (e.g., deletions in chromosome 1q), somatic mutations that activate prostatic oncogenes such as c-*myc*, *MKP-1, bcl-2,* and telomerase (e.g., mutations in the 7p and 8q regions), and somatic mutations that inactivate tumor suppressor genes such as *PTEN/MMAC-1, Mxi1, GSTP1, TGF-β1,* and *Rb* (e.g., mutations in the 8p, 10q, 12q, 13q, and 17p regions). Such mutations accumulate over time, thus accounting for the strong correlation between age and disease prevalence.

The degree of malignancy may be graded according to several different scales. One method (Jewett system) utilizes the following stages:

A1–A2 and B1–B2 neoplasms are confined within the capsule.
C1 has extension of the carcinoma beyond the capsule.
C2 has malignancy that involves the seminal vesicles
D1 involves metastatic disease in the regional lymph nodes, and
D2 involves metastatic disease in bone or other organs.

The left and right posterior lobes of the prostate are most predisposed to malignant transformation. Extensive carcinoma may involve the capsule and the periprostatic tissues. Carcinomas of the prostate usually extend to the base of the bladder and the region of the seminal vesicles to form a shelf or a plateau. Usually, the periprostatic spread is limited by Denonvilliers' fascia, but once this area has been invaded, circumferential extension about the rectum occurs.

The lethality of malignant prostate cancers is a direct function of the heterogeneity in their cellular composition, which consists of both androgen-sensitive and androgen-insensitive cells. Anti-testosterone therapies work by suppressing androgen which itself represses pro-apoptotic genes in cancer cells that would otherwise lead to cellular death. However, the apoptosis (non-necrotic or programmed cell death) of androgen-insensitive cancer cells is not induced by anti-androgen therapies. Through progressive genetic mutations, the androgen receptors on cancerous prostatic tissue are increased in number, level of androgen-independent activity, and resistance to apoptotic death signals from tumor suppressor genes. This accounts for the progressive and inevitably increased androgen insensitivity of malignant prostatic tissue and, in turn, the persistent spread of disease.

Clinical Presentation

Subjective

Men with prostate cancer are usually asymptomatic early in the disease and may also be asymptomatic late in the disease. Latent symptoms include bone pain, weight loss, anemia, shortness of breath, lymphedema, and lymphadenopathy. Neurologic symptoms (inability to perceive touch, pain, and temperature in the perineal or scrotal areas and a lack of sensation of bladder distension) occur with epidural metastasis and cord compression. Patient complaints also include bladder-outlet symptoms or acute urinary retention with very large or locally extensive tumors, but are most often due to BPH.

Objective

Rectal exam reveals a palpable hard prostate that may be localized or diffused; several hard areas may be present or the nodules may be limited to one hardened area. An induration of the prostate may also be noted. Hematuria and hemospermia are signs that appear late in the course of the disease; they are very rarely detected in early prostate cancer. Evaluation of the rectal sphincter, and the anal and bulbocavernosus reflex, directs attention to the possible lesion at the level of the conis.

Diagnostic Reasoning

Diagnostic Tests

PSA is prostate specific but not cancer specific (found only in the cytoplasm of benign and malignant prostate cells). The effectiveness of using PSA in screening programs for prostate cancer has been questioned because of the lack of evidence that routine screening for PSA can improve the quality and quantity of life for the overall population. The American Cancer Society (ACS) and American Urological Association (AUA) recommend the use of PSA-based screening programs in conjunction with DRE to detect prostate cancer in men age 50 years or older. The predominant age range for onset of prostate cancer is 50 to 60 years, which influences the recommendations for screening. Although approximately 67 percent of men 80 years of age have prostate cancer, only about 3 percent are expected to die from it.

Research continues on PSA levels as a viable means of identification and the goal is to increase the specificity of this test. Recent studies indicate that any level of PSA may be a warning sign for cancer, but what is apparently more important is how rapidly the PSA rises. In one recent study, the risk of dying from prostate cancer was directly related to the rate of increase the year preceding the diagnosis. A PSA level greater than 4.0 ng/mL is considered positive. A level of 4.1 ng/mL is the threshold for performing prostate biopsy, however at this threshold 82 percent of prostate cancer in men younger than 60 years is missed and 65 percent is missed in older men. There is some suggestion that the biopsy threshold be lowered to 2.6 ng/mL for younger men but this could lead to unnecessary biopsies because the sensitivity of the PSA is low, anywhere from 18 to 68 percent. Utilizing age-specific PSA norms (shown in Table 12.4) may increase the accuracy of the PSA test for diagnosis of prostate cancer. If serial screening for PSA levels shows an increase greater than 20 percent or 0.75 ng/mL in 1 year, this is considered a positive finding; serial PSAs are thought to be more accurate than a single test.

In any case, the ACS, AUA, and the American College of Physicians (ACP) all recommend that the health-care provider have an open discussion with patients about the pros and cons of prostate cancer screening, as discussed in this section, and decide on a mutually agreeable course of action based on the patient's individual risk of developing

Table 12.4 Age-Specific Reference Ranges for Prostate-Specific Antigen (PSA)

Age	Reference Ranges PSA
40–49	0–2.5 ng/mL
50–59	0–3.5 ng/mL
60–69	0–4.5 ng/mL
70–79	0–6.5 ng/mL

prostate cancer and the implications of such a diagnosis (morbidity and mortality of both cancer and its treatment). If screening is agreed to, it should begin at 50 years for most men, and at age 45 for African American men or those with a strong family history, especially in a father or brother. Screening may stop by 75 years or in those with severe health problems, as prostate cancer is unlikely to be the cause of death for the large majority of these patients.

If prostate cancer is suspected (PSA greater than 10), the patient should be referred to a urologist for a TRUS (transrectal ultrasound) and a transrectal biopsy of the prostate. The identification of any malignancies using TRUS-guided biopsy is not only a conclusive finding; this diagnostic procedure also provides information that is helpful in staging the disease and planning subsequent treatment, which may include radiation and chemotherapy. Prostate screening using a combination of DRE, TRUS, and PSA with age-related values provides the most positive, predictive value of diagnosing prostate cancer. The potential complications of the TRUS-guided biopsy are hematospermia, hematuria, fever, hematochezia, or rectal bleeding. Biopsy may be repeated if initial results are negative and cancer is highly suspected. Free PSA levels in the bloodstream have also been tested as a screening tool and criteria for patients to have a follow-up TRUS. Free PSA occurs in greater concentrations in men without prostate cancer. Alternatively, the ratio of complex PSA to a total PSA is greater in individuals with prostate cancer. Complex PSA is PSA bound to the protease inhibitor alpha-1-antichymotrypsin, which is the form that is most elevated in prostate cancer. The predicted value is 24 percent, based on patients who underwent biopsies after having had the free PSA test.

Another group of researchers has been using the prostate-specific antigen density (PSAD) to screen for prostate cancer. PSAD can help differentiate BPH from prostate cancer because it is calculated by dividing the PSA by the volume of the prostate that is estimated by TRUS. Alkaline phosphatase is typically elevated in patients with metastases, but this finding is not specific for cancer of the prostate. Further studies that are done in patients with prostate cancer include a bone scan, which may show the presence of metastases. CT of the pelvic lymph nodes, ultrasound of the prostate, lymphoscintigraphy, and magnetic resonance imaging (MRI) are alternate techniques that show metastases. On the horizon are molecular diagnostic tests on the urine postprostatic massage that detect highly specific genetic markers of prostate cancer, such as DNS hypermethylation (i.e., inactivation) of the genetic promoter for the tumor suppressor gene glutathione *S*-transferase (*GSTP1*).

Differential Diagnosis

BPH is the number one differential diagnosis in someone with suspected prostate cancer because the urinary outlet symptoms of nocturia, frequency, hesitancy, and weak urinary stream can be seen with both conditions but are far more commonly due to BPH. New-onset ED, hematuria, or hematospermia are less common presentations of prostate cancer. Other differential diagnoses for prostate cancer include a benign nodule, prostate stones, nodular whorls, and seminal vesicle enlargement.

Management

Unfortunately, neither chemotherapy nor immunotherapy can cure prostate cancer once it has spread beyond the gland. If the findings are positive on both DRE and PSA, the patient should be referred to a urologist for a definitive diagnosis (biopsy) and staging.

Staging

Prostate tumors are classified according to the Gleason system in which first a "grade" is applied to the architectural pattern of the cancer in the largest segment of the specimen and then a second "grade" is given to the next largest area. The pathologist adds the two scores together to produce the Gleason score, which is on a scale of 1 to 10. Accurate staging provides an indication of the best treatment options.

Gleason score 1–4: Indicates a well-differentiated cancer that is likely to be slow growing.
Gleason score 5–7: Indicates a moderately differentiated cancer.
Gleason score 8–10: Indicates poorly differentiated cancer cells that are likely to be aggressive and rapid growing.

Prostate cancer is further staged according to the extent of the tumor, based on additional diagnostic studies or findings at the time of surgery. The most commonly used staging system is the American Joint Committee on Cancer tumor–node–metastasis (TNM) system, which grades tumors numerically within more detailed subcategories: "T" describes *tumors* according to their degree of differentiation; "N" describes the extent of *node* involvement; and "M" describes the degree of *metastasis*. For example, T1 tumors are microscopic, nonpalpable, and not visible by TRUS. Tumors classified as T2 are palpable but not beyond the prostate itself, and T3 tumors go beyond the capsule or into the seminal vesicles. T4 tumors are fixed and extend far beyond the prostate. Prostate cancer extending beyond the prostate itself is often fatal and treatment is typically only palliative, as opposed to localized disease, which is often curable by surgery, radiation therapy, and/or chemotherapy.

Patients Older than Age 70

Patients older than age 70 years are usually offered conservative treatment as an alternative to surgery. Radiation external beam therapy or brachytherapy with implants and total androgen ablation are the general measures that are used to treat prostate cancer in older men.

Patients Younger than Age 70

If the patient is younger than 70 years of age, aggressive surgery is recommended for a prostate cancer cure. Surgical interventions may be used for Jewett stages A and B and selected C stages. If the patient is in agreement, an orchidectomy may be warranted for the ablation of the hormonal effects.

The standard treatment options for prostate cancer include radical prostatectomy, radiation therapy, and watchful waiting. Treatment decisions are based more often on the adverse effects, long-term risks, and financial and emotional costs of different therapies. Young healthy patients often are encouraged to undergo the most radical treatment, whereas older patients are often directed to watchful waiting (observation) or radiotherapy.

Other treatments for prostate cancer include hormonal therapy to inhibit cancer growth by testosterone deprivation, or administration of endogenous estrogen to block the release of luteinizing hormone (LH) from the hypothalamus. Unfortunately, estrogen therapy is associated with hypocoagulopathy, cardiomegaly, and gynecomastia. Newer hormone preparations include leuprolide (Lupron) and goserelin acetate (Zoladex), which also block the release of follicle-stimulating hormone (FSH) and LH. These agents are administered IM monthly. Adverse affects include loss of libido and hot flashes. Oral anti-androgens are also available, including asflutamide (Casodex) or flutamide (Eulexin), which inhibit the binding of testosterone to the cancer cells. Finasteride (Proscar) is used to block the enzyme 5-alpha-reductase, which converts testosterone into dihydrotestosterone.

Cryosurgical ablation of the prostate is used to destroy cancer cells in patients who have had negative bone scans for metastatic prostate cancer. Cryosurgery destroys the prostate cancer cells through freezing. Unfortunately, the major adverse effects of this ablation technique include possible destruction of nerves and/or circulation, which can cause incontinence and ED.

Some research indicates that lifestyle modification in conjunction with "watchful waiting" improves the attitudes of men with early stage prostate cancer. (See Nursing Research-Based Practice 12.1.)

Follow-Up and Referral

Patient follow-up is determined by the radiation oncologist and urologist. Without fail, the patient should have a clinical examination every 3 months for a year; with PSA screening every 3 months and then every 6 months. Chest x-ray studies and bone scans should be done every 6 months for a year and yearly thereafter. Potential complications of treatment may include cardiac failure, phlebitis, and pathologic fractures secondary to the hormonal changes (testosterone suppression), as well as those mentioned in the previous section. With early diagnosis and treatment, the expected

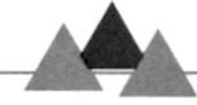

NURSING RESEARCH-BASED PRACTICE 12.1

The Prostate Cancer Lifestyle Trial

Kronenwetter, C, et al: A qualitative analysis of interviews of men with early stage prostate cancer. Cancer Nurs 28(2):99–107, 2005.

There is no conclusive evidence that any one treatment for early prostate cancer is better than the others. There have been studies that indicate the quality of life for those undergoing prostatectomy have better quality of life scores in non-cancer–related areas, whereas those in the "watchful waiting" group scored lower in these areas but scored higher in the areas of sexual and urinary function.

This article reports the results of the Prostate Cancer Lifestyle Trial (PCLT) which included men who opted for watchful waiting and improving their diet, exercise, and stress management and also included attending a support group. The patients were prescribed an intensive lifestyle program including a very low fat vegan diet with supplemental soy, fish oil, and vitamin E; an exercise program that included 30 minutes of aerobic exercise 6 days a week; stress management techniques that included yoga, breathing, meditation, imagery, and progressive relaxation of 1 hour every day; and a 1-hour support group once a week.

The researchers found that the PCLT participants began with feelings of anxiety, fear, distress, and vulnerability after hearing of the cancer diagnosis, but with the program they found a sense of hope, optimism, and fighting spirit. The researchers attribute these positive emotions to the peer community that was built during the study. The improvement in lifestyle behaviors was related to enhanced quality of life and reduced perceived stress. Change to a healthy lifestyle was an important adjunct to watchful waiting contributing to a positive quality of life.

prognosis is good and lesions should be curable, especially in young, healthy males.

Once prostate cancer has been diagnosed and treatment regimens have been chosen and implemented, the patient will be followed by the specialist, but will be seen by the primary-care clinician for regular health maintenance, reassurance, positive outlook, and laboratory test follow-up.

Patient Education

Support groups and other organizations for prostate cancer patients are available, along with books on the subject, including reports from prostate cancer survivors. Even churches are being used as a forum for patient education. It is extremely important for the clinician to be knowledgeable regarding the latest diagnostic and treatment options for prostate cancer, as well as aware of patients' desires and fears.

Testicular Cancer

Primary testicular neoplasms may arise from any testicular or adnexal cell component. Each testes is covered externally by two layers of fascia: the outer layer, the tunica vaginalis; and the deeper albuginea layer, which extends internally and divides the testis into 250 to 300 lobules. Each lobule contains seminiferous tubules (the site of spermatogenesis), and the interstitial cells that produce androgens including testosterone. The epididymis lies along the external surface of each testes and is the site of sperm maturation and storage. Tumors of the germ cells and the seminiferous tubules are the most common testicular carcinomas.

Epidemiology and Causes

Although testicular malignancies comprise only 1 to 2 percent of all neoplasms in males, the psychologically and physically debilitating effects of testicular cancer affecting young men between ages 15 and 35 years deserve mention, as testicular cancer is the most common solid malignancy in the age group. Fortunately, it is also one of the most curable of solid cancers.

In the United States, there are two to three new cases of testicular cancer per year per 100,000 males. It is less common in African Americans, at 0.9 cases per 100,000. In adults, germ-cell types comprise 90 to 95 percent of testicular cancers, and in boys they represent 60 to 75 percent. The peak age at onset is between age 20 and 40 years. Smaller peaks occur between birth and 10 years of age and in men older than age 60 years.

No clear cause-and-effect relationships are identified for testicular cancer. Risk factors for testicular cancer include HIV infection, Caucasian race (especially Scandinavian background), with a much lower incidence among African Americans. Men who have experienced undescended or partially descended testes (cryptorchidism) are at a much higher risk for testicular cancer. Prior cryptorchidism is the only undisputed risk factor for this type of cancer, with 10 percent of testicular tumors associated with this condition. Importantly, a fourth of these tumors occur in the contralateral, descended testis.

Other possible risk factors that have been identified for testicular cancer include higher social status, being unmarried, or living in a rural area. Weak associations demonstrate that hormonal imbalances associated with in utero exposure to estrogen may increase the risk for testicular cancer later in life. One study of mothers who used diethylstilbesterol (DES) during the first trimester found a 2.5- to 5-fold increase of testicular cancer in a son.

Pathophysiology

Primary testicular neoplasm may arise from any testicular adnexal cell component. These are divided into germinal (90 to 95 percent) and nongerminal (sex cord–stromal) tumors. For treatment purposes, the germinal tumors are further divided equally based on histology into seminomas and nonseminomas (i.e., embryonal carcinomas, teratomas, choriocarcinomas, and yolk sac tumors), which are epithelial in nature. In contrast, far rarer are the sex cord-stromal tumors, which consist primarily of Leydig cell variants that produce estrogen due to increased aromatase activity and Sertoli cell tumors which may also present with estrogenic overload.

Only a small number of molecular markers have been consistently associated with testicular cancers, for example, an isochromosome of chromosome 12p, activating mutations in c-*kit*, increased p53 and telomerase expression. Abnormal DNA ploidy is also common in germ cell tumors. Although certain genetic alterations differ in germ cell tumors found in prepubertal males, all germ cell tumors are believed to arise from pluripotential primordial germ cells. One exception to this is the relatively rare spermatocytic seminoma, the pathogenesis of which appears to be fundamentally different based on unique molecular markers.

Except for spermatocytic seminomas, all germ cell tumors may be preceded by a premalignant condition known as intratubular germ cell neoplasia of unclassified type (ITGCNU) or testicular carcinoma in situ. It is found adjacent to 90 percent of germ cell tumors, implying that genetic mutations lead to gonadal dysfunction and subsequent malignancy over a large area of tissue—a phenomenon known as a field defect. At least half the cases of untreated ITGCNU will progress to invasive malignant disease within 5 years, predictably spreading to the retroperitoneal draining lymph nodes. Men with a history of cryptorchidism are recommended to have empiric testicular biopsy between the ages of 18 to 20 years to evaluate for ITGCNU.

Clinical Presentation

Subjective

Typically, the patient with testicular cancer presents with a hard lump or nodule on his testis that he felt while performing a testicular self-exam. He may also note scrotal swelling, heaviness in the scrotum that may be interpreted as pain, a sensation of fullness, or a previously small testis that has enlarged to the size of a normal testis or the contralateral testis. Generally, testicular cancer presents as a painless enlargement of the testis.

Objective

During routine physical exams (sports physical) a scrotal nodule or swelling is most commonly detected in men with testicular cancer. A firm, nontender mass within the confines of the tunica albuginea is usual, palpable, and distinct from the spermatic cord structures. Acute or chronic epididymitis or epididimo-orchitis may result in delay of diagnosis of testicular cancer in about 10 percent of the cases. Gynecomastia may be present in 5 percent of patients with testicular malignancies. Hydroceles (seen in 5 to 10 percent of patients) may be secondary to testicular cancer.

As many as 10 percent of patients with testicular cancer will be asymptomatic and another 10 percent will present with manifestions of metastasis. Symptoms of metastases include respiratory symptoms (cough) due to lung metastases; low back pain and nerve root or psoas muscle irritation due to retroperitoneal metastasis; or lower extremity swelling from vena cava obstruction

Diagnostic Reasoning

Diagnostic Tests

Several biochemical markers can aid in the diagnosis of testicular carcinoma, but their main use is in following disease progression or remission post-treatment (looking at trends). These tests include human chorionic gonadotropin (hCG), alpha-fetoprotein (AFP), and lactate dehydrogenase (LDH). AFP levels are elevated by the pure embryonal carcinoma, teratocarcinoma, yolk sac tumor, or combinations of these three malignancies, but not by pure choriocarcinoma or seminoma. However, AFP may be elevated in benign liver disease, telangiectasis, tyrosinemia, and malignancies of the liver, pancreas, stomach, and lung. Heavy marijuana smoking can also elevate levels of alpha-fetoprotein. HCG levels are elevated by all choriocarcinomas and occasionally in seminomas, however, it is also elevated in liver, lung, pancreatic, and stomach malignancies, as well as by kidney, breast, and bladder tumors. Forty to 60 percent of patients with an embryonal carcinoma, and 5 to 10 percent of patients with seminomas have detectable levels of hCG (usually under 500 ng/mL). Testing for lactate dehydrogenase (LDH) has fallen into disfavor because of the ubiquitous nature of the test. An elevated LDH level may be the sole biochemical abnormality in 10 percent of patients who have persistent or recurrent seminomatous tumors, and other liver function tests are elevated in the presence of hepatic metastases. In general, elevated AFP, hCG, or LDH is a poor prognostic sight and prognosis worsens with the level of elevation. Elevated placental alkaline phosphatase (PLAP) may be the marker of choice for seminomas in 70 to 90 percent of patients. Patients with recurrent or disseminated seminomas have elevated PLAP levels. PLAP may also be elevated by heavy tobacco smoking.

Scrotal ultrasound is also a useful diagnostic tool for testicular cancer. The mass can be seen clearly originating within the testis. Using an echo-texture (hypoechoic) pattern, the mass will appear distinct from the surrounding normal testicular tissue on ultrasound. Uniformly cystic or fluid-filled masses are not likely to be testicular cancer, which is a solid tumor. However, ultrasound is not accurate for staging and should not replace orchiectomy as the procedure of choice. MRI is not usually more informative than scrotal ultrasound and pelvic/abdominal CT for staging and identifying enlarged retroperitoneal lymph nodes, implying the need for lymph node dissection. Positron emission tomography (PET) scanning is usually used only to identify residual masses post-treatment.

Chest x-ray studies, with both posterior–anterior (PA) and lateral views, are important for identification of metastasis. They will also rule out spread of malignancy above the diaphragm. A CT scan is accurate and able to define pelvic retroperitoneal and mediastinal lymphadenopathy, as well as to detect metastases to the abdominal viscera.

Differential Diagnosis

Definitive diagnosis of testicular cancer may be made with a transinguinal scrotal exploration and biopsy, and/or radical orchidectomy (excision of the testicle and spermatic cord). Transscrotal open or cutaneous biopsy and transscrotal orchidectomy are contraindicated because of the potential for anatomic trespassing into the various lymph-drainage systems. The differential diagnosis for testicular cancer should include epididymitis, hernia, hydrocele, hematoma, spermatocele, syphilitic gumma, and a varicocele; however, testicular cancer is typically a painless mass in the testis.

Management

The main principle of management for testicular cancer is a radical orchidectomy, which is also the major diagnostic tool, because the whole testis is removed for biopsy. Testicular cancer is very treatable, with fewer than 400 deaths per year in the United States at the present time. Treatment does, however, leave the patient with a high possibility of being infertile. Sperm-banking (semen cryopreservation) should be done prior to radiographic diagnostic studies, if desired. Many of these men have gonadal dysgenesis with baseline sperm count and morphology problems, but banking in general works well and future children do not have higher rates of congenital defects fathered by this banked sperm.

Staging

Testicular carcinoma is divided into two main categories when considering treatment. The first category, nonseminomas, includes embryonal cell carcinomas (20 percent), teratomas (5 percent), choriocarcinomas (less than 1 percent), and mixed cell types (40 percent). The second category is seminomas (35 percent). Nonseminoma germ cell tumors are staged as:

Stage A—lesion confined to testis
Stage B—regional lymph node involvement in retroperitoneum
Stage C—distant metastasis
Seminomas are staged using the M.D. Anderson system:
Stage I—lesion confined to testis
Stage II—spread to retroperitoneal lymph nodes
Stage III—supradiaphragmatic nodal or visceral involvement

The TNM classification of the American Joint Cancer Committee is also used for testicular cancer. The primary tumor (T) is classed from T0 (no evidence of primary tumor) to T4 (invades scrotum). Lymph node assessment (N) is from N0 (no regional lymph node metastasis) to N3 (metastasis in lymph node greater than 5 cm). Distant metastasis (M) is classified from M0 (no distant metastasis) to M1b (distant metastasis to sites other than nonregional lymph nodes or lungs).

Seventy-five percent of nonseminomas can be cured with orchiectomy alone, usually with modified retroperitoneal lymph node dissection. This is done to preserve the sympathetic innervation so the patient will still have ejaculatory function. The serum markers are monitored postorchiectomy and those that return to normal have an excellent prognosis. For patients with nonseminomas that have metastasized or who have significant lymph node involvement (greater than 3 cm), combination chemotherapy is used following orchiectomy. Commonly used chemotherapeutic agents include cisplatin (Platinol) and etoposide (VePesid) and bleomycin (Blenoxane), or paclitaxel (Taxol). If the serum tumor markers do not normalize after chemotherapy, then salvage chemotherapy is needed. Salvage chemotherapy includes cyclophosphamide (Cytoxan)- or ifosfamide (Ifex)-based protocols, with mesna (Mesnex) to protect against hemorrhagic cystitis.

The 5-year survival rate for those with stage A nonseminomas is 96 to 100 percent after treatment. Patients with stage B nonseminomas have almost a 90 percent 5-year survival rate after treatment. For those patients with stage C nonseminomas the 5-year survival rate is between 55 and 80 percent.

Seminomas are chemosensitive and have good chemotherapeutic response and are also extremely sensitive to radiation therapy. All patients with seminomas will have radical orchidectomy surgery and then, depending on the stage, irradiation and chemotherapy will be used. For patients with stage I and stage IIa (retroperitoneal disease less than 10 cm) surgery and radiation are the treatments of choice and are associated with a 5-year survival of 98 percent and 92 to 94 percent, respectively. More advanced stage II (retroperitoneal disease greater than 10 cm) and stage III seminomas received primary chemotherapy either with etoposide and cisplatin or a combination of cisplatin, etoposide, and bleomycin. If enlarged lymph nodes (more than 3 cm in diameter) persist after chemotherapy, then a retroperitoneal lymph-node resection is done. In 40 percent of cases there is residual carcinoma in these lymph nodes. Ninety-five percent of patients with stage III seminoma have a complete response to orchiectomy and chemotherapy. A viable tumor is present in more than 40 percent of cases. Primary chemotherapy is a last resort.

As with all chemotherapeutic agents, the precautions are specific for each. Cisplatin causes ototoxicity, nephrotoxicity, and neurotoxicity. Etoposide may cause thrombocytopenia. Cyclophosamide and ifosfamide may cause hemorrhagic cystitis. Patients must be well hydrated to minimize the risk of hemorrhagic cystitis. Patients receiving ifosfamide should also receive mesna to reduce the risk of hemorrhagic cystitis. Bleomycin causes pulmonary fibrosis. One alternative drug may be carboplatin (Paraplatin), which can cause ototoxicity. Ondansetron (Zofran), dronabinol (Marinol), and metoclopramide (Reglan) and other medications may be used to control nausea. Follow-up is extremely important for patients with testicular malignancies.

Follow-Up and Referral

For the first 2 years, tumor markers and chest x-ray films are assessed every month, and a physical exam emphasizing the lymph nodes should be performed monthly. After the first 2 years, tumor markers and chest x-ray films are checked every 2 months and the physical exam should be done every 2 to 4 months for another year. CT scans are usually done every 3 to 4 months for the initial 3 years. After year 3 with no further symptoms, the tumor markers, chest x-ray studies, and physical exams should be done every 6 to 12 months. If a patient had a diagnosis of teratoma, he will need to have a follow-up for at least 5 years, however, and a CT scan every year for 3 years. Radiation therapy can cause extreme fatigue and interfere with sperm production; it can also cause diarrhea, vomiting, and skin reaction at the treatment site. Adverse effects of chemotherapy include hair loss, immunosuppression, loss of appetite, and nausea and vomiting. Complications from retroperitoneal lymph node dissection include loss of seminal emission and/or hypoalbuminemia. Radiation treatment may cause nephritis or enteritis. Nonseminotamous tumors are more likely (50 to 70 percent) to metastasize than seminomas (25 percent). Men who have been cured of testicular cancer in one testicle have a 2 to 4 percent chance of developing cancer in the remaining testicle. If cancer develops in the other testicle, it is almost always a new cancer, however, and not a metastasis from the first episode.

Patient Education

The question of life after testicular cancer becomes extremely important to the patient. The patient must be able to cope with the way testicular cancer affects his self-image. A low sperm count may occur after the loss of a testis. Patients need to be informed that losing a testis will not affect their ability to have a prosthesis to simulate the weight and feel of a testicle. Although surgery to remove lymph nodes does not compromise a man's ability to have an erection or reach orgasm, it can interfere with ejaculation. Some men naturally regain the ability to ejaculate; others require medication. A patient should also be educated about sterility and hormone supplements. The option of sperm banking should be discussed with patients when the diagnosis of testicular cancer is first confirmed. Open discussions and reassurance are extremely important in patients diagnosed with testicular cancer.

The importance of a monthly testicular self-exam (TSE) cannot be stressed enough. Males ages 15 to 40 should be instructed on TSE at each primary care visit and the technique should be demonstrated. Advanced Practice Nursing Interventions 12.1 presents information on how to teach the patient to perform a TSE.

Sexually Transmitted Diseases

Sexually transmitted diseases (STDs) are on the rise. In response to that rise, the Centers for Disease Control and Prevention (CDC) has published Guidelines for Sexually Transmitted Diseases, which include information on prevention, diagnosis, and treatment for all known STDs and are available online at http://www.cdc.gov.

STDs are a costly addition to the health-care burden in the United States, not only for the treatment of primary symptoms but also because of the increased risk of further complications from STDs. Open, frank discussions with patients about sexual practices is warranted from the teenage years through old age. The primary care clinician who is proactive and informative is the greatest resource that a patient can have. Pamphlets, posters, and patient education materials including videos and informational handouts are extremely helpful as a way to open a discussion on the topic.

ADVANCED PRACTICE NURSING INTERVENTIONS 12.1

Teaching the Patient to Perform a Testicular Self-Exam

Teach the patient the symptoms of testicular cancer. No symptoms may occur in the early stages. When symptoms do occur, they may include:

- Lumps on the testicle
- Slight enlargement of one of the testes
- Heavy sensation in the testicles or groin
- Dull ache in the lower abdomen or groin

Advise the patient that if hard lumps or nodules are found, or if any of the above symptoms occur, to contact his health-care provider immediately.

Teach the patient when to perform the exam. The exam is best performed after a shower or warm bath, as the fingers glide more easily over soapy skin, making it easier to concentrate on the texture underneath. The heat causes the skin to relax, making the exam easier. The exam takes only about 3 minutes and should be performed once a month.

Teach the patient how to perform the exam:

1. Start by examining one of the testicles. Slowly roll the testicle between the thumb and fingers, applying slight pressure. Try to find any hard, painless lumps.
2. Now examine the epididymis. This comma-shaped cord is behind each testicle. It may be tender to the touch. It is also the location of the most noncancerous problems.
3. Continue by examining the vas (the sperm-carrying tube that runs up from the epididymis). The vas normally feels like a firm, moveable smooth tube.
4. Now repeat the exam on the other side.

Epidemiology and Causes

It is estimated that approximately one in five Americans is infected with a viral STD other than HIV. Perhaps even more alarming is that the United States, with the most educated and highest standard of living, has the highest STD rates in the world. Increased risks for STDs may be influenced by gender, marital status, race and ethnic background, level of education, number of sexual partners, and lack of availability of health care. The long-term effects of STDs can be devastating and, at times, lethal. Improved advances in treatment, screening tests, and diagnostic procedures aid in discussion of the patient's symptoms and treatment therapies.

Pathophysiology

STDs consist of a heterogeneous collection of causative infectious agents (see Table 12.5). However, the unifying principle of these disorders is their propensity for spread by intimate person-to-person sexual contact, particularly after exposure of the mucous membranes to infected bodily fluids. This typically occurs within the genitalia, however, the oral and anal mucosa are also highly susceptible entry points, as exemplified by the incidence of gonococcal pharyngitis after receptive oral intercourse.

Given the length of the male urethra and the relatively smaller area of exposed genital mucosa via the urethral meatus, men had traditionally been thought of as being less susceptible to STD infection. However, microabrasions in the outer skin of the penile shaft sustained during sexual intercourse have been well documented as another important entry site for sexual transmitted organisms to reach the subcutaneous tissue. Moreover, the presence of one STD increases the chances of becoming infected with another—especially HIV. This is likely due to compromise of mucosal and outer skin barriers, as well as interactions on the molecular level, e.g., human papilloma virus (HPV) as a cofactor for HIV infection. Infectious organisms themselves may also express various genetic virulence factors that render them more susceptible to sexual transmission, including surface proteins that facilitate epithelial adherence to the urethral lining.

Clinical Presentation/Diagnostic Reasoning/Management

Table 12.5 presents the treatment of male reproductive system infections and STDs commonly seen by primary-care providers. STDs are typically distinguished from one another by their clinical presentation, although many STDs are asymptomatic in men or present with milder symptoms than in women. (Chapter 13 presents information on infections and STDs that are commonly seen in women.)

It is critical that all patients receiving treatment for one STD should also be screened for syphilis with a serum rapid plasma reagin (RPR), as well as offered screening for HIV infection. In addition, given the frequent asymptomatic nature of *Chlamydia* infection in both men and women, all persons being treated for *Neisseria gonorrhoeae* should be concurrently treated for *Chlamydia trachomatis*, as these two STDs often occur concurrently.

It is a basic tenet of STD treatment that all sexual partners must be notified of their potential for infection (regardless of the original source of infection or index case) and the need for testing and/or empiric treatment with an appropriate regimen. Reporting of many STDs to public health authorities is mandatory, but these laws differ on a state-by-state basis.

Follow-Up and Referral

STDs have traditionally been treated in the primary care outpatient setting, unless clinical symptoms meet criteria for hospital admission, such as severe pelvic inflammatory disease in women or initial presentation of HIV infection with or without the presence of opportunistic infection. Advancement in public health practices gave rise to the development of specialized, high-volume STD clinics to serve urban areas with high STD prevalence rates. However, cases that are refractory to established treatment guidelines may be referred to an infectious disease specialist for further diagnostic testing and individually tailored therapeutic regimens. Regardless of the treatment setting, beginning in the teenage years, patients need to be asked at every visit about sexual practices, the consistent use of condoms, and the benefits of abstinence. Patients with previous STD infection or those practicing high-risk sexual practices should be screened on a regular basis for common STDs including HIV, syphilis, *Chlamydia*, and *Neisseria gonorrhoeae*.

Patient Education

A resurgence in public education through public health is probably the most effective and efficient way to decrease the risk of this contagion. The clinician, while providing direct treatments, must also accept the responsibility for educating the patient about the need to seek treatment as soon as any symptoms appear. Persons most at risk are those with multiple sexual contacts, adolescents, and individuals who need further education. Patients should understand that active STD infection increases the chance of becoming infected with HIV, as well.

Table 12.5 Sexually Transmitted Infections

Infectious Agent	Clinical Presentation	Diagnostic Reasoning	Management
Bacterial Infections			
Chancroid (*Haemophilus ducreyi*)	Single painful ulcer (irregular, erythematous, and undermined edges) with a unilateral painful abcess. Painful lymphadenopathy.	Probable diagnosis is made if: patient has one or more painful genital ulcers; no evidence of syphilis on serologic test performed at least 7 days after onset of ulcers; the clinical presentation is typical for chancroid; and test for HSV is negative.	Azithromycin (Zithromax) 1 g PO × 1 OR Ceftriaxone (Rocephin) 250 mg IM × 1 OR Ciprofloxacin (Cipro) 500 mg PO bid for 3 days OR Erythromycin (E-mycin) 500 mg PO qid for 7 days
Chlamydia (*Chlamydia trachomatis*)	Most commonly, no reported symptoms. Patient may note an increase in mucopurulent discharge and bleeding with intercourse.	Yellow, mucopurulent discharge. Wet mount: >10 WBCs per high-power field (hpf). DNA probe—concurrent testing for *Neisseria gonorrhoeae* can be done with the same probe. Direct chlamydia enzyme immunoassay	Azithromycin (Zithromax) 1 g PO × 1 OR Doxycycline (Vibramycin) 100 mg PO bid for 7 days *Alternate:* Erythromycin base (E-mycin) 500 mg PO qid for 7 days OR Ofloxacin (Floxin) 300 mg PO bid for 7 days

(continued)

Table 12.5 **Sexually Transmitted Infections** (continued)

Infectious Agent	Clinical Presentation	Diagnostic Reasoning	Management
			OR Levofloxacin 500 mg PO for 7 days.
Gonorrhea (*Neisseria gonorrhoeae*)	Usually asymptomatic; partner may have an infection. Purulent yellow/green discharge. Gonococcal pharyngitis manifests as any bacterial pharyngitis, but 60% are asymptomatic	Gonococcal culture, DNA probe Urine DNA (initial 15 mL of a urinary void) Urine will typically have WBC or epithelial cells infected with *Neisseria gonorrhoeae*.	Cefixime (Suprax) 400 mg PO × 1 OR Ceftriaxone (Rocephine) 125 mg IM in a single dose OR Ciprofloxacin (Cipro) 500 mg PO × 1 OR Ofloxacin (Floxin) 400 mg PO × 1 OR Levofloxacin 250 mg PO × 1 IF CHLAMYDIAL INFECTION IS NOT RULED OUT THEN ALSO Azithromycin (Zithromax) 1 g PO × 1 OR Doxycycline 100 mg PO bid for 7 days. Follow CDC guidelines for complicated or refractory gonorrhea.
Granuloma inguinale (*Klebsiella granulomatis*)	Chronic, progressive papule that ulcerates to a beefy red, painless granular area with clean, sharp rolled edges; inguinal swelling; late painful abscesses (buboes).	History of travel and sexual contact in endemically infected area. Cannot be cultured; stained tissue sample may show Donovan bodies (bacteria-filled vacuoles).	Doxycycline (Vibramycin) 100 mg PO bid for 1–4 weeks OR Trimethoprim 80 mg/ sulfamethoxazole 400 mg (Bactrim) 1 tablet PO bid for 14 days OR Erythromycin (E-mycin) 500 mg PO bid for 4 weeks (during pregnancy)
Lymphogranuloma venereum [LGV] (*Chlamydia trachomatis*)	Lymphadenopathy, anorectal swelling, and fistula formation	History of travel and sexual contact in endemically infected area. Serologic LGV complement fixation test: suspect disease if titer is above 1:16; test is diagnostic if titer is above 1:64.	Doxycycline (Vibramycin) 100 mg PO bid for 21 days OR Erythromycin (E-mycin) 500 mg qid for 21 days OR Azithromycin (Zithromax) may be effective if given for 2–3 weeks; no recommended dosage from CDC.
Nongonococcal urethritis [NGU] (*Chlamydia trachomatis*)	Dysuria and urethral discharge (40% of patients); sparse, mucoid penile discharge, usually only after "milking" penis.	Gram stain smear of urethral exudate; culture for sugar fermentation reaction for NGU. Chlamydial DNA probe	Azithromycin (Zithromax) 1 g PO × 1 OR Doxycycline (Vibramycin) 100 mg PO bid for 7 days *Alternate:* Erythromycin (E-mycin) 500 mg PO qid for 7 days

Infectious Agent	Clinical Presentation	Diagnostic Reasoning	Management
			OR Erythromycin ethylsuccinate (EES) 800 mg PO qid for 7 days OR Ofloxacin (Floxin) 300 mg PO bid for 7 days
Syphilis (*Treponema pallidum*)	*Primary:* Painless ulcer at initial site of contact (chancre), adenopathy *Secondary:* Maculopapular rash on palms and soles, condylomalata/ moist, flat wartlike lesions, adenopathy *Tertiary/late:* Cardiac, neurologic, ophthalmic, auditory, and gummatous lesions	Dark field microscopy: Positive for spirochetes Direct microhemagglutinatin-treponema pallidum (MHA-TP): Antibody test Fluorescent treponemal antibody absorption (FTA-ABS): Antibody test reported as positive Venereal Disease Research Laboratory (VDRL) rapid plasma reagin (RPR): Reported as reactive with a titer; indicate degree of infection	*Early (less than 1 year duration):* Benzathine penicillin G 2.4 million units IM × 1 *Latent or Late (duration longer than 1 year or unknown length):* Benzathine penicillin G 2.4 million units IM once a week for 3 weeks *Neurosyphilis (CSF) (infection confirmed):* Aqueous crystalline penicillin G 3–4 million units IV q4h for 10–14 days *Penicillin-allergic patients:* Doxycycline 100 mg PO bid for 2 weeks OR Tetracycline 500 mg PO qid for 2 weeks.
Viral Infections			
Herpes simplex virus (HSV) infection	*First Outbreak:* Flu-like symptoms with adenopathy, tingling of the site prior to outbreak, and very painful vesicular lesions. Ulcers form, with circumscribed erythematous edges and white exudate centrally; lesions may last up to 12 days. *Recurrent Outbreaks:* Symptoms may be similar but are usually less severe and of shorter duration (4–5 days).	Viral culture of vesicle fluid most accurate if done within 48 hours of outbreak. Tzanck smear from the base of an early vesicle. DNA probe from lesion scraping.	*First Outbreak:* Acyclovir (Zovirax) 400 mg PO tid for 7–10 days OR 200 mg PO 5 times a day for 7–10 days OR Famciclovir (Famvir) 250 mg PO tid for 7–10 days OR Valacyclovir (Valtrex) 1 g PO bid for 7–10 days. *Recurrent Outbreaks:* Acyclovir 200 mg q4h 5 times daily for 5 days Famciclovir: 125 mg q12h for 5 days Valacyclovir: 500 mg q12h for 5 days *Suppressive:* Acyclovir 400 mg PO bid Famciclovir 250 mg PO bid Valacyclovir 1 g PO qd Evaluate after 1 year for recurrent episodes.
Human immunodeficiency virus (HIV) infection	Fever, malaise, adenopathy. Rash may occur in first few weeks after infection (acute retroviral syndrome).	Positive enzyme immunoassay (EIA) Positive Western blot (WB)	Treat infections as recommended by CDC. Refer to specialist. Long-term counseling and management.

(continued)

Table 12.5 Sexually Transmitted Infections (continued)

Infectious Agent	Clinical Presentation	Diagnostic Reasoning	Management
	Bloody diarrhea. Opportunistic infections. Increased HPV infections.		HAART (highly active anti-retroviral therapy) is key for the treatment of HIV. Initiation of therapy is a function of T-cell count, viral load, and concurrent symptoms. Treatment is heavily influenced by the ability to comply with various treatment regimens.
Human papillomavirus (HPV) infection	History of multiple partners or sexual abuse. Positive history of HPV. Itching, foul discharge. May be asymptomatic. Fleshy, soft, pale-colored keratinized growths.	Acetic acid test: lesions turn white with application of vinegar.	*Patient-Applied Treatments:* Podofilox (Condylox) 0.5% applied thinly bid for 3 days, then rest for 4 days; may repeat up to 4 cycles OR Imiguimod (Aldara cream) 5% applied 3 times a week for 16 weeks. *Clinician-Applied Treatments:* Cryotherapy and liquid nitrogen treatments—repeat every 1–2 weeks. Podophyllin resin (Podofin) 10–25% in benzoin—apply thinly, allow to dry; patient should wash off in 1–4 hours. TCA/BCA (trichloroacetic acid and bichloroacetic acid, Tri-Chlor) 80–90% applied by clinician every 4–7 days. Other therapies: laser therapy, surgery, interferon lesion injections.
Mulluscum contagiosum (large DNA virus from the Poxviridae family)	Domed papules (2–5 mm) with central umbilication Papules are pearly white, flesh-colored or yellow. Several found at a time in the inguinal area or inner thighs around external genitalia.	Diagnosis is made by clinical examination. Microscopic analysis of papule contents with Giemsa stain show characteristic "inclusion bodies."	No treatment. Lesions may last months to years and often heal spontaneously. Once healed, the person has a lifetime immunity to the virus.
Protozoa			
Trichomoniasis (*Trichomonas vaginalis*)	Heavy, odorous, yellow-green watery discharge. May have complaints of itching, swelling, and redness.	Discharge may be frothy. Wet mount: motile protozoa and WBCs.	Metronidazole (Flagyl) 2 g PO × 1 OR 500 mg PO bid for 7 days.

Bibliography

General

Barker, LR, Burton, JR, and Zieve, PD: Principles of Ambulatory Medicine, ed 6. Lippincott Williams & Wilkins, Philadelphia, 2003.

Bascom, A: Incorporating Herbal Medicine into Clinical Practice. FA Davis, Philadelphia, 2002.

Braunwald, E, et al (eds): Harrison's Principles of Internal Medicine, ed 16. McGraw-Hill, New York, 2005.

Dambro, MR: Griffith's 5-Minute Clinical Consult. Lippincott Williams & Wilkins, Philadelphia, 2003.

Kee, JL: Laboratory and Diagnostic Tests with Nursing Implications, ed 6. Prentice-Hall, Upper Saddle River, NJ, 2002.

McCance, KL, and Huether, SE: Pathophysiology: The Biologic Basis for Disease in Adults and Children, ed 5. Elsevier Mosby, St. Louis, Mo., 2006.

Stoller, ML, and Carroll, PR: Urology. In Tierney, LM, et al (eds): Current Medical Diagnosis and Treatment, ed 44. Lange/McGraw-Hill, New York, 2005, pp 902–943.

Tierney, LM, McPhee, SJ, and Papadakis, MA: Current Medical Diagnosis & Treatment, Lange/McGraw-Hill, New York, 2005.

Youngkin, E, et al: Pharmacotherapeutics: A Primary Care Guide, ed 2. Pearson/Prentice-Hall, Upper Saddle River, N.J., 2005.

Prostate Cancer/Prostatitis/Benign Prostatic Hyperplasia

Bill-Axelson, A, et al: Radical prostatectomy versus watchful waiting in early prostate cancer. N Engl J Med 352(19):1977–1984, 2005.

Burt, J, Caelli, K, Moore, K, and Anderson, M: Radical prostatectomy: men's experiences and postoperative needs. J Clin Nurs 14(7):883–890, 2005.

Colella, J, and Scrofine, S: High-dose brachytherapy for treating prostate cancer: nursing considerations. Urol Nurs 24(1):39–52, 2004.

Diaz-Parker, C, and Bratslavsky, G: Male genitourinary disease: Urethritis, epididymitis, and prostatitis. Clin Rev 15(3):40–45, 2005.

Gilchrist, K: Benign prostatic hyperplasia: Is it a precursor to prostatic cancer? Nurse Pract 29(6):30–37, 2004.

Incrocci, L: Radiotherapy for prostate cancer and sexual functioning. Hosp Med 65(10):605–608, 2004.

Johnson, BK: Prostate cancer and sexuality: Implications for nursing. Geriatr Nurs 25(6):341–347, 2004.

Kirby, M, and Kirby, R: The management of hypertension in patients with benign prostatic hyperplasia and erectile dysfunction. Br J Cardiol 12(2):107–116, 2005.

Kronenwetter, C, et al: A qualitative analysis of interviews of men with early stage prostate cancer: the prostate cancer lifestyle trial. Cancer Nurs 28(2):99–107, 2005.

Murthy, GD, Byron, DP, and Pasquale, D: Underutilization of digital rectal examination when screening for prostate cancer. Arch Intern Med 164:313–316, 2004.

Peters, N, and Armstrong, K: Racial differences in prostate cancer treatment outcomes: A systematic review. Cancer Nurs 28(2):108–118, 2005.

Sachs, H, and Stone, A: Benign prostatic hyperplasia: When to treat—and how. Consultant 43(3):297–300, 2003.

Wallace, M: Prostate cancer update: When to screen, how to treat. Clin Rev 14(8):46–51, 2004.

Watkins-Bruner, D, Moore, D, Parlanti, A, et al: Relative risk of prostate cancer for men with affected relatives: Systemic review and meta-analysis. Int J Cancer 107:797–803, 2003.

Impotence/Erectile Dysfunction

Gades, NM, et al: Association between smoking and erectile dysfunction: A population-based study. Am J Epidemiol 161(4):346–351, 2005.

Gray, M: Andropause and the aging man. Adv Nurse Pract 4:22–28, 2005.

Katz, A: Androgen replacement therapy in aging men. Nurse Pract 29(10):58–64, 2004.

Kellogg-Spadt, S: Sex Rx. Erectile dysfunction: What you patients should know. Am J Nurse Pract 9(9):62–63, 2005.

Lewis, JH: Clinical practice. Challenges in the assessment of erectile dysfunction and treatment with oral therapies: Review with case examples. J Am Acad Nurse Pract 16(10):428–440, 2004.

Lewis, JH, Rosen, R, and Goldstein, I: Erectile dysfunction. Nursing 35(2):64, 2005.

Lewis, JH, Rosen, R, and Goldstein, I: Erectile dysfunction in primary care. Nurse Pract 29(12):42–46, 2004.

Noviasky, JA, Masood, A, and Lo, V: Steps. Tadalifil (cialis) for erectile dysfunction. Am Fam Phys 70(2):359–360, 2004.

Stipetich, R, Abel, LJ, Anderson, RL, Butler, WM, Wallner, KE, and Merrick, GS: Nursing considerations in brachytherapy-related erectile dysfunction. Urol Nurs 25(4):249–254, 259, 2005.

Stoller, ML, Carroll, PR: Urology. In Tierney, LM, et al (eds): Current Medical Diagnosis and Treatment, ed 44. Lange/McGraw-Hill, New York, 2005, pp 921–925.

Thethi, TK, Asafu-Adjaye, NO, and Fonseca, VA: Erectile dysfunction. Clin Diabetes 23(3):105–113, 2005.

Tino, MD, and Noyes, DT: Advisor forum: Clinical pearls. Testosterone replacement for erectile dysfunction. Clin Advisor 8(8):63, 2005.

Wyllie, MG: The underlying pathophysiology and causes of erectile dysfunction. Clin Cornerstone 7(1):19–27, 2005.

Sexually Transmitted Diseases

Centers for Disease Control: CDC. STD treatment guidelines. Morb Mortal Wkly Rep, May 10, 2002.

Morgan, K: Sexually transmitted infections. In McCance, KL, and Huether, SE (eds): Pathophysiology: the Biologic Basis for Disease in Adults & Children, ed 5. CV Mosby, St. Louis, Mo., pp. 863–891, 2006.

Testicular Cancer

Fuentes, EE: Hidden danger: Detection and diagnosis of scrotal masses. Adv Nurse Pract 4:35–38, 2005.

Morgan, K, and McCance, KL: Alteration of reproductive systems. In McCance, KL, and Huether, SE (eds): Pathophysiology: The Biologic Basis for Disease in Adults and Children, ed 5. CV Mosby, St. Louis, Mo., pp 771–855, 2006.

Mullen, BA: Testicular complaints and the young man. J Am Acad Nurse Pract 16(11):490-496, 2004.

Stotts, RC: Cancers of the prostate, penis and testicles: Epidemiology, prevention and treatment. Nurs Clin North Am 39(2):327–340, 2004.

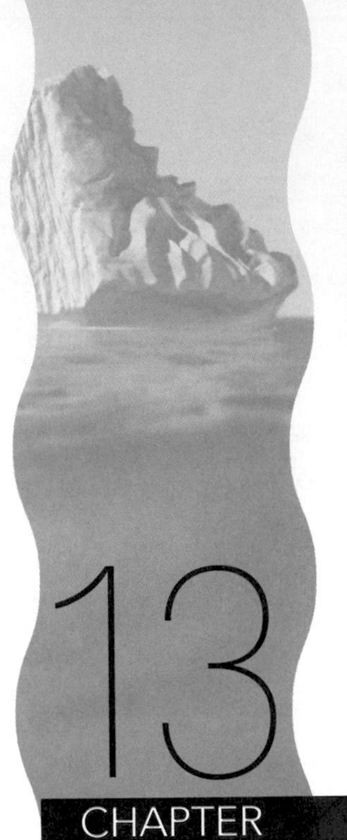

Women's Health Problems

Debera J. Thomas, DNS, APRN, BC
Brian O. Porter, MD, PhD, MPH
Jill E. Winland-Brown, EdD, MSN, APRN, BC

Common Complaints

Dysfunctional Uterine Bleeding

A change in the pattern or volume of menstrual blood flow is a common health concern of women from puberty to menopause. The literature suggests that 10 to 20 percent of women have abnormal uterine bleeding (AUB) at one or several times during their reproductive lives. Women may describe abnormal bleeding episodes as infrequent, prolonged in duration, occurring between regular menstrual periods, and/or excessive. There may be no evidence of genital tract lesions. The causes of AUB are divided into two major categories: organic and dysfunctional (endocrine). The diagnosis of dysfunctional uterine bleeding (DUB) is considered only after organic, systemic, and iatrogenic causes are eliminated.

Abnormal vaginal bleeding is, therefore, considered DUB if it arises from the endometrium of the uterus with no demonstrable organic cause. It is frequently the result of an endocrine abnormality of anovulation or short ovulatory cycles in which estrogen stimulates the growth of the endometrium without the stabilizing effect of progesterone and is not the result of a normal menstruation. In adolescence, anovulatory DUB is commonly caused by an immature hypothalamic–pituitary system that does not respond to the positive feedback effect of estrogen. In contrast, perimenopausal women experience variable menstrual cycle durations and bleeding episodes secondary to a decrease in ovarian response to gonadotropin stimulation. In addition, DUB is commonly seen during the reproductive years of women who are experiencing stress, are participating in a strenuous exercise program, or have undergone a large weight change.

Differential Diagnosis

Anovulatory bleeding is the cause of DUB in approximately 95 percent of women under age 20 years and in 90 percent of perimenopausal women who experience DUB for 2 to 3 years before the onset of menopause. In contrast, ovulatory cycles are associated with certain features such as midcycle pain, specific vaginal mucus changes, dysmenorrhea, and premenstrual breast tenderness. Although approximately one half of ovulating women experience midcycle spotting, it is self-limiting. Irregular endometrial shedding may occur with the prolonged production of progesterone with a persistent corpus luteum resulting in DUB; however, DUB is a diagnosis of exclusion. Emphasis on a thorough history, physical and pelvic examination, and selected laboratory tests usually will yield the appropriate diagnosis. One must inquire about the woman's age, date of last menstrual period (LMP), birth control method, frequency of menses, amount of menstrual blood flow (e.g., the estimated number of pads or tampons used daily), duration of menses, and if there is a menstrual pattern change. In women who report profuse acute bleeding episodes, the diagnosis of pregnancy (e.g., passing tissue, nausea, vomiting, breast tenderness) must be excluded. In an ectopic pregnancy, the woman may complain of abdominal pain. Complaints of fainting spells may be indicative of a ruptured ectopic pregnancy.

Up to 10 percent of patients who use oral contraceptives report irregular bleeding episodes. Any woman who presents with abnormal uterine bleeding who is age 35 years or older should be evaluated for cervical and uterine cancer.

Malignancy must also be excluded. Endometrial sampling is an office procedure to rule out unchecked proliferation of the endometrium that can lead to hyperplasia and potentially endometrial adenocarcinoma. Similarly, a colposcopy, cervical biopsy, and endocervical curettage are used to diagnose cervical cancer. Women with a history of an abnormal Pap smear test or ulcerated or friable lesions on the cervix should be referred for colposcopy. In addition, benign neoplasms such as uterine leiomyomas (fibroids), endometrial polyps, and adenomyomas are commonly seen in patients age 25 to 45 years. Trauma and foreign bodies are seen more commonly in children. A less common cause of uterine bleeding is blood dyscrasia, such as von Willebrand's disease or thrombocytopenia purpura.

Laboratory workup is directed by the history and physical examination findings and usually consists of hematocrit (Hct), hemoglobin, platelet count, and Papanicolaou (Pap) and pregnancy tests. In severe bleeding, partial thromboplastin time (PTT), prothrombin time (PT), and bleeding time tests are indicated. Hysteroscopy may be performed immediately before a dilation and curettage (D&C) to assist in diagnosis of polyps, exophytic endometrial cancer, or fibroids. Prolactin level and thyroid function tests are ordered to rule out hyperprolactinemia and hypothyroidism, respectively.

Treatment

Management of DUB is directed toward controlling bleeding and preventing a recurrence. For teenagers, management includes observation for those with mild cases and no anemia, medroxyprogesterone (if the patient is not sexually active), or oral contraceptives (OCs) for sexually active teenagers. For women of reproductive age, treatment is based on the woman's desire for fertility or contraception. For women who cannot take OCs, medroxyprogesterone is offered. OCs containing ethinyl estradiol (EE) are used in acute bleeding episodes. For women with severe acute bleeding, but who remain hemodynamically stable, conjugated estrogen is used until bleeding stops.

Breast Mass

A breast mass is a lump in the breast and is one of the most anxiety-producing events a woman may encounter in her lifetime. Seventy percent of patients with breast cancer present with a lump in the breast; 90 percent of these breast masses are discovered by the woman herself. Benign breast disorders are referred to as *fibrocystic disease* or *mammary dysplasia* and are the most frequent breast lesions. In benign breast disorders, the breast masses or lumps are tender and usually bilateral. There may be a rapid fluctuation in the size of benign masses compared to breast cancer, which slowly increases in size. Typically, the tenderness and size of the mass may increase before menses. Fibrocystic breast disease is most common in women ages 30 to 50 years or in postmenopausal women on hormone replacement therapy (HRT).

Differential Diagnosis

The symptoms that differentiate a breast cyst from breast cancer are the tenderness, the fluctuations in size, and the multiplicity of lesions. It is difficult to distinguish a breast cyst from cancer based on clinical findings alone; therefore, aggressive testing is warranted. A mammogram is usually the first test performed; however, the breast tissue in patients with fibrocystic breast disease may be too radiodense to provide a conclusive diagnosis. A breast ultrasound will differentiate a cystic mass from a solid mass. A definitive diagnosis is made by breast biopsy. Aspiration of a cystic lesion will relieve the pain and will assist in the diagnosis.

Treatment

Treatment of fibrocystic breast disease consists of avoiding trauma; wearing a firm bra day and night; eliminating coffee, tea, and chocolate from the diet; and taking 400 IU vitamin E daily. For patients with severe pain, danazol (Danocrine), 100 to 200 mg bid has been found helpful. Danazol is an androgen derivative that suppresses pituitary gonadotropins. With its androgenic effects, such as acne, edema, and hirsutism, most women find that the treatment is worse than the condition itself and prefer to try milder forms of pain relief.

Patients with benign breast lumps tend to become complacent about examining their breasts because they know the lumps are there. Breast self-exam (BSE) is just as important with fibrocystic breast disease as it is for women without breast lumps and should be stressed along with instruction on how to perform BSE.

Dyspareunia

Dyspareunia is painful sexual intercourse that can occur as a result of either introduction of the penis into the vagina or deep penile penetration. The pain a patient experiences can be a consequence of vaginal inflammation, structural (anatomic) abnormalities, vaginal atrophy or insufficient lubrication, pelvic pathology, or psychological issues.

Because patients tend not to report painful sexual intercourse, it is difficult to determine the incidence; however, one study of 313 patients documented that more than 60 percent had experienced dyspareunia at some point in their lives. Risk factors include history of sexual trauma, history of sexually transmitted infections (STIs), recurrent candidiasis infection, poor hygiene, menopause, psychological issues, and difficulties in the relationship.

Differential Diagnosis

Obtaining a thorough history from the patient is essential in ascertaining the cause of dyspareunia. As noted earlier, pain

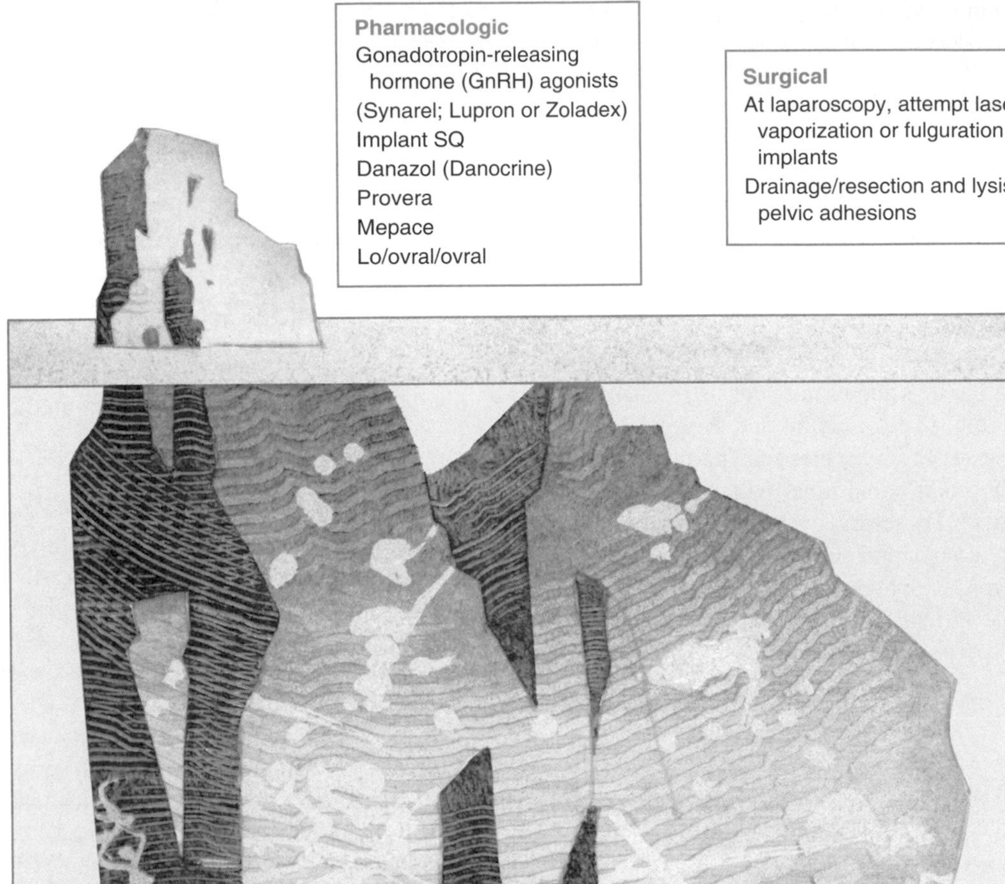

may occur with initial or deep penile penetration and may occur with initial intercourse or after a long time of pain-free experience. The patient may complain of vaginal discharge or irritation. There may be a history of unrelated pelvic pain, recent pregnancy and childbirth, trauma, or surgery. The patient may, on questioning, reveal difficulty in using tampons or difficulty with prior pelvic exams.

On physical exam the patient may present with signs of vulvar or vaginal mucosal irritation, inflammation, lesions, discharge, atrophy, hymenal remnants, Bartholin's cyst or abscess, or vestibulitis. *Vaginismus*, the involuntary contraction of perineal muscles, may occur during the speculum exam, impeding full visualization and examination of the vaginal vault and cervix. The clinician must proceed with sensitivity, allowing the patient control over the pelvic exam. The bimanual exam may reveal pelvic mass, cervical motion tenderness, uterine prolapse, rectocele, or cystocele.

The laboratory workup is directed by findings from the history and physical exam and usually consists of urinalysis, wet mount of vaginal discharge, and cervical cultures. Urinalysis is useful in identifying any urinary tract conditions that may be a contributing factor to the source of the pain. The presence of white blood cells (WBCs), red blood cells (RBCs), or bacteria may indicate a urinary tract infection (UTI). Wet mount examination of vaginal discharge can reveal the presence of bacterial vaginosis (*Gardnerella vaginalis*), trichomoniasis, or candidiasis. Cervical cultures are useful in determining the presence of *Chlamydia* and gonorrhea.

Treatment

Management of dyspareunia depends on the symptoms and etiology. If the cause is atropic vaginitis, HRT and use of a water-soluble lubricant (Astroglide®, KY Jelly) may facilitate vaginal lubrication. STIs are treated with appropriate antibiotic therapy. Progressive dilation and muscle awareness exercises such as Kegel's exercises are recommended for treatment of vaginismus, hymenal strands, anatomically narrow introitus, and scar tissue. If psychological factors, such as sexual trauma, relationship conflicts, stress, and a restrictive sexual attitude, appear to be the cause, referral to a psychotherapist is indicated.

Pelvic Pain

Pelvic pain is seen in 1 to 2 percent of patients in primary-care practice. Pelvic pain is categorized as acute, chronic, or recurrent and presents as both pelvic or lower abdominal pain. Genitourinary (GU), gastrointestinal (GI), or musculoskeletal system diseases or dysfunctions may cause sudden, acute pain in both areas. Chronic or recurrent pelvic pain is described as less urgent. Recurrent pain can be associated with menstruation or unrelated to menses. The origin of chronic pain can be related to benign or malignant neoplasms or characterized as psychogenic.

Differential Diagnosis

An acute onset of pelvic pain may be the result of pelvic disorders including pelvic inflammatory disease (PID), ruptured ovarian cyst, torsion of ovarian cyst, ovary, or fallopian tube, and ectopic pregnancy with rupture. PID accounts for about 20 percent of acute pelvic pain in women, ovarian cysts for up to 40 percent, and adnexal torsion for about 16 percent of acute pain in women. Ten percent of women who report acute pelvic pain may have extrapelvic disease such as appendicitis.

Women reporting recurring pain with menstruation may have primary or secondary dysmenorrhea, endometriosis, adenomyosis, chronic PID, and/or pain related to intrauterine devices (IUDs). Endometriosis is seen in up to 50 percent of women with chronic pelvic pain. Recurrent pain that is not associated with menses may have many causes including Mittelschmerz (release of mature ovum from ovary), leaking ovarian cysts, incompletely treated or recurrent pelvic infections, or UTIs. Nongynecologic pathology includes adhesions, inflammatory bowel disease, and irritable bowel syndrome. However, for as many as 37 percent of women with chronic or recurrent pelvic pain no physiologic cause of the pain can be determined.

Treatment

Differential Diagnosis Flowchart 13.1 presents common differential diagnoses and treatments of pelvic pain.

Vulvovaginitis (Vaginal Itching, Burning, and Discharge)

Vulvovaginitis is defined as the simultaneous inflammation of the vulva and vagina. The patient complains of vaginal itching, burning, and vaginal discharge, which comprise the triad of vulvovaginitis symptoms and account for some of the most common reasons patients seek health care. Although frequently the result of infection, vulvovaginitis may also have noninfectious causes including allergic reactions, foreign body, atrophic vaginitis, traumatic vaginitis, or collagen vascular disease.

Differential Diagnosis

The delicate vaginal environment can be easily altered by numerous internal and external influences. In addition to the effects of normal changes in the body's hormonal condition, such as ovulatory midcycle mucus production, menstruation, or the atrophic mucosal changes that occur after menopause, the use of antibiotics, presence of diabetes mellitus or glycosuria, and stress can also cause symptoms of vulvovaginitis.

A thorough history should include time of symptom onset and a full description of the vaginal discharge and the relationship of the symptoms to the menstrual cycle, coitus, and use of medications (especially antibiotics). A detailed sexual history helps to identify whether the patient is at increased risk for the development of an STI. It is important to determine whether the patient's partner has symptoms of infection (penile discharge or lesion) and if the woman has used spermicidal preparations, douches, bubble bath, or feminine hygiene deodorants and if she has done any self-treatment.

The most common cause of symptomatic complaints of abnormal vaginal discharge, itching, and burning

(Text continued on page 648)

DIFFERENTIAL DIAGNOSIS FLOWCHART 13.1

PELVIC PAIN

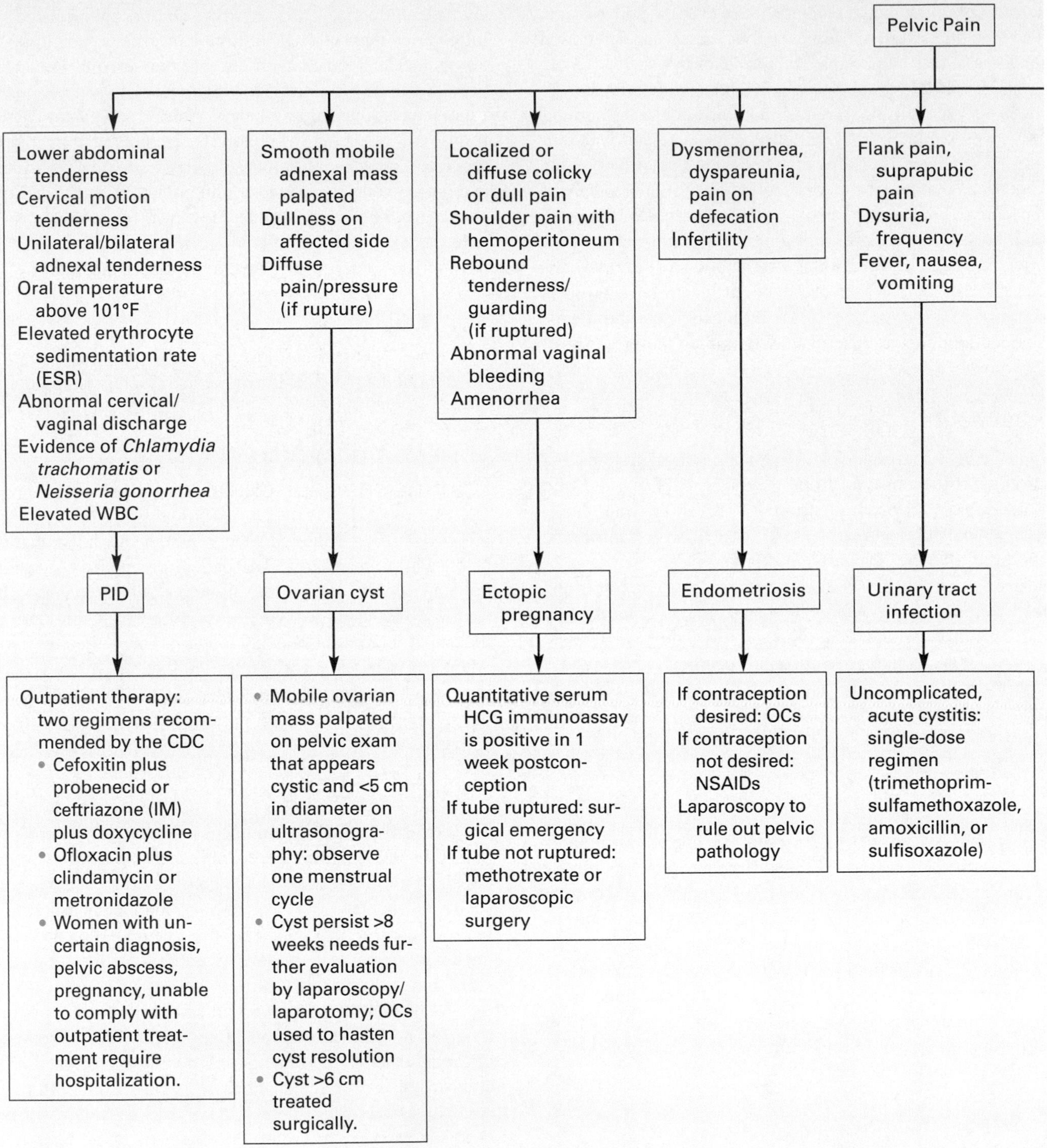

Pelvic Pain

Lower abdominal tenderness; Cervical motion tenderness; Unilateral/bilateral adnexal tenderness; Oral temperature above 101°F; Elevated erythrocyte sedimentation rate (ESR); Abnormal cervical/vaginal discharge; Evidence of *Chlamydia trachomatis* or *Neisseria gonorrhea*; Elevated WBC

→ PID

→ Outpatient therapy: two regimens recommended by the CDC
- Cefoxitin plus probenecid or ceftriazone (IM) plus doxycycline
- Ofloxacin plus clindamycin or metronidazole
- Women with uncertain diagnosis, pelvic abscess, pregnancy, unable to comply with outpatient treatment require hospitalization.

Smooth mobile adnexal mass palpated; Dullness on affected side; Diffuse pain/pressure (if rupture)

→ Ovarian cyst

- Mobile ovarian mass palpated on pelvic exam that appears cystic and <5 cm in diameter on ultrasonography: observe one menstrual cycle
- Cyst persist >8 weeks needs further evaluation by laparoscopy/laparotomy; OCs used to hasten cyst resolution
- Cyst >6 cm treated surgically.

Localized or diffuse colicky or dull pain; Shoulder pain with hemoperitoneum; Rebound tenderness/guarding (if ruptured); Abnormal vaginal bleeding; Amenorrhea

→ Ectopic pregnancy

→ Quantitative serum HCG immunoassay is positive in 1 week postconception
If tube ruptured: surgical emergency
If tube not ruptured: methotrexate or laparoscopic surgery

Dysmenorrhea, dyspareunia, pain on defecation; Infertility

→ Endometriosis

→ If contraception desired: OCs
If contraception not desired: NSAIDs
Laparoscopy to rule out pelvic pathology

Flank pain, suprapubic pain; Dysuria, frequency; Fever, nausea, vomiting

→ Urinary tract infection

→ Uncomplicated, acute cystitis: single-dose regimen (trimethoprim-sulfamethoxazole, amoxicillin, or sulfisoxazole)

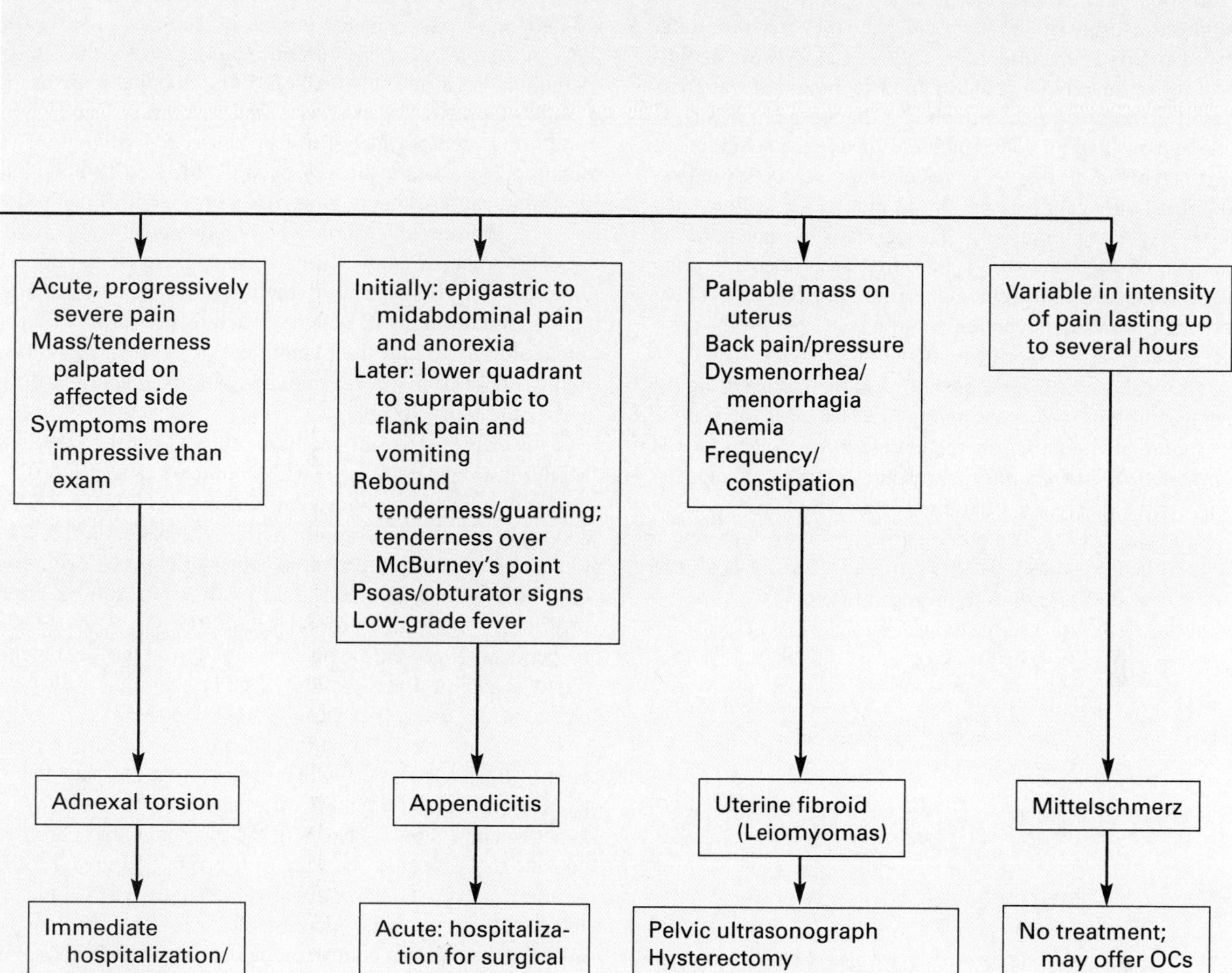
Acute, progressively severe pain
Mass/tenderness palpated on affected side
Symptoms more impressive than exam
Adnexal torsion
Immediate hospitalization/ operative intervention
Initially: epigastric to midabdominal pain and anorexia
Later: lower quadrant to suprapubic to flank pain and vomiting
Rebound tenderness/guarding; tenderness over McBurney's point
Psoas/obturator signs
Low-grade fever
Appendicitis
Acute: hospitalization for surgical evaluation
Palpable mass on uterus
Back pain/pressure
Dysmenorrhea/ menorrhagia
Anemia
Frequency/ constipation
Uterine fibroid (Leiomyomas)
Pelvic ultrasonograph
Hysterectomy
Uterine artery embolectomy
Variable in intensity of pain lasting up to several hours
Mittelschmerz
No treatment; may offer OCs to inhibit ovulation

is infection from either bacteria, yeast, or parasites. Bacterial vaginosis caused by *Gardnerella* accounts for almost 50 percent of all vaginal infections, followed closely by candidiasis (approximately 25 percent) and trichomoniasis (approximately 20 percent). Each infection is diagnosed based on the clinical presentation, which includes the type, amount, color, odor, and pH of discharge. Physical exam includes visualization of the vulva and vagina for the presence of lesions, discharge, erythema, or atrophy. The cervix is examined for the presence of lesions, erosion, friability, or erythema. During the bimanual exam, the clinician should pay particular attention to the presence of cervical motion tenderness or the presence of adnexal and uterine tenderness or masses.

Laboratory workup is directed by findings from the history and physical exam and usually consists of a saline wet mount of vaginal discharge to determine the presence of *Gardnerella, Trichomonas,* or atrophic vaginitis and a potassium hydroxide (KOH) wet mount to determine the presence of *Candida.* A Gram stain of vaginal discharge can reveal the presence of gonorrhea. In addition, a urinalysis should be performed to rule out the presence of a UTI.

Treatment

Differential Diagnosis Flowchart 13.2 presents the differential diagnoses and treatments of vulvovaginitis.

Common Problems

Family Planning

From menarche to menopause, a woman's health concerns may include controlling fertility. Women need to be able to prevent pregnancy, plan intervals between pregnancies, and find help if a desired pregnancy is not achieved. These decisions are related to one's values, professional role, friends, family, cultural and religious beliefs, self-perception, health status, economics, sexual lifestyle, options accessible, and partner status. Ideally, the birth control option should be affordable, easy to use, easy to obtain, 100 percent effective, safe, mutually acceptable, and reversible. The most popular birth control methods are oral contraceptives (OCs), the diaphragm, and condoms. Other popular choices include Depo-Provera injections and the copper IUD.

Although preventing pregnancy is a major concern, some lifestyle behaviors may also cause concern for acquiring an STI. To control both pregnancy and disease, routine health care is important. The gynecologic history and physical examination are essential to address both issues.

The gynecologic history reviews risks for STIs and history of birth control methods, and identifies needs for health promotion. It also identifies sexual dysfunction or sexual concerns. Reviewing anatomy and physiology with the patient may help her understand her body and result in healthier lifestyle choices. Other items important in history taking include menstrual cycle information; menarche; use of tampon or pads; change in menses; number of sex partners in the past year and lifetime; initiation of coitus; dyspareunia; orgasms; history of STIs; medications used; results of previous Pap smears and resolutions; and cigarette, drug, and/or alcohol use or abuse. It is important to obtain a basic health history as well, to identify potential contraindications to new or previous birth control methods.

Wording questions in a nonjudgmental, supportive, accepting manner enables the patient to be open and honest in an area of great sensitivity and possible pain. The clinician addresses areas of concern, such as poor body image, depression, poor nutrition, emotional or physical problems, myths, abuse from others, smoking, obesity, alcohol or drug abuse, and family problems.

Physical exam includes blood pressure, weight, height, last menstrual period (LMP), breast cancer and BSE teaching, bimanual pelvic, a Pap smear, and culture for STIs and other infections as appropriate to the patient's risk factors and presenting information. During the initial examination, baseline lab studies should be done including a lipid profile and complete blood count (CBC). Other tests (dependent on presenting history) are thyroid profile, fasting blood sugar, or liver profile. In addition, after a 10-year period of OC use, a liver profile should be obtained.

Some facilities require signed consent for the birth control method selected which ensures that the patient has been given, in writing, full information on the use, risks, benefits, and follow-up needs of the method. Other facilities educate the patient at the time of the visit and give her the product insert and educational material to read at home. Ideally, both partners, if possible, need comprehensive information on birth control methods, so that their choice is an educated decision based on their lifestyle and needs. The success or failure of any birth control method depends on the woman's motivation, adherence, partner support, consistency and comfort. The main methods of birth control are listed in Table 13.1.

Barrier Methods

Barrier methods include male and female condoms, the diaphragm, and cervical cap. Some barrier methods have the dual advantage of preventing pregnancy and STIs. The most common STIs are caused by herpes simplex virus (HSV), human papilloma virus (HPV), human immunodeficiency virus (HIV), *Neisseria gonorrhoeae,* and *Chlamydia.* Controlling HPV also reduces the risk of cervical cancer. Adverse effects of barrier methods are similar in some ways: messiness, handling of genitalia, precoital interruption of spontaneity, and allergy or contact dermatitis. The use of barrier methods requires motivation on the part of both partners.

Male Condom

The *male condom* is the most common barrier method and is most effective when combined with a spermicide such as

Table 13.1 **Methods of Birth Control**

Method	Type	Prevention	Protection	Rate (%)*
Barrier methods	Male condom	Prevents sperm from entering vagina	Each use	3–12
	Female condom	Prevents sperm from entering cervix	Each use	5–21
	Diaphragm	Prevents sperm from entering cervix	Each use	2–20
	Cervical cap	Prevents sperm from entering cervix	48 hours	2–20
	Vaginal contraceptive sponge	Prevents sperm from entering cervix	24 hours	18–28
	Spermicide nonoxynol-9	Immobilizes and kills sperm	Each use	2–30
Hormonal methods	Combination oral contraceptives	Inhibits ovulation, hostile environment, slows tubal transport	Continuous	0.1
	Progestin-only pills	Inhibits ovulation, hostile environment, slows tubal transport	Continuous	1–4
	Depo-medroxyprogesterone (Depo-Provera)	Blunts LH, inhibits sperm penetration, endometrium unreceptive	90 days	0.3
Intrauterine devices (IUDs)	Copper T-380A Mirena	Prevents fertilization and implantation	10 years	0.8
Regulated abstinence	Calendar calculation	Prevents fertilization	Each cycle	9
	Temperature and mucous changes	Prevents fertilization	Each cycle	4
Postcoital controls	Chance	No protection	0	85
	Withdrawal	Prevents sperm from entering vagina	Each use	18
	Postcoitus douche	Flushes sperm from vagina	0	—
	Emergency contraception	Interferes with fertilization or implant	Each use (Plan B)	2
Sterilization	Female	Fallopian tubes cut/tied to prevent ovum moving to uterus or sperm entering tube	Permanent	0.4
	Male	Vas deferens cut to prevent sperm from leaving male	Permanent	0.15

*Percentage of women experiencing an accidental pregnancy in the first year of use.

nonoxynol-9. Condoms are available in various sizes, colors, flavors, strengths, and lubrication. They should not be applied tightly. The tip should extend one-half inch beyond the penis to collect ejaculate. Care must be taken during withdrawal of the penis to prevent the condom from coming off and spilling the semen. Other adverse effects include irritation, allergic reaction, unfavorable oral sex, and accidental splitting of the condom. Condoms are very effective and when used with a spermicide the failure rate is equivalent to that of OCs. However, condoms may not be the best choice for the under-age-25-year-old group because of noncompliance, inconsistent use, and low motivation.

Female Condom

The *female condom* is a device that is disposable and made of seamless polyurethane. It fits loosely inside the vagina and covers the perineum. There are flexible rims on both ends. The inner rim sits on the closed end and is compressed for placement into the vagina over the cervix. This prevents contact between body secretions. The condom is soft, lubricated by spermicide, inexpensive, and may be purchased over-the-counter (OTC). Many patients state that it is difficult to handle, however. Adverse effects include irritation and allergic reaction. The failure rate of the female condom is 5 to 21 percent when used correctly and comparable to the efficacy of the diaphragm.

Diaphragm

A *diaphragm* is a latex hemisphere with a flexible rim that fits over the cervix. The failure rate is 2 to 20 percent when used with spermicidal jelly. This method allows the woman control and has no systemic side effects. The largest size that covers the cervix comfortably is best. Once the device has been fitted, the patient should insert and remove the diaphragm, then return for a recheck after 1 week of practice using a backup contraceptive method. Before insertion, 1

(Text continued on page 652)

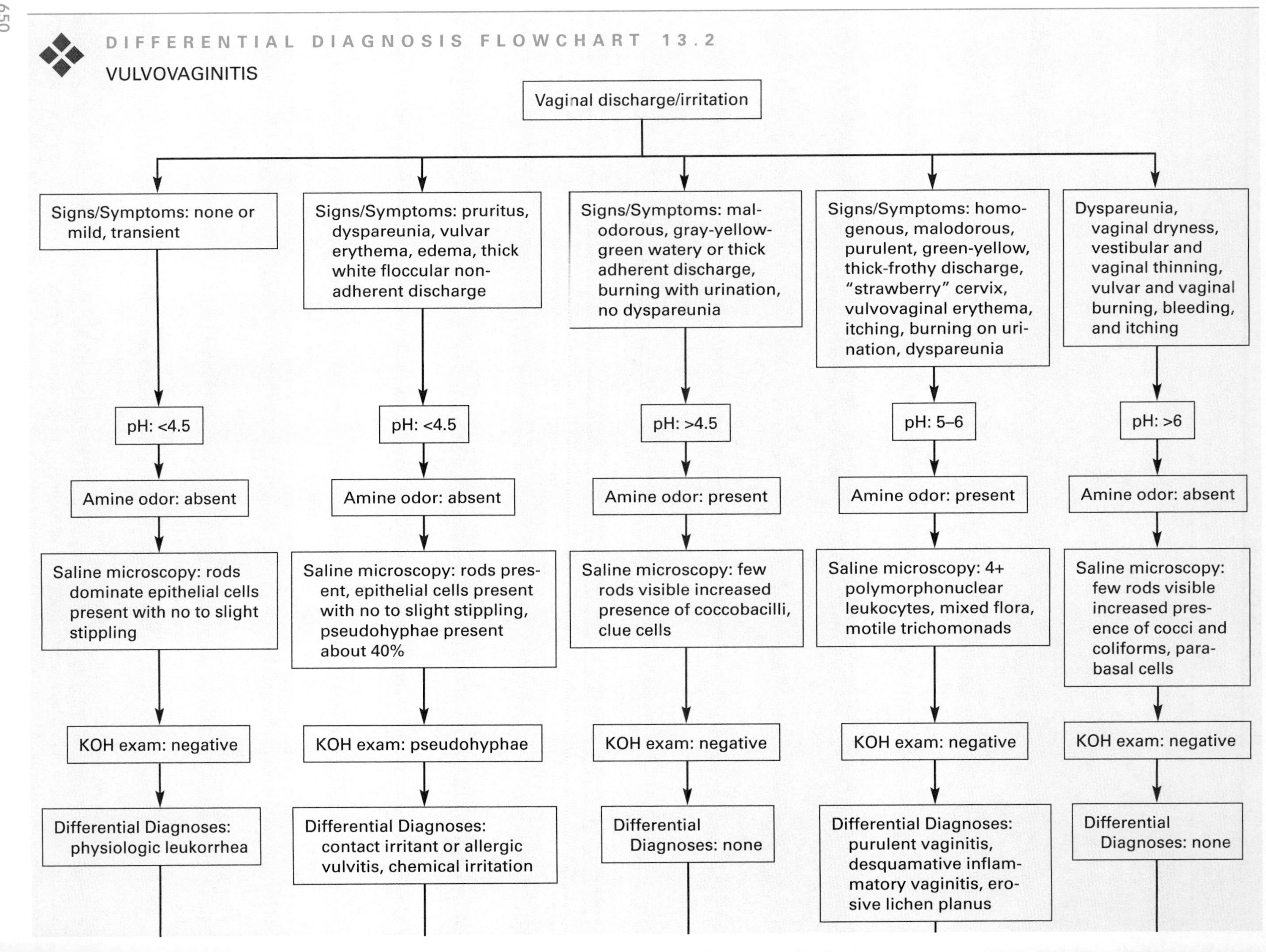
DIFFERENTIAL DIAGNOSIS FLOWCHART 13.2
VULVOVAGINITIS
Vaginal discharge/irritation
Signs/Symptoms: none or mild, transient
pH: <4.5
Amine odor: absent
Saline microscopy: rods dominate epithelial cells present with no to slight stippling
KOH exam: negative
Differential Diagnoses: physiologic leukorrhea
Signs/Symptoms: pruritus, dyspareunia, vulvar erythema, edema, thick white floccular non-adherent discharge
pH: <4.5
Amine odor: absent
Saline microscopy: rods present, epithelial cells present with no to slight stippling, pseudohyphae present about 40%
KOH exam: pseudohyphae
Differential Diagnoses: contact irritant or allergic vulvitis, chemical irritation
Signs/Symptoms: malodorous, gray-yellow-green watery or thick adherent discharge, burning with urination, no dyspareunia
pH: >4.5
Amine odor: present
Saline microscopy: few rods visible increased presence of coccobacilli, clue cells
KOH exam: negative
Differential Diagnoses: none
Signs/Symptoms: homogenous, malodorous, purulent, green-yellow, thick-frothy discharge, "strawberry" cervix, vulvovaginal erythema, itching, burning on urination, dyspareunia
pH: 5–6
Amine odor: present
Saline microscopy: 4+ polymorphonuclear leukocytes, mixed flora, motile trichomonads
KOH exam: negative
Differential Diagnoses: purulent vaginitis, desquamative inflammatory vaginitis, erosive lichen planus
Dyspareunia, vaginal dryness, vestibular and vaginal thinning, vulvar and vaginal burning, bleeding, and itching
pH: >6
Amine odor: absent
Saline microscopy: few rods visible increased presence of cocci and coliforms, parabasal cells
KOH exam: negative
Differential Diagnoses: none

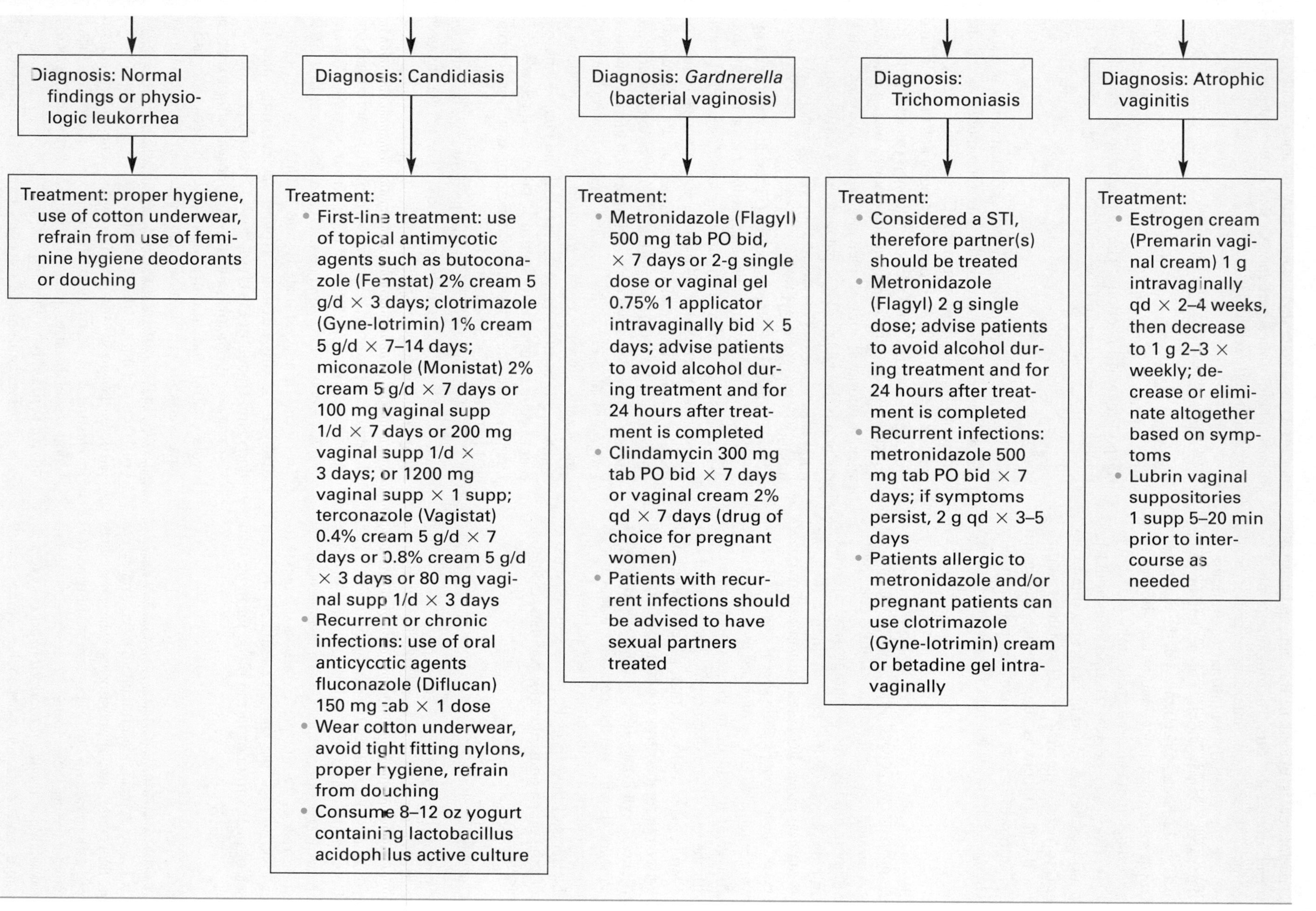

Diagnosis: Normal findings or physiologic leukorrhea
Treatment: proper hygiene, use of cotton underwear, refrain from use of feminine hygiene deodorants or douching
Diagnosis: Candidiasis
Treatment:
• First-line treatment: use of topical antimycotic agents such as butoconazole (Femstat) 2% cream 5 g/d × 3 days; clotrimazole (Gyne-lotrimin) 1% cream 5 g/d × 7–14 days; miconazole (Monistat) 2% cream 5 g/d × 7 days or 100 mg vaginal supp 1/d × 7 days or 200 mg vaginal supp 1/d × 3 days; or 1200 mg vaginal supp × 1 supp; terconazole (Vagistat) 0.4% cream 5 g/d × 7 days or 0.8% cream 5 g/d × 3 days or 80 mg vaginal supp 1/d × 3 days
• Recurrent or chronic infections: use of oral anticycotic agents fluconazole (Diflucan) 150 mg tab × 1 dose
• Wear cotton underwear, avoid tight fitting nylons, proper hygiene, refrain from douching
• Consume 8–12 oz yogurt containing lactobacillus acidophilus active culture
Diagnosis: Gardnerella (bacterial vaginosis)
Treatment:
• Metronidazole (Flagyl) 500 mg tab PO bid, × 7 days or 2-g single dose or vaginal gel 0.75% 1 applicator intravaginally bid × 5 days; advise patients to avoid alcohol during treatment and for 24 hours after treatment is completed
• Clindamycin 300 mg tab PO bid × 7 days or vaginal cream 2% qd × 7 days (drug of choice for pregnant women)
• Patients with recurrent infections should be advised to have sexual partners treated
Diagnosis: Trichomoniasis
Treatment:
• Considered a STI, therefore partner(s) should be treated
• Metronidazole (Flagyl) 2 g single dose; advise patients to avoid alcohol during treatment and for 24 hours after treatment is completed
• Recurrent infections: metronidazole 500 mg tab PO bid × 7 days; if symptoms persist, 2 g qd × 3–5 days
• Patients allergic to metronidazole and/or pregnant patients can use clotrimazole (Gyne-lotrimin) cream or betadine gel intravaginally
Diagnosis: Atrophic vaginitis
Treatment:
• Estrogen cream (Premarin vaginal cream) 1 g intravaginally qd × 2–4 weeks, then decrease to 1 g 2–3 × weekly; decrease or eliminate altogether based on symptoms
• Lubrin vaginal suppositories 1 supp 5–20 min prior to intercourse as needed

teaspoon of spermicide is placed in the cup and a small amount is spread around the rim. The diaphragm must be left in place for 8 hours after intercourse and if additional intercourse is desired, additional spermicide is instilled in the vagina, but it should not be left in place for more than 12 to 18 hours. Once removed, the diaphragm is washed with a mild soap, dried, and stored. Before the diaphragm is used again, it should be held up to the light to check for holes, tears, and breaks. The patient should be instructed to urinate before inserting and after removing the diaphragm, to reduce the risk of UTIs. Under normal circumstances, the diaphragm is fitted during the annual gynecologic visit; however, if the patient has pelvic surgery or a weight change of 10 to 20 pounds, the diaphragm must be refitted.

Cervical Cap

The *cervical cap* is a cup-shaped plastic or rubber device that fits snugly around the cervix with a failure rate similar to that of the diaphragm. Like the diaphragm, the cap is used with a spermicide. Because the cap is smaller than the diaphragm, it may be more difficult to insert and remove. The advantage of the cervical cap is that it can be used in women who are unable to use a diaphragm because of a relaxed anterior vaginal wall or in those who have recurrent UTIs with the use of the diaphragm. The cervical cap should not be left in place for longer than 12 to 18 hours and should not be used during menstruation because of the slight risk of toxic shock syndrome (TSS). Only women with normal Pap smears should use the cap, and a repeat Pap smear should be obtained 3 months after its use is initiated. Adverse effects of the cervical cap are similar to those associated with the diaphragm: allergic reactions, irritation, and displacement.

Spermicidal Methods

Vaginal Contraceptive Sponge

A *vaginal contraceptive* sponge is a one-size-fits-all disposable sponge of polyurethane treated with nonoxynol-9, which protects against pregnancy but not against STIs. The sponge is placed under tap water and rinsed, then inserted into the vagina. Adverse effects include displacement, irritation and a slight risk of TSS (1 per 2 million sponges). To minimize the risk of TSS, the sponge should not be used during menses or puerperium or left in place for more than 24 hours.

Contraceptive Foam, Cream, Film, Jelly, and Suppository

Nonoxynol-9 is the spermicide contained in contraceptive foam, cream, film, jelly, and suppositories. These products have an overall failure rate of 2 to 30 percent when used correctly. The advantage to these forms of contraception are that they are available without a prescription, are easy to use, readily available, and relatively inexpensive. Nonoxynol-9 may have some virucidal and bactericidal activity, but does not offer any protection against HIV as once thought. The disadvantage of these products is that they can cause irritation and allergic reactions.

Hormonal Methods

Hormonal methods include oral contraceptives—both combination and progestin-only pills and medroxyprogesterone (Depo-Provera) injections. The implantable progestin contraceptive levonorgestrel (Norplant) is no longer available in the United States.

Oral Contraceptives

Oral contraceptives contain either a combination of estrogen and progestin or progestin only (commonly called the "mini-pill"). The most popular OCs are the 4-week cycle combination pills. These contain estrogen and progestin and are taken each day for 3 weeks, with inert (placebo) pills for the fourth week. The nonhormonal (fourth) week is the time when withdrawal uterine bleeding occurs. A recent introduction is the cycle of OCs that contain 84 active and 7 inert pills (Seasonale). This results in menses only every 3 months (4 times a year).

The estrogen–progestin OC prevents pregnancy by: suppressing the hypothalamic releasing factor that inhibits the release of follicle-stimulating hormone (FSH) and luteinizing hormone (LH) from the anterior pituitary, thereby preventing ovulation; estrogen in the pill inhibits implantation by changing normal uterine lining maturation; and the progestins slow ovum transport and uterine motility. Progestins also cause the cervical mucus to become thick and scanty, slowing sperm transport and capacitation. In addition, pH is altered and the cervical and uterine environment becomes hostile to sperm. If taken as directed, OCs have a failure rate of less than 0.5 percent, however, the typical failure rate is 3 percent.

Ethinyl estradiol (EE) is the most popular estrogen used in OCs in the United States today. The progestins used today include desogestrel (found in Mircette, Cyclessa, Ortho-Cept, Desogen), levonorgestrel (found in Alesse, Nordette, Seasonale, Trivora, Triphasil), norethindrone (found in Estrostep, Norinyl 1/35, Ortho-Novum 1/35 and 7/7/7, Necon, 1/35, Modicon, Ovcon 35, Loestrin 1.5/30, Tri-Norinyl), norgestimate (found in Ortho-Cyclen, Ortho-TriCyclen), drospirenone (found in Yasmin), and dl-norgestrel (found in Lo-Ovral, Low-Ogestrel).

All progestins, even in low doses, offer excellent cycle control and minimal metabolic changes. Progestins have variable estrogenic, androgenic, and progestational effects. The third-generation progestins (desogestrel, drospirenone, norgestimate) are the least androgenic and are particularly good for women with acne or hirsutism. Progestins may also affect plasma levels of clotting factor, blood vessel disease, diabetes, lipids, and other changes discussed separately in the chapter.

The amounts of estrogen and progestin in OC pills have been greatly reduced since their inception. The lower the effective dose, the lower the adverse effects, and the lowest acceptable dose is guided by the ability of the pill to prevent breakthrough bleeding. Breakthrough bleeding is an undesirable adverse effect. Estrogen content is usually 20 to 35 μg of EE per tablet, with no more than 50 μg available in the United States. Progestin content ranges from 0.1 to 1.5 mg. Both the estrogen and progestin doses may either be constant in a cycle pack (in monophasic contraceptives) or vary (in multiphasic contraceptives). The ratio of estrogen to progestin in combination pills can be 1:5 or 1:50, most commonly, it is 1:10 to 1:30. In the normal menses cycle, the ratio is 1:10 (early follicular), 1:5 (preovulation), and 1:30 (luteal phase). Multiphasic OCs are used in an attempt to emulate the menstrual cycle but may be associated with a higher incidence of breakthrough bleeding than monophasic pills.

To prevent ovulation, the OCs should be started either with the onset of menses (same-day start) or on the first Sunday of the week the menses starts, on the same Sunday if that is the menses start date (Sunday start). In a Sunday start, a backup method (e.g., condom or abstinence) should be used for at least 7 days.

Oral contraceptive effectiveness is dependent on patient adherence. Each pill must be taken at the same hour, every day. Once the start date is established and the pack started, there is no waiting or menstrual impact to start the subsequent pack. As soon as the initial pack is completed, the next day the next pack is started. Patients may need suggestions on how to take the pill on time and every day, whether it is when brushing teeth or at meal time or bedtime, as long as it is the same hour, every day. For women who experience nausea when taking OCs, taking them at bedtime can minimize this adverse affect.

The combination pills are provided in 28-day pill packs, color-coded by dose and time, and include the 21 active and 7 inert tablets. Some manufacturers include iron supplements in the 7 inert (placebo) pills; some eliminate the 7 inert pills and provide a 21-day pack. To keep a patient adherent and on time, it is usually best to recommend the habit of a pill a day and not stopping the last 7 days, only to forget when to restart again.

If the patient forgets to take one or more doses of the OC, the following guidelines are recommended:

- ▲ One dose missed at any time in the cycle: Take the missed dose as soon as remembered and the next dose at the usual time.
- ▲ Two doses missed during the first 2 weeks of the cycle: Take two doses daily for 2 days, then resume one dose a day. Use a backup form of birth control for the balance of the cycle.
- ▲ Two doses missed during the third week of the cycle: Take one dose daily until the last day (day 21), dispose of the remaining pills, and begin the new OC pack that day. Use a backup form of birth control for 7 days.
- ▲ Three or more doses missed at any time in the cycle: Take one dose daily until the last day (day 21), dispose of the remaining pills, and begin the new OC pack that day. Use a backup form of birth control for 7 days.

Some patients experience breakthrough bleeding with missed pills and doubling of pills. Some practitioners do not advocate using the three or more methods but rather to discontinue the pack, use a barrier method, and restart with a new pack when the regular menses begins. If menses does not occur as usual, a pregnancy test must be performed.

Patients need special instructions when starting OCs if they had a recent full-term delivery, are nursing, had a recent abortion or miscarriage, have infrequent or irregular menses, or are using other medications.

Many patients inquire about starting or restarting OCs postpartum. The Food and Drug Administration (FDA) package insert indicates that because the postpartum period lends itself to a higher risk of thromboembolism, OCs should be started no earlier than 4 to 6 weeks after delivery in nonnursing mothers. Ovulation rarely takes place before 4 weeks postpartum of a full-term pregnancy; however, if a patient is using drugs (such as bromocriptine [Parlodel]) to suppress lactation, ovulation may occur earlier and the pill should be started by day 14 postpartum.

Similarly, many patients who are breastfeeding inquire about starting on OCs. Breast milk has been found to contain the hormones of OCs, and their presence may inhibit lactation; therefore, nursing mothers should wait until the infant is weaned to use combination OCs. The World Health Organization (WHO) recommends no restrictions on using progestin-only OCs after 6 weeks postpartum in nursing mothers. This mini-pill has less or no effect on breast milk and may or may not affect the newborn. It is doubtful if the mini-pill needs to be started before 14 days postpartum.

Because ovulation is a possibility within 14 days after either a recent abortion or miscarriage, and because OCs reduce the risk of thromboembolism, the OC should be started either immediately or no later than 7 days after a first-trimester (5 to 13 weeks) abortion. After a mid-trimester abortion, the OC should be started the same way as a postpartum full term pregnancy.

If a patient is not pregnant (as confirmed by test), the pill may be started at any time, with backup contraception for the first cycle of pills. In women with amenorrhea or infrequent cycles, discontinuance of the OC may leave them anovulatory or fully amenorrheic if their history includes secondary amenorrhea, oligomenorrhea, or irregular cycles. These patients should, therefore, consider another method of birth control.

Ineffective contraception and breakthrough bleeding may occur as the result of an interaction between the OC and drugs taken simultaneously. Table 13.2 presents common drug interactions. The exact mechanism of action is not clear, but it may be the result of the alteration of the GI tract's absorption ability or alteration of enzymatic action on medication either accelerating or decelerating metabolism. It is often difficult to modify drug prescriptions in illness and far simpler and safer to consider another form of birth control.

Table 13.2 **Oral Contraceptives: Drug Interactions**

Drug Interactions	Effectiveness	Drugs
Drug Effect on OCs	Increased effectiveness	None
	Decreased effectiveness	Barbiturates, griseofulvin, phenytoin, primidone, rifampin
	Possible decreased effectiveness	Carbamazepine
OC Effect on Drugs	Decreased effectiveness	Acetaminophen, benzodiazepines, guanethidine, methyldopa, oral anticoagulants, oral hypoglycemics
	Increased effectiveness	Alcohol, antidepressants, benzodiazepines, beta-blockers, corticosteroids, theophylline

The combination OC is the most effective reversible form of birth control, relatively inexpensive, and least invasive method of correcting painful and irregular cycles. Some of the other benefits include reduced blood loss, resulting in lower incidence of anemia; less risk of ectopic pregnancy and salpingitis; fewer ovarian cysts; reduction in dysmenorrhea; reduction in risk of ovarian and endometrial cancer; improvement in acne; decreased risk for developing myomas in long-term (greater than 4 years) users; and a beneficial effect on bone mass. In general, these benefits reduce the need for costly hospitalizations.

The benefits and safety of OCs are dependent on adherence, but also to other factors such as smoking. There is an increased risk of cardiovascular disease and thromboembolic disease in women who are older than 35 years of age and who smoke while taking OCs. Women older than 40 years of age who are nonsmokers may safely continue low-dose OCs. OC use is safest throughout the menstrual life in women who are of normal weight, nonsmokers, have normal blood pressure (BP) and cholesterol, have no diabetes, and have no family history of heart disease. Consequently, a full history, gynecologic exam, Pap smear, infection checks, lipid profile, and CBC lab tests should be performed before an OC is prescribed. Evaluation of the history, physical exam, and lab results is necessary to prevent adverse effects.

OCs have a wide range of adverse effects, from simple to more serious. Primarily, the constant presence of low-level hormones creates a pregnancy-like environment in the body. Thyroid hormone and cortisol levels may be elevated. Progestins may alter the lipid profile. Estrogens decrease glucose tolerance and women with diabetes should be monitored closely if using OCs. Estrogen-related increases in clotting factors result in an increased risk of thromboembolism. Women who will be undergoing surgery and postoperative bed confinement should discontinue OCs at least 4 weeks before surgery.

The risk of developing hypertension in OC users increases with the duration of use and also in older women. If a woman develops hypertension while taking OCs, the pills should be stopped and another form of contraception adopted. However, if a woman is younger than 40 years of age and has mild hypertension that is controlled with medication, and who does not smoke, OCs may be used as long as blood pressure is closely monitored.

Other adverse effects of OC use is an increased risk of cervical dysplasia and cancer in long-term (greater than 3 to 4 years) users. There is some evidence that there is a higher incidence of liver (usually benign) tumors, or gallstones, but this is usually associated with higher dosages, long-term use, and older age. The use of OCs can precipitate migraine or vascular headaches or make existing migraines worse. Another form of contraception should be used if headaches increase in severity or frequency. Other problems that have been reported with OC use are depression and fluid retention.

It is unclear whether OCs contribute to breast cancer. FDA packaging inserts infer an association related to duration of use and history. Fibrocystic breast discomfort has been found to be less in OC users. Breast swelling and tenderness are common premenstrual complaints. Low-dose OCs seem to decrease this complaint, as does reducing caffeine intake, avoiding smoking, and reducing sodium intake.

Because the cervical mucus is affected by the progestin component and estrogen can cause cervical mucorrhea, it is not uncommon for OC users to experience mucus-causing irritation, including *Candida,* of the vagina and vulva. Antibiotic therapy may also cause this condition.

Patients who use OCs may have increased pigmentation of the face and forehead. Combination pill users find this in the areola and perineum as well. Weight gain may or may not be an OC effect; it may be simply overeating, lack of exercise, fluid retention, thyroid problems, or poor nutrition, but a gain of 2 to 5 pounds is not uncommon.

To metabolize OCs properly, certain vitamins are utilized and not necessarily stored. Women should be instructed to take a daily multivitamin and extra vitamin C while taking OCs to prevent deficiency of these nutrients.

When combination OCs are discontinued, 90 percent of women resume ovulation and menses within 3 months. A pregnancy test should be done to ensure the patient is not pregnant if normal cycles are not established after 3 months. If a woman does not wish to become pregnant, another form of contraception should be used when the OC is discontinued. If a woman becomes pregnant while using the OC, most studies show no increased incidence of congenital defects. However, it is best not to use OCs if a patient believes she is pregnant but to use another method until it is established whether or not she is pregnant.

The progestin-only pill, the "mini-pill," contains progestin only and has a reported failure rate of 1 to 4 percent, slightly higher than that of combined OCs. Progestin-only pills contain either 0.35 mg norethindrone (Ortho Micronor, Nor-QD) or 0.075 mg dl-norgestrel (Ovrette) and are taken continuously beginning on the first day of the menstrual cycle. The progestin inhibits ovulation inconsistently but does cause thickening of the cervical mucus (makes it hostile to sperm), alters ovum transport (higher risk of ectopic pregnancy), and inhibits implantation. The advantages of the mini-pill are that it is safe during lactation and may actually increase the flow of milk; can be used in women older than 35 years of age; can be used in women with sickle cell disease; and can be used in women with myomas. The progestin-only pill is less likely to cause headache, high BP, depression, cramps, premenstrual syndrome (PMS), or glucose elevation than combination OCs.

Disadvantages of the mini-pill include contraceptive failure and ectopic pregnancy. Irregular bleeding (amenorrhea, breakthrough bleeding, prolonged flow) are common in progestin-only users and may necessitate frequent pregnancy tests. Absolute contraindications include pregnancy, current or past history of thromboembolic disorders, stroke or heart disease, breast cancer, liver mass, and undiagnosed abnormal vaginal bleeding.

If the woman taking OCs complains of any of the adverse effects typically associated with OCs (nausea, abdominal bloating, hair changes, weight gain, leg pain, cramps, swelling), often switching the patient to a pill with a lower estrogen dose or one with a less androgenic progestin will relieve the problem. For example, switching to an OC with less progestational activity relieves hypoglycemia. If the patient complains of abdominal bloating, a lower estrogen dose or different progestin may relieve this problem. Bowel irregularity can also cause bloating, so this should be evaluated. If a patient complains of nausea, she should be instructed to take the pill with food or at bedtime. If the nausea persists or worsens, the patient may need to consult a gastroenterologist.

Regarding hair changes, excessive facial and body hair is usually less obvious in OC users. Hair loss is not usually related to OC use and should be referred to a dermatologist for evaluation.

Progestin, especially at high androgenic activity levels, and estrogen may cause weight gain. The patient should be switched to an OC with lower progestin/androgenic activities and provided with a diet that is lower in calories. If the gain is mainly in breasts, hips, and thighs; is cyclic; and causes bloating, a pill with lower estrogen content should be tried.

Leg pain, cramps, and swelling usually disappear after three cycle packs. A severe pain, especially unilateral pain, can indicate a thrombosis and requires immediate discontinuation of the OC and immediate medical evaluation.

Medroxyprogesterone Acetate Injections

Medroxyprogesterone acetate, or Depo-Provera injectable, consists of 150 mg of deep IM injections given every 3 months and has an efficacy rate of 99.7 percent. The initial injection is given on day 5 of the menses and once injected, it may take 8 to 9 months for fertility to be restored. The mode of action, adverse effects, and contraindications are the same as those for progesterone only OCs. After 5 years of use, bone density loss has been observed, and patients should be advised to have adequate calcium intake daily (1200 to 1500 mg) at the onset of use. The thinning of the uterine lining tends to lend some protection against endometrial cancer but also makes it more difficult for the patient to conceive for up to a year after discontinuing the injection. Depo-Provera may be used for patients who smoke and who are not candidates for the oral combination pill. All patients, however, should stop smoking as soon as possible.

Intrauterine Device

The *intrauterine device* (IUD) is a highly effective method for most women, and contrary to previous thought, nulliparity is not a contraindication to IUD use. Available in the United States today are the Mirena IUD, which releases levonorgestrel slowly, and the copper TCu380A. The Mirena is effective for about 5 years and the TCu380A is effective for about 10 years. The mechanism of action of an IUD is not totally understood, but it is believed to act either as a spermicidal or to have inhibitory effects on sperm capacitation and transport. Clearly, however, the IUD is not an abortifacient.

The IUD is inserted by a clinician trained in the procedure and is done either during or at midcycle to prevent implantation. A 6- to 8-week wait is customary postpartum before insertion. The IUD has two long, off-white monofilament tails that project from the cervix into the vagina. The patient should be instructed to check this string after each menstrual period to ensure the IUD is still in place. A Pap smear and cultures are done during pelvic exam before insertion to be sure there are no abnormalities or infections.

Adverse effects include heavier menstrual periods, bleeding between periods, and cramping, and women with these problems should seek an alternative form of contraception. In 10 to 20 percent of cases during the first year of use there is spontaneous expulsion of the IUD. During the first month following insertion, there is an increased risk of pelvic infection. There does not appear to be any greater risk for infection other than that for acquiring an STI. Fertility is not affected by the use of an IUD.

Absolute contraindications for the use of an IUD include pregnancy, acute pelvic inflammatory disease, and purulent cervicitis. An IUD should be used with caution in women with a history of pelvic inflammatory disease, menorrhagia or severe dysmenorrhea, cervical or uterine neoplasia, or an abnormal uterus.

Regulated Abstinence

Regulated abstinence is another form of birth control. Abstaining from sexual intercourse during the days of the menstrual cycle when the ovum is most vulnerable to fertilization is one way of avoiding pregnancy. There are several techniques used to predict the best time for abstinence. The *rhythm method* or *calendar method* is based on the assumptions that the ovum is viable 24 hours after ovulation, spermatozoa are viable 48 hours after coitus, and ovulation occurs 12 to 16 days before menses. The woman records the length of her cycle for several months and establishes her fertile period by deducting 18 days from her shortest cycle and 11 days from her previous longest cycle. Each subsequent cycle, abstinence occurs during this calculated fertile period. The patient must have regular cycles to use this method.

The *natural family planning method* is another technique used to predict the best time for abstinence. There are three types: the basal body temperature method, the cervical mucus method, and the symptothermal method. In the *basal body temperature method*, the patient measures basal body temperature daily. Abstinence is observed from menses to 3 days of elevated temperature. The lengthy abstinence plus abstinence in anovulatory cycles make this an unfavorable method.

In the *cervical mucus method*, an interpretation and recognition is made of changes in the cervical mucus consistency, which occurs in response to the changes in estrogen and progesterone levels. Abstinence begins in menses (and every other day thereafter to reduce risk of confusing mucus with semen) until the first day of slippery, copious mucus. Abstinence is observed every day thereafter until 4 days after the last day that mucus is present, or the peak mucus day.

In the *symptothermal method*, the fertile period is determined by calendar calculation and cervical mucus changes to decide on the fertile period; changes in mucus and basal temperature are used to decide on the end of this period. This method is difficult to learn but is the most effective natural method to prevent pregnancy.

The greatest obstacle to acceptance of these techniques is the need to avoid sexual relations for many days each cycle. Some couples use the barrier method during fertile times for greater acceptance and reduced failure rate.

Recent developments have produced self-administered tests (ovulation prediction kits) for the detection of hormone changes, reducing abstinence to several days per cycle. Urine evaluation for hormones is another method of family planning.

Postcoital Controls

Postcoital controls are another method of birth control. There are three different types: withdrawal, postcoitus douche, and emergency contraception. The simplest, most practical method of preventing pregnancy after unprotected sex is the administration of emergency contraception. Several regimens are effective in preventing implantation if the ovum has been fertilized, and all have about the same failure rate, 1 to 3 percent. The first method is to give two doses 12 hours apart of levonorgestrel 0.75 mg (called plan B in the United States). An alternative is levonorgestrel 1.5 mg in a single dose. Both of these methods must be instituted within 72 hours of intercourse. Another regimen is ethinyl estradiol 50 μg with 0.5 mg of norgestrel and is prepackaged as Preven. Two tablets are given and then two more 12 hours later. A regimen that is comparable is to give two tablets now and two more 12 hours later of Lo/Ovral, Nordette, or Levlen. An alternative to this is to instruct the patient to take the yellow pills of either Triphasil or Tri-Levlen in the same regimen, two pills followed by two pills 12 hours later. The third regimen is for the patient to take ethinyl estradiol 2.5 mg bid for 5 days, but this method tends to cause more nausea, vomiting, and breast tenderness than the other regimens. It is good practice to check for pregnancy pretreatment in the event that the woman inadvertently became pregnant earlier in her cycle and then posttreatment because the effects on the fetus worsen as the treatment and pregnancy continue, although it is uncertain that birth defects are directly related to steroid exposure in early pregnancy. Again, careful menstrual history should be reviewed and a consent form may be obtained before prescription. Some women elect to continue the pregnancy if the treatment fails, and 10 percent of such cases have been later diagnosed with ectopic pregnancies. Contraindications to emergency contraception are pregnancy and those as listed for oral contraceptive pills.

Sterilization

The most permanent method of birth control is sterilization. After risks and benefits of sterilization are reviewed with the patient, consent is obtained. The presence of two witnesses is recommended for patients younger than age 25 or those who are childless and older than 40 years of age. One percent of 1000 patients who undergo the procedure later request reversal of sterilization.

Male sterilization consists of vasectomy performed on an outpatient basis; the procedure typically takes 20 minutes under local anesthesia. The major complication is hematoma (5 percent), sperm granuloma, and spontaneous reanastomosis. After vasectomy, the man is not considered sterile until two sperm-free ejaculates have been produced. Semen analysis should be performed 1 to 2 months after the procedure. About 15 to 20 ejaculations are required postvasectomy for absolute sterility.

Female sterilization is performed under general anesthesia by transperitoneal incision for tubal ligation. If sterilization is performed postpartum, a small infraumbilical incision is made and a tubal ligation is performed in the delivery room immediately or in the operating room the next day. Failure rate is 1 per 1000. Complications are hemorrhage, puncture, and cautery of the bowel (0.6 percent).

Abortion

An elective abortion is one of the most common gynecologic procedures in the United States and has been legal since 1973. In accordance with the landmark *Roe v. Wade* Supreme Court decision, the state may not interfere with the practice of abortion in the first trimester. To protect the health of the mother, a second-trimester abortion may be performed, and limiting restrictions have been declared unconstitutional. In fact, since legalized abortion in the United States, the maternal mortality rate has fallen considerably.

The primary method used for elective abortion in the first trimester is vacuum aspiration under local anesthesia. Dilation and evacuation can be used in the second trimester and is done under either local or general anesthesia. For pregnancy after 18 weeks hypertonic saline solution is instilled into the amniotic cavity or prostaglandins may also be used to induce labor. The prostaglandins used most often are E_2, as a vaginal suppository; and 15-methyl prostaglandin $F_{2\text{-alpha}}$, as an IM injection. They are given at 2- to 3-hour intervals until evacuation. Instillation of hypertonic saline or prostaglandin administration are both difficult for the patient. Abortions are rarely performed after 20 weeks, as fetal viability is considered to be at 24 weeks.

Complications from abortions increase as gestation increases and include retained products of conception and unrecognized ectopic pregnancy. Currently, most abortions (90 percent) are performed before 12 weeks of gestation and there is an overall mortality rate of 1:100,000. Patients should be counseled to obtain an abortion as early as possible if this is their choice.

Recently, the U.S. FDA approved mifepristone (RU486), a synthetic antiprogestational–antiglucocorticoid pill as an oral abortifacient. RU486 is used to induce abortion during the first 9 weeks of pregnancy. RU486 is given as a single dose of 200 mg and has a success rate of 85 percent but if it is followed in 36 to 48 hours with a prostaglandin vaginal suppository the success rate in terminating pregnancy is 95 percent. Adverse effects include nausea, vomiting, bleeding, and abdominal pain.

Patient Teaching

Contraception is not just a method, it is part of a life decision and future plan. There is no ideal method for every woman, but because so many options are available today, contraception can be tailored for each person's lifestyle, motivation, and partner's participation. Research in reproductive biology may provide less invasive and more effective methods in the future. Maximum outcome still depends on consistent and accurate use—the human element.

Every (heterosexual) woman should consider contraception as part of her overall personal health maintenance just as she should consider an annual gynecologic exam, BSE, balanced nutrition, smoking and alcohol cessation, weight control, mental health, exercise, and risk reduction. Fertility control and good health work hand in hand for the patient and her future plans.

Amenorrhea

The average age of menarche in the United States today is 12.7 years, and usually occurs between ages 11 and 15 years. Absence of menstruation is considered amenorrhea and can be primary or secondary. *Primary amenorrhea* is the failure to menstruate by age 14 in girls with no secondary sex characteristics (breast development) or failure to menstruate by age 16 years in girls who may or may not have developed secondary sexual characteristics. *Secondary amenorrhea* is the absence of menstruation for 3 or more consecutive months in a woman who has achieved menarche.

Epidemiology and Causes

Primary amenorrhea occurs in about 0.3 percent of women and may result from hypothalamic or pituitary failure, ovarian failure, or from chromosomal or enzymatic abnormalities. Amenorrhea is a manifestation of a pathological process and is not a diagnosis itself. Causes of primary amenorrhea include congenital defects of gonadotropin production, genetic disorders (Turner's syndrome), congenital central nervous system (CNS) defects such as hydrocephalus, congenital anatomic malformations of the reproductive system (absence of vagina or uterus), abnormal outflow tract (vaginal aplasia or imperforate hymen), and acquired CNS lesions, including trauma, infection, and tumors. Females without a uterus or vagina usually have normal ovarian function in which skeletal growth and secondary sex characteristics develop in the proper sequence, but menses does not occur. In cases of uterine hypoplasia, the uterus does not respond to hormonal stimulation during puberty.

If a woman is not pregnant (most common cause), secondary amenorrhea is usually associated with anovulation caused by neuroendocrine dysfunction. Secondary amenorrhea occurs in approximately 1 to 3 percent of women, with a higher incidence among college students (3 to 5 percent) and athletes (5 to 60 percent). Amenorrhea reflects a disruption in the normal physiologic or anatomic function of the hypothalamus, pituitary gland, and ovary or outflow tract. Hormones produced by these structures play major roles in ovulation and any slight change in production may result in anovulation and absence of menstruation. Women taking anabolic steroids (weight lifters, body builders) may present with secondary amenorrhea.

Pathophysiology

The hypothalamic–pituitary–ovarian-uterine axis needs to function in a coordinated manner for menstruation to occur.

The most frequent cause of primary amenorrhea is dysfunction of the ovaries resulting from gonadal dysgenesis. This may be caused by various chromosomal abnormalities that result in a depletion of oocytes and ovarian follicles, subsequently impairing the regulated cycle of menses. Turner syndrome characterized by an XO (single X-chromosome) genotype is one of the most common chromosomal disorders. In this condition, the ovaries are replaced by fibrous tissue (known as streak ovaries), which has a very limited or absent capacity for estrogen production. In addition, premature ovarian failure (menopause occurring before age 40 years), polycystic ovary syndrome (characterized by concurrent hyperandrogenism), and estrogen- or androgen-secreting tumors may all produce amenorrhea. Secondary amenorrhea is nearly universally a hormonal problem, as by definition, normal female sexual development has already occurred. By far, the most common cause of secondary amenorrhea are the normal hormonal changes associated with pregnancy, that is, increased progesterone production needed to maintain the pregnant uterus.

Under normal conditions, the hypothalamus produces gonadotropin-releasing hormone (GnRH) in a pulsatile fashion. In response to GnRH, the anterior pituitary gland produces the gonadotropins: FSH and LH. In response to FSH and LH, the ovaries produce estrogen and progesterone, which subsequently drive secondary sexual development and cyclic menstruation. Factors such as stress, weight changes, nutritional deficiencies, strenuous exercise, or infiltrative CNS lesions including hypothalamic tumors (e.g., lymphoma, histiocytosis) or sarcoidosis may all disrupt the normal pulsatile release of GnRH. Pulsatile production of GnRH may also be affected by rare pituitary tumors including macroadenomas and microadenomas, which consist primarily of hyperprolactinomas and account for 20 percent of secondary amenorrhea cases. Amenorrhea may occur before or after the treatment of such tumors (i.e., surgical resection), depending on the underlying production of pituitary gonadotropins. Functional hypothalamic amenorrhea (which may be primary or secondary) is characterized by an absence of histologic CNS pathology, despite an under- or overproduction of GnRH that leads to a decrease in gonadotropin surges and amenorrhea. In contrast, a complete absence of hypothalamic GnRH production may occur congenitally, inherited in an autosomal dominant, autosomal recessive, or X-linked fashion.

While acquired endometrial scarring known as Asherman's syndrome is the only anatomic uterine etiology of secondary amenorrhea, nearly a quarter of primary amenorrhea cases are due to structural abnormalities that prevent menstrual outflow including imperforate hymen, vaginal agenesis, absent or abnormal uterus, or the presence of a transvaginal septum between the hymen and the cervix. Such conditions may not be connected to any specific event or environmental exposure. However, some conditions may result from biochemical abnormalities in hormone receptor functioning, manifested on either an XX or XY genetic background. Thus, an advanced workup of patients with primary amenorrhea should also include karyotyping to confirm that the patient is an XX genetic female.

Complete androgen insensitivity syndrome (testicular feminization syndrome) is the prototype for primary amenorrhea occurring in a genetic male who appears outwardly female on clinical exam. In this disorder, the external genitalia of XY males are unable to respond to testosterone because of a receptor defect and thus fail to undergo differentiation into a phenotypically male form, despite their XY karyotype. Internally, however, the testes do produce functional Müllerian inhibiting factor, causing the regression of all internal female reproductive organs, thus leading to primary amenorrhea. A congenital lack of 5-alpha-reductase enzymatic activity causes a similar phenomenon of external sexual ambiguity in which XY males do not undergo full secondary sexual development at puberty, as testosterone cannot be converted into its more potent metabolite dihydrotestosterone.

Clinical Presentation

Subjective

Amenorrhea is a symptom, so this is usually the reason the patient seeks health care. Other subjective data from the patient usually are obtained during the history. The detailed history must include a complete menstrual history including age at menarche, date of LMP and last normal menses, cycle regularity and flow; obstetrical history, including number of pregnancies, lactation, and birth control methods; developmental data, to evaluate for short stature, or growth hormone or thyroid deficiency; nutritional history, including anorexia, diet, stress, sports activities; family history, especially the mother's onset of menopause; symptoms that may arise from systemic disorders (diabetes, thyroid); the presence or absence of any secondary sex characteristics; and any medications being taken, such as hypertensive medications or OCPs. Cyclic pelvic pain in a young teen or preteen could indicate müllerian outflow tract obstruction.

Objective

The physical exam should include a neurologic exam to assess for headaches and visual field abnormalities to rule out pituitary tumor; olfactory testing to screen for Kallmann's syndrome (hypothalamic or pituitary tumor); a pelvic and rectal exam (to assess for the presence of a vagina, condition of hymen, and presence of uterus); the existence of skin lesions, acne, needle marks, and skin darkening, to rule out adrenal insufficiency; and a breast exam, to observe for galactorrhea, which may be a sign of hyperprolactinemia.

Diagnostic Reasoning

Diagnostic Tests

A urine pregnancy test should be the first test performed in the patient with amenorrhea, because it is inexpensive and easy. It should be done despite what the patient tells you about her sexual history. If the test is positive, a serum beta-human chorionic gonadotropin (hCG) for approximate staging of pregnancy should be done. Other tests should include baseline blood chemistry profiles to evaluate for renal or hepatic disease, thyroid function tests (TFTs), vaginal smears for estrogen effect, and FSH, LH, and prolactin levels.

Tests to include for secondary amenorrhea include androgen studies of total testosterone and dehydroepiandrosterone sulfate, which are specifically done in women who also have clinical signs of hyperandrogenism (acne, hirsutism, etc.); a progesterone challenge test, and the measurement of prolactin and FSH levels, which evaluate the hypothalamic–pituitary–ovarian axis.

A progestin (or progesterone) challenge indirectly provides information regarding outflow tract patency. This test, given once the pregnancy test is negative, consists of giving medroxyprogesterone acetate (MPA) 10 mg PO for 5 to 10 days to induce withdrawal bleeding or spotting which should occur within 14 days after the last dose. If withdrawal bleeding occurs this indicates pituitary–gonadal function and amenorrhea is probably the result of anovulation. The test is negative if no withdrawal bleeding occurs and suggests low levels of estrogen (premature ovarian failure or hypothalamic pituitary failure) or a nonpatent outflow tract.

Differential Diagnosis

Differential diagnoses include pregnancy (intrauterine or ectopic), menopause, premature ovarian failure, hyperprolactinemia related to tumor, stress, or thyroid dysfunction; and some genetic or chromosome-related problems. Outflow-tract abnormalities include Asherman's syndrome, which is characterized by endometrial adhesions and scarring as a result of aggressive dilation and curettage, uterovaginal malignancies, cervical stenosis, or imperforated hymen.

A genetic disorder of male pseudohermaphroditism may result in primary amenorrhea. The patient is male genetically but female morphologically. No male genitalia develop because androgen receptors are absent in undifferentiated target organs.

Management

The goal of management for amenorrhea is to initiate or restore menses while determining the cause. Treatment of amenorrhea is dependent on its etiology and the patient's wishes. For primary amenorrhea, estrogen therapy is indicated for patients to develop secondary sex characteristics and prevent osteoporosis.

For a patient with secondary amenorrhea whose progestin challenge test is negative, treatment consists of oral estrogen 1.25 to 2.5 mg daily for 21 to 25 days, along with oral progesterone 10 mg daily during the last 5 to 10 days of the estrogen doses. The patient should experience bleeding if the endometrium is normally responsive to estrogen and the outflow tract is patent.

For a patient with secondary amenorrhea who is anovulatory and has adequate endogenous estrogen, the common practice is to administer periodic or cyclic progesterone 10 mg PO daily for 10 days each month. These patients must experience withdrawal bleeding for at least 3 months to prevent endometrial hyperplasia or endometrial carcinoma related to unopposed estrogen. If the patient is anovulatory and wants to conceive, ovulation may be induced with clomiphene citrate (Clomid) 50 mg PO on days 5 to 9 of the cycle after induction of bleeding with progesterone.

If the patient wants contraception, OCs are beneficial for monthly cycle regulation. For patients with hyperprolactinemia, bromocriptine (Parlodel) is the drug of choice. Once hypothalamic failure is established, GnRH may be given in a pulsatile fashion. GnRH is given as a combination with estrogen and calcium because these patients are hypoestrogenic and at high risk for osteoporosis. In patients with thyroid dysfunction, replacement therapy should be initiated and the amenorrhea should correct itself.

Surgical intervention is possible for women with endometrial scarring (Asherman's syndrome) from endometritis. Diagnosis and treatment are accomplished in the same way, through hysteroscopic inspection and lysis of adhesions. After this procedure, antibiotics are given and a small Foley catheter is placed in the uterus and left for 1 week. When the catheter is removed, an IUD is inserted and left in place for 2 months while the patient receives cyclic estrogen and progesterone to build the endometrial lining. This treatment usually restores normal menses and fertility, but complications of pregnancy are common, including spontaneous abortions.

Follow-Up and Referral

A gynecologist as well as an endocrinologist should be consulted for further testing. If a CNS problem is detected, computed tomography (CT) scanning or magnetic resonance imaging (MRI) should be performed to rule out pathology. The gynecologist may also consider an endometrial biopsy for patients who are at high risk (those with diabetes, hypertension, and obesity) for endometrial hyperplasia and adenocarcinoma before prescribing medications. Pelvic ultrasound may also be used to measure the endometrial strip and rule out ovarian masses.

Once the workup is completed, the patient should be evaluated annually. Patients with primary amenorrhea should be referred to a gynecologist. Patients with secondary amenorrhea may need to be referred if initial treatment is unsuccessful.

Patient Education

Frequently, teenagers and their parents are apprehensive when menses do not start "on schedule," but reassurance and watchful waiting may be all that is needed. Patients should be taught about their medication regimen and the importance of taking medications exactly as prescribed. Patients must be aware of the need to notify their health-care provider if they take any new medications, because many drugs interact with others and have a potentiating effect as well as a negative effect on the action of some medications.

Dysmenorrhea

Dysmenorrhea is painful menses. It may be primary, with no pelvic pathology, or secondary, usually accompanied by pelvic pathology.

Epidemiology and Causes

Primary dysmenorrhea usually begins within 1 to 2 years of the onset of menstruation, is associated with ovular cycles, and lasts 1 or 2 days each month. The menstrual pain associated with primary dysmenorrhea may lessen for some women as they age or after the birth of children, or it can last until menopause. There is no associated pathology and from 50 to 75 percent of women experience this at some time.

Secondary dysmenorrhea is caused by a physical condition. Women who experience this type tend to be older than those who have primary dysmenorrhea, sometimes beginning when a women is in her 30s or 40s. Menstrual pain is the predominant symptom, as in primary dysmenorrhea. Possible conditions responsible for secondary dysmenorrhea include endometriosis, pelvic inflammatory disease (PID), fibroids (uterine leiomyomata), adenomyosis, and endometrial polyps. Secondary dysmenorrhea is most common in women 40 to 50 years of age.

It is estimated that more than 140 million lost work hours are a result of dysmenorrhea. It is the most common gynecologic complaint of women and the main cause of missed work, school, or other activities. An estimated 42 million women in the United States suffer from painful menstrual symptoms each month. Risk factors for primary dysmenorrhea include obesity, nulliparity, cigarette smoking, and a positive family history for dysmenorrhea. Risk factors for secondary dysmenorrhea include pelvic infection, endometriosis, and STIs.

Pathophysiology

Dysmenorrhea is caused by the production of prostaglandins and leukotrienes, chemical substances that are released when uterine tissue breaks up and is sloughed off during menstruation. Prostaglandin F_2 (PGF_2) and PGE_2 are two of the most important players. Elevated uterine levels of these arachidonic acid metabolites, and more specifically an increased ratio of PGF_2 to PGE_2, have been directly correlated with increases in subjective pain. Increased prostaglandin levels found in uterine tissue, but not in plasma, cause dysrhythmic uterine contractions and increased resting tone by stimulating smooth muscle tissue to contract, which compromises blood supply and oxygenation to uterine muscle, thus causing severe pelvic pain known as "cramps."

These uterine contractions may last for several minutes at a time, producing maximal pressures up to 400 mm Hg, with resting pressures as high as 80 mm Hg. In turn, if uterine muscle tone is consistently higher than systemic arterial pressure, uterine ischemia ensues, resulting in the production of anaerobic metabolites which stimulate small type C pain fibers. In turn, pain relief has been directly correlated with decreases in uterine contraction pressure. Because smooth muscle is found in the stomach, intestines, and blood vessels as well as in the uterus, the excessive stimulation accounts for nausea, diarrhea, and headache which often accompany dysmenorrhea. Cramps facilitate the release of menstrual tissue, and because the cervical opening is usually widened after childbirth or years of menstruation, cramps may lessen in the older patient. In contrast, worsened cramps are associated with anovulatory menstrual cycles—a common phenomenon in young women, affecting up to half of adolescents within 2 to 4 years following the start of menses.

Clinical Presentation

Subjective

Description of the pain is an important factor. The type and severity as well as duration of pain should be noted. A patient with dysmenorrhea may present with sharp stabbing pain and cramping, low back pain, nausea and sometimes vomiting, bowel changes, and fatigue. The pain with primary dysmenorrhea usually starts within 24 hours of menses and may last for 48 to 72 hours. Secondary dysmenorrhea may have the onset of pain a week or more before the onset of menses and continue after cessation of flow for a few days. She may state that she is immobilized by her period every month for the first day. Her pain may be so severe that at times she cannot do anything except stay in bed with a heating pad on her abdomen. She may lose her appetite and eat very little during this time. She may complain of pain during intercourse.

Diagnostic Reasoning

Diagnostic Tests

The physical exam (revealing no signs of pathology) and a history of consistent symptoms for 1 or 2 days each month will usually substantiate the diagnosis of primary dysmenorrhea, as the symptoms are fairly typical. Secondary dysmenorrhea may have a slightly varying description of symptoms; some menses are more painful than others and the level of discomfort may be progressive. If the complaint of painful intercourse is present, a diagnosis of secondary dysmenorrhea, possibly related to endometriosis, should be explored.

Laboratory studies in the evaluation of dysmenorrhea are ordered to rule out potential causes of pelvic pain. They include quantitative hCG and CBC, urinalysis, erythrocyte sedimentation rate (ESR), and stool for occult blood. Serum CA-125 levels are known to be elevated in women with endometriosis (a common cause of dysmenorrhea) as well as ovarian pathology; however, this test is not sufficiently sensitive to serve as a reliable screening tool.

Imaging studies are the choice for the initial evaluation of suspected pelvic disease. Gynecologic consultation with visualization of pelvic organs via ultrasound is the definitive procedure of choice for evaluation of pelvic pathology. If such testing does not produce a definitive diagnosis, it may be followed up by laparoscopic exploration to directly visualize pathologic conditions such as endometriosis.

Differential Diagnosis

The ultimate goal of the differential diagnosis of dysmenorrhea is to exclude underlying pelvic pathology to differentiate between primary and secondary dysmenorrhea. This includes diagnosing conditions that may produce or mimic dysmenorrhea such as endometriosis, ovarian cysts, ectopic pregnancy, UTI, vaginitis, dysfunctional uterine bleeding, uterine leiomyomata, appendicitis, lower back pain, trauma from sexual assault, and PID. Endometriosis is the most common cause of secondary dysmenorrhea.

Management

The principle of management for primary dysmenorrhea is to relieve the menstrual pain as much as possible. For secondary dysmenorrhea, the goal is to find a diagnosis.

Ordinary aspirin 325 mg two tablets PO q4h, started a day or 2 before menstruation, is helpful because of its antiprostaglandin activity as an inhibitor of the enzyme cyclooxygenase which converts arachidonic acid into prostaglandin metabolites. Dietary changes such as the avoidance of caffeine during the first few days of menstruation have been shown to be helpful. Exercise may be of some benefit because it raises levels of beta-endorphins, chemicals in the brain associated with pain relief. Cigarette smoking has been linked to increasing the duration of dysmenorrhea.

Interestingly, in clinical studies placebo treatments have been shown to improve symptoms of dysmenorrhea, albeit often only transiently. Thus, the NSAID ibuprofen (Advil, Motrin) 400 to 800 mg PO tid–qid prn remains the mainstay of dysmenorrhea therapy and is considered the most effective OTC pain reliever for cramps. Several studies have demonstrated that if ibuprofen fails to relieve a patient's symptoms, it is appropriate to try an alternative NSAID agent such as naproxen (Naprosyn; 250 to 500 mg PO tid prn), indomethacin (Indocin), fenoprofen (Nalfon), or mefenamic acid (500 mg PO initially, followed by 250 mg qid for up to 3 days). The latter agent not only inhibits new prostaglandin formation but also inhibits the activity of preformed prostaglandins. In contrast, acetaminophen (Tylenol) appears to be less effective, as it does not inhibit prostaglandin formation and is not considered an anti-inflammatory agent.

Application of a hot water bottle to the abdomen or hot baths may help relieve discomfort and in some studies has been shown to be as effective as NSAID therapy. However, interestingly, the combination of heat therapy and NSAIDs together has been shown to be counterproductive. Acupuncture, transcutaneous electric nerve stimulation (TENS) therapy, and specific herbal teas (e.g., mint tea, certain yogic preparations) have all been shown to decrease uterine spasms in small clinical trials. Relaxation or yoga-type exercises may also help to relieve pain. Dietary restriction of both caffeine and salt is also recommended, while vitamin E, vitamin B_1, vitamin B_6, and fish oil supplements have all been shown in limited trials to confer some benefit.

For some women, even prescribed prostaglandin inhibitors are ineffective. Combined estrogen–progestin OC agents may be considered for these patients, as OCs relieve cramping by inhibiting arachidonic acid production and ovulation, in turn hindering high levels of prostaglandin production. These therapies may be given daily as 21-, 63-, or 105-day continuous courses, each followed by 7 days off medication, prior to repeating the cycle. Longer cycles of OC therapy decrease the frequency of menstruation occurring during the off-therapy week. However, small volumes of breakthrough vaginal bleeding on several days of the week are more common with these longer cycles.

If no relief is achieved following NSAID and OC therapy, ultrasonography and even exploratory laparoscopy may be appropriate to rule out pelvic pathology. If endometriosis (the most common cause of secondary amenorrhea) is found, a gonadotropin-releasing hormone (GnRH) analogue may be prescribed in continuous fashion to inhibit menses (see section on Endometriosis).

Follow-Up and Referral

Each patient with a case of pelvic pain should have follow-up care because treatment is ongoing and requires further evaluation of relief of symptoms or additional diagnostic evaluation for continued symptoms. Prognosis for primary dysmenorrhea is good with the use of antiprostaglandins, with an 70 to 80 percent relief of symptoms in some cases.

Patient Education

Advise the patient that ordinary aspirin, two tablets q4h 1 to 2 days before menstruation begins can significantly reduce prostaglandin levels. Education about changes in exercise and diet may also be useful. Dietary supplementation with omega-3 fatty acids has been shown to help provide relief in adolescents. Patients should be encouraged to stop smoking and decrease alcohol intake. Symptomatic treatment with a warm bath or locally applied heat may be helpful.

Endometriosis

Endometriosis is a painful, chronic disease, characterized by the presence and proliferation of abnormally placed endometrial tissue, which responds to hormone changes in the woman's body. Abnormally placed endometrial tissue has been found outside the uterus, usually in the abdomen, on the ovaries, fallopian tubes, and ligaments that support the uterus; in the area between the vagina and rectum; in the outer surface of the uterus; and in the lining of the pelvic cavity. Other sites for these endometrial growths may include the bladder, bowel, vagina, cervix, vulva, and in abdominal surgical scars. Rarely, endometrial tissue may be located in the lung, arm, thigh, brain, and other locations.

This tissue reacts as correctly placed endometrial tissue would during the menstrual cycle. The bloody discharge produced by such tissue has no outlet. The presence of such discharge may cause severe pain with each menstrual cycle, either during ovulation, menstruation, or both. The accumulation of the discharge may form dense fibrous tissue, leading to adhesions, sterility, and destruction of ovarian tissue.

Epidemiology and Causes

Endometriosis affects an estimated 5.5 million women in the United States and Canada. Women at all levels of society and of all races may be affected. A study of 3684 premenopausal women undergoing laparoscopy or laparotomy found a prevalence of endometriosis varying from 12 to 45 percent, depending on the indication for surgery. Delay in diagnosing endometriosis is common. Statistical analyses place the predominant age group of those diagnosed between 30 and 40 years; however, the disease can be found in adolescents. Research conducted by the Endometriosis Association found that the recognition and diagnosis of endometriosis is still taking a combined average of 9 years (4.67-year delay in seeking medical help and 4.61-year delay in physicians' diagnoses). From the sample of 4000 respondents, almost half said that they had to see a doctor five times or more before they were diagnosed, referred, or treated. Japanese women are twice as likely to have endometriosis as Caucasian women.

The cause of endometriosis is unknown. The retrograde menstruation and implantation theory suggests that during menses, some amount of menstrual tissue backs up through the fallopian tubes, implants in the abdomen, and proliferates in response to ovarian steroids. In turn, conditions that lead to genital tract obstruction and impede menstrual outflow contribute to reflux through the fallopian tubes. However, this theory has been found inadequate to explain all of the possible sites of endometriosis, and some experts believe that all women experience some menstrual tissue backup. Direct transplantation may account for endometriosis that develops in uterine surgical scars after a Cesarean section or episiotomy. Another theory suggests that endometrial tissue is distributed from the uterus to other parts of the body through either the lymphatic or hematologic circulatory systems. The coelomic (peritoneal) metaplasia theory suggests that undifferentiated cells lining the peritoneal cavity are triggered to differentiate into endometrial tissue by hormonal irregularities. There may also be a genetic predisposition to endometriosis; in addition, research by the Endometriosis Association has recently linked dioxin exposure to the development of endometriosis.

Pathophysiology

In addition to the etiologic theories discussed in the preceding text, a link to immune system dysfunction and the pathogenesis of endometriosis has also been suggested. Reduced T-cell and natural killer cell function are thought to impair the ability of the body to recognize and destroy abnormally implanted endometrial tissue, that is, immunosurveillance. Interestingly, however, an increased number of peritoneal leukocytes and macrophages have been identified within ectopic endometrium. Increased levels of cytokines and chemokines produced by these cells have been identified, including interleukin (IL)-1, IL-6, IL-8, tumor necrosis factor (TNF), and RANTES. These mediators act as growth factors for ectopic endometrium, while vascular endothelial growth factor (VEGF) stimulates capillary proliferation into this tissue. Interestingly, women with endometriosis are also more likely than controls to suffer from autoimmune inflammatory diseases.

Any pelvic organ may be a possible site of abnormal endometrial tissue known as endometriosis. The cyclical production of ovarian sex hormones allows for the proliferation and maintenance of these implants. Thus, endometriosis occurs primarily during a woman's active reproductive phase, rather than during premenstrual, immediately postmenarchal, or postmenopausal phases. This bleeding may cause severe pelvic pain and dyspareunia, infertility, and debilitation. In addition, inflammation of pelvic tissues may lead to adhesions and cyst development.

Endometrial may be progressively staged from minimal (stage I: isolated implants without adhesions), mild (stage II: superficial implants less than 5 cm in aggregate without adhesions), moderate (stage III: multiple superficial and invasive implants with or without tubo-ovarian implants), to severe (stage IV: multiple superficial and invasive implants with large ovarian endometriomas and dense adhesions).

Clinical Presentation

Subjective

The primary symptom of endometriosis is recurrent abdominal and/or pelvic pain, which may range from very mild to completely incapacitating. The pain may be associated with menstruation (dysmenorrhea) or it may occur slightly before the menstrual period. Pain may be experienced as generalized abdominal or pelvic pain or pain associated with sexual intercourse (dyspareunia), urination, and defecation. Fatigue, diarrhea, constipation, or nausea may accompany the pain. The patient may complain only of premenstrual spotting.

A careful history of menstruation should be taken, with significant attention to any complaints of pain. A history of allergies, chemical sensitivities, and recurrent yeast (*Candida*) infections may be present. Infertility is associated with endometriosis; 30 to 40 percent of women diagnosed with endometriosis are infertile.

Subjective

On physical exam, tenderness in the posterior fornix is the most common symptom. Lateral deviation of the cervix may be due to internal scarring, and bimanual examination may reveal palpable nodules on supporting ligaments and on affected ovaries. However, definitive diagnosis cannot be made via history and physical exam.

Diagnostic Tests

Direct visualization of endometrial implants through laparoscopy is the preferred diagnostic method, as most implants are located on the pelvic organs. A CBC may be done to diagnose anemia associated with blood loss resulting from endometriosis and an elevated WBC may also show evidence of an infection. This would tend to make endometriosis less likely, although it would not exclude abnormal endometrial tissue. Serum CA-125 levels are more likely to be elevated with advanced (stage III to IV) endometriosis, but this serum marker is not particularly sensitive and not a good screening tool.

Differential Diagnosis

The clinical manifestations of endometriosis are associated with many genitourinary disorders. The pain experienced is often discounted because it is a frequent (normal) accompaniment to menstruation. Pelvic and abdominal pain can be caused by gastroenteritis, appendicitis, ovarian cysts, fibroids, or ectopic pregnancy and these diagnoses must be ruled out. Specific differential diagnoses that must be considered are adenomyosis and endometrial polyps.

Adenomyosis is the presence of ectopic endometrial glands and stroma within the musculature of the uterus, which induces hypertrophy and hyperplasia of the myometrium in response to estrogen (and possibly progesterone); may be microscopic or nodular on gross inspection, but endometrial biopsy typically negative because changes in the myometrium. Adenomyosis seems to be more associated with childbearing, but the pathogenesis is unknown. Although a third of women are asymptomatic, adenomyosis may present with abnormal uterine bleeding, dysmenorrhea, and menorrhagia—just as with endometriosis. Abdominal ultrasound may be able to identify these differential diagnoses, but the laparoscopy is necessary to diagnose endometriosis.

Endometrial polyps are hyperplastic pedunculated/sessile growths of endometrial glands and stroma at the endometrial surface (mm to cm in size) and are common in middle-aged women. Metrorrhagia (irregular uterine bleeding) occurs in 50 percent of cases, while less frequently, menorrhagia, postmenopausal bleeding, prolapse through the cervical os, and breakthrough bleeding on hormonal treatments occur as symptoms. Definitive diagnosis is made on microscopy (after D&C, biopsy, or hysterectomy), but sonohysterography (instillation of saline into uterus prior to ultrasound) is preferred to transvaginal ultrasound for noninvasive evaluation (but it cannot be diagnostic). Curettage via hysteroscopy, rather than blindly, is preferred for best detecting polyps.

Management

Currently, there is no cure for endometriosis. Management is linked to relieving or reducing pain, shrinking or slowing endometrial growths, preserving or restoring fertility, and preventing or delaying the recurrence of the disease. In women with mild disease or those who are perimenopausal and will soon stop ovarian cycling and the hormonal fluctuations that trigger bleeding endometriosis, expectant management (observation) is an important option.

Frequently, OCs may provide adequate relief for women with mild disease, and are a good option because they have fewer side effects than other hormonal treatments. In addition, pain relief is often achieved with NSAIDs and other prostaglandin inhibitors. OCs and NSAIDs are usually sufficient only for disease with minimal pain. Typically, the medications include ibuprofen (400 to 600 mg qid), naproxen sodium (250 mg qid), indomethacin, and mefenamic acid (Ponstel) (250 mg qid to 500 mg tid). Medication administration should begin with the onset of menstruation to avoid the possible influence of medications on pregnancy. Prescription pain medications may be necessary to control symptoms. Conservative management is to use the least powerful medications first. With consistent reevaluation of symptom reduction, the risks associated with medications can be minimized.

For women with moderate to severe disease, hormonal therapy may help relieve symptoms. Drugs such as nafarelin nasal spray (0.2 to 0.4 mg bid), long-acting leuprolide acetate (3.75 mg IM once a month), or goserelin (3.6 mg SQ once a month) are GnRH analogs and suppress ovulation by suppressing pituitary gonadotropin secretion and thus ovarian estrogen secretion. These drugs are used for 3 to 6 months, although the optimum length of therapy is unclear. Adverse effects of this medication are vasomotor symptoms (hot flashes), vaginal dryness, dyspareunia, decreased libido, insomnia, breast tenderness, headache, depression and bone demineralization, which can be mediated by "add back" therapy with norethindrone, 5 to 10 mg qd.

Another hormonal treatment is danazol (200 to 400 mg bid) which is used for 6 to 9 months. Danazol is a testosterone derivative that acts like progesterone and suppresses menstruation. Adverse effects are androgenic and include weight gain, acne, hirsutism, muscle cramps, lower HDL, and decreased breast size.

Continuous combination OCs may also be given, but are most effective in mild disease. Any of the combination OCs discussed earlier in this chapter can be used. Breakthrough bleeding may occur and is treated with conjugated estrogens 1.25 mg qd for 1 week or estradiol 2 mg qd for 1 week. Adverse affects are discussed earlier in the chapter.

Progesterone alone in the form of medroxyprogesterone acetate 100 mg IM every 2 weeks ×4 doses, then 100 mg every 4 weeks can be given to inhibit endometrial tissue growth and initiate decidualization and atrophy of the endometrium. Oral therapy of medroxyprogesterone 10 mg tid or norethindrone 5 mg qd can also be used. These treatments provide 80 percent of women with complete or partial relief of symptoms. These treatments are used for 6 to 9 months. Oral estrogen can be added to control breakthrough bleeding.

Aromatase inhibitors, which decrease estrogen production, are still investigational. Regimens may be developed that combine these drugs with progestins or GnRH analogues.

Laparoscopy is used to ablate endometrial implants, which greatly reduces pain. Some women require removal of ovarian endometriomas along with ablation of implants and this procedure improves fertility. For women who no longer desire to have children, a total abdominal hysterectomy and bilateral salpingo-oophorectomy (TAH-BSO) will treat the endometriosis definitively, but in women with deep implants, TAH-BSO may not be sufficient.

Medical treatment alone is inappropriate for moderate to severe disease, and in addition, in these women it does not improve fertility. Only surgical interventions are shown to improve fertility. For example, some reviews have shown that with observation alone, pregnancy rates in mild, moderate, and severe disease are 50 percent, less than 25 percent, and only 5 percent respectively. With surgery, pregnancy rates are 50 percent and 39 percent in patients with moderate and severe disease, respectively. However, in vitro fertilization (IVF) is usually needed postoperatively, for women with severe disease in whom hysterectomy can be avoided. Infertile women who are trying to improve their chance of pregnancy typically benefit from laparoscopic ablation of endometrial implants.

Alternative therapies are gaining acceptance in the treatment of endometriosis. Visualization techniques, patterned breathing, massage therapy, and others may each have their place in the treatment of this disorder. Diet therapy and therapy to maximize the immune system may also be useful. Therapies must be evaluated for an appropriate match between patient and therapy. Financial issues may be of concern. Hormonal therapies are significantly more expensive than dietary changes and massage therapy. See Complementary Therapies 13.1.

Follow-Up and Referral

The signs and symptoms of endometriosis are related to the menstrual cycle. Follow-up visits should be timed to allow prescribed treatments to have affected the symptoms associated with the next menstrual cycle. The patient should be referred to a gynecologist experienced in laparoscopic diagnosis and treatment of endometriosis if the most conservative medical treatments are not sufficient to ameliorate the symptoms.

Patient Education

Each patient must receive appropriately formulated educational materials about endometriosis, including its signs and symptoms and the effects they may produce, as this is usually a lifelong condition. (See The Patient's Voice 13.1.)

Premenstrual Syndrome

Premenstrual syndrome (PMS) is a cyclic recurrence of a constellation of physical and psychological symptoms that arise during the second or luteal phase of the menstrual cycle, starting at day 14 after menses, immediately following ovulation and the mid-cycle LH and FSH gonadotropin surge. The original term for these symptoms was *premenstrual tension syndrome* (PMT). Most women experience minor physical symptoms before their menstrual cycle; however, about 5 percent of women present with symptoms severe enough to disrupt their daily lives.

Epidemiology and Causes

Premenstrual dysphoric disorder (PMDD) is the term given to a severe form of PMS in the fourth edition of the Diagnostic and Statistical Manual (DSM-IV). While PMS may affect up to 75 percent of women with regular menstrual cycles, only 3 to 8 percent of women suffer from true PMDD. To apply the DSM-IV criteria for PMDD, women must chart symptoms daily for two cycles. Chief complaints must include one of the four core symptoms (irritability, tension, dysphoria, and lability of mood) and at least 5 of the 11 total symptoms that are listed under the subjective heading in clinical presentation section later in this chapter. More than 150 distinct signs and symptoms have been ascribed to PMS within the medical literature, but the 22 most common are those listed in the PMS diary shown in Table 13.3.

The psychiatric hypothesis regarding etiology of PMDD centers around a woman's denial of her body and femininity and negative imprinting about menstruation and poor coping skills. This associates PMS with other psychiatric disorders. There does not appear to be any difference in the prevalence of this disorder between racial or ethnic groups. PMS usually disappears at the time of menopause.

Many believe that PMS is a physical response to organic changes that occur during the luteal phase of the menstrual cycle and, therefore, is not a psychiatric diagnosis at all. Research has postulated that mood and anxiety disturbances arise from ovarian steroid hormones that affect the synthesis, release, and reuptake of neurotransmitters. Several neuroendocrine processes are also affected during this period that may affect mood. Other diseases that present with mood and mental status changes, such as thyroid disease and vitamin B_{12} deficiency, are not classified as psychiatric disorders, and many believe that PMS should be placed in this category.

COMPLEMENTARY THERAPIES 13.1

Women's Health Problems

Problem	Therapy	Dosage	Comments
Premenstrual Syndrome (PMS)	Black cohosh	Dried rhizome/root: 0.3–2 g dry (capsule) or in tea tid	May affect diabetes and hypertension medication; doses more than 5–10 mg cause vomiting, headache, dizziness, limb pains, and hypotension
	Evening primrose oil	250 mg capsules up to tid 2–3 days before menses	Rare adverse effects: headache, nausea, diarrhea
	Calcium	1500 mg qd	Should be taken with optimal daily allowance of vitamin D (400 IU qd) for better absorption
	Vitamin B6	150 mg qd	Those taking levodopa must consult their provider before taking
	Vitamin C	1500–3000 mg qd	Take in divided doses for better absorption and to avoid diarrhea
	Vitamin E	400–800 IU qd	Can interfere with anticoagulant therapy; consult with provider before taking or if taking warfarin or heparin
	Essential oils; chamomile, basil, lavender, marjoram	Use as directed on label	Aromatherapy
Menopausal symptoms	Black cohosh	As above or 40–200 mg daily	Not recommended for more than 6 months
	Chaste tree berry	Extracts or tinctures to provide 20 mg of crude fruit or 30–40 mg of fruits decoction	Possible adverse GI effects; contraindicated in pregnancy
	Vitamin B complex	50 mg qd	High levels of estrogen, related to hormone fluctuations can deplete vitamin B6, resulting in anxiety, irritability, and depression
	Vitamin C	1500–3000 mg qd	Take in divided doses for better absorption and to avoid diarrhea
	Vitamin E	400–800 IU qd	Can interfere with anticoagulant therapy; consult with provider before taking or if taking warfarin or heparin
Breast tenderness	Chaste tree berry	As above	
	Evening primrose oil	As above	
Candidiasis (yeast infection)	Vitamin C	3000–6000 mg qd	Take in divided doses for better absorption and to avoid diarrhea
	Vitamin E	400 IU qd	Can interfere with anticoagulant therapy; consult with provider before taking or if taking warfarin or heparin
Decreased sexual desire	Essential oils: jasmine, neroli, rose, sandlewood, ylang-ylang, clary sage, patchouli	Use as directed on label	Aromatherapy; aphrodisiac

THE PATIENT'S VOICE 13.1

Endometriosis

I had a very painful menstruation from day 1. As long as I can remember, every month I was in bed doubled over in pain. Nothing seemed to relieve the intensity of the pain . . . even taking birth control pills. My periods were not heavy, but I always had pain and even a little spotting, especially after my period every month. About 1 year after the delivery of my third child, I began experiencing great discomfort with intercourse. My gynecologist suggested that since I was almost 40 years old, a surgical intervention was needed. He explained that laparoscopy or laparotomy and eventual hysterectomy was the usual treatment for women with severe pain. My first surgery did reveal that I had endometriosis . . . a small amount . . . but my surgeon said that some of the locations of the endometriosis made it even more painful. I had a difficult time with the hysterectomy... a lot of pain. But, since they removed my uterus, the pain I had for almost 27 years is finally gone. Why did it take so long for someone to give me relief?

Pathophysiology

PMS is difficult to define, as there is no universally accepted definition. As discussed, the American Psychiatric Association has established diagnostic guidelines for PMDD, which are more stringent than criteria for PMS. PMS is a complex clinical somatic entity, and no specific list or number of symptoms has been established that would enable a definitive diagnosis of PMS to be made. However, certain basic facts have been agreed upon. Although the medical literature states PMS is a complex disorder linking ovarian steroid hormones and neurotransmitter release, some feminist authorities feel PMS may be caused in part by the stressors on women within modern society and the need for women to masculinize their work lives to meet the standards of Western society.

The influence of cyclical ovarian hormones on various neurotransmitters has been cited, including the beta-endorphins and gamma-aminobutyric acid (GABA). In fact, the progesterone metabolite allopregnanolone, which potentiates GABA receptor function, is lowered in concentration in women suffering from PMS. However, the majority of evidence supports a deficiency in the tryptophan-derived neurotransmitter serotonin as the primary factor in the pathogenesis of PMS. Serum serotonin levels and serotonin uptake by platelets are both reduced during the luteal phase of the menstrual cycle in women suffering from PMS. Moreover, the serotonin agonist fenfluramine and selective serotonin reuptake inhibitors (SSRIs) both improve PMS symptoms, while tryptophan depletion and the serotonin antagonist metergoline both worsen the syndrome.

Fluctuations in ovarian steroids are believed to underlie these abnormalities in neurotransmitter levels, as demonstrated by the efficacy of gonadotropin-releasing hormone (GnRH) treatments (e.g., leuprolide) which suppress ovarian hormones and relieve the symptoms of PMS. Interestingly, however, the concentrations of serum estrogen and progesterone do not differ between women suffering from PMS and controls; thus, it is the cyclical nature of the sex hormones that appears to be key.

Several subcategories of PMS have been suggested. PMT-A is categorized by the symptoms of anxiety, irritability, and nervous tension. PMT-B is categorized by fluid retention, abdominal bloating, mastalgia, and weight gain. PMT-C is categorized as premenstrual cravings for sweets, increased appetite, and food binges. PMT-D is categorized by depression, withdrawal, insomnia, forgetfulness, and confusion. These categories have some overlap.

Clinical Presentation

Subjective

Usual cognitive symptoms during the premenstrual period are crying spells, depression, hostility, anxiety, irritability, relationship conflict and feelings of inadequacy, increased or decreased libido, and inability to cope with ever-recurring symptoms. These symptoms often persist for years and women tend to seek help from a health-care professional only when adverse events are linked with these alterations in mood. A recent crisis or threat from a significant other may precipitate a perceived need for professional help. Often, women seek relief from a sense of desperation. The delay in seeking help could come from a fear of being labeled a hypochondriac or mentally unstable.

A variety of physical symptoms may accompany these alterations in mood, ranging from mild to severe, and may change from month to month. The following is a comprehensive list of symptoms by body system:

Gastrointestinal: abdominal bloating (most common [more than 90 percent of women]), nausea, vomiting, constipation, increased thirst

Respiratory: colds, hoarseness, rhinitis, asthma, sinusitis, sore throat

Urologic: oliguria, urethritis, cystitis

Ophthalmologic: conjunctivitis, visual changes, glaucoma, styes

Mammologic: breast tenderness (more than 50 percent of women), swelling, heaviness

Dermatologic: acne, boils, urticaria, spot bruising, recurrence of herpes

Neurologic: headaches/migraines (more than 50 percent of women), aggravation of epilepsy, vertigo, syncope, fainting, paresthesias of hands or feet

Miscellaneous: fatigue (affecting more than 90 percent), backache, joint pain, edema of extremities, weight gain, palpitations, pelvic or low abdominal pain, cold sweats, hot flashes, food cravings, compulsive eating

Table 13.3 PMS Diary

A key factor in the diagnosis of PMS is that these symptoms occur on a cyclical basis, tied to your menstrual cycle; typically, part of your month will be symptom free. By completing the chart below, you will be able to aid your health-care provider in determining if your symptoms are PMS. If any one or more of these symptoms apply to you on any given day, write the number or abbreviation on that line. Start on the first day of your menstrual cycle and at the same time in next month's cycle, start month two. Make an entry for each day, even if there are no symptoms.

1. No symptoms	7. Tender breasts	13. Fatigue	19. Joint swelling
2. Headaches	8. Clumsiness	14. Fluid retention	20. Confusion
3. Food cravings	9. Crying	15. Forgetfulness	21. Migraine
4. Anger	10. Depression	16. Bloating	22. Mood swings
5. Anxiety	11. Dizziness	17. Hostility	23. Tension
6. Backaches	12. Feeling faint	18. Irritability	24. Other (specify)

Date	Symptoms: Month 1	Symptoms: Month 2	Symptoms: Month 3
1			
2			
3			
4			
5			
6			
7			
8			
9			
10			
11			
12			
13			
14			
15			
16			
17			
18			
19			
20			
21			
22			
23			
24			
25			
26			
27			
28			
29			
30			
31			

Other changes perceived as "positive" have been reported by patients during the premenstrual period, including increased libido, more energy, more creative ideas, and increased ability to accomplish tasks. Although physical symptoms may be the presenting complaints when patients first seek medical treatment, mood alterations are the most incapacitating and distressing.

All of the symptoms that any one patient may exhibit and believe to be resulting from PMS will present in one of four cycle patterns:

1. Symptoms appear at midcycle, disappear, and reappear the week before menstruation.
2. Symptoms begin at midcycle, with subtle changes that gradually escalate until menses.
3. Symptoms appear the week before menses and intensify until menstruation ensues.
4. Symptoms appear in the first or second luteal weeks and do not disappear until the end of menstruation.

Objective

Increased age and parity are important indicators when assessing whether symptoms are genuinely PMS related, as both of these factors increase the possibility of PMS. A 3-month diary of symptoms, such as the one shown in Table 13.3, which includes the timing of symptoms in relation to menses and severity, should be obtained from the patient. This diary should also list treatments and what makes symptoms better or worse. The diary should also contain a description of the effect the symptoms have had on a patient's family and colleagues. The patient should be asked, after this diary has been compiled, about her expectations concerning evaluation and therapy.

Diagnostic Reasoning

Diagnostic Tests

The most commonly accepted method to diagnose PMS uses a diary during at least two menstrual cycles (three is preferred). If the intensity of whatever symptoms are present increases at least 30 percent in the 6 days before onset of menses (compared with days 5 through 10 of the cycle), and if the symptoms occur in 2 consecutive months, a diagnosis of PMS is made. This is a rather subjective method of diagnosis, as women are asked to assess the percentage of increase subjectively, and there is no objective means of comparison with other patients. Other questions relevant to this diagnosis include those asked during the sexual, reproductive, family, medical–surgical, and psychiatric histories. This enables the health-care professional to rule out other possible diagnoses. Dietary habits, drug and alcohol consumption, exercise, and social and occupational histories are also important. Once the diary of symptoms and impairment can be pinpointed to the luteal phase of the menstrual cycle, with abatement of symptoms during other parts of the cycle, a presumptive diagnosis of PMS can be made.

A complete physical exam including a gynecologic exam is necessary to assess the health of women with PMS symptoms. This will enable the provider to rule out other possible causes for these symptoms. Diagnostic tests that may be useful to rule out other illnesses are a CBC, Pap smear, and urinalysis. Other blood tests can rule out thyroid abnormalities (TSH, T_4), menopause (FSH), hypoglycemia or hyperglycemia (FBS), and hyperprolactinemia (prolactin level).

Depression scales are also part of a complete workup for PMS. These enable the practitioner to rule out depression during the follicular stage of the menstrual cycle and, therefore, to pinpoint the depression and its manifestations to the luteal phase of the menstrual cycle.

Differential Diagnosis

One of the most important assessment parameters in making a diagnosis of PMS is that symptoms occur only during the luteal phase of the menstrual cycle. If symptoms appear during the follicular phase, this may reflect a mood or anxiety disorder. It is important to note that there is a lifetime incidence of psychiatric disorders, especially depression, of nearly 80 percent in women diagnosed with PMS. Differential diagnoses that are possibly related to the symptoms of PMS are cyclothymic disorder; dysfunctional marital situation; depression; bipolar depression; perimenopausal status; poor diet; endocrine abnormalities, such as hypoglycemia, diabetes, hypothyroidism, hyperprolactinemia, and hyperandrogynism; alcoholism; drug abuse; and tumors of the brain, breast, and ovaries. These must all be ruled out before a definitive diagnosis of PMS can be made. Often it is easy to dismiss vague symptoms and use "PMS" as a catch-all term. This can lead to misdiagnosis, which could have serious consequences. The DSM-IV criteria for diagnosing PMDD specifies that a woman must have 5 of the 11 symptoms listed and at least one of them must include one of the first 4 on the list. In addition, to be considered as PMDD, the symptoms must occur during the week before menstruation and end a few days after onset of menses. The symptoms must interfere with work, school, usual activities or relationships and not be merely an exacerbation of another disorder. This must be established for 2 consecutive menstrual cycles. The symptoms are:

1. Depressed mood or dysphoria (a feeling of low mood, irritability, anxiety and/or despair)
2. Anxiety or tension
3. Affective liability
4. Irritability
5. Decreased interest in usual activities
6. Concentration difficulties
7. Marked lack of energy
8. Marked change in appetite, overeating or food cravings
9. Hyperinsomnia or insomnia
10. Feeling overwhelmed
11. Other physical symptoms, i.e., breast tenderness, bloating

Management

The principle of management is to assist the patient in developing strategies to gain control over the symptoms, alleviate them as much as possible, and to normalize life. Once an accurate diagnosis of PMS is made, appropriate interventions can be individualized. There are two principles to keep in mind when developing this plan. First, PMS is a chronic disorder that lasts until after menopause. This makes cost and adverse effects important issues when planning treatment. Second, patients have different degrees of severity of symptoms and different symptom profiles. Treatments should match both the symptoms and the severity of symptoms. Lifestyle changes should be recommended as first-line therapy.

Lifestyle Changes

Lifestyle changes include regularly scheduled meals that are relatively high in complex carbohydrates and low in salt, sugar, and caffeine; regular aerobic exercise (shown to decrease depression); and stress reduction techniques. Aerobic exercise can cause an increase in endorphin levels and thereby improve mood. Epidemiologic studies comparing the severity of premenstrual symptoms in patients who exercise to those who do not have suggested that those who exercise have fewer symptoms. This is especially true for premenstrual depression. Moreover, it appears that the benefits are independent of the intensity of exercise; therefore, low levels of exercise intensity may be beneficial. An exercise as simple as sitting quietly for 20 minutes twice a day and deep breathing while listening to relaxation music was shown to reduce mood symptoms of PMS twice as effectively as no active therapy.

Specific dietary interventions that are effective include a reduction in salt, sugar, alcohol, and caffeine intake and an increase in complex carbohydrate. It is hypothesized that carbohydrates are involved in the serotonergic pathway, and an increase in serotonergic activity caused by increased complex carbohydrate consumption may help to relieve symptoms. In one trial, patients were given a carbohydrate-rich beverage during the late luteal phase of the menstrual cycle. The control group was given an isocaloric control beverage. The patients who drank the carbohydrate-rich beverage reported lower adverse mood symptom scores, whereas the control group reported no effect on mood.

Calcium and magnesium supplements have been shown to help control the emotional and physical symptoms of PMS. In several large clinical trials, 1000 mg of calcium per day decreased all PMS symptoms as well as any other medication or treatment. Women taking magnesium also experienced a reduction in total symptoms. This effect is thought to be due to the reversal of lower than average mononuclear blood cell magnesium concentrations in patients with PMS.

Other dietary supplements have also been tried, but the results are not conclusive. For example, micronutrients such as pyridoxine (vitamin B_6) and tocopherol (vitamin E) have been used to treat menopausal symptoms. Because the adverse effects of vitamins are minimal, a daily supplement may be helpful as long as the dosage does not exceed the recommended daily allowance. Vitamin E has been prescribed as a treatment for mastalgia (breast tenderness). Trials have demonstrated that vitamin E (at doses of 150, 300, or 600 IU/qd) has made little difference in the mastalgia of patients with PMS. Vitamin E can be toxic in high doses so it is important to prescribe appropriate doses to patients with mastalgia; 400 IU is the most commonly available dose, which gives a minimum effect without danger of toxicity.

Medications

In addition to lifestyle changes, selective serotonin reuptake inhibitors (SSRIs) such as fluoxetine 20 mg qd (most common), are effective in relieving tension, irritability, and dysphoria. Sertraline (Zoloft) may be used in doses up to 150 mg qd, paroxetine (Paxil) 20 to 30 mg qd and citalopram (Celexa) 20 to 30 mg qd. These are relatively inexpensive and have limited adverse effects which include nausea, headache, jitteriness, and decrease in libido. Lowering the dose of the SSRI may eliminate some of the adverse affects. If a therapeutic response is not reached within several cycles, the dose may be increased. Although SSRIs are generally administered daily, these drugs were effective when administered only during the luteal phase. SSRIs can then be used advantageously from a cost and adverse effect aspect.

Other antidepressants that inhibit serotonin reuptake but are not selective have also been used. These include clomipramine, nefazodone, and venlafaxine (50 to 200 mg qd), which inhibit both serotonin and norepinephrine reuptake. But they are definitely not first-line therapies, given their side effect profiles. In fact, several studies have shown that antidepressants outside of the SSRI class are not consistently effective for PMS control.

Benzodiazepines (BZDs) such as alprazolam 0.25 mg tid or qid are usually reserved for patients who fit the strict criteria of PMDD, occurring only during the luteal phase. Alprazolam is given starting on day 14 and continued through day 28. This will reduce the chances of developing BZD dependence. Thus, BZDs are considered only as a second-line therapy, after SSRIs and only in patients with documented PMDD.

Patients who do not respond to the above measures are candidates for a trial of ovulation suppression therapy with danazol 200 to 800 mg qd. Danazol is a GnRH agonist; a nortestosterone hormone derivative with progestin-like effects that induces ovarian suppression. It works by continuously suppressing pituitary gonadotropin secretions (LH/FSH). It must be given continuously because pulsatile administration leads to FSH/LH secretion. When this therapy is used, "add back" therapy is also used to provide some of the hormones suppressed by the GnRH agonist. Estrogen and progestin are given in low doses. For patients on GnRH agonist therapy, long-term alendronate is given to help prevent bone mineral density loss. Danazol has several undesirable adverse effects such as weight gain, increased facial hair, and acne.

Fluid retention is commonly reported during the luteal phase of the menstrual cycle and accounts for some of the physical symptoms of PMS. Spironolactone (Aldactone) 100 mg daily during the luteal phase has been shown to significantly reduce physical and psychological symptoms of PMS over placebo. With the use of spironolactone, participants reported improvement in irritability, depression, feeling of swelling, breast tenderness, and food cravings. Other forms of diuretics such as thiazides do not demonstrate effective reduction of the symptoms of PMS.

NSAIDs administered during the luteal phase significantly reduce physical symptoms of PMS. Naproxen sodium (Naprosyn) 500 mg bid, begun 1 week before the onset of menses and continued through the first few days of bleeding, is effective for both PMS symptoms and dysmenorrhea. Although this may not be first-line therapy for patients with PMDD, for patients with moderate symptoms, especially if associated with dysmenorrhea, headaches, or other musculoskeletal symptoms, NSAIDs may be beneficial. This is a relatively inexpensive and safe form of therapy for younger patients and may provide them with the help that they need to function normally during this period of the menstrual cycle.

Many folk remedies and complementary therapies have also been tried by women for centuries with varying degrees of success. Complementary Therapies 13.1 presents some of these measures.

Surgery (bilateral oophorectomy, usually with hysterectomy) is an option for women who respond only to GnRH agonist therapy for documented PMDD, but these women should be shown to tolerate estrogen or estrogen replacement therapy, along with GnRH treatments. This option should be reserved for women who no longer desire childbearing, and is most appropriate for women who are not near menopause, and will likely need therapy for several more years.

Follow-Up and Referral

The first follow-up visit should be in 2 months, to evaluate the data collected by the patient between visits to assess symptom patterns, enabling the diagnosis of PMS to be made and to begin treatment. Frequent visits may be required after that time to evaluate the effectiveness of treatments and to encourage patients to continue to examine and develop treatment plans. Eventually, once symptoms have been controlled, yearly visits should be sufficient.

Referrals to a specialist may be required, depending on findings from the diagnostic tests and physical exam. The diagnosis of PMDD requires referral to a psychiatrist for treatment. The use of certain treatments for severe PMS, such as GnRH agents, is handled by a gynecologist.

Patient Education

It is important to listen to and evaluate the concerns of patients when they present with symptoms typically associated with PMS. PMS must not be identified with weakness on the part of the patient but rather recognized as a disease entity that must be investigated and treated. It may take time and energy to resolve the symptoms and help the patient return to a life free of symptoms. When a patient is able to reduce PMS symptoms, whether severe or mild, it helps her to function within her societal role at a higher level and, therefore, benefits everyone.

Menopause

Menopause has occurred when a patient has not menstruated for a period of 1 year. This takes place most often between the age of 48 to 55 years (average is 51.5 years), but the normal age range for the onset of menopause is wide—anywhere between ages 40 and 60 years. Menopause is not a disease state, but it portends a change in the hormonal, emotional, and reproductive life of women. Many patients have an increased awareness of and respect for the wisdom of nature; they have philosophical and personal concerns about treating the symptoms and consequences of menopause not as a disease but as a normal part of their life cycle. Patients need to be aware of what is happening to their bodies so that they can make rational decisions about how to manage this stage of their lives.

The management of menopause and its symptoms has received a great deal of attention in recent years. As the life span for women lengthens—currently to an average of 84 years—menopause does not signal the end but rather another phase of life, with its own issues, challenges, and opportunities. Most women spend 30 years of their lives postmenopausal.

Epidemiology and Causes

Perimenopause is a triad of phases that include the climacteric or menopausal transition, menopause, and postmenopausal periods in a woman's reproductive life span. Throughout perimenopause, physical changes occur. The years immediately before and the decades after menopause are of much greater clinical significance than the cessation of menses, which identifies menopause itself.

The menopausal transition, or climacteric, is the phase that signals the nearing of menopause; it occurs approximately 10 years before the onset of menopause, usually between ages 38 and 42 years. The period of menopausal transition may have either an insidious or relatively abrupt onset. During this time, ovulation becomes less frequent, and the number of ovarian follicles have decreased and are less likely to mature. Women note the beginnings of this phase usually with changes in the menstrual cycle, which can be a shortening of the menstrual cycle and an increase in menstrual bleeding.

Immediately before menopause, menstrual bleeding may occur after a short luteal phase or after an estradiol peak without ovulation. In approximately 70 percent of patients, menses then become lighter and farther apart until they stop. Another 10 percent of patients simply stop menstruating without any other symptoms.

The remaining 20 percent of patients experience heavier bleeding, which is often unpredictable. This group of patients is at risk for anemia and endometrial hyperplasia, a precursor for endometrial cancer. The diagnosis of endometrial hyperplasia is made by an endometrial biopsy. Other reasons for abnormal bleeding in this age group can be endometrial cancer, endometrial polyps, uterine leiomyomata, and systemic clotting disorders. In the past, many patients were treated for increased menstrual bleeding with hysterectomies.

Premature ovarian failure is cessation of ovarian function before age 35 years. To determine true ovarian failure, two FSH levels must be above the normal limit of 40 mIU/mL.

Pathophysiology

Menopause is the permanent cessation of menses and ovarian function in a woman. To properly understand menopause, however, knowledge of normal ovarian development is required. This is first characterized by germ cell differentiation (i.e., oocyte development) and primordial ovarian follicle formation, both of which begin during embryonic development, with a peak of 6 to 7 million oocytes present in a growing fetus at just 5 months in utero. FSH drives this process by stimulating granulosa cell formation in ovarian follicles and inducing LH receptor formation, which will eventually allow for ovulation to occur later in life in response to surges in LH at the time of menarche. In a sexually mature ovulatory female, follicular release of an oocyte leads to transformation of the follicle into a corpus luteum cyst which produces less estrogen but increasing amounts of progesterone, capable of maintaining a pregnancy following fertilization and implantation of an oocyte into the uterine lining.

However, even during the fetal stages of development, follicular atresia and destruction of oocytes within the ovary itself are normal, continuous processes, which account for the reduction in oocyte number from its peak to 1 to 2 million at the time of birth and down to approximately 300,000 at the onset of puberty. Animal and human studies have shown this may be driven by reductions in FSH, decreased androgen production by ovarian thecal cells (reducing substrate for estrogen production via androgen aromatization), the upregulation of pro-apoptotic genes such as *Bax*, and the downregulation of anti-apoptotic genes such as *bcl-2* in both oocytes (primarily a fetal process) and follicular granulosa cells (primarily in adults).

Perimenopause, which is the period of time 2 to 8 years before and 1 year after the complete cessation of menses, is characterized by the waxing and waning of ovarian function, reflected in both ovulatory and anovulatory (estrogen-only) menstrual cycles of unpredictable duration and intensity, extended periods of estrogen deficiency, and heightened FSH/LH secretion with occasional follicular development and estradiol production. Over time, estrogen feedback to the hypothalamic–pituitary axis declines. In some women, estrogen positive feedback no longer leads to an LH surge capable of triggering ovulation, while in others, estrogen negative feedback fails to suppress LH production during the follicular phase. Moreover, the failure of corpus luteum cysts to form after ovulation leads to a decrease in progesterone and increased exposure to unopposed estrogen, which accounts of the increase in dysfunctional uterine bleeding (DUB) and endometrial hyperplasia observed during this period.

While some degree of follicular atresia occurs continuously throughout a woman's reproductive lifetime and increases rapidly after age 37 years, the permanent cessation of both ovarian function and menses known as menopause is an event rather than a period of time. Occurring on average at age 51 years, factors that influence the timing of menopause have been the subject of much research. While the age of menarche has steadily declined over recent decades (having been linked to nutritional status, environmental factors, and general health), the average age at menopause has remained remarkably constant since ancient times. Today, several factors have been well documented to lower the age at menopause including smoking (which decreases the onset of menopause by 2 years on average), nulliparity, menstrual regularity and a shorter cycle length, a family history of early menopause, increased galactose intake, concurrent type 1 diabetes mellitus, and certain genetic variants in the estrogen receptor and galactose-1-phosphate uridyl transferase gene. Menopause occurring past age 55 years is defined as late menopause.

With the depletion of ovarian follicles that are able to respond to gonadotropins, both follicular development and cyclical estrogen production cease during menopause. FSH levels rise as the body tries unsuccessfully to stimulate follicular production of estrogen. FSH levels above 40 mIU/mL signal the approach of menopause, even though a patient may still experience occasional menstrual bleeding. LH concentration is also elevated, but menopausal levels are difficult to distinguish from LH elevations seen during preovulatory gonadotropin surges in the normal menstrual cycle. Persistently high LH levels lead to continued androgen production by ovarian thecal cells, namely androstenedione, contributing to some of the undesirable physical changes experienced by postmenopausal women such as increased facial hair. Biochemical studies have revealed that the gonadotropins in older women have a longer half-life (contributing to their increased serum levels), but also contain higher levels of carbohydrate which tend to render them less biologically active. Moreover, while residual oocytes and differentiating follicles have been identified in postmenopausal women, the follicles are typically atretic and eventually become cystic in the absence of viable oocytes.

Without a follicular source, circulating levels of estrogen fall significantly during menopause—particularly the active form estradiol, produced from the aromatization of testosterone. High gonadotropin levels stimulate the ovarian stroma to produce the less potent hormone estrone, rather than estradiol, while androstenedione produced by the adrenal glands is converted to estrone by aromatization in the periphery, particularly within adipose tissue which contains significant levels of the aromatase enzyme. In addition, serum levels of the hormone inhibin B also decline, closely correlating to the rise in FSH, implying an inhibitory action of inhibin B on FSH. Estrone and androstenedione levels remain relatively constant as the patient ages, while testosterone levels decline. Obese women with larger amounts of adipose tissue typically display higher levels of circulating estrogens; however, they are still subject to vasomotor symptoms triggered by estrogen deficiency. Patients who are thin tend to experience vaginal dryness and other symptoms associated with low estrogen levels, while obese patients are at greater risk of experiencing symptoms associated with unopposed estrogen, such as dysfunctional uterine bleeding (DUB), endometrial hyperplasia, and endometrial neoplasms. In turn, women who do not experience the vasomotor symptoms of estrogen deficiency during menopause (e.g., hot flashes) should be monitored yearly for endometrial pathology with vaginal ultrasound and biopsy as appropriate.

Clinical Presentation

Subjective

Many women do not seek medical attention while going through menopause; they simply stop monthly menstrual bleeding. Their first presentation may be for a yearly gynecologic exam. If the patient has not menstruated for 12 months, she can be considered to be menopausal. Women should be counseled about the risks and benefits of hormone replacement (HRT), calcium supplementation, and other steps necessary to remain healthy during the postmenopausal decades. If less than 12 months has passed, a reevaluation should occur at the next yearly gynecologic exam.

Several factors have been identified that may alter menopause timing. Genetics and family history are factors that influence the age at which a woman experiences menopause. There is a similarity in menopausal age between mothers and daughters. Hysterectomy (removal of the uterus but not the ovaries) hastens the cessation of follicle stimulation and ovulation by 1 to 2 years. Women who smoke tend to have an earlier menopause. Menopause can also be induced with chemotherapy and radiation treatments.

Most patients go through menopause without experiencing symptoms debilitating enough to make them seek medical attention. About 20 percent of patients seek attention for one or more symptoms related to menopause. The most common symptoms of menopause are the vasomotor symptoms of hot flashes, night sweats, and insomnia. Vasomotor symptoms are caused by thermoregulatory dysfunction in which inappropriate peripheral vasodilation, cutaneous blood flow, and perspiration lead to a rapid heat loss and a fall in core body temperature with chills/shivering as an involuntary reaction to increased body temperature, and up to 75 percent of menopausal patients experience this symptom (and more likely after surgical menopause). Hot flashes contribute to sleep disturbances commonly experienced by perimenopausal women, and this has been linked to mood disorders including depression, irritability, and fatigue, although many studies have failed to show a direct connection between menopause and depression. It is postulated that menopause makes preexisting depression worse, rather than creating it de novo. Ten to 15 percent of all postmenopausal patients report frequent, severe episodes of symptoms that completely disrupt their lives.

Vaginal dryness or atrophy is a common complaint among menopausal women. Vaginal dryness results from decreased blood flow to the vaginal mucosa and vulva caused by estrogen deficiency contributing to the complaints of dyspareunia, or painful intercourse. Lack of estrogen also leads to thinning of the vaginal epithelial lining, decreased rugae, loss of elasticity, and decreased vaginal mucus. Atrophy can become so severe that a woman may complain of postmenopausal bleeding. Although an endometrial biopsy is needed to rule out hyperplasia, the bleeding may be a result of the vaginal dryness.

Five areas of change involving sexual relations have been described: diminished sexual responsiveness, dyspareunia, decreased sexual activity, decline in sexual desire, and a dysfunctional male partner. A decrease in estrogen influences peripheral blood flow responses to sensory stimulation, affecting the timing and degree of vasocongestive response during sexual activity.

Vaginal atrophy is a major contributor to both stress and urge incontinence in the menopausal woman, particularly atrophy of the urethral epithelium with atrophic urethritis, loss of compliance, and irritation interfering with adequate seal of the urethral meatus. Atrophy of the bladder trigone (outlet tract) and decreased responsiveness of alpha-adrenergic receptors at the bladder neck and urethral sphincter all impair continence as well. Detrusor instability is also a cause of urinary symptoms. Patients will report that they either leak urine when they laugh, cough, or sneeze, or that when they feel the urge to urinate they cannot make it to the bathroom in time. This can be very disconcerting and uncomfortable and lead to UTI and urinary odor problems. Done correctly, Kegel exercises (described on page 573) reduce incontinence in 50 to 90 percent of patients within a few months.

Objective

The only documented objective manifestation of menopause is bone demineralization and resultant osteoporosis. Postmenopausal osteoporosis is one of the most common and disabling diseases affecting North American patients today. During the climacteric, patients may lose 2 to 5 percent of bone mass per year. Predisposition to falling created by an unsteady gait and poor eyesight are significant factors equal to low bone density as cause for hip fractures in postmenopausal patients. (See Nursing Research-Based Practice 13.1.)

Up until 2001, it was widely believed that hormone therapy would prevent heart disease in the menopausal woman. As a result of the Heart and Estrogen/Progestin Replacement Study (HERS) and the more recent Women's Health Initiative Randomized Control Study (WHI), it is fairly clear that hormone replacement does not prevent cardiovascular disease and in some cases can precipitate an

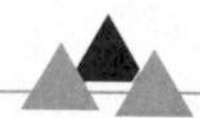

NURSING RESEARCH-BASED PRACTICE 13.1

Twiss JJ, et al: The relationship of actual height loss with health-seeking behaviors and risk factors in perimenopausal and menopausal women. J Am Acad NP 14(3):131–138, 2002.

In both dollars and quality of life, osteoporosis is a costly condition in the United States. A major focus of health-care today is preventing bone loss in perimenopausal and menopausal women. Investigators explored whether there was a difference in perimenopausal and menopausal women's perception of their height and their actual height. They questioned whether each woman's perception of height affected her health-seeking preventive health measures and that if by regularly assessing height, this would be an indicator of osteoporosis and women would exhibit more health-seeking preventive behaviors.

The researchers administered the Osteoporosis Questionnaire, which included the Osteoporosis Risk Questionnaire, Health-O-Meter height measureing stick, tape measure with inch-rule for arm span measurements, and balance scale for weight on 73 women between the ages of 45 and 70 years who presented at a Midwestern clinic for annual exam. The study revealed a significant relationship between actual height loss and osteoporosis risk factors. They concluded that simple height measurements and osteoporosis risk assessment was an effective screening tool for osteoporosis.

adverse cardiac event, especially in the first 5 years of treatment. Critics of these studies, argue that the women in the study were well past menopause when the study began, but clearly indicated that hormone replacement had deleterious effects on older women, whereas the effect on younger women remains unclear. Current research on the relationship between menopause and cardiovascular disease remains controversial at best.

Diagnostic Reasoning

The diagnosis of menopause is based on a history of amenorrhea and the presence of associated symptoms including hot flashes, flushes, night sweats, and sleep disturbances in age-appropriate women. If these symptoms are present, laboratory testing is not necessary. Other causes of amenorrhea must be considered whenever the history is not consistent with estrogen deficiency. Such history would be amenorrhea without vasomotor symptoms. A FSH level above 40 mIU/mL in the face of prolonged amenorrhea is diagnostic.

Diagnostic Tests

The first test that should be done in a woman whose menses has ceased is a pregnancy test, since an elevated beta-hCG level could reflect pregnancy, molar pregnancy, ectopic pregnancy, or even certain germ cell tumors. It is simple and inexpensive.

The serum FSH and LH are elevated in menopause. FSH levels greater than 10 to 25 mIU/mL suggest relative ovarian resistance consistent with menopausal transition. FSH levels of greater than 40 mIU/mL are consistent with complete cessation of ovarian function. LH levels are less sensitive for hormonal and ovarian function. During the menopausal transition, LH levels begin to elevate; however, LH may also be elevated during the midcycle surge and in cases of chronic anovulation.

In patients with amenorrhea who do not have menstrual bleeding after progestin withdrawal, measurement of a serum estradiol may be helpful. Normal estradiol levels range between 40 and 300 pg/mL. A level of greater than 30 pg/mL may indicate some degree of residual ovarian function. Levels less than 30 pg/mL indicate cessation of ovarian function.

Patients on combined OCs should have levels drawn on days 5 to 7 of the placebo-pill week to get accurate FSH and estradiol levels. Patients on progestin-only contraceptive pills can have levels drawn at any time because these pills do not affect FSH and estradiol levels.

Menopausal status can also be determined by vaginal cytologic examination. On microscopic examination parabasal cells will predominate, indicating a lack of epithelial maturating resulting from low estrogen levels.

Differential Diagnosis

The differential diagnoses for patients presenting with menopausal symptoms are pregnancy, spontaneous abortion, anovulation, endometrial hyperplasia, carcinoma, infection, and abnormalities of the uterus such as fibroids or polyps, endometriosis, adenomyosis, injury, and ovarian abnormalities such as tumors or cysts.

Management

Management of menopause focuses on symptom management and includes lifestyle modifications and a variety of medications.

Lifestyle Modifications

Vasomotor Symptoms. Lifestyle modification can assist in the management of vasomotor symptoms. These modifications include aerobic exercise, dietary, vitamin, and mineral therapies, and herbal therapies.

The North American Menopause Society (NAMS) recommends aerobic exercise, since physically active women have 50 percent fewer hot flashes than their sedentary counterparts. As with any strenuous activity, this may precipitate perspiration and hot flashes until the woman becomes physically fit or conditioned. The insomnia that often accompanies these vasomotor problems may be relieved with exercise. Physical conditioning also decreases cardiovascular risk.

In addition to aerobic activity, weight loss for women who are overweight may be beneficial. Women with a high body mass index (BMI) report having more hot flashes than those with a lower BMI. This too, is beneficial for cardiac risk reduction.

Other lifestyle changes that can be helpful for hot flashes and night sweats include dressing in layers, avoiding becoming overheated, limiting intake of alcohol and caffeine, reducing stress, and smoking cessation.

Dietary habits are very personal and often very difficult to change. It is prudent to recommend a diet that is high in complex carbohydrates and fiber (25 to 30 grams qd), low in fat (less than 30 percent of calories from fat), particularly animal fat, and high in antioxidants (fresh fruits and vegetables).

Herbal therapies include those that are similar to estrogen. Isoflavonoid phytoestrogens are contained within plant fibers and are functionally similar to estradiol. They produce estrogenic effects that may reduce vasomotor symptoms. This type of estrogen-like substance is found in soy products such as tofu and soy milk. An alternative herbal preparation that may alleviate vasomotor symptoms is black cohosh (40 mg qd), which has an estrogenic effect and reduces hot flashes.

Vaginal Dryness. For patients who complain of vaginal dryness, a Pap smear and urine analysis should be done to make sure the symptoms are a result of cellular changes and not infection. If positive for infection or cellular abnormalities (other than parabasal cells), these must be addressed and then symptoms must be reassessed. The most effective treatment for vaginal dryness or atrophic vaginitis is topical vaginal application of an estrogen product. The estradiol vaginal ring has little systemic absorption and is suitable for long-term use and is effective for vaginal atrophy and dryness. Progesterone therapy is not necessary with the ring, because there is little systemic absorption of estradiol and therefore is not needed to protect the endometrium. Estrogen vaginal cream can be used for short-term therapy. Creams are inserted into the vagina daily for 4 to 6 weeks and can be continued for a few months if necessary to resolve symptoms. After initial therapy, use of 1 to 2 grams of the cream twice a week will prevent recurrence. Because absorption is variable, the vaginal ring is preferable.

Water-soluble vaginal lubricants are alternatives to topical estrogen or may be used in conjunction with the estradiol ring or estrogen creams as needed. Lubricants (Astroglide, KY-Jelly) used before intercourse to decrease dyspareunia do not alleviate the symptoms of vaginal atrophy. Other alternative therapies that may be useful for vaginal dryness include sitz baths, vinegar douches, and intercourse.

For the symptoms of urinary frequency and incontinence, Kegel exercises remain the first line of therapy for this problem. These exercises are a natural nonpharmacologic therapy that improve the tone of the urethral sphincter in patients with stress incontinence.

Psychological Problems. Many women experience emotional problems with menopause including depression, irritability, and anxiety. As previously stated, depression occurs more often in menopausal women who have experienced depression at other times in their lives. In addition to relieving symptoms of depression, many antidepressants also have a favorable effect on other symptoms such as hot flashes. For example, SSRIs may relieve hot flashes as well as hormone therapy can. Paroxetine 12.5 mg qd or venlafaxine (Effexor) 75 mg qd are given. The antiseizure medication clonidine 100 to 150 μg qd can be given orally or transdermally to relieve hot flashes, but the adverse effects of dry mouth, drowsiness, and hypotension make is less desirable.

Regular aerobic exercise improves cognitive function, enhances mood, and promotes daytime alertness and nocturnal sleepiness. Recent studies have shown that a brisk walk every day on most days enhances wellness and promotes a sense of well-being.

Hormone Replacement Therapy

Because of recent research, hormone replacement therapy is not a first-line treatment for menopausal symptoms, and certainly is not prescribed to prevent heart disease. Hormone therapy (HT) can be estrogen therapy (ET) alone or estrogen plus progestin therapy (EPT). These are the new nomenclature promoted by NAMS to clarify different therapies. In mid-2001 the EPT arm of the Women's Health Initiative (WHI) was halted prematurely because of evidence that it increased women's risk for a cardiac event. However, the ET arm of the study is ongoing with no increase in cardiovascular disease noted. In the WHI, there was definitive evidence that EPT decreased the risk of postmenopausal osteoporotic fractures, but the ET did not show this. Also, these results are in postmenopausal women. Improvement in osteoporotic fracture rates for perimenopausal women has not been established in clinical trials. From these results, it is clear that HT is not a first-line treatment for osteoporosis; there are other nonhormonal therapies with proven efficacy in improving bone mineral density.

NAMS recommends HT only for women with moderate to severe menopausal symptoms, particularly hot flashes and sleep disturbances, but only for a short period, no longer than 5 years. In addition, NAMS clearly states the HT should NOT be used for prevention of heart disease or stroke, or prevention of dementia, but do state that not all data apply to all women.

If after reviewing the benefits and risks with the patient, the patient and clinician decide that HT would be the best option then factors such as frequency of dosage, mode of delivery, and convenience should be considered and the appropriate drug prescribed. See the Common Drugs Prescribed 13.1 table for different forms of HT and dosage. Different types of HT are:

- Estrogen therapy (ET)—start with the lowest dose of estrogens. Estradiol can be given in a transdermal skin patch. The patch is changed once or twice a week. This is usually limited to women who no longer have a uterus.

Drugs Commonly Prescribed 13.1: Menopause

Estrogen Therapy (ET) [oral]	Dosage available
Conjugated estrogen (Premarin)	0.3, 0.625, 0.9, 1.25, 2.5 mg; can be given cyclic or continuous (0.625 mg usual if continuous)
Micronized estradiol (Estrace)	0.5, 1.0, 2.0 mg; can be given cyclic or continuous (1.0 mg usual if continuous)
Esterified estrogens (Estratab, Meneset)	0.3, 0.625, 1.25, 2.5 mg; used mostly for cyclic hormone therapy
Estropiapate (Ogen, Ortho-Est)	0.625, 1.25, 2.5, 5.0; can be given cyclic or continuous (0.625 mg usual if continuous)
Estrogen Therapy (ET) [topical]	Dosage and form
Transdermal estradiol	Released in mg/day
Climara	0.025, 0.05, 0.074, 0.1 mg; change once weekly
Estraderm	0.05, 0.1 mg; change twice weekly
Alora	0.05, 0.075, 0.1 mg; change twice weekly
Vivelle	0.0375, 0.05, 0.075, 0.1 mg; change twice weekly
Vaginal estrogen creams and tablets	
Estradiol	
Vagifem	25 mcg tablets; inserted vaginally qd for 2 weeks then 1 tablet twice weekly.
Estrace	0.01 mg/g cream; given cyclically—3 weeks on, 1 week off.
Estropipate	
Ogen	1.5 mg/g cream; given cyclically—3 weeks on, 1 week off.
Conjugated estrogen	
Premarin	0.625 mg/g cream; given cyclically—3 weeks on, 1 week off.
Estrogen ring	
Estring	7.5 mcg released per 24 hours; remains in place for 3 months
Estrogen plus Progestin Therapy (EPT)	Dosage available
Continuous-sequential (CS-EPT)	
Estrogen	
See the ET above	Estrogens given as above on days 1–25 of cycle
Progestins	
Medroxyprogesterone acetate [MPA] (Amen, Cycrin, Provera)	2.5, 5.0, 10.0 mg; on days 14–25
Norethindrone	2.5, 5.0 mg; on days 14–25
Norethindrone acetate (Aygestin)	5.0, 10.0 mg; on days 14–25
Continuous combined (CC-EPT)	
Estrogen	
Conjugated estrogens	0.625 mg daily
Estropipate	0.625 mg daily
Micronized estradiol	1.0 mg daily
Progestins	
Medroxyprogesterone acetate	2.5, 5.0 mg daily
Norethindrone	0.35 mg daily
Norethindrone acetate	1.0 mg daily
Micronized progesterone (Prometrium)	100, 200 mg daily
Combination Products	Dosage available
Premphase	Conjugated estrogens 0.625 mg for 14 days; conjugated estrogens 0.625 and MPA 5 mg for 14 days
Prempro	Conjugated estrogens 0.625 and MPA 2.5 mg or conjugated estrogens 0.625 and MPA 5.0 mg; continuously
Ortho-Prefest	Estradiol 1.0 mg and estradiol 1.0 mg with norgestimate 0.09 mg in alternating sequence of 3 tablets each
FemHRT 1/5	Ethinyl estradiol 5 mcg and norethindrone acetate 1.0 mg
Activella	Estradiol 1.0 mg and norethindrone acetate 0.5 mg

- Estrogen plus progestin therapy (EPT) [used to be refered to as HRT]—this therapy can be delivered either continuous-sequential (CS-EPT) or continuous combined (CC-EPT). In the case of CS-EPT, estrogen is given days 1 to 25 of each month, and a progestin is given on days 14 to 25. Hormones are withheld from days 26 to 30 causing endometrial sloughing and bleeding. Many women find this method unacceptable. In CC-EPT estrogen and a progestin are given every day continuously. There may be some spotting initially, but after a few months, the endometrium is atrophic and will not bleed.

Exogenous estrogen is contraindicated in patients with estrogen-dependent cancers, such as breast, endometrial, and ovarian cancer, or undiagnosed vaginal bleeding. Patients with liver disease, active thrombosis, or history of stroke should not take estrogen. Pregnancy is another absolute contraindication for estrogen or progestin therapy. Migraine headache is a relative contraindication for the use of estrogen because of the vasoactive properties of estrogen in some patients. Estrogen use has also been associated with a small increased risk of gallbladder disease. Recently, studies have demonstrated an association between estrogen therapy and adult-onset asthma. Increased risk for development of systemic lupus erythematosus exists when taking estrogen; however, the incidence is low.

There are many types of estrogen products. These are 17 beta-estradiol, estrone, and estriol. Conjugated equine estrogens (Premarin) are commonly prescribed. Conjugated equine estrogen is derived from the urine of pregnant mares. It contains naturally occurring estrogens such as estradiol and estrone as well as products not native to humans. Synthetic estrogens used for replacement therapy have a higher potency and increased deleterious effects on hepatic globulins.

Levels of androgens decrease slowly in patients who experience natural menopause and more rapidly in patients who have undergone oophorectomy, because the majority of androgens are produced in the ovary. Androgens are also produced in skin, muscle, and bone tissue. A positive correlation may exist between reduced androgen production and decreased libido in postmenopausal patients. Androgens have been shown to decrease HDL levels, an undesirable effect; however, they have also been shown to decrease triglyceride levels, a factor in cardiovascular disease. Because the effects of androgen depletion on libido occur only in patients with testosterone levels of less than 20 to 60 ng/dL, a testosterone blood level is indicated before initiation of therapy. Androgens are available in synthetic form, either alone as methyltestosterone (Oreton, Android), or combined with estrogen. A natural micronized testosterone may be procured from a compounding pharmacy. The long-term effect of testosterone administration in postmenopausal patients is unknown.

Raloxifene HCl (Evista) is a selective estrogen receptor modulator and is a first-line therapy for prevention and treatment of postmenopausal osteoporosis. It protects patients from bone loss associated with decreased levels of estrogen. It does not affect breast or uterine tissue and, therefore, cannot cause breast tenderness, spotting, and other symptoms that can occur with the initiation of estrogen therapy. In initial studies, raloxifene did not demonstrate an increased risk for breast or uterine cancer. Raloxifene does not decrease hot flashes and may actually cause hot flashes in early treatment.

Bisphosphonates are a relatively new class of medications that are first-line therapies for the prevention and treatment of postmenopausal osteoporosis and include alendronate and risedronate. These drugs have been shown to increase spine and hip bone mineral density and decrease the risk of postmenopausal fracture. The patient should be instructed to take these drugs on an empty stomach in the morning and wait at least 30 minutes before eating or drinking. The patient must remain upright for 30 minutes after taking the medication. If heartburn or difficulty swallowing occur, the patient should be instructed to stop the medication and seek medical attention.

Calcitonin can be used to decrease bone resorption in postmenopausal women. It can be used alone or in conjunction with hormone therapy. It is the drug of choice for women who cannot take HT, bisphosphonates, or raloxifene. The dose of calcitonin is 100 IU/day subcutaneously or 200 IU intranasally daily.

Bone mineral density can also be increased with teriparatide (Forteo, Parathar) which is an analogue of parathyroid hormone (PTH). It is administered subcutaneously in 20 mg/day doses. A serious adverse effect is osteosarcoma when teriparatide is administered in high doses.

Vitamin D and calcium should be taken as supplements by most women, because it is difficult to get the 1200 to 1500 mg recommended to maintain bone health. The form of vitamin D should be ergocalciferol (vitamin D_2). Calcium should be taken with vitamin D since it has only a small effect on preventing osteoporosis. Calcium supplements can be either calcium citrate or calcium carbonate. Some sources indicate that calcium citrate is better absorbed from the GI tract.

Bioflavonoids are thought to have estrogenic activity. One study showed that grapefruit juice increased bioavailability of administered estradiol and estrone. Black cohosh, blue cohosh, ginseng, and wild yam have all demonstrated estrogenic effects. These compounds may result in endometrial hyperplasia, however, if unopposed with progesterone in patients with intact uteri.

Follow-Up and Referral

When therapies recommended for the abatement of symptoms are followed without relief of symptoms, a referral to a gynecologist is recommended. Any patients with suspected abnormalities, especially carcinoma, should be referred to a gynecologist. Any perimenopausal or postmenopausal bleeding requires further evaluation with endometrial surveillance and biopsy to rule out endometrial hyperplasia or other pathology. Vaginal ultrasound may be used first, however, to avoid biopsy in women whose endometrial thickness is 4 mm or less. Estrogen–progestin therapy usually treats DUB, but intermittent ovulation may call for low-dose OCs as well. In smokers or women with contraindications to OCs (blood clots, breast or uterine cancer history) and no significant symptoms of estrogen deficiency, progestin therapy with MPA 5 to 10 mg qd for 2 weeks a month can induce withdrawal bleeding and prevent endometrial hyperplasia. A depressed patient who does not respond to lifestyle changes and medications should be referred to a mental health specialist for counseling. Patients who are not responsive to therapy for insomnia may be referred to a sleep disorder clinic.

Patient Education

Pregnancy is still possible during perimenopause. When a patient presents with amenorrhea, it is important to perform a pregnancy test before assuming that the patient may be menopausal. Patients should be counseled about methods of birth control during this time so that undesired pregnancies do not occur.

The decision about the type of menopausal symptom treatment is made in conjunction with the patient. The following tests should be performed before a final decision to initiate therapy: Pap smear, blood chemistry, lipids, BP, mammogram, endometrial biopsy in patients with breakthrough bleeding, and FSH and thyroid hormone levels.

Patients undergoing menopause may have deep feelings about what is happening. The clinician must assess and evaluate these feelings to better understand how to assist the patient. Studies show that fear, lack of knowledge about menopause, and the lack of an informed decision-making process are some of the factors leading to a woman's reluctance to seek treatment for menopausal symptoms. With much conflicting information in the media and among clinicians, patients may be especially interested in clarification risks and benefits of all the treatments for menopausal symptom relief.

Leiomyomas (Uterine Fibroids)

Leiomyomas are most commonly called *uterine fibroids*. Fibroids are benign tumors (most common benign tumor of the uterus) and arise from the smooth muscle cells in the myometrium. Most are small and asymptomatic.

Epidemiology and Causes

Leiomyomas are extremely common, and the prevalence increases in women between 30 and 50 years of age. However, the prevalence decreases with menopause. By age 50 years, 50 percent of African American and Asian American women have leiomyomas and about 30 percent of white women will have them.

The cause of leiomyomas is unknown, but clearly, there is a hormonal link. Girls before menarche do not have leiomyomas and they shrink after menopause, implicating estrogen. If a pregnant woman has a fibroid, it dramatically increases in size during pregnancy, but decreases after. Risk factors for the development of leiomyomas include nulliparity, age between 30 and 50 years, obesity, and sedentary lifestyle. Interestingly, smoking seems to decrease the risk for developing fibroids.

Pathophysiology

Leiomyomas develop from a single neoplastic smooth muscle cell with abnormal chromosomal patterns. Leiomyomas are classified by location within the uterine wall and can be subserous, submucous, and/or intramural. Rarely, leiomyomas can be intraligamentous, cervical, or parasitic (deriving its blood supply from an organ to which it becomes attached). Most uterine fibroids are surrounded by compressed (otherwise normal) myometrium. When leiomyomas outgrow their blood supply, they can become necrotic and ulcerate.

Clinical Presentation

Subjective

Most leiomyomas are asymptomatic. When symptoms are present, abnormal uterine bleeding is the most common symptom. The woman may also complain of pain, particularly with intercourse. If the fibroid is large enough, it can cause pressure on the bladder, resulting in urinary frequency, urgency, and possibly dysuria. The complaint of abdominal or genital heaviness is also common with large fibroids.

Objective

Pelvic exam will reveal one or more uterine masses. Leiomyomas are usually firm and nontender. If there are multiple fibroids (most of the time), the uterus will feel irregular nodular in shape.

Diagnostic Reasoning

Diagnostic Tests

Because most women with leiomyomas have abnormal uterine bleeding, a CBC is ordered. The hemoglobin is decreased because of the increased amount and frequency of menstrual bleeding. Occasionally polycythemia may be present. A pregnancy test should be done to rule out intrauterine pregnancy.

Pelvic ultrasound or MRI will confirm the diagnosis of leiomyoma, but TVS is used most often. Occasionally, hysterography or hysteroscopy is used to confirm cervical or submucous myomas.

Differential Diagnosis

Differential diagnoses should include other disorders that cause uterine enlargement and abnormal uterine bleeding, including pregnancy, adenomyosis (presence of endometrial glands and stroma in the myometrium), ovarian neoplasm, tubo-ovarian inflammatory mass, uterine cancer, and possibly diverticulitis.

Management

No treatment is necessary for women with asymptomatic or very small myomas. If the patient is severely anemic, measures should be undertaken to stop the prolonged, heavy menstrual periods and boost her hemoglobin. Medroxyprogesterone acetate 150 mg IM given every 28 days or Danazol 400 to 800 mg PO qd will usually slow or stop the bleeding. The woman should be instructed to take over-the-counter iron preparations 300 mg (ferrous sulfate, ferrous gluconate, or ferrous fumarate) daily. Folic acid 400 mcg orally qd will help boost red blood cell production as well.

The goal of conservative medical management is to shrink the leiomyomas. OCs may be effective for some women, but for others, the estrogen in the OC causes enlargement, so frequent monitoring is important. GnRH agonists are given to decrease the LH and FSH level, thereby producing a hypoestrogenic effect which usually causes the leiomyomas to shrink. This is frequently used before surgery, as the risk of surgical complications is increased with large tumors. The GnRH agents that are used are leuprorelin (Lupron) either 0.5 mg SQ daily or depot injection of 3.75 to 7.5 mg every 28 days; or nafarelin (Synarel) 0.2 to 0.4 mg intranasally BID. Treatment lasts 8 to 12 weeks and is very costly. Because these drugs induce a menopausal state the adverse effects reflect those of menopause (see section on menopause). These medications are contraindicated in women with undiagnosed abnormal uterine bleeding and in women who are breastfeeding.

There are several surgical approaches for problematic leiomyomas. Myomectomy is removal of the myoma and is done when preservation of fertility is desired and the tumor is larger than 12-week gestational size. Hysterectomy (with or without removal of the ovaries) is the definitive treatment for very large fibroids, particularly when bleeding is very heavy and the patient is markedly anemic. Few adverse effects occur as a result of hysterectomy, infection, bleeding, and damage to surrounding organs are always possible with any surgical procedure. Other possible effects are depression, sexual dysfunction, and menopausal symptoms.

Uterine artery embolization (UAE) is a relatively new alternative to surgery. The uterine arteries are embolized producing end-organ ischemia and necrosis with subsequent shrinkage. This procedure is effective in reducing menorrhagia, pain, and uterine volume in 80 percent of patients. However, a large number of women report severe pelvic pain, fever, malaise, nausea and vomiting, resulting from the infarcted uterine tissue.

Follow-Up and Referral

Any woman with severe bleeding, marked anemia, and palpable leiomyomas should be referred to a gynecologist for evaluation and treatment. Women with small uterine myomas should be reexamined at 3- to 6-month intervals or more often if symptoms increase. If menorrhagia is present, hemoglobin and hematocrit should be monitored frequently.

Patient Education

Women with leiomyomas should be reassured that this does not increase their chances of developing uterine cancer. If increased bleeding is a problem, the woman should be instructed to take an iron supplement daily and to increase iron-rich foods in her diet. She should report any shortness of breath, palpitations, or increase in fatigue or pain immediately.

Fertility Problems

Fertility is the quality of being productive or fertile. Although science has begun to perfect some techniques that facilitate fertility, chance continues to play a large role in conception. *Infertility* is defined as lack of conception despite unprotected sexual intercourse for at least 12 months, as studies have shown a 93 percent cumulative probability of pregnancy in normal fertile couples after this period of time. A woman younger than age 35 is considered infertile if no conception occurs after 1 year of unprotected intercourse. This time frame is shortened to 6 months in women age 35 or older. A man is considered infertile if he does not produce and deliver enough quality sperm to initiate a pregnancy. Infertility is divided into two categories. *Primary infertility* refers to a woman who has never had a child, whereas *secondary infertility* applies to a woman who has delivered at least one child. *Sterility* is a term applied when there is an absolute factor preventing reproduction. Fecundability is the probability of successful pregnancy within one menstrual cycle.

Epidemiology and Causes

Approximately 10 percent of couples in the United States have difficulty conceiving a child after a year or more of trying. The American Society for Reproductive Medicine estimates that there are more than 6 million couples with infertility problems in the United States. Twenty-five percent of fertile couples conceive during 1 month of unprotected intercourse. Sixty percent conceive after 6 months, and 85 percent conceive after 12 months. These conception rates are averages and vary among couples. Primary infertility occurs in about 1 of 12 couples (8.3 percent). The incidence of infertility increases as the woman ages. For example: one in seven couples age 30 to 34 are infertile; one in five age 35 to 39, and one in four age 40 to 44. These declines reflect the natural aging process and emphasize the need for rapid evaluation and treatment of infertility, especially in a patient older than 35 years of age.

Fertility patterns are dependent on many factors, including age, sex, and health. A major difference between male and female reproductive potential is that women have a finite reproductive life span (approximately 35 years), whereas men, after puberty, have the capacity to reproduce for the rest of their lives. However, fertility decreases in both men and women with aging. The causes of infertility are divided into categories. Male factor is a major cause, being a component in over 40 percent of cases and results from testicular defects, 10 to 20 percent from posttesticular defects (obstruction and disorders of sperm transport), 1 to 2 percent from hypothalamic–pituitary disease, and 40 to 50 percent from unidentifiable causes. Female causes are ovarian disease (failure to ovulate), 20 percent; tubal disease (obstruction), 25 percent; cervical factor (sperm cannot effectively pass the cervix), 5 percent; uterine abnormalities, less than 1 percent, and unexplained, 10 percent. In practical terms, infertility is caused by one of four conditions: the inability to produce healthy gametes (sperm or eggs); the failure of healthy gametes to come into close physical proximity, thus preventing fertilization; the inability of the fertilized egg to attach to the uterine lining successfully; and the inability to carry a pregnancy to term.

Infertility is a complex disease and is often caused by numerous factors. Couples should be referred for infertility evaluation if they have been unable to conceive after at least 1 year of attempting to achieve pregnancy. If the woman is older than 35 years of age, the couple should be referred after only 6 to 9 months of unprotected intercourse without conception. At age 25, the age at which couples are the most fertile, the average length of time needed to achieve conception is 5.3 months. The average 20- to 30-year-old American couple has intercourse one to three times a week, a frequency that should be sufficient to achieve pregnancy if all other factors are satisfactory. The number of women who give birth to their first child after age 30 continues to increase. Delaying parenthood appears to increase the possibility that one or more physiologic processes necessary for conception will be adversely affected.

Even though fertility is defined as no pregnancy after 12 months of trying, evaluation should be initiated after 6 months in women between 35 and 40 years and immediate evaluation in women over 40 years, given the rapid increase in follicular atresia that occurs after age 37.

Pathophysiology

The following essential components must be presented for normal fertility in women. The cervical mucus must be favorable to the survival of spermatozoa and allow passage to the upper genital tract. There must be clear passage between the cervix and the fallopian tubes. The fallopian tubes must be patent and have normal fimbria with peristaltic movements toward the uterus to facilitate normal transport and interaction of ovum and sperm. The ovaries must produce and release normal ova in timely manner, and there must be no obstruction between the ovaries and fallopian tubes. Finally, the endometrium must be in a normal physiologic state to allow implantation of the blastocyst and to sustain normal growth and development.

The most common cause of tubal infertility is antecedent pelvic inflammatory disease, caused most commonly by *Neisseria gonorrhoeae* and *Chlamydia trachomatis*. In addition, tubal endometriosis, pelvic tuberculosis, and adhesions from previous pelvic surgery or infection affecting any portion of the fallopian tubes may lead to obstruction. Hydrosalpinges may form due to obstruction, which are large, elongated typically fluid-filled cystic masses located anywhere along the adnexa. These significantly interfere with the success of in vitro fertilization (IVF), thought to be due to components in the hydrosalpinx fluid that are toxic to developing embryos.

Uterine anatomic abnormalities have not been consistently identified as causal sources of infertility, as many women with abnormal uteri are able to conceive and carry pregnancies to term. However, septate uteri, synechiae (severe endometrial scarring), and polyps are all more common in infertile women, particularly those exposed in utero to diethylstilbestrol (DES), a synthetic estrogen that was used between 1940 and 1970 to help prevent miscarriages but was eventually shown to cause defects in uterine anatomy (e.g., bicornuate or T-shaped uterus). Similarly, uterine leiomyomata or fibroids (benign smooth muscle monoclonal tumors), which are the most common form of pelvic tumors in women, are observed in greater frequency in infertile women. However, it appears that only those with an intracavitary or submucosal component are associated with lower oocyte implantation and pregnancy rates.

Several other factors may affect the ability of the uterus to maintain a normal pregnancy. Endometriosis is more common in infertile women and, even when located outside the fallopian tubes, may contribute to infertility in a number of ways: pelvic adhesions affecting the reproductive tract, direct damage to ovarian tissue by endometrial implants or subsequent surgical removal, cytokine and growth factor production by endometrial implants which interferes with ovulation, fertilization, or oocyte implantation. Cervical stenosis may occur congenitally, following trauma, or from infection and subsequent scarring. This, along with alterations in cervical mucus, may impair entry of sperm into the uterus. Following implantation of the fertilized oocyte, impaired corpus luteum development may lead to inadequate progesterone production and delayed endometrial maturation, as demonstrated by endometrial biopsy. Likewise, in the presence of adequate progesterone, the endometrium may not be adequately responsive to this hormone. However, the importance of luteal phase defects as a direct cause of infertility is controversial.

Systemic factors also exist that affect the ability to initiate or maintain pregnancy. Hypercoagulable states, such as from antiphospholipid antibody syndrome, systemic lupus erythematosus, or other autoimmune and connective tissue disorders are well known to be associated with early, first-trimester miscarriages—likely due to immunologic rejection of the developing embryo or microthrombosis of placental vessels leading to placental insufficiency. Genetic anomalies in both women and men have been associated with infertility, the most common being Turner's syndrome (XO) in women and Klinefelter's syndrome (XXY) and Fragile X syndrome in men. Defects in several genes capable of affecting fertility have been identified including *KAL1,* which leads to congenital hypothalamic hypopituitary hypogonadism (Kallmann's syndrome), the FSH receptor, FMR1, which leads to Fragile X syndrome; *DAX1*, *FGFR1*, and *GPR54*.

For normal fertility to occur in men, the testes must produce an adequate number of morphologically normal, motile sperm. The male genital tract secretions from the seminal vesicles and prostate gland must be normal. The genital tract must not be obstructed, as sperm travel from the testis through the epididymis and vas deferens to the urethra. Finally, ejaculated spermatozoa must be deposited in the female genital tract in such a manner that they reach the cervix and enter the uterus where they may contact oocytes either within the uterus or more commonly within the fallopian tubes.

Primary hypogonadism is the most commonly identifiable cause of male infertility, resulting from congenital causes including chromosomal disorders (e.g., Klinefelter's and Fragile X syndrome), azoospermia from cryptorchidism (i.e., failure of testicular descension from the abdominal cavity during in utero development), defects in androgen production (5-alpha-reductase deficiency) or receptor activity, as well as Y chromosome deletions, especially in the long arm at the Yq6 region. Acquired disorders such as testicular infection (e.g., viral orchitis from mumps paramyxovirus, echovirus, or arbovirus), drugs toxic to sperm (e.g., alkylating immunosuppressants such as cyclophosphamide, antiandrogens such as spironolactone, ketoconazole), radiation exposure, tobacco smoking, and hyperthermia have all been associated with decreased male fertility, as well as underlying systemic disease such as chronic renal insufficiency and cirrhosis. Antisperm antibodies have also been identified in some infertile men which presumably affect fertility, but it is not clear whether these form spontaneously or as a result of testicular injury which compromises the testicular–blood barrier.

In far fewer cases, defects exist higher up on the hypothalamic–pituitary–gonadal axis. A failure of hypothalamic gonadotropin releasing hormone (GnRH) secretion and/or pituitary gonadotropin production may result from congenital defects (e.g., Kallmann's syndrome) or acquired conditions such as secreting or nonsecreting pituitary macroadenomas, prolactinomas, craniopharyngiomas, or infiltrative processes such as sarcoidosis, histiocytosis, or tuberculosis.

Sperm transport may be inhibited anywhere along the male reproductive tract. Intrauterine estrogen exposure may lead to epididymal defects, while infection (e.g., epididymitis caused by *Neisseria gonorrhoeae, Chlamydia trachomatis,* or tuberculosis) and certain chemical toxins (e.g., chlorhydrin) may affect spermatozoal function within the epididymis. The vas deferens may similarly be affected by infection, intentional ligation as in surgical vasectomy, inspissation of thick mucoid secretions (Young's syndrome), or congenital absence due to defects in cAMP-regulated chloride ion channels, as in cystic fibrosis. While secretions from the prostate and seminal vesicles (e.g., fructose) contain several components that contribute to sperm viability and motility, defects in glandular secretion have not been causally related to infertility. In addition, erectile dysfunction and ineffective ejaculation may result from spinal cord damage or disease, as well as defects in autonomic function from diabetes mellitus. Varicoceles (venous dilation of the pampiniform plexus proximal to the testicle) are also far more common in infertile men, but they may also be present in men with normal fertility. Although no definitive evidence exists, they are thought to impair spermatogenesis via increased testicular temperature, hypoxia, or vascular stasis with delayed clearance of toxic serum metabolites.

Clinical Presentation

Subjective

The patient presents with the complaint of inability to conceive and the desire to have a child.

Objective

Assessment of persons seeking evaluation and treatment of infertility should begin with a detailed comprehensive history. Before tests to determine the cause of infertility are made, a detailed medical, social, and family history must be obtained from both partners. Often the history uncovers important information. The history should elicit information about the duration of the infertility and whether it is primary or secondary; the frequency of sexual intercourse; the regularity, the duration, and frequency of menstruation; and any premenstrual signs and symptoms. It should also include information on any vaginal discharge, cervicitis, pelvic infections, surgery, and trauma. General physical condition, illness, allergies, and drug intake (prescription and illicit) should be noted, as should any significant family history. Prior use of contraceptives, including type, duration, and complications, should be recorded. Information on maternal use of DES should also be noted, as this can affect fertility.

Necessary information from the man includes any history of mumps, orchitis, trauma, diabetes mellitus, herniorrhaphy, or exposure to x-rays or toxic substances, such as lead, iron, zinc, or copper. The male should also be questioned about exercise patterns, drug intake (prescription and illicit), exposure to heat (from the environment or from wearing tight underclothes), duration of infertility, whether the fertility is primary or secondary, frequency of coitus, and history of maternal use of DES (can affect a son's fertility). A complete physical examination of both partners is essential, particularly a thorough pelvic examination of the woman. The male examination should include testicular volume (below 15 mL is small) and testicular length less than 3.6 cm is small. Certain laboratory tests, such as CBC, TSH, T_4, and urinalysis should also be included. If findings are negative, an infertility workup is begun.

Diagnostic Reasoning

Diagnostic Tests

The easiest and least intrusive infertility testing should be used first. Extensive testing should be avoided until data confirm that the timing of the intercourse and the length of coital exposure have been adequate. The couple should be informed of the most fertile times to have intercourse during the menstrual cycle. Teaching the couple the signs and timing of ovulation and the most effective times for intercourse within the cycle may solve the problem before extensive testing needs to be initiated. Primary assessment, including a comprehensive history and physical examination for any obvious causes of infertility, is done before a costly, time-consuming, and emotionally trying investigation is initiated. Because infertility is a couple's issue, it is important for both partners to be present. One basic test of ovulatory function is the basal body temperature (BBT) recording, which aids in identifying follicular, ovulatory, and luteal-phase abnormalities. With the additional documentation of coitus, serial BBT charts can be used to indicate retrospectively, if, and approximately when, the woman is ovulating and if intercourse is occurring at the proper time to achieve conception. A proposed schedule for intercourse, based on serial BBT charts, might be to recommend sexual intercourse every other day in the period of time beginning 3 to 4 days before and continuing for 2 to 3 days after the expected time of ovulation.

The semen analysis is the single most important diagnostic study of the male and should be done early in the couple's evaluation and before invasive testing of the female. Semen analysis must be done within 1 day of donation and normal sperm morphology may be as low as 15 to 20 percent with good results. Also, at least 25 percent of sperm should have rapid progressive mobility (not just moving in place). Sperm viability should be tested if motility is insufficient. Semen pH is also important (low pH is correlated with decreased fertility). Cellular debris and agglutination are of concern for antibody-mediated autoimmune destruction of sperm. Antibodies may be detected and are considered concerning if they coat over 50 percent of spermatozoa. The presence of immature germ cells may represent a maturation defect, and the presence of sperm leukocytes (greater than 1 million/mL) reflects infection within the reproductive tract. Semen culture is often sent, but this is usually not diagnostically useful. It is important to note that an absence of sperm may be due to spermatic duct obstruction, rather than a lack of sperm production by the testes. Patients lacking sperm in the semen should be referred to urology to rule out retrograde ejaculation, congenital absence of the vas deferens, or other forms of obstruction. A postejaculatory urine specimen will reflect retrograde ejaculation if sperm are present, while an absence of sperm may reflect obstruction or impaired spermatogenesis.

It is important to assess both partners because of the high incidence of multifactorial infertility. A thorough female evaluation includes assessment of the hypothalamic–pituitary axis in terms of ovulatory function. Progesterone levels are measured at different points along the luteal phase to confirm ovulation. In addition, LH levels can be measured in the serum and with home urine tests to help predict ovulation (as the surge occurs 1 to 2 days ahead of ovulation) to facilitate the timing of intercourse, but home urine tests are not as sensitive (85 percent) as serum tests done during formal fertility evaluation, since once-a-day testing can miss the surge because of variations in renal clearance of LH. Examination of vaginal discharge for increased volume, and clear, slippery mucus that stretches into strings (Spinnbarkheit) is a strong indicator of preovulatory estrogen effect. The progesterone challenge test using MPA 10 mg qd for 5 days and check for induction of uterine bleeding in the week after treatment confirms adequate production of estradiol (estrogen). An FSH level should be drawn on day 3 of the cycle to check for adequate ovarian reserve—a value less than 15 mIU/mL is suggestive of adequate reserve. Prolactin and THS levels should also be checked to rule out hyperprolactinemia (which may be treated with a dopamine agonist like bromocriptine, pergolide, or cabergoline), especially in women with galactorrhea, and thyroid disorders. MRI and hysterosalpingogram imaging are done to evaluate the structure and function of the cervix, uterus, fallopian tubes, and ovaries. Laparoscopy is more sensitive for detecting tubal abnormalities than hysterosalpingogram alone, but may be unnecessary if the finding from the hysterosalpingogram are normal. Also, the performance of the hysterosalpingogram itself (flushing the tubes with oil-based contrast medium) increases the likelihood of pregnancy.

Evaluation of the man may include at least two semen analyses to confirm or rule out a seminal deficiency. Endocrine evaluation of men includes serum LH, FSH, and testosterone levels. If the LH and FSH are high and the testosterone level is low, this is consistent with primary hypogonadism, while a normal to low LH and FSH reflect secondary hypogonadism. In men with low testosterone and normal to low LH levels, prolactin should be measured to rule out prolactinomas.

If the results of both the male and female infertility workups are negative, a laparoscopic evaluation may be necessary. Table 13.4 outlines different fertility tests and favorable clinical findings that indicate that the couple is capable of conceiving.

Table 13.4 Fertility Tests and Favorable Clinical Findings

Gender	Test	How Obtained	Favorable Clinical Findings
Male	Semen analysis	48–72 h after abstinence from ejaculation	Normal amount of ejaculate (3–5 mL; range 1–7 mL). No agglutination of sperm. (Agglutination suggests infection or autoimmunity.) Normal seminal fluid. Sperm count greater than 20,000,000 cells with at least 50% motility 2 h after ejaculation and more than 60% normal appearing cells.
	Karyotyping (in men with severe oligospermia or azoospermia)	Blood sample/bone marrow	Chromosomal abnormalities can be detected
Female	Basal body temperature (BBT) measurement	Oral temperature taken daily before arising throughout several menstrual cycles	Biphasic pattern with persistent temperature elevation for 12–14 days before menses.
	Postcoital test	Vaginal exam within 8 h after intercourse, during time of presumed ovulation	Cervical mucus suggestive of ovulation. Microscopic ferning pattern present. Watery, slippery, abundant mucus. Spinnbarkheit is present. (the act of pulling out a string of cervical mucous and measuring how far it can be stretched before breaking) Presence of normal live and motile sperm in cervical mucus.
	Serum progesterone measurement	Blood sample	3–4 ng/mL in early luteal phase. 10 ng/mL at midluteal phase.
	Serum LH (predict ovulation)	Blood sample	6.17–17.2 IU/Latovalation
	Karyotyping (in women with ovarian failure or repeated spontaneous abortion)	Blood sample/bone marrow	
	Immunoassay tests	Semen and male/female serum	Absence of antibody reaction. Evidence of normal pelvic anatomy and tubal functioning.
	Hysterosalpingogram	Dye injected through cervix into uterus then fluoroscopic visualization of the spread of dye through fallopian tubes. Done during first half of menstrual cycle before ovulation	Patency of fallopian tubes and absence of abnormalities in uterine cavities and fallopian tubes.
	Laparoscopy	Direct visualization of pelvic structures through a small abdominal incision	Normal pelvic structures and absence of signs of infection, adhesions, endometriosis, or lesions.

Management

The principle of management is to assist the couple to achieve pregnancy before or during the natural age-related decline in female fecundity. Several lifestyle changes can increase the chances that a couple will become pregnant. Caffeine intake should be no more than 250 mg (2 cups of coffee) per day. In addition, alcohol intake should be limited to no more than 4 drinks per week. Increasing sexual intercourse to 2 to 3 times a week is also advisable. These measures should be recommended before any other interventions. If the woman's BMI is less than 20 or greater than 27, attempts should be made to get the body weight to a normal level. Loss of just 5 to 10 percent of body weight in obese anovulatory women with polycystic ovarian disease (PCOS) can restore ovulation within 6 months and should be a first-line therapy. For women with PCOS, in addition to weight loss, insulin sensitization with metformin has been shown to improve fertility.

A low percentage of body fat resulting from eating disorders (anorexia nervosa/bulimia) or from extreme exercise can lead to anovulation through GnRH or gonadotropin suppression and must be addressed. Pulsatile GnRH therapy may restore ovulation in these women, but this treatment is available only in Europe at this time.

If an ovulatory defect has been identified during fertility testing, the treatment depends on the specific cause of the problem. In the presence of normal ovaries, a normal prolactin level, and an intact pituitary gland (normogonadotropic normoestrogenic anovulation [WHO Class II anovulation] which is 70 to 85 percent of cases), clomiphene citrate (Clomid), a selective estrogen receptor modulator (SERM) with both agonist and antagonist effects at the estrogen receptor level is effective. Ovulation occurs in approximately 80 percent of properly selected women and conception rates approach 40 percent. The risk of multiple gestation with clomiphene is 5 percent and is almost exclusively with twins. The woman takes a 50-mg dose of clomiphene each day from day 5 to 9 of the cycle. Ovulation can be expected to occur 5 to 10 days after the last dose. If ovulation is not achieved in the first cycle of therapy, the dose may be increased in 50-mg increments to a maximum of 200 to 250 mg qd for 5 days. After the first treatment cycle, a pelvic exam should be done to rule out ovarian enlargement or hyperstimulation. Ovarian enlargement and abdominal discomfort may result from follicular growth and the formation of multiple corpus lutea. Other adverse effects include hot flashes, nausea and vomiting, vision problems, headache, and dryness or loss of hair. Clomiphene citrate should not be used for more than six cycles as it is unlikely to work after this many tries. Tamoxifen is another SERM that works with fewer anti-estrogen effects, but it has no added fertility benefit over clomiphene citrate.

Aromatase inhibitors such as letrozole (Femara) and anastrozole (Arimidex) have a shorter half-life than the SERMs and fewer anti-estrogen effects, producing fewer follicles and lower estradiol levels, reducing the risk of multiple gestations and miscarriage. These agents may be used for patients who do not respond to clomiphene.

Treatment with gonadotropins requires much closer monitoring, is more costly, and has a higher risk of multiple gestations. A laparoscopic technique called ovarian drilling may be used in which a laser is used to induce ovulation. This technique seems to work no better than gonadotropins, but it carries less risk of multiple gestations.

Cervical stenosis can be treated via catheter dilation for several days with concurrent antibiotic prophylaxis (doxycycline 100 mg PO bid). Women with systemic clotting disorders may also benefit from aspirin and heparin anticoagulation therapy to improve the likelihood of pregnancy.

Intrauterine insemination (IUI) just prior to ovulation (based on LH measurements) is often effective when other methods have failed. IUI may be tried before in vitro fertilization (IVF) because it is often effective and less expensive. IUI done high in the uterus is more effective than intracervical injection (ICI), which approximates normal intercourse. With high IUI, the probability of pregnancy is improved through concurrent treatment with clomiphene for three to six cycles, and if this fails, IUI with gonadotropin injections for at least three cycles can be tried.

The last resort for infertile couples is IVF and embryo transfer, or, if the tubes are patent and normal, gamete intrafallopian transfer (GIFT). In some cases of tubal occlusion in which the rate of success with tubal repair is low (less than 30 percent), IVF appears to be preferable to surgery because of the more rapid conception rate. IVF has the highest pregnancy rate in the shortest amount of time, but it is also the costliest intervention, with a price tag of $50,000 to $100,000 per attempt. Intratubal transfer of embryos may improve the success rate over transcervical transfer, but this is unclear and may depend on how good the results are at the particular center with the regular IVF procedure.

The pregnancy rate with IVF has been highly variable from center to center, owing to the complexity of the techniques required, whereas the pregnancy rate with GIFT has been more consistent. The mean live delivery rates per retrieval with IVF and GIFT are approximately 21 and 28 percent, respectively. Ectopic pregnancy occurs in about 4 to 5 percent of these pregnancies, whereas the rate of fetal abnormalities is not increased. There are many ethical considerations associated with assisted reproductive technologies; some of these are presented in Table 13.5.

It is also possible to achieve pregnancy with IVF and embryo transfer using donor eggs, with a higher rate than with regular IVF and embryo transfer (47 percent per retrieval). The eggs generally come from young fertile women (sisters or anonymous volunteers). The recipient can be programmed for optimal uterine receptivity by replacement doses of estradiol and progesterone.

Treatment of male infertility from hypogonadotropic hypogonadism can be done with gonadotropin therapy consisting of human chorionic gonadotropin (hCG) injection 1500 to 2000 IU SQ or IM three times a week for at least 6 months. hCG acts similarly to LH. If this does not work, human menopausal gonadotropin or hMG 37.5 to 75 IU 3 times a week is added which contains FSH. Thus, this treatment can last more than a year. This combination treatment is typically needed for Kallmann's syndrome (congenital hypogonadotropic hypogonadism). Recombinant LH/FSH are also now available. Pulsatile GnRH treatment delivered via IV pump is also available for hypothalamic hypogonadotropic hypogonadism.

Sperm autoimmunity may be treated with high-dose steroids (prednisone 40 to 80 mg PO qd) for up to 6 months, but this may be poorly tolerated. Thus, intracytoplasmic sperm injection (ICSI) is an important IVF alternative with a clinical pregnancy rate of up to 20 percent. Retrograde ejaculation may be treated with IUI, traditional IVF, or ICSI as well. Repair of varicoceles is controversial and is usually recommended only with large defects or in younger men, as prolonged damage to the testes—indicated by testicular atrophy, epithelial damage, and severe oligospermia or azoospermia—is unlikely to be reversed by surgical ligation of the varicocele. Reversal of vasectomy can result in successful

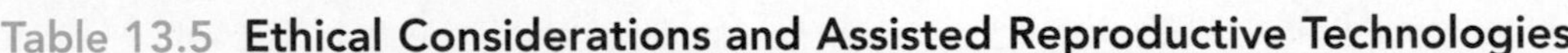

Table 13.5 Ethical Considerations and Assisted Reproductive Technologies

In vitro fertilization (IVF) has been a welcome solution for many couples who have been unable to conceive. Recently, advances in the application of IVF technology have spurred the emergence of even more new avenues of achieving pregnancy and parenting. With hormone replacement therapy (HRT) and donor egg embryos, women past menopause can achieve pregnancy. Other options include cryopreservation, fertilization of donor gametes (donor eggs, sperm, or both), IVF with the use of a gestational carrier, embryo adoption, and the use of surrogacy. All of these options are complicated by the introduction of a third party into the reproductive process and ethical concerns. Some of the issues raised in connection with these techniques include the following:

1. Is it a constitutional right for individuals or couples to be able to utilize donor gametes or to contract with a woman to carry their embryo to treat their infertility?
2. With a multiple pregnancy rate approaching 20% in couples undergoing IVF procedures, the potential (<3%) of having a grand multiple gestation forces some couples to consider embryo reduction to avoid an adverse obstetrical and/or fetal outcome (selective abortion).
3. If excess embryos are frozen and kept, how long can and should they be stored? What should be done in cases of death of one or both of the partners, divorce, or when couples choose not to claim their embryos?
4. Do providers have the right to decide who can participate in using donor gametes, embryos, gestational carriers, and surrogates? What about single women, lesbian couples, or crossing generational lines (daughter being a donor for mother)?
5. Does use of the assisted reproductive technologies take into consideration the best interests of the parties involved, including those of the resulting offspring? For example, what are the effects on a child of knowing or not knowing the identity of the donor?
6. How can the potential for consanguinity (having an ancestor in common) be controlled in the case of gamete and/or embryo donation?
7. Does the existence of new technologies make it more difficult to accept childlessness by increasing pressure on women to follow every avenue in an attempt to conceive?
8. To what extent should health insurance policies cover these modes of treating infertility at a time of growing health-care costs?

pregnancy in a female partner in up to 50 percent of cases. In cases of obstruction along the reproductive tract, sperm may be retrieved for ICSI via direct microsurgical aspiration from the epididymis or the seminiferous tubules of the testes. In all cases of congenital reproductive tract defects such as absent vas deferens, however, genetic counseling must take place prior to microsurgical aspiration and ICSI, given the risk of passing genetic defects, such as the cystic fibrosis gene, Klinefelter's, or deletions in the Y chromosome, onto these men's offspring.

Follow-Up and Referral

After the initial exam and counseling regarding the frequency and timing of intercourse, if couples wish to proceed with fertilization testing and/or treatment, referral to a fertility clinic is indicated. Infertile couples need a great deal of support and advocacy as well as education and help in decision making. The options must be presented in a nonjudgmental way to facilitate the couple's own decision making. Providing referral to other sources of assistance is another way in which the clinician supports the infertile person or couple. One important source of information is RESOLVE, a national organization composed of self-help groups that provide support and information about infertility. Providing anticipatory guidance for the battery of tests to which patients are subjected during infertility evaluation is important.

Patient Education

An important part of care for infertile persons is emphasizing and teaching self-care. Infertility is often experienced as being "out of control." Identifying and using successful coping strategies help the patient regain a sense of control. Stress-reduction techniques, such as exercise, relaxation techniques, and meditation may be especially useful both for those with general concerns about fertility and for those concerned about specific diagnostic or treatment procedures. Infertility can become an all-encompassing concern, resulting in alterations in health and recreation patterns and a loss of interest in other aspects of life. It should be emphasized that one can be creative, productive, and successful in other areas even if unable to produce children. The emotional problems surrounding infertility illustrate the need for emphasis on family-centered care. Infertility is a highly emotional issue that has far-reaching implications for many family members.

Vulvovaginal Infections and Sexually Transmitted Infections

Several different sexually transmitted infections (STIs) affect the female reproductive tract and genitalia. STIs are transmitted through sexual intercourse between heterosexual or homosexual persons by intimate contact with the genitalia, mouth, or anus. STIs, called venereal diseases in the past, include infection by herpes simplex virus (HSV), *Chlamydia trachomatis*, *Neisseria gonorrhoeae*, *Treponema pallidum* (syphilis), human papilloma virus (HPV), trichomoniasis, and human immunodeficiency virus (HIV). Other vulvar lesions include chancroid, lymphogranuloma venereum (LGV), granuloma inguinale, and molluscum contagiosum lesions. Cervical infection known as mucopurulent cervicitis is also largely caused by community-acquired sexually transmitted agents, namely *C. trachomatis* and *N. gonorrhoeae*.

In contrast, vulvovaginal infections affecting the female genitalia that are not officially considered STIs include both vulvar disorders and selected vaginal and cervical infections. Painful vaginal disorders (vulvodynia) go by several names including vulvar pain syndrome, chronic vulvar pain, vestibulitis, focal vulvitis, vestibular adenitis, and burning vulva syndrome. These may be caused by candidiasis (yeast infection), bacterial vaginosis (BV), atrophic vaginitis, allergic vaginitis, and irritation from foreign bodies or chemicals found in soaps, shampoos, or lotions.

Epidemiology and Causes

STIs are the most prevalent communicable diseases in the United States, with the exception of upper respiratory infections. STIs affect more than 12 million patients annually in the United States alone, with 25 percent being adolescents. Although STIs disproportionately affect adolescents and young adults more than any other age group (largely because of increased sexual encounters and risk-taking behaviors), no age group is considered "safe." It is estimated that approximately one American out of five is infected with a viral STI other than HIV. Perhaps even more alarming is that the United States, with one of the most educated populations and highest standards of living, also has the highest STI rates in the world.

The causative agents of the most common vulvovaginal infections and STIs, as well as the clinical presentation, diagnostic reasoning, and recommended management, are presented in Table 13.6. Inadequately treated STIs have far-reaching implications for future health, including long-term fertility. Mucopurulent cervicitis may extend retrograde through the uterus and out the fallopian tubes to the ovaries and throughout the pelvic cavity, causing widespread inflammation, scarring, and adhesions. Known as pelvic inflammatory disease (PID), this condition may occur in up to 15 percent of mucopurulent cervicitis cases, requiring hospitalization and IV antibiotics in its most serious form and leading to obstruction anywhere along the reproductive tract. PID is the most common cause of tubal infertility (see section on Infertility). Untreated syphilis may lead to a tertiary form of infection with serious CNS insult (general paresis and dorsal motor column defects known as tabes dorsalis), aortitis, and nodular, granulomatous lesions on the skin, bone, and solid organs known as gummas. Untreated HIV infection progresses to clinical AIDS over 2 to 10 years, destroying the immune system and leading to increasing numbers of opportunistic infections of the lungs, genitourinary tract, and CNS, which eventually prove fatal. Even BV has been shown to be a risk factor in pregnant women for preterm delivery of low-birth-weight infants.

Pathophysiology

The female reproductive tract is normally protected from infection by several mechanisms, including a low, acidic pH resulting from vaginal secretions and the presence of commensual, nonpathogenic microbial flora, namely hydrogen peroxide–producing *Lactobacillus*. The normal flora environmentally compete and protect against the overgrowth of potentially pathogenic anaerobic and gram-negative bacteria. Disruptions of the mucosal surface either by trauma or preexistent infectious lesion predispose the reproductive tract to infection. In addition, while BV is not considered sexually transmitted, as it is caused by overgrowth of pathogenic vaginal flora, vaginal intercourse may raise intravaginal pH and predispose to the development of BV. Ascending cervical infections, as seen in PID, also appear more common in the week following menses, possibly owing to the absence of endometrial sloughing mechanisms that protect against retrograde infection.

Although the pathogenesis of some vulvar and vaginal pain syndromes has not been fully elucidated, STIs are known to stem from a heterogeneous collection of causative infectious agents (see Table 13.6). However, the unifying principle of these disorders is their propensity for spread by intimate person-to-person sexual contact, particularly after exposure of the mucous membranes to infected bodily fluids. This typically occurs within the genitalia. However, the oral and anal mucosa are also highly susceptible entry points, as exemplified by the incidence of gonococcal pharyngitis after receptive oral intercourse.

Given the length of the vaginal canal and the relatively larger area of exposed genital mucosa, women appear more susceptible to STI infection. They are also more likely to display symptoms of infection. The presence of one STI increases the chances of becoming infected with another—especially HIV. This is likely due to compromise of mucosal and outer skin barriers, as well as interactions on the molecular level, for example, HPV as a cofactor for HIV infection. Infectious organisms themselves may also express various genetic virulence factors that render them more susceptible to sexual transmission, including surface proteins that facilitate epithelial adherence to the vaginal or cervical mucosa.

Clinical Presentation

Subjective

The patient with a vulvar lesion may present with a complaint of a painful lymph node. With vaginal disorders, the patient typically complains of burning and itching of the vulva, along with tenderness at the vaginal opening. Usually there is a long-standing history of complaints with little or no response to treatment. There is increased pain with tight clothing such as jeans and panty hose, sitting, and external pressure. The discomfort can be so great that it interferes with or stops intercourse. Frequently described as "shards of glass" or "pins and needles" on the vulva and at the introitus, the patient may complain of vulvar soreness for days following intercourse.

Sixty to eighty percent of STIs are asymptomatic; therefore, most are detected on routine exam. Other patients present with burning, itching, and a vaginal discharge that

(text continued on page 690)

Table 13.6 **Vulvovaginal Infections and Sexually Transmitted Diseases**

Problem	Clinical Presentation	Diagnostic Reasoning	Treatment: As Recommended by CDC
Vulvar Lesions • Chancroid (*Haemophilus ducreyi*)	Single painful ulcer (irregular, erythematous, and undermined edges) with a unilateral bubo If vaginal lesion, may be asymptomatic. Painful lymphadenopathy	Risk factors: coinfection with HIV, HSV, and syphilis	Azithromycin (Zithromax) 1 g PO × 1 OR Ceftriaxone (Rocephin) 250 mg IM × 1 OR Ciprofloxacin (Cipro) 500 mg PO bid for 3 days OR Erythromycin (E-mycin) 500 mg PO qid for 7 days
• Lymphogranuloma venereum (LGV) (*Chlamydia trachomatis*)	Lymphadenopathy, anorectal swelling and fistula formation	History of travel and sexual contact in endemically infected area Serologic LGV complement fixation test; suspect if titer above 1:16; diagnostic if above 1:64	Doxycycline (Vibramycin) 100 mg PO bid for 21 days OR Erythromycin (E-mycin) 500 mg qid for 21 days OR Azithromycin (Zithromax) may be effective if given for 2–3 weeks; no recommended dosage from CDC.
• Granuloma inguinale (granuloma venereum, Donovanosis) (*Klebsiella granulomatis*)	Chronic, progressive papule that ulcerates to a beefy red, painless granular area with clean, sharp rolled edges; inguinal swelling; late painful abscesses (buboes)	History of travel and sexual contact in endemically infected area Cannot be cultured; stained tissue sample may show Donovan bodies	Doxycycline (Vibramycin) 100 mg PO bid for 1–4 weeks OR Trimethoprim 80 mg plus Sulfamethoxazole 400 mg (Bactrim) 1 tablet PO bid for 14 days OR Erythromycin (E-mycin) 500 mg PO bid for 4 weeks (during pregnancy)
• Molluscum contagiosum (large DNA virus from the Poxviridae family)	Pearly, raised, painless lesions with umbilicated center; diffuse or singular; may be self-limiting	Based on characteristic lesions	No treatment. Lesions may last months to years and often heal spontaneously. Once healed, the person has a lifetime immunity to the virus.
Vaginal Disorders • Vulvodynia	Burning and itching of vulva; tenderness at vaginal opening; dry and swollen vulva; associated with inflamed and painful Bartholin's, vestibular, and Skene's gland	Diagnosis of elimination Changes in touch test Vulvar biopsy for inflammation Colposcopy for microfissures	Treat symptomatically Mild pain: topical lidocaine (Xylocaine) Antidepressants such as amitriptyline 50–100 mg hs or fluoxetine 20 mg q AM or 20 mg AM and noon. Surgery (50% success rate)
• Candidiasis	Pruritus, redness, swelling, "curdy" vaginal discharge (white, thick); occasional burning with urination, vaginal wall redness	Risk factors: previous antibiotic therapy, chronic vulva moisture, diabetes, HIV infection, immunosuppression	Fluconazole (Diflucan) 150 mg PO × 1 OR Butoconazole 2% cream 5 g intravaginally qhs × 3 days

Problem	Clinical Presentation	Diagnostic Reasoning	Treatment: As Recommended by CDC
		Wet prep with saline, KOH, pH 4–5	OR Miconazole 2% cream 5 g intravaginally qhs × 7 days
• Bacterial vaginosis (BV)	Thin discharge, malodorous, increased odor after intercourse, pruritus, edema, erythema	Based on symptoms, including homogenous white discharge with "fishy" odor, pH >4.5, clue cells on microscopic exam and a positive amine test (KOH applied to discharge releases fishy odor—"whiff" test)	Metronidazole 500 mg PO bid × 7 days OR Metronidazol gel 0.75% one full applicator (5 g) intravaginally qd × 5 days OR Clindamycin cream 2% one full applicator (5 g) intravaginally at bedtime × 7 days
• Atrophic vaginitis	Dry, thin vaginal tissue; dyspareunia	History of perimenopause or menopause, pH 6.5–7, wet prep: negative for pathogens	Treat symptoms Vaginal lubricants Estrogen vaginal cream—inserted vaginally daily for 4–6 weeks and can be continued for a few months if necessary to resolve symptoms. After initial therapy, use of 1–2 g of the cream twice a week will prevent recurrence.
• Allergic vaginitis	Excessive or malodorous vaginal discharge, pruritus, external dysuria	Obtain accurate history, pH normal (3.8–4.2)	Avoid offending substance Sitz baths
Cervical Disorders • Mucopurulent cervicitis (MPC)	Yellow mucous discharge, possible bleeding with intercourse, cervical tenderness, "beefy red" friable cervix	Wet prep: increase in WBCs	Azithromycin (Zithromax) 1 g PO × 1 OR Doxycycline (Vibramycin) 100 mg PO bid for 7 days *Alternate:* Erythromycin (E-mycin) 500 mg PO qid for 7 days OR Erythromycin ethylsuccinate (EES) 800 mg PO qid for 7 days OR Ofloxacin (Floxin) 300 mg PO bid for 7 days
STIs • HSV Infection	*First Outbreak:* Flu-like symptoms with adenopathy, tingling of the site prior to outbreak, and very painful vesicular lesions Ulcers form with circumscribed erythematous edges and white exudate centrally; may last 12 days *Recurrent Outbreaks:* Symptoms may be similar, usually less severe and shorter length 4–5 days	Viral culture of vesicle fluid most accurate if within 48 hours of outbreak Tzanck smear from the base of an early vesicle DNA probe from lesion scraping	*First Outbreak:* Acyclovir (Zovirax) 400 mg PO tid for 7–10 days OR 200 mg PO 5 times a day for 7–10 days OR Famciclovir (Famvir) 250 mg PO tid for 7–10 days OR Valacyclovir (Valtrex) 1 g PO bid for 7–10 days.

(continued)

Table 13.6 **Vulvovaginal Infections and Sexually Transmitted Diseases** (continued)

Problem	Clinical Presentation	Diagnostic Reasoning	Treatment: As Recommended by CDC
			Recurrent Outbreaks: Acyclovir 200 mg q4h 5 times daily for 5 days Famciclovir: 125 mg q12h for 5 days Valacyclovir: 500 mg q12h for 5 days *Suppressive:* Acyclovir 400 mg PO bid Famciclovir 250 mg PO bid Valacyclovir 1 g PO qd Evaluate after 1 year for recurrent episodes.
• *Chlamydia*	Most commonly no reported symptoms. Patient may have an increase in mucopurulent discharge and bleeding with intercourse	Yellow mucopurulent discharge on cervix Cervix friable and inflamed May or may not have cervical motion tenderness Wet mount: >10 WBCs per high-power field (hpf) DNA probe (cervical swab)	Azithromycin (Zithromax) 1 g PO × 1 OR Doxycycline (Vibramycin) 100 mg PO bid for 7 days *Alternate:* Erythromycin base (E-mycin) 500 mg PO qid for 7 days OR Ofloxacin (Floxin) 300 mg PO bid for 7 days OR Levofloxacin 500 mg PO for 7 days.
• *Syphilis*	Primary: painless ulcer at initial site of contact (chancre), adenopathy Secondary: maculopapular rash on palms and soles, condylomata/moist flat wartlike lesions, adenopathy Tertiary/Late: cardiac, neurologic, ophthalmic, auditory, and gummatous lesions	Dark-field microscopy: positive for spirochetes Direct microhemagglutination-*Treponema pallidum* (MHA-TP): antibody test Fluorescent treponemal antibody absorption (FTA-ABS): antibody test reported as positive Venereal Disease Research Laboratory (VDRL), syphilis test, rapid plasma reagin (RPR): with titer indicating degree of infection	*Early (less than 1 year duration):* Benzathine penicillin G 2.4 million units IM × 1 *Latent or Late (duration longer than 1 year or unknown length):* Benzathine penicillin G 2.4 million units IM once a week for 3 weeks *Neurosyphilis (CSF) (infection confirmed):* Aqueous crystalline penicillin G 3–4 million units IV q4h for 10–14 days *Penicillin-Allergic Patients:* Doxycycline 100 mg PO bid for 2 weeks OR Tetracycline 500 mg PO qid for 2 weeks.
• *Gonorrhea*	Usually asymptomatic; partner may have an infection. Purulent yellow/green discharge May have Skene's and Bartholin's gland inflammation	Gonococcal culture, DNA probe (cervical swab)	Cefixime (Suprax) 400 mg PO × 1 OR Ceftriaxone (Rocephine) 125 mg IM in a single dose OR

Problem	Clinical Presentation	Diagnostic Reasoning	Treatment: As Recommended by CDC
			Ciprofloxacin (Cipro) 500 mg PO × 1 OR Ofloxacin (Floxin) 400 mg PO × 1 OR Levofloxacin 250 mg PO × 1 IF CHLAMYDIAL INFECTION IS NOT RULED OUT THEN ALSO Azithromycin (Zithromax) 1 g PO × 1 OR Doxycycline 100 mg PO bid for 7 days. Follow CDC guidelines for complicated or refractory gonorrhea.
• *HPV*	History of multiple partners or sexual abuse Positive history of HPV Itching, foul discharge May be asymptomatic Fleshy, soft, pale-colored keratinized growths on the vagina, cervix, vulva, or perianal area	Acetic acid test: lesions turn white with vinegar application	*Patient-Applied Treatments:* Podofilox (Condylox) 0.5% applied thinly bid for 3 days, then rest for 4 days; may repeat up to 4 cycles OR Imiguimod (Aldara cream) 5% applied 3 times a week for 16 weeks. *Clinician-Applied Treatments:* Cryotherapy and liquid nitrogen treatments—repeat every 1–2 weeks. Podophyllin resin (Podofin) 10–25% in benzoin—apply thinly, allow to dry; patient should wash off in 1–4 hours. TCA/BCA (trichloroacetic acid and bichloroacetic acid, Tri-Chlor) 80–90% applied by clinician every 4–7 days. Other therapies: laser therapy, surgery, interferon lesion injections.
• *Trichomoniasis*	Heavy, odorous, yellow-green watery discharge May have complaints of itching, swelling, and redness on the vulva	Discharge may be frothy, with occasional characteristic "strawberry cervix" pH > 5 Wet mount: motile protozoa and WBCs	Metronidazole (Flagyl) 2 g PO ×1 OR 500 mg PO bid for 7 days

(continued)

Table 13.6 **Vulvovaginal Infections and Sexually Transmitted Diseases** (continued)

Problem	Clinical Presentation	Diagnostic Reasoning	Treatment: As Recommended by CDC
• *HIV Infection*	Fever, malaise, adenopathy, rash may occur in first weeks after infection (acute retroviral syndrome) Bloody diarrhea Opportunistic infections Frequent vaginal infections Increased HPV infections	Positive enzyme immunoassay (EIA) Positive Western blot (WB)	Treat infections as recommended by CDC. Refer to specialist. Long-term counseling and management. HAART (highly active anti-retroviral therapy) is key for the treatment of HIV. Initiation of therapy is a function of T cell count, viral load, and concurrent symptoms. Treatment is heavily influenced by the ability to comply with various treatment regimens.

may range from clear to yellowish-green. Table 13.6 presents specific symptoms.

Objective

The primary lesions of some STIs may be painless and blisterlike, or the patient may have severe pain, causing depression. All lesions of an ulcerative or wartlike nature should be serologically tested for syphilis. Any ulcer may become secondarily infected and may confuse the diagnosis. Manifestation of vaginal infections may include a slightly dry and swollen vulva with small splits present. There may be chronic inflammation, with possible glandular involvement. Bartholin's, vestibular, and Skene's glands may be inflamed and painful, with reddened areas. Scarring and muscle contracture may be present.

Diagnostic Reasoning

Diagnostic Tests

Diagnostic testing for some vulvovaginal infections is not available; therefore, the diagnosis is made by exclusion. Diagnosis of vaginal infections is made by eliminating other diseases as the cause and honing in on the patient's symptoms. Frequently there will be a history of treatment for chronic yeast infections. Table 13.6 presents specific diagnostic tests.

If initial treatment is ineffective, an incorrect diagnosis may have been made initially. The vaginal exam should be repeated and any tests repeated to confirm the diagnosis. For vulvodynia, vulvar biopsy for inflammation, colposcopy for microfissures, and assessing for uneven hips caused by muscle contraction may confirm the diagnosis. Vulvodynia is not sexually transmitted or a condyloma. External events or irritants can trigger vulvodynia, so a comprehensive history should be obtained.

Differential Diagnosis

Differential diagnosis should include evaluation for chronic dermatitis, bacterial vaginosis, precancerous changes of the vulva, UTI, and vaginitis, along with assessing for any STI. The patient should be evaluated for allergies, urinary calcium oxalate, and increased sensitivity to touch, which may indicate a vaginal infection.

Management

The principle of management is to make the correct diagnosis, prescribe the correct treatment, and sufficiently educate the patient and partner so that there will not be a repeat occurrence. In response to the progressive rise in incidence of STIs, the Centers for Disease Control and Prevention (CDC, 2002) published Guidelines for Sexually Transmitted Infections, which include information on prevention, diagnosis, and treatment for all known STIs. Table 13.6 presents the specific management of vulvovaginal infections and STIs.

All of the patient's sexual contacts from the 10 days before the onset of symptoms (30 days for STIs) should be treated. A recheck of symptoms is recommended in 3 to 7 days after the start of treatment. Improvement of objective symptoms is usually evident in 3 days and physical improvement within seven days following treatment. The patient should be advised to apply warm compresses to promote healing of vulvovaginal infections. Treatment of LGV may include needle-aspirating enlarged lymph nodes to prevent rupture.

The use of the touch test is helpful for patients with vulvodynia to assess concretely the success of their treatment. To perform the touch test, the clinician lightly touches the vulvar area with a saline-moistened, cotton-tipped applicator and asks the patient to rate the pain on a scale from 0 to 5 (5 being the worst pain). A record should be kept of the pain scale and changes noted. Treatment should focus on eliminating the cause and reducing patient discomfort. Evaluate the patient for suicide risk secondary to the severe pain. Educate patient about long-term therapy and resources available, such as the Vulvar Pain Foundation.

If there is no improvement after treating vulvar lesions, the following questions should be considered: Is the patient HIV-infected? Does the patient have a coexisting infection? Was the medication taken correctly? Is the diagnosis correct? Inform the patient that scarring may occur even with adequate treatment. Incision and draining of many lesions will increase scarring and is generally not recommended.

Diagnosis with any genital ulcer can be difficult. With chancroid (*Haemophilus ducreyi*), screening for HSV and syphilis are negative. Dark-field microscopy of bubo aspirate may be positive for the chains of gram-negative bacilli. Cultures are expensive and limited in availability. Polymerase chain reaction (PCR) testing may be available soon. Preventing long-term sequelae and promoting the patient's optimum health depends on the patient's understanding and adequate treatment. Developing a trusting, compassionate relationship can make all the difference to a patient who may have a problem diagnosis.

Follow-Up and Referral

Follow-up and referral depend on the specific diagnosis, cause, and management.

Patient Education

Treatment options have improved and simplified over the last few years, and some treatments are now available OTC, which may lead to patient self-treatment that can confuse the diagnosis. Education is, therefore, most important.

Lesions of the vulva can be both painful and embarrassing for the patient. Frequently the patient may not realize that a lump or sore can be contagious as well as evidence of a more serious disease. Another problem exists in the fact that the patient may not perform genital self-exam regularly, if at all. The first line of defense is prevention and is best done through regular exams. Other preventative measures include patient education, abstinence, monogamy, use of condoms, and screening for infections. Education should include prevention of transmission and treatment of partners, along with medication use. Follow-up patient education can prevent transmission and promote adequate medication adherence for prevention of serious sequelae.

If the patient has HSV infection, long-term education, counseling, and compassion are indicated. Learning how to live with a lifelong disease is critical to decrease transmission of this STI. (See also discussion of HSV in Chapter 12.) The principal treatment for HSV focuses on the immune system, preventing outbreaks, and treating at the first sign of an eruption. Further study on herbal immune system treatments may provide additional help for a patient with HSV.

Genital warts (HPV infection) need aggressive partner follow-up to help decrease the spread of HPV. The patient should be educated to provide understanding that this infection can cause Pap smear changes and (if the patient is pregnant) that HPV can be transmitted to a newborn if the virus is active at the time of delivery but the incidence is low.

Patients with molluscum contagiosum should be cautioned that scratching and picking can spread the infection. This also increases the chance of secondary infection. Patient education focuses on treatment, including that of the partner. Follow-up in 1 month for evaluation of all lesions is indicated.

General patient teaching should include the following. The patient should use unscented, hypoallergenic care products and wear loose clothing that is made of all-natural fibers, like cotton. Basis® soap (very mild soap), daily sitz baths with baking soda, and vitamin E skin oil can decrease the pain associated with vulvovaginal lesions. Topical lidocaine/benzocaine may help mild pain. Dietary management should include a low–calcium oxalate diet, vitamins, and calcium citrate (Citracal) supplements to decrease urinary burning. Other treatments have had less success and can be disfiguring. The patient should be advised before any surgery for vulvar lesions that historically, surgery has less than a 50 percent success rate and a second opinion is advised. Patient considerations for all these diseases include cost, convenience, lifestyle, pregnancy, other disease conditions, and medication use. Follow-up and testing for HIV and diabetes should be encouraged for patients with recurrent candidiasis.

Considerations when treating pregnant women who have STIs, UTIs, and BV/candidiasis are to plan treatment to prevent adverse effects (dosage should be decreased) and partner evaluation, especially with repeated infection. For foreign bodies, patient education about toxic shock syndrome (TSS) and careful use of tampons should be included. Any infection may interfere with the patient's Pap smear, so the patient needs to know that the smear may have to be repeated. For mucopurulent cervicitis, follow-up in some practices is 3 to 4 weeks posttreatment to evaluate cervical healing. The Centers for Disease Control and Prevention (CDC) recommend treating for the identified STI; however, the tests are frequently negative and some *Chlamydia* tests are only 60 percent accurate. Patient education should discuss partner treatment, medication use, and sexual abstinence during treatment. At every visit, safer sex practices should be encouraged.

Cervical Cancer

Cervical intraepithelial neoplasia (CIN) has been explored and studied more than any other premalignant lesion of the genital tract. The accessible anatomic location of the upper vagina and cervix facilitates investigation. In addition, the development and use of colposcopy to identify sites of potential dysplasia and assist in directing biopsy have positively affected patient outcomes in the management of CIN.

Several terms have been used to describe premalignant lesions of the cervix. These changes are described on a continuum from mildly atypical with a potential to progress to invasive carcinoma.

The grades of severity are CIN I (mild dysplasia), CIN II (moderate dysplasia), and CIN III (severe dysplasia to carcinoma in situ). Alternate nomenclature, as noted, is used to describe similar histologic characteristics by using the term *dysplasia.* Hence, early premalignant changes in cervical epithelium are described as mild, moderate, or severe dysplasia. Mild involvement includes one-third of the cervical epithelium, moderate involvement includes two-thirds of the epithelium, and severe involves the full thickness of the epithelium. Carcinoma in situ is considered the most advanced premalignant change.

Epidemiology and Causes

Cervical cancer is the 14th most common cancer in women in the United States, and the most common cancer in women worldwide. With the prevalence of Pap test screening in the United States, mortality rates have fallen by more than 45 percent since the 1970s. The American Cancer Society estimates that there will be more than 10,000 new cases of invasive cervical cancer and more than 3700 women will die of the disease in 2005 alone. The incidence and mortality rate of cervical cancer in African American women (11.2 per 100,000) is higher than that in white women (7.3 per 100,000).

Precancerous dysplasia or CIN occurs more often in younger women, with the incidence peaking in the early 30s. About 12 percent of women will have cervical dysplasia by age 20. It is believed that this is caused by human papilloma virus (HPV). The prevalence of CIN is increasing and is much more common than invasive cancer.

The cause of CIN remains unknown; however, studies implicate several factors that may be related to the development of CIN. In particular, the HPV virus is believed to support the development of premalignant cervical lesions. Several different HPV types have been associated with various genital lesions. Three specific types have been associated with neoplasia (higher grades of dysplasia and cervical cancer). Condom usage is promoted based more on general principles than on epidemiologic data, and protection against HPV transmission is not 100 percent effective. HPV can be found in many genital areas (e.g., genital tract skin and mucous membranes). Hence, condoms do not protect the vulva from microscopic HPV particles on the skin. Although flat HPV cervical lesions are strongly associated with cellular transformation to CIN, most HPV infections are subclinical. Women may be unaware of their HPV status. In addition, women who have a history of early intercourse (age 14 or 15 years) begin to have children at an early age, and/or have a history of multiple sexual partners are at a greater risk for developing carcinoma of the cervix. A list of cofactors that may contribute to enhanced risk for cervical cancer is shown in Risk Factors 13.1.

RISK FACTORS 13.1

Cervical Neoplasia

History

Early intercourse
Early marriage
Multiple sex partners (more than two)
Early childbearing
Prostitution
Immunosuppression
Prior exposure to radiation
Intrauterine DES exposure
OC use
Cigarette smoking
Vitamin A, B, C, and folic acid deficiencies

Male Partner

History of genital cancer, especially penile carcinoma; STIs, especially penile or urethral condylomas; CIN or cervical cancer in a previous partner; low socioeconomic status; multiple sex partners

Infections

STIs (venereal infection)
HPV infection (serotypes 16 and 18)
HSV infection
HIV infection
Chlamydia trachomatis
CMV infection

Pathophysiology

A normal transformation zone includes columnar epithelium and squamous metaplasia. The squamocolumnar junction (SCJ) of the cervix is viewed via the colposcope, which magnifies the epithelium of the transformation zone. Colposcopic examination of this landmark site is important because this area is most vulnerable to neoplastic changes.

Examination of the exocervix reveals where the cervical glandular, grape-like in appearance, columnar epithelium meets the native squamous epithelium distal to the external os in young adult women. After childbirth this area may enlarge and move farther away from the os. The junction usually recedes after menopause into the endocervical canal. Throughout a woman's reproductive life, squamous metaplasia, a physiologic process involving squamous tissue replacing columnar tissue, occurs. This process is most active during fetal development, adolescence, and pregnancy. The SCJ is first delineated *in utero*; however, metaplasia is an estrogen-dependent process that accelerates during puberty and pregnancy. As noted, SCJ cells are more vulnerable and especially prone to damage at these particular times in a woman's reproductive life. Abnormal colposcopic patterns that characterize an abnormal transformation zone are caused by neoplastic squamous epithelium, thus explaining why exophytic tumors are the most common presentation of cervical cancer.

HPV infection may also alter morphology of the cervical epithelium, leading to nuclear enlargement and multinucleation, hyperchromasia, and perinuclear cytoplasmic halos. Cellular findings of HPV infection on biopsy can be histologically similar to dysplasia, and misdiagnosis can occur. However, the diagnosis of HPV does not imply clinical disease. Thus, treatment is limited only to symptomatic patients (e.g., those with condylomata) or those with demonstrated evidence of neoplasia (e.g., positive colposcopy findings). Two anti-HPV vaccines against serotypes HPV-16 and -18 are currently in development and have been shown to reduce infection incidence, but these have yet to be licensed for widespread use.

In some worldwide studies, the epitheliotropic HPV infection has been identified in greater than 99 percent of cervical neoplasias. Certain viral serotypes that undergo vegetative episomal replication without integrating into the host genome typically lead to condylomata acuminata or LSIL (e.g., HPV-6, -11), while more oncogenic forms of the virus (HPV-18, -16, -58, -52, and -31) which integrate into host DNA are more likely to contribute to malignant transformation—HSIL, invasive squamous cell carcinoma, or adenocarcinoma. The HPV E6 protein degrades the cell cycle inhibitory protein p53, while the HPV E7 protein interacts with the retinoblastoma protein Rb, causing dissociation of E2F which also leads to dysregulated cell cycle progression. E7 protein also leads to upregulation of interleukin (IL)-6 and IL-8, both of which contribute to cervical cancer progression. Importantly, HPV serotypes HPV-16 and -18 are most strongly correlated with invasive squamous cell carcinoma, with HPV-18 portending a worse prognosis. It is clear, however, that HPV infection alone is insufficient to lead to cervical neoplasia, and further insult by cigarette smoking, immunosuppression, or other risk factors appears necessary.

While squamous cell carcinoma comprises 80 percent of all cervical cancers, at least 15 percent are attributed to adenocarcinomas, with another 3 to 5 percent being of a mixed adenosquamous phenotype. The incidence of adenocarcinoma of the cervix has steadily increased in women younger than 35 years since the 1970s, but this may be due to improved screening and early treatment of squamous cell disease. In addition, however, a greater association of adenocarcinoma with oral contraceptive use seems to imply the importance of underlying hormonal mechanisms in its pathogenesis. Far rarer forms include neuroendocrine tumors, small cell carcinomas, or rhabdomyosarcomas.

Clinical Presentation

Subjective

Patients with premalignant cervical lesions may present with one or more of the following: a history of one or more epidemiologic risk factors associated with the development of cervical cancer; a concurrent vaginal infection with symptoms; a history of no recent gynecologic care; and no Pap smear for a long time.

In contrast, women with invasive carcinoma may describe a brownish discharge or a history of abnormal vaginal bleeding occurring spontaneously or after intercourse. Women with a history of postcoital bleeding or irregular vaginal bleeding that cannot be explained should be referred to a gynecologist for further evaluation. Only with an extensive disease spread would other symptoms be manifested (e.g., weight loss, decreased appetite, and back pain).

Objective

Women with abnormal Pap smears are usually asymptomatic with normal cervical, vaginal, and abdominal findings on physical exam. Even if Pap smear findings are normal, any cervical or vaginal lesion that appears abnormal or is friable, raised, or has the appearance of condyloma requires a referral for colposcopy. The location of the dysplasia directs the treatment.

The Pap smear report should include a statement on the adequacy of the specimen for examination, a general categorization, and the descriptive diagnosis.

Pap smear results are described as:

- ▲ Satisfactory but limited (less than optimal; may be secondary to partially obscuring inflammation)
- ▲ Unsatisfactory (not acceptable for diagnostic evaluation and may require a repeat Pap or follow-up)
- ▲ Within normal limits
- ▲ Other (may require follow-up care; the report will have an additional notation if further action is required).

Protocol for triage of the patient with abnormal cytology is presented in Advanced Practice Nursing Intervention 13.1.

Diagnostic Reasoning

Diagnostic Tests

The American Cancer Society's (ACS) Pap smear screening guidelines are supported by the American Medical Association, National Cancer Institute, American Nurses Association, American College of Obstetricians and Gynecologists (ACOG), and the American Academy of Family Physicians. An issue that is the subject of ongoing debate concerns the mandated frequency for performing Pap smears. The ACS recommends screening begin 3 years after the first vaginal intercourse or at age 21 years, whichever comes first. They also recommend that women older the age of 30 be screened at longer intervals after three consecutive annual normal/negative Pap smear results, unless the woman has a history of DES exposure in utero, is HIV-positive, or is immunocompromised (organ transplant, chemotherapy, corticosteroid therapy). The ACS also recommends that screening be discontinued in women older than the age of 70 if they have had not abnormal Pap smears in the previous 10 years. If women have had a hysterectomy with removal of the

ADVANCED PRACTICE NURSING INTERVENTIONS 13.1

Pap Smear Results: Treatment Protocols

Pap Smear Results	The Bethesda System (TBS) Category	Treatment Protocol
Sufficient number of cells were present to determine normalcy: within normal limits	Within normal limits	Repeat Pap test annually
Sample was not prepared correctly or too few cells to be evaluated: inadequate	Less than optimal Unsatisfactory	Repeat Pap test in about 8 weeks
Benign cellular change; may be caused by infectious agent such as *Trichomonas*, fungal organisms, *Gardnerella and Chlamydia* or HSV	Infection	Treat infections that present as symptoms or identified with Pap smear results, or do confirmatory study Repeat Pap test after infection in 3–6 months; repeat annually if results are normal
Benign cellular change secondary to inflammatory process and repair by body of injured tissue; may be caused by mechanical or chemical irritations (inflammation, atrophy, IUD use), trauma, or bacterial or viral infections	Reactive/reparative	For inflammatory changes of unknown cause, repeat Pap test in 6–12 weeks For repeated inflammatory changes on Pap test, refer to possible colposcopic examination For *Chlamydia* or gonorrhea, treat as recommended and repeat Pap test in 1 year For postmenopausal women with atrophic vaginitis and Pap test result of ASCUS or low-grade squamous intraepithelial lesion (LSIL), treat with topical estrogen cream for 4–6 weeks, then repeat Pap test
Cellular changes from HPV or mild to moderate dysplasia	Squamous epithelial cell abnormalities: atypical squamous cells of undetermined significance (ASCUS) Squamous intraepithelial lesion: LSIL or high-grade squamous intraepithelial lesion (HSIL)	Refer for colposcopic examination
Cellular changes from high-grade or squamous cell carcinoma	Squamous cell carcinoma Adenocarcinoma	Refer to gynecologist
Glandular Cell findings–atypical glandular cells (AGC); considered less severe than adenocarcinoma but associated with a greater risk for cancer	AGC	Refer to gynecologist
Atypical gladular cells from endocervical, endometrial or glandular not otherwise specified in origin (AGC-NOS); considered at lower risk for neoplasm than AGC women	AGC-NOS	Refer to gynecologist
Atypical glandular cells–favor neoplasm(AGC, favor neoplasm); high risk for high grade CIN	AGC–Favor neoplasia	Refer to gynecologist
Endocervical adenocacinoma in situ (AIS); high risk for invasive cervical adenocarcinoma	AIS	Refer to gynecologist

cervix, they do not need to be screened if the reason for the surgery was for a condition other than cancer or precancer.

It is important that the cytology laboratory comply with state and national regulations, utilizes a sufficient number of reputable cytologists, maintains a quality assurance program, and supports open, clear communication between health-care professionals and the lab. Historically, several reporting systems have been developed to enhance communication between the cytopathologist and the clinician performing the Pap test. The oldest system was the class system that provided limited information and did not reflect the newer risk factors such as HPV infections.

The Bethesda System (TBS) currently uses only two terms to describe the wide spectrum of squamous cell precursors: *low-grade squamous intraepithelial lesion* (LSIL) and *high-grade squamous intraepithelial lesion* (HSIL). TBS has also established a category called *atypical squamous cells* (ASC) and this is further qualified into two categories: *atypical squamous cells of undetermined significance* (ASC-US) and *atypical squamous cells; cannot exclude high-grade SIL* (ASC-H). TBS has also developed classification for *atypical glandular cells* (AGC) which may be of endocervical, endometrial, or glandular cells. There is *atypical glandular cells not otherwise specified* in origin (AGC-NOS) and these women are at lower risk for neoplasia than women with AGC. Of greater concern, the PAP show AGC, Favor Neoplasia. More worrisome is endocervical adenocarcinoma in situ (AIS) or true adenocarcinoma. These glandular findings are associated with a high rate of premalignancy or true neoplasia and thus these women should be referred for colposcopy; women older than 35 years of age and those with significant anovulatory unexplained bleeding should also get endometrial biopsy. If all cells are endometrial in origin only, colposcopy may be avoided in favor of initial endometrial biopsy.

LSIL is a combination of cytologic changes consistent with HPV without evidence of dysplasia and changes consistent with mild dysplasia (CIN I). ASC-US is delimited to epithelial abnormalities of uncertain significance and usually represents about 5 percent of the smears in most populations screened. When cells are described as atypical further evaluation is necessary. (Table 13.7 presents a comparison of cytopathology reporting systems.)

Obtaining endocervical cells becomes more difficult as the patient ages and the squamous columnar junction (SCJ) migrates inwardly with age. An optimal smear contains squamous cells, endocervical cells, and potentially metaplastic cells. Absence of endocervical cells may indicate an inadequate sample and needs to be repeated. Table 13.8 presents factors affecting Pap smear results.

Use of a cytobrush enhances the capture of endocervical cells. The brush or swab should be rotated 180 to 360 degrees. Light scraping of the cervix with a spatula follows. Samples may be placed on the same slide or on two slides according to the requirements of the cytopathologist. The specimen is preserved by spraying the slide with a cytology fixative. Spray directly with moderate pressure, making sure that spraying too close to the slide does not disturb the cells. See Therapeutic Procedures 13.1 for the technique of obtaining a routine Pap smear. Newer technologies for Pap smears such as liquid-based cytology and computerized rescreening have not been validated through prospective randomized studies yet, but liquid-prep system (ThinPrep or SurePath) appear acceptable, according to several expert organizations. The use of HPV screening has not yet been demonstrated as a primary screening for cervical cancer, however, despite the clear association between HPV and cervical cancer.

Cervical cytology is helpful only for screening. Pap smear results are not considered a definitive diagnosis, and

Table 13.7 Comparison of Cytology Reporting Systems for Pap Smears

Class System	World Health Organization (WHO) System	Cervical Intraepithelial Neoplasia (CIN) System	The Bethesda System (TBS)
I	Normal	Normal	Within normal limits
II	Inflammation	Normal	Other: Infection, reactive and reparative
III	Dysplasia		Squamous epithelial cell abnormalities Atypical squamous cells of undetermined significance
	Mild	CIN-1	Squamous intraepithelial lesion Low grade (includes cellular changes associated with HPV)
	Moderate	CIN-2	High grade
	Severe		High grade
IV	Carcinoma in situ	CIN-3	High grade
V	Invasive squamous cell carcinoma	Invasive squamous cell carcinoma	Squamous cell carcinoma
	Adenocarcinoma	Adenocarcinoma	Adenocarcinoma Nonepithelial malignant neoplasma

Table 13.8 Factors Affecting Pap Smear Results

Patient History
Previous treatment and/or surgery of reproductive tract
Previous abnormal Pap test
Diethylstilbestrol (DES) exposure in utero
Current or recent vaginal or cervical infection and PID
Any medications, especially hormones
Bleeding abnormalities
History of any malignancy
Pregnancy suspected or current
Partner history of genital or urological problems (e.g., discharge, infection, or bumps on penis or scrotum)
Patient Factors
Intercourse
Douching
Birth control methods
Menses
Infection
Accurate history
False-Negatives
Rate for properly performed cytology smears is 1–80%
Rate of sample error (diagnostic cells not on the slide) is 60%; 40% for screening error (cells present on slide but missed by cytotechnologist)
False or less than optimal reports are caused by clinician, patient, or cytopathologist factors
False-Positives
Rate is <1%.

false-negative and false-positive results may occur. The only definitive way to diagnose cervical abnormalities is to perform a colposcopic examination and biopsy of the abnormal area. Additional indications for colposcopy include cervical abnormalities such as dysplasia, squamous cell carcinoma, adenocarcinoma, visible cervical abnormality, HPV on external genitalia or cervix, and persistent inflammation even in the presence of a normal Pap smear. A colposcopic examination may be indicated because of the potentially high false-negative rate of Pap smear results. Diagnosis and treatment options are directed toward preserving fertility in women of childbearing age, detecting early lesions, and preventing cervical cancer.

In colposcopic evaluation, a colposcope that magnifies the cervix 6- to 40-fold is used to visualize the cervix. Vascular changes are noted because of the high-intensity illumination and use of a green filter. Application of acetic acid to the SCJ (transformation [T] zone) accentuates the difference between squamous epithelium and columnar epithelium. The latter epithelium turns white, permitting identification of the SCJ, visualization of the contrasting pink-colored squamous epithelium, and any abnormal tissue in the T zone that also turns white. Areas of punctuations, mosaicism, and atypical vessels are identified and biopsies are performed on these.

THERAPEUTIC PROCEDURE 13.1

Technique for Obtaining a Routine Pap Smear

1. Complete the cytology request form with all pertinent data.
2. Label the slide.
3. Insert the dry or water-lubricated speculum. Direct the speculum in a downward posterior direction.
4. Expose the cervix.
   - Avoid sampling if a vaginal infection is present.
   - Take the Pap smear sample before any other cervical sample.
5. Insert the cytobrush or cotton-tipped applicator in cervical os.
6. Use a vigorous rotary endocervical technique (clockwise fashion).
7. Use a paintbrush motion to place the sample on the glass slide.
8. Scrape the external os area with the cytology spatula.
9. Note the individual topography of squamocolumnar juncture.
10. Obtain a vaginal specimen if needed (e.g., DES exposure, hormone evaluation, history of hysterectomy).
11. Smear the slide and fix immediately.

Technique for Obtaining a Liquid-Based Cervical Cell Collection

1. Complete the cytology request form with all pertinent data.
2. Label the container.
3. Insert the dry or water-lubricated speculum. Direct the speculum in a downward posterior direction.
4. Expose the cervix.
5. Insert cervical broom with central portion into the cervical os.
6. Rotate $^{1}/_{4}$ turn only
7. Place broom in fixative container and vigorously move about to dispel all particles into solution.

An endocervical specimen is obtained by endocervical curettage. Lugol's iodine solution may be applied to the cervix when no lesion is noted. The iodine solution stains cells with a high glycogen content (mature squamous epithelium) a deep mahogany brown. Abnormal cells (atrophic squamous epithelium, undifferentiated metaplastic epithelium, dysplastic epithelium) and columnar cells remain unchanged and do not appear dark in color. Lesions extending into the canal are visualized by use of an endocervical speculum. The entire SCJ and T zone must be visualized. A colposcopy is considered satisfactory only when this entire area is viewed.

Definitive diagnosis of cervical cancer is done by cervical biopsy and endocervical curettage or conization to determine the extent and depth of invasion of the cancer. After diagnosis, cervical cancer is then "staged" or the estimate of gross spread of the cancer. Cervical cancer is clinically staged, although surgical staging may be used for treatment planning if indicated. The International Federation of Gynecologists and Obstetricians (FIGO) system is based on clinical evaluation only and is used for disease beyond CIN. Stage 0 is carcinoma in situ. Stage I is cancer confined to the uterus and is graded according to depth of stromal invasion. Stage II disease goes beyond the uterus but not as far as the pelvic wall or the lower third of the vagina; it is progressively graded based on parametrial invasion. Stage III extends to the lower third of the vagina (IIIA) or pelvic wall (IIIB). Stage IV extends beyond the pelvis or to the bladder or rectum (IVA), stage IVB of which involves distant metastases. There is also a corresponding TNM system, but the FIGO system is used most often. Disease staging is the most important prognostic factor, followed by number of positive lymph nodes.

Differential Diagnosis

Some conditions, mostly infections, may lead to PAP results that mimic dysplasia (CIN). In addition, benign growths may be mistaken for cancers, such as Nabothian cysts, glandular hyperplasia or reactive changes, and endometriosis. As previously noted, TBS lists on the Pap smear report a statement of adequacy, a general categorization, and a descriptive diagnosis. If the specimen is not adequate for testing or the results are not normal, a descriptive diagnosis is included.

Management

The principle of management is to detect cervical dysplasia in the early stages and prevent cervical cancer and its spread.

Initially, a colposcopy is performed first as previously described as a follow-up to an abnormal Pap test. Not all clinicians are trained in this procedure, so the patient may need referral to a gynecologist.

There are four treatment modalities that a specialist may perform for CIN. These include cryosurgery, loop electrosurgical excision procedure (LEEP), laser therapy, and cone biopsy. Cryosurgery involves directing a probe onto the cervical os and destroying the lesion by freezing the tissue. There is usually a 90 percent cure rate. The patient should be advised that a vaginal discharge will occur for 2 to 3 weeks after the cryosurgery. LEEP is a similar technique that uses a thin hot wire to incise and destroy diseased tissue. Although this has a 95 percent cure rate, it should be used only when the lesion is definitively diagnosed as CIN. Postoperative bleeding may occur with this treatment. Laser treatments effectively destroy diseased tissue with milder adverse effects than the aforementioned two therapies. A cone biopsy removes a portion of the tissue by either LEEP or laser therapy and is usually reserved for higher-grade lesions.

Early stage squamous cell carcinoma (or adenocarcinoma) disease up to stage IIA is treated with radical hysterectomy and para-aortic lymph node dissection or radiotherapy (external beam or brachytherapy) with chemotherapy. If the patient is at intermediate or high risk for recurrence (large tumor size, deep stromal invasion, lymphovascular invasion, close or positive resection margins, positive lymph nodes, or microscopic parametrial involvement), she will need postoperative radiation and a platinum-based chemotherapy. Neoadjuvant (preoperative) chemotherapy may also be used for bulky disease before surgical resection. Disease beyond IIA is treated with primary radiation therapy plus cisplatin-based chemotherapy. Most recurrences happen within 2 years. Local recurrence in women previously treated with radiation may be treated surgically; otherwise, if radiation has not previously been used, this is now a viable option. Radiation treatment is also sometimes palliative for severe pain or bleeding from advanced disease. Metastatic disease may be treated with palliative chemotherapy, either single-agent or combination therapy. Microinvasive adenocarcinoma is usually treated with simple hysterectomy, while invasive adenocarcinoma (or adenosquamous disease) is treated in the same manner as squamous cell carcinoma.

Follow-Up and Referral

Management of abnormal Pap smear results continues to be a controversial topic. The patient should be referred to a gynecologist who specializes in the treatment of cervical cancer and is one whom the patient feels she can trust. Posttreatment surveillance is every 3 months for 2 years, then every 4 months for a year, followed by every 6 months for the next 2 years. After this time (5 years) the patient is followed annually. Patients with significant physical or historical findings with recurrence then undergo imaging studies.

Patient Education

The importance of regular screening Pap tests must be stressed, as the identification and treatment of cervical dysplasia is critical in the prevention of cervical cancer. Early treatment can cure cervical dysplasia and prevent cervical cancer. Risk of cervical dysplasia can be decreased if the onset of sexual activity is delayed, number of sexual partners decreased, condoms are used consistently, and tobacco use eliminated. Patients should be knowledgeable about STIs, their prevention, and treatment.

Ovarian Cancer

Tumors of the ovary are quite common and most are benign. But malignant ovarian tumors are the leading cause of reproductive system death. *Ovarian cancer* has three main classifications; surface epithelial–stromal tumors, sex cord–stromal tumors, and germ cell tumors. The classifications are based on ovarian embryology and the differences in tissue origin.

Epidemiology and Causes

The cause of ovarian cancer is unknown. The risk factors for developing ovarian cancer include advancing age (more than half are older than 65 years of age); family history of a grandmother, mother or sister with ovarian, breast, or colon cancer; father or brother with colon cancer (5 to 10 percent are familial); nulliparity, early menarche, and late menopause ("incessant ovulation" increases possibility of ovarian epithelial damage and inactivation of tumor suppressor genes); lifestyle (high-fat diet, smoking history, lack of exercise); and a history of prolonged use of fertility drugs.

Ovarian cancer is quantitatively the rarest but most deadly of the gynecologic cancers. In the United States, more than 25,000 cases of ovarian cancer are diagnosed annually, with approximately 14,500 deaths. It is the seventh most common woman's cancer in the world, with the greatest incidence in industrialized countries. It is most commonly diagnosed in white women with a northern European background and a strong family history. This familial predisposition may be strictly genetic or multifactorial, including environmental causes. The highest incidence occurs in the postmenopausal years, with a gradually rising incidence after age 45 years. Ovarian cancers have been associated with the number of ovulations in a woman's lifetime; therefore, nulliparity increases the number of ovulations and thereby the risk of a cell mutation occurring. Likewise, infertility drugs, which are known to hyperstimulate the ovaries, increase the chances of cancerous mutation.

Although the public is aware that early detection is crucial for cancer in general, no mass screening test has proved effective enough to be recommended at this time. For women who have risk factors for ovarian cancer, however, a pelvic examination, a cancer antigen 125 (CA 125) assay test, and a transvaginal pelvic ultrasound can be used at yearly intervals to increase the chance of early detection.

Pathophysiology

There are several distinct types of ovarian malignancies: epithelial cell, germ cell, and sex-cord stromal cell. By far the most common and life threatening are the malignancies of epithelial origin (80 to 90 percent of ovarian tumors), which are derived from the epithelial layer of cells covering the surface of the ovary, continuous with the peritoneal mesothelium. These in turn are divided into several types, including papillary serous cystadenocarcinoma which resemble the cells lining the fallopian tubes (75 percent), mucinous cystadenocarcinoma which simulate the endocervical epithelium (10 percent), endometrioid tumors (10 percent) which are similar to endometrial cancers, as well as the much rarer clear cell, Brenner transitional cell, undifferentiated, and mixed cell-type tumors. Germ cell tumors comprise 20 to 25 percent of ovarian tumors, with fewer than 5 percent of these being malignant. Dysgerminomas are most common (30 to 50 percent), followed by yolk sac (endodermal sinus) tumors and immature/mature teratomas—each of which accounts for approximately 20 percent of germ cell tumors. Much rarer forms of germ cell tumors include embryonal carcinoma, polyembryoma, choriocarcinoma, and carcinoid tumors.

Stromal cell tumors are less common, comprising only 5 to 8 percent of primary ovarian neoplasms. Neoplasms of stromal cells originate from the cells of the supporting structure of the ovary. These can be divided into gonadal support structures, which are the cells that support the ova or egg and nongonadal stromal cells that are the nonspecialized support structures of the ovary. The gonadal cells are further divided into two specialized subgroups called the granulosa-theca and the Sertoli-Leydig cells. Granulosa-theca cells surround the site on the ovary where the ovum is released and produce the female hormones. The second subgroup, the Sertoli-Leydig cells, is responsible for producing the male hormones. The nongonadal stromal cell tumors are derived from the smooth muscle and ligaments that give the ovary its basic structure and form.

Various germline mutations have been associated with epithelial ovarian tumors, such as *BRCA1, BRCA2,* and the hereditary nonpolyposis colorectal cancer gene, but only in a small minority of cases with serous ovarian adenocarcinomas predominating. These cancers, which appear to run in families, have an earlier age at onset than those in the general population. Mutations in well-characterized oncogenes including *HER-2/neu,* c-*myc, Akt,* and the tumor suppressor genes *p53, p16,* and *PTEN* have also been cited in noninherited forms of ovarian cancer. However, the precise pathogenetic mechanisms implicating these mutations as well as most ovarian cancer risk factors have yet to be determined.

A likely mechanism appears to be the increased frequency of genetic mutations associated with repeated injury and repair to the ovarian epithelium that occurs with cycled ovulation, thus explaining the correlation of ovarian cancer with nulliparity and early menses and the protective effect of OCs that suppress ovulation. Hormonal stimulation of ovarian tissue by high estrogen and possibly also androgen levels has also been cited as a factor in malignant transformation, while progesterone has been shown to have protective effects. Interestingly, some case-controlled studies have demonstrated a connection between ovarian carcinogenesis and environmental agents believed to enter through the genitourinary tract that travel retrograde to the ovaries (e.g., perineal talc).

Clinical Presentation

Subjective

Symptoms can be vague or nonexistent in the early stages of the disease or seemingly unrelated to the ovaries. Such early symptoms include back pain, bloating, and constipation. As the tumor enlarges and the disease progresses, commonly expressed symptoms include a sense of pelvic pressure or discomfort; urinary frequency, pressure, and urgency; abdominal swelling and bloating; nausea and vomiting; gas and indigestion; rectal pressure; painful intercourse; diarrhea or constipation; abnormal vaginal bleeding; unexplained weight loss; and jaundice.

Objective

During the pelvic examination, a pelvic mass, decreased mobility of the cervix and uterus, fullness in the adnexal areas of cul-de-sac, and pain on palpation of the ovaries may be detected. A rectal exam may confirm a pelvic mass as well.

Diagnostic Reasoning

Diagnostic Tests

A comprehensive diagnostic workup begins with a complete history and must include questions and discussions regarding the woman's current complaints, past health experiences, obstetrical history, family history, and dietary habits. Further information that could be useful would be bowel and bladder habits and menstrual history.

If an ovarian neoplasm is suspected, a bimanual pelvic examination is the first step in the diagnostic workup. Malignant ovarian tumors are usually large with irregular contour and decreased mobility, unlike benign tumors and cysts, which usually have smooth borders, are relatively small (less than 5 cm), and are mobile.

When a mass is palpated and suspicious of malignancy, subsequent diagnostic testing should include a pelvic ultrasound to evaluate the size, shape, and consistency of the mass. A serum CA 125 level is done. If the CA 125 is greater than 35 units, there is a greater likelihood that the ovarian mass is malignant, but the level may also be elevated in postmenopausal women with benign disease (i.e., endometriosis). CA 125, however, is most helpful for following the response to therapy and to help determine prognosis, but is not an effective screening tool. A transvaginal ultrasound (TVS) can help differentiate malignant ovarian masses from those that are benign. An intravenous pyelogram (IVP) shows if the mass is impinging on the ureters or bladder. A barium enema determines involvement of the rectum or colon. In some cases a diagnostic laparoscopy can be used for direct visualization of the mass. Abdominal/pelvic CT and MRI are not useful to establish the diagnosis for pelvic masses, but these imaging tests are helpful in establishing the presence or degree of metastases from ovarian cancer of determining whether a primary cancer site exists outside the ovaries.

As part of a preoperative evaluation to further rule out other nonovarian primary cancer sites, a colonoscopy or barium enema should be done if the Hemoccult is positive or if the patient is obstructed. An upper GI series is done if an upper GI site is suspected, bilateral mammography if any breast mass is present, and endometrial biopsy with curettage if uterine bleeding is present.

Differential Diagnosis

Differential diagnoses include ovarian cysts, benign tumors, ectopic pregnancy, hydrosalpinx, GI masses, pelvic kidney, endometriosis, tuboovarian abscess or adhesions, and intrauterine pregnancy. Other differentials include metastases to the ovaries from other primary sites, such as breast, uterus, or GI tract.

Management

The principle of management is early diagnosis and referral for treatment (surgery and oncological). Ovarian cancer is surgically staged, and the staging determines the specific treatment approach. Staging is done using the FIGO staging and this guides treatment. Stage I is confined to the ovaries. In stage II, there is extension to pelvis, and stage III indicates spread beyond pelvis to peritoneal cavity or para-aortic/inguinal lymph nodes (but within abdomen). Stage IV is distant metastasis. Seventy-five percent of women with epithelial disease present in stages III to IV, while 25 percent present in stage I and II. The 5-year survival rate for stage I ovarian cancer is 90 percent, but only 25 percent are diagnosed at this early stage. The 5-year survival rate declines rapidly as the stage increases. For example, 5-year survival for stage II is 40 percent to 60 percent, stage III is 15 to 20 percent, and 5-year survival for stage IV is less than 5 percent.

Unlike other cancers, surgical resection for optimal cytoreduction is standard of care for both early and advanced ovarian cancer. Therapy is based on appropriate surgical staging, unless there are clear contraindications to surgery. Surgery improves disease-related symptoms, improves response to chemotherapy (if cytoreduction leaves tumor of less than 2 cm in the widest dimension), and decreases tumor-produced immunosuppressive cytokines. Surgical staging is done via laparotomy, checking for fluid in the cul-de-sac, as well as exploring the entire abdomen for disease. The para-aortic and pelvic lymph nodes are dissected as well, to look for microscopic extension into the nodes (stage III disease), which can occur in up to a third of cases which initially appear to be stage I.

Surgical removal usually includes hysterectomy and bilateral oophorectomy (since there is a large risk of contralateral disease) with appendectomy (which may be a site of isolated metastasis), and then additional resection of pelvic/abdominal structures as needed (especially the omentum). In very early stage disease, unilateral oophorectomy may be performed only if future fertility is desired, but endometrial biopsy should be done.

Following surgical treatment, the patient is usually given a course of chemotherapy, with or without radiation. The amount and type of chemotherapy is based on the surgical finding and staging and subsequent pathologic diagnosis and grading. Carboplatin plus paclitaxel is the standard of care for stage III to IV epithelial cancers. This same chemotherapy regimen may also be used for stage I to II epithelial cancers after surgery. It may suffice to just observe low-grade stage I disease after surgical resection, rather than treat with chemotherapy, as long as higher grade 2 or 3 disease is not noted. Chemotherapy is started 4 to 6 weeks after surgery and continues for three to six cycles, depending on extent of disease and response to therapy (follow with physical exam/history, CA 125, imaging via CT scan, etc.). Most patients respond with first-line chemotherapy, but if recurrence occurs, chemotherapy may be used for palliative care. Patients with bulky residual disease survive a median of 26 months, while for those with small-volume residual disease, median survival is 60 months. Both maintenance chemotherapy (longer regimens of single or combination chemotherapeutic agents), as well as intraperitoneal (IP) chemotherapy are NOT current standards of care and are under investigation. IP chemotherapy has the advantage of direct contact with cancer cells, less systemic adverse effects, and less collateral damage to nonmalignant tissue. At present for stage III and IV disease, surgery followed by systemic chemotherapy is indicated, but a trial is currently ongoing to evaluate neoadjuvant (preoperative) chemotherapy before surgery. Currently, it is used for patients with poor performance status who would not tolerate surgery before treatment. Secondary cytoreduction after initial surgery and first-line systemic chemotherapy might be beneficial, however.

Follow-Up and Referral

When an adnexal mass is detected, the patient should be referred to a surgeon for prompt treatment. Patients who have been diagnosed with ovarian cancer and have undergone surgical and chemical treatment often are encouraged to have a second-look surgical procedure to assess the results of the prior treatments, both surgical and medical.

Patient Education

As mentioned before, the number of ovulations in a patient's lifetime increases the risk of ovarian cancer; therefore, both pregnancy and use of OCs lower the risk of ovarian cancer. Patients should be aware of screening techniques, especially if they have any risk factors. Annual gynecologic exams should be encouraged and the importance of a low-fat diet and weight control should be stressed.

Endometrial Cancer

Endometrial cancer arises from the lining of the uterus, known as the endometrium. The majority are pure adenocarcinomas. Endometrial cancer accounts for at least 20 percent of cases of postmenopausal uterine bleeding.

Epidemiology and Causes

Cancer of the endometrium is the most common (50 percent) of all gynecologic cancers. There are approximately 36,000 cases of endometrial cancer per year, with 6000 annual deaths in the United States. The overall 5-year survival rate is 80 to 85 percent, but is as high as 98 percent if the cancer is detected early and the depth of invasion is less than 66 percent. The 5-year survival drops to 78 percent if the depth of invasion is more than 66 percent. The average age at diagnosis is 60 years, and about 25 percent of all cases occur before menopause. African American women are at greater risk for most forms of endometrial cancer, and their stage-for-stage survival rates are also worse compared to those for Caucasian women. OC pills have shown to have a protective mechanism against ovarian and endometrial cancer. Patients who use OCs have half the risk of developing these cancers. Women who use OCs for at least a year have this protective effect, which remains even after the OCs are discontinued. Risk factors for endometrial cancer include unopposed estrogen, early menarche, advancing age, a high-fat diet, nulliparity, obesity, hypertension, and diabetes mellitus. Routine screening is neither cost-effective nor warranted, except in extremely high-risk women (40 to 60 percent risk) with certain familial malignancy syndromes such as Lynch syndrome II (i.e., endometrial, ovarian, and colorectal cancers) who are at risk for hereditary nonpolyposis colorectal cancer (HNPCC). However, endometrial cancer screening has rarely been shown to be justified in asymptomatic women, even those on unopposed estrogen hormone replacement or the estrogen agonist tamoxifen.

Pathophysiology

The precursor of endometrial cancer is a hyperplastic state that may progress to invasive carcinoma. Endometrial hyperplasia of glandular tissue occurs when estrogen does not have progesterone as a counterbalance, resulting in a greater gland-to-stroma ratio. The mitogenic effect of estrogen on endometrial tissue appears to result from upregulation of the cell cycle protein cyclin D, as well as various protooncogenes, cellular growth factors and their receptors. These findings are also consistent with the protective effects of progestin-containing OCs or continuous progestin therapies. An unopposed estrogenic state may occur from multiple etiologies, including chronic anovulation such as in polycystic ovarian syndrome (PCOS), an estrogen-secreting ovarian tumor, obesity which causes increased aromatization of androstenedione to estrone and testosterone to estradiol in peripheral adipose tissue with decreased levels of sex hormone binding globulin, or iatrogenic estrogen exposure from older HRT regimens of estrogen monotherapy (10-fold increase in risk) or the selective estrogen receptor modifier (SERM) tamoxifen (2- to 3-fold increase in risk), which is used as adjuvant therapy for breast cancer. The potential for cytologic atypia similarly increases with chronic unopposed estrogenic stimulation, creating a persistent proliferative phase within the endometrium, rather than the normal cycling of proliferative and progesterone-induced secretory phases.

This premalignant condition is characterized by either a simple (i.e., cystic dilation of the glands with occasional outpouching) or complex (more abundant and adjacent glands with outpouching and minimal stroma) architectural pattern of the endometrium, as well as the presence or absence of nuclear atypia and glandular mitoses. Simple hyperplasia without atypia is unlikely to develop into endometrial carcinoma (1 percent of cases), while complex architecture with atypia is most likely to progress to malignancy (30 percent of cases). Atypia is the key negative prognostic factor, as 25 percent of women with atypia on biopsy have coexistent malignancy on further evaluation. In fact, some pathologists group complex architecture with atypia together with differentiated adenocarcinoma under the common heading of endometrioid neoplasia. Indeed, 75 to 80 percent of all endometrial cancers are estrogen-dependent endometrioid carcinomas (type I).

However, not all endometrial malignancy arises from hyperplastic tissue. For example, papillary serous endometrial tumors (5 to 10 percent of cases) arise from atrophic rather than hyperplastic tissue and, as with clear cell (1 to 5 percent of cases), mucinous and squamous cell (fewer than 2 percent of cases) endometrial cancers, are estrogen independent (type II). These rarer forms of endometrial cancer tend to be more poorly differentiated (higher nuclear grade) than type I cancers, are highly aggressive with lymphatic invasion, and portend a worse prognosis. Uterine sarcoma is a rare form of cancer (5 percent of uterine malignancies) which may be completely nonepithelial in origin or of a mixed epithelial–nonepithelial phenotype. Most commonly arising from the uterine myometrium (e.g., mixed Müllerian carcinosarcomas of fibrous, vascular, or lymphatic tissue; leiomyosarcoma), uterine sarcoma may also arise from the endometrium and invade the myometrium (e.g., endometrial stromal sarcoma). These cancers are more aggressive than more common hyperplastic endometrial forms, are prone to metastasis to the retroperitoneal and intra-abdominal nodes and hematogenously to the lungs, and carry a poorer prognosis (e.g., 50 percent 5-year survival for stage I disease versus 90 percent for more common forms of endometrial cancer). They are more common in African American women (except the endometrial stromal form), in women aged 40 to 60 years, and there appears to be a correlation with prior pelvic irradiation and, possibly, tamoxifen use.

Endometrial cancers may be mediated by mutations in a host of genes, such as the *p53* tumor suppressor gene which is a late mutation in 20 percent of endometrioid carcinomas, an early mutation in 90 percent of serous adenocarcinomas, but rarely mutated in endometrial hyperplasia. Estrogen-dependent cancers also demonstrate mutations in *PTEN* (an early mutation seen in 80 percent of cases), microsatellite DNA (20 to 30 percent of cases), and K-*ras* (a late mutation seen in 20 percent of cases). The cancerous cells lining the endometrium may extend directly into the cervix and through the uterine serosa. Both the pelvic (paravaginal) and para-aortic lymph nodes may become involved. While endometrial cancer metastasizes slowly, malignant cells can be found in the peritoneal cavity.

Clinical Presentation

Subjective

The patient, usually postmenopausal, presents with abnormal bleeding in 80 percent of cases. Typically, this is the only patient complaint. Patients who are perimenopausal tend to have irregular periods of bleeding; however, irregular uterine bleeding must not be discounted in these women without further exploration.

Objective

The patient does not demonstrate any pain on the exam unless metastasis has already occurred and the pelvic organs are affected.

Diagnostic Reasoning

Diagnostic Tests

Any postmenopausal patient with abnormal uterine bleeding should be referred for endometrial biopsy. Most cases of abnormal bleeding (80 percent) are from benign causes. A Pap test is not a reliable diagnostic indicator for endometrial cancer. Any atypical glandular cells reported on the Pap smear should be followed up by endometrial biopsy to rule out hyperplasia or carcinoma; the same may be done for women older than 40 years of age with normal endometrial cells on Pap smear, but this is more controversial. If endometrial biopsy reveals hyperplasia with atypia, a more extensive hysteroscopy with curettage should be done to rule out coexistent endometrial cancer. If abnormal bleeding persists after an otherwise normal endometrial biopsy (i.e., showing only atrophy, proliferative or secretory endometrium, or disordered/dyssynchronous endometrium reflecting irregular shedding of the endometrium seen with unopposed estrogen exposure and endometritis), further assessment should be done with TVS, hysteroscopy, and directed biopsy/curettage. TVS is helpful in ruling out carcinoma in women NOT on HT. A biopsy is done if the endometrial thickness is greater than 4 mm or in ANY woman with persistent uterine bleeding, irregardless of endometrial thickness. However, TVS cannot replace biopsy as a means of ruling out cancer. CA 125 should be checked to predict extent of extrauterine spread of the cancer. Depending on the results of the endometrial biopsy, the patient should be referred to a surgeon.

Differential Diagnoses

Differential diagnoses may include benign tumor (leiomyomata [fibroids]), ectopic pregnancy, intrauterine pregnancy, GI masses, endometriosis, adenomyosis, and pelvic abscess or adhesions. Endometrial polyps should also be considered because they present mostly in middle-aged women, but account for 25 percent of cases of abnormal bleeding in pre- and postmenopausal women. They are hyperplastic pedunculated/sessile growths of endometrial glands and stroma at the endometrial surface (mm to cm in size). They are only rarely neoplastic (benign in 70 percent, hyperplasia without atypia in 25 percent, atypia in fewer than 5 percent, and cancer in fewer than 1 percent). Metrorrhagia (irregular uterine bleeding) occurs in 50 percent of cases of endometrial polyps, while less frequently, menorrhagia, postmenopausal bleeding, prolapse through the cervical os, and breakthrough bleeding on hormonal treatments occur as symptoms. The only definitive diagnosis for endometrial polyps is microscopy (after D&C, biopsy, or hysterectomy), but sonohysterography (instillation of saline into uterus prior to ultrasound) is preferred to transvaginal ultrasound for noninvasive evaluation (but it cannot be diagnostic). Curettage via hysteroscopy, rather than blindly, is preferred for best detecting polyps.

Adenomyosis is the presence of ectopic endometrial glands and stroma within the musculature of the uterus, which induces hypertrophy and hyperplasia of the myometrium in response to estrogen (and maybe progesterone); may be microscopic or nodular on gross inspection, but endometrial biopsy typically negative because of changes in the myometrium. It seems to be more associated with childbearing, but pathogenesis is unknown (perhaps invagination of the endometrium or arises de novo from müllerian remnants?). The uterus is large and boggy (as opposed to firm with fibroids) and not related to endometriosis, although this is another form of ectopic endometrium. Although a third of women are asymptomatic, adenomyosis may present with abnormal uterine bleeding, dysmenorrhea, and menorrhagia.

Management

The primary principle of management is to obtain a correct diagnosis as early as possible, as the cure rate for endometrial cancer is very high if treated early.

Since primary prevention is the best management, women with chronic anovulation may benefit from the protective effects of progestin or progesterone-containing regimens (protects against hyperplasia and carcinoma [doses may be decreased from standard recommendations in women with significant side effects from this]). Women with hyperplasia without atypia can be given medroxyprogesterone acetate 10 mg qd for 12 to 14 days each month for 3 to 6 months, while women with atypia (premalignancy) need hysteroscopy with D&C, and hysterectomy (preferred if childbearing is no longer an issue). If no cancer is found, then women can receive megestrol acetate 40 mg bid–qid continuously to suppress the hyperplasia or hysterectomy (if fertility is no longer an issue and the patient can tolerate the surgery). Obviously, any estrogen therapy should be stopped in these cases. In postmenopausal women NOT on HT who have hyperplasia without atypia, a hysteroscopy and D&C is done to find source of the estrogen (such as a tumor or obesity). Women can be given medroxyprogesterone acetate 10 mg qd for 3 months, then reevaluated by biopsy as a guide for further management. If the woman is taking HT, it should be stopped immediately and a similar assessment done. In postmenopausal women with atypia, a hysteroscopy with D&C is done to rule out carcinoma and hysterectomy (preferred) considered. As an alternative, megestrol acetate 40 mg bid–qid can be given with a repeat biopsy in 3 months and hysterectomy done if atypia persists. Otherwise, if the atypia regresses, megestrol can be given and repeat biopsies done every 6 to 12 months for the rest of the woman's life.

Treatment of endometrial cancer is based on the FIGO staging. Stage I is confined to the uterine corpus, stage II involves the cervix, stage III is regional spread to the pelvis, while stage IV is spread outside the pelvis (20 to 25 percent 5-year survival). Node biopsy (lymphadenectomy) is done for clinically suspicious nodes, for anything beyond stage I disease, a tumor greater than 2 cm, type II endometrial cancer, or myometrial invasion beyond 50 percent—as all these indicate an increased risk of metastasis. Peritoneal cytology is also sent as a part of surgical staging, as a positive result with nonendometrioid tumors may indicate the need for postsurgical adjuvant chemotherapy. The bilateral salpingo-oophorectomy (BSO) is done to check for adnexal micrometastases and to eliminate endogenous estrogen production.

In contrast to the treatment of early stage type I endometrial CA above, uterine sarcoma is treated with total abdominal hysterectomy and bilateral salpingo-oophorectomy (TAH-BSO) with adjuvant radiotherapy (either external beam or brachytherapy). Although adjuvant chemotherapy has not been shown to be effective for uterine sarcoma, recurrent disease is treated with chemotherapy. Stage II or higher uterine adenocarcinoma is also treated with TAH-BSO, if the patient can tolerate surgery. Pelvic irradiation is an alternative to hysterectomy, but entails significant comorbidities from fibrotic tissue damage that is progressive and nonreversible. Adjuvant postsurgical radiation may be used for women at intermediate to high risk of recurrent disease (grade 1 or 2 disease extending greater than 50 percent beyond the myometrium [stage IC] or stage II to IV disease) or reserved as salvage treatment for recurrent disease. Disease at high risk of recurrence (grade 2 disease extending to the cervix with greater than 50 percent myometrial involvement, grade 3 disease, involvement of the lymphatic or vascular system or other metastases) should be treated with surgery and adjuvant therapy—either chemotherapy or pelvic irradiation; the choice is individualized depending on potential side effects and patient tolerance. Recurrent or highly advanced disease is treated with a combination of chemotherapy and hormonal therapy, although the choice of regimen is controversial. Localized relapse may be treated with salvage surgery or pelvic irradiation.

Follow-Up and Referral

If endometrial cancer is suspected in a postmenopausal patient with abnormal uterine bleeding, an immediate referral should be made to a gynecology/oncologist for an endometrial biopsy.

Patient Education

The American Cancer Society recommends an endometrial biopsy at menopause for all patients, and then occasionally for those patients at risk. Healthy postmenopausal patients should be encouraged to seek care at the first sign of any abnormal bleeding. In addition, obese women should be encouraged to lose weight because it may prove protective and possibly therapeutic for women with chronic anovulation. The use of HT for any indication is controversial in women with prior endometrial cancer. All women should be encouraged to follow treatment regimens for any existing diseases such as hypertension and diabetes mellitus.

Vaginal Cancer

Cancer of the vaginal wall as a primary site is extremely rare. A vaginal tumor may be a secondary site, local invasion, or metastasis from cervical or endometrial cancer.

Epidemiology and Causes

Fewer than 0.2 percent of all genital cancers are primary vaginal cancers and 75 to 85 percent are squamous cell. About 15 to 20 percent are adenocarcinomas with sarcomas and melanomas occurring very rarely. The incidence of vaginal cancer is 1 in 100,000 women with a mean age of 55 years. As with cervical cancer, vaginal cancer is associated with HPV infection. Other risk factors include intrauterine exposure to DES, multiple sex partners, early age at first intercourse, smoking, and history of STIs

Pathophysiology

Typically, in situ primary vaginal cancer develops from a vulval lesion and is of squamous cell origin; however, adenocarcinoma (arising from glandular tissue), sarcoma (arising from muscle or stromal tissue), and melanoma (arising from mucosal melanocytes) may also occur as primary cancers. Either or both of the anterior and posterior vaginal walls may be affected, but disease is most common in the upper one-third of the posterior wall. They may spread by direct extension to the parametria, bladder and urethra, and rectum, lymphatically to the pelvic and para-aortic lymph nodes, or hematogenously to the lungs, liver, and bone in highly advanced cases. A rare warty, fungating form of squamous cell vaginal cancer exists that simulates clusters of vaginal warts (i.e., condyloma acuminata) called verrucous carcinoma, which is locally aggressive with deep margins, but rarely metastasizes.

Exposure to DES in utero causes clear cell adenocarcinoma of the vagina or cervix (1 in 1000 exposed women through age 34 years), which accounts for nearly all cases of vaginal cancer in women younger than 20 years of age. In contrast to squamous cell carcinoma, more than two-thirds of vaginal adenocarcinomas present in the earliest stage of disease. The most common form of vaginal sarcoma is embryonal rhabdomyosarcoma or sarcoma botryoides, a highly malignant tumor occurring in infancy to childhood that has a nodular, exophytic appearance similar to a cluster of grapes (*botrys* is the Greek word for grapes). Vaginal melanomas are highly aggressive and prone to metastasis, but are also far rarer than squamous cell carcinoma. They are thought to arise from atypical melanocytic hyperplasia or foci of melanosis within the vaginal mucosa, although they are not always pigmented. Interestingly, nearly all cases occur in Caucasian women.

A premalignant lesion called vaginal intraepithelial neoplasia (VAIN) exists that is defined as squamous cell atypia of varying depths within the vaginal epithelium, but without actual invasion through the epithelium. VAIN I involves the lower one-third of the epithelium or less; VAIN II up to the lower two-thirds; and VAIN III between two-thirds and the full epithelial thickness, the latter also being known as carcinoma in situ. The most common predisposing factor to VAIN is infection of the genital epithelia by human papilloma virus (HPV) serotypes 16 or 18, although others may be involved. However, unlike cervical intraepithelial neoplasia (the premalignant lesion for cervical cancer) which displays a stronger relationship with HPV infection and is far more common, VAIN is less likely to progress specifically to primary squamous cell cancer of the vagina. Progression rates have been assessed only through retrospective studies and have ranged from 8 to 28 percent for VAIN III. This may be a function of the greater propensity of the cervical epithelium to undergo constant squamous metaplasia, particularly at the transformation zone (see Cervical Cancer).

Despite the increased stability of the vaginal epithelium, however, the presence of VAIN is strongly associated with prior or concurrent neoplasia in other genital structures, such as the cervix or vulva, seen in 50 to 90 percent of cases. This may simply reflect an extension of CIN into the vagina. However, VAIN is often multifocal, occurring several years posthysterectomy or in the absence of cervical disease. Thus, a more likely pathogenetic mechanism involves a carcinogenic field effect in which the various lower genital tract epithelia (cervical, vaginal, and vulvar), being of common embryologic origin, react similarly to a common carcinogen, such as HPV infection. A distinct histologic entity called intraepithelial glandular dysplasia (atypical vaginal adenosis) also exists that may be a premalignant lesion for clear cell carcinoma, similarly displaying a strong association with intrauterine exposure to diethylstilbestrol (DES) and subsequent squamous metaplasia of the vaginal epithelium. Given its potential for malignant transformation, the presence of VAIN on Pap smear calls for full colposcopic evaluation of the entire vagina with biopsy, followed by treatment with either surgical excision, CO_2 laser ablation, or topical chemotherapy with 5-fluorouracil, with intravaginal radiation used for refractory cases, given its higher rate of morbidity. This eliminates the lesion in 80 percent of women, but also carries a 20 percent recurrence rate.

Clinical Presentation

Subjective

The lesions of vaginal cancer are typically well advanced before the patient complains of any symptoms, thus the low cure rate. The patient eventually complains of foul vaginal discharge, painless vaginal bleeding, pruritus, and pain. If the mass is compressing the bladder, pain and frequency on urination may be reported.

Objective

The only physical signs of vaginal cancer may be the vaginal discharge and possibly the presence of a vaginal mass or lesion. As part of the pelvic exam, the speculum should be withdrawn very slowly and the walls of the vagina carefully examined for lesions, as well as careful palpation of the vaginal canal and are described as nodular, ulcerative, or fungating (exophytic). Often lesions in the early stages are missed.

Diagnostic Reasoning

Diagnostic Tests

About 20 percent of vaginal tumors are detected incidentally on Pap smear, but the Pap test is NOT a screening tool for vaginal cancer (as lesions are often advanced once it picks them up). A colposcopy identifies areas to be submitted for biopsy to identify the types of cells involved. Acetic acid is applied during colposcopy followed by Lugol's iodine solution, which aids in the identification of abnormal areas.

Differential Diagnosis

Because of the symptoms, STIs need to be ruled out, as well as any urinary disorders, cystocele, rectocele, and uterine prolapse. Also, because metastatic lesions (or direct extension) from the endometrium, cervix, vulva, ovary, or breast to the vagina is much more common than primary vaginal cancer, these diagnoses should be considered in the differential diagnosis.

Management

Management depends of the stage of vaginal cancer. The FIGO staging of vaginal cancer, which is done clinically through exam, cystoscopy, proctoscopy, and chest and skeletal radiography. Stage O—carcinoma in situ; stage I—confined to the vaginal mucosa in 26 percent of cases with about a 75 percent 5-year survival rate; stage II—extension to the parametrium, but not to the pelvic wall, in 37 percent of cases with about a 50 percent 5-year survival rate; stage III—extension to the pelvic wall in 24 percent of cases with about a 45 percent 5-year survival rate; and stage IV—extension beyond the pelvis in 13 percent of cases with only about a 15 percent 5-year survival rate. Overall survival rates are lower than for cervical or vulvar cancer, likely owing to a higher rate of diagnosis at more advanced stages of disease.

Superficial early stage disease less than 2 cm can be treated with surgery or only brachytherapy (especially if in the mid to lower vagina), while lesions greater than 2 cm or stage II to IV disease are treated with external beam irradiation with or without brachytherapy. Concurrent chemotherapy may be used with irradiation, but it has not been validated with prospective randomized trials. Radiation therapy and radical surgery are associated with many adverse effects, including radiation burns to surrounding tissue and disfigurement which can complicate or prohibit more aggressive treatment. In more advanced stages of vaginal cancer, recurrent metastases, or when the bladder or rectum is involved, a pelvic exenteration is performed.

Follow-Up and Referral

When vaginal cancer is suspected, the patient should be referred to a surgeon for immediate treatment. The treatment depends on the type of cells involved, the stage of the disease, and the size and location of the tumor.

Patient Education

It is of crucial importance when obtaining a history from a new patient to ask about her mother's use of DES when she was pregnant. DES-exposed women should have their first pelvic exam and colposcopy at menarche and then yearly, and gynecologic exams every 6 months. Patients undergoing vaginal surgery are concerned about the possibility of sexual relations postsurgery. Unless they have reconstructive vaginal surgery, intercourse is not possible.

Breast Cancer

Cancer of the breast is the most common cancer in American women and accounts for approximately 30 percent of all cancers in women in the United States. An estimated 211,240 new breast cancer cases were diagnosed among American women in 2005, which will eventually result in 40,410 deaths. Breast cancer is second only to lung cancer as the leading cause of cancer death among women and is the main cause of death in women aged 40 to 44 years. During the 1980s there were yearly increases in breast cancer incidence rates, probably as a result of an increase in screening, but this rise has slowed over the past few years. Mortality rates are decreasing since 1990, most likely because of earlier detection and advances in treatment.

Epidemiology and Causes

For a woman living in North America, the lifetime odds of getting breast cancer are 1 in 6 for non-Hispanic white women, 1 in 14 for African American women, 1 in 21 for New Mexican Hispanics, and 1 in 40 for New Mexican American Indians. The risk increases with age: it is low in women in their 20s and 30s, continues to rise each decade, with the median age for breast cancer diagnosis at 64 years of age. Increasing age and other risk factors (see Risk Factors 13.2) have been associated with the development of breast cancer, but explain only 50 percent of cases. All women have the potential for the development of breast cancer. Screening recommendations and guidelines are presented in Screening Recommendation/Guidelines 13.1.

Pathophysiology

Breast cancer is a disease of various cell populations, with different growth rates, cell surface markers, and tendencies

SCREENING RECOMMENDATIONS/ GUIDELINES 13.1

Breast Cancer

The American Cancer Society (ACS) recommends the following screening for the early detection of breast cancer in those who are asymptomatic (ACS does not specify an age at which screening should be terminated):

Women age 20 to 39

- Clinical breast examination performed by the practitioner every 3 years.
- BSE performed by the patient monthly.

Women age 40 and older

- Clinical breast examination performed by the practitioner annually. (This should be performed close to the scheduled mammogram.)
- Mammogram performed annually.
- BSE performed by the patient monthly.

The National Cancer Institute (NCI) recommends screening (mammogram and clinical breast examination) every 1 to 2 years for women in their 40s. A review of clinical trials by the NCI showed there to be insufficient data to evaluate the effectiveness of screening mammography in women age 70 and older.

RISK FACTORS 13.2

Breast Cancer

Major Risk Factors

Female gender
Increasing age (>age 50)
Personal history of breast cancer (in situ or invasive)
Family history of breast cancer in a first-degree relative (parent, sibling, or child)
Residing in North America or Northern Europe

Moderate Risk Factors

Biopsy-confirmed atypical hyperplasia
Early menarche (<age 12)
Late menopause (>age 55)
Nulliparity or first live-birth at a late age (>age 30)
Long-term use of postmenopausal hormone therapy especially unopposed estrogen
Exposure to high-dose radiation
History of ovarian or uterine fundus cancer
Higher education and socioeconomic status

Possible Risk Factors

High-fat diet and weight gain
Alcohol consumption (two or more drinks/day)
Physical inactivity
Cigarette smoking, especially during adolescence
Exposure to pesticides and other chemicals
Induced abortion or miscarriages

to metastasize. It is often considered a systemic disease at the time of first diagnosis, as many patients with "early" breast cancer already have established but clinically occult micrometastases, reflecting the importance of adjuvant hormonal therapy (e.g., tamoxifen, anastrozole). Invasive breast cancer is often preceded by carcinoma in situ (CIS) lesions of either ductal or lobular distribution, as discussed in the section on Prognosis. However, a malignant breast mass may be present for many years before the initial diagnosis, and it is not uncommon for invasive disease to be identified at the time of diagnosis, rather than a premalignant lesion. Breast cancers spread by contiguous, lymphatic, and/or vascular channels. The most common areas of metastasis are the regional lymph nodes, lung, skin, bone, liver, and brain.

The development of frank breast cancer may also be preceded by a variety of benign breast conditions (see Differential Diagnosis), characterized by multicentric proliferation of breast tissue. Several genetic mutations have been recognized in both precancerous and cancerous lesions, including genes affecting cellular proliferation, DNA mismatch repair, or the conversion of procarcinogens to carcinogenic compounds. Two of the most widely publicized breast cancer susceptibility genes are the tumor suppressor genes *BRCA1* and *BRCA2,* first cloned in the mid 1990s. These gene products are involved in the repair of double-stranded DNA breaks, and mutations predispose not only to breast cancer in women and men, but also to cancers of the ovary, pancreas, and even prostate. However, *BRCA1/BRCA2* mutations are quite rare, accounting for only one fifth of familial breast cancer cases.

The Knudsen hypothesis of malignant transformation is often credited with the pathogenesis of breast cancer. In this model, at least two sequential genetic "hits" or mutations that interfere with DNA repair are thought to underlie malignant transformation of normal breast tissue, which ultimately loses its capacity for programmed cell death (apoptosis). In familial cancers, the first of these hits is thought to be the inherited germline mutation, while the second mutation may be induced by an environmental carcinogen or related to one of many other predisposing risk factors.

Clinical Presentation

Subjective

History and risk assessment should include age, ethnicity, education and socioeconomic status, and breast lump or area that feel denser (with or without pain), tenderness, dimpling, nipple retraction, nipple ulceration, erythema, or peau d'orange ("orange peel"), change in breast shape, breast enlargement, and/or an alteration in the vein pattern of the breast tissue, nipple discharge, and one or more palpable enlarged axillary lymph nodes. The date of onset, location, and duration and if trauma occurred should also be elicited.

Assessment should also include any systemic symptoms, especially those that may indicate metastases to the skeleton (bone pain, fracture), spinal cord (localized and radicular back pain, lower extremity weakness, paresthesias, paralysis, bladder/bowel dysfunction), brain (headache, seizure, mental status changes, vision and speech defects, sensory loss/muscle weakness, ataxia, persistent nausea/vomiting), bladder or bowel (incontinence), lungs (chest pain, dyspnea on exertion, shortness of breath, cough), and liver (abdominal pain or distension, jaundice, weakness, fatigue, nausea, vomiting, appetite, weight loss, lower extremity edema).

The medical history should include illnesses, especially a previous breast cancer, a benign or preinvasive breast condition or another cancer such as ovarian cancer; prior radiation exposure; medications; allergies; diet and other health habits (fat intake, alcohol consumption, cigarettes, weight gain, exercise); and past surgical history, especially breast biopsy and/or surgery. Questions should be asked regarding gynecologic and obstetrical history: age at menarche; age at menopause; LMP; pregnancy history (age when first full-term pregnancy occurred, abortions, miscarriages); and use HT, particularly unopposed estrogen. Frequency of mammograms and date of last mammogram; results of previous mammograms, noting any abnormalities; other related diagnostic tests and results; and frequency of clinical breast examinations and BSE should be determined. Family history questions should include a first-degree relative with a history of breast cancer (note age at diagnosis and bilaterality of disease) and a family history of ovarian cancer associated with breast cancer.

Objective

A thorough physical examination with a focus on the breasts and axillary and supraclavicular lymph nodes should be performed. In premenopausal women, this assessment should be done during the follicular phase of the menstrual cycle, when hormone levels are low and less likely to affect the breast tissue. Examination of the breasts include inspection and palpation in the upright and supine posi-tions. The size, location, mobility, and consistency of any palpable breast mass or dense area and lymph nodes should be documented. Any breast changes noted on inspection and the characteristics of any nipple discharge are also recorded.

Clinical manifestations of breast cancer include those stated above, but some patients may present only with an abnormality detected on a mammogram. The Patient's Voice 13.2 illustrates the individuality of symptoms.

THE PATIENT'S VOICE 13.2

A Breast Mass

One Patient's Voice

It was on my 48th birthday that I noticed a slightly tender enlargement in my left breast. I had consistently checked my breasts for years during my period. I had no family history for breast cancer and never experienced breast tenderness or lumps on a regular basis. Even before my one pregnancy at age 34, I had never experienced significant breast soreness. My nurse practitioner saw me the next day and stated that she could feel something. She sent me for a mammogram. I had one 2 years ago, so I was sent to the same place. Two days later, I was told there are "changes" and I was referred to a surgeon. I did not know what that meant, except I knew it could be serious. I wanted to do everything they told me to do. I wanted to get better. I had a biopsy and then shortly after, a "lumpectomy." I was told I was very lucky because although the biopsy was positive for cancer, they said my "nodes" were cancer free. I was told I would need radiation therapy since I only had the lump removed. I experienced too much stress and fear at that time in my life. My yoga classes were very important to me then because they helped me relax and heal. I have been going for 7 years since the surgery and now teach yoga too. I know I was lucky and grateful that my nurse practitioner could see me the day after I felt the lump. Waiting is so stressful.

Another Patient's Voice

I felt a lump. After my mammogram and biopsy and diagnosis, I didn't go through the "why me" phase. I knew that things just happened, but I also knew I was going to "beat it." I wasn't going to leave my son and daughter without a mother. So I told my friends about it . . . even invited them to an "I'll beat it" party where I had a ceremony to say good-bye to my breast . . . and celebrate my life. Yes, I've had my "down" days. Facing the possibility of my life ending before I wanted it to has made me take charge of my life and has made me look at the things around me so differently. Life is truly a miracle.

Diagnostic Reasoning

Diagnostic Tests

A diagnostic mammogram is necessary in any woman with a palpable breast mass, suspicious nipple discharge, or a suspicious area on a screening mammogram. A spot compression flattens and isolates a lesion. A diagnostic mammogram determines the needs for subsequent testing, and it determines if other suspicious nonpalpable areas are present in one or both breasts.

Suspicious areas on a mammogram include (1) asymmetry with definitive borders or discernible masses, (2) architectural distortion (a "pulling in" of breast structures) not resulting from previous surgery, (3) a nodule that is more radiodense, irregularly shaped, and has unclear margins, (4) calcifications that are irregularly shaped, clustered, and of varying sizes, (5) skin changes such as a thickening or retraction, (6) spiculations (needle-like), and (7) axillary lymph nodes more than 2 cm and/or intramammary lymph nodes more than 2 cm in diameter.

Additional studies that may be scheduled to further delineate the abnormality are ultrasound, ductal lavage, and galactography or ductography. An ultrasound, which differentiates solid from fluid-filled masses, may distinguish between benign and malignant disease. It may better visualize abnormalities in patients with dense breast tissue (women under age 30 to 35 years) and is used in place of mammography in pregnant patients. Genetic testing for the *BRCA1* and *BRCA2* gene is expensive and done only in women with a high suspicion of a familial breast–ovary cancer syndrome who have undergone extensive pre- (and post-) test counseling.

Mammography views, using the Eckland technique, are used in a patient with a breast implant to provide additional views behind the implant. Galactography or ductography is used in the presence of serous or bloody nipple discharge without a palpable mass to visualize an intraductal lesion; however, it cannot distinguish between benign and malignant disease.

A biopsy is performed next. Suspicious areas noted on a mammogram or ultrasound must be submitted for biopsy for a definitive tissue diagnosis. A mammogram may not always result in a visible lesion; therefore, all clinically suspicious palpable masses must be submitted for biopsy whether or not seen with mammography.

The patient should be referred to a surgeon for further evaluation at this point. One or more of the following biopsy techniques may be done in the outpatient setting, usually under local anesthesia:

1. *Fine-needle aspiration* (FNA). FNA may be performed by a primary-care provider experienced in the procedure. A 21- or 22-gauge needle is used to aspirate a cyst or extract cells from a palpable solid lesion for analysis. It is easy to perform and provides rapid results with little trauma to the tissue. It is highly reliable when used as an adjunct to the clinical exam and mammogram. On the negative side, it requires an experienced cytopathologist, may yield false-negative results, and does not differentiate in situ from invasive cancer. A stereotactic or ultrasound-guided biopsy can be performed on nonpalpable lesions.
2. *Core-needle biopsy.* A large-gauge cutting needle is used to provide a large core of tissue from the lesion for histologic examination. The results of a core-needle biopsy are as accurate as a surgical biopsy, but the procedure is less invasive with better cosmetic results. A stereotactic or ultrasound-guided biopsy can be performed on nonpalpable lesions.
3. *Incisional biopsy.* This procedure may be done when a mass is very large and cannot be removed without major surgery. A wedge of tissue is removed for histologic examination.
4. *Open surgical excisional biopsy (lumpectomy).* This procedure involves the entire removal of a palpable mass or a nonpalpable lesion (after stereotactic or ultrasound-guided biopsy or mammographic needle localization). To qualify as a lumpectomy, lesions suggestive of cancer should be removed with a margin of at least 1 cm of normal tissue. X-ray films of needle-localization specimens are obtained to confirm removal of mammographically detected abnormality. A postexcision mammogram should confirm complete excision. The open surgical excisional biopsy provides complete pathologic assessment but may result in poor cosmesis.

If there is suspicion of inflammatory breast cancer or Paget's disease, a skin biopsy or nipple biopsy should be done at the time of the breast mass biopsy.

Prognosis. Preinvasive breast cancers include ductal carcinoma in situ (DCIS) and lobular carcinoma in situ (LCIS). DCIS has malignant potential but infrequently disseminates; therefore, approximately 98 percent of patients are cured with local–regional therapy (total mastectomy or breast-conserving surgery and radiation therapy). The addition of tamoxifen (Nolvadex) decreases the incidence of subsequent invasive disease. LCIS has a propensity for bilaterality, multicentricity, and a 25 to 40 percent risk for development of subsequent invasive cancer. It is managed with close surveillance, a bilateral mastectomy, or chemoprevention (tamoxifen).

Invasive breast cancers have the potential to disseminate through lymphatic and vascular channels to other organs. Most of these cancers are adenocarcinomas. Approximately 80 percent are infiltrating ductal carcinomas, and 10 percent are invasive lobular carcinomas. Their prognosis is identical. Invasive lobular carcinoma differs in its slightly greater tendency toward bilaterality and metastasis to meningeal and serosal surfaces. Other histologic subtypes are pure mucinous, tubular, medullary, and papillary carcinomas. These subtypes have a slight to somewhat better prognosis resulting from a smaller risk of dissemination. Paget's disease of the breast and inflammatory breast carcinoma are rare. Paget's disease of the breast, unilateral eczema of the nipple, is always associated with DCIS or invasive ductal carcinoma. Inflammatory breast carcinoma has the poorest prognosis of all breast cancers.

Prognostic factors, or tumor-related features, are biologic measures done on the breast tissue specimen. They serve as guides for the oncologist in determining systemic adjuvant therapy for the breast cancer patient. In addition to the histologic types of invasive breast cancer, lymph node status (0, 1 to 3, 4 or more, or 10 or more [range of good to poor prognosis]), tumor size (1 cm or less in diameter [good prognosis]), and histologic differentiation (range of well differentiated [low grade] to poorly differentiated [high grade]) are the standard predictors of risk of recurrence and survival. High-grade tumors are less (poorly) differentiated and carry a worse prognosis, versus lower grade better (well) differentiated tumors. With reference to these factors, patients with breast cancer have an excellent prognosis if they have the following features: DCIS, negative lymph nodes with an invasive tumor size less than 1 cm in diameter, and special histologic subtypes of breast cancer (e.g., pure tubular) less than 3 cm in diameter.

Those patients who have potentially high recurrence rates and who would, therefore, greatly benefit from systemic therapy have the following features: positive regional lymph node(s) and negative lymph nodes with invasive tumors more than 2 cm in diameter. Breast cancer patients who have a tumor that is poorly differentiated have an increased risk of recurrent disease, but they may also have a greater response to chemotherapy.

Hormone receptor status—for example, the presence or absence of estrogen and progesterone receptors—is another important prognostic factor especially in guiding the oncologist in the selection of hormonal therapy. More patients with breast cancer respond favorably if estrogen receptor levels are high and if both estrogen and progesterone receptors are positive. Also, a positive status of the pS2 protein (an estrogen-regulated secretory protein expressed mainly by estrogen receptor–positive tumors) is indicative of a better prognosis in women with both negative and positive lymph nodes.

Other prognostic factors such as those indicative of the proliferative capacity of the tumor (mitotic index, thymidine labeling index, S-phase fraction, ploidy, and Ki-67), nuclear grade, tumor necrosis, tumor microvessel density, peritumoral lymphatic vessel invasion, the protease cathepsin D, and proto-oncogenes (*ERBB2* [*HER-2/neu*, c-*erbB-2*] and c-*myc*), and *p53* (a tumor-suppressor gene) expression may be helpful in predicting response to treatment. For example, the overexpression of c-*erB-2* may predict that a breast cancer patient may be resistant to certain chemotherapy agents and possibly to hormonal therapy. It may also predict a shorter disease-free interval.

Reference to these additional prognostic factors, along with the standard ones, may be valuable in determining the need for systemic therapy in those women who have an intermediate prognosis, such as node-negative patients with invasive tumors 1 to 2 cm in diameter.

Staging. After the diagnosis of breast cancer is confirmed, the stage of the disease is evaluated (see Table 13.9). Certain laboratory tests may determine distant metastasis. A CBC may show an abnormality of WBCs and platelets, and a low hematocrit may indicate bone marrow infiltration and occult metastatic disease. Liver enzymes and calcium and phosphorous abnormalities may indicate occult liver metastasis

Table 13.9 TNM Staging of Primary Breast Cancer

Stage	TNM Staging	Description
	TX, NX, MX	Primary tumor (T), regional lymph nodes (N), or distant metastasis (M) respectively cannot be assessed (X)
0	Tis, N0, M0	Carcinoma in situ or Paget's disease of nipple with no tumor
I	T1, N0, M0	Tumor ≤ 2 cm; no regional lymph node metastasis; no distant metastasis
IIA	T0, N1, M0	No evidence of tumor, metastasis to moveable ipsilateral axillary lymph node(s); no distant metastasis
	T1, N1, M0	Tumor ≤ 2 cm; metastasis to moveable ipsilateral axillary lymph node(s); no distant metastasis
	T2, N0, M0	Tumor > 2–5 cm; no regional lymph node metastasis; no distant metastasis
IIB	T2, N1, M0	Tumor > 2–5 cm; metastasis to moveable ipsilateral axillary lymph node(s); no distant metastasis
	T3, N0, M0	Tumor > 5 cm; no regional lymph node metastasis; no distant metastasis
IIIA	T0, N2, M0	No evidence of tumor, metastasis to ipsilateral axillary lymph node(s) fixed to one another or to other structure; no distant metastasis
	T1, N2, M0	Tumor ≤ 2 cm; metastasis to ipsilateral axillary lymph node(s) fixed to one another or to other structure; no distant metastasis
	T2, N2, M0	Tumor > 2–5 cm; metastasis to ipsilateral axillary lymph node(s) fixed to one another or to other structure; no distant metastasis
	T3, N1 or N2, M0	Tumor > 5 cm; metastasis to ipsilateral axillary lymph node(s) fixed to one another or to other structure; no distant metastasis
IIIB	T4, any N, M0	Tumor of any size with direct extension to chest wall (excluding pectoral muscle) and/or edema (including peau d'orange) or ulceration of the skin or satellite skin nodules confined to the same breast, or inflammatory carcinoma; any nodal status as described above; no distant metastasis
	Any T, N3, M0	Any tumor status as described above; metastasis to ipsilateral internal mammary node(s); no distant metastasis
IV	Any T, Any N, M1	Any tumor or nodal status as described above; distant metastasis, including metastasis to ipsilateral supraclavicular lymph nodes

and/or bone metastasis. Tumor marker (e.g., CEA, Ca 27.29) abnormalities may indicate occult metastatic disease. If the tumor marker is abnormal, it will be useful in later assessing response to treatment (disease progression or recurrence). These radiology exams also determine distant metastasis: A chest x-ray abnormality may indicate lung metastasis, and a bone scan/skeletal survey or liver scan, if signs, symptoms, or laboratory tests warrant, may suggest an abnormality.

Differential Diagnoses

Several differential diagnoses should be considered. With breast cancer, a palpable mass is usually persistent, unilateral, solitary, discrete, firm, irregularly shaped, nontender, and may or may not be fixed to the skin or underlying tissue. Breast distortion and skin changes such as diffuse erythema, edema, peau d'orange, dimpling, nipple retraction, or nipple ulceration are also indicative of cancer. If present, nipple discharge is spontaneous, persistent, unilateral, localized to a single duct, watery or sticky, and clear, sanguineous, serosanguineous, or serous in color. Lymph nodes suggestive of a malignancy are large, firm, or fixed.

Fibrocystic changes (cystic breast disease, chronic cystic mastitis, or mammary dysplasia) may be difficult to distinguish from breast cancer by palpation alone. *Fibrocystic changes* are so common that they are considered a normal variant of breast tissue. However, if accompanied by significant pain, nipple discharge, or palpable physical exam findings that raise suspicion for breast cancer, the condition is termed *fibrocystic disease*. Cystic areas are unilateral or bilateral, somewhat more diffuse, 1 mm to many centimeters in diameter, soft, and mobile; they may also be tender and painful due to stromal edema, dilation of ducts, and accompanying inflammation. These cysts are hormonally regulated and may be worse premenstrually; this variation with menses usually distinguishes fibrocystic changes from fibroadenomas and breast cancer. Aspiration of clear fluid with complete disappearance of the cyst on follow-up examination or the appearance of a fluid-filled cavity on ultrasound confirms the diagnosis. These changes are most common in patients 30 to 55 years of age.

Fibroadenomas are benign, solid masses of fibrous and glandular tissue that are often confused with breast cancer. These masses may be isolated or multiple and are typically firm, nodular, usually well-defined, freely mobile, and possibly tender. Growth of the tumor is hormonally stimulated; thus, it may grow rapidly during pregnancy, lactation, or hormonal manipulation. These are most common in younger patients and are not associated with an increased risk of breast cancer if in their simple form. However, *complex fibroadenomas* (i.e., containing cysts greater than 3 mm in size, calcification on mammography, or histologic evidence of sclerosing adenosis or papillary apocrine changes) have been associated with a greater risk of breast cancer when accompanied by proliferation of surrounding glandular tissue.

Hamartomas composed of stromal and epithelial tissue and *tubular adenomas* consisting of ductal tissue are less common benign tumors of the breast that may present similarly on physical exam but are not considered cancerous. Fat necrosis or *panniculitis* is another benign condition which is typically trauma induced. The mass is firm and possibly tender, often with calcification seen on mammography. *Diabetic mastopathy* results in a breast lump with a dense mammographic appearance but benign histology consisting of keloidal scar tissue and a lobular, lymphocytic inflammation. This is most often seen in women with type 1 diabetes mellitus who also suffer from additional end-organ microvascular damage such as retinopathy or neuropathy.

Intraductal papilloma is a benign condition with a small, usually solitary and nonpalpable mass in one mammary duct with an associated spontaneous sanguineous or serosanguineous nipple discharge. If large enough to palpate, the mass is most often close to or beneath the areola, soft, mobile, 1 to 3 cm in size, poorly delineated, nontender, and sometimes associated with skin dimpling. It is most common in patients 35 to 55 years of age. Solitary papillomas are not considered premalignant; however, diffuse papillomatosis characterized by the formation of multiple papillomas carries with it a greater risk of eventual breast cancer.

Duct ectasia is a benign condition involving inflammation of a subareolar duct, which may produce subareolar erythema and swelling, a mass with nipple retraction and/or dimpling, dull nipple pain, tenderness, burning, and itching. Nipple discharge is pasty and straw-colored, cream-colored, green, or brown. It is most common in perimenopausal or postmenopausal patients who have had children and have nursed.

Ductal hyperplasia without atypia is distinguished from ectasia, in that it is the most common benign breast lesion clearly associated with an increased risk of breast cancer. Epithelial cell proliferation along the basement membranes of the ducts, while benign histologically, varies in size and shape. *Atypical ductal hyperplasia* is associated with an even greater risk of breast cancer (up to sixfold in women with a strong family history of breast cancer), especially in premenopausal women. It is characterized by a loss of apical-basal cellular organization within ductal tissue. *Atypical lobular hyperplasia* is even more concerning, as it is qualitatively (albeit not quantitatively) equivalent to LCIS, which is considered a precursor lesion to invasive breast cancer.

Sclerosing adenosis, most common in patients age 35 to 45, is a benign proliferation of the breast epithelium with increased fibrous and glandular tissue, with hard, pea-sized nodules throughout the affected area. There is mild-to-moderate pain and swelling premenstrually. The presence of this condition has also been associated with an increased risk of breast cancer. *Radial scars* are another benign histologic finding consisting of a fibroelastic core from which ducts and lobules radiate outward. If large, these lesions may appear similar to spiculated carcinoma on mammography and are indeed associated with an increased risk of breast cancer.

Mastitis, a benign infectious condition of the breast that may or may not include formation of an abscess, presents with redness, induration, pain, possible purulent nipple discharge, fever, chills, and myalgias. It is more common during lactation.

Management

The patient diagnosed with breast cancer is referred to oncology specialists, such as a surgeon, medical oncologist, and/or a radiation oncologist for treatment of the disease (see Table 13.10). The choice of treatment is influenced by such factors as tumor stage, estrogen and progesterone receptor levels and other prognostic factors, patient age, menopausal status, and the patient's general health. When detected in early stages, invasive breast cancer that is treatable with surgery, radiation therapy, chemotherapy, and/or hormonal therapy may be highly curable.

Surgical Management

The initial surgical management of stage I and stage II breast cancer includes one of several types of surgery. Breast-conserving surgery involves a partial mastectomy, lumpectomy, wide excision, segmental mastectomy, or quadrantectomy with a separate axillary node dissection and radiation therapy to the breast. A modified radical mastectomy is a

Table 13.10 Management of Invasive Breast Cancer

Stage	Surgery/Radiation Therapy	Adjuvant Therapy
I	Breast-conserving surgery with separate axillary node dissection and radiation therapy (RT) to the breast, OR Modified radical mastectomy (MRM)	Suitable ER-negative patients: adjuvant chemotherapy ER-positive patients: adjuvant chemotherapy or tamoxifen 20 mg qd
II	Breast-conserving surgery with separate axillary node dissection and RT to the breast, OR MRM Consider RT to the chest wall and regional nodes for patients at high risk of local-regional recurrence, including those with known residual disease or 4 or more involved nodes	*Node-positive patients:* Premenopausal and postmenopausal (ER-negative) patients: adjuvant combination chemotherapy with or without tamoxifen Postmenopausal patients with positive hormone receptors: tamoxifen alone *Node-negative patients:* ER-negative or ER-positive patients with large tumors: adjuvant chemotherapy ER-positive patients: adjuvant chemotherapy or tamoxifen 20 mg qd
IIIA	*In operable cases:* MRM with or without RT or radical mastectomy (removal of breast tissue, all axillary lymph nodes, and underlying chest muscle) with or without RT RT should be given because of the high risk of local recurrence; postop external beam RT to chest wall with or without boost as necessary for positive or close margins	Combination chemotherapy with or without hormones Neoadjuvant therapy: chemotherapy may be given preoperatively if primary resection is not feasible or technically difficult
IIIB	Biopsy for diagnosis and estrogen/progesterone receptors (ER/PR) If good response to chemotherapy or hormonal therapy: local therapy with surgery and/or RT If poor response to chemotherapy or hormonal therapy: palliative RT	Chemotherapy/hormonal therapy: combination chemotherapy with or without hormones, OR tamoxifen (if ER/PR receptors positive)
IV	Biopsy for diagnosis and ER/PR receptors External beam RT or palliative mastectomy to control local disease	If visceral disease minimal or absent and ER/PR receptors positive: hormonal therapy (as initial therapy): For premenopausal patients: tamoxifen or oophorectomy For patients who relapse after a period of response or prolonged stability on initial hormone therapy: megestrol 40 mg qid or anastrozole 1 mg qd or letrozole 2.5 mg daily If visceral disease present or ER/PR receptors negative: combination chemotherapy
Inflammatory Breast Cancer	Refer to options for stage IIIB or IV	Refer to options for stage IIIB or IV

total mastectomy with an axillary node dissection. Breast-conserving surgery removes a portion of the breast tissue, while a total mastectomy removes all but approximately 2 to 3 percent of the breast tissue. The survival rates for these two surgical treatment options are equivalent.

The type of initial surgery for a particular patient usually depends on the location and size of the tumor, breast size, characteristics of the disease on mammography, patient age, and the patient's feelings regarding breast preservation. Breast-conserving surgery may not be an option if there is a tumor beneath the nipple, a large tumor-size-to-breast-size ratio, multicentricity, extensive intraductal carcinoma, diffuse malignant-appearing calcifications on the mammogram, or contraindications to radiation therapy such as pregnancy, collagen-vascular disease, or prior radiation therapy to the breast or chest wall.

Following a mastectomy, the patient may choose immediate or delayed breast reconstruction with a submuscular saline implant or expander, a transverse rectus abdominis myocutaneous (TRAM) flap, or a latissimus dorsi flap. Depending on the type of breast surgery, the adverse effects may be wound infection, seroma, bleeding or hematoma, phantom breast syndrome (pain, numbness, or nipple itching), paresthesias, muscle atrophy, arm or shoulder weakness or stiffness, lymphedema, phlebitis, or a winged scapula (protruding scapula resulting from intraoperative injury to the long thoracic nerve). A new technique under investigation, lymphatic mapping and sentinel lymph node (SLN) biopsy may eliminate the need for an axillary lymph node dissection in some patients and thus prevent some of these adverse effects. The sentinel node (the first lymph node along a lymphatic drainage pathway) is identified after peritumoral injection with a radioisotope or vital blue dye. If the sentinel node is negative for metastatic disease a complete axillary lymph node dissection is not indicated.

Radiation Therapy

Radiation therapy is indicated for local–regional control of the primary breast cancer or palliation of metastatic disease. Following breast-conserving surgery, primary treatment includes external-beam radiation to the entire breast with or without a boost (interstitial radioactive implant or external-beam radiation) to the primary site. After a modified radical mastectomy, radiation therapy to the chest wall and regional lymph nodes is considered in those women at high risk of local-regional recurrence, including those with known residual disease or four or more involved lymph nodes. Patients undergoing an axillary lymph node dissection generally do not require radiation therapy to the axilla. Internal mammary lymph nodes may be treated and those patients with four or more positive lymph nodes may require supraclavicular radiation therapy to reduce the risk of supraclavicular lymph node recurrence. The pregnant patient with breast cancer can begin radiation therapy after delivery. Potential adverse effects of radiation therapy include fatigue, edema, breast pain or tenderness, skin reactions, brachial plexopathy, radiation pneumonitis, and myocardial damage if the left breast is treated. Secondary malignancies, such as sarcomas, leukemias, and lung cancer, are rare, although smokers have an increased risk of lung cancer in the ipsilateral lung.

Breast surgery or radiation therapy may make subsequent mammograms difficult to interpret. Masses (postoperative fluid collections and scarring), edema, skin thickening, and calcifications may be seen on these mammograms especially during the first 6 months after treatment. During the next 6 to 12 months, slow resolution of these changes takes place and stability occurs within 2 years.

Chemotherapy

Antineoplastic chemotherapy as adjuvant therapy is indicated for the eradication of micrometastatic disease that may be present at the time of the original diagnosis. It should be initiated within 6 weeks (preferably less) of surgery (radiation therapy would follow the chemotherapy). Combination chemotherapy is the standard of care for the treatment of primary breast cancer because it most likely would overcome the potential for drug resistance. The most widely used regimens are CMF (cyclophosphamide [Cytoxan], methotrexate [amethopterin], and fluorouracil [Adrucil]), CAF [FAC] (cyclophosphamide, doxorubicin [Adriamycin], and fluorouracil), and AC (doxorubicin and cyclophosphamide) with or without sequential paclitaxel (Taxol). Other regimens are CMFVP (CMF and vincristine [Oncovin] and prednisone [Deltasone]), CFM [CNF, FNC] (cyclophosphamide, fluorouracil, mitoxantrone [Novantrone]), NFL (mitoxantrone, fluorouracil, leucovorin [Wellcovorin]), sequential Dox-CMF (doxorubicin followed by CMF), VATH (vinblastine, doxorubicin, thiotepa [Thioplex] and fluoxymesterone [Halotestin]), and vinorelbine (Navelbine) and doxorubicin.

Second-line or later therapy, in the event of disease progression or recurrent disease, includes agents such as vinorelbine, paclitaxel, docetaxel (Taxotere), or gemcitabine (Gemzar). Some of the more common, potential adverse effects of chemotherapy include myelosuppression, nausea and vomiting, anorexia, mucositis, alopecia, fatigue, and neurotoxicity. Less common toxicities include hemorrhagic cystitis (alkylating agents), cardiomyopathy (anthracyclines), thromboembolic events, and early menopause (in premenopausal patients). Paclitaxel and docetaxel may also produce myalgia and rare allergic reactions; docetaxal may cause cumulative fluid retention and symptomatic pleural effusions. A rare complication of antineoplastic chemotherapy may be the development of secondary leukemia. Hematopoietic growth factors (erythropoietin, G-CSF [Neupogen], GM-CSF [Leukine], and oprelvekin [Neumega]) and cytoprotective agents such as amifostine (Ethyol) and dexrazoxane (Zinecard) may help to prevent or reduce some of the chemotherapy-related complications. Pamidronate (Aredia), a second-generation aminobisphosphonate, is used in cases of osteolytic bone metastases to prevent pathologic fractures, cord compression, the need for radiation therapy or surgery to the bone, and hypercalcemia, and it significantly reduces bone pain. Pregnant breast cancer patients may receive antineoplastic chemotherapy during their third trimester or after delivery.

Monoclonal Antibodies

The newest treatment for metastatic breast cancer, trastuzumab (Herceptin), a recombinant DNA–derived humanized monoclonal antibody, is used as a single agent in second-line or later therapy for those patients with metastatic breast cancer whose tumors overexpress the HER2 protein. The combined regimen of trastuzumab and paclitaxel is used for the same patient population who have not previously received chemotherapy for their metastatic disease. Potential adverse effects include cardiomyopathy, anemia and leukopenia, diarrhea, and infection.

Hormonal Therapy

Hormonal therapy includes the use of antiestrogens (tamoxifen), progestins (e.g., megestrol acetate), luteinizing hormone–releasing hormone (LHRH) agonists (e.g., leuprolide), or aromatase inhibitors (anastrazole and letrozole). Tamoxifen is the most prescribed of these agents, and the treatment period is 5 years. Because of its antiestrogenic effect, it is beneficial in those breast cancer patients whose tumors have positive hormone receptors, and with its greatest effect being in those who have both ER (estrogen-receptor)-positive and PR (progesterone-receptor)-positive tumors. Tamoxifen also exhibits an estrogenic effect on the endometrium; therefore, it may increase the incidence of endometrial cancer. Potential adverse effects include mild nausea, hot flashes, menstrual irregularities, vaginal discharge, vaginal dryness and irritation, benign ovarian cysts, thromboembolic events, and ophthalmologic toxicities.

Local Recurrent Disease

Local recurrent disease is usually indicative of widespread recurrence, especially in the postmastectomy patient. Some patients initially treated with breast-conserving surgery and radiation therapy, who later develop a local recurrence in the ipsilateral breast, may be cured with surgery and/or radiation therapy. Prolonged survival is more likely if there is a chest wall recurrence less than 3 cm in diameter, axillary and internal mammary (not supraclavicular) lymph node recurrence, and a disease-free interval of more than 2 years after initial therapy. Treatment options for recurrent disease include surgery, radiation therapy, chemotherapy, and/or hormonal therapy. Surgery and/or radiation may be used for a local or visceral recurrence. In the asymptomatic patient with a positive or unknown ER/PR status, and with absent or minimal visceral disease in one organ, tamoxifen in the pre- and postmenopausal patient or oophorectomy (or LHRH agonists) in the premenopausal patient may be the treatment option. In the event that a patient had an initial response to hormonal therapy but had a subsequent relapse, another type of hormonal therapy may be prescribed, such as tamoxifen, anastrozole or letrozole, Megace, androgens, LHRH agonists (for premenopausal patients), or aminoglutethimide. A subset of patients may respond to hormonal therapy withdrawal for approximately 10 months before switching to another form of hormonal therapy. Patients with positive visceral disease and a negative ER/PR status should receive chemotherapy. If a patient relapses a year or more after receiving adjuvant treatment with CMF, this same regimen may be readministered. If the patient relapses after treatment with an anthracycline-containing regimen, she may be retreated with other agents mentioned earlier. Recurrent breast cancer treatment may be palliative in nature, such as the use of radiation therapy to relieve the pain of bone metastases.

Clinical Trials

At any stage of breast cancer, patients may be eligible for clinical trials designed to improve survival or decrease the morbidity associated with current standard therapy. Some patients with stages II, III, or IV may be considered as candidates for clinical trials of high-dose chemotherapy with bone marrow transplantation or hematopoietic stem cell support.

Follow-Up and Referral

Depending on the breast cancer patient's risk for both local and distant recurrence, a history and physical examination may be done according to the following schedule: every 3 to 6 months during the first 3 years (more frequently during adjuvant therapy), every 6 months for the next 2 years, and annually after the fifth year (more frequently for patients at very high risk for recurrence).

A baseline mammogram should be done 3 to 9 months after tumor excision and at the completion of all treatment. Thereafter, it should be done at least annually to detect a recurrence in the ipsilateral breast of those patients who had breast-conserving surgery or to detect a second primary in the contralateral breast of most breast cancer patients. Further testing such as bone scans, chest x-ray films, CT scans, and liver function tests are ordered for symptomatic patients as indicated. Patients treated with tamoxifen should have routine pelvic examinations. If abnormal uterine bleeding occurs, further evaluation is warranted.

The 5-year relative survival rate for patients with localized breast cancer is 97 percent, for regional spread it is 76 percent, and for distant metastases it is 21 percent. The 10-year survival for localized breast cancer declines to 67 percent, and 15-year survival declines to 56 percent.

Patient Education

The primary care clinician may be involved at various phases of the patient's care, for example, prediagnosis, diagnosis, treatment, and posttreatment. Therefore, the clinician is in a valuable position to teach the patient and significant others regarding breast cancer prevention and detection and to reinforce information about a breast cancer diagnosis and treatment options (including benefits and potential complications).

The patient should be taught the breast self-exam (BSE) technique, which can be found at www.breastcancer.org. Screening recommendations should also be reviewed. If diagnosed at an early stage, breast cancer may be curable with standard treatment.

The breast cancer patient needs to learn how to prevent potential postsurgical and/or radiation therapy complications such as lymphedema. In this situation, the patient should be taught range of motion exercises for the involved arm and shoulder. The need to avoid infections, injuries, strains, and constrictions of the arm is stressed. Antineoplastic chemotherapy and other forms of breast cancer treatment can be teratogenic; therefore, the patient must be advised to use effective contraception during treatment.

The breast cancer patient should be taught about the pharmacologic and nonpharmacologic management for the adverse effects of potential chemotherapy, radiation therapy, or hormonal therapy. For example, the patient may be instructed to take medication such as ondansetron (Zofran) and Decadron to prevent delayed chemotherapy-induced nausea and vomiting, and to perform techniques such as relaxation with guided imagery to prevent or minimize these symptoms. The patient may also be directed in the purchase of a breast prosthesis, mastectomy bra, or wig.

The patient diagnosed with breast cancer may face many physical and psychosocial issues, such as an alteration in body image and sexuality, a role change, anxiety, denial, anger, and depression. The clinician is in a prime position to counsel and support the patient and significant others, and to direct them to the many breast cancer resources available to the public that offer individual and group counseling, among other services.

Mastitis

Mastitis is a general term which refers to inflammation of the breast. The terminology for the various types of mastitis can be confusing. There are overlapping definitions and contradictions in the literature. For purposes of this discussion there are three general categories: puerperal mastitis, nonpuerperal mastitis, and periductal mastitis. Each category is further defined by an explanation of the cause of the mastitis.

Puerperal mastitis is a cellulitis that develops in the lactating or nonlactating breast after parturition. Epidemic puerperal mastitis is a hospital-acquired infection most commonly seen in the preantibiotic era. The most common contagion for epidemic puerperal mastitis is *Staphylococcus aureus*. *S. aureus* is spread by cross transmission of neonate to mother as well as cross transmission in the nursery. There is multiple duct involvement, which results in inflammation of several nonadjacent lobes of the breast. With the progression of rooming-in and the introduction of antibiotics, epidemic puerperal mastitis has become a rare occurrence. Sporadic puerperal mastitis is an acute process that is far more common in women who breastfeed rather than in those who bottlefeed. It usually occurs in the second to sixth week postpartum; however, it has been reported in patients even after breastfeeding for 1 year. It is hypothesized that the higher occurrence of mastitis in the earlier postpartum period is due to the prevalence of nipple and feeding problems at this time, a risk factor for the disease. Feeding problems are more likely to occur in first-time breastfeeding mothers.

Nonpuerperal mastitis is a rare disease, which is usually found in patients who are immunocompromised, have undergone radiation therapy, or have had an autoimmune disorder. It can also occur in neonates. It is common in late adolescence or early adulthood. Nonpuerperal mastitis is a ductal abnormality or a local manifestation of a systemic problem. Several pathological pathways may be involved including squamous metaplasia of the lactational ducts, periareolar abscesses, and cellulitis. Squamous metaplasia is the most common nonpuerperal mastitis. Mastitis can also be caused by several obscure pathogens or by a substance in the breast such as silicone. This disease usually presents a clinical picture of a palpable mass and known infectious process such as tuberculosis (TB) or syphilis. Nonpuerperal mastitis must always be examined for the risk of carcinoma.

Periductal mastitis has been referred to and cross-referenced under several other names, such as mammary duct ectasia, mastitis obliterans, plasma cell mastitis, comedomastitis, and secretory disease of the breast. The term *duct ectasia* refers to the dilated lactiferous ducts of the breast being filled with keratin and secretions. Periductal mastitis is the inflammatory process that occurs around these ducts. Some degree of duct dilation normally occurs with aging. Some researchers have suggested that periductal mastitis seen in younger patients represents a different disease from the more chronic clinical presentation seen in older women. The primary event of periductal mastitis is controversial. Some hypothesize that duct ectasia precedes the inflammatory process and vice versa. The disease is characterized by dilation of the subareolar ducts. The ducts become thick walled and surrounded by plasma cells. Inside the ducts there is a pasty, yellow-brown secretion, which is lipid-rich. The periductal regions become fibrotic and inflamed. This may be caused by rupture and leaking of the ducts themselves. Fat necrosis is often evident.

Epidemiology and Causes

The incidence of mastitis in breastfeeding women has been reported from 1 to 9 percent. One study found an incidence of 26 percent in a population of long-term breastfeeding mothers.

The causative organism of sporadic puerperal mastitis is *S. aureus* in at least 50 percent of reported cases. *S. aureus* is frequently found on skin and cultured from the neonate's mouth. Other organisms implicated in the infection are *Escherichia coli,* group A and group B *Streptococcus*, and *Mycobacterium tuberculosis*. TB mastitis occurs in populations in which TB is endemic.

There is a multitude of contributing factors for puerperal mastitis. Cracked, abraded, or otherwise damaged nipples provide a portal of entry for the microorganism. Patients who are having latch-on and positioning difficulty during feeding also increase their risk for both nipple skin disruption and milk stasis, which can lead to mastitis. Slow milk ejection reflex, engorgement, failure to empty the breast adequately, waiting too long between feedings, supplemental feedings, use of pacifiers, wearing a tight and restrictive bra, sleeping positions that constrict the breast, and weaning also contribute to a woman's risk of developing mastitis. Each of these situations can lead to blocked ducts and milk stasis. Unresolved milk stasis provides a medium for bacterial overgrowth.

Physiologic and psychological stress are both significant risk factors for puerperal mastitis. Fatigue, improper nutrition, and life stress are predictors for breast infections. These situations lead to lower maternal immune defenses and an increased likelihood for the illness.

Periductal mastitis/mammary duct ectasia is seen primarily in perimenopausal and postmenopausal women. The peak incidence is between 40 and 49 years of age, but it can occur at any time after the menarche. The inflammatory process has been observed on microscopic exam in 30 to 40 percent of women older than age 50; however, clinical disease occurs much less frequently. The actual incidence of the disease is unknown. Duct ectasia has a reported incidence of 5.5 to 25 percent as demonstrated on postmortem exams. A risk factor for periductal mastitis is cigarette smoking. The mechanism by which smoking increases the incidence of this disease is unknown, but there is a clear statistical link. Inverted nipples have been suggested to be a source of duct obstruction, which could lead to ectasia, but it has not been shown to be a risk factor.

The cause of periductal mastitis and ectasia is unknown. There may be an autoimmune explanation, but this has not been clarified. Infection by anaerobes and other bacteria may play a role but this has not been verified either. Some patients with this mastitis do have bacteria in their nipple discharge.

Pathophysiology

The causative mechanism of the various forms of mastitis (puerperal, nonpuerperal, and periductal) have been discussed above. However the pathophysiology of the infectious process in the most common form, in puerperal mastitis, is a classic example of a breakdown in the body's protective outer epithelial barriers. This results in entry of bacteria from the infant's mouth or mother's skin into her breast through cracked nipple skin or the nipple pores. With one or more lobes of the breast seeded, infection develops. Moreover, the symptoms of the disease, which include pain, tenderness, and maternal fatigue, contribute to further decreases in effective feeding practices and adequate emptying of the breast, thus, worsening the infection. Milk of a mastitic breast is found to have a higher than normal sodium and chloride content, and it is not unusual for an infant to refuse to nurse on that breast.

The infection of puerperal mastitis is primarily in the extraductal tissue, and thus, breastfeeding through the infectious process generally poses no harm to the infant, provided skin breakdown has not resulted in frank bleeding from the nipples and there is no evidence of purulent nipple discharge. Purulent material may be present within the ducts, however. In addition, although bilateral infection is possible, mastitis is usually unilateral and localized to the upper outer quadrant of the affected breast. The incidence of mastitis progressing to a subareolar breast abscess has been reported to be as high as 4 to 11 percent in patients treated for the disease. It is much higher for those who do not seek treatment for mastitis.

Clinical Presentation

Subjective

The clinical presentation is acute in nature. The patient's first complaint is fatigue followed by the onset of flu-like symptoms. The involved breast segments may be red and warm. Patients describe the affected area with a range of being tender to painful. A fever of at least 100.0°F (37.8°C) can be expected with myalgias, malaise, and chills. Nausea and vomiting can accompany these symptoms.

Many patients with periductal mastitis are asymptomatic. Others present with breast pain, a breast mass, nipple discharge, nipple retraction, a nonpuerperal breast abscess, or a mammary fistula. The pain is usually subareolar and noncyclical. The nipple discharge varies in color and may contain occult blood. It is most frequently green and sticky and occurs spontaneously. The mastitis can be unilateral or bilateral. Nipple retraction and noninflammatory masses occur more commonly in older women. Pain and abscesses tend to occur in younger women. Periductal mastitis and ectasia account for 3 to 12 percent of benign breast lumps. The pain is usually focused behind the areola and tends to be more severe in younger patients.

Objective

On examination, there are varying degrees of erythema and edema of the affected breast. The erythema is most commonly in a V-shaped distribution and may or may not feel hard. Sometimes there is purulent nipple discharge. There may or may not be a palpable blocked duct.

Diagnostic Reasoning

Diagnostic Tests

Milk cultures are rarely done in first-occurrence cases of mastitis because they are costly and may delay treatment.

They are warranted with a recurrence or failure of initial treatment. A breast milk culture can be obtained by manual expression of a midstream, clean-catch specimen. Washing the nipple with water and sterile gauze preps the breast. The first 2 to 3 mL of milk expressed should be discarded. The specimen needs to be fresh when sent to the lab. Breast milk is rarely found to be sterile and naturally has leukocytes present. A normal leukocyte count is 1000 to 4000/mL.

With patients symptomatic for mastitis, there are three diagnostic categories when cytology and cultures are performed on breast milk samples. Milk stasis is present with a WBC of less than 106/mL with a bacterial count less than 103 colony-forming units (CFU)/mL. Noninfectious breast inflammation is considered with a WBC more than 106/mL and bacterial count less than 103 CFU/mL. A WBC of more than 106/mL and a bacterial count of more than 103 CFU/mL is indicative of infectious mastitis. With the help of a milk culture and sensitivity, appropriate antibiotic treatment can be initiated. There are occasionally situations in which a patient develops a chronic puerperal mastitis. These patients may have anatomic strictures of some lactiferous ducts, which lead to chronic plugged ducts. Long-term antibiotic therapy and impeccable breastfeeding management can improve the outcome.

Ultrasound examination of the breast or mammogram may be helpful in making the diagnosis of periductal mastitis. The mammogram shows tubular dilated ducts. Calcification may be present in the lumen and walls of the affected ducts. Intense periductal mastitis may simulate carcinoma on the mammogram. Because carcinoma and mastitis can coexist, a biopsy may be warranted with such findings. In older patients, the mass from the ectasia can be hard to differentiate from carcinoma. Both masses can be hard, irregular, fixed or not to the surrounding tissue, and have the presence of skin or nipple retraction. When the nipple discharge is bilateral and multiple ducts are involved, the likelihood of malignancy is reported to be remote. Another diagnostic tool can be needle aspiration and culture of areas of inflammation. Fine-needle aspiration may show polymorphs, plasma cells, lymphocytes, and giant cells.

Differential Diagnosis

The first differential diagnosis to consider when presented with a patient symptomatic for puerperal mastitis is to identify that a condition of milk stasis or plugged ducts has led to an infectious process. The clinical presentation is invaluable in this judgment. There have been several cases of breast cancer in patients who are lactating or pregnant. Inflammatory breast cancer is a rare disease, but it can present with some of the same symptoms as a traditional puerperal mastitis. The patient with inflammatory breast cancer may have a red, swollen breast, and sometimes (but rarely) a fever. The patient commonly has no palpable breast mass and may or may not have peau d'orange (resembling orange peel). Reports differ on infants rejecting a breast later diagnosed with a cancerous disease. When inflammatory cancer is present, these symptoms do not respond to antibiotic treatment as mastitis generally does. With any suspicion of a cancerous process, the patient must be referred for biopsy and a definitive diagnosis.

Breast engorgement is often mistaken for mastitis, but does not have the accompanying systemic symptoms of infection (e.g., fever, erythema, myalgias). If the infant has signs of poor "latch-on" during feeding (infant showing sunken cheeks, clicking sounds signifying breaking of suction, contact between the upper and lower lips at the corners of the mouth while feeding, etc.), can also predispose the mother to mastitis. Galactoceles (milk retention cysts), which may result from plugged ducts, appear hard and red and be quite painful (soreness, as opposed to the shooting pains of mastitis), but lack the systemic signs of mastitis, should be considered as a possible diagnosis. Interestingly, hard, tender breasts with shooting pains, but without redness or fever may be more associated with fungal infection of the breasts.

Management

The principle of management in puerperal mastitis is to decrease contributing factors and generally improve breastfeeding management.

Flu-like symptoms should always be treated as mastitis in postpartum patients unless proved otherwise. With a first occurrence the diagnosis can be made by clinical symptoms alone. If there is no response to antibiotic treatment, or if there is recurrent mastitis, further diagnostics are indicated.

It is vital that the infant continue to breastfeed to avoid milk stasis. Because the infection is extraductal, there is no risk to the infant on continuing breastfeeding. Massage of the breasts during feeding helps to better drain the breast, and additional pumping may be needed, particularly if the infant is not nursing effectively on the affected side. Pumping breasts in addition to frequent infant feeding decreases the duration of symptoms and sequelae of the disease, notably breast abscess. Breastfeeding management should include correction of any latch-on or positioning difficulties and aggressive discovery and care of cracked or sore nipples.

Bed rest is imperative during the acute phase of the illness. The mother should be assisted with her household duties and rest in bed with her infant. Moist heat to the affected breast can be useful before feeding and pumping to increase milk expression. Cold application may be comfortable between feedings. Of course, stress management should be explored.

Antibiotic therapy is traditionally recommended to treat the infection. With no treatment at all, only 15 percent of patients recover without recurrent infection or breast abscess. Approximately 50 percent improve with pumping alone for treatment and over 95 percent recover completely with combination therapy of pumping and antibiotics.

The best response is when antibiotics are started within the first 24 hours of symptom onset. A broad-spectrum antibiotic such as dicloxicillin or cloxacillin 500 mg PO q6h is recommended for 10 to 14 days. If there is no response in the first 48 hours after initiation of antibiotic therapy, then cephalexin or amoxicillin + clauvulanate (Augmentin) is given for broader coverage. In addition, antibiotic sensitivity should be obtained from the milk culture. For those with a penicillin allergy, erythromycin (E-Mycin) (500 mg PO q6h) can be prescribed. The patient must be instructed to continue her pharmacologic therapy for the duration of the prescription to avoid a partially treated disease. Pain and other uncomfortable symptoms can be treated with nonsteroidal analgesics such as acetaminophen.

In the management of periductal mastitis, broad-spectrum antibiotics have been successful. They tend to treat the periareolar inflammation associated with this condition and reduce pain. If a mass is present it must be biopsied to rule out carcinoma. If the nipple discharge is suspicious a duct excision is necessary to confirm the diagnosis. Symptomatic treatment simply includes good nipple and areolar hygiene. Some have recommended no oral nipple stimulation.

The wound infection rate after breast biopsies where periductal mastitis and/or ectasia is present is high. The infection rate is 2 percent after biopsies with no evidence of this disease but 10.2 percent when it is present. This appears to be unrelated to trends in culture results.

Notable sequelae of this mastitis are breast abscesses and fistulas. Nonpuerperal breast abscesses are seen more frequently than those associated with lactation. The incidence of periareolar abscess is 10 percent in patients who are symptomatic with duct ectasia. The bacteria cultured are usually *S. aureus* and anaerobes. Surgical excision and broad-spectrum antibiotic coverage is the treatment of choice. Needle aspiration may be performed if the risk of malignancy is low, but this treatment frequently needs to be done repetitively.

Abscess is one of the more common sequelae of puerperal mastitis. It can occur when the disease progresses either with or without treatment. The patient presents with worsening local symptoms and may or may not have systemic manifestations. A breast ultrasound can be useful to confirm the diagnosis. Most abscesses are surgically incised and drained under anesthesia. Biopsy of the cavity has been recommended to check for the presence of carcinoma. A drain is put in place, and broad-spectrum parenteral antibiotics should be started with anaerobic coverage pending culture results. A polymicrobial infection is common. The drain can be covered with a sterile gauze. It is not unusual for breast milk to leak around the drain because of severed lactiferous ducts. There are occasions when a breast abscess is treated with recurrent needle aspiration, but this is not currently the treatment of choice.

A recurrence of mastitis may happen for several reasons including inadequate antibiotic therapy. When a recurrence is evident, a breast milk culture is indicated as well as further exploration of the patient's breastfeeding management. Chronic mastitis may be treated with low doses of erythromycin (E-Mycin) 500 mg PO qd for the duration of lactation.

After antibiotic therapy, infection of the nipples with *Candida albicans* is not unusual. Topical treatment for the patient and concomitant oral nystatin for the infant is necessary. A fungal or *Candida* mastitis may develop, which is characterized by fiery pain shooting up the duct system. Oral antimycotic treatment would thus be indicated.

Follow-Up and Referral

The patient may best be served by referral to an International Board–Certified Lactation Consultant for professional evaluation and assistance with infant feeding. The lactation consultant evaluates and corrects problems related to the infant's feeding, which may be causing or contributing to the occurrence of infection. If a patient's symptoms are not resolved after reasonable treatment attempts, or if there is no change in the size or condition of a breast lump presumed to be a plugged duct after 48 hours of care and treatment, the patient must be referred for further diagnostic evaluation.

Patient Education

Appropriate patient teaching and breastfeeding management in the early postpartum period can be the best prevention tool for puerperal mastitis. Early and frequent infant feedings with correct latch and positioning is necessary. No harsh substances such as soaps and lotions should be put on the nipples, and correct bra sizing, rest, and diet instruction can all help with disease prevention.

Patients with periductal mastitis and duct ectasia need much support. The fear of carcinoma in this age group is high, and the patient must be reassured that this diagnosis has been considered and ruled out. Because of the prevalence of this condition, unclear cause, and uncertain absolute recovery, the patient only learns palliative and symptomatic treatment with a clear understanding of the disease process.

Bibliography

General

Alper, BS, and Forman, PD: Dysmenorrhea. Clin Advisor, Sept:68–75, 2004.

American Cancer Society. Cancer Facts & Figures 2003. Available at: http://www.cancer.org (Accessed December 15, 2005).

Barker, LR, Burton, JR, and Zieve, PD: Principles of Ambulatory Medicine, ed 6. Lippincott Williams & Wilkins, Philadelphia, 2003.

Bascom, A: Incorporating Herbal Medicine into Clinical Practice. FA Davis, Philadelphia, 2002.

Braunwald E, et al (eds): Harrison's Principles of Internal Medicine, ed 16. McGraw-Hill, New York, 2005.

Centers for Disease Control: CDC. STD treatment guidelines. Morb Mortal Wkly Rep, May 10, 2002.

Dambro, MR: Griffith's 5-Minute Clinical Consult. Lippincott Williams & Wilkins, Philadelphia, 2003.

Freeman, SB, Moore, A, and Wysocki, S: Menopause hormone therapy: Where do we go from here? Womens Health Care Pract J Nurse Pract 3(4):8–20, 2004.

Kee, JL: Laboratory and Diagnostic Tests with Nursing Implications, ed 6. Prentice-Hall, Upper Saddle River, N.J., 2002.

MacKay, HT: Gynecology. In Tierney, LM, et al (eds): Current Medical Diagnosis and Treatment, ed 44. Lange/McGraw-Hill, New York, 2005, pp 704–738.

McCance, KL, and Huether, SE: Pathophysiology: The Biologic Basis for Disease in Adults and Children, ed 5. CV Mosby, St. Louis, Mo., 2006.

Schettler, AE, and Gustafson, EM: Osteoporosis prevention starts in adolescence. J Am Acad Nurse Pract 16(7):274–282, 2004.

Smith, PE: Menopause: Assessment, treatment, and patient education. Nurse Pract 30(2):33–43, 2005.

Twiss, JJ, Dillon, AL, Konfrst, JM, Stauffer, J, and Paulman, A: The relationship of actual height loss with health-seeking behaviors and risk factors in perimenopausal and menopausal women. J Am Acad Nurse Pract 14(3):131–137, 2002.

Utian, WH: NAMS publishes hormone therapy recommendations. Female Patient 29(2):46–48, 2004.

Youngkin, E, and Davis, M: Women's Health: A Primary Care Clinical Guide, ed 3. Pearson/Prentice-Hall. Upper Saddle River, N.J., 2004.

Youngkin, E, et al: Pharmacotherapeutics: A Primary Care Guide, ed 2. Pearson/Prentice-Hall, Upper Saddle River, N.J., 2005.

Contraception

Bosarge, PM: Triphasic oral contraceptives: An alternative to monophasic formulations. Female Patient 29(Dec):19–27, 2004.

Cothran, MM, and Engberg, S: Vaginal Ring, an HT alternative. Nurse Pract 29(7):54–55, 2004.

Johnson, MJ, and Morgan, KW: Intrauterine contraception benefits extend beyond birth control. Nurse Pract 30(2):50–55, 2005.

Lakha, FH, and Glasier, A: Emergency contraception: What primary care clinicians need to know. Womens Health Primary Care 7(6):301–305, 2004.

Moore, A, and Clark, B: The transdermal contraceptive system: A unique look at patch users. Female Patient 29(July):7–11, 2004.

Nelson, AL, and Zieman, M: Emergency contraception: Not yet over the counter but still available. Female Patient 29(3):20–22, 2004.

Nelson, AL: Contraception doesn't work if you don't use it. Female Patient, April (Suppl):3–5, 2005.

Zieman, M, and Nelson, AL: Beyond forty: Do contraceptive needs change? Female Patient 29(July):45–46, 2004.

Ovarian Disorders

Luce, TL, Dow, KH, and Holcomb, L: Early diagnosis key to epithelial ovarian cancer detection. Nurse Pract 28(12):41–49, 2003.

White, M, Bradbury, A, and Olopade, OI: Breast and ovarian cancer risk assessment: Strategies for the primary care clinician. Womens Health Primary Care 5(8):519–526, 2002

Uterine/Cervical Disorders

ASCUS-LSIL Triage Study (ALTS) Group: A randomized trial on the management of low-grade intraepithelial lesion cytology interpretation. Am J Obstet Gynecol 188:1393–1400, 2003.

Arleo, EK, Masheb, RM, and Tal, MG: Uterine fibroids and sexual dysfunction: True, true, and related? Female Patient 29(July):47–50, 2004.

Berman, NR: Update on primary screening for cervical cancer prevention: Pap and HPV DNA testing. Womens Health Primary Care 7(10): 497–505, 2004.

Bradley, LD: Abnormal uterine bleeding. Nurse Pract 30(10):38–49, 2005.

Cooper, AS, and Boardman, LA: Diagnosing and treating vulvar pain syndromes: A clinical update. Womens Health Primary Care 8(1):37–43, 2005.

Hiller, JY, Miller, MJ, and Stavas, JM: Uterine artery embolization. Adv Nurse Pract Oct:20–26, 2005.

Israel, R: Uterine tumors: A new look at an old problem. Clin Advisor Aug: 34–41, 2004.

Khan, N, and Carr, BR: Endometriosis, Part 2: Treatment options. Female Patient 29(July):21–27,2004.

Majeroni, BA: The differential diagnosis of abnormal uterine bleeding: Changes through the life cycle. Womens Health Primary Care 8(1): 45–50, 2005.

Mancho, P, and Edwards, QT: Chaste tree for premenstrual syndrome. Adv Nurse Pract May:43–44, 2005.

Stemler, K: Abnormal uterine bleeding: A case study of menorrhagia. Nurse Pract 29(12):8–23, 2004.

Resources

American Society for Reproductive Medicine
1209 Montgomery Highway
Birmingham, AL 35216
Phone: (205) 978-5000
http://www.asrm.org

Centers for Disease Control and Prevention
http://www.cdc.gov

Fertilitext
http://www.fertilitext.org

International Council on Infertility Information Dissemination (INCIID)
P.O. Box 91363
Tucson, AZ 85752
Phone: (520) 554-9548

Internet Health Resources: Infertility Resources
http://www.ihr.com/infertility/

Resolve
1310 Broadway
Somerville, MA 02144
Phone: (617) 623-1156
Helpline: (617) 623-0744
http://www.resolve.org

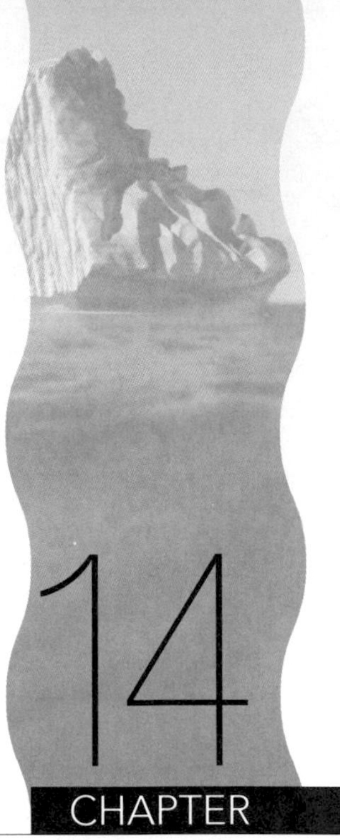

Musculoskeletal Problems

Lynne M. Dunphy, PhD, MSN, APRN, BC
Lori Martin Plank, MSPH, MSN, APRN, BC

Common Complaints

Musculoskeletal Pain and Dysfunction

Musculoskeletal pain and dysfunction accounts for approximately one out of every seven visits to a primary-care provider, which equates to approximately 315,000 million outpatient visits per annum. Because of the complex and ill-defined nature of this problem, and the variable differential diagnosis involved, the actual number of people affected is difficult to ascertain with true accuracy. Musculoskeletal problems in general are known to be the most frequent cause of disability in workers, and population surveys show a greater than 50 percent prevalence of musculoskeletal disorders among older Americans. Musculoskeletal problems may be acute (less than 6 weeks), chronic (more than 6 weeks in duration, i.e., Osteoarthritis [OA]), intermittent (gout), and additive (rheumatoid arthritis [RA]).

Musculoskeletal complaints are generally self-limiting. However, some musculoskeletal complaints, if left untreated, can lead to a cycle of progressive joint instability and a higher risk of subsequent injury if recovery is not complete. It is essential to rule out any musculoskeletal emergencies (Table 14.1). Delayed recognition of certain

Table 14.1 Musculoskeletal Emergencies

Clinical Manifestations	Musculoskeletal Emergencies: Differential Diagnoses
History	
Significant trauma	Soft tissue injury, internal derangement, fracture
Constitutional signs and symptoms (fever, weight loss, malaise)	Infection, sepsis, systemic rheumatic disease
Hot, swollen, painful joint	Infection, systemic rheumatic disease, gout, pseudogout
Physical Examination	
Weakness	
Focal	Compartment syndrome, entrapment neuropathy, mononeuritis, motor neuron disease, radiculopathy
Diffuse	Myositis, metabolic myopathy, paraneoplastic syndrome, degenerative neuromuscular disorder, toxin, myelopathy, transverse myelitis
Neurogenic pain (burning, numbness, paresthesia)	
Asymmetric	Radiculopathy, reflex sympathetic dystrophy, entrapment neuropathy
Symmetric	Myelopathy, peripheral neuropathy
Claudication pain pattern	Peripheral vascular disease, giant cell arteritis (with jaw pain), lumbar spinal stenosis

diagnoses may lead to permanent disability or death. Once these diagnoses have been excluded, proceed with an orderly evaluation of other diagnostic possibilities.

A useful approach to the initial patient encounter is to determine whether the musculoskeletal complaint is (1) articular or nonarticular in origin; (2) inflammatory or noninflammatory in nature; (3) acute or chronic in duration; and (4) localized or systemic in distribution. Musculoskeletal complaints can be a diagnostic challenge for the primary-care provider. There are no routine tests that can be employed in clinical practice to determine the presence of inflammation or muscle spasm. Much of the diagnosis is dependent of patient self-reporting of symptoms. Often, musculoskeletal problems present with the patient's chief complaint being one of "aches and pains" in one body part or another, or as a generalized phenomenon. In addition, some patients will not fit immediately into any clear diagnostic category. Many musculoskeletal disorders resemble each other at onset, and some may take weeks or months to evolve into an identifiable diagnosis. Differential diagnoses of musculoskeletal problems include trauma, infection, metabolic or circulatory disorders, tumors, synovial conditions, congenital or developmental problems, or degenerative disorders.

Identifying the anatomic location of the musculoskeletal complaint is important, but can be difficult. Wrist pain, for example, may be a manifestation of any number of pathologic conditions that involve a variety of anatomic structures. This may include gonococcal arthritis, fracture, cellulitis, neuropathies, carpal tunnel syndrome (classified as an "overuse" syndrome), gout, and tumor. First distinguish between articular and nonarticular structures (Table 14.2). Articular structures include the synovium, synovial fluid, articular cartilage, intraarticular ligaments, joint capsule, and juxtaarticular bone. Disorders of these structures tend to be characterized by deep or diffuse pain, limited range of motion (ROM) on active and passive movement, swelling (caused by synovial proliferation, effusion, or bony enlargement), crepitation, instability, "locking," or deformity. Nonarticular (or periarticular) structures are identified as supportive extra-articular ligaments, tendons, bursae, muscle, fascia, bone, nerve, and overlying skin. Nonarticular disorders are characterized by painful on active but not passive ROM, demonstrated point or focal tenderness in regions distinct from articular structures, and physical findings far from the joint capsule. It is unlikely to see crepitus, instability, or deformity associated with these disorders.

Inflammatory disorders may be infectious or idiopathic. These may be identified by the presence of all or some of the four cardinal signs of inflammation (erythema, warmth, pain, or swelling), systemic symptoms (fatigue, weight loss, morning stiffness, fever), or laboratory evidence of inflammation (elevated erythrosedimentation rate [ESR] or C-reactive protein, anemia of chronic disease, hypoalbuminemia, or thrombocytosis). Noninflammatory disorders tend to be related to trauma (meniscus tear), ineffective repair (OA), neoplasm, or pain amplification (fibromyalgia). There may be pain without swelling or warmth, absence of inflammatory or systemic features, minimal or absent morning stiffness, and normal (for age) laboratory testing (Table 14.3).

The differential diagnoses may be narrowed by the identification of the underlying pathologic process and the exact site of the complaint. This helps to determine whether there is need for immediate diagnostic or therapeutic intervention, or for continued observation.

The clinical history should include the patient profile, including age, sex, race, and family history. The chronology of the complaint gives important diagnostic clues and may be divided into onset (i.e., abrupt), evolution (chronic, intermittent, migratory), and duration. The number and distribution of involved articulations should be noted. Articular disorders are classified based on the number of involved joints: monoarticular (one joint), periarticular (two to four joints), or polyarticular (more than four joints). Nonarticular disorders are classified as either focal or widespread. Precipitating events such as trauma or drug ingestion must be documented, as well as antecedent or current illnesses that may contribute to the patient's complaint. A review of systems may provide useful diagnostic information, eliciting systemic features of diseases such as fever (SLE, infection). Musculoskeletal complaints may be associated with other organ systems, for example, such as the nervous system (Lyme disease, vasculitis), eye (sarcoidosis, Reiter's syndrome), and gastrointestinal tract (scleroderma, inflammatory bowel disease), to name just a few. (See Focusing the History 14.1.)

Guided by the history, the physical examination helps to distinguish between mechanical problems, soft

Table 14.2 Comparison of Articular and Nonarticular Structures

Articular Structures	Nonarticular Structures
Synovium and synovial fluid	Supportive extra-articular ligaments
Articular cartilage, intra-articular ligaments	Bone
Joint capsule	Nerve, overlaying skin
Juxta-articular bone	Muscle, tendons, fascia

Table 14.3 Examples of Disorders of Inflammation versus Noninflammation

Inflammatory MS Disorders	Noninflammatory MS Disorders
Infectious	Ineffective repair (OA)
Crystal-induced	Pain amplification (fibromyalgia)
Immune-related (RA, SLE)	Trauma
Idiopathic	Neoplasm

FOCUS ON HISTORY 14.1

Musculoskeletal Problems

Questions to ask:

1. Have you injured yourself?
2. Describe exactly how your injury occurred:
   When the injury occurred, did it make a noise or sound? If so, describe the sound.
3. Where does it hurt? Does the pain radiate, or is it localized, or diffuse?
4. Do you have numbness or tingling.
5. Is there loss of function?
6. Is there swelling?
7. When did the pain first occur?
   What relieves it?
   What exacerbates it?
   What time of day does it occur?
   Does the pain awaken you at night?
8. Is there joint stiffness?
   Does activity make it worse or better?
9. Do you have any other symptoms (or systemic processes)?
   Do you have a fever?
   Do you have a rash?
   Do you have general fatigue?
   Have you recently been traveling or camping?
   Have you recently been immunized?
   Have you recently been treated with antibiotics?
   Do you have a history of upper respiratory infection? Sexually transmitted disease? Chronic disease?
   Were you ever treated with steroids?
10. Describe your daily activities—work, hobbies, home.

tissue disease, and noninflammatory and inflammatory joint disease. A major goal of the examination is to detect warmth over a joint, joint effusion, and pain on joint motion. These are hallmarks of synovitis. Limitations in movement and instability are also important to assess and are of particular concern in knee and ankle pain. The medial and lateral collateral ligaments of the knee can be assessed by valgus and varus stress of the joint. Excess laxity of the knee on anterior drawer test may indicate an anterior cruciate ligament tear.

If the patient complains about a specific anatomic area, examine that area initially to recognize, for instance, a frozen shoulder, or hip trochanteric bursitis with pain over the greater trochanter. If the patient reports a history of hand numbness that awakens the him or her at night, this clearly suggests carpal tunnel syndrome even with no physical findings. Foot pain that begins the first thing in the morning when the patient puts his or her foot out of bed is suggestive of plantar fasciitis or early RA.

The combination of point tenderness, reduced active ROM, and preserved passive range of motion suggests soft tissue disorders, including bursitis, tendinitis, or muscle injury. If both active and passive ROM are limited, soft tissue contracture, synovitis, or a structural abnormality of the joint is possible. Tendinitis may be suggested by tenderness to palpation along the course of the tendon, or pain or rub produced when the tendon is stretched or stressed during active ROM against resistance. Inability to actively abduct the shoulder fully is suggestive of a rotator cuff tear. Crepitus (joint noises or palpable grinding during joint motion) may be due to articular surface abnormalities or synovitis. Crepitus not associated with pain or limitation of motion is generally of no clinical significance.

If there was a target area, after it has been examined—or if the patient reports diffuse generalized musculoskeletal pain—a simple evaluation may begin with gentle palpation of the hands. Bony enlargements of the distal interphalangeal (DIP) joints or Heberden's nodes are indicative of OA, or soft-tissue swelling of inflammatory arthritis that may indicate RA; inflammation may also be indicated by swelling of the metacarpophalangeal (MCP) joints. If symmetrical swelling has been present for longer than 6 months, a presumptive diagnosis of RA may be made, regardless of laboratory results. Limitations of flexion and/or extension of the wrist are a sign of prior inflammation and a clue to earlier chronic RA.

The shoulders can be examined by asking the patient to raise his or her arms above the head, put hands behind the head, and hands behind the back. Tender points in the muscles of the neck, shoulders and back—a characteristic sign of fibromyalgia—are easily recognized by an experienced examiner. Ask the patient to rise from a chair without holding on. If the patient cannot do this, there is an abnormality of the joints, nerves, or muscles, which requires further examination usually by a specialist. Ask the patient to walk a few steps across the room and back and observe the gait. This should be included in all evaluations.

Have the patient lie down to review motion of the hips, knees, ankles, and feet. It is important to recognize flexion contractures in which a patient cannot fully extend to 180 degrees the PIP joints, elbows, hips, or knees and has limited motion of the wrists, which if not congenital or due to injury (ask the patient), is a sign of prior inflammation. All maneuvers described should take less than 2 minutes and should be included in the "general" physical exam. Note any endocrinopathies (irregular heart rhythms, weight gain, and thyromegaly) and malignancy (severe pain, weight loss, or palpable masses). In addition, muscle strength and function should be systematically evaluated. (See Advanced Assessment 14.1.) On physical exam, evidence of tender points and trigger points, as well as the absence of inflammation or swollen joints, increases the likelihood of a soft tissue problem.

Extra-articular abnormalities such as oral/nasal ulcers, iritis, rash, nodules, pericardial or pulmonary rub, enlargement of liver, spleen, or lymph nodes, and neurologic abnormalities suggest a systemic disease.

ADVANCED ASSESSMENT 14.1

Grading of Manual Muscle Testing

Numeric Grade	Descriptive Grade	Description
5	Normal	Complete ROM against gravity with full or normal resistance
4	Good	Complete ROM against gravity with some resistance
3	Fair	Complete ROM against gravity
2	Poor	Complete range of motion with gravity eliminated
1	Trace	Muscle contraction but no or very limited joint motion
0	Zero	No evidence of muscle function

An accurate diagnosis of injury and/or rheumatic diseases can best be accomplished with careful history and physical exam by an experienced clinician. At the same time, it should be recognized that in some patients—perhaps as many as 10 percent—a definitive diagnosis sometimes cannot be established, particularly at the first visit, and sometimes even over time. This is especially true in cases of chronic musculoskeletal pain. The diagnosis is not as important as the approach to treatment, which typically is similar for a range of diagnoses within three primary categories of rheumatic disease based on (1) inflammation (e.g., RA); (2) structural damage (OA); or (3) muscle tension (fibromyalgia) (see Table 14.3).

Diagnostic Reasoning

Diagnostic Tests

Laboratory tests may be of limited use. One problem with using laboratory tests in the diagnosis of rheumatic diseases is the fact that many, if not most, people who have been told that they have systemic lupus erythematosus (SLE), gout, and Lyme disease do not have the disease at all, but simply an abnormal laboratory test such as a positive ANA, elevated uric acid, or positive Lyme antibody test. These tests are abnormal in at least 5 percent of the general population, while the diseases identified are seen in fewer than 1 percent. Therefore, most individuals with positive laboratory tests do not have the associated disease. In contrast, many people with RA for example often have normal blood tests and x-ray findings, particularly in early disease, when aggressive treatment might be most effective. Some of these tests are useful to research laboratories in the identification and understanding of pathogenic mechanisms, but do not add anything to the meaningful diagnosis and management of the patient. A review of associated laboratory tests is presented here.

- Complete blood count (CBC)—the presence of anemia may be a clue to inflammation and leukopenia is seen in active SLE
- Erythrocyte sedimentation rate (ESR) and C-reactive protein—nonspecific indicators of inflammation. A highly elevated value indicates a likelihood of inflammatory rheumatic disease, infection, or malignancy. ESR increases with age, as does CRP, and some people (as many as 5 to 10 percent of the general population) have elevated values with no explanation. Up to 40 percent of patients who present with RA have normal ESRs and CRPs. The ESR is almost always markedly elevated, and therefore diagnostically useful in patients with giant cell arteritis and polymyalgia rheumatica.
- Rheumatoid factor (RF)—25 percent of patients with RA never have an elevated RF. It may also be elevated with other inflammatory conditions (e.g., SLE, subacute bacterial endocarditis, vasculitis, viral infection) and may also be RF positive. Diagnosis of RA should never be based solely on the results of RA testing, although the higher the RF titer the greater the likelihood of a positive RF being related to RA.
- Fluorescent antinuclear antibody (ANA) test—this test is positive in 99 percent of patients with SLE; however, it is also positive in 5 to 10 percent of normal blood donors, meaning only 1 in 100 people with a positive ANA has SLE. A positive ANA may also develop as a result of drug use (procainamide, hydralazine); it may be transiently positive in people with a severe infection; and it is positive in a high percentage of people with other inflammatory rheumatic conditions including RA (30 to 50 percent), scleroderma (20 to 50 percent), polymyositis (10 to 30 percent), and idiopathic pulmonary fibrosis (10 to 20 percent).
- Lyme borreliosis antibodies—Lyme disease is identified serologically by antibodies to the Lyme *Borrelia* organism. From 5 percent to 10 percent of normal individuals have a positive Lyme borreliosis titer, even in the best laboratories. A test for Lyme disease is not appropriate in patients with unexplained arthritis.
- Uric acid—Uric acid measurement is often included in evaluation of patients with musculoskeletal symptoms, as elevated uric acid resulting from either overproduction or underexcretion is seen in more than 90 percent of people with gout. However, most people with elevated uric acid levels do not have gout. A test for uric acid therefore should be reserved for patients who have clinical evidence of episodic or atypical inflammatory arthritis. Alcohol and diuretics may cause moderately elevated uric acid levels. Asymptomatic hyperuricemia should not be treated. Further, some individuals with gout have normal serum acid levels, particularly at the time of the

acute attack. A definitive diagnosis of gout requires identification of uric acid crystals in synovial fluid.

- ▲ Screening panels—these tests are available from all national laboratories and are marketed as "rheumatology screening panels" to rule out an inflammatory rheumatic disease. The simplest include rheumatoid factor, ANA, and uric acid although more elaborate tests are available. These screens tend to be a major source of potential false-positive information in patient evaluations and not advised for use by the general practitioner.

Imaging studies are indicated when examination cannot localize the anatomic structure that is causing symptoms; after a significant trauma; when there is a loss of joint function (e.g., unable to bear weight); when pain continues despite conservative management; when a fracture or bone infection is suspected; or when there is a history of malignancy. Plain radiographs will be unrevealing or unhelpful (and are therefore not indicated) for most patients with acute and new symptoms of RA, SLE, gout, mechanical back pain, or tendinitis/bursitis.

Radiographs may confirm the diagnosis of OA and assess its severity, but normal findings on radiographs do not rule out the presence of OA. The earliest radiographic changes in RA are nonspecific and include soft tissue swelling and periarticular osteoporosis, but these features are often absent at the initial presentation. In established RA or long-standing gout, erosions may be diagnostic: marginal erosions in the former, and evidence of reparative process in the latter. Radiography (plain x-ray films) can reveal the following:

- ▲ Erosions
- ▲ Calcifications and cysts
- ▲ Osteopenia
- ▲ Narrowing of joint spaces
- ▲ Deformity of bones
- ▲ Separations (fractures, dislocations)

Repeat radiographs after 7 to 10 days are appropriate when a fracture is suspected despite an unrevealing initial examination; because callus formation or abnormal alignment may be evident. Repeated imaging over time in patients with established rheumatic disease may be useful in assessing structural damage. For patients with typical acute mechanical low back pain, a plain radiograph adds little to the management decisions.

Ultrasonography may be useful in the detection of soft tissue abnormalities, but is the preferred method of evaluation in only a few circumstances. The foremost application of ultrasound is in the diagnosis of synovial (Baker's) cysts, although rotator cuff tears and various tendon injuries may be identified by ultrasound.

Computed tomography (CT) has proved most useful in the evaluation of the axial skeleton because of its ability to visualize in the axial plane. CT has been demonstrated to be useful in the diagnosis of low back pain syndromes (herniated intervertebral disk, spinal stenosis, spinal trauma), intra-articular osteochondral fragments, and advanced osteonecrosis. Helical or spiral CT can be useful in the detection of obscure fractures.

Magnetic resonance imaging (MRI) or radionuclide bone scanning is useful when specific disorders are suspected and the management could be altered according to findings. Rotator cuff tear, spinal stenosis, avascular necrosis of bone, or mechanical derangement of the knee are some conditions that may be revealed with an MRI. A bone scan may be useful when osteomyelitis, stress fractures, or bony metastases are a concern. In general, MRI is useful for assessing soft tissue and spinal cord elements, whereas nuclear medicine studies are best for assessing bone turnover. MRI and bone scanning are expensive and the latter exposes patients to significant radiation. Rotator cuff degeneration and disk abnormalities are quite common in older patients. These studies should be reserved for patients in whom specific disorders are suspected, when the diagnosis cannot be made in a less costly manner, and only after a thorough history and physical examination.

Nerve conduction studies (electromyography [EMG]) may be indicated when neurologic abnormalities or paresthesias are present.

Differential Diagnosis

Joint symptoms of one and up to a few joints may be due to trauma, infection, crystal-induced inflammation (gout, pseudogout), or primary inflammatory arthritis (including spondyloarthropathies and atypical presentation of RA). In acute monoarthritis, it is essential that infection of a joint be diagnosed or excluded, and this can be done only via joint aspiration (see Therapeutic Procedure 14.1) and synovial fluid analysis and culture (see Advanced Assessment 14.2). Chronic monarticular symptoms with little or no effusion are usually from OA. Tendinitis and bursitis generally involve one joint region and physical exam is usually diagnostic. Common syndromes include de Quervain's tenosynovitis, olecranon bursitis, medial and lateral epicondylitis, bicipital and rotator cuff tendinitis, rotator cuff teat, trochanteric bursitis, patellar bursitis and prepatellar bursitis, anserine bursitis, plantar fasciitis, posterior tibial tendinitis, and Achilles tendinitis.

Polyarthritis has an extensive differential diagnosis. The presence of prolonged morning stiffness, systemic symptoms, Raynaud's phenomenon, rash, or sicca symptoms, and manifestations of other organ involvement suggest a rheumatic disease. The specific evaluation is guided by the clinical manifestations and should screen organ symptoms that can be involved without overt signs, such as the lung, heart, liver, kidney, and bowel, for potential involvement. Precise diagnosis and management usually requires referral.

Arthralgia and/or myalgia without physical findings has an extensive differential diagnosis. Often, no definitive diagnosis is possible at the initial presentation. Common causes include fibromyalgia, viral infection, an overuse syndrome (tendon strain associated with repetitive motion injuries or muscle fatigue), a neuropathy (e.g., carpal

THERAPEUTIC PROCEDURE 14.1

Arthrocentesis

Joint	Technique
Ankle	*Patient position:* Supine, with foot in plantar flexion *Needle size:* 20–22 gauge $1^1/_2$" *Syringe size:* 10–30 mL and 2–5 mL *Procedure:* Locate the space between the medial malleolus and extensor hallucis tendon. Using an anteromedial approach, enter lateral to the medial malleolus, medial to the tendon, and aim the needle downward, laterally. Insert the needle $1^1/_4$"(3 cm).
Elbow	*Patient position:* Sitting, with elbow flexed to 90 degrees with the palm pronated on a table *Needle size:* 20–22 gauge $1^1/_2$" *Syringe size:* 10–30 mL and 2–5 mL *Procedure:* Locate the space between the lateral epicondyle of the humerus and olecranon process ($^3/_8$" below the epicondyle). Using a posterolateral approach, insert the needle and direct it medially and slightly toward the hand. Insert the needle $^5/_8$" (1.5 cm).
Knee	*Patient position:* Supine, with knee fully extended or bent slightly to 20 degrees over a rolled towel under the knee *Needle size:* 18–20 gauge $1^1/_2$" *Syringe size:* 10–30 mL and 2–5 mL *Procedure:* Locate the joint space by moving medially from midpatella to a point halfway between the patella and underlying the femoral condyle. Using an anteromedial approach, aim the needle posteriorly (downward) and laterally. Insert the needle $^3/_8$"–$^5/_8$".
Knee (patient unable to extend knee)	*Patient position:* Sitting, with knee flexed 90 degrees over edge of examining table *Needle size:* 18–20 gauge $1^1/_2$". *Syringe size:* 10–30 mL and 2–5 mL *Procedure:* Locate the triangle formed by the tendon and condyles. Using an anteromedial or lateral approach, enter distal to apex of patella medially or laterally to the tendon. Direct the needle slightly cephalad to a depth of $1^3/_8$"–$1^3/_4$".
Wrist	*Patient position:* Sitting, with palm pronated over a rolled towel, wrist flexed 20–30 degrees and with a slight ulnar turn *Needle size:* 24–26 gauge $^5/_8$" *Syringe size:* 10–30 mL and 2–5 mL *Procedure:* Locate the space between the bony processes of the radius and ulna and just lateral to the tendon. Using a dorsal approach, enter distal to the space and perpendicular to the skin. Insert the needle downward $^3/_8$"–$^3/_4$".

ADVANCED ASSESSMENT 14.2

Synovial Fluid Analysis

	Normal	Grade I: Noninflammatory	Grade II: Inflammatory	Grade III: Infectious
Visual analysis	Clear, straw-colored	Clear or slightly bloody and turbid	Turbid	Turbid, gray or yellow
Viscosity	Normal	Decreased	Decreased	Decreased
WBC per mm^3	30–150	<2500	2500 to 25,000	>50,000
PMNs (%)	<20	20–50	50–70	70–90
Protein (g/dL)	1–4	1–5	3–6	3–7
Examples		OA, SLE, mechanical derangement	RA, gonococcal arthritis, rheumatic fever, gout, pseudogout, Reiter's syndrome	Septic arthritis, tuberculosis

tunnel syndrome) or hypothyroidism. If the history and physical exam do not provide a diagnosis, symptomatic management and reassessment over several weeks is more productive initially than is laboratory testing or diagnostic imaging.

After ruling out joint pain, trauma, overuse syndromes, and vascular components, primary differential diagnoses for muscle pain (myalgia) typically include infectious causes, such as viral syndromes, mononucleosis, Rocky Mountain spotted fever, or Lyme disease; systemic disorders such as fibromyalgia (FM) or polymyalgia rheumatica (PMR); or psychogenic causes. More than one syndrome may occur concomitantly. For example, a bursitis may coexist with pain from FM. If the inflammation from the bursitis is overlooked, the patient may not receive the treatment indicated for the acute disorder (Fig. 14.1).

Acute Musculoskeletal Injury

Acute musculoskeletal injury encompasses a number of common conditions characterized by acute pain and/or muscular spasm (persistent, painful, and reversible contracture of striated muscle). These symptoms any be caused by specific syndromes, such as low back pain and ankle sprain with well-documented and tested treatment guidelines; specific syndromes such as torticollis and "tennis elbow" with less well tested management guidelines; and a large group of disorders characterized by nonspecific musculoskeletal trauma, which results in tissue derangement that can lead to pain, limitations of movement, spasm, and the inability to perform activities of daily living. Sometimes a traumatic injury, such as from a car accident, or other significant precipitating factor, such as lifting a heavy object, may be identified as the initiating factor. In some cases a trivial movement such as bending over to tie a shoe, or coughing, may precipitate the injury. Acute musculoskeletal injury implies pain of less than 6 weeks' duration. (See Differential Diagnosis 14.1.)

The following are management principles in acute musculoskeletal pain/injury:

- ▲ Reassurance—most injuries self-limiting and improvement should occur within approximately 2 weeks.
- ▲ Limitation of activity—immobilization of injury is appropriate during diagnostic phase; if appropriate at all, bedrest should be limited to the most acute period (2 days or less) to control spasm and promote healing.
- ▲ Physical therapy—may include heat or cold application with the goal being to return patient to full function as soon as possible with minimal limitation. Commonly cold/ice is recommended × 48°; then heat.
- ▲ Skeletal muscle relaxants—a 1- to 2-week course is valuable when injury is accompanied by spasm or tightness. Be aware of potential for sedation and abuse. (See Drugs Commonly Prescribed 14.1).
- ▲ Nonsteroidal anti-inflammatory drugs (NSAIDs)/acetaminophen—first-line choices (see Drugs Commonly Prescribed 14.2). Need to be started asap; if no relief in 2 to 3 days, probably will not be effective.
- ▲ Opioids—useful for moderate or severe pain or if sedation desired—monitor adverse effects such as constipation, abuse potential.
- ▲ Other treatment choices—topical analgesia, antiepileptic agents, manual therapy (massage, chiropractic care), antidepressants may be useful adjunctive therapy in chronic pain syndromes.
- ▲ Referral—to pain specialist as appropriate; no relief with conventional methods, high risk of drug interactions.
- ▲ Imaging studies—radiograph, CT, MRI are *NOT* indicated for acute musculoskeletal NSAIDs/acetaminophen—first-line choices.

Muscle Cramps

Muscle cramps may be described as sudden, involuntary, painful contractions of a muscle or muscle part that last from seconds to several minutes. Cramps may occur spontaneously, while at rest, or may be precipitated by a brief muscle contraction. The cause is usually related to some hyperexcitability of the motor neurons supplying the muscles. In many cases, the reason for episodic, recurrent muscle cramps may remain unclear, even after complete diagnostic evaluation. Muscle cramps may also occur related to vigorous exercise and during sporting events. Monitor for dehydration.

Differential Diagnosis

The initial history should elicit whether the cramps occur with exercise or at rest. In pregnant women and children, leg cramps tend to occur at rest, and are most often benign, requiring no treatment. Certain medications (e.g., some diuretics, some of the statin drugs, and clofibrate [Atromid-S]) may cause muscle cramping. Leg pain and cramps in adults that are precipitated by exercise and relieved by rest are usually caused by peripheral vascular disease. Blood chemistry tests may be necessary, including serum enzymes, to rule out causes such as dehydration (from diarrhea or sweating) (See Differential Diagnosis 14.2.)

Paresthesias

Paresthesia is the sensation of numbness, prickling, or tingling experienced in central and peripheral nerve lesions. Frequently, the patient's understanding and use of the terms will differ from the clinician's; therefore, it is necessary to clearly establish the character of the patient's complaint. During the history, take time to differentiate between the lack of use of a limb from the sensation of tingling and numbness and the total loss of sensation. It is also important

(Text continued on page 728)

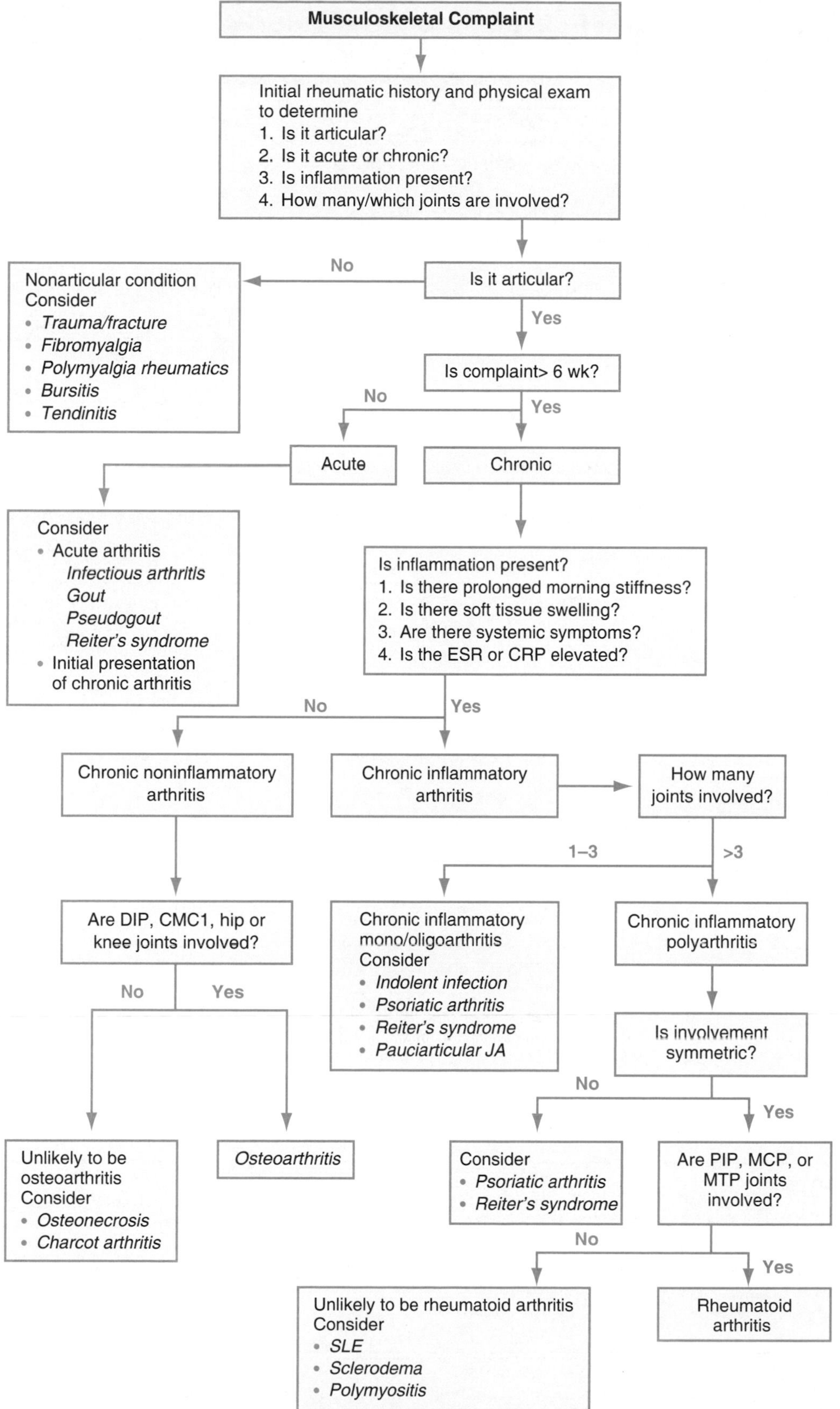

FIGURE 14.1 Diagnosis of musculoskeletal complaints. (*Source*: Kasper, DL, et al: Harrison's Principles of Internal Medicine, ed 16. McGraw-Hill, New York, 2004.)

DIFFERENTIAL DIAGNOSIS 14.1

Classification of Sprains

Grade	Degree of Injury	Treatment
Grade I	Partial tear; no instability, or opening of the joint on stress maneuvers	Symptomatic only
Grade II	Partial tear with some instability indicated by partial opening of the joint on stress maneuvers	Immobilization to protect injured part, but full healing expected
Grade III	Complete tear with complete opening of joint on stress	Immobilization; possible repair

Drugs Commonly Prescribed 14.1: Skeletal Muscle Relaxants

Drug Name	Dose	Comments
Equagesic—meprobamate (200 mg) and aspirin (325 mg)	One to two tablets three to four times daily For short-term use only	Musculoskeletal pain, anxiety, tension CNS depressant
Cyclobenzaprine HCl (Flexeril)	5–10 mg PO three times daily Maximum of 2–3 weeks	Non-neurogenic acute muscle spasm, as adjunct to rest and physical therapy Drowsiness
Orphenadrine—Norflex (anticholinergic muscle relaxant [central])	100 mg twice daily PO (morning and evening) 60 mg IM/IV q12h	Painful musculoskeletal conditions Potentiates anticholinergics, alcohol, other CNS depressants.
Norgesic Forte—orphenadrine citrate 50 mg, aspirin 770 mg, caffeine 60 mg	One-half to one tablet up to four times daily (maximum dose)	Muscle relaxant Increased risk of GI bleed
Chlorzoxazone (Parafon Forte DSC)	500 mg four times daily	Muscle relaxant (central) May potentiate alcohol, other CNS depressants.
Methocarbamol (Robaxin)	500 mg tablets; also Robaxin 750 tablets initially 1.5 g four times daily times 2 to 3 days; maintenance 4 g daily; also injectable (10 mL IM/IV three times daily for 2–3 days)	Muscle relaxant (central) May potentiate alcohol, other CNS depressants.
Metaxalone (Skelaxin)	800 mg three to four times daily	Muscle relaxant (central) May potentiate alcohol, other CNS depressants.
Carisoprodol (Soma)	350 mg four times daily	Muscle relaxant (central) May potentiate alcohol, other CNS depressants.
Diazepam (Valium)	2–10 mg three to four times daily Also injectable 5 mg/mL 5–10 mg IV (slow) or IM Do not use longer than 6 months	Skeletal muscle relaxant May potentiate alcohol, other CNS depressants.
Tizanidine HCl (Zanaflex)	Tablets/capsules Initially 4 mg; may increase by 2–3 mg PRN q6–8h To a maximum of three doses in 24 hours; maximum 12 mg/dose and 36 mg/day	Muscle spasticity May potentiate alcohol, other CNS depressants.

Drugs Commonly Prescribed 14.2: Types of NSAIDs

Drug	Dose	Comments
	Salicylates	
Aspirin—available in 300-, 325-, 600-, 650-mg tablets	325 mg qid	SE: tinnitus, GI irritation (take with food)
Choline magnesium trisalicylate (Trilisate)—available in 500-, 750-, 1000-mg tablets	1500 mg bid	SE: as above
Salsalate (Disalcid)—500-, 750-mg tablets	1000 mg tid; 1500 mg bid	SE: as above
Diflunisal (Dolobid)—500-mg tablet	250 mg bid or tid; 500 mg bid	SE: as above
	Propionic Acids	
Naproxen sodium (Aleve)—220 mg tablets; (Naprelan)—375-, 500-mg tablets—(Anaprox)—275-, DS 550-mg tablets	Aleve—220 mg bid Naprelan—750–1000 mg/day Anaprox—275 mg bid or tid; 550 mg bid	SE: GI irritation (take with food)
Naproxen (Naprosyn)—250-, 375-, 500-mg tablets	250, 375, or 500 mg bid	
Flurbiprofen (Ansaid)—50-, 100-mg tablets	100 mg bid	
Oxaprozin (Daypro)—600-mg tablets	600–1200 mg/day	
Ibuprofen (Motrin)—400-, 600-, 800-mg tablets	400–800 mg bid or tid	
Ketoprofen (Orudis)—25-, 50-, 75-mg tablets	50 mg qid, 75 mg tid	
Ketoprofen extended release (Oruvail)—100-, 150-, 200-mg tablets	200 mg/day	
Ketorolac tromethamine (Toradol oral)—10-mg tablets	10 mg qid; 5 days maximum of oral and IM combined	
	Indoleacetic Acids and Related Compounds	
Sulindac (Clinoril)—150-, 200-mg tablets	150–200 mg bid	Side effects: increased risk GI toxicity with aspirin, other NSAIDs, alcohol, smoking.
Indomethacin (Indocin)—25-, 50-mg tablets	25–50 mg tid	Side effects: GI irritation—take with food; avoid salicylates, other NSAIDs; increases serum lithium levels.
Indomethacin sustained release (Indocin SR)—75-mg tablets	25–50 mg tid	Side effects: GI irritation—take with food; avoid salicylates, other NSAIDs, increases serum lithium levels.
Etodolac (Lodine)—200–500-mg tablets	200–400 mg tid, 500 mg	Side effects: dyspepsia, edema; avoid salicylates; monitor anticoagulants, cyclosporine, lithium, digoxin.
Meloxicam (Mobic)—7.5-, 15-mg tablets	7.5–15 mg qd	Side effects: increased risk GI bleed with aspirin, oral corticosteroids, anticoagulants.
Nabumetone (Relafen)—500-, 750-mg tablets	1 g per day in divided doses	Side effects: take with food—GI irritation; monitor oral anticoagulants; monitor hypertension.
Diclofenac sodium (Voltaren-XR)—100-mg tablets	100 mg qd	Side effects: peptic ulcers—take with food; SGPT/SGOT in 4 weeks, then periodically. Can interact with digoxin, methotrexate, cyclosporine, lithium.
Piroxicam (Feldene)—10-, 20-mg caps	20 mg daily; may give in two divided doses	Side effects: may potentiate oral anticoagulants; GI bleed—take with food.

DIFFERENTIAL DIAGNOSIS 14.2

Muscle Cramps

Symptom	Possible Diagnosis
Cramp-like symptoms	Intermittent claudication related to ischemia; drug-induced (such as statin-induced myopathy)
Contracture	Thyroid disease, McArdle's disease
Tetany	Hypoglycemia, hypomagnesia, respiratory alkalosis, hypokalemia
Dystonia	Occupational (such as writer's cramp) Drug-induced (antipsychotics, anti-Parkinsonian) metabolic/neurologic
True cramps	Ordinary (nocturnal), dehydration, drug-induced (nifedipine, beta-agonists), lower motor neuron, hemodialysis (volume and electrolyte shifts), heat induced (volume depletion, hyponatremia)

SOURCE: Adapted From McGee SK: Muscle cramp. Arch Intern Med 150:571, 1990.

to ascertain if the loss or altered sensation ascends onto the abdomen or thorax.

The location of the paresthesia may be focal or generalized. It may also be nonspecific, as in multiple sclerosis, in which the initial presentation may be bilateral diminution of sensation or paresthesia in the upper or lower extremities, or unilateral, as in stroke or transient ischemic attacks (TIAs), in which unilateral extremity or face paresthesias may occur.

Paresthesias are also likely to be a result of anatomic or mechanical peripheral nerve injury, such as entrapment and compression neuropathies. These are most likely to occur at sites that are more susceptible to damage from an increase in pressure and mechanical forces, such as entrapment or compression of the medial nerve at the wrist (carpal tunnel syndrome), the ulnar nerve at the elbow, and the peroneal nerve at the knee.

Paresthesias also occur as a result of nerve-root injury, chlorinated hydrocarbon exposure, respiratory alkalosis, and the use of certain drugs, such as carbonic anhydrase inhibitors (which are used in the treatment of glaucoma).

The physical examination must determine if the sensory abnormality follows the distribution of a peripheral nerve or nerve root. Commonly affected nerves are cervical nerve roots 5 to 8 (C5 to C8); ulnar and radial nerves of the hand; lumbar nerves 3, 4, 5, and S1; obturator, sciatic, and femoral nerves in the thigh; and peroneal and tibial nerves of the foot. (See Advanced Assessment 14.3.)

Differential Diagnosis

Cervical Radiculopathy

Cervical radiculopathy is commonly caused by compression of the cervical nerve roots, when the cervical disks place stress on the vertebral bodies. It usually is the result of age-related changes, cervical spondylosis, or a herniated disk. The most commonly involved nerve roots are C6 and C7, which produce paresthesias into the lower lateral arm, thumb, and middle finger.

Diagnostic tests include radiologic assessment of the cervical spine, and, if radicular pain is severe or if there is motor or sensory deficit or hyporeflexia, MRI is indicated. If only radiculopathy is present, a conservative trial of cervical traction as in the use of a soft cervical collar is occasionally used. In severe cases, a myelogram may be necessary to rule out neoplasm and to define the extent of compression. Surgery may be considered, but no long-term outcome studies have compared the benefits of surgery to nonoperative treatments such as heat and cold, ROM exercises, and limiting activity during acute outbreaks.

Brachial Plexus Neuritis or Radiculitis

Brachial plexus injuries include a broad array of neurologic dysfunction ranging from momentary paresthesias to completely flail extremities. The mechanism of injury is equally diverse, from high-energy motor vehicle crashes, falls from a height, and gunshot wounds, to lower-energy injuries such as most athletic injuries. "Burners" or "stingers" (transient brachial plexopathy) are transient injuries to the upper trunk

ADVANCED ASSESSMENT 14.3

Paresthesias and Affected Nerve Roots

Nerve Root	Paresthesia
C6 (6th cervical)	Thumb: dorsal and lateral aspects
C7 (7th cervical)	Fingers: index and middle
C8 (8th cervical)	Fingers: fifth and ulnar half of fourth Hand: ulnar side
L4 (4th lumbar)	Thigh: anterior, just above knee
L5 (5th lumbar)	Foot: dorsal aspect Great toe: dorsal aspect
S1 (1st sacral)	Foot: lateral aspect Small toe: lateral aspect

of the brachial plexus involving the C5 and C6 nerve roots. The most common mechanism of injury is a traction force when the shoulder is forcefully depressed and the head and neck are tilted toward the opposite side or compression of the upper plexus between the shoulder pad and the scapula. These injuries are relatively common among college and professional athletes in professional sports, especially contact sports such as football and basketball.

Brachial plexus injuries involving axonal disruptions can be further categorized as occurring proximal to the dorsal root ganglion in the spinal foramen (preganglionic) or anywhere distal to the ganglion (postganglionic). This distinction is important because operative repair is impossible, and the prognosis is poor for preganglionic root recovery.

The symptoms are severe, burning upper arm and shoulder pain that radiates down the arm, followed by weakness affecting C5 and T1 (thoracic) nerve root distributions. The patient is often seen holding the arm on the affected side, which often hangs limply at the side.

A detailed neurologic assessment is required, with examination of the neck and shoulder. Plain radiographs including the cervical spine should be obtained. If radiographs are abnormal, or if symptoms persist, progress to MRI. Cervical spine instability would be evident on radiograph. Depending on the location and severity of the brachial plexus injury, persistent pain, sensory loss, and paresthesias, weakness or paralysis are possible.

An athlete should not return to play while symptomatic. Athletes with prolonged or bilateral involvement should be referred. Treatment options vary from strengthening and stretching exercises, to splinting, to surgical intervention in some cases. Cervical spine precautions should be followed if cervical spine injury is suspected.

Thoracic Outlet Syndrome

Thoracic outlet syndrome (TOS) is compression of the brachial plexus and/or subclavian vessels as they exit the narrow space between the superior shoulder girdle and the first rib. These structures can be affected individually or in combination. Women between the ages of 20 and 50 years are most commonly affected. Etiology may be secondary to congenital abnormalities such as cervical rib or abnormally long transverse process of C7, or an anomalous fibromuscular band in the thoracic outlet. Posttraumatic fibrosis of the scalene muscles is also a possibility.

Symptoms may be vague and variable. Common symptoms are color changes in the hand along with sensory changes and weakness in the fourth and fifth fingers. Cervical spine (C-spine) films are necessary to document cervical rib placements and EMG help to delineate the specific nerve involvement. Ultrasound of the subclavian artery with the arm in different positions helps define the extent of compression.

Conservative treatment consists of shoulder exercises to improve posture. Orthopedic referral may be helpful to evaluate for surgery to remove the offending bony structure.

Peripheral Polyneuropathy

Peripheral polyneuropathy is "stocking-glove" or distal sensorimotor paresthesia, with diminished or variable deep tendon reflexes. Diabetes is a frequent cause; early symptoms may respond to a regimen with tighter glucose control. A rapid onset of motor polyneuropathy is seen in Guillain-Barré syndrome, in which an ascending weakness occurs after a viral illness. Other etiologies include alcoholism, vitamin B deficiencies, vitamin B_6 excess, Sjögren's syndrome, AIDS, hypothyroidism, amyloidosis, and renal failure.

A complete history and physical exam to exclude muscle disease or weakness is necessary. Paresthesias result in weakness, sensory loss, and altered deep tendon reflexes, whereas primary muscle pathology produces only weakness. A CBC, ESR, blood glucose, liver function, blood urea nitrogen (BUN), creatinine, thyroid-stimulating hormone (TSH), and immunoelectrophoresis tests are indicated. A chest x-ray film and EMG will help confirm the diagnosis. A neurologic consult is suggested.

Sciatic Nerve Syndrome

Sciatic nerve syndrome is back pain that radiates into the buttocks and produces tingling in the posterior thigh and posterolateral calf to the lateral malleolus. Often the cause is a herniated disk, spinal stenosis, obturator neuritis, sciatic nerve irritation, direct trauma, or osteoarthritis. The pain may also be secondary to lumbar sacral strain, but does not necessarily indicate disk herniation or prolapse. Sciatic nerve compression may result from tumors in the pelvis or from prolonged sitting or lying on the buttocks. The history may reveal twisting, bending, or heavy lifting.

The physical exam includes evaluating for point tenderness and ROM in the back. With the patient supine, perform straight-leg raising. A positive finding is radicular pain that occurs below the knee at less than 60 degrees of limb elevation, with pain in the buttock or posterior thigh. It is essential to note that bowel and bladder functions remain normal in sciatic nerve syndrome. Treatment is usually conservative.

Femoral Neuropathy

Arising from the second, third, and fourth lumbar nerve roots, the femoral nerve innervates the quadriceps and terminates as the saphenous nerve. Onset of femoral neuropathy is sudden and painful, and is followed by wasting and weakness in the quadriceps, sensory impairment of the anteromedial thigh, and loss of the deep tendon reflex of the knee. Causes include nerve infarction due to diabetes, retroperitoneal compression by tumor, or hematoma from entrapment. Although improvement may occur, residual weakness is common.

Neck Pain

Discomfort and limited ROM arising from the structures in the neck is a common complaint. The pain may originate from any of the musculoskeletal structures, including muscles, ligaments, tendons, cervical vertebrae, nerves, and vasculature. Pain referred to the neck from the temporomandibular joint (TMD), pleura, or mediastinum may also be seen. Causes of neck pain are generally structural in nature and most often are the result of trauma, degenerative changes, or muscle spasms. Stress, sedentary occupations, and biomechanics are frequently found to be contributing factors; questions regarding these factors should be asked during the history taking. The onset (rapid or insidious), location (arm, shoulder, head, or back), and character (sharp, dull, or aching) of the pain are essential in the differential diagnosis. Of particular note is pain (in the absence of trauma) that begins gradually and improves with rest, because infection and malignancy in the vertebrae do occur.

Physical examination of the neck begins with the evaluation of ROM, including flexion, extension, rotation, and side bending to determine limitations and the pain-producing movements. Spurling's maneuver should be used to assess nerve-root compression. (See Advanced Assessment 14.4.) Palpation of the neck must be done thoroughly, checking for tenderness, muscle spasm, and lymphadenopathy. Lymph nodes in the supraclavicular and axillary regions should be examined carefully; enlarged nodes in the absence of infection may indicate malignancy. Evaluate the vascular structures and the thyroid. The examination must also include a musculoskeletal and neurovascular assessment of the extremities, including assessments of the muscle strength of biceps, triceps, and handgrips. (See Advanced Assessment 14.1.) Abnormalities in sensation of any dermatome and altered deep tendon reflexes indicate cervical nerve-root compression.

Laboratory studies such as ESR, RF, or ANA are necessary only if systemic or bone disease is suspected.

Differential Diagnosis

Torticollis

Often referred to as "wryneck," *torticollis* is a self-limiting condition that usually occurs after excessive exposure to the cold or activities that require unusual or prolonged rotation or twisting of the neck musculature. Torticollis most often occurs in young adults. Pain arises from acute muscle spasm and serves a protective function.

Questioning the patient about sleep positions and the number of pillows used may elucidate the cause of the condition. Physical examination findings in torticollis include limitation of neck flexion away from the affected side. Spasms of the sternocleidomastoid or trapezius areas are common.

Radiographic evaluation is not routinely needed, but x-ray studies may be useful if the symptoms continue past the time when improvement is expected.

Treatment involves decreased activity (which may be easiest to obtain with a soft cervical collar), moist heat, and any of the NSAIDs. Resolution is expected in 1 week.

Cervical Ligamental Sprain

A common condition, *cervical ligamental sprain* is often referred to as "whiplash." The cause is hyperextension of the cervical ligaments around C7, resulting in stretching or tearing. Automobile accidents, especially rear-end collisions, are often responsible for whiplash, but the injury may also be seen in certain sports. Other symptoms may include interscapular pain, arm pain, and occipital headache. A severe injury may result in dizziness, tinnitus, diplopia, and cognitive impairment. Neurologic impairments are rare unless there is an accompanying cervical spine fracture that leads to nerve-root or spinal cord compression.

A full C-spine x-ray study—including lateral flexion and extension views—should be done regardless of the physical findings.

Treatment generally includes a soft cervical collar, rest, application of ice for the first 24 hours, then alternating ice and heat, and NSAIDs. Patients with severe injuries should be referred to an orthopedic surgeon. Occasionally, bed rest (to remove the weight of the head from the neck muscles and ligaments), physical therapy, and a low dose of an antidepressant may be used to limit chronicity and disability.

Cervical Muscle Strain and Spasm

See the section on Cervical Muscle Sprain and Spasm later in this chapter.

Cervical Spondylosis

Cervical spondylosis (also known as *degenerative arthritis in the cervical vertebrae*), is a common cause of neck pain in older patients. Degenerative changes on radiography are found in 40 percent of the population at age 50 and in 70 percent of the population at age 65. These changes are usually asymptomatic, meaning that a finding on x-ray study does not necessarily account for the patient's pain. Progression of the osteoarthritismay result in subluxation, osteophyte formation, and disk protrusion.

Common symptoms are recurring neck stiffness and mild aching discomfort. There is pain and limited ROM with lateral rotation and lateral flexion of the neck toward the affected side. Paresthesias may also occur.

ADVANCED ASSESSMENT 14.4

Spurling's Maneuver

To perform Spurling's maneuver (neck compression), follow this procedure:

1. With the patient's neck in extension, rotate the neck to the affected side.
2. Apply downward pressure on the head.
3. Assess for patient complaint of or accentuation of limb pain or paresthesia (a positive finding). Also observe for obvious atrophy in the neck.

Radiographs will determine if subluxation and other osteoarthritic components are present, but an MRI will be necessary to identify disk herniation and soft tissue or spinal cord abnormalities.

Hallmarks of treatment are the use of NSAIDs, a conditioning program, and reeducation to result in better care of the neck.

When the secondary bony changes of cervical spondylosis encroach upon the spinal cord, a pathologic process called *myelopathy* develops. If this process involves both the nerve roots and spinal cord, it is called *myeloradiculopathy.* Regardless of its etiology, radiculopathy causes shoulder and/or arm pain, as well as numbness and/or tingling ("pins and needles"). Fewer than 5 percent of patients with cervical spondylosis develop myelopathy, and they are usually between age 40 and 60. Acute myelopathy is most often the result of central soft-disk herniation that produces a high-grade block, which may be visualized on myelogram. This herniation may require surgical decompression and is a medical emergency. If pain is unremitting and cervical nerve-root compression is present, a neurosurgical consult should be sought immediately.

Myofascial Pain

Regional musculoskeletal pain or tender muscles are often the result of minor muscle tears following injury and are referred to as *myofascial pain,* meaning inflammation of a muscle and its fascia. Although the cause may not be readily identifiable, the pain is as a result of local inflammation and produces a tender "trigger point" when a particular muscle group is palpated. The pain may radiate to surrounding structures. Even though this is a common cause of nonarticular rheumatic pain, it is often misdiagnosed. The trigger points are not visualized on routine imaging studies and cannot be objectively substantiated.

Treatment includes identifying and eliminating aggravating factors, injections of the trigger points with 1 percent procaine, and passive stretching of the muscle involved immediately after the local anesthetic has taken effect.

Shoulder Pain

Pain and dysfunction localizing in and around the shoulder girdle are common presenting musculoskeletal complaints. Shoulder pain affects patients of various ages and activity levels. Although shoulder pain can be referred from the neck, chest, or diaphragmatic region, it is most commonly caused by a local process. The shoulder joint includes three large bones (the clavicle, the scapula, and humerus) and four joints (sternoclavicular, acromioclavicular, glenohumeral, and thoracoscapular). The shoulder is a ball-and-socket joint, like the hip, but the two joints differ significantly in that the hip is a weightbearing joint, and the shoulder is a suspension joint, maximizing mobility. The two chief presenting complaints are usually related to pain and/or instability. Symptoms of decreased motion, power, or function can accompany complaints of pain or instability, but they are rarely the chief complaint.

Common conditions affecting the shoulder include acute injuries (less than 2 weeks' duration; common in younger patients) which include fractures, dislocations, and acute tendon rupture; chronic or repetitive injuries (impingement syndromes, most rotator cuff tears and biceps tendon ruptures); and degenerative, inflammatory, or idiopathic conditions (glenohumoral and acromioclavicular arthritis, frozen shoulder). While there have been many technological advances in diagnostic aids, most shoulder disorders can be diagnosed with careful history, clinical exam, and plain radiographs.

In the history, inquire about any precipitating injury and onset of pain. Obtain specific information about the location of the pain, along with the factors that aggravate or alleviate it. The relationship of the pain to the time of day, to active or passive movement, and to body position is significant. The patient's age, occupation, activities, medical history, and social factors will also be important in making a diagnosis. Patients with an acute symptoms (less than 2 weeks' duration) usually have an injury, such as a fracture, a dislocation, or a rotator cuff tear. For patients with chronic shoulder pain, evaluate the activities related to the onset of symptoms.

Instability, another common complaint, can be classified by the frequency of symptomatic episodes, as well as the direction and degree of instability. Acute injuries may be a first time dislocation or a recurrent episode. Instability can be classified by the frequency of symptomatic episodes, as well as the direction or degree of instability. The instability episode may be partial (subluxation) with spontaneous reduction or may be complete (dislocation). The instability may be anterior, posterior, inferior, or multidirectional. Most traumatic dislocations are anterior. Multidirectional instability should be considered in patients who present with recurrent episodes of subluxations or dislocations and no history of significant trauma.

Determine if there is a discrepancy between active and passive motion. Disuse can cause some passive ROM; equal losses of active and passive ROM can be secondary to soft-tissue contracture, as in frozen shoulder, or the result of joint incongruity from trauma or arthritis.

Muscle strength should be assessed and compared with the opposite shoulder. Pain can affect the accuracy of muscle testing. Tears of rotator cuffs and neurologic injury can produce weakness. Assess functional status although this may be impacted by motivation and ability to adapt to impairment. The level of functional disability will depend on the normal intensity of activities that the patient performs.

A concise differential diagnosis is often obtained by evaluating the patient's chief complaint in the context of its chronicity and the patient's age. Patients younger than 30 years of age, for example, commonly present with traumatic injuries or instability such as glenohumeral dislocations and acromioclavicular (AC) joint separation. Impingement syndromes and rotator cuff tears are more commonly seen in middle-aged patients. These must be distinguished from frozen shoulder, which produces a global loss of passive and active ROM. Glenohumoral dislocations are much less common and must be treated with a high index of suspicion for a concomitant rotator cuff tear (50 percent of patients older than 40 years of age will have an acute tear). Older patients (over 55) are more likely to have rotator cuff tears or degenerative arthritis. Fractures and dislocations also occur in this age group that are related to falls.

Physical examination of the shoulder should begin with inspection of the shoulder for swelling, color, edema, and symmetry, followed by palpation for tender areas, crepitus, temperature, and deformity. Both active and passive ROM movements should be tested while comparing the painful shoulder to the unaffected side.

The most common ROM movements tested include:

- Internal in extension: Have the patient touch the back of his or her hand to the opposite scapula.
- Internal/external in flexion: With the patient's elbow flexed at the side, thumb pointing up, internally and externally rotate the elbow, taking care to keep the elbow against body.
- Internal/external in abduction: Abduct the patient's shoulder to 90 degrees, keeping the elbow flexed at 90 degrees, then have the patient lower his or her forearm from the horizontal plane, then raise the forearm, keeping the upper arm parallel to the ground.

Pain with abduction from 45 degrees to 120 degrees (painful arc) indicates supraspinatus tendinitis or subacromial bursitis, which are the early rotator cuff injuries. Muscle and bursae involvement produces pain only on active motion, whereas pain with passive ROM may involve tendons, bursae, or restricted joint movement and is generally indicative of more pathology. Muscle testing, with resistance, reflex testing, and an assessment of the neurosensory and neurovascular status, completes the exam.

Specific findings can include inability to shrug the shoulders, which indicates trapezius muscle weakness, and weakness of forward flexion, which is associated with rotator cuff impingement. Because shoulder pain can be referred from other areas, the patient should be evaluated for cardiac, pulmonary, and abdominal causes as well as neurologic disease or injury. Pain caused by bony malignancy is usually gnawing, constant, and unrelated to movement. Malignant tumor is usually evident by a lytic lesion in the bone on x-ray film.

Plain x-ray films, including the anteroposterior (AP) projection and an axillary lateral view, are sufficient to reveal most fractures and dislocations. Additional views may include a transthoracic lateral, which images the glenohumeral joint at a 45-degree posterior oblique, or a 60-degree anterior oblique (Y view). A new view—the apical oblique—is suggested to reveal shoulder instability. This view is simple to obtain and painless for the patient. In addition to the standard x-ray studies, other diagnostic tests used in diagnosing shoulder pain include MRI, arthrography, and (if nerve involvement is suspected) EMG. Although the standard x-ray studies will often be normal, they should be done to rule out structural abnormalities, especially if there is history of trauma or if the problem is persistent. C-spine films and chest films may also be necessary if involvement in those areas is suspected. Laboratory studies should be done in accordance with the patient's history.

Differential Diagnosis

Shoulder disorders may be separated into acute versus chronic and traumatic versus nontraumatic. Problems in young adults are frequently the result of instability and traumatic injuries and tendinitis. The mature adult usually suffers with degenerative conditions of the tendons and joints.

Adhesive Capsulitis

Often referred to as a "frozen shoulder," adhesive capsulitis is defined as idiopathic loss of both active and passive ROM, with no clear predisposition based on gender, arm dominance, or occupation. Patients between 40 and 60 years of age are more likely to be affected; diabetes mellitus (especially type 1) is the most common risk factor. Patients with diabetes tend to be refractory to treatment, and 40 to 50 percent will have bilateral involvement. Other underlying conditions related to frozen shoulder include hypothyroidism, Dupuytren disease, cervical disk herniation, Parkinson's disease, stroke, and tumors. In a short period of time, immobility will result in a tight painful shoulder joint that has limited active ROM (a "freezing" phase of pain) and then typically progresses to a "thawing" phase of decreasing discomfort associated with a steady improvement in function. This process may take anywhere from 6 months to 2 years. Although adhesive capsulitis may result from any condition that produces pain and immobility, in older patients and individuals without predisposing factors, the possibility of underlying organic or neoplastic disease should be considered.

Physical exam typically reveals a 50 percent or more reduction in both active and passive ROM. Pain and tenderness are common with motion and at the deltoid insertion. Diffuse tenderness about the shoulder may also be present. AP and axillary radiographs of the shoulder are indicated to ensure that smooth, concentric joint surfaces with an intact cartilage space are present and to rule out other pathology such as osteophytes, loose bodies, calcium deposits, or tumors. Other studies, such as arthrography, CT, or MRI are rarely indicated if radiographs are normal.

Adhesive capsulitis is differentiated from chronic posterior shoulder dislocation, tumor, and OA on radiograph. Posttraumatic shoulder stiffness is, obviously, related to a history of trauma. Rotator cuff tear is differentiated because of the presence of normal passive ROM.

Treatment consists of the application of moist heat, use of analgesics (NSAIDs and non-narcotic analgesics), followed by a gentle stretching program, performed at home three to four times a day (should not cause significant pain). Advise patient of lengthy recovery time and potential for chronic stiffness and residual pain.

Rotator Cuff Syndrome

Rotator cuff syndrome may include impingement problems, calcific tendonitis, and subacromial bursitis (shoulder bursitis). The term *impingement syndrome* refers to pathologic changes that result when the subacromial bursa and/or rotator cuff become inflamed as a result of compression under the acromion or "roof" of the shoulder joint (rotator cuff tendinitis). It is the leading cause of shoulder pain, ranging from bursitis to rotator cuff tendonitis, and eventually, degenerative tears of the rotator cuff. In addition, the biceps tendon may be impinged (in bicipital tendinitis).

The rotator cuff covers the anterior, superior, and posterior aspects of the humoral head and is formed by the coming together of four muscles. These muscles assist in the elevation of the arm. Inflammation of the subacromial bursa and underlying rotator cuff tendons is a common cause of shoulder pain in middle-aged patients. Rotator cuff pathology presents a continuum from edema and hemorrhage to chronic inflammation and fibrosis to microscopic tendon fiber failure progressing to full-thickness rotator cuff tears. The etiology is multifactorial. A loss of microvascular blood supply to the tendon and repeated mechanical insults as the tendon passes under the coracoacromial arch combine to cause damage over time.

The history is usually one of gradual onset of anterior and lateral shoulder pain exacerbated by overhead activity is characteristic. Night pain and difficulty sleeping on the affected side are also common. Atrophy of the muscles about the top and back of the shoulder may be apparent if the patient has had problems over a period of several months, although this may also indicate a full-blown rotator cuff tear.

On physical exam, palpation over the greater tuberosity and subacromial bursa commonly elicits tenderness and crepitus with shoulder motion. Pain will be elicited by having the patient slowly lower the abducted arm against downward resistance. Neer and Hawkins signs are generally positive. Impingement testing involves locally anesthetizing the shoulder. If the patient is then stronger and without pain after subacromial injection, pain inhibition from inflammation and fibrosis is likely rather than full-blown tear. AP and axillary radiographs are usually negative; narrowing of the space between the head of the humerus and the undersurface of the acromion suggests a long-standing rotator cuff tear.

Frozen shoulder is ruled out if active and passive ROM loss is not present; a rotator cuff tear will not improve with subacromial injection of local anesthetic; glenohumeral arthritis is evident on radiograph and there is pain on motion; acromioclavicular (AC) arthritis presents with tenderness over the AC joint.

Treatment includes resting from the offending activity and NSAIDs. The patient should begin a stretching program with emphasis on posterior capsule stretching. If home therapy of three to four times a day over a period of 6 weeks does not result in improvement, a subacromial corticosteroid injection can be administered, followed by continued stretching. Steroid injections should not be repeated if the previous injection does not produce significant and sustained (more than 2 months) relief. Significant weakness of the rotator cuff or failure after 2 to 3 months of rehabilitation (with or without subacromial steroid injection) are indications for further evaluation and operative consideration.

Calcific Tendonitis

Calcific tendinitis is a degenerative process accompanied by a local deposit of calcium that develops in the rotator cuff. The calcified material often creates inflammatory changes in the subdeltoid bursa, and is frequently asymptomatic until an acute event or overuse exacerbates the condition. The symptoms of calcific tendonitis are severe, localized pain that occurs with any movement of the shoulder. With the arm in a dependent position, the pain is absent or minimal. The shoulder is acutely tender and can be warm to the touch or swollen. X-ray films usually demonstrate the deposit. A transaxillary view is necessary if the deposit is anterior or posterior to the joint in the subscapularis muscle.

Minor or mild cases of calcific tendonitis rarely need invasive treatment. Anti-inflammatory medications, ultrasound, physical therapy, and rest are usually effective in ameliorating the pain. Some deposits appear soft, fluffy, or irregular on x-ray examination. Aspiration to remove some of the material while concurrently injecting an anesthetic with corticosteroid preparation can provide immediate relief. In more severe cases or those that fail to respond to conservative treatment, consider injection of corticosteroid.

Rotator Cuff Tear

Rotator cuff tear may occur secondary to trauma, or from degenerative, calcific changes, chronic mechanical impingement, and altered blood supply to the tendons over time. The rotator cuff muscles insert into the tuberosities of the humerus, and tightly hold the ball-and-socket joint of the shoulder together. Rotator cuff injuries are considered to be more serious than other soft tissue injuries of the shoulder. Most full-thickness rotator cuff tears occur spontaneously in patients older than 50 years of age, presumably as a result of age-related changes in vascularity and tissue degeneration. The supraspinatus tendon is most often affected. Most older people with rotator cuff tear may have only mild, disabling symptoms, or may even be asymptomatic. This injury can occur in individuals younger than 40 years of age, usually as a result of aggressive physical injury and repeated trauma from contact sports (e.g., football).

The patient will usually report a lateral deltoid pain and weakness may be present in the setting of a tear. There may be a history of reaching overhead and feeling "something give" in the shoulder, and then noting that the ipsilateral arm drops to the side. Thereafter it is difficult and very painful to abduct the arm. The pain is often worse at night and the patient may report difficulty sleeping. To reach behind to scratch their back causes extreme pain. The "empty can" test also isolates the mechanism of the rotator cuff. A suspected rotator cuff tear can be confirmed by performing the "drop arm" test: If the arm drops to the side, the test is considered positive. Most tears are relatively small, however, and the patient is often able to maintain some control. It is clinically very difficult to differentiate tendinitis from a tear. The back of the shoulder may appear sunken, indicating atrophy of the supraspinatus and infraspinatus muscles following a long-standing cuff tear.

Soft tissue injuries do not show up on plain x-rays; therefore, findings are usually reported as within normal limits even though the films may demonstrate calcification from previous or chronic injuries. There may be spurring of the acromion process or calcium deposits in the soft tissue, as well as bony deformities from previous dislocations. Lytic lesions indicating metastatic disease can also show up on radiography. More aggressive diagnostic testing such as MRI, ultrasonography, or arthrography may be indicated in patients with a history of acute trauma or if there is no response to conservative treatment.

Nonoperative treatment includes icing shoulder (most commonly in cases of acute injury), NSAIDs, physical therapy with stretching and strengthening exercises, and avoiding overhead activities. Ice the entire shoulder 15 to 20 minutes twice daily. Corticosteroid injections should be used judiciously. Over time, steroid injections further weaken the tendon, and can actually accelerate propagation of the rotator cuff tear. Patients should never receive more than three subacromial injections. Patients with significant failure and failed rehabilitation should be considered candidates for surgery. The exception to this rule is the patient younger than age 60 who has an acute traumatic cuff tear and is best accomplished within 6 weeks of the injury.

Degenerative Arthritis

Arthritis of the glenohumeral or acromioclavicular (AC) joints can occur, but it generally is not isolated to the shoulders unless there is a history of old injury such as a dislocation or fracture. The common complaint is diffuse or deep-seated pain, aggravated by any strenuous activity. As the disease progresses any movement can cause the shoulder pain, and rest and night pain become prominent complaints. ROM may become progressively limited. As a result, activities of daily living, such as dressing, combing hair, and reaching overhead are increasingly difficult. OA typically involves a single joint in an older patient, and generally there is no apparent relationship between the development of OA in the shoulder and the patient's previous activity level. Physical exam may reveal atrophy of the shoulder muscles; palpation elicits tenderness over the front and back of the shoulder. Crepitus is commonly present with rotation or flexion; ROM is usually decreased.

AP and lateral radiographs are indicated. The axillary view will demonstrate joint space narrowing that is indicative of cartilage destruction; there may flattening of the humeral head, an inferior osteophyte, and posterior erosion of the glenoid. Treatment includes NSAIDs and application of heat and/or ice to relieve symptoms, and gentle stretching exercises to preserve motion. A trail of glucosamine and/or chondroitin sulfate can be considered although their efficacy needs further evaluation. Activity modifications are beneficial in reducing pain. For advanced arthritis, total shoulder replacement may offer a very satisfactory solution.

Shoulder Dislocations

Shoulder dislocations are a common injury, occurring most commonly in younger adults. The mechanism of injury may be direct or indirect, usually with the arm in extension. There is often an obvious fullness of the anterior capsule on exam and a positive sulcus sign (space under the acromion). In an acute anterior dislocation, pain is severe and ROM is limited. The patient will usually hold the arm slightly abducted and externally rotated. There may be associated neurovascular and/or neurosensory trauma; therefore, the clinician should check the distal pulses and sensation, especially over the deltoid. Posterior dislocations are less common (2 percent) and less apparent. Deformity is minimal, but any motion of the extremity will cause severe pain. Recurrent dislocations can occur and do not require as severe a force as the initial injury. Reduction is usually the treatment of choice; occasionally, surgery is necessary.

Shoulder Fractures

Fractures of the humerus, clavicle, or acromion are common. Fracture of the clavicle typically occurs from a moderate fall (such as from a bicycle or down stairs) or from blows during a contact sport. Patients complain of sharp shoulder pain and are reluctant to move the upper extremity. It is important to verify that no neck pain or upper extremity paresthesias are present. These fractures usually best heal spontaneously after proper immobilization; they rarely require surgery.

Shoulder Sprains

Acromioclavicular joint (ACJ) sprain is classified as first, second, or third degree, depending on severity. These shoulder sprains often occur in young men, and are typically associated with a fall while the arm was adducted, causing trauma to the ACJ, although the injury may occur as a result of indirect trauma also. The patient will present with pain, especially on adduction or abduction past 90 degrees, point tenderness over the ACJ, swelling, and possible deformity. First-degree sprains involve a partial tear of the ACJ, whereas second-degree sprains involve a complete tear of the AC ligament and a partial disruption of the coracoclavicular ligament. In a third-degree ACJ sprain, both the AC and coracoclavicular ligaments are torn, and there is obvious displacement of the distal clavicle. Weighted x-ray views of the ACJ help confirm this by distracting the joint, revealing widening of the joint spaces. Treatment includes ice, NSAIDs, and a sling or figure-8 splint for 2 to 4 weeks, with daily gentle assisted ROM exercises. Patients with third-degree sprains should be referred to an orthopedic specialist.

Shoulder–Hand Syndrome

Shoulder–hand syndrome, also referred to as *reflex sympathetic dystrophy,* occurs as a complication of minor or major trauma, hemiplegia, MI, pneumonia, or peripheral neuropathy. It is more common in elderly patients and is manifested by pain and stiffness in the affected hand. The pain is described as burning and is worsened by light touch and improved with application of cool moisture. The hand or shoulder is often mildly swollen and discolored, and abnormal diaphoresis of the affected areas may be noted. Treatment is early active and passive mobilization and use of NSAIDs. If necessary, a brief course of corticosteroids can be considered.

A summary of common differential diagnoses for shoulder pain is provided in Differential Diagnosis 14.3.

Arm (Elbow, Wrist, and Hand) Pain

Pain in the upper extremity can be caused by problems in the elbow, wrist, or hand. These can be caused by trauma, nerve impairment, joint, muscle, bursa, or tendon disruption or inflammation. Infection is always a possibility, and gout (which can sometimes affect the elbow) is another consideration.

DIFFERENTIAL DIAGNOSES 14.3: SHOULDER PAIN

Musculoskeletal problems	Adhesive capsulitis (frozen shoulder) Rotator cuff syndrome Impingement Calcific tendinitis Subacromial bursitis Degenerative arthritis: glenohumeral, acromioclavicular
Trauma	Fractures: humerus, clavicle, acromion Acromioclavicular joint sprains Rotator cuff tear Dislocation: glenohumeral Nerve injuries: compression
Neurovascular problems	Reflex sympathetic dystrophy (shoulder hand syndrome) Thoracic outlet syndrome Cervical root compression Brachial plexus injury
Systemic disease	Inflammatory disease Cancer

Elbow Problems

Usually, elbow complaints in the adult occur as a result of overuse. The most commonly seen complaint is lateral epicondylitis of the humerus. Although this condition is often called "tennis elbow," it occurs frequently in patients who do not play tennis. It is associated with repeated extension of the wrist and pronation and supination of the forearm, particularly against resistance, which occurs in movements such as opening jars, hammering, and turning doorknobs. The common complaint is pain in the elbow that radiates into the forearm. There is pain and weakness with gripping objects ("coffee cup" sign). Tenderness is present over the lateral epicondyle, and wrist extension against resistance produces the pain. Rest, ice, NSAIDs, and physical therapy are generally effective, although corticosteroid injections and wrist splinting may be considered in some cases.

Medial epicondylitis is less common; this condition is often referred to as "golfer's elbow." It is a result of overuse or strain of the muscle group arising from the medial epicondyle, which is used in wrist flexion. Tenderness and pain is over the medial epicondyle and is exacerbated by wrist flexion. Diagnosis is by clinical exam only, and treatment is the same as for lateral epicondylitis.

Bursitis of the olecranon is often the cause of pain and swelling in the posterior aspect of the elbow. This may occur with forced extension of the elbow joint. ROM is generally normal, but caution is needed to rule out a septic bursitis. Monitor for fever, redness, heat, and warmth at the site. Synovial fluid aspiration can provide evidence of infection. Radiography is indicated to exclude bone infection.

Treatment may include ice for 15 to 20 minutes several times a day and rest. Assessment of position of computer keyboards or other work station corrections may be helpful. NSAIDs are useful, and splinting with an elbow strap may ease pain by exerting counterpressure on the soft tissue below the lateral epicondyle, or short-term use of a wrist splint may reduce pain from lateral epicondylitis. An anterior elbow splint may be useful for medial epicondylitis management. Corticosteroid injection may be necessary. Refer to physical and/or occupational therapy. The above measures are effective in 80 percent of cases. If the patient is still symptomatic, referral to a specialist is warranted. Surgical procedures are a last resort.

Wrist Problems

Wrist and hand problems may be assessed using Allen's test, Phalen's maneuver, the percussion test for Tinel's sign, and/or Finkelstein's test (see Advanced Assessment 14.5).

ADVANCED ASSESSMENT 14.5

Tests for Wrist and Hand Problems

Test	Comments
Allen's test	*Purpose:* Assesses patency of radial and ulnar arteries and the arterial arch. *Procedure:* Compress the radial artery at the wrist. Have patient rapidly open and close his or her hand several times. Then have the patient open the hand. (Hand should be pale, or white.) Release pressure from the artery. The hand should flush, indicating patency.
Phalen's test	*Purpose:* Assesses for median nerve compression. *Procedure:* Have the patient maintain forced flexion of the wrist for 1 minute or more, with the dorsal surface of each hand pressed together. If the patient complains of numbness and paresthesias in fingers, the test is considered positive.
Tinel's sign	*Purpose:* Assesses for compression neuropathy. *Procedure:* Percuss the median nerve at the wrist. If the patient complains of tingling in the digits (positive Tinel's sign), compression at the site of percussion is likely.
Finkelstein's test	*Purpose:* Assesses for de Quervain's disease. *Procedure:* Have patient touch thumb into palm and make a fist. Test is positive if moving the wrist into ulnar deviation causes pain.

Wrist Injuries

Wrist injuries are common after falling on an outstretched hand. Patients present after trauma with pain and swelling in the distal forearm or wrist. Numbness may be present if the medial nerve is affected. The mechanism of injury will often provide important clues to the diagnosis. The examination begins with gentle palpation to locate the area of point tenderness, and includes a thorough neurovascular assessment. A radiograph of the wrist (including an oblique view) will be necessary to rule out fracture. Common fractures are the Colles' fracture of the distal radius and the navicular (scaphoid) fracture of the anatomic "snuff box." It is not unusual to have a navicular fracture missed on radiography, so an orthopedic referral should be provided when the presenting complaint is pain and trauma to the soft tissue area of the "snuff box."

A common wrist ligamental injury is an ulnar collateral ligament tear at the base of the thumb. Often seen with ski-pole injury, related to repetitive gripping, surgery is necessary to repair a tear in this area. Therefore, when the presenting complaint is pain and trauma to the proximal thumb, an orthopedic referral for stress testing is appropriate even if the x-ray result is negative.

Ganglion

A *ganglion* is a cyst that develops on or in a tendon sheath. It is filled with a thick, gel-like material that leaks from the joint into the weakened tendon sheath and forms a cyst sac. A ganglionic cyst is usually caused by frequent strains and contusions, resulting in joint inflammation. The most common sites are on the dorsum of the wrist over the radiocarpal joint or on the volar surface of the wrist near the flexor carpi radialis tendon. The ganglion can be asymptomatic, or it may be associated with dull aching and weakness. It can be distinguished from a tumor by its soft consistency and transillumination. Treatment includes aspiration or surgical removal, although a conservative approach is appropriate because spontaneous disappearance may occur.

Hand Problems

When assessing and/or treating a patient with an injured hand, have the patient remove all rings as soon as possible. Inflammation secondary to most injuries will precipitate edema, making removal of rings difficult. A tight-fitting ring may cause arterial compression and ischemia if not removed. Usually soap or lubricant jelly will be sufficient to remove the ring. If this does not work, several other techniques may be used. (See Therapeutic Procedures 14.2.)

Osteoarthritis and Rheumatoid Arthritis

Although both OA and RA affect the phalanges, the different types of arthritis occur in different locations. *Rheumatoid arthritis* usually presents as bilateral pain, swelling, and stiffness of the metacarpophalangeal (MCP) and proximal interphalangeal (PIP) joints. Generally other systemic complaints will occur, and joints other than just those in the hand will be affected as well. *Osteoarthritis* affects the interphalangeal joints and presents with swelling, stiffness, pain, and deformity.

Carpal Tunnel Syndrome

Carpal tunnel syndrome is a commonly occurring problem resulting from median nerve compression in the wrist. See the section on Carpal Tunnel Syndrome later in this chapter.

THERAPEUTIC PROCEDURE 14.2

Removing Rings

Equipment: 2–0 or 3–0 nylon suture (string technique), rubber tourniquet (tourniquet technique), lubricant (tourniquet technique), mechanical ring cutter (ring cutter technique)

String Technique:

1. In a distal direction, wrap 2–0 or 3–0 nylon suture tightly around the finger just distal to the ring.
2. Slip the proximal end of the string under the ring.
3. Pull the proximal end of the suture over the ring and firmly retract it distally over the axis of the finger. As each coil of suture unwinds, it pulls the ring slightly over the coiled suture until it is free.

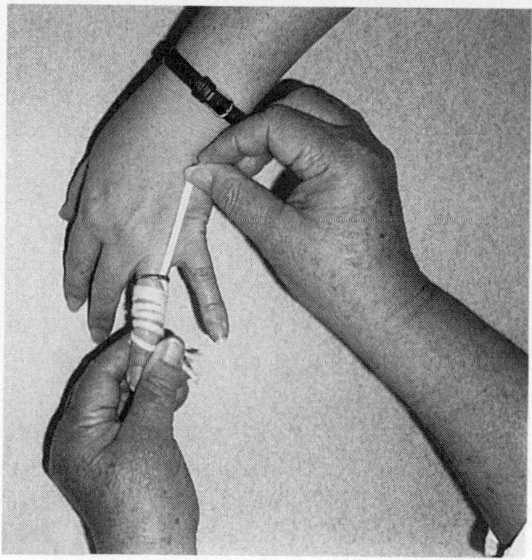

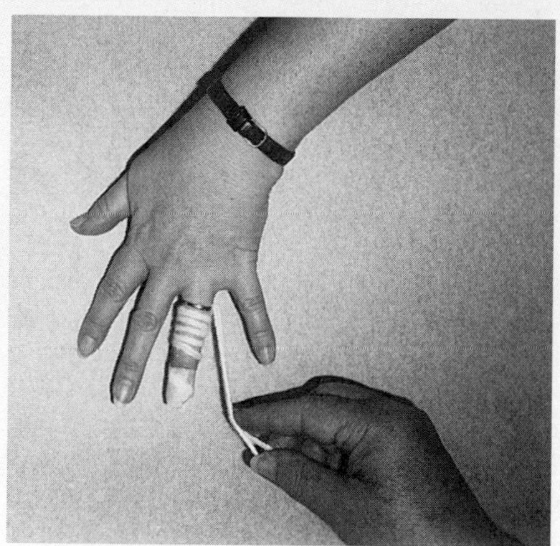

Tourniquet Technique:

1. Carefully wrap the finger with a rubber tourniquet, starting at the fingertip and working up to the edge of the ring.
2. Have the patient lie supine on the exam table, with his or her arm pointed straight upward at the ceiling for about 5 minutes.
3. As soon as the patient lowers his arm, remove the tourniquet, apply copious amounts of lubricant, and slide the ring off.

Mechanical Ring Cutter Technique:

1. Advise patient that the ring will be cut and obtain his or her consent.
2. Follow the manufacturer's directions.

Post-Procedure: Give ring to patient, or secure as per institution policy and document.

Gout

Gout typically occurs in the first metatarsophalangeal joint of the foot, but it may affect the wrist, elbow, or finger. Usually only a single joint is involved, with erythema, swelling, heat, and exquisite pain, but 10 to 15 percent of the patients with gout present with polyarticular symptoms. Attacks spontaneously resolve in 1 week but will recur with more frequency and severity. Diagnosis is made by joint aspiration.

De Quervain's Tenosynovitis

De Quervain's tenosynovitis (stenosing tenosynovitis) is characterized by pain at the base of the thumb or at the radial styloid process on abduction and extension of the thumb. Within the wrist, there are six dorsal tunnels that transport the extensor tendons. The first tunnel transports the abductor pollicis longus (APL) and the extensor pollicis brevis (EPB) tendons. These tendons form the radial border of the anatomic snuffbox. De Quervain's tenosynovitis occurs when the synovial lining of the tunnel becomes inflamed, thus narrowing the opening of the tunnel. This results in pain when the tendons move. The APL and EPB tendons are responsible for thumb flexion and extension, as well as establishing a grip. This condition is seen in patients who perform pinch-grip activities such as using hand tools with extreme pressure, carrying trays with a pinch grip, assembly work, and sewing/cutting activities. It is more common in middle-aged women and is often precipitated by repetitive use of the thumb.

De Quervain's tenosynovitis presents with pain at the radial side of the wrist, usually with lifting. This pain is aggravated by attempts to move the thumb or make a fist. Patients may complain of pain while turning a key or a doorknob, or while attempting to open a jar. Often the condition occurs as the result of lifting infants with the second metacarpals (web bewteen the thumb and the index finger) under the baby's axillae. Chronic pain, loss of strength, and loss of thumb motion can occur.

The history and physical examination should proceed as described for carpal tunnel syndrome. In addition, assess for crepitation over the radial styloid. On palpation, the tendon sheath may feel thickened. Allen's test, Phalen's maneuver, and Tinel's sign (see Advanced Assessment 14.5) should be negative. The confirmation test for de Quervain's tenosynovitis is Finkelstein's test. To perform this test, have the patient grasp the thumb in the palm while you deviate the wrist to the ulnar side. If this motion is painful, the test is considered positive. There is usually no need for additional diagnostic testing. Wrist x-ray studies are indicated only if there is a history of trauma. Calcification associated with tendinitis occasionally can be seen on radiographs.

Ask the patient to bring any work tools to the office visit to better evaluate risky hand and wrist positions. Observe if the patient has attempted to modify the tool (wrapping the handle in duct tape, adding a sleeve of rubbery material) to try to reduce the pressure on the hand surfaces. If it is expected that there is a relationship to the patient's occupation/hobby, ask about the specifics of these activities.

The differential diagnoses include carpal tunnel syndrome, carpometacarpal joint arthrosis of the thumb, and scaphoid fractures, and arthritis of the thumb and/or wrist.

Noninvasive treatment includes rest, splinting, and NSAIDs. Splints that are used are either a radial gutter splint or a customized long opponens splint. The splint should immobilize both the wrist and the thumb. Splinting is used for 3 to 6 weeks. A 2-week course of NSAIDs is usually helpful (see Drugs Commonly Prescribed 14.2).

Invasive treatments include corticosteroid injections into the tendon sheath. If the symptoms are not relieved with two to three injections, then referral should be made for surgical release of the tendon sheath. Patients with unremitting symptoms after 6 to 8 weeks of conservative treatment should be referred for tendon release.

Patients should be educated regarding the cause of de Quervain's tenosynovitis. Modifications to hand tools or the work environment should be made. For example, hand tools may be retrofitted with a larger grip surface, so that pressure is more evenly distributed over the palmar surface of the hand. Avoidance of the precipitating factor is often enough to permanently resolve early symptoms.

Trigger Finger

"Trigger finger" or "locked finger" is often referred to as *stenosing tenosynovitis of the flexor tendons*. This problem can be painful and functionally limiting. Any digit can be affected, although it most commonly affects the ring or middle finger. Inflammation at the MCP joint pulley causes a size discrepancy between the tendon and the pulley. Because the tendon no longer slides freely through the pulley, there is a snapping or locking phenomenon. The digit remains flexed or extended till the tendon pops through the pulley, causing severe pain. Tenderness with palpation of the flexor tendon over the MCP joint is noted. There is a higher prevalence of trigger finger in patients with carpal tunnel syndrome and de Quervain stenosing tenosynovitis.

Trigger finger may be idiopathic (more common in middle-aged women) or associated with RA or diabetes. Patients typically report pain and catching when they flex the finger and may describe the finger as going "out of joint." They may awaken with the finger locked in the palm, although the finger gradually unlocks during the day. Physical exam reveals tenderness in the palm at the level of the distal palmar crease, usually overlying the MP joint. A nodule may also be palpable. The nodule moves, and the finger may lock when the patient flexes and extends the affected finger. This movement is almost always painful. Full flexion of the finger may not be possible.

The most effective therapy for this problem is local anesthetic and corticosteroid injection into the tendon sheath, plus a modification of activities for about a month. A small number of patients require surgical release of the tendon. Splinting and NSAIDs have not proven effective.

Dupuytren's Contracture

Sometimes referred to as "Viking disease," or palmar fibromatosis, this condition affects the palmar tissue between the skin and the distal palm and fingers, most often in the fourth and fifth fingers but also in the thumb–index finger web space. Visible, palpable fibrous bands, reminiscent of tendons, can extend from the palm to the proximal interphalangeal joint of Dupuytren-affected fingers. It is a progressive condition that results in flexor contracture while not affecting the flexor tendons. As the contractures increase, patients have trouble grasping objects, pulling on gloves, and putting hands in pockets. Sensation in the affected fingers usually is normal. It occurs most frequently between the ages of 40 and 60, and is a familial disorder, most commonly affecting males of northern European ancestry. It is dysfunctional and disfiguring, although it does not cause pain. Surgery is the only therapeutic option; recurrence is not uncommon.

Boutonniere Deformity

Another term for this disorder is "jammed finger," or "central slip extensor tendon injury." This deformity is caused by a rupture of the central portion of the extensor tendon at its insertion into the middle phalanx. Patient typically reports a history of trauma; the finger is held partially flexed at the PIP joint and extended or hyperextended at the DIP joint. With a recent injury, the PIP joint is painful and tender.

Boutonniere deformity may not be apparent initially but can develop in 7 to 21 days as the intact lateral bands of the extensor tendon slip inferiorly. Ask the patient to extend the injured finger and observe the position of the DIP and PIP joints. The PIP joint will be flexed more than 30 degrees and the DIP joint will be extended or hyperextended. A radiograph can rule out fracture. Flexion contracture of the PIP joint and extension contracture of the DIP joint is possible.

Splint the PIP joint in extension for 6 weeks in a young patient and for 3 weeks in an elderly patient. The DIP joint is left free. Initiate active and passive ROM at the DIP joint. If the injury is already 1 to 2 weeks old, this may not be possible.

Back Pain

A sharp or aching sensation between the lower rib cage and the gluteal folds is referred to as *low back pain.* More than 80 percent of adults have had at least one episode of back pain sometime during their lifetimes, and many have had recurrent episodes since adolescence. Back pain is the most common cause of disability in patients under age 45, and by age 50, 80 to 90 percent of the population show evidence of degenerative disk disease at autopsy.

Low back pain is a symptom that is rarely attributable to a specific disease or pathologic lesion. The presence of neuromotor deficits, in the distribution of lumbar-sacral nerve roots, is not uncommon. Some patients with local or radicular signs have no evidence of morphological abnormalities, however, even after testing with all appropriate diagnostic technologies. On the other hand, 50 to 60 percent of asymptomatic individuals reveal degenerative changes, and 20 percent have disk herniation without symptoms. In addition, a patient may manifest varying low back syndromes at different times, from acute lumbosacral (LS) strain and spasm to sciatica to chronic low back pain.

The typical history for the patient with back pain often includes the sudden onset of pain without precipitation by an event or injury. Obtain information on the overall health and previous history of the patient, such as a history of cancer and corticosteroid use or fever, which will alert the practitioner to the possibility of infection, tumor, or fracture. The presence of any neurologic deficits, saddle anesthesia, bladder or bowel dysfunction, or pain that is unresponsive to bed rest will reveal whether there is a risk of potentially serious problems. Have the patient point out any areas with neurosensory deficits and note the dermatome affected.

The clinical examination should include inspection, palpation, and ROM for the spine and paravertebral muscles. Lateral bending, touching the toes, and limitations in rotation may indicate muscle spasm, neoplasm, or bony deformity. Straight-leg raising assesses sciatic L5 (fifth lumbar) and S1 (first sacral) nerve roots and has an 80-percent sensitivity rate. This test should be performed on the supine patient by cupping the heel of the dorsiflexed foot with one hand and (while supporting the calf with the other hand) raising the leg by flexing at the hip. Pain below the knee at less than 60 to 70 degrees of flexion, aggravated by dorsiflexion or internal rotation, is a sign of L5 or S1 nerve-root tension, which is suggestive of disk herniation. Check the hip for ROM and muscle strength, because gluteal muscle weakness may occur if L5 nerve-root compression on the gluteal nerve is present. Beware of any limitations of sensation or decreased deep tendon reflex. L3 or L4 disk herniation causes a diminished knee jerk, and a decreased ankle jerk results from S1 nerve-root lesion. Perform an abdominal exam to rule out visceral pain and a rectal exam to assure normal sphincter tone.

For most cases of mechanical back pain, even when it is associated with sciatica, the chance for spontaneous recovery within a 3-week period is high (90 percent). Spontaneous recovery is more likely if the patient hurt his or her back while performing a very strenuous task that will not be repeated than if the back was hurt while doing an activity that is repeated many times daily. In the case of repetition injury, patient education will be key to improvement. If no improvement is seen within a reasonable time, physical therapy may be helpful. Back pain of more than 6 weeks' duration needs to be reevaluated for a more detailed diagnostic workup. Diagnostic examination includes LS spine radiography. Situations that warrant early radiography include age greater than 50, focal persistent bone pain, history of malignancy, women who are postmenopausal, patients who have been on prolonged corticosteroid therapy, severe trauma, fever and focal tenderness, men who have focal tenderness with limited spinal movement and sacroiliac pain, major neurologic deficits, and limited spinal motion. Computed tomography (CT) and MRI are used for patients with extreme symptoms, those under consideration for surgical intervention, or those who are suspected of having systemic disease. Laboratory studies and EMG are used when appropriate.

Differential Diagnosis

Most cases of back pain arise from mechanical causes. These regional causes include acute and chronic LS strain, postural backache, and degenerative LS arthritis.

Back pain can be associated with a herniated intervertebral disk, producing sciatica and in rare cases cauda equina syndrome (a medical emergency), or it can be caused by nonspecific causes such as spinal stenosis, spondyloschises, ankylosing spondylitis, and Scheuermann's disease. Neoplasia, infection, and spinal fracture are potentially serious causes of low back pain that need immediate attention.

Conditions occurring outside the spine that can cause back pain include aortic aneurysm, gallstones, pancreatitis, peptic ulcers, pyelonephritis, renal disease, pleuritis, pelvic inflammatory disease (PID), endometriosis, and prostatitis. Psychogenic causes include depression, somatization, or malingering.

Chronic low back pain occurs more often in patients with social and psychological factors; the physical findings in these patients are less likely to account for the severity of the pain. Patients older than age 50 with back pain are most likely to have OA, compression fractures, visceral pain, or malignant neoplasms.

Common differential diagnoses for back pain are presented in Differential Diagnosis 14.4.

Hip Pain

Hip pain is discomfort within or around the hip. The largest joint in the body, the hip is subject to stress from ambulation and weightbearing; it may suffer trauma and chronic mechanical stress. Possible causes are processes in the hip joint, the surrounding muscles, the soft tissues, or the neurovascular system. Diagnosis needs to consider the patient's age, because certain problems are more prevalent in different age groups. In adults, common problems include OA, RA, fractures, referred pain, bursitis, meralgia paresthetica, avascular necrosis, and malignancy.

Pain in and around the hip can often be felt in the groin or the buttock, or it can be referred to the thigh or knee. Conversely, pain may be referred to the hip if irritation to the femoral, sciatic, or obturator nerve roots occurs. These may be the result of herniation of lumbar disk, spinal stenosis, retroperitoneal tumor, or femoral hernia. Vascular insufficiency of the aortoiliac area may result in hip and buttock pain as well. The history should ascertain if pain is focal, as in bursitis, or diffuse, such as in synovitis. The presence of stiffness should raise the suspicion

DIFFERENTIAL DIAGNOSES 14.4: BACK PAIN

Differential Diagnosis	Characteristic Findings
Ankylosing spondylitis	Back pain and stiffness over several months; relief with exercise; reduced mobility of spine; painful or ankylosed sacroiliac joints; reduced chest wall expansion
Cauda equina syndrome	Acute urinary or rectal incontinence, with or without paraplegia
Dissecting aortic aneurysm	Sudden onset of severe low back pain in older adults; pain that is not relieved with rest; pallor, diaphoresis and confusion may be present; possible asymmetric pulses and blood pressure in extremities
Gallstones	Pain follows ingestion of a fatty meal and radiates around trunk to right scapula; belching, bloating, and acid stomach is present, along with right upper quadrant pain
Gynecologic disorders	Vaginal discharge; pain worse around menstruation or ovulation
Herniated disk	Often preceded by years of recurrent episodes of localized back pain; leg pain overshadows back pain
Infection	Unremitting or progressive pain at rest; tender spinous process at level of involvement; fever; history of drug use; diabetes; immunosuppression or suspected systemic infection; previous genitourinary or spinal surgery
Musculoskeletal strain	Often no precipitating event; pain is over low back spine and muscles without sciatica; aggravated by sitting, standing, and certain movements; alleviated with rest. Palpation localizes pain and muscle spasms may be seen. Insidious onset; progressive improvement
Prostatitis	Constant low back pain; urinary hesitancy; change in sexual frequency
Pyelonephritis	Ill-appearing patient with nausea and vomiting; back and flank pain excruciating with direct percussion
Sciatica	Pain radiating into the buttocks, thighs, and/or below the knees as the result of L5 or S1 nerve-root irritation, compression or disk prolapse
Spinal fracture	Pain felt near the site of injury; history of major trauma to back or (in older adults) a history of strenuous lifting or a minor fall
Spinal stenosis	Gradual onset in older adults; often mimics intermittent claudication, except pain is usually in buttocks, thigh, or calf, worsens with exertion and back extension (leaning backward or walking downhill) and is relieved with sitting, walking uphill, or leaning forward; weakness, bowel and bladder dysfunction may be present
Spondylolisthesis	Systemic inflammatory condition of the vertebral column and sacroiliac joints; most frequently affects males age 20 to 30; chronic low back pain, worse in morning; excessive thoracic kyphosis is present
Tumor	Unremitting or progressive pain at rest, night pain; tender spinous process at level of involvement; variable neurologic findings; weight loss, fever, or other systemic symptoms; known or suspected malignancy

of degenerative disease. Inquire about trauma, involvement of other joints, infection, fever, and relation of pain to activity.

Physical examination of the hip must first assess position at rest, because fracture of the femoral head results in external rotation and flexion, and an internally rotated shortened leg may be a posterior dislocation. These patients should not have the hip moved until radiographic studies have ruled out fracture or dislocation. Performing palpation of the joint allows recognition of focal tenderness and swelling.

The ROM examination begins with assessment of gait, if possible. Next, the extremity should be put through passive ROM to detect crepitus, limitation of movement, muscle spasm, flexion contracture, or guarding. Flexion and extension need to be performed with the knee straight as well as flexed. Abduction, adduction, and internal and external rotation are assessed. Femoral and pedal pulses are auscultated for strength and bruits. Neurologic testing for sensation and deep tendon reflexes concludes the exam. Diagnostic testing should include hip x-ray films. Other x-ray studies, such as spine or sacroiliac films or weightbearing films, may be indicated in special circumstances. MRI, ultrasonography, and joint aspiration are other diagnostic techniques to be considered in special circumstances.

Differential Diagnosis

Osteoarthritis

OA usually causes pain with use that is painful or stiff in the morning and improves during the day. Pain referred to the groin, thigh, knee, and lateral side of the leg may occur. Often pain or stiffness affects other joints as well. For more information, see the section on Osteoarthritis that follows later in this chapter.

Trochanteric Bursitis

The hip area contains multiple bursae. The incidence of trochanteric bursitis peaks between the fourth and sixth decades of life; it is more common in women than in men. It is commonly associated with pain and limited ROM. Onset may be acute or insidious. Bursitis can be associated with trauma or overuse, and may be inflammatory, hemorrhagic, infectious, or calcific. Inflammatory bursitis of the hip is the most common type. Trochanteric bursitis is often associated with lumbar spondylosis, degenerative arthritis of the hip, and lower limb-length discrepancy. It is characterized by chronic, intermittent, aching pain over the lateral aspect of the hip, and some patients report numbness in the upper thigh. Pain will increase with movement, especially external rotation and abduction, and can be triggered by prolonged standing or lying on the affected side. Other signs and symptoms include pain on forced hip abduction, distinct tenderness around the greater trochanter, and pain extending down the lateral aspect of the thigh. Trochanteric bursitis is treated with NSAID therapy (e.g., naproxen [Naprosyn] 375 to 500 mg PO bid for 1 to 2 weeks). Persistent cases may require corticosteroid injections.

Rheumatoid Disease

With rheumatoid disease, the hip pain is bilateral and characteristics include morning stiffness and limited ROM that does not resolve with activity. The hip is generally not the first joint affected. During an acute phase there is tenderness and fullness or thickening seen in the joint.

Proximal Femoral (Hip) Fracture

Hip fractures are one of the most common of all adult fractures, accounting for at least half of all hospital days related to fracture care in the United States. The two primary types of hip fractures are *femoral neck* (intracapsular) and *intertrochanteric,* both of which occur most frequently in older adults who have sustained a fall at home or similar low-energy trauma. The incidence of hip fractures doubles for each decade of life after age 50 years, with women affected twice as often as men are.

Risks for hip fractures include physical activity, previous fracture, visual impairment, institutionalization, and osteoporosis. Pain in the hip area after trauma, such as a fall or motor vehicle accident (MVA), especially in patients older than age 50, should give rise to the suggestion of fractures. Neither a lack of trauma nor the presence of long-standing history of hip pain rules out a fracture. In some cases, a fracture may occur as a pathological fracture secondary to an underlying neoplasm or chronic corticosteroid usage. The patient should be admitted to the hospital.

Obtain a history of how the injury occurred and whether the fall was witnessed by anyone other than the patient. A loss of consciousness (LOC) for any period would necessitate a cardiac and neurologic referral, as well as referral for orthopedic care. Determine the patient's mental status, and try to obtain a realistic assessment of the preinjury functional status.

Physical exam typically reveals an externally rotated and shortened injured leg. Any motion to this extremity will produce severe pain centered around the affected groin. Examine the pelvic bony prominences for tenderness because pubis ramus fractures may also be present or confused with the hip injury. It is important to check for lower-extremity pulses and neurologic function. The entire limb should be assessed for points of tenderness or deformity that may indicate the presence of other fractures at sites such as the femur, tibia, or ankle. An AP view of the pelvis and "shoot-through" lateral views of the affected hip can provide definitive radiographic evidence to confirm the diagnosis. In most cases, surgical repair of the fracture is the treatment of choice.

Meralgia Paresthetica

Caused by compression of the lateral femoral cutaneous nerve, meralgia paresthetica is commonly seen in overweight middle-aged men. Symptoms include pain or paresthesias over the anterior superior iliac spine and the anterior lateral thigh, with decreased touch and pinprick sensation. Treatment includes avoiding tight clothing around the waist, and analgesics.

Avascular Necrosis

Avascular necrosis appears as abrupt hip pain followed by progressive, intermittent episodes. Pain is worsened with motion, activity, and often is worse at night. A limp along with limited abduction and internal rotation is present. MRI is needed for diagnosis, and an orthopedic referral is indicated. It often occurs as a serious complication of hip trauma, but it may occur unrelated to trauma.

Malignancy

Initially, no signs may be present with malignancy, however, tenderness and palpable swelling may develop later over bony prominences. Night pain, systemic symptoms, and fractures may be seen.

Knee Pain

The knee is a complex, modified hinge joint consisting of three bones, three articulations, five major tendons, four major ligaments, and two menisci. The lateral and medial articulations are between the femoral and tibial condyles. The intermediate articulation exists between the patella and the femur. The knee is a relatively weak joint that gains its strength from the strong ligaments that attach the femur to the tibia. There are five intrinsic ligaments that assist in strengthening the articular capsule. The cruciate ligaments connect the femur and tibia within the articular capsule, crossing each other in the form of an X.

As a major weightbearing joint, the knee is susceptible to many injuries. Torsion is limited in the joint, and any motion that extends beyond the defined range results in a ligamentous injury. Because the knee joint depends on the integrity of the ligaments to provide it with stability, an injury to the knee may be a calamitous event.

The arrangement of three articulations allows a combination of rolling, gliding, and rotation, in addition to flexion and extension. Although it is attached to the lateral tibia, the fibula does not articulate with the knee joint. The anatomy of the knee includes bony structures, ligaments, tendons, bursae, and cartilage. The femoral condyles and the tibial plateaus are capped by the patella and cushioned by the menisci, whereas the ligaments, muscles, tendons, and bursae provide stability.

The knee joint is a common site for discomfort due to trauma (24 percent of all activity-related musculoskeletal injuries in men, the highest of all sites), degenerative disease, and/or rheumatologic conditions. Acute pain in the knee may be related to:

▲ Fractures
▲ Meniscal injuries
▲ Ligamentous injuries
▲ Musculotendinous strains
▲ Extensor mechanism injuries; and
▲ Contusions

Many knee complaints by adults are the result of overzealous exercise and sports activity. Fractures can involve the distal femur, patella, proximal tibia, and fibula. Inspect for swelling and deformity, palpate for tenderness in the bone itself, and obtain appropriate radiographs. Patellar fractures can result from indirect forces, such as falls, but fractures of the tibia and femur at the knee usually result from major trauma. Patellar dislocations are often reduced at the scene of injury when the knee is extended for transport.

Obtaining a history of the mechanism of injury is key in diagnosing meniscal tears. A history of a twisting injury sustained with the foot planted on the ground and locking (inability to extend the knee completely) with localized pain and tenderness along the joint are indicative of meniscal pathology. Some patients report that manipulating or pushing on the knee enabled them to "unlock it."

Patients with ligamentous injuries have acute pain, swelling, and instability. Strains of various musculotendinous structures around the knee also cause acute pain and swelling, but most do not result in instability. Patients with an injury to the extensor mechanism report a fall with a sudden weakness or collapse. Contusions are from direct blows and cause localized pain and tenderness.

Knee complaints are categorized as *injury* (trauma) or *overuse,* and are either acute or chronic. Often chronic knee pain cannot be related to any recognized injury or overuse. Conditions that cause chronic knee pain are:

▲ Arthritis
▲ Tumors
▲ Sepsis
▲ Overuse syndromes (including bursitis/tendinitis and anterior knee pain)

Tumors are characterized by night pain and often can be palpated or identified on radiograph. Sepsis in the knee joint is rare; it is more commonly located in the prepatellar bursa. Inspection and palpation of the involved area easily determine the location of the infection. Bursitis/tendinitis and anterior knee pain have similar characteristics: both usually are chronic, often secondary to overuse, and often bilateral. The pain typically is worse with rising or walking after sitting, at night, and with prolonged exercise or use.

The physical exam of the knee begins with the patient standing. Inspect the knee anteriorly and posteriorly. Observe the gait. Inspect the knees for swelling, ecchymosis, erythema, abrasions, puncture wounds, and active ROM. Assess the popliteal space for swelling that may occur with popliteal aneurysm, Baker's cyst, and tumors. It is important to assess movement in both the standing and supine positions, and to note any limping, pain, locking, or giving way of the knee. As the patient lies supine, should palpate the joint line, muscles, tendons, ligaments, and bones in an attempt to localize tenderness. An effusion may be demonstrated by eliciting the *bulge sign*: As the patient lies supine, massage the medial knee toward the head, then stroke the lateral aspect of the knee toward the medial aspect. A bulge sign or effusion is indicated if fluctuance occurs over the medial aspect. Palpation for crepitus while the knee is passively flexed and extended helps to determine if meniscal injury is present. Do muscle testing of the quadriceps and hamstrings.

A complete physical examination is also important to rule out the presence of systemic disease associated with knee pathology.

There are a number of specialized assessment techniques. To evaluate patellar instability, look for the apprehension sign; when evaluating for meniscal tear, perform the McMurray circumduction test; to assess medial collateral ligament stability, do the valgus stress test; when testing the lateral collateral ligament, perform the varus stress test. When testing the anterior cruciate ligament, do the Lachman test; the posterior cruciate ligament calls for the thumb sign; and the anterior and posterior cruciate ligament stability is evaluated with the drawer test. The prone rectus femoris test assesses the tightness or contracture of the rectus femoris; and the popliteal angle assesses hamstring tightness. (See Advanced Assessment 14.6.)

Contusions are injuries to the leg by a direct blow. Disability may be minor; however, contusions can be quite painful, with significant swelling and tenderness. There may be ecchymosis, and active and passive stress will be painful.

Diagnostic testing includes the use of radiographs if mechanical injury or trauma is suspected. Specific weightbearing views as well as sunrise or skyline views can be performed. MRI is helpful in diagnosing a torn meniscus or cruciate ligament injury. Arthrography is used for diagnosis of a Baker's cyst, and effusions can be aspirated for diagnostic purposes.

Differential Diagnosis

Inflammatory Arthritis

Knee arthritis, which may cause an inflammatory effusion, may be a primary manifestation in a number of conditions. It is one of the most common manifestations of OA. Often more than one joint is affected and there is recurrence or chronicity. Gout, pseudogout, Lyme disease, septic arthritis, and avascular necrosis can also be responsible for the inflammatory response. It may be necessary to aspirate the joint and culture the synovial fluid to rule out infection. Treatment will depend on the underlying condition.

Fracture

A fracture is most likely to occur with direct trauma and result in acute onset of pain. Fractures of the knee and leg

ADVANCED ASSESSMENT 14.6

Assessing Knee Ligaments—Special Tests

Test	Comments
Valgus stress test—assess the medial collateral ligament (MCL) stability	Support thigh to relax the quadriceps muscle. Apply stress initially with the knee extended and then flexed to 25 degrees. With the thigh supported and the knee extended, place one hand on the lateral side of the knee, grasp the medial distal tibia with one hand on the lateral side of the knee, grasp the medial distal tibia with the other hand, and abduct the knee. If the knee opens up in a valgus direction more than the opposite knee, the patient has either a complete or partial tear of the MCL.
Varus stress test—assess the lateral collateral ligament (LCL) stability	Assess LCL stability with the knee in extension and 25 degree flexion by reversing the stress pattern used for the MCL. If the knee opens up more than the opposite knee in a varus direction, the patient has either a complete or partial tear of the LCL.
Lachman test—anterior cruciate ligament (ACL)	With the patient supine and the knee flexed 20 to 30 degrees, anchor the patient's foot to the table then pull the tibia forward. Anterior motion is a sensitive test for ACL laxity. Positive test is a mushy or soft feel when the tibia is moved forward, indicating damage to the ACL.
Thumb sign—posterior cruciate ligament (PCL)	With the patient supine, flex the knee to 90 degrees with the foot supported. Normally, the anterior tibial plateaus sit 1 cm anterior to the femoral condyles, and you may place your thumbs on top of the medial and lateral tibial plateaus. If the PCL is injured, the proximal tibia falls back and the area available to your thumbs decreases. When the tibial plateaus are flush with the femoral condyles, there is 10 mm or more of posterior laxity, consistent with a complete tear of the PCL.

include those of the patellar, tibial plateau, fibular head and shaft, and tibial pilon. Most, but not all, knee fractures are the result of fairly significant trauma; fractures of the knee are often present in conjunction with injury to associated structures. Most fractures around the knee are associated with a large effusion. If the joint is tapped, the presence of hemarthrosis with fat globules is clinically indicative of a fracture. Swelling and significant pain on movement will be present. It is important to ensure that no neurovascular compromise is present in the lower leg. Radiography should be obtained and immediate referral is indicated.

Patellar fractures are usually the result of a direct blow from a blunt object or can be attributed to a fall or MVA. The patient with a patellar fracture is usually unable to flex the knee. Marked joint effusion is usually present.

Stress Fractures

Stress fractures are common in patients who experience bone pain after initiating or increasing high-impact activity. Stress fractures are a result of repeated subtle bone trauma over a period of time that causes a gradual loss of bony substance. New bone is fragile until it calcifies. The cortex, temporarily weakened, is then susceptible to fracture. Common sites for stress fractures are the legs and feet.

There is point tenderness over the bone on physical exam. There may be ecchymosis and soft tissue swelling. Often the patient has altered his or her gait, often causing pain to the knee. Resistive motion of the joint is painless. Radiographs may reveal a periosteal reaction or a hairline radiolucency but are usually negative until 2 to 3 weeks after the injury has occurred. Bone scans may be helpful.

Rest is the best treatment for a stress fracture. Once the patient is pain free, gradually resume activity. The best treatment of stress fractures is prevention. Exercise programs should begin slowly and the patient should avoid the "weekend warrior" syndrome.

Runner's Injuries

Lateral knee pain frequently plagues runners, whether they are novice or seasoned ones. When there is an inability to "run through the pain," runners will often seek care. Sometimes the pain occurs when the average time running has been increased, or the distance.

"Runner's knee," or *ilotibial band tendinitis,* may be related to improper footwear, uneven and bumpy paths, running on very hard surfaces, and lack of warmup. The pain is based at the lateral edge of the patella, at the point where the ilotibial band crosses over the anterior aspect of the joint. Most runners with this condition have feet that supinate, meaning that they do not get a good push-off. Pain during a run suggests injury; pain after a run suggests an overuse problem.

Treatment includes rest, ice packs or ice massage, and NSAIDs. For runners with foot problems, orthotics may be indicated. Alternate low-impact activities should be encouraged (e.g., swimming, biking, or running in water). The symptoms should resolve in 10 to 14 days; at that time the individual may resume running at half the distance that he or she was running before. After 3 weeks, if the runner is pain free, the distance may be increased.

Collateral Ligament Sprains

Knee sprain or ligament tears often occur as a result of athletic injuries. Joint laxity will be present to a varying degree, depending on the injury. The two collateral ligaments, the medial collateral ligament (MCL) and the lateral collateral ligament (LCL), provide lateral stability to the knee. The MCL attaches to the medial condyle of the femur and the tibia. The LCL attaches to the lateral femoral condyle and extends to the lateral tibial plateau. The MCL and the LCL are injured when the valgus (MCL) or varus (LCL) stress to the joint extends beyond the defined range. MCL injuries are more common than LCL tears and often include an injury to the medial meniscus. Football players and skiers are more prone to ligamentous injuries, but they may occur just as easily on the dance floor or in the bathroom.

Wrenching the knee with the foot firmly planted causes injury to the MCL. In these injuries, the knee is in flexion and in a slight internal rotation. LCL injuries occur when the varus stress applied to the knee causes a "bend" toward the outside. The knee is painful and often swollen and may be ecchymotic over the body of the ligament. Some patients will report the feeling that the knee is "bent the wrong way." The knee swells within 20 to 30 minutes; more rapid swelling is an ominous sign and should be considered a "red flag."

Examining the knee immediately after the injury is easier and helps to ascertain the severity of the injury. The examination is more difficult once the joint swells. In a suspected collateral ligament sprain, there is tenderness along the body of the ligament, and point tenderness at the attachment sites is frequently present. In the MCL injury, there may be tenderness at the medial joint because the MCL attaches to the medial meniscus. Pain at the lateral joint line is equivalent to a joint injury.

Varus or valgus stress on the knee joint will determine joint laxity. The practitioner should always examine the unaffected knee first, to establish the baseline and to allay anxiety about the evaluation.

Obtain plain radiographs to rule out fractures and dislocations. More extensive radiologic examinations such as stress films, CT scans, and MRIs are obtained in consult with an orthopedist. In an acutely swollen joint, an MRI is often inconclusive. As in all musculoskeletal injuries, it is important to include fractures, dislocations, and tumors in the differential diagnoses.

Isolated first- and second-degree sprains can be managed with **r**est, **i**ce, **c**ompression [or immobilization], and **e**levation ("RICE"). The unstable knee requires an external knee mobilizer. No weightbearing should be allowed on an acutely swollen or painful knee. Once the injury is past the acute stage, the patient should begin adductor-strengthening exercises. Once the swelling and pain subside, a more progressive rehabilitation program should begin.

All severe strains and fractures should be referred to an orthopedic specialist. Referral to a physical therapist to assist in complete rehabilitation should also be considered. An incompletely rehabilitated knee will be weak and potentially unstable. Without accurate diagnosis and treatment, the injury can become more extensive, jeopardizing joint stability and other structures. Traumatic arthritis can be the sequela to any joint injury.

Adherence to the rehabilitation process is imperative. In some instances, a knee support is necessary for sports. Pain and swelling are indicators that the knee is being overstressed or reinjured.

Cruciate Ligament Injuries

The two cruciate ligaments—the anterior cruciate ligament (ACL) and the posterior cruciate ligament (PCL)—provide rotational stability to the knee. The ACL attaches to the anterior part of the intercondylar area of the tibia, posterior to the medial meniscus. It rises superiorly, posteriorly, and laterally to attach to the posterior section of the medial side of the lateral condyle of the femur. The ACL restrains the anterior to the posterior translation of the knee, keeping the proper relationship of the femur to the tibia. It is loose when the knee is in flexion and tight when it is fully extended. It is the weaker of the two cruciate ligaments. The ACL is the most commonly involved structure in severe knee injuries. In 70 percent of the patients presenting with acute, traumatic hemarthrosis, the ACL is the injured structure. The ACL injury frequently occurs in combination with ruptures of the MCL and the medial meniscus ("O'Donaghue's Terrible Triad"). Once the ligament is torn, the knee is unstable. Swelling occurs rapidly in ACL or PCL injuries because of bleeding of the ligament tear.

The PCL originates in the posterior part of the intercondylar area of the tibia. It crosses superiorly and anteriorly on the medial side of the ACL and attaches to the anterior portion of the lateral surface of the medial femoral condyle. The PCL is tight in flexion. The PCL is injured less frequently than the ACL. It is usually injured by trauma to the anterior surface of the proximal tibia, as in hitting the dashboard in an MVA.

With either ACL or PCL injuries, the patient often reports hearing a "pop" or feeling the knee "snap." An instantaneous sensation of something being "terribly wrong" is also commonly reported. Pain from the injury prevents a return to activity. The patient may report a "distrust" of the knee during activities—the knee may give out, especially during exertion.

On exam, the knee is swollen and the patient is unable to fully flex or extend the knee. There are four standard tests to perform to ascertain the integrity of the ligaments: the valgus stress test, the varus stress test, the Lachman test, and the thumb sign (see Advanced Assessment 14.6). Hamstring spasms and the posterior horn of the meniscus can stabilize the knee, so it is important for the patient to relax throughout the examination. Examine the normal knee first to allay anxiety and to establish a baseline, because most people have some degree of laxity in the ligaments.

Obtain radiographs of the knee. Plain films will demonstrate effusions, loose bodies, and avulsion fractures. The Segond fracture—an avulsion off the lateral aspect of the tibial plateau—is pathognomonic of an ACL tear. The ligaments can be definitively evaluated by MRI.

Any trauma to the knee can cause fractures and cartilage, meniscus, ligament, and muscle damage. The clinician should consider all these injuries when evaluating the knee. The degree of the tear and presence of instability should direct the treatment plan. Partial tears and tears without concurrent fracture or meniscus tear can often be managed conservatively. Immobilize the acutely injured knee to decrease swelling and pain. The patient should avoid weightbearing on the knee. The quadriceps muscle begins to atrophy with inactivity, so it is important to begin strengthening exercises as quickly as tolerable. The quadriceps muscles are adjunct stabilizers to the ACL, and rehabilitation should stress regaining full ROM and strength.

All patients who have sustained an injury to the cruciate ligaments require an evaluation by an orthopedic surgeon. An unstable knee is in jeopardy of fracture, worsening the initial injury, or falls as a result of the instability, resulting in other injuries. A knee that has sustained severe trauma is susceptible to developing arthritis. It is important that the patient understand that despite reconstruction and rehabilitation, the knee will never be perfectly normal. Nonetheless, it can be functional, although it may require the use of a custom-made brace.

Cartilaginous Injuries or Meniscal Tears

Cartilaginous injuries or meniscal tearspresent with acute or subacute pain. The patient may complain of the knee "locking" or "giving way." Conservative therapy of rest, application of ice, and use of NSAIDs should be the initial treatment. If no improvement occurs, diagnostic evaluation of x-ray films (to rule out fractures and OA), an MRI, and orthopedic referral are indicated. (See Advanced Assessment 14.7.)

Patellofemoral Dysfunction

Patellofemoral dysfunction encompasses a continuum of disorders, including chondromalacia patellae and patellofemoral arthralgia. It is an overuse syndrome. Pain typically occurs when climbing stairs, or when standing up after a period of sitting. Pain is often reproduced by direct pressure on the patella when the patient is supine with knee extended. X-ray films may reveal irregularity of the patella. Management is conservative; NSAIDs and quadriceps-strengthening exercises, such as tensing of quadriceps and straight-leg raising, are indicated.

ADVANCED ASSESSMENT 14.7

Assessing the Meniscus and the Patella—Special Tests

Test	Comments
McMurray circumduction test—to test for meniscal tear	Flex the knee to the maximum pain-free position. Hold that position while externally rotating the foot, and then gradually extend the knee while maintaining the tibia in external rotation. This maneuver stresses the medial meniscus and often elicits a localized medial compartment click and/or pain in patients with a posterior tear. The same maneuver performed while rotating the foot internally will stress the lateral meniscus. Pain-free flexion beyond 90 degrees is necessary for this test to be useful.
Apprehension sign—to test patellar instability	Have the patient seated with the quadriceps relaxed. Place the knee in extension. Displace the patella laterally and then flex the knee to 30 degrees. With instability, this maneuver displaces the patella to an abnormal position on the lateral femoral condyle. The patient often perceives pain and demonstrates apprehension.
Bulge sign—to assess for effusion	Apply lateral pressure to the area adjacent to the patella. Medial bulge will appear if fluid is in the knee joint.
Inspect/palpate—to assess for effusion	First, inspect the suprapatellar region. A large knee effusion will be visible. Subtle knee effusions can be demonstrated by "milking down" the joint fluid from the suprapatellar pouch. Hold the fluid wave in place with one hand and ballot the patella. Excessive fluid will create a spongy feeling as the patella is pushed down.

Bursitis

Overuse may cause *anserine bursitis,* which produces pain over the inferomedial aspect of the patella, or *prepatellar bursitis,* which is usually a result of direct pressure and produces pain, swelling, erythema, and limited flexion. Initial treatment is the application of ice for 24 hours (then heat), rest, and use of NSAIDs. It is important to rule out infection with fluid aspiration and culture if infection is suspected.

Synovial Growths and Tumors

Pigmented villonodular synovitis is a benign neoplastic disorder, most often affecting young adults. Inflammation of the synovium, which lines the joints, bursae, and tendon sheaths, occurs causing recurrent unilateral pain, erythema, tenderness, and swelling, with intermittent knee locking. An orthopedic referral is necessary for diagnosis.

Ankle Pain

Most ankle pain is the result of ankle injury that results in ligamental damage (a *sprain*). A sprain occurs when the ankle is positioned in an unstable way, causing the ligaments to overstretch. A *first-degree sprain* involves stretching of ligamentous fibers; a *second-degree sprain* involves a tear of part of the ligament, with pain and swelling; and a *third-degree sprain* results in complete ligamentous separation (Table 14.4). The inversion injury is most common, causing damage to the lateral ligaments of the ankle. By contrast, the medial ligaments are very tight and allow for much less motion than the lateral ligaments.

Initiate the history by asking an open-ended question about how the injury happened. Ask what happened after the injury: Was the patient able to get up and walk and continue activity? If so, a serious ligamental injury or fracture is less likely. If the ankle became swollen and discolored within minutes after injury, a severe soft tissue injury or even a fracture can be suspected.

The physical examination should include inspection and palpation. Look for swelling in the area of the internal and external malleoli and compare the landmarks with those of the opposite foot. The location of a deformity helps to localize the injury, and the degree of discoloration is associated with the extent of the injury. The ankle and foot should be palpated to localize the tenderness. It is also helpful to compare the passive ROM in one leg with the opposite extremity. It is important to note crepitus, because it is often a sign of fracture. The anterior drawer test should be performed to test the stability of the anterior talofibular ligament, and the varus stress test to test the stability of the calcaneofibular ligament. (See Advanced Assessment 14.8.)

Radiographic examination of the injured ankle is necessary only in the following:

- ▲ The patient is not able to bear weight immediately after the injury.
- ▲ The ankle develops marked swelling and discoloration soon after the injury.

Table 14.4 Ankle Pain: Sprains

Classification	First Degree	Second Degree	Third Degree
Type of Pain	Stretching, minor tearing of ligament fibers	Partial tearing of ligament fibers	Complete tear of ligament
Clinical Manifestations			
Pain	Minimal	Mild to moderate	Severe
Swelling	Mild	Moderate	Significant; occurs rapidly, usually within the first 30 minutes
Ecchymosis	Mild	Moderate	Severe; occurs rapidly, usually within the first 30 minutes
ROM	Full, nonpainful	Slightly limited, painful	Limited; loss of function
Point tenderness	Mild	Point tenderness	Severe
Joint stability	Stable	Mild joint laxity	Abnormal
Weight-bearing	Able to bear weight	Painful or inability to bear weight	Inability to bear weight
Management	RICE Active ROM Nonweight-bearing activity Return to sports in 2–3 weeks with ankle support	RICE Active ROM Partial weight-bearing activity as tolerated Gradual return to sports with Aircast or taping	Refer to orthopedic specialist; surgery may be required Cast for 4–6 weeks No weight-bearing; rehabilitation Return to sports in 4–8 weeks with support
Complications	Recurrent sprains within 1 month if not fully rehabilitated	Recurrent sprains Joint instability Traumatic arthritis	Persistent instability Traumatic arthritis

- ▲ Pain occurs with ROM and manipulation of the areas most likely to be stressed in a particular injury.
- ▲ Crepitation occurs with palpation or movement of the ankle.
- ▲ There is a high risk for litigation.

Management includes application of ice or immersion in an ice water bath immediately after injury and every few hours for 48 hours after the injury, an elastic bandage or splint to stabilize the ankle against inversion and eversion stresses, limited activity until the pain and swelling subsides, and the use of NSAIDs. Strenuous exercise should not be resumed until 2 weeks after the pain and swelling have ceased.

Differential Diagnosis

Nerve Entrapment

Nerve entrapment may occur secondary to ankle fracture, dislocation, or traction injury. If the tibial nerve is affected, there would be a loss of ankle plantar flexion, toe flexion, and weak ankle inversion.

Posterior Impingement Syndrome

Posterior impingement syndrome is most commonly seen in ballet dancers. It manifests with pain and swelling of the posterior ankle, and worsens with plantar flexion or dorsiflexion of the great toe. Os trigonum is present on lateral x-ray film.

ADVANCED ASSESSMENT 14.8

Assessing Ankle Ligaments—Special Tests

Test	Comments
Anterior Drawer Test—to test stability of anterior talofibular ligament, place the ankle in approximately 20 degrees of plantar flexion.	Stabilize the tibia, grasp the hindfoot, and pull forward. Asymmetric or excessive motion will occur with chronic ankle laxity and severe ankle sprains.
Varus stress test—to test the stability of the calcaneofibular ligament	With the tibia stabilized and the ankle in neutral, grasp the calcaneus and invert the hindfoot. Excessive or asymmetric motion will occur with chronic laxity of the calcaneofibular ligament.

Referred Pain

Ankle pain may be referred pain, secondary to disk herniation at the level of L5 to S1. Signs and symptoms include a sensory deficit over the malleolus, weak eversion, and a decreased Achilles reflex.

Peroneal Tendon Subluxation

Peroneal tendon subluxation may occur secondary to trauma; it will present with pain, and a "snapping" over the posterior distal fibula. Pain will increase with active eversion of dorsiflexed foot, and there may be palpable/visible movement of tendons.

Tendon Rupture

Achilles tendon rupture causes pain and inability to walk normally. Closed tendon ruptures usually result from a sudden excessive load applied to the musculotendinous unit, with failure occurring either within the tendon's substance (torn fibers) or at its insertion into the bone. A tendon rupture can occasionally occur spontaneously in healthy individuals from relatively minor trauma.

Physical examination will usually reveal swelling, tenderness, and often bruising over the site of rupture. Test the tendon's continuity by performing Thompson's test. To do so, (1) have the patient lie prone, (2) bend the knee so that the leg is vertical, and (3) squeeze the calf. The test is positive if squeezing the calf does not produce plantar flexion of the ankle. This means the tendon is ruptured. Treatment is either surgical repair or immobilization with cast with the foot plantar-flexed.

Bursitis

Inflammation of the bursae of the ankle most commonly affects the retrocalcaneal bursa. There will be pain anterior to the Achilles tendon, just above its insertion into the calcaneus; the pain is aggravated by squeezing the area anterior to the tendon, as well as by dorsiflexion of the ankle. This injury is related to repetitive trauma.

Chronic Ligamentous Laxity

Chronic ligamentous laxity may produce few symptoms other than an aching and tenderness over ligaments after prolonged activity. Rest and NSAIDs are the treatment of choice.

Fracture

There will be pain, swelling, or inability to bear weight, decreased ROM, and obvious bony disruption on x-ray film. Stress fractures of the ankle may occur.

Foot Pain

The foot contains 26 bones, 33 joints, and more than 100 ligaments. Foot pain is usually related to an inflammatory process resulting from trauma (13 percent of activity-related musculoskeletal injuries in men), a deformity, or a foot–shoe incompatibility. The feet are subjected to numerous forces: For example, when an individual is standing, forces exerted on the foot are equivalent to four times the individual's body weight. Any alteration in ability to use the feet for any reason, such as pain secondary to hammer toe or corns and calluses, will have a significant effect upon the health and well-being of the patient.

General treatment measures for foot pain include the use of footwear with roomy toes, supportive arches, and low heels. Heel lifts, cushioned inner soles, and arch supports can provide significant relief when used appropriately. Referral to a podiatrist may be necessary.

Differential Diagnosis

Forefoot Problems

Common problems in the forefoot are calluses, corns, plantar warts, bunions, neuromas, and stress fractures. The history in patients with calluses, corns, and warts would reveal discomfort related to pressure, whereas stress fractures cause pain of acute onset involving the metatarsals. An interdigital neuroma causes tenderness in the third and fourth intermetatarsal space with radiation into toes. Physical examination findings in patients with stress fractures include point tenderness and swelling over the involved bone. The hyperkeratotic lesions of calluses and corns may be indistinguishable from each other, but plantar warts can be distinguished by the punctate bleeding associated with the wart. Interdigital neuromas may sometimes produce a tender nodule in the intermetatarsal space. A *bunion* or *hallus valgus* is the deformity of the first metatarsophalangeal (MTP) joint associated with the lateral drift of the toe. This presents as a painful swelling on the dorsomedial aspect of the first metatarsal head. Foot–shoe incompatibility may produce physical findings such as the toe deformities of hammer toe and mallet toe.

Midfoot Problems

Midfoot problems are generally the result of pes planus, or flat foot. This is likely to produce pain and stiffness in the midfoot region, often associated with degenerative arthritis or laxity of the posterior tibial tendon. Tenderness to palpation usually occurs along the medial plantar border of the sole with flat foot. Flattening of the medial longitudinal arch of the foot and often a valgus deflection of the heel are indicative of this condition.

Hindfoot Problems

Common hindfoot conditions include plantar fasciitis, infracalcaneal bursitis, and posterior heel problems such as Achilles tendinitis and posterior bursitis. The history of individuals with plantar fasciitis includes subcalcaneal pain that sometimes radiates to the arch of the foot while the person is running or walking. The pain is worse in the morning. Infracalcaneal bursitis produces an aching sensation in the midplantar region of the calcaneus that becomes worse the longer the heel is weightbearing. The pain associated with Achilles tendinitis is at or proximal to the insertion of the Achilles tendon onto the calcaneus. In this condition, the physical exam reveals swelling and erythema. The pain is increased with dorsiflexion of the ankle, and crepitus may be palpated. Infracalcaneal bursitis produces pain and tenderness to palpation in the midplantar aspect of the calcaneus. Plantar fasciitis findings typically include tenderness along the medial plantar aspect of the calcaneus, with forced dorsiflexion of the digits increasing the pain.

Differential Diagnosis 14.5 presents common differential diagnoses and their treatment.

Common Problems

Osteoarthritis

Osteoarthritis, also known as *degenerative joint disease* (DJD) or "wear and tear" arthritis, is the most common articular disease in adults older than age 45. It is the most widespread form of arthritis and is a significant cause of functional impairment, chronic pain, and disability in the older population.

OA actually encompasses a group of subtypes with different etiologic factors but a common response pattern in joint tissues. This type of arthritis is primarily noninflammatory and involves a combination of biomechanical stresses and biochemical changes in articular cartilage and synovial membrane. There is erosion and fibrillation of cartilage, with joint space narrowing and osteophyte formation. Principal sites for OA are the distal interphalangeal (DIP) joints, proximal phalangeal (PIP) joints, and the carpometacarpal (CMC) joint of the thumb in the hand, the first MCP or great toe joint, the hips, knees, and cervical and lumbar spine. Although hand joints associated with the pincer grasp, and lower-extremity weightbearing joints are affected, the ankle, wrist, shoulder, and elbow are usually not, unless the cause of the arthritis is traumatic or occupational.

Epidemiology and Causes

OA affects approximately 60 million Americans. Radiographic evidence of OA is present in about 33 to almost 90 percent of people older than age 65. Gender differences are not apparent before age 45. After age 50, however, women

DIFFERENTIAL DIAGNOSES 14.5: FOOT PAIN

Differential Diagnosis	Management
Forefoot	
Hallus valgus or bunion Enlarged bone on the medial side of the first metatarsal	Avoid pressure on the tender bunion, NSAIDs, protective shields, orthotic devices, appropriate footware; if no relief, consider surgery
Corns and calluses with keratinized skin	Moleskin protection, gentle rubbing with pumice, separating toes with cushions or orthotics; if unrelieved, consider surgery
Sesamoid disorders Localized pain and swelling over first MTP joint	Protect the injured part by limiting weight bearing, wearing protective padding or strapping, and NSAIDs
Neuromas	Shoe modification: wide toe box, metatarsal bar, and soft inner soles; NSAIDs; and in severe cases, corticosteroid injections to reduce inflammation.
Stress fractures	Rest and efforts to disperse weight bearing away from the fracture such as stiff-soled shoe, metatarsal bar, walking cast
Infection	Treatment as appropriate
Flat feet	Orthotics
Bunion	Pad; surgery
Peripheral neuritis	Investigate cause
Midfoot	
Pes planus	No treatment if asymptomatic; if symptomatic: flexible arch support, heel-cord stretching, and toe exercises such as picking up objects with toes and spreading toes
Hindfoot	
Achilles tendinitis	Initial treatment: rest, ice and use of NSAIDs, and immobilization. Heel lifts and heel-cord stretching exercises. Corticosteroids are contraindicated.
Plantar fasciitis Infracalcaneal bursitis	Heel lifts, padded heel cups, and orthotic devices. Acute treatment is rest, ice, NSAIDs and local corticosteroid injections. Heel-cord stretching exercises and use of a nighttime dorsal splint to maintain ankle dorsiflexion and toe extension may be beneficial; surgical release of the plantar fascia is the measure of last resort.

are more likely to have OA, with women representing 74 percent of cases, according to the Arthritis Foundation. The actual numbers are probably grossly underreported, since many older adults are asymptomatic or do not report symptoms, which they mistakenly believe to be an inevitable consequence of aging, or for which there is no treatment. Also, the definition of OA may differ among various authorities, leading to variations in reporting prevalence and incidence. Some health-care providers consider symptomatology alone, whereas others use radiographic (x-ray) evidence without symptoms; some include both. Studies stemming from autopsy analyses establish degenerative joint changes occurring as early as the second decade of life. Another confounding factor in interpreting prevalence and incidence is the fact that some sources list breakdowns by anatomic site, whereas others do not.

There is conflicting information on racial differences in rates of OA in African Americans and white Americans. Asian counterparts have a very low prevalence of hip OA, although hand OA is equally prevalent in Hong Kong Chinese and Europeans. Age is a risk factor, with a sharp increase in the middle to late years of life. The Framingham Osteoarthritis Study and the English twin study have identified a genetic component in hand arthritis in women.

Genetic research on families with a preponderance of arthritis has demonstrated mutations of the *col2A1* gene, the precursor to type II collagen. Other genetic influences have been identified also, but the current approach to the study of genetics and OA is fraught with inconsistencies in defining the disease. Patients who have parents who developed OA at middle age or earlier or parents with polyarticular disease are considered at high risk for developing the disease themselves.

Obesity is a risk factor for arthritis of the knee, and to a lesser extent, the hip. Exercise, including recreational jogging, has not been shown to increase the risk of OA. Muscle weakness around the joints, abnormal gait pattern or weightbearing, local joint injury, and repetitive occupational joint use are contributing factors. Cruciate ligament damage or meniscal tears, particularly when accompanied by partial or total meniscectomy, increase the risk of knee OA. Low levels of vitamin C and/or vitamin D have also been implicated as a risk factor for OA. Estrogen replacement therapy is associated with a reduced risk of knee and hip OA; it was also shown to have a moderately protective but not statistically significant effect against worsening of radiographic knee OA in a group of white American women enrolled in the Framingham study. Although all of the above factors have been cited as having a role in OA, the definitive cause of the disease is not known. In general, biomechanical, biochemical, inflammatory, and immunological factors are all implicated in the pathogenesis of OA.

Often, osteoarthritis is classified as "primary" or idiopathic, resulting from:

- ▲ Advancing age
- ▲ Obesity
- ▲ Occupational overloading of joints
- ▲ Familial type II collagen gene polymorphisms

This is contrasted to "secondary" OA, which may develop at varying intervals after trauma, infection, osteonecrosis, congenital malalignment, or in the setting of inflammatory arthritis or metabolic disease. In reality, both primary and secondary OA may coexist.

Pathophysiology

The exact pathophysiology of OA is still under study, with many promising developments on the horizon. Normal cartilage derives its viscoelastic and compressive characteristics from cellular and matrix components. Chondrocytes synthesize type II collagen and glycosaminoglycans to maintain the integrity of the extracellular matrix. These chondrocytes are also responsible for balancing cartilage degradation and repair. In contrast to the autoreactive inflammatory pathology associated with rheumatoid arthritis, systemic lupus erythematosus, and other inflammatory arthritides, in OA articular cartilage is thought to be initially damaged due to repetitive microtrauma or a single inciting macrotraumatic event. Bone and joint malalignment, ligamentous laxity, weakness in muscle groups that provide counterforce against the involved joint (e.g., quadriceps for the knee joint), and any type of underlying structural defect may magnify the damage imparted by this repetitive physical trauma. Proprioception is also impaired in affected knee joints. This diminishes muscular reflexes which normally provide compensatory mechanical mechanisms to counter destructive load-bearing forces on arthritic joints. In addition, underlying genetic defects in cartilage formation (e.g., type II collagen defects, ochronotic cartilage with abnormal pigment deposition) may lead to tissue damage from normal wear and tear in the absence of inciting physical trauma.

Mechanical loading of the joint has been shown to increase macromolecule formation by the chondrocyte within the extracellular matrix as a function of both load intensity and frequency of load-bearing, affecting not only the concentration of matrix proteoglycans but also the integrity of the collagen meshwork. The act of mechanical forces triggering biochemical reactions has been termed mechanotransduction and is only now beginning to be characterized within the chondrocyte. Although much of this pathogenesis is poorly understood and stems from preclinical animal studies, we know that cartilage matrix degradation predominates in OA, with greater fluid loss from joint cartilage in response to mechanical loading. In turn, attempts at repair by chondrocytes are ineffectual.

Current focus centers on the role of matrix metalloproteinases (MMPs) in mediating cartilage degradation. This family of proteolytic enzymes includes collagenase-1

(MMP-1), collagenase-2 (MMP-8), collagenase-3 (MMP-13), stromelysin (MMP-3), and gelatinase-A (MMP-2). They are secreted by chondrocytes and synovial cells and are regulated by plasmin, nitric oxide, interleukin-1 (IL-1), and other cytokines such as IL-6 and possibly tumor necrosis factor-alpha (TNF-α). Normally, these substances are tightly controlled by counter-regulatory substances including tissue inhibitors of MMPs (TIMPs). However, in OA, proinflammatory cytokines, namely IL-1, stimulate MMPs and suppress cartilage self-repair by interfering with chondrocyte proliferation, collagen production, TIMP formation, and MMP inactivation. These processes are normally mediated by transforming growth factor-beta (TGF-β) which is found in decreased levels in OA patients. Dysregulated levels of anabolic cartilaginous growth factors including insulin-like growth factor-1 (IGF-1) and IGF-1 binding protein are also evident, as some studies have revealed lower levels of these factors in OA patients, as well. All these processes result in increased production of type 1 fibrous cartilage, rather than type 2 articular cartilage.

In addition, the disease process of OA includes sclerosis of underlying subchondral bone and abnormalities in the juxta-articular bone marrow. Abnormal bone deposition within the degenerating joint, which impinges upon the joint space, is known as osteophyte formation. These osteophytes may give the impression of external bulging within the joint space, which may sometimes be mistaken for the inflammatory joint pathology of rheumatoid arthritis. However, if spinal osteophytes impinge upon nerve roots, they may produce radicular symptoms, similar to those seen in intervertebral disk herniation.

Crystal deposition into the synovial fluid of osteoarthritic joints, particularly calcium pyrophosphate dihydrate and basic calcium phosphate crystals, also correlates with worsening degrees of radiographic joint pathology and cartilaginous fissuring. Although evidence for the pathophysiologic nature of these crystals is primarily circumstantial, these crystals appear to initiate an inflammatory synovitis, MMP secretion, and synovial proliferation with subsequent cartilaginous destruction. Moreover, patients with an inherited predisposition to calcium pyrophosphate dihydrate deposition also develop severely degenerative osteoarthritis.

Clinical Presentation

Subjective

Patients typically present with slowly developing, localized pain in the affected joint or joints that interferes with their usual activities. The onset is subtle and the pain may be ignored initially. Patients with OA in the weightbearing joints may have early morning stiffness or stiffness after inactivity, which subsides after 30 minutes, also referred to as the "gel phenomenon." Pain and stiffness are also present in hand OA, often accompanied by bony deformities such as Heberden's nodes, which affect the DIP joints, and Bouchard's nodes, which affect the PIP joints. Internal derangement in weightbearing joints may cause them to "lock" or "buckle," increasing the risk for falls; patients often report that their knee "gave way" or "wouldn't bend." In the later stages of OA, pain may be also present at rest. OA may present as monoarticular or polyarticular.

The history should include information on the onset, location, and duration of pain, any self-care measures the patient has taken to alleviate pain and the effectiveness of these measures, and associated symptoms such as joint stiffness, swelling, or deformity. Does the pain interfere with sleep or awaken the patient at night? Inquire if there is a family history of OA. An occupational history should be explored for evidence of overuse; any trauma or surgery to the joint should be noted. Elicit a history of activity/exercise patterns, any changes in activities of daily living (ADLs) or instrumental ADLs (IADLs), and weight changes, especially a gain in weight. Socioeconomic factors and vocational issues should be explored. It is also important to obtain a past or present history of any systemic illness or chronic disease state, along with a list of current medications, including over-the-counter (OTC) preparations, herbal remedies, and nutraceuticals. OA of the wrists, ankles, and shoulder is usually related to trauma or other secondary causes.

Objective

Typical clinical findings of OA include minimal or no swelling of affected joints, tenderness on direct palpation, crepitus, and reduced passive and active ROM. Crepitus is a common, although late, finding, and a sensitive criterion for OA. There may be effusions in the large joints.

Physical exam findings include:

- Hands: Enlargement of the DIP and/or PIP joints. The CMC joint of the thumb may also be enlarged and in general there may be pain on motion.
- Feet: Swelling (bunion) of the big toe and DIP joints.
- Knees and hips: Possible pain and crepitus on passive ROM. There may be tenderness to palpation along the joint line and some muscle atrophy may be present. Hard swelling, if present, is usually a result of bone spurs, whereas soft swelling is related to effusion. There may be significant decreased ROM, both active and passive. Carefully examine the hip of any patient who complains of knee pain; pain referred to the knee may be the only symptom of hip OA.
- Spine: Degenerative changes are common. There may be limited motion and stiffness of the neck and/or lower back. Bony spurs at the facet joints may produce pain and compression of spinal root nerves.

Physical examination should include a functional status evaluation in the older adult. Gait abnormalities such as a limp are significant. Evaluation for spinal and hip alignment and leg length discrepancy is helpful initially to detect contributing factors. Affected joints should be examined for tenderness, bony deformities, swelling, redness, warmth, and ROM. Tenderness along the joint line, crepitus, and limited ROM are typical but nonspecific findings. Knee joint effusion may also be seen, as well as Baker's cysts in the posterior popliteal area. Muscle strength, especially that of the quadriceps muscles, and joint stability should be assessed. The presence of fever or weight loss, especially when accompanied by fatigue and poor appetite, is suggestive of a systemic problem rather than OA; these symptoms need further investigation.

Diagnostic Reasoning

Diagnostic Tests

The diagnosis of OA is primarily clinical. Findings in the history and physical examination are often sufficient to diagnose OA in the knees, spine, hands, and feet. Radiographic testing may be useful in the following situations:

- To establish diagnosis at the hip
- To assess disease severity at other joints
- To screen for other types of bone and joint pathology if pain is severe enough and disrupts sleep
- To determine baseline status to assess change over time

Early changes often do not appear, but as the disease progresses, x-ray findings include asymmetric joint space narrowing, bony cysts and osteophytes, and subchondral sclerosis. Radiographic findings are poorly correlated to symptomatology. Further x-ray studies may be ordered to document progression of the disease if symptoms increase markedly, ADL levels change dramatically, or the patient is being evaluated for surgical intervention. MRI and CT scans may be ordered on patients with suspected spinal stenosis.

Laboratory testing is helpful in ruling out other conditions such as RA, gout, lupus, sepsis, or PMR, but has little place in establishing a diagnosis of OA. CBC, C-reactive protein, and ESR are usually normal; the ESR in older patients is more likely to be elevated. RF, ANA, serum uric acid, or 24-hour urinary uric acid levels may be ordered to rule out RA, lupus, or gout, depending on the clinical presentation, but again may yield significant false-positives.

Synovial fluid analyses may be useful in ruling out inflammatory and/or infectious arthritis.

The American College of Rheumatology (ACR) has identified criteria for the diagnosis of OA of the hand, knee, and hip (Table 14.5).

Differential Diagnosis

Differential diagnosis for OA includes soft tissue and periarticular conditions such as bursitis and tendonitis, lupus erythematosus, Lyme disease, septic or crystalline arthritis, RA, gout, PMR, vasculitis, neuromuscular disease, neuropathy, Parkinson disease, osteopenia or osteoporosis, Paget's disease, or bone malignancy.

Table 14.5 Diagnostic Criteria for Osteoarthritis (OA)

Osteoarthritis	Diagnostic Criteria
Hand OA	Hand pain, aching, or stiffness AND three or more of the following: • Hard tissue enlargement of 2 or more of 10 select joints (second and third DIP, the second and third PIP, and the first CMCs of both hands) • Hard tissue enlargement of two or more DIP joints • Swelling in less than three MCP joints • Deformity in at least one of 10 selected joints
Hip OA	Hip pain AND 2 or more of the following: • ESR <10 mm/h • Radiographic evidence of acetabula osteophytes • Radiographic evidence of joint-space narrowing
Knee OA	Knee pain AND radiographic evidence of osteophytes AND one or more of the following: • Age ≥50 • Morning stiffness <30 minutes • Crepitus on motion

Management

The principles of management of OA are to control pain and other symptoms, to maximize functional independence and mobility, to minimize disability, and to preserve quality of life. A variety of modalities are utilized to achieve this, including patient education and self-care strategies, nonpharmacologic and pharmacologic interventions, and surgical management (Table 14.6).

Pharmacologic Management

Acetaminophen. The goal of pharmacologic management is pain control, with acetaminophen (e.g., Tylenol) as the first-line agent. Tylenol—regular strength (325 mg) or extra strength (500 mg)—two tablets may be taken q4 to 6h as needed, or Tylenol Arthritis Extended Relief Caplets (650 mg), two tablets q8h as needed, not to exceed 4000 mg/24 hours. The maximum daily dose of acetaminophen in patient's receiving warfarin therapy should not exceed 2500 mg PO. Several controlled studies have established the efficacy of acetaminophen although other studies demonstrate that NSAIDs are more effective. However, recommendations begin therapy with Tylenol, as this is a viable strategy for a long-term treatment plan. Patients should be cautioned about using alcohol with acetaminophen. Hepatotoxicity is a serious potential adverse effect.

Table 14.6 **Management of Osteoarthritis**

General Management	
Pharmacologic	Non-narcotic analgesics Topical agents (e.g., capsaicin) Nonacetylated salicylates NSAIDs Intra-articular corticosteroids
Nonpharmacologic	Activity modifications Exercise (biking, walking, swimming) Physical therapy Application of heat/cold Psychosocial support Pain management Self-help programs
Surgical	
Specific Management	
OA of the hand	Pharmacologic: Analgesics Nonpharmacologic: Occupational therapy
OA of the hip	Pharmacologic: Analgesics, NSAIDs (at analgesic or anti-inflammatory doses) Nonpharmacologic: Occupational therapy, physical therapy Surgical
OA of the knee	Pharmacologic: Analgesics, NSAIDs (at analgesic or anti-inflammatory doses), intra-articular corticosteroids (intermittent) Nonpharmacologic: Occupational therapy, physical therapy Surgical

Nonsteroidal Anti-Inflammatory Drugs. NSAIDs actually comprise several categories of pharmacologic agents, all sharing comparable anti-inflammatory properties. Although each class acts in an individual manner, all inhibit the production of prostaglandins, which are inflammatory mediators. Cyclooxygenase (COX), or prostaglandin endoperoxide synthase, is the first enzyme in the prostaglandin synthesis pathway. This enzyme transforms arachidonic acid to other prostaglandin breakdown products. Two forms of COX are present: COX-1 is normally present in blood vessels, stomach, and kidney and promotes the normal functioning of those systems; COX-2 is generated in inflammatory settings by cytokines and inflammatory mediators. Aspirin and NSAIDs inhibit cyclooxygenase enzyme and prostaglandin production, but they have no effect on the arachidonic–lipoxygenase pathway resulting in the formation of leukotrienes. NSAIDs are nonselective COX inhibitors. All possess antipyretic, analgesic, and anti-inflammatory properties. Inhibition of COX-1 is largely responsible for the adverse effects associated with NSAID therapy, including GI bleeding, ulcerogenic activity, fluid retention, and blockade of platelet aggregation. Patients on NSAIDs are four to five times more likely to suffer GI bleeding than individuals who are not taking the drugs. The risk of bleeding is increased during the first month of treatment, and with increased dosages of the NSAID; older age and polypharmacy are also risk factors. It was hoped that the use of the COX-2 inhibitors would be equally effective for pain while curbing gastrointestinal side effects or platelets; however, subsequent data regarding the increased risk of vascular events such as MI or TIA/stroke, have resulted in withdrawal of several of these agents from the market. NSAIDs also interact with several other classes of medication. In addition, NSAIDs are well known to cause fluid retention, as well as having the potential to cause nephrotoxicity.

When initiating NSAID therapy, it is best to begin with the lowest dose possible and increase as needed. It is important to question the patient about use of OTC medications, because many patients with OA take ibuprofen (e.g., Advil, Nuprin, Motrin IB) in a nonprescription strength for headache, fever, or other minor discomforts, and do not associate the OTC form with prescribed medication. If the patient is intolerant of one medication in a specific class, another one in the same class may prove to be satisfactory. Individualization of therapy is the key to successful management.

Because of emerging data indicating that COX-2 inhibitors celecoxib and valdecoxib may be associated with increased risk of serious cardiovascular events (MI, TIA) especially when they are used for long periods of time or at very high risk settings (such as after surgery), the U.S. Food and Drug Administration (FDA) has issued a recommendation that prescribers consider this emerging information when weighing risks versus benefits for individual patients. According to the FDA, patients who are at high risk of gastrointestinal (GI) bleed, have a history of intolerance to nonselective NSAIDs, or are not doing well on nonselective NSAIDs may be appropriate for candidates for COX-2 inhibitor therapy, and individual patient risk for cardiovascular events and other risks commonly associated with NSAIDs should be considered for each prescribing information. Rofecoxib (Vioxx) and valdecoxib have been removed from the market. There is considerable variability among patients in both effectiveness and tolerance of NSAIDs. If one particular drug proves ineffective or unacceptable, benefit may be obtained by changing to a drug of a different class. The doses of these drugs should be individualized. The addition of the prostaglandin analogue misoprostol to NSAID therapy helps protect against gastroduodenal ulceration. In addition, Meloxicam (Mobic) is a preferential inhibitor of COX-2, but it is not a true COX-2 inhibitor according to FDA criteria. It seems to be well tolerated with few side effects of drug–drug interaction. Certain of the traditional anti-inflammatory drugs, such as choline salicylate–magnesium salicylate (Trilisate), etodolac (Lodine), salsalate (Disalcid), diclofenac–misoprostol (Arthrotec), and nabumetone (Relafen) allegedly have fewer GI problems associated with their use. They might be considered if the patient will be on long-term therapy.

Additional Pain Relievers. Tramadol hydrochloride (Ultram) is a nonopioid pain reliever that is indicated for moderate to moderately severe pain. It is available as a combination drug with acetaminophen that works synergistically; it can be taken with NSAIDs also. It is contraindicated with alcohol, hypnotics, and narcotics, and should be used with caution in patients with the potential to abuse it. There is no evidence that this medication is any more effective than NSAIDs. Likewise, although there are times when the prescription of opioids might be appropriate, no evidence exists that these medications provide any more relief than NSAIDs; given the side effects and abuse potential, they should be used only in selected situations. Likewise, there is no clear evidence that muscle relaxants or benzodiazepines are helpful adjuncts, although some clinicians continue to prescribe these, as actual spasms of the paraspinous muscles are elicited on physical exam in the case of vertebral OA.

Other medications such as gabapentin (Neurontin), selective serotonin reuptake inhibitors (SSRIs), and tricyclic antidepressants (TCAs), have also proven effective in the management of patients with OA who have chronic pain.

Glucosamine with or without chondroitin, a dietary supplement not regulated by the FDA, has been shown in limited studies to be effective for OA of the knees. The patient should start with glucosamine sulfate 500 mg three times a day. If that is not effective, glucosamine with chondroitin may provide some improvement in symptoms. There are few drug–drug interactions and few side effects; because the quantity and quality are not regulated, one brand may be more effective in one patient than another. If one brand is not helpful, the patient may try another with good benefit.

Topical agents such as capsaicin (Zostrix) cream, applied three to four times daily to the painful areas, either alone or in concert with oral pharmacotherapy, may be helpful. The patient should be cautioned to avoid rubbing the cream in the eyes and to wash hands carefully after using capsaicin, to avoid irritation. Some redness and burning at the site of application is normal initially, but it should disappear after 3 to 5 days. If irritation persists, the medication should be discontinued. Other topical agents, such as Ben Gay, Icy Hot, and similar preparations, are menthol-based and have a temporary, local effect. Topical preparations also give the patient a sense of control over his or her own treatment. (See Drugs Commonly Prescribed 14.3.)

Intra-articular Agents. Two groups of drugs are injected intra-articularly, particularly in arthritis of the knee. Intra-articular steroids have been used for some time in the treatment of OA of the knee. Several controlled studies document their efficacy for up to 4 weeks, although some patients report a response for up to 6 months after injection. Agents include triamcinolone hexacetonide, triamcinolone acetonide, or methylprednisolone (Solu-Medrol). A 1 percent lidocaine solution is usually mixed with the steroid before injection. Patients are instructed to rest the joint for a day and to limit physical activity for 48 to 72 hours postinjection. The hip may also be injected. Joint injection is also used in these and other joints for bursitis or tendonitis.

The use of intra-articular injections of corticosteroids should be judicious: No more than three to four injections should be done per year and up to a maximum of 12 injections per joint, and they should be used only in episodes of acute flareup. If steroid injections are administered excessively, they can accelerate joint deterioration.

Viscosupplementation. Viscosupplementation with intra-articular hyaluronic acid is also used for treatment of osteoarthritis of the knee. Hyaluronic acid is a naturally occurring component of synovial fluid; its purpose is to lubricate the joint for low-impact activities and potentially to prevent mechanical joint damage during high-impact activities. In patients with OA, the viscosity and elasticity of synovial fluid are decreased; there may be a lower concentration and limited distribution of hyaluronic acid. Consequently, all of the rheologic features of synovial fluid, such as shock absorption, lubrication, and protection, may be decreased. This further increases damage to synovial tissue and the articular cartilage surface. Hyaluronan (Hyalgan), hylan G-F 20 (Synvisc), and hyaluronic acid (Orthovisc, a highly purified, high molecular weight form of hyaluronic acid, approved for use of the United States only fairly recently) are intended to restore all of the protective functions found in normal synovial fluid. They are indicated for pain relief of OA of the knee that has failed to respond to conservative measures. Intra-articular injections of hyaluronic acid are marketed as medical devices, not medications, and may be used in conjunction with NSAIDs. It is injected once a week for 3 to 5 weeks depending on the preparation, and it may provide benefit for 6 months or longer. Both hyaluronan and hyalin are produced from chicken combs, so patients should be screened for any allergy to avian proteins, feathers, and egg products before injection of hyaluronic acid. Other contraindications for intra-articular injections include knee joint infections, skin diseases, or skin infections at the injection site. If there is joint effusion, aspiration of synovial fluid before injection is advised. Adverse effects of hyaluronic acid injections include transient, localized pain, burning, and swelling at the injection site. Several studies have demonstrated the efficacy of viscosupplementation as equal to or better than continuous NSAID therapy, with significant improvement in pain at night or at rest as well as pain on motion, including walking pain. Duration of benefit was 8 to 12 months. Intra-articular injection is not 100 percent effective; one study suggested that the benefit was confined to patients with mild degenerative arthritis. Other conflicting information about viscosupplementation indicates the need for more studies and more rigorous methodology.

Drugs Commonly Prescribed 14.3: Pharmacologic Treatment of OA

Drug/Usage	Dose	Comments
Acetaminophen—still considered first-line therapy although more recent trials find NSAIDs more effective.	1 g q4–6h; up to 4 g/day	Monitor use of ETOH; low cost, easy availability, overall safety profile.
Capsaicin Cream	0.025% Cream qid	Naturally occurring substance that seems to interfere with transmission of painful stimuli.
NSAIDs—(see Drugs Commonly Prescribed 14.2) Some theoretic evidence that NSAIDs inhibit joint repair by interfering with prostaglandin synthesis.	Start at low dose; try as needed *Topical NSAIDs have similar profile	Renal and/or platelet dysfunction; GI bleeding *Risk Factors for GI Bleed: greater age, comorbidity, history of peptic ulcer, history GI bleed, glucocorticoids, anticoagulation, combination NSAID therapy and increase dose
Tramadol HCl/Ultram—mild—moderate pain; available with Tylenol as Ultracet—centrally acting analgesic; does not inhibit prostaglandin synthesis.	50–100 mg q4–8h, not to exceed 400 mg in 24 hours; Ultracet—37.5 mg q4–8h, not to exceed 8 in 24 hours (200–400 mg/day = ibuprofen 1200–2400 mg/day)	Low abuse potential; nonscheduled; Ultracet may be more effective if patient can take two tablets at once. *Start at low dose (e.g., 25 mg/day).
Propoxyphene (Darvon)—mild to moderate pain	100 mg every 4 hours as needed. Max: 600 mg/day	Weak narcotic. *May increase risk of hip fracture by 60%.
Codeine (Tylenol with codeine #3, #4) #3 = 30 mg of codeine; #4 = 60 mg of codeine; Tylenol = 300 mg per tablet	#3—One to two tablets q4h #4—One tablet q4h	Weak opioid; SE profile not good for older adults; *also increased risk of hip fracture. Use with caution in head injury; constipation.
Oral glucosamine and chondroitin sulfate—OTC, dietary supplements	Daily dosage 1500 mg/day and 1200 mg/day, respectively Combination does not appear beneficial.	Evidence of pain relief with both agents; requires additional study.
S-Adenosyl-L-methionine (SAM)—OTC, dietary supplement used to treat OA and depression	200–400 mg tid	Some studies support effectiveness as equal to NSAIDs without the SE; needs further study.
Hyaluronic acid (Viscosupplement injection)—used as joint injection for pain relief for OA of knee only	Either three injections over 15 days or weekly injections for 5 weeks	Expensive; mild adverse effects include injection site inflammatory/allergic reaction, transient worsening of symptoms; systemic include occasional muscle cramps (not common); always risk of infection with intra-articular injection.
Corticosteroids—symptom relief for weeks or months— Hydrocortisone (Cortisol) Prednisolone tebutate (Hydeltra) Methylprednisolone acetate (Depo-Medrol) Triamcinolone acetonide (Kenalog) Triamcinolone hexacetonide (Aristospan) Betamethasone (Celestone)	Intra-articular injection—dose depends on anatomic site and medication. *No more than two injections should be given in any weightbearing joint.	Duration of relief may be short (1–2 weeks) in lower extremities, shoulder, or elbow; may be effective in hand for several months; always risk of infection with intra-articular injection.

Surgical Management

If nonsurgical strategies fail to provide sufficient pain relief and maintenance of function, referral to a rheumatologist or an orthopedic surgeon for surgical evaluation is indicated. Arthroscopic procedures can include joint lavage, partial medial or lateral meniscectomy or chondroplasty as indicated, lateral patellar retinacular release, fracture drilling of full-thickness defects, or chondral grafts. Large or open surgical procedures could include osteotomy and partial or total joint arthroplasty. For maximum success, ongoing communication between patients, medical and surgical providers, and physical therapists is essential in identifying appropriate candidates for surgery, treating comorbidities, and establishing rehabilitation goals. A recent study of outcomes following total hip and knee replacement demonstrated a higher level of postoperative function and better quality of life in candidates who had surgery earlier rather than waiting until the pain was intolerable and functional abilities had declined. In another study, psychosocial factors such as motivation and emotional and social functioning (measured at baseline) were strong predictors of postoperative recovery. Once a patient has undergone total joint replacement, prophylactic antibiotics for dental work and other procedures is recommended by some authorities. Annual radiographs to evaluate the position and fixation of the prosthetic components may also be recommended.

Long-Term Pain Management

For patients who are not candidates for surgery and who have intractable pain, long-term pain management is necessary. Goals of long-term pain management are to maximize quality of life and minimize pain and functional loss. Consultation with a pain management specialist for collaborative management may be beneficial; the use of alternative treatments, including massage therapy, acupuncture, or acupressure, can further enhance pain management and promote a feeling of relaxation and well-being. Pharmacologic management should be individualized; it should take into consideration comorbidities, other medications, age, and functional abilities.

New technologies continue to be developed for this disabling disorder. Newer medications, complementary therapies, different prosthetic joint components, osteochondral replacement procedures, and gene therapy for rare hereditary forms of OA are some promising new directions.

Nonpharmacologic Management

Self-Care Strategies. Initial management of OA includes patient education about the nature of the disease, the role of the patient in self-management, and sources of information and support for the patient. The Arthritis Foundation is an excellent resource and offers information sheets, local support groups, and an arthritis self-help course that includes exercise, joint protection, and relaxation techniques, along with information on medications that are typically used to manage symptoms. Weight loss is often an important component of the plan of care (Table 14.7).

Involvement of the patient's spouse or significant other in the education and support of the individual with arthritis, specifically in helping him or her to develop coping skills, has proven superior to working with the patient alone. In a recent study of patients with OA, an informal network of social support appeared effective in mitigating the depression and functional limitations imposed by the disease and significantly enhancing quality of life. Trials of regular monthly phone calls by trained lay personnel to patients,

Table 14.7 Nonpharmacologic Therapies for OA

Nonpharmacologic Therapies	Comments
Continued reassurance and support	Simply telephoning patients periodically can be helpful; support group
Patient education	Provide materials
Protection from overuse	Educate
Exercise—only 24% of patients with OA report a level of activity consistent with health; >75% sedentary	Gentle, regular joint exercise help maintain function and manage pain; water exercise especially effective; other non-weightbearing, bicycling, for example, preserve muscle support; isometric exercises to maintain strength; moderate to vigorous exercise three times a week can lead to dramatic improvements.
Weight loss—BMI should be 25 or lower	Especially important for patients with lower extremity problems; needed after joint replacement also to preserve joint implant
Surgery—indicated if patient has pain at rest, at night, unable to sleep, unacceptable loss of joint function	Joint replacements (hip and knee replacement especially effective in pain and function); patients who have undergone earlier preemptive procedure such as arthroscopic joint débridement, or osteotomy may eventually require joint replacement
Acupuncture	One study showed decrease in pain of about 40% and improved function.
Heat/ice	Application of heat to the OA joint effective—hot shower, bath; ice occasionally
Shoe inserts, patellar taping, bracing (knee), gait aids (cane)	A variety of mechanical aids useful for support

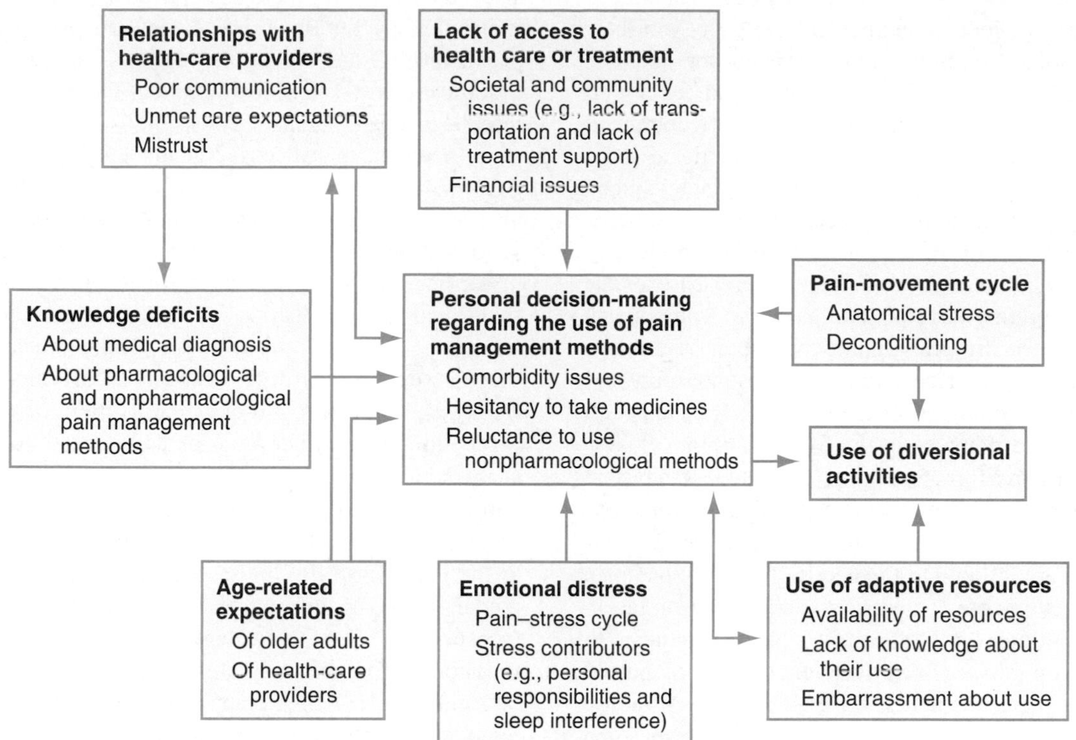

FIGURE 14.2 Theoretical models of barriers to chronic pain management by older adults with arthritis. (From Davis, GC, Hiemenz, ML, and White, TL: Barriers to managing chronic pain of older adults with arthritis. J Nurs Scholar 34(2):121–126, 2002.)

discussing issues such as pain, medication, and treatment adherence, access to medical services, and functional concerns, were also effective. Patients experienced improvement in pain status and function with specific counseling; medical costs were negligible.

Nursing research (see Nursing Research-Based Practice 14.1) demonstrates a variety of impediments to effective pain management. Being aware of the many psychosocial factors that can influence the management of the patient's symptoms (Fig. 14.2) can assist the clinician in helping the patient toward more effective self-care.

Physical Therapy. Nonpharmacologic management strategies include weight loss (when appropriate) and physical

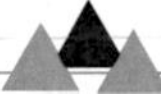

NURSING RESEARCH-BASED PRACTICE 14.1

Davis, GC, Hiemenz, ML, and White, TL: Barriers to managing chronic pain of older adults with arthritis. J Nurs Scholar 34 (2):121–126, 2002.

This research study explored barriers to pain management experienced by older adults with arthritis via a grounded theory methodolgy. Data were collected from 57 older-adult participants with self-reported arthritis via focus groups. Nine themes were identified. The central theme was identified as *Personal Decision-making Regarding the Use of Pain Management Methods* with associated properties of comorbidity, hesitancy to take medication, and reluctance to try nonpharmacologic methods as the major factors, perceptions, and beliefs that influenced participant's decision-making. This theme was central to the associated themes identified which included: (1) relationship with health-care providers, (2) lack of access to health-care treatment, (3) pain-movement cycles, (4) use of diversional activities, (5) use of adaptive resources, (6) emotional distress, (7) age-related expectations, and (8) knowledge deficits.

A better understanding of barriers to pain management can enhance an independent older person's ability to manage chronic pain, as well as knowledge for all health care providers. This understanding can be used in assessments and in planning individualized interventions that include client's as active participants in managing pain.

therapy for muscle strengthening, particularly quadriceps strengthening for patients with knee OA. The physical therapist also evaluates mobility and the need for assistive devices such as canes or walkers to reduce load bearing on the arthritic joint. The physical therapist may recommend environmental modifications to maximize functional independence and safety. Other orthotic devices, such as shoe lifts, splints, or bracing, may be prescribed to improve biomechanics. Heat, ice, or ultrasound may be applied locally to decrease pain. Whenever feasible, a supervised exercise program incorporating aerobic and resistive components should be instituted. Several significant studies of arthritis patients utilizing comparison groups attest to the safety and efficacy of fitness training programs versus ROM and health education alone. Participants in the fitness program experienced better task performance and reported less physical disability, less pain, and improved psychological functioning. Aquatic exercise programs are also excellent, particularly those that are tailored to the needs of arthritic patients.

Transcutaneous electrical nerve stimulation (TENS) is sometimes used for arthritic pain, but studies to date have not established its effectiveness. Use of pulsed electric and electromagnetic fields (PEMF), more commonly for the treatment of nonunion fractures, has shown some promise in preliminary studies of patients with knee OA, but further studies are needed before PEMF can be recommended as adjunctive treatment for OA.

Occupational Therapy. Short-term occupational therapy to maximize ADL abilities and evaluate the need for adaptive devices is often overlooked, but it can be very valuable to the patient with arthritis. Devices such as a raised toilet seat, toilet siderails, elastic shoe laces, reachers, and various kitchen accessories can enhance functional capacity and independence.

Complementary Therapy. Acupuncture and nutritional therapy (including vitamin supplementation) are other therapies used for the management of OA and other musculoskeletal problems. (See Complementary Therapies 14.1.) A growing body of evidence suggests that acupuncture may be beneficial as adjunctive treatment for OA. Methyl sulfonyl methane (MSM) and *S*-adenosyl methionine (SAM-e) are other dietary supplements some patients find beneficial, although at present, no evidence exists to support this. Therapeutic magnets also appear helpful to some patients anecdotally.

Follow-Up and Referral

Patients with OA may be referred to a rheumatologist or orthopedic surgeon for collaborative management. When conservative measures fail, the patient's quality of life can be markedly diminished. Frequent or constant disabling pain, especially pain at rest, and functionally limiting symptoms are the most important criteria for orthopedic referral. They may also be referred to physical therapy or occupational therapy for functional evaluation, education in joint preservation, and recommendations for environmental modifications to maximize function. Other options include referral to a pain management specialist, a professional massage therapist, or a licensed acupuncturist. Referral to the Arthritis Foundation for patient education and support is also valuable. The patient should be seen for follow-up at 3- to 6-month intervals, and should be instructed to contact his or her primary health-care provider if pain increases or functional status declines. ROM and functional status should be assessed at each visit. There are a number of scales, such as Arthritis Impact Measurement Scale-2 (AIMS2), that allow the clinician to monitor the patient's perception of his or her progress with greater accuracy. This scale can be viewed at htpp://www.qolid.org/public/aims/cadre. A short version of this scale is available also. A variety of other scales measure function and disability, such as the Pain Disability Index (PDI) available at htpp://www.medal.org/ch37.html, and the Stanford Health Assessment Questionnaire (HAQ), available at htpp://www. aramis stanford.edu/HAQ.html. It is important to monitor all patients on aspirin or NSAID therapy for GI blood loss and cardiac, renal, and mental status. Practitioners should order periodic CBC, renal function tests, and stool for occult blood.

Patient Education

Education of the patient and support persons is essential to successful management of OA. The Arthritis Foundation is an excellent resource for patient education, as well as a variety of services that are provided at the local and national level. Courses such as the Arthritis Self-Help Course (ASHC) and People with Arthritis Can Exercise (PACE) are available. Research has shown that patients who complete the ASHC show a decrease in pain and physician visits, even with increased physical disability. The improvements, sustained over a 4-year period, are attributed to these patients' feelings of enhanced self-efficacy.

Exercise programs should be individualized, with protection of the weightbearing joints. Swimming or water exercise (which minimizes impact on joints) is especially recommended. Rest after exercise is also important.

The patient with OA needs to be aware of potential adverse effects of medications and drug interactions. Key areas for education include acceptance of the chronic nature of OA and lifestyle management to maximize function and minimize pain, and the preservation of joint function. Vocational rehabilitation may also be necessary.

Low Back Pain

Low back pain (LBP), also referred to as low back sprain, or lumbar sprain, strictly speaking is an injury to the paravertebral spinal muscles. The term also is used to describe lig-

COMPLEMENTARY THERAPIES 14.1

Osteoarthritis and Musculoskeletal Problems

Acupuncture/Acupressure, Massage, and Bodywork Therapy

Acupuncture is used for treatment of OA in Asia, and is being used more frequently in other countries as a complementary modality for OA. Uncontrolled studies in which patients were treated with standard medical therapy and acupuncture have demonstrated significant improvement in functional status and pain relief. These findings have not been replicated in controlled studies using sham acupuncture; both groups in the controlled studies experienced marked improvement. Although further controlled studies on efficacy are needed, acupuncture can be used and is safe and well tolerated.

Acupressure is also used as an adjunct, as are various types of massage and bodywork therapy. Building upon prior studies of spa therapy, a European randomized, controlled study utilized 3 weeks of spa therapy for older patients with OA of the lumbar spine, hip, or knee. Participants experienced significant improvement in function, decreased pain, and decreased use of analgesics and NSAIDs for 24 weeks after the final treatment. Tai-chi has also been studied as an intervention for OA.

Herbals may be used to treat the pain associated with cervical muscle sprain/strain and spasm. Vervain acts like mild aspirin, relieving minor pains and inflammation. White willow is considered nature's aspirin and has been used in China since ancient times to relieve pain and inflammation. These herbs can be made into teas by using powder to brew. Care must be taken to follow directions regarding the amount needed and how often they are used, as renal and gastrointestinal side effects may occur. Massage may be especially helpful. Acupuncture or acupressure may also be considered as adjunctive therapy for patients with chronic cervical spine pain.

The following describes complementary therapies for different musculoskeletal problems.

Problem and Therapy	Dosage	Comment
Arthritis		
Turmeric	400 mg tid with meals (95% curcumin) Once symptoms have improved cut the daily dose in half.	Anti-inflammatory and antioxidant properties. May interfere with cancer chemotherapy agents.
Niacin (vitamin B_3; niacinamide)	500–2000 mg bid	Anti-inflammatory properties; decreases joint inflammation.
SAMe (*S*-adenosylmethionine)	200–400 mg bid	Mechanism of action unknown but preliminary studies show it may have a role in repairing cartilage and lubricating joints. Should not be taken with MAO inhibitors.
Selenium	200–400 mcg qd	Controls free radicals which may destroy cartilage
Chondroitin	400–600 mg tid	May slow cartilage loss, increase joint mobility; mechanism unknown but may encourage water retention in cartilage and inhibit enzymes that break down cartilage.
Glucosamine	500 mg tid	May protect and strengthen cartilage; studies are ongoing.
Green tea	100 mg qd (extract) or 4 cups of brewed tea	Antioxidant and possibly anti-inflammatory
Cayenne pepper (*Capsicum annuum*)	400–500 mg tid or Cream containing 0.02–0.05% capsaicinoids up to qid	Stops Substance P and contains antinociceptive substances which relieve pain.
MSM (methylsulfonylmethane)	500 mg bid–tid	May inhibit transmission of pain impulses and has anti-inflammatory properties.
Carpal tunnel syndrome		
Turmeric	400 mg tid with meals (95% curcumin) Once symptoms have improved cut the daily dose in half.	Anti-inflammatory and antioxidant properties. May interfere with cancer chemotherapy agents.
Fibromyalgia		
Magnesium with malic acid	150–250 mg tid (Mg) 400–800 mg malic acid tid	Relieves aching associated with fibromyalgia. Malic acid enhances absorption of magnesium.

(continued)

COMPLEMENTARY THERAPIES 14.1 (continued)

Osteoarthritis and Musculoskeletal Problems

Problem and Therapy	Dosage	Comment
SAMe (*S*-adenosylmethione)	400–600 mg bid	Studies show that SAMe helps minimize muscle pain, depression, and fatigue that are associated with fibromyalgia. Should not be taken with MAO inhibitors.
Muscle cramps		
Magnesium	400 mg bid	Necessary for muscle contraction and relaxation
Musculoskeletal pain		
White willow bark (Salix alba)	40–80 mg tid (salicin is white willow barks active ingredient)	Has analgesic and anti-inflammatory properties. Salicin is the active ingredient which the body converts to salicylic acid.
SAMe (*S*-adenosylmethioine)	400 mg bid 1 hour before or 2 hours after eating.	May have a part in repair and restoration of intervertebral discs and cartilage.
Osteoporosis		
Calcium	500–800 mg bid–tid	Needed for building and maintaining bone mass
Magnesium	250–400 mg bid	Helps in the activation of vitamin D needed for calcium absorption.
Sprains/strains		
Arnica	Gel, cream, or ointment applied topically q3–4h	Do not take internally. May hasten healing of acute joint injuries and prevent future injury
Glucosamine	500 mg tid	May strengthen joints and hasten healing of acute joint injuries such as sprains and strains.

amentous injuries to the facet joints or anulus fibrosus. The disk may not herniate into the spinal canal, but substances can leak from the nucleus pulposus that induce inflammation and cause irritation of the lumbosacral nerve roots. Owing to the deep location of the lumbar soft tissues, localizing an injury to a specific structure is very difficult if not impossible. Whether muscle or ligamentous structures are involved, the treatment is similar.

LBP is also defined as activity intolerance because of lower back or back-related leg symptoms of less than 3 months' duration. LBP occurs in almost 70 percent of adults at some point in their lives. About 90 percent of patients with acute LBP will spontaneously recover activity tolerance within 1 month. However, back pain associated with a neurologic deficit, decreased or absent pulses, or bowel and bladder dysfunction are potentially life-threatening and warrant immediate referral. Acute low back pain (ALBP) is pain that persists for less than 3 to 6 weeks. Chronic low back pain (CLBP) is defined as pain lasting longer than 3 months; symptoms are typically recurrent and episodic, but may be unremitting.

Epidemiology and Causes

LBP occurs in almost 70 percent of adults at some point in their lives. LBP is one of the most frequent reasons that patients visit primary-care providers and is the most common reason for loss of work time and disability in adults younger than 45 years. Most symptoms are of limited duration, with 85 percent of patients demonstrating significant improvement and returning to work within the month. The 4 percent of patients whose symptoms persist longer than 6 months generate 85 to 90 percent of the costs to society for treating low back pain. Repetitive episodes, however, are common. It is second only to headache as the reason for a complaint of pain. At any given time, 31 million Americans will be experiencing some sort of ALBP. ALBP occurs most frequently in adults between their 20s and 40s; CLBP typically is seen between and the third and sixth decades of life, or even older for women.

The overall incidence of LBP is equal in men and women, but women report more LBP after age 60, most likely due to osteoporosis; these women are at risk for vertebral compression factor. In addition, a woman's likelihood of experiencing LBP is increased after two or more pregnancies. Approximately 2 percent of patients with ALBP have lumbar radiculopathy, or "sciatica" and/or disk herniation (see next section on Herniated Disk).

There are two divisions of risk factors that influence LBP: The first group of risk factors is occupational and the second is patient-related. Occupations that require hard labor and heavy exertions have been associated with increased risk of LBP. Lifting, pulling and pushing, twisting, slipping, sitting for an extended period, and exposure to prolonged vibration (such as driving or riding in a motor vehicle for long periods of time, as truck drivers do) have been attributed to the development of LBP. In addition, patients who view their occupations as boring, repetitious, or dissatisfying have been associated with a higher rate of LBP. LBP is the most frequent cause of lost workdays in the United States.

There is a higher risk of LBP in obese persons and in tall persons. No studies have proven posture as a definite risk factor for LBP, but spine pain from scoliosis is well known and is the basis of this risk factor. Many studies have shown decreased strength of abdominal and spinal muscles in patients with LBP. Physical fitness and conditioning has been found to have a preventive effect on low back injuries. Smoking has been shown to increase one's risk of LBP. Aging increases the risk for CLBP. Finally, psychosocial factors such as depression, anxiety, and alcoholism, among others, have been reported with higher frequency in patients with chronic LBP.

The cause of back pain is not always clear, but it may be related to ligamentous or muscular strain resulting from either a specific traumatic episode or an incompetence of the soft-tisse structure (ALBP). Degeneration of the intervertebral disk, a physiologic event of aging, modified by such factors as injury, repetitive trauma, infection, heredity, and tobacco use, may lead to CLBP. As the hydrophilic properties of the nucleus pulposus degrade, the disk loses height and formerly tight ligaments become loose. Motions such as sliding and twisting create tears in the annulus fibrosus. Osteoarthritis and CLBP may develop.

Pathophysiology

The lumbosacral spine supports the upper body in a balanced, upright position while allowing locomotion. In a static, upright position, maintenance of erect posture is achieved through a balance among the expansile pressure of the intervertebral disks, the stretch placed on the anterior and posterior longitudinal and facet joint ligaments, and the sustained involuntary tone generated by the surrounding lumbosacral and abdominal muscles. The balance of the spine is also related to the reciprocal physiologic curves in the cervical, thoracic, and lumbosacral areas of the vertebral column. The balance in curvature results in an individual's posture. Proper alignment is also influenced by structures in the pelvis and lower extremities. Movement of the lumbar spine is associated with a lumbar pelvic rhythm that results in the simultaneous reversal of the lumbar lordosis and rotation of the hips. During flexion and extension of the lumbar spine, tension is produced in the paraspinous, hamstring, and gluteal muscles, the fasciae that surround the muscles, and the ligaments that support the vertebral bodies and disks. In addition to the normal stresses placed on these structures with lowering and raising of the torso, the stresses on these anatomic structures are increased to an even greater degree when an individual is required to lift a heavy object.

LBP that is associated with back strain may be related to anatomic structures that are tonically contracted in the resting position. LBP may also occur during motion if the stress is greater than the supporting structures can sustain, or if the components of the lumbosacral spine are abnormal. Although the precise pathophysiology of uncomplicated lumbar strain (back strain) is not well characterized, damage may occur in lumbosacral spinal structures if the amount of force generated exceeds the stress capacity of the spine for an individual patient. If the lumbosacral spine is in a mechanically disadvantaged position (e.g., rotated or flexed) the force may not need to be that great to cause a disruption of annular fibers. These fibers may tear when stressed, which in turn causes degeneration of the disk. An annular tear is associated with the production of pain, and may account for the frequent episodes of LBP in patients who eventually rupture a nucleus pulposus. Protruding or bulging intervertebral disk material may then impinge on a spinal nerve root, imparting specific radiculopathic symptoms depending on the spinal level affected. Disk herniation (herniated nucleus pulposus) is discussed as a separate entity in the next section of this chapter.

Far less common than uncomplicated lumbar strain, several other spinal conditions exist that produce LBP. Spinal stenosis results in nerve impingement with back and lower extremity (calf) pain on extension of the spine owing to the narrowed spinal canal, as this maneuver lengthens and further narrows the canal. Osteoarthritis typically produced erosions with irregular bony deposition known as osteophytes at the articular sites of the vertebrae which may also result in nerve impingement and pain as a result of degeneration of the joint. Significant scoliosis can predispose to osteoarthritis and may result in chronic LBP resulting from a fundamental derangement of vertebral biomechanics, that is, the ability of the axial musculoskeletal system to appropriately distribute mechanical loads placed on the spine. Spondylolisthesis is a slipping (displacement) of one vertebral body either anteriorly or posteriorly relative to another which may be a congenital or acquired condition, most often due to increased or repeated stress on the bilateral pars interarticularis from spinal hyperextension, the posterior bony plate connecting the superior and inferior articular facets of an intervertebral joint. A lesion or fracture of the pars interarticularis which causes the facet to separate without actual anterior or posterior slippage of a vertebral body is known as spondylolysis. Either of these conditions may result in nerve impingement with lower back and extremity pain. Although spondylolysis may be asymptomatic, this condition may progress to spondylolisthesis. Importantly, however, all of these conditions may be identified as incidental findings on spinal imaging (plain film or CT scan) in the absence of actual symptoms. Thus, these anatomic and pathologic findings must always be correlated with clinical presentation.

Clinical Presentation

Subjective

An acute onset of LBP often follows a lifting episode, or may be precipitated by something as minor as a sneeze or cough. Patients may have difficulty standing erect and often change position frequently for comfort. The pain often radiates into the buttocks and posterior thigh. The condition often occurs for the first time during the young adult years. There may be associated grimacing and generalized hypersensitivity to light touch. Initial assessment of a patient with activity intolerance resulting from LBP consisting of a focused medical history, including a history of the present illness, past medical history, family history, occupational and social history. A review of systems, especially description of any injury, is essential and may alerts the provider to possible "red flags" warranting immediate attention. A history of recent trauma, recent lumbar puncture, concurrent infection, or chronic use of high-dose corticosteroids will help establish an accurate diagnosis. (See Focusing the History 14.2.) Some questions to consider while evaluating the patient's responses include:

- Is there a serious systemic disease causing the pain?
- Is there neurologic compromise that might require surgical evaluation?
- Is there social or psychological distress that may amplify or prolong pain?

The hallmark symptom of CLBP is recurrent low back pain that often radiates to one or both buttocks. The pain may be described as "mechanical" in that it is aggravated by activities such as bending, stooping, or twisting. There may be stiffness and a history of intermittent sciatica (i.e., pain radiating down the back of the leg), but discomfort in the lower back remains the predominant symptom. This may be relieved with lying down or a good night's sleep, although if the pain is severe enough it may awaken the patient at night. Psychosocial indicators should be assessed as they can be barriers to recovery in all cases of LBP, both acute and chronic. Consider factors such as fear, financial problems, anger, depression, job dissatisfaction, family problems, or stress that can contribute to prolonged disability.

> **FOCUS ON HISTORY 14.2**
>
> **Low Back Pain**
>
> For the patient who complains of low back pain, focus the history by asking questions that will obtain the following information:
>
> - Mode of onset (abrupt or insidious?)
> - Characteristics:
>   Provoking factors
>   Aggravating factors
>   Relieving factors
> - Effects of activities
>   Posture
>   Coughing, sneezing, straining
>   Exercise, exertion, rest
>   Sleep
> - History:
>   Similar or different pains
>   Course (progressive, decreasing, increasing, fluctuating, episodic?)
>   Associated limb and/or neurologic symptoms (pain, paresthesias, numbness, weakness, atrophy, cramps, fasiculations?)
> - Associated symptoms:
>   Urinary problems (frequency, urgency, retention, incontinence?)
>   Bowel problems (incontinence or constipation?)
> - Previous back pain history and treatment (medications, types of surgery, nonpharmacologic management, lifestyle and work modifications, litigation or compensation issues?)

Objective

There is often diffuse tenderness to the lower back. ROM of the lumbar spine, particularly flexion, is typically reduced and elicits pain. Patients may exhibit a side or forward list from muscle spasm. The degree of lumbar flexion and the ease with which the patient can extend the spine are helpful parameters by which to evaluate progress. While not characteristic, nonorganic findings, such as widespread sensitivity to light touch, nonanatomic localization of symptoms, inappropriate grimacing, inconsistent actions, exaggerated pain behaviors may be seen. In most cases of uncomplicated LBP, the motor and sensory functions of the lumbosacral nerve roots and reflexes of the lower extremities are normal. Negative straight-leg raise rules out surgically significant disc herniation in 95 percent of cases. (See Advanced Assessment 14.9.)

Diagnostic Reasoning

Diagnostic Tests

In cases of CLBP, AP and lateral radiographs often show age-appropriate change, such as anterior osteophytes and reduced height of intervertebral disks on the lateral view. ALBP does not warrant radiographs except on the following circumstances:

- Unrelenting night pain or pain at rest
- Fever above 38 degrees C or 100.4 degrees F for greater than 48 hours
- Progressive neuromotor defect
- Pain with distal numbness or leg weakness
- Loss of bowel or bladder control (retention or incontinence)
- Significant trauma
- History of suspicion of cancer
- Osteoporosis
- Chronic oral steroids
- Immunosuppressed or immunosuppressive medication
- Drug or alcohol abuse
- Clinical suspicion of ankylosing spondylitis

ADVANCED ASSESSMENT 14.9

Assessing the Lower Back—Special Tests

Test	Comments
Straight-leg raising—places L5 and S1 nerve roots and the sciatic nerve under tension.	With the patient supine and relaxed, elevate the leg until either the leg begins to bend or the patient reports severe pain in buttock or back. Record degree of elevation at which pain occurs. It is considered positive when the pain is elicited below the level of the knee when the leg is raised less than 60 degrees. Next, dorsiflex the ankle to determine whether this motion increased pain (further stretch of the L5 and S1 nerve roots). Plantar flexion of the ankle relieves sciatic tension. Increased back pain with this maneuver is probably nonorganic. The straight-leg raising test is very sensitive, but not very specific. To increase specificity, raise the leg until pain is felt below the knee, then lower the leg about 5 degrees which should eliminate the pain. Then, have patient dorsiflex the ipsilateral foot while the leg is raised. This should cause more traction on the sciatic nerve and reproduce the symptoms.
Reverse straight-leg raising—places the L1–4 nerve roots under tension.	With the patient prone, lift the hip into extension while keeping the knee straight. Increased pain suggests compression of the upper lumbar nerve roots.
Prone Rectus femoris test—places L1–4 nerve roots under tension.	With the patient prone, maintain the hip in a neutral position while flexing the knee. Increased pain suggests compression of the upper lumbar nerve roots.

- ▲ Consider a complete blood count and erythrocyte sedimentation rate if suspicion of cancer or infection.

Differential Diagnosis

LBP is a diagnosis of exclusion. The diagnosis of back strain is based on the history of localized LBP, and a compatible physical examination demonstrating localized pain, muscle spasm, and a normal neurologic examination. CLBP is recurrent, has lasted for a longer period of time, and the patient may also demonstrate mildly restricted straight leg raising and spinal motion. (See Advanced Assessment 14.9.) Differential diagnoses for ALBP/CLBP are listed below:

- ▲ Ankylosing spondylitis (family history, morning stiffness, limited mobility of the lumbar spine)
- ▲ Drug-seeking behavior (exaggerated symptoms, inconsistent and nonphysiologic exam)
- ▲ Extraspinal causes (ovarian cyst, nephrolithiasis pancreatitis, ulcer disease, abdominal aortic aneurysm)
- ▲ Fracture of the vertebral body (major trauma or minimal trauma with osteoporosis)
- ▲ Herniated nucleus pulposus or ruptured disk (unilateral radicular pain symptoms that extend below the knee and are equal to or greater than the back pain)
- ▲ Infection (fever, chills, sweats, elevated erythrocyte sedimentation rate (ESR)
- ▲ Myeloma (night sweats, men older than 50)

Differential diagnoses for CLBP that are different than ALBP are listed below:

- ▲ Depression (abnormal Beck Depression Inventory, sleep disturbances)
- ▲ Illness behavior (multiple surgeries, multiple illnesses)
- ▲ Inflammatory arthritides (morning stiffness for more than 30 minutes, positive HLA-B27, increased ESR)
- ▲ Intervertebral disk infection or vertebral osteomyelitis (history of excruciating pain, recent IV drug use, fever, recent infection/hospitalization, open wound)
- ▲ Metastatic tumors myeloma, lymphoma (pathologic fractures, severe night pain, weight loss, fatigue)
- ▲ Osteoporosis with compression fractures (female gender, previous fracture)
- ▲ Spinal tuberculosis (lower socioeconomic groups, history of AIDS)
- ▲ Workplace dissatisfaction (discontent with boss, job)

See Differential Diagnosis 14.6.

Management

Stress to the patient that most episodes of ALBP are mild and self-limited; almost 90 percent are resolved within 1 to 6 weeks. Symptom control is considered an adjunct to helping the patient to overcome a specific activity intolerance. The management of the patient with LBP, especially if pain is recurrent and/or chronic, requires a Circle of Caring by the practitioner. Multiple approaches are required to address

DIFFERENTIAL DIAGNOSES 14.6: LOW BACK PAIN

Diagnosis	Spondylolisthesis	Muscle Strain	Scoliosis	Herniated Nucleus Pulposus	Osteoarthritis	Spinal Stenosis
Age	20	20–40	30	30–50	>50	>60
Pain location	Back	Back (unilateral)	Back	Back (unilateral)	Back (bilateral)	Leg (bilateral)
Pain onset	Insidious	Acute	Insidious	Acute (prior episodes)	Insidious	Insidious
Pain increases	When standing, bending	When standing, bending	When standing, bending	When sitting, bending	When standing	When standing
Pain decreases	When sitting	When sitting	When sitting	When standing	When sitting, bending	When sitting, bending
Straight leg raising	Negative	Negative	Negative	Positive	Negative	Positive (stress)
X-ray (plain film)	Positive	Negative	Positive	Negative	Positive	Positive

the "iceberg" of LBP and the ways that it can interfere with the lives of patients and families.

Pharmacologic Management

The oral medications used to control the discomfort of LBP primarily include acetaminophen, NSAIDs, muscle relaxants, and opioids. There is fair to good evidence that NSAIDs are effective for reducing pain in patients with LBP. Acetaminophen has also been found to be comparable in efficacy to NSAIDs for treating LBP, with fewer adverse effects. Health-care providers need to be aware that the long-term use of NSAIDs can lead to serious GI disease such as ulcers and hemorrhage, thus patients with GI histories should use this drug cautiously. Using the lowest possible effective dose can help to prevent this problem. Older adults are more sensitive to the adverse effects of NSAIDs, so it is important to use caution when prescribing NSAIDs for this age group. NSAIDs affect the renal prostaglandins and may cause fluid retention and edema, so it is also important for patients to monitor for weight gain. The risk of fluid retention and edema may be very significant in elderly patients and in those with CHF. In addition, there is the potential for nephrotoxicity.

There is moderate research evidence showing that muscle relaxants are more effective than placebo but no evidence that they are better than NSAIDs in relieving symptoms of acute LBP. Patients need to be aware that this class of drugs is for short-term use because the risk–benefit ratio for prolonged use of muscle relaxants is not known. Muscle relaxants cause drowsiness and dizziness, so patients need to avoid hazardous activities. This class of drug is a CNS depressant, so patients need to avoid taking muscle relaxants with alcohol or other CNS depressants, because the combined use will cause additive effects. Dry mouth is another side effect from this antimuscarinic class of drugs, so frequent mouth rinsing is recommended to prevent dental disease.

Research has shown that opioid analgesics did not enhance the patient's ability to return to full activity sooner than patients taking NSAIDs or acetaminophen. In addition, the adverse effects of opioid analgesics were found to be substantial, including the risk for physical dependence.

Activity

It should be stressed that rest has been proven to have little to no effect on the resolution of LBP. Patients should do whatever activities are tolerable. Weight loss, physical activities, and exercise for 30 minutes a day (walking, or biking with lumbar flexion and/or extension exercises) are also important. De-conditioning is a real phenomenon that occurs increasingly quickly with increasing age. Then, lack of activity, leading to de-conditioning, becomes a vicious cycle. Reassurance is always appropriate after ruling out more serious causes of back pain. These patients should not smoke. Do not label patients "disabled."

Follow-Up and Referral

The course of patients with back strain is one of gradual improvement, usually over a 1- to 2-week period. The recovery is usually complete, without any lasting impairment. The small percentage of patients who do not make a complete recovery may continue to experience LBP associated with muscle strain. Pain may continue for months or years. These patients are experiencing CLBP, which must be evaluated and treated in a manner that takes into account the special difficulties of individuals with chronic pain. Patients with more severe symptoms can have limited vocational and avocational activities, recreation, and sleep disturbances. Mood, sexuality, and concentration can be adversely

The Iceberg of Low Back Pain

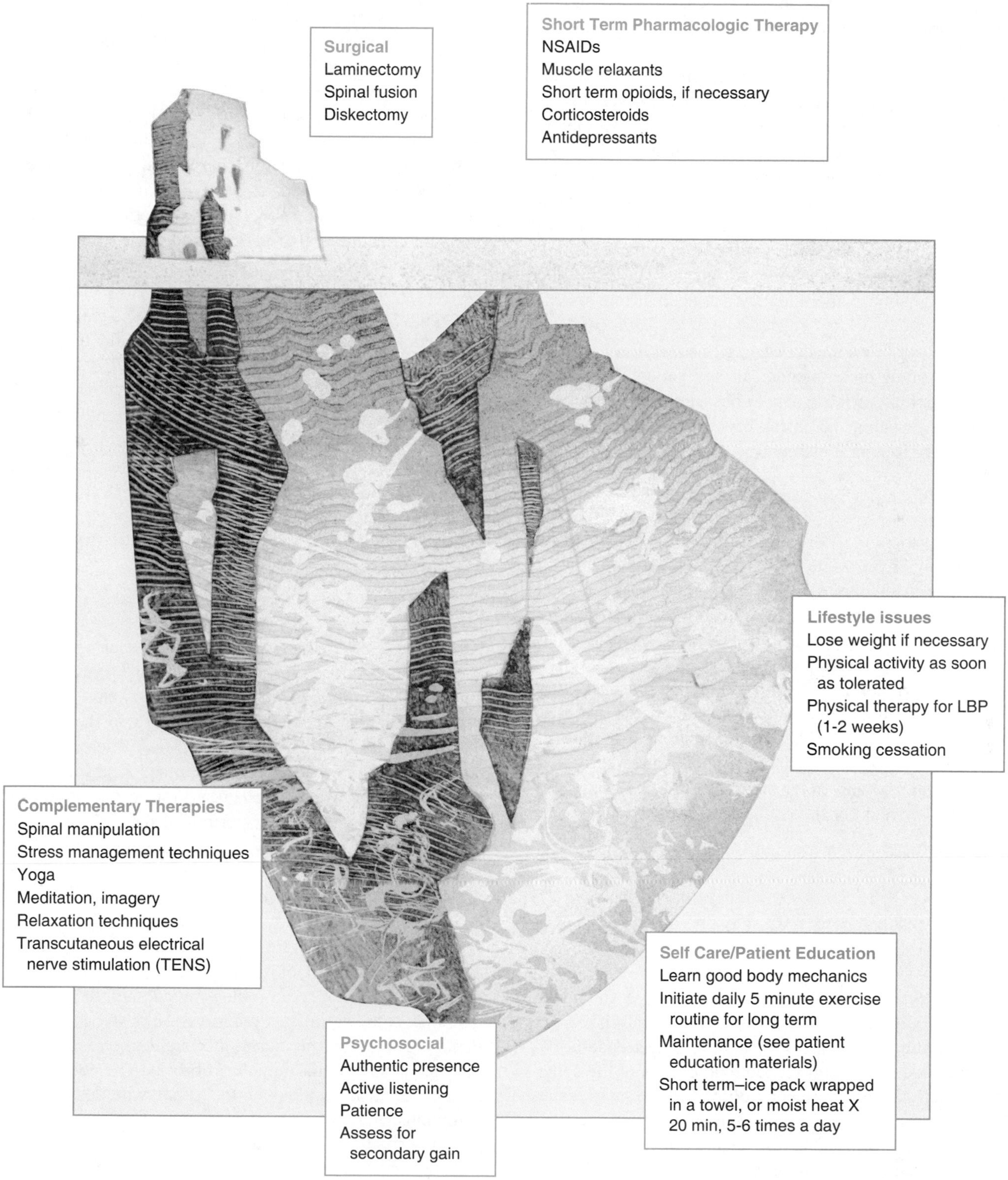

Surgical
Laminectomy
Spinal fusion
Diskectomy

Short Term Pharmacologic Therapy
NSAIDs
Muscle relaxants
Short term opioids, if necessary
Corticosteroids
Antidepressants

Lifestyle issues
Lose weight if necessary
Physical activity as soon as tolerated
Physical therapy for LBP (1-2 weeks)
Smoking cessation

Complementary Therapies
Spinal manipulation
Stress management techniques
Yoga
Meditation, imagery
Relaxation techniques
Transcutaneous electrical nerve stimulation (TENS)

Self Care/Patient Education
Learn good body mechanics
Initiate daily 5 minute exercise routine for long term
Maintenance (see patient education materials)
Short term–ice pack wrapped in a towel, or moist heat X 20 min, 5-6 times a day

Psychosocial
Authentic presence
Active listening
Patience
Assess for secondary gain

affected. De-conditioning can be the result of reduced activities, making both symptoms and and any occupational dysfunction worse. Suggest a modified work schedule and more recreational activities that improve general conditioning. Narcotic abuse and dependency can be a problem for patients with chronic pain.

In all patients, preventing recurrence of back pain is another important consideration. The first episode of back pain is usually the briefest and least severe. The vast majority of individuals with an episode of back pain are at risk of developing another episode of back pain that will be more severe and of greater duration. Patients with recurrence are usually resistant to therapies that are beneficial in management of acute back pain, and therefore may require chronic pain assessment and management strategies (including the use of complementary therapies such as acupuncture or acupressure.)

Referral to a specialist (e.g., neurosurgeon, orthopedic surgeon) is recommended in any patient who has a neurologic deficit, or if the patient has a trauma history with x-ray exam revealing an instability or fracture that could cause damage to neural elements.

Patient Education

Instruct the patient to carefully introduce activities back into his or her day as he or she begins to recover from the worst of the back pain episode. Gradual stretches and regular walking are good activities. Ice or heat, whichever provides more comfort, will help decrease the inflammation. OTC anti-inflammatory medications may be used (e.g., aspirin, NSAIDs) or Tylenol. Provide information on safe back exercises such as modified situps and low back stretches. Encourage patients to make them a regular part of their lifestyle. Emphasize the need to relax. Patients should call if symptoms persist, worsen, or progress; significant pain persists beyond 1 week; or there is no improvement with home management.

Herniated Lumbar Disk (Herniated Nucleus Pulposus)

The most common cause of radicular pain to the lower extremities is a herniated lumbar intervertebral disk. Over time, the lumbar disks are subjected to repeated deformations and large loads with physiologic motion of the spine. In some individuals, fragmentation of the disk may result, followed by annular rupture, and finally a herniation of the nucleus pulposus into the lumbar canal. The resultant herniated disk syndrome (commonly called sciatica or lumbar radiculopathy) may cause pain and/or numbness and/or weakness in one or both lower extremities. In part the pain results from direct mechanical compression of the nerve root and in part from chemical irritation of the nerve root by substances in the nucleus pulposus.

Epidemiology and Causes

Low back pain affects a significant portion of the population at some time in their lives, most commonly between ages 30 and 50. The lifetime incidence of low back pain is between 60 and 90 percent. Among patients with acute back pain, approximately 2 percent have nerve-root symptoms, but only 10 to 25 percent of those patients have symptoms that persist for longer than 6 weeks. Because fewer than 10 percent have symptoms after 3 months, only a limited number of patients require surgical treatment. Disk herniation occurs most commonly at the L4 to 5 or L5 to S1 levels with subsequent irritation of the L5 and S1 nerve root. Herniations at more proximal intervertebral levels constitute only 5 percent of all lumbar disk herniations. Fewer than 2 percent of patients with low back pain have infections, neoplasms, or inflammatory spondyloarthropathies. Spinal stenosis is more likely to be the etiology of radicular pain in patients older than age 55. Disk disease affects males and females equally.

Risk factors are normal aging (often difficult to distinguish between normal aging of the spine and pathologic changes), cigarette smoking, a narrowed lumbar vertebral canal, obesity, osteoporosis, stress, and muscle tension. Causes include trauma (sudden or over time), frequent lifting without proper utilization of body mechanics, and vibration, such as driving and/or riding in a motor vehicle for prolonged periods of time.

Pathophysiology

An intervertebral disk is located between each vertebra and is connected to the vertebral body. The disks have a strong outer layer, the *annulus fibrosus,* and the *nucleus pulposus,* which is a jelly-like material that moves in the center of the annulus and redistributes itself as different stresses are placed on the disk, acting like a shock absorber. Disk anomalies begin when there is injury or degeneration of the annulus fibrosus—the outer portion of the disk. Bulging is an initial indication that the disk is showing signs of wear and tear.

The size of the individual's spinal canal becomes an important consideration when diagnosing a disk problem. A small canal will tolerate less disk material that is bulging, or herniated, ruptured, or extruded. A small herniated disk in one patient will not be a problem; in another, the same size disk may cause significant compression of the neural structures. When a disk herniates, the nucleus pulposus pushes through a tear in the annulus fibrosis. The location and amount of disk material in the canal will determine the symptoms. A small amount of nucleus pulposus in a congenitally small canal can cause significant symptoms. Most disks will rupture more to one side than the other, producing more symptoms in the affected side via compression of a unilateral nerve root. Significant herniations may also bulge bilaterally, producing symptoms on both sides of the body. Thus, the nature of the symptoms is determined by the vertebral level of disk herniation.

In turn, radicular symptoms are the hallmark of disk herniation, and their absence makes this diagnosis highly unlikely. Lesions involving the L5 nerve root produce symptoms extending to the dorsum of the foot with weakened dorsiflexion of the large toe and weakened heel walking. Lesions involving both L5 and S1 nerve roots manifest with symptoms in the lateral and posterior calf, with S1 nerve root lesions extending to the heel as well as gastrocnemius weakness, impaired toe walking, and a reduced or absent ankle reflex. Less common lesions affecting the L4 and L3 nerve roots include a diminished patellar reflex with symptoms extending to the anterior shin and thigh, with quadriceps weakness and difficulty rising from a squatted position.

The *cauda equina* is a continuation of the spinal cord below the first lumbar level in the adult. Referred to as the "horse's tail," it consists of an array of nerves that exit the conus of the spinal cord and continue down the lumbar spine, exiting at different lumbar and sacral levels through foramina. These nerves are responsible for specific sensory and motor functions including perineal sensation and both bladder and anal sphincter function. In some instances, an acute herniation of the disk at the L5 to S1 level may cause acute cauda equina compression characterized by bilateral lower extremity weakness, anesthesia or paresthesia of the perineum and buttocks (saddle anesthesia), and bowel or bladder retention and/or incontinence. This is a medical emergency and requires immediate decompression.

Clinical Presentation

Subjective

The onset of symptoms may be abrupt but is more likely to be insidious. Unilateral radiculopathy is frequently accompanied by low back pain. Some patients report that preexisting back pain disappears when leg pain begins signaling the herniation. The pain is often severe and exaggerated by sitting, walking, standing, coughing, and sneezing. Most often, the pain radiates down from the buttock to the posterior or posterolateral leg to the ankle or foot. These patients typically cannot find a position of comfort. Lying on their side in a fetal position or on their back with a pillow under the knees may afford some relief. Upper or midlumbar radiculopathy (L1 to L4 nerve root compression) refers pain to the anterior aspect of the thigh and often does not radiate below the knee.

Compression of the root may also cause paresthesias, loss of deep tendon reflex, and weakness of specific muscle groups. A herniated nucleus pulposus is most commonly seen in patients from 20 to 50 years of age.

Objective

Most disk ruptures are posterolateral and press upon a lumbar nerve root, which produces radiating pain. There may be paraspinal muscle spasm and lumbar scoliosis, with the trunk tilted away from the affected side. Look for a list with the patient standing. With the patient sitting, look for pain and spinal extension (leaning back) when the leg is raised (flip sign). When coupled with reproduced back pain with supine straight-leg raising limited to less than 45 degrees of leg elevation, these signs are highly reliable for herniated disk.

Evaluate motor and sensory function of the lumbosacral nerve roots as well as the deep tendon reflexes. Evaluate straight-leg raising on both the involved and uninvolved limbs with the patient in the supine position. This test places stress on the L5 and S1 nerve roots. Ipsilateral restriction on straight-leg raising is common with a variety of lumbar spine problems, but a positive crossed straight-leg raising test (pain in the involved leg or buttock that occurs when lifting the uninvolved leg) is highly specific for nerve root entrapment. To stretch the upper lumbar nerve roots, perform a reverse straight-leg raising test. With the patient prone, either extend the hip or do the prone rectus femoris test. With the patient in the prone position, flex the knee. Limited knee flexion is this position compared with supine flexion indicates tightness of the rectus femoris portion of the quadriceps muscle. With severe tightness, the pelvis will elevate as the hip moves into flexion. (See Advanced Assessment 14.10.)

Diagnostic Reasoning

Diagnostic Tests

Age-appropriate changes are usually demonstrated on radiograph. MRI might be useful if there is an unclear diagnosis

ADVANCED ASSESSMENT 14.10

Classic Findings of Disk Herniation

Nerve Root	Findings
L3–4 (L4 nerve root)	Weakness in the anterior tibialis, numbness in the shin, thigh pain, and an asymmetric knee reflex (5% of all herniations)
L4–5 (L5 nerve root)	Weakness in the great toe extension, numbness top of the foot and first web space, and posterolateral thigh and calf pain
L5–S1 (S1 nerve root)	Weakness in the great toe flexor as well as gastrocnemius with inability to sustain tiptoe walking, numbness in the lateral foot, posterior calf pain and ache, and an asymmetric ankle reflex

or if the patient is being readied for surgery, but otherwise is not indicated.

Differential Diagnosis

Cauda equina syndrome (perianal numbness, urinary overflow incontinence or retention, reduced anal sphincter tone, bilateral involvement) can lead to permanent motor loss if not immediately treated. The following lists differential diagnoses:

- ▲ Demyelinating conditions (clonus)
- ▲ Extraspinous nerve entrapment (abdominal or pelvic masses)
- ▲ Hip or knee arthritis (decreased internal rotation of hip, knee deformity or effusion)
- ▲ Lateral femoral cutaneous nerve entrapment (sensory only, lateral thigh)
- ▲ Spinal stenosis (older population)
- ▲ Thoracic cord compression (clonus, spasticity, high sensory pattern, abdominal reflexes)
- ▲ Trochanteric bursitis (no tension signs, pain down lateral thigh and leg, exquisite tenderness over trochanter)
- ▲ Vascular insufficiency (absent posterior tibial pulse, claudication, trophic changes)

Management

Control of symptoms, relief of pain, and improved mobility are all goals of management. Most episodes improve with conservative treatment.

NSAIDs should be given for pain with 1 to 3 days of bedrest. If the pain is severe in the acute phase, which it can be, consider muscle relaxants and/or narcotics but for no longer than 7 to 10 days. Limit sitting, prolonged standing, or walking, and take frequent rest breaks when resuming activity. Reassure patients that most disk herniations resolve without residual problems. Even ruptures with a significant inflammatory component should improve within 3 to 6 weeks. Refer if the problem persists longer than that or if pain increases, or there is evidence of any "red flags." A short course of oral steroids (5 days) or an epidural injection may reduce leg pain within the first 2 weeks after herniation, although some recent studies have indicated that epidural steroids do not significantly alter pain that has persisted for more than 2 weeks or influence the outcome of the syndrome. Persistent numbness, progression of neurologic deficits, and weakness can occur despite treatment.

Surgical options may need to be considered if symptoms persist for more than a 3-month period and other underlying causes are ruled out. Intolerable pain, multiple episodes of radiculopathy, severe postural tilt, and persistent dysfunctional pain are all indications for surgery. If cauda equina compression is confirmed, surgical lumbar decompression is the treatment of choice to halt neurologic deterioration, unless surgery is contraindicated for other medical reasons.

Follow-Up and Referral

The patient should return in about 10 days for evaluation of pain and function. Monitor the patient every 2 weeks until he or she is fully functional. After pain is controlled (usually within 7 to 10 days), the patient should begin a progressive walking program. It is best to start with short walks initially, up to four times per day, then lengthen the walks as tolerated. The patient should return to full activity as soon as possible, while avoiding high-risk activities such as heavy lifting and long car rides.

Most cases of acute back pain (90 percent) and/or radiculopathy (60 to 80 percent) recover with conservative treatment; the same is true of most cases of chronic back pain and radiculopathy.

Progression of any neurologic deficits, such as loss of ankle jerk; bladder and rectal sphincter weakness with retention or incontinence; foot drop with weakness of the anterior tibial, posterior tibial, or peroneal muscles; narcotic addiction in cases of chronic pain; limitation of movement; and restricted activity all warrant referral for further evaluation and treatment.

Patient Education

Cessation of smoking, weight reduction, good posture and body mechanics, and adherence to an exercise regimen are all ways to improve health and prevent recurrence. Modification of work environment may be necessary. Manipulation (chiropractic) and/or physical therapy may prove helpful.

Lumbar Spinal Stenosis

Lumbar spinal stenosis is narrowing of one or more levels of the lumbar spinal canal and subsequent compression of the nerve roots. In the order of descending likelihood, L4 to 5, L3 to 4, and L1 to 2 are the levels most commonly involved. At L1 to S1, the stenosis is usually not central but foraminal, involving the same root (L5) as central canal stenosis at the L4 to 5 level. Typically, the stenosis must be severe before symptoms occur.

Epidemiology and Causes

Anatomically, as many as 30 percent of the population may have spinal stenosis after the age of 60, yet only a portion of this population has symptoms. Obesity is a predisposing factor, as is osteoporosis.

Pathophysiology

Lumbar spinal stenosis is defined as narrowing of the spinal canal with compression of the nerve roots. It may congenital or acquired. It most frequently results from enlarging osteophytes at the facet joints, hypertrophy of the ligamentum flavum, and protrusion or bulging of the intervertebral disks. Lumbar spinal stenosis may produce symptoms by directly compressing nerve roots or by compressing nutrient arterioles that supply the nerve roots.

Clinical Presentation

Subjective

Onset of symptoms may follow a lifting incident or minor trauma or may gradually emerge. Often there is pseudoclaudication causing radicular complaints (with or without associated back pain) in the calves, buttocks, and upper thighs of one or both legs. Symptoms progress from a proximal to distal direction. Walking or prolonged standing causes pain and weakness in the legs and buttocks. In cases of vascular claudication, the pain stops when the patient stops walking, but pseudoclaudication does not immediately subside when walking stops. The patient may obtain short-term relief by leaning forward (manifested as "stooping"); when grocery shopping, the patient will be leaning on the cart. Relief after sitting is variable, depending on the degree of neural compression. Patients who sleep on their backs, meaning with the spine extended, might awaken after several hours with back and leg pain. Lumbosacral pain is associated with walking and standing. A vague aching in the legs or leg weakness may also be present. Spondylolisthesis (degenerative or spondylolytic), vascular insufficiency, and osteoarthritis of the hips are often associated with spinal stenosis, as well as obesity.

Objective

Muscle weakness of the legs is a subtle phenomenon. This may be best elicited after walking on a treadmill. Proprioception can be impaired; there may be a positive Romberg test (mild). There may be sensory changes and these are usually segmental and may involve more than one spinal level. Reflexes are often diminished. Some patients will have a lumbar scoliosis. With bowel or bladder symptoms, sphincter tone may be decreased. However, because many elderly patients have concomitant prostate problems or urinary incontinence, genitourinary evaluation may be necessary to differentiate these processes.

Diagnostic Reasoning

Diagnostic Testing

Radiographs may provide some evidence of spinal stenosis. AP and lateral view radiographs (up to L10 in the lateral view) may show significant narrowing of the intervertebral disk or spondylolisthesis. There may be osteopenia, or an old burst fracture of the vertebral body.

Differential Diagnosis

The following is a list of differential diagnoses:

- ▲ Abdominal aortic aneurysm (palpable pulsatile mass)
- ▲ Arterial insufficiency (distance to claudication constant, recovery after rest, absent or diminished pulses)
- ▲ Diabetes mellitus (abnormal glucose metabolism, nonsegmental numbness, skin changes)
- ▲ Folic acid or vitamin B_{12} deficiency (confirmed by laboratory tests, anemia)
- ▲ Infection (fever, elevated ESR, intervertebral disk narrowing)
- ▲ Tumor (patchy neurologic deficit, bone destruction, severe night pain)

Management

Any neurologic deficit, gait disturbance, or bowel and bladder dysfunction should be evaluated further. These changes may not be reversed following surgery for decompression; thus the goal of the treatment is to prevent progression.

Intermittent use of NSAIDs may be helpful, as well as folic acid or vitamin B_{12} supplementation in some cases depending on results of laboratory tests. However, most management revolves around physical therapy or an exercise program that focuses on flexing the spine. Flexion of the spine increases intraspinal volume. Bicycling is one exercise that is done with the spine in flexion. Improving abdominal muscle tone lifts the pelvis anteriorly and flexes the lumbar spine. Reduction of intra-abdominal fat is critical to achieving the objective. Thus, weight loss may be pivotal. Lumbar flexion exercises increase spinal canal volume. Examples include exercise on all fours, arching the back, or on the fetal position. Exercises that extend the spine should be avoided (swayback).

Lumbar epidural corticosteroid injection may provide some immediate relief for approximately 50 percent of patients and more sustained relief for approximately 25 percent. When disabling symptoms persist, decompression laminectomy provides at least short-term relief in some patients, but does not always rehabilitate lost function.

Referral and Follow-Up

The rate of progression is variable from rapid to none. Many patients never develop any neurologic deficits and overall tolerate the condition well. Pain and limited function, however, can become severe and lead to a secondary depression. Standing erect may become impossible and the patient may be forced to adopt a stooped posture. Claudication may develop after walking only a few feet. Cauda equina syndrome develops in some patients, leading to loss of bowel and bladder function.

Any neurologic deficit, gait disturbance, or bowel and bladder dysfunction should be evaluated further. These changes may not be reversed following surgery for decompression; thus the goal of the treatment is to prevent progression. In nonoperative treatment is ineffective, specialty consultation is warranted. Night pain that disturbs sleep tends to be a sign of advancing disease which also indicates a need to refer and/or consult. Prolonged use of NSAIDs can cause renal failure, hepatotoxicity, and gastrointestinal ulcer disease.

Patient Education

Educate the patient and family as to any potentially serious symptoms such as changes in bowel and bladder function, change in neurologic status, and gait disturbance. Educate as to side effects of NSAIDs or narcotic usage. Support weight loss if necessary with dietary instructions as well as clear guidelines for activity and exercise. Since many of these patients are older adults, they may need a range of services arranged to accomplish these goals.

Osteoporosis

Osteoporosis is a generalized skeletal disorder characterized by normal bone mineralization but low bone mass (bone mineral *density*) and disruption of the bony architecture, both of which result in an increased risk of fragility fractures. Its chief clinical manifestations are vertebral and hip fractures although fractures can occur at any skeletal site. This is contrasted with osteopenia, which is a less severe form of decreased bone mineral density, and osteomalacia, which denotes a decrease in actual bone mineralization. Osteoporosis is now recognized as a significant public health concern with potentially devastating consequences in both human and economic terms. Increasing attention to women's health issues, the application of epidemiologic research in prioritizing public health problems, and the need to minimize health-care expenditures have all contributed to recent efforts aimed at the prevention, identification, and effective treatment of this condition, to avoid fractures. Fractures associated with osteoporosis are not only a physical stress to the individual and a burden for the health-care system; they also inflict great strain on the psychosocial well-being of individuals who suffer fractures and on the family or friends who take on the role of caregiver.

Epidemiology and Causes

Osteoporosis is characterized by microarchitectural deterioration of bone tissue, which leads to low bone mineral density (BMD) and fragility, and a consequent susceptibility to fractures. Epidemiologic studies in Europe, Japan, and the United States reveal that an estimated 75 million people are affected by osteoporosis. Roughly 4 out of 10 white women older than the age of 50 in the United States will experience a hip, spine, or wrist fracture during the remainder of their lives. Looking ahead, the lifetime risk of fractures will increase for all ethnic groups as people live longer. Approximately 10 million individuals older than the age of 50 in the United States have osteoporosis of the hip. An additional 33.6 million individuals older than the age of 50 have low bone mass or "osteopenia" of the hip and thus are at risk of developing osteoporosis and its potential complications later in life. Common consequences of osteoporosis are vertebral fractures and fracture of the hip and distal radius. In addition, a diagnosis of osteoporosis can lead to depression, a change in role, loss of independence, body deformities, and a real fear of initial or subsequent osteoporotic fractures.

As a result of both the aging of the population and the rise in the age-specific incidence of osteoporosis, the number of osteoporotic fractures has been increasing annually. Approximately 1.5 million osteoporotic fractures of the vertebral body, proximal femur, or distal radius occur each year in the United States, with an estimated annual cost in excess of $12 to $18 billion per year in 2002 dollars. Proximal femur fractures are associated with the greatest health-care costs, are accompanied by a 20 percent risk of dying within 1 year of the fracture, and impair the ability to perform ADLs in up to 75 percent of patients who survive. Women are more likely to have osteoporosis but men also suffer from this. White woman are more susceptible than black women; the prevalence of osteoporosis in Hispanic and Asian women is similar to that of white women.

Unless comprehensive prevention, screening, and treatment programs are initiated, as the average age of the American population continues to increase over the next 30 years, costs related to bone fragility could more than double. Women have a two to four times greater lifetime risk of sustaining an osteoporotic fracture than men do, as a result of the loss of BMD following the cessation of ovarian function at menopause. Bone loss after menopause is caused predominantly by estrogen deficiency, and is most rapid (up to 7 percent per year) in the first decade after menopause. Postmenopausal osteoporosis is more prevalent in white and Asian women than in women of other races, with the majority of white women developing osteoporosis by the end of the first postmenopausal decade. By age 65, one-third of women will have had a vertebral fracture, and by the ninth decade of life, one in three will have had a hip fracture. The incidence, prevalence, and pathogenesis of bone loss in men are incompletely understood, and more research is called for in this area. Fractures of any type from osteoporosis are associated with a significantly higher likelihood of both physical and functional limitations. Patients who have already sustained a fracture from osteoporosis have a more than a fivefold increase in the risk of sustaining another fragility fracture.

The cause of osteoporosis is multifactorial. Although genetic factors are important determinants of bone density, other lifestyle, disease-related, and medication-related factors also contribute to an individual's risk for having osteoporosis, as shown in Risk Factors 14.1.

Although genetic factors may account for up to 70 percent of the variance in peak bone mass, many lifestyle factors play a significant role and are most amenable to interventions aimed at primary and secondary prevention and treatment of osteoporosis. Regular exercise has been shown to preserve BMD, whereas a sedentary lifestyle probably contributes to osteopenia. Weightbearing exercise, such as walking, is considered the best form of activity, and is associated with higher bone density. There is increasing evidence that muscle strength training may prevent further loss

RISK FACTORS 14.1

Osteoporosis

Lifestyle	Low body weight Cigarette smoking Excessive alcohol intake Low dietary calcium intake Vitamin D deficiency
Disease-related risk factors	Thyrotoxicosis Hyperparathyroidism Cushing's disease Hypogonadism RA Inflammatory bowel disease Chronic renal insufficiency Malabsorptive diseases Secondary estrogen deficiency resulting from anorexia or overexercise
Medication-related risk factors	Glucocorticoids Excessive thyroxine Long-term use of phenytoin
Other risk factors	Advanced age Family history of osteoporosis Postmenopausal Genetic predisposition

of BMD in postmenopausal women. Further, the improved mobility, agility, and muscle strength that occur in people who engage in regular exercise may help to prevent falls and associated fractures.

The primary dietary risk factor for osteoporosis is lack of adequate calcium intake throughout the life cycle. The majority of cross-sectional studies support the supposition that long-term inadequate dietary calcium has a deleterious effect on skeletal mass. The importance of adequate calcium, phosphorus, and vitamin D intake for children, adolescents, and young adults should not be underestimated, as studies have indicated women begin losing bone mass (albeit at a rate of less than 1 percent a year) in their early thirties. There is increasing evidence that vitamin D deficiency may be more prevalent than previously thought, particularly among individuals at increased risk, such as the elderly; those living in northern latitudes; and in individuals with poor nutrition, malabsorption, or chronic liver or renal disease. Modest vitamin D deficiency can lead to a compensatory, secondary hyperparathyroidism and is an important risk factor for osteoporosis and fractures.

Cigarette smoking is an established risk factor for loss of bone density, with the proposed mechanism of action being a reduction in circulating estrogen levels, as well as toxic effects on osteoblasts.

Genetics are important determinants of the risk for developing osteoporosis. Although the specific genes that determine bone mass remain largely unknown, some investigators claim that polymorphisms in the vitamin D receptor gene may be associated with up to 75 percent of the variance in bone density.

A variety of disease-related conditions may be associated with an increased risk for osteoporosis. GI diseases such as inflammatory bowel disease, among others, that lead to malabsorption of minerals and/or vitamin D are associated with low BMD. Other generalized inflammatory diseases that elevate levels of cytokines—substances believed to induce bone resorption—have also been associated with lower bone density. Younger women with eating disorders and women athletes who have altered menstrual function secondary to a hypoestrogenic state are at increased risk for lower bone densities earlier in life, and should be targeted for primary prevention interventions as early as possible, as well as treatment of the underlying disease when indicated. Finally, chronic renal impairment with parathyroid dysfunction and vitamin D metabolism abnormalities can lead to bone loss.

Among the medications associated with the development of osteoporosis, long-term use of glucocorticoids (steroids) has been shown to cause bone loss both rapidly and dramatically. Patients who take 7.5 mg or more of prednisone per day for more than 1 month have been identified as being at particular risk. Long-term excessive thyroid hormone may also potentiate bone loss, reinforcing the need to routinely monitor TSH levels in patients who require thyroid hormone replacement. Cyclosporine, cytotoxic drugs, anticonvulsants, excessive alcohol intake, heparin, and lithium are medications that have potentially detrimental effects on the skeleton

In men, testosterone deficiency from primary or secondary hypogonadism is a common cause of osteoporosis, although few large-scale studies have been done in this area. One small cross-sectional study found that men who had undergone orchiectomy for prostate cancer had significantly higher rates of severe osteoporosis, some of which developed before castration. Research identifying the causes of and treatment for osteoporosis in men is both increasing and necessary, as preliminary data have shown a higher mortality in men with hip fractures when compared to women.

Pathophysiology

Normal bone contains an abundance of intracellular mineral salts (calcium phosphate and calcium carbonate) referred to as *hydroxyapatites.* As hydroxyapatites are deposited in collagenous fibers within immature bone cells (osteoblasts), the tissue becomes hardened, or ossified. Essentially, two types of bone are formed—cancellous or dense. Cancellous bone tissue is spongy, containing many open spaces filled with marrow. It consists of an irregular latticework of thin plates of bone called *trabeculae* and provides some skeletal support. Overlying spongy bone is dense bone which is much more compact, providing substantial skeletal support.

There is a continual remodeling process of bone tissue throughout life, in which osteoclasts release proteolytic enzymes that are responsible for breaking down osseous tissue, and new bone tissue is formed in its place by osteoblasts. At menopause, the remodeling process becomes less homeostatic, and osteoclastic activity begins to predominate, while the rate of bone turnover increases. Bony spicules are reduced in number and size, while horizontal spicules acting as struts do not fully extend to contralateral supporting structures from their sites of origin, thus drastically reducing structural support. This leads to a decrease in cortical thickness and both the number and size of trabeculae in cancellous bone, leading to a decrease in bone density.

Osteoporosis is likely to be a multifactorial process, relating to increased bone resorption, decreased bone formation, and an overall decrease in peak bone mass at baseline (largely determined by genetic predisposition). Each of these physiologic processes may predominate to a different extent in different osteoporotic individuals. Studies exploring the genetic basis for osteoporosis have not yet proved definitive, but polymorphisms in the genes of several proteins have been implicated, including collagen, bone morphogenetic protein (BMP)-2, apolipoprotein E, transforming growth factor (TGF)-β, and the estrogen receptor. Normal estrogen function is important in preventing osteoporosis in both men and women, as it has been shown to inhibit osteoclastogenesis, induce osteoclast apoptosis, and decrease the erosive activity of osteoclasts. These activities are likely mediated through estrogen's inhibition of macrophages and osteoclasts to secrete tumor necrosis factor (TNF)-α, IL-1, and their binding proteins. New bone formation also appears to be impaired in estrogen-deficient states, as estrogen has been shown to mediate TGF-β secretion by osteoblasts. Interestingly, androgen (e.g., testosterone) deficiency similarly results in increased bone turnover and can predispose to osteoporosis as well.

As serum hormone levels often do not differ between osteoporotic individuals and age-matched controls, changes in bone resorption and formation appear to be mediated largely by local factors, including mechanical loads on the bones themselves, as well as changes in the concentrations of local growth factors and their receptor proteins. Excesses in both exogenous (therapeutic) and endogenous (stress- or disease-related) glucocorticoids are well known causes of osteoporosis, but unlike the role of sex hormones, glucocorticoids appear to be most involved in the regulation of new bone formation by osteoblasts. This growth effect is mediated largely by the inhibition of local growth factors including insulin-like growth factor (IGF) and its cognate receptor binding proteins, as well as prostaglandins.

Research on the effects of prostaglandins and NSAIDs on osteoporosis is not definitive. It appears as though excess prostaglandin production, especially that of PGE_2, may increase bone resorption, while significant inhibition of prostaglandins may lead to reduced bone formation in response to mechanical weightbearing. IL-6 produced by osteoblasts and other marrow-derived cells has been shown to increase osteoclastogenesis via a prostaglandin-dependent mechanism, leading to increased bone resorption in osteoporotic individuals. In contrast, IL-4 and IL-13 appear to inhibit bone resorption by decreasing prostaglandin synthesis, while IL-7 may contribute to bone loss. Finally, excess production of parathyroid hormone (PTH) (as seen in primary hyperparathyroidism) as well as PTH-related protein (produced by bone and cartilage cells and the mammary gland in lactating women), both lead to increased bone resorption via their effects on downstream growth factors, possibly including fibroblast growth factor. Importantly, however, this complex set of interactions by secreted growth factors on bone resorption and formation has yet to be fully characterized, and the importance of the aforementioned cytokines and growth factors can only be suggested by the current literature.

Clinical Presentation

Subjective

Most often, there are no clinical symptoms with the onset of osteoporosis until a fracture occurs. The only "early" symptom that may be noticed is the gradual development of upper or midthoracic back pain associated with activity or long periods of sitting or standing, which is relieved with rest in the recumbent position. To emphasize the importance of taking a comprehensive history, a strong predictor for future osteoporosis-related fractures is a history of previous fractures, notably those occurring from minimal trauma.

Objective

Acute vertebral compression fractures generally occur in the thoracic or high lumbar region, with the patient experiencing a more sudden, severe onset of pain. With acute compression fractures, point tenderness in the specific area of the fracture can be elicited during the physical examination. As bone density decreases, microfractures of the anterior vertebral bodies in the thoracic spine are likely to accumulate over time, leading to the characteristic dorsal kyphosis (or "dowager's hump"). The resultant exaggerated kyphosis produces a loss of height, which is generally not a "complaint," per se, but may be only casually mentioned by a patient during the course of a health-care visit. This may be the only verbal cue the practitioner receives to help identify that patient as being at risk for having osteoporosis. As the kyphosis worsens over time, impairment of rib mobility, a decrease in lung volumes, and an increase in respiratory complaints may develop.

Diagnostic Reasoning

Diagnostic Tests

Although it is important for identifying patients who may be at particular risk for developing osteoporosis, clinical assessment alone cannot accurately identify patients who do or do not have this condition. For the practitioner, assessing a patient's risk for osteoporosis and signs of the disease based on the physical exam can provide support for the decision to proceed with further diagnostic testing. Risk assessment tools are currently available, and may be used by clinicians as a quantitative means to support the need for additional diagnostic testing. The Simple Calculated Osteoporosis Risk Estimation (SCORE) instrument, for example, is estimated to have a 90 percent sensitivity and approximately a 40 percent specificity for identifying individuals with low BMD at the hip.

The American Association of Clinical Endocrinologists (AACE) recommends BMD testing in all perimenopausal or postmenopausal women who are willing to accept interventions should a low BMD be found. In the current health-care environment, insurance companies are increasingly requiring quantitative justification (e.g., in the form of risk assessments and/or other physical findings) from practitioners before paying for further diagnostic BMD testing. Standard radiographs are considered extremely insensitive for detecting bone loss, with films typically indicating bone loss only when it exceeds 30 percent or more. No biochemical marker currently exists that is used to detect bone loss; however, preliminary evidence from clinical trials suggests such markers may be used in the future to evaluate early response to therapy.

The physiologic process of bone turnover may be assessed with a variety of serum or urinary markers, allowing the monitoring of bone loss and reformation, although these markers do not provide bone mass density, which is considered the definitive test for diagnosis. However, these markers are useful in monitoring treatment and can serve as useful adjuncts in the original diagnosis of osteoporosis. In general, serum markers provide information about bone formation, whereas urinary markers supply evidence of bone resorption.

Bone alkaline phosphatase (BAP) is the most commonly available serum indicator of osteoblastic activity. These levels should be obtained prior to the initiation of therapy and then at 3- to 6-month intervals to monitor response. BAP levels that drop significantly may indicate lack of compliance with treatment.

The urinary biochemical marker for bone resorption that is most commonly available is deoxypyridinoline (Dpd). Urinary levels of Dpd are highly specific for bone activity, and the value of Dpd in initial assessment and therapeutic monitoring of postmenopausal women has been well established. The normal reference range for Dpd is 3.0 to 7.4 nM/mM for women. Values that exceed normal represent increased bone resorption; values within or below the range indicate normal bone remodeling. The urine sample should be an early morning voiding.

Urinary N-telopeptide (Ntx) is the most specific and newest urinary bone resorption marker available. This assay, which measures the urinary excretion of cross-linked N-telopeptide of type I collagen, is useful in identifying individuals with osteoporosis who have high rates of bone resorption and who might be good candidates for antiresorption therapy.

BMD measurement by densitometry is currently considered the gold standard diagnostic test for definitively diagnosing either osteopenia or osteoporosis. *Osteopenia* is the diagnostic term used when BMD is found to be less than normal but not severe enough to be considered osteoporotic. BMD densitometry is noninvasive and can be completed in 5 to 15 minutes. A number of BMD measurement technologies are available, including dual-energy x-ray absorptiometry (DXA, or DEXA)—the "gold standard" for documenting osteoporosis of the proximal femur and lumbar spine; single-energy x-ray absorptiometry (SXA) and peripheral DXA for the radius and calcaneus (heel); ultrasonography for the heel, fingers, and tibia; and quantitative computed tomography (QCT), including peripheral QCT (PQCT) for the spine, hip, and radius.

These technologies use a variety of anatomic sites from which to measure BMD and emit very low radiation doses (less than or equal to a standard chest x-ray study). Although all methods are considered accurate, the DEXA method is most widely accepted, because prospective epidemiologic studies have found it to be most precise for reproducibility in both the short and long term, making it an excellent method for monitoring responses to interventions over time. DEXA densitometry measures BMD at the central skeletal sites of the lumbar spine and hip (including both the femoral neck and greater trochanter).

BMD measurement reports are interpreted by using the calculated *Z*-scores and *T*-scores. Both use a normally distributed bell curve in determining how any one individual compares to a reference population, with *Z*-scores representing age- and sex-matched distributions, and *T*-scores representing mean peak bone mass of a young adult distribution. The *T*-score is the most clinically relevant value on the BMD report, and is used to confirm the presence of osteoporosis as well as determine fracture risk. For every standard deviation (SD) below the young-adult matched mean, there is a significant increase in fracture risk.

Medicare-approved indications for BMD testing include: (1) estrogen-deficient women at risk for osteoporosis; (2) patients with vertebral abnormalities; (3) patients receiving or needing to be on long-term glucocorticoids; (4) patients with primary parathyroidism; and (5) patients being monitored for response or efficacy of an approved osteoporosis drug therapy.

Secondary causes of osteoporosis should be considered in all patients with low BMD. The following routine laboratory tests are considered appropriate by the AACE for excluding secondary causes of osteoporosis: CBC, serum chemistry panel (calcium, phosphate, liver enzymes, total alkaline phosphatase, creatinine, electrolytes), and urinalysis, including pH.

Also based on AACE guidelines, additional laboratory analysis may be warranted if there are abnormalities in the aforementioned tests, or if there is sufficient other evi-

Table 14.8 World Health Organization Diagnostic Criteria for Osteoporosis

Diagnosis	Diagnostic Findings
Normal	BMD within 1 standard deviation of young adult reference mean
Osteopenia	BMD >1 standard deviation below young adult reference mean (−1)
Osteoporosis	BMD >2.5 standard deviation below young adult reference mean (−2.5)
Osteoporosis (severe)	BMD >2.5 standard deviation below young adult reference mean (−2.5) AND presence of osteoporotic fractures

dence to suspect specific secondary causes for bone loss. These include sensitive TSH, 24-hour urinary calcium excretion, ESR, parathyroid hormone concentration, 25-hydroxyvitamin D concentration, dexamethasone suppression and other tests for hyperadrenocorticism, acid–base studies, serum or urine protein electrophoresis, and bone marrow examination or bone biopsy.

The World Health Organization's diagnostic criteria for osteoporosis are presented in Table 14.8.

Differential Diagnosis

If a fracture has occurred, it is important to distinguish the underlying cause. Was it related to trauma, or was there an underlying pathologic condition such as osteoporosis, or neoplasm? Similarly, skeletal changes could result from a variety of underlying conditions, including a neoplasm such as multiple myeloma or other neoplasias, osteomalacia, osteogenesis imperfecta tarda (type I), skeletal hyperparathyroidism (primary and secondary), and hyperthyroidism.

Management

The goals for either the prevention or treatment of osteoporosis are to prevent fractures, to stabilize or improve bone mass, to maximize physical functioning, to relieve symptoms of fractures and resulting skeletal deformity, and to maximize psychosocial functioning and coping.

The ability to meet these goals is dependent on both the patient and the practitioner's dedication to work as a team, first in determining what therapeutic regimen will be most beneficial and acceptable to the patient. Following this is the long-term commitment to continuing treatment, evaluating the therapeutic response, and assessing for the need to redirect the management plan based on the response. An algorithm outlining prevention, detection, and management strategies for osteoporosis is presented in Treatment Flowchart 14.1.

In addition to the physical and functional limitations that can be quantified, practitioners must also address the human and emotional aspects of being diagnosed with osteoporosis. Nursing research has contributed to our understanding of the experience of women who suffer osteoporotic vertebral fractures. One study identified an essential structure of this experience was an abrupt descent into disease, disability, and deformity—essentially perceiving oneself as a specter or a crone. Feeling vulnerable, isolated, and uncertain of the future were also characterized as hallmarks of the experience. (See Treatment Flowchart 14.1.)

Lifestyle Management

For both the prevention and treatment of osteoporosis, smoking cessation, moderation of alcohol use, weightbearing exercise, and adequate calcium and vitamin D intake are advised. In addition, avoidance of falls by eliminating hazards in the home, as well as gait training or other exercises that improve strength and agility through physical therapy are important considerations. Nursing research has found that women with osteoporosis seek interventions that promote the ability to better care for themselves, reduce stress and isolation, and prevent further disability. Weight training and walking are effective interventions for prevention and/or treatment. An active lifestyle, including safe and appropriate exercise, should be actively encouraged by the provider. Protective pads worn around the outer thigh, which cover the trochanteric region of the hip, can prevent hip fractures in elderly residents in nursing homes. Patients with pain from osteoporotic fractures may find therapies such as massage, music, or acupuncture helpful.

Pharmacologic Management

Calcium and Vitamin D Supplements. Optimal calcium intake varies according to age, sex, and other conditions. The recommended daily calcium intake as based on the National Institutes of Health (NIH) Consensus Development Conference is as follows:

- Children: 800 to 1200 mg/day
- Adolescents and young adults: 1200 to 1500 mg/day
- Adults age 25 to 65: 1000 mg/day
- Adults over age 65: 1500 mg/day
- Postmenopausal women:
  65 years or younger taking estrogen or hormone replacement therapy (HRT): 1000 mg/day
  65 years or younger not taking estrogen or HRT: 1500 mg/day
- Men and women over 65: 1500 mg/day – up to 2000 mg/day seems safe in most individuals

An adequate calcium intake of 1000 to 1500 mg/day and sufficient amounts of vitamin D are necessary for both the prevention and treatment of osteoporosis. Supplementation is advised when dietary intake does not consistently meet the recommended amount. Fracture reduction in women 75 years and older who use only calcium and vitamin D supplementation has been previously demonstrated. There are many available forms, and patients

TREATMENT FLOWCHART 14.1
OSTEOPOROSIS

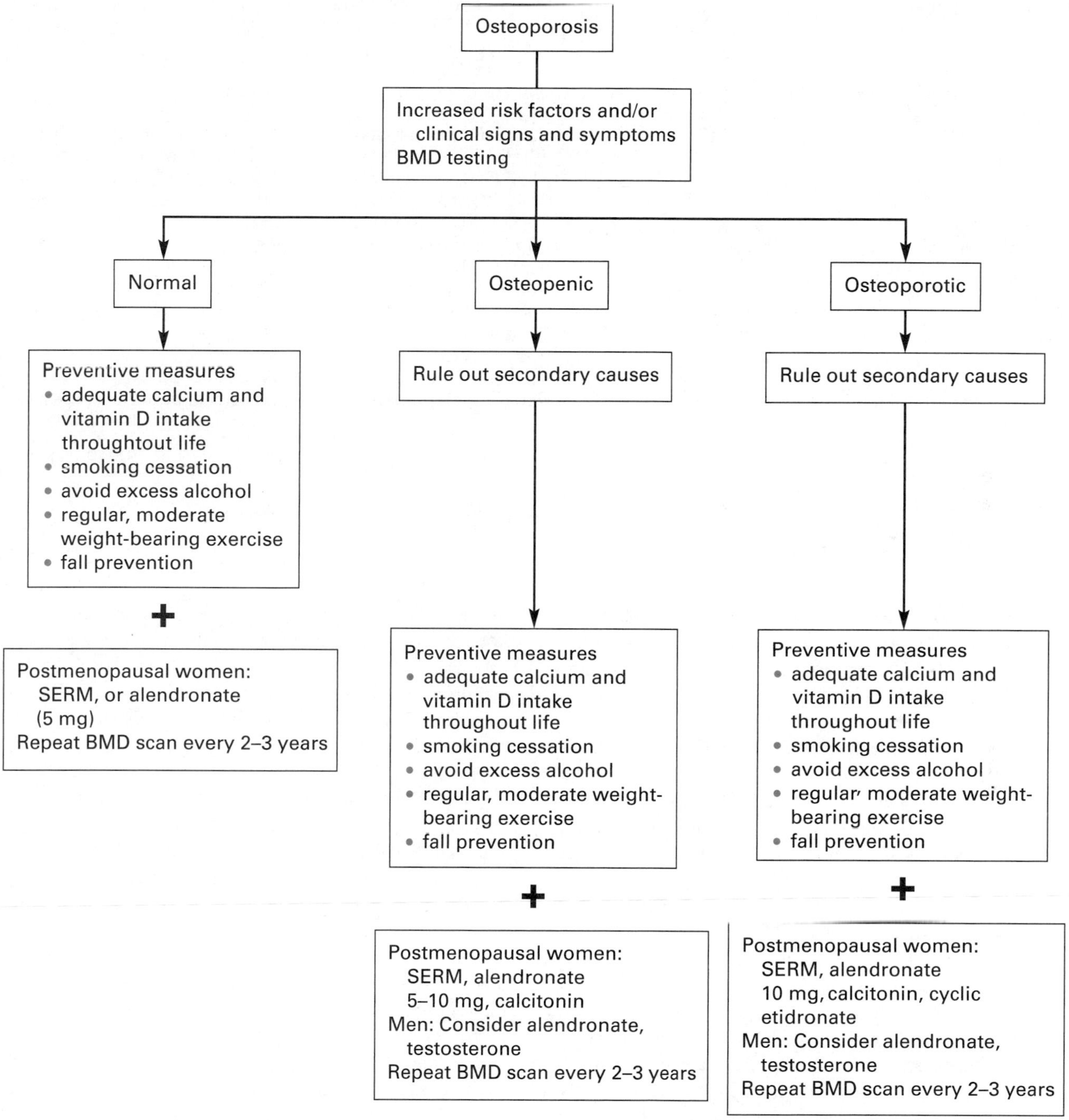

Osteoporosis

Increased risk factors and/or clinical signs and symptoms
BMD testing

Normal

Preventive measures
- adequate calcium and vitamin D intake throughtout life
- smoking cessation
- avoid excess alcohol
- regular, moderate weight-bearing exercise
- fall prevention

\+

Postmenopausal women:
SERM, or alendronate (5 mg)
Repeat BMD scan every 2–3 years

Osteopenic

Rule out secondary causes

Preventive measures
- adequate calcium and vitamin D intake throughout life
- smoking cessation
- avoid excess alcohol
- regular, moderate weight-bearing exercise
- fall prevention

\+

Postmenopausal women:
SERM, alendronate 5–10 mg, calcitonin
Men: Consider alendronate, testosterone
Repeat BMD scan every 2–3 years

Osteoporotic

Rule out secondary causes

Preventive measures
- adequate calcium and vitamin D intake throughout life
- smoking cessation
- avoid excess alcohol
- regular, moderate weight-bearing exercise
- fall prevention

\+

Postmenopausal women:
SERM, alendronate 10 mg, calcitonin, cyclic etidronate
Men: Consider alendronate, testosterone
Repeat BMD scan every 2–3 years

may be confused about which type or brand is best. In general, the majority of commercially available supplements contain similar amounts of elemental calcium per calcium weight in milligrams (mg), and patient choice should be dependent on affordability, number of tablets per day necessary, and whether it is convenient for the patient to take them with food or not. Most patients will benefit from taking calcium with meals, as this tends to reduce GI side effects. (See Drugs Commonly Prescribed 14.4.)

Estrogen Replacement Therapy. Estrogen was the mainstay of treatment for osteoporosis for many years, until the Women's Health Initiative, showing increased risk of cardiovascular disease and breast cancer from hormone

Drugs Commonly Prescribed 14.4: Calcium Supplements

Drug	Indication	Dosage	Comments
Calcium Supplements		Weight in mg (elemental calcium)/Tablets per day to supply 1000 mg elemental Ca^{2t}	
Calcium carbonate (40%) (generic; chewable)	Prevention and/or treatment of osteoporosis	500 (200)/five tablets	Available OTC
		600 (240)/four tablets	Most commonly used calcium preparation for osteoporosis
		650 (260)/four tablets	
		1260 (500)/two tablets	Food improves absorption
		1500 (600)/two tablets	
(Caltrate 600)	As above	1500 (600)/two tablets	As above
(Equilet chewable)	As above	500 (200)/five tablets	As above
(Os Cal 500 chewable)	As above	1250 (500)/two tablets	As above
(Titralac chewable)	As above	420 (168)/six tablets	As above
(Titralac extra-strength)	As above	750 (300)/four tablets	As above
(Tums chewable)	As above	500 (200)/five tablets	As above
(Tums E-X)	As above	750 (300)/four tablets	As above
(Tums 500)	As above	1250 (500)/two tablets	As above
Calcium citrate (21.2%) (Citracal 950)	As above	950 (200)/five tablets	As above; better absorbed in fasting state than calcium carbonate
(Ultracal liquitabs)	As above	2376 (500)/two tablets	As above
(Nutravelcent)	As above	1000/two tablets	As above
Calcium phosphate (138%) (Posture)	As above	1565.2 (600)/two tablets	As above

replacement therapy (HRT). Despite a risk/benefit ratio that is not favorable according to recent, large-scale clinical trials, women may still choose to take estrogen based on their own risk-factor profile.

Selective Estrogen-Receptor Modulators. One of the most recent developments in osteoporosis prevention has been the introduction of a selective estrogen-receptor modulator (SERM; e.g., Evista). The approval of this drug by the FDA represents a new class of drugs that are nonhormonal but modulate selective estrogen-receptor sites in skeletal tissue that decrease resorption of bone that occurs after menopause. The advantage of a SERM over traditional HRT is that it does not stimulate estrogen receptors found in the breast or uterus, and therefore does not increase the risk for breast or uterine cancer associated with estrogen use (over 39 months of trials). Although SERMs do not adversely affect lipid profiles, whether they provide any cardiovascular benefit is under investigation. SERMs are currently approved for use in postmenopausal women only for the prevention of osteoporosis but not its treatment. For many women, the addition of this class of drug into the market may provide an appealing alternative. Tamoxifen is another SERM that, although not FDA approved for osteoporosis, has shown promise in some research.

Bisphosphonates/Diphosphonate. Alendronate sodium (Fosamax), a third-generation bisphosphonate, has been approved by the FDA for the prevention and treatment of osteoporosis. It is an aminobisphosphonate that binds to bone hydroxyapatite and specifically inhibits the activity of osteoclasts, thus reducing bone turnover. Treatment with alendronate sodium has been shown to increase BMD of the vertebrae, femoral neck, and femoral trochanter by 5 to 10 percent, and to reduce hip, vertebral, and wrist fractures by approximately 50 percent over a 3-year study period, making it an effective alternative to ERT/HRT for treating osteoporosis in women who either cannot or will not take estrogen therapy.

Like other bisphosphonates, alendronate sodium has the potential to irritate upper GI mucosa, and is contraindicated in patients who have abnormalities of the esophagus that delay esophageal emptying, or in patients who are unable to take the medication exactly as directed. Because of the very specific manner in which alendronate sodium needs to be taken, some individuals initially perceive it as an inconvenience they would rather avoid; with careful patient teaching and the willingness to try this medication, however, many patients find no difficulty incorporating it into their daily routine. Risedronate (Actonel) is another drug in this category, also available in weekly dosing, as is ibandronate (Boniva), which is available in monthly dosing. Only bisphosphonates have been demonstrated in large clinical trials to reduce the risk of fractures in patients being treated with glucocorticoid therapy. Risedronate (Actonel) prevents bone loss and reduces vertebral fractures risk by about 70 percent. Similar effects have been noted in alendronate (Fosamax) and etidronate disodium (Didronel).

Organic bisphosphonate compounds strongly adsorb to hydroxyapatite crystal in bone and inhibit osteoclast-mediated bone resorption. Etidronate disodium (Didronel) is the first-generation diphosphonate used "off-label" (i.e., not FDA approved) for the treatment of osteoporosis. Although it has been shown to increase spinal BMD by 4 to 5 percent and to decrease vertebral fractures by 50 percent over 2 years, it remains a relatively weak antiresorptive agent when compared with newer-generation bisphosphonates. It is given as intermittent, repeated-cyclical therapy, which may be confusing to patients unless clear, written instructions are provided (optimally, on a calendar).

Few studies have examined the effectiveness of bisphosphonates for fracture reduction in men, although they have been shown to increase BMD. Currently, few well-designed trials have examined the effects of pharmacologic therapy on BMD in men.

Calcitonin. Calcitonin is another antiresorptive agent approved for the treatment of osteoporosis. It may be used for women who cannot or will not take estrogens or a bisphosphonate. Although it produces small increases in bone mass, there are conflicting data regarding whether calcitonin reduces fractures as the quality of bone formed is in question and currently under further investigation. Calcitonin is available for SC or IM injection as well as in a nasal spray preparation. Studies evaluating nasal spray calcitonin have documented an increased lumbar vertebral BMD after 1 year, but no difference from the placebo in BMD at the forearm or hip. Calcitonin has also been found to produce an analgesic effect in the treatment of bone pain, and may be useful during the immediate postfracture period. (See Drugs Commonly Prescribed 14.5.)

Androgen Supplementation. Few studies have examined pharmacologic therapy effectiveness in osteoporotic men. Preliminary data from one study showed an increase in BMD in men with idiopathic primary osteoporosis when treated with testosterone IM over 6 months. Although no adverse cardiovascular events were found in the treatment group, studies of longer duration are indicated in this area, to better estimate the risks versus benefits of testosterone supplementation in men.

Fluoride. Oral sodium fluoride has been used extensively in Europe for the treatment of osteoporosis, and has been found to significantly increase vertebral bone density by increasing the number of osteoblasts. Large, prospective studies have not shown a concurrent reduction in fractures, however, and until future research shows otherwise, it is believed the quality of bone produced by fluoride is more brittle than that formed by antiresorptive agents. Therefore, in the United States sodium fluoride is currently not approved for the prevention or treatment of osteoporosis by the FDA.

Follow-Up and Referral

Perhaps the most important part of managing the treatment of osteoporosis is improving adherence to treatment by individualizing the plan of care according to what is most effective in terms of increasing BMD and preventing fractures, and what is most acceptable to the patient. There are currently no well-accepted guidelines for monitoring treatment of osteoporosis. Medication-induced increments may require several years to produce changes. Monitoring the response to treatment in osteoporotic patients by using repeat BMD tests is should not be monitored at intervals $<$ than 2 years. For patients with less-than-normal BMD (but who are not osteoporotic) or normal baseline BMD, repeat measurement every 2 to 3 years is indicated to monitor for either stabilization or progression of the disease. Referral to an endocrinologist is warranted any time secondary causes of osteoporosis cannot be excluded, or if the response to treatment is less than expected for the type of therapy instituted.

Patient Education

A number of informative patient education materials are available from a variety of sources, including sources from pharmaceutical companies. Extensive, individualized education should be given to individuals when BMD results are available. This is particularly true for patients who are found to be osteoporotic and to have an array of interventions available to them. The amount of information about osteoporosis required for teaching can be overwhelming for patients; therefore, written information is essential. In addition, a number of resources are available to patients through both federal and national organizations. (See the Resources listed at the end of this chapter.)

Reviewing potential hazards that may lead to falls and reinforcing the importance of maintaining agility are equally important in the ongoing care and management of patients who are at increased risk for fractures. Referral to a physical therapist and/or a home-care nursing evaluation is often of value in this area. Referral to local support groups, national osteoporosis education groups, and mental health counseling may also be of benefit for patients who seek further assistance in either learning about their condition, or for individuals who require additional help in coping with their situation.

Active exercise, either weight training and/or walking, should be encouraged and supported.

Overuse Syndrome (Repetitive Motion Syndrome)

Overuse syndrome describes a constellation of cumulative soft-tissue trauma disorders that develop in the absence of acute injury. All major tissues in the musculoskeletal system are subject to overuse injuries. Overuse syndromes may be

Drugs Commonly Prescribed 14.5: Osteoporosis, Paget's Disease

Drug	Dose	Comments
	Bisphosphonates	
Risedronate (Actonel) 5-mg, 30-mg, 35-mg tablets	Prevention and treatment: 5 mg qd or 35 mg once weekly *Paget's disease	Swallow whole; take in the morning with a full glass of water before other food or drink; remain in upright position for at least 30 minutes; caution with other GI irritants such as aspirin.
Alendronate (Fosamax) 5-, 10-, 35-, 40-, 70-mg tablets 70 mg/75 mL (oral solution)	Prevention: 5 mg qd or 35 mg once weekly Dose: 10 mg qd or 70 mg/week	Take on an empty stomach at least 30 minutes before a meal; drink full glass of water and remain upright for at least 30 minutes. Can increase toxic effects of aspirin; can decrease absorption of calcium supplements and vitamin D.
Alendronate + Cholecalciferol (vitamin D) (Fosamax Plus D)—70 mg + 2800 IU tablets	Treatment: 70 mg/2800 IU once weekly	Take on an empty stomach at least 30 minutes before a meal; drink full glass of water and remain upright for at least 30 minutes. Can increase toxic effects of aspirin; can decrease absorption of calcium supplements and vitamin D.
Ibandronate (Boniva) 2.5-mg, 150-mg tablets	Prevention: 2.5 mg qd; consider 150 q month Treatment: 5 mg qd or 150 mg monthly	Swallow whole; take in the morning with full glass of water; remain upright and eat or drink nothing additional for 60 minutes; take on same day each month.
	Diphosphonate	
Etidronate disodium (Didronel) 200-, 400-mg tablets	Treatment: Paget's disease: initially 5–10 mg/day (max 6 months)	Give qd (preferred) or in divided doses at least 2 hours before or after food; ensure adequate calcium and vitamin D.
	Calcitonin	
Calcitonin-salmon (Fortical) 200 U/nasal spray	Treatment: 1 spray in nostril qd	Alternate nostrils—Must receive 1.5 g of calcium plus 400 U vitamin D qd
Calcitonin-salmon (Miacalcin) 200 U/nasal spray; 200 U/mL (injectable)	Treatment: 1 spray in nostril qd 100 U SQ/IM qd for osteoporosis; 100 U SQ/IM qd for Paget's; also for hypercalcemia (check dosing)	Alternate nostrils—Must receive 1.5 g calcium + 400 U vitamin D qd Injectable—give test dose of 1 IU and observe for 15 min
	Selective Estrogen Receptor Modulators (SERMs)	
Raloxifene (Evista)—60 mg tablets	Prevention and Treatment: 60 mg qd *Has not been shown to decrease hip fractures	May be taken anytime of day, regardless of meals Decreased effects of warfarin Discontinue 72 hours before immobilization.
	Parathyroid Hormone	
Teriparatide (Forteo)—250 mcg/mL (injection)	Treatment: 20 mcg SQ qd For postmenopausal women at high risk for fracture	Stimulates bone formation more than bone resorption; caution with digoxin; expensive.
	Hormone Replacement Therapy	
	Use as second-line therapy only	

referred to as *repetitive strain injury, chronic microtrauma, cumulative trauma disorders, soft tissue rheumatism,* and *work-related pain disorder*; all of these terms refer to syndromes that result in chronic localized pain and dysfunction. It may manifest itself as well-defined pathology of a single periarticular site or a regional myofascial pain syndrome. Examples of single-site periarticular pain generators include bursitis, tendonitis, or fasciitis (i.e., plantar fasciitis). Finding several pain generators in the absence of articular involvement suggests a chronic, low-grade, repetitive trauma disorder or an acute overexertion syndrome that one may find in "weekend warrior" athletes.

Proper diagnosis of overuse syndromes may be difficult and often involve more than one type of tissue. Most commonly overuse problems develop in the muscles and tendons. Although it is common to divide the muscles and tendons for ease of presentation, it is important to remember that they function together as a unit—the musculotendinous unit. Other soft tissues, including the bursa, fascia, synovium, and nerves, may also be affected by overuse. *Muscle overuse injuries* may be divided into muscle strains and muscle soreness (acute and delayed); there are overuse injuries of the tendons and bursa; any joint that is subject to abnormal loads, ranges of motion, or activity may develop a reactive synovitis. Chronic compartment syndromes may occur related to entrapment of fluid in the fascial sheath. Common anatomic sites and types of overuse syndromes are described in Table 14.9.

Epidemiology and Causes

Overuse injuries are common in both athletes and nonathletes. It is difficult to determine the true incidence because frequently overuse injuries are not brought to the attention of a health-care provider. Despite this, such injuries account for more than 50 percent of the injuries seen in a primary-care setting and are the most frequently encountered athletic injury. While individuals seem aware of the benefits of exercise, they do not always seem aware that these same activities can also bring problems with injury. Overuse injuries of soft tissue include damage to tendons, muscles, bursa, fascia, and nerves. They include impingement and snapping syndromes, and compartment syndromes.

Given that repetitive stress can traumatize tissue, the potential for injury is enhanced by a wide variety of predisposing factors. Female sex, youth and old age, pregnancy, smoking, menopause, diabetes, poor physical conditioning, underlying anatomic imperfections aggravated by exercise or repeated motions, and obesity have all been identified as risk factors. In addition, poor cardiovascular or musculoskeletal conditioning, underlying cardiovascular disease, arthritis (OA or RA), gout, and stress may all contribute to the development of overuse syndrome. In athletes, overtraining, running on uneven surfaces, poor equipment, inadequate footwear, and leg-length discrepancy may all contribute; in workers, unhealthy work environments both physically and emotionally are thought to contribute. Repeatedly performing arm and hand movements with a very short repetitive cycle of less than 30 seconds in the course of one's daily job is a risk factor. Repeatedly performing the same task over and over in a short period of time in a factory can impose the same level of risk. Dancers, musicians, grocery clerks, computer keyboard operators, and dental hygienists are all particularly susceptible. Vibration, cold environment, and use of some specific hand tools also are considered risk factors. (See Risk Factors 14.2.)

Sitting all day in an awkward body position may lead to muscle fatigue, for example. This may lead to generalized muscle inflammation and nerve compression throughout the upper extremities. Poor neck and shoulder posture places skeletal bone pressure on the nerve and blood supply to the arms, wrists, and hands, thereby diminishing circulation and nerve conduction to these areas. Fresh nutrient blood supply is diminished thereby slowing recovery from microtrauma. Independent of whether muscle, tendon, cartilage, or hard tissue is involved, injury results from a simple mismatch between stress on a given tissue and the ability

Table 14.9 Common Anatomic Sites: Overuse Syndrome

Anatomic Site	Overuse Syndrome
Shoulder	Rotator cuff tendinitis
	Thoracic outlet syndrome
Forearm	Lateral epicondylitis
	Medial epicondylitis
	Ulnar nerve entrapments
Hand and wrist	Carpal tunnel syndrome
	de Quervain's syndrome
	"Trigger finger"
Leg and foot	Chondromalacia patellae
	Iliotibial band syndrome
	Shin splints
	Achilles tendinitis
	Plantar fasciitis
	Stress fracture

RISK FACTORS 14.2

Overuse Syndrome

Arthritis (OA and RA)
Congenital defects
Diabetes mellitus
Ganglia
Gout
Hobbies (knitting, musical instruments, electronic games)
Hormonal factors (pregnancy, oral contraceptive use, menopause, thyroid disorders, hysterectomy with bilateral oophorectomy)
Hypertension
Impaired circulation
Inflammation of tendons and tendon sheath
Obesity
Occupational activities (computer usage, cash registers)
Paget's disease
Raynaud's phenomenon
Renal disease
Sports (racquet sports, golf, softball, running)
Underlying anatomic abnormalities

of that tissue to withstand the stress. There are two basic mechanisms behind tissue trauma: single-impact macrotrauma and repetitive microtrauma (damage at the microscopic or molecular level). Overuse injuries therefore can be defined as the level of repetitive microtrauma sufficient to overwhelm the tissue's ability to adapt, or in other words, its healing ability.

Pathophysiology

Overuse syndrome results from repetitive microtrauma to bones, ligaments, and musculotendinous units. This repetitive microtrauma causes a local inflammatory process, leading to pain and loss of function. *In vitro* studies have demonstrated that tendinous fibroblasts produce elevated concentrations of prostaglandin E_2 and leukotriene B_4 in response to repetitive stretch maneuvers. Thus, repetitive microtrauma is believed to lead to repeated cycles of inflammation and tissue regeneration, characterized by fibroblast proliferation, collagen production, and resultant tissue contraction.

Overuse syndrome most commonly involves the musculotendinous unit, resulting in tendonitis or tenosynovitis. Repetitive mechanical trauma to a joint may result in synovitis or arthritis, and repetitive overuse stress on bones can result in periostitis or stress fractures. Bone has the ability to constantly remodel and repair itself. However, if the degree of repetitive microtrauma exceeds the bone's capacity for repair, an overuse injury in the form of a stress fracture may occur. Stress fractures occur most commonly in the weightbearing bones of the lower extremities, such as the tibia and metatarsals, but are sometimes seen in the upper extremities of athletes who throw (e.g., baseball pitchers).

Histopathologic studies of muscle biopsies have also revealed differences in limbs affected by overuse syndrome. These include an increased number of type 1 muscle fibers (smaller, slow-twitch or red fibers) with a decreased number of hypertrophied type 2 fibers (larger, fast-twitch or white fibers). Muscle fibers affected by overuse syndrome also display mitochondrial changes with an increased number of muscle cell nuclei. These changes become increasingly evident at higher grades of overuse syndrome. Decreased blood flow to affected muscles has also been noted in some studies.

Clinical Presentation

Subjective

In general, overuse injuries are insidious in onset. Typical complaints include pain, fatigue, numbness, or any combination of the same. Patients often have difficulty localizing the pain, and may report swelling and sensation not apparent on physical exam.

Often, the symptoms have existed for some time; it is when the symptoms occur more frequently, or have become more intense, and last longer, that they may begin to interfere with function. This is most likely the point that the patient seeks help.

Objective

Specific findings will vary depending upon the joints and body area involved. However, in general, overuse syndrome may be categorized by grade. (See Advanced Assessment 14.11.)

Diagnostic Reasoning

Diagnostic Tests

The diagnostic tests indicated will vary depending on the body part involved. Radiographs are necessary with a history of trauma. A bone scan may be necessary to rule out stress fractures. Likewise, nerve conduction velocity studies can be ordered to rule out carpal tunnel syndrome or ulnar nerve entrapment at the elbow, but the results are usually negative. X-ray results are usually negative. MRI may help to visualize soft tissue injury.

ADVANCED ASSESSMENT 14.11

Grading Overuse Syndrome

Grade	1	2	3	4
Pain history	Hours after activity; soreness	Late, or just after activity	Early, or in middle of activity	At rest
Clinical manifestations	Tenderness (generalized)	Tenderness (localized)	Point tenderness Erythema Swelling	Point tenderness Erythema Swelling ROM decreased Function impaired
Management	Ice	Ice Decrease activity (25%)	Ice Decrease activity (50%)	Ice Rest NSAIDs

Differential Diagnosis

The differential diagnoses will vary, depending on the joints and body area involved. Some specifics are listed below:

- ▲ Angina with referred arm pain (abnormal EKG)
- ▲ Claudication (decreased peripheral pulses)
- ▲ Deep vein thrombosis (abnormal venogram)
- ▲ Fibromyalgia (11 of 18 pressure points in four body quadrants)
- ▲ Herniated cervical or lumbar disk (abnormal spine radiograph, myelogram, and MRI)

Management

There are two primary goals in the management of overuse injuries: reducing inflammation and improving vascular blood flow. Overuse injuries can be very difficult to treat. Treatment should be initiated as early as possible, because once chronic, they become even more difficult to treat both physically and psychologically. Exercise and physical therapy are the keys to successful recovery. Initial management should include *protection* from further injury, abstaining from the irritating activity, and in some cases, splinting for immobilization; *rest; ice* applied for 10 to 30 minutes with an equal period without ice; *compression*, such as with an elastic bandage to provide support to injured tissue; and *elevate* to decrease swelling (*PRICE*). An individualized rehabilitation program should be designed and implemented as soon as possible. Flexibility, strength, proprioception, and endurance must be addressed and encouraged.

Pharmacologic approaches may include NSAIDs during the acute phase, and in some cases, muscles relaxants, and occasionally antidepressant therapy in chronic situations. Acupuncture is often effective, and some patients may benefit from the use of transcutaneous electrical nerve stimulation (TENS). Injured muscles, tendons, and nerves may require significant amounts of rest to allow healing to take place.

Follow-Up and Referral

The degree of follow-up will depend on the location and severity of the injury. Once a diagnosis is made, treatment by a team of health-care professionals may be warranted, a Circle of Caring. Considerable psychologic sequelae may be involved. Better results are obtained when there is a specific, clearly identifiable syndrome such as carpal tunnel syndrome. Lack of job satisfaction and depression are also important predictors of recovery. Poor prognosis is associated with both long-standing disability (longer than 6 months) and litigation. With these disorders, patients often lose time from work and experience psychological changes. They may change occupations or never return to work.

Patient Education

The patient needs to be educated as to the precipitating activity and the need to refrain from that activity for a certain period of time. This can be especially difficult to reinforce with athletes. Patience and assistance in designing alternate activities will help, so that the patient may remain active. If the cause is work related, monitor for chronicity and issues of secondary gain.

Carpal Tunnel Syndrome

Carpal tunnel syndrome (CTS) is the most common cause of peripheral nerve compression. Pain and/or numbness affects some part of the median nerve distribution of the hand, and in some cases, may radiate into the arm. Symptoms tend to affect the dominant hand, but more than half the patients experience bilateral symptoms. Women are three times more likely than men are to be diagnosed with CTS.

Epidemiology and Causes

CTS is the most common entrapment neuropathy. It is most common between the ages of 40 and 60 and affects females significantly more frequently than males, and most commonly, middle-aged and pregnant women. Roughly, 80 percent of patients are older than age 40. Any condition that reduces the size or space of the carpal tunnel can cause compression of the medial nerve. Any movement that causes the wrist to repeatedly flex or extend out of the neutral position, or places pressure on the median nerve, may contribute to the development of CTS. Direct compression may result from neoplasms, a misaligned fracture, or trauma to the carpal tunnel. The greatest risk is found in occupations that require repeated flexion or extension of the wrist, use of hand tools that require forceful gripping, or use of hand tools that vibrate. CTS has been reported to occur spontaneously, most often during conditions that affect hormone balance (e.g., pregnancy, menopause, myxedematous hypothyroidism, diabetes mellitus) or in patients with other underlying musculoskeletal disorders (e.g., gout, rheumatoid arthritis, acute injury, acromegaly). Although the mechanism is unclear, it is thought that the generalized fluid increase or deposition of matrix substances (e.g., myxedema, amyloidosis) in the body tissues causes impingement on the median nerve within the carpal tunnel. This is also likely to underlie the association of CTS with fluid overload in end-stage renal disease and chronic dialysis.

Past history of wrist trauma or Colles' fracture, degenerative (and inflammatory) joint disease, ganglionic cysts, obesity, fibromyalgia, and scleroderma are other risk factors for this disorder. There is no universal agreement that CTS is work-related. Although no genetic mutations have been identified other than a rare chromosome 17 deletion that leads to an autosomal dominant neuropathic disorder prone to pressure-related nerve palsies, carpal tunnel syndrome is well known to occur in families. In fact, up to half the risk of developing CTS is thought to be attributable to genetic factors.

Pathophysiology

The anatomy of the wrist extends from the distal radius and ulna to the carpometacarpal joint. The eight small carpal bones of the wrist, arranged in two rows, account for numerous articulations and enable the wrist to perform a wide range of motion (ROM). The wrist is the second most mobile joint in the body, allowing for the exceptional mobility of the hand. Radial ligaments and the triangular fibrocartilage complex maintain the stability of the carpal bones. The carpal tunnel is formed by the arrangement of the wrist bones and the inelastic flexor retinaculum ligament. Through this tunnel run the finger flexor tendons as well as the median nerve. Any source of inflammation or pressure within this canal can result in symptoms of carpal tunnel syndrome.

Patients with carpal tunnel syndrome are exquisitely prone to developing increases in pressure within the carpal tunnel during wrist flexion and extension. In turn, this may lead to edema within the nerve tissue. Some studies have also demonstrated increased connective tissue proximal to the median nerve with a notable reduction in nerve fiber caliber, following nerve impingement. These mechanisms may also result in venous congestion and stasis, compression of the median nerve, and resultant ischemia, leading to the pain and paresthesias associated with carpal tunnel syndrome.

Clinical Presentation

Subjective

Typically, the patient will present with an aching sensation that radiates into the thenar area; it may also be perceived in the proximal forearm, and occasionally the pain can extend to the shoulder. Paresthesias and numbness in the median distribution (thumb and index, long, and radial half of ring fingers, or some combination thereof) typically accompanies the pain. Patients often report that they frequently drop objects, that they cannot open jars or twist off lids. Repetitive motions of the hand, or stationary tasks with the wrist held flexed or extended for a period of time (such as when driving) worsens pain and numbness. A hallmark symptom is night-time awakening with pain and numbness. Patients report that they must rub or shake the hand to "get the circulation" going. Persistent numbness and thenar atrophy can occur when the compression is severe and/or longstanding.

Objective

Examination of the patient with suspected carpal tunnel syndrome should include inspection of the wrist and hand for swelling, redness, nodules, deformity, and muscle atrophy. The thenar eminence (at the base of the thumb) is the best location to assess for atrophy. If the thenar eminence is atrophied or flattened, then chronic carpal tunnel syndrome should be suspected. Palpation of the hand and wrist should be done to check for swelling, bogginess, or tenderness. Each DIP, PIP, and MCP joint should be palpated, as well as the wrist bones. Capillary refill time should be determined, and the radial and ulnar arteries should be assessed for patency. Allen's test should be performed to determine individual patency of both the radial and ulnar arteries.

ROM of the fingers and wrists should be assessed as follows:

- ▲ Have the patient make a fist with the thumb across the knuckles.
- ▲ Have the patient extend and widely spread the fingers.
- ▲ Have the patient touch each finger with the thumb of the same hand.
- ▲ With the palms facing down, passively move the fingers laterally and medially.
- ▲ Have the patient flex and extend the hands, with and without resistance.

Assessment may also include:

- ▲ Phalen's maneuver: Have the patient acutely flex the wrists by pressing the backs of the hands together for 60 seconds. An abnormal or positive Phalen's maneuver is present when the patient reports numbness and tingling in the thumb or first two digits.
- ▲ Tinel's sign: Lightly percuss the palmar surface of the wrist with a percussion hammer. An abnormal or positive Tinel's sign occurs when the patient reports tingling or a shocklike sensation that travels across the palm into the thumb and first two digits, a sign of nerve compression.
- ▲ Carpal compression test: Place the thumbs over the flexor retinaculum and apply even pressure over the area of the median nerve for 30 to 60 seconds. A positive test is indicated by the occurrence of paresthesia in the hand or first three digits.

The performance of sensory testing to aid in the diagnosis is of little clinical value. Many patients who do not have carpal tunnel syndrome have diminished ability to differentiate sharp and dull sensations on the fingers, and therefore yield a high false-positive rate for this testing. Also remember that occupation and handedness may affect the muscular symmetry of the hands and wrists in the absence of a musculoskeletal condition.

Diagnostic Reasoning

Diagnostic Tests

Radiographs should be done if the patient has limited wrist movement; however, the most useful diagnostic test is a median nerve conduction velocity study. By measuring the velocity of sensory conduction, nerve entrapment may be conclusively validated. It is important to remember that this is an invasive test and that it is considerably more expensive than other diagnostic methods. In addition, a patient may have an abnormal nerve conduction velocity study but have no clinical symptoms; conversely, 5 to 10 percent of patients with CTS have normal test results.

Differential Diagnosis

The following is a list of differential diagnoses:

- ▲ Arthritis of the carpometacarpal joint of the thumb (painful motion)
- ▲ Cervical radiculopathy affecting C6 nerve root (neck pain, numbness in the thumb and index finger only)
- ▲ Diabetes mellitus with parathesias (determine on history)
- ▲ Median nerve compression at the elbow (tenderness at the proximal forearm)
- ▲ Wrist arthritis (limited motion, evident on radiograph)

Management

Conservative treatment is recommended for patients who present with acute symptoms. It has been reported that 50 to 75 percent of conservatively treated patients will attain symptom relief. The goal of treatment is to prevent the flexion and extension movements of the wrist. This is best accomplished through use of a splint that allows free movement of the fingers and the thumb while maintaining the wrist in the neutral position. Recommendations for wearing of the splint vary from constantly (day and night) to nighttime only. Some providers recommend using the splints day and night for 3 weeks, then nightly only for 3 more weeks. Splinting can be a cost-effective method for symptom control. Maximum results from splinting are attained if it is instituted within the first 3 months of symptom onset.

Oral NSAIDs are another conservative measure that can be used in conjunction with splinting. These drugs are often prescribed for patients who experience pain as part of the syndrome, but they may have some general usefulness in controlling edema in the carpal tunnel.

Corticosteroid injections, although used by some providers, are discouraged for treatment of CTS. Although the injections provide temporary relief, there is a concern that the median nerve could sustain damage, as well as the side effects of scarring or infection. When paients present with acute CTS with pain as the predominate symptom, they may respond well to corticosteroids. One recent study reported that steroid injections (two) were as effective as surgery.

The use of vitamin B_6 (pyridoxine) has been reported in the literature over the past several years. Although there are no conclusive studies on the utility of this medication in treating or preventing carpal tunnel syndrome, use of this vitamin is becoming more prevalent. Care should be taken with dosing, as larger doses may result in neuropathies. It is also important to determine whether the patient is on any other medications that may be affected by pyroxidine: For example, serum concentrations of phenytoin and phenobarbital may be decreased with pyridoxine.

Management of concurrent disease (e.g., hypothyroidism, diabetes mellitus) is an important aspect of the conservative treatment of CTS. Treatment that diminishes fluid retention, when used with other conservative methods, will produce better results in relieving the symptoms of CTS.

CTS that occurs during pregnancy, usually resolves when the pregnancy terminates. Treatment should consist of splinting and other nonoperative measures such as corticosteroid injections. CTS that is work related may be improved with ergonomic modifications.

Follow-Up and Referral

The presence of thenar atrophy or unremitting symptoms with conservative treatment warrant referral for surgical evaluation. Carpal tunnel release is one of the most commonly performed hand surgeries; it is usually done under local anesthesia, on an outpatient basis. The surgery may be performed by a hand specialist, plastic surgeon, or neurosurgeon. Although small incisions are being used more frequently, some surgeons state that visual inspection of the entire carpal space is necessary. The use of a longitudinal incision must be weighed against the risks of wound infection, scarring, and diminished motor abilities.

Postoperatively, patients can expect to have the hand splinted for 8 to 14 days while the sutures remain in place. Depending on the type of surgical intervention, healing will occur within 4 to 10 weeks. Passive and active ROM exercises are encouraged to promote healing. Patients should be cautioned that subjecting themselves to the same risks that caused the carpal tunnel syndrome may curtail healing and cause the problem to return. Modification of the work environment may be necessary to reduce this possibility.

Patient Education

Workers who are exposed to occupational risks for carpal tunnel syndrome should be educated on the causes and prevention of CTS. The work environment should be assessed for ergonomic risks to workers; often an ergonomic specialist is needed to perform these assessments. *Ergonomics* means fitting the job to the worker, as opposed to the worker accommodating to the workspace. Special attention should be paid to jobs with a known ability to produce extreme or repeated flexion of the wrist. Ergonomic evaluations and recommendations include, for example:

- ▲ Evaluating the workstations of computer keyboard workers in regard to the height of the keyboard, chair, and monitor.
- ▲ Teaching lifting techniques and reviewing them annually.
- ▲ Rotating jobs for workers who perform repetitive tasks.
- ▲ Resting frequently or wearing specially designed hand wear; for example, workers who use vibrating tools should wear antivibration gloves or should be given frequent, short rest breaks.

Outside of workplace risks, patients should be educated to consider the stress on the wrist during everyday activities such as gardening and cleaning. Knitting, sewing, and playing musical instruments may put tension on the wrist. Patients should be advised to avoid carrying heavy briefcases, packages, or purses with the hands. Bags with shoulder straps or backpacks should be recommended to patients with risk factors for CTS.

Paget's Disease

Paget's disease (*osteitis deformans*) of the bone, first diagnosed by Sir James Paget in 1877, is a disease of the osteoclast and is the most exaggerated example of disordered bone remodeling. It is characterized by excessive osteoclastic bone resorption followed by excessive bone formation from osteoblasts, resulting in bone that is architecturally unsound. This can lead to bone pain, bone deformity, and skeletal fragility, and can involve a single bone or multiple bones.

Epidemiology and Causes

Prevalence of the disease is difficult to determine because it is often asymptomatic (70 to 90 percent of cases). Older adults are most commonly affected; it is the second most common bone disorder after osteoporosis in older adults. It is estimated that the disease affects more than 10 percent of people older than 80 years of age. Ethnic and geographic clustering of cases has been well described for Paget's disease, while 40 percent of patients report a family history of the condition. This disease is common in England, with statistics indicating a prevalence as high as 5 percent of the general population in some areas. Australia, New Zealand, and Argentina are also high prevalence areas. In the United States, the prevalence varies between 1 and 3 percent.

Although Paget himself felt the disease was caused by chronic inflammation, the etiology remains unknown to date. Bone biopsy data has identified various viral antigens which suggest that a "slow virus" infection by a member of the paramyxovirus family (e.g., rubeola which causes measles, respiratory syncytial virus, canine distemper) may be responsible for the disease.

Pathophysiology

The disease affects all aspects of bone metabolism and may be divided into three phases: lytic, mixed, and sclerotic. It begins with the lytic phase characterized by increased activity of multinucleate (up to 100 nuclei compared to 5 to 10 normally) osteoclasts, which leads to greatly increased resorption of bone (up to 20-fold). Hypercalcemia may manifest, particularly if the patient experiences prolonged immobilization. The mixed phase then follows in which bone remodeling is abnormally increased, due to a greater number of osteoblasts, although they are of normal morphology. This leads to an abnormal, irregular deposition of collagen fibers. The final phase, known as the sclerotic phase, is notable for a predominance of abnormal bone formation. This is characterized by disorganized bone that takes on a mosaic pattern known as "woven bone," which is recognizable on x-ray exam. Eventually osteoblastic activity quiets, leaving sclerotic lesions. As the hypercellularity decreases, this bone becomes known as burned-out Paget's disease.

There are no Haversian systems within pagetic bone, and the bone marrow is eventually replaced by hypervascular fibrous tissue. Bones that are commonly affected with these sclerotic lesions include the cranium, long bones, and clavicles. These affected bones will change in shape, enlarge in size, and undergo changes in predominant direction of growth due to increased osteoid volume—all of which lead to considerable morbidity. Pagetic bone is weaker and less compact than normal adult lamellar bone, and bones affected by this change may be painful and, over time, may develop deformities, fractures, or nerve entrapment. Cytokines and growth factors which have been implicated, albeit inconclusively, in the pathophysiology of Paget's disease include IL-6, RANK-ligand (a member of the TNF-α superfamily), and macrophage-colony stimulating factor (M-CSF).

A rarer juvenile form of Paget's disease also exists. However, this form is fundamentally different from the adult form, as it is typically polyostotic with widespread skeletal involvement. In addition, both histological and radiological findings differ from the adult form and may be readily distinguished.

Clinical Presentation

Subjective

The clinical presentation of Paget's disease is a function of the actual extent of disease, bones involved, and any complications present. Most (70 to 90 percent) patients are asymptomatic. Although the affected bone may be larger than other bones, pagetic bones are weaker and more susceptible to fracture. The bones most commonly affected, in order of decreasing frequency, are the femur, sacrum, vertebrae, skull, tibia, and pelvis. Involvement of the tibia and humerus is less common, but the disease may occur at any site and may involve one (monostotic) or many (polyostotic) bones. Hands and feet are rarely involved.

The most typical complaint is one of pain at the involved site. The pain is usually dull or boring, but it can be shooting or knife-like, and often occurs at night. In some cases, a swelling or deformity of a long bone is noticed or the development of a change in gait. Back pain, with radiation to the buttocks or lower extremities, is another common complaint. Headache is a common complaint when the skull is involved.

Pagetic bone is of a highly vascular nature, and there may be increased warmth of the skin over the affected bones. The incidence of high-output cardiac failure may be tied to the increased vascularity of the involved bone, manifesting the classic symptoms of "dropsy" (generalized fluid overload). While rare, this condition correlates with greater than 15 percent of skeletal involvement.

In patients with involvement of the ossicles of the inner ear or impingement of bone on the eighth cranial nerve, hearing loss may occur. Vertigo and tinnitus may also develop with skull involvement, as well as cranial nerve involvement resulting from compression by deformed bone. Spinal cord compression has also been observed with resultant cauda equina syndrome or paraplegia. Pathologic fractures of vertebrae may also produce spinal cord lesions and pain. Articular complications, including both asymptomatic hyperuricemia and classic gout, pseudogout, and degenerative arthritis, may occur. Fractures of the long bones occur most commonly in the femur, tibia, and humerus. Significant morbidity may result from heavy bleeding which may result from pathologic fractures in these hypervascular bones.

Complications include cardiovascular problems, arthritic and osteoporotic problems, and neoplastic problems. When Paget's disease becomes widespread in the body, blood flow increases and may be associated with high cardiac output. The end result in this situation may be congestive heart failure (CHF). Arthritic changes in weightbearing joints may result in pathologic fractures. One dreaded complication is that of sarcoma. Incidence of sarcoma is approximately 1 percent; it may be in the femur, humerus, skull, facial bones, or pelvis. The extent of neoplastic involvement may be detected by CT and/or MRI.

Objective

Bowing of the long bones may be apparent, as well as enlargement of the skull (e.g., frontal bossing, maxillary enlargement). The sacrum, pelvis, and spine, particularly the lumbar spine, are the most common areas involved. Other less frequently involved sites include the femur (right more than left), cranium, sternum, and pelvis. Erythema and warmth is often noted over affected bone sites due to the increased hypervascularity.

Diagnostic Reasoning

Diagnostic Tests

Paget's disease is most commonly diagnosed through radiographs, radionuclide bone scanning, biochemical testing of bone resorption parameters, or biochemical testing of bone formation parameters. Biochemical tests reflecting osteoclast activity and resultant bone collagen resorption include measurements of urinary hydroxyproline/creatinine as well as measurements of urinary and serum deoxypyridinoline, N-telopeptide and C-telopeptide. Elevated 24-hour urinary deoxypyridinoline and type I collagen N-telopeptide excretion reflect bony destruction (resorption). As a marker of osteoblast activity, the measurement of serum alkaline phosphatase activity provides a general indication of bone turnover and disease activity in Paget's disease. Serum bone specific alkaline phosphatase activity is helpful in patients who also have liver disease. At least one measurement of bone metabolic activity and x-ray films of affected bones are the minimum recommended level of evaluation to track and monitor the progression of treatment in Paget's disease.

Radiographs may illustrate three distinct stages of Paget's disease. In the earliest stage of the disease, an osteolytic lesion may be observed in the skull or a long bone. In the second stage of the disease, x-ray films reveal both osteolytic and sclerotic changes in the same bone. In the last stage of the disease, the sclerotic lesion demonstrates the bone and here may be an increase of the bone itself.

Although it is not a specific test, a radionuclide bone scan, using a radiolabeled bisphosphonate, is the most efficient means of detecting Paget's disease in a skeleton. The bisphosphonate is injected intravenously and is concentrated in areas of increased blood flow and high levels of bone formation, both common characteristics of Paget's disease. The test is used primarily to establish the full extent of skeletal involvement.

Diagnosis is often made when x-ray studies are performed or a high level of bone-specific alkaline phosphatase (a marker of bone formation) is found on routine screening. Immobilization in patients with Paget's disease is a primary risk factor for significantly elevated serum calcium and phosphorus, but immobilization alone will not necessarily result in hypercalcemia without underlying pathology. Occasionally, an associated hyperthyroidism can also lead to hypercalcemia. Quantitative histomorphometry of bone biopsies confirm the extent of remodeling present. Imaging studies to rule out malignancy should be performed whenever pathologic fractures or elevated bone-specific alkaline phosphatase levels are detected.

Differential Diagnosis

When lesions are noted on x-ray film, metastatic cancer should be considered. Disseminated breast and prostate cancer are the cancers most likely to resemble Paget's disease radiographically, and need to be ruled out. Occasionally, a hemangioma of bone may be sclerotic and mistaken for pagetic bone.

When making a diagnosis of Paget's disease, differential diagnoses such as osteoporosis, osteomalacia, hypercalcemia, and compensatory, secondary hyperparathyroidism should be considered. As with Paget's disease, osteoporosis involves the imbalance between bone formation and bone resorption. When bone formation exceeds resorption, the circulatory levels of parathyroid hormone may become increased, thus resulting in compensatory, secondary hyperparathyroidism.

Management

If Paget's disease is discovered incidentally and the patient is asymptomatic, no treatment may be necessary. However, there is an increasing trend to treat even if the patient is asymptomatic. This is based on evidence that failure to treat leads to further bone destruction, that successful treatment has been associated with restoration of normal patterns of new bone deposition, and a study that showed that facial and skull deformities improved after successful treatment. However, there is no direct evidence that aggressive treatment of Paget's disease is associated with prevention of progression or reduction in the risk of future complications.

There are four main approaches to treatment for a patient with Paget's disease: nonpharmacologic therapy, focusing mainly on physical therapy as a way to improve muscle strength; pharmacologic therapy using either bisphosphonates or calcitonins; pain management using analgesics; or surgery.

Currently, bisphosphonates are approved by the FDA for the treatment of Paget's disease. Bone resorption is suppressed or reduced by bisphosphonates. They hinder the recruitment and function of osteoclasts and they are thought to indirectly stimulate osteoblasts to produce an inhibitor of osteoclast formation.

The bisphosphonates alendronate and risedronate have been shown to reduce biochemical indices for bone turnover into the normal range in many patients with a moderate to severe form of Paget's disease. Aldendronate (Fosamax) is taken as a daily 40-mg tablet for 6 months; risedronate (Actonel) is taken as a daily 30-mg tablet for 2 to 3 months. Calcium and Vitamin D supplementation is also recommended for patients using either of these drugs. Etidronate (Didronel) is less potent than alendronate and risedronate but is recommended for treatment of symptomatic Paget's disease. Given once daily (preferred) or in divided doses at least 2 hours before or after food; initially 5 to 10 mg/kg per day for a maximum of 6 months.

Subcutaneous injection of salmon calcitonin was the first widely used therapy for Paget's disease. Salmon calcitonin (Fortical, Miacalcin) has been shown to reduce elevated indices of bone turnover by 50 percent, decrease symptoms of bone pain, reduce warmth over affected bones, improve some neurologic complications, and promote healing of lytic lesions. It is available in a nasal spray as well as an injectable (Miacalcin) form. The recommended dosage for the injectable form is 100 units per day as subcutaneous or intramuscular injection. Its use today is primarily limited to patients who do not tolerate bisphosphonates. In the case of secondary resistance to salmon calcitonin, a switch to bisphosphonate therapy is necessary.

Pain directly attributable to Paget's disease is generally relieved through anti-osteoclast therapy as described earlier. Pain that is a result of bone deformity or arthritic or neurologic complications may be treated additionally with acetaminophen, NSAIDs, and depending on the circumstances, cox-2 inhibitors.

Surgical intervention is indicated in the face of significant bony deformities, nerve compression, or pathologic fractures. Severe osteoarthritis of major joints such as the hip or knee may require artificial joint replacement with preoperative bisphosphonate therapy. Neurologic sequelae from vertebral abnormalities may call for laminectomy for spinal decompression in lesions refractory to medical therapy. Osteosarcomas arising in pagetic bone may also require amputation to improve prognosis. In all these cases, extended physical therapy will follow.

Follow-Up and Referral

Follow-up will depend on symptomatology, as will referral. Pain status needs to be monitored, as well as any laboratory abnormalities. If started on medication, the patient will need to be followed for therapeutic effects as well as any adverse effects that may occur secondary to therapy. Serum and urinary markers of disease activity should be followed 2 to 3 months after initiation of therapy and periodically thereafter. Any suspicion of malignancy warrants full evaluation and referral, as prognosis is particularly grim with the development of sarcoma with only a 1- to 3-year survival. Appropriate referrals may include an orthopedic surgeon, neurosurgeon, physical therapist, and/or oncologist.

Patient Education

Patient education is important because so many people are asymptomatic. The canine distemper virus has been postulated to be an etiologic agent for Paget's disease; therefore, owners of dogs that are not vaccinated against this virus are at increased risk. Many of the medications prescribed for Paget's disease have significant adverse effects. Calcitonin analogues produced from other species may induce anaphylaxis and should be used with caution. Hypocalcemia may also result and should be monitored periodically. The bisphosphonates require ingestion on an empty stomach and the ability to stay in an upright position anywhere from 30 to 60 minutes. They can all cause GI irritation and other medication such as ASA and NSAIDs should be used concurrently with caution. Adequate calcium and vitamin D intake must be maintained as the bisphosphonates interfere with their absorption. These medications also interfere and interact with a wide variety of other drugs, blocking tetracycline, fluoroquinolone, and levothyroxine absorption. Warfarin must be monitored also.

Costochondritis

Costochondritis, also called *anterior chest wall syndrome*, is an inflammation of one or more costochondral junctions that manifests with chest wall pain. The pain may be sharp and acute or dull and persistent in nature. It is the most frequently occurring nontraumatic type of chest pain in adolescents and young adults. Pain is located over the costochondral and costosternal areas of the anterior chest.

Epidemiology and Causes

Costochondritis accounts for 10 percent of chest pain complaints in the United States. In the adolescent population, more than 20 percent of reported chest pain may be due to costochondritis. It is more common in women than in men, with a peak age range of 20 to 40 years. The cause of the problem is poorly understood, although trauma and overuse have been implicated in some cases. It is also sometimes seen in association with upper respiratory infection.

Pathophysiology

Costochondritis is an inflammation of the costochondral junctions manifesting only with pain in the absence of erythema, heat, or swelling. Repetitive minor trauma is currently believed to be the most likely etiology. However, epidemiologic research has revealed an increasing incidence of costochondritis resulting from bacterial or fungal infections of the costochondral joints in injection drug users due to needle contamination or in people with postoperative thoracic wound infections.

When symptoms of costochondritis are accompanied by localized nonsuppurative swelling, this condition is termed Tietze's syndrome, which is characterized by a firm, palpable, tender fusiform swelling in the sternoclavicular joints or upper costal cartilages.

Clinical Presentation

Subjective

The patient presents with chest pain, which may be sharp and fleeting or intermittent. The patient may report previous episodes and may be concerned that there is something wrong with his or her heart. The onset of the pain is typically insidious and located at the costochondral junctions, most commonly involving the second to fifth costochondral joints. More than one site is involved in 90 percent of cases. There may be some radiation to the arm, but the pain is unrelated to position, respiration, or activity, although some patients report an increase in pain with trunk movements or deep breathing. The pain may persist for several months, causing the patient to return to the clinician for reassurance that nothing else is responsible for it. Chest tightness or localized muscle spasm may accompany the pain. There may be a history of recent upper respiratory infection, trauma, or unusual activity involving the chest or pectoral muscles.

Objective

In most cases, there are no objective physical findings other than sharply localized tenderness to palpation. These same sites may not be painful without direct palpation. In a few cases, inspection may reveal an area of redness, warmth, and nonsuppurative edema; however, this condition is more appropriately termed Tietze's syndrome and is seen most often in teenage girls. It is imperative in the examination of all patients with chest pain that the examiner apply pressure on the pectoralis muscles and each costochondral and costosternal junctions. This maneuver will reproduce the pain of costochondritis.

Diagnostic Reasoning

There are many causes of chest pain, ranging from life-threatening and acute to troublesome but benign etiologies. All of these must be considered in arriving at an accurate diagnosis.

Diagnostic Tests

The diagnosis of costochondritis is based on a thorough history and physical examination which reveal no red flags for more serious pathology. There are no specific diagnostic tests. However, testing may be initiated to rule out other conditions that manifest with chest pain and are part of the differential diagnosis. A chest radiograph is often helpful in this regard to evaluate for more serious lung, cardiac, or bony pathology. ESR is elevated in some instances of costochondritis, but inconsistently. Moreover, the lack of specificity of a positive ESR means that it cannot be used to exclude other conditions and rule in costochondritis. However, a nonelevated ESR may assist in ruling out more serious pathology.

Differential Diagnosis

Differential diagnosis includes cardiac-related chest pain such as mitral valve prolapse, myocarditis, pericarditis, left ventricular outflow obstruction, tachyarrhythmias, aortic aneurysm, and acute coronary syndrome resulting from coronary artery disease or sympathomimetic drugs of abuse such as cocaine. Respiratory causes of chest pain include asthma, pneumonia, pleuritis, pneumothorax, pulmonary embolism, and chronic cough. Gastrointestinal causes of chest pain include gastroesophageal reflux disease (GERD), esophagitis, gastritis, peptic ulcer disease (PUD), and esophageal spasm. Musculoskeletal causes of chest pain include muscle strain, trauma, hypersensitive xiphoid pain (xiphodynia or xiphoidalgia), slipping rib syndrome (pain originating in the lower, floating ribs), subacromial bursitis, and fibromyalgia syndrome (FMS). Psychogenic disorders manifesting with chest pain include panic attacks and generalized anxiety disorder. Other diagnostics considerations with cutaneous pain include early herpes zoster (characterized by dermatomal clustered skin lesions) or pain related to chest wall tumors.

Management

Management consists of reassurance and patient education regarding the benign and self-limited nature of the problem. Application of heat to the area may alleviate discomfort. NSAIDs may be prescribed for pain management, given the inflammatory nature of costochondritis. However, patients should be cautioned of the potential gastric and renal toxicities of NSAID overuse and contraindications should be stressed (e.g., PUD, gastritis, acute or chronic renal insufficiency). Drugs from these classes should be taken with food or milk. In addition, to avoid aggravating costochondritis, patients should be cautioned to avoid overuse or trauma.

Follow-Up and Referral

The patient can be seen for reevaluation in a week to 10 days or can be contacted by phone. The patient should be instructed to call the office if pain intensifies or other symptoms appear. One of the most important considerations when making the diagnosis of costochondritis is to rule-out pathology of greater morbidity or potential mortality, as discussed earlier. A complete history and physical examination are the most important tools in guiding this evaluation; however, a complete work-up may require follow-up visitations to complete the diagnostic evaluation or assess changes in signs and symptoms over time.

Patient Education

The most critical point in many cases is convincing the patient that his or her condition is benign and self-limited despite the sharp nature of the pain. The patient is often fearful and requires reassurance. The clinician should educate the patient regarding the need to avoid overuse injury if any repetitive motion appears to be involved. It is important to stress the importance of avoiding any sudden, significant changes in activity.

Tendonitis/Tenosynovitis

Tendonitis is the inflammation of a tendon, which usually occurs at its point of insertion into bone or at the point of muscular origin. The term *tenosynovitis* refers to inflammation involving synovial sheaths surrounding the tendon in addition to the tendons. Common tenosynovitis syndromes, also referred to as "overuse" syndromes, include supraspinatus tendonitis, lateral epicondylitis or "tennis elbow," bicipital tendonitis, de Quervain's tenosynovitis (inflammation of the abductor pollicis longus and extensor pollicis longus and brevis tendons), "trigger finger" (volar flexor tenosynovitis), patellar tendonitis (patellar tendinosis or "basketball player's knee"), and Achilles tendonitis (see section on Overuse Syndrome in this chapter).

Epidemiology and Causes

This problem occurs commonly, with a slightly increased frequency in males, most likely related to sports. It occurs at all ages. Professional athletes and manual laborers are especially prone to tendonitis as a result of repetitive use. Painful areas of tendon are often labeled *tendonitis,* implying an inflammatory nature of the lesion; however, it is unclear whether inflammation is truly present in all forms of the pathology, especially in more chronic situations, which tend to have a more degenerative component. Some sources advocate the use of the term *tendinosis* for this reason. *Tenosynovitis* may result from inflammatory arthropathies such as rheumatoid arthritis or from gout. Tenosynovitis from amyloidosis is also common in renal dialysis patients. It also may occur for no discernible reason. Adults who overuse a joint with repeated motion are most likely to develop a *tendonitis*. Some classifications are based on degree of function and whether there is a partial or complete rupture of the tendon.

Pathophysiology

Exact pathophysiologic entities involved with tendonitis and tenosynovitis have not been clearly established. It is understood that tenosynovitis involves inflammation of the synovial-lined sheath around one or more tendons, while tendonitis involves inflammation of the tendinous tissue itself. Because flexor tendons typically run in tight fibroosseous tunnels, thickening of the surrounding sheath caused by inflammatory changes may in turn limit movement and cause pain as the trapped tendon attempts to glide within the thickened, tight sheath. The parietal and visceral layers of the synovium that surround flexor tendons typically provide nutrition and stability to the tendons, while allowing for smooth movement of these connective tissues without extensive friction. However, infection may spread to these areas from nearby mucosal tissues, by direct extension from the skin through a puncture wound, or even hematogenously (as is the case with gonococcal tenosynovitis, which complicates 1 to 3 percent of patients with mucosal infection of the pharynx or genitalia), as these synovial compartments normally offer little resistance. Tenosynovitis may also be associated with an inflammatory, infectious arthritis of large joints resulting from similar spread of infectious organisms (especially bacteria).

Tendonitis is usually associated with some degenerative changes in the tendon including cell atrophy along with the presence of fibrinoid, mucoid, or hyaline degeneration of the connective tissue, which is visible under microscopic examination. Peritendinous scarring is not unusual, as tendons are relatively avascular and particularly sensitive to increased pressure within their synovial sheaths. Calcium deposits may also be noted along the length of the tendon, known as calcific tendonitis; this is especially common in the shoulder joint. These tendons tend to stiffen without treatment. Loss of function often follows, as they become progressively weaker and may eventually rupture.

Clinical Presentation

Subjective

Frequently insidious in onset, patients typically complain of pain and swelling over a localized area of tendon, usually in a region where the tendon passes through a tunnel. Pain is usually worse with motion, especially motion that stretches the involved tendon. A squeaking or rubbing and sometimes a triggering or catching sensation will be described by patients who have significant tenosynovitis. Tenosynovitis around the finger flexor tendon in the carpal tunnel region can have the associated symptoms of fingertip numbness from median nerve compression, as noted previously. A good history is essential, including all extracurricular activities.

Objective

The diagnosis of tendonitis is clinically driven. Early imaging is usually of minimal benefit. Perform a thorough physical exam that includes palpating any tender areas and ruling out any articular involvement of pain. One may see minimal swelling in tendonitis, although it can be impressive in cases of infection or with inflammatory causes of tenosynovitis. Examination may reveal localized pain, swelling, and tenderness. The pain will be worsened with certain motions, such as stretching the involved tendon, or with active work or activity that involves use of the tendon, especially against a resisting force. Crepitus and sometimes triggering can be palpated if a significant tenosynovitis has developed. These signs vary depending on anatomic site of the tendonitis.

For example, tendonitis of the shoulder includes the bicep tendon as well as the tendons of the rotator cuff. This is similar to impingement syndrome. When patients have shoulder tendonitis, one will note tenderness with palpation of the subacromial space. These patients will have tenderness when one palpates the long head of the biceps tendon in the bicipital notch. To do this, have the patient keep his or her elbow at the affected side and externally rotate the shoulder to palpate the bicipital notch anteriorly and medially in the humeral head. When examining these patients one can also elicit pain with resisted supination or flexion of the forearm. There is often an overlap of impingement syndrome with tendonitis of the shoulder.

If an inflammatory disease is present, then associated redness, soft tissue swelling, and warmth may be present. Inflammatory processes of the tendon sheaths most commonly involve the dorsum of the hands, feet, and ankle and may cause marked soft tissue swelling. The ROM of contiguous joints may be limited by pain.

Diagnostic Reasoning

Diagnostic Tests

Diagnostics involve a thorough history and complete physical examination. Plain films may be useful to rule out other potential causes of pain in areas in question, but they will not show a tendinitis. An MRI scan will show any significant tenosynovitis and tender nodules that sometimes develop. However, the diagnosis can almost always be made clinically without the need for an MRI. Other options may include arthrography and MRI. In cases of tenosynovitis, there may be an associated anemia or elevation of the ESR.

Differential Diagnosis

Differential diagnoses to rule out include fracture, avulsion of the tendon, inflammatory arthritis, RA, and compartment syndrome. In the case of Achilles tendonitis, one must also consider a gastrocnemius strain, soleus strain, or tarsal tunnel syndrome. Tendonitis can be practically impossible to differentiate from bursitis and the two conditions commonly occur together. The pain in tendonitis is localized to the side of the joint where tendon insertion occurs. Infectious tenosynovitis occurs primarily in the hand. In addition, the tenderness and swelling are located along the synovial lines proximally instead of at the insertion site and the pain is more marked, as is swelling and erythema. The ESR and WBC count are more likely to be elevated in the case of infection.

Essentially, definitive diagnosis of tenosynovitis requires careful musculoskeletal examination, confirming the tendon source of the symptoms and excluding pathology from other contiguous musculoskeletal structures, including joints, bursae, and nerves. However, an inflammatory tenosynovitis of the dorsum of the hand or foot may require aspiration of synovial fluid, examination, and culture to confirm the diagnosis.

Management

Specific treatment requires an exact diagnosis to prevent further injury. An aggressive exercise program for example would be inappropriate for a compartment syndrome, complete tendon rupture, or nerve entrapment. Treatment will also depend on the stage of healing of the damaged tissue of the musculoskeletal system. There are essentially three phases of healing: (1) inflammation, (2) proliferation of new collagen and ground substance, and (3) scar remodeling and maturation.

Initial management should include rest, protection, ice, compression, and elevation. The injury should be protected and rehabilitated in parallel with the healing process. The injured tissue needs to be stressed in order to activate collagen remodeling and realignment but also protected from overstress, which will cause re-injury and incite a further inflammatory response. Taping and bracing can both be helpful in providing protection. Ice is useful for treating pain, hemorrhage, and edema. It induces vasoconstriction, which results in a decrease in local blood flow. Ice acts as a topical anesthetic agent to control pain and decrease reflex muscle spasms by reducing the conduction velocity in peripheral nerves. Ice bags compared with cold gel packs elicit the greatest decrease in tissue temperature over the longest period of time, and application for 15 to 20 minutes is recommended. Treatment may be repeated every 1 to 2 hours in acute cases. In lowering the temperature, ice decreases metabolism and enzymatic function; further, it slows down the inflammatory process. It is useful during the first 48 hours in acute cases and in chronic cases it can be applied post-activity for 30 to 50 minutes.

Compression in concert with cold therapy helps to reduce the swelling. Elevation decreases edema by aiding lymphatic and venous return. In acute ankle sprains, elevation has been shown to be the most effective method of reducing swelling, for example. The objective is to treat the initial symptoms with the above techniques to prevent prolonged inflammation and avoid new tissue disruption. In addition, measures of relative rest are used to protect the tissue from further injury. In some cases, specifically carpal tunnel syndrome, for example, splinting may be effective. Ideally, the splint should be custom-made and fitted for the individual patient; an occupational therapist may assist with this.

In stage 2 of the healing process, the objective is to gradually introduce stress and apply modalities to increase collagen production, size, cross-linking, and alignment. The rate of collagen fiber formation is directly related to the functional state of the affected area. The collagen fibers reorient themselves in line with the tensile force applied to the tissue. In stage 3, the objective is to make the collagen as elastic as possible and decrease formation of scar tissue. Progressive stress is placed on tissue to promote an increase in collagen fibril size and to increase cross-linking in tissues. Flexibility training is needed to decrease cross-linking in the joint capsule.

Immobilization may be counterproductive and absolute rest should be limited to 1 to 2 days at most until the inflammation response has settled or in the most severe, chronic cases of tendonitis after active rest has failed. *Active rest* means that the injured area can be used, but it should be protected from significant stress, which may cause further damage. The frequency and intensity of an activity may be decreased or altered, for example, but all activity should not be completely eliminated. Physical therapy is a cornerstone of treatment and can aid in the development of an individualized plan for the patient. Ice plays an important role once exercise and activity is resumed. It should be applied at the end of every exercise session to help prevent recurrence of inflammation and swelling.

Heat is effective after 48 hours in the acute phase and in the chronic phase. After the acute phase of the healing process, heat is useful in improving blood flow, relieving muscle spasm, and decreasing tissue stiffness, allowing greater ease of deformation. The most beneficial form of deep heat is ultrasound because the high-frequency waves render the tissues less stiff and more susceptible to remodeling by applied tensile forces. Ultrasound also increases local circulation and has been shown to speed wound healing. Lasers are another modality that has positive effects on wound healing, but unlike ultrasound, they also decrease inflammation.

Two types of electrical stimulation may be used in treatment. Transcutaneous nerve stimulation (TENS) is used for pain relief and can be a useful adjunctive modality. High voltage galvanic stimulation (HVGS) not only produces heat in the tissue but also has been reported to be effective in retarding the formation of edema. Deep friction massage is a modality used by physiotherapists to prevent the formation of adherent scars early in healing and later to break down scar tissue. It should be avoided in the first couple of days after injury because it can produce microtrauma, induce inflammation, and have a deleterious effect on healing.

NSAIDs are useful in the treatment of acute overuse injury, especially if used early, when they can decrease the production of arachidonic acid derivatives in the inflammatory pathway. They are probably best prescribed at maximum dose for 10 to 14 days. If no benefit is noted in the first 3 days it is unlikely further benefit will be gained. They probably do not have a major anti-inflammatory role in the treatment of chronic injuries because there is scant histologic evidence of true inflammatory response. Although widely prescribed, they have not been shown to effectively shorten recovery time; they may be useful in their analgesic effect in supporting patient's compliance with physical therapy.

Corticosteroids are occasionally indicated in cases of chronic overuse syndromes. They should never be injected directly into a tendon, as this can lead to rupture. In addition, activity needs to be decreased for 5 to 10 days after injection. Tendon sheath injections by contrast are quite effective in treating tenosynovitis of the ankle or wrist. Steroid injections can also be given intra-articulately when there is significant reactive synovitis with effusion.

Follow-Up and Referral

As noted under the section on *Overuse Syndromes* in general, soft-tissue injuries cause considerable pain, discomfort, and potential dysfunction. A comprehensive, team approach, structured in a Circle of Caring model is what is needed for these patients to avoid significant sequelae. As noted under *Management,* interventions need to be geared toward the stage of healing to be effective. The balance between rest and healing and the danger of erring in either direction can be great without thoughtful consideration by a team of providers as well as maximum hearing of the patient's voice. Athletes may be over-anxious and over-do; unhappy employees might have more of a psychogenic component to their pathology.

Referral to physical therapy is essential as is referral to orthopedic specialist if there is any question as to nature of pathology. Treatment must be individualized and the patient must be a chief architect in the plan of care. Patients requiring corticosteroid injections should be referred. Occupational therapists can assist with fitting of splints if necessary. Adequate sleep is essential to the overall treatment plan and may require follow up also. Aggressive intervention will potentially offset the possibility of the development of chronic pain syndrome.

Patient Education

It is important that patients understand the nature of their injury and be involved in the plan of care. In the case of athletes, careful evaluation of training schedules and circumstances surrounding the injury are essential so appropriate preventive measures can be put in place to support healing and avoid future injury. In the case of a work-related repetitive motion injury, evaluation of the workplace may be necessary.

All risk factors should be assessed. In the case of a patient with obesity, nutritional counseling may be necessary. A diabetic patient may need additional assistance in controlling their disease and likewise with a patient with hypertension and cardiovascular disease. Managing household chores may be a challenge for individuals with tendonitis. Carrying groceries in a paper bag rather than a plastic bag, driving a car with an automatic transmission, placing hands properly on the steering wheel (at 9 o'clock and 3 o'clock) and using electric kitchen appliances such as a food processor or electric can opener can dramatically reduce strain on injured muscles and nerves. Some hobbies, such as quilting, knitting, gardening, playing certain musical instruments, computer games, frequent internet usage, and needlepoint may have to be altered during the healing process and in some cases permanently. For many patients, stress management techniques such as yoga or meditation may be effective in promoting relaxation of injured, inflamed, and tense muscles.

In cases in which the patient's job is the source of repetitive strain injury, restrictions on work activity may be necessary. A careful and through occupational history can help make determinations about the contributing factors in the patient's job environment. A comprehensive ergonomic worksite evaluation may be conducted by a physical or occupational therapist in identifying specific problems. Ultimately, however, patients with severe forms of repetitive strain injury may be forced to change occupations.

Likewise, a severe tendonitis can potentially spell the end of a promising athletic career. From this vantage point, hearing the patient's voice—his or her concerns, feelings—is critical.

Bursitis

Bursitis, which is inflammation of a bursa, is a common cause of painful musculoskeletal syndromes. Bursae are sacs filled with synovial fluid, located between muscles, tendons, and bony prominences. Bursae cushion bony prominences from overlying muscles (deep bursae) or surface skin (superficial bursae); they may or may not communicate with the adjacent joint space. The bursa provides lubrication for movement of tendons over bones and can be affected by trauma, as in overuse, as well as by infection, inflammation, and neoplasms. The total number of bursae vary from person to person, but on average, this figure approaches 160. Some cases of bursitis may result from rheumatic afflictions and others from a pathologic condition of adjoining tissues. It may be acute or chronic.

Epidemiology and Causes

Bursitis is a common complaint, seen most often in patients who are skeletally mature. It is more common in males, and tends to be more commonly associated with trauma (including overuse syndrome) in patients younger than 35 years of age. Interestingly, up to 85 percent of septic bursitis cases are in men. It is one of the most common reasons for visits to the primary-care setting; the incidence is clearly related to increasing age. The incidence of bursitis of the lower extremities is increased by obesity.

Bursitis commonly develops in the subdeltoid and subacromial bursa of the shoulder, the olecranon bursa of the elbow, the greater trochanteric bursa that is lateral to the hip, the ischial bursa, the prepatellar bursa of the knee, the anserine bursa, and the heel. The anserine bursa lies between the pes anserine tendons, which insert into the sartorius, gracilis, and semitendinosus muscles, and the medial collateral ligament which lies over the medial aspect of the tibia.

Trauma in the form of repetitive motion injury is probably the most common cause of bursitis, as a result of constant friction between a bursa and musculoskeletal tissues surrounding it. Friction in turn causes irritation, edema, and over time, inflammation and subsequent degeneration. The end result is an engorged bursal sac with surrounding tissue that has become tender and painful. Movement around the bursa may result in increased pain and pressure. In turn, flexion and extension of the closest joint may be limited by the affected bursa. Aging connective tissues are at a higher risk for microtears with bursitis.

Pathophysiology

Bursitis is an inflammatory process that may be acute or chronic; the exact etiology is often unknown. Bursitis may be caused by an infectious process, trauma (more common in patients under age 35 years), repetitive movement disorders, pseudogout, gout, or neoplastic disease. Less often, it may be attributed to rheumatoid disease (especially with nodular or bilateral bursitis) or infection by Mycobacteria tuberculosis (TB) or Candida fungal infection. Far more commonly however, septic bursitis is due to bacteria infection.

Up to 80 percent of septic bursitis cases are due to infection by Staphylococcus aureus, with 5 to 20 percent due to Streptococcus and other gram-positive skin flora, which are typically introduced via direct trauma which compromises the protective skin barrier. Immunocompromised conditions such as diabetes mellitus, HIV infection, chronic steroid use, or autoimmune conditions such as rheumatoid arthritis may all predispose to septic bursitis, and causative trauma to the overlying skin surface may even be microscopic in nature.

Bursitis is essentially a soft tissue problem rather than a joint problem such as arthritis, and often coexists with tendonitis or tenosynovitis. Overuse injury is characterized by repeated cycles of degeneration and regeneration with new collagen deposition. Synovial cells increase in thickness, and the normal bursal lining may be replaced by granulation tissue before eventual fibrosis. In turn, the bursa may become filled with transudative fluid with a high concentration of fibrin. At the conclusion of this inflammatory process, calcium deposition may occur proximal to the affected bursa.

Clinical Presentation

Subjective

The presenting symptoms are usually pain and sometimes swelling over the known locations of bursal sacs, which may be accompanied by swelling and warmth over the involved bursa. When the subcutaneous bursal sacs (olecranon and prepatellar) are inflamed by systemic illnesses such as RA, gout, or infection, additional clues to diagnosis may include fever, chills, and arthralgias. The prepatellar and olecranon bursae frequently present with local redness, swelling, and warmth that must be distinguished from septic arthritis. Patients who develop subcutaneous bursitis may have a family history of articular problems. An occupational history may provide a clue to diagnosis. Some examples include "weaver's bottom" (ischial-gluteal bursitis), "miner's elbow" (olecranon bursitis), and "housemaid's knee" (prepatellar bursitis). Bursitis of a deep bursa is manifested by pain over the bursa with activity or direct pressure. The pain may radiate some distance, as in the case of gluteal bursitis, in which the patient may complain of pain in a sciatic distribution.

Objective

Pain may be referred to other musculoskeletal structures contiguous to the bursa; therefore, careful examination is necessary to identify the source of the pain. Clinical signs and symptoms include induration, erythema, and effusion over the olecranon and prepatellar bursae. Gross distension of the bursal sac may be apparent. If there is significant limitation of ROM or pain on flexion, then a coincident arthritis must be suspected. Bursitis may also develop from repeated microtrauma, leading to effusion and thickening of the bursal sac. When irritation and inflammation continue, the bursa is at risk for calcification as well as development of adhesions around the bursa, thereby limiting tendon movement.

Diagnostic Reasoning

Diagnostic Tests

Laboratory findings will usually be normal. The ESR may be elevated by gout, rheumatoid arthritis, or infection. In cases of gout, uric acid levels would be elevated. In infectious leukocytosis, the WBC count may be elevated

Differential Diagnosis

When formulating a diagnosis, RA, gout, or pseudogout, and septic arthritis must be ruled out. A diagnosis is generally determined from an x-ray film showing the involved joint or bursa, with or without calcified deposits. Further diagnosis is determined from the aspiration of fluid in the affected joint. The fluid is cultured, and a WBC count done to assess the presence of bacterial infection. An elevated red blood cell (RBC) count is associated with trauma.

Management

Medical management and treatment of bursitis includes avoidance of activities that can lead to constant irritation of the bursa, and application of moist heat or ice to the affected area q4h for 20 to 30 minutes. The use of moist heat versus ice is an individual preference. Immobilization of the affected area to reduce edema and provide support is recommended, along with ROM exercises to prevent loss of mobility and to help maintain motion. It has also been recommended in certain cases that an NSAID along with ultrasound therapy be used. If symptoms recur and fluid re-accumulates, then an injection of a long-acting corticosteroid (triamcinolone 2 to 10 mg, hydrocortisone 25 to 37.5 mg, methylprednisolone 20 to 40 mg, or dexamethasone 4 to 16 mg, each mixed with an equal volume of lidocaine hydrochloride 1 percent) into the affected bursa is recommended, followed by application of ice for 10 to 20 minutes. Injections should not be repeated more than every 6 to 8 weeks, and most clinicians limit the number of intrabursal injections to two to the same site, before referral for more invasive interventions is initiated, such as surgery. In severe cases, surgery may be performed to excise the inflamed portion of bursa and calcified deposits, and to aspirate bursal fluid

Follow-Up and Referral

Follow-up is determined by the response to therapeutic interventions. Follow-up is determined by the response to therapeutic interventions.

Patient Education

Patient education is vital to ensure a rapid recovery. Encouraging a patient to decrease certain activities will speed up recovery. Encourage preliminary stretching and warm-up exercises before activities, to maintain flexibility and strength. If medications are a part of the treatment regimen, reinforcement of proper administration and a discussion of their side effects is recommended.

Fibromyalgia Syndrome

The name "fibromyalgia" is made up from "fibro-," for fibrous tissues such as tendons and ligaments, "my-," indicating muscle, and "-algia," meaning pain. *Fibromyalgia*—previously referred to as *fibrositis*—is a diffuse "muscular rheumatism" of a noninflammatory nature. It is characterized by an extremely common pain phenomenon that occurs in a defined pattern, which can be reproduced by pressure on "tender points." Fibromyalgia syndrome (FMS) is a chronic condition, characterized by general pain, fatigue, and tender areas in the soft tissue that persists for longer than 3 months. The joints however are spared. The cause is unknown, and a cure is no available. FMS is usually manifested by a disturbed sleep pattern and reduced functional ability. There may be accompanying irritable bowel syndrome, paresthesias, restless leg syndrome, cold sensitivity, interstitial cystitis, and often migraine-type headaches. Chronic fatigue is a hallmark of this syndrome.

Fibromyalgia remains poorly understood, despite abundant attention in the scientific and lay press. Perhaps there is also significant overlap between fibromyalgia syndrome (FMS), and chronic fatigue syndrome (CFS), another controversial chronic pain syndrome. There continues to be a lack of agreement as to the cause of CFS, laboratory markers, and clinical course and explains why the syndrome is not named in many medical texts even to this day. The majority of patients with CFS meet criteria for FMS; at least 70 percent of patients with FMS meet criteria for CFS. Both these disorders have been widely recognized in persons with comorbid psychiatric illness, as nearly two-thirds of CFS patients and 30 percent of FMS patients meet criteria for depression, dysthymia, or anxiety disorders. Many authors have criticized the historical and physical examination diagnostic criteria for both conditions as having a strong potential for overlap with somatization disorders.

Epidemiology and Causes

Using the 1990 American College of Rheumatology (ACR) criteria, the prevalence of FMS is reported as 0.5 percent for men, 3.4 percent for women (some studies claim an increased prevalence in women of 10:1), and 2 percent in the general population. It is estimated that up to 20 percent of all visits to a rheumatology practice are for patients with FMS, and is the second most common musculoskeletal disorders seen by rheumatologists. The prevalence increases with age, being 7.4 percent in women between the ages of 70 and 79. Most patients present with FMS between 30 and 50 years of age. Several studies have shown that up to 50 percent of patients with FMS have a history of either sexual and/or physical abuse, and a high incidence of eating disorders. Approximately 30 percent of patients fit a psychiatric diagnosis, the most common being anxiety, depression, somatization, and hypochondriasis, although FMS also occurs in patients without concurrent psychiatric problems. There is disagreement as to whether some patients have psychiatric problems preceding the development of FMS, or whether they develop as a sequela to the FMS.

Ten to 25 percent of patients with FMS will not be able to work at all; others will need significant modifications in their work. FMS is a growing source of work-related disability and results in health-care costs in excess of $10 billion. Currently, 16 percent were receiving Social Security benefits compared to 2.2 percent of the general population. As many as 70 percent see themselves as disabled. FMS may be triggered by emotional stress, infections, other medical illnesses, surgery, hypothyroidism, and trauma.

Chronic fatigue is a presenting complaint in up to 25 percent of patients presenting to ambulatory care settings, and it is estimated that approximately 10 percent of these individuals meet diagnostic criteria for CFS. Numerous books in the popular press have advanced the belief that women are affected two times more often than men are. The same books tend to agree that younger women are more often affected. Causes of CFS have been hypothesized to be autoimmune and infectious; however, the causes for the syndrome have yet to be determined. Importantly, like FMS, it is a diagnosis of exclusion.

Pathophysiology

After much investigation, the pathophysiology of FMS and CFS is still unclear. It has been hypothesized that both syndromes may be a disorder of muscle energy metabolism, an inflammatory or immunopathologic disease of muscle, a generalized disorder of pain perception, neuronally mediated hypotension, a neuroendocrine disturbance, dysregulated serotonin secretion, a sleep disturbance, or a result of sexual abuse or domestic violence. However, it is important to note that none of these etiologies has been consistently confirmed through randomized, well-controlled studies. While depression and anxiety disorders demonstrate great overlap with both CFS and FMS, it is a matter of great debate as to whether these conditions occur concurrently, whether CFS and FMS lead to psychiatric sequelae, or whether these chronic conditions are simply somatic manifestations of underlying mood disorders. While psychologic dysfunction has been documented in patients with FMS, the extent and incidence of dysfunction does not appear to vary from the general population. In turn, patients with CFS and FMS commonly experience accusations of malingering, which, by definition, would be unfounded.

Extensive work explored a potential infectious etiology of CFS, focusing on Epstein-Barr virus, retroviruses, and human herpesvirus (HHV)-6 as causative agents. However, promising data from certain research groups could not be reproduced by other laboratories. Moreover, no consistent serologic profile could distinguish patients with CFS from control groups across multiple studies. There is some support to the theory that FMS may be triggered by infection. Some studies have linked infection with *Borrelia burgdorferi* (which causes Lyme disease), *Brucella* (the bacterial agent of brucellosis), or parvovirus to the development of FMS.

Several studies have demonstrated qualitative and quantitative differences in immune function between patients with CFS and controls, including reduced numbers of natural killer cells with depressed function, reduced levels of Ig molecules and immune complexes, and increased numbers of cell surface adhesion molecules, among others. However, these differences are of questionable clinical significance and have been inconsistent (even conflicting) between different studies.

Research that has examined neuroendocrine differences between affected patients and controls has produced similar inconclusive results. While some evidence points to undersecretion of adrenocorticotropin hormone (ACTH) and reduced serum cortisol levels, these findings are not specific for CFS and have been observed in FMS as well as in healthy subjects with altered sleep patterns related to overnight work shifts. This collection of inconclusive studies has also demonstrated upregulation of the hypophyseal-adrenal axis with an overproduction of ACTH but blunted cortisol production. In either case, FMS may be seen as belonging to the spectrum of stress-related disorders. A low level of growth hormone and abnormalities of the thyroid and gonadal axes have also been described. However, it is unclear whether these abnormalities develop primarily as a consequence of genetic predisposition, exposure to adverse life experiences, or both.

For many years, FMS was considered a disorder of muscle metabolism, possibly related to chronic hypoxia of muscular tissue. Changes have been documented in the muscles of patients with FMS, yet it remains possible that such changes are a result of deconditioning. Some researchers postulate that repetitive microtrauma of daily living may play a significant role in FMS and that fatigue and physical inactivity may lead to unfit muscles, which are more susceptible to microtrauma. However, studies of lactate levels, muscle force studies, and postexertional pain have demonstrated a marked similarity between patients with FMS and sedentary controls. An inflammatory component to the myalgias of FMS has also never been shown, which likely explains the lack of efficacy of NSAID and steroid therapies.

Thus, the most current theories suggest patients with FMS suffer from disproportionate perceptions of pain, exacerbated by muscle inactivity and deconditioning. In fact, lower pain perception thresholds have been documented in first-degree relatives of patients with FMS. Some studies have also demonstrated elevated levels of substance P and lower levels of 5-hydroxyindoleacetic acid in the cerebrospinal fluid of patients with FMS, as well as spinal fluid deficits of serotonin, norepinephrine, and dopamine, along with serotonin gene abnormalities. These monamine deficits have established associations with depressive syndromes. The functional brain activity in persons with FMS appears to be decreased; however, there is increased activity of cerebral pain processing areas on fMRI. It is felt that this is related to increased nociceptive stimuli and occurs in other populations that are subject to this increased input, as well.

Although no studies have been conclusive, altered pain perception is likely a central rather than peripheral nociceptor phenomenon. Central sensitization is thought by many to be the primary dysfunction manifested in FMS. Sensory impulses are amplified at the level of the spinal cord. Impulses are "gated" at this level by changes in the sensitivity of the dorsal horn neurons directly and indirectly via descending pathways from the brainstem. During central sensitization, peripheral pain nerves—the nociceptors—such as those in skeletal muscles are repeatedly stimulated by stretching or pressure. They can become sufficiently sensitized to cause the release of pain mediating neurotransmitters in the spinal cord (e.g., substance P). The resulting nerve impulses are carried to the central nervous system, where central sensitization reduces the pain threshold, increases nociceptor response to painful stimuli, increases the duration of pain after the stimulation, and results in an expansion of the receptive fields of pain.

This is supported by observations in FMS patients of altered patterns of sleep and mood, decreased blood flow to pain centers in the brain (e.g., thalamus, caudate nucleus), as well as alterations in serotonin secretions and the pituitary–hypothalamic–adrenal neuroendocrine axis as previously discussed. In addition, autonomic dysregulation of heart rate and systemic blood pressure have also been implicated on the basis of tilt table testing for orthostatic hypotension. However, again, these findings have not been consistently reproduced.

Clinical Presentation

Subjective

The typical patient with fibromyalgia is a menopausal, overweight women with proximal muscle pain (rated as 7/10 in severity), mostly in the neck and shoulders or proximal thighs. They often complain of morning stiffness and joint pain, typically lasting 1 hour, and thus suggesting inflammatory disease initially. Heat is often described as helpful to loosen up. The major presenting complaints are diffuse musculoskeletal pain, disordered sleep, headache, mood and cognitive disturbances, stiffness, and fatigue in various combinations. Pain can be present on the left and right sides of the body, above or below the waist. Axial skeletal pain, which is present in the cervical spine or anterior chest, thoracic spine, or low back, will be reported in most cases. Patients state that the pain "travels." There are select times when an individual may have a "regional fibromyalgia" that does not encompass the entire body. This is an unusual presentation, but it does happen.

Sleep disturbance, although not usually the presenting complaint, is present in most cases. The patient usually awakens feeling tired, with a sense of nonrestorative sleep. Some describe a "fibro-fog"; short-term memory loss may be present, as well as impaired concentration. Headaches are commonly associated, including in some patients, migraines. The patient may complain of frequent diarrhea and/or constipation, sometimes accompanied by gas in the abdomen or nausea. These are all symptoms of irritable bowel syndrome, which may accompany FMS. Some sources note that taken collectively, this has been referred to as the "irritable everything syndrome." Symptoms are made worse by stress and anxiety, overexertion, and cold and damp weather. The course of the disorder is variable; the symptoms may wax and wane.

Objective

The patient will appear tired. The skin may be pale. The physical exam may be remarkably normal except for highly tender muscle–tendon junctions, the classic "tender points" (Fig. 14.3). For a diagnosis of FMS to be made, the patient must have widespread muscular pain that has been present for at least 3 months; the pain should be present in 11 of 18 trigger points (or tender points) on digital palpation with an applied pressure of 4 kg (9 lb), which is the degree of force required to whiten the examiner's nailbed. The 18 trigger points are bilateral sites at nine key locations: (1) insertion of the suboccipital muscle, (2) lower border of the sternocleidomastoid muscle, (3) mid-upper trapezius muscle, (4) origin of the supraspinatus muscle, (5) second costochondral junction, (6) 2 cm distal to the lateral epicondyle, (7) upper-outer quadrant of the gluteus muscle, (8) prominence of the greater trochanter, and (9) medial fat pad of the knee. Pain at these sites should be significantly greater than at control sites that are not expected to be tender, such as the patient's thumbnail or mid-forearm. Patients who exhibit fewer tender points may be diagnosed with fibromyalgia as long as they have had widespread pain in all four quadrants of the body for at least 3 months. Subcutaneous nodules may be felt at the sites of tenderness or pain, but the number of tender points is more diagnostic.

The strength exam is normal, as is ROM in the joints except for some loss of external hip rotation and back flexion. Osteoarthritic pain sites may also be identified, as two-thirds of patients have so-called secondary fibromyalgia, that is, they have some identifiable painful condition that becomes augmented.

Diagnostic Reasoning

Diagnostic Tests

Typically, all laboratory studies are normal. The CBC, ESR, creatinine phosphokinase (CPK), ANA, rheumatoid factors, TSH, T3 resin uptake, and T4 are normal or absent. X-ray films and bone scans are also normal, as well as EMG. Advanced imaging tests such as CT and MRI are not indicated in the absence of significant physical findings.

Differential Diagnosis

As a diagnosis of exclusion, other disorders must be systematically ruled out. Other diseases and disorders that may present initially like FMS are AIDS, polymyalgia rheumatica (PMR), bursitis or tendinitis, SLE, RA, polymyositis, Lyme disease, carpal tunnel syndrome, multiple sclerosis, myofascial pain, temporal arteritis, hypothyroidism, complex regional pain syndrome, and CFS. Virus-specific serologies against Lyme disease for example are also not recommended without a strong suspicion by history or physical exam findings, since any positive result is likely to be false positive in the setting of low suspicion.

AIDS is ruled out by blood testing

PMR is frequently seen in elderly patients. This disorder is characterized by pain symptoms that are proximal, but not distal. Pain is located in the neck, shoulders, back, and upper thigh. The ESR is usually high in rheumatic disease.

Bursitis or tendinitis typically involves a single joint or extremity

SLE is seen in young women with fatigue; affected patients have a positive ANA 95 percent of the time. SLE has other signs and symptoms, which include a malar or discoid rash, photosensitivity, and oral ulcers. Arthritis involving two or more peripheral joints, serositis, and a renal disorder with persistent proteinuria or cellular casts are also common in SLE. Neurologic disorders involving seizures or psychosis, hematologic disorders (including hemolytic anemia, leukopenia, lymphopenia, or thrombopenia), and immunologic disor-

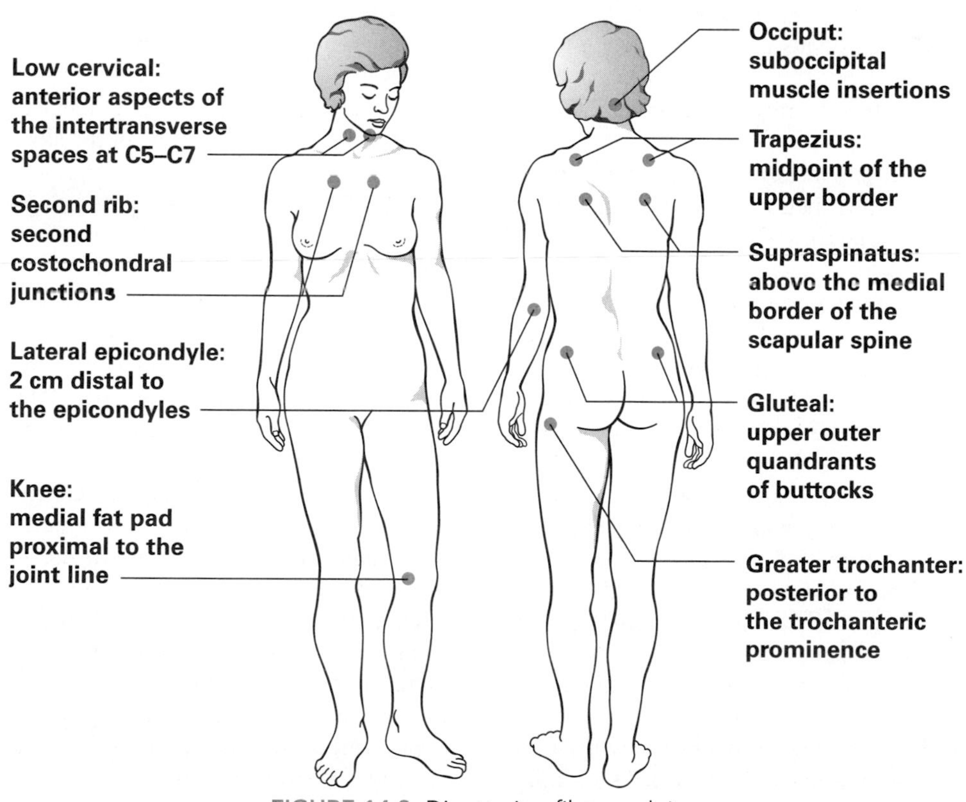

FIGURE 14.3 Diagnosing fibromyalgia.

ders, such as positive lupus erythematosus cell preparation or anti-DNA antibody to native DNA in abnormal titer or anti-SM or false-positive serologic test for syphilis for at least 6 months, are also common signs and symptoms of SLE.

RA is characterized by prodromal systemic symptoms of malaise, fever, weight loss, and morning stiffness. Onset is usually insidious and in small joints. Deformity is common. There is usually a positive rheumatoid factor, which is not present in FMS. Radiographic (x-ray) findings show joint erosion and narrowing of joint spaces. These signs and symptoms, along with a definite persistent joint swelling, rule out FMS.

Polymyositis is a systemic disorder of unknown origin whose presenting symptom is primarily muscle weakness, especially in the extremities. Usually, skin manifestations are noted with polymyositis: This feature causes the diagnosis to be called *dermatomyositis.* There is a characteristic dusky red rash on the malar area of the face, neck, shoulders, upper back, and chest. Other findings include periorbital edema, and a purplish (heliotrope) suffusion over the eyelids. Patients typically have a high CPK level. Patients may also experience significant stiffness and weakness of the muscle structure.

Lyme disease may be verified on serology, although false-positive rates are high for this disease; look for coexisting positive IgM.

Carpal tunnel syndrome is characterized by paresthesias, which are also common in FMS, but the EMG and nerve conduction studies are normal in patients with FMS. Cervical and lumbar radiculopathy must be ruled out in such a presentation. In addition, patients with FMS have diffuse trigger points and paresthesias, not a localized phenomenon such as CTS.

Multiple sclerosis is verified by abnormal MRI of brain.

Myofascial pain is a localized, unilateral muscular pain that has an equal sex distribution. This condition is seen by some as a regional version of FMS.

Temporal arteritis is a systemic granulomatous disease, most commonly affecting the branches of the cranial arteries. Signs and symptoms include headache, jaw or tongue "claudication" upon mastication, visual disturbances, scalp tenderness, swollen or red temporal artery, decreased temporal artery pulse, sore throat, and neurologic manifestations.

Hypothyroidism is a clinical state resulting from decreased circulating levels of free thyroid hormone or from resistance to hormone action. The signs and symptoms are weakness, fatigue, lethargy, cold intolerance, decreased memory, constipation, muscle cramps, depression, and carpal tunnel syndrome, to name a few.

Complex regional pain syndrome usually involves a single extremity.

Chronic fatigue syndrome is defined as a disabling fatigue of at least 6 months, usually accompanied by flu-like symptoms. CFS demonstrates a tremendous amount of overlap with FMS except that FMS is a pain syndrome.

Tenosynovitis is a phenomenon with a single focus, and is associated with tendon motion.

The diagnosis of FMS is a clinical diagnosis of exclusion, made after numerous other causes of diffuse aches and pains have been excluded. The ACR criteria include chronic, diffuse musculoskeletal pain and the presence of soft tissue tender points in at least 11 of 18 defined anatomic sites. The criteria, it should be noted, were not developed as a diagnostic aid, but rather for the purpose of studying subjects with this condition in a systematic fashion. Thus there is no rationale for making this diagnosis strictly on the basis of tender points. These specific symptoms must be looked at as part of the whole constellation of the patient's presentation.

Management

The optimal treatment program is multifaceted. Treatment is directed toward controlling discomfort, improving sleep, maintaining function, and should be predicated on an optimistic and holistic approach. Patients should be advised that there is no "cure," but stress that symptom relief is possible. (See Nursing Research Based Practice 14.2.)

Clinicians can manage "milder" presentations of FMS with low-dose pain and sleep medication, exercise, weight loss, and behavioral strategies. However many patients with FMS are more challenging to manage and require a variety of approaches and multiple medications. Multiple symptoms require multiple medications, making it difficult sometime to distinguish symptoms from side effects. With all FMS patients, it is important to initiate medications at lower dosages and gradually increase. Doing so decreases the "amplification" of the side effects. (See Drugs Commonly Prescribed 14.6.)

Pain is the primary presenting symptoms in these patients and must be adequately treated. This approach begins with nonscheduled medications and schedule II short-acting agents to schedule III long-acting narcotics (both oral and transdermal) and methadone. With break through pain, short-acting agents may be added to long-acting agents. This may be especially true during a pain "flare," a common, and difficult to control, occurrence in patients with FMS. Appropriate use of scheduled drugs are supported by increased functional ability and enhanced activities, both vocational and otherwise. Patients need to understand that they cannot abruptly stop these medications. NSAIDs overall are not effective except perhaps for HA. Some reports suggest that agents such as Gabapentin (Neurontin) and Zonisamide (Zonegran), typically used to treat neuropathic pain, have also proved useful. If the pain is particularly strong in a confined region, an injection of lidocaine or lidocaine with a low-dose corticosteroid may be helpful. This technique is specifically effective for chest wall pain (or cos-

NURSING RESEARCH-BASED PRACTICE 14.2

Sturge-Jacobs, M: The experience of living with fibromyalgia: Confronting an invisible disability. Res Theory Nurs Pract 16 (1):19–31, 2002.

The purpose of this phenomenological study was to describe and enhance the understanding of the experience of living with fibromyalgia. Nine women between the ages of 30 to 56 were interviewed. Thematic analysis was conducted using van Manen's methodology and eight themes were identified: (1) pain—the constant presence, (2) fatigue—the invisible foe, (3) sleep—the impossible dream, (4) thinking of a frog, (5) dealing with a flare-up, (6) longing for a normal life, (7) the power of naming—seeking a diagnosis, and (8) living within the boundaries. Through the interrelationships of these themes, the essence *confronting an invisible disability* was captured. While the results of such a study are not generalizable, an understanding of the women's experience can enable nurses to provide care that would serve to empower women diagnosed with fibromyalgia to elicit their own strengths to manage and control their own lives. The author concludes with the following statement:

"Women suffering from fibromyalgia must be encouraged and supported if they are to meet the challenge of controlling fibromyalgia, rather than letting fibromyalgia control them" (p 29).

tochondritis), which is found with high frequency in patients with FMS. Complete pain control is rare. Patients often must settle for pain reduction to the 4/10 levels.

Disturbed sleep was one of the first objective findings in FMS. Insomnia may include difficulty falling asleep (sleep latency), staying asleep or both. Poor sleep is a leading cause of fatigue. The tricyclic Amitriptyline (Elavil), has proven effective in studies over time in improving sleep. Cyclobenzaprine (Flexeril), a muscle relaxant, has a sedating effect when taken at bedtime, and may additionally provide relief throughout the next day, although over time will prove less effective. Trazodone (Desyrel) or zolpidem (Ambien) may also improve sleep, and some favor Clonazepam (Klonopin).

FMS patients may have sleep apnea and often have restless leg syndrome (30 to 60 percent of all FMS patients). For all male patients and overweight/obese female patients with FMS, consider sleep studies. A diagnosis of Sleep Apnea may need to be treated with CPAP. It often takes careful trial and error to come up with an effective sleep regimen which may vary greatly from patient to patient.

The selective serotonin reuptake inhibitors (SSRIs) that have been demonstrated as effective for depression in patients with FMS in controlled studies include Fluoxetine (Prozac), Citalopram Hydrobromide (Celexa), and Sertraline HCl (Zoloft), however, they do not help with either the pain or fatigue that are often the symptoms precipitating the depression.

Exercise is pivotal to symptom control. As many as 25 percent of patients report a decrease in overall symptomatology with gentle exercise from two to five times a week, and often require less prescription medication. However, it is difficult to get these patients to start and continue because of fatigue, depression, and postexertional pain. It has been theorized that this pain is due to muscle microtrauma which is worsened related to inadequate growth hormone release during exercise. A traumatized muscle sends nerve impulses to the spinal cord and these impulses are amplified by central sensitization at the spinal cord level. People with FMS may interpret muscle soreness as pain. Some theorize that administration of growth hormone may prove effective in decreasing pain during exercise; this has yet to be proven. (See Drugs Commonly Prescribed 14.6.)

People with FMS are de-conditioned. De-conditioning is part of the constellation of symptomatology that patients with FMS experience. It is a vicious cycle that must be broken for the patient to feel better. They need to stretch all major muscle groups to a point of gentle tension, not pain, several times a day. Yoga may be an effective approach, although it has not been evaluated in controlled trials. Likewise, patients should counter their "head forward" position, a rounded pain posture that tends to develop in those with chronic pain. They need to "breathe deeply" and open up the chest several times a day. Deep breathing may also reverse the oxygen deficit muscles and decrease stress, and also, indirectly, improve sleep. Warm pool exercise is easiest on de-conditioned muscles. Slow graduation of intensity is critical; as many as 40 percent of all FMS patients may discontinue exercise related to pain and fatigue.

Eccentric contractions of muscle should be minimized. All 12 major muscles groups can be tailored to minimize eccentric work. Advise patients to take smaller steps when walking downhill, using short strokes when vacuuming or sweeping and placing the body's midline near any object that they are lifting or manipulating.

In addition to stretching and minimizing the potential of microtrauma in eccentric work, patients with FMS need aerobic exercise. Performing aerobic exercise in a chair or in water may be helpful for those patients who have lower body pain syndromes such as plantar fasciitis, ankle tendini-

Drugs Commonly Prescribed 14.6: Pharmacologic Treatment for Fibromyalgia

Drug	Dose	Comments
Alprazolam/Xanax—used for panic attacks, common comorbidity.	0.25–3 mg/day	Extremely short half-life; rebound effect; potential for abuse; not usually useful for sleep.
Amitriptyline/Elavil—may assist with pain control and sleep.	25–75 mg one bedtime dose per day (may begin as low as 10)	Use supported by recent JAMA meta-analysis; good support for efficacy of this agent.
Bupropion HCl/Wellbutrin—good for fatigue, and "fog" of FMS	Slow release 150–300 SR bid or 300 XL qd—begin with half dosage and titrate gradually.	May augment SSRI/SNRI. Takes several weeks for full effects as with most antidepressants.
Carbidopa, levodopa/Sinemet—used for restless leg syndrome, another comorbidity.	10/100–20/200, 1 tablet qhs	Inexpensive
Capsaicin cream—depletes local sensory nerve endings of substance P.	0.025% Cream qd—apply to trigger points for pain.	Effective in small group of FMS patients.
Carisoprodol/Soma—muscle relaxant, pain	350 mg, 1–4 per day	Use at bedtime if causes daytime sleepiness.
Clonazepam/Klonopin, Clonapam—anxiety, sleep	0.25–2 mg hs, tablets or fast-dissolving wafer	Excellent adjunct for sleep but not tested in FMS at present.
Cyclobenzaprine/Flexeril—muscle relaxant, mild pain, sleep	5–30 mg hs	Good effect, especially at bedtime; abuse potential; daytime sleepiness.
Dextromethorphan—pain; use as adjunct to Ultram before moving to scheduled narcotics	30–120 mg in 24 hours	"Out of body feeling" reported in some patients; can increase "fog" of FMS in some patients.
Dicyclomine HCl/Bentyl—for IBS, another common comorbidity in some	20 mg oral qd	Inexpensive, well tolerated; fairly benign, may assist with pain.
Eszopiclone/Lunesta—sleep	2–3 mg hs	Precursor of zopiclone.
Gamma hydroxybutyrate/Xyrem—sleep	4.5–6 mg hs, repeat 3–4 hours later	Abuse potential; available only through manufacturer. Multicenter FMS trial in process.
Gabapentin/Neurontin—for neuropathic pain	900–3600 mg/day in three divided doses	Try nighttime dosing—often causes daytime fatigue.
Growth hormone—depression, fatigue, pain	Dependent on growth factor levels and body weight.	Approved only for use for adult growth hormone deficiency syndrome—anecdotally has proved useful in some patients with FMS.
Hydrocodone Bitartrate/Vicodin—short-acting, for moderate pain	Several short-acting narcotics available and dosage depends on half-life of drug selected.	If patient is using 90–120 tablets/month consider move to long-acting agent.
Lidocaine/Lidoderm patch—used in myofascial pain syndrome	Apply patch directly to FMS trigger point.	Lidocaine can be directly injected into trigger points. Acupuncture has not been proven effective.
Loperamide/Imodium—mild IBS/diarrhea	2–4 mg initially, up to 16 mg in 24 hours	OTC—can cause constipation.
Metaxalone (Skelaxin)—muscle relaxant for painful muscle conditions	800 mg three to four times/day	Least sedating; potentiates alcohol.

Drug	Dose	Comments
Methadone/Dolophine—moderate to severe pain	5–20 mg bid	Used in heroin withdrawal—patient may resist usage.
Modafinil/Provigil—severe daytime fatigue; FMS "fog"	200–400 mg qAM	Anecdotal evidence of positive results in FMS; side effects include headache, insomnia.
MS Contin/Kadian—moderate to severe chronic pain	15–60 mg bid	Not for use in opioid-naïve patients.
NSAIDs—chronic HA, tendonitis, concurrent OA	Depends on agent selected *See Drugs Commonly Prescribed 14.2.	Of minimal use in FMS; can help associated headaches.
Oxycodone/Percocet, Percodan—moderate pain	Varies with half-life of selected drug.	Try if hydrocodone ineffective; constipating; rebound headache.
Oxycodone HCl/OxyContin—moderate to severe chronic pain	10–30 mg bid	Do not chew or break any long-acting opiate.
Pramipexole (Mirapex)—dopamine agonist—for restless leg syndrome	0.125–1.0 mg qd—take several hours before bed.	Daytime sleepiness.
Ropinirole (Requip)—restless leg syndrome	0.25–2.0 mcg qd approximately 3 hours before bedtime	Higher doses of dopamine agonists in general are being studied including daytime use for muscle pain relief.
SSRI—those tested for FMS include fluoxetine (Prozac), citalopram hydrobromide (Celexa), sertraline HCl/HCl (Zoloft)—depression, anxiety	Depends on agent chosen.	Although mood may improve, ineffective for pain and sleep disturbance.
Tegaserod maleate/Zelnorm—IBS, constipating-type	6 mg bid before breakfast and after dinner	Efficacy questioned in some patients with long-term usage.
Tiagabine HCl/Gabitril—neuropathic pain, sleep	4–56 mg/day given in two to four doses	Side effects: fatigue, may worsen "fibro fog."
Tizanidine HCl/Zanaflex—muscle relaxation, mild pain, sleep	4–8 mg hs	Monitor liver enzymes at baseline, and at 1, 3, and 6 months. Avoid abrupt cessation.
Tramadol HCl/Ultram—mild—moderate pain; available with Tylenol as Ultracet	50–100 mg q4–8h, not to exceed 400 mg in 24 hours; Ultracet—37.5 mg every 4–8 hours, not to exceed 8 in 24 hours.	Low abuse potential; nonscheduled; Ultracet may be more effective if patient can take two tablets at once.
Transdermal fentanyl (Duragesic Patch)—moderate to severe pain	25 mcg/h; change every 3 days	Need constipation prophylaxis; considered chronic opioid therapy.
Trazodone HCl/Desyrel, Trazon, Trialodine—depression, sleep	50–150 mg hs	Causes headache in some patients; potentiates ETOH and other CNS depressants.
Zolpidem/Ambien—sleep *Overall favorite of many FMS patients	5–15 mg hs—tolerance uncommon	May need to request "quantity override" for patients to receive more than 14 tablets per month.
Zonisamide/Zonegran—neuropathic pain	100–400 mg qhs	Side effects: fatigue, dizziness when taken in daytime may occur; FDA approved for epilepsy only but may help neuropathic pain.

tis, or knee or hip OA. However, exercises should minimize repetition (can increase microtrauma), overhead work, and allow for a 50 percent reduction in intensity, especially during a pain flare.

Other therapies for muscle tension such as biofeedback, pleasant imagery, meditation, and even hypnotherapy, have shown promise in individual studies. Anxiolytics may prove helpful, especially for the subgroup of patients with FMS who have concurrent panic attacks. Muscle relaxants may also be helpful, with Metaxalone (Skelaxin) being the least sedating (see Drugs Commonly Prescribed 14.1). Preventing stress, and the aberrant response that often occurs in FMS patients, may be more effective than treating the aftermath. Self-care is critical.

Cognitive behavioral therapy (CBT) has been proven effective in minimizing pain and fatigue. Refer patients to Web sites and FMS support groups. CBTs work to change erroneous beliefs that influence and underlie behaviors that may be non-productive. CBT may include strategies for pacing, fatigue control, establishing realistic expectations given the chronic and recalcitrant nature of the disorder, and boundary setting. All of these strategies, as well as an active lifestyle, biofeedback, stress reduction, job modifications, and deep breathing exercises, may help decrease the pain of FMS. They will also aid the patient to sleep more restfully, and help with depression. Not all therapies will work with each patient, but a variety of these therapies in some combination should help most patients. Trial and error can be used until the proper care plan can be adjusted for the patient; however, such an approach requires much patient direction, so that the patient will not get discouraged. Patience, courage, active listening and humor are valuable adjunctives. (See The Patient's Voice 14.1.)

Follow-Up and Referral

For efficacy, it is best to schedule a follow-up visit at 2 to 4 weeks, initially. The practitioner will find persons with FMS to be highly sensitive to medication: In most cases, they will require more frequent monitoring of response to medications. After this, see the patient every 1 to 2 months for approximately three visits, and then every 3 to 4 months, depending on symptomatology.

THE PATIENT'S VOICE 14.1

Fibromyalgia

"There's always crazy signals going through your body. Everything hurts, everything feels as if a truck ran over you. I feel like my body has been through a major physical exhaustion...I feel like I've abused my body. I feel like I've been, shook, and twisted, everything hurts."

Research has shown FMS to be a greater source of work loss and dysfunction than RA. With resolution of sleep disturbance, FMS may resolve totally. In actuality, the long-term prognosis for FMS is better than the short-term prognosis. Approximately 5 to 10 percent of patients do not respond to any modality. Hypnosis may be attempted with this refractory group, although this modality is questionable, not scientific, and generally not utilized.

Chronicity may occur in some patients. Adequate sleep and general conditioning exercise helps to slow down or prevent a relapse of the FMS syndrome. Increased social interaction and supportive counseling is very helpful in such patients. Physical therapy is critical in those who do not respond to therapeutic modalities. Sleep disorder counseling is always appropriate. Likewise, psychological counseling referral may be necessary for many of these patients, specifically for cognitive-behavioral therapy. Table 14.10 summarizes nonpharmacologic treatments for FMS.

Patient Education

An optimistic approach is crucial; although there is no cure for the disorder, the clinician should emphasize the many ways available to reduce symptoms. Self-help and support groups are available and important. These can prove extremely beneficial in assisting the patient and family to

Table 14.10 Nonpharmacologic Treatments for FMS

Nonpharmacologic Therapies	Comments
Exercise; all studies that include aerobic or strength-training exercises show decreased pain, increase in overall well-being	Begin with stretching exercises for flexibility; increased evidence supports aerobic exercise as beneficial. Must break cycle of de-conditioning; begin when patient has improved sleep, less pain and fatigue
Cognitive–behavioral therapies—behavioral modifications	See Chapter 17 Elaborates therapeutic approaches
Heat/ice	Moist heat, especially in morning; ice effective during "flare" in specific location
Nutrition	Weight loss if BMI >25; nutrition consult
Stress management	Identify stressors; discuss; strategize to avoid stressful situations
Support groups	Useful source of information and encouragement
Hypnotherapy	Occasionally effective
Biofeedback	Occasionally effective
Relaxation exercises	Deep breathing

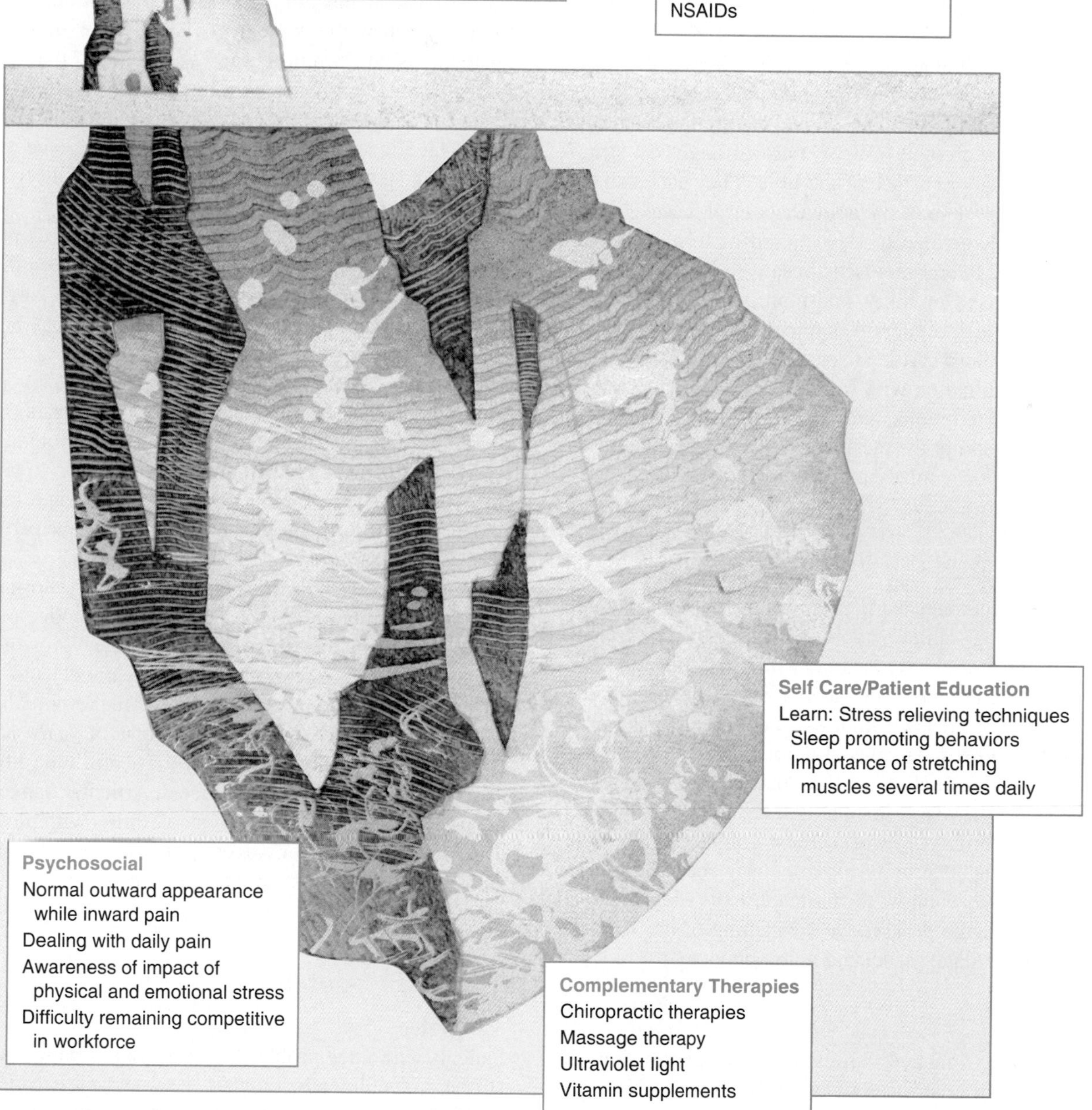

cope. Treatment approaches require individualized, multiple-treatment approaches. Educate the patient and family regarding any potential adverse effects of medications and should encourage exercise such as walking and stretching, and swimming. The patient should gradually increase the level of exercise as tolerated; overexercising may worsen symptoms. Heating pads, warm baths and showers, whirlpools, and moist, hot packs may help relieve symptoms. Gentle massage may be helpful and also helps provide relaxation and stress reduction. FMS can be aggravated by stress, depression, anxiety, and overexertion; therefore, the lifestyle and daily activities of the patient should be discussed. Encourage frequent rest periods, to help minimize pain and fatigue. The treatment plan must be multifactorial and individualized, based on the needs of the individual patient. Complementary therapies are an important component of care, as are the qualities of patience, active listening, and advocacy.

Meniscal Tears

Knee injuries are the most frequent sports-related injury. The knee is an inherently unstable joint held together by ligaments, cushioned by the menisci, and covered by muscles. The menisci are crescent-shaped fibrocartilaginous structures on the articular surface of the tibia. They act as shock absorbers for the knee and help to control normal knee motion. The medial meniscus is injured or torn more frequently than the lateral meniscus because of its more rigid structure, decreased mobility, and more vulnerable sites of attachment which render it subject to greater stress. Meniscal tears ("torn cartilage" or "locked knee") can occur alone or in combination with ligament injuries such as cruciate ligament disruptions, and/or collateral ligament tears. Meniscal tears disrupt the mechanics of the knee, leading to varying degrees of symptoms and predisposing the knee to degenerative arthritis.

Epidemiology and Causes

Meniscal and ligament tears affect two groups of patients primarily—young, athletic adults with a history of trauma and middle-aged or elderly patients with osteoarthritis (OA). Several case series have indicated meniscal tears are the most common of all knee injuries, accounting for an estimated 52,000 knees damaged by football injuries alone. Moreover, an estimated 1.7 million people undergo meniscal surgery each year. Traumatic tears may not always involve contact injury; however, most commonly, they are due to sports-related activities, particularly soccer, football, and basketball. In contrast to traumatic tears, degenerative tears result from the progressive weakening of the menisci and articular cartilage associated with aging.

Pathophysiology

The menisci are C-shaped fibrocartilaginous partial rings of tissue that line the surfaces of opposing bones within the mobile knee joint, maintaining the distance between the involved bones—the tibia and the femur. The medial and lateral menisci lie on the tibial plateau, with their curved portions facing outward. They consist of two phases: a liquid interstitial phase and a solid, extracellular collagenous (predominantly type I) matrix phase that is secreted by meniscal fibrochondrocytes. This dense viscoelastic structure allows them to provide nutrition and lubrication to the articular cartilage, as well as serve a cushioning and stabilizing function, given their cup-like form. As the knee is fully extended from a flexed position, the distal end of the femur normally rotates slightly medially, with its bilateral bony prominences (femoral condyles) coming to rest within the cupped forms of the two menisci, essentially screwing into place when in the highly stable, fully extended position. When extended, the menisci support 50 percent of the load placed on the knee joint and when the knee if fully flexed, they support up to 85 percent of the load.

The menisci of the knee joint are particularly prone to injury when the knee is twisted while in the flexed position, as the femur compresses against the tibia and grinds against the meniscus. This grinding motion tears the meniscus as the force exceeds the strength of the fibrocartilage. The adult meniscus is poorly vascular, except for the peripheral 10 to 25 percent; thus, it is particularly slow to heal once torn.

Menisci tear either as a direct result of injury or indirectly because of the normal wear and tear on the knee. Traumatic tears are most commonly vertical, longitudinal tears (called bucket-handle tears when displaced), but transverse (radial) tears are also common. They are often associated with anterior cruciate ligament (ACL) or less commonly posterior cruciate ligament (PCL) tears. The second type of meniscal tear is known as a degenerative tear which usually occurs in persons over the age of 40 years and is not preceded by trauma. Horizontal cleavage tears and flap tears are most common. These injuries have particularly poor healing capacity.

Microtears in the menisci heal via the formation of a fibrin clot, containing fibronectin, chemotactic, and mitogenic growth factors (e.g., platelet-derived growth factor) which cause undifferentiated mesenchymal cells to migrate into the tear, producing a meniscal scar that eventually transforms into fibrocartilage over the course of years. Meniscal chondrocytes act in concert with the scaffolding fibrin clot to contribute to this healing process. Articular damage from the meniscal tear may lead to osteoarthritis with progressive degeneration of the involved joint. Further, because the menisci stabilize the knee, loss of their integrity can lead to more extensive joint injuries.

Clinical Presentation

Subjective

Patients with knee problems usually report pain, instability, stiffness, swelling, locking or weakness. The patient with traumatic tears typically report a "twisting injury" to the knee. Older patients with a degenerative tear may report a history of minimal or no trauma—they may simply stand from a different position, or walk on an uneven surface. The patient may experience the knee "giving way," as well as a painful popping or locking. Typically patients can ambulate after an acute injury and may continue to participate in athletics.

In acute knee pain, obtaining a history of the mechanism of injury is essential to proper diagnosis.

Traumatic tears are typically followed by the insidious onset of knee swelling and stiffness over 2 to 3 days. Mechanical symptoms such as locking, catching, and popping may continue. Patients usually experience pain on the medial or lateral side of the knee, particularly with twisting or squatting activities. Motion is often limited by a feeling of "tightness" secondary to effusion. In some cases, large fragments of meniscal tissue can become incarcerated in the kee joint, leading to a "locked knee." The mechanical symptoms and degree of pain tend to wax and wane.

Objective

The most common finding on physical examination is tenderness over the medial or lateral joint line. Young patients who have traumatic tears that disrupt the peripheral blood supply typically present with a large effusion or hemarthrosis. In degenerative tears or tears that involve the avascular central body of the meniscus, effusions are typically small or absent. Knee motion may be limited secondary to pain or effusion in either instance. During provocative testing forced flexion and circumduction (internal and external rotation of foot) pain is frequently elicited on the side of the knee with the meniscal tear. The McMurray test is positive when the flexion-circumduction maneuver is associated with a positive click.

Diagnostic Tests

AP, lateral, tunnel, and axial views are indicated for patients with a history of trauma or effusion. For patients with chronic conditions, the AP and lateral view should be weightbearing. The definitive diagnostic test for a meniscal or ligamentous tear is MRI, which should be done only if the diagnosis is in doubt or if surgery is anticipated. MRI has also effectively supplanted invasive knee arthrography with intra-articular contrast media, except in contraindicated circumstances (e.g., preexisting metallic clips, severe claustrophobia, etc.). Aspiration generally yields noninflammatory fluid that may be bloody, depending on the extent of the tear.

Differential Diagnosis

In cases of acute knee pain, the following are diagnostic considerations:

- ▲ Fractures (distal femur, patella, proximal tibia, and fibula) may be ruled out on radiograph.
- ▲ Meniscal injuries are preceded in most cases by a twisting injury and "locking," inability to extend the knee completely, with localized pain and tenderness along the joint line.
- ▲ Ligamentous injuries show acute pain, swelling and instability.
- ▲ Musculotendinitis strains demonstrate acute pain and swelling but rarely instability.
- ▲ Extensor mechanism injuries may cause a fall or collapse related to a sudden weakness.
- ▲ Contusions present with a history of a direct blow, localized pain, and tenderness

Conditions that cause chronic knee pain include arthritis, tumors, sepsis, and overuse syndromes (including bursitis/tendinitis and anterior knee pain). Arthritis is relatively easy to diagnose because symptoms localize to the joint line and are associated with loss of motion and radiographic changes. Tumors are characterized by night pain (relentless and causing sleeplessness), often can be palpated, and should be identifiable on radiographs. Sepsis in the knee is rare in adults; it is more commonly located in the prepatellar bursa. Inspection and palpation of the involved area should determine the location of the infection. Bursitis/tendinitis and anterior knee pain have similar characteristics: both usually are chronic, often secondary to overuse, and often bilateral. The pain typically is worse with rising or walking after sitting, at night, and with prolonged exercise or use.

Management

In the absence of mechanical symptoms and particularly when a degenerative tear is present, initial therapy should be conservative. RICE and the use of crutches help quiet the acute phase. A short course of oral analgesics, such as acetaminophen or NSAIDs, can facilitate return to normal activities. Rehabilitation to improve the strength of the quadriceps muscle is imperative. Straight-leg raises with the knee extended, but not locked, can be started immediately. Gradually increase weightbearing, although nonweightbearing activities such as swimming and riding a stationary bicycle are excellent for increasing ROM and strength.

Traumatic tears on younger patients should be treated aggressively. Sports activity should be restricted until MRI evaluation is made or symptoms resolve. Surgical débridement or repair is indicated in younger patients with significant tears or older patients who do not respond to conservative treatment.

Follow-Up and Referral

A patient with traumatic effusion, mechanical symptoms, or ligamentous instability requires further evaluation. Patients who do not respond to nonoperative treatment and have persistent joint tenderness or effusion may require further evaluation. Recurrent episodes of locking and damage to adjacent articular cartilage with subsequent osteoarthritis are possible sequelae. With the exception of the outer rim, the blood supply to the meniscus is poor. Although small peripheral tears can heal, most tears are more central and cannot heal. Patients with recurrent stiffness, locking, or pain have a mechanically significant tear, which suggests ongoing internal damage. Failure to recognize and treat and traumatic tear can lead to progressive damage and a lost opportunity for surgical repair.

Patient Education

Maintaining quadriceps strength is key to minimizing disabilities from this injury. These include "closed-chain" exercises in which the bottoms of the feet are stabilized as they push directly against resistance, e.g., squats, stationary bicycle riding, leg presses. Although following healing, the knee will not return to 100 percent of baseline, participation in sports with proper warm-up exercises and protective equipment can still be enjoyed. Achiness and swelling after a particularly strenuous work-out may occur, reflecting the need for increased quadriceps strengthening, as well as the need to return to RICE therapy, as ice and NSAIDs will only help control the symptoms but not address the underlying pathology. Persistent swelling, pain, or episodes of instability should be further evaluated.

Cervical Muscle Sprain/ Strain and Spasm

Muscle sprain/strain, ICD-9 code 847.0, defined as "sprains and strains of other and unspecified parts of back and neck," is a muscle injury in the neck, a common and largely self-limited condition. The soft-tissue muscles of the neck are deeply buried and protected, and it is often difficult to differentiate injuries to the neck by either physical exam or more sophisticated imaging modalities. Thus, this term is also used to describe ligamentous injuries of the facet joints or intervertebral disks. After ruling out neurologic dysfunction and unstable injuries, the treatments for a neck sprain or strain are similar.

"Whiplash" describes an acceleration–deceleration of the neck with rapid flexion–extension and is a common sequelae of motor vehicle accidents. Despite no apparent instability, these injuries may cause prolonged disability, probably related to a combination of relatively severe ligamentous/muscle injury with nonorganic overlay.

Epidemiology and Causes

Cervical pain is common in both men and women and is usually described as lasting 2 weeks or longer. Mechanical disorders of the cervical spine are the most common cause of neck pain. Information on the prevalence and incidence of cervical pain is available from multiple sources but varies across a wide range. Consistent reporting of occurrence rates is also hampered by the lack of a reproducible definition of cervical pain across multiple studies. Terms such as *whiplash*, *acute neck sprain*, *neck spasm*, and *cervical strain* are frequently used to describe what seems to be a single condition. The prevalence of cervical pain in men and women is approximately 8 percent among persons 25 to 74 years of age. The highest prevalence (10 percent) is among persons 45 to 64 years of age. Rates are higher for whites than for blacks and other racial groups.

It has been estimated that 85 percent of all neck injuries presenting to primary-care providers result from automobile accidents. The National Safety Council estimates that 20 percent of all automobile accidents are rear-end impacts that can cause *whiplash*—an acceleration–deceleration injury related to cervical hyperextension, most commonly caused by a rear-end motor vehicle crash (MVC) occurring when the driver of a stationary car is struck from behind by another vehicle. The driver is usually relaxed and unaware of the impending collision. The sudden acceleration of the struck vehicle pushes the back of the car seat against the driver's torso. This force pushes the driver's torso and shoulders forward, while the head remains static but moves posteriorly, causing hyperextension of the neck. This injury is most common in Western societies and metropolitan areas, where there are more automobiles. Approximately one-third of people will develop neck pain within 24 hours of the injury. The natural history of hyperextension cervical muscle strain and spasm injuries (commonly referred to as whiplash) is that 60 percent get better within the first year, 32 percent get better in the next year, and 8 percent have permanent problems.

The relationship between occupational factors and cervical pain is difficult to study, because exposure to those factors is usually difficult to quantify. Workers may be exposed to multiple risk factors both on the job and at home. The majority of work-related cervical injuries are diagnosed as a sprain or strain, and certain occupations appear to have a predisposition to cervical symptoms. Workers who have been required to do repetitive tasks with their upper extremity as well as prolonged sitting with their head in a flexed position are at risk of developing mechanical neck pain; these include machine operators, carpenters, office workers, dentists, and keyboard operators.

Pathophysiology

Cervical sprain is a clinical condition describing a nonradiating discomfort or pain in the neck area associated with a concomitant loss of neck motion and stiffness. The major biomechanical function of the cervical spine is to support the skull and provide movement in flexion, extension, and rotation. The supporting structures of the cervical spine are relatively unprotected; thus, injury to the muscles and ligaments that provide these motions can easily occur. Specific abnormalities in cervical strain can almost never be identified, except in traumatic injury to a specific structure.

Trauma to the cervical muscles that results in a strain may occur from elongation of muscle fibers with subsequent edema to rupture of muscle tissue and secondary hemorrhage. The response of the muscle to injury is contraction, with reflex recruitment of surrounding muscles for protection (splinting) of the injured muscle. The contracted state may also occur because of poor posture, increases in muscle tension, or environmental trauma.

A *spasm* is caused by increased muscle tone that may be demonstrated by rigidity or spasticity. When a muscle cannot relax, it cannot recover from contracting, which allows for restoration of internal blood flow, removal of metabolic byproducts, and the influx of nutrients. Chronically contracted muscles develop subsequent ischemia and pain.

Normal posture should be effortless and painless. Abnormal forward posture of the head results in chronic strain on the posterior structures of the neck. A variety of daily activities may result in chronic abnormal posture, such as the prolonged use of a computer with a screen below eye level, a faulty sitting position, or the use of bifocal glasses. Muscle tension is controlled by the interaction of spindle organs, Golgi's tendon organs, and extrafusal nerve fibers. A balance exists between these structures, as this system coordinates muscular length, rate of contraction, and tension and relaxation of opposing muscles. A coordinating system in the spinal cord and the cerebral cortex influences the set point of this balance.

Muscle tone control is a multifactorial process, and the balance can be easily upset. In addition, a variety of factors extraneous to the muscles affect muscle tension, including include fatigue, pain, anger, emotional stress, anxiety, and depression. Environmental trauma may lead to an acceleration–deceleration mechanism of energy transfer to the neck. The impact may result in bony or soft tissue injuries. The sternocleidomastoid, scalene, and the longus coli muscles may be mildly or severely stretched, or at worst, torn. In an MVC, the neck is subject to forced flexion, extension, and lateral flexion, as well as shear forces parallel to the direction of impact.

Clinical Presentation

Subjective

Pain is the most common presenting symptom, although the associated complaint of a headache, usually occipital, which may persist for months, is not unusual. The pain is usually located in the middle to lower part of the posterior neck. The area of pain may be limited or it may cover a large area. The pain may radiate toward the shoulders, but usually will not radiate down into the arm. The pain associated with a cervical strain is most often a dull, aching pain that is exacerbated by neck motion and alleviated by rest or immobilization. The pain may follow a significant trauma or may be spontaneous in onset; pain following trauma often persists longer than sprains of spontaneous onset. Nonradicular, nonfocal neck pain is most common, and noted anywhere from the base of the skull to the cervicothoracic junction. Pain is often worse with motion and may be accompanied by paraspinal spasm and discomfort in the region of the trapezius muscle. Pain may be accompanied by fatigue, sleep disturbance, irritability, and difficulty concentrating. Work tolerance may be impaired.

Cervical pain from an automobile accident usually does not appear for about 12 to 14 hours after the accident. The driver is often unaware at first of having been injured, then later begins to feel stiffness in the neck. The pain at the base of the neck increases and is made worse by head and neck movement. Pain patterns should be evaluated carefully to differentiate muscular pain from radicular symptoms which typically radiate down the upper extremities.

Objective

Physical examination shows decreased neck ROM with poor quality of movement. With typical cervical muscle strain or spasm, Spurling's sign (radicular pain reproduced when the examiner exerts downward pressure on the vertex while tilting the head toward the symptomatic side) is usually negative.

Frequently, there is tenderness to palpation over both the anterior and posterior structures of the cervical spine, specifically the paraspinous muscles, spinous processes, interspinous ligaments, or medial border of the scapula. Pain is often noted at the extremes of motion. The neurologic examination is normal in uncomplicated cases. The intensity of pain is variable and the loss of cervical motion correlates with intensity of pain. The presence of true spasm (continuous muscle contraction) is rare. Active motion of the cervical spine against any type of resistance causes an increase in pain. Shoulder examination, as well as the remainder of the physical examination, is typically normal.

Diagnostic Reasoning

Diagnostic Tests

Any evidence of neurologic deficit merits further diagnostic testing (such as EMG or nerve conduction studies) to determine the cause. By definition, hyperextension cervical injuries cause only soft tissue damage, but plain x-rays films of the cervical spine should be obtained in all instances. It is important to include radiographic studies so that unsuspected fractures or dislocations of the cervical spine, facet fractures, odontoid fractures, or spinous process fractures that might otherwise be missed in the neurologically intact patient can be identified or ruled out. Any evidence of neurologic deficit merits further diagnostic testing (such as EMG or nerve conduction studies) to determine the cause.

All seven cervical vertebrae must be seen. Anterior displacement of the pharyngeal air shadow indicates soft-tissue swelling and possible disruption of the intervertebral disk or anterior longitudinal ligament and requires further evaluation. The width of the prevertebral soft tissue at the level of C3 should not exceed 7 mm in normal adults. The normal lordotic curve may be straightened or reversed with muscle spasm, but this limited finding is noted in approximately 10 percent of normal adults. Preexisting degenerative disease may be noted most frequently at C5 to 6 or C6 to 7 and are usually age related. In a patient with severe pain, the screening radiographs should be examined for signs of instability.

Differential Diagnosis

The diagnosis of cervical muscle strain is based on the history of localized neck pain and a compatible physical examination demonstrating localized pain, muscle spasm, and a normal neurologic examination. Trauma to the cervical spine may result in major neural damage with paralysis; if the history reveals a significant trauma, then a thorough evaluation with x-ray exam should be performed. Because of the significant consequences of potential damage to the spinal cord, it is recommended that the expertise of an orthopedic surgeon or neurosurgeon be sought. Potential differential diagnoses are listed below:

- Cervical disk herniation presents with associated radicular pain and neurologic findings.
- Cervical spine tumor is accompanied by night pain, weight loss, history
- Cervical spine infection is accompanied by fever, sweats, and chills.
- Dislocation or subluxation of the spine would be evident on radiographs.
- Inflammatory conditions of the cervical spine (rheumatoid arthritis) would be accompanied by abnormal radiographs.
- Spinal fracture would also have abnormal radiographs.
- Malingering is accompanied by exaggerated symptomatology and evidence of secondary gain.

Management

Reassurance is a cornerstone of treatment in uncomplicated cases. The treatment of cervical muscle strain includes controlled physical activity and immobilization in a soft cervical collar It is important the collar be worn at night during sleep, as the neck is at greatest risk of undergoing abnormal movements or assuming unnatural positions during sleep. A decrease in activity allows the injured tissues to heal. Collars should be worn for no more than 2 to 4 weeks, because the recovering muscles start weakening from disuse. Recommendations from the Quebec Task Force on Whiplash-Associated Disorders suggest restricting the use of cervical collars to a minimal period.

Non-narcotic analgesics such as NSAIDs are helpful in making the patient more comfortable (see Drugs Commonly Prescribed 14.2). NSAIDs can be continued until symptoms have resolved. Long-term use of NSAIDs can lead to serious gastrointestinal disease, however, such as ulcers, gastritis, and hemorrhage. Thus, patients with gastrointestinal histories should use this drug cautiously. Using the lowest possible effective dose can help to prevent this problem. It is particularly important to use caution in recommending doses for elderly patients who are more sensitive to the adverse effects of NSAIDs. This class of medicines affects renal as well as gastrointestinal prostaglandins and may cause fluid retention, edema, and increases in blood pressure; thus, patients should be monitored for weight gain. These problems may be very significant in elderly patients and in people with congestive heart failure.

Muscle relaxants may be helpful if palpable spasms are seen on physical examination, but the practitioner should use caution when prescribing them, as they have a potential for addiction, while several studies have failed to show their efficacy beyond NSAIDs alone. Patients need to be aware that this class of drugs is for short-term use, as the risk–benefit ratio for prolonged use of muscle relaxants is poorly established. Muscle relaxants cause drowsiness and dizziness, so patients need to avoid hazardous activities such as driving or operating machinery while using these medicines. Because these drugs are central nervous system (CNS) depressants, patients need to avoid taking them with alcohol or other CNS depressants to prevent additive effects. Dry mouth is another side effect of this anticholinergic class of drugs, so frequent mouth rinsing is recommended to prevent dental disease. Topical application of creams such as capsaicin may also help to relieve pain. Narcotic analgesics should be avoided if at all possible, as very little research supports the use of narcotics in the treatment of soft tissue injuries.

Manipulation of the cervical spine is contraindicated in patients with osteoporosis, rheumatoid arthritis, carotid or vertebral atherosclerosis, or tumors. It is also contraindicated in the elderly, in patients with associated radiculopathy or myelopathy, or those on anticoagulants.

Herbals may also be used to treat the pain (see Complementary Therapies 14.1).

Neck pain and mobility are improved with physiotherapy. The goal of therapy is to maximize function of the cervical spine. Physical therapy modalities may take the form of cold (ice) initially or heat (warm bath) to help relieve pain and spasm. Activity should be encouraged as determined by the severity of the symptoms. Cervical traction may also be used to diminish pain and spasm if no improvement is seen with heat and medication. After 2 to 4 weeks of treatment with drugs and rest, if there is no significant improvement, a patient may benefit from an anesthetic injection, with or without the addition of corticosteroids. Administered only by experienced personnel, these injections can relieve pain and block reflex muscle spasms. Aerobic activity, such as walking, should be started as soon as possible. Once improvement is seen, a course of isometric exercises should begin. Encourage an early return to work and activities.

Follow-Up and Referral

Usually the course of cervical muscle strain is one of progressive improvement with complete resolution of symptoms over several weeks. Recovery is usually complete without any lasting impairment; however, a small percentage of patients may continue to experience cervical spine pain, despite adequate treatment.

If symptoms persist longer than 4 weeks postinjury, further evaluation with CT scans or MRI is indicated. If these tests are normal, the patient can be assured that no compression of neural structures is present and can be strongly encouraged to increase activity. If imaging findings are abnormal, a referral to a neurologist, neurosugeon, or orthopedic surgeon should be made for further evaluation.

If neck pain and restricted ROM are still present after patients have received analgesics and physical therapy while the findings on CT scan or MRI are normal, referrals for psychiatric support or vocational rehabilitation may be indicated to assist in recovery.

Patient Education

Knowing how a healthy neck works can help patients understand their cervical spine problems and how to care for them. It is important for patients to understand the concepts behind their treatments in order to receive the greatest benefits. They must also learn appropriate body mechanics to help protect the cervical spine from further damage by preventing its misuse or overuse. Stress from home or work can also lead to muscle tension and other symptoms, so the patient may also need professional guidance in relieving or controlling these stressors.

Bibliography

General

Bazzo, E, et al: Conducting the preparticipation sports examination. Womens Health Primary Care 7(5):237–255, 2004.

Bazzo, E, et al: Interpreting the preparticipation sports examination. Womens Health Primary Care 7(6):287–295, 2004.

Blazar, P, and Simmons, B: Treating carpel tunnel syndrome. Womens Health Primary Care 5(12):738–748, 2002.

Coylar, M: Ganglion cyst aspiration. Adv Nurse Pract 19, 2005.

Dambro, M: Griffith's 5-Minute Clinical Consult. Williams & Wilkins, Baltimore, 2005.

Duke, JA: The Green Pharmacy. Rodale Press, Emmaus, Penn., 1997.

Eliopoulos, C: Integrating Conventional and Alternative Therapies: Holistic Care for Chronic Conditions. CV Mosby, St. Louis, Mo., 1999.

Epstein, O, et al: Clinical Examination. CV Mosby, London, 1997.

Kasper, DL, et al: Harrison's Principles of Internal Medicine, ed 16. McGraw-Hill, New York, 2004.

King, S: Chronic pain control: What's adequate and appropriate. Consultant 1558–1573, 2003.

Meagher, K, et al: Special concerms in caring for the female athlete. Female Patient 29:7–18, 2004.

Messier, E: Diagnosis and management of repetitive strain injury. Adv Nurse Pract 32–50, 2001.

Rakel, RE: Conn's Current Therapy. WB Saunders, Philadelphia, 2005.

Rapuri, V, et al: Postsurgical management of total hip arthroplasty. Womens Health Primary Care 7(1):27–34, 2004.

Rudy, DR, and Kurowski, K: Family Medicine. Williams & Wilkins, Baltimore, 2003.

Shahady, E, et al: Lower leg pain in a runner. Consultant 1357–1360, 2004.

Snyder, M, and Lindquist, R (eds): Complementary/Alternative Therapies in Nursing, ed 3. Springer, New York, 1998.

Stitik, T: Sports Injuries: Part 2: When—and how—to apply the heat. Consultant 144-158, 1999.

Stitik, T, et al: Joint and soft tissue corticosteroid injections: A practical approach. Consultant 1469–1475, 2000.

Verst, A: Get in the game. Adv Nurse Pract 66–68, 2000.

Waldrop, J: Screening for female athlete triad. Clin Advisor 116, 2004.

Musculoskeletal Pain (General)

Connelly, J: Hazards of immobilizing musculoskeletal injuries: Why ice is nice and motion is lotion. Consultant 602–612, 1998.

Fedutes, B: A targeted approach to musculoskeletal pain, Part 1: Mechanisms and diagnosis. Female Patient 29:8–12, 2004.

Kempen, PM: Managing pain in elderly patients [letter]. JAMA 281(7): 605–606, 1999.

Pincus, T, and Holm, G: A practical approach to the patient with chronic musculoskeletal pain. Clin Advisor 2–22, 2005.

Ruoff, GE: Strategies to control chronic musculoskeletal pain: A guide to drug therapy. Consultant 2773–2781, 1999.

Ruoff, GE: Strategies to control chronic musculoskeletal pain. I. Work-up and nondrug therapy. Consultant 2561–2571, 1999.

Szer, I: Musculoskeletal pain in adolescent, Part 3: Psychogenic rheumatism. Consultant 1253–1258, 2000.

Rotator Cuff Tear

Blair, B, et al: Efficacy of injections of corticosteroids for subacromial impingement syndrome. J Bone Joint Surg Am 78(11):1685–1689, 1996.

Blevins, FT, et al: Biology of the rotator cuff tendon. Orthop Clin North Am 28(1):1–16, 1997.

Eustace, JA, et al: Comparison of the accuracy of steroid placement with clinical outcome in patients with shoulder symptoms. Ann Rheum Dis 56(1):59–63, 1997.

Frieman, BG, Albert, TJ, and Fenlin, JM Jr: Rotator cuff disease: A review of diagnosis, pathophysiology, and current trends in treatment. Arch Phys Med Rehabil 75(5):604–609, 1994.

Fukuda, H, et al: Pathology and pathogenesis of the intratendinous tearing of the rotator cuff viewed from en bloc histologic sections. Clin Orthop 304:60–67, 1994.

Goupille, P, and Sibilia, J: Local corticosteroid injections in the treatment of rotator cuff tendinitis (except for frozen shoulder and calcific tendinitis). Groupe Rhumatologique Francais de l'Epaule (GREP). Clin Exp Rheumatol 14(5):561–566, 1996.

Guckel, C, and Nidecker, A: Diagnosis of tears in rotator-cuff injuries. Eur J Radiol 25(3):168–176, 1997.

Iannotti, JP: Evaluation of the painful shoulder. J Hand Ther 7(2):77–83, 1994.

Kleinhenze, J, et al: Randomised clinical trial comparing the effects of acupuncture and a newly designed placebo needle in rotator cuff tendinitis. Pain 83(2):235–241, 1999.

Lyons, PM, and Orwin, JF: Rotator cuff tendinopathy and subacromial impingement syndrome. Med Sci Sports Exerc 30(Suppl 4):S12–S17, 1998.

Miniaci, A, and Salonen, D: Rotator cuff evaluation: Imaging and diagnosis. Orthop Clin North Am 28(1):43–58, 1997.

Onieal, ME: Problems of the shoulder. J Am Acad Nurse Pract 6(6):283–285, 1994.

Rodgers, JA, and Crosby, LA: Rotator cuff disorders. Am Fam Physician 54(1):127–134, 1996.

Romeo, AA, et al: Repair of full thickness rotator cuff tears. Gender, age, and other factors affecting outcome. Clin Orthop (2):243–255, 1999.

Snyder, SJ: Evaluation and treatment of the rotator cuff. Orthop Clin North Am 24(1):173–192, 1993.

Tempelhof, S, Ruff, S, and Seil, R: Age-related prevalence of rotator cuff tears in asymptomatic shoulders. J Shoulder Elbow Surg 8(4):296–299, 1999.

Uhthoff, HK, and Sano, H: Pathology of failure of the rotator cuff tendon. Orthop Clin North Am 28(1):31–41, 1997.

Vecchio, PC, Hazleman, BL, and King, RH: A double-blind trial comparing subacromial methylprednisolone and lignocaine in acute rotator cuff tendinitis. Br J Rheumatol 32(8):743–745, 1993.

Yocum, LA: Assessing the shoulder. History, physical examination, differential diagnosis, and special tests used. Clin Sports Med 2(2):281–289, 1983.

Foot and Ankle Pain

Little, D, et al: Ankle sprain. Clinical Advisor 56–62, 2004.

Shahady, E, et al: Acute ankle pain in a runner. Consultant 1529–1533, 2004.

Shahady E, and Mills, T: Severe foot pain in a runner. Consultant 585–531, 2004.

Walker, MJ: Pearls for practice: Overuse running injuries. J Am Acad Nurse Pract 10(6):261–265, 1999.

Back

Diamond, L: Treatment of vertebral compression fractures. Clin Advisor 40-45, 2004.

Knee

Adams, J, and Dahm, D: Nonoperative management of knee osteoarthritis in middle-aged women. Womens Health Primary Care 8(4):175–194, 2005.

Shahady, E, et al: A runner with knee pain. Consultant 170–176, 2005.

Shoulder

Le, T, et al: Common shoulder problems: A "hands-on" approach to adhesive capsulitis. Consultant 1481–1490, 2004.

Wilson, C: Rotator cuff versus cervical spine making the diagnosis. Nurse Pract 30(5):45–50, 2005.

Yen, Y, and Hame, S: Preventing ACL injuries in women. Womens Health Primary Care 7(3):146–155, 2004.

Arthritis

Alper, B: Evidence-based medicine. Clin Advisor 98–99, 2004.

Bellamy, N, et al: Recommendations for a core set of outcome measures for future phase III clinical trials in knee, hip, and hand osteoarthritis. Consensus development at OMERACT III. J Rheumatol 24(4):799–-802, 1997.

Berman, BM, et al: Effectiveness of acupuncture as adjunctive therapy in osteoarthritis of the knee: A randomized, controlled trial. Ann Intern Med 141:901–910, 2004.

Block, JA, and Schnitzer, TJ: Therapeutic approaches to osteoarthritis. Hosp Pract (Off Ed) 32:159–164, 1997.

Brandt, KD: Nonsurgical management of osteoarthritis, with an emphasis on nonpharmacologic measures. Arch Fam Med 4(12):1057–1064, 1995.

Bruce, M, and Peck, B: New rheumatoid arthritis tretaments. Nurse Pract 30(4):29–41, 2005.

Campbell, JM, and Linc, LG: Managing osteoarthritis pain. Adv Nurse Pract 7(4):57–60, 1999.

Chao, S, and Vega, C: Alternative approaches to relieving the pain of osteoarthritis. Clin Advisor 21–25, 2004.

Clegg, DO, et al: Glucosamine, chondroitin sulfate, and the two in combination for painful knee arthritis. N Engl J Med 354:795-808, 2005.

Davis, G, et al: Barriers to managing chronic pain of older adults with arthritis. J Nurs Scholar 121–126, 2002.

Fung, HB, and Kirschenbaum, HL: Selective cyclooxygenase-2 inhibitors for the treatment of arthritis. Clin Ther 21(7):1131–1157, 1999.

Grober, DL: Osteoarthritis: Practical nondrug steps to successful therapy. Consultant 53–60, 2003.

Huch, K, et al: Osteoarthritis in ankle and knee joints. Semin Arthritis Rheum 26(4):667–674, 1997.

Kagen, L: An update on the newer therapies for rheumatoid arthritis. Clin Advisor 10–16, 2004.

Lane, NE, and Thompson, JM: Management of osteoarthritis in the primary-care setting: An evidence-based approach to treatment. Am J Med 103(6A):25S–30S, 1997.

Leslie, M: Hyaluronic acid treatment for osteoarthritis of the knee. Nurse Pract 24(7):38–48, 1999.

Lipman, AG: Rheumatoid arthritis: Newest strategies to control the pain. Consultant 1228–1244, 1999.

Malemud, CJ: Fundamental pathways in osteoarthritis: An overview. Front Biosci 4:D659–D661, 1999.

McAlindon, TE, et al: Level of physical activity and the risk of radiographic and symptomatic knee osteoarthritis in the elderly: The Framingham study. Am J Med 106(2):151–157, 1999.

Michel, BA, et al: Chondroitins 4 and 6 sulfate in osteoarthritis of the knew: A randomized, controlled trial. Arthritis Rheumatol 52:779–786, 2005.

Mochan, G: Rheumatoid arthritis: Clues to early diagnosis. Consultant 545–555, 2005.

Neville, C, et al: The needs of patients with arthritis: The patient's perspective. Arthritis Care Res 12(2):85–95, 1999.

Poole, AR: An introduction to the pathophysiology of osteoarthritis. Front Biosci 4:D662–D670, 1999.

Puppione, AA: Management strategies for older adults with osteoarthritis: How to promote and maintain function. J Am Acad Nurse Pract 11(4):167–171; quiz, 172–174, 1999.

Rehman, Q, and Lane, NE: Getting control of osteoarthritis pain. An update on treatment options. Postgrad Med J 106(4):127–134, 1999.

Ruoff, SG: Rheumatoid arthritis: Emerging treatments. Consultant 297–305, 2002.

Schnitzer, TJ: Osteoarthritis treatment update. Minimizing pain while limiting patient risk. Postgrad Med J 93(1):89–92, 95, 1993.

Schwartz, ST, and Zimmermann, B: Update on osteoarthritis. Med Health R I 82(9):321–324, 1999.

Sharma, S, Prasad, A, and Anand, KS: Nonsteroidal anti-inflammatory drugs in the management of pain and inflammation: A basis for drug selection. Am J Ther 6(1):3–11, 1999.

Sims, K: Assessment and treatment of hip osteoarthritis. Manual Ther 4(3):136–144, 1999.

Sims, K: The development of hip osteoarthritis: Implications for conservative management. Manual Ther 4(3):127–135, 1999.

Stitik, T: Osteoarthritis of the glenohumeral joint: A "hands-on" approach. Consultant 154–160, 2005.

Stitik, T, Foye, PM, and Nadler, SF: Osteoarthritis of the knee and hip. II. Keys to successful nondrug therapy. Consultant 1975–1982, 1999.

United States Senate Committee on Health, Education, Labor and Pensions, Subcommittee on Aging. Center for Disease Control's role in combating the burden of arthritis. Department of Health and Human Services, Washington, D.C., 2004.

Vecchio, P, Thomas, R, and Hills, BA: Surfactant treatment for osteoarthritis. Rheumatology (Oxf) 38(10):1020–1021, 1999.

Whyte, TT: Exercise programs for your arthritis patients: A quick guide. Consultant 341–349, 2005.

Zagaria, MAE: Osteoarthritis in older women. Womens Health Primary Care 17–23, 2006.

Osteoporosis and Osteopenia

Abbruzzese, A: Danger zone ,osteoporosis in young female athletes. Adv Nurse Pract 61–65, 2005.

Bone, HG, et al: Ten years experience with alendronate for osteoporosis in postmenopausal women. N Engl J Med 346:653–661, 2003.

Department of Health and Human Services: Bone Health and Osteoporosis: A Report of the Surgeon General. U.S. Department of Health and Human Services, Public Health Service, Office of the Surgeon General, Rockville, Md., 2004, pp 1–35.

Freeman, SB: Tailor Made: Today's hormone therapy is all about fit. Adv Nurse Pract 57–62, 2006.

Greenwald, L, et al: The who, why, and how of bone density reports. J Muscuoloskel Med Nov:452–457, 2002.

Hudson, T: Nutritional influences on osteoporosis. Female Patient 29:42–46, 2004.

Kleerekoper, M: Choosing the right therapy for postmenopausal osteoporosis. Council Horm Educ 4(2):1–16. [Publisher is University of Wisconsin School of Medicine and Public Health]

Licata, A: An updated look at therapies for osteoporosis. Clin Advisor 10–19, 2003.

National Institutes of Health. NIH Consensus Development Panel on Osteoporosis Prevention, Diagnosis, and Therapy. Osteoporosis prevention, diagnosis, and therapy. JAMA 285:785–795, 2001.

Moussa, J, et al: Osteoporosis: Prevention and treatment in the primary care setting. Primary Care Rep January 13, 1997.

National Osteoporosis Foundation: Physician's guide to prevention and treatment of osteoporosis. National Osteoporosis Foundation, Washington D.C., 2003.

Orr-Walker, B, et al: Effects of prolonged bisphosphonate therapy and its discontinuation on bone mineral density in postmenopausal osteoporosis. Clin Endocrinol (Oxf) 46(1):87–92, 1997.
Predergast, K, and Dalkin, A: Therapeutic options in the management of osteoporotic patients. Womens Health Primary Care 7(4):185–193, 2004.
Ralston, SH: The genetics of osteoporosis. QJM 90(4):247–251, 1997.
Research Report: The telltale T score: Should osteopenic women be treated for bone loss? Womens Health Primary Care 7(6):297–298, 2004.
Rossouw, JE, et al: Risks and benefits of estrogen and progestin in healthy postmenopausal women: Principal results from the Women's Health Initiative randomized controlled trial. JAMA 288:321–333, 2002.
Rubin, SM, and Cummings, SR: Results of bone densitometry affect women's decision about taking measures to prevent fractures. Ann Intern Med 116(12 pt 1):990–995, 1992.
Schafer, M: Orthopedic surgery: vertebroplasty and kyphoplasty offer new hope. Adv Nurses 13:13–17, 2003.
Schieber, L, and Torregrosa, L: Postmenopausal osteoporosis: when—and how—to measure bone mineral density. Consultant: 781–789, 2000.
Simmermacher, N: Osteoporosis" case study. Adv Nurse Pract 32–34, 2004.
Takada, M, et al: Assessment of osteoporosis: Comparison of radiographic absorptiometry of the phalanges and dual x-ray absorptiometry of the radius and lumbar spine. Radiology 202(3):759–764, 1997.
The telltale t score: Should osteopenic women be treated for bone loss?. Womens Health Primary Care 7(6):297–298, 2004.
Whyte, J, and Marting, R: Osteoporosis prevention: What kind of exercise is best? Consultant 1002–1011, 2004.
Yates, J, Barrett-Connor, E, and Barlas, S, et al: Rapid loss of hip fracture protection after estrogen cessation: Evidence from the National Osteoporosis Risk Assessment. Obstet Gynecol 103:440–446, 2004.

Paget's Disease

Delmas, PD, and Meunier, PJ: The management of Paget's disease of bone. N Engl J Med 336(8):558–661, 1997.
Fraser, WD: Paget's disease of bone. Curr Opin Rheumatol 9(4):347–354, 1997.
Lewis, T, Tesh, AS, and Lyles, KW: Caring for the patient with Paget's disease of the bone. Nurse Pract 24(7):50–65, 1999.
Oai, CG, and Fraser, WD: Paget's disease of bone. Postgrad Med J 73(856):69–74, 1997.
Papapoulos, SE: Paget's disease of bone: Clinical, pathogenetic and therapeutic aspects. Baillieres Clin Endocrinol Metab 11(1):117–143, 1997.
Wallach, S: Identifying and controlling Paget's disease: Localized enlargement and weakening of bone is characteristic. J Musculoskel Med 14(6):66–68, 74–76, 79–82, 1997.

Hand

Brandenburg, TF: Hand injuries, Part 1: Initial evaluation and wound care. Consultant 242 254, 2005.
Brandenburg, TF: Hand injuries, Part 2: When nerves, vasculature, tendons, or ligaments are traumatized. Consultant 361–368, 2005.
Brandenburg, TF: Hand injuries, Part 3: Fractures, dislocations, nail bed trauma and bites. Consultant 393–402, 2005.
Shahady, E, et al: Limited finger movement after an injury. Consultant 1766–1772, 2004.

Tendinitis

Brandenburg, M, et al: How to "wring" the ring safely from your patient's hand; the string technique. Consultant 202, 2005.
Haupt, G: Use of extracorporeal shock waves in the treatment of pseudovanthrosis, tendinopathy, and other orthopedic diseases. J Urol 158(1):4–11, 1997.

Bursitis

Brooks, CB, and Berras, BL: Elbow pain: Olecranon bursitis and epicondylitis. Hosp Med 33(4):47–50, 1997.
Buindo, JJ Jr, et al: Sports-related and other soft tissue injuries, tendinitis, bursitis, and occupation-related syndromes. Curr Opin Rheumatol 9(2):151–154, 1997.
Handy, JR: Anserine bursitis: A brief review. South Med J 90(4):376–-377, 1997.
Jones, DJ, and Erhard, RE: Diagnosis of trochanteric bursitis versus femoral neck stress fracture. Phys Ther 77(1):58–67, 1997.
Vassilopoulos, D, et al: Musculoskeletal infections in patients with human immunodeficiency virus infection. Medicine (Baltimore) 76(4):284–294, 1997.

Fibromyalgia

Alarcon, GS: Fibromyalgia: Dispelling diagnostic and treatment myths. Is this common condition organic or affective? Womens Health Primary Care 2(10):775–784, 1999.
Alarcon, GS, and Bradley, LA: Advances in the treatment of fibromyalgia: Current status and future directions. Am J Med Sci 315(6):397–404, 1997.
Arslan, S, and Yunus, M: Fibromyalgia: Making a firm diagnosis, understanding its pathophysiology. Consultant 1233–1243, 2003.
Clark, S, and Odell, L: Fibromyalgia syndrome. Clin Rev 10(5): 57–83, 2000.
Harding, SM: Sleep in fibromyalgia patients: Subjective and objective findings. Am J Med Sci 315(6):367–376, 1998.
Jones, K, and Burckhardt, C: A multidisciplinary approach to treating fibromyalgia syndrome. Pain Manage 7–14, 2004.
Maurizio, SJ, and Rogers, JL: Recognizing and treating fibromyalgia. Nurse Pract 22(12):18, 1997.
Mountz, JM, Bradley, LA, and Alarcon, GS: Abnormal functional activity of the central nervous system in fibromyalgia syndrome. Am J Med Sci 315(6):385–396, 1998.
Olsen, NJ, and Park, JH: Skeletal muscle abnormalities in patients with fibromyalgia. Am J Med Sci 315(6):351–358, 1998.
Russell, IJ: Advances in fibromyalgia: Possible role for central neurochemicals. Am J Med Sci 315(6):377–384, 1998.
Russell, IJ: Fibromyalgia syndrome: Approaches to management. Bull Rheum Dis 45(3):1–4, 1996.
Simms, RW: Fibromyalgia is not a muscle disorder. Am J Med Sci 315(6):346–350, 1998.
Sturge-Jacobs, M: The experience of living with fibromyalgia; confronting an invisible disability. Res Theory Nurs Pract 16(1):19–31, 2002.
Yunus, M, and Arslan, S: Fibromyalgia syndrome: Can it be treated? Consultant 289–302, 2004.
Weigent, DA, et al: Current concepts in the pathophysiology of abnormal pain perception in fibromyalgia. Am J Med Sci 315(6):405–412, 1998.

Low Back Pain

Andersson, GB, et al: A comparison of osteopathic spinal manipulation with standard care for patients with low back pain. N Engl J Med 341(19):1426–1431, 1999.
Barlyn, S: Pain in the back. NJ Med 96(1):29–31, 1999.
Birrer, TG: Low back pain: A focused approach. Consultant 993–996, 2003.
Birrer, JT: Low back pain: A quick guide to exercises. Consultant 1029–1035, 2003.
Borenstein, DG: A clinician's approach to acute low back pain. Am J Med 102(1A):16S–22S, 1997.
Borenstein, DG: Epidemiology, etiology, diagnostic evaluation, and treatment of low back pain. Curr Opin Rheumatol 11(2):151–157, 1999.
Braddom, RL: Perils and pointers in the evaluation and management of back pain. Semin Neurol 18(2):197–210, 1998.
Cherkin, DC, et al: A comparison of physical therapy, chiropractic manipulation, and provision of an educational booklet for the treatment of patients with low back pain. N Engl J Med 339(15): 1021–1029, 1998.
Clinical Practice Guidelines No. 14: Acute Low Back Problems in Adults. US Department of Health and Human Services, Agency for Health Care Policy and Research, Rockville, Md., December, 1994, AHCPR publication 95-0642.
Connelly, C: Low back pain: Management of thc psycological component. Consultant 84–92, 2003.
Della-Giustina, D: Acute low back pain, Part 1: Recognizing the "red flags" in the work-up. Consultant 995–1002, 1998.
Deyo, RA, and Phillips, WR: Low back pain. A primary care challenge. Spine 21(24):2826–2832, 1996.

Garfin, J, and Garfin, S: Low back pain: A quick guide to exercise as acute therapy. Consultant 350–353, 2002.
Garfin, J, and Garfin, S: Low back pain: Exercise to prevent recurrence. Consultant 357–359, 2002.
Jones, AK: Primary care management of acute low back pain. Nurse Pract 22(7):50–52, 61–63; quiz, 74–75, 1997.
Laird, N: Evaluating and managing chronic low back pain. Womens Health Care 2(1):13–16, 2003.
Low back prescriptin pad. Patient Information Network, 1987.
McGregor, AH, and Hughes, SP: Initial assessment of back pain: An overview. Hosp Med 59(6):492–495, 1998.
Padfield, N: When should you investigate in back pain? Practitioner 242(1592):770–774, 776, 1998.
Rauck, RL, et al: Chronic low back pain: New perspectives and treatment guidelines for primary care. Part II. Managed Care Interface 11(3):71–75, 1998.
Sponseller, PD: Back pain in children. Curr Opin Pediatr 6(1):99–103, 1994.
Stevens, RJ, and Mathews, JA: A new protocol for back pain. Practitioner 241(1575):351–354, 1997.
Tacci, JA: et al: Clinical practices in the management of new-onset, uncomplicated, low back workers' compensation disability claims. J Occup Environ Med 41(5):397–404, 1999.
van Tulder, MW, et al: Management of chronic nonspecific low back pain in primary care: A descriptive study. Spine 22(1):76–82, 1997.

Resources

American Academy of Orthopedic Surgeons
http://www.aaos.org
American Association of Clinical Endocrinologists (AACE)
(904) 353-7878
American Orthopedic Foot and Ankle Society
http://www.aofas.org
American Academy of Physical Medicine and Rehabilitation
http://www.aapmr.org
American Academy of Physical Therapy
http://www.aaptnet.org
Arthritis Foundation
http://www.arthritis.org
The Arthritis Source
http://www.orthop.washington.edu/arthritis
Association of Hip and Knee Surgeons
http://www.aahks.org
California Center for Minimally Invasive Spine Surgery
http://www.spinecenter.com
Creighton University Osteoporosis Research Center
http://creighton.edu/org
Fibromyalgia
http://www.fmagw.org
Fibromyalgia Network
PO Box 31750
Tucson, AZ 85751
Fitness Partner
http://www.primusweb.com/fitnesspartner
Mayo Health Oasis Back Care
http://www.mayohealth.org/ivi/mayo9401/htm/backcare.htm
National CFS and Fibromyalgia Association
3521 Broadway, Suite 222
Kansas City, MO 64111
816-931-4777
National Fibromyalgia Research Association
PO Box 3000
Salem, OR 97302
National Institute of Arthritis, Musculoskeletal & Skin Diseases
http://www.nih.gov/niams
National Library of Medicine
http://www.nim.nih.gov/melineplus
National Osteoporosis Foundation
http://www.nof.org
National Women's Health Resource Center (NWHRC) women.org
@REF:http://www.healthywomen.org/
Osteoporosis and Bone Disease
http://www.osteo.org
Osteoporosis and Related Bone Diseases National Resource Center (ORB-NRC)
http://www.osteo.org/
Osteoporosis Society of Canada
http://www.osteoporosis.ca/
A Patient's Guide to Low Back Pain
http://www.sechrest.com/mmg/back/backpain.html
Physical Therapy Association
http://www.apta.org
Physician's and Sports
http://www.physsports.org
Rehabilitation Foundation
http://www.rfi.org
Spine Center
http://www.spinenet.com
Virtual Hospital: Acute Low Back Problems in Adults
http://www.vh.org/providers/clinguide/backphysician/ back physician.html

Endocrine and Metabolic Problems

Debera J. Thomas, DNS, APRN, BC
Brian O. Porter, MD, PhD, MPH
Susan L. Folden, PhD, APRN, BC

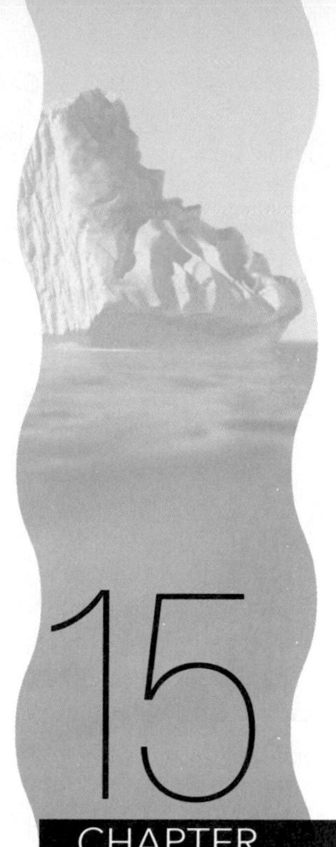

15
CHAPTER

Common Complaints

Carpopedal Spasm

Carpopedal spasm is a violent, painful contraction of the hands or feet. It is one of the neuromuscular signs indicating hypocalcemia and is a significant sign of tetany. Neuromuscular signs and symptoms occur in the presence of hypocalcemia, because calcium is an important mediator in neurotransmission and other intracellular biochemical activity. In response to hypocalcemia, there is an increased secretion of parathyroid hormone, which leads to immobilization of calcium stores from the bone and an increase in the absorption of calcium in the intestines.

Trousseau's sign (carpal spasm) is one of two neuromuscular signs indicative of hypocalcemia. It is often preceded by muscle cramps in the legs and feet. Carpal spasm consists of a flexed elbow and wrist, adducted thumb over the palm, flexed metacarpophalangeal joints, adduction of hyperextended fingers, and extended interphalangeal joints. The response is elicited by inflation of a blood pressure cuff to 20 mm Hg above the level of the systolic blood pressure. Inflation is maintained for 3 minutes to elicit the response, which is secondary to ulnar and median nerve ischemia. In severe hypocalcemia, spontaneous spasms may occur in the lower extremities. *Chvostek's sign* is the second neuromuscular sign associated with hypocalcemia. It is an abnormal unilateral spasm of the facial muscle when the facial nerve is tapped below the zygomatic arch anterior to the ear lobe.

Differential Diagnosis

Acute neuromuscular irritability producing carpopedal spasm occurs when the serum calcium drops abruptly by 2 to 3 mg/dL. Parathyroid disease or inadvertent damage to the parathyroid glands during neck surgery may cause acute severe hypocalcemia. Acute transient hypocalcemia may occur in burns, severe sepsis, pregnancy, extensive blood transfusions, acute pancreatitis, and acute renal failure.

Patients with carpopedal spasm should be immediately assessed for hypocalcemia. Normal serum calcium values in adults range from 9 to 11 mg/dL. Immediate medical treatment is indicated in patients with marked hypocalcemia (less than 6.5 mg/dL).

A focused history, clinical examination, and subsequent laboratory tests may determine the cause of hypocalcemia. In absence of a clearly identifiable etiology such as a medication, chronic liver or renal disease, or an acute disease process, additional laboratory studies are needed. Further laboratory evaluation should begin with serum magnesium, serum phosphorus, and albumin levels. Depending on these findings, the practitioner should initiate treatment if indicated. A serum parathyroid hormone (PTH) level will assist in the diagnosis of parathyroid disease. A direct measure of serum vitamin D levels is the 25-hydroxycholecalciferol (25-[OH]D_3) assay.

Aggressive treatment of hypercalcemia with plicamycin (Mithracin), bisphosphonates, and calcitonin (Cibacalcin, Calcimar) may result in acute hypocalcemia. Other drugs that may produce hypocalcemia include radiographic contrast dyes that contain a calcium chelating agent, EDTA, and foscarnet (Foscavir).

Chronic hypocalcemia is usually caused by the absence of PTH, ineffective PTH, vitamin D deficiency, chronic renal failure (CRF), hypomagnesemia, or hypoalbuminemia. Other potential causes of chronic hypocalcemia include alkalosis, malabsorption syndromes, chronic pancreatitis, laxative abuse, chronic liver failure, phosphate excess, and osteomalacia.

Patients exhibiting either Trousseau's sign or Chvostek's sign accompanied by respiratory distress (e.g., stridor, loud crowing noises, and cyanosis) require immediate referral for emergency care, because the neuromuscular irritation produced by hypocalcemia may progress rapidly to laryngospasms, seizures, and dysrhythmias. If the serum calcium levels have gradually declined, symptoms are usually subtle.

Other symptoms of hypocalcemia include various neuropsychiatric disorders, including irritability, emotional instability, problems with memory, and psychosis. Complaints of parasthesias, fatigue, muscle cramps, or muscle weakness may be elicited on history. Gastrointestinal (GI) manifestations include dysphagia, nausea, vomiting, biliary colic, and abdominal pain or cramping. Patients may also complain of chronic constipation or diarrhea. Cardiovascular symptoms include hypotension, bradycardia, congestive heart failure (CHF), and dysrhythmias. Prolonged QT intervals may be seen on the electrocardiogram (ECG).

Chronic hypocalcemia may cause the skin to be coarse, dry, and scaly. Alopecia may present with thinning of the eyebrows and eyelashes. Nails are often rigid, brittle, and thin, with transverse grooves. Subcapsular cataracts, optic neuritis, intracranial calcification, papilledema, and parkinsonian-type movements may also be present in chronic hypocalcemia.

Management

Emergency treatment of hypocalcemia is IV replacement of calcium. Patients with hypomagnesemia also require IV magnesium replacement. During acute therapy and the initial therapy of chronic hypocalcemia, patients must be monitored closely for signs of hypercalcemia such as confusion, abdominal pain, dehydration, weakness, polydipsia, anorexia, nausea, vomiting, constipation, pancreatitis, peptic ulcer, polyuria, hypertension, and a shortened QT interval.

The goal of treatment for chronic hypocalcemia is to restore the serum calcium level to the low to normal range.

Gynecomastia

Gynecomastia is the enlargement of glandular breast tissue in men, resulting in increased breast size. True gynecomastia involves enlargement of the stromal and ductal tissues; it may present unilaterally and progress to bilateral symmetrical or asymmetrical enlargement. Gynecomastia results from an imbalance of androgen and estrogen or an increase in prolactin. Growth hormones, estrogen, and corticosteroids stimulate ductal growth in the breasts. Progesterone and prolactin stimulate alveolar lobular growth of the breasts.

Gynecomastia is estimated to affect 12 to 40 percent of the male population in the United States and is present in 40 to 60 percent of men older than age 50 years. Transient gynecomastia occurs in male neonates and at puberty.

Differential Diagnosis

Asymptomatic gynecomastia may be an incidental finding on routine examination. It may also present as an acute unilateral or bilateral painful tender mass beneath the areola or as a progressive painless enlargement of breast tissue. The enlargement may be obvious by observation alone; however, less severe cases are noted only during palpation. Pain in the nipple or breast and tenderness often accompany gynecomastia. Gynecomastia lasting longer than 1 year is usually asymptomatic. Nipple discharge is rare (present in fewer than 5 percent of cases).

Gynecomastia that presents before or after puberty and cannot be associated with physiologic aging, a drug, or chronic disease requires further investigation by an endocrinologist. Associated symptoms may assist in identifying the cause.

When gynecomastia is accompanied by other breast abnormalities, especially if they are unilateral, a mammogram is indicated to rule out a neoplasm. A disk that is greater than 4 cm in diameter should be evaluated by mammography.

True gynecomastia must be differentiated from pseudogynecomastia, which is fatty enlargement of the breast. The patient is examined in a supine position, while the examiner grasps breast tissue between the thumb and forefinger and gently moves the two digits toward the nipple. A firm or rubbery, mobile, disklike mound of tissue at least 2 to 4 cm in diameter arising concentrically from beneath the nipple and areolar region confirms gynecomastia. The glandular enlargement of gynecomastia is usually resistive and ropy in texture. Severe cases present with more extensive enlargement. Lack of a disk of tissue suggests the enlargement is the result of adipose tissue deposition (pseudogynecomastia). Mammography will distinguish between the two if clinical examination is inconclusive.

When true gynecomastia has been established, the patient is evaluated for physiologic (developmental) or pathologic causes. The most common causes of gynecomastia are puberty (25 percent), idiopathic (25 percent), drug related (15 percent), cirrhosis or malnutrition (10 percent), and testicular failure (10 percent). Other causes include renal failure, thyroid disease, neoplasms, hyperprolactinemia, Klinefelter's syndrome, and gonadotropin deficiency. Although physiologic development of gynecomastia is the most common cause of gynecomastia, pathological causes should always be considered and ruled out via a thorough history and physical examination.

Malignant breast tumors (which represent about 3 percent of all cases of gynecomastia) in men are typically unilateral, firm, and immobile; grow rapidly and are often painful. Nipple retraction and discharge, skin dimpling, and axillary lymphadenopathy also may accompany breast neoplasms. Mammography and fine-needle biopsy are essential for confirming the diagnosis.

Decreased libido and impotence may accompany gynecomastia and may indicate the presence of chronic pulmonary, renal, or liver disease, testicular failure, or endocrine pathology.

Management

Idiopathic and pubertal gynecomastia should resolve spontaneously within 1 to 2 years. The patient should be followed biannually and the size of the disk measured until it has resolved. Tamoxifen (Nolvadex) 10 mg bid (twice daily) may be useful in treating painful gynecomastia. Cold compresses and analgesics may also relieve discomfort. Attention to any impact on body image, especially in adolescents, is important. In refractory cases, surgical resection (mastectomy) or liposuction may provide cosmetic improvement. Low-dose radiation may prevent gynecomastia in men receiving estrogen therapy for prostate cancer.

A referral to an endocrinologist is required for all cases in which gynecomastia appears before puberty, if gynecomastia does not resolve 2 years following puberty, if it occurs in the presence of abnormal serum levels of free testosterone and luteinizing hormones (LH), or when gynecomastia is accompanied by abnormal presence or the absence of secondary sex characteristics, undermasculinization, or small, asymmetric testes. In a pubertal male, a referral is indicated at any time when physical findings are not consistent with normal growth and development.

The patient should be provided with information about gynecomastia and its cause. Reassurance is very important in a pubertal male. Patients should receive instruction on breast and testicular self-examination.

Hirsutism

Hirsutism is an increase in terminal hair growth on the face, chest, back, lower abdomen, pubic area, axilla, and inner thighs. It is present in approximately 5 percent of the female population in the United States. Almost 25 percent of these women have terminal hair growth on the face, especially on the upper lip. Hirsutism is caused by increased secretion of androgens by the ovary or adrenal glands or an increased sensitivity to androgens. It is often accompanied by menstrual irregularities.

There are two major types of hair: vellus and terminal. Vellus hair is found over most of the body and is fine, soft, and unpigmented. During puberty vellus hair often changes to terminal hair in the presence of an increase in androgen. Terminal hairs are characteristically dark, coarse, pigmented, and thicker compared to vellus hair. Terminal hairs are found on the scalp, eyebrows, and the axillary and pubic areas following puberty. They are found in a lesser extent on the extremities.

Differential Diagnosis

The characteristic increase in terminal hair growth occurs in areas most sensitive to androgen: the upper lip, chin, chest, upper arms, upper abdomen, lower abdomen, thighs, and upper and lower back. Accompanying signs of virilization, hoarseness of the voice, clitorimegaly, receding temporal hair line, acne, loss of body fat, and breast atrophy may be due to an ovarian or adrenal tumor. Markedly increased levels of plasma androgens often accompany virilization.

Although most cases (95 percent) of hirsutism are idiopathic or result from polycystic ovary disease, more serious underlying disease entities must be ruled out. A targeted history with emphasis on when hirsutism was first recognized and how rapidly it has progressed, a detailed menstrual history, and a review of associated symptoms may provide some insight into the cause of hirsutism. The physical examination should focus on signs of adrenal disease and virilization that may further clarify possible causes.

Laboratory evaluation of hirsutism is indicated in women with menstrual irregularities, a history of sudden onset or rapid progression of hirsutism, associated symptoms of ovarian or adrenal pathology, and moderate to severe presentations. Evaluation of free testosterone levels, androstenedione, and dehydroepiandrosterone (DHEA) will provide insights into possible causes or the need for further evaluation. Testosterone levels greater than 200 ng/dL (in women) suggest adrenal or ovarian pathology and are rarely seen in idiopathic hirsutism or in polycystic ovary disease. Slightly elevated levels of serum androgens (free testosterone) are found in 40 percent of women with idiopathic hirsutism.

The basic workup includes a total testosterone, DHEA, urine 17-hydroxycorticosteroids (17-OHCS), thyroid stimulating hormone (TSH), and prolactin levels. A testosterone level greater than 200 ng/dL indicates the need for an ovarian tumor workup. If the DHEA is above 700 ng/dL, an adrenal tumor workup is indicated. The LH/FSH (follicle-stimulating hormone) level is increased in 75 percent of cases of polycystic ovarian disease.

Androgen-dependent terminal hair growth may be caused by pathology in the adrenal glands or ovaries or by exogenous androgen administration. The age, associated symptoms, and rapidity of onset are critical factors in differentiating potential causes.

Idiopathic hirsutism in women is the result of excessive androgenic activity and begins during puberty. There is a gradual development over 2 to 3 years followed by a period of stability. There is a familial tendency toward hirsutism. Women of eastern European or Mediterranean descent are likely to have increased terminal hair growth. Idiopathic hirsutism usually occurs in women between ages of 15 to 25 years without symptoms of virilization. It is usually mild and not accompanied by menstrual irregularities. Hirsutism may present in pregnancy owing to production of androgens by the placenta and corpus luteum. Postmenopausal women experience an increase in androgen production, with 75 percent experiencing noticeable facial hair growth.

Management

When the cause of hirsutism is determined to be of adrenal or ovarian origin, the patient is referred to an endocrinologist for treatment. Discontinuing a drug that is determined to be the cause or substituting an alternative may stop the rapid progression of terminal hair growth.

Treatment of idiopathic hirsutism and hirsutism resulting from polycystic ovary syndrome (POCS) is dependent on the severity and treatment preferences of the patient. Hirsutism is often perceived as a loss of femininity and sexuality; women affected will need reassurance. Idiopathic hirsutism does not frequently interfere with fertility.

Mild cases of hirsutism can be managed by cosmetic therapy, including physical removal, chemical depilatories, and bleaching. Electrolysis and laser therapy are more permanent solutions but are costly. Androgen production may be reduced with weight loss if the woman is obese.

Pharmacologic therapy may be indicated in women with more severe hirsutism, such as those caused by a tumor. After the tumor has been removed, oral contraceptives, either monophasic or triphasic, may be effective. Estrogen-dominant medications, such as the Ortho brands of contraceptives, are effective and will increase sex steroid–binding globulin. Progesterone-dominant medications, such as the Wyeth brands of contraceptives, will increase clearance of testosterone. Medroxyprogesterone (Depo-Provera) is also effective. Hormonal therapy will stop further hair growth but will not reverse the present hair growth, which must be treated cosmetically. It may take 6 to 24 months to see results of hormonal treatment, which may need to be lifelong.

Increased Neck Size

The neck contains 75 lymph nodes, the trachea, larynx, pharynx, the submandibular and salivary glands, cervical vertebrae, and the parathyroid and thyroid glands. Pathology in one of these structures or in an area that is drained by one of the many lymph nodes may increase neck size.

A patient with increased neck size may present with complaints that shirt collars are tight. The patient should be evaluated immediately for difficulty swallowing or breathing problems. An immediate referral is indicated in the presence of either symptom. Some patients may complain of pain.

Differential Diagnosis

Increased neck size may be caused by a mass in any structure in the neck, including glands, lymph nodes, larynx, or pharynx. Cysts may also develop in the neck and increase the size of the neck. Blockage of the salivary glands produces neck enlargement. The most common cause of increased neck size is an enlarged thyroid gland. Other potential causes include trauma, masses, neoplasms, cysts, and lymph node enlargements.

The history can assist in diagnosing the cause of increased neck size. Patients reporting a recent fall, automobile accident, or injury may have sustained cervical trauma. History of a recent infection may cause lymph node enlargement. The patient should be questioned about a history of thyroid problems or recent surgeries; allergies, sinus problems, as well as any complaints of headaches. Symptoms of dysphagia, dyspnea, chest tenderness, cough, and hoarseness should be addressed. Complaints of pain should be investigated including if the pain is aggravated by range of motion movements, breathing, swallowing, or chewing.

The physical examination should assess whether the swelling (enlargement) is focal or diffuse. One or more focal masses may be enlarged lymph nodes related to Hodgkin's disease, sarcoidosis, a thyroglossal cyst, thyroid adenoma, or carcinoma. If the swelling is diffuse, venous distension of CHF, Graves' disease, subacute thyroiditis, superior vena cava syndrome, or subcutaneous emphysema (which would usually be accompanied by subcutaneous crepitus) is suspected. If the swelling is focal, it should be noted if the lesion is midline or lateral because midline masses can be indicative of thyroglossal cysts or adenoma of the thyroid; lateral masses are more likely related to Virchow's node, Hodgkin's lymphoma, bronchial cysts, a pharyngeal pouch, or a stone of Wharton's duct. Intermediate swelling suggests venous congestion of CHF, a bronchial cyst, a stone of Warton's duct, or an aneurysm.

A technique for detecting thyromegaly is to have the patient sit upright for examination. During examination, the neck is exposed down to the sternal notch while the examiner stands directly in front of the patient with the thyroid gland at the examiner's eye level. The patient should take several sips of water while the examiner observes for an enlarged thyroid gland. Following visual examination, the thyroid is palpated anteriorly and posteriorly.

Thyroid nodules can be palpated in about 5 percent of Americans. Women are more likely to have palpable thyroid nodules, and the frequency of nodules increases with age. Fewer than 10 percent of singular nodules are malignant. TSH and thyroxine (T_4) levels should be obtained on the patient with enlargment or any abnormalities in the thyroid.

A single enlarged lymph node is unlikely to result in a significant increase in neck size. Sudden complaints of a lymph node enlargement suggest an infectious process. Patients who present with enlargement of a node over several months or multiple node involvement are more likely to have neoplastic disease. A hard, immobile mass is also suggestive of a neoplastic process. A referral is indicated for biopsy of the nodes. Laryngeal cancer produces cervical lymphadenopathy and increases neck size. Pain, dyspnea, dysphagia, hemoptysis, stridor, and hoarseness may also be present.

Management

Management of the patient with increased neck size is to treat the underlying cause.

Polydipsia, Polyphagia, and Polyuria

Polydipsia is excessive thirst; it is associated with several endocrine diseases and certain drugs. Polydipsia may accompany increased urine output (polyuria), which can be related to excessive loss of water and salt.

Polyphagia refers to excessive eating before satiety. This symptom can present as a persistent or intermittent condition, resulting from endocrine and psychological disorders. Certain drugs are also known to cause polyphagia. Elevated T_4 levels increase metabolism and thus the body's need for calories, often causing polyphagia.

Polyuria is a condition associated with increased urine production; it is defined as excretion of more than 3000 mL (3 L) per day. Any condition that increases hyperosmolar states will increase urination as a consequence of osmotic diuresis. The patient with polyuria is at risk for fluid volume deficit that could result in hypovolemia.

Differential Diagnosis

Differential diagnoses for the patient with symptoms of polyuria, polydypsia, or polyphagia include diabetes mellitus, diabetes insipidus, diuretic abuse, head trauma, and psychiatric disorders. See Differential Diagnosis Flowchart 15.1 for other causes of these symptoms.

The patient should be questioned about any history of head trauma, weight changes, thyroid disease, hypertension, and family history of diabetes. The patient should also be questioned about any history of psychiatric illnesses or changes in mental status, for example, alertness or memory, as well as symptoms of fatigue. A detailed 48-hour history of intake and output should be obtained, including the type of fluid intake over 48 hours, as well as the characteristics of the urine output. A weight history should be obtained.

The patient should be assessed for signs of dehydration and malnutrition. Weight and vital signs are assessed. Initial laboratory testing includes urinalysis, urine specific gravity, electrolytes, blood urea nitrogen (BUN), serum creatinine, complete blood count (CBC), and a blood glucose.

Polydipsia, polyphagia, and polyuria are the classic symptoms of diabetes mellitus. Blood glucose level should be evaluated in patients who experience these three symptoms. Positive fasting blood glucose levels greater than 126 mg/dL on two separate occasions and a random blood glucose level greater than 200 mg/dL confirmed by a fasting blood glucose level of 126 mg/dL on a subsequent day confirm the diagnosis of diabetes mellitus. Accompanying symptoms indicating diabetes mellitus include weight loss, weakness, fatigue, increased susceptibility to infections, and nocturia.

Management

Management of the patient with polydipsia, polyphagia, and/or polyuria is dependent on treating the underlying cause.

Weight Gain

Weight gain is a common complaint in clinical practice. It may be assessed as a risk factor, such as in coronary artery disease; as a symptom of another disorder, such as the edema seen with CHF; as a "sign of aging"; or it may indicate a problem such as hypothyroidism, Cushing's disease, or obesity.

Energy expenditure is composed of the resting energy expenditure, the thermic effect of food, and physical activity. Weight gain results from the ingestion of more calories than are expended. Most often, weight gain is a result of a combination of genetic and environmental factors. However, endocrine disorders, nephrotic syndromes, cardiovascular disease, and some drugs may be the cause of weight gain.

Differential Diagnosis

The history of weight gain, a 24- to 48-hour diet recall, and assessment of activity may provide insight into potential causes. Weight gain, when not associated with pathologic disease, results from a complex combination of genetic and environmental factors. The incidence of weight gain increases with age. Several factors account for this weight gain, including a decrease in metabolic rate, decreasing muscle mass, and decreased physical activity. Without reductions in caloric intake, weight gain results.

Multiple complex factors interacting simultaneously within the individual usually lead to weight gain. These include biologic, genetic, metabolic, psychological, environmental, and social factors. Americans tend to have high-fat diets and put taste and convenience ahead of nutritional content. A sedentary lifestyle and a variety of psychological factors, including depression, anxiety, guilt, and seasonal affective disorder all contribute to weight gain.

The major differential diagnoses that present with weight gain include hypothyroidism, Cushing's syndrome, renal or hepatic disease, CHF, premenstrual syndrome, pregnancy, medication use, depression, and excessive caloric intake (see Differential Diagnosis Flowchart 15.2).

The patient's history may reveal a family history of obesity, recent weight changes, precipitating psychosocial factors, or a past dieting experience. Food intake (including

DIFFERENTIAL DIAGNOSIS FLOWCHART 15.1

POLYDIPSIA, POLYPHAGIA, AND/OR POLYURIA

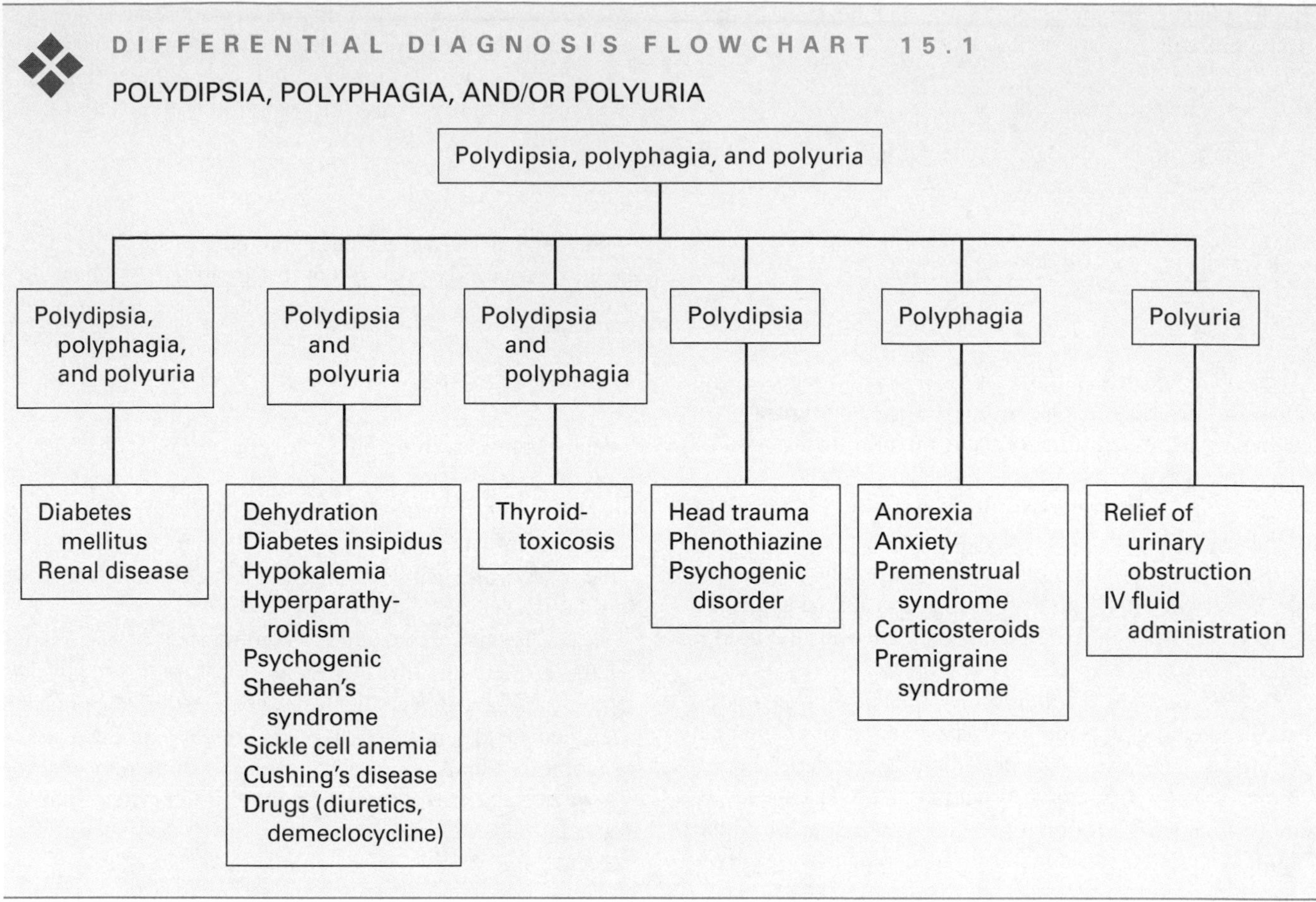

alcohol) and exercise behaviors should be examined, as well as tobacco and drug use.

A complete physical examination may be needed to evaluate potential pathological causes for weight gain. The weight is recorded and abdominal girth measured, as well as vital signs taken. Thyroid function tests (TSH and T_4), a serum blood glucose level, and a CBC are done in the initial evaluation of patients first presenting with weight gain. Serum cholesterol level, triglycerides, and a lipoprotein panel should be obtained to assess the patient's risk factors for cardiovascular disease.

In addition to the complaint of weight gain, patients may present with fatigue, inability to engage in physical activity, dyspnea on exertion, and pain in weight-bearing joints or spine. Patients may also present for the treatment of hypertension, diabetes, cholecystitis, or cardiovascular complaints.

Management

Treatment requires a variety of approaches and depends on the cause. Assessing the patient's motivation is crucial in assisting the patient to set realistic goals. The patient may require in-depth counseling and close follow-up. Many commercial and community programs exist to assist the individual with weight control. If an endocrine disorder is suspected, referral to an endocrinologist is indicated.

Weight Loss, Unintentional

Unintentional weight loss of more than 5 percent of usual body weight within 6 to 12 months may reflect a physical or psychological illness and a 10 percent loss of body weight in 1 to 2 months is predictive of a poor clinical outcome. Underweight is defined as being 15 to 20 percent or more below ideal body weight or a body mass index (BMI) of 18 or less.

Unintentional weight loss is often a presenting symptom for many underlying pathologies. It may result from a decrease in intake, an increase in metabolic needs, or a combination of the two.

Differential Diagnosis

History and physical examination may provide initial clues to the cause of the weight loss. The patient's height, weight, and BMI should be recorded, as well as the details about the onset and progression of the weight loss. Actual weight loss needs to be confirmed, because it cannot be substantiated in up to 50 percent of all patients with this complaint. History should include a 3- to 5-day diet record; use of cigarettes, alcohol, over-the-counter (OTC) and street drug use, any active medical problems, prescribed medication use, and previous surgery.

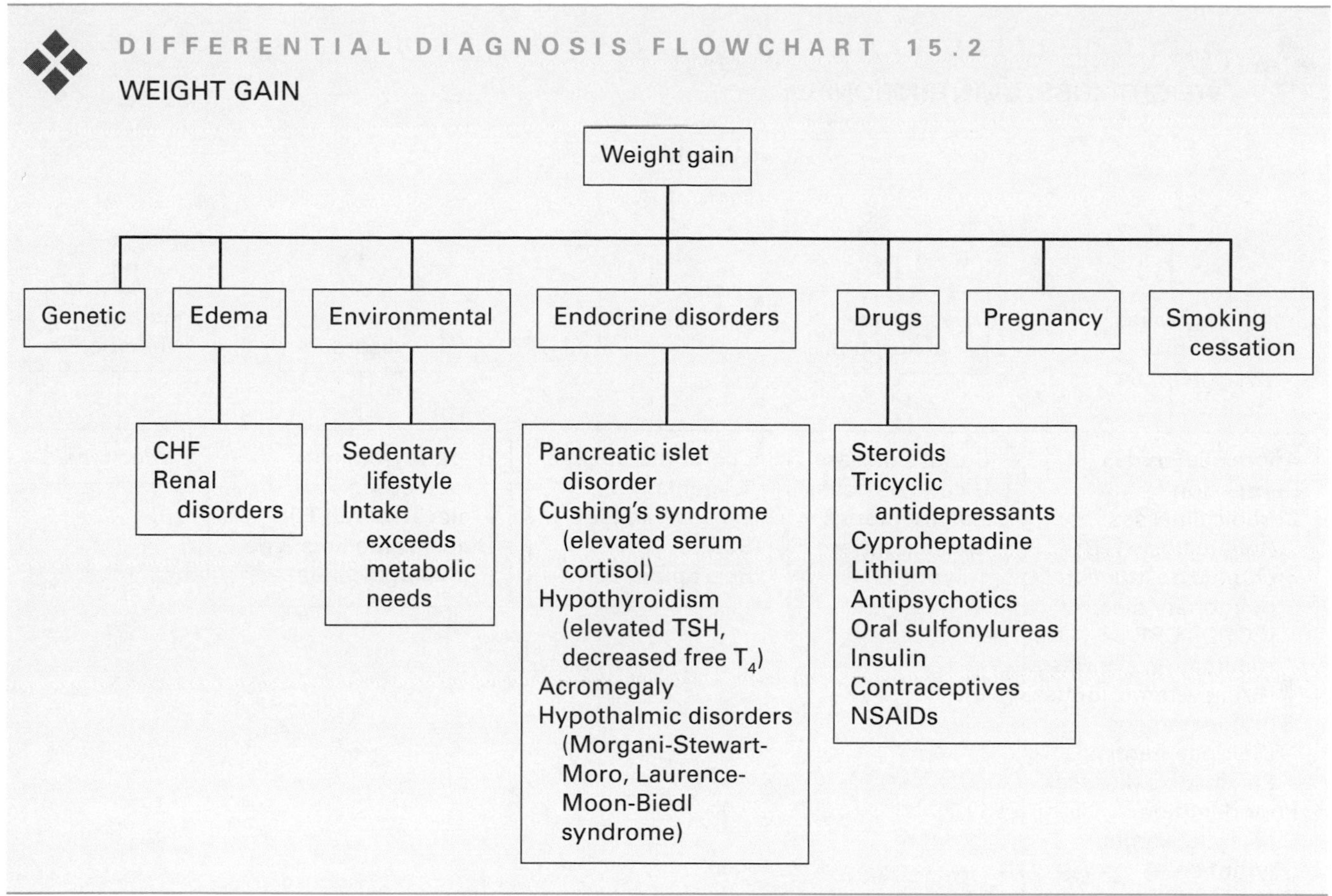

Diagnostic testing should be based on the findings of the history and physical exam. Basic screening should include a CBC, chemistry profile, thyroid function studies, urinalysis, chest x-ray film, and stool for occult blood.

A physical cause of weight loss can be found in about 65 percent of patients, psychiatric cause in 10 percent, and no identifiable cause in approximately 25 percent of cases. Physical causes of weight loss are almost always apparent after a brief evaluation or within 6 months of the first evaluation, even when the initial diagnosis is elusive. Many prescription medications, as well as poor dentition, oral lesions, irritation, and infection have the potential to cause weight loss (see Differential Diagnosis Flowchart 15.3).

Management

The underlying medical or psychiatric causes of weight loss should be treated. Neurologic causes may respond to medications or rehabilitation. Nutritional deficiencies must be corrected with oral or parenteral supplements; an additional 500 to 1000 calories per day may be indicated.

Megestrol (Megace) 800 mg/day is used as an appetite stimulant in patients with anorexia associated with human immunodeficiency virus/acquired immune deficiency syndrome (HIV/AIDS). Thalidomide is under FDA consideration as an appetite stimulant for patients with AIDS. Tricyclic antidepressants (amitriptyline [Elavil], imipramine [Tofranil], doxepin [Adapin, Sinequan]) are effective in patients with weight loss associated with depression and stimulate appetite.

Follow-up is determined by underlying cause and plan of management. If no cause is found, the clinician should reevaluate the patient thoroughly in 2 to 3 months. The patient should be referred for systemic medical problems or for psychiatric evaluation. Referral to a nutritionist, a dentist for oral problems, or a social worker may also be indicated. The patient needs to understand the nature of the problem and participate in the development of the treatment plan.

Common Endocrine Problems

Hyperthyroidism

Hyperthyroidism, a common clinical condition, includes a heterogeneous group of conditions characterized by the excessive secretion of one or both of the thyroid hormones: thyroxine (T_4) and triiodothyronine (T_3). Although many clinicians use the terms interchangeably, *thyrotoxicosis* is a larger term which encompasses hyperthyroidism, as well as exogenous thyroid hormone intake and subacute thyroiditis, in which acute inflammation of the thyroid gland results in

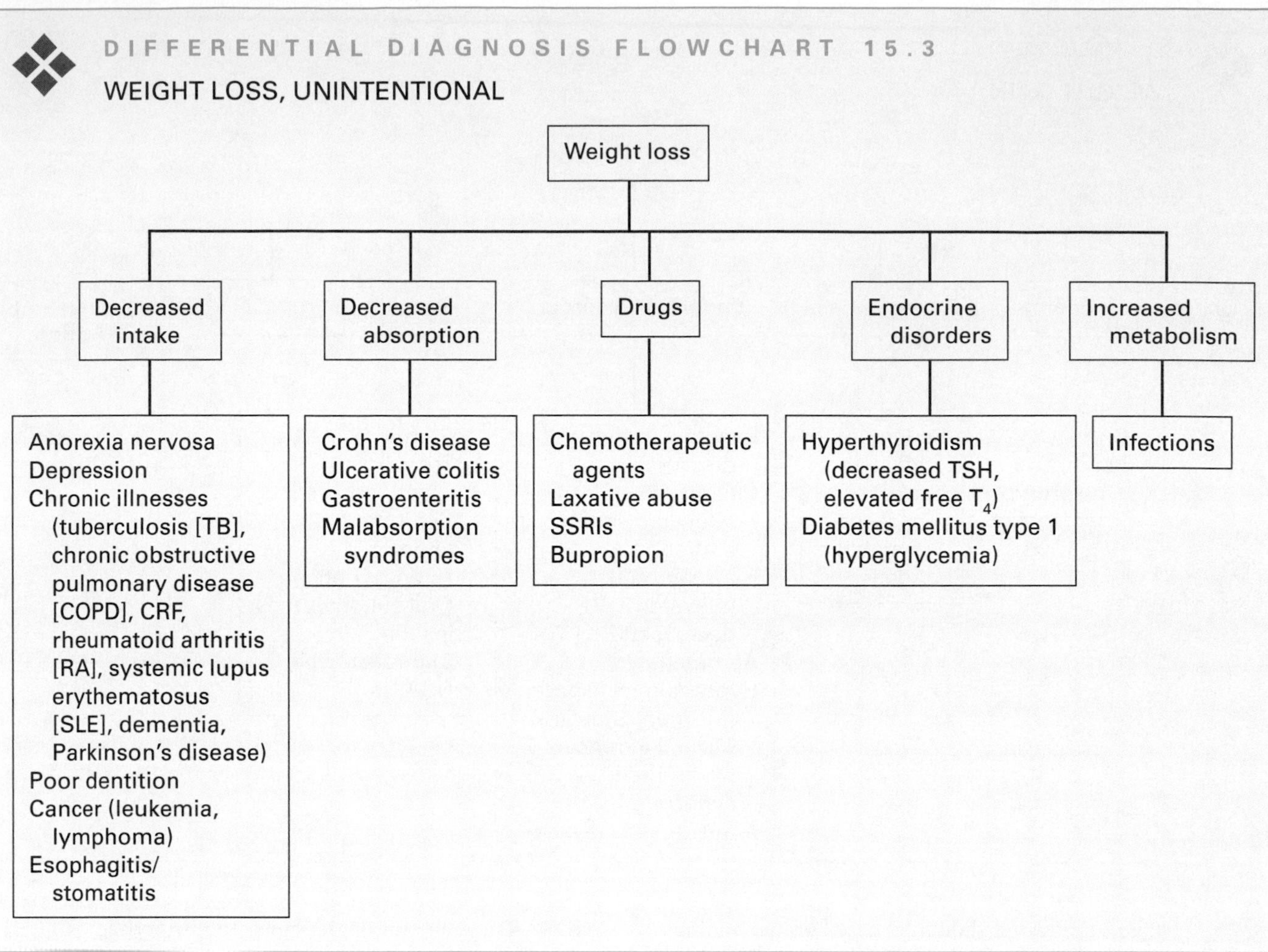

the rapid excretion (rather than overproduction) of stored thyroid hormones.

The clinical manifestations of hyperthyroidism result from the effects of excessive thyroid hormone on body tissue, resulting in alterations in growth, metabolism, and development. These manifestations are sometimes mistaken for signs of psychiatric illnesses. The long-term effects of inadequately treated overt hyperthyroidism are heart disease, osteoporosis (in post-menopausal women), mental illness, and infertility.

Epidemiology and Causes

Hyperthyroidism occurs in 1 in 1000 women and 1 in 3000 men. It may occur at any age but peaks between the ages of 20 to 40 years. Only 10 to 15 percent of hyperthyroidism is diagnosed in older adults. The prevalence of hyperthyroidism is 2 percent in women older than 70 years and 4 percent in women between ages 40 and 60 years, with an overall prevalence of 1 to 3 percent. Hyperthyroidism is much more common in women than men (8:1).

The American Thyroid Association recommends routine screening in asymptomatic women beginning at age 35 years and every 5 years thereafter. However, the American Academy of Family Physicians does not recommend routine screening in women until age 50 years. If the patient is symptomatic or in a high-risk category, such as having a family history of thyroid disease or previous history of thyroid disease or autoimmune disorders, then screening is appropriate. The sensitive TSH level should be followed by a free T_4 assay when the TSH level is either undetectable or 10 mU/L or higher.

Hyperthyroidism often occurs spontaneously and can result from the excessive intake of thyroid hormones. Graves' disease is by far the most common cause of spontaneous hyperthyroidism in the United States. An autoimmune disorder characterized by autoreactive, agonistic antibodies to the TSH receptor, Graves' disease accounts for 80 to 90 percent of hyperthyroid cases, peaking in young adults aged 20 to 40 years. It is also the most common form of hyperthyroidism occurring in pregnancy.

Subacute thyroiditis is the most common cause of thyrotoxicosis, accounting for 15 to 20 percent of cases. Characterized by glandular inflammation and follicular cell destruction, it is thought to be of viral etiology, frequently occurring following an acute viral infection. More common in middle-aged adults between 40 and 50 years, women are more likely to develop subacute thyroiditis than men. Silent thyroiditis is a form of subacute thyroiditis in which the thyroid gland is moderately enlarged and nontender. It usually occurs in adults between 30 and 40 years and is also more common in women.

Toxic multinodular goiter (Plummer disease) is as common as subacute thyroiditis, accounting for 15 to 20 percent of thyrotoxicosis cases. This type of goiter is more common in older adults and is a complication of chronic, inactive nodular goiter. This condition is more common in other parts of the world where dietary iodine deficiency is prevalent. A single, toxic thyroid adenoma is the next most common cause of thyrotoxicosis, accounting for 3 to 5 percent of all cases.

The inappropriate use of thyroid replacement or treatment errors may also produce symptoms of hyperthyroidism. Thyrotoxicosis factitia is a form of thyrotoxicosis in which a patient takes excessive amounts of either thyroxine (T_4) or triiodothyronine (T_3). This condition should be considered in a patient with access to hormone supplements or with a psychiatric problem. An excess of dietary iodine may also precipitate symptoms of hyperthyroidism.

A tumor of the pituitary gland causing hypersecretion of TSH (thyrotropin) is a rare cause of hyperthyroidism. Other uncommon causes include metastatic follicular thyroid carcinoma, ingestion of iodine-containing drugs (e.g., certain expectorants, amiodarone, seaweed-containing health food supplements) or iodinated radiocontrast media, choriocarcinoma or hydatidiform molar pregnancy producing high amounts of human chorionic gonadotropin (HCG) which is capable of weakly activating the receptor for TSH, struma ovarii (ectopic thyroid tissue) which is associated with dermoid tumors and ovarian teratomas, and testicular embryonal carcinoma (Table 15.1).

Pathophysiology

All types of hyperthyroidism are a result of overproduction or secretion of thyroid hormones, and the clinical manifestations of hyperthyroidism are a direct result of the effect of excessive thyroid hormones on essentially all organ systems and bodily tissues. While thyroid hormones are required to regulate normal growth and development, excessive release of T_4 and T_3 from the thyroid into the circulation upregulates metabolism, leading to an increase in total body heat production, heart rate and contractility, and vasodilatation. This explains the clinical manifestations of thyrotoxicosis, which include palpitations, diaphoresis, heat intolerance, and anxiety. T_3 is normally 20 to 100 times more biologically active than T_4, which is converted to T_3 in peripheral tissues. Interestingly, degree of symptomatology does not consistently correlate with the extent of thyroid hormone overproduction. In general, younger patients tend to have symptoms more reflective of sympathetic activation (tremors, anxiety, and hyperactivity), while older patients manifest more cardiovascular symptoms including atrial fibrillation and dyspnea, as well as weight loss.

Graves' disease is believed to result from an autoimmune response that may reflect a defect in suppressor T-cell function. Serum evaluation usually reveals the presence of antibodies to the thyroid-stimulating hormone receptor (TSH-R), known as thyroid-stimulating immunoglobulin (TSI). This antibody reacts with the TSH-R on thyroid follicular cells and allows release of thyroid hormones independent of the effects of pituitary TSH. Thyroid hormone levels are typically highest with this form of thyrotoxicosis. Excessive thyroid hormone levels result in thyroid growth (hypertrophy), hypermetabolism, and sympathetic overactivity. Circulating antithyroperoxidase (anti-TPO) is another common finding. A diffusely enlarged goiter involving both thyroid lobes, hyperthyroid ophthalmopathy (periorbital edema, conjunctival edema and injection known as chemosis, proptosis, lid lag, and even diplopia), as well as excessive uptake of radioactive iodine on diagnostic testing are all common characteristics. Graves disease has a higher prevalence in people with human leukocyte antigen (HLA)-DRw3 and HLA-B89. It is also strongly correlated with other autoimmune conditions including vitiligo, type 1 diabetes mellitus, pernicious anemia, myasthenia gravis, or adrenal insufficiency.

Table 15.1 Hyperthyroidism: Common and Rare Causes

	Disorder/Problem	Etiology
Common causes	Graves' disease	Autoimmune disease
	Toxic nodular goiter	Unknown development of nodules that progress from nontoxic to toxic over time
	Subacute thyroiditis	Thought to be caused by viral infection
	Thyrotoxicosis factitia	Excessive ingestion of thyroid hormones
	Jod-Basedow phenomenon	Large intake of iodine in diet in person with thyroid disease
Rare causes	Pituitary adenoma	Rare tumor of the pituitary gland
	Struma ovarii	Rare secretion of thyroid hormones by thyroid tissue located in ovarian dermoid tumors
	Metastatic thyroid cancer	Very rare cause
	High-dose amiodarone	Excessive dosage of iodine containing amiodarone
	Pregnancy and trophoblastic tumors	Very high serum levels of HCG

In contrast, subacute thyroiditis produces symptoms of thyrotoxicosis via the release of preformed thyroid hormones, in response to an inflammatory response following an acute viral infection. Thus, unlike other common causes of thyrotoxicosis including toxic multinodular goiter and an isolated toxic adenoma which involve increased production and hypersecretion of thyroid hormones, subacute thyroiditis demonstrates decreased uptake of radioactive iodine on diagnostic testing. Subacute painful or granulomatous thyroiditis is associated with HLA-Bw35.

Toxic multinodular goiter typically arises in areas on dietary iodine deficiency. As scattered portions of the thyroid gland increase in activity in an attempt to compensate for insufficient iodine, hormonal excess develops slowly over time. In fact, this condition may be asymptomatic at the time of diagnosis, especially in older individuals in whom the classic symptoms of hyperthyroidism may be blunted (a condition termed "apathetic hyperthyroidism").

Nuclear scintigraphy demonstrates scattered areas of both increased and decreased iodine uptake, which reflect the increased thyroidal activity which manifests in the setting of adequate dietary iodine. In contrast, a single hyperfunctioning monoclonal follicular adenoma will demonstrate only a single focus of increased uptake on a radioactive thyroid scan. Such nodules tend to be functional only once they reach at least 2.5 cm in size. As pituitary TSH production is suppressed by the adenoma, the remaining glandular tissue becomes hypofunctional and actually demonstrates decreased uptake on nuclear scintigraphy.

Autoregulation of the thyroid normally prevents thyrotoxicosis in the face of dietary iodine excess, a phenomenon known as the Jod-Basedow effect. However, in the setting of a particularly concentrated iodine load (such as with iodinated radiocontrast media), patients with one or more autonomous thyroid nodules may lose this adaptive capability and be thrown into thyrotoxicosis (Jod-Basedow syndrome).

Clinical Presentation

The clinical presentation of hyperthyroidism depends on the duration and the amount of excessive thyroid hormone secretion. Symptoms are varied and depend on the cause and the multiple organ systems affected. Patients may be asymptomatic in the presence of mild elevations of thyroid hormones; they are more likely to remain asymptomatic at increasing levels if the increased secretion has been gradual.

Subjective

Because thyroid hormones have effects on most organ systems, a complete history and review of systems is indicated. Most patients with hyperthyroidism will complain of some combination of anxiety, nervousness, diaphoresis, fatigue, heat intolerance, palpitations, weight loss, and insomnia. In situations in which the thyroid tissue has become enlarged, the patient may complain of fullness or pressure in the neck. Additional symptoms include weakness, exercise intolerance, tremors, lower extremity edema, weight loss in the presence of an increased appetite, menstrual irregularities, frequent bowel movements or diarrhea, and exertional dyspnea.

Eye complaints include blurred vision, proptosis (downward displacement of the eyeball), photophobia, and double vision. Patients may also report that they are unable to concentrate, extremely irritable, and emotionally labile. Older patients may present with vague symptoms such as unexplained weight loss, apathy, worsening of angina, depression, change in bowel habits, and weakness. A summary of potential signs and symptoms of hyperthyroidism is presented in Table 15.2.

Patients should be questioned about current and prior endocrine diseases (in the patient and family), as well as a personal or family history of thyroid nodules, goiter, use of iodide-containing drugs, and thyroid neoplasms. Radiation to the head and neck increases the risk of thyroid cancer which can produce hyperthyroidism. A weight history should be obtained, including recent and long-term weight patterns. If the patient is currently taking thyroid hormone replacement medication, how the medication is being taken should be assessed. Patients should also be questioned about any recent viral infections or the possibility of pregnancy as well as use of other medications.

Objective

Signs of thyrotoxicosis on physical examination are associated with the various forms of hyperthyroidism and range from overt manifestations in young adults with an acute onset to a more subtle presentation in older adults. Often, the older adult will present with symptoms typically diagnosed as failure to thrive.

On physical examination, the thyroid may be enlarged, nodules may be palpable, and a bruit may be heard over the thyroid gland with the bell of a stethoscope. The neck should be examined for visual enlargement of the thyroid and palpated for lymphadenopathy. The thyroid must be palpated thoroughly, noting any nodules or enlargement, both anteriorly and posteriorly. While the goiter of Graves' disease is often somewhat firm, the thyroid in toxic multinodular goiter may be softer, but with several palpable nodules. The neck should be moderately extended during examination, and water should be provided to the patient to aid swallowing. The thyroid gland moves with swallowing; however, a very large goiter or a large thyroid mass may prevent movement.

In subacute thyroiditis, the patient will present with a firm, painful, thyroid gland enlargement, and possibly a low-grade fever. An enlarged painful thyroid gland is also consistent with degeneration or hemorrhage into a thyroid nodule, as well as either granulomatous or suppurative thyroiditis. In contrast, in silent thyroiditis or subacute lymphocytic thyroiditis, the gland is swollen but not usually tender.

Table 15.2 Hyperthyroidism: Clinical Presentation

Body System	Subjective	Objective
General	Fatigue Weight loss Increased appetite	Muscle atrophy Tremors
Integumentary	Diaphoresis Heat intolerance	Warm, flushed, moist skin Onycholysis Hyperpigmentation Fine and silky hair Thinning hair Dermopathy of legs Pretibial myxedema urticaria Pruritus vitiligo
Gastrointestinal	Diarrhea Increased bowel movements Increased appetite	Increased liver function
Eye	Blurred vision Increased tearing Double vision Decreased visual acuity Photophobia Feelings of increased orbital pressure	Increased exophthalmos Lid lag and edema Corneal ulceration
Neurologic	Tremors of hands	Hyperactive reflexes Tremor
Cardiopulmonary	Palpitations Exertional dyspnea	Sinus tachycardia Elevated blood pressure Symptoms of congestive heart failure Dysrhythmias (atrial fibrillation)
Genitourinary	Menstrual irregularities (decreased menstrual flow)	Gynecomastia
Head and neck	Pressure in neck Increased neck size	Enlarged thyroid gland
Psychosocial	Anxiety Nervousness Insomnia Irritability Emotional lability Restlessness	Increased pulse rate Increased respiratory rate Increased blood pressure
Musculoskeletal	Weakness	Proximal muscle weakness Loss of muscle tone Osteoporosis (post-menopausal women)
Hematologic	Fatigue Breathlessness Palpitations	Normochromic normocytic anemia
Metabolic		Hypercalcemia Potassium wasting Increased alkaline phosphatase

Cardiovascular manifestations include tachycardia (resting heart rate greater than 90 beats per minute), irregular pulse, systolic murmurs, and widening of the pulse pressure. Although rare, an infiltrative dermopathy may be present in the lower extremities, which includes myxedema (deposition of glycosaminoglycan material in the dermis of the lower extremities causing non-pitting pretibial edema), erythema due to an inflammatory cell infiltrate, and skin thickening along the ankles and pretibial areas.

Visual acuity is tested and the patient is assessed for lid lag. Lid lag is assessed by instructing the patient to slowly gaze up and down. As the patient gazes downward, the upper lid will lag behind the globe. Lid lag can also be detected by the globe lagging behind the lower lid as the patient gazes upward. Hyperthyroid ophthalmopathy occurs in 40 percent of patients with Graves' disease and is rare in patients with subacute thyroiditis. The conjunctiva may be inflamed and visual acuity may be affected. Exophthalmos, excessive lacrimation, lid retraction, and lid lag may be present.

The examiner should assess the skin for edema, general appearance, and signs of thinning hair. The skin may be moist and velvety to the touch, with increased pigmentation, spider angiomas, and vitiligo. Onycholysis (splitting and spooning of the nails) may be present.

Deep tendon reflexes (DTR) may show a rapid relaxation of the reflex and the most predominant hyperactive reflex is usually the Achilles tendon reflex. The patient may have decreased strength in the extremities and fine tremors, especially of the hands when the arms are fully outstretched. Lymphadenopathy and splenomegaly may also be present. A few patients may also have nonpitting pretibial edema.

Patients with long-standing hyperthyroidism may also have clubbing of the digits and signs of new bone growth in the hands, termed *thyroid acropachy.* Older adults with hyperthyroidism often appear apathetic. Physical examination may reveal atrial fibrillation (present in one-third of all older adults with hyperthyroidism), fine skin, brittle nails, and symptoms of CHF. The thyroid gland is often not enlarged in older adults.

Thyroid storm or crisis is a severe, sometimes fatal form of hyperthyroidism and requires immediate emergency medical care. Assessment, contributing factors, and treatment are listed in Table 15.3.

Diagnostic Reasoning

Diagnostic Tests

Initial Testing. Laboratory examination is undertaken with the understanding that in many situations, levels of thyroid hormone often do not correlate reliably with Clinical Presentation. The initial screening tests for hyperthyroidism are measurement of the serum TSH and the free thyroxine immunoassay (FT_4).

In most cases of hyperthyroidism, a TSH level less than 0.35 μIU/mL usually accompanies an elevated FT_4 measurement (above 12.5 μg/dL). Although some laboratories have only recently acquired the ability to measure free T_4, measures of free thyroxine is generally preferred over total T_4 because it measures the level of T_4 unbound to carrier proteins, which is, therefore, biologically active. In turn, a significant number of medications may alter the laboratory results due to alterations in protein binding. These include anabolic steroids, androgens, estrogens, heparin, iodine-containing compounds, phenytoin (Dilantin), rifampin (Rimactane, Rifadin), and salicylates.

If the FT_4 is normal, a T_3 level should be obtained because about 5 percent of hyperthyroid patients have normal T_4 levels, but elevated T_3 levels.

Subsequent Testing. Subsequent testing includes more sophisticated measurement of TSH levels. These tests (third generation) can detect TSH levels as low as 0.01 μIU/mL. In Graves' disease, antithyroglobulin and antimicrosomal antibodies are elevated. A TSH receptor antibody test is usu-

Table 15.3 Thyroid Storm/Crisis

Contributing factors	Acute infection Trauma Stress in patient with hyperthyroidism Uncontrolled diabetes mellitus Severe drug reaction Following withdrawal of antithyroid medication or radioactive iodine therapy
Symptoms: initial	Fever (usually initial symptom), often >100.4°F Nausea Abdominal pain Vomiting
Symptoms: progressive	Severe agitation, occasional psychosis Elevated temperature Diaphoresis Tachycardia, congestive heart failure Dysrhythmia (atrial fibrillation or flutter) Confusion Cardiovascular collapse Malignant exophthalmos Elevated free thyroid hormone (T_4) levels but no more increased than in hyperthyroidism; clinical diagnosis, not biochemical
Management	Hospitalization and aggressive reversal of thyrotoxins 1. To block thyroid hormone synthesis, give propylthiouracil (PTU) 300–900 mg/day in 4 divided doses (q6h), then as symptoms resolve give 50–600 mg PTU qd (2–4 divided doses) 2. To alleviate the beta-adrenergic symptoms of hyperthyroidism, give propranolol (Inderal) 60–80 mg q4–6h IV, or 0.5–1 mg/min. 3. To block T_4 and T_3 conversion, give hydrocortisone 50 g IV q8h. If radioactive iodine is prescribed but is not to be given in the next few days, potassium iodide oral solution (SSKI) 5 gtts q6h or telepaque 500–1000 mg q12h may be given. 4. Supportive measures—decrease fever, treat underlying infection, give fluids (3–5 L/day) and glucose.

ally elevated in Graves' disease and is part of subsequent testing. The diagnosis of thyrotoxicosis is considered in cases of hyperthyroidism when TSH levels are depressed and measurements of T_4 are normal.

Nuclear scintigraphy with radiolabeled iodine (^{123}I) or technetium (^{99}Tc) helps in assessing the functional status of the thyroid gland. A 24-hour radioadsorbed iodine uptake (RAIU) test can differentiate Graves' disease from subacute thyroiditis and toxic nodular goiters, thereby refining treatment recommendations. It identifies areas of increased and decreased thyroid function, often termed "hot" and "cold" spots, within the gland. Patients with a toxic nodular goiter and Graves' disease have a high RAIU, while in subacute thyroiditis, iodine uptake is low. Importantly, however, toxic adenoma and toxic multinodular goiter both present with areas of decreased isotope uptake as well, as the hyperfunctioning nodules lead to suppression of TSH via negative hormonal feedback. A thyroid scan is critical to determining functionality of any dominant thyroid nodule in a patient presenting with thyrotoxicosis, as cold nodules are highly suspicious for concomitant malignancy and must be evaluated further.

An ultrasound of the thyroid will assist in differentiating a cyst from a nodule. A pure thyroid cyst is less likely to be malignant than a nodule. A fine-needle biopsy is the preferred initial diagnostic technique for evaluation of thyroid masses, particularly solid masses, to rule out malignancy. Magnetic resonance imaging (MRI) is the preferred test to assess for ophthalmopathy resulting from Graves' disease. It is especially beneficial in ruling out an orbital tumor.

Differential Diagnosis

Thyrotoxicosis, with high levels of TSH, is seen in a rare pituitary tumor. Excessive exogenous thyroid administration will produce the same symptoms seen in thyrotoxicosis. Thyroid cancer must be considered when the thyroid gland is hard and enlarged or when nodules are palpated.

T_4 levels may be elevated in acute illnesses such as hepatitis, in the presence of elevated estrogen levels, acute psychiatric problems, hyperemesis, familial thyroid hormone binding abnormalities, and autoimmunity. Dopamine (Intropin, Dopastat) and high dosages of glucocorticoids may decrease TSH levels. Drugs that may increase T_4 levels are amiodarone (Cordarone), amphetamines, clofibrate (Atromid-S), glucocorticoids in high doses, heparin administered during dialysis, heroin, levothyroxine (Synthroid), methadone (Dolophine), and perphenzine (Trilafon).

Management

Treatment of hyperthyroidism differs depending on the cause and patient characteristics. A euthyroid state is the goal of treatment, while minimizing the adverse effects of treatment and decreasing the incidence of hypothyroidism.

Emergency treatment is necessary if the patient presents in thyroid storm (Table 18.3). The patient should be hospitalized for oral and intravenous hydration, if needed, and immediately begin thyroid-blocking medications, beta-adrenergic blockers, and corticosteroids if signs of ophthalmopathy are present. Patients intolerant of beta-blockers (asthmatics, patients with COPD) may be treated with calcium channel blockers as an alternate therapy. Supportive measures include treating any underlying infection, managing fever with antipyretics, hydration, and correcting any fluid and electrolyte imbalance.

Multinodular and uninodular goiters should be referred to an endocrinologist for evaluation of possible malignancy. Nonmalignant thyroid nodular disease with laboratory evaluations indicating hyperthyroidism are most often treated with radioactive iodine.

Management of Graves' Disease

The three treatment options for Graves' disease include antithyroid drugs, radioactive iodine, and surgery. None of these treatments alters the underlying autoimmune process of Graves' disease. The most successful treatment in achieving a permanent euthyroid state is surgery; however, it is rarely the preferred method of treatment unless the thyroid gland is extremely enlarged and is pressing on other structures in the neck. Many patients treated with radioactive iodine will experience a relapse and require a second treatment. Radioactive iodine also may worsen ophthalmopathy if present.

Pharmacologic Therapy. Patients experiencing tachycardia, palpitations, or tremor benefit from the introduction of a beta-blocker during initiation of therapy. Beta-blockers provide effective, short-term relief of hyperadrenergic symptoms. Use of a beta-blocker is contraindicated in patients with bronchospasm or uncompensated heart failure. It is used cautiously in patients who take insulin for diabetes mellitus (DM) because it may block symptoms of hypoglycemia. Propranolol (Inderal) 10 to 60 mg q6h is usually given initially to control symptoms at the start of radioactive iodine therapy. Response to initial treatment is evaluated weekly or more often if symptoms are not relieved on initial dose. The average dose is 80 mg qd. Other alternatives include atenolol (Tenormin) 50 to 200 mg qd or a long-acting beta-blocker, propranolol HCl (Inderal LA) 80 to 160 mg, given once daily. As stated previously, calcium channel blockers are an option in patients for whom beta-blockers are contraindicated; however, this class of drug should also be avoided in patients with uncompensated heart failure, given their propensity to decrease inotropy (cardiac contractility).

Antithyroid medications work by inhibiting thyroid hormone synthesis at multiple steps. They are used as a primary treatment to reduce the level of hormone on initiation of radioactive iodine therapy, as well as preceding and following thyroid surgery. These drugs take time to achieve their peak effect, however, and hormone levels may not be significantly decreased for up to 2 to 8 weeks.

Two antithyroid drugs are presently being used—propylthiouracil (PTU) and methimazole (MMI). These drugs are the treatment of choice for pregnant women, especially PTU, because it is less likely to cross the placenta than MMI. They are often used in persons awaiting surgical intervention and in patients of childbearing age. Antithyroid drug treatment is often the preferred treatment in the patient without significant thyroid gland enlargement. PTU has an added therapeutic effect of inhibiting T_3 activity and preventing peripheral conversion of T_4 into T_3—the more biologically active of the two main thyroid hormones. Thus, it is useful in cases of thyrotoxicosis to rapidly reduce hyperthyroid symptoms.

PTU is usually started at doses of 50 to 100 mg PO tid. MMI (Tapazole) is given at an initial dosage 10 to 20 mg q8h or 30 to 60 mg PO qd. The dosage is titrated every 3 to 4 weeks based on thyroxine levels and TSH levels. TSH and T_4 levels are evaluated every visit and a targeted history and physical is performed to monitor therapeutic response. (See Drugs Commonly Prescribed 15.1 for hyperthyroidism.)

Because of the amount of thyroid hormone stored in the thyroid gland, it may take 2 to 8 weeks to see a therapeutic response to antithyroid medication. These drugs are not indicated for long-term use because more than one-half of patients on these drugs alone experience resumption of symptoms. Once the patient has achieved a euthyroid state, the frequency of follow-up visits is extended to every 4 to 6 weeks for a period of 3 to 4 months. If the TSH and free T_4 remain stable during this time, the follow-up is extended to every 3 to 4 months. Patients taking antithyroid medication should have a serum FT_4 level evaluated with TSH levels, because the TSH level may remain suppressed due to chronic hyperthyroidism long after T_4 levels are decreased.

Common adverse reactions to antithyroid medications include rash, urticaria, and arthralgias which may occur in 1 to 5 percent of patients. Rare but serious adverse reactions include agranulocytosis, aplastic anemia, and hepatitis, which may occur in up to 0.5 percent of patients taking antithyroid medications. Except for agranulocytosis which is more common with MMI, these reactions are more likely to occur with PTU. Thus, patients taking these drugs should be instructed to report immediately any signs of infection, especially a fever, sore throat, malaise, or mouth sores. The antithyroid medication must be discontinued immediately if any of these symptoms are experienced. The patient is often changed to a regimen of radioactive iodine to produce a euthyroid state. Agranulocytosis may take up to 10 to 14 days to fully resolve after the medication is stopped and may require concommitant administration of granulocyte-colony stimulating factor (filgrastim).

Before initiation of antithyroid therapy, a baseline CBC and liver function tests (LFTs) including hepatic aminotransferases (AST, ALT) should be obtained. During therapy, the white blood cell count (WBC) is checked every 2 weeks during the first month and then every 4 to 6 months after than. Liver enzymes should be evaluated every 3 to 6 months.

Antithyroid drugs (Drugs Commonly Prescribed 15.1) are used for 6 to 24 months following achievement of a euthyroid state. The dosage is then gradually decreased until the drug is withdrawn. The patient is followed every 1 to 2 months initially following cessation of therapy for a possible relapse. Many patients will experience a permanent remission following a 1- to 2-year course of antithyroid medications.

Radioactive Iodine. Radioactive iodine-131 (^{131}I; Iodotope) is the treatment of choice for hyperthyroidism in the United States, especially in middle-aged or older adults. Typically, a 24-hour radioiodine uptake dose of 75 to 150 µCi per gram of estimated thyroid tissue is administered orally, which concentrates in overactive thyroid cells where it emits radiation, causing inflammation and the ultimate destruction of the pathologic cells. It is less invasive than thyroidectomy, is

Drugs Commonly Prescribed 15.1: Hyperthyroidism

Drug	Indication	Dosage	Adverse Reactions
Propylthiouracil (PTU)	Hyperthyroidism	Dose: 300–900 mg PO qd or in 3 divided doses initially Maintenance: 100–150 mg qd or in divided doses	Common: pruritus, drowsiness, allergic dermatitis, nausea, vomiting, arthralgia Rare: agranulocytosis Onset of PO: 10–21 days Peak of PO: 6–10 weeks Duration of PO: 1–4 weeks
Methimazole (MMI) (Tapazole)	Hyperthyroidism	Initial: 15–60 mg PO qd in three divided doses depending on severity of disease	Common: pruritus, drowsiness, allergic dermatitis, nausea, parotitis, arthralgia Rare: agranulocytosis Onset: 1 week Peak: 4–10 weeks Duration: 36–72 hours

a targeted therapy that is focused solely on the thyroid, and does not require hospitalization. Although response to this therapy is slower than with antithyroid drugs or surgical excision, radioablation is indicated in patients who have a poor response to antithyroid medication, as well as in cases of toxic multinodular goiter. It is contraindicated in pregnancy and during breast-feeding, however.

Women receiving radioactive iodine therapy should refrain from becoming pregnant for 4 months after therapy. T_4 levels need to be checked monthly for 3 months after the administration of radioactive iodine in patients receiving radioactive thyroid ablation therapy. Euthyroid patients should be assessed every 3 to 6 months for hypothyroidism by monitoring the FT_4 and sensitive TSH levels. Hypothyroidism may occur at any time, but is most likely to present during the first year. Some patients will fail treatment and require a second dose. First-time failure rates may be as high as 45 percent but about 70 percent of patients receiving radioactive iodine therapy eventually develop hypothyroidism.

Hyperthyroid ophthalmopathy is often exacerbated with radioactive iodine treatment; however, research has found that the incidence of ophthalmopathy is reduced when prednisone (0.4 mg/kg) is given concurrently with radioactive iodine treatments. If ophthalmopathy occurs, the patient requires referral to an ophthalmologist. Treatment often includes diuretics and ophthalmic prednisone. Methylcellulose eye drops (Tear Naturale) are useful to protect against excessive eye dryness.

A nonradioactive alternative to thyroid radioablation for severe Graves' disease or subacute thyroiditis involves administering a large quantity of concentrated iodine as a saturated solution of potassium iodide (SSKI, 35 to 50 mg iodide per drop, 1 to 2 gtts in water PO bid; Lugol solution, 8 mg iodide per drop, 3 to 5 gtts in water PO tid) or iopanoic acid (Telepaque, 1 to 3 g PO or 0.5 g PO bid). These concentrated iodine therapies effectively block the conversion of T_4 to T_3 and inhibit the release of thyroid hormones. SSKI and Lugol solution should not be used when autonomous thyroid nodules are present, however, such as in toxic multinodular goiter or toxic adenoma, as they may worsen thyrotoxicosis. In addition, these therapies are generally only used in severe cases of thyrotoxicosis, as their use precludes definitive therapy with radioactive iodine for several months, as the thyroid must first process out the iodine load.

Surgery. Surgery (subtotal or total thyroidectomy) is required for patients with compressive symptoms of the neck such as hoarseness (from compression of the recurrent laryngeal nerve) or respiratory stridor, which indicates displacement of the trachea. It may also be considered for cosmetic reasons and for patients who have failed other treatment options. Surgery is often recommended in a patient with a large gland, multinodular goiter, or when thyroid cancer is suspected. It is also indicated in individuals who cannot tolerate antithyroid medication; however, an antithyroid medication may be administered during the initiation of therapy to prevent excessive release of stored thyroid hormones. In addition, propranolol is typically used to decrease the resting heart rate to below 80 beats per minute, and SSKI may be administered (1 to 2 gtts PO bid) for 2 weeks before surgical resection. Before the development of these preoperative pharmacotherapies, thyroidectomy was one of the most common causes of thyroid storm. Today, important complications of surgery include permanent hypothyroidism, which will require lifelong thyroid hormone replacement, and laryngeal paralysis via damage to the recurrent laryngeal nerve. Hypoparathyroidism may also result if one or more of the parathyroid glands are inadvertently resected during surgery.

Management of Subacute Thyroiditis

Subacute thyroiditis is a self-limiting condition treated with anti-inflammatory agents and prednisone. It often follows a viral illness. Following the thyroiditis, some patients may experience a transient hypothyroid state. These patients will need thyroid hormone until they return to a euthyroid state. The use of propanolol (Inderal) and antithyroid medications is not necessary unless the patient has overt thyrotoxic symptoms. For the patient with severe pain, a nonsteroidal anti-inflammatory drug (NSAID) may help. Short-term use of oral prednisone (Deltsone) may be indicated for severe inflammation and pain. Doses of 20 to 40 mg bid are usually effective.

Management of Subclinical Hyperthyroidism

The treatment of subclinical hyperthyroidism remains controversial. Subclinical hyperthyroidism is characterized by undetectable TSH levels and normal levels of T_4 and T_3. Consultation with an endocrinologist is indicated. If treatment is not initiated, the patient should be monitored annually for overt hyperthyroidism.

Patients experiencing symptoms of infiltrative ophthalmopathy will need to be followed by an ophthalmologist. Glucocorticoids, diuretics, and methylcellulose eye drops may provide symptomatic relief. Radiation or surgical decompression may be initiated by the ophthalmologist in severe cases.

Follow-Up and Referral

The complex nature of thyrotoxicosis requires referral to an endocrinologist for effective management and close follow-up. Importantly, up to half of all patients with Graves' disease who go into remission after starting antithyroid pharmacotherapy without definitive thyroid ablation will have a second attack of thyrotoxicosis within 1 year. In addition, all patients with Graves' disease should be referred to an ophthalmologist for full evaluation, as up to half of these patients have some form of ophthalmopathy, which may present subclinically. In contrast, Graves' disease ophthalmopathy may present prior to developing symptoms of full-blown thyrotoxicosis.

Specific time frames for follow-up are dependent on the treatment and patient response. TSH and T_4 levels should be monitored at each follow-up visit as well as measurement of blood pressure, pulse, weight, and character of the thyroid gland. General guidelines include the following:

1. Monitor thyroid function tests at least twice a year.
2. Initial treatment should be evaluated at 1 month and at 3 months or more frequently if the patient is symptomatic.
3. Therapy with antithyroid medications should continue for 3 to 12 months.
4. After radioiodine therapy, thyroid function tests should be performed at 6 weeks, 12 weeks, 6 months, and annually thereafter.

Patient Education

After diagnosis, the patient with hyperthyroidism must be provided with the various treatment options available. The risks and benefits of each treatment must be explained. The importance of strict adherence to provider guidelines for follow-up must be stressed to each patient. If the treatment regimen has produced a state of hypothyroidism, the patient is informed that thyroid replacement therapy must continue for life.

Patients must be instructed that it takes 4 to 6 weeks after medication begins to notice an improvement in symptoms because of the amount of stored hormone in the thyroid gland. Patients who are unaware of this phenomenon may not comply with the treatment regimen. Patients need written instructions for the signs and symptoms of thyroid storm, as well as signs of hypothyroidism once treatment is initiated. The patient should be informed of all potential adverse reactions of all medications, particularly those of antithyroid preparations and to discontinue the medication and to call their primary-care provider if a fever, sore throat, or malaise develops.

Persons receiving radioactive iodine therapy should avoid contact with infants, children, and pregnant women for 7 days following ingestion. Women who receive this treatment postpartum must not breast-feed for at least 3 to 6 months, as radioactive iodine is excreted in breast milk and can ablate the infant's thyroid.

The need for adequate rest and exercise should be stressed. Patients will need adequate sleep as well as relaxation time and should be taught methods to promote relaxation, such as biofeedback, music, or guided imagery. Patients should be encouraged to express their concerns regarding psychosocial implications of their disease and the physiologic basis for their symptoms should be reinforced.

Patients who complain of heat intolerance may benefit from wearing or sleeping on natural fabrics during the summer months and should remain adequately hydrated. Patients who have experienced significant weight loss may benefit from a high-carbohydrate, high-caloric diet. A patient with Graves' disease may benefit from dividing food intake into six smaller meals daily. If diarrhea is a problem, discourage foods that increase peristalsis such as highly seasoned foods and bulky or fibrous foods. The patient should check his or her weight daily and report any weight loss of more than 4 pounds in 1 day immediately. A consistent weight loss of 1 to 2 pounds daily should also be reported. A supplemental multivitamin, particularly with vitamin B complex, is needed to prevent deficiencies in times of severe hyperthyroidism because of a high level of vitamin consumption during states of elevated thyroid hormones.

Once treatment is initiated and the patient is euthyroid, caloric needs decrease but the patient may still have an increased appetite. A sensible diet low in fat and sugar with adequate protein may avoid a significant unwanted weight gain during this period. The patient should be instructed to check his or her weight frequently and to adjust intake to maintain an ideal weight. Stimulants such as caffeine should be avoided. A multivitamin is often indicated for the patient who has sustained thyrotoxicity. Patients suspected of having long-standing hyperthyroidism may benefit from vitamin D and calcium supplementation since osteoporosis is a complication of elevated thyroid hormones.

Some patients may experience depression as the levels of thyroid hormones change and this should be explained. The patient should be instructed to report any worsening of symptoms of depression. If the patient presents with signs or symptoms of depression or anxiety, they should be evaluated for depression or anxiety. If reassurance does not relieve anxiety, temporary symptomatic treatment may be indicated.

Patients with exophthalmos should wear dark lenses outdoors during the day. The use of artificial tears may relieve feelings of dryness and provide some corneal protection. Glasses or eye protection should be worn during any activity that may introduce dust or dirt into the eyes. A sleeping mask should be worn at night if the patient cannot close the eyes adequately. Elevating the head of the bed at night and restricting sodium intake may relieve edema.

Patients taking antithyroid medications should wear a medical identification bracelet.

Hypothyroidism

Hypothyroidism is a common, treatable disorder in which there is a slow progression of thyroid hypofunction, followed by signs and symptoms indicating thyroid failure. It is a disease of various causes that lead to inadequate amounts of thyroid hormone being produced and/or secreted, resulting in a slowing of many body functions and metabolic processes. Because hypothyroidism has an insidious onset and progresses slowly, the clinical manifestations may go unrecognized.

Thyroid hormone deficiency present at birth was historically called *cretinism* but is now known by the less pejorative term *congenital hypothyroidism.* Affecting 1 in 4000 newborns, the causes of congenital hypothyroidism include developmental abnormalities of the thyroid gland, enzymatic defects, iodine deficiency, maternal antibodies to thyroid hormones, and excessive intake of goitrogens by the mother. In such instances, the mother may also suffer from thyroid deficiency. Thyroid hormone deficiency beginning in early infancy and childhood is characterized by growth retardation, mental deficiency, and delayed dentition. Adolescents with primary hypothyroidism may manifest an enlarged sella turcica and, rarely, precocious puberty, in addition to growth retardation. Growth retardation is treatable with hormone replacement therapy, but mental retardation persists.

Epidemiology and Causes

The incidence of hypothyroidism varies with age, gender, and geographic and environmental factors. The incidence from numerous surveys ranges from 3 to 14 cases per 1000 women, with significantly fewer cases reported in men. In fact, the incidence in women is 2 to 8 times greater than it is in men. It is estimated that as many as 4.6 percent of the United States population has an elevated TSH with a higher incidence in whites (5.1 percent) than either Hispanic (4.1 percent) or African American (1.7 percent).

The most common worldwide cause of thyroid disorders is iodine deficiency with worldwide prevalence of 2 to 5 percent. In the United States, where iodine ingestion is usually adequate, autoimmune processes are the primary cause of thyroid disease. Hashimoto's thyroiditis, a type of primary hypothyroidism, is the most common form of autoimmune thyroid disease. This type of hypothyroidism occurs at least four times more often in women than men, with the average age of onset from 30 to 60 years.

Iatrogenic hypothyroidism, which occurs following treatment with radioactive iodine (for hyperthyroidism) or surgery (for hyperthyroidism, thyroid nodules, or carcinoma) is the next most common cause of hypothyroidism, accounting for 30 to 40 percent of the cases. Hypothyroidism also becomes increasingly common with age; in individuals over age 50, up to 10 percent may have elevated TSH levels.

More than 95 percent of patients with hypothyroidism have primary or thyroidal hypothyroidism, involving dysfunction or atrophy of the thyroid gland. When the thyroid dysfunction is caused by failure of the pituitary gland, the hypothalamus, or both, it is known as central hypothyroidism. More specifically, secondary hypothyroidism refers to the failure of the pituitary gland to secrete adequate amounts of TSH. Tertiary hypothyroidism is a type of hypothyroidism resulting in inadequate secretion of thyrotropin-releasing hormone (TRH) by the hypothalamus or failure of TRH to activate its cognate receptors within the pituitary (peripheral resistance). Table 15.4 summarizes the causes of hypothyroidism.

Although one in five women will develop an alteration in thyroid function in her lifetime, recently published clinical guidelines do not recommend routine screening of asymptomatic women before age 50 years. Many clinicians, however, still use age 40 years as their criterion to begin screening. All patients with a prior history of any medically or surgically treated thyroid disease should be screened with a serum TSH measurement yearly. In addition, patients with other autoimmune diseases and those with unexplained depression, DM, cognitive dysfunction, prior external radiation to the head and neck, hypercholesterolemia, or other risk factors should be screened with TSH measurements. Women experiencing unexplained infertility should be screened for thyroid dysfunction, and

Table 15.4 Causes of Hypothyroidism

Cause	Etiology
Loss of functional thyroid tissue	• Idiopathic hypothyroidism: atrophy (probably autoimmune), TSH receptor-blocking antibodies • Chronic autoimmune thyroiditis (Hashimoto's disease), subacute, postpartum, treatment with cytokines or amiodarone, external radiation • Status post (S/P) ^{131}I treatment • S/P thyroidectomy • Infiltrating disorders: malignancy, granulomatous disease • Thyroid dysgenesis
Biosynthetic defects in thyroid hormone production	• Inherited defects in hormone synthesis • Iodine deficiency • Antithyroid agents: thioamides, lithium, iodide
Central hypothyroidism	• TSH deficiency caused by pituitary disease: postpartum infarction, tumors, granulomatous disease (sarcoidosis), irradiation, idiopathic • TRH deficiency caused by hypothalmic disease: tumor (e.g., craniopharyngioma), irradiation, and transiently occurring nonthyroidal illness • Peripheral resistance to TRH by the pituitary
Transient hypothyroidism	• Postpartum thyroiditis • Subacute thyroiditis (usually viral) • Withdrawal of thyroid hormone therapy in a euthyroid patient.

postpartum women with vague complaints may benefit from screening.

Risk factors for thyroid failure include a family history of thyroid disease; personal history of thyroid disease; presence of antithyroid antibodies; radiation treatment to the head, neck, or chest; other autoimmune disease; old age; and use of lithium, amiodarone (Cordarone), or iodine.

Although production of T_4 decreases with age, serum T_4 and TSH levels remain stable, whereas T_3 levels may decrease in persons older than age 80 years. In many cases, hypothyroidism in the older adult is characterized by symptoms that may be subtle and similar to the normal signs of aging, thus making it easy to overlook. Common symptoms include hoarsenss, deafness, confusion, frank psychosis, dementia, ataxia, depression, constipation, intolerance of cold temperatures, dry skin, or hair loss. As many as 15 percent of patients older than age 65 years, as well as many other adults, have normal FT_4 and elevated TSH levels, but few report hypothyroid symptoms or they report nonspecific symptoms. This condition is called *subclinical hypothyroidism.*

Pathophysiology

Normal thyroid function is required for every metabolic process in the human body. Growth and development, protein synthesis, and cell metabolism are all dependent on an adequate supply of thyroid hormone to the peripheral tissues. The thyroid plays an essential role in fetal development, oxygen consumption, heat production, sympathetic nervous system function, and cardiovascular, hematopoietic, pulmonary, and renal system function. Because of the multiple physiologic effects of the thyroid gland, a deficiency of the T_4 hormone can lead to a complex array of clinical findings.

Localized thyroid disease is the most common cause of hypothyroidism in the United States, namely Hashimoto's autoimmune thyroiditis, while worldwide, iodine deficiency is the primary etiology, as this element is a critical component of all thyroid hormones and incorporation of iodide molecules is a critical step in thyroid hormone synthesis. Under normal circumstances, the thyroid secretes 100 to 125 μg of thyroxine (T_4) per day, but only minute amounts of triiodothyronine (T_3). T_4 is converted to T_3 in peripheral tissues, and T_3 is 20 to 100 times more biologically active than T_4.

When the production of T_4 is inadequate, the thyroid gland enlarges in response to increasing levels of pituitary TSH. This stimulates hypertrophy and hyperplasia of the thyroid gland, resulting in a *goiter*. In addition, deiodinase activity within the thyroid is increased, allowing for greater conversion of T_4 to T_3. Thus, the thyroid attempts to compensate by secreting increased amounts of T_3. However, in areas where the soil and water are deficient in iodine, inadequate substrate exists for these compensatory mechanisms, and endemic goiter results. Thus, a simple (nontoxic) goiter is the most common type of thyroid enlargement.

Hashimoto's thyroiditis is the most common etiology of hypothyroidism in the United States. This autoimmune form of hypothyroidism results when the body pathologically recognizes thyroid antigens as foreign, leading to a chronic immune response involving lymphocytic infiltration, vacuolization, and fibrosis of the parenchyma, which eventually leads to atrophy of the thyroid follicles. Autoantibodies may be undetectable early on in the disease process. However, over the course of the disease, up to 95 percent of these patients demonstrate serum antibodies to thyroid tissue including antimicrosomal (antithyroperoxidase) antibodies (95 percent of patients) and antithyroglobulin antibodies (60 percent of patients). Over time, however, these autoantibodies usually become undetectable.

Inflammatory hypofunctioning thyroiditis may also result from other etiologies. Destructive thyroid inflammation may occur due to immune cross-reactivity following viral infections, producing transient forms of hypothyroidism including de Quervain or painful thyroiditis, as well as subacute thyroiditis. In addition to a painful and tender thyroid gland, these patients are often significantly fatigued. Lymphocytic thyroiditis and transient hypothyroidism also occurs in up to 10 percent of new mothers 2 to 10 months postpartum. This figure may rise as high as 25 percent in those with other autoimmune conditions such as type 1 diabetes mellitus. While this condition is usually transient lasting less than 4 months and responds well to short courses of thyroid hormone replacement, postpartum thyroiditis predisposes these women to long-term hypothyroidism in the future.

Several iatrogenic causes of hypothyroidism have been recognized. Amiodarone (Cordarone), an iodinc-containing anti-arrhythmic, is one of the best known offenders because of its direct effects on the thyroid gland. However, both dopamine and lithium are associated with central (secondary or tertiary) hypothyroidism owing to their effects on the hypothalamic–pituitary axis and the secretion of either thyrotropin-releasing hormone (TRH) from the hypothalamus or thyroid-stimulating hormone (TSH) from the pituitary gland. Interferon-α, thalidomide, and the antiretroviral agent stavudine have also been associated with primary hypothyroidism.

Central hypothyroidism may also result from direct impingement by tumors on the pituitary gland (e.g., a pituitary adenoma that fails to produce TSH) or the hypothalamus. Brain irradiation has also been associated with subsequent defects along the hypothalamic–pituitary hormonal axis. However, by far the most common reason for iatrogenic hypothyroidism is the therapeutic result of previously treated hyperthyroidism (see previous section on Hyperthyroidism in this chapter). Radioactive iodine treatment (^{131}I, Iodotope), concentrated iodine therapy (SSKI, Lugol solution), therapeutic surgical resection, or treatment for head and neck cancer involving external beam irradiation to the neck or surgical excision of a cancerous mass may all result in permanent hypothyroidism. Thus, these patients require close follow-up to detect clinical or biochemical evidence of hypothyroidism.

Low levels of thyroid hormones affect virtually every bodily system, resulting in an overall decrease in basal metabolic rate. An insufficient amount of thyroid hormone causes abnormalities in lipid metabolism, with an increase in total cholesterol, low-density lipoproteins, and triglycerides. These increases are associated with the development of atherosclerosis and cardiac disease in the hypothyroid patient. The gastrointestinal tract may be slowed in both gastric emptying and intestinal transit time, while gastric parietal cell dysfunction may result in achlorhydria and impaired digestion. Endocrine abnormalities of hypothyroidism include menstrual irregularities, infertility, delayed onset of puberty, and insulin resistance. Adequate amounts of thyroid hormone are also necessary for optimal erythropoiesis, and anemia is common in patients with hypothyroidism. Deficiencies in vitamin B_{12}, iron, and folate may also occur.

A characteristic pathophysiologic change of hypothyroidism is the accumulation of hydrophilic proteoglycans within the interstitial space, which causes an increase in interstitial fluid. Pleural, cardiac, and peritoneal effusions are a common result of this process, as is the characteristic mucinous edema seen in long-standing hypothyroidism, known as myxedema. In a general sense, myxedema denotes infiltration of various bodily tissues with glycosaminoglycan substances, which may have widespread effects. In the heart, this infiltration decreases both chronotropy and inotropy, leading to cardiac hypertrophy as the body attempts to compensate for the decreased cardiac output.

Untreated hypothyroidism may progress steadily for 10 to 15 years before resulting in *myxedema coma*—a life-threatening state of multiorgan failure, characterized by progressive respiratory depression, decreased cardiac output, and fluid and electrolyte abnormalities including hyponatremia—or even death. Table 15.5 presents the assessment and management of the patient with myxedema coma.

Clinical Presentation

Subjective

The clinical presentation of the patient with hypothyroidism varies with the age at onset, duration of illness, and severity of disease. Regardless of the type or cause of hypothyroidism, the signs and symptoms are similar. Because this can be an insidious disease, the early symptoms are often subtle and nonspecific, increasing the risk of a missed diagnosis. The severity of symptoms may be related to the

Table 15.5 Assessment and Management of Myxedema Coma

Untreated hypothyroidism may progress steadily for 10–15 years before resulting in myxedema coma (a life-threatening condition characterized by progressive respiratory depression, decreased cardiac output, and fluid and electrolyte abnormalities) or death. Myxedema coma is severe hypothyroidism, most commonly seen in older adult women, presenting with altered mental status (profound lethargy or coma), hypothermia, bradycardia, hypoventilation, hypoglycemia, and adrenal insufficiency. It is usually triggered by a precipitating factor such as noncompliance with levothyroxine therapy, ingestion of narcotics or analgesics, sepsis, cerebral vascular accident (CVA), myocardial infarction (MI), trauma, or severe stress. The mortality rate can be greater than 50% despite emergency medical intervention.

Assessment

The patient is usually pale with periorbital edema, dry skin, decreased temperature, macroglossia, distant heart sounds, bradycardia, and delayed deep tendon reflexes. The patient may have hyponatremia, seizures, and hypotension, with secondary respiratory acidosis, hypoxia, retention of CO_2. Clinical diagnosis, not laboratory diagnosis, is required, but T_4 is usually low and TSH is high.

Management

Give ventilatory support if indicated, treat hypothermia and give levothyroxine (Synthroid, Levothroid) IV 300–500 μg over 15 min; then IV 100 μg q24h to bring thyroxine concentrations back to normal quickly. Glucocorticoids should also be administered until coexistent adrenal insufficiency can be ruled out. Hydrocortisone hemisuccinate 100 mg IV bolus is initially given, followed by 50 mg IV q12h or 25 mg IV q6h until plasma cortisol level is confirmed as normal. Administer IV hydration to correct hypotension and hypoglycemia (if present). Avoid overhydration because clearance of free water is impaired in these patients. Rule out and treat precipitating factors (if septic, treat with antibiotics). Patients with myxedema coma need emergency medical intervention and should be treated by an endocrinologist in an intensive care setting.

- Idiopathic hypothyroidism: atrophy (probably autoimmune), TSH receptor-blocking antibodies
- Chronic autoimmune thyroiditis (Hashimoto's disease), subacute, postpartum, treatment with cytokines or amiodarone, external radiation
- Status post (S/P) ^{131}I treatment
- S/P thyroidectomy
- Infiltrating disorders: malignancy, granulomatous disease
- Thyroid dysgenesis
- Inherited defects in hormone synthesis
- Iodine deficiency
- Antithyroid agents: thioamides, lithium, iodide
- TSH deficiency caused by pituitary disease: postpartum infarction, tumors, granulomatous disease (sarcoidosis), irradiation, idiopathic
- TRH deficiency caused by hypothalamic disease: tumor (e.g., craniopharyngioma), irradiation, and transiently occurring nonthyroid illness
- Peripheral resistance to TRH by the pituitary
- Postpartum thyroiditis
- Subacute thyroiditis (usually viral)
- Withdrawal of thyroid hormone therapy in a euthyroid patient.

duration of hypothyroidism. A rapid onset of hypothyroidism is associated with more recognizable symptoms than is a gradual onset. The signs and symptoms are directly related to the inadequate amount of thyroid hormone at the peripheral tissue level.

Early classic symptoms include fatigue, dry skin, slight weight gain, cold intolerance, constipation, and heavy menses. Myalgia, muscle cramps, headaches, and weakness may also be present. Later symptoms include very dry skin, coarse hair, loss of lateral eyebrows, alopecia, hoarseness, continued weight gain, slight impairment in mental ability, depression, decreased libido, and hypersomnia. Many of the symptoms are common complaints, which are not specific by themselves but together make up the manifestations of clinical hypothyroidism. Subclinical disease may be even more subtle or asymptomatic.

A complete review of systems is needed because symptoms are often subtle and may involve every body system. The presense of pain and swelling or enlargement in the neck, a history of radiation to the neck, and previous endocrine problems in the past medical history or family history should be elicited. It is also important to obtain a complete medication history and for women, a complete menstrual history is essential, including the most recent date, characteristics, and duration of last menstrual period. Some findings are more specific for Hashimoto's thyroiditis including painless thyroid enlargement, neck pain, sore throat, feeling of fullness in the throat, low-grade fever, and exhaustion.

Decreased motility of the gastrointestinal (GI) system is often experienced by patients with hypothyroidism, so constipation may be present. Although the exact mechanism of the effect of thyroid hormone on the GI tract is not fully understood, many patients experience atrophic gastritis and pernicious anemia.

Objective

Physical exam should begin with observation of the overall appearance of the patient, noting slow movements and dull facies. The blood pressure, resting pulse, respiratory rate, and weight should be compared to previous exams.

The hair may become coarse and thin, and thinning of eyebrows may occur. Patients with hypothyroidism frequently have a thickened tongue, evident by the indentation of the teeth around the edges. The thyroid may be enlarged and tender or not palpable. The consistency, size of thyroid, and nodules (focal or diffuse) should be noted, as well as any scars present on the neck. A visible goiter may also be present.

The heart may be hypertrophic which may be assessed by identifying the point of maximal impulse (PMI). The patient is usually bradycardic and may have a pericardial effusion.

The lung exam may reveal a pleural effusion. Abdominal exam usually reveals diminished or hypoactive bowel sounds. On neurologic exam, the patient may be hypotonic and hyporeflexic with a prolonged relaxation phase and/or ataxic.

The patient with hypothyroidism may have facial puffiness; periorbital edema; dry, coarse, thick skin and hair; brittle nails; slow speech; bradykinesia; hoarseness; large tongue; bradycardia; mild diastolic hypertension; psychological disorders; and pitting edema of the lower extremities. Myxedematous changes occur in the later stage with thickened, scaly, and "doughy" skin, enlarged tongue, muscle weakness, joint complaints, hearing impairments, and ascites. Table 15.6 summarizes the clinical presentation of hypothyroidism.

Diagnostic Reasoning

Diagnostic Tests

Initial Testing. Although there are no universally accepted screening recommendations for hypothyroidism, the American Thyroid Association recommends a baseline screening at 35 years, with close attention to high-risk patients (pregnant women, women older than 60 years, persons with other autoimmune diseases). The American Association of Clinical Endocrinologists recommends checking the TSH in women of childbearing age even before pregnancy and then in the first trimester. Congenital hypothyroidism is routinely screened for in neonates, as mandated in most states, as not treating hypothyroidism in this group has devastating effects (mental retardation).

The diagnosis of hypothyroidism is made by measuring serum TSH and FT_4. When autoimmune thyroiditis is the suspected underlying cause, it is helpful to confirm this with antithyroid antibody titers, either antimicrosomal antibody (antithyroid peroxidase [TPO] antibody) or antithyroglobulin antibody. The antimicrosomal antibody test is more sensitive and specific. If the TSH is low, inappropriately normal, or insufficiently elevated in the presence of low T_4 values, central hypothyroidism caused by hypothalamic or pituitary disease should be excluded before starting thyroid replacement therapy.

The sensitive thyrotropin assay is the most specific test for diagnosing primary hypothyroidism. A rise in the TSH will precede any other abnormality of thyroid function as the first evidence of primary hypothyroidism. Hypothyroidism caused by primary thyroid failure can be confirmed by a concomitant finding of a decrease in serum FT_4. Patients in an early stage of hypothyroidism may present with an increase in serum TSH together with a normal or low normal serum FT_4.

Primary hypothyroidism is associated with low FT_4 by radioimmunoassay with an elevated TSH level. The normal range of TSH is 0.35 to 5.5 μIU/mL. An elevated TSH (up to 15 to 20 μIU/mL) may be temporarily seen in euthyroid patients with a systemic illness. In this situation, the TSH and T_4 should be repeated in 2 to 3 weeks for confirmation. Patients with secondary or tertiary (central) hypothyroidism, show a low, normal, or mildly elevated TSH level

Table 15.6 Clinical Presentation: Hypothyroidism

Body System	Subjective	Objective
General	Fatigue Lethargy Mild weight gain Cold intolerance Mild depression Decreased libido Hypersomnia Muscle weakness and cramping	Slowing of mental processes Dull facial expression Periorbital puffiness Hypothermia Yellow skin (carotenemia) Facial pallor/swelling (myxedema)
Integumentary	Decreased sweating Hair loss Ankle swelling	Dry, cool, rough skin Alopecia Dry, coarse, thick hair Nonpitting edema
Gastrointestinal	Constipation Nausea	Hypoactive bowel sounds Large tongue Ascites
Neurologic	Memory deficits Personality changes	Hyporeflexia Bradykinesia Delayed relaxation of reflexes Slowing of mental processes
Cardiopulmonary	Inability to exercise	Bradycardia Cardiac enlargement Pleural effusion
Genitourinary	Menorrhagia, irregular menses	Decrease in fertility
Head and neck	Enlargement of the neck	Enlarged tongue (late) Hoarseness

with low FT_4 and T_3 by radioimmunoassay. The laboratory values for patients with subclinical hypothyroidism show a mildly increased TSH (5.5 to 15 μIU/mL) with a normal FT_4 level. Measurement of free T_4 is always preferred over total T_4, owing to alterations in hormone protein binding that may result in large fluctuations in total serum T_4 levels. Free thyroxine index (FTI), although not the test of choice, may be used since not all labs have the capacity to measure FT_4. FTI uses a T_3 resin uptake test to calculate the percentage of hormone binding sites available and multiplies this by the total T_4 level to give an estimation of the free T_4 level.

The antimicrosomal antibody (anti-TPO antibody) is diagnostic for Hashimoto's thyroiditis when found in high titers (1:400). The degree of elevation of this antibody correlates directly with clinical hypothyroidism. When hypothyroidism is present for a long period of time, the antibody titers fall. The antithyroglobulin antibody is also increased, but it is not as specific for Hashimoto's thyroiditis. If no antibodies are identified at the time of diagnosis, the condition is called *idiopathic hypothyroidism,* a form of autoimmune thyroiditis.

Medications such as metoclopramide (Reglan) increase the TSH level. Dopamine (Intropin), glucocorticoids, NSAIDs, and somatostatin decrease the TSH level. Other medications, such as phenytoin (Dilantin), amiodarone, cordarone, and lithium carbonate can also affect thyroid function tests. Smoking (nicotine) can also affect thyroid hormone levels. There are many mechanisms by which medications affect thyroid function. It may be because the drug binds with albumin and displaces the thyroid hormones off the carrier proteins or they may prevent albumin from binding with T_3 or T_4, in each case resulting in more active hormones in circulation. Some drugs may cause an upregulation in processing proteins (different cytochrome P [CYO] oxidase isomers). These normally inactivate thyroid hormones so the upregulation can lead to more rapid processing of thyroid hormones, in turn affecting TSH levels.

Subsequent Testing. Once a diagnosis of hypothyroidism is confirmed, additional testing may be necessary to determine the effect of the disease on other body systems. Because T_3 is nonspecific and not sensitive, it is not routinely used as an initial diagnostic tool. In the early stages of hypothyroidism, T_3 levels may be normal because of TSH-induced hyperstimulation. T_3 levels may not fall until late in the disease. Because the T_3 level correlates well with clinical status, the patient will not be as severely hypothyroid clinically until the T_3 falls to significantly low levels. In addition, the T_3 level may be below normal or elevated in patients with chronic disease.

Because anemia is a frequent complication of hypothyroidism, a CBC should be done. A complete blood chemistry profile should be done to assess for alterations in electrolytes, BUN, creatinine, serum osmolarity, and glucose, because a decreased glomerular filtration rate (affecting renal function) can occur. A complete urinalysis should also be performed, with specific attention to the presence of protein (indicating possible renal impairment). Changes in

THE PATIENT'S VOICE 15.1

Karilee's Story

I led a normal life until the birth of my second daughter. I was 32, professionally accomplished, and enjoying myself except for one problem—I was so tired, I could hardly get out of bed. I felt constantly exhausted. I blamed it on having young children and perhaps a touch of postpartum depression. The doctors I saw tried to convince me that this was normal, although I couldn't understand how other mothers could live like that. I had no energy for life, and felt depleted and irritable. I had no interest in recreation or sex, which eventually began to affect our marital relationship. I was too tired to even care!

I was also experiencing some strange symptoms that no one could explain. In addition to weight gain, I had exceptionally dry hair and skin, and brittle nails. Around that time, I also began to suffer from migraine headaches which incapacitated me for 24 to 48 hours once a month and left me feeling completely drained. Another most unsettling symptom, which plagued me for many months, was a thick tongue that I would bite many times a day, without knowing why or what to do about it.

Fortunately, one practitioner caring for me had the wisdom to consider the possibility of thyroid problems and did some testing. My levels of thyroid hormones were low. We began to experiment with Synthroid, a synthetic thyroid pill, and after several months of trying different doses, hit upon one that made a definite difference. I began to feel human again.

SOURCE: Shames, R, and Shames, KH: Thryoid Power: Ten Steps to Total Health. HarperCollins, New York, 2002.

the chemistries may be an indication of deteriorating thyroid function leading to myxedema.

Patients with mild to moderate hypothyroidism have a tendency to develop hypertension (especially diastolic hypertension); therefore, the blood pressure should be monitored. Interestingly, patients with long-standing or severe hypothyroidism tend to be normotensive or hypotensive. Depression of the biosynthesis of cholesterol causes a decreased rate of cholesterol catabolism and leads to hypercholesteremia. These patients tend to have elevated triglycerides and elevated low-density lipoprotein (LDL) cholesterol. The combination of hypertension and hyperlipidemia increases the risk of atherosclerotic heart disease in a hypothyroid patient. Thus, an annual lipid profile and an ECG should be done. As the cardiac system continues to deteriorate, the ECG may show nonspecific ST and T wave changes or low-voltage QRS complexes.

Unless there is reason to suspect a nodule or to confirm multinodular goiter, radioactive iodine scans and uptake are not usually necessary. As part of the complete examination, patients should have an annual chest x-ray exam to rule out the complications of hypothyroidism including cardiomegaly, CHF, and pleural effusion.

Ultrasound studies of the thyroid may be useful if a nodulary thyroid is detected or if infiltrative disease is suspected (amyloidosis, sarcoidosis, or tuberculosis). Fine-needle aspiration is indicated for suspicious nodules which may be found in patients with hypothyroidsim, hyperthyroidism, or euthyroidism. In fact, 5 to 6 percent of isolated nodules are malignant, especially larger ones, and ultrasound may reveal suspicious findings such as irregular margins or microcalcifications.

Differential Diagnosis

Marked variations in TSH may occur in the setting of an acute illness or psychiatric disorder when the body's metabolic demands are altered. TSH levels normally peak in the evening and are at their lowest in the afternoon. Nonthyroid illness is often associated with decreased TSH, T_3, and free T_4 levels without clinical hypothyroidism, with a reduction in the conversion of T_3 from T_4. In addition, usually the TSH level is normal or mildly increased during recovery from nonthyroid illness.

In euthyroid hypothyroxinemia, the patient is euthyroid with a decreased T_4 level due to increased thyroid-binding globulin concentration caused by nephrotic syndrome, exogenous testosterone, or high-dose steroids. Also, drugs that inhibit T_4 binding, such as phenytoin, phenobarbital, and salicylates may decrease the total T_4 level.

Management

The goal of thyroid hormone replacement in primary hypothyroidism is to normalize, not suppress, the TSH. Suppressed TSH, particularly in postmenopausal women or individuals with levothyroxine overreplacement, causes decreased bone mineral density after several years, leading to osteoporosis. The replacement goal in central hypothyroidism is to normalize the FT_4 because the TSH is not reliable. Hypothyroidism is typically treated medically; however, surgery may be indicated for particularly large, nonfunctional goiters that impair tracheoesophageal functioning.

Management of Hypothyroidism

The treatment for hypothyroidism is the daily administration of thyroid hormone to restore the patient to a euthyroid state. The usual medication is levothyroxine (Synthroid, Levothroid, Levoxyl), a synthetic preparation of T_4, which has generally replaced a desiccated thyroid preparation. Levothyroxine preparations are manufactured in numerous dosages, allowing for specific, precise titration to meet individual patient requirements.

According to the Treatment Guidelines developed by the American Thyroid Association Standards of Care

Committee, the usual dose is 1.7 μg/kg per day for full replacement. Healthy patients younger than age 60 years may receive 50 to 100 μg daily (full replacement dose). Patients who are older or have coronary artery disease should begin with one-half of the expected replacement dose or 25 to 50 μg/day PO, increasing the dose gradually by 25 μg/day once every 4 to 6 weeks. The TSH level should be measured every 6 to 8 weeks after initiating therapy and before each dosage increase. The optimum dose is 75 to 150 μg/day. Dosing is best done in the morning to avoid nighttime insomnia. Many other medications and mineral supplements interfere with GI absorption, including iron, calcium carbonate, aluminum hydroxide, sucralfate, and tube feedings. Thus, these medications require separation of dosing in time, while patients receiving continuous tube feedings require IV thyroxine dosing.

Replacement with T_3 preparations (liothyronine; Cytomel, Triostat) is usually not indicated; however, anecdotal reports exist that indicated combination T_3/T_4 therapy may be helpful in patients who do not respond adequately to T_4 replacement alone. Although T_3 is better absorbed via the GI tract than T_4, the appropriate ratio of triiodothyronine preparations versus thyroxine in combination therapy has not been well established, and such treatment decisions require expert input from an endocrinologist.

Another treatment of historical importance that is still used today in some settings owing to its relative lower cost is desiccated bovine thyroid (Armour Thyroid). Obtained from pooled thyroid extracts from cows, these preparations contain multiple foreign antigens, and the specific levels of active hormone are difficult to control. Some manufacturers standardize preparations based on bioassays, while others use iodine content as a surrogate measure of activity. T_3 and T_4 are both present, usually in a 1:4 ratio. While some older patients who have been treated for many years with desiccated thyroid are wary of changing medications after decades of replacement therapy at stable doses, few clinicians in the United States will start new patients on these preparations. They should not be used for patients with underlying cardiac disease, given the varied concentrations of highly active T_3 which poses a greater risk of overreplacement and iatrogenic thyrotoxicosis.

Regardless of choice of replacement therapy, all patients should be monitored for signs of thyrotoxicity, especially angina pectoris and arrhythmias, as optimizing thyroid replacement dosing can be difficult and time-consuming. If significant adverse symptoms occur during levothyroxine replacement, the dose should be decreased and the patient should be referred to an endocrinologist for evaluation prior to re-attempting replacement therapy at the original higher dose.

Concurrent severe illness or major surgery may alter dosing requirements in either direction in the hypothyroid patient. Pregnancy is also well known to increase replacement therapy requirements. Some clinicians suggest increasing replacement dosing by 30 percent upon confirmation of pregnancy, with subsequent adjustments per TSH levels, as untreated hypothyroidism in pregnancy is associated with preeclampsia, postpartum cardiac dysfunction, anemia, miscarriage, and low birth weight. The levothyroxine dose should be returned to the prepregnancy dose after delivery and a serum TSH level should be obtained 6 to 8 weeks postpartum.

Management of Subclinical Hypothyroidism

Treatment for subclinical hypothyroidism is still controversial and an endocrinologist should be consulted. The American Thyroid Association recommends treating subclinical disease when the TSH level is greater than 10 μIU/mL, there is presence of antithyroid antibodies, serum lipid levels are abnormal, if the patient smokes, and if the patient is symptomatic at this TSH level. However, data regarding the treatment of asymptomatic patients with TSH levels between 4.5 and 10 μIU/mL are inconclusive.

Some patients with subclinical hypothyroidism feel better when treated with levothyroxine. Medication therapy has potentially dangerous adverse effects but may improve subtle abnormalities, prevent goiterous growth, and prevent the development of frank hypothyroidism. Therapy is advisable especially if thyroid autoantibodies are positive, because overt hypothyroidism frequently develops.

In young patients or patients with goiter, consider initiating levothyroxine therapy. If the decision is made not to treat these patients, then they should be evaluated at 6- to 12-month intervals for evidence of more severe clinical and biological loss of thyroid function. A lower dose (0.5 to 1.0 μg/kg) could be given in the treatment of subclinical hypothyroidism. If the diagnosis of hypothyroidism is uncertain in a patient who is already on levothyroxine, the dose can be reduced by one-half and the FT_4 and TSH levels can be reassessed in 6 to 8 weeks. If the TSH level is increasing, the patient should resume the previous dose. If the TSH is normal, the patient should discontinue the levothyroxine and the TSH level should be rechecked in 6 to 8 weeks for any increase.

Follow-Up and Referral

After therapy has been initiated with levothyroxine, the practitioner should check the patient's levothyroxine levels in 4 to 6 weeks by evaluating the TSH level to determine whether adjustment of the levothyroxine dose is necessary. Increasing the levothyroxine dose more often than at 6 week intervals will probably lead to overreplacement. Once a stable dose of levothyroxine has been established, the TSH level in primary hypothyroidism or the FT_4 level in central hypothyroidism can be checked biannually or annually.

The patient should be examined annually for manifestations of thyrotoxicity (e.g., tachycardia, nervousness, or tremor) before increasing dosages. Laboratory values (FT_4 and TSH levels) within normal limits and a satisfactory clinical examination suggest that treatment is adequate. For

Drugs Commonly Prescribed 15.2: Hypothyroidism, Lifelong Pharmacuetical Treatment

Drug	Indication	Dosage	Adverse Reactions
Synthetic L-thyroxine*, T_4 (Levothroid, Levoxyl, Synthroid)	Patients with increased TSH levels, usually 3 times the upper limit of the assay. Overt hypothyroidism, pharmaceuticals lifelong treatment. Goal: to give enough thyroid supplement orally to result in normal free T_4 and TSH levels	Start 0.025–0.05 mg/day; increase by 0.025 mg/day every 3–6 weeks/to a maximum of 0.3 mg/day. Usual maintenance 0.1–0.2 mg/day. In older adults begin with a slightly higher dose.	Monitor antihyperglycemics, oral anticoagulants, and potential sympathomimetics Wait 4–5 hours after cholestyramine ingestion Not for prescription of obesity Use with caution in patients with cardiovascular disease, diabetes, adrenal insufficiency Increased sensitivity in myxedema and severe hypothyroidism.

*Synthetic T_3 supplements (cytomel) are not recommended as the drug of choice.

maintenance treatment, the medication should be titrated to the lowest dosage required to maintain euthyroidism, with a normal TSH and a normal or slightly elevated T_4.

Undetectable TSH levels suggest overtreatment; medication should be decreased in these patients. TSH levels greater than 20 μIU/mL indicate undertreatment and medication should be increased.

Referral to an endocrinologist is necessary if the patient has cardiac disease, symptoms of myxedema, or central (secondary or tertiary) hypothyroidism. After starting hormone replacement therapy, if signs or symptoms of myxedema, chest pain, or thyrotoxicosis occur, the endocrinologist should be consulted. These patients are at high risk for serious complications related to hypothyroidism or its treatment. Hypothyroid patients with severe illness or those who present with unusual or confusing laboratory findings should be referred to an endocrinologist. Referral to an endocrinologist is indicated in patients younger than age 16, when there is evidence of pituitary disease, in pregnant and postpartum patients, and in those taking lithium or amiodarone (Cordarone).

For asymptomatic patients with subclinical hypothyroidism, who (after consultation) are not being treated with medication, a TSH should be performed yearly, along with a focused history and physical examination.

Patient Education

During the follow-up visits, emphasis should be placed on compliance with lifelong thyroid replacement therapy (if indicated), reviewing the symptoms of hypothyroidism and hyperthyroidism, and stressing the importance of follow-up.

Instructions should be simple and repeated frequently until the patient's mental status improves. An older adult with hypothyroidism may need additional emotional support, reinforcement, and follow-up teaching. Support in the home setting may be necessary until the symptoms of slowed mental processes and depression abate. Initially, a family member may be needed to remind the patient to take his or her daily dose of medication.

Patients should be encouraged to wear an extra layer of clothing if they have cold intolerance and should be warned not to use a heating pad. The patient is at risk for burns owing to diminished mental status and slowed responses. If psychomotor symptoms are present, the patient should be cautioned against operating dangerous machinery or driving a motor vehicle until the symptoms have resolved.

Because heredity is implicated in hypothyroidism, patients with children should be instructed to advise their child's primary-care provider of their diagnosis.

Patients who are at high risk for hypothyroidism (those who have had thyroid surgery, radioactive iodine treatments, history of thyroiditis, and postpartum women) should be taught the common symptoms of hypothyroidism (lethargy, fatigue, cold intolerance, constipation, weight gain, dry skin). The patient and family should also be instructed that hypothyroidism is a chronic, sometimes progressive disease requiring monitoring every 6 to 12 months. Patients and their families should be reassured that as the treatment progresses, the symptoms will resolve.

Patients should be instructed to continue with the same brand of thyroid preparation because the bioavailability, stability, and content of the medication may vary with the different brands. Patients should be given the rationale for treatment, adverse effects, and dosage for their medication. Emphasis should be on the fact that medication use is lifelong. The patient needs to understand that as the body ages or there are changes in body weight, the dosage of medication may need to be adjusted.

The patient should be taught the signs of hyperthyroidism (thyrotoxicity) in the event of thyroid replacement overdosage—for example, nervousness, palpitations, insomnia, and tremor. It is important to explain that it will take 1 to 2 weeks for the medication to be effective. During this time, patients may experience an increase in urination and a decrease in periorbital puffiness.

The absorption of levothyroxine from the GI tract may be slowed by concurrent use of certain drugs, such as ferrous sulfate, sucralfate (Carafate), or antacids. The dose of thyroid hormone should be taken 2 hours before or

THE PATIENT'S VOICE 15.2

Hypothyroidism

Onley Cahill, age 57, came down with what she thought was the flu 3 years ago, but the fatigue hung on. She would drive home from work and have to rest in her car before mustering the energy for the climb to her second-floor apartment. She stopped going out at night. She spent entire weekends in bed, only to feel even more tired come Monday morning. At work she would close her office door and collapse on the floor. At meetings, where she had once been quick with suggestions, she was having trouble speaking.

"I felt like an absolute idiot," she says. "I kept wondering if something was wrong with my mind."

A cluster of symptoms—constipation, constantly feeling cold, and difficulty swallowing, among others—had her hopping from doctor to doctor. Finally, Cahill checked into a hospital where a number of specialists, including a psychiatrist, examined her. The psychiatrist wondered if her problems weren't rooted in depression, though she felt too much of a physical mess for the problem to be entirely psychological.

"I said, 'Listen, you'd be depressed too if you didn't have the energy to get out of bed,'" she recalls. The doctors also gave her a battery of tests, among them, a thyroid-stimulating hormone (TSH) assay. That was when Cahill learned that she had an underactive thyroid, that her thyroid had shut down almost entirely. A timely thyroid test would have saved her years of grief.

SOURCE: Adapted from Kelley, BB: Running on empty. Hippocrates: J Health Med (Nurse practitioner edition). p 24, September 1997.

4 hours following ingestion of these medications. Because levothyroxine supplements may increase blood glucose levels, patients with diabetes mellitus should carefully monitor their blood sugar levels; their dose of insulin or oral hypoglycemic agents may need to be adjusted. Thyroid hormones may also affect the levels of phenytoin (Dilantin), lithium, tricyclic antidepressants, estrogen, digitalis, anticoagulants, and indomethacin (Indocin). The appropriate blood tests and screenings should be performed and patients should be instructed on the important adverse reactions to report should they occur.

Because of increased sensitivity to certain medications in hypothyroid patients, patients should be cautioned against the use of analgesics and sedatives. Even in small dosages, these medications can cause severe somnolence and respiratory depression. Infrequently, a patient with normal TSH levels may continue to feel fatigued, but the patient should be discouraged from increasing the dose of medication, since some patients may be tempted to do this. This symptom warrants further investigation as to the underlying cause and should be discussed during an office visit. In cases where patient compliance may be a problem, weekly dosages can be given, because the half-life of T_4 is approximately 1 week.

Patients should be taught to follow a healthy diet, with an emphasis on low-fat, high-fiber foods. Some patients may need to follow a diet that promotes weight loss once medication has been started. Because many patients with hypothyroidism experience constipation, they should increase their intake of raw fruits and vegetables, bran or high-fiber cereals and breads, and add unprocessed bran (two tablespoons/day) to cereal or liquids. A bulk-forming laxative containing psyllium may be taken on a daily basis. Increasing water intake to six to eight glasses a day is often beneficial in reducing constipation, as is increasing physical activity. A low-fat diet is recommended because there is a high incidence of atherosclerotic heart disease in patients with hypothyroidism.

Once therapy with levothyroxine is initiated, the patient should be able to resume all previous activities. Initially, rest periods with a gradual increase in exercise and activity, as tolerated, may be indicated. The patient must be instructed that if he or she develops any signs or symptoms of cardiac or respiratory difficulty, it is essential to seek medical attention.

Thyroid Cancer

Thyroid cancer is classified as differentiated (papillary and follicular) and undifferentiated (medullary and anaplastic). Most thyroid cancers (60 percent) are papillary; 20 percent are follicular; and the remaining tumors are medullary or anaplastic. Medullary thyroid cancer is more likely to be familial. Anaplastic tumors are the fastest growing of all thyroid neoplasms; they are more common in older adults and are associated with a high mortality rate. A rare type of thyroid cancer is non-Hodgkin's lymphoma, which should be considered in persons with a rapidly growing goiter. Hürthle cell carcinoma is a rare type of thyroid malignancy (2 to 3 percent of thyroid cancers) which is often considered a variant of follicular carcinoma. Consisting almost exclusively of Hürthle cells (also called oxyphilic or oncocytic cells) that contain abundant granular acidophilic cytoplasm, these malignancies are highly aggressive, metastasize in more than half of cases, and are difficult to follow because they do not respond to TSH or take up radioiodine.

Epidemiology and Causes

The incidence of thyroid cancer in the United States is small, with only 0.4 percent of the population diagnosed with this type of cancer, however, 13 percent of people in the United States are found to have thyroid cancer on autopsy. Most thyroid cancers are small and slow growing. Thyroid cancer accounts for 0.5 percent of all cancer deaths per year.

The incidence increases with age and it is more common in adults ages 20 to 54, but it can occur at any age.

Thyroid cancer is more common in women than in men (3:1). Thyroid nodules found in persons younger than 20 years of age or initially found in adults older than age 60 years are more likely to be cancerous. Nodules are often found on routine physical examinations, by the patient, or during imaging for other purposes.

The major risk factor for development of thyroid cancer is exposure to ionizing radiation. Several historical incidents resulting in high-dose radiation exposure have been linked to an increased incidence of thyroid papillary malignancies in children, including the atomic bombings of the Japanese cities of Hiroshima and Nagasaki, military atomic testing near the Marshall Islands, and the nuclear power plant meltdown in the Russian city of Chernobyl. Moreover, until the 1950s, radiation treatments were given to children for an enlarged thymus, enlarged tonsils, and acne. It is estimated that 1 to 2 million individuals were exposed to this risk factor. Studies have estimated that one-third of patients who received radiation therapy to the head and neck will develop a thyroid nodule, and one-third of these patients will later develop a malignancy. It may be advisable for patients who received head and neck irradiation as a child to have an ultrasound for screening purposes.

Importantly, low-dose radiation exposure associated with routine radiographic imaging studies has not been shown to be tumorigenic. Interestingly, ^{131}I radioablation therapy for thyrotoxicosis and high-dose external beam radiotherapy have also not been associated with papillary thyroid carcinoma, presumably because of the greater amount of cellular apoptosis associated with these doses of radiation.

There is also an increased incidence of follicular and anaplastic thyroid carcinoma in areas where iodine deficiency and goiter are more prevalent. Thyroid cancer is also more common in persons with autoimmune disease. Medullary carcinoma is an inherited form of thyroid cancer, with 90 percent of those inheriting the autosomal dominant gene ultimately developing cancer.

Metastatic cancer of the thyroid is less common, but renal cancer, breast cancer, lung cancer, and malignant melanoma may metastasize to the thyroid gland.

Pathophysiology

While thyroid carcinomas are relatively rare in the United States, benign thyroid disease is significantly more common. An estimated 4 to 7 percent of the general population develops thyroid nodules, and while the vast majority of these represent benign disease, it is estimated that 5 to 6 percent of isolated nodules are malignant. Thus, distinguishing malignant from nonmalignant cases requires careful clinical evaluation.

As with all types of cancer, thyroid cancer is believed to develop from a series of mutational events producing a cell that is genetically different from its source. This explains the strong association of thyroid cancer with radiation exposure, which increases the incidence of DNA mutation and transformation of normal thyroid cells into malignant clones. Similarly, germline mutations in the RET proto-oncogene have been associated with the inherited cancer syndromes multiple endocrine neoplasia (MEN) 2A, MEN 2B, familial adenomatous polyposis (FAP), and familial medullary thyroid carcinoma (FMTC) syndrome—all of which are associated with medullary thyroid carcinoma.

Thyroid cancers range from those that are well differentiated and slow growing to those that are poorly differentiated and aggressive. As with other malignancies, poorly differentiated thyroid cancers have an unfavorable prognosis. Cancers of the thyroid gland are typically classified into primary and secondary (metastatic) tumors. Primary tumors include papillary (80 percent of cases), follicular (10 percent of cases), anaplastic (2 percent of cases), and medullary tumors (5 to 10 percent of cases), and rarely primary thyroid lymphomas (2 to 5 percent of cases) and sarcomas. Papillary, follicular, and anaplastic tumors derive from the endodermally derived thyroxine- and thyroglobulin-producing follicular epithelium, while medullary tumors arise from the neuroendocrine-derived parafollicular or C cells. Thyroid lymphomas arise from intrathyroid lymph tissue and is strongly associated with chronic lymphocytic thyroiditis (Hashimoto's autoimmune thyroiditis), while sarcomas are derived from the vascular and connective tissue interwoven throughout the thyroid gland.

Clinical Presentation

Subjective

The major symptom of thyroid cancer is a lump or nodule in the neck, which are usually painless. Patients may also complain of a tight or full feeling in the neck, difficulty breathing or swallowing, hoarseness, hemoptysis, and swollen lymph nodes. New onset of hoarseness with hemoptysis is strongly suggestive of a malignant growth. Progressive dysphagia and shortness of breath may indicate invasiveness. Pain in the neck is usually a late symptom. History may reveal exposure to radiation as a child.

Objective

Four to seven percent of the United States population have a palpable thyroid nodule, making clinical examination of the thyroid an ineffective method of screening. Differentiated thyroid carcinomas most commonly present as a thyroid mass or nodule. Although malignant neoplasms are more likely to be fixed, nontender, firm, and irregular in shape, only a biopsy can rule out malignancy. Physical examination should include examination of the tongue, oropharynx, and cervical spine for swelling, nodules, or tenderness.

Diagnostic Reasoning

Although there are some typical presentations of benign versus malignant nodules of the thyroid, many malignant lesions have an atypical presentation. A biopsy is the only reliable method of differentiating a benign from a malignant lesion; therefore on palpation of a nodule, the patient should be referred to an endocrinologist. Early referral of patients with nodules to an endocrinologist for evaluation and treatment reduces costs, decreases patient hospital time, and increases the precision of the diagnosis.

Nodules that develop in men, in persons younger than age 20 years or older than age 60 years, in persons with a family history of thyroid cancer, or in those with a personal history of exposure to radiation are suggestive of malignancy. Malignant growths are more likely to be irregular in shape, fixed, firm, and nontender. Multiple nodules of the same consistency are more likely to be benign. Fewer than 5 percent of nodules are malignant. The prognosis is good for thyroid cancer found early, is less than 2 cm in diameter, is a favorable histologic type, and has not invaded locally or metastasized.

Diagnostic Tests

Initial Testing. High-resolution ultrasonography is beneficial in identifying thyroid nodules but is not reliable in differentiating a benign from a malignant lesion. It is indicated when there is suspicion of multinodular disease or when the thyroid is difficult to evaluate clinically.

Subsequent Testing. A fine-needle aspiration (FNA) biopsy is usually successful in differentiating a benign from cancerous lesion of the thyroid gland and has an 83 percent sensitivity and a 92 percent specificity. Thus, the FNA will not capture all cases, and repeat biopsy may be necessary. The sensitivity of FNA is increased when it is ultrasound guided. Nondiagnostic FNA biopsies may require surgical lobectomy to confirm that the nodule is not in fact malignant. Psammoma bodies are found in 50 percent of papillary carcinomas; they are circular, laminated bodies found in the stroma of the tumor.

Elevated serum calcitonin is a strong tumor marker of medullary thyroid carcinoma, but these cancers are somewhat rare overall, so this test is not usually used in the initial work-up. For the inherited cancer syndromes MEN 2A, MEN 2B, and FMTC, polymerase chain reaction (PCR) assays are used to detect germline mutations in the *RET* oncogene. Also, give a brief discussion of radioiodine uptake testing as a means of determining functionality of a thyroid nodule.

Computerized tomography (CT) and magnetic resonance imaging (MRI) are used when the tumor is large, recurrent, or when there is expected extrathyroidal extension of the tumor, but are not helpful for evaluation of a simple, isolated nodule. However, they can be used to assess for distant metastases and regional lymph node involvement. Spread to lymph nodes is more common with papillary than with follicular carcinomas, but if metastases do occur, lung and bone are the most common sites. Interestingly, lymph node metastases are not an important prognostic factor, but distant metastasis is associated with nearly a 70-fold increase in death.

Thyroid neoplasms are often painless and thyroid function tests may show levels within the normal range unless the patient has thyroiditis.

Differential Diagnosis

Differential diagnoses include lymphocytic thryoiditis, multinodular goiter, benign thyroid nodule, cystic nodules, and regional lymphadenopathy. Mass-related effects may be similar to those associated with laryngeal or other forms of neck cancer, e.g., dysphagia or hoarseness due to recurrent laryngeal nerve involvement with vocal cord paralysis, hemoptysis due to local invasion through the trachea.

If medullary thyroid carcinoma is diagnosed, it is critical to take a thorough family history to assess whether this presentation occurs as a component of several inherited cancer syndromes including multiple endocrine neoplasia (MEN) 2A or Sipple syndrome (which may present with concurrent pheochromocytoma and hyperparathyroidism), MEN 2B (which may present with concurrent pheochromocytoma, tall and slender Marfanoid body habitus, and ganglioneuromas), and familial medullary thyroid carcinoma (FMTC) syndrome.

Management

Initial Management

Any swelling suggestive of malignancy should be referred to an endocrinologist, with subsequent referral to an oncologist for surgery if indicated (and possibly a radiation or medical oncologist) once a diagnosis of cancer has been established. Thyroidectomy or near-total thyroidectomy is the treatment of choice. The decision is based on the type of tumor, the size, and whether the tumor is compressing other structures. A surgeon with expertise in thyroid surgery should perform the procedure because of the potential of damage to the laryngeal nerves and the parathyroid glands. For small, noninvasive tumors, some surgeons prefer to perform a lobectomy, a more conservative approach. However, if there is local invasion there is a greater possibility of recurrence. Radical neck surgery may be indicated for tumors with extensive local invasion.

Subsequent Management

Following a total thyroidectomy, patients are often treated with radioactive iodine therapy to ablate any remnant thyroid tissue. Thyroid replacement therapy is initiated to suppress TSH to a goal of 0.1 μIU/mL, and patients are monitored closely for response to therapy. They are subsequently followed every 6 to 12 months by an endocrinologist. A thorough neck examination, a chest x-ray exam, and physical examination are performed with observations for thyrotoxicosis. Thyroglobulin levels may also be measured for well-differentiated carcinomas. The endocrinologist may perform a follow-up ^{131}I scan 6 to 12 months after a total thyroidectomy and may initiate further radioactive iodine ablation therapy if indicated. A follow-up ^{131}I scan is not useful in medullary cancer because medullary carcinoma does not take up the radioactive isotope.

Some forms of malignancy have unique treatments. In addition to thyroidectomy and postoperative radiation therapy, thyroid lymphomas may also require chemotherapy directed by a medical oncologist. Sarcomas are particularly aggressive and, following thyroidectomy, are poorly responsive to chemotherapy and carry a poor prognosis.

Long-term prognosis of thyroid malignancy depends on cell type of tumor, size of the primary growth, gender (men are twice as likely to die from thyroid cancer than women), age at diagnosis (death is more common in those diagnosed younger than 20 years or older than 40 years of age), and extent of metastasis at the time of excision. Fortunately, papillary thyroid cancer is rarely fatal.

Follow-Up and Referral

Follow-up is directed by the knowledge that no single diagnostic tool is sufficient to evaluate for recurrent disease. The follow-up of patients who have been treated for thyroid cancer includes periodic clinical examinations, serum thyroglobulin measurements, chest x-ray films, and ultrasound examination to assess for recurrence. The patient is followed more closely during the first 3 to 4 years following surgery because recurrence is more likely within this time.

The patient with a total thyroidectomy will require thyroid hormone replacement for life. See Management of Hypothyroidism for specific guidelines.

Patient Education

Patients with a family history of thyroid cancer should be advised to perform a "neck check" monthly. Patients with a history of goiter or irradiation should also perform this screening technique. The check is performed at home with a glass of water and a hand-held mirror. The patient should be instructed to hold the mirror to visualize the area between the Adam's apple and clavicle. Then the head should be tilted backward, enough to adequately visualize the area without producing coughing or choking. As a sip of water is taken and swallowed, the patient should observe the area for any bulging. The maneuver should be repeated several times. Any signs of bulging should be reported immediately.

Free copies of the *Neck Check* can be obtained at http://www.aace.com/public/awareness/tam/2006/.

Cushing's Syndrome

Cushing's syndrome includes a myriad of symptoms and physical features produced by persistent inappropriate hypercortisolemia. The condition was named after Harvey Cushing, a physician who found pituitary adenomas in six of eight patients with symptoms of adrenocortical hyperfunctioning in 1932. Cushing's syndrome may be caused by cortisol hypersecretion by the adrenal cortex due to cortical hypertrophy or a tumor of the adrenal gland. However, the prolonged administration of large doses of exogenous glucocorticoid hormones will also cause this cluster of signs and symptoms and simulate disordered adrenal function. The term *Cushing's disease* refers specifically to pituitary adrenocorticotropic hormone (ACTH) excess caused by a pituitary tumor (adenoma), which, in turn, causes oversecretion of cortisol by the adrenal gland.

Epidemiology and Causes

Cushing's syndrome may be classified mechanistically as ACTH-dependent or ACTH-independent hypercortisolemic states. The former mechanism results in adrenocortical hyperplasia and is most frequently due to an ACTH-secreting pituitary adenoma (70 percent of cases). Known as Cushing's disease, this condition occurs more commonly in women. The tumors are usually small (microadenomas) and may not be recognizable on pituitary imaging, with some patients demonstrating only hyperplasia of pituitary corticotrophs. Fewer than 10 percent of affected patients have a tumor greater than 10 mm in diameter. The tumors are not encapsulated and present in the anterior pituitary gland. Spontaneous cases of Cushing's syndrome are rare, occurring in 2.6 persons per 1,000,000 per year. Malignant pituitary tumors are, fortunately, rare.

Nonpituitary tumors account for ectopic ACTH secretion in 10 to 15 percent of ACTH-dependent cases of Cushing's syndrome. In contrast, excessive administration of exogenous ACTH and ectopic secretion of corticotropin-releasing hormone (CRH) by nonhypothalamic tumors each account for fewer than 1 percent of ACTH-hypersecretion cases.

The majority of ACTH-independent cases of Cushing's syndrome are due to iatrogenic administration of glucocorticoid hormones for therapeutic purposes. However, tumors of the adrenal cortex account for up to 20 percent of ACTH-independent cases, and both micronodular and macronodular dysplasia of the adrenal gland have been observed, although these etiologies are both quite rare, accounting for fewer than 1 percent of cases.

Pathophysiology

A basic knowledge of the hypothalamic–pituitary–adrenal neurohormonal axis is required to properly understand the Pathophysiology of Cushing's syndrome. Ultimately regulated by the central nervous system, CRH is first produced by the hypothalamus and released into the hypophyseal portal circulation, where it stimulated the production of proopiomelanocortin (POMC) by corticotrophs in the anterior pituitary gland, from which ACTH (also called corticotropin) is derived as a cleavage product. ACTH then acts directly on the adrenal cortex to stimulate the production of cortisol and other adrenal hormones that act at peripheral tissue sites as intranuclear transcription factors for steroid-responsive genes. Cortisol is then metabolized by the liver and kidneys, and its breakdown products are secreted in the urine as 17-hydroxycorticosteroids, 17-ketogenic steroids, and 17-ketosteroids.

A key regulatory mechanism of this neuroendocrine axis is the negative feedback exerted by each downstream product on its preceding hormone—namely, the inhibitory effects of ACTH on CRH secretion, as well as serum cortisol on the secretion of ACTH and CRH at the level of the pituitary and hypothalamus, respectively. The pituitary is also likely subject to other forms of positive feedback from additional secretagogues. For example, pituitary corticotrophs have been shown to express receptors for growth hormone–releasing peptide (GHRP) and increase ACTH production in response to GRP secretion.

The secretion of ACTH (and, hence, serum cortisol) is normally pulsatile in nature in terms of frequency and remains constant. However, with the extent of ACTH release with each pulse varies according to the body's circadian rhythms (sleep–wake cycles), which accounts for the variation in serum cortisol levels observed through serial measurements at different times of the day. Physical and emotional stressors that increase the body's metabolic demands also increase ACTH and cortisol secretion. In the normal diurnal sleep–wake cycle, levels are highest in the early morning on awakening and are lowest late in the evening and during the very early morning hours after midnight.

In patients with Cushing's disease, pituitary adenomas secrete excessive amounts of ACTH. The hypersecretion is random, episodic, and does not follow the usual circadian rhythm of ACTH secretion in terms of amplitude and duration. ACTH stimulates the secretion of glucocorticoids, mineralocorticoids, and androgenic steroids from the adrenal cortex. As cortical hyperplasia increases, the adrenal glands secrete increasing amounts of cortisol in response to each incremental pulse of ACTH. Moreover, in the presence of an adenoma, the usual negative feedback mechanism of excessive glucocorticoid secretion does not suppress ACTH production to the same extent as in unaffected persons, possibly owing to a defect in the glucocorticoid receptor in adenomatous corticotrophs. In turn, these patients present with hypercortisolemia and elevated levels of ACTH—particularly those with macroadenomas.

Importantly, however, in contrast to the ACTH-producing cells of relatively rarer ectopic, nonpituitary adenomas which remain virtually unresponsive to negative feedback mechanisms, pituitary adenomatous corticotrophs appear to still retain a threshold level, albeit a higher one than in normal corticotrophs, for cortisol-mediated negative feedback. This allows a high-dose dexamethasone suppression test to differentiate between pituitary and nonpituitary sources of ACTH hypersecretion. With ectopic, nonpituitary ACTH secretion, both hypothalamic CRH secretion and pituitary ACTH secretion from normal corticotrophs are suppressed. A number of different tumor types have been implicated with ectopic ACTH hypersecretion, most commonly small oat-cell carcinoma of the lung and carcinoid tumors of the thymus or pancreas, all of which arise from neuroendocrine cell precursors. Interestingly, most of these tumors secrete a greater proportion of POMC precursors than ACTH itself.

In patients with Cushing's syndrome, cortisol measurements taken at various times during a 24-hour period will demonstrate prolonged elevations of cortisol levels, even though some readings may be within the normal range. The normally tight regulatory relationship between ACTH and cortisol secretion is lost, with late evening levels being particularly high. This excessive production of cortisol over the entire 24-hour sleep–wake cycle results in the clinical signs and symptoms of Cushing's syndrome.

The most frequent cause of Cushing's syndrome, however, is prolonged administration of exogenous glucocorticoid hormones—an iatrogenic etiology which is considered ACTH-independent. Thus, any medical problem requiring the prolonged use of corticosteroids predisposes the patient to develop this syndrome. Examples include autoimmune disorders, reactive airway disease, and COPD—all of which may involve long-term systemic steroid use as maintenance therapy or for recurrent exacerbations. Rarely, megestrol acetate (Megace), which has intrinsic glucocorticoid activity, may also lead to Cushing's syndrome. Exogenous steroid administration leads to suppression of CRH and ACTH excretion, as well as steroid production by native adrenal tissue. This results in bilateral adrenocortical atrophy and low salivary and urinary levels of 17-hydroxycorticosteroid and cortisol, unless cortisol itself is the steroid being administered.

Primary adrenocortical disease including cortical tumors and both micro- and macronodular hyperplasia is much less common. Adrenal tumors may be benign adenomas or malignant carcinomas. Both types of tumors demonstrate altered expression of genes involved in apoptosis and telomeric function, which appears to underlie clonal immortalization. However, a number of significant differences exist between benign and malignant tumors. Adrenal adenomas produce cortisol from cholesterol backbones very efficiently, secreting relatively low levels of the cortisol precursors dehydroepiandrosterone (DHEA-S) and 17-ketosteroids. Adenomatous cells have also been shown to respond to beta-adrenergic agonists and multiple cytokines, including IL-1, gastric inhibitory peptide, vasopressin, and serotonin.

In contrast, adrenal carcinomas are far less efficient at producing cortisol, secreting cortisol precursors at disproportionately higher concentrations. Adrenal carcinomas are still capable of leading to Cushing's syndrome, however, owing to their size and secretory cell mass. They are also more likely than adrenal adenomas to produce elevated levels of the aldosterone precursor corticosterone and its hydroxy and deoxy variants. Adrenal carcinomas also produce high levels of vascular endothelial growth factor A

(VEGF-A), insulin-like growth factor (IGF)-1, IGF-2, IGF-2 receptor, cell cyclins, cyclin-dependent kinase, and the chemokines IL-8 and epithelial neutrophil-activating protein-78. In contrast, levels of the antiangiogenic factor thrombospondin-1 are reduced.

With primary adrenocortical tumors, hypercortisolemia allows for negative feedback of both CRH and ACTH secretion. Thus, pituitary corticotrophs atrophy, as do the normal adrenal cells of the zona fasciculata and zona reticularis. In contrast, macronodular adrenal hyperplasia results in glands weighing from 25 to 500 grams or more, with multiple benign nodules greater than 5 mm in diameter and a hypertrophic (rather than atrophic) internodular cortex.

Clinical Presentation

Subjective

The clinical presentation of Cushing's disease is usually gradual, developing over months or years. Signs and symptoms of Cushing's disease are those of hypercortisolism and androgen excess.

The presentation of patients with Cushing's syndrome is similar. Common complaints include weight gain, back pain, headaches, skin changes (see below), and muscle weakness. Women may complain of menstrual irregularities and hirsutism, and men often report decreased libido and impotence. Patients may also complain of emotional lability, increased appetite and weight gain, increased irritability, anxiety, poor concentration and memory, and sleep disturbances.

Objective

Patients with Cushing's syndrome predominantly present with generalized or central obesity. In fact, obesity is the most common and often the first clinical manifestation of this disorder. Excessive accumulation of fat in the face leads to the typical "moonface" appearance. Facial plethora often accompanies the moon facies. The "buffalo hump" appearance is caused by excessive accumulation of fat in the supraclavicular and dorsocervical area.

Most patients will have readily recognizable skin changes. There is atrophy of the epidermis and connective tissue, producing a thinning of the skin and easy bruising. Additional skin changes include hirsutism, acne, and striae. Striae are typically red to purple and usually are present on the abdomen, but may be present on the hips, buttocks, thighs, breast, and axilla. Hyperpigmentation, commonly found in some types of Cushing's syndrome, is rare in patients with Cushing's disease.

Fungal infections of the skin, nails, and oral mucosa are common. Skin wounds heal slowly in the presence of excessive cortisol.

Most patients have muscle weakness, which is more prominent proximally and in the lower extremities. The extremities are usually thin, with muscle wasting. Osteoporosis is common in patients with prolonged elevated cortisol levels, and pathological fractures may be evident on radiographic examination.

Other manifestations include glaucoma, leukocytosis, granulocytosis, lymphopenia, and psychiatric symptoms. Less common clinical findings include renal calculi and edema. Hypokalemic alkalosis is rare in Cushing's disease, but is often seen in Cushing's syndrome.

Hypertension is often present secondary to sodium and water retention. Glucose intolerance and hyperglycemia result because cortisol interferes with the transfer of insulin across the cell membrane.

Diagnostic Reasoning

Cushing's disease is diagnosed via a combination of laboratory testing and radiographic examinations.

Diagnostic Tests

Initial Testing. Patients with Cushing's disease will most often have moderate elevations of cortisol levels and slightly elevated ACTH secretion. Normally, plasma cortisol levels range from 5 to 23 μg/dL in the morning and from 3 to 13 μg/dL in the afternoon. The afternoon level is usually one-half the morning level. Additional laboratory tests should include a CBC, blood glucose levels, and electrolytes. Hypercortisolemia impairs glucose tolerance, and often produces hypokalemia and leukocytosis.

Initial tests to assess cortisol levels include serum cortisol levels and urinary cortisol. The overnight dexamethasone suppression test assists in the confirmation of hypercortisolemia. To do the overnight dexamethasone test, the patient takes 1 mg of dexamethasone (Decadron) orally at 11 P.M. and the plasma cortisol level is measured at 8 A.M. the next morning. A normal finding is a value below 5 μg/dL, as an elevated morning cortisol level would indicate the patient's endogenous cortisol secretion is insensitive to the negative feedback imparted by the exogenous dexamethasone dose. False-positive results may occur in patients who are obese, depressed, or under extreme stress. Medications that may also produce high cortisol levels are estrogens, antiseizure medications, and rifampin. Phenytoin (Dilantin), phenobarbital (Luminal), and primidone (Mysoline) accelerate the metabolism of dexamethasone and can also produce a false-positive dexamethasone test.

The 24-hour urinary free cortisol test is the best test for initial screening since false-positive results can occur with plasma cortisol screening. Some studies recommend the 24-hour urinary free cortisol and creatinine examination in addition to the overnight dexamethasone suppression test because it is the most sensitive (95 to 100 percent) and specific (98 percent) screening test for Cushing's syndrome.

The 24-hour urinary excretion test requires good compliance on the part of the patient. Because alcoholism can result in similar clinical findings, the test is not reliable if the alcoholic patient does not refrain from drinking for at least 1 month before testing.

If either of the tests is positive for Cushing's syndrome, the patient should be referred to an endocrinologist. A high-dose dexamethasone suppression test is necessary to differentiate between the possible types of Cushing's syndrome. However, it is not useful for distinguishing the source of ACTH secretion. If symptoms of Cushing's syndrome are present, but the tests do not confirm the diagnosis of hypercortisolism, the low-dose dexamethasone suppression test should be performed.

Subsequent Testing. The low-dose dexamethasone suppression test involves administration of dexamethasone 0.5 mg PO q6h for 48 hours. Urine is collected on day 2 of the test. Urine free cortisol above 20 μg/dL or a 17-hydroxycorticosteroid (17-OCHS) over 4.5 μg/dL confirms the diagnosis of hypercortisolism. Many medications, including corticosteroids, phenothiazines, phenytoin, diuretics, quinidine, penicillin G, oral contraceptives, lithium, acetylsalicylic acid (ASA), and monoamine oxidase inhibitors (MAOIs) may affect the accuracy of test results.

Baseline plasma ACTH levels should be assessed once hypercortisolism is confirmed. Levels are highest between 7 and 10 A.M. (8 to 80 pg/mL) and lowest right before bedtime (<10 pg/mL). Generally, levels below 20 pg/mL indicate a possible adrenal tumor, and levels exceeding 20 pg/mL are indicative of a pituitary or ectopic secreting ACTH tumor.

Following completion of hormonal studies, radiological studies are performed to localize the possible source of excess cortisol production. Most microadenomas of the pituitary gland are detected by imaging. An abdominal CT scan of the adrenal glands is done to detect adrenal tumors. In Cushing's disease, the adrenal glands are enlarged. A CT scan of the chest and abdomen is also beneficial in detecting possible sites of ectopic secretion. Because the lung is the most likely source of ectopic secretion, special attention to the chest is indicated. If the source is determined to be the pituitary gland, an MRI is indicated.

Patients should also be assessed for other sequelae of Cushing's syndrome such as hypokalemia, anemia, metabolic alkalosis, hyperglycemia, and hypercholesterolemia. Except for initial testing, the diagnosis of Cushing's syndrome and the differentiation as to cause is best accomplished under the direction of an endocrinologist.

Differential Diagnosis

Pregnancy, obesity, and excessive activity may produce elevated serum cortisol levels. Other conditions that may produce elevated cortisol levels are alcoholism, severe depression, obesity, hypertension, diabetes mellitus, glucocorticoid therapy, estrogen replacement therapy, and oral contraceptives. There are also various familial (genetic) predispositions to hypercortisolemia. Type 1 multiple endocrine neoplasia (MEN 1) syndrome presents with pituitary corticotroph adenomas in 2 percent of cases, while Carney's syndrome is a rare autosomal dominant complex consisting of bilateral micronodular dysplasia, pigmented lentigines and blue nevi on the head and trunk, as well as multiple endocrine and nonendocrine neoplasms.

Management

The goals of treatment are to reduce the cortisol levels to normal and treat the underlying cause. The initial clinical management of patients with Cushing's syndrome should be handled by an endocrinologist. Despite successful treatment, some patients may relapse, so the patient must be evaluated for recurrence of hypercortisolemia.

Initial Management

Transsphenoidal pituitary microsurgery is the treatment of choice for pituitary adenoma causing Cushing's disease. If surgery is unsuccessful, irradiation of the pituitary may be considered. Complications from surgery include transient diabetes insipidus, visual disturbances, cerebrospinal rhinorrhea, and meningitis. After microsurgery, 75 percent of patients will experience dramatic decreases in cortisol and will require exogenous glucocorticoid therapy for 6 to 36 months after surgery. For patients who fail to respond or who have a recurrence, treatment may include stereotactic pituitary radiosurgery (gamma knife) or laparoscopic bilateral adrenalectomy. Conventional pituitary irradiation therapy has a 23 percent cure rate. Failure rates with both types of treatment increase over time. Diagnostic errors (depression and lack of a pituitary adenoma) increased failure rates of patients treated with surgery.

Twenty-five percent of patients following a transsphenoidal pituitary microsurgery have persistent signs and symptoms. This is more likely to occur if the tumor was not completely removed and in those patients with corticotrophic hyperplasia. These patients require a second pituitary operation, radiotherapy, or bilateral total adrenalectomy.

In younger patients who are not surgical candidates, mitotane (Lysodren) or alternatively ketoconazole (Nizoral) 200 mg q6h may be used alone or in combination to reduce cortisol overproduction. Older adults who are not surgical candidates may tolerate the use of ketoconazole, however, liver enzymes may be elevated with this treatment and need to be monitored by an endocrinologist.

Subsequent Management

Following resection of a pituitary adenoma, normal corticotrophins are suppressed and temporary cortisone replacement therapy is indicated for 9 to 12 months, but may be as long as 36 months. The drugs of choice for replacement therapy are hydrocortisone (Cortef), prednisone (Deltasone), and fludrocortisone (Florinef). Dexamethasone (Decadron) is an alternative. The lowest dose effective in maintaining hormone levels is recommended. Complications of untreated or inadequate treatment of Cushing's disease are increased susceptibility to infections, nephrolithiasis, hypertension, and osteoporosis. Inadequate treatment may also lead to psychosis or uncontrolled diabetes mellitus.

Medications for Cushing's syndrome are listed in Drugs Commonly Prescribed 15.3.

Follow-Up and Referral

The follow-up for each patient depends on the therapy. The patient should be followed monthly for the first year and checked for signs of adrenal hypofunction, and then every 6 to 12 months thereafter. Excessive corticosteroid treatment should be avoided as much as possible. The patient may need education to cope with lifelong symptomatology, specifically information on the importance of early interventions for infections, a prevention of emotional lability mechanism to cope with overwhelming stress, use of potassium supplements, and maintenance of a high-protein diet.

The disorder is usually chronic, characterized by periods of cyclic exacerbation and rare remissions. Complications are osteoporosis, increased susceptibility to infection, hirsutism, and metastases of malignant tumors (depending on causality).

Referrals are suggested for surgical intervention for the following conditions associated with Cushing's syndrome:

1. *Primary hypersecretion of ACTH.* Transsphenoidal microsurgery is recommended and is often followed by radiation and sometimes by medication (adrenocortical inhibitors).
2. *Adrenocortical tumors.* Surgery is recommended, but prognosis is still poor. Replacement therapy is used but usually for only 3 to 12 months. The patient may need treatment with adrenocortical inhibitors if not treated with surgery, and this should definitely be managed by an endocrinologist.
3. *Ectopic ACTH production.* Surgery is recommended for removal of neoplastic tissue to manage symptoms, although surgical cure is unlikely. Sometimes a bilateral adrenalectomy is performed. Follow-up for these

Drugs Commonly Prescribed 15.3: Cushing's Syndrome

Drug	Dosage and How Supplied	Glucocorticoid Activity	Mineralocorticoid Activity
Prednisone (Deltasone, Meticorten)	Dosage: 5–60 mg PO qd How supplied: 2.5-mg, 5-mg, 10-mg, 20-mg, 50-mg tablets	Moderate	Weak
Prednisolone (Delta-Cortef, Prelone)	Dosage: 5–60 mg PO qd How supplied: syrup	Moderate	Weak at 5 mg/5 mL and 15 mg/5 mL
Methylprednisolone (Medrol) or Depo-Medrol IM or IV	Dosage: 4–48 mg PO qd How supplied: Medrol dose pack, Methylprednisolone 4 mg tablets; unit-of-use scored tablets: oral 2-mg, 4-mg, 8-mg, 16-mg, 24-mg, and 32-mg (scored) tablets Dosage: Depo-Medrol 4–120 mg IM/week for 1–4 weeks Solu-Medrol IV may be given 10–40 mg IV	Moderate	Minimal to none
Hydrocortisone (Cortef, Hydrocortone)	Dosage: 20–240 mg qd How supplied: oral; 5-mg, 10-mg, 20-mg tablets Intramuscular; 100, 250, 500 mg for IV or IM injection Also intraarticular, topical, ophthalmic preparations	High	Yes
Cortisone acetate (Cortone)	Dosage: 25–300 mg/day as a single dose or in divided doses How supplied: oral, IM; 20–300 mg/day	High	Yes
Dexamethasone (long-acting) (Decadron)	Dosage: 0.75–9 mg/day How supplied: oral 0.5-mg, 0.75-mg, 4.0-mg scored tablets IM: 24 mg/ml, 0.5–9 mg IV qd	Very High	Weak
Fludrocortisone (Florinef)	Dosage: 100 μg/day; range 100 μg three times/week to 200 μg/day How supplied: oral	None	High

patients would depend on causality and recommended treatment.

Patient Teaching

Although patients with Cushing's syndrome will be managed initially by an endocrinologist, the primary-care clinician often manages other aspects of the patient's health. A caring relationship between the primary-care clinician and the patient is essential in the management of this multifaceted disorder. It is important to work collaboratively with the patient in managing symptoms successfully.

Patients need a thorough understanding of the medications and warning signs of undermedication or overtreatment with cortisone. Cortisone preparations should be taken with food. Patients need to be told that they should consult with the primary care clinician when initiating additional medications. Patients on high doses should wear a medical identification bracelet. Because these patients are prone to infections, they should be instructed on how to avoid common infections, both bacterial and fungal. Patients cannot rely on elevated temperature to indicate the seriousness of any infection; therefore, they need to report any initial signs of infection.

Nutritional counseling may be indicated, including information on avoidance of excessive sodium and on a well balanced low-fat diet. Many patients are obese, and the importance of weight loss must be addressed.

Patients should monitor their glucose levels at least weekly. During periods of stress or medication adjustment, glucose levels will need to be tested more frequently. Patients should assess their glucose levels daily during periods of medication adjustment. If levels are stable and within normal levels, they may continue testing glucose levels until at least 1 week after final dose adjustment. They should resume daily glucose testing in times of stress or if any signs of infection are present. If the morning glucose level at any time is above normal, more frequent testing is indicated. The patient should be given a log to record the glucose testing, and instructed to bring the log for each primary care visit.

Patients with Cushing's syndrome will need to have their blood pressure monitored weekly. As with glucose monitoring, the frequency will depend on their symptoms and coexisting cardiovascular disease. More frequent monitoring will be needed during times of stress. The patient should obtain a sphygmomanometer for home use.

The patient should be instructed about fall prevention. Because of the potential for osteoporosis, the patient should avoid those activities that are likely to cause falls. Simple environmental changes can be made in the home to increase safety, such as removing small rugs, placing rails around the bathtub, and using a shower chair.

Patients should also report any symptoms of gastrointestinal upset (nausea, bloating, vomiting) and monitor themselves for signs of gastrointestinal bleeding (vomiting blood, tarry stools, increasing fatigue).

Instructions on skin care are essential. Research indicates that older adults with a history of long-term corticosteroid use are more prone to pressure ulcers. Thin, easily traumatized skin must be protected. These individuals should avoid applying tape and adhesive bandages directly to their skin. They should wear protective clothing for outdoor activities such as gardening.

There is potential for failure of the surgical intervention. Instruct the patient to report any return of symptoms if he or she has been asymptomatic for a period following the operation.

Diabetes Mellitus

Diabetes mellitus (DM) is a syndrome of disordered carbohydrate, fat, and protein metabolism and hyperglycemia resulting from deficits in insulin secretion, insulin action, or a combination of both. There are two distinct types of diabetes mellitus, type 1 and type 2 (each with a distinct epidemiology and etiology), but impaired fasting glucose (IFG) and impaired glucose tolerance (IGT) are used to describe a fasting glucose between 110 and 126 mg/dL or a 2-hour postglucose load blood glucose 140 to 200 mg/dL. Some sources state that IGT and gestational diabetes are now considered under the IFG category.

DM is the most common endocrine disorder, affecting 16 to 18 million people in the United States, up to 5 million of whom may be undiagnosed. In 2002, DM affected 8.7 percent of the U.S. adult population. The complications of DM include cardiovascular and peripheral vascular disease, decreased immune system functioning, renal failure, and retinopathy. Diabetic nephropathy is now the leading cause of end-stage renal disease. DM also is the leading cause of acquired blindness in the United States. Tight control of blood glucose levels reduces the morbidity and mortality associated with DM, but control is not without its costs. The costs of long-term management of diabetes has serious implications on the quality of life of those affected and their families.

Diabetes Mellitus Type 1

Diabetes mellitus type 1 is a metabolic disorder characterized by a severe insulin deficiency resulting from beta-cell destruction and producing hyperglycemia. The lack of insulin alters lipid, carbohydrate, and protein metabolism. Chronic hyperglycemia of DM results in damage to various body organs, especially the eyes, kidneys, nerves, heart, and both small and large blood vessels. Loss of vision, renal failure, loss of a lower extremity, and chronic foot ulcers caused by peripheral neuropathy are common sequelae of long-term hyperglycemia. Chronic hyperglycemia affects all body systems and places significant social, economic, and psychological demands on patients and their families.

Diabetic retinopathy remains the leading cause of new-onset blindness among adults ages 20 to 74 years. After 20 years of type 1 DM, nearly all patients have some retinopathy. Impairment of growth, an increased susceptibility to infection, and autonomic neuropathy, resulting in gastrointestinal, genitourinary, and cardiovascular symptoms including sexual dysfunction, also occur. Persons with DM have an increased incidence of atherosclerotic heart disease, peripheral vascular disease, and cerebrovascular disease. Diabetic ketoacidosis (DKA) and hyperosmolar hyperglycemia syndrome (HHS) produced by hyperglycemia are life-threatening sequelae of hyperglycemia. HHS is more commonly seen in type 1 DM, however. Tables 15.7 and 15.8 provide more information on these conditions.

Epidemiology and Causes

DM type 1 occurs in approximately 700,000 Americans and accounts for about 10 percent of all cases of diabetes in the Western world. It is more common in whites (1.5 to 2 times higher than in nonwhites) with the peak onset between age 11 and 13 years. While there is no gender predisposition, marked variations have been observed across ethnocultural groups, which correlates with differential expression of human leukocyte antigen (HLA) haplotypes (see below). Type 1 DM was previously known as insulin-dependent diabetes mellitus (IDDM) or juvenile onset diabetes. However, cases may occur at any age with a fairly abrupt onset. It is uncommon in children younger than 1 year of age and in adults older than 30 years. In nonpediatric patients, this condition is sometimes known as latent autoimmune diabetes of adults (LADA).

Currently, the American Diabetes Association (ADA) does not recommend screening for type 1 diabetes in apparently healthy individuals. Current clinical trials are being conducted to evaluate prevention strategies to delay clinical disease, and the ADA is hopeful that effective preventive therapies will eventually be found.

Type 1 DM has two forms—immune-mediated DM and idiopathic DM. *Immune-mediated diabetes mellitus* accounts for 90 percent of type 1 diabetes and results from an autoimmune destruction of the beta cells. It typically occurs in childhood or adolescence but can arise at any age. Current thinking on the etiology of type 1 is that it results from an infection or toxic insult in persons with a genetic predisposition. It is believed that there is an autoimmune response against either pancreatic B cell antigens or against molecules of the B cell. The infectious agents most commonly identified are the mumps virus or coxsackie B4 virus. Sensitized immunocytes may release destructive cytotoxins and antibodies that contribute to the development of type 1 diabetes. Patients with immune-mediated diabetes are rarely obese and are also prone to other autoimmune diseases such as Graves' disease, Hashimoto's thyroiditis, Addison's disease, vitiligo, and pernicious anemia. *Idiopathic diabetes*

Table 15.7 Diabetic Ketoacidosis

DKA represents an acute decompensation in diabetes and requires immediate medical attention. The cardinal features of DKA are hyperglycemia (blood glucose > 350 mg/dL), ketonemia (plasma ketone level > 5 mmol/L), and acidosis (plasma bicarbonate levels < 9 mEq/L). It is often caused by a lack of insulin but may result from physical (e.g., infection) or emotional stress despite continued insulin therapy. As insulin levels drop, the concentrations of glucagon rise. Glucagon is a pancreatic hormone that acts to increase glucose levels.

Additionally, epinephrine inhibits glucose transport in the peripheral tissues. These hormonal changes have two critical effects: (1) they stimulate the production of glucose in the liver, called gluconeogenesis, causing even greater hyperglycemia, and (2) they activate the ketogenic process. Free fatty acids from adipose (fat) stores are oxidized in the liver, causing a release of ketones and resulting in acidosis.

Clinical Presentation

DKA begins with anorexia, increased thirst, nausea, vomiting, abdominal cramping, and increased urine formation. Later signs include Kussmaul respiration, signs of dehydration (usual fluid deficit is 3–5 L), oliguria, and altered consciousness. If left untreated, coma, vascular collapse, and renal shutdown can occur and blood glucose increases from 300 to 800 mg/dL.

Initial diagnostic testing begins with determinations of serum glucose, sodium, potassium, phosphate, bicarbonate, beta-hydroxybutyrate, and osmolarity. Unfortunately, plasma ketone levels are not helpful; therefore, the key indicators of treatment success are the pH and calculated anion gap (AG = sodium − (cloride + bicarbonate)).

Management

Treatment goals are to correct the dehydration, normalize electrolytes, and correct acidosis. This is accomplished first with insulin. Most cases can be reversed with a low, continuous-dose insulin infusion of approximately 0.1 to 0.2 U/kg per hour. To correct dehydration, between 1 to 2 L of normal saline or Ringer's lactate solution is rapidly given intravenous based on the clinical assessment of the fluid state. Potassium replacement is usually needed, but the administration time varies. The initial level is often high, which reflects depleted tissue stores that have shifted to the plasma. Potassium administration generally begins 3–4 hours after initiation of therapy, when acidosis begins to reverse and the insulin causes an intracellular shift of potassium. If the potassium levels are normal or low on admission, potassium therapy should not be delayed. Bicarbonate therapy is indicated if the pH is 7.0 or below and is not used routinely in less ill patients.

The patient should be monitored for amounts of insulin, fluid administration, urine volume, blood chemistries, and vital signs. After recovery, events that lead to the development of DKA should be explored with the patient. Occasionally, a patient may theorize that insulin therapy should be discontinued when ill with a "flu," the rationale being that if they are too ill to eat they should not inject insulin. Providing educational guidelines for "sick days" can prevent future occurrences of DKA.

Table 15.8 Hyperosmolar Hyperglycemic Nonketotic Syndrome (HHNKS)

HHNKS is characterized by severe hyperglycemia (>600 mg/dL) in the absence of significant ketosis, with hyperosmolality and dehydration. It is a syndrome of profound dehydration that results from prolonged hyperglycemia. It is associated with a high mortality rate and is seen in older adults who have developed an infection or other illness, undiagnosed diabetics, and patients with diabetes diagnosed after a long period of hyperglycemia. Certain therapeutic procedures such as peritoneal dialysis, hemodialysis, tube feeding with high-protein formulas, and the use of mannitol, phenytoin (Dilantin), steroids, immunosuppressive agents, and diuretics have been known to precipitate its development. There may be an underlying condition, such as renal insufficiency or CHF, or it may be precipitated by an event such as sepsis, an MI, or surgery.

Clinical Presentation

The onset of HHNKS may be insidious; symptoms may be subtle at first. A history may indicate decreased fluid intake. Patients may present with polyuria, polydipsia, and weakness extending over several days to weeks. Symptoms of ketoacidosis are absent, subsequently often delaying a clinical diagnosis. Lethargy and confusion develop as serum osmolality exceeds 310 mOsm/kg, and coma can occur if it goes higher.

On laboratory examination, there is severe hyperglycemia—blood glucose levels may exceed 600 mg/dL. Initially, sodium levels are decreased, followed by elevated sodium levels as dehydration progresses. Serum osmolality levels can exceed 400 mOsm/kg (normal adult levels are 280–300 mOsm/kg).

Management

Treatment consists of fluid replacement, insulin, and treatment of electrolyte imbalances. The incidence of this condition in older adults and a delay in treatment, often because of unrecognizable signs in its early stages, result in an overall poor prognosis. Provide hemodynamic support as needed and institute seizure precautions.

Fluid replacement is essential, usually with hypotonic saline (0.45%). In cases of hypovolemia, isotonic saline (0.9%) should be used. As much as 4 to 6 L may be required in 8–10 hours. Careful monitoring is required for proper sodium and potassium replacement. The sodium is typically hyponatremic initially and is corrected using the following equation: corrected sodium = measured sodium + (0.8 × every 50 mg/dL increment of plasma glucose above 100 mg/dL). Once blood glucose reaches 250 mg/dL, fluid replacement should be changed to 5% dextrose in 0.45% saline solution or 0.9% saline solution. An important end point of fluid therapy is to return urine output to 50 mg/h or more. Fluids alone may be enough to reduce hyperglycemia. Less potassium is needed than in diabetic ketoacidosis (DKA). Potassium chloride (10 mEq/L) can usually be added to the initial bottle of fluids administered if the patient's serum potassium level is not elevated.

mellitus has no known cause and has no evidence of autoimmunity and accounts for less than 10 percent of type 1 diabetes. It is a rare form of diabetes, is inherited, and is more common in people of Asian or African origin. The need for insulin replacement therapy in these patients is variable.

Pathophysiology

Type 1 DM is characterized by a reduction or absence of functioning beta cells in the pancreatic islets of Langerhans. Although the exact process is not well understood, it is speculated that the sequence begins with a genetic susceptibility which has been mapped to the HLA region on chromosome 6p. Specifically, an increased risk of type 1 DM has been associated with the presence of at least five genetic polymorphisms: HLA-Dqα, HLA-Dqβ, HLA-DR, preproinsulin (a promoter of the insulin gene), and PTPN22 (a lymphocyte-specific tyrosine phosphatase involved in T-cell receptor signaling, which also confers susceptibility to other autoimmune disorders). Inheritance of type 1 DM appears to be polygenic, however, as expression of a particular HLA allele alone is insufficient to lead to autoimmune beta-cell destruction.

While other genes located within major histocompatibility complex (MHC) genetic loci, as well as non-MHC genes such as cytotoxic T lymphocyte-associated antigen 4 (*CTLA-4*), influence diabetes risk, class II HLA genes have the greatest effect. In fact, certain non-MHC genes confer an increased risk of type 1 DM only in the presence of particular HLA haplotypes, implying the importance of polygenic interactions.

Much of our understanding of the pathogenesis of autoimmune DM stems from studies in diabetogenic murine models, including NOD (nonobese diabetic) mice and BB rats. Some triggering mechanism such as a viral infection or other environmental factor is believed to stimulate an inflammatory response and initiate autoimmune infiltration of the pancreatic beta cells within the islets of Langerhans—a process termed insulitis. Strongly associated with IL-18 (interferon-γ–inducing factor or IGIF) and IL-12 expression, as well as interferon-γ–positive Th1 T cells in NOD mice, insulitis involves autologous beta cells being recognized as foreign by the body's immune system. Islet cell antigens are presented by macrophages and other antigen-presenting cells within the context of class II MHC proteins to autoreactive T cells which mediate much of the subsequent beta islet cell destruction. Alterations in just one or two amino acid positions within certain class II MHC proteins can markedly increase their capacity to present autoantigens to autoreactive T cells. In turn, more than 90 percent of patients with type 1 diabetes express HLA-DR3,DQB1*0201 or HLA-DR4,DQB1*0302, while persons expressing both of these HLA haplotypes are most susceptible to developing this disease. By contrast, other HLA polymorphisms confer a protective effect against type

1 diabetes, presumably due to their decreased affinity for binding autoantigen.

It is known that type 1A DM is clearly associated with an increased incidence of other autoimmune disorders, including thyroid, adrenal, and gonadal insufficiency. The coexistence of all these conditions has been termed polyglandular autoimmune disease type 2. Other rare autoimmune syndromes which involve insulitis shed further light on the importance of genetic pathogenic mechanisms. Autoimmune polyendocrine syndrome type 1 results from a mutation in the *AIRE* gene, an autoimmune regulatory gene that controls the subsequent expression of multiple peripheral autoantigens within the thymus (including insulin itself) which is believed to mediate T-cell self-tolerance. The IPEX syndrome involves mutations in *foxp3*, which is considered a master control gene for regulatory T cells. T suppressor cells are subsequently reduced in activity, allowing for the development of autoimmune disease in affected infants, including DM and fulminant enteritis, which is often fatal.

Both Th1 and Th2 cells are capable of inducing beta-cell destruction, underscoring the importance of both cell-mediated and humoral immune processes in the pathogenesis of type 1 DM. Indeed, the presence of functional autoreactive B lymphocytes and islet cell autoantibodies has been shown both to increase the incidence and shorten the time to progression of type 1 DM. Interestingly, however, autoantibodies are not absolutely required for the development of type 1 diabetes, as demonstrated by documented cases of the disease occurring in humorally immunodeficient persons with X-linked (Bruton's) agammaglobulinemia.

Nonetheless, islet-specific antibodies may be identified in 70 to 80 percent of prediabetic and newly diagnosed type 1 diabetic patients. Multiple species of autoantibodies have been identified, including immunoglobulins specific for the islet cell enzyme glutamic acid decarboxylase (GAD), the tyrosine phosphatase insulinoma-associated protein 2 (IA-2), and the insulin molecule itself. It has not been fully determined whether these antibodies are themselves pathogenic or simply formed as a consequence of immunologic upregulation. For example, although anti-GAD antibodies are found in 70 percent of human patients with type 1 DM, they do not play a significant role in the pathogenesis of diabetes in NOD mice.

However, even before GAD-specific immunoglobulins form, anti-insulin antibodies may be detected. Studies in NOD mice and humans have confirmed the role of both pathogenic CD8+ and CD4+ T-cell clones that recognize peptide epitopes of the insulin B chain. IA-2-specific immunoglobulin is typically detected after antibodies to insulin and GAD. Identification of two of these three classes of autoantibodies is strongly predictive of progression to type 1A DM in genetically predisposed individuals.

Genetic predisposition alone, however, does not fully account for disease pathogenesis. Identical (monozygotic) twin studies reveal only a 30 percent lifetime risk of developing type 1 DM in twin siblings of probands; however, this compares to only a 5 percent risk in nonidentical siblings. Moreover, twin studies also demonstrate that autoantibodies against islet cells may be present for years in the unaffected sibling of a proband before autoimmune diabetes develops in this twin as well. Thus, destruction of a significant amount of beta-cell mass may take months to years but will eventually lead to a lack of insulin.

It is this lack of insulin that disturbs the regulatory mechanisms which control the metabolism of glucose in the body. Hyperglycemia typically develops once 80 to 90 percent of a patient's beta cells have been destroyed. However, there are animal (baboon) models of autoimmune diabetes which demonstrate insulin deficiency with as much as 50 percent of beta-cell mass still intact. Moreover, inflamed islet cells from NOD mice explanted to isolated cell cultures slowly regain their ability to secrete insulin after 1 week of incubation. Thus, external factors such as the inflammatory cytokine milieu are believed to play an important role in diabetic pathogenesis, despite the presence of adequate beta-cell mass. The treatment implication of this is that some patients with autoimmune DM may have a reversible component to their disease, if the autoinflammatory process can be stopped early enough and an adequate number of beta cells salvaged. For example, insulin-like growth factor (IGF)-1 has been cited as a cytokine that plays an important role in preserving beta-cell function.

However, progressive beta-cell destruction with hyperglycemia remains the hallmark of type 1 DM. In turn, it is this hyperglycemia that leads to both microvascular and macrovascular complications, which underlie long-term diabetic damage. Vascular endothelial dysfunction and inflammation result in fibrosis and intimal thickening, leading to progressive narrowing of the vascular lumen. In turn, blood flow through the microvasculature is reduced, leading to tissue ischemia throughout the body, which results in functional impairment of multiple end organs. Several clinical trials have demonstrated that careful glycemic control reduces the development and delays the progression of microvascular manifestations of diabetes, including nephropathy and retinopathy. Thus, patients with type 1 DM universally require exogenous insulin to maintain glycemic homeostasis.

Identifying the triggering event or events that are capable of inducing the pathogenesis of autoimmune diabetes has been the subject of much research and debate. Molecular mimicry is often sited as the mechanism by which seemingly innocuous environmental (e.g., food-based epitopes) or infectious (e.g., viral) antigens that share homology with islet cell antigens initiate a destructive autoimmune process with the development of cross-reactive antibodies (e.g., the association of coxsackie B viral infection with anti-GAD antibodies and the shared homology between the FC2 protein of the coxsackievirus B4 and human GAD). Another proposed mechanism of pathogenesis observed in BB rats involves delayed expression of islet cell antigens which is thought to eliminate self-tolerance mechanisms associated with thymic T-cell education early in development, i.e., negative thymic selection of autoreactive T lymphocytes. How this mechanism may relate to autoimmune diabetes in humans is less clear, however.

Some research has identified certain perinatal factors as increasing the risk of type 1 DM (e.g., maternal age greater than 25 years, preeclampsia, neonatal respiratory disease, neonatal jaundice secondary to ABO incompatibility). However, the increase in risk noted in this study was small. In contrast, a significant body of research has established viral antigens and certain dietary influences as having the strongest impact on the development of autoimmune DM. Direct viral infection of pancreatic beta islet cells may play a role, but evidence for this mechanism is lacking. However, acute IgM titers to coxsackie B virus are known to be elevated in the mothers of children with type 1 DM. In addition, enteroviral infections are also more common in type 1 diabetics, as compared to their nondiabetic siblings. Congenital rubella syndrome has also been associated with the development of type 1 DM and other autoimmune syndromes up to 5 to 20 years later, especially in individuals with the HLA-DR3 haplotype.

Contrary evidence also exists, however, that appears to exonerate viral infection as a triggering mechanism. Human immunization with either viral or bacterial antigens has never been shown to increase the risk of developing autoimmune diabetes. Moreover, when NOD mice and BB rats are raised in pathogen-free conditions with no viral contact, they display an increased incidence of autoimmune DM. In fact, infection of either of these animal strains by the lymphocytic choriomeningitis virus (LCM) early on in development actually protects against type 1 DM. The precise mechanism is poorly understood, however.

The impact of dietary influences on the development of type 1 DM has been heavily studied. While food epitopes may not mimic beta-cell antigens directly, similar proteins from other animal species are thought to trigger autoimmune reactions leading to type 1 DM. Epidemiologic research from at least 10 countries has implicated key protein components of cow's milk including bovine serum albumin and beta-casein as the most likely triggers of these autoimmune responses. However, cross-sectional and prospective studies have not confirmed these associations. In fact, some work has even suggested vitamin D confers protection against autoimmune DM. In contrast, one epidemiologic study indicated the risk of developing type 1 DM was 30 percent higher in regions of the United Kingdom where drinking water contained high levels of nitrates (14.8 mg/L vs. 3.2 mg/L).

The timing of the introduction of gluten- and rice-containing cereals into an infant's diet has also been implicated in increasing type 1 DM risk, specifically, when cereals are introduced prior to 3 months or after 7 months of age. The early introduction of rice cereals prior to 3 months is also associated with the development of celiac disease. Fortunately, these parameters correspond with the current American Board of Pediatrics recommendation to begin rice cereals (ostensibly, for their iron content) at 4 to 6 months of age.

Finally, secondary causes of diabetes may mimic either type 1 or type 2 DM, depending on whether the primary disease mechanism is destruction of beta islet cells with subsequent insulin deficiency or, rather, peripheral insulin resistance in which the body still produces insulin but the peripheral tissues utilize it less efficiently. Nonimmune mechanisms of beta-cell destruction which produce a type 1B diabetes-like state include hemochromatosis, cystic fibrosis, and pancreatitis.

Clinical Presentation

Subjective

The manifestation of symptoms varies, but the majority of patients seek medical attention because of symptoms related to hyperglycemia. The diagnosis of DM type 1 is often made when a patient presents with diabetic ketoacidosis.

The classic symptoms of type 1 DM are polydipsia, polyuria, polyphagia, anorexia, and weight loss. Nocturnal enuresis is often a disturbing symptom reported by many patients. Visual changes, especially blurred vision, weakness, and fatigue are frequently present.

Polyuria or increased urination results from osmotic diuresis secondary to sustained hyperglycemia. The loss of glucose, free water, and electrolytes induces a hyperosmolar state, which causes thirst (polydipsia). Blurred vision results from the lenses and retina being exposed to hyperosmolar fluids. There may be a decreased plasma volume, which causes dizziness. Weakness is due to the catabolism of muscle and potassium loss.

The patient may also complain of nausea or abdominal pain. Urinary tract infection and pyelonephritis should be ruled out, especially in patients with abdominal pain, as diabetics are more likely to experience serious complication of pyelonephritis including renal papillary necrosis, emphysematous (necrotizing) pyelonephritis, or progression to gram-negative sepsis.

Patients with DM have impaired immunity and may present with repeated infections, decreased wound healing, or infections that are uncommon in the general public including staphylococcal and *Klebsiella pneumoniae* infections. Hyperglycemia worsens humoral immunity and leukocyte function. In fact, infections such as malignant (necrotizing) otitis externa (due to *Pseudomonas aeruginosa*) and rhinocerebral mucormycosis occur almost exclusively in patients with DM. Patients may present with complaints of pruritus caused by an infection such as vulvovaginitis. Patients with poorly controlled DM may have chronic pyogenic infections of the skin. Necrobiosis lipoidica diabeticorum is rarely seen in any patient without DM and consists of plaques with demarcated borders and a shining yellow surface occurring on the anterior surfaces of the legs or dorsal aspect of the ankles. Because most patients with DM also have micro- and macrovascular complications that decrease the blood flow to the tissues, pathogens are able to multiply rapidly because the increased glucose in body fluids is a good source of energy for them.

Diabetic foot ulcers result from a combination of factors including decreased circulation, infection, decreased immune response, and peripheral neuropathy. Occasionally, the patient may present with a complaint of paresthesia, which is related to a temporary dysfunction of peripheral sensory nerves. The patient with peripheral neuropathy presents with a stocking-glove distribution of anesthesia, leading to missed foot ulcers or burns on the hands (from cooking or smoking).

Objective

Weight loss despite normal or increased appetite occurs as water, glycogen, and triglyceride stores are depleted. There is a reduced muscle mass as amino acids are used by the liver for gluconeogenesis with resultant ketone bodies formed. Signs of dehydration such as poor skin turgor and dry mucous membranes may be present. Genital or urinary tract infections may be present as a result of the hyperglycemic state. Ketoacidosis is usually present and may be mild to severe. Hyperosmolar hyperglycemic nonketotic acidosis is a second complication of prolonged hyperglycemia.

Patients with long-standing DM frequently develop diabetic retinopathy, which is a result of retinal ischemia. There are five stages of retinopathy that are evident on physical exam and include: (1) dilation of retinal venules and retinal capillary microaneurysms; (2) increased vascular permeability; (3) retinal ischemia due to vascular occlusion; (4) angiogenesis with proliferation of new retinal surface blood vessels; and (5) retinal hemorrhage with fibrovascular proliferation and contraction which may lead to retinal detachment. These patients must be referred to an ophthalmologist for evaluation.

Physical exam also requires a detailed neurologic exam because DM can have neurologic complications. For example, diabetics may have third cranial nerve palsy, or the sixth (abducens) and fourth (trochlear) cranial nerves can also be affected in cranial neuropathy.

Diagnostic Reasoning

Immediate testing in the office can be accomplished by utilizing a portable monitor to test capillary blood glucose level. This test is referred to as a random plasma glucose measurement and is given without regard to time of last meal. It is important to consider that certain drugs, including glucocorticoids, furosemide (Lasix), thiazide diuretics, estrogen-containing products, beta-blockers, and nicotinic acid can produce hyperglycemia. If the random plasma glucose level is elevated, the urine should be tested for ketones and additional blood plasma glucose testing should be done.

Diagnostic Tests

Initial Testing. Current recommendation for the diagnosis of diabetes are:

1. Symptoms of diabetes (e.g., polyuria, polydipsia, weight loss) plus a random (casual) plasma glucose level of 200 mg/dL or higher
2. OR fasting plasma glucose level of 126 mg/dL or higher
3. OR a 2-hour plasma glucose of 200 mg/dL or higher during an oral glucose tolerance test (OGTT) with a 75-gram glucose load (not for routine use)

These criteria should be confirmed by repeat testing on a different day except in the case of unequivocal hyperglycemia with acute metabolic decompensation.

Adult-onset autoimmune diabetes or patients at risk for developing type 1 DM can be given the acute insulin response test to a known injected dose of glucose (AIRg). This test along with immune studies (e.g., measurements of islet cell glutamate decarboxylase antibodies) can aid in diagnosing the above conditions, but it is not universally available.

Another test that may be helpful in assessing beta-cell function in a patient with type 1 DM is the C-peptide level. Pro-insulin is cleaved into insulin and C-peptide, which is biologically inactive. So that a patient with some residual pancreatic beta-cell function may have decreased levels of C-peptide (normal fasting = 0.51 to 2.72 ng/mL or 0.17 to 0.90 mmol/L).

Subsequent Testing. A glycated hemoglobin (Ghb or HbA_{1c}) determination gives valuable insight into the mean plasma glucose concentration over the preceding 2 to 3 months and is helpful in documenting the degree of glycemic control at the time of diagnosis and as part of continuing care. The American Diabetes Association (ADA) recommends that the treatment goal should be a HbA_{1c} below 7.0 percent. The HbA_{1c} level roughly correlates to the mean plasma glucose: 6 percent = glucose of 135 mg/dL; 7 percent = 170 mg/dL; 8 percent = 205 mg/dL; 9 percent = 240 mg/dL; 10 percent = 275 mg/dL; 11 percent = 310 mg/dL; and 12 percent = 345 mg/dL.

Additional laboratory tests that are appropriate to the evaluation of the patient's general medical condition should be performed. They include fasting lipid profile (total cholesterol, high-density lipoprotein (HDL), low-density lipoprotein (LDL), and triglyceride levels), urinalysis, microalbuminuria, thyroid function tests, and serum creatinine if protein is present. Urine cultures are obtained if indicated.

Differential Diagnosis

With the classic symptoms of DM confirmed by blood plasma glucose testing, a diagnosis of DM is confirmed; however, other potential causes of hyperglycemia should be considered. Hyperglycemia and glucosuria are present in patients with Cushing's disease, pheochromocytoma, or acromegaly. Extreme stress or trauma, such as that seen in extensive burns, may produce transient hyperglycemia. Renal tubular disease may produce glycosuria without concurrent hyperglycemia. Several pharmacologic agents can cause hyperglycemia including glucocorticoids, sympathomimetic agents, and niacin.

Management

Type 1 diabetes is a chronic illness that requires ongoing health care and education to prevent acute and chronic complications. The complexity and lifelong management regimens necessitate that the patient and clinician work as a team to develop and implement the treatment plan. The ADA recommends a team approach to care, including the primary-care provider, an endocrinologist periodically when indicated, a certified diabetes educator, a dietitian, the patient, and the patient's family. Essential to successful implementation of the treatment plan is the plan's fit with the patient's lifestyle to the extent possible. This is where a diabetes educator is of the most assistance.

To be effective, the treatment program requires insulin regimens, frequent self-monitoring of blood glucose (SMBG), medical nutrition therapy (MNT), regular exercise, continuing education in the prevention and treatment of complications, and periodic assessment of treatment goals. The principles of management are summarized in Table 15.9. The Insulin Management Diabetes Self-Efficacy Scale is shown in Advanced Assessment 15.1, and complementary therapies in Complementary Therapies Box 15.1.

A diagnosis of diabetes, as with any chronic illness, requires the incorporation of the diagnosis and ultimate management into the patient's lifestyle. It may take a traumatic event or "turning point" in a patient's management to break the complacency of management to one that focuses on lifestyle changes.

Initial Management

Insulin Therapy. The initial goal of treatment for type 1 diabetes is to normalize the blood glucose level. This is best accomplished by intensive insulin regimens to accomplish the following goals: plasma glucose levels at 80 to 120 mg/dL before meals, plasma glucose levels of 100 to 140 mg/dL at bedtime and an HbA1c below 7 percent. The new type 1 diabetic often presents in crisis and requires hospitalization. These patients should be managed by an endocrinologist or a diabetologist. It is beyond the scope of primary care.

When patients present in acute hyperglycemia, it is essential not only to treat the hypoglycemia, but also to determine the underlying cause of the hyperglycemia (medication nonadherence, underlying infection [most common cause of DKA), dietary indiscretion). See Table 15.7 for the management of DKA.

Recent studies (Diabetes Control and Complications Trial, Diabetes Prevention Trial-1) conclusively demonstrated that in patients with type 1 DM, the risk of development or progression of retinopathy, nephropathy, and neuropathy is reduced 50 to 75 percent by intensive insulin regimens when compared with conventional treatment regimens. Individual treatment goals should, however, take into account the patient's capacity to understand and carry out the treatment, the risk for severe hypoglycemia, and any other factors that increase risk or decrease benefit. However, tight control does increase the chance of hypoglycemic episodes and is probably not appropriate for many elderly type 1 diabetics, patients with cornary artery disease who may be prone to hypoglycemia, or those with diabetic neuropathy who may lack the early neurologic (adrenergic) warning signs of hypoglycemia.

Some patients may experience early morning hyperglycemia due to complete absorption of the evening insulin dose prior to the early morning hours (dawn phenomenon). In addition, humans have an increased insulin requirement in the morning because of early morning secretion of growth hormone and cortisol. Thus, increasing nighttime insulin may just lead to late evening hypoglycemia, so that the evening dose should be given later, or switching to a longer acting form (Ultralente or Glargine rather than NPH) may be more effecting in preventing early morning hyperglycemia.

Patients requiring initiation of insulin therapy should be referred to an endocrinologist. The majority of insulin used today is made chemically identical to human insulin by recombinant DNA technology or by chemical modification of pork insulin; however, beef and pork insulins are still available. Insulin is available in rapid, short, intermediate, and long-acting forms. The optimum dosage is highly individual and can depend on site and depth of injection, skin temperature, and exercise. Human insulin is preferred for patients newly beginning insulin therapy, pregnant women, and persons with allergies.

In the United States, insulin is available in concentrations of 100 or 500 units (U)/mL but the higher concentrated preparations are only used in rare cases of insulin resistance, when the patient requires large doses. Many patients achieve better glycemic control with doses of regular insulin before meals with an evening dose of neutral protamine Hagedorn (NPH). This requires diligent and frequent blood glucose monitoring by the patient and should be chosen only if appropriate for the patient. Commercially mixed NPH and regular insulins are available, or the patient can custom mix his or her insulin. Dose amount and timing should be individualized to the patient according to his or her health needs and lifestyle (see Drugs Commonly Prescribed 15.4).

Self-Monitoring of Blood Glucose. Self-monitoring of blood glucose (SMBG) is the testing of capillary blood to determine the blood glucose level. Typically, plasma venous glucose measurements are within 15 percent of the results of whole blood capillary test results. SMBG is recommended for patients with type 1 diabetes to evaluate the effectiveness of the insulin regimen, medical nutrition therapy, and exercise. Used properly, it is the most useful mechanism to

ADVANCED ASSESSMENT 15.1

Insulin Management Diabetes Self-Efficacy Scale

When used with subjects, the 28 items are arranged as per the sample item; the Likert choice and scoring system is added in the right columns. The Likert scale ranges from (1) strongly agree to (5) strongly disagree. The codes for identifying subscales (G = general, D = diet, I = insulin) are at the end of the item that constitutes the subscale. An asterisk (*) beside the number indicates items that are reverse-scored. Both should be removed before using the scale.

1. *I can carry out practically all of the self-care activities in my daily diabetes routine. (G)
2. *I am confident in my ability to manage my diabetes. (G)
3. I feel unsure about having to use what I know about diabetes self-treatment every day. (G)
4. I don't think I can follow my diabetes routines every single day. (G)
5. *I can eat my meals at the same time every day. (D)
6. *I can stay on my diabetic diet when I eat in familiar places away from home (such as a friend's house). (D)
7. *I can stay on my diabetic diet when I eat in unfamiliar places. (D)
8. I'm not sure I'll be able to stay on my diabetic diet when the people around me don't know that I have diabetes. (D)
9. I'm not sure I'll be able to follow my diabetic diet every day. (D)
10. *I can correctly exchange one food for another in the same food group. (D)
11. *When I go to parties, I can follow my diet plan. (D)
12. *I can exercise several times a week.
13. I can't exercise unless I feel like exercising.
14. *I can figure out when to call my doctor about problems with my feet.
15. *I can routinely apply the recommended lotion to my feet. (G)
16. I cannot test my blood or urine when I am away from home. (I)
17. *I can recognize when my blood sugar is too high. (I)
18. *When I feel sick, I can test my blood or urine more than I routinely do. (D)
19. *I can take my insulin using the recommended procedure. (I)
20. I may have difficulty taking my insulin when away from home. (I)
21. *I can adjust my insulin dose based on the results of my urine or blood tests. (I)
22. I'm not sure I can figure out what to do about my insulin dose when changes occur in my usual routine. (I)
23. *I can do what was recommended to prevent low blood sugar reactions when I exercise. (I)
24. *I can figure out what self-treatment to administer when my blood sugar gets higher than it should be. (I)
25. I'm not sure I can recognize when my blood sugar is low. (I)
26. I'm not sure I can adjust my diabetes self-treatments if I get a cold or the flu. (I)
27. *I can fit my diabetes self-treatment routine into my usual lifestyle. (G)
28. *I think I'll be able to follow my diabetes plan even when my daily routine changes. (G)

Do you have any comments you wish to add about confidence in your ability to self-manage your diabetes?

Thank You

maintain glucose levels as close to normal as possible and prevent the single most common complication of therapy, hypoglycemia.

The frequency and timing of monitoring are dependent on the needs and goals of the individual patient. Optimal monitoring for patients with type 1 DM is three to four times a day—before each meal and before bedtime. Barriers to frequent monitoring in all patients with type 1 DM are cost, inconvenience, and the discomfort produced by the finger-prick. The benefit versus cost ratio must be thoroughly explored with each patient as a treatment plan is developed and goals are established. Table 15.10 presents the goals of glucose management in the patient without symptoms of hypoglycemia.

There are many different types of blood glucose meters and one should be selected that best fits the needs and resources of the patient. Many of the meters have the ability to download records into personal computers, which allows the clinician to view the data. This can provide helpful information on trends of blood glucose control. The patient should, nevertheless, be instructed to keep a log of results along with insulin doses so that adjustments can be made to the treatment plan. The glucose meter, as well as the individual patient's technique, should be assessed at each visit for accuracy initially, then annually once the patient is stabilized.

Management of Hypoglycemia. Hypoglycemia (plasma glucose less than 60 mg/dL) is a common occurrence in patients with type 1 diabetes. It can occur for a variety of reasons: excessive exogenous insulin, missed meals or inadequate food intake, exercise, alcohol ingestion, drug interactions, and a decrease in liver or kidney function. Signs and symptoms include diaphoresis, tachycardia, hunger, shakiness,

COMPLEMENTARY THERAPIES 15.1

Problem and Therapy	Dosage	Comment
Diabetes mellitus		
• Cinnamon (*Cinnamomum cassia*)	1–2 tsp qd	In one study, the ingestion of 1–6 g of cinnamon for 20 days reduced blood glucose, LDL cholesterol, triglycerides, and total cholesterol.
• Fenugreek (*Trigonella foenum-graecum*)	0.5 g of seeds in 150 mL of boiling water; steep for 3 hours and strain. Do not exceed 6 g/day	Contains soluble fiber that decreases blood glucose. Has anti-inflammatory properties.
• Zinc	15 mg qd	May improve effectiveness of insulin.
• Niacin	500 mg tid	May slow the progression of type 1 diabetes and may prevent complications of the disease.
• Alpha-lipoic acid	200 mg bid	Used in Europe for decades for the treatment of diabetic neuropathy. Prevents nerve damage by toxic free-radicals and may improve the action of insulin.
Biofeedback-assisted relaxation for type 2 diabetes		Patients enrolled in a biofeedback relaxation therapy group were found to have decreased blood glucose levels significantly.

altered mentation (ranging from inability to concentrate to coma), slurred speech, and seizure. The signs and symptoms exhibited by the patient are highly individual and can vary from mild to severe.

The goal of treatment is to normalize the plasma glucose promptly. If the patient is conscious and able to swallow, this is best accomplished by the ingestion of 15 g of carbohydrate. Examples include one-half cup of any fruit juice (no additional sugar added), 6 ounces of regular soda (not diet), 1 cup milk, or glucose tablets. Candy (no chocolate) can be used but is not recommended because the patient may eat it when it is not needed. Blood glucose should be checked 15 minutes after treatment and additional carbohydrate should be given if the blood glucose results remain less than 60 mg/dL. For severe hypoglycemia and if the patient is unconscious or unable to swallow, 1 mg of glucagon can be given subcutaneously. Another treatment alternative is 50 mL of 50 percent dextrose solution given intravenously.

Nocturnal hypoglycemia can occur if the predinner, intermediate-acting insulin dose is too high or if the patient skips dinner or eats an inadequate amount. The patient may not awaken with symptoms but on arising may note an increased fasting glucose level. This is due to a compensatory mechanism in the liver, which responds in the event of sustained hypoglycemia. After hypoglycemia has been resolved, the possible causes should be reviewed with the patient and preventative measures discussed. The Somagyi effect, for example, is a unique combination of hypoglycemia during the night with rebound hyperglycemia in the morning. Although several studies failed to confirm the validity of this pathologic process, many clinicians still feel the Somagyi effect exists and is most common in children with type 1 DM. This possibility should be investigated whenever fluctuations in blood sugar levels are serious.

Once the patient has been educated in insulin therapy, SMBG, and hypoglycemia, subsequent management should include education in meal planning and assistance in developing a regular exercise program. Most patients will benefit from a referral to a certified diabetic educator for a group program or individual counseling. A referral to a dietitian should be ordered for all patients.

Diet. Meal planning or medical nutritional therapy (MNT) is one of the most challenging aspects of diabetes management because achievement of treatment goals may require substantial lifestyle changes. The goals of nutritional therapy are to maintain normal blood glucose level, prevent hypoglycemia, maintain normal serum lipid levels, attain or maintain reasonable body weight, and promote healthy eating patterns. The meal plan should be based on the patient's food choices, exercise, medical history, weight, lifestyle, and cultural, ethnic, and financial factors. The first step of the nutritional consult should be an initial assessment of the patient's nutritional status, including a diet history. Recommendations for change should not be made until the patient's current eating patterns are determined. Most patients with type 1 diabetes are lean, so weight loss is generally not a factor in meal planning. The following formula can be used to determine the total number of kilocalories needed to maintain current weight:

For men: 66 + 13.7 (weight in kg) + 5 (height in cm) – 6.8 (age)

For women: 65 + 9.6 (weight in kg) + 1.7 (height in cm) – 4.7 (age)

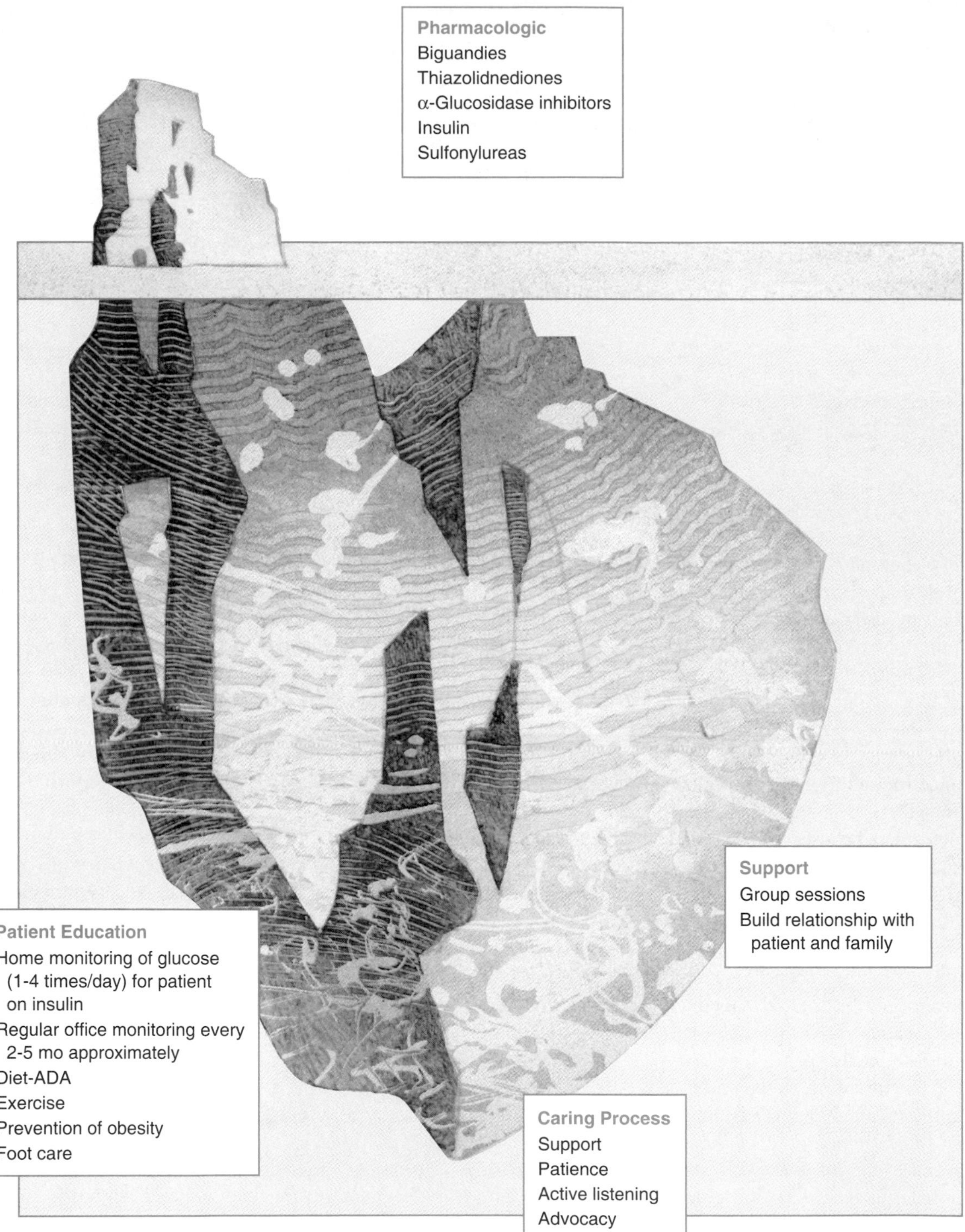

Multiply the result by 1.2 for a fairly active person and up to 1.5 for an ill person. Individuals on insulin should eat at consistent times that are synchronized with their insulin administration.

A nutritionally balanced meal plan is important for the patient with type 1 diabetes and should take into account the higher prevalence of atherosclerosis. The ADA guidelines recommend that the meal plan consists of the following:

- ▲ Protein: 10 to 20 percent of daily caloric intake from protein

Table 15.9 Outpatient Management of the Patient with Diabetes Mellitus Type 1

Every visit:
Question:
- Symptoms of hypoglycemia and hyperglycemia
- Results of SMBG
- Any self-adjustments based on SMBG or symptoms
- Problems with adherence
- Symptoms of complications
- Any other medical illnesses
- Medications (prescription and OTC)

Clinical examination to include:
- Height and weight
- Blood pressure
- Cardiovascular assessment
- Thyroid examination
- Ophthalmic examination (with an annual dilated retinal eye exam)
- Peripheral vascular assessment
- Feet and skin assessment
- Neurological assessment
- Oral examination

Laboratory monitoring to include:
- HbA_{1c} every 3 months during the first year of initiation of insulin therapy and during periods of insulin dosage adjustment. In patients who have met treatment goals, measure biannually.
- Initially and annually:
  Lipids (cholesterol, triglycerides, HDL, and calculated LDL)
  Urinalysis (protein, glucose, ketones, and sediment)
  Serum creatinine
  Microalbuminuria screening
  Method 1: measurement of albumin-to-creatinine ratio (can be performed in office; first morning void is preferred because of the diurnal variation in albumin excretion; >30 μg/mg creatinine indicates microalbuminuria)
  Method 2: 24-hour urine collection (creatinine can also be measured at this time; >30 mg in 24 h indicates microalbuminuria)
  Method 3: timed collection (collection of urine for 4 h or overnight; excretion of >20 μg/min indicates microalbuminuria)

General health maintenance to include:
- Pneumococcal vaccine
- Influenza vaccine (annually)
- Aspirin prophylaxis in patients over age 40 years

Patient education to include:
- Preconceptive or contraceptive counseling (initial and quarterly when applicable)
- Smoking cessation recommendations if applicable

▲ Fat: 10 to 20 percent of daily caloric intake from fat (less than 8 to 9 percent saturated fat with no more than 300 mg of cholesterol).

▲ Carbohydrates: a minimum of 60 to 70 percent of daily caloric intake from carbohydrates (with 20 to 35 grams of fiber).

Previously, it was a widely held belief that simple sugars should be avoided based on the assumption that sugars (simple carbohydrates) are more rapidly digested and absorbed than starches (complex carbohydrates) and can therefore aggravate hyperglycemia. There is very little scientific evidence to support this. Although various simple and complex carbohydrates do have different glycemic responses, the first priority should be given to the total amount of carbohydrate consumed rather than the source of the carbohydrate. This means that sucrose and sucrose-containing foods must be substituted for other carbohydrates gram for gram. Other nutritive sweeteners (such as fructose, dextrose, and maltose) and sugar alcohols (such as sorbitol, mannitol, and xylitol) do not have any significant advantage over sucrose in improving overall diabetes control and sugar alcohols in excessive amounts may have a laxative effect. The calories and carbohydrate content of all these sweeteners should be taken into account in the meal plan. Non-nutritive sweeteners such as saccharin, aspartame, and acesulfame K are noncaloric and do not affect the blood glucose level. The majority of patients with type 1 diabetes can safely use them.

Although soluble fiber can inhibit the absorption of glucose from the small intestine, the amount contained in most foods will not have a significant effect on blood glucose levels. Fiber recommendations for individuals with diabetes, therefore, are the same as for the general population (20 to 35 grams).

Vitamin and mineral supplementation is not generally recommended for persons whose dietary intake is adequate. Chromium replacements have no known benefit except for the patient who may be chromium deficient as a result of long-term parenteral nutrition. Magnesium and sodium replacement should be given only if medically warranted.

The same recommendations used for the general population concerning alcohol ingestion are appropriate for the patient with type 1 diabetes. Moderate consumption does not adversely affect blood glucose control if the patient has overall good control, but calories from alcohol should be included as part of the total calorie intake. Heavily sweetened drinks should be avoided and alcohol should be taken with and in addition to the meal plan.

Exercise. Before beginning an exercise program, the patient should be screened for the presence of macro- and microvascular complications that may be worsened by exercise. These include coronary artery disease (CAD), peripheral arterial disease, retinopathy, nephropathy, and peripheral or autonomic neuropathy. The patient with type 1 diabetes can perform all levels of exercise as long as glycemic control is good and there is no evidence of the complications that would preclude exercise. The ADA recommends that patients with diagnosed CAD should undergo a supervised evaluation of exercise tolerance before beginning an exercise program.

Because the metabolic adjustments that occur to maintain blood glucose levels during exercise in a nondiabetic individual are absent in patients with type 1 diabetes, exercise can exacerbate hyperglycemia if the patient has too

Drugs Commonly Prescribed 15.4: Diabetes Mellitus Type 1

Insulin Regimens

Single-Dose Therapy:

Single injection

- Intermediate or long-acting insulin with or without regular insulin in the morning OR Intermediate or long-acting insulin at bedtime
- Recommend minimal SMBG in morning and at bedtime

Conventional Split-Dose Therapy:

Two injections

- Mixture of NPH and regular insulin in the morning and evening
- Recommend minimal SMBG monitoring before each dosing and at bedtime

Intensive Insulin Therapy:

Three injections

- NPH and regular insulin in the morning; regular insulin at dinner; NPH insulin at bedtime
- Monitor for increased risk of hypoglycemic episodes

Four injections

- Regular or Lispro insulin before meals and long-acting insulin to maintain basal insulin levels
- Monitor for increased risk of hypoglycemic episodes

Types of Insulin	Species	Onset, Peak, and Duration	Route
Lispro Insulin			
human insulin Lispro (Humalog)	Recombinant DNA technology (usually used in combination with other insulins)	>15 min, 30–60 min, 3–4 h	SC
Regular Insulin			
Humulin R	Human	30–60 min, 2–6 h, 6–8 h	SC, IM, IV
Iletin II Regular	Pork	30–60 min, 2–6 h, 6–8 h	SC, IM, IV
Novolin R	Human	30–60 min, 2–6 h, 6–8 h	SC, IM, IV
Purified Pork Regular	Pork	30–60 min, 2–6 h, 6–8 h	SC, IM, IV
Velosulin	Human	30–60 min, 2–4 h, 6–8 h	SC, IM, IV
Insulin Isophane Suspension (NPH) Insulin/Regular Insulin			
Humulin 70/30	Human	30–60 min, 2–12 h, 24 h	SC
Humulin 50/50	Human	30–60 min, 3–5 h, 24 h	SC
Novolone 70/30	Human	30–60 min, 2–12 h, 24 h	SC
Insulin Isophane Suspension (NPH)			
Humulin N	Human	1–1.5 h, 4–12 h, 18–24 h	SC
Iletin II NPH	Pork	1–1.5 h, 4–12 h, 18–24 h	SC
Novolin N	Human	1–1.5 h, 4–12 h, 18–24 h	SC
Purified Pork NPH	Pork	1–1.5 h, 4–12 h, 18–24 h	SC
Insulin Zinc Suspension (Lente)			
Humulin L	Human	1–2.5 h, 7–15 h, 24 h	SC
Iletin II	Pork	1–2.5 h, 7–15 h, 24 h	SC
Novolin L	Human	2 h, 7–15 h, 24 h	SC
Purified Pork Leute	Pork	2 h, 7–15 h, 24 h	SC
Insulin Extended Zinc Suspension (Ultralente)			
Humulin	Human	4–8 h, 10–30 h, > 36 h	SC
Insulin Glarygine (Lantus)			
Lantus	Insulin analog	Slowly absorbed with gradual onset, peakless, lasting up to 24 h	SC

Table 15.10 Goals of Glucose Management*

Time	Goal
Before meals	80–120 mg/dL
Bedtime	100–140 mg/dL
Postprandial	<180 mg/dL

*Goals are for glucose management without symptoms of hypoglycemia.

little insulin. Conversely, if there is too much insulin, hypoglycemia may occur. The patient must, therefore, use the following general guidelines regarding exercise to regulate the glycemic response:

- Check blood glucose before, every 30 to 60 minutes during, and after exercise.
- Avoid exercise if the fasting glucose is more than 250 mg/dL and ketosis is present or if the glucose level is more than 300 mg/dL, regardless of whether ketosis is present.
- Consume additional carbohydrate if the glucose is less than 100 mg/dL and as needed to avoid hypoglycemia.
- Identify when changes in insulin or food are necessary.

Any exercise prescription should be individualized to take into account the patient's interest, lifestyle, physical condition, and motivation. The program should include 30 minutes of aerobic activity most days and include flexibility exercises to warm up and cool down. Muscle-strengthening exercises can also be added. With careful instructions, the patient with type 1 diabetes can enjoy the benefits of an exercise program.

Urine Ketone Testing. Urine ketone testing is recommended for patients with type 1 diabetes and should be performed when the patient is experiencing stress and when SMBG levels are greater than 300 mg/dL. During an acute illness, especially if the patient is nauseated and vomiting, urine ketones should be monitored. Since pregnancy is a stress on the diabetic patient, pregnant women should assess urine for ketones periodically. Ketonuria can reflect dehydration and the need for extra fluid, as well as an increased insulin requirement.

Follow-Up and Referral

Continuing care is essential in the management of type 1 diabetes. Long-term surveillance for potential complications of DM demands almost as much daily attention of the patient and office time of the provider as do the daily regimens needed to effectively manage this disease.

The frequency of patient visits depends on the degree to which blood glucose levels are controlled, changes in therapy, and the presence and degree of complications or other medical conditions. If the patient is performing SMBG, telephone consultations instead of office visits may be possible. Once regulated, the patient should be seen at least quarterly. These visits should include a discussion on results of SMBG; adjustments to therapy made by the patient; symptoms of medical illnesses; problems with adherence to the treatment plan; changes in lifestyle; medications; and frequency, causes, and severity of hyperglycemia or hypoglycemia.

The NIH has set up a multicenter program called Trialnet which accepts referral of relatives of patients with type 1A DM for screening with islet cell antibody measurements. They offer treatment with various agents that are being investigated as potentially preventing the development of the disease. The Web site is www.diabetestrialnet.org.

Complications

Risks of type 1 diabetes complications (retinopathy, nephropathy, and neuropathy) are significantly reduced when HbA_{1c} levels are maintained below 7 percent. HbA_{1c} determination should be performed at least twice a year in patients with good control and quarterly in patients whose therapy has changed or who are not meeting glycemic goals. The physical exam should include a comprehensive foot exam and a fundoscopic exam.

Referral to a specialist for the following complications may be indicated:

- Retinopathy: The ADA reports that after 20 years, almost all patients will have some degree of retinopathy, documenting the need for annual ophthalmic evaluations. Comprehensive dilated eye and visual exams should be performed annually by an ophthalmologist who is knowledgeable and experienced in the management of diabetic retinopathy for all patients age 10 years and older who have had diabetes for 3 to 5 years, all patients diagnosed after age 30 years, and any patient with visual symptoms or abnormalities.
- Hyperlipidemia: Adults with type 1 DM should be retested annually for lipid disorders with a complete fasting lipid profile because there is an increased risk in these individuals for cornary artery disease.
- Nephropathy: Adults with type 1 DM should have a routine urinalysis performed annually. Screening for microalbuminuria should begin with puberty and after 5 years duration of the disease. Persistent microalbuminuria (greater than 30 mg/24 h) has been shown to be the earliest stage of diabetic nephropathy. Overt nephropathy (albuminuria greater than or equal to 300 mg/24 h) will develop over a period of 10 to 15 years in approximately 80 percent of patients who develop microalbuminuria, many of whom will also develop hypertension. Transient elevations of albumin excretion occur during acute febrile illnesses, marked hypertension, short-term hyperglycemia, exercise, urinary tract infections, and in heart failure. Angiotensin-converting enzyme (ACE) inhibitors

have been found to postpone progression of microalbuminuria and ultimately nephropathy in patients. They have few adverse effects and are suggested as part of the initial therapy for diabetic patients with nephropathy. Their use is contraindicated in women who are pregnant, and they should be used with caution in women of childbearing age. ACE inhibitors may also exacerbate hyperkalemia in patients with advanced renal insufficiency or hyporeninemic hypoaldosteronism. Older adults with advanced renal disease and patients with renal artery stenosis may experience a decline in renal function with ACE inhibitors. If a patient does not tolerate the use of ACE inhibitors, angiotensin receptor blockers (ARB) can be used. Some studies suggest that they be used together in all diabetic patients for the benefit in nephropathy, because the medications act by different mechanisms.

- Hypertension: In a patient with type 1 diabetes, hypertension is often a manifestation of nephropathy. Control of hypertension has been demonstrated to reduce the rate of progression of nephropathy and to reduce the complications of cardiovascular disease. ADA guidelines recommend that the goal for blood pressure control in nonpregnant adults is to maintain the systolic blood pressure less than 120 mm Hg and the diastolic less than 80 mm Hg. Studies have shown that the closer patients with DM get to the target blood pressure, the less likely they are to develop cardiac sequelae. The goal for patients with isolated systolic hypertension is the above target blood pressure, but a more realistic goal may be for a patient with a systolic pressure of 180 mm Hg or higher to decrease the systolic blood pressure to less than 140 to 160 mm Hg and for those patients with isolated systolic blood pressure of 160 to 170 mm Hg by 20 to 30 mm Hg. Recommendations include that initial treatment for patients with hypertension, unless contraindicated, should be ACE inhibitors. Patients with signs of congestive heart failure (CHF) but with a normal or higher than normal ejection fraction should be screened for diastolic dysfunction and treated to target accordingly.
- Macrovascular disease: Diabetic patients are at risk for developing marcrovacular complications including stroke/CVA, peripheral vascular disease (PVD), and CAD/CVD. Evidence of uncontrolled angina, carotid bruits, and ECG abnormalities may require advanced intervention. Daily intake of aspirin has been shown to reduce cardiovascular events in patients with diabetes. Patients with disabling claudication or nonhealing ulcers require a vascular consultation for their PVD. All diabetic patients should be screened for these diseases, as symptoms may not be present until late in the course of the disease process.
- Neuropathy: Foot ulcers and problems are a major cause of morbidity and mortality in the patient with DM. Half of the patients with hyperglycemia extending over 15 years will develop some degree of neuropathy. Peripheral neuropathy may result in pain, loss of sensation, and muscle weakness. The feet and ankles are affected most often, but many patients also complain of pain in the knees and upper extremities. Severe pain from neuropathy can lead to sleep and mood disturbances. A thorough initial and annual foot examination is indicated in asymptomatic patients. A 10-g Semmes-Weinstein monofilament should be used to assess sensation at least annually. Abnormal findings indicate the need for a thorough vascular, neurologic, musculoskeletal, and soft tissue evaluation. Many patients take several medications to control the pain or discomfort of neuropathy. Analgesics, narcotic analgesics, tricyclic antidepressants, antiarrhythmics, and local anesthetics are frequently prescribed. Tricyclic antidepressants are commonly prescribed for painful neuropathies and are often the first-line drug in patients for whom they are not contraindicated. Gabapentin (Neurontin) may be an alternative choice for patients who cannot take tricyclic antidepressants. Patients suffering from chronic pain syndromes may benefit from a referral to a chronic pain clinic. Patients with neuropathy require professional nail and callus care, because most ulcers begin at the site of a callus. Supportive, athletic shoes are recommended for all patients for walking. Extra-depth shoes and custom-molded shoe inserts are indicated for patients who are at high risk for foot ulcers. Patients at high risk include those with neuropathy; structural deformities of the feet, skin, or nails; or a history of previous ulcers. Charcot foot disorders occur in 9 percent of patients with neuropathy, and its symptoms may be confused with those of cellulitis. It leads to bony destruction, joint subluxation, and bony remodeling of the foot. Patients with abnormal findings on radiologic examination should be referred to an orthopedist for initial evaluation.
- Other: Autonomic involvement can affect gastrointestinal, cardiovascular, and genitourinary function. Sexual dysfunction, particularly impotence, may occur. The demands of glycemic control on lifestyle often lead to depression. Patients should be evaluated for depression initially and annually (see Nursing Situation 15.1).

Patient Education

Insulin administration involves the use of subcutaneous syringes marked in insulin units. Regulations governing the purchase of syringes vary greatly from state to state. Although syringe manufacturers recommend that syringes be used only once, it appears safe and practical for the patient to reuse the syringe if needed, but it should be discarded if the needle integrity is compromised. Syringes should be recapped by the patient using a one-handed technique, and they should be discarded according to the state requirements. Patients with visual or dexterity difficulties may benefit from prefilling syringes. Prefilled insulin

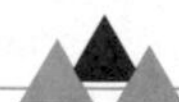

NURSING SITUATION 15.1

Depression in the Patient with Diabetes Mellitus Type 1

Depression is at least twice as prevalent among diabetics as in the general population. Patients with depression and those with diabetes both have heightened levels of the hormone cortisol. Patients treated for depression may achieve better diabetes control.

Mrs. H, 51, is a high school math teacher in a small town in New England. Diagnosed with diabetes type 1 at age 14, she developed retinopathy. The condition worsened and was no longer amenable to laser therapy. Her blood sugar levels began rising and falling in "violent arcs" and she found herself contemplating suicide. Mrs. H began seeing a therapist and started on an antidepressant drug therapy, paroxetine (Paxil). As her mood improved, so did her blood sugar.

An especially interesting finding is the effect that psychotherapy can have on depressed patients with diabetes. A 1998 study in the *Annals of Internal Medicine* reported that a 10-week course of cognitively based therapy helped relieve depression in 85% of diabetics so treated, compared with only 27% of patients receiving standard care. Glucose levels in the patients who received the therapy were significantly lower than in controls when both groups were examined 6 months after the therapy ended.

SOURCE: Laulin, PA: Depressed mind, sick body. Hippocrates: J Health Med (Nurse practitioner edition). pp 20–26, February 1999.

syringes may be stored in a vertical position in the refrigerator for up to 30 days with the needle pointing upward.

Alternatives to syringes include jet injectors and penlike devices. Jet injectors are useful for patients who have needle phobias, but they are expensive. Penlike devices hold insulin cartridges and are useful if the patient is visually or neurologically impaired, and they help to increase the accuracy of insulin administration. Another alternative is the insulin pump, which is a small device (about the size of a pager) that is worn externally. Continuous subcutaneous insulin is delivered via tubing attached to the pump. Use of the insulin pump requires care by skilled professionals, careful selection of patients, frequent blood glucose monitoring, and comprehensive patient education.

Insulin should be injected at room temperature, and bottles not in use should be stored in the refrigerator. It should be injected into the subcutaneous tissue of the upper arm, anterior and lateral aspects of the thigh, the buttocks, or the abdomen. Rotation of the site within one area is recommended rather than rotating to a different site with each injection.

Foot care should be reviewed at each visit. Patients at high risk for foot ulcer development need continued education to follow through with professional foot care and daily foot hygiene. Patients at low risk should be encouraged to continue good hygiene, wear proper footwear, avoid trauma to the feet, stop smoking if they do, and report any blisters, macerated skin, or hemorrhage into a callus immediately and limit weightbearing on affected extremity.

Any illness maximizes stress, and this is especially true for diabetics. When ill, all diabetics must continue to take their insulin and increase blood glucose monitoring to every 2 hours. Supplemental dosages of regular insulin may be needed to control blood glucose levels. If blood sugar is higher than 240 mg/dL, the urine should be checked for ketones every 4 hours. A caloric intake of 50 g of carbohydrates every 4 hours should be maintained. A variety of clear fluids, including some with glucose, should be encouraged, as well as gelatin, ice pops, regular soda, soups, and toast, if tolerated. Patients should be encouraged to maintain an oral fluid intake of 6-9 oz/h to avoid dehydration.

If vomiting or diarrhea persists over 2 hours, a fever of 101°F or higher is present, or blood glucose is 240 mg/dL or higher and ketones continue to appear in the urine despite additional insulin, the patient should be instructed to seek medical attention immediately.

Signs of DKA to be alert for include extreme fatigue, abnormal cramping, and alterations in breathing pattern.

Diabetes Mellitus Type 2

DM type 2 is the fifth leading cause of death in the United States, however, it contributes to many other diseases, particularly heart disease, which is the leading cause of death. Type 2 diabetes is a group of heterogeneous forms characterized by sufficient circulating endogenous insulin, resistance to insulin action, and an inadequate compensatory insulin secretion response. Approximately 90 percent of all Americans diagnosed with diabetes have this type of DM. Type 2 DM reduces life expectancy because of complications, which are affected by the duration of diabetes, the degree of blood glucose control, and other cardiovascular risk factors such as smoking and hypertension.

Epidemiology and Causes

The prevalence of *DM type 2* in the United States today is 6.6 percent. About 18 million Americans have type 2 diabetes, but only one-third of individuals with it are aware that they have the disease. The disease is often asymptomatic in its early stages; as a result, individuals can remain undiagnosed for many years. The chronic hyperglycemia, however, is associated with long-term damage and dysfunction of various organs, including the kidneys, eyes, nerves, heart, and blood vessels. The comorbidities associated with type 2 DM are thus quite extensive, as reflected in the per capita health-care costs for diabetics in the United States which are five times higher than those of nondiabetics.

Numerous risk factors are associated with the development of type 2 diabetes (see Risk Factors 15.1). At risk are those with a first-degree relative with type 2 diabetes, who demonstrate a 5- to 10-fold higher lifetime risk of developing the disease than age-matched controls with no family history. Moreover, nearly 40 percent of patients have at least one affected parent with the disease, and monozygotic twin studies further demonstrate between 60 and 90 percent concordance.

Racial and ethnic variations also affect the prevalence of type 2 DM. A disproportionate number of African Americans, Hispanic Americans, Native Americans, Asian Americans, and Pacific Islanders have diabetes. The prevalence of type 2 diabetes in Native Americans and Alaskan natives is approximately two to six times that found in non-Hispanic whites. Pacific Islanders living traditionally have a prevalence of 2.9 percent while those who immigrate to the United States and adopt Western ways have a prevalence rate of 12 percent. Along with genetic differences, there are a host of factors that may underlie this disparity in disease prevalence, including socieoeconomic factors, differential health-care practices, unequal access to health-care resources, as well as ethnocultural influences in diet and activity and the impact of institutionalized racism. However, the overall prevalence rate of type 2 DM appears to be increasing in the general population, as well as among specific ethnic minority groups.

The incidence of diabetes increases with age, especially in those 45 years of age and older. However, it is important to note the condition may be diagnosed at any age. Paralleling the marked increase in childhood obesity over the last several decades, rates of newly diagnosed cases of type 2 DM among children are on the rise. Prevalence rates in adolescents and young adults are increasing faster than in any other age group.

Those previously identified as having an elevated fasting glucose, impaired glucose tolerance, a history of gestational DM, or past delivery of an infant weighing more than 9 pounds are also at greater risk. Gestational DM is defined as any degree of pregnancy-associated glucose intolerance which affects 2 to 4 percent of all pregnancies in the United States. It is associated with significant fetal morbidity including macrosomia, congenital heart defects, hypoglycemia, hyperbilirubinemia, hypocalcemia, and sepsis. At the other end of the spectrum is polycystic ovarian syndrome—a condition characterized by obesity, infertility, and insulin resistance in women, which is also a major risk factor for type 2 DM.

Several pharmacologic agents are associated with iatrogenic hyperglycemia and the eventual development of overt DM. These include glucocorticoids, hormonal therapies such as oral contraceptives, the immunosuppressants tacrolimus and cyclosporine, nicotinic acid (niacin), antiviral HIV protease inhibitors (which also cause central fat redistribution known as lipodystrophy syndrome), several atypical antipsychotic agents including clozapine and olanzapine, and certain antihypertensives including beta-blockers, calcium channel blockers, clonidine, and thiazide diuretics. In contrast, both angiotensin-converting enzyme (ACE) inhibitors and angiotensin II receptor blockers (ARBs) appear to improve insulin sensitivity and reduce the development of type 2 DM in hypertensive nondiabetics.

Increasing evidence points to linkage between CAD, hyperlipidemia, obesity, and DM, as discussed extensively under Pathophysiology. Because early detection and prompt treatment may reduce the complications of type 2 DM, screening for diabetes as part of routine medical care is appropriate under certain circumstances. Testing for diabetes should be considered in all individuals age 45 and older, and if normal, should be repeated at 3-year intervals. Testing should be considered in younger individuals who are obese (more than 20 percent over desired body weight), have a first-degree relative with diabetes, are members of high-risk ethnic populations, have delivered a baby weighing more than 9 pounds, or have an impaired facting glucose during pregnancy.

RISK FACTORS 15.1

Diabetes Mellitus Type 2

- Family history (first-degree relative)
- Age over 45 years
- Impaired fasting glucose
- Delivery of baby weighing more than 9 pounds
- Hypertension
- Hyperlipidemia (high-density lypoproteins [HDL] < 40 mg/dL in men and <50 mg/dL in women, triglycerides > 250 mg/dL)
- Obesity
- Ethnicity/racial

African American
Hispanic American
Native American
Asian American
Pacific Islander

Pathophysiology

Type 2 DM is associated with two physiologic abnormalities: insulin resistance and impaired insulin secretion. It is believed that insulin resistance is an inherited feature that is nonetheless associated with acquired traits, such as obesity and aging. In fact, a stronger heritable component has been established for type 2 DM than for type 1 DM. This genetic tendency has been confirmed in studies of lean, nondiabetic offspring of type 2 diabetic parents, who demonstrate decreased glycogen synthesis and reduced nonoxidative glucose metabolism in muscle tissue, despite maintaining a euglycemic state. Intracellular lipid content is also increased in these subjects, which was suggested in one study to be due to a defect in mitochondrial function. Indeed, other studies have demonstrated that increased levels of plasma free fatty acids (as observed in obese individuals) predispose patients to developing type 2 DM by inhibiting insulin secretion and impairing insulin-mediated glucose uptake.

Initially, as insulin resistance increases, insulin levels begin to rise and the glucose level remains normal, causing a state of hyperinsulinemia. In turn, both fasting and postprandial hyperinsulinemia are predictors of future weight gain, which, in turn, predisposes to hyperglycemia. Thus, this compensatory hyperinsulinemia fails to keep pace, if blood glucose begins to rise as in a postprandial state. Moreover, hyperglycemia itself is toxic to pancreatic beta cells, possibly via decreased expression of the insulin gene. As a result, over time, this hyperinsulinemia actually progresses to relative hypoinsulinemia.

Unlike the pattern in type 1 DM, there is no autoimmune destruction of pancreatic beta cells. Rather, there is a decline in their endocrine function, with impaired insulin secretion in response to a glycemic load, which produces elevated plasma glucose levels. This appears to occur at the level of proinsulin, the secreted precursor form of insulin. In nondiabetic individuals, 10 to 15 percent of secreted insulin may be detected via immunoassays as proinsulin or one of its conversion intermediates. However, in diabetic patients, this value may be as high as 40 percent. While the resultant hyperglycemia drives increased insulin secretion even further, obesity and insulin resistance alone do not appear to account for the increased fraction of proinsulin, thus implicating a potential defect in the conversion of proinsulin to insulin or the premature, dysregulated secretion of proinsulin.

Amylin, an islet cell–produced amyloid polypeptide, is also present in beta-cell secretory granules. Serum levels of amylin decrease in concert with those of insulin in type 2 diabetics, whereas pancreatic concentrations of the polypeptide are markedly increased in type 2 diabetics. These observations, along with amylin antagonist studies performed in rat models, have suggested that amylin may be a negative regulator of insulin secretion in type 2 DM; however, this hypothesis has yet to be confirmed in rigorous human studies.

Regardless, in conjunction with hyperinsulinemia, insulin resistance worsens, manifesting first as postprandial hyperglycemia and eventually as fasting hyperglycemia, once hepatic gluconeogenesis increases. The sequence of impaired insulin secretion preceding worsening insulin resistance has been documented in prospective studies. However, several other studies have indicated that these two pathophysiologic mechanisms are independent risk factors for the development of type 2 DM and, in fact, occur in concert with one another, rather than in a sequential manner. Indeed double-knockout mouse models lacking activity in both the glucokinase (involved in insulin secretion) and IRS-1 (involved in insulin sensitivity) genes develop DM, while single-knockout mouse strains lacking only one of these genes do not. Although insufficient to cause DM alone, insulin resistance appears to be the strongest predictor of type 2 DM development, an observation that is reinforced by the importance of insulin resistance as a component of the insulin-resistant metabolic syndrome (syndrome X).

There is a strong non-Mendelian genetic component to type 2 DM. Only about 5 percent of type 2 DM cases can be attributed to single-gene mutations that decrease insulin secretion or function, e.g., glucokinase (a probable beta-cell glucose sensor), insulin promoter factor (IPF)-1 (an insulin gene transcription factor), and beta-3-adrenergic receptor (a regulator of lipolysis). However, several other genetic defects have been associated with insulin resistance, including mutations in the genes encoding the protein components of the insulin receptor, which is a tetramer consisting of two extracellular alpha subunits and two transmembrane/intracellular beta subunits with inherent tyrosine kinase activity that initiates intracellular signaling on binding of the insulin molecule. In addition, genes not directly involved in insulin secretion or function, such as the hepatocyte nuclear factors 1-alpha, 1-beta, and 4-alpha, have each been associated with different forms of maturity-onset diabetes of the young (MODY)—a rare form of type 2 DM that may first manifest in a patient's early 20s.

However, the most common forms of type 2 DM most likely involve insulin resistance that is due to postreceptor genetic defects. Candidate genes that may play an important role include those for glycogen synthase (needed for hepatic glucose stores), insulin-receptor substrate (IRS)-2 (a cell signaling mediator downstream of the insulin receptor), calpain-10 (a cysteine protease particularly important in diabetic Mexican Americans), and peroxisome-proliferator–activated receptor (PPAR)-γ-2 (the target molecule of the thiazolidinedione class of antihyperglycemic drugs, which plays an important role in adipocyte differentiation).

Obesity is a major modifiable risk factor for developing type 2 DM, affecting up to 90 percent of type 2 diabetics. Moreover, patients who are not obese but have an increased percentage of body weight distributed in the abdominal area rather than the hips (also known as central obesity, upper body obesity, or male-type obesity) are also at greater risk. Although this mechanism has not been fully elucidated, obesity is known to contribute to peripheral insulin resistance, both impairing glucose uptake and decreasing pancreatic beta-cell sensitivity to plasma glucose levels, thereby decreasing reactive insulin secretion. The aforementioned beta-3-adrenergic receptor and the c-Jun amino-terminal kinase (JNK) intracellular signaling pathways have both been implicated. Moreover, adipocyte-derived tumor necrosis factor-alpha (TNF)-α has been positively correlated with increasing insulin resistance, as has the adipocyte hormone resistin. In contrast, the adipocyte hormone adiponectin appears to be negatively correlated with insulin resistance. However, the bulk of the evidence for all these hormones comes primarily from rat and mouse studies, while human data are lacking. Whatever the case, physical exercise with a corresponding weight loss of just 10 to 20 percent of total body weight confers protection against the subsequent development of type 2 DM in overweight individuals, generating marked improvement in glucose tolerance.

Elevated plasma glucose levels may be well tolerated for many years by the diabetic patient, who may not seek treatment until chronic complications result. Eventually, however, insulin secretion will become insufficient to compensate for insulin resistance. Moreover, hyperinsulinemia and hyperglycemia increase lipid synthesis, raising the serum levels of fatty acids, triglycerides (greater than 150 mg/dL), and low-density lipoprotein (LDL) cholesterol, while lowering HDL cholesterol. As a result, increased lipids are deposited on vessel walls more readily.

Hyperglycemia thus leads to both microvascular and macrovascular complications, which underlie long-term diabetic damage. Vascular endothelial dysfunction and inflammation result in fibrosis and intimal thickening, leading to progressive narrowing of the vascular lumen. In turn, blood flow through the microvasculature is reduced, leading to tissue ischemia throughout the body, which results in functional impairment of multiple end organs. This explains how DM can simultaneously reign as the leading cause of acquired blindness (due to retinopathy), ESRD (due to nephropathy), and nontraumatic lower extremity amputation (due to PVD and infection), as well as its major contribution to heart disease and stroke. In turn, several clinical trials have demonstrated that careful glycemic control reduces the development and delays the progression of microvascular manifestations of DM, including nephropathy and retinopathy.

Sympathetic tone and cardiac contractility are increased by hyperinsulinemia due to increases in the plasma catecholamines epinephrine and norepinephrine. With high levels of circulating glucose caused by cellular resistance to insulin, the distal nephron of the kidney absorbs increased amounts of sodium and water, expanding the intravascular volume and increasing the blood pressure. The triad of disturbed glucose metabolism, hypertension (>140/90 mm Hg), and dyslipidemia with obesity is variably referred to as insulin resistance syndrome, syndrome X, obesity dyslipidemia syndrome, or the metabolic syndrome. This condition may exist in prediabetic, glucose intolerant, or overtly diabetic states. Typically, this syndrome culminates in significant CAD and PVD and is strongly associated with the development of full-blown type 2 DM in prediabetics.

Clinical Presentation

Because the onset of diabetes may occur years before a diagnosis is made, individuals who are asymptomatic tend to be diagnosed during a routine physical examination or during treatment for another condition.

Subjective

Because the onset of type 2 diabetes is usually insidious, only a minority of patients are initially symptomatic. The patient may, however, present with pruritus or neuropathic complaints such as numbness and tingling. Some patients present with increased urination, nocturia, thirst, or polydipsia. In many cases, type 2 diabetes first presents as an infection, especially vaginitis (candidiasis) or a skin infection. Cardiovascular symptoms such as angina may prompt the patient to seek health care. The symptoms of type 1 and type 2 DM are basically the same. See the sections for type 1 DM for a complete discussion.

Clinical Presentation

Objective

There may be no dramatic change in objective findings, although the patient is often obese, with a history of dyslipidemia, hypertension, and CAD. Abnormal healing and an increased occurrence of infection, especially yeast infection, may be present.

Hyperosmolar hyperglycemia syndrome (HHS) is profound dehydration that results from prolonged hyperglycemia (Table 15.8). Formerly known as hyperosmolar hyperglycemia nonketotic coma (HHNC), HHS is associated with a high mortality rate and is seen in older adults who have developed an infection or other illness. It is commonly recognized in the older adult with pneumonia. Patients with undiagnosed DM may develop this condition because of prolonged hyperglycemia without treatment. Other risk factors for development include peritoneal dialysis, hemodialysis, tube feedings with high protein formulas, and the use of mannitol, phenytoin, steroids, immunosuppressive agents, and diuretics. Symptoms are dramatic, including severe hyperglycemia (more than 600 mg/dL), plasma or serum hyperosmolality (more than 340 mOsm), and profound dehydration. Ketosis may or may not be present, while neurologic symptoms range from clouded sensorium to coma. The condition requires immediate referral for acute care management.

Diagnostic Reasoning

Diagnostic Tests

Initial Testing. Immediate testing in the office can be accomplished by using a portable monitor to test capillary blood glucose level. This test is referred to as a random capillary glucose measurement and is given without regard to time of last meal. A result of 200 mg/dL or more should be evaluated by screening for blood glucose with whole blood. It is important to consider that certain drugs, including glucocorticoids, furosemide (Lasix), thiazides, phenytoin (Dilantin), estrogen-containing products, beta-blockers, and nicotinic acid can produce hyperglycemia. If the random plasma glucose level is elevated, the urine should be tested for ketones and additional blood glucose testing should be done. There are three ways to diagnose diabetes:

1. Symptoms of DM plus random plasma glucose concentration 200 mg/dL or more on two occasions.
2. Fasting plasma glucose 126 mg/dL or more on two occasions. Fasting is defined as no caloric intake for at least 9 hours.
3. Two-hour postload glucose 200 mg/dL or more during an oral glucose tolerance test on two occasions. The test should be performed using a glucose load containing the equivalent of 75 g of anhydrous glucose dissolved in water. This test is not recommended for routine clinical use or in pregnancy.

Subsequent Testing. A glycated hemoglobin (Ghb or HbA_{1c}) determination gives valuable insight into the mean glycemia over the preceding 2 to 3 months and is helpful in documenting the degree of glycemic control at the time of diagnosis and as part of continuing care. An HbA_{1c} value less than 7 percent indicates good control, however, a value less than 6 percent has been shown to significantly decrease the occurrence of complications.

Additional laboratory tests that are appropriate to the evaluation of the patient's general medical condition should be performed. They include fasting lipid profile and serum creatinine in adults; in children, if proteinuria is present, a urinalysis for microalbuminuria should be performed, along with urine culture if indicated.

Correct classification of patients with diabetes can be difficult. A determination of the C-peptide level may be helpful in determining the extent to which exogenous insulin is being produced. Proinsulin, a precursor of insulin, is produced in the pancreas and is split into insulin and C peptide. Unlike insulin, C peptide is not metabolized in the liver; its serum concentration thus reflects insulin secretion. If the basal (fasting) C-peptide level is more than 0.5 nmol/L (greater than 1 ng/dL), then the patient most likely has type 2 diabetes. In type 1 diabetes, the basal C-peptide level is less than 0.2 nmol/L. Intermediate results require further evaluation with a Sustacal stimulation test.

Differential Diagnosis

Differential diagnosis includes type 1 DM, IFG, genetic defects in insulin action, diseases of exocrine pancreas, drug- or chemical-induced DM, immune-mediated infections, and neurologic disorders that mimic diabetic neuopathy.

Management

Type 2 diabetes is a chronic illness that requires ongoing health care and education to prevent acute and chronic complications. To be effective, the treatment program requires frequent SMBG, medical nutritional therapy with weight reduction when indicated, use of oral glucose-lowering agents and/or insulin, regular exercise, continuing education in the prevention and treatment of complications, and periodic assessment of treatment goals. Careful attention should be given to the control of cardiovascular risk factors, such as hypertension, smoking, and dyslipidemia.

Research confirms the benefits of improved glycemic control in the improvement in overall work and disability outcomes, improved quality of life, decreased symptomatology, and health-care cost savings. Research also provides beginning evidence in the benefits of intensive blood-glucose control on many complications of type 2 diabetes. The lifestyle behavioral changes needed to improve glycemic control are best accomplished with frequent and concise direction. Diet and exercise therapy must be addressed with specific instructions.

Although the primary-care provider's focus is often on glycemic control, the patient's focus is on the need to fit control into an acceptable lifestyle. Research has identified that dietary modifications, the need for constant monitoring, and the subsequent follow-up with health-care providers place a financial and psychological burden on patients and families.

Initial Management

Diet and Weight Loss. Meal planning or nutritional therapy is one of the most fundamental and challenging components of diabetes management. The goal of nutritional therapy is to achieve and maintain blood glucose level, lipid, and blood pressure goals. Most patients with type 2 diabetes are overweight, so weight loss is generally a significant factor in meal planning. Although hypocaloric diets and weight loss usually improve blood glucose control, traditional dietary strategies have not been very effective in achieving long-term weight loss. As research continues to explore why weight loss and maintenance is so difficult, the emphasis should be on controlling glucose and promoting healthy eating patterns. The meal plan should be based on the patient's food choices, exercise, medical history, weight, lifestyle, cultural, ethnic, and financial factors.

If weight loss is indicated, a moderate caloric restriction (250 to 500 calories less than average daily intake as calculated from food history) and a nutritionally adequate meal plan with a reduction of total fat, especially saturated fat, is recommended. A hypocaloric diet, independent of weight loss, is associated with increased sensitivity to insulin and improvement in blood glucose levels. Moderate weight loss, irrespective of starting weight, has significant benefits especially in decreasing the morbidity and mortality. In fact, weight loss is a primary intervention because it improves the serum lipid profile, reduces blood pressure, decreases insulin resistance, and ameliorates glucose intolerance.

Individuals on oral glucose-lowering agents and/or insulin should eat at consistent times that are synchronized with their medication administration. A nutritionally balanced meal plan is important for the patient with type 2 diabetes and should take into account the higher prevalence of atherosclerosis.

Specific diets for patients with diabetes are no longer recommended by the ADA; however, their recommendations for the composition of a healthy diet are 10 to 20 percent of daily intake from protein, 10 to 20 percent from fat (less than 10 percent being saturated fat), and 60 to 70 percent from carbohydrates.

Self-Monitoring of Blood Glucose. The optimal frequency of SMBG in patients with type 2 DM has not been clearly established. The frequency, however, is dependent on the attainment of blood glucose goals. SMBG is recommended in patients being treated with sulfonylureas and in patients who have not consistently achieved blood glucose treatment goals. The patient should, nevertheless, be instructed to keep a log of results along with oral glucose-lowering agents.

Urine glucose testing provides only a rough estimate of blood glucose levels and is infrequently recommended; however, in patients who cannot or will not implement SMBG, urine glucose testing is an alternative. Urine glucose testing does not reflect blood glucose levels until the renal threshold of 180 mg/dL of blood glucose is exceeded.

Exercise. Exercise is an integral component of management of type 2 DM. Before beginning an exercise program, the patient should be screened for the presence of macro- and microvascular complications that may be worsened by exercise. These include coronary artery disease, peripheral arterial disease, retinopathy, nephropathy, and peripheral or autonomic neuropathy. The patient with type 2 diabetes can perform all levels of exercise as long as glycemic control is good and there is no evidence of the complications that would preclude exercise. If the patient is taking oral antidiabetic agents or is on insulin, exercise can cause hypoglycemia. The patient, therefore, must use the following general guidelines on exercise to regulate the glycemic response:

- ▲ Check blood glucose before and after exercise.
- ▲ Avoid exercise if the fasting glucose is more than 250 mg/dL and ketosis is present, or if the glucose level is more than 300 mg/dL, regardless of whether ketosis is present.
- ▲ Consume additional carbohydrate if the glucose is less than 100 mg/dL and as needed to avoid hypoglycemia.
- ▲ Identify when changes in insulin or food are necessary.

Any exercise prescription should be individualized to take into account the patient's interest, lifestyle, physical condition, financial situation, and motivation. The program should include an aerobic activity, such as walking, for at least 30 minutes most days of the week and should include flexibility exercises to warm up and cool down. Muscle-strengthening exercises can also be added. With careful instructions, the patient with type 2 diabetes can enjoy the benefits of an exercise program.

Subsequent Management

If fasting plasma glucose measurements are less than 200 mg/dL and presenting symptoms are not severe, a course of diet and exercise should be initiated to control hyperglycemia. The patient with type 2 DM will need frequent follow-up during the trial period. Symptomatic patients and patients with marked hyperglycemia (fasting plasma glucose 300 mg/dL or more) will show significant improvement in both with initiation of an oral agent.

Pharmacologic Therapy. Pharmacologic therapy for type 2 diabetes is required when dietary modification and exercise do not result in blood glucose control. Drug therapy should always be considered an adjunct therapy to diet and exercise and not as a substitute. Oral medication is initiated when 3 months of nutritional therapy and exercise alone have not achieved and maintained fasting plasma glucose levels less than 120 mg/dL and a HbA_{1c} level of less than 7 percent. Current therapy for type 2 diabetes includes drugs that primarily stimulate insulin secretion (first- and second-generation sulfonylureas), drugs that alter insulin action (metformin [Glucophage] and rosiglitazone [Avandia]), drugs that affect the absorption of glucose (acarbose [Precose]), drugs that mimic the effects of incretin (exenatide [Byetta]), drugs that act as an insulin secretagogue (repaglinide, [Prandin]), and drugs that suppress postprandial glucagon release (pramlintide [Symlin]).

Sulfonylureas work by stimulating pancreatic insulin secretion, which then reduces hepatic glucose output and increases peripheral glucose metabolism. First-generation sulfonylureas include acetohexamide (Dymelor), chlorpropamide (Diabinase), tolazamide (Tolinase), and tolbutamide (Orinase). Second-generation sulfonylureas include glimepiride (Amaryl), glipizide (Glucotrol), and glyburide (DiaBeta, Glynase, Micronase). The benefits of second-generation sulfonylureas are that they are more potent, tend to produce fewer adverse effects, and have fewer interactions with other drugs.

Sulfonylureas are not recommended for use during pregnancy or for women who are planning a pregnancy. Sulfonylureas are metabolized in the liver, and their use should be avoided in persons with significant hepatic dysfunction. Patients with severe insulin resistance may respond better to metformin or thiazolidinedione therapy than to the use of sulfonylureas (see Drugs Commonly Prescribed 15.5).

Therapy with sulfonylureas should be initiated at the lowest possible dose and usually begins with a once-

Drugs Commonly Prescribed 15.5 Diabetes Mellitus Type 2

Drug	Dosage	Duration of Action	Comments
First-Generation Sulfonylureas			*Applicable for all first-generation sulfonylureas*
• Tolbutamide (Orinase)	0.5–2 g in two to three doses Maintenance range: 0.12–2 g PO in divided doses Maximum dose: 3 g/ day PO in divided doses	6–12 hours	For use as adjunct to diet and exercise in type 2 diabetes. Contraindicated in keto-acidosis. Reduce dose in older adults; potentiated by NSAIDs, alcohol, salicylates, sulfonamides, probenecid, MAOIs, tricyclics, beta-blockers.
• Tolazamide (Tolinase)	0.1–1 g in one to two doses 100 mg to 1 g in single or divided dose (above 500 mg) Maximum dose: 1 g/day	Up to 24 hours	Antagonized by diuretics, steroids, phenothiazines. NIH precautions: monitor urine and blood glucose; discontinue if jaundice or persistent rash occurs.
• Chlorpropamide (Diabanese)	0.1–0.5 g in one dose 250–750 mg in single or divided doses Maximum dose: 750 mg/day in single or divided doses	24–72 hours	Secondary failure may occur with prolonged usage.
Second-Generation Sulfonylureas			*Applicable for all second-generation sulfonylureas*
• Glyburide (DiaBeta, Micronase)	1.25–20 mg in single or divided doses Maximum dose: 20 mg/day in single or divided doses	24 hours	For use as an adjunct to diet and exercise in type 2 diabetes mellitus Same as for 1st-generation sulfonylureas
• Glyburide, micronized (Glynase Pres Tabs)	0.75 mg–12 mg in single or divided doses Maximum dose: 12 mg/day in divided doses	24 hours	
• Glipizide (Glucotrol)	5–15 mg once daily or 5–40 mg in divided doses Maximum dose: 15 mg once daily or 40 mg in divided doses	6–12 hours	
• Glipizide (Glucotrol XL)	5–10 mg once daily Maximum dose: 20 mg/day	24 hours	
• Glimepiride (Amaryl)	1–4 mg once daily Maximum dose: 8 mg/day	24 hours	
Biguanides			
• Metformin (Glucophage)	500 mg–2.50 g in two or three divided doses Maximum dose: 2.55 g/day	7 12 hours	Monotherapy; may be used as an adjunct to diet in type 2 diabetes or with a sulfonylurea or insulin Contraindicated in renal disease; check renal function before starting prescription. Monitor for hypoglycemia, especially in older adults. Adverse reactions: GI disturbances, metallic taste, many drug interactions.
Thiazolidinediones			*Applicable for all thiazolidinediones*
• Rosiglitazone (Avandia)	4–8 mg PO in single or two doses Maximum dose: 8 mg/day	24 hours	Insulin resistance reducer. Adjunct to diet and exercise in type 2 diabetes; used as monotherapy or added to metformin.

(continued)

Drug	Dosage	Duration of Action	Comments
• Pioglitazone (Actos)	15–30 g/day PO Monotherapy: maximum dose: 45 mg/day Combination: 30 mg/day	24–30 hours	Not for use with type 1 diabetes or in ketoacidosis. Do not give to patients with liver disease or if ALT is greater than 2.5 × upper limits of normal (ULN) Monitor transaminases—obtain baseline and check every 2 months for first 12 months, then periodically. Discontinue drug if levels increase or jaundice occurs. May cause resumption of ovulation in an anovulatory patient (and thus may result in an unintended pregnancy).
Alpha-Glucosidase Inhibitors • Acarbose (Precose)	50–100 mg tid Maximum dose: 60 kg or less: 150 mg/day in divided doses; more than 60 kg: 300 mg/day in divided doses	2–4 hours	*Applicable to all drugs in this class* Adverse reactions: asthma, dizziness, hepatic injury. Adjunct to diet and exercise in type 2 diabetes; used as monotherapy, or with insulin, metformin, or a sulfonylurea. Do not use if serum Cr is greater than 2 mg/dL.
• Miglitol (Glyset)	25–100 mg tid PO Maximum dose is 300 mg/day (take with first bite of each meal)	4–6 hours	Use glucose not fructose to treat hypoglycemia. Monitor serum transaminases. Adverse reactions: occasional diarrhea, flatulence, abdominal pain—advise patient to take with first bite of main meal.
Meglitinides • Repaglinide (Prandin)	0.5 mg–4 mg within 30 min of meals 2–4 times daily Maximum dose: 16 mg/day		This class stimulates the release of insulin from islet cells. Adjunct to diet and exercise in type 2 diabetes; used as monotherapy or in combination with metformin. Use with caution in older adults and patients with renal or hepatic dysfunction. Interacts with many drugs. Adverse reactions: hypoglycemia, URI, headache, diarrhea, arthralgia.
Phenylalanines • Nateglinide (Starlix)	60–120 mg tid PO (give 30 minutes prior to meals)		Resembles sulfonylurea agents. This agent has fewer side effects than biguanides or alpha-glucosidase inhibitors.
Other agents • Exenatide (Byetta)	5 mcg bid SQ starting dose after 1 month increase to: 10 mcg bid SQ		Action is to mimic incretin: slows gastric emptying and mimic glucose-dependent insulin secretion.
• Pramlintide acetate (Symlin)	60 mcg SQ before meals initially then titrated to 120 mcg SQ before meals If using with insulin, the insulin dose should be decreased by 50 percent.		Suppresses postprandial glucagon release, gastric emptying, and appetite, thereby lowering postprandial glucose.

daily dose before breakfast, although twice-daily dosing is an option. The dose can be increased every 2 weeks until the desired response is achieved or the maximum dose is reached. Common adverse reactions are mild GI upset and skin rashes. Numerous drugs can interfere with sulfonylureas and can alter their effects. The first-generation sulfonylureas are relatively inexpensive, with a monthly cost of \$33 to \$120.00 and second-generation drugs costing \$35 to \$94.00.

Metformin (Glucophage) is a biguanide that works by suppressing excessive hepatic glucose production and by increasing glucose utilization in peripheral tissues. Metformin reduces fasting and postprandial hyperglycemia and reduces hepatic gluconeogenesis. It may also improve glucose levels by reducing intestinal glucose absorption. Metformin does not stimulate endogenous insulin secretion but does lower triglyceride and LDL cholesterol levels while increasing HDL-cholesterol.

Metformin can be used as a monotherapy or in combination with sulfonylureas and insulin. It is beneficial in persons with type 2 diabetes who remain hyperglycemic despite maximum doses of sulfonylureas. It is also beneficial to patients who are obese. Metformin should be used only in patients with adequate renal function (serum creatine less than 1.4 or creatinine clearance greater than 50 mL/min). Because metformin can cause fatal lactic acidosis, although rarely, it should not be used in patients with liver impairment alcoholic patients, or patients who may develop hypoxia due to cardiopulmonary insufficiency. The risk for lactic acidosis increases if contrast dyes for radiologic procedures are used in patients taking metformin. In this case, and in the case of any surgical procedure (decreases kidney function and increases risk of lactic acidosis), metformin should be discontinued 24 to 48 hours before diagnostic and surgical procedures. Metformin administration should not be resumed for at least 6 hours after these procedures or until the patient is adequately hydrated. Initial dosing is 500 mg/day with dinner for 1 week, then twice daily with breakfast and dinner. The dosage should be titrated toward a maximum dose of 2500 mg. Several weeks are needed to achieve the maximum effects of the dose. Common adverse reactions are diarrhea, nausea, anorexia, and abdominal discomfort, which usually resolve with gradual increase of dosage. At the maximum dose, the monthly cost of metformin is about \$108.00.

Acarbose (Precose) and miglitol (Glyset) are alpha-glucosidase inhibitors that slow down the breakdown of complex carbohydrates into monosaccharides. This causes a delay in the absorption of glucose and reduces postprandial blood glucose levels. They do not stimulate insulin secretion, and if used as single therapy, they usually do not produce hypoglycemia. However, if used with insulin or sulfonylureas, the potential for hypoglycemia is present. The recommended initial dose of acarbose is 50 mg/day; it should be titrated slowly up to the maintenance dose of 50 to 100 mg tid with meals. Miglitol also delays absorption of carbohydrates, thereby lowering the postprandial glucose. Therapy is initiated with the lowest effective dose of 25 mg tid, but the maintenance dose is 50 mg tid. Both drugs have similar adverse effects, which are flatulence and diarrhea, thought to be caused by the osmotic effect of undigested carbohydrates in the distal bowel. The cost of monthly therapy with these medications is between \$79 and \$84.00.

Two thiazolidinediones, pioglitazone (Actos) and rosiglitazone (Avandia) are a newer class of antihyperglycemic agents. They work by sensitizing peripheral tissues to insulin and can be used either alone or in combination with sulfonylureas, metformin, or insulin. Neither of these agents should be used in any patient with liver disease or if the ALT level is greater than 2.5 times the upper limit of normal. Liver enzymes should be monitored every 2 months for the first year of therapy and then periodically after that. If the ALT level is 1 to 2.5 times the upper limit of normal, then the patient should be monitored closely or the drug discontinued. As of this writing, no significant cases of liver failure have occurred with either of these drugs, as they have with troglitazone (Rezulin), which has since been pulled from the market.

Several very new drugs for type 2 DM are exenatide (Byetta) and pramlintide acetate (Symlin). Exenatide is an incretin mimetic and has the same effects as human incretin hormone GLP-1. It enhances glucose-dependent insulin secretion and slows gastric emptying, possibly leading to a decreased food intake. Exenatide is given initially in a dose of 5 mcg bid subcutaneously and can be increased to 10 mcg after 1 month. Pramlintide acetate (Symlin) is an amylin (hormone secreted by beta cells) analogue that suppresses postprandial glucagon release, gastric emptying, and appetite, thereby lowering postprandial glucose levels when given before meals. It can be used in both type 1 and type 2 DM and is used in conjunction with insulin. Symlin is given at a dose of 60 mcg sq initially just prior to each meal and then titrated up to 120 mcg. It is important to note that the dose of insulin should be reduced by 50 percent when given with Symlin.

The patient who fails to respond to the use of sulfonylureas or other agents should be evaluated for the possibility of type 1 diabetes. Although type 1 diabetes infrequently presents in older adults, it should be considered in patients with other autoimmune disorders, patients without a family history of type 2 diabetes, and patients of normal weight.

When nutritional therapy, exercise, and oral antidiabetic agents have failed to control blood glucose levels, the addition of insulin is recommended. The guidelines for insulin administration in type 2 diabetics are essentially the same as for type 1 diabetics and the reader is referred to this section under the previous discussion of type 1 DM. Patients should be referred to an endocrinologist for evaluation for possible addition of insulin to the treatment regimen. Individual treatment goals should take into account the patient's capacity to understand and carry out the treatment, the risk for severe hypoglycemia, and any other factors that increase risk or decrease benefit.

Because there are several different types of oral antidiabetic agents that can be used as monotherapy or in combination with each other or with insulin therapy treatment decisions can be complex. The following is a synopsis of treatment recommendations:

- Immediately on diagnosis of type 2 diabetes begin nutritional therapy and exercise.
- If glycemic goals are not met in 3 months, initiate monotherapy with oral antidiabetic agents.
- If glycemic goals are still not met 3 months later, begin combined therapy with oral antidiabetic agents.
- If glycemic goals are not met in 3 additional months, start combined therapy with oral antidiabetic agents and insulin.
- If glycemic goals are not met in 3 additional months, begin insulin therapy alone.

Insulin therapy alone or in combination may be needed sooner if glycemic levels significantly exceed goals. When glycemic control is not adequate with a combination of metformin, sulfonylurea, and a thiazolidinedione, a single nighttime injection of NPH insulin or insulin glargine can be added and titrated to get the desired blood glucose level. If daytime glycemic control is inadequate, the patient may be changed to an insulin only regimen (see discussion in section on type 1 DM). Metformin and thiazolidinediones can be used with insulin therapy, but sulfonylureas should be discontinued. Metformin and thiazolidinediones facilitate lower doses of insulin in maintaining glycemic control.

Monitoring for Hypoglycemia. Hypoglycemia (plasma glucose less than 60 mg/dL) may occur in patients with type 2 diabetes for a variety of reasons: excessive exogenous insulin, excessive dose of oral antidiabetic agents, missed meals or inadequate food intake, exercise, alcohol ingestion, drug interactions, and a decrease in liver or kidney function. When using two oral antidiabetic agents, the potential for hypoglycemic episodes is greater, and the patient and family should be aware of this. Signs and symptoms include diaphoresis, tachycardia, hunger, shakiness, altered mentation (ranging from inability to concentrate to coma), slurred speech, and seizure. The signs and symptoms exhibited by the patient are highly individual and can vary from mild to severe. When the patient becomes ill, blood glucose will need closer monitoring and parenteral insulin may be necessary if oral agents cannot be tolerated.

Follow-Up and Referral

On initial diagnosis, the patient should be referred to a dietitian and a certified diabetes educator. Because type 2 diabetes is a chronic disease, continuing care is essential and the goal of treatment is to prevent or slow the chronic complications. The frequency of patient visits depends on the degree to which blood glucose levels are controlled, changes in therapy, and the presence and degree of complications or other medical conditions. If the patient is performing SMBG, telephone consultations may be possible instead of office visits. Once regulated, the patient should be seen at least quarterly. These visits should include a discussion on the results of SMBG; patient adjustments to therapy; symptoms of illnesses; problems with adherence to the treatment plan; changes in lifestyle; medications; and frequency, causes, and severity of hyperglycemia or hypoglycemia if the patient is on insulin or oral antidiabetic agents.

HbA_{1c} determination should be performed at least twice a year in patients with good control and quarterly in patients whose therapy has changed or who are not meeting glycemic goals. The physical exam should include a comprehensive foot exam and a funduscopic exam.

Research indicates that patients are more successful in accomplishing lifestyle changes when there is regular contact with the health-care provider. This can be expensive and inconvenient. Community-based telemedicine programs can be helpful. (See Nursing Research-Based Practice 15.1.)

Complications

Referrals for the following complications are indicated:

- Retinopathy. Comprehensive dilated eye and visual exams should be performed annually by an ophthalmologist who is knowledgeable and experienced in the management of diabetic retinopathy for all patients who are diagnosed with type 2 DM, as most individuals have had diabetes for several years before they are diagnosed. Type 2 DM is the leading cause of acquired blindness in adults aged 20 to 74 years, and up to 25 percent of newly diagnosed patients may present with retinopathy at the time of diagnosis.
- Hyperlipidemia. Adults with type 2 diabetes should be retested annually for lipid disorders with fasting lipid profile including serum cholesterol, triglyceride, HDL, and calculated LDL cholesterol measurements. ADA guidelines suggest that emphasis in clinical management should be directed toward lowering of the LDL, increasing the HDL, and lowering elevated triglyceride levels. Aggressive therapy is indicated because it is suggested that it will lower the risk of CAD. LDL levels should be less than 100 mg/dL in patients with diabetes and preexisting cardiac disease. If behavioral therapy and medical nutritional therapy fail to achieve this goal in an individual patient, statin (HMG CoA-reductase inhibitor) antihyperlipidemic therapy should be initiated. In patients with diabetes without a history of coronary vascular disease, behavioral therapy is indicated when the LDL is 130 mg/dL or more. If behavioral and medical nutritional therapy is unsuccessful, the use of statins is indicated.
- Nephropathy. A routine urinalysis should be performed annually for all patients. Screening for microalbuminuria in the patient with type 2 diabetes should begin at the time of diagnosis because it is not known how long the patient has had diabetes. Microalbuminuria is found in a

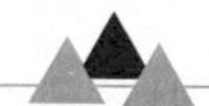

NURSING RESEARCH-BASED PRACTICE 15.1

Chan, W, Woo, J, Hui, E, Lau W, Lai, J, and Lee, D: A community model for care of elderly people with diabetes via telemedicine. Appl Nurs Res 18(2):77–81, 2004.

Diabetes self-management programs have been shown to be effective in lifestyle changes including diet and exercise with results of better blood sugar control. A study to assess the feasibility and acceptability of a telemedicine diabetes care program for seniors in a community center setting was conducted in Hong Kong. The program included education about diet, ideal body weight, glucose monitoring, signs of hypoglycemia, foot care, and an exercise regimen. There was 100% adherence with the program. Participants significantly decreased caloric intake and body mass index. Subjects had better control of blood sugar and demonstrated an improved understanding of their illness.

Seniors can benefit from a diabetic telemedicine program. Reinforcement of knowledge and the patient's proactive role in the process aids in retention of the information. The community-based model assists patients in access to health-care providers while preserving resources. However, this model is best used in an urban community where access to such a center is more feasible. The pilot study revealed an improvement in diabetes control and lifestyle changes and that a telemedicine community program should be further evaluated for broad-based use.

high proportion of patients when first diagnosed with type 2 diabetes. The ADA recommends screening at the time of diagnosis of type 2 diabetes followed by annual screening because 20 to 40 percent of patients with type 2 diabetes will progress to overt hyperalbuminuria and 15 to 20 percent progress to renal disease. The use of ACE inhibitors to slow the progression of microalbuminuria to overt disease in normotensive patients has not been as extensively studied as in patients with type 1 diabetes, but appears to improve morbidity. Type 2 DM is the leading cause of end-stage renal disease (ESRD).

- ▲ Hypertension. In a patient with type 2 diabetes, hypertension is often a part of a syndrome that includes glucose intolerance, insulin resistance, obesity, dyslipidemia, and CAD. It is present in one-third of patients diagnosed with type 2 DM. Isolated systolic hypertension may occur with long duration of diabetes and is due in part to inelasticity of atherosclerotic large vessels. Control of hypertension has been demonstrated to reduce the rate of progression of nephropathy and to reduce the complications of cardiovascular disease. As with patients with type 1 diabetes, ACE inhibitors should be the initial treatment unless there are contraindications to their use. If a patient does not tolerate the use of ACE inhibitors, angiotensin receptor blockers (ARBs) can be used. Some studies suggest that they be used together in all diabetic patients for the benefit in nephropathy, since the medications act by different mechanisms.
- ▲ Macrovascular disease. Evidence of uncontrolled angina, carotid bruits, and ECG abnormalities may require advanced intervention. An ECG is indicated in patients older than 40 years of age. Daily intake of aspirin has been shown to reduce cardiovascular events in patients with diabetes. Diabetic patients are at risk for developing macrovascular complications including stroke/CVA, peripheral vascular disease (PVD), and CAD/CVD. Patients with disabling claudication or nonhealing ulcers require a vascular consultation for their PVD. All diabetic patients should be screened for these diseases, as symptoms may not be present until late in the course of the disease process. Type 2 DM is the leading cause of nontraumatic lower extremity amputation due to PVD and peripheral neuropathy. Problems involving the feet may require care by a podiatrist, orthopedic surgeon, vascular surgeon, or rehabilitation specialist. Assessment guidelines are addressed in the section on type 1 DM.
- ▲ Neuropathy. Peripheral neuropathy may result in pain, loss of sensation, and muscle weakness. Its incidence increases over time in patients with type 2 diabetes and is more prevalent in patients with low serum insulin concentrations and poor glycemic control. Autonomic involvement can affect gastrointestinal, cardiovascular, and genitourinary function. Patients with significant urinary symptoms or impotence should be referred to a urologist.
- ▲ Pregnancy. To reduce the risk of fetal malformation and maternal and fetal complications, every pregnancy in a woman with type 2 diabetes should be planned in advance. Pregnancy is contraindicated in women taking oral antidiabetic agents, and, if receiving this treatment, the patient must switch to insulin. The pregnant woman with type 2 diabetes requires excellent blood glucose control and should be monitored closely by a multidisciplinary team, which includes the obstetrician.
- ▲ Psychosocial. The complex management of DM places stress on the patient and family. Research has shown that obese women with type 2 diabetes reported stress, anxiety, and guilt. The complex self-management skills required to manage DM and its impact on well-being

may affect the quality of life and contribute to depression. Patients should be monitored for problems with treatment adherence and for depression.

Patient Education

Successful diabetes management involves a team effort to achieve mutually agreed upon treatment goals. To achieve these goals, it is crucial that the patient and family or significant other be educated in all aspects of the treatment plan. The following list is a synopsis of the salient topics for patient education:

- Introduction: definition of type 2 diabetes, causes of diabetes, and function of the pancreas and insulin.
- Regulation of blood glucose: role of diet, exercise, insulin; signs and symptoms of hyperglycemia; causes, treatment, and prevention of hyperglycemia; signs and symptoms of hypoglycemia; causes, treatment, and prevention of hypoglycemia; when to contact the practitioner.
- Blood glucose monitoring and urine testing: how to perform SMBG, how often to test, recording and reporting results, and urine ketone testing.
- Medication and insulin administration: actions and adverse reactions of oral antidiabetic agents; actions of insulin; types of insulin, effects on blood glucose; storage of supplies; drawing, mixing, and injecting insulin; site selection and rotation; and needle disposal.
- Meal planning: types of nutrients (carbohydrates, proteins, fats), timing of meals, portions, use of sweeteners, eating out, use of alcohol, and sick-day management.
- Exercise: benefits, types of exercise, effects on blood glucose, planning and measuring exercise, snacks
- Prevention of long-term complications: importance of blood glucose control, vision exams, foot care, prevention of infection, and signs and symptoms of complications.

Metabolic Syndrome

Metabolic syndrome is a constellation of conditions and/or risk factors that lead to an increased incidence of type 2 diabetes and related cardiovascular disease. Each condition is independently associated with an increased risk of heart disease and diabetes but together, they have an affect that is more than the sum of the conditions. The characteristics of metabolic syndrome include abdominal obesity, hypertension, lipid abnormalities, insulin resistance, and a proinflammatory state.

Epidemiology and Causes

The CDC estimates that 31.9 percent of adults in the United States, or roughly 64 million individuals, have metabolic syndrome. One million adolescents have been diagnosed with this disorder. There has been a 33 percent increase in the prevalence of both metabolic syndrome over the last 10 years, principally because of the obesity epidemic. Estimates are that 45 percent of the population older than the age of 60 has metabolic syndrome and many of these will go on to develop type 2 diabetes. Mexican Americans are at a very high risk for developing metabolic syndrome and type 2 diabetes and are twice as likely as non-Hispanic Americans to develop these conditions. African American and Hispanic women are much more likely to develop metabolic syndrome than their male counterparts.

The cause of metabolic syndrome is unclear. There is a strong relationship between abdominal obesity and insulin resistance, type 2 diabetes, hypertension, and endothelial inflammation/dysfunction. Visceral adipose tissue is more resistant to the action of insulin, but more sensitive to lipolytic hormones, causing release of free fatty acids which provides a substrate for the synthesis of triglycerides.

Pathophysiology

Metabolic syndrome is a common disease characterized by a combination of atherogenic and diabetogenic factors. Increased body mass index (BMI), elevated systolic BP, hypertriglyceridemia, hyperglycemia, and low levels of protective HDL-cholesterol are found in affected persons. Any three of the above conditions occurring together can establish the diagnosis (see Diagnostic Reasoning).

Metabolic syndrome is also a proinflammatory and prothrombotic disorder causing endothelial injury, as evidenced by serum elevations in C-reactive protein (CRP), interleukin (IL)-6, and plasminogen activator inhibitor (PAI)-1, as well as increased platelet aggregation and plasma fibrinogen levels. In addition to hyperglycemia and deranged lipid metabolism, peripheral tissues are resistant to insulin. The pancreas oversecretes insulin to overcome tissue resistance, which results in hyperinsulinemia. Obesity enhances insulin resistance and predisposes the individual to type 2 DM.

Obesity and advanced age are believed to significantly contribute to the development of the metabolic syndrome. As a modifiable risk factor, the National Cholesterol Education Program (NCEP) recommends obesity as the primary target for intervention. Weight loss improves serum lipid profiles, reduces blood pressure, decreases insulin resistance, and ameliorates glucose intolerance.

Clinical Presentation

Subjective

Patients with metabolic syndrome are most often asymptomatic. They may report a history of gradual weight gain, especially around the abdomen. History often reveals a sedentary lifestyle and a diet that is high calorie, highly refined, and nutrient poor.

Objective

Objective findings usually consist of an abdominal measurement that is more than 40 inches in men and more than 35 inches in women. The individual may or may not be overweight and he or she will usually have a blood pressure of 130/85 mm Hg or higher.

Diagnostic Reasoning

The National Cholesterol Education Program (NCEP) Adult Treatment Panel (ATP) III has developed criteria for diagnosing metabolic syndrome. To be diagnosed with metabolic syndrome the patient must have any three of the following:

- ▲ Abdominal obesity (waist circumference)
  Men: greater than 40 inches
  Women: greater than 35 inches
- ▲ Fasting HDL level
  Men: less than 40 mg/dL
  Women: less than 50 mg/dL
- ▲ Fasting triglyceride level of 150 mg/dL or higher
- ▲ Blood pressure of 130/85 mm Hg or higher
- ▲ A fasting serum glucose level of 110 mg/dL or higher

Diagnostic Tests

The patient who is suspected of metabolic syndrome should have a fasting lipid profile. Although the patient may have a normal LDL cholesterol, this can be misleading because it is a calculated value. If the triglyceride level is above 200 mg/dL, the calculated LDL is not valid. When there is a high triglyceride and a low HDL-cholesterol, this usually means there is a high concentration of small, dense LDL cholesterol particles. These small dense LDL particles are highly atherogenic and lead to cardiovascular disease.

A fasting blood sugar should be done. Patients with metabolic syndrome may have a fasting level of 100 mg/dL or higher, but it frequently is below 126 mg/dL. The range between 100 to 126 mg/dL indicates impaired fasting glucose (IFG). Most patients with metabolic syndrome have a normal or near normal HbA_{1c}, so this test is of little help. Because a proinflammatory state is also implicated in metabolic syndrome, the patient should also have a test for C-reactive protein (CRP). A value of more than 3 mg/L in a high sensitivity CRP would indicate high risk for cardiovascular disease. In fact, this may be a better predictor of future heart disease than either LDL or HDL. However, if the results of the high sensitivity CRP are more than 10 mg/L, this indicates a noncardiovascular inflammatory problem and the test should be repeated in 2 to 3 weeks.

Differential Diagnosis

Differential diagnoses include type 2 diabetes, obesity, and any condition that results in increasing abdominal girth, hypertension, or IFG. Some of these conditions are cirrhosis, Cushing's syndrome, acromegaly, and ingestion of certain medications (cortisol).

Management

The ultimate goal of management is to prevent type 2 diabetes and cardiovascular disease. Treatment is largely with lifestyle change. Weight loss is the key to successful management, in fact, a loss of 5 to 10 percent of body weight improves all facets of metabolic syndrome and significantly reduces morbidity and mortality. Smoking cessation is also another key to reduce the risk associated with metabolic syndrome.

Most patients will benefit from nutrition counseling. Counseling should consist of several (three to six) 30-minute sessions and discuss the importance of weight loss and eating a diet that contains mostly fruits, vegetables, and complex, unrefined carbohydrates. Patients should eat at least 5 servings of vegetables and four servings of fruit every day. Simple carbohydrates (sugar, white flour, white rice) should be limited as much as possible. Patients should be counseled to eat 20 to 35 grams of fiber per day and include three servings of low-fat or fat-free dairy products. In addition, the diet should contain limited saturated and trans fats (less red meat, more fish).

For patients with a BMI between 27 and 35, a simple reduction (300 to 500 kcal) in calories can produce a 1- to 2-pound weight loss per week. If the BMI is greater than 35, then a daily reduction of 500 to 1000 calories is recommended. Portion control is the key to calorie reduction. Studies have shown that the average American eats 7 to 20 percent more calories today than in 1971, with women consuming the most. Also, Americans are 25 pounds heavier on average than they were in 1960.

Treatment of metabolic syndrome is dependent on increased physical activity. Exercise should be moderately intense (50 to 80 percent of maximal heart rate) and should be an activity that the patient will enjoy and more likely to continue for life. Walking is a good activity to begin. The patient should start with about 10 to 15 minutes a day and work up to a minimum of 30 minutes, and this should be done most days of the week. The goal is to make activity a normal part of everyday living.

For patients who are unable to lose weight with diet and exercise, pharmacologic therapy may help, but surgery may be an option. Usually, this is reserved for patients who have a BMI greater than 40, but is considered in patients with a BMI of 35 if they also have comorbid conditions. Surgery should be suggested only in patients who have truly failed at weight loss through conventional methods, as the complication rate with surgery is about 20 percent.

Patients who exhibit some degree of dyslipidemia usually benefit from pharmacologic therapy. Statins are the drugs of choice for dyslipidemia because they also have an effect on the inflammatory cascade created by metabolic syndrome. See Chapter 9 on cardiovascular disease for specific drugs and dosages.

Hypertension is an important cause of cardiovascular morbidity and mortality. Even in normotensive individuals, a decrease of 2 mm Hg in systolic blood pressure can produce as much as a 7 percent decrease in mortality from heart disease and 10 percent reduction in stroke mortality. The JNC 7 recommends treating patients with a BP above 140/90 mm Hg. See the chapter on cardiovascular disease for specific drugs and dosages.

Follow-Up and Referral

Patients with metabolic syndrome should be followed closely for hypertension and the development of type 2 diabetes. Studies indicate that when patients have frequent contact with the clinician, they are more successful in making lifestyle change and weight loss, keys in the treatment of metabolic syndrome. Measurements of BMI and abdominal girth should be done at every visit.

Patient Education

The importance of lifestyle change cannot be stressed enough. Patients need to be encouraged to find an activity that they enjoy and will do most days for the rest of their lives. It is also important to stress that weight loss is best accomplished by a change in lifestyle rather than viewing it as a diet.

Hypoglycemia

Hypoglycemia is a clinical syndrome of subnormal plasma glucose concentration that may affect infants through the elderly, although the primary etiology of the disorder differs markedly among various age groups. Adult hypoglycemia is characterized by blood glucose levels of less than 60 mg/dL of blood, while neonatal hypoglycemia is typically defined as a level below 30 mg/dL in the first 24 hours of life and below 45 mg/dL. Universal agreement does not exist as to these thresholds, however, with some research supporting a level of less than 50 mg/dL for men, 45 mg/dL for women, and 40 mg/dL for infants and children as indicative of hypoglycemia.

Regardless, hypoglycemia is the most commonly occurring endocrine emergency, producing symptoms that are typically relieved by the intake of sugar. There are two major types of hypoglycemia: fasting and reactive. Fasting hypoglycemia is a low blood sugar level more than 5 hours after eating; it can be subacute or chronic. Reactive or postprandial hypoglycemia is less common and is most often acute in nature. Reactive hypoglycemia usually produces symptoms 2 to 4 hours following a meal rich in carbohydrates and symptoms rarely occur in a fasting state.

Epidemiology and Causes

Hypoglycemia as a separate disease entity is most common in the elderly, as well as young diabetic adults. It is more prevalent in women. About 1 percent of the nondiabetic population is affected. Hypoglycemia in persons with DM is more common with type 1 diabetes and in patients following a regimen of intensive glycemic control. Although endocrine disorders are the most frequent cause of hypoglycemia, lifestyle patterns also contribute to this condition. In adults, hypoglycemia is most commonly due to iatrogenic phenomena caused either by administration of exogenous insulin or another plasma glucose–lowering medication. In childhood, hypoglycemia is most commonly observed in children affected by autoimmune, insulin-dependent type 1 DM. In contrast, hypoglycemia in neonates is a unique phenomenon, largely related to the immature developmental stage of the neonatal endocrine system, as discussed in the Pathophysiology section below.

Classic hypoglycemia denotes a low plasma glucose level in the setting of insulin-dependent DM. Inconsistent subcutaneous absorption of insulin, decreased food intake, missed meals, and increased insulin secretion during exercise produce hypoglycemia in patients with DM. Moreover, physical and emotional stress may alter the body's reaction to insulin. Sulfonylureas also can produce hypoglycemia in patients with type 2 DM, but it occurs less commonly than with type 1 DM.

Hypoglycemia often occurs during the early stages of adrenal stress and blood sugar imbalance problems. It is an early sign of pancreatic and diabetic problems. In persons with DM, hypoglycemia is often precipitated by stress, pregnancy, intensive control of hyperglycemia, and in diabetic gastroparesis.

The symptoms of fasting hypoglycemia occur when the patient has not eaten for 5 or more hours. The possible causes of fasting hypoglycemia include pancreatic beta-cell tumor, extrapancreatic tumors, hypopituitarism, myxedema, ethanol-induced hypoglycemia, severe malnutrition, septicemia, and renal failure which results in decreased clearance of insulin from the body. The list of drugs that can cause fasting hypoglycemia is lengthy: insulin and sulfonylureas, propanolol (Inderal), salicylates, quinidine, pentamidine (Pentam 300, Nebupent), coumarin, sulfonamides, tricyclic antidepressants, disopyramide (Norpace), didanosine, ritodrine, chlorpromazine, isoniazid (INH), selective serotonin reuptake inhibitors (SSRIs), clofibrate, thiazide diuretics, lithium, and angiotensin converting enzyme (ACE) inhibitors. Poisoning with organophosphate and carbamate-based pesticides also results in hypoglycemia. In adrenocortical insufficiency, there is a decreased production of cortisol which is required for gluconeogenesis, thus leading to hypoglycemia. Liver diseases, including hepatitis, cirrhosis, hepatomas, and hepatic congestion, interfere with the uptake and release of glycogen from the liver and ultimately may lead to hypoglycemia.

Postprandial hypoglycemia or reactive hypoglycemia may be caused by gastrointestinal surgery, or any other alimentary tract disorder that affects absorption, congenital deficiency of enzymes necessary for carbohydrate metabolism, and late insulin release caused by B-cell dysfunction. It is an early manifestation of DM and has been seen with extreme exertion in untrained, physically unfit persons, as well as in patients with sepsis or heart failure. Idiopathic or functional postprandial hypoglycemia also exists which cannot be ascribed to any discrete cause.

Hypoglycemia may be factitious or self-induced by the excessive intake of sulfonylureas or insulin. Timing of these types of hypoglycemic events is not related to food intake. If this type is suspected in patients with known access to these drugs (health-care workers and caregivers of diabetic patients), serum and urine sulfonylurea levels should be obtained. A very low or non-existent serum C-peptide level confirms that insulin is being injected exogenously.

Lifestyle patterns may contribute to hypoglycemia as well. The excessive consumption of simple sugars, an excessively refined and processed diet, excessive exercise, stress, irregular eating patterns, or missing meals may cause abnormal fluctuations of blood sugar levels. Nutrient deficiencies, food allergies, and poor digestion may also contribute to hypoglycemia. Cigarette smoking and high caffeine intake produce instability of blood glucose levels. (Table 15.11 lists the causes of hypoglycemia.)

Pathophysiology

To understand the clinical and biochemical phenomenon of hypoglycemia, it is important to grasp the mechanics behind the body's careful regulation of euglycemic plasma glucose levels between 80 and 90 mg/dL. After a carbohydrate-containing meal in which glucose is absorbed from the gut into the bloodstream, plasma glucose levels transiently increase to 120 to 140 mg/dL. Glucose subsequently enters pancreatic beta cells via the GLUT1 and GLUT2 cell membrane transporters, where the enzyme glucokinase phosphorylates it to glucose-6-phosphate, thereby acting as a glucose sensor and triggering the passive entry of calcium into beta cells, causing insulin secretion. Insulin lowers plasma glucose levels by decreasing hepatic glycolysis (glycogen breakdown) and gluconeogenesis (de novoglucose synthesis), driving glucose uptake by skeletal muscle and adipose tissue via the translocation of intracellular glucose transporter molecules to the cell membrane surface, and decreasing both proteolysis and lipolysis which decreases the number of gluconeogenic precursors. In turn, plasma glucose levels typically return to normal within several hours following a carbohydrate-containing meal.

Table 15.11 Causes of Hypoglycemia

Type of Hypoglycemia	Causes
Fasting hypoglycemia	Renal failure (decreases rate at which insulin is secreted contributing to hypoglycemia) Hepatic disease Insulinomas Pancreatic tumors Autoimmune disease Hypopituitarism Extrapancreatic tumors Ethanol intake Septicemia
Reactive hypoglycemia	Postgastrectomy Gastric bypass surgery Hereditary fructose intolerance Congenital enzyme deficiency Pancreatic beta cell dysfunction Meals high in carbohydrates Exercise Pregnancy
Drug-induced hypoglycemia	Exogenous insulin Sulfonylureas Propranolol Salicylates Quinine Pentamidine Disopyramide

Hypoglycemia is sensed by central nervous system receptors in the hypothalamus as well as peripheral receptors that act via afferent nerves to trigger an appropriate hormonal response to maintain glucose homeostasis. The body counters low glucose levels below 80 mg/dL by decreasing pancreatic insulin production, eventually secreting several counterregulatory hormones at levels below 70 mg/dL, including glucagon from pancreatic alpha cells which acts directly on the liver and epinephrine from the adrenal medulla which acts similar to glucagon via hepatic beta-adrenergic receptors, as well as mediating the autonomic (sympathetic, adrenergic) symptoms of hypoglycemia (e.g., diaphoresis, anxiety). Epinephrine also directly inhibits insulin secretion via alpha-2-adrenergic receptors. If hypoglycemia is severe ($<$ 60 mg/dL) or persists for several hours, additional counterregulatory hormones are mobilized, including cortisol from the adrenal cortex and growth hormone from the pituitary gland.

These counterregulatory hormones increase hepatic glucose production via a number of mechanisms, including glycogen breakdown into individual glucose monomers (glycogenolysis) and, once intrahepatic glycogen stores are depleted, *de novo* glucose synthesis from amino acid, pyruvate, glycerol, and free fatty acid precursors (gluconeogenesis). In turn, the body also metabolically shifts away from glucose utilization toward alternate sources of fuel to maintain euglycemia, e.g., proteins, ketone bodies converted from fats. Increased lipolysis is thus reflected in increased plasma free fatty acids while increased protein breakdown is reflected in higher concentrations of the amino acids alanine and glutamine.

The brain utilizes glucose almost exclusively as its sole fuel source; however, it is not capable of synthesizing or storing it. Thus, the brain is particularly sensitive to dramatic changes in blood glucose concentration. Hypoglycemia in which plasma glucose falls below 60 mg/dL prevents the brain from receiving an adequate supply of blood glucose, thereby impairing function. Even asymptomatic hypoglycemia has been associated with neurocognitive impairment in infants and children. Type 1 diabetics with a history of recurrent hypoglycemia have been shown to display more frontal lobe deficits and impairments in motor and visuospatial skills than control diabetics. In adults, cognitive dysfunction can be detected in otherwise normal individuals at plasma glucose levels between 50 and 55 mg/dL; older men are particularly prone to this type of neurologic impairment. At levels between 45 and 50 mg/dL, lethargy and obtundation follow, with coma occurring at levels below 30 mg/dL, followed by convulsions below 20 mg/dL and eventual death. Severe hypoglycemia has also been associated with cardiovascular dysfunction.

The histologic structure of the pancreas is uniquely designed to prevent these events. Within the pancreas, each islet of Langerhans consists of several hundred cells, including a core of insulin-producing beta cells surrounded by glucagon-secreting alpha cells and an outer layer of somatostatin-producing delta cells and PP cells, which make pancreatic polypeptide. As arterial blood enters the islet core, the beta cells are the first to encounter plasma glucose concentrations. Thus, the function of alpha cells is determined largely by the normal activity of beta cells. For example, insulin directly inhibits glucagon secretion by pancreatic alpha cells.

In adults, reactive hypoglycemia occurs when these counterregulatory responses fail after consuming a carbohydrate load, causing blood glucose to fall 2 to 5 hours after eating. However, hypoglycemia more commonly occurs owing to iatrogenic medication effects, particularly exogenous insulin administration in diabetic patients or the use of a sulfonylurea secretagogue, since the suppression of insulin release cannot be utilized as an effective regulatory mechanism in these patients. This mechanism is also common in children with insulin-dependent type 1 DM if they miss a meal (intentional or unintentional fasting) or mistakenly overdose on their insulin.

In addition, although the mechanisms are poorly understood, persons with DM have impaired secretory responses of both glucagon and epinephrine to hypoglycemia, which only aggravates this condition, as the secretion of counterregulatory hormones is the main defense against hypoglycemia in these patients. Persistently elevated insulin levels suppress glucagon secretion. However, even in patients with type 1 DM and an absence of endogenous insulin, glucagon secretion is markedly impaired to absent after several years of the disease. Thus, these patients are relatively more dependent on epinephrine secretion as a counterregulatory mechanism; however, epinephrine secretion in these patients is eventually impaired as well, after several more years of the disease.

Thus, these patients can experience hypoglycemic unawareness in which they lose the early autonomic manifestations of low plasma glucose. Patients with decreased glucagon and epinephrine responses to low blood glucose levels have up to a 25-fold greater risk of experiencing hypoglycemia, particularly during sleep, as sleep itself decreases counterregulatory hormonal responses. Hypoglycemia is less common in patients with type 2 DM, as the defects in counterregulatory mechanisms are less severe in these patients, as compared to those with type 1 DM. In addition, the glucose thresholds for counterregulatory hormone secretion in type 2 diabetics are quantitatively higher by 7 to 23 mg/dL versus those in type 1 diabetics. In fact, glucose thresholds for counterregulatory hormone secretion are generally higher in poorly controlled diabetic patients as compared to normal controls, emphasizing that chronically hyperglycemic patients are prone to adrenergic and neuroglycopenic symptoms at relatively higher plasma glucose levels than nondiabetic patients. This may be due to a decrease in central nervous system glucose transporters in chronically hyperglycemic patients, which would result in a higher glucose activation threshold.

Unfortunately, an initial hypoglycemic episode appears to contribute to a vicious cycle of hypoglycemia, as recurrent hypoglycemia has been associated with autonomic failure and a delay in the early warning signs associated with a subsequent hypoglycemic episode. This may relate to an increased production of cortisol, which decreases glucagon and epinephrine responses, as well as upregulation of glucose transport in the brain, which renders the central nervous system less sensitive to producing neuroglycopenic symptoms. However, in contrast, tight glycemic control with strict avoidance of hypoglycemia is capable of restoring early hypoglycemic warning signs and neuroendocrine homeostatic responses in as little as 2 days, early on in the disease course in diabetic patients. Two other factors have been suggested to mediate hypoglycemic unawareness: a slow rate of decrease in plasma glucose concentration and diabetic autonomic neuropathy. However, neither of these mechanisms has been confirmed to play a significant role in well-controlled studies.

Hypoglycemia in infants has an extensive differential diagnosis of potential etiologies, as a number of congenital genetic defects exist that may initially present with neonatal hypoglycemia. These include disorders of glucose utilization related to hyperinsulinemic states (e.g., persistent hyperinsulinemic hypoglycemia of infancy, macrosomia associated with maternal diabetes, insulinoma), disorders of glucose metabolism (e.g., Krebs cycle or oxidative respiratory chain defects), genetic defects in the metabolism of alternate fuel sources (e.g., carnitine acyl transferase deficiency, long- and medium-chain acyl-coenzyme A dehydrogenase deficiency), and hypermetabolic states such as sepsis, severe burns, hyperthermia, polycythemia, or congenital hyperthyroidism. Persistent hyperinsulinemic hypoglycemia of infancy is the most common etiology of hyperinsulinemia during the first 3 months of life. This primary disorder of the pancreas is more commonly observed in infants who are small for gestational age and those born to mothers with toxemia (maternal sepsis).

Infants may also suffer from inadequate glucose stores (e.g., prematurity, malnutrition, intrauterine growth restriction), congenital hormonal deficiencies (e.g., growth hormone, cortisol, panhypopituitarism), or disordered gluconeogenesis (e.g., glucose-6-phosphatase deficiency, glycogen synthase deficiency, galactosemia, maple syrup urine disease, or any one of several glycogen storage diseases). Perinatal asphyxia potentiates hypoglycemia, worsening the resulting neurologic impairment that is associated with sustained or recurrent hypoglycemia.

Clinical Presentation

The clinical presentation of hypoglycemia, especially subjective symptoms, varies depending on the physical status of the person. Older adults with neuropathy may lack awareness of its symptoms unless they are severe. In an accidental exposure to hypoglycemic agents, the symptoms are often not recognized or associated with this disease.

Subjective

Symptoms of hypoglycemia may be present when the blood glucose level falls below 60 mg/dL. Brain function is often impaired when levels fall below 50 mg/dL. Some patients may exhibit symptoms with abnormal fluctuations of glucose and insulin. Symptoms vary from very mild to severe and are classified into adrenergic and neuroglycopenic.

Adrenergic symptoms include sweating, tremulousness, dizziness, confusion, anxiety, and palpitations. Neuroglycopenic symptoms include headaches, seizures, fatigue, weakness, drowsiness, syncope, diplopia and blurred vision, and personality changes. The neurologic manifestations of hemiparesis, convulsions, confusion, and coma are more common in patients with DM. Symptoms are often relieved with ingestion of carbohydrates. Seizures and coma are severe complications.

The history should focus on eating habits, meal times, and exercise habits, including alcohol intake and any history of liver or renal disease. A focus on family history of DM and hypoglycemia is essential.

Objective

Objective findings are tachycardia, with or without premature ventricular contractions, diaphoresis, hypothermia or hyperthermia, coma, seizures, Babinski's sign, aphasia, and hemiparesis. Diaphoresis, trembling, and an increased heart rate may be present.

A physical examination with special attention to objective signs of endocrine disease is indicated initially. Assess for an enlarged liver and neurologic indications of chronic alcohol abuse. Observe the skin for needle marks to indicate possible insulin injection.

Infants prone to hypoglycemia have a unique physical presentation. Hyperinsulinemic babies (e.g., those born to diabetic mothers or babies with insulin-producing tumors) have large body size, given the growth effects of insulin. In contrast, those with decreased body fat are more likely to suffer from insufficient glucose stores. Poor linear growth reflects growth hormone deficiency, while midline craniofacial defects may indicate more global pituitary hormone defects. Hepatomegaly is a common sign of glycogen storage diseases. In more general terms, neonatal hypoglycemia presents with jitteriness, hypotonia, lethargy, poor feeding, cyanosis, apnea, or hypothermia.

Diagnostic Reasoning

Diagnostic Tests

Plasma blood glucose levels are used to diagnose hypoglycemia. Hypoglycemia is suspected if the plasma blood glucose level is between 45 and 60 mg/dL or if an overnight fasting glucose level is less than 60 mg/dL. Hypoglycemia is present if the plasma blood glucose level is 45 mg/dL or less. Evaluation of the etiology, when not attributed to treatment of DM, requires subsequent laboratory evaluations.

Initial Testing. Initial testing includes a blood glucose level. The best time to obtain a blood glucose level is when the patient is experiencing symptoms. If hypoglycemia and symptoms occur concurrently and if both are relieved with eating, the diagnosis of postprandial hypoglycemia is confirmed. However, fingerstick monitors are not very accurate at extremes of high and low glucose concentrations. They are a helpful tool in detecting high and low blood glucose, but the number itself may not be accurate. An oral glucose tolerance test may be done; however, overinterpretation of glucose tolerance test may lead to an overdiagnosis of hypoglycemia. More than one-third of normal patients have hypoglycemia with or without symptoms during a 4-hour fasting test. For definite diagnosis, the patient should have (1) documented occurrences of blood glucose levels, (2) symptoms that occur when the blood glucose level is low, (3) evidence that symptoms are relieved by sugar or other foods, and (4) identification of the particular type of hypoglycemia. It is important to remember that whole blood glucose levels are 10 to 15 percent lower than serum glucose levels, as RBCs consume glucose. The most reliable method of diagnosing hypoglycemia is with a plasma glucose 72-hour fast. During this test, the patient is allowed calorie-free, caffeine-free fluids and the patient fasts at least overnight, but may be as long as 72 hours. Before and after the fast, a baseline serum glucose, insulin, proinsulin, and C-peptide measurement is obtained. Urine is tested for ketone throughout the test and capillary glucose measurements are taken every 4 hours. The test is terminated when symptoms of hypoglycemia appear and a blood glucose is measured immediately. Positive test results for men is considered a blood glucose less than 55 mg/dL and in women it is less than 45 mg/dL. If after 72 hours of fasting and light exercise, hypoglycemia (less than 60 mg/dL) is not demonstrated, the test is negative. This test is performed in a hospital under close observation. Chronic hypoglycemia may be evident by a low glycohemoglobin level.

Subsequent Testing. The following laboratory tests assist in the diagnostic reasoning during a hypoglycemic episode: plasma insulin level, insulin antibodies, plasma and urine sulfonylurea levels, and C-peptide. Other tests include a BUN, creatinine, alcohol levels, and liver function tests. To rule out endocrine pathology, if suspected as a possible cause, obtain cortisol and ACTH levels. The first void in the morning can be tested to detect ketones; a lack of them would imply a defect in the fatty acid oxidation pathway, since ketone bodies are not formed. In infants, urine may also be sent for organic acid analysis.

Fasting insulin levels range from 8.0 to 15.0 μU/mL or 3.0 to 0.6 ng/mL. An abnormally elevated insulin level is seen in patients with insulinomas, exogenous insulin administration, insulin resistance syndrome, and reactive hypoglycemia in developing DM. An elevated insulin level in the absence of blood glucose variation is suggestive of insulinomas, exogenous insulin administration, insulin resistance syndrome, and reactive hypoglycemia in developing DM. An elevated insulin level in the absence of blood glucose variation is suggestive of insulinoma. Elevated insulin levels in response to glucose fluctuations suggests a functional or reactive hypoglycemia.

C-peptide analysis is done with radioimmunoassay techniques and provides an index of beta cell function. Normal values range from 0.9 to 4.2 ng/mL. A low C-peptide level with an elevated insulin level confirms insulin administration. C-peptide levels are elevated in insulinomas. To differentiate insulinoma from factitious hypoglycemia the ratio of insulin to C-peptide is done. If the ratio is less than 1.0, then the hypoglycemia is a result of endogenous insulin secretion; if greater than 1.0, then exogenous insulin is confirmed.

Differential Diagnosis

Differential diagnoses include generalized anxiety disorder, panic attacks, hyperventilation, pheochromocytoma, drug or alcohol intoxication, transient ischemic attack, cerebral vascular accident, and psychosis. Causes of reactive hypoglycemia include meals high in refined carbohydrates; certain nutrients such as fructose and galactose cause a burst of insulin secretion. Drugs (e.g., sulfonylureas, salicylates) can cause excess glucose utilization or deficient glucose production. Oral diabetic medications are especially prone to causing reactive hypoglycemia when used in combination therapy. Insulinoma (adenoma of islets of Langerhans), although rare, should be considered in an otherwise healthy adult who is found to have fasting hypoglycemia.

Management

The goal in management of hypoglycemia is to normalize the blood glucose levels and treat the underlying cause. The patient with pathology is referred to an endocrinologist for further evaluation and treatment. In cases of functional and idiopathic hypoglycemia, the initial management plan may be developed in consultation with an endocrinologist.

Initial Management

Treatment of acute hypoglycemia for alert patients is 6 to 12 ounces of orange juice or another fruit juice without sugar. One cup of milk can be substituted if juice is not available. Glucose tablets, if available, can be used. In acute care settings glucose is provided emergently as standardized IV bolus preparations of dextrose diluted to various concentrations in water (e.g., D25 percent or D50 percent), as opposed to the standardized hypotonic saline solutions with lower amounts of dextrose that are used primarily for maintenance glucose requirements (e.g., D5 percent 0.45 percent NaCl). The blood glucose level should be monitored closely following bolus IV administration of dextrose and then periodically while the patient is on a dextrose-containing continuous IV drip. Glucagon hydrochloride (0.03 to 0.1 mg/kg/dose; 1 to 2 mg in adults; 1 mg in children older than 5 years or weighing more than 20 kg; 0.5 mg in children younger than 5 years or weighing less than 20 mg) may be given IM, SC, or IV, if the patient is unresponsive. Doses may be repeated as needed every few hours in adults and even more frequently in children (up to every 20 to 30 minutes initially).

Hypoglycemia is a medical emergency, given the seriousness of the potential sequelae (e.g., seizures, coma, cardiovascular dysfunction, death). Even if euglycemia is readily restored, patients must be evaluated for potential hospital admission for inpatient care and close observation, if there is any concern for symptom recurrence. Patients requiring admission include those with hypoglycemia without an obvious cause, severe or persistent neurologic deficits, or iatrogenic episodes in known diabetics due to oral agents such as sulfonylureas (especially chlorpropamide) or long-acting insulin preparations.

Subsequent Management

Long-term management of hypoglycemia includes treatment of underlying causes and dietary modifications. If hypoglycemia is a result of pancreatic or extrapancreatic tumors, surgical excision is recommended. Although the treatment of choice for insulinoma is surgical resection, there is only an 85 percent success rate with an experienced surgeon. If the tumor is small it may not be found on an exploratory laparotomy. When surgery is unsuccessful, an endocrinologist may initiate diazoxide (Hyperstat, Progylcem; 3 to 8 mg/kg per day PO divided tid or 200 mg q4h in adults) therapy to reduce insulin secretion. If hypoglycemia is caused by rapid gastric emptying following a gastrectomy, an anticholinergic drug may delay gastric emptying, decrease intestinal motility, and provide relief.

In patients with pseudohypoglycemia or idiopathic hypoglycemia, in which the cause cannot be identified, the treatment is primarily with dietary modifications. A high-protein, low-carbohydrate diet divided into six small daily feedings often relieves the symptoms. Caffeine, refined sugars, and alcohol should be restricted. If food allergies are suspected, allergy testing may be indicated to identify offending foods.

In a hyperinsulinemic infant, therapy may be only supportive with glucose infusions if the increased insulin levels are due primarily to maternal diabetes and are transient. However, if increased insulin levels are intrinsic to the infant, diazoxide is typically the first step in pharmacologic treatment (15 to 20 mg/kg/day PO divided tid). Octreotide (Sandostatin; 2 to 10 mcg/kg/day SC divided q4 to 6h), a long-acting analogue of somatostatin, may be used as second-line therapy for short-term management of hypoglycemia. The dihydropyridine calcium channel blocker nifedipine (Adalat, Procardia; 10 mg PO tid initially and titrated up to 80 mg/day) has also been shown to be useful in hyperinsulinemic children, as it interferes with the calcium-dependent secretion of insulin (other calcium channel blockers have not been approved for this indication). There is no role for cortisol in acute treatment.

In patients with pseudohypoglycemia or idiopathic hypoglycemia, in which the cause cannot be identified, treatment is primarily with dietary modifications. A high-protein, low-carbohydrate diet divided into six small daily feedings often relieves symptoms. Caffeine, refined sugars, and alcohol should be restricted. If food allergies are suspected, allergy testing may be indicated to identify offending foods.

If a medication is at fault, an alternative drug is considered. In patients with diabetes who are experiencing hypoglycemia, treatment goals may be relaxed. Some research supports the finding that frequent episodes of hypoglycemia in a patient with diabetes have been shown to lower recognition of subsequent events. Shorter-acting glipizide can be substituted for longer-acting glyburide if sulfonylureas are determined to be the cause. Metformin should be considered as monotherapy in patients with type 2 DM who have frequent episodes of hypoglycemia.

SMBG is the cornerstone of self-management. Patients may need to monitor blood glucose levels frequently during initiation of lifestyle changes to evaluate success. Persons with DM may need to monitor blood glucose levels in the morning, before meals, and at bedtime. This regimen may be altered depending on patient response. Stressing the need for monitoring glucose levels during exercise, eating at regularly scheduled intervals, and the importance of SMBG may prevent severe hypoglycemic reactions. All patients with hypoglycemia will benefit from home blood glucose monitoring.

Infants younger than 3 months who have refractory hypoglycemia that cannot be treated pharmacologically may require pancreatic resection. Usually, a near total resection of 85 to 90 percent of the pancreas is recommended, but development of diabetes is a subsequent risk. In infants between 3 and 6 months, frequent feedings may first be attempted for up to 1 month to see if this addresses a temporary phenomenon.

In patients with inoperable pancreatic tumors or patients in whom resection has been unsuccessful, small frequent feedings that are high in carbohydrates (every 2 to 3 hours) may be effective in preventing acute hypoglycemic episodes. In patients with renal failure, small frequent high-carbohydrate meals may prevent episodes.

Follow-Up and Referral

Diabetic patients with a history of hypoglycemic events need frequent follow-up and evaluation. On each visit, the record of hypoglycemic events should be reviewed. More frequent SMBG may be indicated, especially 12 to 24 hours following a hypoglycemic event. Patients who continue to experience hypoglycemic episodes despite intervention should be referred to an endocrinologist.

Patient Education

The importance of dietary modifications must be stressed. Nondiabetic patients with reactive, functional, and fasting hypoglycemia should eat five or six small meals daily to steady the release of glucose into the blood. The meals should be balanced with carbohydrates, protein, and some fat. Instruct the patient who experiences symptoms following a meal high in refined sugar, but not following a regular meal, to restrict refined sugars in the diet. Patients who cannot eat small meals throughout the day should be encouraged to carry raw seeds and nuts mixed with dried fruits.

Patients with diabetes should be instructed to maintain their glycemic goals, report any episodes of hypoglycemia and to monitor their blood glucose at bedtime and before, during, and after exercise. Alcohol, cigarette smoking, and caffeine should be avoided.

Common Metabolic Problems

Obesity

Obesity is an excess of adipose tissue (body fat) and is manifested by body weight in excess of 20 percent over the ideal body weight or a body mass index (BMI) 30 or more. Recently published clinical guidelines on the identification, evaluation, and treatment of overweight and obesity cite that the complex etiology of overeating makes this chronic illness poorly understood and often intractable to medical management. The two major types of obesity are upper body (apple-shape) and lower body (pear-shape) obesity. Patients with central or upper body obesity have excessive body fat in the abdomen and flank areas and are at a greater risk for type 2 DM, coronary artery disease, stroke, and early death than those with lower body obesity. Patients with lower body obesity have excessive adipose tissue in the buttocks and thighs.

The direct and indirect costs of obesity are more than $100 billion per year in the United States, including the direct medical costs as well as the cost attributable to lost wages, and so on. The psychological cost of obesity in those affected includes stigmatization and discrimination.

Epidemiology and Causes

Overweight and obesity are epidemic in the United States today. According to the National Health and Nutrition Exam

Survey III, 59.4 percent of men and 49.9 percent of women are overweight. Almost 20 percent of men are obese while 25.1 percent of women are obese. African American women are more likely to be obese than are white women. The incidence of obesity is higher in those of lower socioeconomic status regardless of race. Central and upper body obesity is more common in men, whereas lower body obesity is more common in women.

Worldwide, obesity is more prevalent in industrialized countries and the prevalence is increasing worldwide, including in developing countries. The World Health Organization classifies obesity as one of the world's most neglected public health problems.

The causes of obesity are categorized as essential and secondary. Essential obesity is the most prevalent type and is a result of the intake of more calories than are expended. This type of obesity results from the multiple interactions of genetic and environmental factors (cultural, metabolic, social, and psychological factors). It is estimated that 40 to 70 percent of obesity can be explained by genetic influences with environmental factors making up the balance. Five genes have been identified that affect control of appetite and mutations in these genes, along with environmental factors and behavior, result in obesity.

Secondary obesity is rare; possible causes include Cushing's disease, polycystic ovary disease, hypothalamic disease, hypothyroidism, and insulinoma. Some medications associated with weight gain include glucocorticoids, tricyclic antidepressants, and phenothiazines.

Risk factors for development of obesity include diet, lifestyle, environment, and the interaction among the aforementioned causes. A diet high in fat contributes to obesity because dietary fat has more than twice the calories of carbohydrates or proteins. A sedentary lifestyle or a sudden decrease in physical activity without a reduction in caloric intake may cause obesity. An environment that supports sedentary lifestyles and facilitates access to fatty foods, processed foods, and refined sugars contributes to the incidence of obesity today.

Obesity affects almost every body system and is associated with an increased risk of multiple diseases. The consequesnces of obesity are listed in Table 15.12. The different types of obesity are related more closely to specific complications. Central trunk obesity is closely related to DM, coronary heart disease, stroke, and early death. The health risks associated with obesity are directly correlated with the severity of obesity and include metabolic, structural, and psychosocial changes. Mortality increases as complications of obesity develop and approaches 50 percent when weight is 30 to 40 percent over the ideal weight. Reduction in body weight by 5 to 20 percent significantly decreases these comorbid risk factors in obese individuals.

Obesity is also associated with an increased risk of colon, rectal, and prostate cancer in males. In obese females, uterine, gallbladder, biliary tract, breast, and ovarian cancer are more prevalent. Persons who are obese have an increased surgical and obstetrical risk. Psychosocial disability is related to obesity. This is often a result of the societal stigma attached to obesity. Pickwickian syndrome is associated with severe or morbid obesity. This syndrome includes hypersomnolence, congestive heart failure, and hypertension.

Table 15.12 Consequences of Obesity

Coronary heart disease/congestive heart failure
Hypertension
Dyslipidemia/hyperlipidemia
Type 2 diabetes mellitus/metabolic syndrome/insulin resistance
Sleep apnea
Restrictive lung disease
Asthma
Varicose veins and venous insufficiency
Gout and hyperuricemia
Osteoarthritis
Reflux esophagitis
Gallbladder disease
Thromboembolic disease
Cancers: endometrial, breast, prostate, colon

Pathophysiology

Obesity results when one's intake of calories exceeds metabolic needs. The control of appetite and the mechanisms that govern food intake are complex and incompletely understood. The hypothalamus controls certain aspects of appetite and appears to have a role in an individual's food preferences. Other important CNS sites include the tractus solitarius of the hindbrain, the arcuate and paraventricular nuclei, and the amygdala. Mediated by several neurotransmitters including norepinephrine, dynorphin, hypocretin, serotonin, neuropeptide Y, and ghrelin to name just a few, both the central and peripheral nervous systems produce and integrate a complex array of neural inputs that regulate diet and weight. In contrast, other hormones such as cholecystokinin, enterostatin, and the gut hormone peptide YY 3–36 have all been shown to suppress food intake. Whether obesity can be significantly attributed to dysregulation in one or more of these neuroendocrine regulatory mechanisms remains to be seen.

There is, however, a well-documented genetic predisposition to the development of obesity. Twin studies have revealed high correlations in obesity prevalence between siblings raised apart in separate households as well as together by the same set of parents, while the BMIs of adoptees correlate more closely with those of their biological rather than adopted parents. Secondary causes of obesity due to medical conditions are rare, however, and include various endocrine and neurologic diseases.

In many individuals, obesity, overweight, and overeating appear intrinsically tied to a fragile emotional state, poor self-esteem, and dissatisfaction with life circumstances. The stressors and psychological demands that underlie a patient's poor dietary choices may be powerful influences that are capable of defying the counterbalancing knowledge that overeating and obesity lead to ill health. Thus, an addictive behavioral component to overeating appears to be a driving factor in many obese individuals. The complex psychology of obesity has been the subject of extensive study, and the most effective obesity treatment programs typically involve some sort of psychiatric analysis or counseling as primary or adjunctive therapy.

While most individuals tend to underestimate their food intake by 10 to 20 percent, obese individuals underestimate caloric intake even further by 30 percent. However, behavioral choices alone do not explain the entire Pathophysiology of obesity. Basal or resting metabolism required to maintain autonomic body processes (e.g., cardiorespiratory function), ion gradients, and body temperature accounts for 70 percent of total energy expenditure, while the thermic response to food digestion (mediated by the sympathetic nervous system) consumes another 10 percent. Spontaneous, often involuntary physical activity (fidgeting) as well as intentional exercise and physical exertion account for a significant portion of energy expenditure as well, which explains the weight gain associated with sedentary lifestyles.

The body is known to have neuroendocrine homeostatic feedback control mechanisms involving both the peripheral and central nervous systems which seek to maintain nutrient intake and ideal weight. Examples include glycemic levels (hypoglycemia is a trigger to eat), serum leptin concentrations (see below), glucocorticoids which act as appetite stimulants, sympathomimetic hormones that act as appetite suppressants, and the peptide ghrelin—a ligand for the growth hormone secretagogue receptor that increases appetite (ghrelin levels increase in anticipation of a meal and in response to diet-induced weight loss). Differences in fat-free body mass also correlate strongly with differences in energy expenditure among different individuals. In particular, weight gain is associated with increased metabolic demands and energy expenditure which retard further weight gain, while weight loss is associated with reductions in energy expenditure that counter further weight loss. Thus, a formerly obese individual who loses weight will experience a relative decrease in energy expenditure compared to a non-obese individual and will thus require 15 percent fewer calories to maintain his or her reduced weight. In turn, failing to reduce one's caloric intake appropriately may result in progressive weight gain.

On a molecular level, the bulk of our understanding of the Pathophysiology and genetics of obesity stems from preclinical animal models—particularly that of the obese mouse, for which a number of genetically altered strains are available. Through genetically engineered knockout mice that lack one or more target genes, as well as transgenic models that overexpress either a functional or nonfunctional version of a target gene, researchers have identified several single gene defects that result in murine obesity. Some of these genetic findings have been further generalized to humans.

Expressed by adipose, intestinal, and placental cells, the leptin gene has been the subject of much controversy in human obesity. Serum leptin concentrations strongly correlate with body fat content, while leptin-deficient mice demonstrate insulin resistance, hyperinsulinemia, and hyperphagia. Leptin has been shown to reduce levels of neuropeptide Y, a potent stimulus for food intake produced in the brain's arcuate nucleus. Human obesity due to leptin deficiency has been identified in two consanguineous families, as has obesity due to leptin receptor deficiency. However, leptin overexpression has not been shown to reduce appetite or weight, and most obese patients express normal levels of this protein. Thus, decreased leptin levels appear to signal that fat stores are insufficient for growth and reproduction; however, the hormone itself is not a negative regulator of appetite or weight gain.

Other single-gene defects associated with murine obesity include mutations in carboxypeptidase E, the enzyme responsible for the cleavage of proinsulin, and the *tub* gene, which is associated with neurologic deficits, hypothalamic damage, and increased appetite. The *agouti* gene which encodes an antagonist protein for the hypothalamic melanocortin-4 receptor has also been associated with murine obesity and hyperphagia, as have deletions in the melanocortin-4 receptor. Mutations in multiple species of serotonin receptors are associated with murine obesity, a finding that appears to underlie the role of serotonergic pharmacotherapies which reduce appetite.

Mutations in prohormone convertase-I have been associated with human obesity in one family. In contrast, the role of the *agouti* gene in human obesity has not yet been confirmed. Other candidate genes involved in human obesity include the beta-3-adrenergic gene, which is involved in sympathetic autonomic responses that affect appetite, and peroxisome-proliferator-activated receptor (*PPAR*) γ-*2,* a gene involved in adipocyte differentiation. Genome scans have identified other potential DNA regulatory sites (e.g., chromosome 10p), but definitive gene products have yet to be identified.

Obesity is also a presenting feature of at least 24 different genetic syndromes, displaying an entire range of heritability patterns. These syndromes are relatively rare, but the most common are Prader-Willi syndrome, a neurodegenerative disorder resulting from genetic abnormalities in the long arm of chromosome 15q11 to 13, and the autosomal recessive Bardet-Biedl syndrome involving concurrent hypogenitalism, mental retardation, and renal abnormalities.

Clinical Presentation

Subjective

Patients will often present to their health-care provider with some or all of the following symptoms as a result of obesity: fatigue, decreased energy, weakness, joint pain, shortness of breath, increased daytime sleepiness, and depression. Most will seek help for another medical condition or present with one or more of the foregoing complaints. When weight history is obtained, patients often report several attempts at weight loss.

Objective

The diagnosis of obesity is most often made by observation alone. Simple anthropometric measures such as relative weight and height, BMI, diameters and circumferences, and skin fold measurements are used to establish obesity.

Historically, ideal body weight was calculated by comparing actual body weight to the Metropolitan Life Insurance Company's table. Weights for the original and updated tables were calculated based on data from middle-class Americans seeking insurance, and as Americans got fatter, the weights in the table increased.

Measurements of weight and height are used to calculate the BMI for the exact classification of obesity. BMI is calculated by taking the body weight in kilograms divided by the height in meters squared. One problem with BMI measurement is that it fails to consider ethnic or racial differences, nor does it differente the individual with a large percentage of muscle mass.

Despite criticism, BMI remains the measurement most frequently used in research and clinical practice because it is easily calculated without laboratory equipment. In research, BMI correlates with percentage of body fat measurements taken with underwater weighing, but is not as reliable in older adults.

In 1998 the guidelines shifted the index for overweight from a BMI of 27 to 25. An index of 30 is classified as obesity (Table 15.13). The panel proposed that men with a BMI of 25 to 35 with a waist measurement greater than 40 and women whose waist measurement exceeds 35 inches are at increased risk. Owing to differences in complications of different types of obesity, the waist-to-hip ratio should also be calculated using the following formula:

$$\text{Waist-to-hip ratio} = \frac{\text{Waist measurement at smallest part}}{\text{Hip measurement at largest circumference}}$$

A ratio of greater than 1 for males and 0.8 for females indicates central trunk obesity.

Diagnostic Reasoning

Secondary causes of obesity must be ruled out before initiating a treatment plan with the patient. Cushing's syndrome, hypothalamic injury, and hypothyroidism should be considered as potential causes. A complete history and physical with anthropometric measurement are essential elements of the initial assessment. A comprehensive history includes a weight history and attempts at weight loss. Family history of obesity and cultural food preferences must be addressed in the assessment. The amount of control the patient maintains in food purchasing and preparation should be considered.

Table 15.13 Calculating Body Mass Index and Classifying Obesity

Calculating Body Mass Index

The most recent formula for calculating body mass index (BMI) was developed by a panel convened by the National Heart, Lung, and Blood Institute and the National Institute of Diabetes and Digestive and Kidney Disease. Using this formula, BMI is calculated by multiplying the patient's weight in pounds by 704.5 and then dividing the results by the patient's height in inches once and then for a second time (weight [lbs.] × 704.5 ÷ height [in.]^2).

An alternate method calculates BMI by converting pounds to kilograms (1 lb = 0.45 kg) and inches to meters (1 in. = .025 m). The equation for BMI is weight (kg) divided by height (m) squared [kg/m^2].

Classifying Obesity

Classification	*Relative Weight*	*BMI*
Overweight	100–120%	25–27.5 kg/m^2
Mild obesity	120–140%	27.5–30 kg/m^2
Moderate obesity	140–200%	30–40 kg/m^2
Severe (morbid) obesity	>200%	>40 kg/m^2

The patient should be questioned about any periods of rapid weight gain and environmental or psychosocial changes in lifestyle during these periods explored. An exercise history should also be obtained, with special emphasis on the relationship of any weight gain or loss periods to exercise. Specific questions to assess current or past eating disorders are essential.

A past medical history and complete medication profile is necessary, especially the intake of corticosteroids, laxatives, diuretics, and appetite suppressants. Although rarely the cause of obesity, a personal or family history of thyroid disease should be explored.

The complete physical examination with a focus on signs of a possible cause of obesity (Cushing's syndrome or thyroid disease) as well as complications of obesity is done.

Diagnostic Tests

Initial assessment of the patient who is obese should include the following laboratory tests: TSH, CBC, serum electrolytes, glucose, magnesium, calcium, uric acid, liver function tests, and a liver profile. An ECG should also be obtained.

Differential Diagnosis

The diagnosis of obesity is usually straightforward. Acute or chronic fluid retention should be distinguished from increased adiposity, as edematous states and water balance must be considered. The differential diagnosis of obesity is geared toward determining the underlying cause. While the vast majority of cases are due to non-nutritive dietary and sedentary lifestyle choices, certain medical conditions such as hypothyroidism should be ruled out with simple lab tests like TSH. But in general, an extensive laboratory work-up is not necessary. Patients should be evaluated for other risk factors associated with obesity, however—especially those implicated in CAD like hyperlipidemia and insulin resistance associated with DM-II.

Management

Whether weight gain is related to exogenous factors or endogenous factors is an important difference. Clinical management of obesity requires the balancing of energy intake and expenditure. After reviewing the evidence from research in the development of the clinical guidelines, the NIH concurred that successful management must include a combination of diet, exercise, and behavioral interventions. Multidisciplinary approaches to weight loss have a higher success rate. It also appears that continuted close contact with a health-care provider is more important for long-term success than any particular diet program. Because of the chronicity of obesity, the patient must learn long-term management skills. Cognitive therapy in conjunction with education is effective in increasing self-esteem, improving depression, and decreasing women's dissatisfaction with their bodies.

The management plan should focus on reducing comorbidity and reducing visceral obesity, not solely on improving cosmetic outcomes. In fact, dietary instructions are pretty much the same for the obese individual as a healthy nonobese person: low-fat, high-fiber, high complex carbohydrate eating plan with emphasis on portion control. A management plan that is realistic, can fit into the patient's lifestyle, and includes gradual changes in diet and activity is more likely to be accepted.

Assisting the patient to identify reasons for overeating may benefit the patient in managing his or her behavior. Being tired, anxious, and angry are major triggers for overeating. Remember the acronym HALT: hungry, angry, lonely, and tired.

Counseling of patients should include the benefits of weight loss: reduction in blood pressure, serum triglycerides, and blood glucose levels and an increase in HDL-cholesterol. Patients with type 2 diabetes may experience a decreased HbA_{1c} level. Management should be directed toward an initial goal of decreasing the patient's weight by 10 percent over 6 months. Subsequent goals are made following achievement of the initial goal. Treatment guidelines as outlined by the National Institutes of Health (NIH) are shown in the Treatment Flowchart 15.1.

Management of the patient will depend on the patient's motivation and the cause of the obesity. Research has shown that attempts to lose weight almost always follow a major life transition such as an acute life-threatening illness, divorce, or death of a loved one. Other recent research with overweight women found incongruencies in women's beliefs about the causes of their being overweight and how they planned to lose weight. Although many women identified stress as a major factor for overeating, they believed that dieting was the key to management.

Culture and socioeconomic factors affect not only the prevalence of obesity but also attitudes as to acceptable weight and its implications. For example, some cultures view being overweight as a sign of good health and prosperity. In many Western cultures, obesity is seen more as a cosmetic problem than a major health problem.

Dietary Management

Before dietary modifications are initiated, a 3- to 7-day diet history should be evaluated. The patient should keep a diet diary, recording all oral intake, including water and drinks. It is often beneficial for evaluation to have the patient record daily activity along with food intake. Clues as to lifestyle patterns and behavioral eating patterns can be more adequately assessed with both sets of data.

The overall goal of weight loss depends on a calorie deficit. To calculate the energy requirements of patients, the following formula can be used: Multiply body weight by 10 for women and 12 for men. This will provide the amount of calories needed to maintain the current weight. A weight-loss goal of 1 pound per week can be achieved by reducing caloric intake by 500 kcal daily, since 1 pound of fat accounts for about 3500 kcal. The NIH guidelines suggest that the ideal weekly weight-loss goal is 1 to 1.5 pounds. More weight loss can be expected during the first week of a caloric-restricted diet because of excessive loss of water.

The diet should be balanced, and the patient should follow current guidelines for a healthy diet. Total calories eaten should consist of 30 percent or less from fat, 15 percent from protein, and 55 percent or more from complex carbohydrates. Saturated fats should be avoided. Besides restriction of fat intake, dietary recommendations must take into consideration minimum daily requirements, the patient's food preferences, and the patient's lifestyles.

Usual calorie restrictions range from 1200 to 1800 kcal daily. A restriction of 1000 to 1500 kcal per day is classified as a low-calorie diet (LCD). This level of restriction is indicated in patients who are at least 40 percent over the ideal weight.

A very low calorie diet (VLCD) includes 800 kcal daily, or 6 to 19 kcal/kg of body weight. VLCDs have short-term effectiveness and usually do not produce long-term results if used alone. A VLCD should be reserved for patients who are more than 40 percent over ideal body weight and at high risk for serious health consequences. VLCDs are contraindicated in older adults, pregnant and lactating women, and individuals with cardiovascular disease, gout, DM, cancer, severe renal or hepatic disease, and hypertension. Most VLCDs are liquid protein preparations. The major advantage of protein-formula liquid diets is that they remove the patient from the food environment.

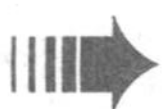

TREATMENT FLOWCHART 15.1

OBESITY

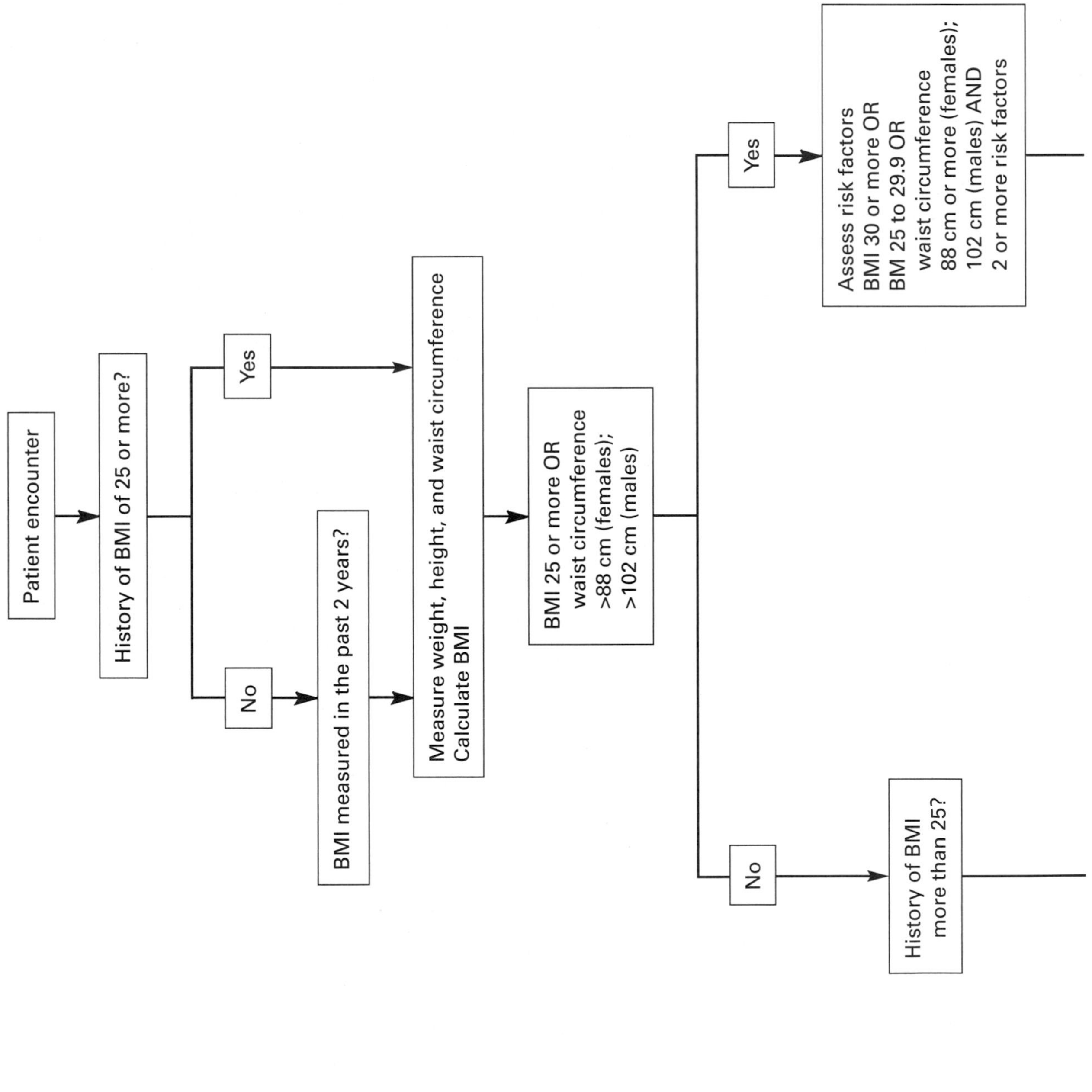

Patient encounter

History of BMI of 25 or more?

No

BMI measured in the past 2 years?

Yes

Measure weight, height, and waist circumference
Calculate BMI

BMI 25 or more OR
waist circumference
>88 cm (females);
>102 cm (males)

No

History of BMI
more than 25?

Yes

Assess risk factors
BMI 30 or more OR
BM 25 to 29.9 OR
waist circumference
88 cm or more (females);
102 cm (males) AND
2 or more risk factors

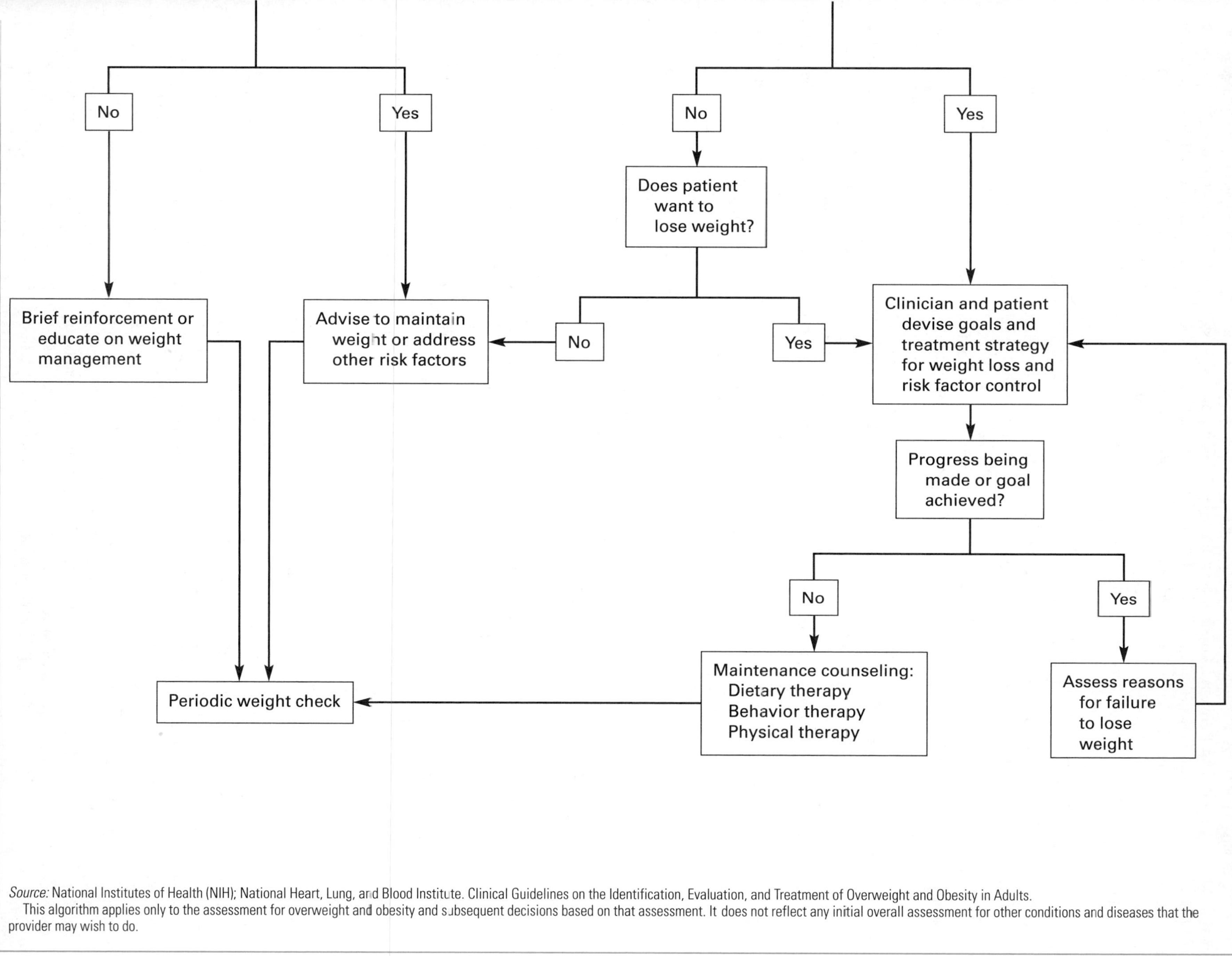

Source: National Institutes of Health (NIH); National Heart, Lung, and Blood Institute. Clinical Guidelines on the Identification, Evaluation, and Treatment of Overweight and Obesity in Adults.

This algorithm applies only to the assessment for overweight and obesity and subsequent decisions based on that assessment. It does not reflect any initial overall assessment for other conditions and diseases that the provider may wish to do.

Patients on VLCDs will need fluid, mineral, and nutritional supplements and frequent laboratory evaluations of potassium, magnesium, and uric acid levels. An initial ECG is done to rule out cardiac arrhythmias. Patients with this level of dietary restrictions will need weekly evaluations by a specialist skilled in weight loss management. Most patients will average a 1.5 to 2.5 kg/week weight loss on this restriction. Men are more likely to respond to a VLCD. VLCDs, although initially very successful, often are not effective in producing long-term maintenance of the weight loss. Fifty percent of patients will gain the weight back within 1 year.

The patient on a VLCD must be monitored for hypomagnesemia, hypokalemia, hyperuricemia, ECG changes, and cardiac arrhythmias. The overall long-term effectiveness of these diets remains controversial and they should be reserved for patients who are extremely obese.

Exercise

Exercise is a significant part of a weight-loss and maintenance program. It is especially beneficial in the long-term management of weight loss, lowering blood pressure, increasing muscle mass, increasing insulin sensitivity, improving the lipid profile, and improving glucose metabolism. Unless specific contraindications exist, exercise should be prescribed for all patients. Including resistance exercises in the exercise prescription will help maintain lean body mass.

Slow, sustained exercise, 45 to 60 minutes daily is more beneficial for weight loss than are high impact exercise routines. Adults should engage in at least 30 minutes of moderate intensity physical exercise on most days of the week. Moderately intense physical exertion is equal to a brisk walk of 3 to 4 miles per hour. Patients are more likely to continue low-intensity exercise than high-intensity exercise. A 20-minute walk is usually acceptable to most patients as a starting point.

Younger patients with mild to moderate obesity may begin an aerobic exercise program if physical examination results are within normal levels. Older, sedentary patients should begin with walking programs. Exercise tolerance testing (ETT) may be indicated for older adults and adults at risk for CAD before beginning an exercise program.

Behavior Modification

Behavior modification is essential for initial weight loss and weight maintenance. Unless the patient can identify eating patterns and lifestyle patterns that have contributed to weight gain and change those within his or her control, long-term weight management will not be achieved.

Restrictive eating behavior control includes cognitive strategies for portion control and healthy food selections. The need to identify impulsive and binge eating is also important. Behavioral management is enhanced by avoiding high-risk environments or altering the environment to reduce triggers to overeating.

Stress has a significant impact on eating behavior. During times of stress, the patient may find it impossible to implement behavior modification techniques. Relaxation techniques can assist in managing stress. Relaxation techniques must be practiced frequently in times of low stress so they can be effectively used in times of excessive stress.

Pharmacologic Management

The NIH guidelines suggest aggressive treatment for patients whose BMI is 30 or greater without concomitant risk factors and for those with a BMI of 27 or greater with two of the major risk factors.

Appetite suppressants are available over the counter and by prescription and are classed as either catecholaminergic or serotonergic. Pharmacologic therapy for obesity has received much press, especially because the combination of fenfluramine (Fen Phen) and dexfenfluramine (Redux) produced an increased incidence of valvular disease in some users. Both of these drugs were classed as serotonergic and they have both been removed from the market. There are no other serotonergic medications approved for weight loss as this time.

Catacholaminergic agents include amphetamines, but also nonamphetamine schedule IV appetite suppressants including phentermine (Fastin), manzidol (Mazanor, Sanorex), and diethylpropion (Tenuate). Phenylpropanolamine is available over the counter under a variety of trade names, although serious adverse reactions continue to be reported.

The potential adverse reactions, the lack of evidence for long-term effectiveness, and the potential for drug dependence for many of the aforementioned pharmacologic agents make their use in the management of obesity debatable. These pharmacologic agents typically reduce weight by 5 to 10 percent but must be administered continually or the weight is regained.

There are two newer weight loss medications approved by the FDA: sibutramine HCl monohydrate (Meridia) and orlistat. Sibutramine is a noradrenergic neuronal reuptake inhibitor that blocks the uptake of serotonin and norepinephrine in the central nervous system. Orlistat works totally differently by blocking the absorption of fat in the GI tract.

Sibutramine 10 mg qd PO is the recommended dose and usually produces an average weight loss of 3 to 5 kg in 6 to 12 months. Adverse reactions include elevated blood pressure, increased heart rate, constipation, insomnia, and headaches. It is contraindicated in persons with a history of hypertension, CHD, congestive heart failure, arrhythmias, or a history of stroke.

Orlistat 120 mg tid with meals is the recommended dose and results in a 2- to 4-kg weight loss maintained for 2 years. Adverse effects of orlistat are diarrhea, gas, and abdominal cramping. Some studies suggest it may also inhibit the absorption of fat-soluble vitamins.

Surgical Intervention

Surgical intervention for obesity should be reserved for those patients who have a BMI over 40, or over 35 if they have complications of the obesity. It is usually not considered until the obese patient has failed more conventional weight loss methods. The incidence of bariatric surgery is booming in the United States today. The most common surgical procedures are the vertical-banded (Mason) gastroplasty and the roux-en-Y gastric bypass and may be done laparoscopically. Some studies have shown that surgery can produce up to a 50 percent loss of initial body weight. Complications following the surgery may occur in up to 40 percent of patients after surgery and include peritonitis, abdominal wall hernia, dumping syndrome, infection, acute cholecystitis, hypoglycemia, pyloric outlet obstruction, chronic diarrhea, nausea, and vomiting. Patients should be counseled regarding these potential complications. They should also be informed of the possiblity of regaining much of the lost weight if lifestyle changes are not also undertaken.

Follow-Up and Referral

Most weight-loss programs require close follow-up. The severity of the problem and the nature of the interventions should govern how frequently the health-care provider sees the patient, but clearly, patients are more successful in maintaining weight loss with frequent follow-up visits. Many patients will benefit from frequent clinician visits that provide medical guidance, goal setting, and emotional support throughout the weight-loss process. In addition, the importance of clinical follow-up once weight loss goals have been achieved should be emphasized, as recurrent weight gain following periods of significant weight loss is quite common. The patient should be seen for weigh-in, blood pressure measurement, and discussion of progress at least monthly, but once a week is often most beneficial until the patient has developed lifestyle change (habituated).

Patient Education

Patient education includes instruction on how to maintain a balance between intake and energy expenditure. Exercise, a low-fat diet, and lifestyle changes should be emphasized. Patients may benefit from a referral to a dietitian. Many patients are unaware of techniques to reduce fat in their diet by cooking methods alone. One suggestion that may help is to use non-stick cookware so that there is no need to use fat or grease in the pan. Other suggestion are to bake, broil, and braise rather than fry foods. Patients with obesity must be educated about the importance of a combination of therapies. They must be guided to set realistic goals. Most obese persons skip breakfast and eat more in the late afternoon and evening, which is not helpful.

Sustaining weight loss requires behavioral changes. Patients should plan out their weight loss strategy in writing. The plan should include diet modifications, exercise routine, and behavioral strategies. A calendar should be developed outlining the schedule. If lapses in the plan are experienced, the patient should explore the reasons for the lapse. Health-care providers should review this outline on each visit.

Some patients will benefit from support groups. A list of support groups for weight loss and overeating are indicated in the reference list. Patients who feel sabotaged by family members will need to explore methods for support outside of the family. Finding a walking partner or walking right after work before going home are some strategies to suggest.

Gout

Gout is a metabolic disease that produces an inflammatory arthritis. Gout was identified in the days of Hippocrates and was often referred to as "the disease of kings" because of its prevalence in the wealthy, who were able to afford the rich foods that sometimes trigger this disorder. Once a disabling chronic disease, current medical diagnostics and treatment modalities have decreased its disabling effects.

An overproduction or underexcretion (or both) of uric acid causes the metabolic disease underlying gout. Most individuals with gout (90 percent) have a problem with underexcretion of uric acid. The arthritis produced by gout is characterized by recurrent, painful attacks of monoarticular joint inflammation caused by the phagocytosis of urate crystals, which deposit in joints, soft tissue, and cartilage.

Epidemiology and Causes

Gout occurs rarely in children, premenopausal women, or men younger than 30 years of age. Ninety percent of people with gout are men with a peak incidence between 40 and 50 years. Gout is more prevalent in black men, possibly because of the increased prevalence of hypertension in this group. The increased incidence in older adults has been associated with the increased use of diuretics.

Twenty percent of patients who present with gout have a family history of the disease. Persons from the United States, the Pacific Islands, and countries with abundant lifestyles have an increased incidence of gout. The prevalence of gout in the United States is 14 per 1000 men and 6 per 1000 females.

Hyperuricemia (uric acid levels exceeding 7 mg/dL in men and 6 mg/dL in women) occurs in 5 to 10 percent of the United States population. Most of these adults, however, are asymptomatic. One in five persons with hyperuricemia will develop urate deposits in a joint, soft tissue, or cartilage.

The risk factors and predisposing factors for development of gout are listed in Risk Factors 15.2. Causes of primary gout include the idiopathic inborn error of purine metabolism, decreased renal clearance of uric acid, and specific enzyme defects such as Lesch-Nyhan syndrome, and glycogen storage disease. Secondary causes of gout include other disease processes and medications that produce an overproduction or underexcretion of uric acid.

RISK FACTORS 15.2

Gout

Primary risk factors	Enzyme defects Decreased renal clearance of uric acid
Secondary risk factors	Excessive daily intake of purine Obesity Starvation Alcohol abuse Medications: thiazide, diuretics, ethambutol, nicotinic acid, pyrazinamide, low-dose salicylates, cyclosporine Paget's disease Chronic hemolytic anemia Psoriasis Cytotoxic drugs Carcinoma and sarcoma Chronic renal disease Hypothyroidism Lead poisoning Hyperparathyroidism Diabetes insipidus Diabetes ketoacidosis

Patients with gout may experience an acute attack with rapid fluctuations of serum urate levels. Surgery, dehydration, an alcohol binge, emotional stress, infection, diuretics, and uricosuric drugs can cause rapid fluctuations.

Pathophysiology

Gout is a direct result of hyperuricemia (high serum uric acid). Gout is characterized by an increased saturation of urate in the plasma and bodily fluids. Supersaturation of bodily fluids results in a precipitation of monosodium urate crystals out of body fluids into the joints, soft tissues, and cartilage. This leads to the symptoms and clinical findings of gout, because the deposition of urate in the joints and its crystallization trigger an inflammatory response. Several mechanisms may trigger an acute attack of gout, the most common being trauma or surgery. Gouty attacks may also be triggered by prophylactic or uricosuric agents which are known to lower serum uric acid levels.

At the time of puberty, serum uric acid levels increase in men; however, most (90 to 95 percent) remain asymptomatic throughout life. Estrogen is believed to protect women from hyperuricemia. Acute attacks are more likely to occur at lower serum uric acid levels in persons with alcoholism due to decreased urinary excretion. There is also an increased incidence of hypothyroidism in persons with confirmed crystal aspirates in synovial fluid. Although gout is frequently cited as a risk factor for the development of CAD, subsequent studies did not confirm previous findings of the Framingham Heart Study.

For unclear reasons, gouty arthritis has a predilection for the first metatarsophalangeal joint (the great toe)—a condition known as podagra. This may result from the relative coolness of this peripheral joint which allows for greater crystal deposition, the constant microtrauma to which this joint is subjected, and the differential impact weightbearing alternating with recumbency has on the resorption of joint fluid and intraarticular urate. Gouty arthritis may extend to several joints and is classified into four stages based on timing and Clinical Presentation (Table 15.14).

In general, urate crystallization is more likely to occur at lower temperatures. Noninflamed synovial fluid in the knee is significantly cooler (90 to 91°F) than core body temperature. Thus, while a serum uric acid concentration of 7 mg/dL appears to be the threshold level above which gout is more likely to develop, crystallization may be more likely to occur at lower concentrations intra-articularly. Hyperuricemia alone is insufficient to lead to crystallization, however. As part of the inflammatory process, urate-specific Ig molecules coat monosodium urate crystals in gouty synovial fluid, likely serving as a promoter of nucleation for urate crystals.

As gout progresses, crystals are deposited into multiple bodily tissues. In severe cases with repeated attacks, monosodium urate monohydrate crystals form into a nodular deposit known as a *tophus*, surrounded by granulomatous inflammation consisting of monocytes and giant cells. In addition to the skin and joints, *tophaceous* swellings may be found in a number of bodily tissues including the heart valves, kidneys, and larynx, capable of leading to significant pathology. Microtophi, consisting of collections of urate crystals surrounded only by a thin fibrocytic ring, may also be present in gouty synovial fluid. Some researchers have suggested that these microtophi release their urate crystals into the joint fluid following the initiation of synovial inflammation in the early stages of a gouty attack.

Urate crystals induce intraarticular inflammation via a number of mechanisms. Synovial lining cells, monocytes, and endothelial cells have all been shown to phagocytose urate crystals in vitro and subsequently increase their production of inflammatory mediators via transcriptional upregulation and mRNA stabilization, including interleukin (IL)-1, IL-6, IL-8, and tumor necrosis factor (TNF). Blockade of IL-8 and TNF activity has been further shown to counter urate-induced inflammation.

However, neutrophilic migration into affected joints and their subsequent phagocytosis of urate crystals appears to play a central role in the pathogenesis of gouty arthritis. Neutrophils undergo an oxidative burst during this process, releasing lysozomal enzymes, superoxide anions, leukotriene B4, and IL-1, among other mediators. In fact, the complexities of neutrophilic chemotaxis and function within gouty joints has been a central focus of gout research. Studies have indicated tyrosine kinases, phospho-

Table 15.14 Stages of Gout

Stage	Subjective Findings	Objective Findings	Diagnostic Findings
I. Asymptomatic	None	None	Microtophaceous deposits of urates in joints and bursae
II. Acute phase (inflammatory phase)	Extremely painful monarticular or polyarticular attack Pruritus and desquamation of the skin surrounding the joint as the inflammation subsides	Affected joints are red, warm, swollen Early acute attack subsides within a few days; may last up to 2 weeks; inflammation gradually subsides 10% of patients experience only one acute attack during their lifespan	Elevated WBC count Elevated temperature Elevated serum uric acid or normouremia
III. Intercritical (the interval between acute attacks)	None; patient is asymptomatic	Intervals between attacks decrease as the disease progresses If a second acute attack occurs, it usually presents within the first year following the initial attack	
IV. Chronic (chronic tophaceous gout phase; occurs as a result of recurrent attacks with multiple sites of urate deposits [tophi] in articular and periarticular tissue)	May restrict movement of affected joints Chronic pain, stiffness, decreased joint function, joint derangement, secondary degeneration	More than 50% of patients progress to this stage within 20 years of the initial attack if not properly managed Occasionally, tophus ulceration and erosion with chalk-textured drainage Uric acid kidney stones (5–10% of patients)	Tophi

lipases, adhesion molecules such as E-selectin, and several chemotactic factors play key roles in neutrophilic recruitment and activation by urate crystals. This explains the efficacy of colchicine in treating acute attacks, as it inhibits neutrophil tyrosine kinase activity in response to both gout and pseudogout crystals, as well as downregulates the activity of adhesion molecules on both neutrophils and endothelial cells.

A number of proteins interact with urate crystals to increase their proinflammatory properties. Immunoglobulins bound to urate crystals lead to a greater release of lysozomal and superoxide enzymes by neutrophils. In turn, neutrophil mediators have been shown to cleave Ig molecules from urate crystals to reduce their inflammatory nature. The inflammatory properties of tophaceous urate crystals are also reduced following protease treatment in vitro. In contrast, lipoproteins (specifically apolipoprotein B) reduce the inflammatory potential of urate crystals after binding, indicating that they may be involved in the self-limited resolution of acute attacks. The complement and kinin systems have also been implicated in urate crystal pathology, but they are not requisite for acute gouty inflammation.

The self-limited nature of an acute gouty attack involves several mechanisms. In addition to the deactivation and death of inflammatory cells and the inactivation of secreted proinflammatory mediators, leukocytes, monocytes, and macrophages have been shown in vitro to alter their cytokine transcriptional activity over time. In turn, they secrete several anti-inflammatory cytokines on resolution of an acute attack, including IL-1 receptor antagonist, transforming growth factor (TGF)-β, and peroxisome proliferator-activated receptor (PPAR)-γ. Although acute attacks of gout typically resolve spontaneously within several weeks, if left untreated or if inadequately treated, gout leads to chronic arthritis and bony erosions within 5 to 10 years, producing joint deformities and ultimately restricting function.

Clinical Presentation

Subjective

A thorough evaluation of the onset, characteristics, and potential potentiating causes of the pain is completed on initial evaluation. The patient will present during an acute attack with pain, tenderness, erythema, and swelling. Usual presentation is monarticular, the joint most frequently affected is the first metatarsal joint; however, the midfoot, knees, fingers, wrists, and elbows may also be affected. The typical presentation is excruciating pain that awakens the patient at night. Patients often describe the pain as throbbing, crushing, and pulsating. The pain is not relieved by rest or position change. Pain prevents any weight bearing on the affected limb. Often the patient cannot tolerate anything coming in contact with the affected part—even bed clothing touching the part is extremely painful. The patient may also report an episode of recent trauma to the affected joint, a recent drinking binge, or an eating binge before the acute attack. Patients may report a recent operation or severe illness, especially one producing a shift in fluid balance.

Objective

The patient's past medical history, including any joint or musculoskeletal trauma, should be reviewed, along with any family history of gout. Because gout is more prevalent in patients with hypertension, obesity, and hyperlipidemia, history taking should focus on these contributing factors. A recent drug history, specific for recent increased intake of aspirin or cyclosporine should be obtained.

Even though the patient initially presents with monarticular complaints, a complete bilateral examination of all joints should be performed. Joints should be assessed for symmetry in appearance and range of motion. Asymmetrical presentation of joint inflammation, redness, tenderness, and limitations in range of motion are typical of gout.

The joint most frequently affected in the initial attack is the first metatarsalphalangeal joint (podagra). Podagra is experienced by approximately 90 percent of patients with gout. Subsequent attacks may progress to include several joints (polyarticular). Other joints that are frequently affected include the instep of the ankle, the heels, knees, wrists, fingers, and elbows. Peripheral joints are more likely to be involved, because central joints are warmer and less conducive to crystal formations. In polyarticular episodes or if a large joint is involved, the patient may have an elevated temperature, tachycardia, anorexia, malaise, headache, and chills. On physical examination, the affected area is warm or hot to the touch. The patient will complain of pain on palpation, and range of motion will be limited. Skin overlying the affected area is often red and taut. Several days following an acute attack, desquamation over affected joints may be evident.

Patients who have progressed to the chronic tophaceous stage will have palpable tophi. *Tophi* are nodular deposits of monosodium urate monohydrate crystals that initiate an inflammatory process. Most tophi are firm and movable, whereas the overlying skin is thin and red. Tophi are most likely to develop on the pinnae, olecranon tips, and the distal joints of the hands and feet. Extensive tissue deposits of urate may also occur on the helix and antihelix of the ear, the eyelids, the sclera, and cornea.

Diagnostic Reasoning

Diagnostic Tests

Clinical Presentation and history are often diagnostic of gout. Serum uric acid levels and radiographic imaging provide some confirmation; however, a definitive diagnosis is made only with identification of sodium urate crystals of aspirate.

Initial Testing. Initial testing for gout includes a serum uric acid level. Most patients will have an elevated serum urate level in absence of an elevated blood urea nitrogen (BUN); however, some patients will have normal levels. Serum urate levels are often above 7.5 mg/dL in 95 percent of all persons with gout. The erythrocyte sedimentation rate (ESR) and white blood cell (WBC) count may also be elevated during an acute attack. The WBC count is typically greater than 10,000, but values to 100,000 may occasionally be present.

The classic radiographic findings of gout are tophi, normal mineralization of bone, joint space preservation, asymmetric polyarticular distribution, overhanging edge cortex, and punched-out erosions of bone. Radiographs of affected joints may show no changes in early stages. The only radiographic evidence in early stages may be asymmetrical soft tissue swelling. With recurrent attacks and progressive disease, however, radiolucent urate tophi and punched-out appearing areas are apparent in bone. Tophi appear as cloudlike increases in density, which may show signs of calcification. Urate crystals may also be seen in subcutaneous tissue, cartilage, joints, and other tissues. In the very late stages of gout, demineralization and loss of articular structures may be apparent on radiographic examination. Most changes are asymmetrical and occur predominantly in the feet, ankles, and knees. Patients with severe disease often have involvement of the hands and elbows.

Subsequent Testing. The definitive test to confirm the diagnosis of acute gout is urate crystals in joint fluid aspirate. The synovial fluid will be turbid during an acute attack. The crystals are identified by compensated polariscopic examination of wet smears of the aspirate and are noted to be negatively birefringent (a diagnostic finding). Aspiration and subsequent examination of the fluid should provide evidence for the diagnosis. Patients who present with gout and comorbid symptoms of abdominal pain, peripheral neuropathy, and proteinuria should be assessed for lead exposure.

Differential Diagnosis

Differential diagnoses include septic arthritis, cellulitis, rheumatoid arthritis, bursitis, fracture, acute trauma, and Reiter's syndrome.

Septic arthritis should be considered when a patient presents with joint pain, swelling, and erythema. Septic arthritis occasionally coexists with gout. It should also be strongly considered when a patient does not respond to initial management for gout. Septic arthritis more commonly occurs in larger joints. Gram stains and cultures of synovial fluids are positive for bacteria in septic arthritis. Patients often present with fever and chills. Radiographic examinations often reveal joint-space narrowing and erosions within 1 to 2 weeks of the onset.

The rheumatoid factor titer may help rule out rheumatoid arthritis. Rheumatoid arthritis may resemble gout but it typically has a symmetrical subjective presentation and radiographic presentation. Joint-space narrowing is also typical of rheumatoid joint disease.

Psoriatic arthritis may resemble gout in its early stages; however, the initial joints affected are frequently the hand, feet, sacroiliac joint, and spine. Fusiform soft tissue swelling is typical of psoritic arthritis and early joint-space narrowing is common.

Presence of symptoms in young adult women may indicate Reiter's syndrome.

Pseudogout presents with many similar characteristics of gout; however, polarized microscopic examination of aspirate reveals a calcium pyrophosphate dihydrate (CPPD) crystal. Pseudogout usually presents at a later age, and the symptoms are characteristically less acute and severe. Pseudogout is usually polyarticular (in approximately 75 percent of patients) and usually affects the knees and larger joints. Pseudogout is associated with hyperthyroidism and hypothyroidism, hypomagnesemia, amyloidosis, hypercalcemia, hypophosphatemia, and hemosiderosis.

Management

The goals of clinical management are to terminate an acute attack, prevent future attacks, normalize hyperuricemia, and prevent potential complications of urate deposits. Management of gout includes pharmacologic treatment of acute attacks and long-term medical and pharmacologic treatment of hyperuricemia. Acute management of gout includes generalized rest, elevation and immobilization of affected joints, and pharmacologic treatment. Prevention of disability due to gout is a reality today because of advances in pharmacologic treatment; however, the patient must become an active participant in the long-term treatment plan (Treatment Flowchart 15.2).

Initial Management

Pharmacologic treatment for an acute attack includes NSAIDs, colchicine, and corticosteroids.

Nonsteroidal Anti-inflammatory Drugs. The medication of choice initially is an NSAID. Traditionally indomethacin (Indocin) has been the most commonly prescribed NSAID for an acute attack of gout, but the other NSAIDs are just as effective. Indomethacin 25 to 50 mg q8h and is given until symptoms subside, usually 5 to 10 days. A good alternative to indomethacin is naproxen (Naprosyn). The first dose of naproxen is 750 mg, followed by 250 mg every 8 hours for 5 to 10 days. NSAIDs are discontinued after the pain has dissipated. Contraindications to the use of NSAIDs are active peptic ulcer disease, impaired renal function, and allergic reactions to NSAIDs. Potential adverse reactions of NSAIDs include gastrointestinal bleeding, nausea, rash, hypertension (especially in the elderly), hepatic impairment, fluid retention, and acute tublur necrosis with subsequent acute renal insufficiency (particularly at high doses or with chronic use).

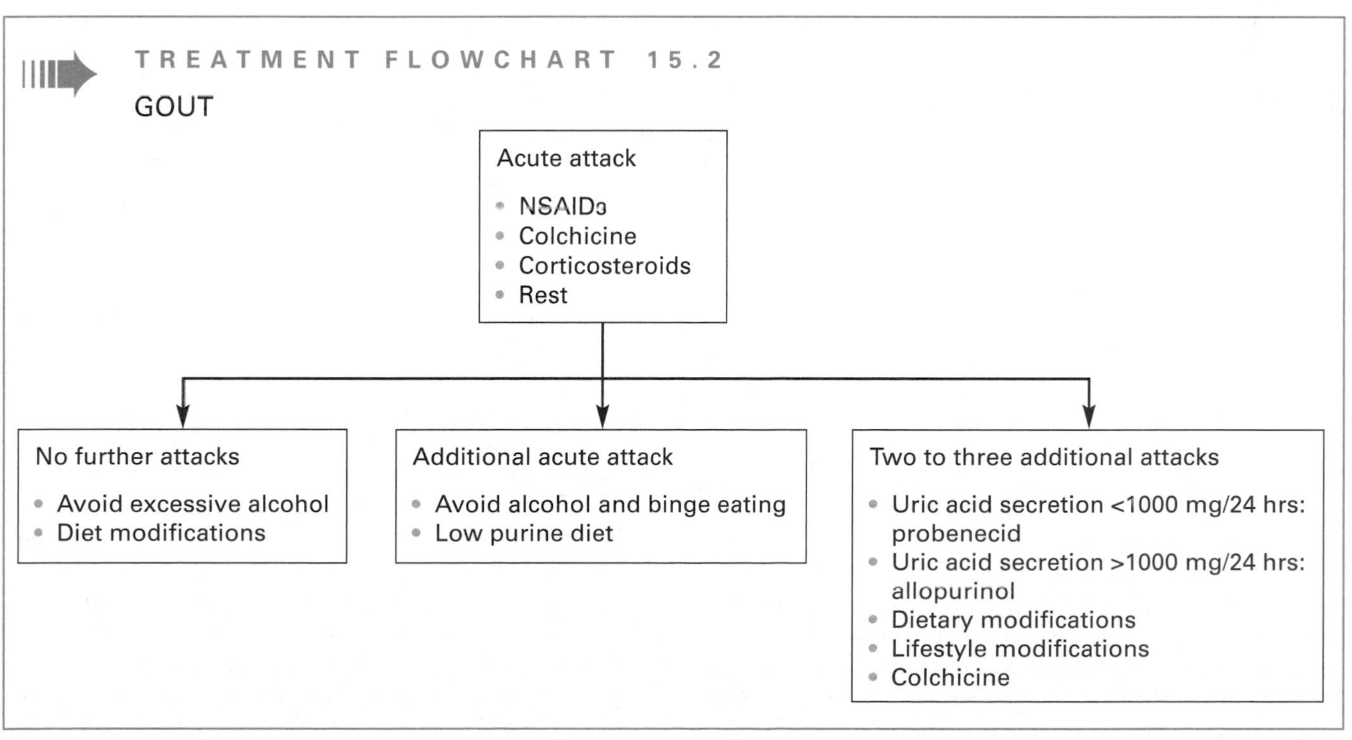

Colchicine. Colchicine is an effective medication to terminate an acute attack if administered within 48 hours of the initial onset of symptoms. If administered within this time frame it is effective in 90 percent of all patients. Colchicine can be administered orally or intravenously. The intravenous route is rarely used due to its low benefit versus toxicity ratio. In acute attacks, administer 1 to 1.2 mg of oral colchicine at the first sign of attack, then 0.5 to 0.6 g every hour or 1 to 1.2 mg q2h, or 0.5 to 0.6 g q2 to 3h until pain is relieved. The cumulative dose of colchicine should not exceed 4 to 6 mg during one course of therapy for an acute attack. Adverse reactions include nausea, vomiting, diarrhea, and abdominal pain and cramping. Colchicine usually provides relief in 18 hours; however, most patients will experience diarrhea or nausea within 24 hours of the first dose. Patients with renal or hepatic disease will need a decreased total dose. Colchicine is contraindicated in patients with a hypersensitivity to colchicine; severe cardiovascular, renal, or gastrointestinal disease; and blood dyscrasias. Colchicine must be used with caution in older adults.

Corticosteroids. Corticosteroids can provide dramatic systematic relief and can be administered orally, intramuscularly, or intra-articular. In most cases, corticosteroids are reserved for refractory cases or cases where the use of colchicine and NSAIDs is contraindicated. Corticosteroids are contraindicated in septic conditions; therefore, they should not be administered before analysis of the synovial aspirate. For polyarticular gout, prednisone, 40–60 mg PO qd usually produces a good response. The dose should be tapered quickly over 5 to 7 days. A referral to a physician is indicated if the patients could benefit from aspiration or an intra-articular steroid injection. Patients with monarticular disease and who cannot tolerate oral corticosteroids or NSAIDs benefit from intra-articular steroid injection. Intra-articular injection is with triamcinolone 10–40 mg and depends on the size of the joint.

Subsequent Management

The long-term management of gout includes pharmacologic agents, dietary modifications, activity evaluation, and educating the patient regarding prevention of gout.

Pharmacologic Management. Pharmacologic prophylaxis should be initiated following the second or third attack. In asymptomatic patients with hyperuricemia and with a history of only one acute attack, modification of lifestyle may prevent further attacks. Lifestyle modifications include limiting high-purine content foods, limiting alcohol to one drink per day, and increasing fluid intake. Alternatives to thiazide diuretics should be addressed. Pharmacologic prophylaxis, however, should be considered in patients with polyarticular gout and patients with consistent hyperuricemia greater than 8 mg/dL. Colchicine and NSAIDs may be continued in lower doses up to 12 months following an acute attack.

Colchicine is often used to prevent further acute attacks triggered by changes in uric acid levels. Colchicine does not correct the underlying causes of an acute attack, however. Adverse reactions to long-term use of colchicine are bone marrow depression, peripheral neuritis, and gastrointestinal symptoms, especially diarrhea. The dosage of colchicine for long-term preventative management ranges from 0.5 to 1.2 mg daily. Colchicine is often used to prevent an acute attack with the initiation of probenecid or allopurinol, because they may precipitate an acute attack by rapidly decreasing the urate serum level. Before scheduled surgery, colchicine 0.5–0.6 mg PO tid 3 days before and 3 days following surgery may prevent an acute attack of gout.

Three agents are currently available to lower uric acid levels—probenecid (Benamid) and sulfinpyrazone (Anturan) are uricosuric agents that block tubular reabsorption of filtered urate; and allopurinol (Zyloprim) which is an xanthine oxidase inhibitor that lowers plasma urate and urinary uric acid concentrations. They should not be started during or within 1 month following an acute attack. Before initiation, a 24-hour urinary uric acid excretion test is performed to differentiate between patients who are hypersecretors from those who are hyposecretors, because pharmacologic management of the two conditions differs.

Before initiation of probenecid therapy a 24-hour uric acid excretion test should be performed. Uric acid excretions greater than 1000 mg in 24 hours are abnormal, and levels between 800 to 1000 mg are considered to be borderline. Probenecid is indicated in patients whose excretion of uric acid is below 700 to 800 mg in 24 hours.

Probenecid is the drug of choice in persons younger than 60 years of age without a history of blood dyscrasias, renal failure, or kidney stones. An initial dosage of 500 mg is recommended, increasing gradually to 1 to 2 grams after 1 week. Dosage is increased based on uric acid levels, with a maximum dose of 2 grams daily. Major adverse reactions of this drug include skin rash, uric acid stones, and gastrointestinal upset. It may also precipitate an exacerbation of gout if it produces rapid shifts in uric acid levels. Probenecid inhibits the excretion of penicillin, indomethacin (Indocin), and acetazolamide (Diamox). Sulfinpyrazone (Anturane) is an alternative uricosuric drug and is started initially at 50 to 100 mg bid and gradually increased to 200 to 400 mg bid. A combination of probenecid and colchicine is now available.

Allopurinol (Zyloprim) is used to decrease uric acid production in patients who are unable to take probenecid. It is indicated in patients whose 24-hour uric acid secretion is greater than 1000 mg. Adverse reactions include gastrointestinal upset, headache, rash, bone marrow suppression, fever, liver or kidney failure, vasculitis, lymphadenopathy, hepatitis, alopecia, and dermatitis. It is contraindicated in persons with idiopathic hemochromatosis and renal and hepatic disease. Serious hypersensitivity reactions to allopurinol may occur but are rare. However, patients should still

Table 15.15 Foods High in Purine

All meats and seafoods (especially organ meats such as liver)
Meat extracts and gravies
Yeast and yeast extracts (brewer's and baker's)
Beer and alcoholic beverages
Beans, peas, lentils, oatmeal, spinach, asparagus, cauliflower, and mushrooms

be cautioned to discontinue use and immediately report any rash or fever which occurs after starting the drug. Twenty percent of patients on both allopurinol and ampicillin develop a rash. The safety of its use in pregnant or lactating women has not been established. The initial dose is 100 to 200 mg daily, with the average daily dose ranging from 200 to 300 mg.

Dosages of 400 to 600 mg daily are indicated only in severe gout. The maximum daily dose is 800 mg. The goal of therapy is to decrease the serum uric acid levels below 6 mg/dL. Dosage should be adjusted based on serum uric acid levels every 2 to 6 months.

Dietary Modifications. Dietary modifications include avoiding high purine-containing foods, maintaining adequate fluid intake, and moderate alcohol intake. The complete restriction of purine in the diet has not proved effective; therefore, a moderation of purine in the diet is now recommended. Foods high in purine content are listed in Table 15.15. Patients who are overweight may benefit from weight loss. Fluid intake should be sufficient to maintain an output of 2000 mL/day. Patients should force fluids to exceed 3000 mL/day, especially if they are prescribed a uricosuric agent.

Lifestyle Modifications. Activity must be restricted during an acute attack, and bedrest should be maintained 24 hours following the acute attack. The joint should be immobilized and if a lower extremity is involved, no weightbearing should be allowed during the acute attack. During intercritical periods, physical therapy may be indicated to maintain or improve function.

Hot compresses may promote comfort following an acute attack but should not be instituted until the acute pain subsides, usually 24 to 72 hours after initiation of therapy. Instruct patient to apply for 20 minutes two to three times daily. Heat can be applied with moist heating pads, warm showers and baths, or moist towels heated in a microwave.

Long-term management includes dietary moderation (one to two servings of purine-rich foods per day), alcohol in moderation, and maintenance of joint mobility.

Surgical Intervention. Patients with extensive or large tophi may benefit from surgical excision and should be referred to a surgeon.

Follow-Up and Referral

The patient should be evaluated 1 to 2 weeks following an acute attack. If antihyperuricemia therapy is initiated, the patient needs to be followed every 4 to 6 weeks to adjust medications and review the goals of treatment.

Annual follow-up is recommended. Special attention is given to previously affected joints as to their range of motion and stability. Joints should be symmetrically evaluated for tophi. Annual serum uric acid levels are indicated in all patients, and evaluation of renal function is indicated for patients on prophylactic antihyperuricemic therapy. An evaluation of the patient's diet (including specific questions about alcohol intake) and exercise regimen should be conducted during the annual examination. Reinforcement of previous education is essential to increase adherence to medication and physical regimens during intercritical periods. Patients who are overweight will need continued reinforcement to lose weight and reduce stress on weightbearing joints. Patients younger than age 35, premenopausal women, patients with frequent acute attacks despite prophylactic treatment, and patients with renal insufficiency should be referred to a rheumatologist for an initial evaluation.

Patient Education

Patients need instructions on avoidance of triggers for acute attacks. Excessive exercise, trauma, and alcohol or eating binges may precipitate an acute attack. Patients need explicit information on the adverse reactions of medication and measures to allay some preventable adverse reactions.

Fluid intake should exceed 3000 mL daily to prevent formation of uric acid kidney stones. Patients should avoid dehydration because it may precipitate an acute attack. Diet modifications must be reviewed with patients in detail and written information provided. Because both wine and spirits in excessive amounts impair the kidney's ability to excrete uric acid, they should be used in moderation. Patients must be aware that binge drinking may provoke an acute attack. If the patient is obese, weight loss should be encouraged because loss of excess body fat may normalize serum uric acid without pharmacologic intervention. Weight loss will also decrease stress on weight-bearing joints. Caution as to severe, rapid weight loss should be given because secondary hyperuricemia may result. A very low caloric-restricted diet may precipitate an acute attack.

Patients may need to take colchicine before having elective surgery if they are not already taking it regularly. They should be instructed to avoid aspirin.

Good posture and protection of weightbearing joints are essential. Because the feet are most frequently affected, the patient should wear supportive and properly fitting shoes. Some patients may benefit from a physical therapist's exercise prescription or a visit to a podiatrist for an evaluation. At first signs of an acute attack, the patient should limit all activity, weightbearing if appropriate, and contact the primary-care provider.

Bibliography

General

Banning, M: Obesity: Pathophysiology and treatment. J Roy Soc Prom Health 125(4):163–167, 2005.

Barker, LR, Burton, JR, and Zieve, PD: Principles of Ambulatory Medicine, ed 6. Lippincott Williams & Wilkins, Philadelphia, 2003.

Baron, RB: Nutrition. In Tierney, LM, et al (eds): Current Medical Diagnosis and Treatment, ed 44. Lange/McGraw-Hill, New York, 2005, pp 1214–1242.

Bascom, A: Incorporating herbal medicine into clinical practice. FA Davis, Philadelphia, 2002.

Braunwald E, et al (eds): Harrison's Principles of Internal Medicine, ed 16. McGraw-Hill, New York, 2005.

Dambro, MR: Griffith's 5-Minute Clinical Consult. Lippincott Williams & Wilkins, Philadelphia, 2003.

DiDiego, ML, Eggert, JA, Pruitt, RH, and Larcom, LL: Unmasking the truth behind endocrine disorders. Nurse Pract 30(10):54–59, 2005.

Fitzgerald, PA: Endocrinology. In Tierney, LM, et al (eds): Current Medical Diagnosis and Treatment, ed 44. Lange/McGraw-Hill, New York, 2005, pp 1068–1156.

Hunter MH, and Carek, PJ: Evaluation and treatment of women with hirsutism. Am Fam Physician 67(12):2565–72, 2461–3, 2629, 2003.

Kee, JL: Laboratory and Diagnostic Tests with Nursing Implications, ed 6. Prentice-Hall, Upper Saddle River, N.J., 2002.

Masharani, U: Diabetes mellitus and hypoglycemia. In Tierney, LM, et al (eds): Current Medical Diagnosis and Treatment, ed 44. Lange/McGraw-Hill, New York, 2005, pp 1157–1201.

McCance, KL, and Huether, SE: Pathophysiology: The Biologic Basis for Disease in Adults and Children, ed 5. CV Mosby, St. Louis, Mo., 2006.

Prisco, MK: Evaluating neck masses. Nurse Pract 25(4):30–51, 2000.

Youngkin, E, et al: Pharmacotherapeutics: A Primary Care Guide, ed 2. Pearson/Prentice-Hall, Upper Saddle River, N.J., 2005.

Cushing's Syndrome

Findling, JW, and Raff, H: Cushing's syndrome. Endocrinol Metab Clin North Am 34(2):xiii–xv, 257–499, 2005.

Kouri, JG, and Oldfield, EH: Clinical picture: A twin with Cushing's disease. Lancet 365(9467):1332, 2005.

Ma, RCW, Chan WB, Som WY, Tong, PCY, Chan JCN, and Chow, CC: Lesson of the week: Carbamazepine and false positive dexamethasone suppression tests for Cushing's syndrome. BMJ 330(7486):299–300, 2005.

Raff, H, and Findling, JW: A physiologic approach to diagnosis of the Cushing syndrome. Ann Intern Med 138(12):980–991, 2003.

Schuff, JG: Issues in the diagnosis of Cushing's syndrome for the primary care physicial. Primary Care Clin Office Pract 30(4):791–799, 2003.

Diabetes Mellitus/Metabolic Syndrome

American Diabetes Association. Physical activity/exercise and diabetes. Diabetes Care 27(Suppl 1):S58–S62, 2004.

Appel, SJ, Jones, ED, and Kennedy-Malone, L: Central obesity and the metabolic syndrome: Implications for primary care providers. J Am Acad Nurse Pract 16(8):335–341, 2004.

Appel, SJ: Calculating insulin resistance in the primary care setting: Why should we worry about insulin levels in euglycemic patients? J Am Acad Nurse Pract 17(8):331–336, 2005.

Appel SJ, Harrell, JS, and Davenport ML: Central obesity, the metabolic syndrome, and plasminogen activator inhibitor-1 in young adults. J Am Acad Nurse Pract 17(12):535–541, 2005.

Aliabadi, Z: Understanding and managing prediabetes. Clin Advisor 8(8):36, 38, 43–45, 2005.

American Diabetes Association: All about diabetes. http://www.diabetes.org/about-diabetes.jsp.

Chan, W, Woo, J., Hui, E, Lau, W, Lai, J, and Lee, D: A community model for care of elderly people with diabetes via telemedicine. Appl Nurs Res 18(2):77–81, 2004.

Deen, D: Metabolic syndrome: Time for action. Am Fam Physician 69 (12), 2875–2882, 2004.

Dodd, K, and Zimmerman, RW: Advisor forum. Convincing a reluctant patient. Clin Advisor 8(8):59, 2005.

Fowler, SB, Moussouttas, M, and Mancini, B: Metabolic syndrome: Contributing factors and treatment strategies. J Neurosci Nurs 37(4):220–223, 2005.

Garg, A: Statins for all patients with type 2 diabetes: Not so soon. Lancet 364:641–642, 2004.

Grundy, SM, et al: Definition of metabolic syndrome: Report of the National Heart, Lung, and Blood Institute / American Heart Association. Circulation 109(3):433–438, 2004.

Harmon, C, Willoughby, DF, and Floyd, C: A lesson in early morning hyperglycemia. Nurse Pract 29(11):58–63, 2004.

Kahn, A, Safdar, J, Ali Khan, MM, Khattak, KN, and Anderson, RA: Cinnamon improves glucose and lipids of people with type 2 diabetes. Diabetes Care 26(12):3215–3218, 2003.

Koch, J: The role of exercise in the African-American woman with type 2 diabetes mellitus: application of the health belief model. J Am Acad Nurse Pract 14(3):126–129, 2002.

Mahdi, OZ: Pre-diabetes: Halting the progression. Geriatr Med 35(8):17–22, 2005.

McCarty, MF: Nutraceutical resources for diabetes prevention—an update. Med Hypotheses 64(1):151–158, 2005.

McGinnis, RA, McGrady, A, Cox, SA, and Grower-Dowling, KA: Biofeedback-assisted relaxation in type 2 diabetes. Diabetes Care 28:2145–2149, 2005.

Meijer, ME: An unusual approach to glycemic control. Clin Advisor 8(3):33–36, 2005.

Misra, A, Wasir, JS, and Vikram, NK: Waist circumference criteria for the diagnosis of abdominal obesity are not applicable uniformly to all populations and ethnic groups. Nutrition 21(9):969–76, 2005.

Nambi, V, Hoogwerf, BJ, and Sprecher, DL: A truly deadly quartet: Obesity, hypertension, hypertriglyceridemia, and hyperinsulinemia. Cleve Clin J Med 69(12): 985–994, 2002.

Nash, DT:. The metabolic syndrome: Early clues, effective management. Consultant May:859–863, 2004.

Shahady, EJ: Type 2 diabetes, the metabolic syndrome, inflammation, and arteriosclerosis: Steps to stem a rising epidemic. Consultant 45(14):1579–1586, 2005.

Unger, J: Screening for type 2 diabetes in primary care. Female Patient 29(Dec):32–34, 2004.

U.S. Preventive Services Task Force: Screening for type 2 diabetes mellitus in adults: Recommendations and rationale. AJN 104(3):83–94, 2004.

Weiss, PM, Finch, FG, and Hess, LW: Insulin delivery system options in diabetes: Novel approaches to an old disease. Female Patient 28(Sept):23–27, 2003.

Whyte, J. The metabolic syndrome: Early clues, effective management. Consultant 45(11):1195–1200, 2005.

Thyroid

Carmichael, KA, and Alper, BS: Hypothyroidism. Clin Advisor (June):107–109, 2004.

Diez, JJ: Hyperthyroidism in patients older than 55 years: An analysis of the etiology and management. Gerontology 49:316–323, 2003.

Fatourechi, V: Subclinical hypothyroidism: When to treat, when to watch? Consultant 44(4):533–539, 2004.

Godfrey, J, Pearce, EN, and Bergman, DA: Conversation with the experts. Toward optimal health: The experts discuss thyroid dysfunction. J Womens Health 13(2):141–146, 2004.

Grubbs, L, and Karioth, S: Hyperthyroidism: Focus on Graves disease. Clin Rev 14(11):34–39, 2004.

Hassel, B: Prenatal thyroid dysfunction: Unmasking a significant threat to mother and baby. Adv Nurse Pract (October):41–44, 2005.

Helfand, M: Clinical guidelines. Screening for subclinical thyroid dysfunction in nonpregnant adults: A summary of the evidence for the U.S. Preventive Services Task Force. Ann Intern Med 140(2):128–141, 2004.

Ralph, CT: Recertification refresher. Finding and treating the cause of hyperthyroidism. J Am Acad Phys Assist 17(2):20, 23–26, 29–30, 2004.

Shames, R, and Shames, KH: Thryoid Power: Ten Steps to Total Health. HarperCollins, New York, 2002.

Surks MI, Ortiz E, Daniels GH, et al: Subclinical thyroid disease: Scientific review and guidelines for diagnosis and management. JAMA 291:228–238, 2004.

Vidt, DG: Thyroid dysfunction and hypertension: What's the connection? Consultant 44(1):136–137, 2004.

White, RD: Hyperthyroidism: Current standards of care. Consultant 44(8):1085–1088, 1089–1090, 2004.

White, RD: Cases in point: Hyperthyroidism: 5 cases to hone you diagnostic skills. Consultant 44(8):1091–1092, 2004.

Resources

General

American Association of Clinical Endocrinologists
http://www.aace.com
American Cancer Society
http://www.cancer.org
Centers for Disease Control and Prevention
http://www.cdc.gov
College of Endocrinology
http://www.aace.com
The Self-Help Sourcebook
http://www.cmhc.com/selfhelp
Dr. Andrew Weil (alternative health)
http://www.drweil.com
Endocrine Society
http://www.endo-society.org
Food and Drug Administration
http://www.fda.gov
National Institutes of Health
http://www.nih.gov
U.S. National Library of Medicine
http://www.nim.nih.gov/
RxList—The Internet Drug Index
http://www.rxlist.com/
Association of Clinical Endocrinologists
http://www.aace.com
Center for Disease Control—Diabetes
http://www.cdc.gov/ncc.dphp/ddt/ddthome.htm
Diabetes Association
http://www.diabetes.org
Indian Health Services Diabetes Program
http://www.ih.gov/IHSMAIN.html
National Diabetic Information Clearinghouse
http://www.aerie.com/nihdb/ndic/dmdbase.html
National Institute of Diabetes, Digestive, and Kidney Disease
http://www.niddk.nih.gov

Gout

http://www.arthritis.org
http://www.rheumatology.org

Obesity

http://www.obesity.org
http://www.tops.org

Thyroid

American Thyroid Association
http://www.thryoid.org

Diabetes

American Association of Diabetes Educators
444 N. Michigan Ave., Suite 1240
Chicago, IL 60611
(800) 338–3633
http://www.aadenet.org
American Diabetes Association
1660 Duke Street
Alexandria, VA 22314
(800) 232–3472
http://www.diabetes.org
American Dietetic Association
(800) 366–1655 (Spanish speaking assistance available)
(800) 745–0775
http://www.eatright.org
Juvenile Diabetes Foundation International
120 Wall Street, 19th Floor
New York, NY 10005
(800) 223–1138
National Diabetes Information Clearinghouse
I Information Way
Bethesda, MD 20892–3560
(301) 654–3327
National Eye Institute
National Eye Health Education Program
Blooding 3 1, Room 6A32
31 Center Drive, MSC-25 IO
Bethesda, MD 20892–2510
(800) 869–2020
http://www.nei.nih.gov

Gout

Arthritis Foundation
PO Box 19000
Atlanta, GA 30325
(800) 283–7800
National Institute of Arthritis and Musculoskeletal Disorders
Building 31, Room 4C05
Bethesda, MD 20892
(301) 496–8188

Obesity

American Society of Bariatric Physicians
5600 S. Quebec Street, Suite 160-D
Englewood, CO 80111
(303) 779–4833
Overeaters Anonymous
World Services Office
PO Box 92870
Los Angeles, CA
(213) 936–4206

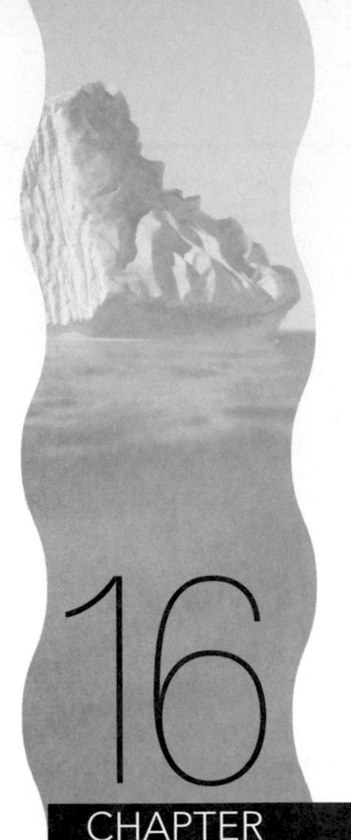

Hematologic and Immune Problems

Brian O. Porter, MD, PhD, MPH
Sande Garcia Jones, PhD, APRN, ACRN, FAAN
Jill E. Winland-Brown, EdD, MSN, APRN, BC

Common Complaints

Bruising

A *bruise* is an integumentary manifestation of extravasated blood. Discoloration of the skin is attributed to a local interstitial pool of erythrocytes, which causes a light to dark blue skin color associated with red pigment. The bruise sets off a local inflammatory event that includes macrophage invasion and histamine release and may be associated with edema. Macrophages engulf red blood cells (RBCs) to clear the area.

Macrophages that contain the RBCs excrete hemosiderin and hematoidin. Hemosiderin is brown and hematoidin is yellow. The release of these molecules from macrophages accounts for the characteristic color changes in bruises during their resolution. Hematomas (larger bruises) require lengthier periods of time to resolve than smaller bruises do.

Bruising may result from blunt trauma or no trauma at all. In the case of spontaneous bruising, the underlying cause is often chronic use of steroid or anticoagulant therapies. Steroids weaken the vascular walls, making them prone to release erythrocytes. Anticoagulants, when their levels exceed the therapeutic range, can permit microvascular ruptures to spill blood into interstitial spaces.

Anticoagulant therapy consists of warfarin (Coumadin) in oral dosages that are intended to keep the international normalized ratio (INR) between 2.0 and 3.0 for most disease-related prophylaxis and between 2.5 and 3.5 for the prevention of valvular thrombus in atrial fibrillation. Initial dosing of warfarin is 10 to 15 mg per day for 3 days, followed by measurement of prothrombin time (PT) and INR. This initial loading dose starts the process of anticoagulation. Dosages thereafter range from 2 to 10 mg, on average, per day. Dosages can be higher than 10 mg if the INR dictates.

If the INR result is above the therapeutic range, several options can be followed depending on how far above range it is. First, the clinician should consider withholding one or more days of anticoagulant therapy. Second, therapy should be restarted at a lower dose after a hiatus of therapy. Finally, the PT and INR should be reevaluated within 1 week of the dosage adjustments.

Differential Diagnosis

The differential diagnoses of bruising include chronic use of steroid and anticoagulant therapies, hemolytic anemia, domestic violence, self-inflicted injury or other blunt trauma, and hypersensitivity vasculitis. A thorough history and physical exam by the clinician should focus on the cause of the bruising.

Fatigue

Fatigue presents as a complaint of tiredness that cannot be explained on the basis of exercise or other activity. It may be either acute or chronic, associated with a disease or independent of other pathophysiology. Acute fatigue is most often associated with viral or bacterial infections and may serve as a harbinger of impending symptoms such as fever. Chronic fatigue that lasts for months is far more complex. A patient seeking relief from chronic fatigue may occupy the clinician's attention during many visits before the causes of the symptoms can be identified. The patient usually cannot explain the cause of chronic fatigue without the clinician asking appropriate assessment questions.

The clinical history of fatigue offers insights into the nature of the cause. Patient reports of fatigue that increases over the course of a day and abates after rest indicates an organic origin for fatigue. Functional fatigue, on the other hand, is characterized by fatigue on awakening and may actually improve after exercise. The close associations of depression and anxiety with fatigue make for a difficult task in distinguishing these functional causes of the fatigue from the fatigue itself.

Differential Diagnosis

Fatigue by itself presents a complicated differential. Fortunately, it seldom presents without other comorbidity.

Acute fatigue is perhaps the simplest type to diagnose and treat. For example, acute fatigue typically appears in a clinical history that is positive for viral or bacterial exposure, combined with examination findings of fever and other systemic abnormalities.

Chronic fatigue has many causes, including chronic anxiety or stress reactions, depression, infectious mononucleosis, hepatitis, tuberculosis (TB), anemia, heart disease, lung disease, electrolyte disturbances, rheumatoid diseases, and cancer.

Fever

Fever is defined as a temperature elevation above normal baseline in which pathology can be identified as the cause. On average, most individuals maintain a body temperature of 98.6°F (37°C). Exertion can elevate the temperature temporarily, followed by a return to baseline after activity ends. Persistent elevation in temperature is clearly pathologic, however.

Fever may be either acute or chronic. If acute, body temperature tends to be greater than 101.3°F (38.5°C). Acute fever is associated with upper respiratory infections (URIs) that are either bacterial or viral in nature, drug reactions, gastroenteritis, or urinary tract infections (UTIs). The ability of the body to elevate the temperature in the event of infection diminishes with advancing age; therefore, acute fever in an older adult might not be comparable to that in a younger patient.

Chronic fevers tend to be low-grade temperature elevations. Temperatures rise to 100.4°F (38°C) in cases of hepatitis, infectious mononucleosis (especially in the third and fourth weeks after onset of symptoms), cancer, sinusitis, dental abscess, prostatitis, and tuberculosis.

The origin of a fever may not be apparent from the patient's history, examination, and laboratory testing. If not evident, the fever should be classified as *fever of unknown origin* (FUO). A FUO is defined as a fever greater than 101.3°F (38.5°C) that occurs on at least three occasions in a 3-week period in an ambulatory patient. A hospitalized patient is diagnosed with FUO if the unexplainable fever persists for 1 week.

Differential Diagnosis

The magnitude of fever elevation may guide the clinician in differentiating its cause. Fever can vary widely, however, based on the patient's age, history of pathogenic exposure, as well as many other factors. Fevers in excess of 104°F (40°C) tend to be associated with pancreatitis, UTIs, and intracranial pathology. Fevers between 101.3°F (38.5°) and 104°F (40°C) are associated with URIs and some acute viral syndromes. Fevers less than 101.3F (38.5°C) are characteristic of hepatitis, some acute viral infections, and TB.

Differentiations in fever elevation guide the decision-making process of which laboratory evaluations to recommend. Correlated with history and physical examination findings, fever elevation determines the type of sampling of blood or other body fluids to be ordered. In addition, in the absence of definitive test results, knowledge of the categories of fever elevation may give the clinician more or less reason for alarm. For example, when a middle-aged women with a 3-day fever of 102.2°F (39°C) presents with a nonproductive cough, chills, and inspiratory chest discomfort, and her lungs are clear but dull to percussion in the bases, the suspicion of a pulmonary consolidative process should cause the clinician to order a chest x-ray exam and complete blood count (CBC), but not blood cultures, because the fever is not high enough to suggest systemic infection, for which blood cultures might be indicated. Moreover, there are focal symptoms that explain the fever.

Environmental toxins may also cause fever. When this etiology is suspected, the history should focus on exposure to industrial chemicals and to potential animal sources of fever. Fevers of environmental origin follow an indolent course, often showing peaks and troughs. Physical signs may also be absent, thus adding to the indolence of the presentation.

Lymphadenopathy

Lymphadenopathy is a term used in clinical practice to designate any abnormality of lymph nodes, but in particular, enlarged lymph nodes. Perhaps the more exact term should be *lymphadenitis,* which suggests that inflammation is the cause of the lymph node enlargement. Lymph node enlargement may be regionally or systemically associated with inflammation. If the inflammation is regional, the lymph nodes that are proximal to a site of infection will show enlargement. If the disease process is systemic, lymph nodes in three or more sites that are dispersed across the body may become enlarged. An example of regional lymph node enlargement is cervical lymphadenopathy associated with pharyngitis. An example of systemic lymphadenopathy is human immunodeficiency virus (HIV) infection, in which there may be three or more extrainguinal lymphadenopathies.

Lymphadenopathy follows the course of the disease. Thus, nodes may be acutely or chronically enlarged depending on the duration of the disease. Acute infection often leaves the regional nodes tender to touch. On the other hand, chronically enlarged nodes may not be tender at all.

Differential Diagnosis

The differential diagnosis for lymphadenopathy depends on the location of involvement and associated findings. Neck masses, for example, involve a differential that is based on node location in the neck, age of the patient, and associated morbidities, such as tobacco use. The clinician should distinguish between slow growth in nodes and rapid or acute onset of lymphadenopathy. Acute onset is characteristic of inflammation, and slow-growing nodes in the neck suggest neoplasm, such as lymphoma; however, there may be exceptions. For example, a young patient with no history of tobacco or ethanol use may present with slow-growth cervical lymphadenopathy, but the possibility of neoplasm is minimal in a patient of this age and with this history. Nonetheless, an adult older than age 70 years with even a remote history of tobacco use is likely to be diagnosed with lymphoma if there is a slow-growth neck lymphadenopathy. Thus, the patient's age contributes to the differential of neck lymphadenopathy.

HIV-associated lymphadenopathy presents challenges to the differential. The average HIV-infected patient is younger than age 50, has a history of alcohol and/or tobacco use, and may be antibody-positive to other sexually transmitted diseases. Lymphadenopathy could occupy the neck, axillae, inguinal region, breasts, and thorax. Reactive lymphadenopathy is characteristic of early and middle stages of the disease, but later disease findings include lymphoma, cytomegalovirus (CMV) and human papilloma virus (HPV) infections, toxoplasmosis, and *Mycobacterium avium* complex. Persistent slow-growth enlargement, therefore, is reason to consider lymph node aspiration and cytologic evaluation.

Sore Throat

Sore throat is defined as discomfort or pain in the throat that is most intense when swallowing. It can be associated with sore mouth, especially if there is a viral infection such as herpes simplex virus (HSV) that erupts as lesions that can cause soreness in both anatomic locations. HSV infection occupies time and resources for diagnosis and treatments and is a primary reason for lost wages because of absence from work.

The most common causes of sore throat are streptococcal and viral infections, such as those of rhinovirus. The onset of pain builds over the course of hours and may be accompanied by fever and malaise. Physical examination offers customary findings such as injected mucosa, patchy exudates (bacterial invasion), tender regional lymphadenopathy, tachycardia, and fever. The clinical history is often positive for known exposure within families.

Differential Diagnosis

The differential diagnosis focuses on the diseases of suspicion. These include infection by *Streptococcus,* HSV, candidiasis, aphthous ulceration, and influenza virus or rhinovirus. Throat culture for group A streptococci and a fourfold rise in the antistreptolysin-O (ASO) titer are indicative of the diagnosis that is commonly called "strep throat." Small, indurated lesions with central cavernous pits are evidence of HSV infection. Initial HSV infection may follow a florid presentation, with ulcerations erupting in 10 or more oral and pharyngeal sites. Candidiasis presents as either white or red exudate, which may be apparent in both the mucous membranes of the mouth and external pharynx. A definitive diagnosis of candidiasis is made with potassium hydroxide (KOH) preparation.

Aphthous ulceration mimics HSV eruptions; however, aphthous ulceration is more prone to present near the opening of the mouth and not in the throat. The central core of aphthous ulcers is not as cavernous as in HSV lesions, nor will these ulcers appear as white in the center. Finally, viral infections of the pharynx are difficult to distinguish by their presentation. They may also be associated with a secondary bacterial infection, which makes them particularly vexing to diagnose. They should, however, present as injection without exudate.

Common Hematologic Problems

Microcytic Anemia

Anemia can mean any of several problems that involve RBCs (Table 16.1). The diagnosis suggests low hemoglobin, low hematocrit (Hct), and a low number of RBCs. All of these problems involve a reduced amount of oxygen circulating in the body, because RBCs carry oxygen to tissues and cells. The World Health Organization (WHO) identifies *anemia* as a hemoglobin level of less than 13.0 grams/deciliter (g/dL) in men (less than 42 percent Hct) and less than 12.0 g/dL in women (less than 36 percent Hct). Slightly higher values of hemoglobin and hematocrit are considered standard in developed versus underdeveloped regions of the world.

As a rule of thumb, the estimated level of hematocrit is three times the value of the hemoglobin: For example, a hemoglobin value of 13.0 g/dL amounts to an estimated Hct of 39 percent.

Microcytic anemia is a category of anemia based on the small size (*micro-*) of the RBCs (*-cytic*). It has been linked to nutritional deficiencies, particularly a deficiency in

Table 16.1 Classification of Anemias

Anemia	Examples of Causes	MCV* (mm^3)	MCH† (pg)	MCHC‡ (%)
Normocytic, normochromic	Sepsis, hemorrhage, hemolysis, drug-induced aplastic anemia, radiation, hereditary spherocytosis	82–92	25–30	32–36
Microcytic, normochromic	Renal disease, infection, liver disease, malignancies	<80	20–25	27
Microcytic, hypochromic	Iron deficiency, lead poisoning, thalassemia, rheumatoid arthritis	50–80	12–25	25–30
Macrocytic, normochromic	Vitamin B_{12} and folic acid deficiency, some drugs, pernicious anemia	95–150	30–50	32–36

Indications for Hemoglobin Electrophoresis

- Suspected thalassemia, especially in individuals with positive family history for the disorder
- Differentiation among the types of thalassemias
- Evaluation of a positive Sickledex test to differentiate sickle cell trait (20 to 40 percent Hgb S) from sickle cell disease (70 percent Hgb S)
- Diagnosis of HgbC or Sickle cell anemia (Hemoglobin SC disease)
- Identification of the numerous types of abnormal Hgb, most of which do not produce clinical disease

Hemoglobin Electrophoresis	Normal Percentage	Comments
Hb A_1 Adult Infants	>95 10–30	Lower in alpha- and beta-thalassemia major and minor
Hb A_2 Cord blood Birth–6 months > 6 months	 0–1.8 0–3.5 1.5–3.5	Elevated—beta-thalassemia minor and major up to 9%
Hb F Adult Neonates 1 month 2 months 3 months 6 months–1 year	<10 70–80 70 50 25 3	Elevated—beta-thalassemia minor up to 9% Elevated—thalassemia minor and major (after 6 months)
Hb H (β_4 tetramers)	Absent	30% of hemoglobin in severe alpha thalassemia with three of four mutated alpha chain genes.
Hb C (β chain 6 Glu→Lys)	Absent	Usually, asymptomatic, but causes a milder form of sickle cell disease when heterozygous with Hgb S.
Hb D Hb E (β chain 26 Glu→Lys)	Absent Absent	Hb D and E rarely occur by themselves. and only cause mild anemia When they occur in combination with sickle cell anemia or thalassemia, disease is more serious.
Hb S (β chain 6 Glu→Val)	Absent	Elevated—sickle cell anemia: <40% sickle cell trait; 85–95% sickle cell disease. Most common hemoglobin variant. If both genes have Hb S = sickle cell anemia—1% of population. If one gene has Hb S = sickle cell trait—8–10% of population

* Mean corpuscular volume.
† Mean corpuscular hemoglobin.
‡ Mean corpuscular hemoglobin concentration.
Glu, glutamine; Lys, lysine; Val, valine.

dietary intake or uptake of iron. The small size of the RBCs is identified by one of the three indices of RBCs known as the mean corpuscular volume (MCV). Microcytosis, therefore, is defined by an MCV value of less than 80 femtoliters (fL). In short, the clinician can make a diagnosis of microcytic anemia by identifying the presence of anemia combined with a low MCV.

Epidemiology and Causes

Microcytic anemia, as related to iron deficiency, is one of the most common anemias throughout the world. The incidence is high among women of childbearing years, accounting for 50 percent of cases among pregnant women. The ratio of incidence between women to men is 4:1. In the United States, 20 percent of adult women are affected by the condition compared with 3 percent of adult men. These statistics have remained constant for the past decade.

The causes of microcytic anemia include (1) an inadequate intake or uptake of dietary iron, (2) anemia of chronic disease (ACD), (3) thalassemia, and (4) sideroblastic anemias.

The incidence of iron-deficiency anemia has been estimated to be 1:2.0 to 2.5 among pregnant women and 1:6 in persons older than age 75. Iron deficiency anemia is often the easiest type to correct and remedy, unless it is caused by a gastrointestinal (GI) malignancy. Iron deficiency is, therefore, less important in the differential even though it remains the most common cause of microcytic anemia.

Most adults in the United States ingest and absorb enough iron in their diets. It is estimated that the average dietary intake of iron in the United States is 10 to 15 mg per day, of which not more than 10 percent is absorbed in the stomach, duodenum, and jejunum. The average healthy adult, therefore, absorbs approximately 1 to 2 mg of iron per day. In addition, the same adult loses an amount of iron equal to that ingested and absorbed, thereby maintaining homeostasis.

ACD, unlike iron-deficiency anemia, presents a more complex diagnostic picture because of the many and varied causes of inflammatory disorders in chronic disease, which include rheumatoid arthritis, malignancies, and serious infections. Given its complex diagnostic picture, ACD is considered more important in the differential than the other three causes. Despite its importance in the differential, the incidence and prevalence of ACD are unknown.

The thalassemias are a group of inherited diseases of alpha- or beta-globin chains. Microcytic anemia is caused by hemolysis that results from the suboptimal synthesis of alpha- or beta-globin chains, hence the categories of thalassemias known as alpha- and beta-. Beta-thalassemia is associated with descendants of groups of individuals who originated around the Mediterranean Sea. Alpha-thalassemia is far more widespread, occurring in individuals with families from the Asian continent, including China and Southeast Asia. Prevalence has also been noted among West Coast Africans.

Sideroblastic anemia may be caused by chronic alcoholism or lead poisoning, or may be a stage in the evolution of a generalized bone marrow disorder that may end in acute leukemia.

Pathophysiology

Normal Hemoglobin Formation

The predominant normal adult hemoglobin (hemoglobin A; $\alpha_2\beta_2$) comprises one pair of alpha-globin chains and one pair of beta-globin chains, accounting for 90-95 percent of total adult hemoglobin. Each of these globin chains is linked to an individual heme group, which consists of a protoporphyrin IX molecule bound to a ferrous (Fe^{2+}) reduced iron ion. It is this heme unit that reversibly binds oxygen, allowing for transport of oxygen by the hemoglobin tetramer to the bodily tissues.

Several other forms of hemoglobin are formed during human development. At least three distinct forms of hemoglobin consisting of different combinations of zeta (ζ), epsilon (ϵ), gamma (γ), and alpha (α) chains present themselves throughout embryonic development in the following order: hemoglobin Gower I ($\zeta_2\epsilon_2$), hemoglobin Portland ($\zeta_2\gamma_2$), and hemoglobin Gower II ($\alpha_2\epsilon_2$). In contrast, the predominant normal hemoglobin form in infancy is hemoglobin F (~80 percent), which has two gamma-globin chains substituted for the beta-chains (hemoglobin F; $\alpha_2\gamma_2$). Hemoglobin F has a stronger affinity for oxygen than hemoglobin A does, allowing for oxygen transport across the placenta from the mother to the developing fetus. As a newborn ages, this form of hemoglobin slowly clears from the circulation, accounting for less than 1 percent of hemoglobin by 6 months of age, with a corresponding increase in Hemoglobin A. Finally, an additional form of adult hemoglobin known as hemoglobin A_2 also exists, which is present in far smaller amounts than hemoglobin A (about 2 to 5 percent of total adult hemoglobin). With a slightly higher oxygen affinity than hemoglobin A, hemoglobin A_2 has two delta (σ)-globin chains substituted for the beta-globin chains ($\alpha_2\sigma_2$).

Iron-Deficiency Anemia

As the reduced ferrous (Fe^{2+}) ion is a critical component of the heme moiety in hemoglobin, adequate iron stores are critical for adequate erythropoiesis in the bone marrow. In low iron states, the production of hemoglobin is severely reduced, resulting in marked microcytosis. Iron deficiency remains the most common cause of microcytic anemia in the United States. Because most adults receive enough iron in their diets to prevent microcytosis (other than strict vegan vegetarians), the clinician's attention should turn to malabsorption or occult loss of blood as the primary causes of iron-deficiency anemia.

The majority of iron uptake occurs in the duodenum and upper jejunum. Thus, malabsorption of iron is linked to underlying GI problems such as celiac sprue, surgical resections involving the stomach, duodenum, or jejunum, inflammatory bowel disease such as Crohn's disease, rapid gastrointestinal motility, gastroenteritis, and selected drugs such as the histamine receptor 2 (H_2) antagonist cimetidine (Tagamet). Decreased levels of iron can also occur as the result of molecular bonds between plasma stores of iron and certain drugs. These bonds develop during the distribution phase of pharmacokinetics, sequestering iron ions and decreasing the plasma pool available for integration into heme molecules. For example, the sulfonamides, such as cotrimoxazole and sulfamethoxazole-trimethoprim (Bactrim), can cause decreased plasma levels of iron.

Iron deficiency resulting from acute or chronic (occult) blood loss is perhaps the most prevalent cause of microcytic anemia. A net loss of blood depletes iron stores and impairs the bone marrow's ability to synthesize new RBCs, due to progressively decreased heme synthesis. Thus, RBCs are decreased not only in number, but also in size, producing a characteristic microcytic anemia. Common sites of bleeding (which may be either painless or painful) include the GI tract (e.g., upper tract lesions such as peptic ulcers or gastritis, lower tract lesions such as colon cancer, ulcerative colitis, Crohn's disease, diverticulosis, ruptured hemorrhoids) and the GU tract (e.g., heavy endometrial bleeding known as menorrhagia, hematuria from bladder cancer). In fact, microcytic anemia may be the first laboratory finding that initiates a line of investigation identifying underlying malignancy. For example, heme-positive stools or melena are strong indications for colonoscopic cancer screening in men and women older than 50 years or in younger individuals with a strong family history.

Anemia of Chronic Disease

Anemia of chronic disease (ACD) may cause microcytic or normocytic anemia. ACD as a cause of microcytic anemia results from mechanisms that involve inflammation, infection, and/or underlying malignancy. Inflammation may lead to occult and progressive blood loss, as microvascular eruptions result from histamine-release and immune complexes that physically invade the involved region. When these eruptions occur in the GI tract, occult blood escapes through the intestines. Thus, of particular concern is the relationship of occult blood in the stool to GI malignancy. Alternatively, chronic use of nonsteroidal anti-inflammatory drugs (NSAIDs), such as ibuprofen (Motrin, Advil) and aspirin, for chronic pain conditions must also be considered as a cause of occult blood loss. NSAIDs and aspirin are used in the routine management of both rheumatoid arthritis and osteoarthritis. Blood loss results from erosion of the protective mucosal lining of the stomach, in particular, due to decreased production of prostaglandin formed by the enzymes cyclooxygenase-1 and cyclooxygenase-2—the molecular targets inhibited by NSAIDs.

Thalassemias

The pathology of thalassemia is related either to depletion or mutation in the genes that code for the subunits of the protein component of adult hemoglobin—the alpha- and beta-globin chains. Alpha-thalassemia is caused by gene depletion that, in turn, creates a reduction of alpha-globin chain synthesis. Because two copies of the alpha-globin chain gene are inherited from each parent on chromosome 16, mutations or deletions may exist in one or more of these four genes, producing distinct clinical manifestations. Mutations or deletions in all four genes results in alpha (O)-thalassemia or alpha-thalassemia major. No hemoglobin A, A_2, or F can form in this disorder, which is incompatible with extrauterine life. Rather, there is an excess of Bart's hemoglobin, which consists of gamma chain tetramers (γ_4). Bart's hemoglobin has an oxygen affinity at least 10-fold greater than that of hemoglobin A, and thus cannot effectively release oxygen to fetal tissues. This causes severe anemia with resultant congestive heart failure, widespread capillary leak, and anasarca known as hydrops fetalis (widespread edema of all fetal tissues), typically with fetal demise by the third trimester of pregnancy.

Mutations in three of the four alpha genes results in hemoglobin H disease, characterized by the widespread formation of hemoglobin H which consists of a tetramer of four beta genes (β_4). This results in moderate to severe lifelong hemolytic anemia, which typically requires repeated blood transfusions. Mutations in only two of the four alpha genes is called alpha thalassemia minor or alpha-thalassemia-1 trait. This results in a mild anemia with only minor clinical manifestations. Mutation in one of the four alpha-globin genes is a silent carrier state called alpha-thalassemia minima or alpha-thalassemia-2 trait and can only be diagnosed through DNA analysis, because it has no clinical manifestations.

In contrast, only one gene for the beta-globin chain is inherited from each parent. Mutation or deletion of one of these genes results in beta-thalassemia minor or beta-thalassemia trait, characterized by a mild anemia that is typically asymptomatic. Deletions or severe mutations in both beta-globin genes result in beta-thalassemia major (Cooley's anemia), characterized by a severe, transfusion-dependent, lifelong anemia with skeletal abnormalities due to bone marrow expansion in attempts to increase hematopoiesis. An intermediate form of the disorder known as beta-thalassemia intermedia also exists in which a patient inherits two mutated, albeit expressed, beta-globin genes, each with a different type of mutation (a compound heterozygote) that results in varied levels of expression or functionality. Clinical manifestations may be worsened by acute illness or infection that impairs erythropoiesis and exacerbates the anemia.

Sideroblastic Anemias

Sideroblastosis and its resulting microcytic anemia are caused by a host of molecular defects that affect the biosynthesis of the heme moiety of hemoglobin. Heme is normally formed first by the creation of 5-aminolevulinic acid (ALA) from glycine and succinyl-coenzyme-A by the erythroid isoform of the mitochondrial enzyme ALA synthase, which requires vitamin B_6 (pyridoxine) as a cofactor. Although the underlying genetic defects in many forms of hereditary sideroblastic anemia have not been characterized, known mutations occur most commonly in the genes for the erythroid form of ALA synthase (located on the X chromosome), the mitochondrial transporter ABC7, pyridoxal 5-phosphate (a reversible form responsive to pyridoxine therapy), ferrochelatase, the copper-dependent enzyme cytochrome oxidase, and pseudouridine synthase-1.

In most forms of sideroblastic anemia, elemental iron is typically delivered appropriately to erythrocyte precursors. However, underlying enzymatic mutations prevent or reduce the ability of heme to incorporate into protoporphyrin IX. A reduced number of RBCs form from ring sideroblast precursors (a diagnostic hallmark) found in the bone marrow, as peripheral reticulocytosis is markedly diminished. Despite an increase in the RBC growth factor erythropoietin, anemia results from the destruction of the abnormal erythroid precursors in the bone marrow via apoptosis and intramedullary hemolysis.

Sideroblastic mutations result in excessive iron deposition in the mitochondria of affected erythrocytes (erythropoietic hemochromatosis) which, nonetheless, are hypochromic and microcytic because this form of mitochondrial ferritin cannot be utilized for cytoplasmic maturation in the developing erythrocyte. Intestinal iron absorption is actually increased in sideroblastic anemia owing to ineffective erythropoiesis, as is also observed in the thalassemias. Thus, iron overload occurs not only in erythroid cells, but throughout the body, similar to genetic (familial) hemochromatosis, with predictable end-organ damage due to iron deposition (e.g., cirrhosis [liver], cardiomyopathy [heart], and endocrine defects [pancreas and adrenals]).

Acquired forms of sideroblastic anemia also exist. The most common causes include chronic alcoholism which results in a multifactorial pathogenesis including many of the hypoproliferative mechanisms previously cited, iatrogenic associations with the antituberculous drug isoniazid and the antibiotic chloramphenicol, zinc toxicity in which zinc ions preferentially bind to protoporphyrin in place of iron, and copper deficiency which leads to decreased intestinal absorption of iron and diminished reduction of iron ions from the ferric (3+) state to the bioavailable ferrous (2+) form as a result of reduced cytochrome oxidase activity. Lead poisoning is also often cited as an acquired cause of sideroblastic anemia, as lead inhibits ALA synthase. However, true ring sideroblasts are typically not seen in the bone marrow, due to the inhibitory effect of lead inhibitory effect on iron transport to ferrochelatase, preventing its subsequent integration into heme. Idiopathic acquired sideroblastic anemia may also occur when a single erythroid progenitor cell develops a mutation affecting the heme synthesis pathway but is also conferred a survival advantage. As clonal proliferation of this precursor cell ensues, the bone marrow is largely replaced by this single sideroblastic lineage prone to apoptosis, resulting in a myelodysplastic anemia.

Clinical Presentation

Subjective

Overall, patients with microcytic anemia present with subjective findings of tachycardia, fatigue, shortness of breath, dyspnea on exertion, palpitations, listlessness, poor concentration, anorexia, and dizziness or lightheadedness. Because similar subjective findings are also associated with many diagnoses in addition to microcytic anemia, the history of subjective findings will not be conclusive.

Objective

As the hemoglobin drops below 10 g/dL (approximately 30 percent Hct), many patients present with a facial mask of fatigue, sallow-colored skin, pale mucous membranes, tachycardia, and tachypnea at rest. It is possible also to note a prolonged blanch response in the nailbeds (more than 3 seconds), although many patients may never present with this sign. Severe iron-deficiency anemia can cause progressive skin and mucosal changes, such as brittle nails, cheilosis (reddened appearance of lips with fissures formed at the angles), and a smooth appearance to the tongue. In addition, pica is considered an objective finding associated with severe iron deficiency. *Pica* is identified as an eating disorder of craving for food substitutes, such as clay, ice chips, and cotton.

Diagnostic Reasoning

Diagnostic Tests

Initial diagnostic testing is focused on obtaining a CBC, from which an RBC count and RBC indices (MCV, mean corpuscular hemoglobin [MCH], and mean corpuscular hemoglobin concentration [MCHC]) are isolated. A low RBC count, hemoglobin level, and/or Hct identify anemia (Table 16.1).

Secondary diagnostic testing for specific causes are listed below.

Iron-Deficiency Anemia. The diagnostic tests for iron-deficiency anemia are relatively simple to perform and are readily available. Serum ferritin is a reliable test of low stores of iron as long as the patient does not have advanced liver disease. A serum ferritin value of less than 30 mg/L is considered pathological. As the ferritin level falls, the total iron-binding capacity (TIBC) rises above the normal range. If the drop in ferritin and rise in TIBC continue untreated, the serum iron level will also fall (to less than 30 mg/L) as will the transferrin saturation (to less than 15 percent). In addition, secondary testing should focus on results of RBC morphology from the CBC. Findings such as anisocytosis (variable RBC size), poikilocytosis (variable RBC shape), and hypochromasia (pale-colored RBCs) are revealed when samples severely deficient in iron are evaluated under the microscope.

Anemia of Chronic Disease. Diagnostic tests for ACD focus on distinguishing ACD from iron-deficiency anemia. Unlike iron-deficiency anemia, ACD presents with a low serum iron level, along with a low TIBC. In addition, the serum transferrin level is either normal or increased in patients with ACD. Finally, the clinician should expect the transferrin saturation to be low, as it is in iron-deficiency anemia.

Thalassemias. The thalassemias, both alpha- and beta-thalassemia, require a CBC and hemoglobin electrophoresis for diagnosis. The CBC is essential to determine the diagnosis of microcytic anemia, and the MCV is low for each group of the thalassemias. In alpha-thalassemia trait, the hemoglobin electrophoresis reveals no increase in hemoglobin A_2 and fetal hemoglobin (F). In addition, no hemoglobin H is present. Plasma iron parameters remain normal. The anemia of alpha-thalassemia is modest, as evidenced by a hematocrit between 27 to 40 percent.

Beta-thalassemia minor patients also have a modest anemia. In these patients, unlike those with alpha-thalassemia trait, hemoglobin electrophoresis reveals an elevated hemoglobin A_2 level and, in some cases, an elevated hemoglobin F. Neither hemoglobin elevation will be greater than 9 percent.

Patients with beta-thalassemia major are very different from the others. Their anemia is severe. Left untreated, their hematocrits will fall to less than 10 percent. Electrophoresis results show little or no hemoglobin A, with variable amounts of hemoglobin A_2 present. The clinician should expect hemoglobin F to be the primary hemoglobin that is detectable in these patients. As with all of the thalassemias, findings in patients with beta-thalassemia will include abnormal RBC morphology such as poikilocytosis, anisocytosis, and related presentations.

Sideroblastic Anemia. A diagnosis of sideroblastic anemia is confirmed by a Prussian blue stain of a bone marrow aspirate. The Prussian blue stain reveals tinged sideroblasts, which have iron deposits located in the mitochondrion that surrounds the red cell's nucleus. In addition, erythroid hyperplasia is present in the aspirate from patients with sideroblastic anemia. A high level of serum iron and a high serum transferrin saturation should accompany these findings. Without a stain of the bone marrow aspirate, the diagnosis could mimic iron-deficiency anemia, with a moderately low Hct of 20 to 30 percent and a low MCV.

Differential Diagnosis

The differential diagnosis depends on the blood work results. For microcytic anemia, it may be summarized by reference to its four causes: iron-deficiency anemia, ACD, thalassemias, and sideroblastic anemia. The goal is to identify the underlying cause of the microcytic anemia, such as GI malignancy, blood loss, menorrhagia, and so forth.

Management

The management of microcytic anemia focuses on treating and eradicating the cause of the anemia. If amelioration of the cause is impossible, then symptomatic care alone is indicated.

The severity of the anemia will direct the intervention. The decision to transfuse a patient with red blood cells is a major clinical step that may be indicated if the HCT is 27 percent or less. The decision requires a thoughtful analysis of the hemodynamic status of the patient, which may not be severely compromised, even at low Hgb levels. Transfusing patients with comorbidities such as CHF calls for great caution (given risks of fluid overload and output heart failure), and the risk of iron overload must be carefully considered.

Iron-Deficiency Anemia

Iron-deficiency anemia is treated first with an increase in dietary iron and thereafter with supplemental iron. Foods rich in iron should be prescribed, such as animal proteins, legumes, and dark-green leafy vegetables, such as spinach. Diet alone may be useful in treating iron deficiency if the patient is either young or middle-aged or the cause of the anemia is short-lived. However, as the patient ages (particularly beyond age 65) and if the cause of the anemia is chronic, then iron deficiency must be treated with either supplemental oral or parenteral iron.

Supplemental oral iron is best given as ferrous sulfate, 325 mg tid; 10 to 20 mg will be absorbed from the total daily regimen if the serum iron is moderately low. In more severe cases, however, the level of absorption will increase. The clinician should recheck the indices of anemia and iron values 2 to 4 weeks after starting the regimen to ascertain the effectiveness of the oral regimen. The patient's adherence to the regimen could be complicated by the requirement that the supplement be taken on an empty stomach to achieve maximal absorption. Therefore, if no measured improvement in anemia (hematocrit elevated by one-half of baseline), MCV, and iron stores appears after 1 month of therapy, the clinician should question adherence to the regimen along with the underlying cause of the iron deficiency. The patient should continue to take supplemental iron for 3 to 6 months after normal levels in the blood and serum indices have been restored. Thereafter, the clinician should recheck laboratory values as indicated by the clinical assessment. If the patient does not respond to supplemental iron, then the clinician should doubt the initial diagnosis of iron-deficiency anemia. In particular, ACD should be suspected as the cause or reconsider whether the rate of GI blood loss might exceed stem-cell deployment from the bone marrow.

Supplemental iron by a parenteral route is indicated only when there is documented failure to therapy with oral iron supplements. The clinician should calculate the daily dose by subtracting the patient's measured MCV from the normal lower range value (which varies by age and gender). This value is considered the total number of milligrams of iron to add according to the MCV. In addition, the clinician must add 1000 mg to the delivered dose to cover the storage of iron in the body. Overall, the daily dosage of supplemental parenteral iron is approximately 1300 to 2000 mg (1.3 to 2.0 g) of iron. The preferred route of administration is IV. Because anaphylaxis is possible with IV iron, the initial dose should be delivered over 4 to 6 hours to prevent adverse effects; some practitioners even advocate giving 50 mg over the first hour as a trial.

Anemia of Chronic Disease

ACD is treated symptomatically. Red blood cell transfusions may become necessary when the Hct falls below 27 to 30 percent. In most cases, however, the Hct will stay above 30 percent. Chronic ACD might require treatment with drugs that stimulate erythropoesis given subcutaneously. Typical ACD causes that require this are chronic renal failure and HIV infection or acquired immunodeficiency syndrome (AIDS). The dosage varies according to patient tolerance and hematological requirements. Darbepoetin (Aranesp) may be given weekly initially then adjusted to every-2-week dosing. Erythropoietin (Epogen, Procrit) is given three times weekly, then adjusted. The patient can learn to self-inject these meds, just as the diabetic learns to self-inject insulin.

Thalassemia

The thalassemias often require no treatment other than vigilance by the clinician concerning hematological markers. If a clinician diagnoses microcytosis with mild anemia, the patient should not be subjected to further and repeated checks for iron deficiency if the cause is something else. Vigilance is all that is required for microcytosis with mild anemia.

Patients with severe anemia, such as is associated with beta-thalassemia major and hemoglobin H disease require regular transfusion with RBCs. In addition, these patients require folate supplementation and possibly oral iron chelation therapy to prevent hemosiderosis and hemochromatosis. Hemosiderosis of chronic standing may also require referral for a splenectomy.

Sideroblastic Anemia

There are few options for treatment of sideroblastosis. Depending on the severity of anemia, RBC transfusions may be required. Large doses (200 mg/day) of vitamin B_6 (pyridoxine, e.g., Beesix) have benefited some patients. Erythropoietin-alpha (Epogen) has proved to be of little aid in supporting these patients.

Follow-Up and Referral

Iron-deficiency anemia that is mild necessitates follow-up every 4 to 6 months. There should be no need to retest iron stores after the first follow-up visit following initial diagnosis, unless indicated by the history and physical examination. Thereafter, testing should consist of a CBC. A referral may be necessary if a thorough work-up has been completed that may identify serious pathology that could account for iron-deficiency anemia, such as GI malignancy or other type of occult blood loss. These patients may require upper and/or lower endoscopy or other type of work-up to exclude serious pathology. Anyone 50 years or older with heme positive stools or evidence of iron-deficiency anemia should be referred for a colonoscopy, unless the risks of colonoscopy outweigh the potential benefits of catching a GI cancer early—such as in elderly patients in whom the risk of perforation is greater and could prove fatal.

In general, the plan of referral for microcytic anemia should go the course of isolating the cause of the anemia, followed by initial treatment in primary care. The clinician, therefore, has the responsibility to perform all screening tests and to seek to diagnose the cause. In particular, referral for iron-deficiency anemia is almost never required unless it is complicated by concurrent diagnoses, including other causes of microcytic anemia.

ACD follow-up can be more complicated than follow-up of iron-deficiency anemia. If the patient requires erythropoietin-alpha injections, then he or she should be maintained on a 30-day follow-up for the first 6 months after initiating therapy. In most cases only a CBC will be required to determine the effectiveness of this therapy. It is exceptional for patients with ACD to require transfusions. The clinician should refer patients with ACD to gastroenterologists and/or hepatologists, oncologists, rheumatologists, or hematologists depending on the suspected pathology of the disease. For example, if the clinician were to detect occult blood in the stool of a patient with microcytic anemia and the history did not contribute a probable cause, then a referral to a gastroenterologist would be warranted.

Once one of the less aggressive thalassemias (alpha- or beta-minor) has been diagnosed, it may only be necessary to monitor the patient's CBC every 3 to 4 months. More frequent observation and intervention is required for the other types of thalassemias, which require transfusions as therapy. The plan of care established by the hematologist will dictate the follow-up schedule.

Patients diagnosed with one of the thalassemias may or may not require referral to a hematologist. Although patients with the more aggressive thalassemias (such as beta-thalassemia major and hemoglobin H disease) must be referred promptly to a hematologist, who will be entrusted with managing the plan of care, patients with alpha-thalassemia and beta-thalassemia minor may be managed by the clinician.

Because sideroblastosis is diagnosed by examination of a bone marrow aspirate, early referral to a hematologist is required. The hematologist may also perform tests to determine lead exposure and lead damage. Follow-up evaluation will become the responsibility of the clinician, however. The CBCs of these patients should be monitored every 2 to 3 months.

Patient Education

Education should focus on self-care and primary care management of the underlying cause of microcytic anemia. Self-care encompasses topics such as drug regimen, dietary changes, level of activity, self-monitoring for signs and symptoms of anemia, and adjustment to requirements that new health-related practices may determine. For example, patients with iron-deficiency anemia must be educated to perform the following self-care behaviors: (1) take ferrous sulfate (supplemental iron) on an empty stomach or at the most with a small snack; (2) eat foods that are rich in iron, vitamin C, and B-complex vitamins, the ingredients for building RBCs; (3) remain as active as can be, and if fatigued, rest before resuming activity; (4) self-monitor for fatigue, shortness of breath, pale-colored stools (before supplemental iron) and palpitations or tachycardia; and (5) share information about iron deficiency so that friends and/or family can assist in adjustments that new health-related behaviors will require.

Additional patient education focuses on primary care management. Patients need to understand the importance of timely clinical laboratory evaluations, return visits, signs and symptoms of anemia that should be reported to the clinician, and proper technique for administering or receiving drugs that must be delivered via a parenteral route, such as erythropoietin-alpha. Most important for patients with severe anemia is the necessity to remain vigilant in receiving transfusions.

Normocytic Anemia

Normocytic anemia is defined as an anemia associated with normally sized RBCs (MCV = 81 to 99 fL), although the ranges of normal vary with age. Many forms of normocytic anemia have normally shaped RBCs as well, although some conditions are recognized by typical morphologic findings on peripheral blood smear. Most commonly, this type of anemia results from chronic disease states, but acute blood loss, hemolysis, and volume overload are other important etiologies of normocytic anemia.

Epidemiology and Causes

Normocytic anemias cover a broad range of diseases and conditions, each with its own epidemiology and prevalence rate. Nonetheless, it is possible to estimate the incidence of normocytic ACD by recognizing that at least half of all patients with underlying chronic disease will develop normocytic anemia over the course of their illness

Pathophysiology

Most chronic diseases create mechanisms that reduce the life cycle of erythrocytes. In addition, chronic diseases may also be myelosuppressive. As discussed earlier, ACD may be microcytic. However, the combination of reduced cell life and impaired stem cell production (hypoproliferation) associated with chronic illness typically results in a normocytic, normochromic anemia. This may be related to a variety of different underlying conditions including infection, inflammation, autoimmune activation, malignancy (with or without marrow invasion), cardiac disease, diabetes mellitus, endocrine disorders (e.g., hypothyroidism, hypoadrenalism, hypopituitarism, hypogonadism), acute renal insufficiency (due to the accumulation of uremic metabolites that decrease RBC lifespan), and chronic renal insufficiency (due to impaired erythropoietin synthesis). Severe trauma, surgery, or major acute disease states such as sepsis and myocardial infarction may result in a similar form of anemia, possibly due to the significant tissue damage and inflammatory response associated with these events.

Hypoproliferation appears to be the major contributing factor to normocytic ACD, resulting primarily from iron sequestration in bone marrow macrophages which effectively decreases the plasma iron pool available for integration into newly synthesized hemoglobin molecules. In addition, patients with ACD are less capable of adequate erythropoietin upregulation in response to their anemic state, as compared to patients with non–iron-sequestering anemias (e.g., iron-deficiency anemia). Moreover, although absolute erythropoietin levels may be increased in ACD compared to non-anemic normal values, the bone marrow demonstrates no erythropoietic response to this growth factor. Animal studies have shown that certain inflammatory cytokines including tumor necrosis factor, interferon (IFN)-β, and IFN-γ may underlie these mechanisms of hypoproliferation in normocytic ACD. In addition, expression of the acute phase reactant protein hepcidin is also increased in ACD. Upregulated by the proinflammatory cytokine IL-6, hepcidin has been shown in animal models to directly inhibit iron absorption by the gut, resulting in decreased plasma iron levels.

Acquired aplastic anemia also results in a normocytic anemia. This may be a primary condition affecting only the erythroid lineage or it may encompass more than one cell line (e.g., WBC or platelet), which would indicate a proliferative defect in an earlier common progenitor cell that gives rise to more than one bone marrow lineage. Aplastic anemia may also be associated with certain types of viral infections in high-risk individuals, such as parvovirus B19 infection in patients with sickle cell disease or hereditary spherocytosis. A failure of erythropoietin production by the kidneys, as is also observed in chronic renal insufficiency, will similarly result in reduced RBC production and decreased reticulocytosis.

Normocytic anemia may also be caused by a relative increase in plasma volume, such as occurs in pregnancy or iatrogenic parenteral overhydration. This results in a dilutional drop in plasma hemoglobin, which may be considered physiologic, as in pregnancy, or which may be reversible via pharmacologic diuresis, as in the case of fluid overload.

Increased blood loss, such as from acute bleeding or hemolysis, is another major cause of normocytic anemia. As bleeding progresses and the marrow undergoes a reticulocytosis, MCV may be transiently increased due to the relatively larger size of reticulocytes. However, once plasma and bone marrow iron stores are exhausted, hemoglobin production decreases, and this anemia transitions into a microcytic anemia characteristic of iron-deficiency anemia.

If hemolysis occurs intravascularly, fragmented RBCs termed schistocytes are seen on peripheral blood smear. This type of anemia is most commonly associated with hemolytic uremic syndrome (HUS), thrombotic thrombocytopenic purpura (TTP), disseminated intravascular coagulation (DIC), or heart valve abnormalities which cause mechanical RBC shearing. Hemolysis may also occur extravascularly with clearance of RBCs by the reticuloendothelial system. This is characterized by rounded RBCs termed spherocytes on peripheral blood smear and occurs most commonly due to splenic removal of RBCs, as seen in hypersplenism or autoimmune hemolytic anemia (AIHA).

Immune-mediated hemolysis typically occurs when RBC-specific antibodies coat erythrocytes, rendering them prone to splenic removal or direct hemolysis by antibody-mediated complement fixation. RBC-specific antibodies may form as a consequence of antibody upregulation from viral infections such as mononucleosis, malignancies (especially chronic lymphocytic leukemia), or autoimmune disorders such as systemic lupus erythematosus. When these antibodies are primarily of the IgG class, they are known as warm agglutinins, since they result in RBC aggregation (agglutination) at warmer temperatures, due to he binding of two RBCs at a time (one to each of the IgG molecule's two antigen-binding sites). In contrast, IgM RBC-specific antibodies, such as those associated with *Mycoplasma* infection, are termed cold agglutinins, as they are capable of causing RBC aggregation at relatively lower temperatures, by virtue of a greater number of antigen-binding and complement fixation sites which results from their tendency to cluster in pentamers (i.e., aggregates of five IgM molecules with a total of 10 antigen-specific binding sites).

Extravascular hemolysis may also result from a whole host of intrinsic RBC membrane defects, such as mutations in the membrane protein spectrin which causes hereditary spherocytosis. In addition, mutations in certain cytoplasmic enzymes render RBCs more prone to hemolysis. A prime example are disorders of glucose-6-phosphate dehydrogenase (G-6-PD), an enzyme critical to the production of glutathione, a powerful reducing agent and the RBC's main protective mechanism against highly oxidizing compounds such as naphthalene (the active chemical agent found in mothballs) or certain drugs such as trimethoprim-sulfamethoxazole (Bactrim), primaquine, and dapsone.

Clinical Presentation

Subjective

The patient presentation will depend on the severity of the anemia. Because normocytic anemia rarely presents with a moderate to severe anemia (less than 30 percent Hct), many patients with the diagnosis do not report subjective findings. Upon closer questioning, however, they might note malaise or fatigue.

Objective

The objective findings are the same as for microcytic anemia.

Diagnostic Reasoning

Diagnostic Tests

Initial testing begins with the CBC. The clinician should expect the finding of anemia not to be accompanied by an alteration in the RBC indices (MCV, Hct, MCHC). In particular, the RBC indices should be within normal limits to establish a diagnosis of normocytic anemia.

Subsequent testing begins with an absolute reticulocyte count (normal range for adults is 0.5 to 2.5 percent of the total RBC count). Reticulocytes are the less mature type of RBCs. They acquire their name from their fine cytoplasmic network, which is called a *reticulum;* this network appears when stained. The reticulum is lost as the RBC matures. The reticulocyte count is always higher than normal in any proliferative condition (proliferative normocytic anemia), but the MCV may be normal in a microcytic anemia with a reticulocytosis, since the average (mean) RBC size may appear normal in the face of both small and large cells. If the count is low, the diagnosis is proliferative microcytic anemia. Additional testing must focus next on thrombocyte and leukocyte counts.

Of the two disorders, proliferative microcytic anemia is far more complex to differentiate in subsequent testing. If the cause of the RBC cell size is hemorrhage, as is the case after trauma, then the diagnosis is probably proliferative microcytic anemia secondary to hemorrhage. However, when no hemorrhage is part of the clinical picture, the attention should turn to diagnosing the cause of hemolysis.

Testing of hemolysis requires a peripheral smear. Based on the morphology of RBCs in a peripheral smear, it is possible to better determine the cause of the hemolysis. Possible morphologic changes include spherocytes, sickle cells, and schistocytes. Spherocytes are erythrocytes shaped like spheres or globes, which are abnormal shapes for an erythrocyte. Sickle cells assume the shape of a quarter moon or the curved metal blade instrument known as the sickle, from which erythrocytes having this shape take their name. Schistocytes are the third type of RBC. The classic term for schistocytes is "fragmented." Schistocytes, therefore, are RBCs that are divided into many and varied shapes.

Although the peripheral smear may reveal morphologic changes in RBCs, the shape of the RBCs may be normal in some patients with hemolysis. Should this be the case, it will then be necessary to check for the enzyme glucose-6-phosphate dehydrogenase (G-6-PD). A low level of G-6-PD in the absence of morphologic changes in the peripheral smear indicates the lack of this enzyme as the cause for the hemolysis.

Should the G-6-PD level be within normal limits, especially when the patient reports voiding dark-red urine in the morning, then it is necessary to consider the Ham acidified serum lysis test. The dark-red urine should raise suspicion that the diagnosis may be paroxysmal nocturnal hemoglobinuria (PNH); the Ham acidified serum lysis test will provide a definitive diagnosis.

G-6-PD levels measured during an acute attack of hemolytic anemia may be artificially elevated due to the relatively higher concentration of G-6-PD found in reticulocytes, which will be upregulated. Thus, serum levels are often normal, and diagnosis must be confirmed by re-drawing levels several weeks after the acute anemia has resolved.

Further testing will be required if spherocytes and schistocytes are isolated in the peripheral smear. The presence of sickle cells on the smear implies a sickle cell diagnosis or one of its variants, such as sickle beta thalassemia, or sickle C disease. The presence of spherocytes necessitates obtaining a Coombs' test. A positive Coombs' test indicates autoimmune hemolytic anemia (AIHA), and a negative test suggests hereditary spherocytosis.

Schistocytes require the clinician to order a prothrombin time (PT) and partial thromboplastin time (PTT). An elevated PT/PTT may reflect disseminated intravascular coagulation (DIC), but only if there is also a thrombocytopenia, as platelet consumption from widespread thrombi/microthrombi is characteristic of this disorder. This results in the characteristic (and often treatment refractory) bleeding and/or oozing seen with the disorder. A normal PT/PTT suggests any one of several diagnoses, including severe hypertension, hemolytic uremic syndrome/thrombotic thrombocytopenic purpura (HUS/TTP), heart valve abnormalities (such as mitral valve stenosis), vasculitis, and hemolysis, elevated liver enzymes, and low platelet count syndrome (HELLP). HELLP is typically associated with pregnancy, especially later-term pregnancies, and often delivery of the baby is the primary intervention.

In patients diagnosed with a hypoproliferative normocytic anemia based on a low result from the absolute reticulocyte count, attention should turn to the white blood cell (WBC) count and platelet count. If both are low, the clinician should suspect pancytopenia. If the WBC and thrombocyte counts are high, then either ACD or renal disease is causing the normocytic anemia. Subsequent tests, therefore, involve renal function studies (e.g., blood urea nitrogen [BUN] and creatinine) and a careful review of the history. Assessing endogenous erythropoietin levels is an important part of this work-up as well.

Differential Diagnosis

The differential for normocytic anemia includes anemias of other classifications. Differentiation should be made between the three mechanisms: deficiency (iron, vitamin B_{12}, folic acid, pyridoxine); central—caused by impaired bone marrow function (anemia of chronic disease, anemia of the elderly, malignant blood disorders); and peripheral (bleeding and hemolysis). Mixed anemias may look normocytic because the MCV is within normal range, even though iron deficient RBCs may be small and vitamin B_{12} or folate deficient RBCs are megaloblastic.

Because ACD is part of the differential for microcytic anemia as well as normocytic anemia, the clinician must distinguish between the RBC indices of the two.

Management

Management of normocytic anemia focuses on the cause for the disorder. Causes of normocytic anemia include ACD, renal disease, pancytopenia, hereditary spherocytosis, AIHA, sickle cell anemia, G-6-PD deficiency, paroxysmal nocturnal hemoglobinuria (PNH), DIC, heart valve abnormalities, HUS/TTP, vasculitis, severe hypertensive nephropathy, and HELLP.

Treatment is defined by the cause of the anemia. In the initial phase of management, treatment should be symptomatic, thereby alleviating the untoward effects of anemia, however unlikely they might be. Subsequent management consists of correcting, stabilizing, or preventing the cause for normocytic anemia. Correcting and/or stabilizing the underlying cause is limited to some cases of ACD, AIHA, heart valve abnormalities, vasculitis, severe hypertension, HELLP, and DIC.

Management of ACD usually requires only watchful waiting; however, if the patient's Hct drops below 30 percent, the clinician should consider using erythropoietin-alpha. With adult patients, the dose of erythropoietin-alpha should start at 3000 units SC three times per week. For the first 3 weeks of therapy, the clinician should check the Hct twice weekly until the dosage level is stabilized. Two to 6 weeks may pass before the Hct undergoes an appreciable elevation.

Toxic levels have not been established for erythropoietin-alpha; therefore, the clinician may increase the dosage and frequency of administration until the Hct rises. As the dosage level rises, however, it is possible that polycythemia (HCT greater than 60 to 65 percent) may develop as a side effect of exogenous erythropoietin usage. If the patient becomes polycythemic, then the drug should be discontinued. Within a week, the Hct should start to decline. Otherwise, in rare cases, it may be necessary to phlebotomize the patient, removing enough volume to cause a drop in the Hct. After the clinician achieves and maintains a normal Hct, the dosage level may be reduced and/or the frequency of administration changed.

The treatment of autoimmune hemolytic anemia (AIHA) consists of prednisone (1 to 2 mg/kg per day) in divided doses. Thus, an adult who weighs 70 kg would receive between 70 and 140 mg of prednisone in two or three divided doses each day. If transfusion is required for severe anemia, the clinician should note that the risk of transfusion reaction is very high owing to cross-match difficulties for these patients and any with a positive Coombs' test. The clinician should expect that the transfused cells will survive no better than the patient's own erythrocytes. Surgical consultation is required for possible splenectomy should prednisone become ineffective or the dosage level remain too high for chronic administration. In emergency situations, short-term hemolytic control of 1 to 3 weeks may be achieved with IV immune globulin (500 mg/kg per day for 1 to 4 days).

Heart valve abnormalities require treatment that is individualized to the problem. Interventional cardiology referral is indicated. The cardiologist will establish the plan of care, which may include surgical correction of the abnormality. Many patients with heart valve abnormalities will have already started taking warfarin sodium (Coumadin) to prevent embolism formation. They should not stop taking the drug unless their platelet counts fall along with the Hct. or active bleeding is present. Even if the platelet counts do not fall along with the Hgb, anticoagulation may be stopped in the face of a rapidly falling Hgb.

Treatment of vasculitis consists of high-dose prednisone. It may be necessary to raise the prednisone dose to 60 mg daily. The clinician should slowly taper the dose as the lesions of vasculitis heal, fever declines, and other symptoms abate. Additional immunosuppressive therapy may also be required to augment the prednisone. Cyclophosphamide (Cytoxan) in a dosage range of 1 to 2 mg/kg per day is then added to the prednisone regimen. If the dosage exceeds 100 mg, the clinician can anticipate that only 75 percent of the dose will be absorbed via the GI tract. Therefore, in doses that exceed 100 mg, the dose should be split. Weekly or biweekly monitoring of the patient's CBC, liver and renal function tests, and uric acid level are necessary. The drug should be taken either along with or following a meal to avoid GI upset.

Severe hypertension (greater than 180 mm Hg systolic and 110 mm Hg diastolic) can be treated with one antihypertensive agent or a combination of agents. Typically, hemolysis that is secondary to severe hypertension will present in a patient that is known to the clinician. Therefore, drug therapy should be adjusted according to the history of treatment for the individual patient. (See the section on management of HTN in Chapter 9.)

HELLP occurs during the third trimester of pregnancy. Because of its late onset in pregnancy, premature delivery of the infant is the treatment of choice. Most hematologic indices return to baseline within 2 to 3 days after delivery; however, thrombocytopenia may persist for a week or more.

DIC requires treatment with heparin and platelet transfusions (replacement therapy). Platelet transfusion parameters run as low as greater than 20 to minimize the risk of spontaneous bleeding or greater than 50 with active bleeding or higher in anticipation of invasive procedures. Platelet transfusions, however, are often futile because of severe consumptive coagulopathy.

Although the role of heparin is controversial, especially preceding or following surgery, heparin is mandated if thrombus is diagnosed in DIC. In addition, fresh frozen plazma (FFP) is an important therapy in DIC. It is often used empirically, rather than waiting for tests that specifically confirm deficits in certain clotting factors. Before symptoms are present, anti-coagultion in the form of low molecular weight heparin such as enoxaparin (Lovenox) is a well accepted therapy for patients at risk of post-operative DVT, provided renal function is normal (because LMWH is renally cleared). There are also recombinant versions of certain human clotting factors such as factor VIII available for use with significant bleeding disorders.

Because patients who require heparin therapy for DIC require around-the-clock nursing care, they should be admitted to a hospital, where they can receive 500 to 750 units/h of heparin. Platelet transfusions should be used to maintain the thrombocyte count. In addition, cryoprecipitate should be given to raise the fibrinogen level to 150 mg/dL.

Prevention of hemolysis caused by low levels of G-6-PD is preferred to treating hemolysis; however, the clinician must understand both prevention and treatment of hemolysis resulting from G-6-PD deficiency. Avoidance of oxidant drugs, such as dapsone (Avlosulfon), quinidine (Quinaglute Dura-tabs), and the sulfonamides (e.g., sulfamethoxazole/trimethoprim) will prevent hemolysis in patients who are G-6-PD deficient. Treatment consists of discontinuing any and all oxidant drugs, increasing oral and/or IV fluids, and transfusions of erythrocytes as indicated by the Hct level. Screening for G-6-PD among patients who may require one or more oxidant drugs has become standard in the management of patients with HIV/AIDS (treatment and prophylaxis for *Pneumocystis jiroveci* pneumonia) and elderly women who are more susceptible to UTIs.

Follow-Up and Referral

If normocytic anemia is not accompanied by a low or elevated reticulocyte count, then follow-up every 6 months is sufficient for most patients. Follow-up should consist of a history and physical examination, along with obtaining a CBC and reticulocyte count. The patient's records should be constructed so that these values are readily retrievable. No referral is required for these patients.

If the peripheral smear is positive for spherocytes, sickle cells, or schistocytes, the clinician should refer the patient to a hematologist. The hematologist will create a plan of care, which the clinician can comanage. Routine follow-up with the hematologist should occur every 3 to 6 months, depending on the severity and chronicity of the hemolysis.

If the reticulocyte count is low and the clinician discovers a low WBC and platelet count, the patient is diagnosed as pancytopenic. A referral to a hematologist is indicated. If the evaluation of bone marrow aspirate suggests a need for treatment, then the hematologist will determine the plan of care. Normal or high WBC and platelet counts indicate referrals to specialists who will treat the cause for ACD and renal disease. These include gastroenterologists, hepatologists, rheumatologists, infectious disease specialists, nephrologists, and cardiologists.

Patient Education

Education should follow the pattern outlined in the section on microcytic anemia; thus, education should address self-care regimens, and primary care management.

Self-care of normocytic anemia is similar to that for other anemias. The patient should be instructed to remain as active as possible, and, if he or she becomes fatigued, to rest. In addition, the patient must remain vigilant for the signs and symptoms of a declining Hct—malaise, fatigue, shortness of breath, tachycardia, and palpitations. If a deficiency in G-6-PD is diagnosed, the patient should be made aware of it and all drugs that must be avoided.

Patient education concerning primary care management addresses topics that are part of the cause for the normocytic anemia. Because of the chronicity of several of the causes of normocytic anemia, patients must be instructed at every visit to adhere to treatment regimens, including laboratory testing. For example, sickle cell disease patients require frequent follow-up, infectious disease prophylaxis, and assistance from their families during crises. Establishing a plan for the management of sickle cell crisis, then, is a good idea in anticipation of an event. The following section on sickle cell anemia includes a discussion of sickle cell crisis management.

Sickle Cell Anemia

Sickle cell anemia is an autosomal–recessive disorder. The disease is caused by a point mutation in the DNA sequence of the gene for the beta-hemoglobin chain (termed the hemoglobin S gene), resulting in a marked hemoglobinopathy in which intracellular hemoglobin molecules form abnormal polymers that lead to gross sickling of RBCs under hypoxic conditions. It is therefore diagnosed by the detection of sickled (scythe-shaped) cells on peripheral blood smear, a positive familial history, recurrent painful episodes of vaso-occlusive pain, and a dominant pattern of mutated hemoglobin S on an electrophoresis profile.

Epidemiology and Causes

Sickle cell anemia and sickle cell trait are inherited conditions. For the most part, they are found among people of West African descent. The disease has also been identified in persons of sole European or Middle Eastern ancestry, although these cases are considered anomalies and are extremely rare. The disease is not prevalent among persons of Asian or Pacific Island descent.

Initial symptoms appear within the first year of life for those born with sickle cell anemia. Given the perinatal manifestations and associated comorbidities, prenatal screening is now available for at-risk couples, consisting of DNA analysis from fetal cells. The procedure should be offered to these couples as part of their prenatal counseling. If both the father and mother have sickle cell trait and each carry one copy of the mutated hemoglobin S gene, their offspring have a 1 in 4 chance of developing true homozygous sickle cell anemia. In more than 40 states, newborns undergo universal neonatal screening for hemoglobinopathies, including hemoglobin protein electrophoresis screening for sickle cell disease, the thalassemias, and variant hemoglobinopathies.

Autosomal recessive genes for hemoglobin S are equally distributed between both sexes. Individuals who are homozygous for the hemoglobin S gene will develop sickle cell anemia, which means that they will spend their lives living with sickle cell crises and will die, on average, between 40 and 50 years of age. Those who are heterozygous for the hemoglobin S gene are said to carry sickle cell trait, which is asymptomatic since hemoglobin A accounts for more than half their hemoglobin. About 8 to 10 percent of persons of West African descent in the United States carry the sickle cell trait. One in 400 to 500 West African descendants suffer from sickle cell anemia, while up to 2 percent of African-Americans are affected.

Pathophysiology

The cause of sickle cell anemia is a point mutation in the genetic sequence of the beta chain gene of hemoglobin which results in the replacement of glutamic acid by valine at the N-terminal amino acid position 6 of this protein chain. The substitution of valine leads to the production of hemoglobin S, which is poorly soluble and prone to rigid polymerization when in its deoxygenated state. This typically occurs under conditions of physiologic stress, such as physical overexertion, muscle tissue ischemia causing lactic acidosis, dehydration, infection, or exposure to cold environmental temperatures. However, the majority of acute sickling events have no identifiable cause.

Polymerized deoxyhemoglobin S takes on a rope-like form, aligning itself with other polymerized strands and transforming erythrocytes into a rigid, sickled, crescent-like shape. In turn, these sickled erythrocytes regularly become lodged in the microvasculature of various organs and bodily tissues, causing small but highly symptomatic infarcts throughout the body. Sickled cells rigidly adhere to the inner membranes lining small blood vessels, inducing intimal hyperplasia which contributes to the obstruction of free blood flow in the smaller capillaries, as well as inducing RBC hemolysis due to this adherence to the inner vessel wall. RBCs in patients with sickle cell disease have an average lifespan of 17 days, versus the normal length of 100 days.

Sickled cells become lodged in the microvasculature as small thrombi. Once the thrombi are situated against the vascular membrane, they attract plasma proteins, leukocytes, and platelets, creating an occlusion to blood flow. The inflammatory process escalates as ischemia to the surrounding tissue unfolds. Ischemic injury and infarcts cause pain as perimeter tissue is increasingly starved for oxygen and other nutrients. The cascade or rate of sickling increases its pace as tissues become more hypoxic and acidotic. Erythrocytes, with or without hemoglobin S, that are lodged in and around the microthrombus lose intracellular water, which results either in hemolysis occurring prior to RBC sickling or in escalated sickle cell formation and plasma hyperviscosity. As hypoxia and acidosis increase, more erythrocytes begin to sickle, and nearly all sickled cells in the area of the thrombus will eventually hemolyze.

The body attempts to compensate for this resultant anemia (which is typically normocytic, unless associated with iron deficiency or a form of thalassemia) with expansion and upregulation of the bone marrow. This has several pathologic implications. Chronically elevated WBC counts result in the production of inflammatory cytokines which further complicate vaso-occlusive crises. The additional blood flow also leads to cardiomegaly and eventual high-output congestive heart failure. This results in greater metabolic and caloric requirements as the affected individual ages, leading to stunted growth and lower than average adult weight if the condition is poorly controlled and nutritional needs are not met with dietary supplements.

Anemia is also worsened by impaired production of the RBC growth factor erythropoietin (which is normally produced in the kidney), owing to the presence of progressive renal disease from microinfarction of the vasa recta capillaries in the renal medulla. Hemolysis results in hyperbilirubinemia which predisposes to the development of pigmented cholelithiasis (gallstones). In turn, cholecystectomy is the most common surgical procedure in sickle cell patients.

The formation of microthrombi occurs in many parts of the body but is especially prone to occur in the chest, vertebrae, and long bones of the legs. In pediatric patients, swelling, tenderness, and inflammation of the hands and feet (especially the fingers) termed dactylitis (hand–foot syndrome) is a common manifestation before the age of 2 years. Leg ulcers are also common among affected patients, typically affecting the skin over the lateral and medial malleoli and subject to infection by *Staphylococcus aureus*, *Pseudomonas*, *Streptococcus* species, or *Bacteroides*. Bone manifestations also occur. As ischemia progresses due to vaso-occlusion, the affected bone eventually infarcts and becomes susceptible to osteomyelitis by *Salmonella* species and, less commonly, *Staphylococcus aureus*. Severely debilitating noninfectious asceptic necrosis of the hip or shoulder joints may also occur due to vaso-occlusion of the arterial supply to the femoral or humeral heads, resulting in eventual loss of the entire joint.

Organs such as the heart, liver, penis, and kidney also tend to be affected by vaso-occlusive crises, particularly during childhood and adolescent years. Priapism (painful and sustained penile erection often lasting several hours) is an emergent condition requiring inpatient treatment with hydration, transfusion, and in some cases surgical intervention, as ischemia of the penis may lead to tissue necrosis. Retinopathies caused by microvascular ischemia increase in prevalence with age as well, including proliferative retinopathy, retinal hemorrhage and detachment, as well as retinal artery occlusion. Such changes may begin in childhood, and in turn, many patients with sickle cell anemia become blind before the age of 40 years.

Splenic sequestration results when large numbers of sickled erythrocytes become lodged in an engorged, functional spleen during early childhood, resulting in severe anemia and potentially fatal hypovolemic shock, carrying a mortality of 10 to 15 percent. As this condition tends to be recurrent, splenectomy is often performed after the first episode. Later in adult life, vaso-occlusive episodes in the spleen lead to autoinfarction, with replacement of splenic parenchyma by fibrotic tissue, which results in functional asplenia. Although this obviates the occurrence of splenic sequestration syndrome, splenic autoinfarction results in an increased susceptibility to infection by encapsulated organisms, such as *Streptococcus pneumoniae* and *Haemophilus influenzae*.

In addition to splenic sequestration, severe anemia may also result from aplastic crises, in which patients experience extreme suppression of bone marrow erythropoiesis. This is often a postinfectious phenomenon that may follow infection with Epstein-Barr virus, *Streptococcus pneumoniae*, *Salmonella*, and especially parvovirus B19, seen classically in pediatric patients, which directly infects erythroid progenitors. The bone marrow is also susceptible to infarction, which may also result in an exacerbation of the chronic anemia.

Sickle cell disease patients are at risk for other life-threatening conditions, as well. In acute chest syndrome, bilateral pulmonary infiltrates occur with fever and significant pleuritic chest pain, resulting in a "splinting" pattern of respirations, consisting of shallow breaths of suboptimal volume, resulting in progressive atelectasis and hypoxia. Respiratory failure may occur if not treated aggressively with hydration, transfusion, pain management, supplemental oxygen, and antibiotics for documented infection (e.g., community-acquired pneumonia or less commonly bacteremia). This condition may be triggered by vaso-occlusion, pulmonic infection, in situ thrombus formation and pulmonary infarction, or pulmonary emboli associated with bone marrow infarction (including fat emboli). Another serious complication of sickle cell disease is the tendency for cerebrovascular accidents (e.g., strokes, transient ischemic attacks). In fact, a significant percentage of these patients have experienced strokes prior to reaching adulthood, some repeatedly, but with the first episode most commonly occurring between 2 and 8 years of age. Myocardial infarction may also occur in the presence of absence of documented coronary artery disease, believed to be due either to occlusion or to severe hypoxemia due to the reduced oxygen-carrying capacity of the blood.

Clinical Presentation

Subjective

Subjective findings are associated with the severity of the anemia and with pain. Pain is evident only when there is a crisis, but the subjective findings of anemia may be apparent without concurrent crisis. In brief, the subjective findings of sickle cell anemia are no different from those of other anemias.

The cardinal subjective symptom of sickle cell crisis is pain. Pain appears suddenly in the back, chest, abdomen, or extremities. Patients characterize the pain as excruciating. It may last for several hours or several days. It is unrelieved by rest and position of the body. Massaging the site is of little value to relieve the pain. Other subjective findings may include nausea, anorexia, light-headedness, panic level of anxiety, palpitations, and shortness of breath.

Objective

The patient may present with a low-grade fever (less than 101.3°F [38.5°C]) during and preceding a sickle cell crisis, point tenderness and guarding at the sites of pain, pinpoint pupils, inability to follow commands, photophobia, tachycardia and systolic murmur, tachypnea, diminished respiratory excursion, hepatomegaly, nonpalpable spleen (it infarcts earlier in life), and pretibial ulcers. These findings are associated with sickle cell crisis. Outside of crisis, if the Hct is less than 25 percent (the average Hct between crises is 20 to 30 percent), objective findings may include tachycardia, tachypnea, systolic murmur, hepatomegaly, nonpalpable spleen, and pretibial ulcers.

The clinician may note characteristic physical findings resulting from chronic bone marrow expansion including a lengthened tower-shaped skull, frontal bossing of the forehead, and fish-mouth deformities of the vertebrae. Also during the objective examination, the clinician may note the chronic effects of hemolysis, such as jaundice or a sallow color to the skin. The patient may appear older than his or her stated years. Personality characteristics of one who has lived with a chronic debilitating disease may also be present.

Diagnostic Reasoning

Diagnostic Tests

Initial testing involves a CBC and a blood smear. It should be clear, however, that adults with sickle cell disease do not present de novo. They have been diagnosed since soon after birth and have learned to cope with sickle cell crises even as they risked delaying their own physical and psychological maturation. Initial testing of infants, therefore, involves a CBC and a blood smear.

Sickled cells will constitute 5 to 10 percent of the blood smear. The elevated reticulocyte count (greater than 10 percent of the total erythrocyte count) is characteristically accompanied by the presence of Howell-Jolly bodies which are small remnants of nuclear material from hemolyzed erythrocytes reflective of hyposplenia or autoinfarction, and target cells (an erythrocyte with a deeply stained core surrounded by a lighter-stained margin; it resembles a target with a bull's eye, hence its name).

The clinician should expect the WBC to be elevated to 12,000 or greater, especially during and following a crisis.

Further testing might include an indirect bilirubin level, which will be elevated following hemolysis. Conversely, the haptoglobin level will be low or absent because it cannot be replaced quickly enough after severe hemolysis. Haptoglobin, a glycoprotein, exists to bind free hemoglobin that is released from hemolyzed erythrocytes.

Differential Diagnosis

The differential diagnoses for sickle cell anemia include anemia resulting from another cause, sickle thalassemia, hemoglobin C disorders, nonspecific abdominal pain, UTI, poisoning, and diabetes mellitus. Each of these mimics some or all of the subjective and objective findings from the history and physical examination.

Sickle cell anemia is differentiated from sickle thalassemia by the MCV. The MCV should be low if there is any combination of sickle cell anemia and beta-thalassemia (a microcytic anemia) and normal if only sickle cell anemia is present. A combination of sickle cell anemia with alpha-thalassemia may cause a slower rate of sickling due to reduced MCHC in the erythrocytes caused by the alpha-thalassemia. Therefore, the sickle cell crises should prove less damaging and possibly less painful for these patients than for those without this combination.

Hemoglobin C disorders are differentiated by a much milder onset and course of anemia than sickle cell anemia. Indeed, some patients with hemoglobin C disorders may pass their lives without any crises caused by the disorder. The underlying pathology is differentiated by the substitution of lysine for valine at amino acid position 6 on the beta-globin chain. Definitive differentiation comes with a blood smear, which reveals rectangular crystals of hemoglobin C. With sickle cell/hemoglobin C disease (sickle C disease or SC disease), adult patients may still be prone to splenic sequestration crises, as their spleens typically do not autoinfarct and fibrose. Sickle beta-thalassemia may also be a milder, but nonetheless significantly morbid, condition than homozygous sickle cell disease, but is usually microcytic. In this condition, there may be no other production from the other beta-globin gene (*sickle beta thal^{o}*) that produces the most symptomatic condition or, alternatively, reduced production (*sickle beta thal^{+}*) that gives a milder condition, since there is still some hemoglobin A present. There are even rarer forms of doubly heterozygous hemoglobinopathies when hemoglobin S is combined with hemoglobins A, G, or O.

Nonspecific abdominal pain will have none of the laboratory markers of sickle cell anemia except for an elevated WBC and possibly a lower Hct. Sickle cell anemia in crisis should manifest with extra-abdominal pain. Urinary tract infection is linked to sickle cell anemia as these patients experience UTIs more frequently than individuals without it. A UTI can present as excruciating abdominal pain, with referred pain to the back and chest. The WBC is elevated, there could be a low-grade fever, and frank and/or microscopic blood may be present in the urine. However, the distinguishing difference between isolated cases of UTI and those associated with sickle cell anemia is the history and the laboratory markers of sickle cell anemia.

Poisoning presents with the hypoxemia and acidosis that are similar to sickle cell crisis. For example, ingestion of strong alkalines, such as those contained in household cleaning compounds, causes nausea, vomiting, acute abdominal pain, and dyspnea. The history and CBC should aid in ready and almost certain differentiation from sickle cell anemia.

Finally, diabetes is in the differential because of the similarities in blood chemistries, such as renal and hepatic function tests, blood pH, urinalysis, and physical examination. Again, as was the case with the other differential diagnoses, the history, CBC, and if necessary, blood smear should resolve any doubt that the clinician might face, even in an emergent situation.

Management

Initial Management

Folic acid (Folvate) supplementation of 1 mg/day by mouth is indicated, along with a diet that is rich in the complex B vitamins and vitamin C. Significant rehydration is needed as a part of management and is a key to reversing sickle cell crises. It aids in keeping the blood pH normal, thereby preventing acidosis with the sequela of sickling. Hydroxyurea, a chemotherapy agent, is a common treatment to increase hemoglobin F levels, an infant hemoglobin form with a higher affinity for oxygen than hemoglobin A or S, which allows for less hypoxemia and less sickling of RBCs. It reduces the frequency of painful crises.

Although packed red blood cell transfusions may be indicated in sickle cell treatment to decrease the fraction of hemoglobin S prone to polymerization, especially in children, they are less commonly used in adults and must always be weighed against the risks of infection (especially with Hepatitis C) and transfusion reactions. Anemia with a hemoglobin less than 7 has been associated with a greater risk of stroke, severe vaso-occlusive episodes, acute chest, and death in children. Chronic transfusions, however, lead to iron overload and iatrogenic hemochromatosis, which can destroy solid organs such as the liver, adrenals, and so forth. Exchange transfusion may be used when the clinical manifestations of sickle cell (e.g., acute chest, priapism) are severe and refractory to initial treatment, in order to decrease hemoglobin S to less that 50 percent of total hemoglobin. If osteomyelitis is confirmed with MRI, which is the diagnostic imaging of choice, then antibiotic therapy will be required. *Salmonella* in osteomyelitis of sickle cell patients predominates over *Staphylococcus aureus* as seen in non-sickle cell patients. Dactylitis (painful swelling of the feet and hands during the first several years of life in children with sickle cell anemia) needs to be treated, as well as aseptic necrosis of the hip, and priapism.

Subsequent Management

Management of sickle cell crisis often requires hospitalization. General goals include symptomatic control of pain with opioid-type drugs, rehydration, oxygen supplementation to reestablish normal or near-normal oxygen tension and to prevent or control acidosis, and vigilance against possible damage to vital organs such as the heart, liver, and kidneys.

Prophylactic penicillin should be used in children 2 months to 5 years and lifelong in children who have had splenectomies secondary to splenic sequestration crises. This will decrease infection by encapsulated organisms (*Streptococcus pneumoniae* and *Haemophilius influenzae*). In addition, patients should have the pneumonia vaccine, Hib vaccine, influenza vaccine, and meningococcal vaccine, and so forth. Parents should also be taught splenic size assessment, so that they can recognize the early signs of splenic sequestration syndrome.

There is a phenomenon of learned helplessness, narcotic addiction, and drug-seeking behaviors which develop in many sickle cell disease patients who are afflicted with chronic pain. There are critical conditions that must be considered when developing a treatment plan for the management of this condition.

Follow-Up and Referral

Follow-up with sickle cell anemia patients should be every 3 months when they have not been in crisis for 6 months or more; however, the frequency and duration of crises may increase the frequency of follow-up examinations. Laboratory evaluations occur periodically in anticipation of clinic visits. Routine clinical markers to be assessed include a CBC, fasting blood sugar, electrolytes, renal and liver function studies, and urinalysis. Annual or biannual 12-lead electrocardiograms (ECGs) are also necessary to rule out cardiac pathology.

Every patient with sickle cell anemia should be evaluated at least twice per year by a hematologist. In addition, retinal examinations should be performed by an ophthalmologist on an annual basis. Retinal photographs may be required once retinopathies have been diagnosed. Other referrals become evident as organs start to fail; therefore, cardiologists, gastroenterologists, nephrologists, orthopedic surgeons, and general surgeons may be enlisted as necessary.

Patient Education

Education involves the subject of the patient's maturation and personality development. Secondary gains (in the form of extra attention) that the patient received from the illness early in life may mean that, during crises, the patient regresses to childish behavior and coping mechanisms. These patients typically have poor coping skills. Patients who exhibit such regressive behaviors need to know that would-be friends and acquaintances, particularly prospective life partners and spouses, may be offended by the behaviors. The patient, therefore, should be educated in ways that provide anticipatory guidance to others who witness such events.

Self-care behaviors that may prevent sickle cell crises should be reinforced on a regular basis. These include adequate hydration, folic acid supplementation, avoidance of situations that tax the patient's physical and emotional stamina, and adequate sleep and rest as part of every day's activities. Additional self-care actions include participation in peer-support groups; the practice of pregnancy prevention unless the patient is prepared for the possibilities of more sickle cell crises during pregnancy and lactation; involvement in prenatal counseling and testing of the fetus for DNA evidence of disease; and avoidance of alcohol and adrenergic dietary elements, such as caffeine, that dehydrate the body.

Self-care also involves the practice of the patient's own spirituality. Spiritual beliefs and practices provide a unique contribution to the course of disease adaptation. In light of the early death of sickle cell anemia patients in contrast with the general population, spiritual practices may enhance personal acceptance of the disease. In addition, spiritual practices can marshall inner resources to resolve feelings of hopelessness and helplessness during sickle cell crises.

As sickle cell disease is a lifelong condition, problems unique to children and adolescents with chronic disease are abundant. There is an important transition period in which these patients typically transition their specialty care from a pediatric setting to an internal medicine setting. Thus, these patients are often shocked to find that they are treated differently in an adult medicine setting, with more stringent requirements for adhering to a chronic treatment plan—especially regarding patient compliance and its relationship to the emergent treatment of chronic pain exacerbations. Peer support groups can be particularly helpful for their patients.

Macrocytic Anemia

Macrocytic anemia is defined as having an MCV equal or greater than 100 femtoliters (fL). These conditions are typically normochromic and may be megaloblastic with large erythroid precursors or normoblastic. Macrocytic anemias results most commonly from defects in DNA metabolism or changes in RBC membrane structure. Macrocytic anemia has four general categories of causes: (1) vitamin B_{12} deficiency, (2) folate deficiency, (3) antimetabolite drugs such as methotrexate, and (4) miscellaneous etiologies.

Epidemiology and Causes

Both sexes are equally affected by macrocytic anemia. Prevalence is greatest among people of northern European lineage and Caucasians. Its incidence increases past age 60 years, but it has been observed in all age groups. The most common cause of megaloblastic anemia is a hereditary autoimmune disorder called pernicious anemia, which results in vitamin B_{12} deficiency, a critical component to the RBC maturation pathway and effective erythropoiesis. Pernicious anemia affects women over men at a rate of 5:1, and onset occurs in midlife, often after age 40 years.

Pathophysiology

Vitamin B_{12} Deficiency

Pernicious anemia is a macrocytic anemia caused by a hereditary autoimmune disorder in which destructive antibodies are directed against intrinsic factor, a 45-kDa protein produced by gastric parietal cells that binds to dietary vitamin B_{12} (cobalamin) during the digestion and absorption of nutrients and is critical to DNA synthesis and RBC maturation.

Under normal conditions, dietary vitamin B_{12} is cleaved from carrier proteins in the acidic environment of the stomach by the protease pepsin. However, it is then rapidly bound by cobalamin-binding factors known as R-proteins, which are found in gastric secretions and the saliva. As these complexes are not absorbable, they pass out of the stomach and into the duodenum. However, the alkaline environment produced by pancreatic proteases in the duodenum allows for the release of vitamin B_{12} from R-factor and its subsequent rapid, high-affinity binding to intrinsic factor. This newly formed complex then binds to receptors in the ileum which are specific for the vitamin B_{12}-intrinsic factor complex (e.g., cubulin), where absorption into ileal enterocytes is mediated primarily by transcobalaminase II (complexes bound to transcobalaminase I and transcobalaminase III are metabolically inert).

Vitamin B_{12} is essential to the maturation of erythrocytes via the conversion of homocysteine into methionine via the demethylation of tetrahydrofolate. In turn, demethylated tetrahydrofolate is a key component in the conversion of deoxyuridate to thymidylate and in purine synthesis involved in DNA metabolism. Anti-intrinsic factor antibodies are present in up to three-fourths of all patients with pernicious anemia and act either by blocking the binding of vitamin B_{12} to intrinsic factor or by blocking the binding of the cobalamin-intrinsic factor complex to ileal enterocyte receptors. In addition, autoantibodies produced against the parietal cells themselves and pathogenic CD4+ T cells act in concert to destroy gastric parietal cells, producing a morphologic change known as atrophic gastritis.

A subsequent decrease in gastric acid production compounds vitamin B_{12} deficiency, as cobalamin cannot be freed from its carrier proteins in the stomach, preventing subsequent binding to intrinsic factor in the duodenum.

Prolonged use of medications that counter gastric acid production such as histamine-2 blockers (e.g., ranitidine, famotidine, cimetidine) and proton pump inhibitors (e.g., esomeprazole, omeprazole, pantoprazole) have a similar effect. The widely used diabetic drug metformin (Glucophage) also decreases vitamin B_{12} absorption in up to one-third of patients taking this medication.

Thus, insufficient levels of vitamin B_{12} cause erythrocytes to expand in size compared to normal RBCs, thereby producing a characteristic megaloblastic anemia. In turn, pernicious anemia is characterized by a macrocytic anemia, a low serum level of vitamin B_{12}, atrophic gastritis, achlorhydria secondary to gastric atrophy, and a greater probability of other autoimmune diseases, such as hypothyroidism and vitiligo.

Normally, the complex of vitamin B_{12} and intrinsic factor is absorbed through the terminal ileum and then travels to the liver, where it is stored. Studies have estimated that the liver may store up to 5000 μg/day of B_{12}. Because the body requires no more than 10 μg/day, liver stores of vitamin B_{12} typically last for several years before anemia ensues. Therefore, megaloblastic anemia is insidious in onset. In patients with HIV disease and liver dysfunction, both depletion of liver stores of vitamin B_{12} and the destruction of storage sites within the liver have been identified as underlying causes of megaloblastic anemia.

Dietary deficiency of vitamin B_{12} is practically nonexistent because of its rich supply in animal proteins. However, because meats and dairy products are the only dietary source, vegetarians and in particular vegans (who completely avoid all meat and dairy products) are prone to consume inadequate amounts of vitamin B_{12}. Other reasons for poor absorption include a number of mechanical causes, such as those associated with surgical gastrointestinal resections (e.g., partial or total gastrectomy, terminal jejunum or proximal ileum resections). Crohn's disease can also cause a mechanical disturbance by destroying sections of the small intestine where absorption of vitamin B_{12} might otherwise occur.

Folic Acid Deficiency

Folic acid is a critical nutrient that acts in concert with vitamin B_{12} to further erythrocytic nuclear maturation, as folate deficiency leads to decreased levels of tetrahydrofolate, an important building block of DNA. As with vitamin B_{12} deficiency, abnormal erythroid precursors deficient in folate are prone to intramedullary hemolysis within the bone marrow, leading to a characteristic anemia clinically indistinguishable from that of vitamin B_{12} deficiency. Animal models have also demonstrated these RBC precursors are more prone to apoptosis or programmed cell death, although human studies are less definitive. Unlike vitamin B_{12} deficiency, folic acid deficiency does not produce neurologic sequelae.

Folate deficiency as a cause of macrocytic anemia presents with a low serum folate level and a normal level of vitamin B_{12}. It is almost always related to inadequate dietary intake of the esterol (pteroylmonoglutamic acid), a nutrient found in citrus fruits and dark-green leafy vegetables; folate is also present in animal proteins. Adequate intake is 50 to 100 μg/day, except for pregnant women, who need 800 μg/day. Even in developed countries such as the United States, pregnant patients may not consume adequate amounts of folate in their diets, and folic acid deficiency increases in incidence in multigravid patients and in multigestational pregnancies.

A second cause of folic acid deficiency is metabolic interruption or impairment of folate storage. The liver should store enough folic acid as N^5-methyltetrahydrofolic acid (approximately 5000 μg) to serve the body's needs for several months, given the body's use of 50 to 100 μg/day, as long as hemolysis and increased erythrocyte production are not issues, as in sickle cell anemia. There are many causes of impaired folate metabolism and hepatic storage, including chronic alcohol use due to decreased enterohepatic cycling, drugs such as phenytoin (Dilantin), sulfamethoxazole/trimethoprim (Bactrim), methotrexate, and oral contraceptives.

Poor absorption of folic acid is the third cause of folic acid deficiency. Tropical sprue, GI resections, Crohn's disease, and a few intestinal parasitic infections are the primary causes of impaired or interrupted absorption of folic acid. Unlike vitamin B_{12}, folic acid can be absorbed along the entire GI tract.

Drugs

Any chemical that serves as a potential inhibitor of DNA or RNA synthesis is a potential cause of macrocytic anemia. Drugs such as hydroxyurea (an inhibitor of ribonucleotide reductase), the antiviral zidovudine, and the chemotherapies methotrexate, azathioprine, and 6-mercaptopurine can all cause macrocytosis, with methotrexate being best known for leading to anemia. Methotrexate interrupts purine metabolism in the liver by preventing molecular binding with dihydrofolate reductase, an enzyme required for the storage of folic acid. Thus, less folic acid can be stored, thereby leading to a reduction in serum folate levels.

Miscellaneous Etiologies

Various unrelated causes for macrocytic anemia include thiamine- or pyridoxine-responsive anemias and Lesch-Nyhan syndrome. Macrocytic anemia may also be caused by chronic alcoholism (ingestion of at least 80 grams of alcohol per day), possibly via changes in RBC membranes caused by the alcohol breakdown product acetaldehyde. In addition, liver disease may lead to macrocytic anemia, possibly via increased lipid deposition in RBC membranes, and myelodysplasia, which causes a normoblastic (albeit macrocytic) anemia.

Clinical Presentation

Subjective

Patients with macrocytic anemia typically complain of stomatitis, glossitis, nausea and anorexia, diarrhea, peripheral neuropathies, and malaise if they are deficient in vitamin B_{12}. A deficiency in folate, drug impairment of folate storage in the liver, and miscellaneous disorders will cause similar symptoms, with the exception of peripheral neuropathy. Peripheral neuropathy is part of the differential among subjective symptoms for vitamin B_{12} deficiency alone.

Objective

The clinician should note pale or icteric mucosa, dry and cracked oropharynx, thick and smooth tongue, tachycardia, systolic ejection murmur, tachypnea, diffuse abdominal tenderness without organomegaly, glove/stocking locator signs of peripheral neuropathy, increased or decreased deep tendon reflexes, impaired position sense, position, diminished vibratory sensation in the lower extremities, a positive Romberg's sign, variable Babinski's sign, and pronounced irritability or other mental status changes. Of the megaloblastic anemias, neurologic signs related to myelin defects in the dorsal and lateral spinal columns will be present with vitamin B_{12} deficiency only and not with isolated folic acid deficiency. In fact, even frank dementia may be evident.

Diagnostic Reasoning

Diagnostic Tests

Initial testing involves isolation of a megaloblastic-macrocytic anemia on the peripheral blood smear. Expected findings include anemia and an elevated MCV (greater than 100 fL). The MCHC should be within normal limits, as the anemia is usually normocytic. It is important to note that pathologic processes that underlie macrocytic anemia may occur simultaneously with causes of microcytic or normocytic anemia, such as iron deficiency and thalassemia (microcytic) or anemia of chronic disease (normocytic). In these mixed anemias, MCV may actually be within a normal range, and the RBC indices are difficult to predict, possibly requiring referral to an expert hematologist.

Reticulocytes may be either low or normal in number, depending on the cause of the anemia. If the cause of macrocytosis is a deficiency in vitamin B_{12}, then the serum level should be less than 0.1 μg/mL, and hypersegmented neutrophils will be present on peripheral smear. Macroovalocytes will also be evident. In the case of folic acid deficiency, the serum folate level should be less than 3 ng/mL. Serum folate levels may vary even in patients with chronic deficiency. Even one meal can normalize folate levels in a person with true deficiency. Homocysteine and methylmalonic acid levels can distinguish between these two etiologies, with both values being elevated in vitamin B_{12} deficiency, while only homocysteine is elevated in folic acid deficiency. Common to both etiologies is a high serum iron level and findings consistent with mild hemolysis including low haptoglobin, elevated LDH, and mildly increased unconjugated bilirubinemia.

The Schilling test is rarely performed today, but you still may see it mentioned. The Schilling test measures the ability of the small intestine to absorb vitamin B_{12} and also identifies the source of the problem. It is a two-stage 24-hour urine collection test that needs to be done before any radioactive scans as the materials of the scans will alter the count of the radiolabeled vitamin B_{12}.

When diagnosing iatrogenic etiologies of macrocytic anemia, it is important to recognize that blood levels of specific drugs such as the antimetabolite methotrexate may vary according to individual laboratory standards. In rare cases, the judicious use of transfusion may be used with macrocytic anemia. It is generally avoided, but may be indicated in severe cases. The clinician must consider that patients are often elderly and unable to handle large volume transfusions well.

Additional tests are linked to liver function that could be impaired by drugs. These include the liver transaminases (alanine aminotransferase [ALT] and aspartate aminotransferase [AST] elevations), elevated bilirubin, and lactate dehydrogenase (LDH) elevation. Finally, urobilinogen may be identified in the urinalysis.

Differential Diagnosis

The differential diagnoses for macrocytic anemia include all of the causes identified in this section: vitamin B_{12} deficiency, folate deficiency, drug causes, and miscellaneous causes. In addition, the differential diagnosis includes anemia of chronic liver disease and myelodysplasia.

The history will lead the clinician to the cause of the anemia even when the laboratory results might be equivocal. For example, if the patient is pregnant, then the clinician should suspect folate deficiency over vitamin B_{12} deficiency. In addition, megaloblastic anemia due to vitamin B_{12} or folate deficiency is also often characterized by thrombocytopenia and neutropenia due to defects in megakaryocyte and myeloid precursors. This same pancytopenia is also commonly seen in the various types of myelodysplasia.

Management

A general approach to the patient with macrocytic anemia should address the cause of the anemia. The goal is to correct or ameliorate the cause even while addressing the anemia. For example, it might be appropriate to deliver supplemental vitamin B_{12} even while providing red cell transfusions as needed.

If the cause of vitamin B_{12} anemia is not pernicious anemia, then the clinician may follow these guidelines: prescribe up to 1000 μg/day of oral cobalamin until normal serum levels of vitamin B_{12} are achieved (usually 6 to 12 weeks after initiation of therapy). High doses such as these may even be effective in pernicious anemia, despite the lack of intrinsic factor, given the presence of an additional lower efficiency gastrointestinal absorption system which works independently of intrinsic factor and does not require a functional terminal ileum. Daily oral therapy, however, requires a high degree of patient commitment and compliance.

Thus, in most cases of pernicious anemia, and especially if neurologic symptoms are present, more aggressive therapy is warranted. In these cases, the preferred route of administration is parenteral with 1000 μg of vitamin B_{12} intramuscularly (IM) qD for the first 7 days, then weekly for 1 month, followed by once monthly for life. Lower parenteral doses of 100 μg have been advocated, but there are no apparent ill effects of overtreatment, and excess vitamin B_{12} is excreted in the urine. After depleted stores are replaced, patients may transition to oral, sublingual, or nasal preparations of vitamin B_{12} for ease of administration; however, serum levels of vitamin B_{12} and methylmalonic acid should still be followed periodically to ensure compliance with these medication regimens.

For folic acid deficiency, the clinician should prescribe 1 mg/day of supplemental folic acid. The effects of therapy should be reassessed after 2 to 3 months. It is critical to understand that treatment of folic acid deficiency will reverse many of the hematologic defects of vitamin B_{12} deficiency, while the neurologic manifestations of cobalamin deficiency will progress and may be devastating. Thus, it is important to rule out vitamin B_{12} deficiency before starting a folate replacement regimen, and if empiric therapy must be started before testing is available, patients should be treated with both folic acid and vitamin B_{12} supplements. Patients suspected of having either condition who do not respond with a significant reticulocytosis after the week of therapy should be evaluated further for a mixed anemic process originally masked by the megaloblastic manifestations.

It is also important to evaluate serum potassium levels in profoundly anemic patients once they start treatment, as increased erythropoiesis will markedly increase potassium utilization. These patients may become significantly hypokalemic, requiring oral repletion.

If the cause of the anemia is drug effects, the patient should discontinue all suspected drugs. Laboratory tests for elevated drug levels should be ordered; the liver transaminases (AST, ALT) should also be monitored for evidence of liver dysfunction, as well as coagulation times (PT/INR and PTT) as an indication of adequate hepatic synthetic function. The clinician should continue to address the continuation of any experimental or routine drugs that might interrupt purine metabolism. For patients with anemia resulting from miscellaneous causes, the individual disorders must be addressed.

Follow-Up and Referral

Follow-up of the patient with vitamin B_{12} deficiency involves the assessment of the severity of the anemia. Serial CBCs and vitamin B_{12} levels are required on a monthly basis after starting oral cobalamin therapy. If parenteral therapy is required, more frequent testing is in order, such as once every 2 weeks. Additional testing involves liver function tests (LFTs). If LFTs reveal elevated transaminase levels before cobalamin replacement is started, then their course should be evaluated every 2 to 4 weeks. If liver enzymes elevate after the start of therapy, more frequent testing might be required, as well as concurrent testing for underlying hepatotoxicity.

Referral for vitamin B_{12} deficiency is often not required unless the diagnosis is pernicious anemia or the patient suffers from a particularly difficult to diagnose mixed anemic process. A hematologist and gastroenterologist should be consulted in the event of pernicious anemia, as these patients are at greater risk for gastric cancer, carcinoid tumors, and colorectal carcinoma. Thus, stool should be monitored periodically for occult blood as a trigger for colonoscopy. In addition, the hyperhomocysteinemia which accompanies vitamin B_{12} or folic acid deficiency is a risk factor for atherosclerosis and venous thromboembolism and should be addressed as an independent risk factor.

Follow-up of the patient with folic acid deficiency consists of a CBC and serum folate level 2 to 3 months after starting therapy. The problem should be corrected by this point if the patient has adhered to the daily regimen of folic acid replacement. No referrals are indicated unless the anemia does not resolve.

Patient Education

Patients need to learn how to enrich their diets with folic acid and vitamin B_{12}. Increasing dark-green vegetables in one or two meals daily can support supplements and other therapies. In addition, patients should be educated about the basic signs and symptoms of macrocytic anemia so they can self-monitor the effectiveness of therapy.

Polycythemia

Polycythemia involves an increase in erythrocyte volume, which results in an increase in blood viscosity. The disorder may be either relative or absolute. A hematocrit greater than 51 percent in women and 54 percent in men is characteristic. The term "polycythemia" is a bit misleading. It means too many cell lines (*poly* = "many"; *cythemia* = "cell lines"), in general, and not just too many erythrocytes, in particular. Nevertheless, the name is associated with erythrocytes only.

Epidemiology and Causes

The incidence of polycythemia increases with age. It remains more prevalent in older men (older than age 70) than in women of similar age by a 2:1 ratio. On average, the incidence is 1.9:100,000. These statistics have remained stable for the past 60 years, according to three retrospective analyses. The incidence and prevalence of polycythemia increase among persons who reside at high altitudes.

Causes of relative polycythemia include decreased fluid intake, increased fluid loss, and extravasation of fluids. Absolute polycythemia, on the other hand, may be caused by either primary or secondary mechanisms. The primary mechanism for polycythemia involves the proliferation of stem cells independent of erythropoietin. This condition is also called *polycythemia vera.* The secondary causes of absolute polycythemia are technically not called polycythemia vera. Secondary causes of absolute polycythemia include chronic hypoxia, such as associated with residence at high altitudes, carboxyhemoglobinemia, Cushing's syndrome, and erythropoietin-secreting tumors.

Pathophysiology

Relative Polycythemia

Relative polycythemia is a condition in which there is a decrease in plasma volume while the total number of circulating erythrocytes remains the same. The underlying pathology is almost always dehydration. Dehydration may be either acute or chronic. Acute dehydration is associated with vomiting, burns, crushing-type injuries, and fevers, whereas chronic dehydration is an outcome of long-term use of diuretics, such as furosemide. Another chronic cause of dehydration is decreased oral fluid intake, a condition frequently encountered in older adults. Cigarette smoking, while being an important cause of absolute polycythemia, is also known to decrease plasma volume. Interestingly, this reduction reverses on cessation of smoking (with a reduction in hematocrit of four or more percentage points in just a matter of days). Terms such as pseudo- or spurious polycythemia, stress erythrocytosis, and Gaisbock's disease have all been used to label chronic states in which plasma volume is reduced while hematocrit or hemoglobin are elevated.

Absolute Polycythemia

Absolute polycythemia is a condition in which the actual numbers of circulating erythrocytes are increased with a corresponding increase in measured RBC mass. (One exception is inapparent polycythemia in which the increase in RBC numbers is counterbalanced by an increase in plasma volume, often masking the polycythemia on standard blood tests.)

Absolute polycythemia may be divided into primary and secondary categories. Many diagnosticians consider primary disease to be polycythemia vera, which is a chronic myeloproliferative disorder caused by an abnormally dividing pluripotential stem cell that leads to a clonal erythrocytosis that is erythropoietin-independent, as well as a variable leukocytosis (increased myelocytes) and thrombocytosis. The molecular defect underlying polycythemia vera has yet to be fully characterized, but aberrant cell signaling pathways involving tyrosine kinases, tyrosine phosphatases, insulin-like growth factor-1, as well as transcriptional dysregulation have all been suggested. Interestingly, however, the defect does not appear to be in the erythropoietin–erythropoietin receptor pathway, as erythropoietin levels are typically low in these patients.

Physiologically, erythropoietin has many functions: (1) stimulating mitogenicity (cell division) of progenitor cells, (2) protecting progenitor cells from apoptosis, and (3) inducing specific proteins involved in the differentiation and terminal maturation of erythrocytes, such as ankyrin and spectrin (structural membrane proteins) and the oxygen-binding globin chains. In turn, primary polycythemia may result from congenital or acquired mutations in erythroid progenitor cells which affect the erythropoietin–erythropoietin receptor pathway. For example, primary familial and congenital polycythemia (PFCP or benign erythrocytosis) is an autosomal dominant disorder thought to result from mutations in the erythropoietin receptor that lead to a hypersensitivity of erythrocytes to this growth factor. However, the specific molecular defect remains undefined in many patients.

There are several additional causes of secondary absolute polycythemia—chronic hypoxia, carboxyhemoglobinemia, Cushing's syndrome, chronic corticosteroid use, erythropoietin-secreting tumors, and cardiopulmonary diseases (the most common cause of polycythemia) which decrease oxygen saturation or diminish renal blood flow. Acquired forms include polycythemia due to the chronic hypoxia associated with prolonged high-altitude living, where the partial pressure of ambient oxygen is decreased. Carboxyhemoglobinemia is a disease associated with tobacco use, whereby carbon monoxide–containing cigarette smoke increases carboxyhemoglobin levels, preventing the binding of oxygen to hemoglobin molecules and resulting in a leftward shift in the hemoglobin dissociation curve. This shift reflects a decrease in oxygen delivery to the tissues and, in turn, is compensated by polycythemia. Cushing's syndrome (abnormal corticosteroid production arising from the pituitary gland [ACTH overproduction], adrenals, or a hormonally active tumor [cortisol overproduction]) and chronic exogenous steroid use (either corticosteroids or anabolic steroids) are erythropoietic and, when left unchecked, may lead to polycythemia. In addition, the act of blood doping in which RBC infusions are administered prior to sporting events by some athletes to increase oxygen-carrying capacity is an important iatrogenic source of polycythemia. Finally, erythropoietin-secreting tumors tend to be located in the kidneys (e.g., renal cell carcinoma), liver (e.g., hepatocellular carcinoma, hepatoma), uterus (e.g., leiomyomata or fibroids), or as a hemangioblastoma.

Although these congenital forms are quite rare, secondary polycythemia may also be congenital, caused by inborn mutations that alter the oxygen affinity of hemoglobin, leading to decreased oxygen delivery to peripheral tissues with resultant hypoxemia. These include mutations in the alpha- and beta-globin genes which cause a marked increase in oxygen affinity with compensatory polycythemia, congenital methemoglobinemia in which the iron moiety in hemoglobin is trapped in the oxidized ferric form and therefore unable to bind oxygen (mutations in cytochrome b5 reductase prevent reduction of ferric ions back to the oxygen-binding ferrous form), and mutations that lower levels of 2,3-bisphosphoglycerate, a key molecule involved in oxygen delivery to peripheral tissues.

Several other erythroid growth factors have also been shown to exist. Stem cell factor (SCF), granulocyte-macrophage colony-stimulating factor (GM-CSF), and interleukin-3 (IL-3) are responsible for the growth of early pluripotent stem cells that give rise to the erythroid lineage. In addition, insulin-like growth factor-1 (IGF-1) also stimulates erythropoiesis in early progenitors and appears particularly important in patients with end-stage renal disease who no longer produce adequate amounts of erythropoietin due to parenchymal kidney damage. Type 1 receptors for angiotensin II have also been identified on erythroid progenitor cells, and both angiotensin-converting enzyme (ACE) inhibitors and angiotensin II receptor blockers (ARBs) have been shown to counteract erythrocytosis in renal transplant patients. Thus, secondary polycythemia may result from any number of mutations that affect these different growth factors, although these molecular lesions tend to be rare, many of which have only been identified in familial cohorts.

Clinical Presentation

Subjective

Many subjective complaints do not arise until the hematocrit is greater than 60 percent. Because cardiopulmonary disease is the most common cause of polycythemia, the clinician should elicit an effective history of lung or pulmonary symptoms such as chronic cough, cyanosis, hypersomnolence, or shortness of breath and dyspnea on exertion.

Common complaints include headache, blurred vision, weakness, fatigue, irritability, dizziness, and, on occasion, tinnitus. Epistaxis, however, may be the complaint of clinical presentation. Epistaxis is due to mucosal engorgement in the nares and irregularities in clotting. After a warm bath or shower, patients may complain of generalized pruritus, which is caused by the release of histamine from basophils that become released from the vasculature or pool along dilated vascular walls.

Eliciting a detailed smoking history is also crucial. The constellation of symptoms that reflect chronic carbon monoxide exposure, such as in cab and bus drivers, underground tunnel or garage attendants, and so forth needs to be assessed.

Objective

The clinician should assess for erythromelalgia (burning pain in the hands and feet pathognomonic for polycythemia vera), as well as the tendency toward venous and arterial thrombosis or hemorrhage in this condition due to hyperviscosity and thrombocytosis. GI complaints are also common and may be present including peptic ulcer disease and gastroduodenal erosions. These are believed to be from hyperviscosity and increased histamine release. On an ocular examination, the clinician may note new vessel growth on the retinae as well as vascular engorgement. Splenomegaly is almost always present. Tenderness may be elicited from palpation of both upper abdominal quadrants. The left quadrant may be tender because of gastric ulceration and the right quadrant because of hepatomegaly (infrequent) and duodenal ulcers. A ruddy cyanosis might be apparent in the fingers and toes.

Pulse oximetry should be measured after minimal exertion or ABGs for PO_2 (and co-oximetry for carbon monoxide exposure or to detect methemoglobin) as an important part of the diagnostic work-up. The skin, especially the face, and mucous membranes have a dark, flushed (plethoric) appearance. The skin appears purplish or cyanotic as a reasult of inadequate tissue oxygenation. Cushingoid features may be present if Cushing's syndrome or chronic corticosteroid use is the cause of the secondary absolute polycythemia.

Diagnostic Reasoning

Diagnostic Tests

Initial testing always includes a CBC. The CBC results start the process of differentiating absolute from relative polycythemia. If the patient has polycythemia vera or one of the other absolute polycythemias, the Hct should be greater than 60 percent for men and 55 percent for women. In fact, if the Hct is not greater than these percentages, it is reasonable to rule out Cushing's disease and steroid use, because both cause a milder polycythemia. Of course, by definition, there is an elevated RBC count in absolute polycythemia. Nevertheless, the practitioner should anticipate that the RBC morphology will remain normal.

In the absence of a concurrent infection, the WBC count of absolute polycythemia should fall between 10,000 and 20,000, and the differential should prove unremarkable except for occasional basophilia. In addition to the CBC, the platelet count should be added to the panel of initial tests. The clinician should expect the platelet count to be elevated and to vary—at times exceeding 1 million cells.

If the patient has relative polycythemia, the CBC will reveal an elevated RBC mass, but the Hct will often not be as high as 55 to 60 percent. Plasma volume may also be measured to help distinguish relative versus absolute polycythemia, but values are not always as expected. In addition, the WBC and platelet counts are lower for relative polycythemia.

Secondary tests aid in the differentiation of absolute polycythemia. Polycythemia vera is diagnosed by splenomegaly in combination with an elevated Hct and platelet count. Secondary tests will assist the clinician in differentiating polycythemia vera from other causes of absolute polycythemia.

A definitive diagnosis of polycythemia vera may call for bone marrow biopsy, if other biochemical studies are inconclusive. Erythropoietin (EPO) levels are usually low in polycythemia vera and a normal or elevated EPO level necessitates a search for other causes. Polycythemia tends to be suspected when Hct is greater than 48 percent or Hgb greater than 16.5 g/dL in women or Hct greater than 52 percent or Hgb greater than 18.5 g/dL in men. These levels should always be age-adjusted. Carboxyhemoglobin levels greater than 5 percent suggest CO poisoning.

Differential Diagnosis

Spurious polycythemia (where there is a contracted plasma volume rather than a true increase in red cell mass) may be due to diuretic therapy.

The differentials for polycythemia vera include chronic myeloid leukemia, myelofibrosis, and essential thrombocytosis. Chronic myeloid leukemia would have an extremely elevated WBC (30,000/μL); myelofibrosis would have a normal or decreased Hct and abnormal red cell morphology; and essential thrombocytosis would have a normal Hct with a markedly elevated platelet count.

Management

In general, the principles of polycythemia management concern the difference between relative and absolute causes. This section, therefore, presents management of polycythemia according to underlying pathology.

Initial Management

Relative Polycythemia. Relative polycythemia is associated with dehydration; therefore, the clinician's objective is to rehydrate the patient. Rehydration in the primary-care setting consists, generally, of oral therapy and medication adjustment, if the cause of dehydration is related to a pharmaceutical agent, such as diuretics. Should IV rehydration be required, other factors must be considered, such as the patient's age, associated morbidities (e.g., cardiopulmonary diseases), ability to adhere to instructions, and availability of outpatient nursing care. Because of the complexity of care required for IV rehydration, acute care or in-hospital nursing management is often the preferred setting for IV fluid therapy. The clinician must decide whether the patient is able to adhere to instructions regarding oral fluids and changes in drug regimens. Central to the decision is the appreciation of the adequacy of family or friend caregivers in assisting with the patient rehydration interventions.

Absolute Polycythemia. Absolute polycythemia management begins with progressive phlebotomies if the Hct is greater than 55 to 60 percent. Phlebotomy is required to prevent thrombus formation, which is the cause of death from embolus, cerebrovascular accident (CVA), and myocardial infarction (MI) in a polycythemic patient. The goal of phlebotomy is to reach an Hct of 45 percent. This goal can be achieved by the weekly removal of 500 mL of whole blood. For example, if the starting Hct is 65 percent and 3 to 4 percent Hct is lost with each 500 mL of blood, then the goal of a 45 percent Hct can be reached after six phlebotomies. Maintenance of an Hct at or below 45 percent will require subsequent phlebotomies; iron deficiency will develop after repeated phlebotomy.

Patients will report abatement of symptoms as the Hct falls. Should iron deficiency ensue, iron supplementation should not be started because supplements can stymie therapeutic gains achieved by phlebotomy. The fatigue that had been associated with polycythemia should not return because of iron deficiency once an Hct of 45 percent or less has been reached.

Initial management of all absolute polycythemias follows the path of phlebotomy outlined above. Additional guidelines for initial management may be specific to the cause of Cushing's disease or corticosteroid use, erythropoietin-secreting tumor, hypoxia, and carboxyhemoglobinemia. Surgical resection of the pituitary gland may be indicated for Cushing's syndrome depending on where the source of excess corticosteroids actually is—the pituitary, the adrenals, and so forth.

Tapering of steroids, if possible, is the management of steroid-induced polycythemia. Tumor excision or reduction is the management for erythropoietin-secreting tumors. Oxygen supplementation may be the initial management of chronic hypoxia (if the partial pressure of oxygen in arterial blood [PaO_2] is less than 60 mm Hg), and cessation of smoking is the management for carboxyhemoglobinemia.

Hydroxyurea (Hydrea) is particularly useful in patients at risk for thrombosis, and low-dose aspirin should be started in all patients unless contraindicated by another condition, IFN-α is useful in patients refractory to other treatment or in those with significant refractory pruritus. Anagrelide is an antiplatelet agent that reduces platelet count and can be useful in patients with thrombocytosis, although long-term safety studies are not completed and it should be used in caution in patients with CAD. Allopurinol should be used in patients with significantly elevated uric acid levels due to high RBC turnover (provided any acute gout attacks have already been treated with colchicine, since its use may precipitate uric acid deposition in the joints).

Subsequent Management

Subsequent management follows the steps taken in initial management. Patients with polycythemia vera will require repeated phlebotomies. Nonalkylating agents may be employed to suppress stem-cell formation. These include erythropoietin (Epogen) 3000 units SC injection three times per week, hydroxyurea (Hydrea) 60 to 80 mg/kg three times per week, and busulfan (Myleran) 1 to 3 mg/day as maintenance; higher doses are required for induction. Higher dosages of all three agents have been employed, but the risks of myelosuppression, such as systemic infection, increase with dosage escalations.

Secondary maintenance of patients with absolute polycythemia may also include antiplatelet aggregation therapy with aspirin. This course of treatment is considered controversial because the therapeutic goal of reduction in thromboses has been achieved with phlebotomy alone. If aspirin is used, the dosage range of 81 mg to 325 mg/day should be all that is required. No consensus among hematologists and oncologists exists regarding the effectiveness of aspirin or the dosage range in this population.

Follow-Up and Referral

Relative Polycythemia

After dehydration has been converted, usually no follow-up or referral is required. However, follow-up of patients who receive diuretics should be based upon the need to monitor electrolytes and therapeutic aims. Maintaining normal levels of potassium and sodium is the goal of 90-day call-back schedule for patients maintained on non–potassium-sparing diuretics.

Absolute Polycythemia

The follow-up of polycythemia vera is far more complicated than rehydration therapy. Because weekly phlebotomies are required to achieve and maintain an Hct of 45 percent or less, weekly assessments of the CBC and brief office visits are also necessitated. An initial referral to a hematologist is also required to confirm the diagnosis and the plan for care management. If secondary management strategies such as myelosuppression are required, the clinician should rely on the hematologist for recommendations and comanagement. A referral is important to note as polycythemia vera carries a significant risk of transforming in time into myelofibrosis with myeloid metaplasia (MMM) or acute myeloid leukemia (AML).

Referrals to surgeons are required for tumor excision and pituitary resections. A positive finding from computed tomography (CT) of the abdomen or magnetic resonance imaging (MRI) of the brain should involve an immediate surgical consultation. A pulmonary referral may become necessary if the clinician does not detect lower carboxyhemoglobin levels after the patient stops smoking.

Patient Education

Patients should learn that absolute polycythemia reduces the lifespan. On average, patients live for less than 15 years after diagnosis because of the risks of thrombosis. In spite of this grim prognosis, they should be reassured that active participation in their care may extend the quality of their lives and may increase their longevity.

Increased quality of life is associated with improvement in the subjective presentation of the disease. Points to consider in patient education include adherence to fluid intake requirements, drug regimens, exercise, laboratory evaluations, and visits to the clinician and specialists.

Fluid intake requirements may fluctuate according to the stage and longevity of treatment. As the disease progresses and phlebotomies transpire, the daily fluid intake should average 2 L for a 70-kg adult. Earlier in the treatment before blood volume is reduced, the intake is likely to be less—on average, 1 to 1.5 L/day. Drug regimen adherence may require learning how to self-medicate with a parenteral agent such as Epogen. Therefore, teaching the patient and/or loved one how to draw up and deliver the drug is essential to the educational plan.

Instruction regarding exercise is entirely dependent on the patient's level of tolerance for activity. The goal, however, should remain clear that increasing the level of activity can reduce thrombosis formation. Simplest among exercise plans for persons older than age 60 is walking. The clinician should recommend that the patient walk with a friend in a safe place such as an indoor shopping mall. An alternative is walking from side to side in waist-high water. This form of aquatic exercise can be helpful for patients with joint- and bone-related immobilities who otherwise may have an increase in pain when walking out of water.

Adherence to laboratory evaluations may diminish over time as the patient copes with this chronic and indolently fatal disease. Drawing the family and other loved ones into the circle of education may enhance the patient's adherence to regimens. Call-back schedules for laboratory evaluations that fit with the individual's daily activities and provide another rhythm to the patient's life are more likely to meet with improved adherence profiles.

Finally, the visit to the clinician and specialists are times when education should be reinforced. Addressing and treating depression—an anticipated outcome of absolute polycythemia—can enhance adherence to all other elements of the patient's education. Teaching the patient and loved ones to recognize and report depression is, therefore, part of the educational plan.

Leukemia

Leukemia is a neoplastic disease of malignant hematopoietic stem cells that differentiate and proliferate according to classified trajectories that distinguish the types of leukemia as either acute or chronic. Further classification of leukemia specifies the stage of development and type of WBC (immunophenotype) that is involved in the malignant transformation (see Table 16.2). The result of the malignancy is the suppression of nonmalignant blood cells. Thus, the involved leukocytes proliferate and occupy space once filled by nonmalignant cell lines.

Epidemiology and Causes

The incidence of leukemias varies according to childhood and adult groups. Overall, however, there is a slight predominance of male to female incidence. Acute lymphoblastic leukemia (ALL) is predominant in children between age 2 and 15 years. Higher prevalence is among children aged less than 5 years.

Other leukemias strike adults. Acute granulocytic leukemia (AGL) and acute myelocytic leukemia (AML) strike adults of all ages, but the incidence increases after age 40 years. The incidence of acute lymphocytic leukemia increases in adults older than age 60. Chronic lymphocytic

Table 16.2 Types of Leukemia and Treatment

	Age at Onset	Treatment—Meds (Combination Therapy)	Treatment*—Other
Acute Leukemia			
Acute lymphocytic leukemia (ALL)	2–15 years	Daunorubicin (Cerubidine) Vincristine (Oncovin) Prednisone (Deltasone) Asparaginase (Elspar)	CNS intrathecal Methotrexate and cranial irradiation Autologous or allogeneic BMT
Acute nonlymphocytic leukemia (ANLL) or acute myelogenous leukemia (AML) and acute granulocytic leukemia (AGL)	All adults but more prominent >40 years	Daunorubicin (Cerubidine) OR Idarubicin (Idamycin) plus Cytarabine (Cytosar-U)	Autologous or allogeneic BMT
Chronic Leukemia			
Chronic granulocytic leukemia (CGL) or chronic myelogenous leukemia (CML)	All patients, but more prominent >60 years Median age 42 years	Imatinib (Gleevec) Hydroxyurea (Hydrea)	Allogeneic BMT for younger patients, autologous BMT for others
Chronic lymphocytic leukemia (CLL)	>60 years	Cladribine (Leustatin) Chlorambucil (Leukeran) and Prednisone (Deltasone) Second-line treatment: Alemtuzumab (Campath) Rituximab (Rituxan)	Allogeneic BMT

*For all leukemias, the need for epoetin (Epogen, Procrit), darbepoetin (Aranesp), and/or pegfilgrastim (Neulasta) must be assessed.

leukemia (CLL) and chronic granulocytic leukemia (CGL) are more prevalent among adults older than age 60; however, they may appear in persons of any age. CLL is the most common leukemia in developed Western countries, with a median age at onset of 70 years. Chronic myelocytic or myelogenous leukemia (CML) strikes middle-aged persons, at a median age of 42 years.

The etiology of leukemia remains unknown. Nevertheless, researchers have linked leukemia to environmental toxins such as chemical solvents, petroleum products, and insecticides, as well as heredity, although familial leukemias are rare. No study has linked adult-onset leukemias to siblings of prior-affected individuals, as have studies of children. Moreover, it is unclear whether the incidence of leukemia is any higher among adult identical twins than among other adults; however, CLL in particular does appear to have a familial disposition.

Mutagenic pharmacotherapies used to treat lymphoma, rheumatoid arthritis, or post-transplantation show greater promise for providing insight into disease etiology. For example, alkylating agents, such as melphalan (Alkeran) and cisplatin (Platinol) have been implicated in a 5 to 10 percent increased incidence of leukemia among patients who have been receiving them for a prolonged period of time. Likewise, prolonged exposure to high doses of ionizing radiation is also associated with leukemia. In cases of prolonged toxin and radiation exposure, a length of time up to 20 years may pass before a leukemia diagnosis is established. Shorter latency periods are seen following exposure to chemotherapies that inhibit the DNA-splicing enzyme topoisomerase II, such as etoposide, doxorubicin, or mitoxantrone.

Pathophysiology

Acute Nonlymphocytic Leukemia

By far, the largest number of adults with acute leukemia (as high as 80 percent) suffer from acute nonlymphocytic leukemia (ANLL). ANLL is a category that includes the leukemias formerly known as AML and AGL. ANLL presents after age 40 and increases in incidence with each year thereafter. It originates in the malignant transformation of a single stem cell or a few cells. At least 85 percent of all cases have been associated with defined clonal karyotypic abnormalities. Cells in the progenal line are universally affected, thus providing a clue that the leukemia is intrinsic to the cell line following malignant transformation.

ANLL has been divided into eight distinct morphologic classes (M0 to M7), according to the French-American-British (FAB) system, with classes M3 to M5 further subdivided into two subclasses each. Thus, the pathophysiology of ANLL is exceedingly complex, and a full discussion of the complete cytogenetics of this disease is beyond the scope of this discussion. However, each of these subtypes is characterized by one or more cytogenetic abnormalities that may be used to predict prognosis and guide treatment, as they often determine responsiveness to specific chemotherapies. For example, acute promyelocytic leukemia (AML class M3) is associated with a translocation between chromosomes 15 and 17 that juxtaposes the PML and retinoic acid receptor (RAR)-alpha genes, repressing the latter and preventing retinoic acid–induced differentiation of promyelocytes. Nonetheless, this mutation portends a favorable prognosis, as promyelocytic M3 cells are particularly sensitive to therapy with all-trans retinoic acid (ATRA).

In contrast, abnormalities that carry a particularly poor prognosis include mutations with monosomy (entire chromosomal deletion) of chromosomes 5 or 7 or trisomy of chromosome 8. The former monosomies are particularly associated with AML resulting from previous chemotherapy with alkalinizing agents or exposure to ionizing radiation. In contrast, AML associated with past exposure to topoisomerase II inhibiting agents are often associated with mutations in chromosome 11.

Acute myeloblastic leukemia (AML class M2) and acute myelomonocytic leukemia (AML class M4) have both been associated with a balanced translocation between chromosomes 8 and 21, which juxtaposes the transcription factor genes *AML1* and *ETO*, leading to dysregulated transcription of genes directly involved in myeloid cell division (e.g., granulocyte-monocyte colony stimulating factor, interleukin-3, the antiapoptotic gene *BCL-2*). AML class M4 has also been associated with inversions or translocations in chromosome 16, creating a fusion of the genes *CBFB* and *MYH11* which leads to repressed transcription of genes involved in myelocytic differentiation. Acute monoblastic leukemia (AML class M5) is associated with rearrangements of chromosome 11, while mutations in chromosome 3 appear to confer thrombocytosis in the setting of AML.

Acute Lymphoblastic Leukemia

ALL can appear among persons of all ages but is clearly a disease of early childhood as noted earlier. B-cell or, in far fewer cases, T-cell lymphoblasts increase in number after a single hematopoietic stem cell undergoes transformation (immortalization). Interestingly, the cytogenetics of ALL in children are far different from those in adults. For instance, the Philadelphia chromosome (a balanced translocation between chromosomes 9 and 22 that juxtaposes and activates the *BCR* and *ABL* oncogenes) is seen in only 5 percent of childhood cases, while this is the most common abnormality in adult ALL and may be found in up to 40 percent of cases. In contrast, hyperdiploidy (in which greater than 50 chromosomes are found in malignant clones) is seen in up to 30 percent of childhood cases but in no more than 5 percent of affected adults.

In contrast to CML (see next section), the presence of the Philadelphia chromosome is a poor prognostic indicator in ALL, contributing to dysregulated activation of the RAS intracellular signaling pathway that leads to uncontrolled cell division. These patients often have additional karyotypic abnormalities such as monosomy of chromosome 7. Studies have shown that ALL patients with the Philadelphia chromosome may be divided into two subsets that are distinguished by differing translocation breakpoints along the BCR gene—one in which this karyotypic abnormality appears restricted to a B lineage lymphoblastic cell clone and another in which the Philadelphia chromosome is further identified in myelogenous cell lines as well, indicating that these patients may actually have a indolent form of CML that underwent a B lineage lymphoblastic crisis at the time of diagnosis.

As with AML, different forms of ALL have been distinguished on the basis of morphology, with certain cytogenetic profiles correlating with each. For instance, ALL cases of L3-type B-cell origin often share a translocation of chromosomes 8 and 14 which is also seen in B-cell–derived Burkitt's lymphoma, suggesting that these cancers are varied manifestations of the same underlying malignant transformation event. Pre–B-cell ALL has been associated with translocations between chromosomes 1 and 19, which lead to a fusion protein between the highly active transcription factors *E2A* and *PBX1*, with subsequent immortalization of this early B-cell progenitor and a particularly poor prognosis. Infantile ALL has been associated in up to 80 percent of cases with translocations involving the mixed lineage leukemia (MLL) gene at chromosome 11q23, which is thought to regulate a number of downstream genes involved in lymphocyte differentiation, in turn, resulting in extremely poor outcomes. A poor prognosis is also seen in ALL associated with translocations between chromosomes 4 and 11, a mutation that is commonly seen in AML class M5.

Translocations between chromosomes 12 and 21 which produces a fusion protein between the transcription factors *TEL* and *AML1* is the most common mutation seen in childhood ALL. Fortunately, this translocation confers a favorable prognosis in ALL, as does the presence of hyperdiploidy (a cellular complement of 50 to 60 chromosomes) with occasional structural abnormalities such as partial duplications and translocations. Multiple copies of chromosome 21 and the X chromosome are the most common findings in hyperdiploidy, but several others duplications have been noted as well (e.g., chromosomes 4, 6, 10, and 14). The high prevalence of these karyotypic abnormalities in childhood ALL underlies the generally favorable outcomes associated with this leukemia in children.

T-cell ALL is a less common entity that typically strikes young men. Related to T-cell lymphomas, these patients may present with particularly high WBC counts, invasion of malignant cells into the CNS (cerebrospinal fluid), and the presence of a mediastinal tumor. Well over half of these cancers are characterized by mutations in genes coding for the various protein components of the T-cell receptor—either alpha, beta, gamma, or delta subunits. The T cell receptor is a heterodimeric protein composed of either alpha–beta or gamma–delta subunits, expressed on the surface of the T cell, allowing for the recognition of specific antigens. Mutations commonly occur in chromosome 14, which encodes the alpha and delta receptor subunits, or chromosome 7, which encodes the genes for the beta and gamma chains. Translocations at these sites typically juxtapose these genes with various transcription factors that lead to dysregulated expression of the receptor subunit and proliferation of the T-cell clone. Mutations in the same chromosomes that do not involve these receptor subunits as well as others such as chromosomes 6 and 11 have also been identified in T-cell ALL. Interestingly, prognosis does not appear tied to these particular cytogenetics, and outcomes are generally favorable in both adults and children with this condition.

Chronic Myelogenous Leukemia

CML (CGL, chronic myelocytic leukemia, chronic myeloid leukemia), is most commonly associated with the development of the Philadelphia chromosome (Ph) in a hematopoietic stem cell which commits to the myeloid lineage. While differentiation is typically unaffected, the leukemic stem cell is self-renewing and produces a tremendous number of daughter cells, with the same leukemic clone dominating up to 90 percent of the bone marrow at the time of diagnosis. In this mutation, breaks occur in the DNA resulting in an equivalent exchange genetic material between chromosomes 9 and 22. Oncogene activation occurs, as the reciprocal translocation [t(9;22)(q34;q11)] juxtaposes the *BCR* and c-*ABL* genes, creating a BCR–ABL fusion protein which confers a proliferative advantage to the leukemic clone, even in the absence of cellular growth factors.

The functions of the native BCR and ABL proteins are not fully elucidated, and neither gene alone is capable of malignant transformation; however, the fusion protein is oncogenic, giving rise to malignant clones through upregulated tyrosine kinase (phosphorylation) activity within a number of intracellular signaling pathways contributing to cell division (e.g., RAS, c-myc, and JAK/STAT molecular pathways). This explains the effectiveness of treatment with the tyrosine kinase inhibitor imatinib (Gleevec). Depending on the site of the chromosomal breaks, various types of the BCR-ABL fusion protein may be formed. In turn, cells transformed by these different species appear to respond differentially to specific therapies.

While IL-3 and G-CSF mRNA transcripts are both upregulated in leukemic cell clones, the precise role of cytokines in the dysregulated growth of these cells remains unclear. As with other forms of leukemia, leukemic cell clones appear to arise from a self-renewing pool of mutated leukemic stem cells, which are typically less mature than the differentiated granulocytic leukemic clones themselves. In fact, the Philadelphia chromosome has been further identified in a number of cell lineages in CML, including granulocyte, macrophage, erythrocyte, megakaryocyte (platelet), and B-lymphocyte precursor cells, indicating that the mutation first occurs in an early, non-committed, multilineage hematopoietic stem cell.

The creation of the Philadelphia chromosome may predate the onset of disease symptoms by many years, a pattern suggesting that the disease progresses through a latent or asymptomatic phase before becoming active. For example, the karyotypic abnormality may first arise in the third decade of life, with symptom onset as much as 10 to 20 years later. In fact, normal bone marrow function is characteristic of the disease trajectory in the early years after development of the Philadelphia chromosome. The pool of leukemic stem cells may not be expanded in number; however, leukemic daughter cells undergo clonal expansion and eventually crowd out normal bone marrow components. In addition, cell surface adhesion factors (e.g., beta-1 integrin) are downregulated, which eliminates adhesion-dependent growth inhibition in which normal cells are triggered to stop proliferating after coming into contact with one another.

As with any chronic leukemia, a dreaded complication of CML is degeneration into a leukemic blast crisis, in which leukemic progenitor cells develop self-renewing properties as they undergo further mutations resulting in clonal proliferation of either myeloid or lymphoid (almost exclusively B lineage) blasts, given the widespread presence of the Philadelphia chromosome in multiple lineages. Most commonly, the additional mutations described include trisomies of chromosomes 8 or 19, duplication of the Philadelphia chromosome itself, or mutations in the *p53* tumor suppressor gene on chromosome 17. These blast cells may express many of the same proteins as hematopoietic stem cells, such as the transcription factor beta-catenin. Both leukemic stem cells and their progeny appear more resistant to apoptosis than wild-type (nonmutated) cells, but the significance of this to the pathogenesis of CML is not fully known. However, resistance to apoptosis appears to be important, as the lifespan of leukemic cell clones is not significantly greater than that of wild-type granulocytes and does not appear to account for their increase in number.

Finally, CML may also occur in the absence of the Philadelphia chromosome mutation known as atypical CML. Up to 15 percent of CML patients may suffer from this condition, although some hematologist-oncologists have chosen to classify them as having a distinct myeloproliferative disease, rather than a true CML. For reasons that are poorly understood, these patients have a worse prognosis with a poorer response to therapy and shorter survival times.

Chronic Lymphocytic Leukemia

CLL is a chronic lymphoproliferative disorder typically associated with increased numbers of small B lymphocytes. In fact, it is clinically indistinguishable from small lymphocytic B cell lymphoma. After a malignant alteration occurs in a B cell precursor, thus forming a malignant line, the clonal abnormality is passed on to slowly replicating progeny which are functionally incompetent.

The genetics of the malignant alteration are not as well established as they are for CML. Malignant B-cell clones are known to be frozen in a state of differentiation somewhere between the pre-B and mature B-cell phase, with rates of proliferation and cell death varying widely among different individuals. These cells express very low levels of surface immunoglobulin, various B-cell–specific cell surface proteins (e.g., CD19, CD20, CD21), as well as CD5, which is primarily considered a T-cell marker. Variant forms exist that do not adhere to these criteria, although some hematologist-oncologists feel that a proliferation of non–CD5-expressing B cells represents a leukemic phase of non-Hodgkin's lymphoma, rather than true CLL.

The relative percentages of both T cells and natural killer (NK) cells are reduced in CLL, although absolute numbers of T lymphocytes may be increased, given the tremendous expansion of lymphocytes. Moreover, some CLL patients demonstrate unusual forms of T cells with low levels of surface CD4 and CD8 proteins. Such nonclassical T cells are also found in other autoimmune diseases. Moreover, although hypogammaglobulinemia is common in patients with CLL, immunoglobulin receptors on leukemic cells may demonstrate autoimmune specificity, which may explain the increased frequency of autoimmune hemolytic anemia (AIHA), idiopathic thrombocytopenic purpura (ITP), and pure red cell aplasia in persons with CLL. Owing to the lack of protective antibodies, infection by gram-negative or encapsulated organisms is the most frequent cause of morbidity and mortality in persons with CLL.

Cytogenetic analysis of CLL cell clones has revealed chromosomal abnormalities in up to 70 percent of cases. The most frequent karyotypic abnormalities include trisomy of chromosome 12, partial deletions in chromosome 13 that affect the tumor suppressor retinoblastoma gene, and partial deletions in chromosomes 11 and 17 that are associated with a particularly poor prognosis and shorter survival. The *p53* tumor suppressor gene located on chromosome 17 is often affected, either by deletion or expression of a mutated, nonfunctional protein, with both conditions leading to unregulated cellular proliferation. In contrast, the overexpression of survival factors has also been identified in B lineage CLL, including the anti-apoptotic molecules BCL-2 and inducible nitric oxide synthetase.

Clinical Presentation

Subjective

Patients with acute leukemia complain of bone and joint pain. They have gingival bleeding associated with gingival hyperplasia. Fevers, chills, palpitations, and shortness of breath (signs of infection) also constitute the initial subjective presentation. Skin eruptions, easy bruising, or prolonged bleeding time from simple wounds form a significant part of the subjective history.

Patients with chronic leukemia complain of fatigue, night sweats, and low-grade fevers. While there is no clear differentiation in subjective findings between CML and CLL, CML may present with the symptoms of leukostasis, which is associated with a very high WBC count (greater than 500,000). The syndrome of leukostasis is characterized by blurred vision, respiratory distress, and occasionally priapism (prolonged and painful erection that lasts several hours). Nausea and vomiting may be associated with organomegaly in both types of chronic leukemia. Bone and joint pain are limited to myeloproliferative stages of CML.

Objective

The clinician will often note a high fever in patients with acute leukemia. Tachycardia and tachypnea are related findings. Patients appear pale and manifest eruptions such as petechiae and purpura. The patient's confusion—related to hypoxemia and fever—will be manifest on the Folstein Mini–Mental Status Examination (MMSE). (See a description of the exam and the exam itself in the section on Alzheimer's disease in Chapter 5.)

Heart and lung sounds should be within normal limits except during infection, in which case the lungs may reveal adventitious sounds. Splenomegaly is variably associated with hepatomegaly in chronic leukemia patients. They may or may not have enlargement of the spleen, liver, and lymph nodes. Temperature may not be elevated, as with acute leukemia, unless the disease has progressed or there is a concurrent infection. The patient's skin color varies between pale and normal. Few, if any skin eruptions are evident.

Diagnostic Reasoning

Diagnostic Tests

Initial testing for acute leukemia includes peripheral blood smear, platelet count, and CBC. The WBC may be significantly elevated (more than 300,000 cells). Granulocytes (polysegmented and banded cells) are diminished in number as are platelets (often less than 50,000). A hematocrit of less than 30 percent is a common finding, especially if the WBC count is markedly elevated. The peripheral smear reveals a blastocytosis of greater than 25 percent in almost all cases.

Initial tests for chronic leukemia are the same: peripheral blood smear, platelet count, and CBC. The WBC should be elevated in CML and CLL, but more so in CML (elevations greater than 100,000 are common). Lymphocytosis, however, differentiates CLL from CML. Lymphocytes occupy as much as 90 percent of the peripheral smear in CLL. The peripheral smear of CML is characterized by a left-shifted myeloid series, with mature forms of myeloid cells predominant in the smear. Platelets may be elevated, but in any event they are usually not diminished.

Subsequent testing for both acute and chronic leukemia is the bone marrow aspirate. Results should parallel the peripheral blood smear, thus confirming the initial diagnosis with greater accuracy in quantitative and qualitative indices. In acute leukemia, the bone marrow aspirate reveals hypercellular components, which are dominated by blasts. At least 30 percent of the cells must be blasts to diagnose acute leukemia. Auer bodies are rod-shaped structures, present in the cytoplasm of myeloblasts, myelocytes, and monoblasts, found in leukemia. They are typically seen among the myeloblasts in the bone marrow aspirate of people with AML. Serum chemistry profiles also are associated with secondary testing for acute leukemias. Because of rapid turnover in the WBC population, intracellular uric acid is liberated and rises in serum concentration.

In CML, bone marrow evaluation exposes the Philadelphia chromosome along with the left-shifted myelopoiesis. Blasts occupy less than 5 percent of the aspirate sample. Subsequent testing of CML also includes measuring leukocyte alkaline phosphatase (LAP), which is usually low, thus reflecting the abnormal function of neutrophils. Additional testing includes vitamin B_{12} level and serum chemistries. The vitamin B_{12} level should be elevated, as should the uric acid level.

Subsequent CLL bone marrow results confirm the initial peripheral blood smear. Small, mature lymphocytes dominate the field. A surface immunoglobulin on the monoclonal malignant lymphocytes aids in distinguishing these small cells from their normal counterparts. Another secondary test, immune electrophoresis, further supports the diagnosis of CLL in about half of patients. The profile from the electrophoresis shows that the patient is hypogammaglobulinemic.

Cytogenetic analysis (fluorescent in situ hybridization or hypridization or fish, Southern blot, reverse transcriptase-polymerase chain reaction [RT-PCR]) as molecular methods of identifying the Philadelphia chromosome and other karyotypic abnormalities, are critical for predicting prognosis and determining the most effective treatment plan for each type of leukemia. These analyses have revolutionized leukemia treatment with directed therapy.

Differential Diagnosis

Acute Leukemia. The left-shifted (immature) bone marrow aspirate of acute leukemia must be distinguished from the left-shifted aspirates that are associated with recent exposure to toxic chemicals and radiation. The clinician should expect that the full recovery period after toxic exposure will be at least 6 weeks and may extend to 12 weeks. It is possible to rule out so-called false-positive left-shifted aspirates by repeating the procedure several days later. If the exposure to toxins and not monoclonal malignant mutations was the cause, then the subsequent test should reveal maturing cell lines.

Acute leukemias must be distinguished from their chronic counterparts and from similar myeloproliferative disorders, such as polycythemia. ALL resembles lymphoproliferative diseases, such as lymphomas and mononucleosis; therefore, a skilled pathologist is required to distinguish the lymphoproliferative disorders from particular acute leukemias.

Chronic Leukemia. The Philadelphia chromosome of CML distinguishes this disease from myeloproliferative responses to infection, systemic inflammation, and other malignancies. Clinical wisdom will also help the practitioner distinguish the leukocytosis of CML from other reactive states. CML will likely present with more than 50,000 WBCs but reactive states will not mount so great a response. In addition, CML is clearly different from other myeloproliferative diseases; the erythrocyte count, RBC indices, and hematocrit are generally normal in CML.

Microscopic evaluation of a bone marrow aspirate differentiates CLL from lymphocytic disorders, including viral infections. Moreover, viral infections, unlike CLL, will present with flu-like symptoms, which include fever, chills, myalgias, and arthralgias. Thus, CLL is perhaps the easiest among the leukemias to differentiate.

Management

Successful treatment and subsequent cure for acute leukemia decreases with increasing age. In addition, a cure for acute leukemia is less probable if the patient is diagnosed late in the disease trajectory, after several physiologic systems have become involved. In general, treatment begins with combination chemotherapy to induce remission (i.e., induction phase), followed by a stage of chemotherapy called the consolidation phase, and finally a prolonged maintenance phase. Unlike the acute leukemias, the chronic leukemias usually follow an indolent pathway, which means that myelosuppressive chemotherapy may not be initiated until symptoms necessitate action. Symptoms, therefore, are managed as they appear.

Acute Leukemia

ANLL patients receive combination chemotherapy. (Medications are listed in Table 16.2.) The oncologist will set the dosage ranges for at least two drugs—daunorubicin (Cerubidine) or idarubicin (Idamycin) plus cytarabine (Cytosar-U). The clinician is responsible for monitoring hepatic function throughout the course of combination therapy, which may run in 3- to 6-day cycles every 3 to 4 weeks for a total of 3 to 6 months, depending on successful remission and patient tolerance. Combination therapy produces bone marrow aplasia, which abates after 2 weeks following the conclusion of therapy. Aplastic patients, therefore, require supportive antibiotic prophylaxis, vigorous stoma care given severe denuding of mucosal surfaces, and possible red cell transfusions. The clinician's role is to comanage the adverse effects of the chemotherapy and to monitor serum chemistries, including LFTs.

Adult patients with ALL may enter remission in initial management (albeit not as quickly or easily as children with ALL) without the aplastic disorders associated with the initial treatment of AML. Combination chemotherapy is the mainstay for initial management. It includes vincristine (Oncovin), daunorubicin (Cerubidine), and prednisone (Deltasone). Other combinations are under investigation. Comanagement with the oncologist is the same as for patients with ANLL, except that vigorous stoma care and associated weight reduction may not figure as prominently in ALL. Glucose intolerance may be made by prednisone therapy, particularly in patients suffering from diabetes mellitus at baseline. The clinician is responsible for making adjustments to antidiabetic agents during chemotherapy.

After remission has been achieved for the patient with acute leukemia, a consolidation course of management is begun. Consolidation cycles differ for the acute leukemias. ANLL patients receive one complete chemotherapy consolidation cycle. Alternatively, they may receive a bone marrow transplantation (BMT) to consolidate the gains of earlier therapy. Transplantation may be autologous (an individual's own marrow saved before treatment), allogeneic (marrow donated by someone else), or syngeneic (marrow donated by an identical twin). Advanced Practice Nursing Interventions 16.1 presents information that should be provided to the patient who will be undergoing bone marrow transplantation.

Patients with ALL, on the other hand, face different challenges. They must receive central nervous system (CNS) prophylaxis against malignant lymphocytes that may have crossed the blood–brain barrier to hide in meningeal crypts. CNS prophylaxis typically consists of intrathecal methotrexate and cranial irradiation.

Chronic Leukemia

Patients with CML are initially managed with watchful vigilance. Should treatment be required for extreme hyperleukocytosis–related symptoms, such as blurred vision and respiratory distress, leukophoresis may be initiated. In addition, depending upon severity of symptoms, hydroxyurea (Hydrea) may be initiated at 2 to 4 g/day PO, followed by maintenance therapy of 0.5 to 2 g/day. The leukopenic goal of 5000 to 10,000 WBCs requires frequent monitoring.

Symptom management and clinical vigilance are the initial therapies for patients with CLL. Symptoms that require intervention include thrombocytopenia (less than 50,000 platelets), anemia (less than 27 percent Hct), lymphadenopathy that impedes activities of daily living, and fatigue that reduces nutritional intake and immobilizes the patient. While some sources cite a threshold of 50,000 platelets for thrombocytopenia requiring intervention, most oncologists tolerate much lower values before giving transfusions of PLT (even as low as 10,000 provided there is no active bleeding). Combination chemotherapy is required in this event. Chlorambucil (Leukeran), with an alternative regimen of cladribine (Leustatin) is recommended. In either case, the monitoring of platelet and erythrocyte counts is required because of the myelosuppression secondary to chemotherapy.

Exogenous erythropoietin (Epogen, Aranesp, or Procrit) may assist in countering the chemotherapy-induced

ADVANCE PRACTICE NURSING INTERVENTIONS 16.1

Bone Marrow Transplantation

The following information should be provided to the patient undergoing bone marrow transplantation:

What it is

A bone marrow transplantation (BMT) is the administration of 500 to 700 mL of bone marrow. The patient is "conditioned" to receive the bone marrow through a regimen of immunosuppression therapy (chemotherapy or radiation). This conditioning eradicates malignant cells, provides immunosuppression, and creates a space for the bone marrow to engraft the transplanted marrow. The marrow is usually infused 48 to 72 hours after the patient's last dose of chemotherapy or radiation.

The bone marrow is "harvested" from a donor. It may be an autologous transplant (aspirated from the pelvic bones of the patient during a remission), an allogeneic transplant (from a compatible donor such as a parent or sibling with a similar tissue type), or a syngeneic transplant (from an identical twin).

What will happen before the procedure

- The health-care provider should provide complete information about the specific procedure (e.g., treatment, restrictions), answer any questions, and provide emotional support.
- The patient should prepare for an extended hospital stay.
- The patient should prepare for side effects that are anticipated (nausea, vomiting, cataracts, sterility, hair loss).

What will happen during the procedure

- The nursing staff will:
  1. Monitor vital signs and for complications (e.g., allergic reactions, fluid overload, pulmonary embolism)
  2. Provide support and reassurance

What will happen after the procedure

- The nursing staff will monitor:
  1. Routine vital signs
  2. Signs and symptoms of infection (e.g., fever and chills)
  3. Complications from chemotherapy given to prevent graft-versus-host diseases
  4. Signs and symptoms of graft-versus-host disease (e.g., rash, jaundice, joint pain, diarrhea, failure to engraft [pancytopenia])
- Mouth and skin care will be provided every 2 hours to help prevent infection
- IM injections will be avoided because they may lead to increased bleeding into the muscles

What to do after discharge

- Avoid infection by staying away from crowds and people with known infections
- Avoid sharp objects, for example, shave with an electric razor

anemia. In addition, the use of pegfilgrastim (Neulasta) and other colony stimulating factors may counter neutropenia.

Follow-Up and Referral

When suspicion is elevated concerning a diagnosis of leukemia, the clinician should refer the patient to an oncologist. Pertinent laboratory results along with a clinical history should accompany the patient for the oncologist's appointment. It is usually the oncologist's responsibility to request the bone marrow analyses.

For the patient with acute leukemia, comanagement of adverse effects from combination chemotherapies will require primary care follow-up monthly during the course of chemotherapy. The oncologist will direct treatment recommendations and adjustments and supervise laboratory analyses. The clinician will provide oversight of the same laboratory results, along with recommendations for symptom management.

For the patient with chronic leukemia, if clinical vigilance is all that is required, the clinician should order laboratory evaluations of the patient's CBC, platelet count, and peripheral blood smear every 6 weeks. Depending on symptom onset and severity, physical examinations could be as infrequent as every 2 to 3 months. Once chemotherapy intervention begins, the oncologist will make treatment recommendations and alterations.

Patient Education

The patient may not be prepared for education soon after receiving a clinical diagnosis of leukemia; therefore, it is important to involve not only the patient but significant others as well in any education provided. Particular attention should be focused on treatment recommendations and their proposed impact on daily life and state of well-being. Treatment recommendations that include myelosuppressive therapies will require self-care activities that may not be in the patient's repertoire of capabilities. Thus, education should begin with an assessment of the patient's ability to monitor self for infection, adverse effects of treatments, integrity of skin and mucous membranes, and fluid/nutritional status. Any deficits in the patient's ability to follow through with self-assessment should increase suspicion of complications from treatment yet to come; thus, resources that can aid the patient in assessment should be lined up before treatment is started.

In addition to assessment, the patient's education must address the anticipated burden on caregivers. Older patients and family members may not be able to adapt to the demands of treatment schedules, aplastic crises, and the like. The following strategies can assist in this regard: The clincian should plan teaching sessions with the patient and caregivers present. The information should be repeated in subsequent sessions and rehearse instructions provided in earlier sessions. The clinician should monitor not only the patient but also caregivers for signs of strain and possible depression.

Patients need to be reassured that clinical vigilance is a form of treatment just as surely as is chemotherapy. If vigilance is indicated, the patient and caregivers should learn the reasons to withhold pharmacologic interventions while maintaining a watchful eye. Finally, patient education may require referral to support groups in which other leukemia patients have learned to live with cancer, if not beyond. Referrals can include connections to other patients with leukemia within a primary care practice as well as support groups convened by local chapters of the American Cancer Society. The goal of support group referral is to advance the patient's connection with others who can share treatment-related information and advance coping strategies. Caregivers may require a separate support group where they can discuss issues that are unique to their role.

Common Immune Problems

Allergic Reactions

Allergy is defined as an immune-mediated reaction to a foreign environmental allergen. It is characterized by an inflammatory response to allergenic invasion of the body. Typical sites for allergenic invasion are the skin and respiratory tree, where local reactions occur. Allergenic invasion may cause a systemic response, however, whereby multiple organs and the circulatory system may become involved. Allergenic shock or anaphylaxis is an extreme example of this systemic response.

Epidemiology and Causes

Allergies are equally distributed between the sexes, affecting women as often as men, without regard to race. The incidence of allergies is greater in children than adults, perhaps because of the immaturity of immune responses in children and the tendency toward humorally mediated T helper-2 (Th2) type responses.

Seasonal allergies vary according to hemispheric geography, which means that pollens, mold, and spores affect individuals by seasonal patterns of the Northern and Southern Hemispheres. In North America, pollens rise and fall in a May to September pattern, whereas molds follow a March through December pattern; therefore, there are only 2 to 3 months of the year, in the winter, when pollens and molds do not affect the population. During cold weather, however, individuals remain indoors for longer periods of time, which can increase the risk of more frequent exposure to dust mites and other indoor allergens.

Causes of allergies include environmental allergens and their corresponding intrinsic immune complexes formed by the body as it mounts a vigorous response to allergenic exposure. Environmental allergens include natural *inhalants* such as pollens, molds, and spores, *ingestants* such as food and drug allergens, *injectants* such as animal or insect venoms, and *contactants* including dust mites and their feces, animal hair and dander, as well as chemical components in hair- and skin-care products. Regardless of the source, the allergen invades the body, eliciting a complex immune-regulated response that results in either local or systemic effects.

Pathophysiology

All allergens are foreign substances to the body. Cellular and humoral immune responses occur after initial exposure to a foreign substance. Immune responses result from a complex, coordinated set of events requiring several different cell types, cell surface signaling proteins, and secreted regulatory cytokines. Key cell types include histamine-containing mast cells and basophils, as well as highly granular eosinophils. Also important are antibody-secreting plasma cells which are specialized, differentiated cells of the B lineage designed to produce monoclonal antibody of a single antigenic specificity. Just as important are CD4+ T helper cells that are also antigen-specific and produce an array of regulatory cytokines after their T cell receptors come into contact with specific antigens. Helper T cells of the Th2 class produce cytokines (e.g., IL-4, IL-5, IL-13) which upregulate humoral antibody-mediated immune responses, while Th1 helper T cells produce a separate set of cytokines (IFN-γ, IL-12) that upregulate cell-mediated antibody-independent cytotoxic responses.

There are four basic types of immune responses to allergens (sometimes classified as a group as hypersensitivity responses), categorized by whether or not they are dependent on circulating antibodies (types 1 through 3) or cellular immune components (type 4). Only type 1 immune reactions are considered true allergic responses. However, type 3 immune responses often underlie what are erroneously termed drug and food allergies, while type 4 immune reactions mediate contact dermatitis, a pathologic response to certain skin irritants, such as poison ivy and poison oak.

Type 1: IgE-Mediated Immediate Hypersensitivity Response

In the first step of initial exposure to an allergen, the immune system must recognize that the allergen is foreign. IgE is an immunoglobulin class present in relatively low concentration in the circulation. As with all immunoglobulins, IgE molecules are antigen specific in their variable arms, allowing for binding of more than one IgE molecule to a single circulating antigenic molecule. However, the constant portion (Fcϵ) of the IgE molecule allows for its binding to the surface of cells specifically expressing high-affinity receptors for the IgE molecule (FcϵRIII). IgE molecules are bound to tissue-derived mast cells located primarily in the skin, respiratory, and GI tracts, where allergens are most likely to contact or invade the body. In addition, circulating basophils are bound to allergen-specific IgE molecules.

Antibody cross-linking is the process by which two or more IgE molecules bound to the cell surface bind a common antigen and triggering intracellular signaling and degranulation. Such responses do not occur on initial exposure to an allergen. On first exposure, specific IgE molecules are formed via class-switching of antigen-specific B cells from the IgG or IgM classes to IgE, based on the constant portion of the antibody molecule. These molecules then bind to mast cells and basophils, and on reexposure to the same antigen when an allergen binds to cell-bound IgE, a cascade of cellular events occurs dependent on intracellular calcium shifts, which facilitates cyclic nucleotide signaling molecules to trigger leukocytic degranulation.

This leads to the excretion of preformed inflammatory mediators including histamine, heparin, tryptase, and other proteolytic enzymes; thromboxane; arachidonic acid; prostaglandins; superoxides; and several eosinophilic and neutrophilic chemotactic factors, as well as triggering the synthesis of newly formed inflammatory mediators including leukotrienes and key cytokines.

Inflammatory mediators cause venules, capillaries, and arterioles to dilate and become hyperpermeable. The mucous membranes are triggered to increase mucus excretion and the walls of hollow visceral structures to spasm as a result of smooth muscle contraction. Dehydration may result from a relative shift of fluids that follow intravascular proteins out of the vasculature and into extravascular space, thus potentially lowering the blood pressure. Hypotension may be aggravated by other environmental factors such as relative heat and humidity.

IgE activation and cellular excretion of inflammatory mediators takes place only a few seconds after antigenic exposure. Whereas the effects of initial inflammatory mediators may last for 30 minutes, repeated allergenic exposure can prolong the inflammatory cycle for hours. A prolonged and intractable inflammatory cycle is the clinical picture of the atopic (hypersensitivity) diseases such as allergic rhinitis and allergic asthma, which are also heavily dependent on inflammatory cells including mast cells, eosinophils, and T cells. *Atopy* is a term used to characterize an IgE-mediated immune response that is exaggerated or out of character for exposure to what appear to be innocuous environmental allergens. While allergic skin reactions are classically characterized by raised, erythematous wheals termed urticarial plaques, another common allergic skin condition, atopic dermatitis, has several different manifestations whose pathophysiology extends beyond IgE-mediated allergic processes (see Chapter 6).

Atopic diseases are one of the type 1 allergies. A second category is *anaphylaxis.* Unlike atopic diseases, which are characterized by localized effects in the skin or respiratory tract, anaphylaxis is systemic in scope. All of the inflammatory processes of hypersensitivity become exaggerated, leading to life-threatening hypotension, bronchospasm, laryngospasm, angioedema, smooth muscle and visceral organ contractions, and raised inflammatory skin eruptions termed urticaria. Anaphylaxis may follow exposure in susceptible individuals to well-known allergens, such as insect venom (bee or wasp stings) or certain drugs such as penicillin. However, these responses are not limited to individuals with a history of atopic disease and may occur unexpectedly in any individual. Therefore, a history of atopy does not predict anaphylaxis. If left untreated, anaphylaxis is fatal. Advanced Practice Nursing Interventions 16.2 lists the seven-step treatment for anaphylaxis.

Type 2: Antibody-Mediated Cellular Cytotoxicity Response

Type 2 antibody-mediated cellular cytotoxicity responses introduce an immune mechanism different from type 1 immediate hypersensitivity responses. Type 2 responses involves the activation of antigen-specific IgM and IgG molecules. These humoral immune molecules bind to foreign antigens and activate serum immune complement. This leads to destruction of any cell to which an allergen is bound; thus, a type 2 immune response is cytotoxic. Examples of such type 2 responses include neonatal Rh-incompatibility hemolytic disease and immune-mediated hemolytic anemia. In addition, once antibodies bind to foreign antigens such as microbial cell surface proteins, these invading microbes become prone to phagocytosis and destruction by other immune cells, a process known as opsonization.

ADVANCE PRACTICE NURSING INTERVENTIONS 16.2

The Seven-Step Treatment for Anaphylaxis

Step 1: Administer aqueous epinephrine 1:1000 dilution 0.2 to 0.5 mg (0.2–0.5 mL) IM.

Step 2: Repeat epinephrine every 5–15 minutes as required by clinical picture.

Step 3: If the patient is conscious and without laryngospasm, administer diphenhydramine (Benadryl) 25–50 mg to relieve the sequelae of potential vascular damage.

Step 4: Support bronchodilation if patient is without laryngospasm by administering albuterol 0.3 mL inhalation via nebulizer. If hypotensive, position the patient supine with feet elevated.

Step 5: If patient is in laryngospasm or pulmonary arrest, perform emergency endotracheal intubation and support with artificial oxygenation.

Step 6: Start IV fluids using normal saline or Ringer's lactate solution to maintain systolic blood pressure greater than 90 mm Hg. The rate of flow should be determined by the blood pressure reading.

Step 7: Transfer the patient to an acute-care emergency center for continued support and observation.

See text regarding teaching about Epipens.

Type 3: Antibody–Allergen Complex Response

The third category of immune responses also requires immunoglobulin M (IgM) and IgG activation, as is characteristic of a type 2 immune response. However, type 3 responses denote an immune complex that is formed between these immunoglobulins and the allergen. These complexes become deposited into the various tissues of the body, activating serum complement that in turn triggers various inflammatory mediators. These illnesses tend to be systemic, as immune complexes affect multiple organs and tissue types throughout the body. The reaction is not immediate, and in fact, may occur up to 2 to 3 weeks after antigenic exposure. Hypersensitivity-type pneumonitis secondary to inhaled allergen and serum sickness are two examples of type 3 responses. Delayed drug reactions are also classic examples of type 3 responses, with the most common offenders being the antiepileptic drugs phenytoin, phenobarbital, and carbamazepine, as well as various antibiotics.

Type 4: Delayed-Type Cellular Hypersensitivity Response

The fourth category of immune responses is defined as a cell-mediated delayed-type immune response that is unlike the three previous categories, which are all mediated by humoral factors (antibody-dependent). The other three categories directly involve few, if any, T lymphocytes. However, type 4 reactions are T cell dependent and usually begin in the skin, where large numbers of T cells are found. Antigen contacting the skin is endocytosed (taken up) by antigen-presenting cells, which process and relocate small antigenic peptides on the cell surface, coupled to antigen-presenting proteins known as major histocompatibility complexes (MHC).

Antigen-specific T cell receptors recognize and bind to these antigenic peptide–MHC complexes, which leads to a series of inflammatory reactions including cellular lysis of the antigen-presenting cell and cytokine production. Because of this delay in cellular lysis, lasting up to 2 to 3 days after antigenic exposure, skin eruptions do not appear immediately. Contact dermatitis (e.g., poison ivy, chemical irritations, nickel metallic allergies) is the classic example of a type 4 immune response. In addition, the wheal and flare response to *Mycobacteria tuberculosis* purified protein derivative (PPD) used in TB screening is also a type 4 immune response, when positive in persons previously exposed to TB. This explains why the Tuberculin Skin Test (TST) is read at 48 to 72 hours after placement.

Clinical Presentation

Subjective

Patients report fatigue and/or malaise, irritability, itchy and watery eyes, sneezing, rhinorrhea, nasal congestion, coughing without sputum production (unless a secondary bacterial infection accompanies the allergy), and pruritus. Two elements are common to subjective complaints associated with allergies. First, an exposure to an allergen precedes the onset of symptoms. Thus, allergic rhinitis can be distinguished from perennial rhinitis, because environmental exposure precedes the former. Second, patients report attempts to control their symptoms with self-care. For example, their subjective picture has usually been self-medication and somewhat controlled with over-the-counter (OTC) agents. A history of subjective symptoms, therefore, requires accompanying inquiry concerning use of OTC antihistamines and decongestants.

Objective

The sinuses may be tender to percussion. The conjunctivae and mucous membranes in general will be injected. Nasal turbinates should be erythematous. Cervical nodes will feel shoddy, with few greater than 1 cm in size. Postauricular nodes and thoracic nodes may not be involved. Tympanic membranes may appear dull to light but will be otherwise unremarkable.

Tachycardia will accompany OTC drug use, but fever does not contribute to the tachycardia because fever is almost always absent. Lungs will be clear after several deep breaths and cough unless allergic asthma causes wheezing to appear. Except in patients with anaphylaxis or allergenic invasion of the GI tract, the abdominal exam will prove unremarkable. In these exceptional cases, profound abdominal tenderness may inhibit deep palpation.

Skin eruptions will include urticaria, fissures, circumscribed papules, bullae, and petechiae. The clinician should expect no singular picture of skin eruptions that corresponds with the allergenic source; however, there are associations in skin presentation and history that lend themselves to diagnostic conclusions. For example, a history of exposure to poison ivy and multiple circumscribed papules in the anatomic place of exposure provides an association that is diagnostic of specific exposure. Poison ivy is a contact dermatitis, while urticaria is classic for allergic disease.

If the patient's sensorium is affected, the Mini-Mental Status Examination (MMSE) should be administered. (The tool is described in the section on Alzheimer's disease in Chapter 5.) The MMSE could manifest diminished problem-solving ability, impairment in recent recall, and unfocused attention. These signs are particularly evident in older adults and others who practice polypharmacy in combination with OTC agents

Diagnostic Reasoning

Diagnostic Tests

Initial testing begins with the clinical history. The clinician should ask the patient to describe what was different in diet, skin-care products, and activities before the onset of symptoms. Suspicions raised in the history often will prove true or at least supportive in subsequent tests.

Type 1 Response. Initial testing continues with skin tests to diagnose the response to specific allergens. Skin tests involve first pricking the epidermis and later injecting the intradermal layers of the skin. (Patch testing is generally reserved for contact dermatitis and other manifestations of type IV sensitivities.) Pricking is the first stage of testing because of the very slight but potentially fatal chance that the allergen could cause a systemic response. For every negative prick test, an intradermal injection is given.

The selection of antigens to be tested follows a pattern of reasoning based on the question: What are the most likely culprits? The exact composition of skin-test panels is determined by regional and patient-specific determinants. The allergist will inject small amounts of regional and suspected environmental allergens in skin-test panels. If the test is positive, a wheal should appear in 15 to 20 minutes. The reliability and exquisite accuracy of skin testing still makes it the preferred test for initial diagnosis. Skin tests are done with positive (histamine) and negative (inert) controls, and results must be judged against these controls, since some individuals are sensitive to any kind of scratching or pricking of the skin, just by the nature of the insult to the skin, and not due to the antigen itself. Skin tests are definitely more sensitive than serum RAST tests, as more atopic individuals will be positive on the skin tests. Not all atopic individuals will have high levels of allergen-specific IgE, however.

Alternatives to the skin test include in vitro methods, such as the radioallergosorbent test (RAST), the enzyme-linked immunosorbent assay (ELISA), and the fluorescent antibody staining technique (FAST). Each of these can be accomplished by serum testing which, therefore, reduces the risk of hypersensitivity-type reactions from allergens in skin testing as serum tests just measure antigen-specific IgE levels in the blood.

RAST tests are more specific, so non-atopic individuals are really unlikely to have high allergen-specific IgE levels, but they are not as sensitive, so not all atopic individuals will have high levels of allergen-specific IgE. This is particularly important for food challenge testing. While some food allergies may be type 3 immune complex responses, there certainly are anaphylactic food allergy reactions, which are IgE-mediated. These may be tested in an office setting (with ready access to endotracheal intubation supplies and epinephrine) in the presence of physicians or other persons qualified to treat anaphylactic reactions. Set amounts of food are given to persons suspected of food allergy (typically children) in progressively increasing amounts, and these people are monitored for several hours for any reaction. This is a highly specific test, so it is great at ruling out food allergies. Obviously, however, this carries a great risk of anaphylaxis. RAST testing may be done instead, so that if an individual with a high IgE level is identified, he or she will not be subjected to a food challenge test needlessly.

Asthma is an allergen-driven disease and is atopic and characterized by type 1 responses, although it is not a systemic anaphylaxis. Atopic airway hypersensitivity may also be triggered by environmental irritants such as tobacco smoke, which is not a true allergen, as these individuals will not expresses true tobacco-specific IgE levels, but smoke may certainly trigger an asthma attack.

Reactive airway disease may be either allergenic or nonallergenic. Asthma is an allergen-driven disease and is atopic and characterized by type 1 responses, Allergenic sputum will stain positive for eosinophils; therefore, a sputum sample stained with methylene blue dye may reveal eosinophils.

Type 2 Response. Rh testing of blood during pregnancy is the initial test to determine prospective Rh incompatibility. With reference to immune hemolytic anemia, an elevated indirect bilirubin indicates hemolysis. Hemolysis is associated with decreased haptoglobin levels. AIHA is also associated with a positive Coombs' test, which detects anti-RBC specific antibodies in the blood.

Type 3 Response. Initial tests are employed to determine complement activation. A complement ELISA will give specific evidence of complement activation. For example, the ELISA might show lower levels of C_3 and C_4, which are two elements of complement that should not be diminished unless an allergic inflammatory response has activated complement. Skin manifestations in type 3 responses may be biopsied and stained for immune complexes.

Type 4 Response. Skin testing for anergy, associated by example with tuberculin skin testing, is the initial test of preference for cell-mediated hypersensitivity. Allergens are either injected or laid in patches. Results are read at 48 hours. Positive test results are induration (if injected) and erythema and papules (patch results).

IgE serum levels may aid in distinguishing allergenic from nonallergenic disease. In type 4 reactions, these are not IgE-mediated responses. In addition, an elevated eosinophil count from the WBC differential may provide a secondary confirmation of recent IgE-mediated atopic disease.

Differential Diagnosis

The clinical history is the mainstay of differentiating allergenic disease. Allergies are caused by exposure to environmental antigens. The history, therefore, must support allergenic exposure proximal to onset of symptoms, relief or failure from OTC agents, and possibly familial allergic patterns. Additional differentiation of allergy comes from skin-test results and other initial tests.

Alternative irritants that enter the body but do not initiate inflammation include nonallergic sources. For example, asthmatics may experience onset of symptoms associated with barometric changes in the atmosphere that elicit an inflammatory response in susceptible individuals.

Management

While atopic dermatitis is a core atopic disorder, it is covered in Chapter 6. Allergy management requires symptom relief and treatment against specific allergens. In addition, because it is better to prevent than to treat, the first step of management is to identify and avoid allergens. Second, symptom management is important. Third, immunotherapy offers both prophylaxis and treatment for the patient. Initial management is considered avoidance of allergens, whereas subsequent management involves symptom control and immunotherapy.

Initial Management

The patient must become vigilant to avoid allergenic exposure. After skin testing has identified specific allergens, avoidance behaviors should be initiated. For example, individuals diagnosed with hypersensitivity to penicillin must avoid not only penicillin but also cephalosporins because of a likelihood of cross-reactivity. The patient history should focus on whether an anaphylactic reaction to penicillin (PCN) really occurred, as most proposed PCN allergies are not true allergies and certainly not true anaphylaxis. PCN and other antibiotic desensitization can be performed to use the antibiotic to which a patient has a supposed allergy.

Bee venom reactions can be avoided by not disturbing beehives or wasp nests. Allergen avoidance measures like the use of mattress and pillow covers, avoiding dust-collecting ceiling fans and keeping windows closed in favor of air conditioning, as well as hot water washing of plush toys or any potential dust reservoirs should be encouraged. Carpets can be removed from bedrooms to limit dust mite exposure during sleeping hours. HEPA filters and chemical agents to reduce aeroallergens have actually not been shown to be effective. Air conditioning filters should be changed monthly.

Subsequent Management

Subsequent management provides symptom control and immunotherapy. Symptom control can be achieved either through prescribed or OTC agents. There are many groups of drugs as possible therapeutic selections for symptom management in allergenic disease: sympathomimetics, antihistamines, corticosteroids, cromolyn, and theophylline. There are many H1- and H2-histamine receptor antagonists, as well as IV steroids to prevent delayed or secondary phase reactions of anaphylaxis, mediated by the de novo, newly formed inflammatory mediators. Late-phase reactions may occur up to 24 hours later and can also prove fatal, so steroids are almost always used. (Many of these are covered in the Drugs Commonly Prescribed Box 8.1.) The newer antihistamines have less of an anticholinergic effect and do not cause as much tachycardia.

Symptom Control. Many OTC agents are sympathomimetic in activity. Common examples of oral drugs in this class include pseudoephedrine (Sudafed), chlorpheniramine (Chlor-Trimeton), and ephedrine (Vicks Va-Tro-Nol). In addition, epinephrine (Primatene Mist) is available by inhalation in the same class of sympathomimetic drugs.

Sympathomimetic agents provide alpha-adrenergic and beta-adrenergic properties. They vasoconstrict engorged mucosa (alpha-adrenergic property) and dilate the bronchioles (beta-adrenergic property); therefore, they support the antihistamines in drying secretions, open the airways of the nasopharynx and bronchial tree, and speed up the heart rate (another beta-adrenergic effect). Because of their low molecular weight and the small size of the therapeutic proteins, sympathomimetics cross the blood–brain barrier, causing irritability and addictive effects with other psychoactive substances such as ethanol.

Abuse potential with the OTC sympathomimetics remains high for many reasons. They make one feel better and provide symptom control without professional supervision; they are relatively inexpensive and readily available; and they are well known, after having attracted the attention of millions of television viewers in commercial advertisements. Some studies suggest that regular use of beta-adrenergic inhalants, such as albuterol (Proventil), can increase disease morbidities.

A second group of agents used for mild allergic reactions is antihistamines. Available OTC and by prescription, the antihistamines block H_1 receptors, thereby reducing the effects of histamine that is released in the inflammatory cascade. The block of H_1-receptor sites offers the therapeutic effect of drying secretions. Adverse effects include overdryness and sedation. Sedation, particularly in the older adult, requires dose limitation or a prescription drug trial. Among prescription drugs, there are newer generation antihistamines such as desloratadine (Clarinex), fexofenadine (Allegra), and cetirizine (Zyrtec) which are nonsedating. Loratadine (Claritin) is OTC. These drugs dry secretions without causing excessive drowsiness, are not associated with untoward cardiac events that may result from combination therapy with the macrolides, and can be dosed once daily. Other commonly used H_1 antagonists are diphenhydramine (Benadryl) and hydroxyzine (Atarax) which do have sedating effects. Anticholinergic agents such as intranasal ipratropium (Atrovent) are also very effective at drying secretions.

H_2 antagonists such as cimetidine (Tagamet) are also useful in managing mild allergic reactions. In some cases when patients have failed to improve after receiving epinephrine and diphenhydramine, they did respond to cimetidine.

Corticosteroids form a third group of drugs used in symptom control. They may need to be ordered for patients with mild allergic reactions, such as urticaria, besides being given to patients with severe laryngeal edema, bronchospasm, or hypotension. For most hypersensitivity reactions, a dosage of 1 to 2 mg/kg per day of prednisone for 4 or 5 days is usually appropriate. This dosage does not require tapering. The clinician should consider tapering if the patient has received corticosteroid therapy in the recent past or if there are plans to continue therapy for more than several weeks. When given as short-term therapy, prednisone has fairly benign adverse effects. Overuse of oral corticosteroids does have a number of implications, including a Cushingoid syndrome, adrenal insufficiency, and hyperglycemia. Inhaled corticosteroids such as mometasone furoate (Nasonex) are used as a standard prophylactic controller in allergic asthma (see Chapter 8). Intranasal corticosteroids are extremely effective for allergic rhinitis (see Chapter 7). As corticosteroids are immunosuppressant agents, they downregulate the allergic responses characteristic of atopy.

Immunotherapy. Immunotherapy offers the patient long-term control of atopic disease. Its use is usually limited in scope to patients with intractable allergic rhinitis or asthma whose disease fails to be controlled with symptom management or for whom there is no chance of avoiding allergens. Injections are given SC in 0.5-cc allotments of allergenic diluent that progresses from minimal dilutional strength to higher concentrations. The weekly injections continue, increasing in concentration until symptoms are controlled. Immunotherapy may require more than 12 months of treatments before positive effects are observed. There are also "rush immunotherapy" or shorter course regimens that are being evaluated. But in reality, injections may continue for life. For extremely refractory cases of atopy such as allergic asthma with atopic dermatitis, Xolair (anti-IgE specific monoclonal antibody immunotherapy) may be effective.

A clinical scenario offers the picture of a patient who might benefit from immunotherapy. A 55-year-old woman has been diagnosed with allergic rhinitis. Her primary allergens are dust mites, ragweed, chocolate, and *Aspergillus.* She avoids chocolate. She has removed carpeting from her bedroom and substituted blinds for curtains. But she cannot move from her home in the Midwestern United States, where ragweed pollen levels are elevated between July and October. Her husband cleans the bathroom tiles and kitchen cabinets where *Aspergillus* might grow. For the past 3 months she has consulted the clinician on six occasions. Her drug regimen includes a nasal steroid inhalant and an antihistamine. Nonetheless, her symptoms keep her awake at night, and recently she has started to wheeze, requiring the use of an albuterol nebulizer. The clinician referred her to an allergist who made the specific allergen diagnoses. The allergist recommends immunotherapy on the basis of the severity and recurrence of symptoms.

Follow-Up and Referral

Follow-up consists of increased consultations during seasonal allergy periods and regular visits depending on symptoms. Follow-up tests include a CBC, to determine leukocytosis and eosinophilia, and a fasting blood sugar, should systemic steroids be required.

An allergist should be consulted if the symptoms cannot be controlled. The allergist is responsible for ordering and evaluating skin tests and for recommending and evaluating the effectiveness of immunotherapy.

Patient Education

The patient must know what foods and other environmental allergens to avoid. The patient and clinician should decide together how to identify and control allergens that may have been unknown by the patient before the diagnosis. For example, few patients know the places that dust mites hide or understand how to kill *Aspergillus* with simple household chemicals.

Patients must learn how to use nasal inhalants and metered-dose inhalants (MDI). Initial use under the clinician's supervision can provide both the patient and clinician with reassurance that the drug will be delivered correctly. The use of spacers for MDI should be discussed (see Chapter 8). Further attention to drug adherence suggests that the patient should learn which drugs are best taken together, alone, or with food. Therapeutic drug levels, particularly with theophylline, will require vigilance on the part of the patient to report the early symptoms of drug toxicity.

Patients with a history of anaphylaxis must have epinephrine available at all times for emergencies, should they come in contact with the offending allergen. The immediate use of epinephrine following any repeated exposure to an anaphylactic agent is crucial.

The clinician should prescribe a kit for the patient and have the patient demonstrate understanding of its use before leaving the office. There are several brands of epinephrine in kits (Ana-Kit, AnaGuard, EpiPens). The expiration date is 1 year and most kits contain more than one dose of epinephrine, which the patient injects IM. The patient should be instructed that whenever a dose is self-administered, emergency room care should be sought, in case the reaction worsens and the patient requires IV epinephrine. Susceptible individuals must always have access to a ready source of epinephrine if exposure occurs a second time.

Many patients will take OTC agents to help with allergies and should be taught to read the labels for ingredients that might cause tachycardia. Patients should be cautioned to be on the alert for anything containing ephedrine, phenylephrine, phenylpropanolamine, and pseudoephedrine.

Rheumatoid Arthritis

Rheumatoid arthritis is a chronic, progressive, systemic inflammatory process that primarily affects the synovial joints. Joints are destroyed over a long course of disease remissions and exacerbations. Deformities are common as the disease progresses, which create emotional as well as physical trauma for the patient. *Healthy People 2010* has two objectives related to this chronic debilitating conditon. One objective is to increase the proportion of adults who have seen a health-care provider for their chronic joint symptoms; the other is to increase the proportion of persons with arthritis who have had effective evidence-based arthritis education as an integral part of the management of their condition.

Epidemiology and Causes

In the general population of the United States, rheumatoid arthritis (RA) is the second most common connective tissue disease and the most destructive to the joints. Women with the disease outnumber men in a 2.5 to 3.1:1 ratio. Incidence increases with age, with a peak of cases occurring between ages 40 and 60 after an onset of the disease between ages 20 and 40. No associations with any particular racial or ethnic group have been determined. However, the disease follows a familial pattern, and further inquiry is ongoing concerning the genetics of the disease. Immunologists have identified the appearance of a relationship between rheumatoid arthritis and the human leukocyte antigen (HLA) system, a series of linked genes on the sixth chromosome. The cause of the disease, though indicating a genetic factor, to date is unknown. Other multiple factors implicated include infection, autoimmunity, environmental, and hormonal factors.

Pathophysiology

Rheumatoid arthritis destroys the joints in two ways. First, proteolytic enzymes known as proteases digest the tissue components of affected joints. This is speculated to occur due to locally released antigens that evoke the inflammatory cascade; however, the source of these antigens is not fully characterized. These antigens may actually be autoimmune substances (e.g., Type II collagen found only in articular cartilage and the vitreous of the eye, glycoprotein-39 found in cartilage, citrulline containing peptides (CCP) including citrullinated fibrin, and glucose-6-phosphate isomerase), activating self-reactive T cells which initiate the inflammatory cascade.

T cells comprise nearly half the immune cells in a rheumatoid joint and are characterized by an activated T helper phenotype based on surface expression of HLA-DR (MHC Class II) antigens, CD27, CD4, as well as the costimulatory molecules CD28 and CD40. It has been difficult to characterize the antigenic specificity of the initial set of T cells which trigger this immunoresponse, as the subsequent cascade is characterized by widespread recruitment of so-called "bystander T cells" which do not express autoantigen specificity but nonetheless proliferate and contribute to destruction of the affected joint through cytokine expression. Interestingly, some evidence indicates that it may not be the actual peptide antigen that triggers the self-reactive T cell, but rather genetic mutations which alter specific amino acids within MHC Class II antigen-presenting molecules (such as HLA-DRβ1) found on antigen-presenting cells. Other work has implicated superantigen interactions which trigger several different T cell clones independent of MHC Class II molecules.

Cells of the synovial (joint) lining including joint endothelium, T cells, and fibroblast-like cells proliferate, producing cytokines (e.g., IL-1, IL-6, IL-8, IL-15, IL-18, IFN-γ), neuropeptides such as substance P, and chemotactic factors that induce cell adhesion molecules (e.g., intercellular adhesion molecule [ICAM]-1, vascular cell adhesion molecule [VCAM]-1, P-selectin, E-selectin). This leads to recruitment of an array of immune cells into the affected joint, including mast cells that produce histamine, tryptase, leukotrienes, cytokines, and chymase, multinucleated cells and macrophages which are the main source of potentially toxic nitric oxide and destructive matrix metalloproteinases (MMP) (e.g., collagenase [MMP-1], stromelysin [MMP-3], macrophage elastase [MMP-12]), and self-reactive plasma cells capable of producing autoantibodies (e.g., rheumatoid factor). Synovial fibroblasts further produce MMP-13, which has great specificity for type II collagen and is primarily responsible for soft tissue invasion in the affected joint.

Particularly noteworthy in the pathogenesis of RA is the production of rheumatoid factor—polyclonal species of antibody typically of the IgM class which have specificity for the constant Fc region of IgG. Rheumatoid factor thus forms large immunocomplexes capable of activating complement proteins that themselves are cytolytic and chemotactic. The production of these antibodies is enhanced by cytokines secreted by regulatory CD4+ T helper cells. The plasma cell genes that encode rheumatoid factor undergo somatic mutations that increase their affinity for IgG, a process known as affinity maturation. While rheumatoid factor is not pathognomonic of RA (also present in scleroderma, SLE, and even some viral infections) and may be absent in up to 25 percent of cases, the presence of these antibodies in the peripheral circulation correlates with invasive disease of greater severity.

Tumor necrosis factor (TNF)-α appears to be the main cytokine that triggers the proliferative rheumatoid synovium, which explains the efficacy of anti-TNF-α immunotherapies. But in addition to TNF-α, a wide array of cytokines has been implicated in the pathophysiology of the rheumatoid joint in addition to the factors mentioned above, including granulocyte macrophage-colony stimulating factor (GM-CSF), IL-2, IL-13, IL-17, and transforming growth factor (TGF)-β. Moreover, cells of the synovial lining undergo transformation into a rapidly proliferating state (although incapable of true metastasis) in which several type of transcription factors (NF-κB, Fos, Jun, Raf, Myc) and intracellular kinases (e.g., mitogen-activated protein kinase [MAPK]) are upregulated.

Second, joints are progressively destroyed by an invasive rheumatoid pannus. The pathology of RA is widespread, enveloping layers of the heart muscle, cardiac valves, pulmonary visceral pleura, sclera, spleen, larynx, dura matter, and, of course, the synovia of the joints. Similar to a destructive malignancy, the rheumatoid pannus is a creation of the inflamed synovium. It consists of granulated vascular tissue extending from the vascular bed into the joint and is characterized by increased angiogenesis (i.e., new blood vessel formation) which is mediated by the upregulation of several angiogenic cytokines and growth factors, including hypoxia-inducible factor (HIF)-1, vascular endothelial growth factor (VEGF)/VEGF receptor, heparin-binding growth factors, macrophage angiogenic factor (MAF), epithelial neutrophil activating peptide-78 (ENA-78), TNF-α, PGE1, PGE2, and IL-8. This increased vascularity is often inadequate for the level of cellular proliferation in the rheumatoid synovium. In addition, the increased intra-articular pressure manifested by cellular proliferation, fibrin and clotting factor deposition, and fluid accumulation within the affected joint may tamponade articular vessels resulting in progressive joint ischemia.

Mutations and overexpression in certain cell cycle regulatory proteins such as the *p53* tumor suppressor gene have been identified in cells of the rheumatoid synovium which may render them less susceptible to apoptosis (programmed cell death). As discussed, cells in the pannus release proteolytic enzymes (e.g., MMP, glycosidases) that destroy glycosaminoglycans, fibronectin, proteoglycans such as chondroitin sulfate, collagen, and eventually subchondral bony structures. Moreover, the rheumatoid pannus (in particular, regulatory T cells and bone marrow stromal cells) induces differentiation and proliferation of bone osteoclasts which leads to further bony destruction of the joint. Fortunately, however, the pannus remains responsive to antiproliferative immunosuppressant treatments.

Within the synovial fluid, an inflammatory response also ensues but with a notably different distribution of immune cells. Polymorphonuclear neutrophils are the most prominent cellular infiltrate, numbering upwards of one billion in severely inflamed joints. These cells secrete a host of proteolytic enzymes into the joint fluid (e.g., myeloperoxidase, collagenase and other MMP, elastase, and lysozyme), as well as inflammatory cytokines (e.g., prostaglandins, IL-1β), and chemotactic factors (e.g., leukotriene B4, platelet activating factor). As this accumulation of joint fluid distends the joint capsule, contributing greatly to articular pains, aspiration of this exudative fluid may provide instant relief.

Clinical Presentation

Subjective

In the early stages of the disease the patient may complain of malaise, diffuse arthritis, weight loss, anorexia, and low-grade fever. In addition, the patient may complain of neuropathic pain in the extremities, painful eyes, and chest pain on deep inspiration.

The patient awakens in pain but reports that it improves as the day progresses. Not only does pain subside but the swelling associated with joints in the early morning also abates with moderate activity. As the disease progresses, pain and swelling form the subjective picture that becomes associated with diminished activity and a downward spiral of worsening pain and immobility.

Objective

The key physical findings are peripheral symmetric polyarthritis and morning stiffness, especially if the latter lasts longer than 1 hour. The clinician will note that some joints are more involved than others. These include the proximal interphalangeal (PIP) and metacarpophalangeal (MCP) joints in the hands, wrists, and knees. The toes and ankles also tend to be affected. Early disease radiographic markings may prove nondescript even though synovial changes have already begun. The clinician should expect the affected joints to be painful to pressure, edematous, and partially immobile. As the disease progresses, joints will appear more deformed and rigid. Monoarticular arthritis of a large joint is a far less common presentation in RA and is more suspicious for reactive arthritis, which does not include morning stiffness as a symptom.

Physical examination may unfold additional significant findings associated with the disease. A cardiac rub associated with pericarditis may be detected. A pulmonary friction rub or diminished respiratory excursion may suggest inflammation in the visceral pleura as well as involvement of the bony structures of the ribs and sternum.

A finding of injected sclera suggests scleritis. Loss of sensation, especially over lower extremities, indicates peripheral neuropathy. Range of motion in affected joints will be diminished. Ecchymotic lesions may appear on the arms and legs. Rheumatoid nodules, if present, typically appear on the elbows. These microscopic nodules are subcutaneous. It is a granuloma with a central section of fibrinoid necrosis, a surrounding palisade of radially arranged elongated connective tissue cells surrounded by chronic granulation tissue. The clinician may note that they are tender to touch.

Diagnostic Reasoning

Diagnostic Tests

The initial test of preference for diagnosis is rheumatoid factor (RF), which is an IgM that reacts in an autoimmune fashion against IgG. The test result provides both qualitative and quantitative information that is useful in correlation with physical markers. For example, a positive titer of greater than 1:150 indicates a poorer prognosis and is accompanied often by additional findings of severe disease such as rheumatoid nodules. It is necessary to read both the presence of RF (qualitative) with the titer (quantitative), because the factor may be present in other diseases and its incidence increases with age. It is estimated that only 75 percent of patients that have the disease have a positive RF.

Initial testing should also include an erythrocyte sedimentation rate (ESR), which will be elevated if the disease is active. C-reactive protein is another acute phase reactant test that could be drawn in addition to or in place of ESR as a nonspecific indicator of inflammation. Other tests include a CBC to rule out anemia as the cause of the fatigue and indicate whether a leukocytosis might be associated. A platelet count (showing normal or high values) will become more elevated as joints become more inflamed. Joint-fluid analysis may aid in distinguishing rheumatoid arthritis. Aspirates from rheumatoid joints will show between 2000 and 50,000 WBCs/mL and pronounced neutrophils. Advanced Assessment 16.1 compares the results of synovial fluid analysis.

Radiographic changes may not be evident in the initial phases of the disease; however, after the disease has run its course for 6 months or more, radiographs will reveal bone erosions at the joints of the hands and feet. Plain films may show bony erosions in up to 30 percent of patients within one year of diagnosis and up to 90 percent of cases after the first 2 years.

Subsequent tests are used as markers of disease progression. For example, the ESR provides a marker of inflammation that may become invaluable in charting the course of the disease. Quantitative antinuclear antibodies (ANA) may help in differentiating rheumatoid arthritis from

ADVANCED ASSESSMENT 16.1

Analyzing Synovial Fluid

	Normal	Noninflammatory	Inflammatory	Purulent	Hemorrhagic
Clarity/Color	Clear, yellow	Transparent, xanthochromic	Opaque, white or translucent	Opaque, white	Opaque, hemorrhagic
Leukocytes/mL	<200	200–2000	2,000–50,000	50,000–300,000	Variable
Percent of PMN	<25%	<50%	>75%	50–100%	Variable
RBCs	Low	Low	Low	Low	High
Possible Causes	Normal	Osteoarthritis Trauma SLE Polyarteritis nodosa Scleroderma Corticosteroid therapy	Rheumatoid arthritis Rheumatic fever Reactive arthritis Crystal synovitis	Septic arthritis Bacterial infection Fungi Tuberculosis	Trauma Blood dyscrasias Tumor Anticoagulants Sickle cell disease Myeloproliferative diseases

systemic lupus erythematosus (SLE). Lower titers suggest rheumatoid disease.

Differential Diagnosis

In general, connective tissue diseases must be considered in the differential. These include osteoarthritis, gout, chronic Lyme disease, SLE, infection by human parvovirus B 19, polymyalgia rheumatica, Sjögren's syndrome, sarcoidosis, and various neoplasms. Osteoarthritis almost never affects the wrists and the metacarpophalangeal joints. Osteoarthritis is classically known for affecting the distal IP joints with Heberden's nodes in the fingers, while these distal joints are usually not affected in RA and there are no Heberden's nodes in the hands. Within the thumb, the carpophalangeal joint is affected in OA, while the interphalangeal joint is affected in RA.

Osteoarthritis almost never affects the wrists and the metacarpophalangeal joints. Gout is distinguished by its gold standard test, which is a synovial aspirate revealing urate crystals. For crystalline arthritides, gout crystals are negatively birefringent, while pseudogout has positively birefringent calcium pyrophosphate crystals. Chronic Lyme disease often involves a singular joint and not polyarthralgia. More importantly, there are positive serologic markers that are associated with Lyme disease.

SLE arthritic changes are almost never deforming, nor would one expect erosive changes on radiographs. In reference to infection by human papovavirus B 19, serologic evidence of antiparvovirus B 19 IgM antibody and a characteristic rash distinguish this infection from RA. Patients with polymyalgia rheumatica are RF negative or have low titers. This disease strikes persons older than age 50 years, just as qualitative RF also increases with age; however, these patients suffer myalgias but not arthralgias or arthritis. Psoriatic arthritis is much more difficult to distinguish from RA, but a family history of psoriasis helps give this away. Finally, some neoplasms can mimic rheumatoid disease, but again, the RF should remain either negative or quantitatively low. When considering acute viral polyarthritis, other causative infections include Hep C and rubella.

Management

Management of RA progresses from conservative interventions to aggressive symptom management. Because the disease is debilitative over time, primary interest remains in introducing therapies only as required by symptoms, thereby sparing the liver and GI tract from early use of pharmacologic agents and their adverse effects.

The overall goals of management are to reduce pain and inflammation and to spare joint function. It is possible to achieve these goals in early management without pharmacologic agents. This section on management, therefore, addresses nonpharmacologic interventions as subsequent therapy for RA.

Initial Management

Joint swelling and immobility upon rising, which abates or diminishes throughout the day, characterize early rheumatoid disease. Early disease symptoms can be managed by one or a combination of the following: physical and occupational therapies, heat and cold applications, exercise, rest, assistive devices, splints, meditation, chiropractic adjustments, and weight loss.

Physical and occupational therapists are educated to identify strategies that promote function and prevent immobility. Their special skills in motivating patients to remain active should not be underestimated in early management. Often patients attend therapy sessions and derive accompanying educational and emotional benefits from associating with other patients diagnosed with RA.

Heat and cold applications provide analgesia and relaxation to muscles and connective tissue. It is usually necessary to try both heat and cold with individual patients, because some respond better to one than the other. Application in anticipation of exercise may enhance joint mobility during exercise. Particularly helpful to some patients is to remain seated in warm water for 10 to 30 minutes.

Exercise reduces pain and inflammation only if the affected joints are not stressed during an inflammatory period. Outside an inflammatory event, the joints may undergo judicious stress through an increase in resistance exercises to promote strength and endurance. Thus, isometric exercises should be prescribed for inflamed joints and isotonic exercises should be done at other times. Patients may profit from aerobic exercise at the shallow end of a swimming pool.

Rest reduces pain and inflammation by controlling joint movement. One must distinguish between systemic rest and resting the joints. Systemic rest signifies a prescribed period of relaxation that may involve sleep. Patients with mild inflammation may benefit from systemic rest in the prone position for 1 to 2 hours per day; the rest period may extend upwards to 2-hour periods three or four times daily during waking hours, as necessitated by severe inflammation. Like systemic rest, resting the joints should be done in a prone position to avoid hip contractures; however, the duration of rest is much shorter than systemic rest, usually lasting only 20 to 40 minutes. In either case, the patient should prepare a method for awakening to prevent excessive rest. Excessive rest may signal depression or other underlying disease.

Assistive devices involve those that the patient requires to complete activities of daily living. Canes or crutches can relieve stress to affected weightbearing joints during periods of inflammatory involvement. Once the inflammation subsides, the patient may walk free of the device. When the clinician or physical therapist recommends using a cane or crutches, it is important to the patient's self-esteem and inner hope to explain why these may be required only temporarily. Other assistive devices for the home include bars for gripping inside the shower or tub or beside the toilet, a raised toilet seat, retrieval–extension devices for picking up items from the floor or at a distance, and an electronic lift to help the patient manage stairs.

Splints reduce pain, promote function, and stabilize involved joints. The hands and wrists are the preferred regions for splints, which are usually applied at night. Splints of the hips and knees are usually not preferred over lying prone. The position of optimal function should be considered when applying the splint. Moreover, the material of the splint should be lightweight, unabrasive, and durable enough to withstand frequent applications. Because self-application is preferred, the splint should be structured so that the patient can apply it without assistance.

Meditation relieves depression and anxiety associated with chronic disease and disability. In addition, it promotes self-care practices and self-efficacy. Meditation may follow traditional spiritual paths, whereby patients learn from teachers in traditional religious communities. Alternatively, meditation may involve guiding the attention through the use of restful music, images, spiritual charms, and breath-work. Patients with RA should meditate in a prone position to prevent postmeditation joint stiffness and pain.

The role of chiropractic adjustment remains controversial among traditional Western medicine practitioners; however, its benefits to the patient with RA must be considered. Chiropractors can relieve pressure to unaffected joints that compensate for weight or activity from other joints that are affected. Although adjustments may require repeated manipulations and therapeutic benefits may be short lived, other benefits include an increased sense of well-being and an improved quality of life.

Weight loss reduces pressure on weightbearing joints in the lower extremities and enhances activity. Alternatively, overeating may be a sign of depression, so weight gain must be addressed in an overall plan of encouraging weight reduction to achieve the goal of ideal body weight.

Subsequent Management

Drug therapies may involve analgesics, NSAIDs, steroids, DMARDs, or older therapies as described below.

Analgesics. Analgesics such as acetaminophen (Tylenol) or capsaicin cream, gel, lotion or roll-on may be effective even though it has no anti-inflammatory effects. While aspirin has been the mainstay of therapy for RA, acetaminophen as a nonopioid pain reliever may help for mild pain.

NSAIDs. Subsequent management begins with a consideration of arachadonic acid inhibitors, which include aspirin and other NSAIDs. Drugs of this class need not be used daily during the early stages of the disease. Rather, the patient can employ them only when there is pain that is unrelieved by nonpharmacologic means. Sulindac 150 mg PO bid is a good alternative NSAID therapy, as it tends to be less harsh on the stomach.

Extra-strength (1000 mg) aspirin can be used up to four times per day, if baseline liver function studies, platelet count, renal function studies, and hematocrit are within normal limits. Caution must be exercised when prescribing 4 g of aspirin per day to persons older than age 65, as their liver and renal functions may be impaired by age. Dosage reductions may be warranted should adverse effects ensue or laboratory markers dictate.

Aspirin should always be taken with 8 ounces of water or milk to avoid pill erosion or ulceration of the gastric mucosa. Enteric-coated aspirin is preferred to prevent gastric erosion. Concurrent anticoagulant therapy is a relative contraindication for aspirin and other NSAID use. Relative contraindication means that the drug might be employed in lesser amounts relative to subsequent coagulation studies and clinical histories.

Other NSAIDs may be substituted for aspirin, should the adverse effects or diminishing therapeutic effects warrant the switch. It is curious that, over time and with chronic use, individual drugs of the same class of NSAIDs can lose their effectiveness in an individual patient; therefore, the NSAIDs provide a wide range of therapeutic options. The clinician can recommend another drug in the class when treatment effects diminish with a given agent.

The primary adverse effect of the NSAIDs is GI upset. Their inhibition of gastric prostaglandin E (a natural protectant) predisposes the gastric mucosa to erosion. Most of the NSAIDs can be taken with an H_2-blocker such as ranitidine (Zantac) to reduce dyspepsia; however, H_2-blockers do not reduce hemorrhage or mucosal erosion. Proton pump inhibitors (PPI), such as omeprazole (Prilosec) OTC, or esomeprazozle magnesium (Nexium) suppress gastric acid secretion and may be preferred to H_2-blockers for GI prophylaxis.

With reference to liver function, minimal elevations in serum transaminases are to be expected at daily doses of 2400 mg for ibuprofen (Motrin) for adults younger than age 65 years; the maximum dose may go as high as 3200 mg/day if no adverse effects are apparent. Should the transaminase levels exceed two times normal, dose reduction is indicated along with laboratory evaluation for infectious causes, such as hepatitis B and C.

Toxicity of prolonged NSAID use may result in renal impairment and presents quite often with acute renal failure to the ER, as people have a tendency to overuse NSAIDs. It is as important as gastritis and ulcer formation. A rise in serum creatinine or BUN after starting NSAID therapy is an indication for further testing and possibly dose reduction or drug alteration. Should renal failure develop, it is usually reversible.

Steroids. Steroids, up to 7.5 mg of PO prednisone daily or injected intra-articularly such as triamcinolone, may be extremely helpful. Side effects of prolonged steroid use include adrenal insufficiency, hyperglycemia, osteoporosis, and skin discoloration, which explains why it is not recommended to use maximal daily steroid therapy for more than 6 months. Calcium, vitamin D, and bisphosphonates are indicated with prolonged steroid use. (Steroids are thoroughly covered in the atopic dermatitis section in Chapter 6.)

Disease-Modifying Anti-rheumatic Drugs (DMARDs). DMARDs, which are essentially immunosuppressants of various types, include anticytokine and antityrosine kinase immunotherapies such as imatinib (Gleevec) and the anti-TNF-α therapies such as etanercept (Enbrel), adalimumab (Humira), and infliximab (Remicade) (see Table 16.3). Active disease should be treated early with DMARDs within 3 months of disease onset and even more aggressively in severe disease. Potential side effects of these therapies include the risk of reactivating TB with anti-TNF-α therapy, given the inhibition of cell-mediated immunity. Combination therapy with DMARDs is more effective than monotherapy and several different combinations have been tested in randomized trials with no obvious ideal combination. Thus, therapies may be crafted based on tolerance of side effects and the presence of comorbid conditions.

Older Therapies. Many drugs are possible options in the event of treatment failure by aspirin and other NSAIDs, but are used less often now, given their low therapeutic index (higher toxicity risk). These include methotrexate (Mexate), azathioprine (Imuran), gold sodium thiomalate (Myochrysine), antimalarials, penicillamine (Depen), sulfasalazine (Azulfidine), and minocycline hydrochloride (Minocin). Hydroxychloroquine is an antimalarial usually used in milder disease, compared to sulfasalazine used in moderate disease. Methotrexate still seems most effective but is not used in women at risk of pregnancy or with chronic liver disease

Methotrexate is administered to adults younger than age 65 years in an initial weekly dose of 7.5 mg PO. The dosage may be doubled the second week if tolerance and therapeutic aims require. Maximum dosage is 20 mg per week. Toxic effects include interstitial pneumonitis and hepatic cirrhosis. Combined use of methotrexate with NSAIDs, sulfonamides (e.g., sulfamethoxazole/trimethoprim [SMZ/TMP], Bactrim), and sulfonylureas such as glipizide (Glucotrol) increases the chance of hepatoxicity, so concurrent use of these drugs is discouraged. For reasons yet unclear, increased risk of hepatoxicity is associated with diabetes, obesity, and renal disease in association with methotrexate use. Initiation of therapy, therefore, must be weighed against potential risks and alternative therapy options.

Most of the Cox-2 inhibitors, which were the mainstay of therapy several years ago, are off the market because of their cardiovascular risks. Celecoxib (Celebrex) is one of the last remaining.

Therapy should be driven by the severity of the disease, whether mild, moderate, or severe per American College of Rheumatology guidelines.

The C-reactive protein (CRP) blood test is a nonspecific method for evaluating the severity and course of the

Table 16.3 Commonly Used Disease-Modifying Anti-Rheumatic Drugs (DMARDs)

Drug	Usual Maintenance Dose	Comments and Side Effects
Adalimumab (Humira)	40 mg SC every other week	May be used in conjunction with methotrexate. May cause predisposition to infections, worsening of demyelinating syndromes.
Anakinra (Kineret)	100 mg SC once daily	May cause predisposition to infections, headache, GI upset, neutropenia.
Etanercept (Enbrel)	50 mg SC once weekly	May cause infections, worsening of demyelinating syndromes, pancytopenia, aplastic anemia, exacerbation of heart failure.
Hydroxychloroquine (Plaquenil)	400–600 mg PO daily	Irreversible retinopathy, alopecia, blood dyscrasias
Infliximab (Remicade)	3–10 mg/kg IV q4wks	Lupus-like syndrome, worsening of demyelinating syndromes, exacerbation of heart failure.
Leflunomide (Arava)	20 mg PO daily	Monitor LFTs, GI upset, leukopenia, thrombocytopenia
Methotrexate (Rheumatrex)	7.5–20 mg/week, PO or SC	Monitor LFTs, blood dyscrasias, GI upset, hepatotoxicity, opportunistic infections, fatal skin reactions.
Sulfasalazine (Azulfidine)	1 g PO bid	Monitor LFTs, GI upset, leukopenia, thrombocytopenia, urine or skin discoloration.
Rituximab (Rituxan)	Four doses IV over 3 weeks	Stop HTN meds during treatment. Angioedema, GI upset, blood dyscrasias.
Imatinib (Gleevec)	400–600 mg PO daily	Potentiated by CYP 3A4 inhibitors, antagonized by CYP 3A4 inducers, GI disturbances, hypokalemia, renal or hepatotoxicity.

inflammatory process. The normal CRP is less than 0.8 mg/dL. Failure to decrease the CRP level indicates an infection or tissue necrosis; therefore, the CRP should be monitored to determine the effectiveness of therapy.

Follow-Up and Referral

Follow-up of patients with RA requires routine clinical laboratory evaluation and episodic adjustments in interventions. Routine clinical laboratory evaluation is performed every 90 days and includes CBC, platelet count, serum liver and renal function studies, and fasting blood sugar. Most of the adverse effects of drugs used in the management of RA can be monitored with this routine panel. If methotrexate is used, a serum albumin level should be added to the routine panel of tests.

Each visit to the clinician, following scheduled laboratory evaluations, should address the clinical history since the last visit. Attention focuses on the efficacy of relief measures and the onset, duration, and frequency of pain.

The clinician should refer the patient to a rheumatologist when initial management (including aspirin or NSAID therapy) fails. The rheumatologist is responsible for initiating therapies such as methotrexate and gold salts. Comanagement may mean that the rheumatologist will evaluate the patient twice each year.

Patient Education

Patient education focuses on the goals of therapy, which are reduction of pain, control of inflammation, and preservation of function. Much of the education was covered in the initial management section. In addition, education should address the therapeutic and adverse effects of any drugs employed. Finally, because rheumatoid arthritis is a chronic disease, education should envelop the emotional, social, and spiritual sequelae of living with recurrent bouts of pain and disability.

The goals of therapy are best realized by promoting self-care. Education concerning self-care should include caregivers who must share similar beliefs before they can support self care practices. To help keep the patient from sinking into secondary gains from the "sick" role, the caregiver should support normal social role behaviors by encouraging self-care. The caregiver, therefore, becomes integral to achieving the goals of therapy.

Infectious Mononucleosis

Infectious mononucleosis is a viral syndrome characterized by prolonged malaise and fatigue, fever, sore throat, tender cervical lymphadenopathy, and a predominant monocytosis with a reactive lymphocytosis on peripheral blood smear. Also present may be GI manifestations including nausea, vomiting, and anorexia, abdominal organomegaly, headache, and occasionally a morbilliform viral exanthem (rash). Infectious mononucleosis results from acute infection with Epstein-Barr virus (EBV) or, less commonly, cytomegalovirus (CMV). Saliva is the most common source of infectious virions, which explains the traditional adage that refers to this condition as the "kissing disease."

Epidemiology and Causes

Infectious mononucleosis occurs predominantly among sexually active individuals between ages 10 and 35. Sexual activity, in this sense, implies the exchange of bodily fluids between sex partners, particularly the exchange of saliva. Although the disease can occur outside this age range, case reports are rare. Its distribution is equal among genders, economic classes, and educational levels, although the incidence of clinical infection is up to 30 times higher in whites than blacks.

The cause of the disease is recent infection by EBV (90 percent of cases with an incubation period of 30 to 50 days) or, to a much lesser extent, CMV, toxoplasmosis, human herpes virus-6 (HHV-6), or acute HIV infection. Even certain medications such as isoniazid, phenytoin, or carbamazepine may induce a mononucleosis-like illness. However, it is EBV infection that has been best characterized, associated with a prolonged recovery period with persistent symptoms lasting up to a year, and connected most consistently to significant sequelae of infectious mononucleosis.

Pathophysiology

Both EBV and CMV are members of the Herpesviridae family of viruses. Infection by these viruses is particularly widespread, with up to 95 percent of adults being seropositive for EBV-exposure. Humans are the major reservoir for latent EBV infection, which typically spreads through intimate contact with asymptomatic viral shedders. EBV infection may result in a number of conditions, given its tropism for (ability to infect) B and T lymphocytes.

EBV typically enters the body via oropharyngeal epithelial and lymphoid cells, which explains the ability of the virus to be shed in saliva. Migration of B cells throughout the lymphoreticular system allows for widespread dissemination of this virus. Circulating antibodies are soon formed against viral antigens, as well as against unrelated RBC-specific antigens termed heterophile antibodies. These IgM antibodies serve as a primary means of early detection of EBV infection, although they are not highly specific.

An atypical peripheral lymphocytosis occurs 1 to 3 weeks after the onset of clinical symptoms, which is characterized largely by an activated set of HLA-DR+, CD8+ T cells, as well as nonspecific CD16+ NK cells. These cells are key to preventing the acute lysis of virally infected cells (lytic phase of infection) and establishing a nonlytic, subclinical lifelong infection (latent phase of infection). Acute manifestations such as infectious mononucleosis are believed to result from suboptimal lymphocytic immune responses, rather than from ongoing viral replication. In turn, antiviral therapies are ineffective in the treatment of infectious mononucleosis.

While the majority of EBV infections are actually subclinical, significant manifestations include not only infectious mononucleosis, but also relatively benign cases of upper respiratory infection, otitis media, and even potentially fatal cases of Hodgkin's or Non-Hodgkin's lymphoma. Sequelae of EBV infection is largely determined by the age of the infected host, with adolescents and young adults being most susceptible to infectious mononucleosis. The precise reasons for these differential manifestations are not fully understood. However, they are thought to relate to the size of viral innoculum and the extent of the host B-cell immunoresponse, both of which vary with age. In turn, patients with infectious mononucleosis may develop serious sequelae affecting virtually any organ system. In contrast, infectious mononucleosis caused by CMV is typically a self-limited condition without significant complications, except in significantly immunosuppressed individuals.

Clinical Presentation

Subjective

Patients present with an acute history of fever, neuropathies, headache, photophobia, dysphagia, sore throat, diffuse chest pain, dyspnea and cough, nausea, anorexia, myalgias, and arthralgias. They usually cannot identify a known contact with EBV before the onset of symptoms.

Objective

Patients will report fevers, as high as 39°C (more than 102.5°F) among children and teenagers. Cervical and postauricular lymphadenopathy may be painful on examination. Nuchal stiffness (not as rigid as in meningitis) associated with painful nodes may be present. The pharynx should be injected, and there may be exudate across the tonsils or the tonsillar crypt. Tachycardia may accompany arrhythmias, in particular premature atrial contractions. The lungs might reveal fine, scattered inspiratory crackles (rales). Splenomegaly is present in up to 60 percent of patients. While splenic rupture is rare (2 in 1000), it is a potentially fatal sequela. The liver, if not enlarged, may be tender to deep palpation.

A maculopapular rash may be evident across the trunk and upper extremities, although this finding is infrequent. A characteristic maculopapular or morbilliform rash may occur with concurrent use of amoxicillin, ampicillin, or occasionally other antibiotics such as azithromycin and fluoroquinolones, which may be inadvertently started because of suspicion of bacterial infection. This rash can be particularly concerning for parents, although it is often just a consequence of concurrent antibiotic use. While the Pathophysiology of this rash is unclear, it is likely related to circulating antibodies to the antibiotic.

Diagnostic Reasoning

The diagnostic reasoning for infectious mononucleosis should progress step by step according to the complexity of its presentation. The symptoms of mononucleosis mimic those of many diseases; therefore, laboratory findings play an important role in the differential diagnosis.

Diagnostic Tests

The first set of laboratory tests to be ordered includes the CBC, heterophil test (Monospot) rapid plasma reagin (RPR) test (to rule out syphilis), throat cultures, serum liver transaminases, and serum bilirubin. The goal of initial testing is to establish a pattern of results that would indicate infectious mononucleosis. Lymphocytosis predominates—atypical lymphoctes account for at least 10 percent of the total lymphocytes. Mild thrombocytopenia and neutropenia are frequent transient findings. Liver enzyme levels, particularly the transaminase levels, are mild to moderately elevated in about 90 percent of patients with mono.

The Monospot test detects heterophil antibodies, and while not very sensitive, is the characteristic laboratory abnormality. These antibodies are found in 90 percent of patients with acute infectious mononucleosis, although the test may take up to 3 weeks to become positive. Retesting may be necessary if the first test was done early. The heterophil antibodies usually disappear by 3 months but may be present up until 1 year. The test is less sensitive in young people (75 percent sensitivity at 24 to 28 months and 25 percent at 10 to 24 months). The EBV-specific serologies should therefore be checked in children. Anti-EBNA and anti-VCA are two anti-EBV antibody tests that are available. These are also less sensitive in younger children (60 percent in infants, but up to 100 percent in young adults). False-positives for EBV have been noted in HIV-infected individuals but are considered rare. During the first 20 to 30 days after EBV infection, the CBC could show a granulocytopenia but no rise in lymphocytes. By the fourth week after infection, however, the CBC could reveal a lymphocytic leukocytosis, with more than 10,000 WBCs and more than 30 percent of these being lymphocytes. Under microscopic examination, these lymphocytes are larger than normal lymphocytes and they stain more darkly.

Throat cultures will be negative for *Streptococcus* and other bacteria. The RPR should prove negative in most cases, but a transient false-positive RPR result occurs in 10 percent of cases. Serum levels of liver transaminases and the bilirubin will likely be elevated.

Further testing of serum IgM antibodies to EBV may prove useful if a diagnosis based on initial testing is questionable.

Differential Diagnosis

Many diseases present similarly to infectious mononucleosis; however, careful assessment of the patient's signs and symptoms as well as the diagnostic tests will assist in making the diagnosis. Table 16.4 presents a comparison of the signs and symptoms of Epstein-Barr virus-related syndromes. Glandular variant infectious mono, with lympa-

Table 16.4 Epstein-Barr Virus–Related Syndromes

	Infectious Mononucleosis	Oral Hairy Leukoplakia	Duncan's Disease
Malaise	+	+/−	+
Lymphadenopathy	+	+	+
Fever	+	+/−	+/−
Splenomegaly	+ (50%)	+/−	+
Pharyngeal exudate	+	−	−

+, present; −, absent.

denopathy out of proportion to the pharyngitis, differs from systemic variant mono with fever and fatigue with mild or absent lymphadenopathy and pharyngitis.

Positive results from the heterophil (Monospot test) will distinguish infectious mononucleosis from other diseases of similar presentation. In the differential of exudative pharyngitis, streptococcal, adenoviral, diphtherial, gonococcal, and herpes simplex infections should be considered. HIV-infected or other myelosuppressed teenagers and young adults may present with findings similar to those of EBV mononucleosis if they are infected with cytomegalovirus (CMV) or toxoplasmosis, but the heterophil (Monospot) tests should prove negative in these cases. In addition, peritonsillar abscesses should be ruled out by a culture.

Management

Symptom management is all that can be done for someone with infectious mononucleosis. The overall plan of care, therefore, involves supportive measures, including providing a quiet atmosphere where the patient can sleep.

No antivirals are available for initial or subsequent therapy; therefore, initial management focuses on symptom relief with rehydration, NSAIDs, gargling with warm salt water, and OTC throat lozenges. Acetaminophen may be used for supportive, analgesic, and antipyretic treatment. In cases in which the airway is in danger of obstruction, corticosteroid therapy (Prednisone) should be introduced over the course of 5 days (40 mg/day with taper). Steroids may reduce viral shedding but do not affect symptoms duration or the convalescent period duration.

Complications may arise for some patients in the course of the disease. While peritonsillar abscess is rare, the soft palate and tonsils may become so edematous that the airway may be threatened. Therefore, airway obstruction should be assessed. In addition, a mild hepatitis may be seen in 90 percent of cases. Impending splenic rupture necessitates surgical resection of the spleen. Hepatitis requires removal of hepatotoxic medications, if possible, and in extreme cases, IFN-α injections. Other complications are also treated symptomatically.

Acyclovir can reduce the lytic phase, but does not affect the latent phase and has no clear therapeutic role. Human vaccine trials against the gp350/220 viral protein which binds the B-cell CD21 surface receptor to initiate infection were not successful, but recombinant vaccinia virus plus the gp350/220 gene is being tested in China.

Follow-Up and Referral

Patients should be followed up to rule out the development of serious sequelae. Many sequelae can result from infectious mono. Neurologic complications may include: Guillain-Barré; facial nerve palsy; meningoencephalitis; aseptic meningitis; transverse myelitis; and optic neuritis. Hematologic complications include hemolytic/aplastic anemia; thrombocytopenia; TTP/HUS; and DIC. Cardiovascular complications may include myocarditis. Renal and GU complications may include glomerulonephritis or genital ulceration, and GI complications may include pancreatitis.

It is important to provide the patient with a clinical picture of the disease so that follow-up can be self-initiated should the individual stray from the trajectory outlined. Referrals are also rare unless complications ensue. Patients with hemolytic anemia and thrombocytopenic purpura should be referred to a hematologist. Any patient with encephalitis will require an immediate neurology consultation. Patients with pericarditis must be referred to a cardiologist.

Patient Education

Young, school-aged patients must be warned of the dangers of contact sports and rough-housing for at least 4 weeks following the onset of symptoms, as splenic rupture occurs predominantly within 3 weeks of symptom onset and may very well occur in the absence of actual splenomegaly (50 percent of splenic rupture cases). In fact, up to half of cases may occur without any preceding trauma. Rupture does not correlate with symptom severity or abnormal laboratory results. A good rule of thumb is that the patient's energy level must be at baseline before the resumption of strenuous or risky physical activity and this must be greater than 4 weeks. Strict bedrest is not needed, however.

Patients must learn that their fevers usually will disappear long before they feel better. They should learn that the fevers will subside after 10 to 14 days although their energy levels will not rebound to normal until 1 to 3 months postinfection. Therefore, teenagers and young adults, who often manage busy and active lives, will need to learn that they will require rest for a long time.

Other elements to consider in education include giving information about prescribed drugs, including the dosage and adverse effects. The clinician should caution patients to avoid ethanol and cigarettes because they will aggravate coughing and nausea. Alcohol should be avoided for a minimum of 3 months after liver function tests return to normal. If there is a follow-up visit after the fever subsides, the clinician can raise the subject of sex counseling, given the fact that some sexually transmitted diseases (STDs) are fatal, unlike infectious mononucleosis.

Chronic Fatigue Syndrome and Fibromyalgia Syndrome

Chronic fatigue syndrome (CFS) remains poorly understood, despite abundant attention in the scientific and lay press. Perhaps the lack of agreement as to its cause, laboratory markers, and clinical course explains why the syndrome is not named in many medical texts even to this day. There is also significant overlap between CFS and fibromyalgia syndrome (FMS), another controversial chronic pain syndrome. The majority of patients with CFS meet criteria for FMS, while at least 70 percent of patients with FMS meet criteria for CFS. Moreover, both these disorders have been widely recognized in persons with comorbid psychiatric illness, as nearly two-thirds of CFS patients and 30 percent of FMS patients meet criteria for depression, dysthymia, or anxiety disorders. Many authors have criticized the historical and physical examination diagnostic criteria for both conditions as having a strong potential for overlap with somatization disorders.

Epidemiology and Causes

Without a generally accepted working definition of CFS, it is impossible to ascertain its epidemiology. Chronic fatigue is a presenting complaint in up to 25 percent of patients presenting to ambulatory care settings, and it is estimated that approximately 10 percent of these individuals meet diagnostic criteria for CFS. Numerous books in the popular press have advanced the belief that women are affected two times more often than men are. The same books tend to agree that younger women are more often affected. Causes of CFS have been hypothesized to be autoimmune and infectious; however, the causes for the syndrome have yet to be determined. Importantly, it is a diagnosis of exclusion. The incidence of CFS ranges from 4 to 8.6 cases per 100,000 adults.

Researchers have published more data regarding the epidemiology of FMS. The prevalence of FMS is 0.5 percent for men, 3.4 percent for women (some studies claim an increased prevalence in women of 10:1). The prevalence is more than 7 percent for women aged 60 to 79 years. An estimated 11 million people in the United States have FMS and 80 to 90 percent are women. It is estimated that up to 20 percent of all patient visits to a rheumatology practice are for FMS. It is now considered the most common cause of generalized musculoskeletal pain in women aged 20 to 55 years. Several studies have shown that up to 50 percent of patients with FMS have a history of either sexual or violent abuse.

Pathophysiology

After much investigation, the pathophysiology of CFS and FMS is still unclear. It has been hypothesized that both syndromes may be disorders of muscle energy metabolism, inflammatory or immunopathologic diseases of muscle, generalized disorders of pain perception, neuronally mediated hypotension, neuroendocrine disturbances, dysregulated serotonin secretion, sleep disturbances, or a result of sexual abuse or domestic violence. However, it is important to note that none of these etiologies has been consistently confirmed through randomized, well-controlled studies. While depression and anxiety disorders demonstrate great overlap with both CFS and FMS, it is a matter of great debate as to whether these conditions occur concurrently, whether CFS and FMS lead to psychiatric sequelae, or whether these chronic conditions are simply somatic manifestations of underlying mood disorders. In turn, patients commonly experience accusations of malingering, which, by definition, would be unfounded.

Extensive work explored a potential infectious etiology of CFS, focusing on Epstein-Barr virus, retroviruses, and human herpesvirus (HHV)-6 as causative agents. However, promising data from certain research groups could not be reproduced by other laboratories. Moreover, no consistent serologic profile could distinguish patients with CFS from control groups across multiple studies.

Several studies have demonstrated qualitative and quantitative differences in immune function between patients with CFS and controls, including reduced numbers of natural killer cells with depressed function, reduced levels of Ig molecules and immune complexes, and increased numbers of cell surface adhesion molecules, among others. However, the differences are of questionable clinical significance and have been inconsistent (even conflicting) between different studies.

Studies that have examined neuroendocrine differences between affected patients and controls have produced similar inconclusive results. While some evidence points to undersecretion of adrenocorticotropin hormone (ACTH) and reduced serum cortisol levels, these findings are not specific for CFS and have been observed in FMS as well as in healthy subjects, with altered sleep patterns related to overnight work shifts.

Studies attempting to clarify the etiology of FMS have also been less than definitive. For many years, FMS was considered a disorder of muscle metabolism, possibly related to chronic hypoxia of muscular tissue. However, studies of lactate levels, muscle force studies, and postexertional pain have demonstrated a marked similarity between patients with FMS and sedentary controls. Thus, the most current theories suggest patients with FMS suffer from disproportionate perceptions of pain, exacerbated by muscle inactivity and deconditioning. In fact, lower pain perception thresholds have been further documented in first-degree relatives of patients with FMS.

Although no studies have been conclusive, altered pain perception is more likely to be a central rather than peripheral nociceptor phenomenon. This is supported by observations in FMS patients of altered patterns of sleep and mood, decreased blood flow to pain centers in the brain, as well as alterations in serotonin secretions and the pituitary–hypothalamic–adrenal neuroendocrine axis. In addition, autonomic dysregulation of heart rate and systemic blood pressure have also been implicated on the basis of tilt table testing for orthostatic hypotension; however, again, these findings have not been consistently reproduced. An anti-inflammatory component to the myalgias of FMS has never been shown, which likely explains the lack of efficacy of NSAID and steroid therapies.

Clinical Presentation

Subjective

The patient may report postexercise malaise, fatigue, multiple-joint pain, headaches, impaired memory, mood, concentration and cognitive disturbances, sore throat, restless disordered sleep, and myalgias. Often the patient will also report having consulted one or more specialists concerning these vague symptoms.

Objective

The onset of CFS is sudden and may be preceded by a mononucleosis-like illness or by significant GI findings. This same type of preceding event may also herald the onset of FMS.

The patient will appear tired. The skin may be pale. Despite complaints of impaired memory and concentration, the MMSE results will vary in reference to recent recall and problem-solving abilities. (The MMSE is discussed in the section on Alzheimer's disease in Chapter 5.) Cervical lymph nodes, if enlarged, will be shoddy and nontender. Otherwise, the examination may be unremarkable.

For a diagnosis of FMS to be made, the patient must have widespread muscular pain that has been present for at least 3 months; the pain should be present in 11 of 18 trigger points (or tender points) on digital palpation with an applied pressure of 4 kg/cm (enough force to whiten the examiner's nailbed). The 18 trigger points are bilateral sites at nine key locations (see Table 16.5). Pain at these sites should be significantly greater than at control sites, which are not expected to be tender, such as the patient's thumbnail or mid-forearm.

Diagnostic Reasoning

Diagnostic Tests

Chronic fatigue syndrome tends to strike down once active, highly functional adults. The physical exam for CFS is typically normal. Advanced imaging tests such as CT and MRI are not indicated in the absence of significant physical findings. In addition, virus-specific serologies against EBV or Lyme disease are also not recommended without a strong suspicion by history or physical exam findings, as any positive result is likely to be a false positive in the setting of low suspicion.

Table 16.5 Diagnostic Criteria for Fibromyalgia*

History Criteria	Pain is considered widespread when ALL of the following are present: Pain in the left side of the body Pain in the right side of the body Pain above the waist Pain below the waist Axial skeletal pain (cervical spine, anterior chest, thoracic spine, or low back)
Pain Criteria	Pain exists in 11 of 18 tender points (trigger points) on digital palpation (at a force of at least 4 kg): Occiput: bilateral, at the suboccipital muscle insertions Low cervical: bilateral, at the anterior aspects of the intertransverse spaces at C5–C7 Trapazius: bilateral, at the midpoint of the upper border Supraspinatus: bilateral, at origins above the scapula spine near the medial border Second rib: bilateral, at the second costochondral junctions, just lateral to the junctions on upper surfaces Lateral epicondyle: bilateral, 2 cm distal to the epicondyles Gluteal: bilateral, in upper quadrants of buttocks in anterior fold of muscle Greater trocanter: bilateral, posterior to the trocanteric prominence Knee: bilateral, at the medial fat pad proximal to the joint line For a tender point to be "positive," the client must state that the palpation was painful. A statement of "tender" is not considered "painful."

*Client must have a history of widespread pain (present for at least 3 months) in specific anatomic areas and must exhibit this pain during an examination of tender points.

Source: Running, AF, and Berndt, AE: Management Guidelines for Nurse Practitioners Working in Family Practice. FA Davis, Philadelphia, 2003, p 586.

Laboratory testing for FMS should include the same screening tests as for CFS, as well as muscle enzymes (creatine kinase, aldolase). ANA is often not helpful unless autoimmune disorders such as lupus are highly suspected, since it may provide a false positive result which incorrectly labels these patients as having SLE.

Differential Diagnosis

There are many differential diagnoses for both CFS and FMS. The majority can be ruled out via the basic laboratory studies mentioned in the preceding text. The differentials include rheumatic disease, such as SLE, rheumatoid arthritis, and polymyalgia rheumatica; endocrinologic diseases, such as thyroid disease and parathyroid disease, metabolic myopathies, and neuropathies; infectious diseases such as Lyme disease; and other diseases, such as dysthymia, personality disorders, psychotic illness, irritable bowel syndrome, cancer, and parkinsonism. Myofascial pain syndrome is a regional version of FMS.

The patient should be classified as having CFS or idiopathic chronic fatigue if fatigue persists or relapses for 6 months. It should be classified as CFS if the criteria for severity of fatigue are met and four or more of the following symptoms are concurrently present for 6 months: impaired memory or concentration, sore throat, tender cervical or axillary lymph nodes, muscle pain, multiple-joint pain, new headaches, restless sleep, and postexertion malaise.

The CDC's criteria for CFS is based on persistent or relapsing fatigue that had been clinically evaluated without explanation with at least four of the following self-reported symptoms (but no criteria for physical exam findings): impaired concentration/short-term memory, sore throat, tender cervical/axillary nodes, muscle pain, arthralgias without redness or swelling, poor sleep, new-onset headache or headache of a new and worsening pattern, as well as malaise following activity that lasts at least 24 hours. For patients with chronic fatigue who do not fit these criteria, the term idiopathic chronic fatigue is used, but these criteria are still being evaluated for validity. Sjögren's disease should also be considered as a differential diagnosis, as many CFS patients present with anhydrosis.

Management

Management of CFS and FMS remains controversial. The goal of therapy remains to enable the patient to have the best quality of life possible within the limitations of the chronic disability related to pain.

The two therapies that have been shown to be beneficial in terms of symptom relief and increased function (but not in terms of cure) are cognitive behavioral therapy that changes beliefs, and behaviors that are barriers to recovery and graded exercise. Increased bed rest should not be encouraged. A supportive approach to the patient–clinician relationship is critical. This reinforces that this is a genuine diagnosis, if the patient meets criteria and avoids the debate between psychologic and "organic" etiologies.

The following pharmacotherapies have been tried with little consistent success: the Alzheimer's drug galantamine (Reminyl), IVIG, acyclovir (Zovirax), and selective serotonin reuptake inhibitors (SSRIs) such as citalopram (Celexa), fluoxetine (Prozac), and paroxetine (Paxil). Corticosteroids have shown some benefit in uncontrolled studies but with concurrent adrenal suppression. Controlled, blinded studies have not confirmed these benefits.

Positive Lyme titers should not be taken as a definite sign of infection, unless IgM is positive with a strong suspicion of this disorder, as false-positive rates with be high. Antibiotics should not just be given indiscriminately. Long-term prognosis is better than short-term prognosis. Certain factors have been cited as predicting a poor prognosis: (1) having more than eight medically unexplained physical symptoms other than the ones cited as CFS diagnostic criteria, (2) lifetime history of dysthymia, (3) chronic fatigue lasting more than 1.5 years, (4) less than 16 years of formal education, and (5) age greater than 38 years at onset of disease.

For FMS, acetaminophen (650 mg qid) and tramadol (Ultram; 75 mg qid) as combination therapy may be helpful analgesics, but there is little to no evidence for NSAIDs or steroid therapy as being beneficial. Of course, as a narcotic, tramadol has abuse potential, but this is generally considered less than for other narcotic pain meds such as oxycodone or morphine. Amitriptyline (Elavil), 75 mg daily in divided doses, remains one of the medications frequently ordered. Although it helps some patients, research has shown that after 3 months, it has no more effect than a placebo. This and other tricyclics have anticholinergic side effects. A similar transient effect has been seen with cyclobenzaprine (Flexeril), which is effective for the first 3 months, initially 5 mg tid, then increasing to 10 mg tid. The old adage of "start low and go slow" applies to this med as well. Desipramine (Norpramin) is an alternative tricyclic with fewer side effects and may work in patients who respond to Elavil, but cannot tolerate it. Of all the SSRIs, fluoxetine has been most promising in doses from 20 to 80 mg qd. Dual norepinephrine and serotonin reuptake inhibitors such as duloxetine (Cymbalta) (40 to 60 mg qd) have shown some benefit as well. Tramadol should probably be added only after psychotropic meds are tried first. After this, low-doseclonazepam (Klonopin, 0.5 mg qhs) may be helpful, and research is also being done on the usefulness of antiseizure meds.

An ongoing low-impact aerobic (cardiovascular) exercise program (walking, swimming, biking, water aerobics) with cognitive behavioral therapy, hypnotherapy, or EMG biofeedback therapy may be a useful adjunct in certain patients, as these therapies have been shown in limited trials to increase quality of life (although not symptom severity). Chiropractic and massage therapies are only weakly supported. Trials with ultraviolet light (especially blue light) exposure have shown mixed results. Vitamin supplementation also has received mixed results in small clinical trials.

Follow-Up and Referral

Follow-up should occur according to the symptoms reported. Because many of these patients have been treated for affective psychiatric disorders in the past, they know when to seek professional assistance. Typically, patients are referred to rheumatologists initially to assist in confirming the diagnosis. Referral to regional specialists who study and treat CFS and FMS may be required. Psychiatric referral could be necessary if mental-status test results warrant.

Patient Education

For both CFS and FMS, management relies on helping the patient cope with a chronic condition while learning methods to deal with the chronicity of the symptoms. Clinicians should stress that the patient does not have a fatal disease, although symptomatic, it is relatively benign and the patient can live a normal and productive live. Living with the uncertainty of the diagnosis and the chronicity of the problem are continuing challenges for both the patient and clinician. This is illustrated in The Patient's Voice 16.1. Patients should be encouraged to try whatever alternative means they want that might assist them with pain such as chiropractic, therapeutic touch, guided imagery, hypnosis, and so on. There are no right answers or guaranteed treatment. Pain is as the patient perceives it, and any treatment may relieve the pain if the patient believes it to be helpful. Patients should understand that physical and emotional stress can worsen their symptoms. Patient education has been shown in unblinded studies to improve FMS symptoms and quality of life and is a critical component of treatment. The Circle of Caring Model is tested in cases in which patients are frustrated and experience daily pain. It is especially trying when patients appear outwardly to be fine, but are suffering inside. Conditions such as these require all resources available and for all involved with the patient to focus on finding what works for each individual patient.

THE PATIENT'S VOICE 16.1

Chronic Fatigue Syndrome

I have been chronically tired for years. It started out that I would drive the kids to school in my nightgown, then I'd go back to bed. I had given up my job the year before. Thank goodness we could afford it. My husband thought that I was depressed, so I went to doctor after doctor and tried all sorts of antidepressant medications with no relief. One doctor suggested that I needed to see a psychiatrist because the antidepressants were not working and he said I was obviously depressed. I knew "deep down" that I wasn't depressed, but I also knew that something wasn't right. I knew I had to do something when I overheard one of my kids on the phone telling his friend not to come over because his Mom was just "having another lazy day in her pj's."

That same week, I heard an ad on the radio inviting participants for a study on chronic fatigue syndrome. I had heard about the syndrome vaguely and thought it was just a "catch-all term" for tiredness. I didn't really think it was a medical condition. I called the phone number given for the study and just answering a few questions over the phone, I felt 200 percent better! There actually is a medical name for the condition that I know I have. Now, I know that I'm no longer crazy or simply lazy. I can't wait to participate. Even if they don't help me, I feel better knowing that what I have is "real."

Lyme Disease

Lyme disease is a multisystem inflammatory disease of infectious etiology that does not take its name from the spirochete that causes it, *Borrelia burgdorferi.* Instead, it is named for a town in Connecticut (Old Lyme) where it was isolated among the town residents in the 1970s. It is a tick-borne disease that is prevalent among people who live in wooded areas of the eastern United States, with 90 percent of cases occurring in the following nine states: Connecticut, Massachusetts, Rhode Island, New Jersey, New York, Pennsylvania, Minnesota, Wisconsin, and California. In addition, Lyme disease has been isolated in eastern provinces of Canada, central and western regions of the United States, Europe, and Australia.

Epidemiology and Causes

The Centers for Disease Control and Prevention (CDC) report an increasing incidence of Lyme disease. Because of epidemiologic policies at the state level that are not exact, the number of cases has been exaggerated. Not only has over-reporting become a problem, but over-diagnosis has blossomed. It is a curious anomaly that spirochete isolates were available in fewer than one half of states in the United States that reported incidence. Incidence should be correlated with isolates of *B. burgdorferi.*

Vector-borne diseases do not distinguish among races, gender, and other demographic features. Lyme disease in the United States is limited only to individuals with exposure to *B. burgdorferi* via tick bites. In Europe and Asia, other species of *Borrelia* such as *B. afzelii* and *B. garinii* are also causative agents, but these have not been isolated in the United States. These differences in bacteriology may underlie the differing clinical manifestations of this disease by geography, that is, a higher frequency of arthritis and erythema migrans rash seen in the United States.

Pathophysiology

The pathophysiology of the infection concerns the length of time of tick exposure and the likelihood of infection. The infected tick must feed for at least 24 to 48 hours before it can pass along the spirochete to the host. Up to 90 percent of cases are transmitted via bites from ticks in the immature nymph stage, rather than due to bites from adults. Because of the small size of the tick (which is smaller in comparison to the typical wood ticks found on dogs), finding the tick before 24 hours have elapsed may prove difficult. However, vigilant inspection of skin and hair after exposure to wooded areas heightens the success of locating and removing the tick.

Lyme disease is caused primarily by the tick *Ixodes scapularis*. Once hatched from summer leaf clutter blanketing the forest floor, tick larvae acquire spirochetes on taking their first blood meal from infected mice, birds, or other small mammals. The larvae eventually detach from their hosts to molt and emerge the following spring as infected nymphs that are prone to spreading disease in the late spring, summer, and early fall. After this blood meal, these nymphs detach from their hosts and molt into adult forms later in the fall, in turn, seeking blood meals and passing on the infection most often to white-tailed deer throughout the rest of the season and into the winter and early spring, before laying another egg mass the following summer to begin this cycle again. Thus, the 2-year tick life cycle and the ability to identify and avoid bites from larger adult ticks help to explain the seasonal preference for Lyme disease in the summer months, rather than in the winter.

Half of the ticks that occupy the eastern and midwestern United States in localized hotspots of high disease incidence may be infected with the spirochete; therefore, there is a high likelihood of infection by tick exposure in the wooded areas of these regions. Few ticks along the Pacific Coast of the United States are infected (*Ixodes pacificus*), so tick bites in this region are less likely to pass the spirochete to a human host. Although only 30 percent of affected persons can clearly recall an antecedent tick bite, blood meals by infected ticks remain the only well-documented mechanism of spirochete transmission to human hosts. Some evidence exists for transplacental transmission from infected mothers to developing fetuses, but this generally results in good outcomes, and the clinical significance of intrauterine infection is questionable.

The causative organisms of Lyme disease are capable of producing systemic tissue injury with a relatively low microbial load. This occurs despite the absence of any excreted microbial toxins or widespread host inflammatory response such as a lymphocytic infiltrate. At the initiation of infection, spirochetes are believed to bind fibronectin and epithelial cell–derived proteoglycans in the extracellular matrix (e.g., heparin, dermatan sulfate) via glycosaminoglycan receptors. This initiates a mild local inflammatory response that causes cutaneous erythema at sites of spirochetal invasion and centrifugal spread from the original tick bite. Subsequent spirochetemia and tissue-specific binding allows for the development of neurologic sequelae (via glycosphingolipid receptors), a vasculopathy similar to endarteritis obliterans seen in syphilis, and cardiac conduction defects in certain individuals. Arthritis is thought to be due to joint inflammation from localized exposure to spirochetal antigens such as outer surface protein A (OspA) or the heat shock protein groEL.

B. burgdorferi has been shown to exert immunomodulatory influences on host cells, including both decreased major histocompatibility complex (MHC) class II antigen-presenting molecules in Langerhans cells isolated from late-phase cutaneous skin lesions and upregulation of the class II MHC molecules HLA-DRβ1, HLA-DR2, and HLA-DR4 on synovial endothelial cells in arthritic joints. The role of cytokines in this disease has not been fully elucidated, but several studies have demonstrated increased levels of macrophage-derived tumor necrosis factor (TNF)-α, interleukin (IL)-1, and IL-6 in the blood, synovial fluid, and cerebrospinal fluid (CSF) of affected persons.

In addition, an autoimmune pathology has also been implicated in late disease manifestations. Most notably, the predominant T-cell receptor found on activated T lymphocytes after infection is specific for an epitope of OspA presented within certain class II MHC molecules that are upregulated in affected patients. Moreover, this OspA epitope has been shown to be cross-reactive with the leukocyte adhesion molecule human lymphocyte function associated antigen 1 (LFA-1), which is expressed particularly highly on T lymphocytes. Studies of transgenic mice tolerant to OspA suggest that this protein does not fully explain these autoimmune phenomena.

Minimal evidence has suggested the importance of a *Borrelia*-specific superantigen. In addition, IgM antibodies against the spirochete protein flagellin are cross-reactive with human axonal proteins and myelin; these have been suggested to mediate the neurologic sequelae of Lyme disease. Several other types of autoantibodies have been identified in the CSF of Lyme disease patients. However, it is not known whether these antibodies play a role in the actual pathogenesis of the disease or are simply a benign secondary consequence of infection.

Clinical Presentation

Subjective

Early in the course of the disease, the patient typically complains of a flulike illness, including fever, chills, and myalgia. The patient may report having discovered a rash or red spot that grew in size. The report of a rash may be accompanied by objective findings on examination.

Later in the course of the disease, malaise, fatigue, headache, neck pain and stiffness, and generalized pains may constitute presenting symptoms. Left untreated, the disease will progress so that complaints will include multiple joint arthritis. Late in the disease trajectory, the patient may complain of memory loss, cognitive disturbances, mood changes, and peripheral neuropathy in addition to arthritis.

Objective

In the early-localized disease, occurring days to 1 month after the exposure, erythema migrans rashes are seen in 90 percent of cases, accompanied by the nonspecific findings of fatigue, malaise, headache, myalgias and arthralgias, cervical stiffness, and lymphadenopathy. The patient may also present with a low-grade fever. The exanthem is called erythema migrans, which is a rash that is located in parts of the body where the tick selectively feeds, such as the axilla, groin, and waistband. The rash is caused by the tick bite. It grows in size as it spreads ("migrates") from the site of the bite. This classic rash of erythema migrans is occasionally pruritic and/or burning, may develop central clearing, greater than 5 cm in size. The presence of this rash is essentially diagnostic of Lyme disease in the setting of appropriate clinical findings and, in fact, obviates the need for serologic confirmation.

In early-disseminated disease, which occurs days to 10 months after infection, often in the absence of erythema migrans, the patient presents with systemic manifestations including carditis (<10 percent of cases) and neurologic manifestations (10 percent of cases) such as lymphocytic meningitis, cranial nerve palsies [especially CNVII] and radiculoneuritis. This neurologic triad is known as Bannwarth's syndrome and is more common in European cases of Lyme than in the United States.

In late disease, which may be months to years after exposure, the symptoms are characterized by intermittent arthritis (50 percent; which responds to oral antibiotic therapy) and arthralgias (20 percent), with 10 percent having monoarthritis of the knee), neurologic manifestations called tertiary neuroborreliosis (including encephalopathy, neurocognitive impairment, and peripheral neuropathy), and cutaneous manifestations such as solitary lymphocytoma and acrodermatitis chronica atrophicans. These cutaneous manifestations are seen only in European cases due to *B. afzelii*.

Objective findings later in the disease include regional or organ-specific physical abnormalities. Cardiac findings include dysrhythmias and a prolonged P-R interval. Rare would be the finding of third-degree heart block, however. If the neurologic system were to be involved, objective findings might include nuccal rigidity, sensorimotor disturbances, and paresthesias. The MMSE results may be positive for impaired problem resolution. Skin eruptions resembling the erythema migrans of early infection may recur later, as well. Very late in the disease trajectory, musculoskeletal findings dominate. In particular, joints become edematous and are associated with pain to touch. Gait disturbance may occur in association with encephalopathy. URI or GI symptoms are more consistent with viral syndromes rather than with Lyme disease.

Diagnostic Reasoning

Diagnostic Tests

The term "chronic Lyme disease" is not preferred, as it tends to foster fixation on this diagnosis as a cause of chronic, nonspecific complaints. Cultures of the skin lesion or rash can isolate *Borrelia burgdorferi* in half of the cases. Because the culture takes a long time to grow, serologic studies are preferred. Histologic and immunologic staining is low yield in diagnostic testing owing to the low frequency of causative organisms. Positive serologies with ELISA tests against *Borrelia* sonicates containing mixtures of bacterial antigens (which often have suboptimal specificity, giving a number of false positives due to cross-reactivity with normal human proteins, other spirochete infections, EBV infection, or autoimmune disorders such as SLE or RA) must be confirmed by Western blot tests in which specific spirochetal proteins (heat shock proteins, flagellins) are directly detected by antibody staining. Western blot (or immunoblot) tests have lower sensitivity than the ELISA, but have greater specificity (as with HIV tests), so they are useful to confirm Lyme disease. These tests should be measured against CDC testing standards, however, and not just those of an individual lab, as there will be a lot of variation between labs. It is best to send blood samples to a lab associated with an established academic medical center doing research on Lyme disease. A hepatic panel may also be helpful when characterizing the disease, as hepatitis may be apparent.

Patients are often seronegative with early localized (erythema migrans) disease. This is another reason not to do blood testing initially. Patients are usually positive for IgM and IgG by the early disseminated phase (6 to 8 weeks after exposure). Early antibiotic therapy may render serologic tests negative, but for unknown reasons, as spirochetes may still be detected. In contrast, previous vaccination with Lymerix (a Lyme vaccine that is now off the market) can lead to false-positive ELISA tests up to 6 years after vaccination. Also, antibody tests may stay positive even after Lyme disease has been treated and has fully resolved. IgM levels can remain elevated for more than a year, so they cannot be used to make a diagnosis, only to confirm one that is suspected for other reasons. These tests are nearly always positive in late disease, and a negative ELISA in these patients has strong negative predictive value and should not be followed by a Western blot test, as these will have lower sensitivity. *Borrelia*-specific antibody levels should be measured in the synovial fluid and CSF and is useful if there is evidence of localized inflammation in the joints or CNS (closed-space inflammation) to see whether this inflammation is due to *Borrelia* infection or is merely coincidental.

Lyme disease should never be diagnosed based on lab tests alone. Lab tests are only confirmatory, not diagnostic, and they should never be used as screening tools, as the false-positive rates are too high. A diagnosis of Lyme disease should also be made only with findings that clearly suggest this disease, rather than just any nonspecific chronic complaints. The CDC criteria for Lyme disease, which were developed for research purposes, are too narrow to be used for clinical diagnosis, as these will exclude many cases. For a number of reasons, the following tests for Lyme detection are not widely accepted, as they are still experimental and have a number of drawbacks: variable surface antigen (VlsE) ELISA, PCR, urinary antigen testing, T-cell proliferative responses, and immune complex disruption.

These lab tests should not be trusted to confirm a diagnosis of Lyme disease.

Differential Diagnosis

Differential diagnoses for Lyme disease include viral syndromes, Rocky Mountain spotted fever, and relapsing fever. It is important not to confuse FMS or CFS, which are not inflammatory disorders and have never been shown to be clearly infectious in etiology. Although FMS may develop after onset of Lyme disease, it is important not to simply accept a diagnosis of chronic Lyme disease made previously by another clinician, as there is little evidence that this condition actually exists, as opposed to the late manifestations of the disease, which are considered genuine aspects of the disease. Human granulocytic erlichiosis, caused by *Anaplasma phagocytophilum,* is an important consideration as an alternate or a comorbid diagnosis, especially in the setting of high fever and severe constitutional complaints, elevated LENZ, or leukopenia/thrombocytopenia.

Management

The goal of management is not only to stop the manifestations of the disease at the time of diagnosis, but also to prevent progression of the disease. About 90 percent of early-localized disease responds to antibiotic therapy. The duration of treatment depends on the extent of involvement. Regimens for early-localized disease should last for 10 to 14 days, whereas 30 days of therapy are required for cardiac, neurologic, and arthritic manifestation.

Doxycycline (Vibramycin) 100 mg bid may be used in the initial management of erythema migrans. Doxycycline, or any tetracycline, is not recommended for children younger than 8 years of age or pregnant women. The dosage is 2 mg/kg for children older than 8 years. Doxycycline is also effective against erlichiosis, however, which may be a common morbidity. Alternative agents include amoxicillin (Amoxil), cefuroxime (Ceftin), and erythromycin (E-mycin). Cefuroxime is more expensive than doxycycline or amoxicillin. The amoxicillin dose is 500 mg tid (50 mg/kg per day divided q8h, with this same maximum dose in children). The cefuroxime dose is 500 mg bid in adults and up to 30 mg/kg/day divided bid with this same maximum dose for children. Up to 15 percent of patients may display a worsening of symptoms with rigors, fever, or hypotension in the first 24 hours of antibiotic thereapy due to an acute cytokine storm involving TNF-α, IL-6, and IL-8. This is referred to as a Jarisch-Herxheimer reaction and is well documented in tick- and louse-borne relapsing fever conditions. Macrolides such as erythromycin are not as effective as doxycycline, amoxicillin, or cefuroxime, and should be used only for patients intolerant to these other first-line choices. A first-generation cephalosporin such as cephalexin (Keflex) should not be used, as these are not active against *Borrelia*.

Early disseminated disease with mostly musculoskeletal manifestations should be treated with the same oral agents for 2 to 3 weeks total as long as meningitis or third-degree heart block is noted. If neurologic sequelae other than isolated facial nerve palsy or third-degree heart block is noted, IV antibiotic therapy should be started with ceftriaxone (2 grams qd) or cefotaxime (2 grams tid) for 2 to 4 weeks. First- and second-degree heart block and isolated facial nerve palsy can be treated with 3 weeks of oral antibiotics. The patient should have a lumbar puncture done to analyze the CSF for anti-*Borrelia* antibodies or inflammatory cells (WBCs). If subclinical meningitis is suspected with elevated WBCs in the CSF, IV antibiotic therapy is required. Third-degree heart block should be treated with IV ceftriaxone or cefotaxime, and prednisone 40 to 60 mg/day in divided doses may be added if patients do not respond within 4 days, but this approach has not been validated in randomized trials. Late Lyme disease is treated with amoxicillin or doxycycline for at least 4 weeks if arthritis is the primary manifestation. If patients fail one or two courses of oral antibiotic therapy or if late disease presents with neurologic sequelae (or if an LP shows subclinical meningitis with WBC or autoantibodies), IV antibiotic therapy of (ceftriaxone or cefotaxime) for 4 weeks should be used.

All IV antibiotic therapy may be done on an outpatient basis if the patient has reliable IV access (generally a PICC or a C-line, as opposed to a regular IV) and a stable social situation. In addition, the first IV dose should be given in a monitored setting to evaluate for drug hypersensitivity. Weekly CBCs should be done to monitor for leukopenia seen with ceftriaxone and cefotaxime. Ceftriaxone may cause biliary sludging which can be monitored with weekly hepatic panels to look for hyperbilirubinemia. If this occurs, the patient should be switched to cefotaxime. GI effects, including *Clostridium difficile* colitis may also occur. Doxycycline causes photosensitivity, while amoxicillin and cefuroxime can cause drug rashes. Combination antibiotic therapy, an oral course of antibiotics following IV courses, pulse therapy with weekly IV treatments, and extended regimens lasting beyond 2 to 4 weeks have never been validated through randomized trials and should be avoided. These are only likely to increase drug toxicity. There is also no evidence that pharmacologic treatment of asymptomatic seropositive people, found on routine "screening" for instance, is of any benefit. These patients should be thoroughly evaluated, though, to determine whether an asymptomatic phase is actually latent infection that will eventually manifest as late disease, as these individuals typically do not progress through early disease manifestations.

Failure of antibiotic therapy may relate to coinfection by other tick-borne diseases, such as erlichiosis. Headache, fatigue, and malaise may persist after treatment, but continued infection or the presence of a comorbid condition should probably be suspected only if symptoms worsen posttreatment, if new signs of inflammation develop, or if there are documented changes on neuropsychiatric testing.

Follow-Up and Referral

Follow-up before diagnosis is made may require weekly sessions. It is important to start antibiotic therapy after initial laboratory testing. The rash of erythema migrans begins to resolve after the fifth dose of oral antibiotics. Fibromyalgic and CFS-like symptoms (HA, weakness, fatigue, arthralgias) may persist for years after infection, and actual FMS is recognized as a post-infectious complication of Lyme disease. Referral may not be required if the diagnosis is clear and straightforward. In the event that it is not clear, a referral to an infectious disease specialist is indicated for further evaluation and recommendations. Neurologic, cardiac, and other manifestations may necessitate appropriate referrals should the manifestations persist despite primary care management.

Patient Education

People should be encouraged to avoid foliage, especially at ankle level, along wooded paths, and walk in the center of the path to avoid low-lying brush. They should wear clothing that can prevent ticks from attaching to skin. When planning an activity in the woods, the patient should wear long pants and boots, and the pants should be tucked inside the boot lip. Shirt collars should be closed. Tick repellant should be applied to the exposed skin and scalp. After removing clothing, the patient should inspect the axillae, groin, and waistband areas, in particular, for evidence of ticks.

If infection has already occurred, the patient needs to learn the course of the disease, and that recurrence of symptoms after initial treatment might occur. Seropositivity does not equal immunity against reinfection. Re-infection is possible with *Borrelia* of a different strain if the patient remains exposed to high-risk environments, although symptoms do not tend to be worse than those of the initial infection.

Sjögren's Syndrome

Sjögren's syndrome (SS) is a chronic inflammatory autoimmune disorder caused by exocrine dysfunction. It presents as dryness in all areas of the body where there are exocrine glands associated with mucous membranes, most notably the salivary and lacrimal glands. However, SS has the potential for affecting a wide array of organ systems including the skin, lung, kidney, and heart. In addition, the hematopoietic system may be affected with a propensity for lymphoma.

Epidemiology and Causes

SS has a worldwide distribution with an annual incidence of 4 in 100,000; 70 percent of these cases may be primary, while the others are associated with comorbid conditions and are considered secondary. Accurate estimates of disease prevalence are complicated by a lack of agreement as to the defining diagnostic criteria of the disease. However, it is generally agreed that SS strikes women nine times more often than men. Rheumatic diseases often accompany it. The average age range for disease onset is 40 to 60 years. The cause for the syndrome remains under investigation. Because SS typically accompanies underlying rheumatic diseases, investigations evaluating the etiologic links among these are ongoing.

Pathophysiology

SS is believed to be an autoimmune disorder. Lymphocytic infiltration in all affected organs is the pathophysiologic hallmark of the disease. Pooling of lymphocytes and plasma cells in the lacrimal glands causes the characteristic dry eye conjunctivitis of the syndrome called keratoconjunctivitis sicca, while parotid enlargement and diminished salivary excretions result from a similar infiltrate within the salivary glands along with hyperplasia of the ductal epithelium, which produces characteristic dry mouth or xerostomia.

At least three-quarters of these infiltrating cells are T lymphocytes, primarily of the CD4+ T helper subset with classical TCR αβ receptors and expressing a memory cell surface phenotype including the leukocyte adhesion molecule LFA-1. About 10 percent of the cells are B lymphocytes and plasma cells that produce significant amounts of oligoclonal immunoglobulin. The adjacent glandular epithelium expresses high levels of class II MHC (HLA-DR) and costimulatory molecules such as B7, suggesting antigenic T-cell stimulation is central to the pathogenesis of SS. It is unclear whether these antigens are autoantigens and/or certain viral antigens.

Evidence for a genetic predisposition to SS is supported by studies that recognize a familial propensity for specific HLA-DR3, HLA-DR5, and HLA-DRβ3 alleles in affected patients and their relatives. At least one study has also linked primary SS to genetic polymorphisms in regulatory DNA sequences of the IL-10 gene, a cytokine that may potentially influence cell-mediated immunity. However, IFN-γ and IL-2 appear to be the primary immunomodulatory cytokines in SS. Produced by ductal epithelium, IFN-γ upregulates the expression of HLA-DR molecules on epithelial antigen presenting cells and potentiates T lymphocyte cellular cytotoxicity. Cytolytic destruction of exocrine gland tissue does not appear to explain the full pathology of SS, however, as decreased saliva and tear production does not correlate well with the degree of histologic damage on glandular biopsies.

The importance of autoantibodies in the pathophysiology of SS has long been emphasized. Autoantibodies specific for acetylcholine receptors in salivary glands have been suggested to impair the secretion of saliva in histologically normal glands. Far more common, however, are autoantibodies to specific nucleoproteins associated with RNA, including anti-Ro (SSA) antibodies seen in up to 90 percent of SS cases and anti-La (SSB) antibodies seen in up to half of cases. Although the pathogenetic role of these antibodies is unclear, the same antibodies can be found in a variety of other autoimmune disorders, including neonatal lupus in which they are suggested to mediate complete heart block after crossing the placenta from mother to child. Anti-α-fodrin antibodies may be even more sensitive and specific for SS than anti-Ro or anti-La, but their pathologic significance is not yet established.

Infection by various viruses has been suggested to underlie primary SS, including Epstein-Barr virus (EBV), retroviruses such as human T cell lymphotropic virus (HTLV-1), Hepatitis C virus, and coxsackievirus. In vitrostudies and preclinical animal models have demonstrated that infection with these viruses is capable of leading to lymphocytic infiltrates of the salivary and lacrimal glands, recreating many of the same symptoms as SS. Although viral particles are typically not present in high numbers, viral infection has been suggested to break tolerance to autoantigens, in turn leading to SS via autoimmune activation. The relationship between SS and viral infection is not entirely clear, however, and at present, most of the etiologic evidence is indirect and does not predominate for any single virus.

Disorders of estrogen have also been indirectly implicated, as primary SS is seen virtually only in women. Moreover, postmenopausal women taking estrogen-containing hormone replacement therapy (HRT) have a higher incidence of ocular dryness compared to non-HRT controls. This evidence remains circumstantial, however.

Clinical Presentation

Subjective

Patients may complain of dryness of their eyes and feel like something is in them. Keratoconjunctivitis sicca is dryness of the cornea caused by a deficiency of tear secretion in which the corneal surface appears dull and rough and the eye feels gritty and irritated. The patient may also complain of dryness of the mouth (xerostomia) caused by cessation of normal salivary secretions. In addition, the patient may complain of loss of taste and smell, recurrent dental caries, dysphagia, vaginismus, and rectal bleeding. Associated complaints may be those of rheumatoid arthritis (RA), joint swelling and pain, malaise, and low-grade fever.

Objective

The patient appears ill, which is to say that the presentation is of one who has been sick for some time. If RA precedes SS, then the chronic debilitation caused by rheumatic disease can account for the ill appearance.

The patient's breath may smell fetid because of dental caries and mucosal dryness. Mucosal beds of the nose and throat will be pale and may reveal small fissures. The tongue could be beefy red because of dryness. Similar findings are associated with the vagina and anus.

Many other systemic, although rare, manifestations of SS may be assessed: a macular, papular, vesicular, or purpuric skin rash; arthralgias and myalgias; cardiopulmonary manifestations such as pericarditis or pulmonary hypertension from (lymphocytic) interstitial pneumonitis; a tendency for pulmonary emboli due to circulating antiphospholipid/anticardiolipin antibodies; interstitial nephritis leading to renal tubular acidosis or glomerulonephritis (similar to that of systemic lupus erythematosus [SLE]); gastroesophageal reflux disease (GERD); a higher prevalence of hypothyroidism; and rare neurologic sequelae such as peripheral (mononeuritis multiplex or symmetric neuropathies) and autonomic neuropathies and CNS manifestations mimicking multiple sclerosis; transverse myelitis, optic neuritis, or ischemic strokes that may be due to vasculitis, thrombosis, or demyelination. Fatigue is another important aspect of many presentations of SS, due to disrupted sleep patterns from dryness or accompanying systemic symptoms such as arthralgias/myalgias.

Diagnostic Reasoning

Diagnostic Tests

SS is diagnosed by clinical and laboratory findings, rather than identification of a single causative agent. Clinical diagnosis of SS includes six defining criteria: (1) inadequate tear production (using the Schirmer test with filter paper to blot tears on the lateral third of the lower eyelid [less than 5 mm of wetting in 5 minutes is abnormal] or using artificial replacement tears more than tid), (2) signs of corneal epithelial damage from dry eye using Rose-Bengal or fluorescein staining and slit-lamp examination, (3) decreased saliva production, (4) lymphocytic infiltration of labial salivary gland tissue on histopathology following labial gland biopsy (LGB)—the closest test to a gold standard for diagnosis (greater than 50 immune cells surrounding an intact glandular lobule), (5) impaired salivary gland function by objective testing via radionuclide technetium scanning (quantitative salivary gland scintigraphy demonstrating poor uptake), parotid sialography with parotid gland cannulation and injection of oil-based contrast material, or spontaneous salivary production of less than or equal to 1.5 mL/15 min), and (6) autoantibodies including anti-Ro (SSA) and/or anti-La (SSB).

Initial lab tests include a CBC, rheumatoid factor, ANA, and gamma-globulin. The CBC might reveal an anemia of chronic disease, which should be mild; leukopenia; and eosinophilia. The eosinophilia is caused by autoimmune factors and not by external antigens. The RF is positive in three-fourths of samples. ANA will be elevated, as will gamma-globulin levels.

Electrophoresis studies are required to determine whether SS is present alone or in combination with rheumatoid disease. SS alone manifests more specific autobodies—anti-Ro/SSA and anti-La/SSB antigens, whereas SS and rheumatoid disease together reveal antibodies against exocrine ducts and antibodies to RA-associated nuclear antigens (RANA).

Differential Diagnosis

As patients with SS have a higher prevalence of hypothyroidism, this should be screened for with a good history taking and a TSH. Further laboratory work-up to rule out other important disorders include a basic metabolic panel with hepatic function tests (transaminases), rheumatoid factor, and ANA with autoantibody protein electrophoresis. HIV and hepatitis C testing may also be indicated. Sarcoid could be evaluated with a chest x-ray exam to look for hilar adenopathy or interstitial lung diagnosis. An MRI or ultrasound and biopsy should be done if there is unilateral salivary gland enlargement to rule out malignancy or specific glandular pathology such as acute bacterial sialadenitis. Bilateral salivary gland swelling may be due to acute viral infection (mumps, coxsackievirus, echovirus, or EBV) or chronic infection with HIV or hepatitis C, granulomatous disease such as sarcoidosis, amyloidosis, or TB, malnutrition, alcoholism, and eating disorders such as bulimia or anorexia with purging features.

Further differentials for Sjogren's syndrome include other autoimmune disorders which may exist concurrently; such as SLE, scleroderma, or rheumatoid arthritis. In fact, rheumatoid factor (RF) may be positive in up to 75 percent of cases. It is also critical to distinguish SS from patients with fibromyalgia or depression who may have significant anticholinergic toxicities from psychiatric meds, which can include dry eyes and especially dry mouth. Dry eyes may also be from impaired blinking resulting from muscular or neurologic disorders, vitamin A deficiency leading to mucin deficiency (xerophthalmia), conjunctivitis, infiltration of the lacrimal glands (from sarcoidosis, lymphoma, or amyloidosis), or blepharitis from Meibomian gland dysfunction. Dry mouth can also result from sialadenitis from obstructing salivary gland stones, chronic viral infections (hepatitis C, HIV), and iatrogenic anticholinergic drug effects. The following conditions are exclusion criteria in terms of meeting the defining criteria of SS: previous head/neck irradiation or preexisting lymphoma, comorbid infection with hepatitis C or HIV with AIDS, sarcoidosis, graft versus host disease, or recent use of anticholinergic meds. Symptoms of mucosal dryness are also common in liver disease and depression, so these must be considered.

Management

The management of this syndrome cannot be divided into initial and subsequent stages, because it remains poorly understood; therefore, management consists of symptom support. Normal saline eye drops can relieve lacrimal dryness. Hard candies and gum may be used to stimulate salivation but must be sugar-free to avoid worsening dental caries. Dried fruits that contain malic acid may also be helpful in stimulating salivation. In extreme cases of salivary dryness, the patient should be encouraged to apply an artificial salivary gel or use a mouth spray. Fluids can also keep the mouth well lubricated as long as they do not contain caffeine (a diuretic) or ethanol (as used in mouthwash), which can be drying. Special toothpastes and toothbrushes designed for a dry mouth are also available. Quarterly dental evaluations, along with vigorous flossing and regular brushing, may prevent dental caries.

Pilocarpine (Salagen) 5 mg tid or qid and cevimeline (Evoxac) 30 to 60 mg tid are specific cholinergic (muscarinic) antagonists for stimulating aqueous secretions. These drugs are contraindicated in persons with narrow-angle glaucoma or iritis, owing to their mydriatic effects. Cevimeline should not be used if a patient has asthma, as this can worsen respiratory secretions. Artificial tears and salivary gels often contain hypromellose (0.3 percent) or methycellulose (0.3 percent) and may be used every 2 to 4 hours if needed. Several of these can be irritating to certain individuals. Even acetylcysteine can be used as a mucolytic if thick mucous fibers coat the eyes, but this smells like rotten eggs because of its sulfur content. Spreading agents such as polyethylene glycol and dextran-70 0.1 percent drops are also available for dry eyes. If artificial tears prove ineffective, the next step is punctal occlusion in which collagen plugs are placed by an ophthalmologist in the lacrimal puncta on the inferior lid, so that tears (artificial or natural) cannot drain away to the nose. Topical cyclosporine 0.05 percent 1 gtt q12h was recently approved by the FDA to increase tearing, presumably by decreasing T cell infiltration within the conjunctivae. Dry lips may be treated with vaseline and dry skin with moisturizing lotions. Vaginal dryness may be treated with lubricant jelly.

The following are some rarer systemic manifestations of SS with their treatment:

- macular, papular, vesicular, or purpuric skin rashes that may require biopsy and treatment as a vasculitis;
- arthralgias and myalgias that may respond to NSAIDs or hydroxychloroquine;
- cardiopulmonary manifestations such as pericarditis or pulmonary hypertension from (lymphocytic) interstitial pneumonitis which may require treatment with steroids (prednisone) or immunosuppressants (azathioprine, chlorambucil, cyclophosphamide);
- interstitial nephritis leading to renal tubular acidosis or glomerulonephritis (similar to that of SLE) which may require steroid or immunosuppressant therapy (cyclophosphamide, mycophenolate);
- rare neurologic sequelae such as peripheral (mononeuritis multiplex or symmetric neuropathies) and autonomic (confirmed by tilt table tests) requiring mineralocorticoid therapy); and
- neuropathies and CNS manifestations mimicking MS, transverse myelitis, optic neuritis, or ischemic strokes which may be due to vasculitis, thrombosis, or demyelination—requiring treatment with immunosuppressants.

Follow-Up and Referral

Follow-up consists of evaluation of symptom management. On occasion, alterations in symptom management may be required. If SS alone is isolated, follow-up evaluations need not occur except twice per year. More frequent evaluations will be necessitated by concurrent disease. Referrals are not necessary except when this syndrome accompanies other diseases. The clinician may consult with a rheumatologist initially to differentiate the disease from other rheumatoid problems and to finalize the diagnosis.

During follow-up exams, it is important to monitor for dental caries and oral candidiasis which would require antifungal therapy. This can lead to severe mouth pain, as well as screening for infectious conjunctivitis and complications from nasal dryness and laryngotracheal reflux which can stimulate vagal responses and mimic allergic or recurrent sinusitis symptoms, such as repeated throat clearing and postnasal drip–like symptoms. This type of reflux may be treated with proton pump inhibitors (similar to GERD) with referral to an ENT if needed.

Patient Education

The patient should learn that mucosal dryness can be controlled with conservative interventions. Regular application of artificial lubricants can prevent the soreness and untoward effects of dry mucosae. The patient should be encouraged to wear sunglasses to protect the eyes from strong light, wind, and dust, as well as avoid low-humidity environments. If the patient has sore lesions in the mouth, tobacco, alcohol, and spicy, salty foods should be avoided. OTC medications that decrease pharyngeal secretions, such as antihistamines, antidepressants, anticholinergics, and atropine derivatives should be avoided. Patients should be warned that they are at greater risk with surgeries needing general anesthesia, given their increased risk for thick, inspissated mucus and atelectasis.

Systemic Lupus Erythematosus

SLE is an inflammatory autoimmune disease. It tends to affect many organ systems. Spontaneous remissions and exacerbations characterize the clinical picture. SLE can be mild or aggressive and even life-threatening in presentation.

Epidemiology and Causes

The prevalence of SLE is 40 to 50 cases per 100,000 and is associated with age, gender, race, and genetics. Nearly 85 percent of patients with SLE are women, most often in their 20s and 30s. However, 15 percent of cases present after the age of 55 years. Juvenile cases are not uncommon, though, with 20 percent of diagnosed patients younger than the age of 16 years. In children, the female to male ratio is 3:1; in adults, it is 10 to 15:1. Epidemiologic studies have identified sex hormones as potential causative factors for SLE, as onset of the disease in women typically occurs between menses and menopause. Estrogen has been shown to stimulate T cells, B cells, and macrophages, as well as increase expression of cytokines, endothelial cell adhesion molecules, and antigen-presenting major histocompatibility (MHC) molecules. SLE flares have also been associated with hyperprolactinemia. In contrast, androgenic hormones such as testosterone tend to be immunosuppressive, which may also contribute to the gender specificity of SLE.

Descendants of African races are four times more likely to develop the disease, as compared to Caucasians. Several lines of evidence have also demonstrated a genetic component to SLE, for example, a high concordance rate between monozygotic twins, a propensity for specific HLA-DR class II MHC genes in affected individuals and positive gene linkage studies in affected siblings.

Although not causative of SLE, several triggering factors for acute exacerbations have been identified. These include exposure to ultraviolet (UV)-B and UV-A rays, which is believed to cause increased cytokine and cell adhesion molecule expression, microbial infection (e.g., EBV, *Mycobacteria*, trypanosomes) that may stimulate cross-reacting autoantibodies; emotional stress which, although controversial, has been tied to mild disease flares; pregnancy and postpartum hormonal fluctuations; and surgery, which may increase the formation of autoantibody-containing immune complexes via the release of intracellular antigens into the circulation from tissue trauma. Exposure to cigarette smoke or silica dust also increases the risk of developing SLE, which implicates inflammatory lung pathology.

Pathophysiology

The pathophysiology of SLE is best understood by a review of the diagnostic criteria. The diagnosis of SLE is made after 4 or more of the following 11 criteria are met in the absence of medications or other disorders known to induce these effects:

- ▲ Arthritis—nonerosive and usually involving two or more joints
- ▲ Photosensitivity—often triggering skin rashes, exposure to the sun's UV-B rays may be a triggering event for SLE exacerbations.
- ▲ Oral (or nasal) ulcers—typically painless
- ▲ Malar rash—bilateral butterfly formation across the cheeks and nasal bridge
- ▲ Discoid rash—red raised patches, sometimes with denuded central areas
- ▲ Serositis (inflammation) of the pleura or pericardia
- ▲ Renal disease (any one of three indicators: more than 0.5 g/day proteinuria, 3+ or more proteinuria [as detected by dipstick], or cellular casts)
- ▲ Hematologic disorders (any one of four indicators: hemolytic anemia, leukopenia [greater than 4000 WBC/mm^3], lymphopenia [greater than 1500 lympho-

cytes/mm^3, thrombocytopenia [less than 100,000 platelets/mm^3])
- ▲ Neurologic disease (e.g., seizures, psychoses) not otherwise explained by iatrogenic or metabolic causes
- ▲ Positive ANA
- ▲ Immunologic abnormalities (any one of four indicators: positive antiphospholipid antibodies such as anticardiolipin or lupus anticoagulant), antibody to double-stranded native DNA, anti-Sm [Smith] antibody, false-positive serologic test for syphilis [VDRL, RPR])

SLE is, at its core, a condition of disordered immunity in which mechanisms that normally prevent immune cell activation by autoantigens are eliminated. A number of factors have been cited that contribute to this autoimmune activation, for example, an inhibition of suppressor T cells that normally downregulate immune responses; an increase in CD4+ T helper cells, cytokine production (e.g., IFN-α, IL-4, IL-6, IL-10), and polyclonal B cell activation; and dysregulated intracellular signaling (particularly pathways involving cytosolic calcium). These changes contribute to a significant production of autoantibodies that are considered to be a hallmark of the disease. Mouse models of SLE have demonstrated dysregulated apoptosis in which nuclear antigens (e.g., DNA, ribonucleoprotein, histones) are exposed on the cell surface, capable of recognition by autoreactive lymphocytes. In turn, autoantibodies often appear in the serum years before the actual onset of SLE symptoms.

Autoantibodies are also formed against cell surface antigens, including antibodies specific for red and white blood cells, platelets, and neuronal and renal cells. These antibodies mediate cellular destruction via complement activation, antibody-dependent cellular cytotoxicity, and opsonization. While not seen universally, autoantibody-derived immune complexes are believed to underlie the pathology of a majority of clinical manifestations of SLE. Histochemical staining has identified immune complex deposition along the basement membrane in nephritic kidneys, at the dermal–epidermal junction in skin lesions, within the choroid plexus, as well as the pleural cavity and pericardium—all major sites of SLE pathology. The biochemical nature of both the autoantigen and autoantibody (e.g., size, charge, binding affinity, rate of phagocytic clearance, ability to be neutralized by complement proteins) determines where these complexes form and the extent of tissue damage after their deposition.

One of the organ systems most severely affected by immune complex deposition is the kidneys. In addition to the deposition of circulating immune complexes along the glomerular basement membrane, autoreactive IgG1 and IgG3 anti-DNA antibodies also bind directly to autoantigens in the basement membranes, serving as a nidus for complement activation. These chemotactic complement proteins then attract leukocytes and mononuclear cells that phagocytose the immune complexes, releasing cytokines and clotting factors that lead to fibrinoid necrosis, ongoing inflammation, renal scarring, and kidney dysfunction. Diffuse proliferative glomerulonephritis is the most common histologic form of lupus nephritis, which results from this inflammation. In contrast, lupus membranous nephropathy is not associated with inflammation. Rather, in this setting, immune complex activation is separated physically from circulating immune cells by the glomerular basement membrane, resulting in epithelial injury and proteinuria without active inflammation.

A subset of individuals with SLE is also prone to developing antiphospholipid antibodies, including antibodies against the β-2-glycoprotein I complex and cardiolipin, as well as the lupus anticoagulant. These individuals have more severe disease, related primarily to an increased thrombogenic state, which predisposes to both venous and arterial thromboembolism, resulting in a greater incidence of deep venous thrombosis, pulmonary embolism, cerebrovascular accidents (strokes and transient ischemic attacks), and recurrent first-trimester miscarriages due to placental infarcts. Normally, β-2-glycoprotein has an anticoagulant effect, which is abrogated by these antiphospholipid antibodies.

One of the most characteristic physical findings of SLE is a bilateral malar rash. This and other SLE skin rashes are exacerbated by sun exposure, largely due to ultraviolet damage to DNA in skin keratinocytes and alterations in membrane phospholipid metabolism. Thus, anti-DNA, anti-RNA, anti-Ro, anti-La, and antiphospholipid autoantibodies form that mediate keratinocyte destruction and local skin inflammation. IL-1 production from cutaneous keratinocytes and antigen-presenting Langerhans cells potentiates this inflammatory response.

Clinical Presentation

Subjective

The patient may complain of malaise, fever, anorexia, and unplanned weight loss. The patient may also complain of blurred vision and conjunctival swelling. Sleeplessness and depression may be focal complaints. Joints may be reported to be swollen and painful in the history but this may not be evident on examination. Shortness of breath and painful inspiration may also be present. Vague abdominal pains and/or abdominal cramping could enter the history.

Objective

Integumentary assessment findings:

- ▲ The characteristic "butterfly" rash could be present, along with assorted other rashes.
- ▲ Alopecia and scalpal exanthems are typical findings.
- ▲ Splinter hemorrhages, periungual erythema, and fingertip lesions may be observed on the fingers and toes.
- ▲ Lymphadenopathy in several regions of the body indicates systemic disease.
- ▲ There are often scarring and highly inflammatory (even ulcerating) lesions of discoid lupus. This form of lupus often does not present with the familiar autoantibodies

of SLE, including ANA, anti-dsDNA, and anti-Smith antibodies.

- ▲ Raynaud's phenomenon, a vascular condition, may be seen as white-blue skin color changes in response to cold, then red upon rewarming, and may predate other symptoms and present in up to 40 percent of patients.

Musculoskeletal assessment findings:

- ▲ Swollen joints, however, the swelling does not follow a pattern, such as affecting only weightbearing joints.
- ▲ Musculoskeletal joint pains (an asymmetric, nondeforming, migratory arthritis—often in the hands and fingers) occur in 90 percent of cases and are often the presenting complaint.

Neurologic assessment findings:

- ▲ Thought processes may be impaired. Therefore, the clinician should listen to the patient's explanations to establish lapses in logic, but these often are not evident in primary care tests, such as the MMSE.
- ▲ Evidence of peripheral paresthesias and diminished deep tendon reflexes .

Cardiac assessment findings:

- ▲ A systolic murmur may be present.
- ▲ Distended jugular veins suggest cardiac failure.

GI assessment findings:

- ▲ Typically painless oral and nasal ulcers may be seen.
- ▲ Right upper abdominal quadrant tenderness may accompany the finding of hepatomegaly. Hepatitis is a common finding. Right lower quadrant tenderness suggests right colon enlargement, which may be caused by intestinal vasculitis.

Diagnostic Reasoning

Diagnostic Tests

Initial testing should include a CBC with platelet count, basic metabolic panel (serum electrolytes and kidney function tests), serum albumin (which will be reduced in nephropathy), ANA, urinalysis (UA), and antibody screens for double-stranded DNA (highly specific with 75 to 95 percent sensitivity), antiphospholipid antibodies, and anti-Smith antibodies (highly specific with only 25 percent sensitivity). Other common autoantibodies include those against single-stranded DNA and nucleoprotein as also seen in rheumatoid arthritis, antiribonucleoprotein as in scleroderma, and both anti-Ro (SSA) and anti-La (SSB) as in Sjögren's syndrome.

- ▲ The CBC may show either anemia or leukopenia or both. If the patient is leukopenic, the differential may reveal lymphocytopenia. One-third of patients with SLE will be thrombocytopenic. ANA results are likely to be elevated in more than 90 percent of samples; however, this is not specific for SLE. Numerous other inflammatory diseases are also associated with an elevated ANA. Changes in serum levels of autoantibodies (rising anti-double-stranded DNA IgG levels) or complement levels (decreasing CH50, C3, and C4) correlate with active disease. An erythrocyte sedimentation rate (ESR) and C-reactive protein (CRP) may also be used as non-specific markers of active inflammation. Proteinuria is a possible finding from the UA in nephrotic or nephritic patients, with hematuria in the latter. Serum complement levels (CH50, C3, and C4) are measured to assess degree of disease activity (i.e., lower levels reflect greater activity). These tests should be used in conjunction with clinical presentation (history and physical exam) to evaluate for worsening of the disease state, and should not be over- or underinterpreted. These initial tests along with characteristic clinical manifestations should be sufficient to confirm a diagnosis of SLE. RPR tests for syphilis may be falsely positive (due to anticardiolipin antibodies or other SLE-related phenomena).
- ▲ Pertinent imaging tests should be guided by clinical presentation such as a chest radiography for pulmonary symptoms; renal ultrasound in the face of renal failure; and plain films for arthritic joints. Similarly, invasive procedures such as renal biopsy are indicated when histology is needed to determine prognosis and guide therapy. Electrocardiography and echocardiography are indicated to evaluate for pericarditis and other cardiac pathology, while specific tests such as ventilation–perfusion (V-Q) scans or high-resolution spiral computed tomography (CT) scans of the lungs are used to evaluate for pulmonary emboli in prothrombotic patients.
- ▲ Drug-induced lupus is amilder presentation, associated with procainamide, hydralazine, and minocycline.
- ▲ As with SS, keratoconjunctivitis sicca may result, as can pathognomonic, although rare, cotton wool retinal exudates from retinal vasculitis. Scleritis and anterior uveitis may occur but are both uncommon. Mild to moderate cytopenias may affect all three major cell lines (leukopenia, anemia, low PLT), with thrombocytopenia leading to easy bruising and purpura; severe autoimmune hemolytic anemia can also result. In contrast, thrombophilia may also occur, increasing the risk of thrombosis, including DVT and arterial disease, especially if antiphospholipid antibodies are present. This prothrombotic state is the cause of recurrent miscarriages (abortions) early in pregnancy, usually in the first trimester. Thus, such a history should always make the clinician think of antiphospholipid syndrome and SLE.

Differential Diagnosis

The differentials for SLE includes vasculitis, rheumatoid arthritis, scleroderma, SS, JRA (juvenile RA), chronic active hepatitis, drug reactions, drug-induced lupus, and polyarteritis. The diagnostic criteria set forth under pathophysiology in this section should aid in distinguishing SLE from these other diseases. Hypothyroidism needs to be ruled out as a cause of fatigue; the TSH should provide this information.

Management

The principal goal of therapy is symptom control. Many patients require little or no intervention. Their joint pain may be managed with nonpharmacologic interventions, as provided in the section on RA. Emotional support and referral to SLE support groups are both helpful in establishing control over some symptoms. If conservative management fails, the patient may require corticosteroids, cyclophosphamide, or antimalarials.

Fatigue is the most common symptom and tends to be the most debilitating. It can happen even in the absence of signs of active inflammation. Fatigue may be multifactorial, but if due predominantly to SLE, it tends to respond to treatment with steroids, hydroxychloroquine, or even DHEA (dehydroepiandrosterone). In addition to weight loss, weight gain may happen due to generalized edema from hypoalbuminemia from nephrotic syndrome (anasarca), if there are kidney manifestations. If fever is present, it is important to deduce whether it is due to the SLE itself, infection (more likely if fever occurs while on active steroids or immunosuppressant therapies and is episodic), or a drug reaction that may present with a morbilliform rash and be prolonged, without response to NSAIDs or acetaminophen.

Kidney involvement may be clinically apparent in up to half of patients and is the primary reason for lupus-related hospitalization. Renal biopsy may reveal several histologic subtypes of lupus nephritis. Type I is normal. Type II is pure mesangial and carries with it a good prognosis. Type III is segmental and focal proliferative lupus nephritis, and responds to steroids. Type IV is diffuse proliferative lupus nephritis, which is the worst form with HTN and ESRD or death in up to 50 percent of cases and needs to be treated with high-dose steroids and immunosuppressants such as azathioprine (Imuran) mycophenolate mofetil, or cyclophosphamide (Cytoxan). Type V is membranous nephritis with a variable presentation that worsens as complement levels decrease as more immune complex formation leads to more complement deposition. One-third need no treatment other than that for other SLE symptoms, one-third need low to moderate dose steroids, and one-third need high-dose steroids. Type VI is advanced sclerosing lupus nephritis which nearly always leads to ESRD.

Gastrointestinal manifestations usually relate to SLE treatments, rather than the disease itself, such as gastritis and peptic ulcers from chronic NSAID and steroid use. SLE vasculitis can lead to inflammation of the pancreas, large intestine, and peritoneum in the serosal layers, as well as esophagitis and GERD. Both hepatomegaly and splenomegaly may be detected, along with the lymphadenopathy already mentioned. Pulmonary manifestations relate to lung inflammation including pleuritis with a pleural friction rub, effusions, pneumonitis, interstitial lung disease, alveolar hemorrhage, and eventually pulmonary hypertension. In turn, pulmonary function tests often have a restrictive pattern, given all the inflammation and scarring.

The severity of organ damage does not always correlate with severity of inflammation. For instance, kidney dysfunction may relate to scarring from past kidney inflammation that has since resolved. This is an important distinction for the clinician to make, because worsening ongoing inflammation may be treated with steroids or other immunosuppressants, while treating noninflammatory organ damage with this same regimen just increases risks of side effects and iatrogenic complications due to immunosuppression without really addressing the organ damage. Dietary modifications should be made specific to clinical presentation, for example, active inflammatory states may requiring higher calorie diets if weight loss is a concern, steroid-induced surges in appetite may call for low-calorie diets, while steroid-induced hypertension and hyperlipidemia, or that accompanying lupus nephritis, may call for a low-salt and low-fat/low-cholesterol diet, respectively. Likewise, lack of sun exposure because of photosensitivity may require vitamin D and calcium supplements, especially given chronic steroid use, to prevent bone loss. The clinician should be aware of the important side effects of systemic (IV or PO) steroids which include avascular necrosis (cutting off of blood supply to a major joint like the hip which results in joint necrosis), osteoporosis with fractures or vertebral collapse, growth inhibition in children, glaucoma, and hyperglycemia/diabetes, hypertension, early atherosclerosis which can lead to long-term CAD and heart damage, fatigue, and even cognitive dysfunction with chronic use. This is unfortunate because use of higher dose steroids, > 10 mg/day of prednisone for instance, is associated with a delayed time to onset of actual organ damage following diagnosis of SLE.

NSAIDs are good for mild musculoskeletal symptoms or mild serositis (inflammation of the serous layers like the pleura or pericardia). COX-2 inhibitors have been withdrawn from the market except for celecoxib (Celebrex) due to recent information on cardiovascular side effects. This should be used with caution. Cutaneous lupus responds well to antimalarials such as hydroxychloroquine (Plaquenil), which are also second-line agents for joint pains/myalgias. These drugs need to be monitored for ocular toxicity. When other organ systems are involved (such as the kidneys, CNS, or pulmonary vasculitis which leads to alveolar hemorrhage), glucocorticoids may be given alone or in combination with another immunosuppressant such as cyclophosphamide. Prednisone is good at preventing relapses if treatment is started as soon as a marked rise in anti-double-stranded DNA antibodies is observed in the setting of clinical disease manifestations. Disease progression in the face of cyclophosphamide use portends a particularly poor prognosis, and no treatment regimens are well-established for these refractory patients. Several treatments are being explored, with the most promising including immune system ablation (with high-dose chemotherapy), with or without stem cell transplantation, and use of the anti-B cell (anti-CD20) monoclonal immunotherapy rituximab. Five-year survival is much better now than in the past (currently greater than 90 percent), but the course of SLE tends to be relapsing and remitting (recurrent flares with intermittent quiescent periods, sometimes ending up in prolonged periods of remission lasting for several years). CNS and renal involvement, especially diffuse proliferative nephritis or advanced sclerosing nephritis, give the worst prognosis. Most SLE inpatients are admitted for renal issues, while cutaneous and joint/muscle manifestations alone have the best prognosis. Short-term death is also often due to infection related to immunosuppression by medications, in addition to organ involvement in active inflammation in the heart, kidney, or CNS.

Other poor prognostic factors are hypertension, male gender, having active disease at a young age, low socioeconomic status, and being African American. These trends have been seen with so many chronic diseases and are multifactorial in nature. They must not be chalked up solely to "genetic differences between the races," the presence of prothrombotic antiphospholipid antibodies, like the lupus anticoagulant and anticardiolipin, and highly active inflammatory disease. While men have less photosensitivity, they have more serositis with higher 1-year mortality and tend to present with an older age at onset.

The cardiovascular system can manifest pericarditis, a verrucous form of nonbacterial endocarditis known as Libman-Sacks endocarditis. This is associated with antiphospholipid antibodies and can produce emboli due to valvular insufficiency and turbulent blood flow. There is also the well-documented phenomenon of transplacentally delivered anti-Ro (SSA) and anti-La (SSB) anti-single-stranded DNA antibodies from a mother with SLE to her developing fetus which results in a potentially fatal third degree heart block. This is known as neonatal lupus, which is not a manifestation of primary lupus in the fetus, however, and is not the same as pediatric SLE.

CNS and psychiatric manifestations of SLE are quite varied and include cognitive defects, delirium, depression, mania, anxiety, psychosis, which can also be iatrogenic from steroid use, headache, aseptic meningitis, and various neuropathies. Ischemic CNS damage, including thromboembolic CVAs due to an antiphospholipid-mediated prothrombotic state, may underlie these symptoms as well. SLE is also the most common cause of chorea in the United States.

Follow-Up and Referral

Follow-up of SLE patients is critical to track the course of this disease. Patients who require nonpharmacologic management should be seen at least twice per year. Before consultation, they should receive laboratory evaluation of CBC, UA, platelet count, and ANA to follow the course of the disease. In addition, SLE patients have a greater risk of lymphoma. Greater risk of breast CA, abnormal PAPs, and squamous cell skin CA has also been suggested.

Referral to a rheumatologist is indicated if corticosteroids, cyclophosphamide, and antimalarials are to be prescribed.

Patient Education

The patient should receive referral to the national hotline for SLE. The toll-free number (see the Resources section at the end of this chapter) provides the patient with access to materials that support symptom control. In addition, the patient needs to learn the trajectory of the disease, including the prognosis. Rest will become essential during exacerbations. The need for increased oral fluids and correct dosing of NSAIDs are also essential parts of the educational plan. The patient should learn the need for professional intervention when the temperature escalates beyond 101.5°F (38.5°C). Fever elevations can mean the onset of an opportunistic infection, for which the clinician should be consulted immediately.

Immunizations have not been shown to "bring out SLE" and should not be avoided, except for live attenuated vaccines in immunocompromised hosts. Sulfonamide antibiotic therapy like Bactrim should be avoided, as these may bring out exacerbations or have adverse effects in people with SLE. Women should be encouraged to avoid pregnancy as there are high miscarriage rates due to thromboembolus, until the disease is at least 6 months in remission. In addition birth control pills might bring out the disease, although low-dose estrogen pills are less likely to. Steroids, NSAIDs, and hydroxychloroquine are usually used to treat pregnant women, while other immunosuppressants like methotrexate and cyclophosphamide are contraindicated.

Human Immunodeficiency Virus Infection

Infection by HIV results in eventual destruction of the immune system. HIV uses the CD4+ T cell receptor sites to enter and infect cells in the human body. In early HIV infection, the patient's CD4+ count (T4 cell count, T lymphocyte) remains above 500 cells/mL of blood. Over time, the immune system weakens, and the patient's CD4+ count begins to decline. When this occurs, the patient becomes susceptible to opportunistic infections.

Although there is no cure at this time for HIV infection, viral suppression of HIV to undetectable levels in the peripheral blood can be achieved by a combination of potent antiretroviral agents (ARV). With early detection and initiation of treatment, HIV infection can be managed as a chronic but controllable infectious disease.

Table 16.6 presents the Centers for Disease Control and Prevention (CDC) HIV classification system for adults and adolescents.

Table 16.6 CDC HIV Classification System for Adults and Adolescents

This system emphasizes the importance of CD4+ T lymphocyte testing in clinical management of HIV-infected persons. The system is based on three ranges of CD4+ T counts and three clinical categories, giving a matrix of nine exclusive categories.

Criteria for HIV Infection

Persons age 13 years or older with repeatedly (two or more) reactive screening tests (ELISA and specific antibodies identified by a supplemental test such as the Western blot). Other specific methods of diagnosis of HIV-1 include virus isolation, antigen detection, and detection of HIV genetic material by polymerase chain reaction (PCR) or branch DNA (bDNA) assay.

AIDS-Defining Condition

The term AIDS-defining condition refers to any of a list of illnesses that, when occurring in an HIV-infected person, leads to a diagnosis of AIDS, the most serious stage of HIV infection. AIDS is also diagnosed if an HIV-infected person has a CD4+ T count below 200 cells/mm^3, whether or not that person has an AIDS-defining condition. Twenty-six conditions were identified and classified as AIDS-defining conditions in 1993 by the Centers for Disease Control and Prevention (CDC).

Clinical Category	CD4+ Cell Count*	Clinical Manifestations
A1	≥500/mm^3	Category A consists of one or more of the conditions listed below in a person with documented HIV infection. Conditions listed in Categories B and C must not have occurred. • Asymptomatic HIV infection • Persistent generalized lymphadenopathy (noted in two or more extrainguinal sites, at least 1 cm in diameter for ≥3 months) • Acute (primary) HIV infection with accompanying illness or history of acute HIV infection
A2	200-499/mm^3	See A1
A3	<200/mm^3	See A1
B1	≥500/mm^3	Symptomatic HIV infection (but not A or C conditions) Examples include but not limited to: • Bacillary angiomatosis • Candidiasis, vulvovaginal: persistent >1 month, poorly responsive to treatment • Candidiasis, oropharyngeal • Cervical dysplasia, severe, or carcinoma in situ • Constitutional symptoms such as fever or diarrhea >1 month (The above must be attributed to HIV infection or have a clinical course or management complicated by HIV)
B2	200-499/mm^3	See B1
B3	<200/mm^3	See B1
C1	≥500/mm^3	Category C includes the clinical conditions listed below; for classification purposes, once a Category C condition has occurred, the person will remain classified as category C: • Candidiasis: esophageal, tracheal, bronchi • Coccidioidomycosis, extrapulmonary • Cryptococcosis, extrapulmonary • Cervical cancer, invasive • Cryptosporidiosis, chronic intestinal (>1 month) • CMV retinitis or CMV in other than liver, spleen, nodes • HIV encephalopathy • Herpes simplex with mucocutaneous ulcer >1 month, bronchitis, pneumonia • Histoplasmosis: disseminated, extrapulmonary • Isosporiasis, chronic >1 month • Kaposi's sarcoma • Lymphoma: Burkitt's immunoblastic, primary in brain • *M. avium* or *M. kansaii,* extrapulmonary • *M. tuberculosis,* pulmonary or extrapulmonary • *Pneumocystis jiroveci* pneumonia (PCP) • Pneumonia, recurrent (≥ 2 episodes in 1 year) • Progressive multifocal leukoencephalopathy • *Salmonella* bacteremia, recurrent • *Toxoplasma gondii* • Wasting syndrome due to HIV
C2	200-499/mm^3	See C1
C3	<200/mm^3	See C1

Source: Public Health Service Revised Classification System for HIV Infection (Adolescents and Adults) 1993 Revised. In C. Kirton (ed), ANAC's Core Curriculum for HIV/AIDS Nursing, 2nd ed. SAGE, Thousand Oaks, Calif., pp. 351–353.

*There is diurnal variation in CD4+counts, averaging slightly higher in the afternoon, in HIV-positive persons. Blood for sequential CD4+counts should be drawn at about the same time each day.

Epidemiology and Causes

HIV was originally identified in homosexual men in the 1980s, but the virus now affects men and women of all races, ethnicities, and sexual orientation, as well as infants, children and adolescents. An estimated 40 million people globally are infected with HIV, and more than 4 million people were estimated to become newly infected with HIV in 2005. HIV has impacted all regions of the world. According to the Joint United Nations Programme on HIV/AIDS (UNAIDS), as of 2005, two-thirds of all people living with HIV are in sub-Saharan Africa, as are 77 percent of all women with HIV. The Caribbean is the second-most affected region in the world. Growing epidemics are also underway in Eastern Europe, Central and East Asia.

Epidemiologic changes have also occurred in the United States. In 1992, the majority of cases of HIV infection in the United States were among white, non-Hispanic individuals. The face of the epidemic has changed, and minorities and women in the United States have been disproportionately impacted. Reports from the Centers for Disease Control and Prevention (CDC) note that in 2003 blacks accounted for nearly half of all AIDS cases, more than any other racial/ethnic group. Almost two-thirds of all women reported with AIDS were black, and the AIDS case rate among black males was more than eight times greater than the rate for white males. Hispanics have also been affected, representing 20 percent of all reported AIDS cases. In 2003, 18 percent of all women reported with AIDS were Hispanic. These data may reflect differences in socioeconomic factors, such as income and education, rather than race or ethnic background.

The largest decline in reported cases has occurred among homosexual men. The greatest increase in HIV infection is now being seen in individuals with heterosexual contact. Of new concern is the increasing rate of HIV infection in persons older than the age of 50. Concerns are also raised about the incidence of HIV infection in adolescents. Prelimary 2003 data from CDC reveal that in the United States, HIV disease is the 10th leading cause of death among people between the ages of 15 and 24 for all races combined. The CDC estimates that at least 50 percent of HIV infections in the United States are acquired before age 25 and most are acquired sexually.

HIV-1 is the type of virus found in the United States. HIV-2 is relatively rare in the United States, except among immigrants from West Africa. HIV-2 is biologically similar to HIV-1 but shows reduced virulence, with a slower rate of CD4+ decline. Blood banks now routinely test for both HIV-1 and HIV-2. HIV-2 should be suspected in natives of Africa, persons who have traveled in Africa, or persons who have had sexual contact or shared needles with Africans.

Transmission

HIV is transmitted through the exchange of blood and body fluids, and cannot be transmitted by casual contact (handshakes, open-mouth kisses, and hugs). HIV is considered an STD, because CD4+ T cells (T lymphocytes) are abundant in semen and vaginal secretions. During vaginal or anal sex, friction can cause minute tears to these highly vascular mucous membranes. These minute tears can allow the entrance of the HIV-infected body fluids during ejaculation. The use of latex condoms can help prevent the exchange of secretions. Anyone who has had unprotected sex (without a condom) is considered potentially at risk for HIV infection. The risk of HIV transmission from a single episode of unprotected receptive vaginal intercourse with a known HIV-positive sexual partner is estimated to be between 0.08 and 0.2 percent, while the infection risk associated with a similar episode of receptive anal intercourse is 0.1 to 0.3 percent.

HIV can also be transmitted through the sharing of needles with an HIV-infected person; therefore, injection-drug users (IV-drug abusers) are a high-risk group for HIV infection. Needlestick injuries are the most common cause of occupational exposure to HIV. Treatment Standards/Guidelines 16.1 presents the postexposure prophylaxis guidelines for health-care workers, and The Patient's Voice 16.2 presents a health-care worker's viewpoint. The risk of HIV transmission from a single episode of needle-sharing during injection drug use with a known HIV-positive partner has been estimated at 0.67 percent, while the risk from an occupational needlestick from an HIV-positive patient is estimated at 0.4 percent.

Before blood banks began testing for HIV, people who had blood transfusions were at risk for HIV, as were hemophiliacs who might have been given contaminated blood products. Routine testing of all blood products for HIV-1 and HIV-2 has now virtually eliminated this route of transmission. However, given the potential of an HIV-positive individual to donate blood during the asymptomatic and undetectable window period prior to HIV-specific seroconversion, transmission rates as low as 1 in 1,000,000 to 1 in 2,000,000 are typically cited during informed consent procedures for transfused blood products.

HIV can be maternally transmitted from mother to newborn. The AIDS Clinical Trial Group 076, which used oral zidovudine (Retrovir; ZDV; AZT) during pregnancy, with IV AZT during labor and liquid AZT to the newborn, showed a dramatic decrease in HIV maternal transmission from 25 to 30 percent to as low as 8 percent. Current guidelines that employ elective Cesarean section to avoid birth canal exposure, thorough STD screening and treatment, as well as updated prenatal and perinatal antiretroviral regimens for both mother and child, have decreased this rate even further to less than 1 percent in some centers. However, HIV is present in breast milk, so breastfeeding by an HIV-infected woman is still considered a potential route of transmission.

HIV-infected women have poorer survival rates than men, but no difference has been found in the rate of disease progression. Some studies indicate, however, that sur-

Treatment Standards/Guidelines 16.1 **Postexposure Prophylaxis for Health-Care Workers (HCWs)**

Triage the exposure according to the type and severity of injury and the source patient

Type of Injury

Percutaneous

- Less severe: Superficial injury or solid-bore needle
- More severe: Large-bore hollow needle, deep puncture, visible blood on device, or needle used in patient's artery or vein

Mucous membrane exposures or nonintact skin exposure

- Follow-up needed for skin exposure only if compromised skin integrity (abrasions, dermatitis, open wound)
- Small volume: Few drops
- Large volume: Major blood splash

Source Patient: Five categories

- HIV-positive, class 1: asymptomatic HIV infection or known low viral load (less than 1500 copies/mL)
- HIV-positive, class 2: symptomatic HIV infection, AIDS diagnosis, acute seroconversion (time of high viral load) or known high viral load (greater than 1500 copies/mL)
- Unknown HIV status of source patient (i.e., source patient is deceased and no blood samples are available for HIV testing)
- Unknown source (i.e., needle in a sharps container; splash from inappropriately disposed blood)
- HIV-negative source

Determine Need for PEP (four options):

No PEP warranted:

- Percutaneous injury, Less severe: HIV-negative source; unknown HIV status of source or unknown source (also see Consider basic two-drug PEP)
- Mucous membrane/nonintact skin exposure, small volume: HIV-negative source; unknown HIV status of source or unknown source (also see Consider basic two-drug PEP)

Consider Basic Two-Drug PEP

- Percutaneous injury, Less severe and more severe: If source patient has unknown HIV status, consider basic two-drug PEP if source patient has/had HIV risk factors; if unknown source, consider basic two-drug PEP in settings in which exposure to HIV-infected persons is likely
- Mucous membrane/nonintact skin exposure, Small volume: If source is HIV-positive class 1, consider basic two-drug PEP
- Mucous membrane/nonintact skin exposure, Large volume: If source patient has unknown HIV status, consider basic two-drug PEP if source patient has/had HIV risk factors; if unknown source, consider basic two-drug PEP in settings in which exposure to HIV-infected persons is likely.

Recommend Basic Two-Drug PEP

- Percutaneous injury, Less severe: HIV-positive source, class 1
- Mucous membrane/nonintact skin exposure, Small volume: HIV-positive source, class 2
- Mucous membrane/nonintact skin exposure, Large volume: HIV-positive source, class 1

Recommend Expanded Three-or-More Drug PEP

- Percutaneous injury, Less severe: HIV-positive source, class 2
- Percutaneous injury, More severe: If source patient is HIV-positive, class 1 or class 2
- Mucous membrane/nonintact skin exposure, Large volume: HIV-positive source, class 2

Determine PEP Regimen

- Should be done in collaboration with client (assess lifestyle, dietary habits, medication history) to help promote adherence to the PEP regimen.
- Studies have revealed that HCWs may stop taking PEP because of side effects of HIV drugs.
- HIV drug resistance has been transmitted to HCWs; however, do not delay starting PEP while waiting for lab tests.
- Because of the complexity of selection of HIV PEP regimens, consultation with an experienced clinician is advisable; the Resources section of this chapter lists several resources available by telephone or through the Internet.

PEP Regimens

There are several preferred two-drug basic regimens plus alternate basic regimens, and there are several preferred expanded regimens and alternate expanded regimens. All regimens are for 30 days (4 weeks).

Basic Two-Drug Regimens

a. Zidovudine (Retrovir; AZT; ZDV) 600 mg daily with food (300 mg twice a day or 200 mg three times a day) PLUS lamivudine (Epivir; 3TC) 300 mg (300 mg once a day or 150 mg twice a day); Can be dosed as Combivir (combination drug of Retrovir 300 mg and Epivir 300 mg) taken as one tablet twice a day
b. Zidovudine (Retrovir; AZT; ZDV) 600 mg daily with food (300 mg twice a day or 200 mg three times a day) PLUS emtricitabine (Emtriva; FTC) 200 mg (one capsule once a day)
c. Tenofovir DF (Viread; TDF) 300 mg (one tablet once daily) PLUS lamivudine (Epivir; 3TC) 300 mg (300 mg once daily or 150 mg twice a day)

Alternate Basic Regimens

d. Lamivudine (Epivir; 3TC) 300 mg (300 mg once daily or 150 mg twice a day) PLUS stavudine (Zerit; d4T) 80 mg (40 mg twice a day; can use lower doses of 20–30 mg twice a day if toxicities occurs; use 30 mg twice a day if body weight is under 60 kg)
e. Emtricitabine (Emtriva; FTC) 200 mg (one capsule once a day) PLUS stavudine (Zerit; d4T) 80 mg (40 mg twice a day; can use lower doses of 20–30 mg twice a day if toxicities occurs; use 30 mg twice a day if body weight is less than 60 kg)
f. Lamivudine (Epivir; 3TC) 300 mg (300 mg once daily or 150 mg twice a day) PLUS didanosine (Videx; ddI) 400 mg (200 mg twice daily or 400 mg once daily) if weight more than 60 kg (if under 60 kg, Videx dose is 250 mg; can be taken as 250 mg once daily or 125 mg twice a day)
g. Emtricitabine (Emtriva; FTC) 200 mg (one capsule once a day) PLUS didanosine (Videx; ddI) 400 mg (200 mg twice daily or 400 mg once daily) if weight more than 60 kg (if under 60 kg, Videx dose is 250 mg; can be taken as 250 mg once daily or 125 mg twice a day)

Preferred Expanded Regimen

- Basic regimen PLUS lopinavir/ritonavir (Kaletra; LPV/RTV) 800/200 mg (3 capsules of Kaletra 133/33 mg twice a day)

Alternate Expanded Regimens

Basic Regimen PLUS ONE of the following:

- Atazanavir (Reyataz; ATV) with or without ritonavir (Norvir; RTV): ATV 400 mg once daily unless used in combination with tenofovir (Viread); dosage when also

(continued)

Treatment Standards/Guidelines 16.1 Postexposure Prophylaxis for Health-Care Workers (HCWs) (continued)

taking Viread is ATV 300 mg once daily plus Ritonavir (Norvir) 100 mg once daily

- Fosamprenavir (Lexiva; FOSAPV) with or without ritonavir (Norvir; RTV): Lexiva 1400 mg twice daily (two 700-mg tablets taken twice a day); or FOSAVP 1400 mg daily and RTV 200 mg once daily; or FOSAPV 700 mg twice daily with RTV 100 mg twice daily
- Indinavir (Crixivan; IDV) with or without ritonavir (Norvir; RTV): Crixivan 800 mg every 8 hours on an empty stomach; or IDV 800 mg and RTV 100 mg twice daily without regard to food
- Saquinavir (Invirase; SQV) with ritonavir (Norvir; RTV): SQV 1000 mg (comes as 200-mg capsules; take five capsules) with RTV 100 mg (comes as 100-mg capsule) twice daily (daily total of 12 pills, 10 SQV capsules and 2 RTV capsules)
- Nelfinavir (Viracept; NFV) 1250 mg twice daily with a meal (two of the 625-mg tablets or 5 of the 250-mg tablets; daily total of either four of the 625-mg tablets or 10 of the 250-mg tablets)
- Efavirenz (Sustiva; EFV) 600 mg daily, taken at bedtime (one 600-mg tablet at HS)

Begin Postexposure Prophylaxis (PEP)

After occupational exposure:

1. Begin PEP promptly, as soon as possible, preferably within hours rather than days after the exposure.
2. All HCWs with occupational exposure to HIV will need follow-up, even if they do not start PEP. Provide follow-up counseling and medical evaluation, including HIV-antibody tests at baseline and periodically for at least 6 months postexposure (e.g., 6 weeks, 12 weeks, and 6 months), and observe precautions to prevent possible secondary transmission of the virus. Extended follow-up is recommended for HCWs who become infected with Hepatitis C after exposure to a source co-infected with HIV and HCV.
3. Perform drug-toxicity monitoring, including a complete blood count and renal and hepatic function tests, at baseline and 2 weeks after starting PEP. If toxicity is noted, dose reduction or drug substitution should be considered with expert consultation, and further diagnostic studies may be indicated.
4. Provide appropriate medical care for HCWs who become infected with HIV.
5. An occupational exposure is an emotionally charged event for most HCWs, and can have a severe psychological impact. Psychological support is needed to help deal with the stress of awaiting HIV test results, and to assist with coping with side effects of PEP.

vival is not necessarily related to sex or race; rather, it is related to unequal socioeconomic status and thus unequal access to care and appropriate drug therapy.

In response to the changing HIV epidemic, in 2003 the CDC proposed new strategies for advancing HIV prevention: (1) Make voluntary HIV testing a routine part of medical care. (2) Implement new models for diagnosing HIV infections outside medical settings. (3) Prevent new infections by working with persons diagnosed with HIV and their partners. (4) Further decrease perinatal HIV transmission.

THE PATIENT'S VOICE 16.2

HIV Infection

I am furious! I've been a nurse for 20 years and have always been proud of my skills and techniques. I have been stuck by needles, but only a few times during my career...usually when a patient suddenly moved, not through negligence on my part. I thought nothing of it, until last month when I went to my doctor because I was feeling so tired and run down. He asked if I had been tested for HIV and I said no. Just to appease him, I had the test done and it was positive.

The only thing I can relate it to is a needle stick that occurred when I was working in Home Health. I didn't even think anything of it, and didn't even fill out an incident report. I don't know what I'll do if the next test is positive. I'll have no recourse since I can't prove it was contracted "on-the-job." Now, I hear about the needle-less syringes, and if I had them then, I probably wouldn't be in the situation I am! I am angry! What do I do now?

Pathophysiology

Human immunodeficiency virus (HIV) is a member of the Lentivirinae subfamily of "slow" retroviruses, known for their prolonged latent infectious period, persistent viremia, species-specific infectivity, tropism for cells of the immune and nervous systems, and subsequent destruction of host immune defenses including the triggering of autoimmune responses. Evolutionarily conserved members of this family include simian immunodeficiency virus (SIV) and feline immunodeficiency virus (FIV).

HIV was identified as the causative agent of AIDS in 1984. As the predominant strain worldwide, HIV-1 has been genetically divided into subclasses known as clades, designated A through O. In the United States, more than 98 percent of HIV infections are due to HIV-1 clade B. HIV-2, found predominantly in West African nations, Angola, Mozambique, France, and Portugal, results in slower disease progression and appears less readily transmissible.

Studies utilizing quantitative assays of plasma HIV RNA have provided new insights into the pathogenesis of HIV infection. Molecular genetic studies have resulted in a better understanding of the viral genome and its complex replication process, which has led to multiple drug therapy that attempts to suppress viral replication at different stages. The HIV genome consists of several regulatory genes (*nef*, *rev*, *tat*, *vif*, *vpu*, and *vpr*) and three structural genes called *gag* (which encodes several core capsid proteins), *pol* (which encodes reverse transcriptase and integrase), and *env* (which encodes several outer viral envelope surface proteins involved in binding of the virion to target host cells).

These gene products result in an HIV virion consisting of a nucleoprotein core with two copies of single-stranded genomic RNA and several key proteins, including p6 and p7 (nucleocapsid proteins bound directly to genomic RNA), p24 (a capsid protein forming a shell around the genomic core), and p17 (a matrix protein that lines the inner surface of the lipid bilayer, providing structural integrity). Also included in the core are several enzymes involved in viral replication including reverse transcriptase, integrase, and protease. This nucleoprotein core is surrounded by an outer lipid bilayer studded along its surface by two major glycoproteins named for their molecular mass in kilodaltons, gp120 and gp41.

The sequence of events in HIV infection begins with the transfer of the virus from one host to another. Once the virus is transmitted across the mucocutaneous barrier and into the blood stream, HIV attaches to cells at the CD4+ receptor site via gp120. CD4+ receptors are found on many cells of the body, including cells of the CNS, GI tract, and immune system (e.g., CD4+ T cells, monocyte-derived macrophages, and tissue dendritic cells). At the onset of HIV infection, the average number of CD4+ T cells is about 1000 (normal range: 500 to 1500) per mm^3 of blood.

Although CD4+ T cells were first identified as the primary target of HIV infection, it is now known that tissue dendritic cells called Langerhans cells found within the genital mucosal epithelium are believed to be the earliest targets of HIV infection, given their proximity to the initial site of HIV exposure. After infection, dendritic cells fuse with CD4+ T cells and subsequently migrate to draining lymph nodes via regional lymphatic channels. Within these lymph nodes, HIV further infects follicular dendritic cells capable of presenting virus to additional circulating hematopoietic cells. Thus, the lymph nodes are a major site of viral replication and a focus of HIV infectivity.

After attaching to the target host cell, HIV enters the cell by fusion at the plasma membrane. This is a sequential process, which first involves a conformational change in HIV after gp120 binding to CD4 that allows the virion to interact with chemokine receptors on the host cell surface. This initiates another conformational change, which exposes the gp41 viral envelope protein and brings the virion into even closer proximity to the plasma membrane.

Thus, in addition to interactions with gp41, viral adhesion requires the aid of secondary co-receptors, most notably the chemokine receptors CXCR4 (also known as fusin) which binds T cell-tropic HIV strains called X4 viruses and CCR5 which binds macrophage-tropic strains or R5 viruses. Tissue dendritic cells express CCR5 and less commonly CXCR4. In turn, R5 viruses are more common early on in HIV infection, while X4 viruses predominate in the later stages of symptomatic infection. Studies of people who have had multiple exposures to HIV yet remain uninfected have shown that these people have defects or polymorphisms in these coreceptors, which may answer the question of why they have not become infected. In turn, investigational studies are addressing each step in the viral fusion process as a potential target for pharmacologic intervention, as exemplified by the recently approved gp41 fusion inhibitor T-20 (Fuzeon).

Once HIV enters the healthy CD4+ T cell, the cell becomes infected, and HIV begins its replication activities, by converting its own genetic material (RNA) into complementary DNA strands, using the RNA-dependent DNA polymerase enzyme reverse transcriptase (RT). Viral DNA then becomes double stranded and is incorporated into the host cell genome by viral integrase, while the RNA template is digested by viral RNase. This new DNA acts as a blueprint for replication, directing the infected host cell to make new virus particles.

Since mammalian cells do not express reverse transcriptase, this enzyme serves as a viral-specific therapeutic target for the nucleoside (and nucleotide) RT inhibitors (NRTIs) as well as the non-nucleoside RT inhibitors (NNRTIs). These agents either interfere with the DNA template-primer activity of RT or serve as competitive chain terminators of elongating viral DNA strands. Studies are also underway to develop integrase-specific antiretroviral agents.

Importantly, RT lacks the histone repair enzymes characteristic of mammalian DNA polymerases. This results in a high rate of uncorrected mutation during each cycle of viral DNA replication. Unfortunately, this results in the rapid development of resistance by HIV to most antiretroviral agents, particularly if used suboptimally as monotherapy or, alternatively, as combination therapy with a high degree of patient noncompliance.

In addition to genomic replication, a large portion of viral DNA is transcribed and subsequently translated into a large polyprotein, which must then be activated. The HIV protease enzyme, acting like "chemical scissors," catalyzes the cleavage of polyproteins into mature structural proteins and enzymes. This process results in formation of a large number of infectious viral particles, which bud from the host cell and seek out new cells to infect. Given its effect on such a large number of viral proteins, HIV-specific protease serves as a critical target for one of the most potent classes of antiretroviral agents—the protease inhibitors. Table 19.4 reviews the steps of viral replication of HIV.

Once HIV enters the body, a series of stages occur in the infectious process:

- ▲ The acute retroviral stage or syndrome (or primary infection period)
- ▲ The asymptomatic stage (including a "window" period prior to seroconversion)

▲ The symptomatic stage (or HIV infection, which may result in opportunistic infections and acquired immunodeficiency syndrome [AIDS])

The initial period of infection, or acute retroviral syndrome, resembles infectious mononucleosis and is accompanied by high HIV viremia, often in excess of 1 million viral copies/mL. Primary HIV infection refers to the 4- to 7-week period of rapid viral replication immediately following exposure and infection by the virus. About 30 to 60 percent of individuals with primary infection develop an acute syndrome characterized by fever, malaise, lymphadenopathy, pharyngitis, headache, myalgia, and sometimes rash. Importantly, common cold symptoms including rhinorrhea and congestion are typically absent during acute retroviral syndrome.

There is spontaneous recovery from these flulike symptoms in 1 to 3 weeks. Within days after the initial infection, however, there is extension to the regional lymph tissue, presumably by dendritic cells. This is followed by massive viremia with extensive involvement of lymph tissue. Within a few weeks, there is an immune response, ascribed to the complex interplay of HIV-specific cytotoxic T cell responses, a plasma and B-cell–mediated humoral antibody response, and cytokine proliferation. Seroconversion (the development of antibodies to HIV in the blood) usually occurs 1 to 3 months after viral transmission. Once seroconversion has occurred, the ELISA test used to diagnose HIV will be positive in infected individuals. However, there is a "window period" between transmission and seroconversion. Although the infected person will have a negative antibody blood test during this asymptomatic period, the patient is already infectious to others.

HIV infection is a dynamic process characterized by a high rate of viral replication. Complete viral latency, a "quiet time" for the virus, does not exist. Initially, in individuals with acute HIV infection, the viral load is extremely elevated (10^5 to 10^7 copies/mL). Once the host immune response begins, plasma HIV RNA levels decline rapidly. Without treatment, this level fluctuates for the initial 6 months of infection until a set point is reached. "Set point" refers to a steady state of the plasma HIV RNA level that persists for years before it starts to increase progressively. At that time patients begin to deteriorate clinically. Thus, the magnitude of the viral set point predicts the rapidity of disease progression, and chronic therapy is designed to drive this set point down as far as possible.

The half-life of a free HIV virion is less than 1 hour, while the half-life of an acutely infected T cell is approximately 1 day. In HIV infection, an estimated 1 to 10 billion viral particles are produced and cleared each day. Research data suggest that billions of CD4+ T cells may be destroyed every day, eventually overwhelming the immune system's capacity to regenerate. This rapid turnover of virus and CD4+ T lymphocytes is now thought to occur throughout the course of HIV infection. An additional pool of longer-lived macrophages and follicular dendritic cells infected with HIV may persist for up to several weeks. However, it is a smaller, long-lived pool of memory lymphocytes, which numbers approximately 1 million, that may persist for several years in a latent infected stage. Avoiding the antiretroviral activity of current pharmacotherapies, these cells may enter an active lytic stage of viral replication up to several decades later, repopulating the immune system with rapid viral proliferation.

Over a period of time, the replication activities of the virus eventually supersede CD4+ T cell activity. In some patients, the rate of CD4+ T cell loss is extreme, with counts below 200 cells/mm^3 within 2 years, whereas other patients—called long-term nonprogressors—still have CD4+ T cell counts of above 500 cells/mm^3 up to 10 years after infection. Research data suggest that billions of CD4+ T cells may be destroyed every day, eventually overwhelming the immune system's capacity to regenerate.

From the start of infection, there is persistent HIV replication, with plasma viremia and CD4+ T cell depletion. Over time, the immune system appears to "burn out," accompanied by the eventual loss of functioning T cells, as new T-cell production can no longer balance T-cell destruction. This loss of T-cell inducer function also results in dysregulated B-cell activity. After a period of years, if left untreated, HIV results in massive destruction of the immune system, creating susceptibility to opportunistic pathogens and tumors. Once the patient's CD4+ T cellcount drops below 200 cells/mm^3, or the patient develops an opportunistic infection or certain other disease states, the patient becomes symptomatic and moves from being considered HIV positive into the advanced stage—AIDS.

Through the use of blood tests to determine viral activity (often called viral load), it has been shown that the level of plasma HIV RNA is proportional to the rate of viral replication and the rate of CD4+ T cell destruction. Viral load is one of the most useful tests in predicting the risk of progression to AIDS. Because the natural history of HIV infection varies from one patient to another, the plasma HIV viral load can help predict the rapidity with which clinical immunodeficiency will develop. Fortunately, with the initiation of appropriate antiretroviral therapy, the immune system appears to retain the capacity for cellular recovery even in the later stages of HIV infection. Thus, a trend has emerged away from the rapid initiation of antiretroviral therapy at the time of diagnosis in favor of more conservative treatment approaches, which seek to minimize the resistance of HIV to pharmacotherapies.

Clinical Presentation

Subjective

The patient may present with any of the following clinical presentations: flulike symptoms (typically seen in the acute stage of early HIV infection); darkish colored spots on the skin (indicative of Kaposi's sarcoma); nonproductive cough, shortness of breath, and fever that has been present for several days or weeks, suggesting *Pneumocystis carinii* pneumonia (PCP, a fungal infection also known as *Pneumocystis jiroveci*), *Mycobacterium tuberculosis*, or a bacterial pneumonia, seen in the patient who is HIV positive and has a CD4+ T cell count below 200/mL; and constitutional symptoms such as weight loss, night sweats, chronic fever, and/or chronic diarrhea (usually seen in the patient with advanced HIV infection, or AIDS, or who has a CD4+ T cell count below 200/mL).

In acute HIV infection, more than 8 percent of patients have symptoms that include fever (90 percent), sore throat (70 percent), myalgia (60 percent), headaches (60 percent), cervical lymphadenopathy (50 percent), and night sweats (50 percent).

A careful history should be done to determine the patient's risk of HIV infection, as certain behaviors place a patient at higher risk of exposure to HIV than others. Focusing the History 16.1 lists questions the clinician should ask.

Objective

The most common clinical presentations of HIV infection include:

▲ Persistent generalized lymphadenopathy. This is a relatively common feature early in HIV infection when the patient is asymptomatic. During the assessment, the clinician must be alert for enlarged lymph nodes involving two noncontiguous sites other than inguinal nodes. The clinician should measure and record the size if the nodes are palpable and record as negative if not palpable.

▲ Pulmonary symptoms. These are seen with *Pneumocystis carinii* pneumonia, tuberculosis, and bacterial pneumonia. The clinician should be alert for decreased breath sounds and patient's report of shortness of breath, nonproductive cough, fever, and night sweats.

▲ Localized *Candida* infections. Thrush is a common finding in HIV infection. The presence of thrush indicates advanced immunosuppression, with a high probability of a serious or opportunistic infection within 3 years. The clinician should carefully assess the oral cavity, using a high-quality flashlight. Look for the presence of white plaque (thrush), darkish lesions (possibly Kaposi's sarcoma) and a whitish, hair-like growth on the tongue (hairy leukoplakia, seen in advanced immunocompromised states). If white plaque is found, attempt to lightly scrape with a tongue blade. If thrush is present, the plaque will bleed as it is scraped off. *Candida* esophagitis is a late complication of HIV infection; the usual presentation is thrush with odynophagia. *Candida* vaginitis in women with HIV infection is more likely to be recurring or refractory to therapy.

▲ Kaposi's sarcoma. These lesions will appear as nodules or papules—purple in light-skinned patients and dark brown to black in dark-skinned patients. The lesions can be found in any part of the skin or mucous membrane. The clinician should perform a thorough dermatological exam of the back, buttocks, extremities, hands, and feet.

▲ Sexually transmitted diseases. STDs increase the likelihood of HIV transmission or acquisition. The clinician should do a thorough exam of the rectal and genital area.

FOCUS ON HISTORY 16.1

Evaluating Risk of HIV Infection

Sexual History and Sexually Transmitted Diseases

- Describe your sexual relationships.
- Describe your sexual orientation.
- Describe your sexual practices. Have you ever had anal sex?
- Have you ever had a sexually transmitted disease (STD)?
- Have you ever had vaginal discharge or problem (for women)? Penile discharge or problem (for men)?
- Have any of your sexual partners been tested for a STD?
- Do you practice safe sex?
- What form of birth control do you use?
- Have any of your sexual partners been informed that they were HIV positive or had AIDS?
- Would you expect any of your sexual partners to have been exposed to a STD or HIV?

Substance Abuse

- Have you ever self-injected drugs (legal or illegal [street])?
- Have you ever shared needles?
- Have you ever used (in any form) illegal or street drugs?
- Do you drink alcohol? If so, how much?

Transfusion History

- Did you receive any blood or blood products between 1977 and 1985?
- Are you or your partner a hemophiliac?
- Have you received any donor sperm during artificial insemination?

Infection History

- Have you or a sexual partner ever had any form of hepatitis?
- Have you or anyone close to you been diagnosed with tuberculosis (TB)? If so, what is (or was) the treatment?
- Have you ever had a positive test for TB?
- Have you ever taken medications for TB?

Occupational History

- Do you work in the health-care field? In a long-term residential facility? In a jail or prison?
- Are you exposed to blood or other body fluids while on the job?
- Have you ever had a needlestick injury?

Inspect for perianal and genital herpes simplex lesions and check for penile or vaginal discharges.

- ▲ Neurologic and optic symptoms. Headache is a common complaint during the acute retroviral stage. The clinician should conduct a careful funduscopic exam to check for CMV infection.
- ▲ Weight loss. The clinician should document height and weight at the time of the exam and record the patient's description of weight loss (amount lost over what period of time).
- ▲ Cytopenia. Anemia, leukopenia, and/or thrombocytopenia often complicate HIV infection. The clinician needs to check the CBC.

Diagnostic Reasoning

Diagnostic Tests

A diagnosis of HIV infection is based on the presence of antibodies to HIV-1 in the blood. The patient must receive informed consent before HIV testing is done. Some states require that the patient also be informed of his or her right to anonymous testing versus confidential testing. In anonymous testing, the patient is issued a number, and results are given for this number. No names are used, and the results cannot be tracked to a name. Anonymous test results are not reportable to health departments. In confidential testing, the patient's name is used. If the test result is positive, the patient's name and positive HIV status may be reported to the health department, as is done with other sexually transmitted and communicable diseases. Primary care providers should be aware of federal, state, and local HIV reporting requirements, educate the patient about them, and ensure that the patient is aware of the extent and the limits of HIV test result confidentiality.

The preferred method for diagnosis of acute HIV infection is an HIV RNA viral load, since HIV DNA and RNA can be detected 2 to 3 days earlier than p24 (as with a Western blot assay). The ELISA test is useless during this window period prior to seroconversion.

Some state, federal, and managed care companies do not do a viral load until after a diagnosis is made because of the expense. A viral load test costs approximately 15 to 20 times more than an ELISA. For this reason, some clinicians use an ELISA to screen for HIV antibodies.

If the ELISA test is positive, a second, more sophisticated test, the Western blot, is done on the same sample of blood. The Western blot test involves separation of individual viral proteins into defined bands. The presence of any two of the p-24, gp41, or gp 120/160 bands, designates a positive Western blot and serves as the confirmatory test for diagnosing HIV infection. In many states, positive Western blot test results must be reported to the health department. Studies have shown that the frequency of false-negative results in a high prevalence population is about 0.3 percent. The usual cause of false-negative tests is testing during the "window period" (the time between transmission and seroconversion), which is usually no more than 3 months.

OraQuick Advance is the first rapid HIV test for use with oral fluids. The OraQuick Advance HIV 1/2 Antibody Test can be used with oral fluids or plasma specimens. After 20 minutes, the test device indicates if HIV antibodies are present in the solution by displaying two reddish-purple lines in a small window in the device. A reactive HIV test result on oral fluid is a preliminary positive and must be confirmed by a Western blot test. Several other rapid HIV tests for use with serum or plasma have also been approved (such as Uni-Gold Recombigen, Reveal G2, and MultiSpot).

A T-cell subset blood test is done to determine the patient's CD4+ T cell count. A viral load, which is a quantitative assay of HIV RNA in the blood, is also drawn to determine the viral activity. These two tests are looked at together to determine the stage of illness and as a predictor of disease progression. As mentioned earlier, this viral load test is the preferable method of diagnosing acute HIV infection.

A discussion of test results, including HIV status results, is also the beginning of dialogue between the clinician and the HIV-infected client on the need for HIV prevention behaviors, to decrease the possibility of the HIV-infected client transmitting HIV to other persons. Although the plasma viral load (HIV RNA) may be undetectable, the clinician should remember that this test only reflects the level of cell-free virus in the peripheral blood. It is possible that latently infected cells might transmit infection in the absence of viremia.

Additional baseline laboratory work should include a CBC with differential (check for cytopenia), chemistry profile, transaminase levels, BUN and creatinine, urinalysis, Venereal Disease Research Laboratory (VDRL) or rapid plasma reagin (RPR) (tests for syphilis); serum toxoplasmosis plasma IgG titer; hepatitis A, B and C serologies; and a PAP smear for female clients. A tuberculin skin test (TST; PPD) should be done, unless the patient has a history of tuberculosis or positive skin test. Other tests for sexually transmitted diseases should be done as needed as determined from the clinical presentation.

If the patient presents with pulmonary symptoms, the clinician should check the oxygen saturation level and order a chest x-ray exam and arterial blood gas analysis. Hypoxemia and bilateral pulmonary infiltrates on the x-ray film indicate a pulmonary process but cannot differentiate between *Pneumocystis carinii* pneumonia (PCP) and tuberculosis in the HIV-infected patient. The clinician should perform a Mantoux purified protein derivative (PPD) skin test on one arm, and place two anergy controls on the other arm. Although some physicians do not feel anergy testing is necessary, it enables the clinician to disregard a negative PPD as diagnostic for ruling out TB. The patient's vital signs should be checked for fever and tachycardia.

Differential Diagnosis

Immunosuppression can be noted in a variety of situations besides HIV infection, such as the patient on chemotherapy or radiation therapy, or the patient on long-term steroid therapy. Certain cancers can also cause a decrease in the CD4+ T cell count. Differential diagnosis for acute retroviral syndrome includes EBV mononucleosis, CMV mononucleosis, toxoplasmosis, rubella, viral hepatitis, syphilis, primary herpes simplex virus, or drug reactions. Cytopenia and lymphopenia may be due to a primary or infiltrative bone marrow disorder and may require bone marrow biopsy if the HIV test is negative.

Management

Principles of management for early HIV infection include (1) initial disclosure of the HIV status, (2) initiation of drug therapy to suppress the virus, and (3) monitoring of viral activity to determine need to modify or revise drug therapy.

Key components of HIV infection management include prevention of transmission, preserving immune function, prophylaxis against opportunistic infection if the CD4+ T cell level falls, early diagnosis and treatment of opportunistic infection, and optimizing the quality of life. Figure 16.1 presents an algorithm of the management of early HIV infection.

Initial Disclosure

With the advent of rapid HIV testing, and the CDC's emphasis on integrating HIV prevention into medical care, disclosure of HIV results may soon be immediately done by the clinician during the client's office or clinic visit. The disclosure of HIV test results is a critical event in the clinician–patient relationship. Disclosure counseling sets the tone and foundation for the patient's acceptance, knowledge base, and attitudes about his or her HIV infection. Disclosure of HIV test results can be a stressful period for the patient, and the patient may deny a positive test result. Even with a confirmatory Western blot test, some agencies offer to repeat the test to ensure that the diagnosis is correct and help the patient accept the reality of the diagnosis in a timely fashion. Some guidelines and concepts for disclosure counseling are summarized here.

1. Disclosure counseling should be done face to face. In planning the disclosure of the patient's HIV status, the clinician should assess the degree to which the patient or parent or guardian is prepared to receive the results. The clinician should also assess the patient's social, demographic, cultural, and psychological characteristics, which may relate to coping with a positive HIV antibody test. During the disclosure session the provider should discuss the natural history of HIV infection, the potential effects of HIV infection on physical and mental health, the role of health maintenance, the availability of treatment, and the need to attain/maintain HIV prevention behaviors.
2. The disclosure counseling process is an opportunity to provide immediate interventions and to involve the patient in ongoing medical, mental health, social and family support networks. Some immediate interventions should include: assessing the patient for the risk of inflicting violence to themselves or others; ensuring that the patient will receive a thorough evaluation, staging, and initial care; informing the patient of ongoing availability of services; scheduling the next appointment; addressing prevention of further HIV transmission; assessing the availability of an immediate support person and other care providers; providing available local and national sources of information; and making appropriate referrals for any ongoing services that cannot be provided on site.
3. The patient should be informed of the potential for discriminatory practices against persons with HIV. Clinicians should assist patients in understanding the advantages and disadvantages of disclosing their HIV status to others by providing counseling, including factual information, opportunities for patient education and dialogue, and referrals as needed.
4. The patient should be strongly advised and encouraged to disclose their HIV status to significant others, particularly sexual and needle-sharing partners. Some local and state health departments will do partner notification without disclosing the name of the HIV-positive person, to provide the partner with the knowledge that he or she has been exposed to a sexually transmitted disease and that HIV testing is advised.

The prevention of HIV transmission must be discussed at the time of initial diagnosis of HIV infection. The patient's blood and semen become infectious to others shortly after the patient is initially infected, so risky sexual behaviors need to be addressed. The patient should also be advised against donating blood, plasma, tissue, body organs, and sperm.

The patient must also understand that the virus mutates or changes within each person; therefore, the HIV-infected person is at risk of acquiring a slightly different HIV virus from other people. The existence in the patient of a secondary virus can cause problems with medication therapy, can increase the likelihood of complications, and hasten the progression of the disease for the patient.

Initiation of Drug Therapy

Although HIV infection in the 1980s was associated with death, it is crucial to emphasize to the patient that improved and simplified drug therapies have prolonged survival and improved quality of life for many persons who are infected with the virus. The importance of beginning appropriate drug therapy and the need for continual follow-up with a health-care provider must be stressed.

Concepts of Medication Therapy. Concepts that underlie the foundation of antiretroviral (ARV) medication treatment for HIV infection include the following:

- ▲ Eradication of HIV infection cannot be achieved with current HIV drug therapy.

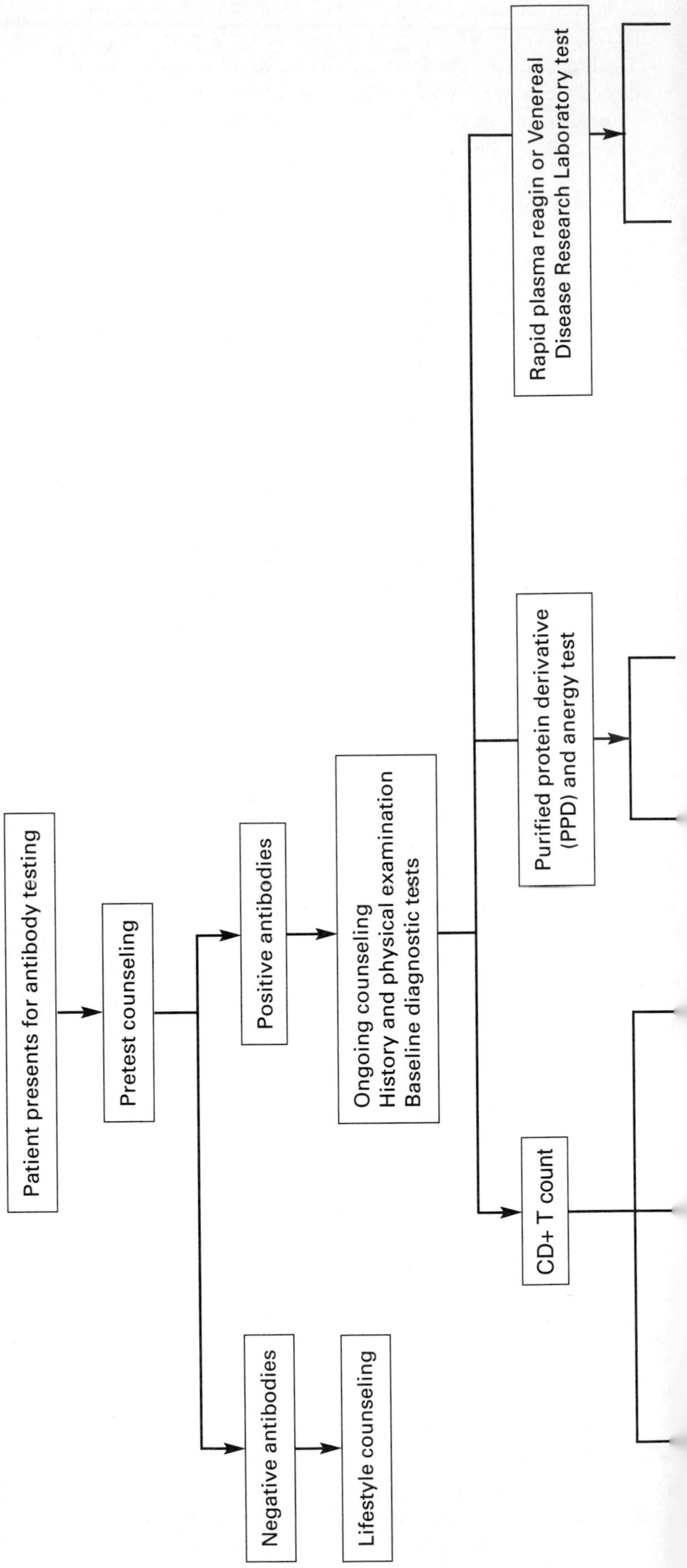

Patient presents for antibody testing

Pretest counseling

Negative antibodies

Lifestyle counseling

Positive antibodies

Ongoing counseling
History and physical examination
Baseline diagnostic tests

CD+ T count

Purified protein derivative (PPD) and anergy test

Rapid plasma reagin or Venereal Disease Research Laboratory test

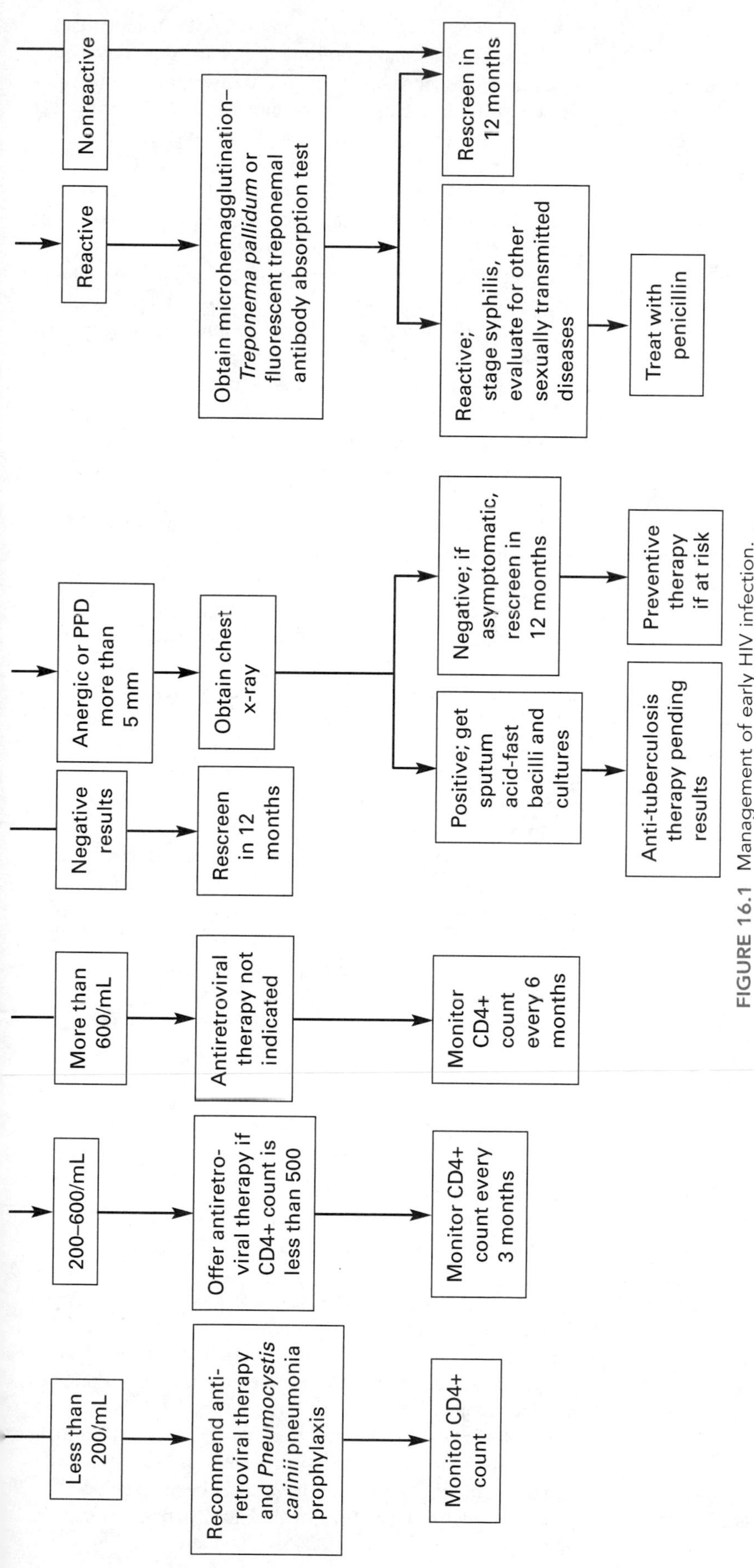

FIGURE 16.1 Management of early HIV infection.

- Complete viral latency does not exist. Viral activity is constant throughout the course of the infection.
- The level of plasma HIV RNA is proportional to the rate of viral replication and the rate of CD4+ T lymphocyte destruction. The plasma HIV RNA level can help predict the rapidity with which clinical immunodeficiency will develop.
- Treatment-induced changes in HIV RNA levels (and, to a lesser extent, changes in CD4+ T lymphocyte counts) correlate with clinical outcome. Studies have demonstrated that greater reductions in viral load are associated with greater improvements in clinical outcomes. These two markers have been shown to strongly predict the likelihood of disease progression, including death.
- Viral replication leads to the generation of viral mutants. Some of these mutants will be resistant to one or more antiretroviral drugs; therefore, the greater the immediate suppression of the virus, the fewer drug-resistant mutants will be available. Incomplete inhibition of viral replication leads to the emergence of drug-resistant populations and to resumption of disease progression. Emergence of drug resistance can be delayed by the maximum suppression of viral replication.
- Complete immune reconstitution, particularly for those who have advanced HIV disease, may not be possible. Regeneration and increases in CD4+ T cell counts have been seen within patients receiving antiretroviral therapy; however, the loss of CD4+ T lymphocyte clones as the disease progresses may not be entirely reversible. Early intervention with antiretroviral therapy is a strategy to preserve immune function.
- There are both benefits and risks to deferring HIV drug therapy.
- Some benefits of deferring therapy include avoiding treatment-related effects that may negatively impact quality of life; avoiding drug-related toxicities; preserving future treatment options; delaying the development of drug resistance related to incomplete viral suppression; and gaining time for the client to understand the demands of drug treatment.
- Some risks of deferring therapy include potential irreversible damage to the immune system; potential progression to AIDS; and the potential for increased risk of transmission of untreated virus to others.
- Although HIV drug therapy has dramatically improved survival time, the long-term impact of drug therapy has not been established. Patients on drug therapy have experienced a wide variety of side effects, including increased cholesterol levels, hyperglycemia, metabolic acidosis, lipodystrophy, and facial wasting. Close and continual clinical monitoring of patients on HIV drug therapy is essential.

Drug Categories. There are four major drug categories for antiviral therapy: nucleoside analogue reverse transcriptase inhibitors (NRTIs), non-nucleoside reverse transcriptase inhibitors (NNRTIs), protease inhibitors (PIs), and fusion inhibitors. Some clinicians further divide the drugs by using the category of nucleotide reverse transcriptase inhibitors (NtRTIs) to describe the unique characteristics of the NRTI drug tenofovir (Viread, TDF). Combination drug therapy is referred to as highly active antiretroviral therapy (HAART).

NRTIs were the first effective class of antiretroviral drugs. The nucleoside analogues work by incorporating themselves into the DNA of the virus, thereby stopping the building process. Because the resulting DNA is incomplete, it cannot create a new virus. Drugs in this category include zidovudine (Retrovir; ZDV; AZT), lamivudine (Epivir; 3TC), didanosine (Videx; ddI), ddI-EC (Videx EC), zalcitabine (Hivid; ddC), stavudine (Zerit; d4T), Combivir (combination drug containing Retrovir and Epivir), abacavir (Ziagen; ABC), Epzicom (combination drug containing Ziagen and Epivir), Trizivir (combination drug containing Ziagen, Epivir, and Retrovir), emtricitabine (Emtriva; FTC), tenofovir (Viread; TDF) and Truvada (combination drug containing Emtriva and Viread).

NNRTIs are called non-nucleoside inhibitors because, even though they work at the same stage as nucleoside analogues, they act in a completely different manner. NNRTIs stop HIV production by binding directly onto reverse transcriptase and preventing the conversion of DNA to RNA. The NNRTIs are generally effective in crossing the blood–brain barrier and may be useful in managing HIV-associated dementia. The drugs included in this category are nevirapine (Viramune), delavirdine (Rescriptor), and efavirenz (Sustiva).

PIs work at the end of the viral reproductive cycle. They prevent HIV from being successfully assembled and released from the infected CD4+ T cell. The drugs in this category include saquinavir (Invirase; SQV), indinavir (Crixivan; IDV), ritonavir (Norvir; RTV), Kaletra (lopinavir/ritonavir; LPV/r), nelfinavir (Viracept; NFV), fosamprenavir (Lexiva; LXV; prodrug of amprenavir [Agenerase]), atazanavir (Reyataz; ATV) and tipranavir (Aptivus; TPV).

The newest category of drugs is fusion inhibitors, which work by stopping the virus from attaching to the cell. Enfuvirtide (Fuzeon; T20) is currently the only FDA approved drug in this category.

Drugs Commonly Prescribed 16.1 presents dosage information on these drugs.

Clinical Guidelines. Clinical practice guidelines have been developed for the use of antiretroviral therapy for HIV-infected adults and adolescents. The guidelines are revised on an ongoing basis by the Panel on Clinical Practices for Treatment of HIV Infection, convened by the Department of Health and Human Services (DHHS). Treatment Standards/Guidelines 16.2 presents these standards. Clinical practice guidelines have also been developed by expert panels on HIV care for pediatric patients and pregnant women.

(Text continued on page 975)

Drugs Commonly Prescribed 16.1: Highly Active Antiretroviral Therapy (HAART)

Drug	Usual Adult Dosage	Adverse Effects	Notes
Nucleoside Reverse Transcriptase Inhibitors (NRTIs) Zidovudine	200 mg tid or 300 mg tid	Headache, GI distress, mild macrocytosis with or without anemia; neutropenia	Take with food or antacids. Hold if WBC falls to below 750. For GI distress or headache, take acetaminophen. Stop if severe anemia develops; persistent anemia may respond to erythropoietin (epoetin [Procrit]). Check CBC on ongoing basis. Long-term use may result in myalgias, muscle wasting and weakness, increased CPK.
Lamivudine (Epivir, 3TC)	150 mg bid		
Compivir (Combination of Retrovir and Epivir)			
Didanosine (ddl, Videx)	200 mg bid	Pancreatitis (alcohol exacerbates toxicity), peripheral neuropathy, retinal depigmentation, optic neuritis, hyperuricemia	Take on an empty stomach, at least 30 minutes before meal. Monitor uric acid levels. If using buffered powder for oral solution, do not mix with fruit juice. Drugs such as ketoconazole or dapsone, whose absorption can be affected by the level of acidity in the stomach, should be administered at least 2 hours before didanosine. Use with caution in patients with impaired renal or hepatic function. Do not give with tetracycline.
Videx EC (didanosine, ddl-EC) (Extended formulation of Videx)	One 400-mg capsule once a day for adults at or more than 60 kg; Is also available as a 250-mg capsule		Take on an empty stomach or at least 30 minutes before or 2 hours after eating.
Zalcitabine (ddC, Hivid)	0.75 mg tid	Peripheral neuropathy, pancreatitis (rare)	Advise patient to watch for abdominal pain, nausea and vomiting, ulcers, mouth sores. Do not give with didanosine. Avoid simultaneous use with antacids.
Stavudine (d4T, Zerit)	40 mg bid	Neuropathy, pancreatitis, nausea, vomiting, chills, fever, diarrhea	Take with or without food. Adjust dose if renal function is impaired.
Abacavir (Ziagen, ABC)	One 300 mg tablet twice a day or two 300 mg tablets once a day	Has caused a severe allergic reaction resulting in death; occurs in about 8% of all patients; reaction	Take with or without food.

(continued)

Drug	Usual Adult Dosage	Adverse Effects	Notes
		usually occurs during the first 6 weeks of taking abacavir but can occur at any time. Hypersensitivity to abacavir is a multiorgan syndrome usually characterized by at least two of the following manifestations: fever; rash; malaise, fatigue, or achiness; GI symptoms of N/V, diarrhea, or abdominal pain; or respiratory symptoms of dyspnea, cough, or pharyngitis. Less common signs and symptoms of hypersensitivity include lethargy, myolysis, edema, abnormal chest x-ray, and paresthesia. Anaphylaxis, liver failure, renal failure, hypotension, ARDS, respiratory failure, and death have occurred in association with hypersensitivity reactions. Inform clients to stop taking the drug and call their APN immediately if they have a skin rash or any two or more of the following symptoms: sudden fever; severe tiredness or achiness; diarrhea N/V or stomach pain; sore throat, SOB or cough; or generally ill feeling. These symptoms are listed on a warning card included with the prescription; tell clients to carry the warning card with them at all times. If these symptoms are caused by an allergic reaction, client should never take abacavir or an abacavir-containing medicine (Epzicom or Trizivir) again because death could occur within hours. If abacavir treatment is stopped for a period of time, it is important that a provider be notified before the individual starts to take it again.	
Epzicom (Combination of Ziagen and Epivir)	One tablet twice a day (Contains abacavir 600 mg and lamivudine 300 mg)	See information on abacavir and lamivudine.	Take with or without food. See information on abacavir and lamivudine.

Drug	Usual Adult Dosage	Adverse Effects	Notes
Trizivir (Combination of Ziagen, Retrovir and Epivir)	One tablet twice a day (Contains abacavir 300 mg, lamivudine 150 mg and zidovudine 300 mg)	See information on abacavir, zidovudine and lamivudine	Take with or without food. See information on abacavir, zidovudine and lamivudine.
Tenofovir (Viread, TDF)	One 300 mg tablet once a day; If baseline creatinine clearance (CrCl) less than 50 ml/min, dosing interval recommendations are as follows: CrCl 30 to 49 mL/min, 300 mg every 48 hours; CrCl 10 to 29 ml/min, 300 mg twice weekly; and hemodialysis patients, 300 mg every 7 days	Most common adverse effects: Asthenia, diarrhea, nausea, and vomiting. Less common S/E: Hepatotoxicity, including lactic acidosis; abdominal pain; anorexia; flatulence; allergic reaction, dyspnea. Fanconi's syndrome, hypophosphatemia, pancreatitis, proximal tubulopathy, renal failure or insufficiency, and acute tubular necrosis. In a study in HIV infected patients, decreases from baseline in bone mineral density were seen at the lumbar spine and hip, along with significant increases in levels of serum bone-specific alkaline phosphatase, serum osteocalcin, serum C-telopeptide, and urinary N-telopeptide; not known if long-term administration of tenofovir DF (greater than 1 year) will cause bone abnormalities.	Take with or without food. Closely monitor patients taking ddl and tenofovir; monitor for ddl-related toxicities; suspend tenofovir if S/S of pancreatitis, symptomatic hyperlactemia or lactic acidosis develop; D/C didanosine in patients who develop ddl-associated adverse events. Hepatic function should be monitored closely with both clinical and laboratory follow-up for at least several months in patients who D/C tenofovir DF and are coinfected with HIV and HBV. If appropriate, initiation of anti-hepatitis B therapy may be warranted.
Emtricitabine (Emtriva, FTC)	One 200-mg capsule once a day	Most frequently reported: Mild to moderate headache, nausea, diarrhea, and skin rash. Skin discoloration on palms and soles was reported with higher frequency in emtricitabine-treated patients than in controls; mechanism of skin discoloration is unknown. 1% of patients had triglycerides greater than 750 mg/dL and creatine kinase over four times the upper limit of normal.	Take with or without food. Have been reports of severe acute exacerbations of hepatitis B after D/C drug in patients coinfected with HIV and HBV; hepatic function should be monitored closely for at least several months after discontinuing emtricitabine in such patients.
Truvada (Combination of Viread and Emtriva)	One tablet once a day (Contains Emtriva 200 mg and Viread 300 mg)	See information on Viread and Emtriva.	Take with or without food. See information on Viread and Emtriva.
Non-nucleoside Reverse Transcriptase Inhibitors (NNRTIs)			
Nevirapine (Viramune)	200 mg bid	Rash (may decrease after initiation of therapy)	

(continued)

Drugs Commonly Prescribed 16.1: Highly Active Antiretroviral Therapy (HAART) (continued)

Drug	Usual Adult Dosage	Adverse Effects	Notes
Delavidine (Rescriptor)	400 mg tid	Skin rash (upper body and arms)	Take medication with water. Advise patient that skin rash usually lasts less than 2 weeks; use Benadryl or cortisone. Advise the patient with achlorhydria to try taking with an acid beverage (orange or cranberry juice). Use with caution in patient with impaired renal function. Do not give at same time as antacids. If patient is also on didanosine, separate administration by 1 hour. Do not give if patient is on phenytoin, phenobarbital, carbamazepine, rifabutin, rifampin, cimetidine, famotidine, nizatidine, ranitidine. Plasma concentrations of the following drugs are increased: indinavir, saquinavir, terfenadine, astemisole, clarithromycin, dapsone, rifabutin, ergot derivatives, alprazolam, midazolam, triazolan, dihydropyrides (nifedipine, cisapride, quinidine, warfarin).
Efavirenz (Sustiva)	600 mg PO HS	CNS symptoms (lightheadedness, inability to concentrate, anxiety, dysphonia) rash; with combination therapy nausea, vomiting, diarrhea, headache	Do not give with terfenadine, astemizole, or cisapride.
Protease Inhibitors (PIs) Saquinavir (Invirase)	600 mg tid		See note below. Take with meals. Do not give with rifampin or rifabutin, terfenadine, astemizole, phenobarbital, phenytoin, dexamethasone, carbamazepine.
Indinavir (Crixivan)	800 mg q8h	Nephrolithiasis, transient increases in bilirubin, abdominal pain, fatigue, weakness, flank pain, feeling unwell, nausea, diarrhea, vomiting, acid regurgitation, loss of appetite, dry mouth, back pain, headache, trouble sleeping, dizziness, taste changes, rash, URI, dry skin, sore throat	See note below. Take on empty stomach and with plenty of fluids; do not take with grapefruit juice. Keep dry in container.

Drug	Usual Adult Dosage	Adverse Effects	Notes
Ritonavir (Norvir)	600 mg bid; Titrate to relieve potential symptoms of nausea, vomiting, diarrhea: day 1 and 2: 300 mg bid; day 3 and 4: 400 mg bid; day 5 and 6: 500 mg bid; day 7: 600 mg bid if no problems; if problems on day 5 and 6, stay on 500 mg bid; day 8 and thereafter: 600 mg bid	Nausea, vomiting, diarrhea, stomach pain, taste change, fatigue, mild to severe skin sensitivity, numbness around the mouth	See note below. Take with meals (full stomach, to improve absorption of the drug). Keep in refrigerator. Available in capsules or oral solution; oral solution may be mixed with 8 oz of chocolate milk, Ensure, or Advera. Females using ethinyl estradiol for birth control will need to have the dosage increased. If on theophylline, may need increased dose.
Nelfinavir (Viracept)	750 mg tid	Mild to moderate diarrhea, nausea, flatulence	See note below. Take with meal or light snack.
Fosamprenavir (Lexiva) Prodrug of amprenavir (Agenerase)	Two 700-mg tablets twice a day or two 700 mg tablets with 200 mg Ritonavir tablet once a day; If previously on PI drugs, one 700 mg tablet with 100 mg ritonavir twice a day	Most common: Mild to moderate diarrhea, N/V and headache. Oral paresthesia, abdominal pain, and depressive symptoms or mood disorders have also been reported. In clinical studies, 19% of patients treated with fosamprenavir developed skin rash. Most rashes were of mild to moderate intensity; fewer than 1% of patients receiving fosamprenavir developed a severe or life-threatening rash (Grade 3 or 4) including Stevens-Johnson syndrome. D/C fosamprenavir in patients with severe or life-threatening rash or with moderate rash accompanied by systemic reactions.	Take with or without food. Use with caution in patients with a known sulfonamide allergy. Fosamprenavir contains a sulfonamide moiety; potential for cross-sensitivity between drugs in the sulfonamide class and fosamprenavir is unknown. Concomitant use with lovastatin or simvastatin is not recommended. Coadministration of fosamprenavir with dihydroergotamine, ergonovine, ergotamine, methylergonovine, cisapride, pimozide, midazolam, and triazolam is contraindicated. Serious or life-threatening drug interactions could occur between fosamprenavir and amiodarone, systemic lidocaine, bepridil, tricyclic antidepressants, or quinidine. If fosamprenavir is coadministered with ritonavir, flecainide and propafenone are also contraindicated. Concomitant use of rifampin or products containing St. John's wort (Hypericum perforatum) is not recommended. Carbamazepine, phenobarbital, and phenytoin should be used cautiously in combination with fosamprenavir: may decrease fosamprenavir effectiveness.

(continued)

Drugs Commonly Prescribed 16.1: Highly Active Antiretroviral Therapy (HAART) (continued)

Drug	Usual Adult Dosage	Adverse Effects	Notes
Lopinavir/ritonavir (Kaletra)	Three soft gel capsules twice a day OR six soft gel capsules once a day (Contains both lopinavir and ritonavir)	Pancreatitis has been observed in patients receiving lopinavir/ritonavir, including those who developed marked triglyceride elevations; in some cases, fatalities have occurred. Although a causal relationship with lopinavir/ritonavir has not been established, marked triglyceride elevation is a risk factor in the development of pancreatitis. Patients with advanced HIV disease may be at increased risk of elevated triglycerides and pancreatitis; patients with a history of pancreatitis may be at increased risk for recurrence during lopinavir/ritonavir therapy. Pancreatitis should be considered if clinical symptoms suggestive of pancreatitis occur (N/V, abdominal pain, or abnormal laboratory values such as increased serum lipase or amylase): Patients who exhibit these S/S should be evaluated and lopinavir/ritonavir and/or other antiretroviral therapy should be suspended.	Take with food. Capsule formulation will be phased out by 2006, in favor of the new tablet formulation; advantages include a lower pill burden, no required dose adjustments for concomitant use of certain NNRTIs in treatment-naive patients, and easier storage requirements. Risk-benefit should be considered if patients also have diabetes mellitus, hepatic function impairment, hepatitis B, hepatitis C, or a history of pancreatitis. Contraindicated in patients with known hypersensitivity to any of its ingredients, including ritonavir. Contraindicated: With drugs that are highly dependent on CYP3A for clearance and for which elevated plasma concentrations are associated with serious and/or life threatening events such as cardiac arrhythmias, prolonged or increased sedation, or respiratory depression. These drugs include antihistamines (astemizole, terfenadine), ergot derivatives (dihydroergotamine, ergonovine, ergotamine, metylergonovine), the gastrointestinal motility agent cisapride, the neuroleptic pimozide, and sedatives (midazolam, triazolam). Use of rifampin with lopinavir/ritonavir is contraindicated, as it may lead to the loss of virologic response and possible resistance to lopinavir/ritonavir, other PIs, or any other coadministered antiretroviral agents. Should not be administered once daily in combination with efavirenz, nevirapine, amprenavir, or nelfinavir; once daily administration has not been evaluated in combination with fosamprenavir, indinavir, or saquinavir.

Drug	Usual Adult Dosage	Adverse Effects	Notes
Atazanavir (Reyataz)	Two 200-mg capsules once a day; if previously on PIs, 300 mg with 100 mg ritonavir once a day (also available as a 100 and a 150-mg capsule); patients with moderate hepatic insufficiency may need reduced dose of 300 mg once a day	Headache, nausea, and skin rash were reported in clinical trials as the most common treatment-emergent adverse effects of moderate or severe intensity. Adverse effects observed with clinical use include: allergic reaction; new onset or exacerbation of existing diabetes mellitus or hyperglycemia; asymptomatic hyperbilirubinemia, including yellow eyes or skin: lactic acidosis; PR interval prolongation; abdominal pain; back pain; increased cough; depression; diarrhea; headache; jaundice; lipodystrophy; and N/V. Microscopic hematuria (greater than five red blood cells per high-powered field) has been observed in patients taking atazanavir. Uric acid crystals were observed in some urine samples. The relationship between these observations and atazanavir therapy is not known. Cases of lactic acidosis syndrome (LAS), sometimes fatal, and symptomatic hyperlactatemia have been reported in patients receiving atazanavir in combination with nucleoside analogues. Nucleoside analogues, female gender, and obesity are all known risk factors for LAS. The contribution of atazanavir to the development of LAS has not been established.	Take with food. Has a unique HIV resistance profile that suggests it may be an appropriate component of antiviral regimens in treatment-naive patients; Patients taking atazanavir on their first antiretroviral regimen develop a characteristic 150L mutation that increases viral susceptibility to other PIs. Unlike other PIs, has a minimal effect on lipid levels (both cholesterol and triglycerides). Coadministration of atazanavir is contraindicated with drugs that are highly dependent on CYP3A for clearance, including benzodiazepines (midazolam, triazolam); ergot derivatives (dihydroergotamine, ergotamine, ergonovine, methylergonovine), gastrointestinal (GI) motility agents (cisapride); and neuroleptics (pimozide). Coadministration of atazanavir is also contraindicated with rifampin, irinotecan, bepridil, lovastatin, simvastatin, indinavir, proton-pump inhibitors including omeprazole, and St. John's wort. Has been shown to prolong the PR interval of the electrocardiogram, risk-benefit should be considered in patients with pre-existing atrioventricular (AV) conduction abnormalities. Concurrent administration of atazanavir with amiodarone, lidocaine, or quinidine may increase antiarrhythmic drug concentrations, resulting in potentially serious or life-threatening adverse events; caution and concentration monitoring is suggested. Risk-benefit should also be considered in patients with obesity, diabetes

(continued)

Drug	Usual Adult Dosage	Adverse Effects	Notes
			mellitus, or hyperglycemia; hepatic function impairment, elevated transaminase levels, or hepatitis B or C infection; or type A or B hemophilia (atazanavir may induce increased bleeding, spontaneous skin hematomas, and hemarthrosis).
Tipranavir (Aptivus)	500 mg of TPV taken with 200 mg of ritonavir twice a day (TPV available as a 250-mg soft gel capsule).	Most frequent: Diarrhea, N/V, fatigue, and headache. TPV coadministered with ritonavir has been associated with clinical hepatitis and hepatic decompensation, including some fatalities. Extra vigilance is warranted in individuals with advanced HIV disease or those with chronic hepatitis B or hepatitis C coinfection, as these individuals have an increased risk of hepatotoxicity. Symptoms of hepatitis include fatigue, malaise, anorexia, nausea, jaundice, bilirubinemia, acholic stools, liver tenderness, or hepatomegaly. Individuals with hemophilia may have increased risk of bleeding. Women using estrogens may have an increased risk of nonserious rash. Other adverse effects include rash, elevated lipid levels, fat redistribution and immune reconstitution syndrome.	Absorption of TPV increases when taken with a high-fat meal. Antacids reduce absorption of TPV, requiring timing adjustments of antacid use. Contraindicated in individuals with moderate to severe hepatic insufficiency. Like other PIs, TPV/ritonavir at the recommended dosage is a net inhibitor of CYP3A and may thus increase plasma concentrations of agents that are primarily metabolized by this enzyme. Coadministration of TPV/ritonavir with drugs that are highly dependent on CYP3A for clearance are contraindicated. These drugs include amiodarone, bepridil, flecainide, propafenone, quinidine, rifampin, dihydroergotamine, ergonovine, ergotamine, methylergonamine, cisapride, St. John's wort, lovastatin, simvastatin, pimozide, midazolam, and triazolam. Alternative methods of nonhormonal contraception should be used when estrogen-based oral contraceptives are coadministered with TPV/ritonavir. Women using estrogens as hormone replacement therapy should be clinically monitored for signs of estrogen deficiency. TPV/ritonavir may have significant interactions with some drugs that require a dosing or timing adjustment: didanosine, amprenavir, lopinavir, saquinavir, itraconazole, ketoconazole, voriconazole, rifabutin,

Drug	Usual Adult Dosage	Adverse Effects	Notes
			desipramine, disulfiram/metronidazole, atorvastatin, meperidine, methadone, sildenafil, tadalafil, and vardenafil. Other drugs coadministered with TPV/ritonavir may require careful monitoring, including diltiazem, felodipine, nicardipine, nisoldipine, verapamil, glimepiride, glipizide, glyburide, pioglitazone, repaglinide, tolbutamide, cyclosporine, sirolimus, tacrolimus, and warfarin.
Darunavir (Prezista; TMC114)	600 mg (two 300-mg tablets) taken with ritonavir 100 mg twice daily with food	Most common: Diarrhea, nausea, headache, nasopharyngitis; Also reported: Abnormal liver and pancreatic function tests, abnormally high cholesterol and triglyceride levels, decreases in white blood cell counts; See ritonavir for ritonavir-associated A/Es	Since Prezista is primarily metabolized by the liver, use with caution for patients with hepatic impairment; patients with pre-existing liver dysfunction, including chronic active hepatitis, can have an increased frequency of liver function abnormalities during HIV drug therapy, monitor according to standard of practice. Both darunavir and ritonavir are both inhibitors of CYP3A. Coadministration of darunavir and ritonavir with drugs primarily metabolized by CYP3A may result in increased plasma concentrations of such drugs, which could increase or prolong their therapeutic effect and adverse effects. See additional notes on Ritonavir and on Protease Inhibitors.
Drug Class: Entry Inhibitors Enfuvirtide (Fuzeon; T20)	90 mg (1 mL) twice daily by subcutaneous injection	Local injection site reactions, associated with mild to moderate pain and discomfort, induration, erythema, nodules and cysts, pruritus, and ecchymosis; hypersensitivity reactions; increased rate of bacterial pneumonia; peripheral neuropathy, sinusitis, conjunctivitis, pancreatitis, skin papilloma, anxiety, decreased appetite, asthenia, cough, depression, herpes simples, pruritis, insomnia, myalgia, and weight loss	Patients developing signs and symptoms suggestive of a systemic hypersensitivity reaction should discontinue enfuvirtide and seek medical evaluation immediately; Therapy with enfuvirtide should not be restarted following systemic S/S consistent with a hypersensitivity reaction.

(continued)

Drugs Commonly Prescribed 16.1: Highly Active Antiretroviral Therapy (HAART) (continued)

Drug	Usual Adult Dosage	Adverse Effects	Notes
Drug Class: Multi-Class Combination Therapy			
Atripla, a fixed-dose combination tablet containing three HIV drugs (Efavirenz/Emtricitabine/Tenofovir disoproxil fumarate); One tablet of Atripla is equivalent to one 600-mg tablet of the NNRTI efavirenz and one tablet of Truvada, a fixed-dose combination tablet containing two NRTIs: emtricitabine 200 mg and tenofovir disoproxil fumarate (tenofovir DF) 300 mg	One tablet once a day, taken on an empty stomach, alone or in combination with other HIV medications	Most common: Headache: dizziness, abdominal pain, nausea, vomiting, rash Nucleoside analog drugs such as Atripla may cause lactic acidosis and liver toxicity. Discontinuation of Atripla in patients with chronic Hepatitis B infection can cause severe flare-ups of Hepatitis B infection. Monitor for liver toxicity, renal impairment and severe depression. Efavirenz: impaired concentration, anorexia, abdominal pain, anxiety, pruritus, and some reports of pancreatitis. Emtricitabine: Mild, asymptomatic hyper-pigmentation of palms and soles. Emtricitabine and tenofovir DF: Anxiety, arthralgia, increased cough, dyspepsia, fever, myalgia, abdominal pain, peripheral neuropathy, rash, pruritis, urticaria, and paresthesia.	See individual notes on each of these drugs: Efavirenz; Emtricitabine; Tenofovir. See additional notes on NRTIs. Atripla has not been evaluated in the presence of food.

NOTE: For all NRTIs and NNRTIs:

1. Lactic acidosis and severe hepatomegaly with steatosis have been reported with the use of nucleoside analogues alone or in combination.
2. Immune reconstitution syndrome has been reported in patients treated with combination antiretroviral therapy (ART), including lopinavir/ritonavir. During the initial phase of combination ART, patients whose immune system respond may develop an inflammatory response to indolent or residual opportunistic infections (such as *Mycobacterium avium* infection, cytomegalovirus, *Pneumocystis carinii* pneumonia, or tuberculosis) which may necessitate further evaluation and treatment.

NOTE: For all protease Inhibitors:

1. May cause hypertension and diabetes. Advise patient to be alert for increased thirst and hunger, unexplained weight loss, increased urination, fatigue, dry itching skin that may start 10 to 11 weeks after starting treatment.
2. Many of the protease inhibitors compete with the P450 hepatic metabolic pathway; do not give with drugs that use the same pathway.
3. Caution should be used when prescribing PDE5 inhibitors for erectile dysfunction (e.g., sildenafil, tadalafil, or vardenafil) to patients receiving PIs; Coadministration of a PI with a PDE5 inhibitor is expected to substantially increase the adverse events associated with PDE5 inhibitors, including hypotension, visual changes, and priapism.
4. Caution should be used when any PI is used concurrently with other HMG-CoA reductase inhibitors (statins) that are metabolized by the CYP3A4 pathway (for example, atorvastatin or cerivastatin). The resulting increased concentration of statins may increase the risk of myopathy or rhabdomyolysis.

GI = gastrointestinal; WBC = white blood cells; CBC = complete blood count; CPK = creatine phosphokinase; CNS = central nervous system; URI = upper respiratory infection.

Treatment Standards/Guidelines 16.2 Antiretroviral Therapy

Department of Health and Human Services

Initiation of Therapy

- HIV drug therapy should be immediately started for all patients with a history of an AIDS-defining illness or severe symptoms of HIV infection regardless of CD4+ T cell count.
- HIV drug therapy is recommended for asymptomatic patients with a CD4+ T cell count less than 200 cells/mm^3.
- Asymptomatic patients with CD4+ T cell counts between 201–350 cells/mm^3 should be offered treatment.
- Asymptomatic patients with CD4+ T cell counts over 350 cells/mm^3 and plasma HIV RNA levels over 100,000 copies/ml: Most experienced clinicians defer therapy: some clinicians may consider initiating therapy.
- Defer therapy for patients with CD4+ T cell counts of over 350 cells/mm^3 and plasma HIV RNA levels under 100,000 copies/ml.

Initial Therapy

For patients who have never been on HIV drug therapy (treatment-naïve):

Preferred regimens

Initial regimen should contain two nucleoside/nucleotide reverse transcriptase inhibitors (NRTI) and either a non-nucleoside reverse transcriptase inhibitor (NNRTI) or a ritonavir-boosted or unboosted (no added ritonavir) protease inhibitor (PI)

NNRTI-based regimen

- Efavirenz* + (lamivudine or emtricitabine) + (zidovudine or tenofovir DF) (2-3 pills)

*Not during first trimester of pregnancy or women with high potential for pregnancy

Alternative NNRTI-based regimens

- Efavirenz* + (didanosine or abacavir or stavudine) + (lamivudine or emtricitabine)
- Nevirapine-based regimens may be used as an alternative in adult females with CD4+ T cell counts at or less than 250 cells/mm^3 and adult males with CD4+ T cell counts at or less than 400 cells/mm^3

NNRTIs NOT RECOMMENDED as initial therapy:

- Delavirdine – because of inferior antiretroviral potency and three times daily dosing
- Nevirapine for adult females with CD4+ T cell counts above 250 cells/mm^3 and adult males with CD4+ T cell counts above 400 cells/mm^3

PI-based regimen

- Lopinavir/ritonavir (Kaletra) + (lamivudine or emtricitabine) + (zidovudine)

Alternative PI-based regimens

- Atazanavir, fosamprenavir, ritonavir-boosted fosamprenavir, ritonavir-boosted indinavir, nelfinavir or ritonavir-boosted saquinavir - all of these used in combination with either zidovudine, stavudine, tenofovir, abacavir or didanosine, plus either lamivudine or emtricitabine
- Lopinavir/ritonavir plus either stavudine, tenofovir, abacavir or didanosine plus either lamivudine or emtricitabine

PIs NOT RECOMMENDED as initial therapy:

- Unboosted indinavir – because of inconvenient three times daily dosing and the need to take this drug on an empty stomach or with a light meal
- Ritonavir as the only PI – because of high incidence of GI intolerance
- Unboosted saquinavir – because of poor oral bioavailability, three times daily dosing, and high number of pills that need to be taken
- Ritonavir-boosted tipranavir – because of lack of clinical trial data in treatment-naïve patients

Triple NRTI-based regimens

- Should only be used when a preferred or alternative NNRTI-based or PI-based regimen cannot or should not be used as first-line therapy
- Abacavir + zidovudine + lamivudine

3-NRTIs regimens NOT RECOMMENDED as sole antiretroviral combination at any time:

- Abacavir + tenofovir + lamivudine
- Didanosine + tenofovir + lamivudine

Designing a Compatible Medication Regimen. The patient's ability to adhere to a potent combination drug cocktail must be discussed in detail before initiating therapy. Once a client is started on drug therapy, there is a risk of developing drug resistance if viral suppression is not maintained. Viral mutation causing drug resistance can rapidly occur within 2 weeks to 2 days of a patient stopping medication, or not taking all prescribed doses. The medications all have varying requirements regarding dosing, dietary requirements, number of pills to be taken each day, and drug interactions. The clinician must prescribe a HAART that is compatible with the patient's day-to-day activities, including lifestyle, eating habits, social habits, and work and home environments.

Monitoring Viral Load. The viral load test directly measures the amount of viral particles that are in the patient's plasma. Viral load test results are reported as either copies or units per milliliter of plasma. If the test result is below 500 copies or units/mL or below the detection threshold of the assay used, the viral load is considered undetectable. This means that the amount of virus in the blood is so minimal that it cannot be measured by the test assay being used.

A baseline viral load is determined by taking two separate viral load tests, about 2 to 3 weeks apart. If the results of the two tests are similar, a stable baseline is established and used to monitor the effects of drug therapy. The viral load should be repeated 4 to 6 weeks after initiation of drug therapy or any changes in the drug therapy. Initiation of drug therapy should correspond with a decrease in viral load. If the viral load results are about the same or higher than the baseline, changes in drug therapy need to be made. Once an effective drug regimen has been established, the viral load should be repeated every 3 to 4 months. Changes in viral load of less than three times higher or lower are not considered significant.

Because the tests measure viral activity, anything that affects the production of virus can influence the results. A sudden rise in viral load can occur after an active infection, such as the flu or a herpes outbreak, because previously HIV-infected, but inactive, CD4+ T cells suddenly "wake up" (are activated by the flu or herpes virus) and start producing HIV. A viral load test can also be affected by the administration of a vaccine, so a test should not be done until 4 to 6 weeks after illness or vaccination.

The goal of HAART is to decrease the viral load to undetectable levels. An undetectable-viral load should be achieved within 4 to 6 months of initiation of therapy. If this does not occur, the patient should be switched to a new medication regimen.

There are presently three test assay methods commercially available to assess viral load: polymerase chain reaction (PCR), branch DNA (bDNA) test, and nucleic acid sequence–based amplification (NASBA). Because the methods of each test are slightly different, the results are not exactly the same. If the test assay method is switched, a new baseline test may be required. Table 16.7 presents information on these tests.

Follow-Up and Referral

Follow-up for the patient infected with HIV will be required for the rest of the patient's life. If an HIV antibody test is done at the initial visit, the patient must come back in 1 to 2 weeks for counseling regarding the results. If results are negative, the clinician should discuss risk reduction behavior with the patient. The patient will also need to know that the test result may be negative as a result of the "window period," so the HIV antibody test should be repeated in 3 months. If any risky behaviors occur before the test is redone, the time period for testing will need to be recalculated, because the window period exists for up to 3 months after all high-risk behaviors.

If the test is positive, the need to begin medications should be discussed. The patient's present clinical condition, along with the viral load and CD4+ T count, will need to be considered in order to prescribe the most appropriate therapy. However, the patient should be educated regarding all aspects of HAART, so that the patient can determine what combination is most compatible with his or her lifestyle and ability to follow the requirements for adherence with the different drugs. The patient may need time to accept the diagnosis, in order to make informed decisions on medical care. A follow-up visit must be scheduled to discuss the patient's decision regarding medication therapy. Follow-up will also be necessary to monitor the affect of drug therapy by the results of the viral load test.

If the patient is having severe pulmonary symptoms, he or she may need to be admitted to the hospital to rule out PCP or TB. If the patient's viral load is high and the CD4+ T count is low, the clinician should refer the patient to a special immunologist or an infectious disease practitioner for follow-up primary care. If Kaposi's sarcoma is suspected, the patient may need to be referred to an oncologist. If there is a suspicion of CMV retinitis, the patient should be immediately referred to an ophthalmologist for a thorough eye exam.

Health maintenance of the HIV-infected patient also requires close attention to preventive immunizations, including pneumococcal vaccine (23-valent polysaccharide

Table 16.7 Viral Load Tests

Viral load monitoring can establish the prognosis of a patient with HIV infection. Rising viral load indicates disease progression; falling viral load indicates a favorable prognostic trend.

Plasma viral load may range from a few hundred virons (also called viral copies or viral equivalents) to more than a million per mL, a 10,000-fold range. Such large ranges are easiest to express in logarithms (logs).

To express a number in logarithmic form, a base is raised to a power. The latter is the logarithm, or exponent. The base 10 is commonly used in medicine without being explicitly specified; often only the power (the exponent, or log) is shown. A viral load of 10,000 copies/mL, or 10^4 copies/mL, is 4 logs. A viral load 10 times as high, or 100,000 copies/mL, is 10^5 copies/mL, or 5 logs.

Changes in viral load are commonly expressed in either numeric or logarithmic terms. For example, a two-fold change is equal to approximately a 0.3-log change.

In viral load measurements, the sum of the laboratory and biologic variation is generally assumed to be 0.3–0.5 log (twofold to threefold). Therefore, only changes greater than this are considered meaningful. The table below gives further information on several of these exams.

Name	Manufacturer	Other Name	HIV Range
PCR (polymerase chain reaction)	Roche Diagnostics	Amplicor HIV-1 Monitor Test 1.5	400–750,000 copies
PCR (polymerase chain reaction)	Roche Diagnostics	Amplicor HIV-1 Monitor Test 1.5 Ultra Sensitive	50–75,000 copies
bDNA (branch DNA test) Signal Amplification	Bayer	VERSANT HIV-1 RNA 3.0 (bDNA)	75–500,000 copies
NASBA (nucleic acid sequence based amplification)	Organon Teknika	NucliSens HIV-1 QT	80–10,000 copies

Pneumovax vaccine) which may be readministered after 6 years, annual influenza vaccination (but never the intranasal attenuated live virus vaccine, which is contraindicated), tetanus toxoid boosters every 10 years, the hepatitis B vaccine series (in patients without preexisting hepatitis B surface antibody), and, in most cases, hepatitis A vaccine (particularly in patients with coexistent HIV and hepatitis B infection). Importantly, live virus vaccines including MMR (measles, mumps, rubella), OPV (oral polio virus), BCG (Bacillus Calmette-Guerin anti-TB vaccine) and those for varicella (chicken pox) and yellow fever are contraindicated in HIV-infected patients with advanced disease and significant immunosuppression. However, the MMR and varicella vaccines may be given early on in the course of the disease to nonimmunosuppressed HIV-positive individuals.

Patient Education

HIV infection is a lifelong chronic disease. Education helps the patient with self-care activities that can decrease the risk of reinfection and opportunistic infections. The patient will need extensive education for his or her specific condition and specific therapy, including specific drug contraindications and interactions, and support to help the patient follow some of the demands of adherence to HAART. In addition, the patient will need continual reinforcement and education on the need to attain and maintain HIV preventive behaviors, such as safer-sex practices, to decrease the potential of transmitting HIV to others. Extensive patient education materials are available from pharmaceutical companies, AIDS support organizations, and government and health-care agencies (see Resources section at the end of this chapter). Educational programs for clinicians are also available through the Association of Nurses in AIDS Care (ANAC) (800) 260-6780. Nursing Research–Based Practice 16.1 presents updates on HIV clinical trials.

Acquired Immunodeficiency Syndrome

If left untreated, HIV infection will eventually undermine the immune system. Once the CD4+ T cell count is below 200 cells/mL of blood, opportunistic infections can occur. These infections can be life threatening unless diagnosed and treated. Once the CD4+ T cell count goes below 200 cells/mL of blood, or if the patient experiences an opportunistic infection, the HIV-positive patient is classified as having progressed from HIV infection to AIDS.

Epidemiology and Causes

AIDS, which is the advanced stage of HIV infection, is a leading cause of death in sub-Saharan Africa. Early detection of HIV and improved HIV drug therapy has dramatically decreased the death rate from AIDS.

There is a tremendous variation in the natural history of HIV infection from one patient to another. Thus, it is impossible to predict when AIDS will occur in a person infected with HIV. Studies from the 1980s to the mid-1990s showed that the usual survival time after the diagnosis of AIDS was 3 years. However, the impact of early HIV diagnosis and care, including drug therapy, has increased survival time and quality of life for many HIV-infected persons, including those with both an HIV and an AIDS diagnosis. Unfortunately, some HIV-infected persons have not responded to drug therapy (referred to as treatment failure). These clients will need to be monitored closely for opportunistic infections and other life-threatening conditions as their immune system deteriorates, manifested by an increasing viral load and a decreasing CD4+ T cell count.

Pathophysiology

HIV is well-recognized for its lengthy latency period in which infected persons remain relatively asymptomatic, despite persistent low-level viremia and progressive CD4+ T cell destruction (approximately 40 to 80 CD4+ T cells/mm^3 per year). However, among individuals, there is wide variability in length to progression to clinical AIDS. While the average latency period in untreated individuals has been estimated at 9 years, a subset of HIV-infected persons will progress rapidly to AIDS within months to less than 2 years, while even in the absence of therapy, approximately 5 percent of infected persons will show little to no progression of disease for more than a decade and are known as long-term nonprogressors. A complex interplay of multiple environmental and genetic factors of both host and virus is thought to underlie this variation.

Anti-HIV immune responses include both humoral and cell-mediated mechanisms. HIV-specific antibodies form in the majority of individuals within several weeks to 3 months of initial infection; however, these antibodies are insufficient to prevent disseminated infection. These neutralizing antibodies appear to have a role in natural killer (NK) cell destruction of HIV-infected cells via antibody-mediated cellular cytotoxicity. In addition, CD8+ cytotoxic T cells also target HIV-infected cells for destruction. However, these mechanisms are unable to fully eradicate HIV infection from long-lived cellular compartments (e.g., follicular dendritic cells, memory T lymphocytes) or cells that are physically sequestered from the lymphatic system (e.g., CNS cells).

Unfortunately, given HIV's tropism for cells of the hematopoietic and immune system, the CD8+ killer T cell activity which is key in clearing the high levels of viremia associated with initial HIV infection also contributes significantly to CD4+ T cell destruction and eventual progression to clinical AIDS. This can occur via single-host cell killing resulting from an accumulation of unintegrated viral DNA and eventual cell lysis or via disruption of normal host cell protein synthesis. However, in vitro studies have also revealed that HIV-infected cells are capable of fusing with large numbers of uninfected CD4+ T cells to create large, multinucleated syncytia. Although not confirmed in vivo,

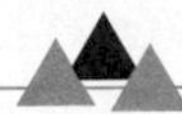

NURSING RESEARCH-BASED PRACTICE 16.1

Clinical Trials

HIV Vaccine and Clinical Drug Trials

Since 1987, researchers have attempted to identify vaccines that can immunize uninfected persons or prevent disease progression in those who are already infected. Obstacles to the development of an effective vaccine have been the genetic variability of the virus and the inability of antibodies raised by vaccines to consistently neutralize viral isolates in laboratory experiments.

One vaccine study that started in 2004 is a two-part study that will evaluate two pairs of matching recombinant HIV vaccines (FPV vaccine and MVA vaccine), which are pox virus vaccines developed for use in this study. The study is called Safety of and Immune Response to Two HIV Vaccine Formulations (rMVA-HIV and rFPV-HIV) Alone or in Combination in HIV Uninfected Adults. Pox viruses are used for investigational vaccines in humans because they can accommodate large amounts of foreign DNA, can infect mammalian cells, and can access the cytotoxic T-cell responses believed to be important in the control of HIV infection and disease. The study will evaluate the safety and immunogenicity of the vaccine pairs.

Part A: Participants will be randomly assigned to one of five different vaccination groups. Within each group, participants will be randomly assigned to receive either vaccine or control injections. Group 1 participants will receive the FPV vaccine pair or FPV control at each vaccine visit. Groups 2, 3, and 4 will receive one of three different doses of the MVA vaccine pair or MVA control at study entry and month 1, then a fixed dose of the FPV vaccine pair or FPV control at months 3, 5, and 7. Group 5 participants will receive the MVA vaccine pair or MVA control at maximum tolerated dose (MTD) at each vaccine visit. Groups 1 and 2 will enroll simultaneously; groups 3, 4, and 5 will enroll as safety data from the previous groups become available.

Part B: Participants will be randomly assigned to receive study vaccine or control vaccine in one of three vaccination groups. Group 6 participants will receive the FPV vaccine pair or FPV control at each vaccine visit. Group 7 participants will receive the MVA vaccine pair or MVA control at study entry and month 1, then a fixed dose of the FPV vaccine pair or FPV control at months 3, 5, and 7. Group 8 participants will receive the MVA vaccine pair at MTD or MVA control at each vaccine visit. Enrollment into groups 6, 7, and 8 will begin simultaneously after the completion of the safety data evaluation of groups 1 and 2.

Study vaccinations will be given at study entry and at months 1, 3, 5, and 7. Tests for cardiac injury will be performed at screening and at each 2-week follow-up visit after vaccination. Participants will have an electrocardiogram (ECG) at screening and 2 weeks after the first and last vaccinations. Study visits will occur at screening, study entry, and at 11 visits over 13 months. Study visits will consist of a physical exam, risk reduction/pregnancy prevention counseling, cardiac symptom assessment, and blood and urine collection. Women will have pregnancy tests at study entry and months 1, 3, 5, 7, and 13.

Leflunomide (Arava)

Leflunomide is currently approved by the FDA for treating rheumatoid arthritis. The drug works by blocking cell division in activated T cells. This study will evaluate the effect of leflunomide (Arava) on the life cycle of a specific immune cell called CD4+ T cell in HIV-infected patients. This study will see if leflunomide can block T-cell division and possibly reduce the number of cells that die, reduce the number of cells in which HIV can reproduce, and lead to a lower level of HIV virus in the body. Participants are randomly assigned to take leflunomide or a placebo every day for 28 days. Participants will come to the clinic three times during the first 29 days of the study (days 1, 15, and 29) for a physical examination and review of any drug side effects. Patients taking placebo end their participation on day 29. Patients taking leflunomide stop taking the drug on day 29 and begin taking cholestyramine three times a day for 11 days out of the next 14 days to clear the leflunomide from their body. On day 43, they return to the clinic to have their leflunomide level checked to make sure that only very little or none of the drug remains in the body. If the level is low, patients end their participation on or around day 57. If the level remains high, they repeat the cholestyramine treatment.

UK-427,857 (Maraviroc)

UK-427,857 (Maraviroc) is a chemokine receptor antagonist that acts as an entry inhibitor. It is designed to prevent HIV infection of CD4+ T cells by blocking the CCR5 coreceptor from binding to HIV. Maraviroc is being studied as an investigational HIV entry inhibitor drug. The drug works by binding to a protein on the membrane of T cells called CCR5. The CCR5-tropic variant of the virus is common in earlier HIV infection, so UK-427,857 may be most useful in acute and early infection. A previous study demonstrated that when UK-427,857 was given as monotherapy for 10 days to HIV-1 infected patients, HIV-1 viral load was reduced by up to 1.6 log, consistent with currently available agents. The goal of the current study is to compare the safety and efficacy of UK-427,857 versus efavirenz, when each are combined with two other antiretroviral agents, in patients who are previously naive to antiretroviral therapy. This study will involve approximately 200 centers from around the world to achieve a total randomized subject population of 1071 subjects. Patients will be randomly assigned to one of three groups: UK-427,857 300 mg once daily added to zidovudine/lamivudine (300 mg/150 mg twice daily), UK-427,857 300 mg twice daily added to zidovudine/lamivudine (300 mg/150 mg twice daily) or efavirenz (600 mg once daily) added to zidovudine/lamivudine (300 mg/150 mg twice daily).

this process has been theorized to contribute to the rapid depletion of the helper T cell compartment in advanced stages of HIV infection.

Shared structural homology between the HIV envelope glycoproteins gp120 and gp41 and major histocompatibility complex (MHC) class II molecules is thought to underlie the cross-reactivity and autoimmune destruction of T lymphocytes and antigen-presenting cells in the HIV-infected individual. However, even before significant CD4+ T cell depletion, dysregulated B-cell activity and autoantibody production caused by regulatory T cell dysfunction may lead to autoimmune damage of additional cell lines and organ-specific tissues, including primary HIV-associated thrombocytopenia (PHAT), HIV nephropathy, and HIV cardiomyopathy.

In addition to destruction at the cellular level, advanced HIV infection is also characterized by destruction of the gross lymphatic architecture over a period of months to years. This includes disruption of the lymph node follicular network, which is critical for immune cell trafficking and exposure to circulating antigens, both of which are necessary to mount an effective immune response.

Moreover, qualitative defects in immune cell function are also important to the pathogenesis of advanced HIV infection. Binding studies with gp120-specific immunoglobulins demonstrated that T cell anergy (inactivation) could be induced on antibody binding of CD4+ T cell surface receptors. In addition, increased rates of apoptosis (non-necrotic programmed cell death) have been demonstrated in T cells repeatedly stimulated by a specific antigen; this mechanism may be particularly relevant to chronic HIV infection.

Because of immunosuppression, the patient with AIDS is at high risk for developing viral, bacterial, fungal, and/or protozoal opportunistic infections. Common viral infections include cytomegalovirus (CMV), herpes simplex, varicella-zoster virus (VZV), and progressive multifocal leukoencephalopathy (PML, due to the JC virus). Common bacterial infections include those of *Mycobacterium avium* complex (MAC; due to *M. avium* and *M. intracellulare*), and *Mycobacterium tuberculosis* (TB). Common fungal infections include candidiasis, *Pneumocystis jiroveci pneumonia* (PCP), and cryptococcosis. Common protozoal infections include cryptosporidiosis and cerebral toxoplasmosis (*Toxoplasma gondii* infection of the CNS). These infections can be life-threatening. Other potential problems include malignancies and AIDS wasting. The most common infections will be discussed in the upcoming section.

Clinical Presentation

Subjective

The patient may complain of visual problems, such as loss of vision, either central or peripheral, blurring of vision, or "floaters," a symptom that is typical of CMV retinitis.

GI problems such as diarrhea may occur along with unintentional weight loss, fevers, chills, night sweats, and abdominal pain as a result of CMV colitis, gastroenteritis, pancreatitis, AIDS wasting, MAC, *Salmonella*, cryptosporidiosis, isosporiasis, or histoplasmosis.

Dermatologic problems may occur, such as papules with burning, rash or bumps in a line or pattern, burning or stinging of the skin, darkish colored lesions, draining lesions, and rectal pain, which may be indicative of herpes, HPV, or Kaposi's sarcoma.

Neurologic problems or alterations or changes in mental status, such as headaches, confusion, mood swings (personality changes), dizziness, stiff neck, fever, lethargy and malaise, photophobia (intolerance of light due to resulting eye pain), nausea, vomiting, seizures, neurologic deficits, hemiparesis, ataxia, and cranial nerve palsies or seizures may be a result of herpes encephalopathy, PML, cryptococcosis, or *Toxoplasma gondii.*

The patient may also complain of pulmonary symptoms, such as shortness of breath and a dry, nonproductive cough. These may be accompanied by fever, chills and night sweats, and/or loss of weight, productive cough with blood-tinged sputum, and chest pain, which may indicate PCP, bacterial pneumonia, or TB. Also nonspecific complaints of fatigue, weakness and fever could be indicative of anemia, leukopenia, and disseminated MAC.

Objective

With CMV retinitis, retinal changes are seen on ophthalmoscopic exam. With toxoplasmosis encephalitis, the most common presentation of toxoplasmosis, the clinician should check for headache, altered level of consciousness, and any stroke-like symptoms. With pulmonary complaints, the clinician should check for the onset of symptoms. PCP is usually insidious, with worsening of symptoms over a day to weeks, whereas pulmonary toxoplasmosis progresses more rapidly than PCP. TB also tends to be insidious. With skin lesions, the clinician must note if the papules are indicative of herpes simplex virus (HSV), or if the lesions are indicative of Kaposi's sarcoma. The clinician should also note if the GI symptoms are sudden or insidious. Advanced Assessment 16.2 presents additional history and physical examination information to be gathered from the HIV-positive patient.

Diagnostic Reasoning

Diagnostic Tests

The patient with AIDS should have had all initial testing done when he or she was first diagnosed with HIV. Once the CD4+ T cell count is below 200 cells/mL of blood, the patient is diagnosed with AIDS. HIV drug resistance testing should be considered for clients who have been on HIV medications and did not respond to drug therapy.

Table 16.8 includes additional lab tests to perform and how to interpret them. For patients with suspected TB or PCP, the clinician should order a PPD, ABG, chest x-ray exam, and sputum samples for smear and culture for acid-

ADVANCED ASSESSMENT 16.2

HIV-Positive Patient

History	
Present Illness	When did you take the HIV antibody test? Why did you take the HIV antibody test? What brought you to the clinic today?
Past Medical History	Have you been to a health-care provider for HIV care? Do you know what your viral load is? What your CD4+ count (T-cell count) is? When were these tests last done? Have you had any opportunistic infections such as *Pneumocystis carinii* pneumonia or thrush? Were you ever hospitalized for these infections? What is your past medical history? Surgical history? Are you using any nontraditional therapies (alternative or complementary therapies)? If so, please explain.
Health History	What is your living situation (e.g., home life, support system [friends, relatives], financial situation, emotional situation, occupational situation, sexual relationships, safe sex)? What do you know about HIV infection?
Medication History	What HIV drugs have you taken in the past? How long were you on them? How long have you been off them? Have you been taking any medications for prophylaxis? Do you take them all the time, or do you take them some of the time? What other medications are you taking (prescription, over-the-counter, herbal)?
Nutritional History	Tell me about your usual diet. Do you eat raw eggs or raw fish? How do you cook your meat? Do you take any appetite enhancers? Do you take any nutritional supplements?
Travel History	Do you travel often? If so, where? Have you traveled or lived in other states or out of the country? If so, when?, where?, for how long?
Physical Examination	
General Overview and Mental Status	Level of consciousness Confusion Difficulty in remembering Change in mental status, mood Fatigue Change in activities of daily living
Neurologic System	Headaches and associated signs and symptoms Neurologic exam; cranial nerve exam
Respiratory System	Shortness of breath or dyspnea and associated signs and symptoms Cough and associated signs and symptoms Hiccups Lung sounds Respiratory rate, rhythm, characteristics; use of accessory muscle
Cardiovascular System	Heart sounds Pulse rate, rhythm, characteristics
Hematologic and Lymphatic System	Swollen, enlarged, or tender glands Night sweats, fever
Gastrointestinal System and Nutrition	Sores or white spots in mouth or lips; dental assessment Problems eating or swallowing Nausea/vomiting Change in weight, appetite Change in bowel habits (diarrhea, constipation) Nutritional intake Anorectal symptoms

HIV-Positive Patient

	Bowel sounds Enlarged liver or spleen Weight, anthropometric measurements
Reproductive System	For women: vaginal changes or discharge; pelvic exam For men: penile changes or discharge; prostate exam
Musculoskeletal System	Change in mobility (e.g., walking differently) Muscle bulk Range of motion Strength
Skin	Changes in skin (e.g., new flaking skin, new moles, new bruises or bumps) Rashes
Hearing	Change in hearing Therapies affecting the ears
Vision	Change in vision Therapies affecting the eyes

fast bacillus (AFB), which will detect the *Mycobacterium* family, a silver stain for PCP, blood cultures, and a bronchoscopy. For patients with neurologic symptoms, a referring physician should order a CT scan or MRI of the brain to check for the presence of ring-enhancing lesions, which could be associated with *Toxoplasma gondii*, or white matter that does not enhance, which could indicate PML.

If diarrhea is present, with or without other GI symptoms, the clinician should send stool cultures for infectious organisms.

Table 16.8 Diagnostic Tests in the HIV-Positive Patient

Test	Interpreting the Results
Complete Blood Count (CBC)	Anemia is common, may be related to HIV, infection, or medication (particularly AZT). Explore to find cause: bone marrow biopsy may be done; check for fungi, *M. avium* or tuberculosis, CMV, parvovirus, and malignancy. If anemia is related to medication, may need to prescribe erythropoietin (ProCrit).
Platelets	Thrombocytopenia is often seen: In early infection idiopathic thrombocytopenia purpura may be seen; in later infection the thrombocytopenia may be because of marrow suppression. Thrombocytopenia may also be seen with Kaposi's sarcoma.
Differential	Leukopenia is common; white blood cell counts less than 2000 are common and by themselves are not a cause for alarm. If using medications that cause neutropenia, may need to prescribe colony stimulating factors such as filgastrim (Neupogen)
Chemistry	Renal function may be impaired because of HIV nephropathy, volume depletion from diarrhea, or wasting. Elevated LDH may be nonspecific or related to PCP, lymphoma, hemolysis, or muscle wasting, or may be caused by HIV or AZT. Elevated triglycerides may be a response to cytokine activation. Low albumin levels may indicate malnutrition.
Purified Protein Derivative (PPD)	PPD induration of 5 mm or more is considered a positive reaction; no reaction may be caused by anergy; check chest x-ray.
CD4+ Cell Count (T cell count)	>500: at low risk for opportunistic infections. 500–200: low to moderate risk for opportunistic infections <200: high risk for opportunistic infections; prophylaxis for PCP, MAC may be needed while awaiting increase in T cell count in response to effective antiretroviral therapy To calculate absolute CD4+ count: number of WBC × % lymphs × %CD4+ = absolute CD4+ count
HIV Viral Load	A decrease in the HIV viral load indicates effective response to antiretroviral therapy: an increase in the viral load indicates disease progression.

Differential Diagnosis

The differential diagnoses are related to the pulmonary, neurologic, and GI systems. For pulmonary differential, consider TB, PCP, MAC, other bacterial, viral, fungal, or protozoal infections of the pulmonary system, and Kaposi's sarcoma. In the neurologic system, the clinician should consider a lymphoma or other malignancy. In the GI system, CMV, and disseminated MAC must be considered.

Management

Identifying the causative organism of the opportunistic infection is crucial for treatment. Therapy for the person with AIDS is both supportive, while trying to extend the patient's lifespan, and educational, in teaching the patient to avoid opportunistic infections. The CD4$^+$ T cell count (T cell count) serves as the major clinical indicator of immunocompetence in HIV-positive clients. When the CD4$^+$ T cell count falls below 200, the HIV-positive client is prone to opportunistic infections. PCP prophylaxis is required for CD4+ T cell counts less than 200 cells/mm^3; *Toxoplasmosis gondii* prophylaxis for counts less than 100 cells/mm^3, and MAC prophylaxis for counts less than 50 cells/mm^3.

Nursing Research–Based Practice 16.2 presents a vignette on caregiving of AIDS patients in a Thai population, which could be used to promote more awareness of the disease globally and encourage greater development of nursing interventions.

CMV

Several options are available for acute treatment. Ganciclovir (Cytovene) may be given 5 mg/kg IV q12h for 14 days (discontinue ZDV during induction); or foscarnet (Foscavir) 90 mg/kg IV q12h for 14 days may be given. The dose of either drug should be reduced in patients with renal failure. In addition, cidofovir (Vistide) 5 mg/kg IV may be given with probenecid (Benemid) for 1 week, then reduce to every 2 weeks. Cidofovir should not be used in patients with renal insufficiency. Also, a combination of foscarnet/ganciclovir, or intravitreal injections or implants of ganciclovir, which treats only the affected area, may be tried. For maintenance, ganciclovir 5 mg/kg IV qd or foscarnet 90 to 120 mg/kg IV qd may be ordered. Oral ganciclovir 1 g PO tid is not as effective but should be considered for systemic CMV coverage for patients with implants.

Herpes Zoster

Herpes zoster should be treated with acyclovir (Zovirax) 800 mg five times daily for 7 to 10 days or famciclovir (Famvir) 500 mg tid plus topical silver sulfadiazine for skin lesions. In severe cases, the patient may need IV acyclovir.

Herpes Simplex

For treatment of acute herpes simplex, the clinician should order acyclovir 200 to 400 mg TID for 7 to 10 days, or famciclovir 250 mg TID or valacyclovir 1 gram bid for 7 to 10 days. For suppressive treatment, acyclovir 400 mg bid for 3 to 7 days/week should be ordered. Foscarnet 40 mg/kg IV q8h for 10 days can be used for acyclovir-resistant herpes.

PML

There is no treatment for this progressively deteriorating disease. The clinician and referring physician should consider discussing hospice with the patient, family, or significant others.

Pneumocystis jiroveci pneumonia

There are two major options for prophylaxis of *Pneumocystis jiroveci* pneumonia. The first is trimethoprim-sul-

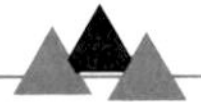

NURSING RESEARCH-BASED PRACTICE 16.2

Kespichayawattana, J and VanLandingham, M: Effects of coresidence and caregiving on health of Thai parents of adult children with AIDS. J Nurs Scholar 35(3):217–224, 2003.

This article talks about caregiving practices performed among Thai parents to their adult children dying from AIDS. The Thai culture views the mother as pure, good, and nurturing. The Thai culture has a strong maternal influence. Therefore it is not unusual for adult children dying from AIDS to return home to be cared for by their parents. The mother is usually the primary caregiver throughout the illness. Caregiving practices such as lifting, bathing, toileting, wound care, laundry, and meal preparations are some of the tasks provided by the caregivers. Parents define the work as strenuous which in turn affects their own health. Caregivers are also at risk for exposure to opportunistic infections. Caregivers experience pain, stress, confinement from taking care of their sick adult child, depression, insomnia, anxiety, feelings of helplessness, and bodily ailments. Despite the difficult work in providing care, the parents are encouraged to care for their dying children because it helps them to transition emotionally after their loved has expired. It is imperative to understand different cultures so that the appropriate nursing intervention can be applied effectively. The experiences of the Thai parents could be used to generate more awareness globally and could be used to assess and establish effective nursing interventions.

famethoxazole (TMP/SMZ, Bactrim, Septra), one double-strength (DS) tablet daily or three times per week. Prophylaxis may be better tolerated when begun with small doses and incremental increases, such as TMP/SMZ suspension 1 mL PO qd for 3 days, then 2 mL PO qd for 3 days, then 5 mL PO qd for 3 days, then 10 mL PO qd for 3 days, then 20 mL PO qd for 3 days, and then 1 DS TMP/SMZ tablet qd. A reported 10 to 40 percent of all patients on this oral course will develop a sulfa reaction and may need to consider a TMP/SMZ rechallenge. Dapsone (Avlosulfont) 100 mg PO qd or inhaled pentamidine (NebuPent) 300 mg every month can also be used for prophylaxis. For treatment of mild to moderate PCP, the clinician may use TMP/SMZ 15 mg TMP/kg qd divided tid PO or IV; pentamidine 4 mg/kg qd IV; dapsone 100 mg qd (check G-6-PD level) plus TMP 15 mg/kg qd divided tid; clindamycin 600 mg PO or IV tid plus primaquine (Primaquine) 30 mg qd; atovaquone (Mepron) 750 mg PO bid with meals plus pyrimethamine (Fansidar) 50 to 75 mg PO qd; or trimetrexate (Neutrexin) plus dapsone plus leucovorin (Wellcovorin), with continuation of therapy for 3 weeks before switching to maintenance therapy. Patients with acute PCP who develop respiratory distress may require hospitalization. The clinician should watch for signs of respiratory failure.

Cryptosporidium

There is no cure at this time. Paromycin may decrease the intensity of the infection and improve intestinal function. Spiramycin or dicalzuril may decrease diarrhea and oocyst number.

Diarrhea

For symptomatic relief of diarrhea, the patient may try loperamide (Imodium) 4 mg PO to start, then 2 mg q6h or after each bowel movement, up to 16 mg/day. Other options are diphenoxylate-atropine (Lomotil) 2.5 to 5 mg tid or paregoric 5 to 10 mL qid, or tincture of opium 0.3 to 1.0 mL qid and PRN, up to 6 mL/day. Alternative/complementary therapy, including acupuncture and moxibustion, have had reported effect on decreasing diarrhea and discomfort associated with diarrhea.

MAC

At CD4+ T cell counts less than 50 cells/mm^3, three drugs may be used for prophylaxis: azithromycin (Zithromax), two 600-mg tablets together (1200 mg) once a week; rifabutin (Mycobutin) 300 mg/day; or clarithromycin (Biaxin) 500 mg bid. However, prophylactic regimens readily induce multidrug resistance in MAC strains. Thus, prophylaxis should never be initiated until active MAC infection has been thoroughly ruled out in any patient who presents with suggestive constitutional symptoms of MAC, such as fever, malaise, fatigue, or chills. For acute treatment, use clarithromycin 500 mg bid or azithromycin 500 to 600 mg qd plus ethambutol 15 mg/kg per day, with or without rifabutin 300 mg qd. If the patient fails to respond, the provider should consider adding amikacin (Amikin) 10 mg/kg per day IV/IM for 1 to 2 months, or try ciprofloxacin or ofloxacin.

Mycobacterium tuberculosis

Several antiretroviral drugs are contraindicated or require dosage adjustments when co-administered with TB medications, so check for current guidelines for each HIV drug the patient is prescribed. For patients with a positive PPD, the provider should place the patient on isonicotinoylhydrazine (INH) (Isoniazid, Laniazid) 300 mg qd with pyridoxine 500 mg PO qd for 12 months. For active TB, start on INH 300 mg qd plus rifampin 600 mg plus pyrazinamide 15 to 30 mg/kg qd plus either ethambutol (Myambutol) 15 mg/kg qd or streptomycin 15 mg/kg IM qd (maximum 1 g). The treatment should be continued for 6 months (and 6 months beyond conversion). Pyrazinamide and ethambutol may be discontinued after 2 months, depending on susceptibility testing.

Cryptococcus

For acute treatment, use amphotericin B (Fungizone) 0.7 to 1.0 mg/kg IV qd for 14 days, with or without 5-flucytosine 100 mg/kg PO qid, then fluconazole (Diflucan) 400 mg qd or itraconazole 200 mg PO bid for 8 to 10 weeks. In milder cases, fluconazole 400 to 800 mg qd for 8 to 12 weeks may be used.

Toxoplasmosis

For acute treatment, use pyrimethamine 75 to 100 mg qd plus folinic acid (Wellcovorin) 10 to 20 mg qd plus either sulfadiazine 1 to 1.5 g PO qid, or clindamycin 600 to 900 mg PO qid, for 6 to 8 weeks. For prophylaxis, use TMP/SMZ DS qd or three times per week or dapsone 100 mg qd plus pyrimethamine 50 mg every week with folinic acid 25 mg per week. For maintenance suppressive therapy, use pyrimethamine 25 to 50 mg qd plus either sulfadiazine 1 g PO bid or clindamycin 300 to 450 mg qid.

Candidiasis

Oral candidiasis can be treated with fluconazole (Diflucan) 3 to 6 mg/kg (maximum of 100 mg/day) PO qd for 14 days. Antifungal prophylaxis is not typically initiated until after an AIDS patient is treated for his or her first fungal infection.

Kaposi's Sarcoma

Local treatment consists of cryotherapy, excision, intralesional vinblastine, or radiation; or systemic chemotherapy with vinblastine, vincristine, doxorubicin, liposomal doxorubicin, liposomal daunorubin, bleomycin, or paclitaxel.

Follow-Up and Referral

Clinical status determines how often a patient needs follow-up appointments. A CD4+ T cell count should be obtained every 3 to 6 months. Viral load should be determined when initiating or switching antiretroviral medication therapy, and a follow-up viral load must be done to determine effectiveness of medication regimen. Resistance testing should be considered if therapeutic response is not noted with HAART.

Referrals should be made depending on patient status. A referral should be made to an ophthalmologist whenever the patient complains of visual problems. Unresolved diarrhea or GI problems may require referral to a gastroenterologist. An oncology referral may be necessary for patients with Kaposi's sarcoma or if there is a suspicion of a malignancy.

Patient Education

Patient education is an ongoing process. It should include an ongoing review of health maintenance and HIV prevention behaviors. Patient education is particularly needed on early detection of visual problems and self-care to avoid opportunistic infections. Table 16.9 presents household infection precaution guidelines.

Because AIDS has taken on a "female face," as an increasing number of women have become affected, the need for women to use effective contraception and infection prevention methods has taken on a new urgency. In addition, women should be encouraged to get a Pap smear every 6 months because there is a higher prevalence of Pap smear, vaginal, and cervical abnormalities among HIV-infected women. If abnormalities are present, they tend to be more severe and progress more rapidly in these women.

All patients should be encouraged to complete advanced directives early in the course of the disease; the later the patient is approached, he or she may think that the clinician has additional information regarding his or her prognosis of which the patient is not aware. Lines of communication need to be keep open between the clinician, patient, significant other, and family.

Complementary Therapies 16.1 lists complementary therapies that may be useful for some conditions cited in this chapter.

Table 16.9 Household Infection Precaution Guidelines

Food and Cooking	• Sharing dishes and silverware is fine; wash them with hot soapy water between use. • Do not eat or drink raw or unpasteurized milk products (because of risk of *Salmonella* infection [food poisoning]). • Do not eat raw or undercooked meat (because of risk of toxoplasmosis or other infections); cook all meat to a temperature of at least 140°F. • Use a separate cutting board for raw meat and fish; all cutting boards should be plastic and have no nicks or scratches. • Cook or peel organic fruits and vegetables; many organic foods are composted with substances like manure that can contain infectious organisms. Avoid organic lettuce. • When cooking for other people, do not lick your fingers or taste food from the cooking spoon. Use a separate spoon to taste and only use it once.
Kitchen Cleaning	• Common mold and fungi found in the kitchen can be very dangerous to people with an impaired immune system. Use a cleansing agent to clean the kitchen counter; rinse area thoroughly. • Keep separate sponges for kitchen and bathroom. Always use clean sponges for washing counters and dishes; disinfect sponges by soaking them in a bleach solution (9 parts water to 1 part bleach) for 5 minutes. • To prevent mold from growing, frequently clean the inside of your refrigerator; use baking soda and water. • Mop the kitchen floor at least once a week and immediately clean up after spills. Pour mop water down the toilet, not the kitchen sink. • Keep the house well ventilated to prevent the spread of airborne infections. • Keep garbage in covered trash cans lined with plastic bags.
Bathroom Cleaning	• Use a bleach solution (9 parts water to 1 part bleach). to clean the shower, bathtub, and sink; mop the bathroom floor at least once a week and immediately clean up after any spills. • If any body fluids are spilled (blood, urine, feces, vomit, semen) clean them up first; then use a bleach solution (9 parts water to 1 part bleach). Do not use the bleach solution directly on body fluids (it may cause a terrible-smelling gas). • Use full-strength bleach to disinfect the toilet. • Do not share washcloths or towels without washing them in between use. • Never share toothbrushes, razors, or other personal equipment.
Pets	• If someone who does not have HIV cannot clean up after the pet, then wear gloves and wash hands thoroughly in hot soapy water afterward. • Change a cat's litter box every day. • Avoid handling turtles or cleaning their cages because of the risk of *Salmonella*.
Gardening	• Always wear gloves and wash hands thoroughly afterward.

COMPLEMENTARY THERAPIES 16.1

Problem and therapy	Dosage	Comment
Allergy		
Nettle	250–500 mg (standard extract) tid on an empty stomach.	May reduce seasonal allergy symptoms by inhibiting the release of histamine. Very little research is done on nettle.
Panthothenic acid (vitamin B_5)	500 mg tid	May help control nasal congestion related to allergies.
MSM (methylsulfonylmethane)	500 mg tid	May block histamine release and has anti-inflammatory properties.
Anemia		
Folic acid	400 mcg qd	Boosts production of RBCs.
Vitamin B complex		
Fatigue		
SAMe (*S*-adenosylmethionine)	400 mg bid	Studies show that SAMe alters the brain's response to pain, improves the quality of sleep, and releaves depression. Should not be taken with MAO inhibitors.
Alpha-lipoic acid	100–200 mg qd	Potent antioxidant and assists B vitamins to produce energy.
Vitamin C	1000 mg bid	Antioxidant, strengthens weakened immune system.
HIV		
Selenium	200 mcg qd	Is an antioxidant that helps prevent cellular damage from free radicals. Studies show that individuals with a low level of selenium had a more rapid HIV disease progression.
Alpha-lipoic acid	100–200 mg qd	Potent antioxidant and assists B vitamins produce energy (studies are ongoing).
General Immune System Boosters		
Coenzyme Q_{10}	100 mg qd	May boost immune system function (little research in this area). Safety during pregnancy and lactation has not been established.
Beta-glucans	500–1000 mg qd	Natural soluble fiber found in many foods. Activates macrophages and may increase immune response (little research). No known drug interactions or adverse effects
Vitamin A	5000 IU qd	Research has shown that patients with/who leukemia have high levels of vitamin A have better survival rates. Do not use with anti-acne medications.
Vitamin E	200–400 IU qd	Studies have shown improved immune responses in older adults who take vitamin E supplements and also acts as an antioxidant.

SOURCES: http://ods.od.nih.gov/factsheets/Selenium retrieved 12/27/2005
Bascom, A: Incorporating herbal medicine into clinical practice. Philadelphia: FA Davis, 2002.
http://www.wholehealthmd.com
Blumenthal, M, Goldberg, A, and Brinckmann, J (eds): Herbal Medicine Expanded Commission E Monographs. American Botanical Council, Austin, Tex; Integrative Medicine Communications, Newton, Mass. 2000.

Bibliography

General

Bishop, ML, Fody, EP, and Schoeff, L: Clinical Chemistry: Principles, Procedures, Correlations, ed 5. Lippincott Williams & Wilkins, Philadelphia, 2005.

Cavanaugh, BM: Nurse's Manual of Laboratory and Diagnostic Tests. FA Davis, Philadelphia, 2003.

Chernecky, CC, and Berger, BJ: Laboratory Tests & Diagnostic Procedures, ed 4. WB Saunders, Philadelphia, 2004.

Kasper, DL, Braunwald, E, Fauci, AS, Hauser, SI, Longo, DI, and Jameson, JL: Harrison's Manual of Medicine. McGraw-Hill, New York, 2005.

Murphy, JL (ed): Nurse Practitioners' Prescribing Reference. Prescribing Reference, New York (a division of Haymarket Media), 2005.

Running, A, and Berndt, A: Management Guidelines for Nurse Practitioners. FA Davis, Philadelphia, 2003.

Tierney, LM, McPhee, SJ, and Papadakis, MA: Current Medical Diagnosis & Treatment, ed 44. Lange Medical Books/McGraw-Hill, New York, 2005.

Anemias

Aggarwal, A, and Carr, PL: Work-up of women with anemia. Womens Health Primary Care 8(7):314–320, 2005.

Huffstutler, SY: Adult anemia. AdvNurse Pract 88–91, 2000.

Justice, KM: A streamlined workup for anemia. Clin Advisor 32–43, 2000.

Payne, SK, Cronk, JW, and Wheby, MS: Anemia: How to streamline the office evaluation. Consultant 2711–2719, 1999.

Fibromyalgia/CFS

Bobadilla, RV, Barnett, EM, and Randeis, CL: Cox-2 inhibitors and the heart–putting risk in perspective. Adv Nurse Pract 13(11):48–50, 2005.

Jones, KD, and Adams, DG: How to diagnose and treat fibromyalgia. Arthritis Pract 15–20, 2005.

Williams, GW: Determining the appropriate use of COX-2 imhibitors in pain management. A Practical Approach to Pain Management: A Therapeutic Update. A Supplement to Clin Advisor 9–14, 2005.

HIV/AIDS

CDC: Incorporating HIV Prevention into the Medical Care of Persons Living with HIV, MMWR Recommen Rep 52(RR-12); 1–24, July 18, 2003.

CDC: Revised Guidelines for HIV Counseling, Testing and Referral. MMWR RecommenRep 50 (RR19); 1–58, Nov 9, 2001.

CDC: Updated US Public Health Service Guidelines for the Management of Occupational Exposures to HIV and Recommendations for Postexposure Prophylaxis. MMWR Recommen Rep 54(RR-9), 1–17, Sept 30, 2005.

How HIV Causes AIDS. NIAID Fact Sheet, November 2004. National Institute of Allergy and Infectious Diseases, NIH, US DHHS. http://www.niaid.nih.gov/factsheets/howhiv.htm Accessed January 29, 2006.

Jones, SG: The other side of the pill bottle: The lived experience of HIV^{+} nurses on HIV combination drug therapy. J Assoc Nurses AIDS Care 13(3):22–36, 2002.

Jones, SG: Primary care: Promoting sexual health and HIV prevention through risk assessment and client education. Nurse Pract Forum 12(4):181–191, 2001.

Kirton, C (ed): ANAC's Core Curriculum for HIV/AIDS Nursing, ed 2. SAGE, Thousand Oaks, 2003.

Panel on Clinical Practices for Treatment of HIV Infection, DHHS: Guidelines for the Use of Antiretroviral Agents in HIV-1-Infected Adults and Adolescents, October 6, 2005. Available at http://www.aidsinfo.nih.gov

UNAIDS: AIDS Epidemic Update, December 2005. Available at http://www.unaids.com

Yen-Lieberman, B: HIV-1 Viral load testing and Roche Diagnostics assay kits. Infect Med 18(9):417–427, 2001.

Rheumatoid Arthritis

Savage, C, St. Clair, EW, and Sundy, JS: Emerging Treatments for Rheumatoid Arthritis: Update. Consultant 984–995, 2005.

Resources

Fibromyalgia/CFS

National Fibromyalgia Association
http://www.fmaware.org
American Fibromyalgia Syndrome Association, Inc.
http://www.afsafund.org
National Fibromyalgia Research Association (NFRA)
http://www.nfra.net
CFIDS (Chronic Fatigue and Immune Dysfunction Syndrome) Association of America
http://www.cfids.org

HIV/AIDS

National Pediatric AIDS Network
http://www.npan.org
AIDS Resource List
http://www.specialweb.com/aids
The Center for AIDS
http://www.centerfor aids.org
American Public Health Association
http://www.apha-hivaids.org
National Pediatric and Family HIV Resource Center
http://pedhivaids.org
HIV Consumer Council
http://www.hivcouncil.org
The H.O.P.E. Foundation
http://www.hopedc.org
HIV/AIDS Treatment Information Service
U.S. Dept. of Health and Human Services
http://www.aidsinfo.nih.gov
Office of National AIDS Policy
The White House
http://www.whitehouse.gov/onap/aids.html
Centers for Disease Control (CDC) and Prevention
National Prevention Information Network
http://www.cdcnpin.org

Allergies and Infectious Diseases

National Institute of Allergy and Infectious Diseases
National Insitutes of Health
http://www3.niaid.nih.gov

Autoimmune Diseases

American Autoimmune Related Disease Association
http://www.aarda.org
The Lupus Foundation of America
http://www.lupus.org

Pain

American Pain Society
http://www.ampainsoc.org
International Association for the Study of Pain
http://www.iasp-pain.org

Sickle Cell Anemia

Sickle Cell Disease Association of America, Inc.
http://www.sicklecelldisease.org

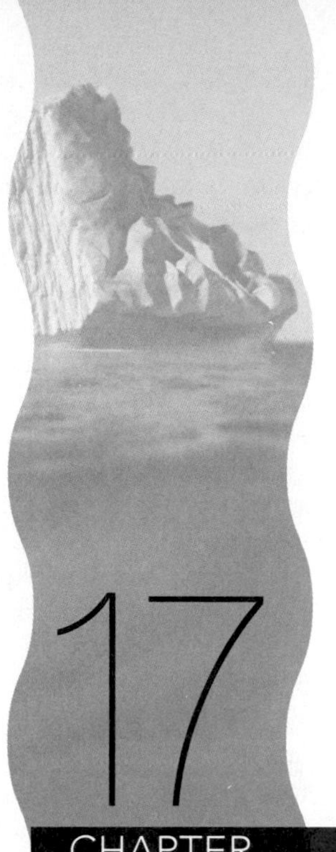

Psychosocial Problems

Lynne M. Dunphy, PhD, MSN, APRN, BC
Linda Denise Oakley, PhD, RN

Common Complaints

Anxiety

For most people, *anxiety* is an unpleasant state of physical and psychological arousal that interferes with effective psychosocial functioning. Mild anxiety is a normal fact of life and can be positive; however, severe or chronic anxiety can become debilitating. Mental defense mechanisms are the first line of protection against increases in anxiety. Defenses make it possible for a person to psychologically defend against and/or reduce anxiety. Effective defense mechanisms can reducc both the physical and psychological arousal symptoms of anxiety. Inadequate or ineffective defenses do not reduce anxiety. A range of unconscious, semiconscious and conscious psychological defense mechanisms have been defined (Table 17.1).

The types of defenses a person employs will vary with age and circumstances. For example, younger people tend to use more immature defenses which are less effective; likewise acutely ill people tend to regress and use fewer mature defenses. Ineffective, immature defenses such as as denial reduce anxiety but undermine effective coping. Over the long run, the person with ineffective defenses becomes more rather than less vulnerable to anxiety. Few people can tolerate anxiety for long; thus those with a lack of effective defenses are more likely to engage in ineffective coping behaviors, or negative anxiety-relief behavior. They strive to escape their anxiety. An anxious person who tends to deny and rationalize reality may use substances such as food, alcohol, or drugs to escape from anxiety. For some people, certain mood states such as apathy, anger, and procrastination are less distressing than anxiety. The long-term effect of negative anxiety-relief behaviors are almost always additional anxiety.

Anxiety symptoms are typically manifested in several dimensions: affective, cognitive, behavioral and somatic. Affectively, anxiety is an experience of dread, foreboding, or panic, often accompanied by autonomic hyperactivity—primarily sympathetic—manifested as bodily symptoms. The affective component is typically countered

Table 17.1 Defense Mechanisms

- *Repression:* Ongoing process of forgetting or pushing thoughts, feelings, experiences into the unconscious.
- *Denial:* Ongoing or selective process of refusing to acknowledge reality that is apparent to others.
- *Rationalization:* Acceptable explanations for the unacceptable
- *Isolation:* To detach or separate thoughts and feelings that are connected.
- *Displacement:* To generalize, disconnect, or redirect a feeling regarding a person, object, or experience, then attribute that feeling to a less threatening substitute person, object, or experience.
- *Projection:* Attributing internal experiences to others or to circumstances.
- *Regression:* To retreat from a later stage of growth and development to an earlier or younger stage.
- *Intellectualization:* Abstract thinking to avoid the experience of intense feelings.
- *Sublimation:* To neutralize intense or unacceptable internal experiences into experiences that are less intense and more acceptable.
- *Humor:* Conscious effort to find the lighter aspects of emotionally heavy experiences or circumstances.
- *Suppression:* Intentional act of excluding disturbing thoughts, feelings, and experiences from awareness.

by cognitions that seek to make sense of or minimize the discomfort. Some other affective symptoms of anxiety are apprehension, fear, irritability, intolerance, frustration, and overreaction or hypersensitivity to personal feelings of shame. Behaviors such as avoidance, distractibility, and restlessness reflect the anxiety or may evolve in response to it. Behavioral symptoms of anxiety may include apathy, compulsions, rigidity, overreactions, preoccupation, and repetitive actions such as hair pulling or nail biting. Somatic symptoms of anxiety range in intensity from a loss of appetite, dry mouth, and fatigue, to diarrhea, sweating, chest pain, hyperventilation, vomiting, and paresthesias. Highly anxious persons may experience the full range of anxiety symptoms or may have only one or two symptoms. The classification of *anxiety disorders* is largely based on clinical presentation (Table 17.2).

Anxiety affects approximately 40 million adults; thus it is the most common psychiatric disorder in the United States. It most commonly presents in the 20- to 45-year-old age group and affects women more frequently than it does men.

Table 17.2 Physiologic Causes of Anxiety

- *Cancers:* Carcinoid syndrome, pancreatic cancer, lung cancer, pheochromocytoma
- *Cardiac:* Mitral valve prolapse, arrhythmia, congestive heart failure (CHF), ischemic heart disease
- *Pulmonary:* Asthma, chronic obstructive pulmonary disease (COPD), sleep apnea, pulmonary embolism, hypercapnia, hypoxia
- *Neurologic:* Ménière's disease, cerebral vascular accident (CVA—"stroke"), transient ischemic attack (TIA), multiple sclerosis, encephalopathy, subdural hematoma
- *Hematologic:* Anemia
- *Metabolic:* Thyroid disease, hyperparathyroidism, Cushing's syndrome, Addison's disease, hypoglycemia, hyperglycemia, hyponatremia, hypokalemia
- *Nutritional:* Folate deficiency, vitamin B_{12} deficiency, iron deficiency

Medications and Medication Side Effects

Significant anxiety can develop as an adverse effect of prescribed or over-the-counter (OTC) medications. Medications commonly associated with drug-induced anxiety include:

- *Prescription drugs:* Aminophylline, digitalis, dopamine, epinephrine, levodopa, lidocaine, neuroleptics, NSAIDs, steroids, SSRIs, theophylline, sympathomimetics, thyroid preparations
- *OTC drugs:* Certain decongestants containing ephedrine and pseudoephedrine, caffeine, certain cough syrups, salicylates (in large doses), nicotine, monosodium glutamate, phenylpropanolamine
- *Herbals:* Ephedrine, ginseng, yohimbine
- *Illicit drugs:* Alcohol, amphetamines, marijuana, cocaine, ecstasy (methamphetamine), hallucinogenics, caffeine
- *Others:* Organic solvents

Differential Diagnosis

The primary care provider must differentiate between patients with a relatively mild and transient anxiety state, often externally situated, and patients with a pervasive and more debilitating anxiety disorder. To do this, all primary-care clinicians should be familiar with the latest (fourth as of this printing) edition of the Diagnostic and Statistical Manual of Mental Disorders, Fourth Edition, Text Revision (DSM-IV-TR), as well as the version prepared for primary care providers prepared by the American Psychiatric Association (APA) in collaboration with a variety of other organizations such as the American Academy of Family Physicians. (See Advanced Assessment 17.1 for an overview of the DSM-IV-TR diagnostic classification system and Advanced Assessment 17.2 for information on how to use in primary care.)

A variety of psychiatric disorders, such as mood disorders, certain psychoses, dementias, and substance-abuse disorders present with anxiety as a prominent part of their constellation of symptomatology. This can pose considerable diagnostic and treatment challenges for the primary-care clinician. For example, anywhere from 42 to 100 percent of depressed patients (average 67 percent) have anxiety symptoms and 33 percent of depressed patients have panic attacks. In addition, 17 to 65 percent (average 40 percent) of anxious patients have depressive symptoms; 33 percent of patients with panic disorder have depressive symptoms.

Many medical conditions in which there is stimulation of the sympathetic nervous system mimic anxiety, complicating the diagnosis. For example, undiagnosed arrhythmias, metabolic conditions, as well as drug reactions, may all manifest as anxiety (Table 17.3). In all cases, potential physical explanations for anxiety symptoms should be evaluated first. The extreme variability of the presentation of the symptom of anxiety in primary care make it one of the most commonly seen complaints. Several of these specific diagnoses are developed and presented later in this chapter.

Depression

Another common psychosocial symptom seen in primary-care settings is depression. Depression is common for many reasons. People use the term *depression* to describe a wide variety of negative emotional experiences, ranging from sadness to disinterest in pleasurable activities to self-hate. The hallmarks of major depression are sadness and apathy. In most cases, the sadness and apathy associated with major depression can be distinguished from ordinary changes in mood.

The variety of experiences that people refer to as depression reflects the complexity of this universal human experience. Experiences of depression include depression as a passing mood, a personality trait, an acute illness episode, and a disabling chronic illness. Moreover, distress

ADVANCED ASSESSMENT 17.1

The Diagnostic and Statistical Manual of Mental Disorders

The DSM-IV-TR is a descriptive manual of mental disorders authored by the American Psychiatric Association to provide clear descriptions of diagnostic categories in order to enable clinicians and investigators to diagnose, communicate about, study, and treat people with various mental disorders. The specified diagnostic criteria for each mental disorder are offered as guidelines for making diagnoses. It has been demonstrated that the use of such criteria enhances agreement among clinicians and investigators. All of the diagnostic codes included in the DSM-IV-TR are all official ICD-9-CM codes. Each clinical axis represents a specific level of assessment. Precise DSM-IV-TR criteria have been defined for each DSM-IV-TR diagnosis, but practitioners will routinely encounter patients with symptoms that, although significant, do not fully meet DSM-IV-TR diagnostic criteria. Comorbid (concurrent) disorders are frequently encountered.

Clinical Axis

Axis I: Clinical Disorder or Focus of Clinical Attention: It is customary to list the Axis I disorder currently being treated first when the patient has a history of disorders or has more than one current disorder. Axis I disorders may be specified as current, partial remission, full remission, or prior history.

Axis II: Personality Disorder and Developmental Disorder: Axis II disorders differ from Axis I disorders in that they have a much longer duration. Symptom onset for Axis II disorders begins in childhood or adolescence and are viewed by some third-party payers as "trait disorders" meaning something not amenable to treatment, and inappropriate for the same. Patients with Axis II disorders frequently also have one or more Axis I disorders.

Axis III: Physical Health: General medical conditions such as diabetes or hypertension and current physical health status are assessed at Axis III. Conditions that require ongoing treatment, recently treated illness, or surgical procedures should also be noted at this axis. When a physical condition is the cause of an Axis I disorder, it is noted as such at Axis I.

Axis IV: Psychosocial and Environmental Problems: Axis IV problems are current problems that have developed within the previous year or in some way currently impact the person or the person's life. Problems that occurred or started a long time ago may be considered if the problem is associated with a current disorder such as post-traumatic stress disorder or alcohol abuse. Axis IV problems are self-defined. Any set of circumstances that is subjectively troubling for the person is considered.

Axis V: Psychosocial Functioning: Clinically significant changes in psychosocial functioning can develop in relation to the onset or persistence of a mental disorder or psychosocial problem. Because psychosocial functioning is such a broad area of assessment, the specific areas of Axis V functioning are social, occupational, and academic which is added up and called the Global Assessment of Functioning (GAF) score, with a scale from 1–100. A score of 40 or lower indicates severe disruption in functioning.

Using DSM-IV-TR Symptom Criteria

Specific symptom criteria are listed and defined for all DSM-IV-TR disorders and problems. In most cases these criteria include symptom type, number, intensity, and duration. To meet the symptom criteria for a particular disorder, the patient must have experienced the minimal number of specified symptoms for a defined period of time and the symptoms experienced should be sufficient to cause distress or impair psychosocial functioning. Persons who have fewer symptoms, of less duration, or less intensity, may have an atypical form of the disorder, or their condition may be described as subclinical. The term subclinical does not imply that treatment is unnecessary. Atypical symptoms and subclinical symptoms can cause significant distress.

Using DSM-IV-TR Distress Criteria

Symptomatic patients typically report subjective distress. However, a patient's distress may also be observed by others or assessed by the practitioner. There are no absolute measures of symptom-induced distress: Symptoms that are highly distressing to one person may be only mildly distressing to another. The experience of distress should not be confused with the manner in which a person expresses his or her distress. It is possible for a highly distressed person who is suffering a great deal to have trouble expressing his or her distress, whereas others may be able to describe their distress in painful detail. Whether or not a distressed person is expressive should not overly influence the assessment. Often, simple verbal statements of symptom-related discomfort and suffering are sufficient.

of any nature, duration, or intensity can cause depression or include elements of depression as a symptom. For example, symptoms of physical exhaustion or boredom can include depression. Intense or chronic sadness or apathy should be considered symptoms of a depressive disorder. Low mood or disinterest that is relieved by a change in circumstances is not likely to be a symptom of a depressive disorder, however.

Elements of depression that make up the core experience of depression, regardless of the form, are presented in Table 17.4.

No description of depression, whether as a symptom or disorder, is complete without addressing the psychological pain and suffering of depression. The pain of depression can become so severe that some depressed persons are willing to go to any length to obtain even a moment

ADVANCED ASSESSMENT 17.2

Using DSM-IV-TR in Primary Care

- DSM-IV-TR Primary Care Version (DSM-IVPC) 1995 emphasizes psychiatric disorders that regularly present in primary care settings.
- Contains 9 *Algorithms for Common primary Care Presentations* with step-by-step procedures for confirming a psychiatric diagnoses.
- Decision tree that matches the patient's presenting symptoms to appropriate algorithm
- Appendix contains "Symptom Index for Common Presentations" arranged in alphabetical and topical order.
- Provides criteria that helps rule out whether symptoms are best accounted for by direct physiologic consequence of substance intoxication or withdrawal, medication effects, toxin exposures, or general medical condition.
- Characterized by a unitary model of psychiatric and physical disorders that replaces what can be an artificial distinction between the realms of "organic" and "functional."
- Psychosocial/Environmental Checklist
- Limited attention to hard-to-diagnose personality disorders
- DSM-IV-TR encompasses a variety of biopsychosocial parameters, but this multi-axial schema is not emphasized in DSM-IVPC.
- Use of DSM-IVPC requires level of familiarity before use.

of relief. Depression-related thoughts of death or suicide are not uncommon. Yet the pain of depression can be difficult to articulate: The depressed person may only be able to make vague references to "hurting" or "feeling bad." The pain and distress of depression can fuel negative coping behaviors. When severely depressed, a person may behave in ways that are intended to relieve the pain and distress, with little regard for the consequences. For example, depressed persons may intentionally avoid work, school, or people. Self-abusive behavior is also common. Depressed persons may abuse food, alcohol, or drugs in an attempt at self-medication to relieve their pain. Reckless gambling, spending, or sexual behavior can also occur. Valued relationships may be neglected or abused. Two common exceptions to this pattern are depressed persons who shut down and become numb to everything, including their depression, and persons who experience depression as a physical illness or somatic symptoms, such as headaches and stomach aches. (See Nursing Research–Based Practice 17.1.)

People learn "appropriate" ways to express sadness or depression. Social groups, families, and communities establish norms that govern important aspects of life. However, each person decides if he or she will conform to, modify, or reject these norms. Individual variations in the clinical presentation of depression can be great, sometimes making the condition difficult to recognize. The more common patient presentation of depression in primary-care settings is the person who has moderate to severe feelings of sadness or apathy that he or she attributes to depression. Common presentations also include complaints of unexplained fatigue, irritability, anger, anxiety, and hyperactivity. Many deeply depressed persons are unaware of their depression. Slowed thinking and emotional numbness—two severe symptoms of depression—can contribute to minimal self-awareness of depression. Gender can affect presentation, but gender should not influence assessment.

Ethnic variations in the presentation of depression are also individualized, based on how traditional or nontraditional the individual's attitudes and behaviors are. For example, Asian, African American, and Hispanic American patients have been described as tending to have a somatic presentation when depressed. The term *somatic* means that the report of depression includes more physical than emotional symptoms. Ethnic variations in the presentation of depression also reflect ethnic differences in the standards of appropriate conduct when interacting with health-care professionals. Members of ethnic groups that endorse formal interactions with health-care professionals may focus less on personal experiences, and more on physical aches and pains. Ethnic norms concerning privacy, embarrassment, and disclosure will have an impact on the patient's presentation.

Differential Diagnosis

Numerous types of depressive disorders have been defined and new disorders continue to be proposed. The current DSM-IV-TR list of depression disorders includes major depression, bipolar II disorder, cyclothymic disorder, mood disorder due to general medical condition, and substance-induced mood disorders. Depression may also be classified as seasonal pattern depression, psychotic depression, depression with catatonic features, depression with melancholic features, and postpartum-onset depression. As noted in the preceding text, there are significant overlaps between depressive and anxiety disorders. Comorbid depression and anxiety is the rule, not the exception, with a worse prognosis and increased suicide risk. Further elaboration of these various differential diagnoses appear later in this chapter. (See Advanced Assessment 17.3 for information on a tool that can help distinguish between various disorders.)

Common Problems

Grief

Grief, mourning, and bereavement are terms that define a universal human response to loss. Specifically, *grief* refers to the individual's multidimensional response to the loss of a loved one and encompasses psychologic, behavioral, and physical reactions with cognitive, emotional, behavioral,

Table 17.3 Classification of Anxiety Disorders

Disorder	Features
Generalized Anxiety Disorder (GAD)	• Occurs more days than not, for at least 6 months • Excessive anxiety and worry about a number of things • Inability to control worry • Associated with three or more symptoms: easily fatigued, difficulty concentrating, inability, muscle tension, sleep disturbance, feeling "hyper," feelings of restlessness
Anxiety Disorder due to a general medical problem	• General anxiety, panic, other manifestations as a direct physiologic consequence of a general medical problem
Substance-Induced Anxiety Disorder	• General anxiety, panic, other manifestations directly related to medication usage, intoxication, or withdrawal
Anxiety Disorder Not Otherwise Specified	• Prominent and persistent anxiety and/or phobic avoidance that does not meet full criteria of any other anxiety disorder
Acute Stress Response	• Exposure to traumatic event or threat of death or serious injury to self and/or others • Response to event is terror, helplessness, intense fear • Three or more dissociative symptoms experienced during or after event: numbing, detachment, depersonalization, amnesia re: aspects of the event, absence of appropriate event response • Event reexperienced • Increased arousal • Disorder lasts 2 days to a maximum of 4 weeks and occur within 4 weeks of event
Posttraumatic Stress Disorder (PTSD)	• Exposure to traumatic events that involved actual or threat of severe injury to self and/or others • Response involves terror, helplessness, intense fear • Event is consistently re-experienced by upsetting dreams, acting/feeling as if event is reoccurring, physiologic reactivity, intrusive image re: event, intrusive thoughts re: event, intense distress on exposure to certain triggers • Numbing • Increased arousal from sleep, sleep disturbances, angry outbursts/instability, hypervigilance, exaggerated startle response • Lasts longer than 1 month
Panic Disorder (with or without agoraphobia)	• Intense fear • Must be manifested by four or more of the following: chills/hot flushes, depersonalization, fear of losing control, fear of dying, fear of going crazy, paresthesias, sweating, palpitations, shortness of breath, choking, chest pain, GI distress
Agoraphobia (with or without Panic Disorder)	• Fear of being in places where the individual cannot escape • Situations causing fear are avoided • Fear of panic symptoms
Obsessive–Compulsive Disorder (OCD)	• *Obsessions:* Recurrent and persistent intrusive and inappropriate thoughts that cause significant anxiety, despite attempts to neutralize such thoughts • *Compulsions:* Repetitive acts and/or behaviors in response to obsessive thoughts, aimed at decreasing anxiety
Specific Phobias	• Unreasonable and excessive fear (not based in reality) in response to a specific object and/or situation • Exposure to specific object and/or situation causes immediate and intense anxiety, fear
Social Phobias	• Unreasonable (not based in reality) excessive fear of social and/or performance situations • Fear of social humiliation

Source: Adapted from the Diagnostic and Statistical Manual of Mental Disorders, ed 4 (DSM-IV-TR). American Psychiatric Association, Washington, DC, 2000.

social, spiritual, and somatic components. *Mourning* describes the process by which grief is resolved. The word mourning tends to imply "normal and uncomplicated" grief. Mourning is a highly personal experience that allows one to achieve acceptance of a loss; grief is a process of well-defined stages. The actual differences between mourning and grief may be more conceptual than clinical, however, in that both begin with shock and distress and end with acceptance and improvement. *Bereavement* refers to the objective situation of having lost a family member or close friend through death and refers to being in a state of mourning. In thinking of these terms as a response to loss,

(Text continued on page 994)

Table 17.4 Elements Influencing the Complaint of Depression

Stress and Depression

An accepted fact of life today is that ordinary people spend most of their time working, leaving very little time for the "rest, relationships, and restoration" needed for mental health and well-being. Among the many factors shown to precede the onset, persistence, and recurrence of depressive disorders, stress or stressful life events are by far the most powerful predictors. A high-demand, low-reward lifestyle can make a person more vulnerable to stress-induced depression. Biochemical and psychosocial models of depression both include acute or chronic stress as a predictor of depression.

Unfortunately, what might appear to be a simple equation is not. Although the relationship between stress and depression has been identified, stress is highly individualized. What is stressful for one person may not be stressful for another. The connection between stress and depression may be mediated by each person's ability to cope with stress effectively. Stressful life experiences can be actual, perceived, or potential events that a person may have full, partial, or no awareness of. Therefore, the relationship between stress and depression should be thought of in the broadest possible terms. For example, a romantic relationship with many problems suddenly becomes a very stressful, failed romance. In this example, the stress that induces depression could be a failed romance, persistent relationship problems, or both. The most powerful and universal stressful life events associated with depression include poverty, loss, illness, abuse, unemployment, isolation, discrimination, substance abuse, and violence.

Biochemistry

Significant advances in biochemical depression research have made it possible to develop sophisticated models of serotonin and norepinephrine (NE) as key mood-manager neurotransmitters related to depression. Experts have also identified critical aspects of the pathophysiology and psychosocial impairments of depression. The most promising biochemical models of depression hypothesize that depression involves a dysregulation of serotonin and NE activity, with concurrent negative physiological alterations in related cellular structures. Neurotransmitter dysregulation may play a part in the psychological interaction between growth and development, learned responses to life stress, and family genetic background as depression risk factors. Prior to these advances, much of what was understood about the biochemical, pathophysiological, and psychosocial processes of depression had been based on clinical observations of depressed patients. Researchers now are able to develop extremely precise explanatory biochemical models of depressive illness. Based on these models, the most effective antidepressant medications appear to be those that can target specific serotonin and NE subgroups and subgroup-subtypes at specific receptor sites in the brain. Presently, newer antidepressants increase serotonin and NE brain activity. Thus, the fundamental biochemical model of depression is neurotransmitter depletion or receptor down-regulation.

Circadian Rhythm Dysregulation

Circadian rhythms can play a role in the onset of depression symptoms and in the ability to recover from depression disorders. However, compared to the biochemical neurotransmitter models of depression, circadian rhythm dysregulation is less well understood. Presently, it is theorized that various biological "clocks" govern various psychological and physical processes, including mood. One of the many functions of the 24-hour circadian clock is to coordinate the biological systems that operate in cycles to produce sleep. The 24-hour circadian sleep-wake cycle is one of the many important interfaces between humans and their various environments.The activity of brain melatonin, a metabolite of serotonin, appears to be affected by exposure to environmental light and darkness within the 24-hour sleep-wake cycle. Seasonal depression may be associated with seasonal disruptions in sleep and serotonin activity. Winter depression may be the result of decreased hours of light causing decreased levels of melatonin.

Family Transmission

Having a family history of mood disorders has long been recognized as a personal risk factor for depressive disorders. A family history of depression is not a predictor of depression disorder, however. Of the family transmission models of depression that have been developed thus far, the genetic inheritance model and the family stress model best address some of the more perplexing aspects of depression disorders in families. Compelling research evidence has established genetic inheritance as the key to the family transmission of bipolar disorder. However, researchers are still grappling with the mechanisms of family history as a risk factor for other forms of depression disorder, such as major depression. Generally speaking, having a family history of any type of mood disorder increases the risk of depression disorder for family members.

Family history as a depression risk factor is nonspecific. An adult with major depression could have a family history of major depression, bipolar disorder, or dysthymic disorder. Fifty percent of adults with bipolar I disorder, for example, are children of at least one parent with a mood disorder, with the most common disorder being major depression. Looking at the same risk in the opposite way, an individual with bipolar disorder has a 25% higher risk of having at least one child with some form of mood disorder. In practice, the individual impact of a family history of depression must be determined on a case-by-case basis. A family history of depression cannot predict which family member will develop a mood disorder, the type of mood disorder a relative may develop, or when symptom onset will occur.

Depression disorders have interpersonal elements that make it possible for a depressed person to communicate the experience of depression to a person who is not depressed. This transmission appears to be greatest when there is a significant relationship between the depressed and nondepressed person. For example, depressed parents can greatly increase the risk of depression in their children because, for the child, interactions with a depressed caregiver can be highly stressful. Or a depressed parent may unintentionally model depression as a normal mood state, in which case the child is at risk for learning to be depressed. Depressed parents can find it difficult, if not impossible, to meet their child's emotional needs, creating a psychological deficit that could increase the child's risk of depression.

Self-Conflict

Each person has a psychological self-view of who they are, who they would like to be, who they feel they should be, and how others view them. When differences between these four self-views are small, the person experiences normal levels of self-conflict. When differences among these self-views are significant, the person can become subject to deep psychological conflict that becomes focused on or aimed against the self. This self-conflict is experienced as severe psychological stress, which, like other forms of stress, can result in the onset of depression symptoms. Sometimes this process is called anger turned inward. This is a gross oversimplification of a complex psychological process. A more accurate description would be to say that such a person is at war with him or herself—a war that cannot be won. Lack of self-acceptance and the resulting "eternal-internal"struggle with oneself is associated with depression. Having an adequate level of self-acceptance based on a realistic self-view decreases the risk of depression associated with psychodynamic self-conflict.

Helpless-Hopelessness

Learned helplessness is a cognitive theory of depression having to do with a specific set of learned negative beliefs that increase susceptibility to depression. Depression has been associated with the belief that hoped-for goals cannot be obtained and feared outcomes cannot be avoided. This hopeless thinking supports helpless behavior. Hopeless thinking and helpless behaviors are thought to represent lessons learned from critical negative life experiences in which the person tried but was unable to exert control over his or her circumstances. For example, a person with internalized learned helplessness may have difficulty meeting important performance goals at school or work. According to learned helplessness theory, school and work are situations that call for effective action, but if a person has learned from previous experience that his or her efforts will not be effective, his or her behavior becomes helpless, leading to performance failures. Performance failures reinforce hopeless thinking and persistent helpless behavior.

A key assumption of learned helplessness theory is that individuals who actively strive to obtain desired goals, regardless of whether or not their efforts are successful, are less susceptible to depression than those who, due to helpless thinking, are unable to strive. Helpless-hopelessness theory does not apply to individuals who consciously choose to avoid meeting ordinary demands. Two drawbacks of this popular model of depression are that helpless behavior can also develop as a symptom of depression, and hopelessness is a common response to horrific life circumstances, such as poverty and family violence.

Negative Cognitive-Behavioral Patterns

The premise of the cognitive theory of depression is that depression is associated with persistent, global negative distortions about life in general, about oneself, and about the future. Negative thinking is stressful. Although fixed patterns of negative thinking such as these have been generally accepted as powerful correlates of depression, the model is not without important limitations. As with the hopeless-helplessness model, negative thoughts may not always represent distortions of reality. Horrific life circumstances produce negative views about life, oneself, and the future without being distortions. For example, a woman who has suffered abuse and poverty may develop highly negative views of herself, life, and the future that increase her risk for depression, but her views should not necessarily be considered distorted.

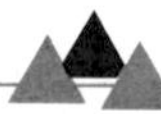

NURSING RESEARCH-BASED PRACTICE 17.1

Postpartum Depression

Beck, CT: Teetering on the edge: A substantive theory of postpartum depression. Nurs Res 42(1):42–48, 1993.

This classic, grounded theory study utilized a qualitative approach to develop theory regarding women's perceptions of postpartum depression. Drawing a sample of 12 from a postpartum support group, the researcher conducted in-depth interviews with the women about their experiences of postpartum depression. What emerged was a rich description of the nature of postpartum depression and how these women managed their depression. "Teetering on the edge" was the hallmark metaphor that the researcher extracted to describe the process that the participants confronted during their depression. They felt "between" sane and insane, and the researcher identified several stages: "Encountering the terror" described the unpredictable nature of feelings that overwhelmed them, anxiety and panic attacks, obsessions, and loss of concentration. In the next stage, called "the dying of self," the women experienced isolation, withdrawal, and feelings of dissociation and depersonalization. Most had suicidal ideation. In the next stage, "struggling to survive," they began to grapple with their feelings. They searched out support groups, used prayer and faith to manage the depression, and began, hesitantly, and with some steps forward and some steps backward, to recover.

Women are at highest risk of developing postpartum depression from a few days to 6 months following childbirth. APNs need to be aware of this type of depression and be alert to it. They need to educate others about the phenomenon and truly understand the meaning of the experience to these women. They need to understand. They need to "hear" the voices of these women, "teetering on the edge."

ADVANCED ASSESSMENT 17.3

Screening and Diagnostic Tool

PRIME-MD

The PRIME-MD is a two-stage instrument that assesses common mood, anxiety, eating, alcohol, and somatoform disorders. It has a self-report *screening/case finding* component, the Patient Questionnaire (PQ) to be administered *PRIOR* to the clinical encounter. It consists of 25 Yes/No questions about signs and symptoms present during the previous month and one question about the patient's overall health. The questions are divided into five groups corresponding to the five categories of mental disorders assessed by the PRIME-MD.

The diagnostic component, the Clinician Evaluation Guide (CEG), is a branching-logic, clinician-administered interview, subdivided into five modules to address the categories revealed by the patient's self-report (PQ). The average time to administer the PRIME-MED CEG and review this tool is 8.5 minutes for all subjects and 11 minutes for those who have a PRIME-MD diagnosis. Overall accuracy is 85%, sensitivity is 75%, and specificity is 90%. This tool is available in a number of different languages.

A current version of the PRIME-MD, the Patient Health Questionnaire (PHQ), increases the efficiency of PRIME-MD by making the entire screening and diagnostic process largely self-report and taking only 3 minutes of the clinician's time. The PHQ is four pages long and contains questions similar to those in PRIME-MD-CEG. However, the PHQ contains questions specific to women, with questions dealing with menstruation pregnancy, and childbirth. The completed PHQ provides the clinician with most of the symptom-based information required to make the diagnoses at the beginning of the interview. This then allows the clinician to take more time for an assessment of the patient's life-situation and personal history. This tool was designed for a low-health-literacy population, but the tool may still prove difficult for some patients to fill in by themselves. This is especially so with the elderly patient, immigrants, and persons with low-educational attainment. These populations are all at risk for mental disorders. Information from the PHQ can provide baseline data for some disorders and may prove useful in tracking the patient's response and progress over time with repeated administrations.

the definitions are broadened to include loss of anything or anyone significant to the person—a job, a limb, the state of health, or a pet. The circumstances and meaning of the loss are always an important consideration. Was this a miscarriage, divorce, or murder? Did the loss involve a spouse, a parent, a chid?

Epidemiology and Causes

More than three million Americans died in 2003, leaving behind 18 to 22 million bereaved family members. There have been more than 2000 deaths as of this writing from the war in Iraq, leaving behind children, wives, husbands, and relatively young parents. In addition, the morbidity burden of the war has been far higher than the mortality rate given improved medical treatment. Between 6,000 and 8,000 servicemen and women and their extended families are currently coping with traumatic injuries and the loss of a normal life, a normal future. They are grieving (Table 17.5).

Pathophysiology and Psychodynamics of Grief

Grieving is both an emotional and a physiologic response. In acute grief, as in cases of other stressful events, there may be a disruption of biological rhythms. It is well documented that grief is accompanied by impaired immune function, specifically decreased lymphocyte proliferation and impaired functioning of natural killer cells although it is not known how clinically significant these changes are. It is established, however, that the mortality rate for widows and widowers following the death of a spouse is higher than in the general population, with widowers at higher risk. Overall, women are less distressed and exhibit fewer instances of depression and perceived poor health than men who have experienced a comparable loss. Manifestations of grief reflect the individual's personality, previous life experiences, the significance of the loss, past psychological history, the relationship with the deceased, existing family and social networks, other life events, resources, educational level, and general state of health.

Some grief is anticipatory; for example, when someone is diagnosed with a terminal illness, both the patient and family grieve, although these processes are different for each. According to Kubler-Ross in her classic 1969 book *On Death and Dying,* preparatory grief is "that [grief that] the terminally ill patient has to undergo to prepare himself for his final seperation from this world." The terms anticipatory grief and anticipatory mourning are terms commonly used to the grief experienced by family members or friends before the death of a loved one.

Stages of preparatory grieving, identified in the classic work of Elisabeth Kübler-Ross, are:

- shock,
- denial,
- anger,
- bargaining,
- depression, and
- acceptance.

Table 17.5 Mourning

The initial reaction to loss is shock, disbelief, and numbness. Psychological pain signals the start of mourning, as the shock of loss begins to wear off. Up until that time, the person may prefer to continue with routine activities. Because the psychological work of mourning is to separate from an attachment, the painful onset of mourning may feel like one is being torn apart. Daily routines soon lose their value or meaning, and even minimal functioning at home, work, or school can require enormous physical and psychological effort. Mourning—as living with the absence of what had been, but is no longer—creates tension, and this tension compels the individual toward recognition and validation of the loss.

The actual expression of grief encompasses a wide range of emotions, depending on cultural norms and expectations. For example, some cultures encourage or even demand an intense display of emotions, whereas other cultures value stoicism. The circumstances of the loss, including how sudden or violent the death was, may also affect the expression of grief.

Feelings of weakness, decreased appetite, weight loss, difficulty in concentrating, breathing, and talking may occur. Sleep difficulties may occur—difficulty falling asleep, waking up during the night, and awakening early are all common manifestations of grief-related sleeplessness. Dreams often occur; the person may awaken, only to realize anew that the loved one is gone—for good. Self-reproach is not uncommon, often related to some small act of omission, such as "I didn't kiss him goodbye this morning!" Survivor guilt may occur in some cases, depending on the circumstances. Denial comes and goes. There may be "linkage" objects: Lynn Caine, in the well-known book *Widow,* talks about wearing her deceased husband's bathrobe for a whole year after his death. As part of what has been labeled an identification phenomenon, the person may take on some of the mannerisms or characteristics of the deceased, which helps perpetuate the deceased in some concrete way. A sense of the deceased person's presence may be so strong that it appears like a hallucination. In normal grief, the person realizes this is not real; in the case of pathological grief, the person may truly believe the deceased is present.

The process of mourning (Rando, 1993) does not move forward until the person is able to start letting go of attachment reexperiences and is able to:

- Recognize the loss
- React to the separation
- Reexperience the attachments
- Relinquish the attachments
- Readjust to the changes
- Reinvest in living

This is a difficult process, made all the more difficult when feelings of attachment are reexperienced as comforting. Examples of adaptive coping behaviors include using interpersonal support, joining a support group, cognitive coping strategies ("I can get through this"), and action-oriented strategies such as keeping busy.

The last two levels of mourning, in which the person makes the changes that complete the separation, are extremely difficult. At this point, each person will struggle to find his or her own way, sometimes by trial and error. It can be difficult to know what kind of change or how much change will be necessary in order to begin to reinvest in life after a painful loss. Few people are prepared to live as though the lost attachment never existed or as though the loss never occurred, but each person must define a way of living with loss that does not diminish the present or refute the past.

Pathological grief can present in a number of different ways. It can range from absent or delayed grief, to excessively intense and prolonged grief, to grief associated with suicidal ideation or frank psychosis. The risk factors for pathological grief reactions include: (1) sudden and/or violent death, (2) social isolation, (3) individuals who believe that they are in some way responsible for the death (real or imagined), (4) individuals with a history of traumatic losses, and (5) individuals who had an intensely ambivalent or dependent relationship with the deceased. In some instances, reduced or absent grief may be an appropriate reaction.

Clinical Presentations

Each person grieves in a manner that is, for him or her, meaningful and effective. Yet the stages of grief vary little from person to person. People are more likely to differ in the way they progress through the stages of mourning and grief. With normal grief, there is consistent progress toward acceptance. When a person reaches acceptance, he or she has become willing to "let go" and able to "go on." Nonetheless, even when a person may be willing to accept a loss, going on can be difficult. For example, parents may accept the death of their child, only to relive the loss as they watch their child's former classmates graduate from high school and go on to college or start families.

Stages of mourning and grief make the most sense when the loss is a person, possession, or an attachment that cannot be regained, such as the death of a loved one or the loss of a job. When the nature of a loss changes over time, the process can be more difficult. Some examples of this are when a loss does not occur as a single event or if the scope of a loss keeps changing, such as the loss of physical or mental health. A person who is newly diagnosed with a severe, chronic condition such as diabetes or bipolar illness may not grieve for his or her loss of health in progressive stages, yet being able to grieve for the loss of one's health would enable a search for a new definition of health and new personal goals. Many people will struggle with the reality of their first important loss.

Grief consists of three distinct phases: avoidance, confrontation, and accomodation. Mourning processes accompany these phases:

- ▲ Acknowledging the loss
- ▲ Reacting to the separation—feeling the pain, expressing reactions

- ▲ Recollecting and reexperiencing the deceased and the relationship—realistically reviewing and remembering the deceased
- ▲ Relinquishing attachment to the deceased while still acknowledging a loving connection to the deceased
- ▲ Readjusting to move adaptively into the new reality without forgetting the old
- ▲ Reinvesting; redirecting one's energy to new goals, pursuits, hopes, causes, beliefs, activities

Grief can be understood as a journey along a well-marked psychological path: Each person travels in his or her own way and at his or her own speed. The way a person grieves, and, consequently, the amount of time a person needs to move from agony to acceptance, is heavily influenced by personal, social, cultural, religious, and spiritual norms. Many different factors influence the process of grieving. Some individuals will also have to deal with serious interpersonal conflict when their grief-related needs conflict with those of their family or community. Take, for example, the conflict that can occur between the parents of a deceased child: One parent might need to take steps to celebrate the child's life, but the other parent might be unable to accept the circumstances of the child's death.

Lifestyle is also a factor to be considered. Individuals who live in social isolation may find it more difficult to grieve a loss without close significant others who can offer comfort and assistance. Grieving for a loss alone can drain psychosocial resources that are needed for day-to-day functioning. An equally difficult modern problem is the overvaluation of immediacy. Living with technology has increased our cultural expectations for speed. Human experiences that require time may appear suspect in this context. Busy employers, families, and friends may support grieving, as long as (in their perceptions) it does not take too long—the implication being that personal grief should not take too much time, or demand too many valuable social resources. After a year has passed, family and friends may begin to ask why the grieving person is not "over" his or her loss yet.

Differential Diagnosis

Cultural, ethnic, religious, and social beliefs, community and family traditions, and personal characteristics all determine how and when a person, a couple, or a family will mourn a loss. For some people, mourning is a well-defined, highly satisfying ritual. For others, particularly those who have never suffered a major loss before, mourning can be confusing and disturbing. In terms of psychosocial health and well-being, the process of mourning should allow the person to experience pain but achieve acceptance. Mourning that is harmful to self or others, or that persists without progressing toward acceptance, requires specialized care. Because of the pain and disturbance associated with mourning, some individuals may present their mourning as an illness that requires treatment rather than as a process.

Grief and depression share many of the same characteristics, and it can sometimes be difficult to evaluate exactly when the scope of normal grieving has slipped into a pathological realm. Obviously, elements of psychosis clearly indicate a need for aggressive treatment: Some patients may even become suicidal; they obviously should be monitored closely. An individual with a history of depression is at risk for becoming depressed at times of major loss. The mood disturbance in depression is typically pervasive and unrelenting, whereas fluctuations of mood in grief are common. Grief is often described as "coming in waves, washing over" the individual affected; even in intense grief, moments of happy reminiscence can surface. In contrast, people suffering from major depression feel hopeless—they cannot imagine ever feeling better. Non-pathological grief, on the other hand, is a normal, although intensely painful, state that is responsive to support, empathy, and the passage of time. The emergence of a major depressive disorder associated with grief is a medical emergency and should be treated as such (Table 17.6).

When the criteria for a comorbid psychiatric disorder are met, a codiagnosis sgould be made to ensure proper treatment. For a patient diagnosed with Major Depressive

Table 17.6 Differentiating Grief from Depression

Component	Normal Grief	Major Depression
Feelings	Able to feel happiness and pleasure at times; mood fluctuates	Unable to feel pleasure
Worthiness	May blame self for not preventing the loss	Feels worthless and bad; is preoccupied with self
Sleep, appetite, and activity	Variations in sleep, appetite, and activity; sometimes is more able to do things than others	Has disturbance of sleep, appetite, and activity
Dreams	Frequently dreams and fantasizes about the lost object/person	Cannot remember dreams; rarely fantasizes
Responsiveness to others	Responds positively to support and warmth	Unresponsive to others; has no interest
Anger	Expresses anger at appropriate times, even if not in appropriate ways	Denies anger or has inappropriate rage

Disorder (MDD), the diagnosis should be coded as such with the bereavement V-Code included to emphasize the reactive nature of the diagnosis.

According to the DSM-IV-TR, symptoms that are atypical of a "normal" grief reaction and that suggest a diagnosis of complicated grief are:

- ▲ Prolonged and marked functional impairment
- ▲ Marked psychomotor retardation or limitation
- ▲ Morbid preoccupation with thoughts of worthlessness
- ▲ Feelings that one would be better off dead and should have died with the deceased
- ▲ Guilt

The accurate diagnosis and treatment of complicated grief is recognizing where symptoms overlap and when multiple diagnoses are warranted. Specific subtypes of depression may occur; a number of other psychiatric disorders share symptoms with complicated grief, including posttraumatic stress disorder (PTSD), adjustment disorder, anxiety disorder, and personality disorder. As under any severe stressor, subclinical pathologies may emerge floridly. The DSM-IV-TR categorizes normal grief under Axis V–V62.82 – under the heading *Other Conditions That May Be a Focus of Clinical Attention.*

Management

All too often, treatment for bereavement occurs within the realm of tertiary intervention, when grief has already emerged as complicated. Early detection and preventive interventions could alleviate suffering and lead to earlier and more effective treatment. Primary care clinicans can assist in the attainment of those goals by:

- ▲ Validating pain and distress related to loss
- ▲ Providing appropriate pharmacologic therapy
- ▲ Making bereaved patients aware of the many supportive therapies available and have a ready list of referrals

In the case of terminal illness, early and ongoing bereavement assessment and a collaborative process are essential components of a preventive approach to bereavement care. Interventions include bereavement education and counseling that assist in facilitating communication with the dying person. There is strong evidence that involvement and caregiving benefits survivors.

Management of grief includes preparing (if possible) the person and family for the normal stages of grieving—normalizing grief. The practitioner should let the person know that feelings of guilt and anger are normal and counsel patience. Encouraging expression of feelings may be helpful. Offering comfort is important but the practitioner must recognize that he or she cannot "fix" things for the patient—efforts to remove emotional pain can actually hinder the grieving process. Word are not always necessary.

Provide medical therapy as indicated depending on symptomatology and past history. A brief course of a short-acting sedative may be appropriate during acute grief to induce sleep or get through the funeral and burial, especially when supportive interventions have not succeeded. Actually, the use of drugs such as tranquilizers or alcohol, which numb emotions, should be discouraged over time. Narcotizing patients with drugs interferes with the normal process of grieving, however painful. Antidepressant therapy may be considered for patients with particularly proloned or complex grief reactions, even when it may be difficult to differentiate depression from a normal grief response. Clinical data suggest that selective serotonin reuptake inhibitors may be beneficial and assist the patient to mobilize the energy necessary to progress through the stages of mourning and grief.

Specific counseling sessions for the bereaved may be extremely valuable and may assist in the prevention of pathologic mourning or depressive reactions. These sessions, with trained counselors, can assist the grieving person in recognizing and expressing angry or ambivalent feelings toward a deceased person. Group counseling, as well as self-help groups, are important adjunctive therapies. More than 30 percent of widows and widowers reported feeling isolated from friends and withdrawing from social activities; self-help groups offer companionship, social contact, and emotional support. This is particularly important given the contraction of the family unit in modern times. Have a referral list available to assist the patient in seeking such psychosocial support.

Follow-Up

The manifestations of grief usually subside over time. Typically, acute grief reactions gradually lessen and within 1 to 2 months the grieving person is able to eat and sleep normally, beginning to return to normal functioning. Traditionally, grief lasts from 6 months to one year as the grieving person experiences the calendar year at least once without the lost person. This varies from person to person and is dependent on circumstances.

Patient Education

It is important to prepare the person and family for the emotional "triggers" that will exacerbate the sense of loss—holidays, birthdays, the anniversary of the death or traumatic event, or at times of future loss. The clinician should encourage good nutrition and health habits, especially in elderly patients. Grieving persons should be encouraged to maintain self-care and not to neglect any active medical problems of their own. The clinician can encourage physical activity as a positive way of dealing with the stress of grieving. The clinician should discourage making major decisions early in the grieving process.

Intimate Partner Violence

Intimate partner violence (IPV) is defined as a pattern of assaultive and coercive behaviors that may include inflicted physical injury, psychological abuse, sexual assault, progressive social isolation, stalking, deprivation, intimidation and threats perpetrated by someone who is, was, or wishes to be involved in an intimate relationship with an adult or adolescent, and aimed at establishing control by one partner over the other. IPV is not associated with any ethnic group, religion, income level, level of education, employment, or sexual orientation. However, typically the victim is a child, a woman, or an elderly person, and the typical perpetrator is a man (in the case of partner abuse), a parent or other trusted adult (in the case of child abuse), or an adult child or other caregiver (in the case of elder abuse). More than one type of violence may occur in any given family; for example, in one study, 45 to 70 percent of battered women reported that their batterer also abused their children. (See The Patient's Voice 17.1.)

Epidemiology and Causes

The incidence of IPV in America is high: Most experts cite the incidence rate for domestic violence as one act every 15 seconds. As many as half of all Americans women have been exposed to domestic violence in their lifetime. Two to four million women are battered each year by their husbands or boyfriends in the United States, and between 21 and 34 percent of all American women will be physically assaulted by a male partner at least once in their lifetime. Ninety-five percent of cases of IPV are perpetrated by men on women; the rates of IPV in same-sex relationships appear to be as high, or higher, than those found in heterosexual populations. Thousands of women and children die as a result of IPV each year. Annual health-care costs are estimated to be 44 million dollars annually, not including money lost from work absenteeism, turnover, and decreased productivity.

Examples of IPV include punching, slapping, kicking, burning, pushing, dragging, choking, restraining, and sexual assault. In one study, 68 percent of domestic assault incidents involved weapons; in 15 percent of these cases the assault resulted in serious injury. Recent research indicates that 82 percent of women killed in their homes are killed by someone that they knew, 55 percent in the context of a quarrel, physical domestic fight, or assault by a spouse, lover, or close relative. Statistics on violent crime indicate that three out of every four American women murdered die at the hands of their male partners. Violent episodes are recurrent: 89 percent of victims in one study reported previous episodes of injury; 34 percent of these victims were battered on a daily basis.

Additional risk factors that increase the potential for violence include financial instability, pregnancy (15 to 25 percent of pregnant women are abused physically while pregnant, with the abuse often leading to birth defects), the birth of a child, and job loss by either partner. Women are at great risk when they leave an abusive relationship. They have a 75 percent greater chance of being killed by their batterers than women who stay.

Numerous studies have documented that women with a history of IPV have greater rates of specific physical symptoms, a higher prevalence of unexplained physical symptoms, a greater number of symptoms, and poorer overall health status than nonabused controls. Similarly, IPV survivors have higher rates of mental health problems, including major depressive disorders, depressive symptoms, dysthmia, generalized anxiety disorder, phobias, PTSD, suicidality, and substance abuse. IPV survivors have been found to have higher health care cost and utilization. However, the U.S. Preventive Taskforce (USPSTF) recently found insufficient evidence to recommend for or against routine screening for IPV in asymptomatic women and children as well as in older adults or their caregivers. However, the review was focused on asymptomatic individuals and the recommendations do in fact encourage clinicans to be alert to physical and behavioral signs of abuse such as trauma or somatic symptoms. Most clinicians will see a number of cases each year and fail to recognize about half of them.

THE PATIENT'S VOICE 17.1

Domestic Violence

as soon as crystal let the baby outta her arms/beau
jumped up laughin & gigglin/a hootin & a hollerin/
awright bitch/awright bitch/you gonna marry me/
you gonna marry me...
i aint gonna marry ya/I aint ever gonna marry ya/
for nothin/you gonna be in the jail/you gonna be
under the jail for this/now gimme my kids/ya give
me back my kids/

he kicked the screen outta the window/& held the kids
offa the sill/you gonna matty me/yeh, I'll marry ya/
anything/but bring the children back in the house/
he looked from where the kids were hangin from the
fifth story/at alla the people screamin at him/&
he started sweating again/say to alla the neighbors/
you gonna marry me/
I stood by beau in the window/with naomi reachin
For me/& kwame screamin mommy mommy from the
fifth
Story/bit I cd only whisper/& he dropped em

SOURCE: Ntozake Shange: "for colored girls who have considered suicide/when the rainbow is enuf." Macmillan, New York, 1977, pp 59–60.

Psychodynamics and Pathophysiology

Domestic violence occurs in families of every racial and religious background and in every socioeconomic strata. Although alcohol/substance abuse and a history of childhood abuse are important correlates of IPV, this does not cause or explain domestic violence. Many individuals with substance-abuse disorders are not violent toward members of their household. However, individuals who abuse alcohol/substance abuse are likely to have other psychosocial problems that make relationships difficult for them. Children who grow up with violence can, as adults, grow up to be adults who do not reject violence. Violent individuals may have strong feelings of inadequacy that their partners and children may not realize this. Violence is self-reinforcing: violence always leads to more violence.

Violent individuals use fear, pain, injury, humiliation, and suffering to establish power and control over their victims. With no warning at all, or after repeated threats, a violent individual can become intent on killing his or her victim. The abused individual often is forced into isolation, which prevents anyone from observing the violence or assisting the victim. The abused adult and/or children can be physically or psychologically isolated from help. The psychologically isolated victim typically is convinced that he or she is alone and that no one cares or is willing to help.

IPV may follow an established pattern or it may be unpredictable. In some cases, the only predictable element of the violence may be the offender's use of violence to establish power and control over the person he or she wants to dominate. This includes stalking behaviors that are intended to display the violent person's skill, strength, and determination. A common pattern, known as the *cycle of violence,* starts with an episode of violence, followed by reconciliation, increasing tension, and the next episode of violence. Typically, the periods of tension and episodes of violence increase in duration while the reconciliation periods become shorter.

Victims of IPV often develop strong dependency needs and may deny the violence. About 50 percent of battered wives grew up in violent homes, and their most common trait is dependency. Victims may rationalize the violence by thinking that they can change the violent individual's behavior by making changes in their own behavior. For example, women with small children and women who are unemployed may deny the violence exists because they feel escape is impossible. Victims of domestic violence, particularly adolescents who feel they cannot escape, may first try to escape psychologically by abusing alcohol or drugs. However, all too often the violence is then blamed on the victim's substance abuse.

Clinical Presentation

Generally there are two times that it is appropriate to routinely assess for IPV: when taking a complete history such as with a new patient or during an annual exam and whenever violence is part of the differential diagnosis. If inquiring is part of a routine history, it is unlikely that there would be a positive response about current violence. However, such screenings will educate the patient and lay the groundwork for future discussions. Always preface IPV questioning with an appropriate and nonthreatening explanation such as "I ask all of my patients these questions because these problems affect many people's health." Avoid using stigmatizing words such as domestic violence or abuse. If a patient is not directly questioned about IPV, he or she may infer that the provider does not want to know about abuse. In some instances, a patient may disclose a past experience with violence which may provide useful information in providing appropriate care.

Women who end an abusive relationship are usually at greater risk for serious injury—and therefore in greater need of intervention—than women who are still involved in an abusive relationship, but these individuals are less likely to seek help.

It is more difficult to know when to include violence in the differential diagnosis. Recognition of IPV continues to be difficult because the victim and the abuser often conspire to conceal it. Potential red flags include evidence of unexplained blunt trauma—particularly of different ages, such as old and new bruises—combined with alcohol abuse, low self-esteem, poverty or other financial stress, mental or physical disability, or social isolation. The partner, if present, may be suspicious. Exposure to IPV is frequently linked with mental health issues such as depression, anxiety, suicide attempts and/or substance abuse. Problems or injuries during pregnancy should raise the level of suspicion, as well as delays in seeking medical care. In addition, abused women have been shown to have a greater number of physical complaints and unexplained symptoms. Often these patients are labeled "difficult" or "somatizing" and are not assessed for IPV. Any patient presenting with multiple complaints or whose symptoms are not consistent with her history should be assessed for violence at least once and reassessed if she fails to respond to therapy appropriately. Behavioral red flags are (1) a patient reluctant to speak in front of her partner or giving evasive answers, and (2) an overly protective or controlling partner.

The first goal of assessment is to determine whether or not an individual is a target of violence. The second goal is to evaluate the level of danger. The patient must be seen alone. Ask the partner, children, and family members to leave the room. If an interpreter is needed use a professional rather than a family member. If the partner refuses to leave, do not confront him or her. This should be considered a strong indicator of IPV and strategize a way to get the patient alone later. Requesting a urinalysis or chest x-ray exam is often an effective approach.

The clinician must communicate concern and caring and tell each woman that all women are assessed for abuse. The seriousness of the issue cannot be underscored enough. Although it may be necessary to obtain specific information, the clinician should try to limit data-gathering to essentials. Some sources suggest "funneling" beginning with innocuous questions and progressing to more direct interrogation. The three questions listed in Focusing the History 17.1, a validated instrument. At least one question should emphasize emotional abuse and control and one question should use specific examples of physical and sexual violence. Athough control issues to do not always

FOCUS ON HISTORY 17.1

Domestic Violence: Three Questions to Ask

By asking the following three questions, the APN may be able to identify approximately 75% of women at risk for domestic violence. A positive response to any of the three questions represents a positive screen for partner violence.

- Have you been hit, kicked, punched, forced to have sex, or otherwise hurt by someone within the past year? If so, by whom?
- Do you feel safe in your current relationship?
- Do you feel threatened or controlled by a partner or ex-partner or anyone else in your life?

SOURCE: Reprinted with permission from Feldman K, et al: Accuracy of three brief screening questions for detecting partner violence in the emergency department. JAMA 277:1357–1361, 1997.

lead to physical violence, controlling behavior is a key feature of IPV and a risk factor for homicide or severe injury. Many patients will disclose emotional abuse long before they are comfortable disclosing physical abuse, even if both are occurring. A key component of the abuse experience is intrusion; many patients who are in an abusive relationship may perceive questioning as intrusive. Again, sensitivity is crucial.

Do not jump to conclusions too quickly. One sign or symptom alone is not sufficient to make a "diagnosis" of abuse. It is important not to pathologize: a person in an abusive relationship may be an essentially healthy individual who has been the victim of a traumatic relationship, perhaps unanticipated. The clinician should be aware that a traumatic experience such as abuse, especially over an extended period of time, will have an impact on the victim's thought processes and belief systems. This must be taken into consideration during the assessment. Some health-care providers may stereotype a woman who is with a violent male, and some may even believe that anything they may do is futile. Those who are not victims of violence feel certain that they would leave a violent partner immediately; this may or may not be true. Some health-care providers may view the problem as a sociolegal and not a health problem. This is not true. Maintaining contact with a patient in the primary-care environment and working within a Circle of Caring may help the clinician make this difficult assessment as well as a viable plan for dealing with the difficult situation. (See Nursing Research–Based Practice 17.2.)

Positive disclosure can trigger intense and conflicting emotions. Being a target of violence triggers feelings of fear that can range from sarcasm to terror to silence. A positive disclosure should ALWAYS elicit a response of empathy and support, prior to even assessing safety. Statements such as "I am really sorry to hear that this has happened to you;" "This is not your fault; no one deserves such treatment;" and "It is unfortunate, but many of my patients have had similar experiences" are critical and should always be clearly communicated.

At this point, ask the patient what change, if any, he or she wants to make. Do *not* expect or even try to "fix" the situation. An abusive relationship is most often a chronic condition. As with any condition that threatens a patient's health, an important step is to determine the urgency of the situation. If there is any recent violence or threat it is essential to assess the level of danger. Listen first to the women's

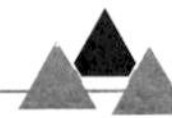

NURSING RESEARCH-BASED PRACTICE 17.2

Domestic Violence

Locsin, R, and Purnell, M: Intimate Partner Violence, Culture-Centrism, and Nursing. Holistic Nurs Pract 16(2):1–4, 2002.

Using the metaphor of "Ring of Violence," these authors use the analogy of the bullfight and bullring to vividly describe a women's experience of domestic violence with a partner of a "different culture." They quote 'Jane Doe': "I suppose he thought he was doing what men were supposed to do in his culture, and what generations before him had probably done" (p. 1). She describes her experience of domestic violence as "…it was like a bullfight, and that I was cornered, like an animal for slaughter, with nowhere to hide. It was either me or him" (p. 1). They note that problems of multiculturism compound problems of domestic violence. Although domestic violence is frequently identified as a family-centered problem, these authors place it in the broader context of culture. They note that cultural values are not easily adjusted or changed, and stress the need for nurses to educate culturally different individuals living intimate lives about intimate partner violence thus may promote the integrity of a relationship, but even more importantly, may save lives. Problems arise with persons living unprepared for life in culturally diverse situations, whether with intimate partners or within the larger context of local and global societies. Conceptualizing persons as "global citizens," their daily conduct should be guided by respect and concern for the culture of others among whom they abide.

own assessment; if she feels she is in danger, she most likely is. But her assessment that she is not in danger may be a misperception. There are a variety of Danger Assessment tools such as the Danger Assessment 2 (DA-2), which is a 20-question instrument; another validated tool is the Spouse Abuse: Assessing Level of Violence in the Home, which includes a revised form of that instrument and its use. (See Advanced Practice Nursing Interventions 17.1.)

If the patient says no to all questions but there is still a suspicion of abuse, avoid confrontation. Make a note of the concerns on the chart, offer resources, and leave the issue open for future discussion. Ask again on future visits. Note that this is a "concern for possible abuse," not the leading diagnosis if unconfirmed.

Management

Careful documentation of assessment findings is critical to effective management of the health-care needs of victims of domestic violence. The clinician should record the history using specific, plain language; record all physical findings; use a body map; and take photographs. The care-provider should preserve physical evidence, if appropriate.

Treatment for a victim of abuse involves more than treating the injuries and providing telephone numbers and referrals. Developing a caring relationship with the patient is essential. This is truly a patient who needs a Circle of Caring. Clinician's can sometimes find themselves in the position of being able to treat a victim's injuries but not the cause of the injuries. Patient mistrust can further complicate what often is already a difficult treatment situation. For some patients, even accepting printed material about domestic violence or abuse can be a dangerous act. False reassurance is to be avoided, but conveying a negative or judgmental attitude toward a victim of violence is equally harmful. Victims of IPV typically look for professionals they feel they can trust, and individuals who are planning their escape may require a great deal of time and support before they act.

Advanced Practice Nursing Interventions 17.1 lists some general interventions clinicians can make, including a danger assessment and counseling concerning the individual danger that is assessed. If the abuse is presently occurring and the batterer has access to the victim, safety is compromised. Referral to Women's or Child's Protective Services or to the appropriate law enforcement or social services agency may be warranted. It may be necessary to develop with the patient a "safety plan," although there is no guarantee that the patient will comply with the plan. In some practice settings, the health-care provider may need to take these actions unilaterally; in others, a team approach is more facilitative.

ADVANCED PRACTICE NURSING INTERVENTIONS 17.1

Domestic Violence

Prevention:

- Teach conflict resolution skills.
- Create a safety plan to remove the individual(s) from the violent situation.
- Inquire about the abuse. Questions to ask include:
  1. Has the physical violence increased in frequency/severity over the past year?
  2. Have you ever been choked?
  3. Has a weapon or threat with a weapon been used?
  4. Have you been threatened with death or do you believe the individual could kill you?
  5. Is there a gun in the house?
  6. Have you ever been forced to have sex when you did not wish to?
  7. For women, have you ever been abused while you were pregnant?
  8. Is alcohol or substance abuse a factor? How often is the alcohol or substances used?
  9. Have your daily activities been controlled?
  10. Is the individual violent and constantly jealous of you?
- Provide community resources.
- Provide counseling and other therapy as indicated (for example, crisis intervention, post-traumatic stress disorder therapy, physical rehabilitation).
- Document findings and interventions.

SOURCE: Adapted from Jezierski, M: Abuse of women by male partners: basic knowledge for emergency nurses. J Emerg Nurs 20(5):361–368 1994.

Follow-Up and Referral

Any evidence of domestic violence requires full compliance with local reporting and referral laws. Local and state agencies for victims of domestic violence have established protocols and systems for providing services that include emergency housing, health care, foster care, and displacement counseling. Despite the significant incidence of domestic violence, there is still a shortage of referral services for violent offenders. Violent individuals who are motivated to stop their violence may benefit from community support groups such as Men Stopping Rape and Parents Anonymous. Local crisis services and police hotlines should be contacted to protect victims of domestic violence. Victims of domestic violence should have the phone number and address for local emergency services and support groups, or at least be informed regarding how to obtain this information. When indicated, specialized psychiatric care for severe depression, anxiety, or substance abuse should be offered repeatedly. A patient who may refuse referrals for domestic violence services may accept a referral to obtain help with abuse-related depression and anxiety.

Participate in prevention by working with local and state coalitions against domestic violence, child abuse, and elder abuse. In addition, the work environment should have clear policies and procedures defining abuse-reporting procedures. This is important in every primary-care office, because health-care providers are often the "first stop" for victims of abuse.

Patient Education

Education regarding who is at risk and information about the cycle of violence is a crucial step. In many states, continuing education on the topic of domestic violence for professionals is mandated on an annual basis. It is important to remember that much knowledge in this area is new. The concept of battering as a social problem did not become widely accepted until the 1960s. Education about the fact that a woman may be *more* at risk *after* she leaves an abusive relationship is also very important. Options for help need to be made available and accessible to the individual at risk. Instrumental support for new mothers, for example, may be important in limiting child abuse or other forms of domestic violence. Careful attention to the risk factors for violence in a relationship is necessary, and most important, the care-provider should provide information on where and how to get help.

Substance-Related Disorders

Overview

All substances in the substance-related disorder category of the DSM-IV-TR are considered brain-altering substances, and are associated with a pathological intoxication state, but the substances vary as to whether the pathological state is associated with withdrawal or persists after the elimination of the substance from the body. Legal substances are not separated from illegal substances. The concept of substance dependence has taken on many meanings although two concepts have been used over time to define aspects of dependence: behavioral and physical. Behavioral dependence emphasizes pathological use patterns and substance-seeking activites, whereas physical dependence refers to the physiologic effects of multiple episodes of substance use.

Substance Abuse

Substance abuse is a pattern of substance use that causes significant distress or impairment of functioning. To meet the criteria for this diagnosis, one or more of the following symptoms of recurrent use should be present within a 12-month period:

- Recurrent substance use that results in work, school, or home obligation failures
- Recurrent substance use in physically hazardous situations
- Recurrent substance-related legal problems
- Continuous or recurrent social or interpersonal problems that are caused by or made worse by substance-use effects

Substance Dependence

Substance dependence is a pattern of substance use that leads to clinically significant distress or impairment of functioning. To meet the criteria for this diagnosis, three or more of the following symptoms need to occur within the same 12-month period:

- Tolerance, defined as a marked increase in the amount of substance needed to achieve intoxication or to achieve the desired effect, or a marked decrease in the effect achieved with the same amount of substance.
- Withdrawal, defined by symptom onset in the absence of substance use, or the use of a substance to relieve or avoid withdrawal-symptom onset.
- Larger than intended amounts of substance are used, or duration of substance use is longer than intended.
- Persistent desire to use a substance or unsuccessful efforts aimed at decreasing or controlling substance use.
- Extensive amounts of time spent obtaining, using, or recovering from the substance.
- Interruption or cessation of important activities because of substance use.
- Ongoing substance use despite acknowledgment of persistent or recurrent problems (physical or psychological) that are caused by or made worse by substance use.

Codependence is a term that has come to mean the behavioral patterns of family members who have been significantly affected by another family member's substance use or addiction. Related concepts of enabling and denial may characterize family members of patients who abuse substances.

Epidemiology and Causes

A recent National Institute on Drug Abuse (NIDA) survey indicated that 40 percent of the population reported using one or more illicit substances in their lifetime; 15 percent had used illicit substances in the year before the survey; 6.37 percent had used them in the month before the survey. The lifetime prevalence of substance abuse is about 20 percent. Lower educational and lower income levels predict a lifetime history of dependence (odds ratio greater than 2), but race, ethnicity, or living in an urban environment do not. Generally, the earlier the age at which substance abuse begins, the longer the duration of substance abuse later in life. Recent NIDA data (2004) reported a slight decrease in use of illegal substances abuse in teenagers, but increased abuse in this age group of prescription drugs. Different substances demonstrate variation in lifetime dependence rates (e.g., for opioids, this rate is 23 percent; for nicotine 32 percent; for alcohol, 17 percent). In the late 1990s, the total annual cost to society of substance use problems was estimated at almost 200 billion dollars. Another important annual survey to track use of illicit drugs, alcohol, and tobacco in the U.S. population by age group, the National

Household Survey on Drug Abuse (NHSDA) is available at http://www.samhsa.gov.

National statistics indicate that the most commonly used legal substances are caffeine, alcohol, and nicotine, and the most commonly used illegal substances are marijuana and cocaine. Different population-based causes for substance abuse have been described. As with all psychiatric disorders, the initial causative theories evolved from psychodynamic models; subsequent models include behavioral, genetic, and neurochemical explanations. According to one NIDA survey, family transmission is a core risk factor for substance abuse. Both social learning and genetic models have been developed to explain the increased risk and incidence of substance abuse in the children of substance-abusing parents. Compared to earlier generations, however, Americans today are more likely to seek the immediate gratification and immediate solutions offered by drugs. In nearly every case, the patient who is abusing drugs and or alcohol will have defined the moment at which their substance abuse began. In practice, the causes a person may describe for his or her substance abuse are always less important than the reasons for stopping.

Comorbidities (also known as "dual diagnosis") are common in persons with substance abuse. The most common comorbidities were substance abuse with more than one substance—for example, both drugs and alcohol. It is estimated that 65 percent of persons with a substance-abuse problem fall into this category of multiple substance usage. Antisocial personality disorder, phobias and other anxiety disorders, major depressive disorder, and dysthymic disorder are common comorbidities (listed in order of frequency) with substance abuse. The most potent and dangerous substances have the highest incidence of comorbidities.

People who abuse substances are about 20 times more likely to die from suicide than are the general population. About 15 percent of people with alcohol abuse or dependency have been reported to commit suicide. The frequency of suicide among individuals in this group is second only to that among patients with major depression; many individuals with alcohol abuse or dependency may have underlying depression, further increasing their risk.

A person may initially consume a drug for any number of reasons. However, many people continue using a drug based on the actual and perceived rewards of substance use. The rewards of substance use vary with the individual but can include social acceptance, changes in mental status, psychological escape, avoidance of stress and problems, and thrill seeking. Denial and rationalization of substance use, substance effects, or consequences of substance use make it possible for an individual to continue to use a substance as though he or she is immune to unexpected or dangerous consequences.

Individuals who have developed psychological and physical needs for a substance often have also formed strong attachments to their substance-use lifestyle and substance-based relationships. It may be impossible to effectively address a person's substance abuse without taking into account his or her substance-based relationships and attachments. A person can become strongly attached to the people, places, and community that make up his or her substance-abuse lifestyle. From friendships among co-workers that develop at designated smoking areas to football parties and alternative lifestyles, for many people, the thought of giving up their attachments may be more painful than the thought of giving up their actual substances of abuse. The fear of losing these valued attachments is frequently used to rationalize continued substance abuse.

Personal losses may increase or decrease the motivation to significantly change substance-use behaviors. Individuals who have not suffered substance abuse-related losses may nevertheless have to deal with significant interpersonal conflicts related to their substance-abuse behaviors. Years of substance abuse can result in the loss of all non–substance-based relationships, significant loss of self-esteem, financial losses, and loss of physical and mental health. These personal losses can have a devastating psychological impact on the individual. The patient may feel that he or she is in a no-win situation: Feelings of hopelessness may manifest as ambivalence about making needed changes in substance-use behaviors or bravado about continued substance abuse.

Substance-abuse disorders that may be seen in a primary-care setting include cannabis, cocaine, amphetamine, nicotine, and alcohol disorders.

Cannabis Disorders

The psychoactive effects of marijuana are produced by cannabinoids, of which tetrahydrocannabinol (THC) is the predominant substance. Specific receptors for cannabis have been identified in the brain, particularly in the basal ganglia, hippocampus, and cerebellum. Tolerance and psychological dependence on cannabis have been reported; and abrupt discontinuation of high daily doses can produce withdrawal symptoms that include irritability, insomnia, and mild nausea. The euphoric effects of marijuana can last for hours. These effects include distortions of time, sound, color, taste, changes in the ability to concentrate, and dreamlike states. Studies of the mental status changes produced by smoking marijuana indicate that the drug affects behavior by increasing brain cell-receptor sensitivity to dopamine. THC can create a mellow mood state by increasing gamma-aminobutyric acid (GABA) activity. THC impairs short-term memory by decreasing brain acetylcholine activity. High doses of marijuana are associated with red eye, mild increases in heart rate; orthostatic hypotension; increased appetite; dry mouth; and disruptions in recall, memory storage, and sensory-input coding. Memory impairment appears to be the most significant long-term effect of marijuana.

Because marijuana is smoked, it is very well absorbed. Behavioral effects tend to develop immediately. Absorbed THC is distributed throughout the body but concentrates in body fat. THC crosses the blood–brain barrier with ease and efficiency. THC also crosses the placenta and affects the fetus. Ingested THC is slowly metabolized and eliminated by the liver over a period of 1 to 4 days. Chronic marijuana smokers can test positive for THC metabolites for weeks, despite brief drug-free periods.

Smoked marijuana has been shown to improve appetite in persons with human immunodeficiency virus (HIV) infection and acquired immunodeficiency syndrome (AIDS) and to reduce nausea and vomiting in chemotherapy patients. U.S. demand for marijuana has resulted in significant increases in the availability and potency of the drug. No longer a sixties symbol of social rebellion, marijuana smokers today equate their drug of choice with tobacco, alcohol, and caffeine. As with nicotine, alcohol, and caffeine, long-term marijuana smokers who wish to stop usually find it extremely difficult to do so. Heavy daily users of marijuana experience significant withdrawal symptoms and cravings.

Cocaine Disorders

Cocaine acts as a stimulant by blocking the reuptake of dopamine, thereby increasing dopamine activity in several areas of the brain. Cocaine may also have dopamine-agonist effects. The dopamine effects of cocaine account for most of the immediate and long-term effects of the drug. Biochemical studies of cocaine have shown that cocaine is an extremely self-reinforcing, or self-rewarding, drug. The euphoria of cocaine intoxication, combined with the dysphoria of cocaine crashing and craving, can lead to compulsive consumption. One of the most important studies of cocaine effects on the brain and emotional states successfully used functional magnetic resonance imaging (fMRI) to study the rush, high, low, and craving experiences of cocaine-dependent adults. Maximum cocaine blood levels were reached in an average of 7 minutes after infusion, dysphoria and paranoia developed about 11 minutes after infusion, and cravings for more cocaine occurred about 12 minutes after infusion. One of the most impressive indicators of the speed and scope of cocaine effects on the brain was that subjects reported maximal feelings of euphoria as cocaine was being infused, before maximal cocaine blood levels had been reached. Cocaine intoxication is characterized by elation, significant increases in self-esteem, and the perception of improved task performance. Intoxication can also produce agitation, irritability, impaired judgment, impulsive sexual behavior, aggression, hyperactivity, and mania. Chronic cocaine use has been associated with the onset of symptoms of thought, personality, and mood disorders.

Over the past few decades, smoked cocaine (crack), an extremely rapid-acting form of the drug, became cheap and easy to obtain. Cocaine has consistently been linked with severe social problems and antisocial behavior, such as gang violence and prostitution. Well-publicized cocaine-related deaths and the emaciated physical appearance associated with chronic cocaine abuse have severely limited the social acceptance of the drug.

Amphetamine Disorders

"Speed kills" was a popular slogan of the 1960s. After having been a relatively popular and cheap drug of abuse, amphetamines quickly came to be associated with violent, bizarre behavior at a time when mellow "highs" were more socially acceptable. Decades later, amphetamines, particularly methamphetamine ("crank"), have once again become popular among older adolescents and young adults. Users describe being high on amphetamines as being "amped" (amplified) or "tweaked." Methamphetamine is a potent, easy-to-make, inexpensive stimulant, which can be snorted or injected. "Crystal-meth" is methamphetamine in a free-base form, and "ice" is a high-grade form of "crystal-meth" that is sold in rocks, like crack cocaine. Because of its purity and potency, "ice" is expensive; one hit can deliver an extreme amphetamine high that can last for hours. CAT (methcathinone) is a low-grade stimulant made from household chemicals. A methamphetamine rush is intense. Intoxication includes elation, increased self-esteem, increased physical endurance, insensitivity to fatigue, and feelings of being invulnerable. The half-life of methamphetamine, 11 hours or more, far exceeds that of cocaine. But like cocaine, amphetamine increases dopamine activity, is self-reinforcing, and is a highly efficient addictive agent. Chronic users experience acute episodes of euphoria and dysphoria that can mimic bipolar disorder (manic–depressive illness). Long-term amphetamine users are subject to symptoms of dopamine depletion that can manifest as psychosis or other mental disorders. Neurologic effects include jaw clenching and facial tics. Ritalin, an amphetamine prescribed to treat attention-deficit/hyperactivity disorder (ADHD), and amphetamine-type weight-loss medications are subject to abuse.

Nicotine Disorders

Nicotine effects are numerous and, because the drug is inhaled, potent. The immediate effects of inhaled nicotine are a brief period of stimulation; mild improvements in alertness, mood, and memory; and feelings of relaxation. Nicotine has immediate brain dopaminergic and acetylcholine effects and it is highly self-reinforcing. The half-life of nicotine is approximately 2 hours. Two hours after smoking, the chronic smoker experiences irritable nicotine cravings, or a "nicotine fit." As a mild stimulant, nicotine effects include alterations in metabolism that can affect (suppress) appetite. Adolescent girls may intentionally become smokers with the hope that using nicotine will help them to stop the normal weight gain associated with puberty or improve their ability to control their appetite. Fear of weight gain keeps many young female smokers from stopping: A temporary weight gain of about 10 pounds is not uncommon when smokers first quit.

The biochemistry of nicotine withdrawal is as complex as the biochemistry of nicotine stimulation, but nicotine withdrawal symptoms make quitting difficult. Management of withdrawal symptoms is the first and foremost goal of smoking cessation treatment. Nicotine withdrawal symptoms start within 2 hours of the last dose of nicotine, peak within 48 hours, and can last for weeks. Symptoms include severe cravings, irritability, decreased concentration, drowsiness, insomnia, decreased heart rate, decreased blood pressure, impaired motor skills, muscle tension, and increased appetite. Practitioners are encouraged to find out if the patient smokes, repeatedly encourage him or her to stop, and repeatedly recommend proven treatments.

Alcohol Disorders

According to the National Institute on Alcohol Abuse and Alcoholism (NIAAA), the younger the age at drinking onset, the greater the chance that at some point in life, an individual will develop an alcohol disorder. The person who begins drinking before age 15 is four times more likely to develop an alcohol disorder as an adult. Researchers have found that the risk of adult alcohol disorders decreases by 14 percent for each additional year of age of drinking onset. Individuals who start drinking at age 21 to 22 years have significantly lower risks for developing adult alcohol dependence. Alcohol disorders are family disorders. It is estimated that one in five adults in the United States has lived with an alcoholic while growing up. Children who grow up with alcoholism are at risk for being abused and becoming adult problem drinkers. Concurrent depression, anxiety, or personality disorder, evidence of a family history of alcohol disorder, or evidence of early age at drinking onset are critical risk factors for alcohol disorder. Although there is little debate about alcohol as an addictive drug, there is a great deal of debate regarding the nature of alcoholism. The core of the debate has to do with significant evidence of alcoholism as a genetic disorder, a biological disease, and as a maladaptive behavior. Alcoholism cannot be fully explained by any one of these models. What is not clear is how these different factors interact. What is clear, however, is that significant exposure to high blood alcohol levels increases the risk of uncontrolled, compulsive, or problem drinking.

The unique biochemical effects of alcohol are the drug's ability to produce both short-term and long-term changes in neuron membranes and the enhancement and inhibition of critical ion channels. As a central nervous system (CNS) depressant, alcohol compares to drugs such as barbiturates and benzodiazepines. Alcohol is readily absorbed from the stomach and small intestine into the bloodstream and is metabolized by the liver.

Alcohol intoxication is greatest when blood alcohol levels are increasing. In other words, alcohol intoxication is a manifestation of the rate at which alcohol is consumed.

- Blood alcohol level of 0.05 causes disruptions in thinking, judgment, and inhibition.
- Blood alcohol level of 0.1 produces obvious intoxication.
- Blood alcohol level of 0.2 results in depression of motor functioning and emotional/behavioral dyscontrol.
- Blood alcohol level of 0.3 produces stupor and confusion. Blood alcohol levels of 0.4 and higher produce coma.

Alcohol affects circulation and cardiac functioning and dilates skin blood vessels, thereby producing flushing and a drop in body temperature. Reduction in risk of coronary artery disease has been proposed as a benefit of low daily doses of alcohol. The rationale for this proposal is based on the finding that in low doses, alcohol can increase high-density lipoprotein (HDL) and decrease low-density lipoprotein (LDL). This benefit is canceled out, however, by common unhealthy behaviors such as poor diet or smoking.

Clinical Presentation

Patients who ask questions about their personal substance use may have used substances for a relatively short period of time, but more often, patient questions are motivated by having recently suffered negative consequences from long-standing substance use. Routine substance use and abuse screening has become a standard of practice in primary care, but fear of disclosure makes effective screening difficult. The most consistent descriptor for substance abuse may be the numerous health consequences of abusing drugs and alcohol. Personal characteristics are not reliable indicators. Persons of all ages, races, religions, and socioeconomic status are susceptible to substance abuse, and substance dependence typically follows substance abuse.

The clinical presentation of a person with substance intoxication, abuse, or dependence will varies depending on the substance abused. Table 17.7 presents a summary of the clinical presentation of an individual with cannabis, cocaine, amphetamine, nicotine, or alcohol intoxication, abuse, or dependence.

Disorders that can be induced by cannabis, cocaine, amphetamine, and alcohol intoxication, abuse, or dependence include anxiety disorders, mood disorders, psychotic disorders with delusions or hallucinations, and delirium. Sexual dysfunction and sleep disorders may be induced by cocaine, amphetamine, or alcohol intoxication, whereas a motivational syndrome may occur with cannabis use, and withdrawal delirium or persisting dementia may occur with excessive alcohol use.

A variety of screening/assessment tools exist to assess risk of substance abuse

Diagnostic Reasoning

DSM-IV-TR Symptom Criteria

The DSM-IV-TR divides substance-related disorders into two groups: the Substance Use Disorders (Substance Dependence and Substance Abuse) and the Substance-Induced Disorders that includes delirium, withdrawal, intoxication, dementia, persisting amnestic disorder, psychosis, mood disturbances, anxiety, sexual dysfunction, and sleep disorders.

Table 17.7 Clinical Presentation: Selected Substance Intoxication, Abuse, or Dependence

Cannabis Disorder

- *Abuse:* Evidence of use that interferes with performance at work or school or in physically hazardous situations. Legal problems associated with possession or use. Conflict with significant others over use and/or effects.
- *Dependence:* Evidence of tolerance and psychological or physical problems associated with compulsive use. Heavy users experience withdrawal that is relieved or avoided by repeated use throughout the day. A great deal of time may be spent in acquiring and using the drug. Use interferes with important relationships and continues despite interpersonal, performance, psychological, physical, financial,or legal problems associated with use.
- *Intoxication:* Cannabis high typically includes euphoria, grandiosity, sedation, lethargy, short-term memory impairment; complex mental processes are impaired; user perceives self and experiences as occurring in slow motion. Intoxication may include anxiety, dysphoria, or withdrawal away from others. Two or more of the following should also be present: conjunctiva injection (red eye), increased appetite, dry mouth, and tachycardia.

Cocaine Disorders

- *Abuse:* Evidence of use-related problems, neglect of important responsibilities, interpersonal conflict, particularly around payday or special occasions when high-dose use occurs for a longer-than-usual period of time that is followed by less frequent use, fewer use-related problems, or abstinence. Legal problems associated with use or possession.
- *Dependence:* Early evidence is significant difficulty resisting cocaine use whenever it is available. Because of the short half-life of cocaine, frequent doses must be taken to maintain intoxication or the "high" effects. Therefore, dependence can require a great deal of time and money to obtain the drug. Dependent individuals engage in illegal activities in order to buy or obtain the drug. Dependence is marked by drug-free periods when the individual seeks sleep or rest. Hallmarks of cocaine dependence include gross neglect of all other activities or responsibilities in order to continue use of the drug, and severe mental and physical effects (e.g., paranoid thinking, aggressive behavior, weight loss).
- *Intoxication:* Significant negative behavioral and psychological changes and two or more of the following: tachycardia or bradycardia, pupillary dilation, increased or decreased blood pressure, sweating, chills, nausea or vomiting, weight loss, psychomotor agitation or retardation, muscular weakness, respiratory depression, chest pain, cardiac arrhythmia, confusion, seizures, dyskinesias, dystonias, or coma.
- *Withdrawal:* Acute withdrawal ("crash") typically occurs following a binge or prolonged use of high doses. There is intense dysphoria and weariness. Suicidal thoughts and behavior can develop. Typical withdrawal symptoms develop within a few hours. Characteristic withdrawal includes severe dysphoria and two or more of the following: fatigue, vivid nightmares, insomnia or hypersomnia, increased appetite, and psychomotor retardation or agitation. Some people may have only mild withdrawal symptoms. Experienced heavy users may plan their drug use to include substances that can prevent or minimize withdrawal.

Amphetamine Disorders

- *Abuse:* Evidence of significant use related legal and social problems typically associated with amphetamine abuse. Characteristic problems tend to be problems associated with behavior while intoxicated, particularly aggressive behaviors.
- *Dependence:* Evidence of significant aggression or violent behavior, particularly when amphetamine is injected. There may be evidence of binges or runs of repeated high doses, followed by drug-free periods or rest. Acute anxiety, paranoid thinking, and psychosis are associated with high-dose use. Tolerance leads to marked dose increases.
- *Intoxication:* Recent use, followed by significant behavioral and psychological changes, impaired judgment, and impaired functioning. Euphoria, blunted affect, changes in interactions with others, interpersonal sensitivity, anxiety, tension, along with two or more of the following: tachycardia or bradycardia, pupillary dilation, increased or decreased blood pressure, sweating or chills, nausea or vomiting, weight loss, psychomotor agitation or retardation, muscular weakness, respiratory depression, chest pain, cardiac arrhythmia, confusion, seizures, dyskinesias, dystonias, or coma.
- *Withdrawal:* Following heavy and prolonged use there is dysphoria and two or more of the following: fatigue, vivid nightmares, insomnia or hypersomnia, increased appetite, psychomotor retardation or agitation. Rather than the weight loss associated with heavy use, withdrawal typically includes significant increase in appetite and rapid weight gain. Amphetamine withdrawal depression can include suicidal thoughts.

Nicotine Disorders

- *Dependence:* Evidence of tolerance to nicotine includes the absence of nausea, dizziness, or other characteristic symptoms of nicotine effects, the use of nicotine to relieve or to avoid withdrawal symptoms, and use of larger amounts than desired. Many people who are nicotine dependent have an expressed desire to stop trying and have tried to stop, unsuccessfully, within the previous year. Dependence is also characterized by decreasing or giving up activities because of smoking restrictions, and continued use despite the experience of chronic nicotine-related health.

Substance dependence may be with or without physiologic dependence. Substance dependence is defined by the DSM-IV-TR as a maladaptive pattern of substance use, leading to clinically significant impairment or distress manifested by tolerance, withdrawal, lack of success in cutting down, spending increasing amounts of time in activities to obtain the substance, other important activities are given up or reduced in favor of pursuing the substance, the substance is taken in larger than intended amounts, and use continues despite awareness of negative consequences. Three or more of these must occur during the same 12-month period.

Substance abuse is defined as a maladaptive pattern of substance use leading to significant impairment or distress, as manifested by one or more occurring in the past 12-month period: failure in significant role obligations (work, school, neglect of children); recurrent use in physically hazardous situations, such as driving an automobile; legal problems related to substance use; and continued use despite significant problems.

A diagnostic label is significant and often necessary for the patient's recovery. However, hearing the voice of the patient is always important. The Nursing Situation 17.1 described in "Jake's Story" illustrates a multifactorial approach to substance abuse, in this case, alcoholism, that is consistent with practice within a Circle of Caring model.

The existence and prevalence of significant comorbidities may make the "primary" disorder difficult to identify. However, it is always necessary to treat the substance-abuse and dependence issues, regardless of the comorbidity; concurrently, the evidence shows that unless the comorbid condition is also addressed and treated, recurrence of the substance abuse is likely.

Management

The first treatment goal in substance abuse is abstinence. Research for many years has shown that moderation in usage is rarely effective for those with a substance-abuse problem. The second goal is restoring the physical, psychological, and social well-being of the person and family. Significant damage has often been done to the patient's support system. The family may have additional co-dependent and enabling issues to address and also may need treatment. Sometimes relationships that have remained intact during the substance-abuse phase ultimately falter and disintegrate when one partner becomes engaged in treatment.

Although some patients with substance-related problems recover without formal treatment, especially as they age, most require a variety of interventions. Approaches include specific procedures or techniques such as individual therapy, family therapy, group therapy, relapse prevention, pharmacotherapy, and treatment programs. Treatment programs tend to be multidisciplinary, and often include a specific set of procedures. However, there is no standardization of terminology for categorizing treatment programs and procedures, and their effects are difficult to measure. Broadly, some programs focus on controlling acute withdrawal (detoxification) and others aim at long-term behavioral change; some use pharmacologic interventions and others are based on individual psychotherapy, Alcoholics Anonymous (AA) or other 12-step principles, or therapeutic community principles. Publicly funded treatment programs for drug dependence are categorized as methadone maintenance (mostly outpatient), outpatient drug-free programs, therapeutic communities, or short-term inpatient programs.

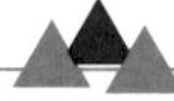

NURSING SITUATION 17.1

Jake's Story

Jake was in his early 60s, was disabled, and lived above a bar. He was an alcoholic, which took me a little while to figure out, but anyway, he was alcoholic and never ate anything much. His refrigerator just had beer in it. . . . We decided ("we"–it was really I who decided) that if he had a microwave, he could actually get some food from the drugstore down the street. He'd be able to pop it in the microwave and have a nice hot meal. So Jake decided that's what he wanted to do, or, so I thought. We got the simplest kind of microwave ever, and I trained Jake and his neighbor, Falstaff, to use it. . . . They practiced and they had a nice meal . . . [but] when I came back the next week, the little microwave plate had a hole burned through it. And Jake and Falstaff both said they would never touch the microwave again. . . . He wanted to do what he'd always done and stop by the pub and get a little something with his beer and that was his lifestyle and a young, brash nurse wasn't going to change any of that.

So he really taught me an important lesson about listening in lots of different ways for what clients really want and need and where they are. I thought I had done that. But I learned a whole new dimension from him. . . . It was after this incident that I actually wanted to talk to him in depth about what his lifestyle was really like and what he wanted. I had never done it in a dialogue kind of way. I think it had been more [in terms of] you assess and ask certain questions and you get certain information. But we had to dialogue, because here was this microwave sitting between us. . . . Here was this hilarious thing that had happened, and I think breaking through more of the professional edge that I maybe kept too shiny made the difference. He talked about what he expected for the rest of his life. He needed help with his scabies and that's why I had come in originally, he needed to make sure that his laundry lady kept coming and washing his sheets, and basically, he didn't need anything else. He was happy to be able to talk about his life; he had worked in a sheltered workshop and felt very proud of that when he was a young man. He needed to be connected and he needed to talk about his life. It helped me understand that's what everybody has a need for (p 80).

SOURCE: Smith-Battle, L, et al: The responsive use of self in community health nursing practice. Adv Nurs Sci 20(2):75–89, 1997.

Substantial reduction in illicit drug use, antisocial behaviors, and psychiatric distress among patients dependent on cocaine or heroin are much more likely following treatment lasting at least 3 months. Such a time-in-treatment effect is seen across very different modalities, from residential therapeutic communities to ambulatory methadone maintenance programs.

After an initial period of detoxification, persons in treatment for substance abuse will need a period of sustained rehabilitation that includes education, support, and in some cases, psychotropic drugs, to discourage patients from using the substance involved or to treat any underlying psychiatric disorder.

Substance-abusing and substance-dependent patients may be resistant and fearful or lack the will and motivation to confront their behavior. In addition to primary care, specialized substance treatment services are needed if the patient's disorder is to be adequately addressed and his or her risk for substance-related disability, morbidity, and mortality are to be decreased. Primary-care practitioners are often the first health-care professionals to observe the health and psychosocial impact of substance abuse; sometimes, the practitioner is the only health-care professional the patient is willing to talk to. Clinicians can take advantage of this by striving to help patients to recognize their substance abuse and to take the first steps toward improvement. Patients with poor physical health or severe legal and interpersonal problems will need improvement in these areas in order to feel able to change their substance-abuse behaviors. Substance-related mental disorders should be treated as well. Patients often already have a great deal of information about their substance abuse and the benefits of stopping. The most useful patient education will address the process of stopping. Some people are able to stop on their first try, but the more typical pattern is repeated efforts to stop until the individual is finally substance-free. An *intervention* is a strategy to get a person who has been resistant to treatment to confront the reality of his or her drug and/or alcohol problem. In a private location, close family and friends confront the individual with the facts of his or her substance abuse and the consequences of actions the individual has taken, or failed to take. The intervention is an attempt to hold the person accountable for his or her actions, using a "tough love" approach. The end result sought is for the person to willingly choose to seek treatment.

Specific management of each case will depend on the substance being abused. General indications for the need for inpatient treatment of substance abuse are presented in Table 17.8. Specific interventions and assessment tools the clinician may use for nicotine or alcohol disorders in the outpatient setting are presented in Table 17.9.

Treatment of the severely mentally ill who are also drug dependent continues to pose problems; specialized addiction agencies have trouble treating such patients. Generally, integrated treatment of both the psychiatric disorder and the addiction is more effective than either parallel or sequential treatment, but facilities able to handle both are rare.

A related issue is the funding of treatment programs for substance-related disorders in general. Managed care organizations tend to assume that the relatively brief course of outpatient counseling will be effective with patients who are dependent on illicit drugs, perhaps suffer from significant comorbidities, and who have minimal social supports. At present, the trend is a short-term view that provides the care that costs the least, ignoring studies that show that more services can produce better long-term outcomes.

Table 17.8 Indications for Inpatient Treatment of Substance Abuse

Current Situation

- Severe illness
- Suicidal, either in ideation or intent
- Lengthy and heavy substance abuse
- Physiologic dependence on a substance (as defined by DSM-IV criteria), such as withdrawal as manifested by the characteristic withdrawal symptoms for the substance OR taking the same (or closely related) substance to relieve symptoms of withdrawal
- Alcohol withdrawal (as defined by DSM-IV criteria), such as (1) cessation (or reduction) in alcohol use that has been heavy and prolonged; (2) two or more of the following, occurring within several hours to a few days of withdrawing the alcohol: autonomic hyperactivity, increased hand tremor, insomnia, nausea and vomiting, transient visual or auditory hallucinations or illusions, psychomotor agitation, anxiety, or grand mal seizures; (3) use as the cause of clinically significant distress or impairment in social, occupational, or other important areas of functioning; (4) the symptoms are not due to another medical condition or mental disorder.

Past History

- History of withdrawal
- History of seizures

Follow-Up and Referral

In addition to primary care, patients being treated for substance abuse will need access to several information and support resources, which should include education services, treatment programs, and support groups. It is unlikely that any single program or support group will be sufficient, so patients are encouraged to make repeated contact with several different types of programs and groups. (See Nursing Situation 17.2.) Referral to a specialist should be made immediately when the patient's behavior represents a danger to self or others. Substance abuse, particularly alcohol abuse, is a factor in motor vehicle accidents, family violence, and suicide. It can also be very helpful for patients to have

Table 17.9 Interventions for Nicotine or Alcohol Disorders in the Outpatient Setting

Nicotine Disorders Ask every patient at every visit if he or she smokes. Write a patient's smoking status in the health record under vital signs. Ask patients about their desire to stop and support their intentions to do so. Motivate patients who are reluctant to quit. Help motivated patients to set a stop date. Prescribe/recommend nicotine replacement therapy. Help patients resolve problems that result from quitting. Encourage relapse smokers to quit again. *Alcohol Disorders* Screen for alcohol abuse using the CAGE questionnaire or the Alcohol Use Disorders Identification Test (AUDIT). *CAGE:* C: Have you ever felt you should *cut* down on your drinking? A: Have people *annoyed* you by criticizing your drinking? G: Have you ever felt bad or *guilty* about your drinking? E: Have you ever had a drink first thing in the morning to steady your nerves or to get rid of a hangover (*eyeopener*)? A score of 1 or more raises a high index of suspicion and warrants further evaluation. See http://www.projectcork.org/clinical-tools/index.html	*AUDIT:* How often do you have a drink containing alcohol? How many drinks containing alcohol do you have on a typical day when you are drinking? How often do you have six or more drinks on one occasion? How often during the last year have you found that you were not able to stop drinking once you had started? How often during the last year have you failed to do what was normally expected from you because of drinking? How often during the last year have you needed a first drink in the morning to get yourself going after a heavy drinking session? How often during the last year have you had a feeling of guilt or remorse after drinking? How often during the last year have you been unable to remember what happened the night before because you had been drinking? Have you or someone else been injured as a result of your drinking? Has a relative or friend or a health-care professional been concerned about your drinking or suggested that you cut down? See http://www.projectcork.org/clinical–tools/index.html for details regarding usage & scoring

at least one appointment with a specialist, in order to develop a comprehensive assessment of the patient's substance use and abuse. For the patient, this assessment is a critical source of information that can reduce his or her ambivalence toward making needed changes in substance-related behaviors. Seeing a specialist can also be motivational, in that one of the most common reasons for failing to try to make required changes in behavior is the patient's unspoken fears of failure.

Patient Education

The clinician should educate patients regarding the effects of drugs, especially during pregnancy, and provide information on substance abuse and treatment to patients and their families. Practitioners should provide information regarding danger of exposure to HIV, hepatitis, and other infections, and to obtain appropriate testing if there is suspicion of exposure. Care providers should teach family members about the dynamics that may continue to enable substance abuse; often they are unaware of these. The clinician can give family members specific feedback in this area about behaviors that he or she has observed; it is also important to discuss the strategy of using an intervention with the family and how to set up one if indicated.

Twelve-step programs should be encouraged—for example, Narcotics Anonymous (NA) or Alcoholics Anonymous (AA) for the individual with the substance-abuse problem and AlAnon for family members. As noted earlier, family members and significant others need treatment also.

Mood Disorders

Overview

Mood (affective) disorders are characterized by abnormalities of the emotional state (attitude, predominant state of mind) that are generally described as elated or depressed. The two major types of mood disorders include major depressive (unipolar) disorder (MDD) and bipolar (manic–depressive) disorder (BPDI and BPDII). The depressive episodes in Bipolar (BD) are essentially indistinguishable from those in major depressive disorder. Patients with underlying BD who present with major depression are likely to be misdiagnosed, especially if depression is the initial manifestation of their illness or they (and their family/friends) are not carefully queried about prior symptoms of mania or hypomania. Moreover, there is no clear boundary between mood disturbances; the Mood (affective) disorder category encompasses a complex continuum of officially recognized and unrecognized subtypes. Some authorities make the case that depression should no longer be regarded as a diagnosis but rather as a presentation of several important disorders that need to be ruled in or out.

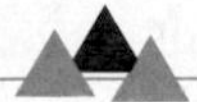

NURSING SITUATION 17.2

Substance Abuse and the Circle of Caring

The following vignette, abstracted from L. Smith-Battle, M.A. Drake, and M. Diekemper, "The Responsive Use of Self in Community Health Nursing Practice," Advances in Nursing Science, 20(2):85, addresses a person with substance abuse. It is a story that highlights the skills of involvement, coordination, and advocacy that helped to reintegrate this mother into the community and the child into the family. The mother's eventual reintegration was contingent upon the APN's responsiveness and perseverance in a situation with an uncertain outcome, which demonstrates practice within a Circle of Caring.

In this situation, an unreceptive new mother tested positive at the birth of her baby for cocaine abuse. The infant was severely injured at 2 months of age in a car accident when, unrestrained, he hit his head against the dashboard. The infant was removed from the mother's care and placed with an aunt. The following account is from a nurse involved with the family:

> [In the year after the accident], I saw the baby at the aunt's house and we got him involved with developmental programs… I hooked them up with all that… Meanwhile, I was visiting mom. [Describes how the mother was in and out of treatment programs.]
>
> I got a phone call from her one morning. She told me that a drug dealer had beat her up and put a gun to her head over a 5-dollar debt. "I'm going to die. I'm either going to get killed or I'm going to die of using cocaine."So I worked with the social worker and we got her into a long-term, 3-month treatment [program] away from the entire environment. And when she came back, I will never forget, I cried when I called her. She had make-up on. She had gained weight… I didn't even recognize her…
>
> A year later, when she came back, she started visiting with her son at the aunt's house, and gradually the whole team, the social worker, myself, the aunt, and all other interventionists, we had huge meetings and we basically started reintegrating the child into the home. And now she has him full-time. And she's been clean… She keeps up with all [her son's appointments] and she goes to Narcotics Anonymous three times a week. She wants to become a treatment counselor and …she finished her GED. She's just a total success story…
>
> … She told me once, "Everyone that ever cared about me has left me or treated me like crap."…[it] was the first time in her life where [although] she was downright obnoxious and hateful [to me], I never bit back or quit coming. I mean, I accepted her behavior because I knew it was the drug use and it wasn't her.

Consensus recommendations from a panel of experts representing psychiatry, primary care, pharmacy, and managed care state that every patient suspected of having unipolar depression be evaluated for bipolar disorder (BD) using a quick screening tool before being treated with antidepressants. Emerging data from a variety of sources have confirmed a typical delay between symptom onset and diagnosis of 5 to 10 years with patients seeing an average of four health-care providers before the correct diagnosis is given. MDD (unipolar depression) is a common misdiagnosis, the treatment for which (e.g., antidepressant monotherapy) may induce mania in BD patients. Over a 5-year period, 85 percent of patients will have a relapse after one affective episode. Half of the patients may experience subsyndromal symptoms during interepisodic periods, such as cognitive impairment and impulsivity, with length of interepisode intervals progressively diminishing with each recurrence.

Further complicating this picture is the typical comorbidity among mood disorders and anxiety disorders. Some studies indicate that 47 percent of patients with a history of major depression also meet the criteria for comorbid anxiety disorder; other studies report 59 percent and higher of the patients who meet DSM-IV-TR criteria for MDD have a history of comorbid anxiety disorders. Typically, MDD has a later age at onset than anxiety, suggesting that MDD may be secondary to anxiety. The fact that anxiety appears to pose a strong predisposition for depression also suggests that early identification and treatment of anxiety may be an important preventive intervention strategy for limiting subsequent development of depression.

In the case of BD, comorbid substance abuse is greater than in any other psychiatric disorder except for antisocial personality. The lifetime prevalence of anxiety disorders in BD patients is approximately 50 percent and associated with worse functional outcomes. Many BD patients demonstrate cognitive impairments. Common medical conditions associated with BD include migraine headaches, asthma, and obesity.

Major Depressive Disorder (MDD)

Major depressive disorder is a primary mood disorder that is characterized by severe negative changes in mood, thinking, and behavior. A person who is severely depressed will have intense feelings of sadness, irritability, or apathy. These feelings may persist at all times and are unrelieved by circumstantial changes. At home, at school, at work, or in recreational situations, the mood of the depressed person basically varies little. In some cases, the mood of the depressed person may vary slightly but without improving significantly. It is not unusual for a depressed person to feel consistently worse at certain times of the day. Many depressed persons may actually experience better moods toward the end of the day and worse moods at the start of the day. This pattern may have to do with depression-induced disturbances in sleep–wake circadian cycles and brain serotonin activity. The thought of facing yet another gloomy day can act as a psychodynamic factor that makes morning moods worse than afternoon moods.

Negative changes in thinking associated with depression are common. Depressed thinking can be described as global, distorted, and circular. Rather than dealing with today, the depressed person may instead focus on distant events or think about the future as if it is a singular, knowable event. With depression, the balance between positive and negative thoughts about self, about life and about the future becomes distorted. Negative views can seem more valid than positive views. Global negative thinking can take on a ruminative or circular pattern, so that the depressed person's negative thinking seems to always depart from and arrive at the same painful conclusions.

Major depression interferes with decision making and concentration. The smallest decision, such as whether or not to make a phone call, becomes difficult. Depression-related negative changes in thinking can be very upsetting. The depressed person may become alarmed by his or her inability to make choices or to concentrate. Although others may recognize negative changes in the depressed person's thinking, the onset of negative thinking can also develop without warning to the patient. The negative thinking associated with major depression may include thoughts of death and suicide. Some people make a clear distinction between passive thoughts of death and active thoughts of suicide, but both patterns are disturbing.

Changes in behavior associated with major depression may occur. The person's behavior may become uncharacteristic. Unlike changes in thinking, there can be very clear, external evidence of changes in behavior. For this reason, significant others may become aware of the depression before the depressed person does. Depression-related changes in behavior range from changes in grooming and in interpersonal interactions to substance abuse, aggression, and social withdrawal.

For some people, depression is made up of vague physical symptoms that are difficult to describe. For example, an acutely depressed man may describe his problem as fatigue rather than depression. He may also complain of headache, backache, or abdominal pain. In Western cultures, physical conditions and psychological conditions are viewed as different and separate states. People are expected to use psychological language to describe their psychological experiences and physical language to describe their physical experiences. Persons with other cultural backgrounds, including individuals of African-American, Asian, or Hispanic descent, may reject this mind–body split.

Epidemiology and Causes

It is estimated that between 5 and 20 percent of the population will experience a significant depression at some time during their lives. Specifically, the lifetime prevalence of a major depressive episode (MDE) is 16.2 percent and 6.6 percent 12-month prevalence. The prevalence of depression in older adults (over 65) can be as high as 40 percent in hospitalized and nursing home patients and as high as 30 percent in community-dwelling elders. Older adults have many risk factors for depression because of the frequent losses experienced within this age group.

Once a person experiences a depressive episode, he or she is at high risk for a recurrence. As many as 50 percent of these individuals go on to experience a recurrence; after two episodes, there is a 80 percent chance of another recurrence. There is a higher incidence of depression in women (21 percent) than in men (13 percent). Researchers have studied this phenomenon for decades, but there does not appear to be a single, universal explanation for women's greater susceptibility to depression. It has been suggested that men and women may in fact be equally susceptible to major depression, but men are taught to value masculinity and therefore may be less likely to express depression directly, whereas women learn to express their negative mood states directly. Significantly, 8–19 percent of patients with MDD severe enough to require hospitalization eventually commit suicide. One out of seven patients with recurrent depressive illness commits suicide, 70 percent of whom have seen their primary care provider within 6 weeks prior to committing suicide, often for somatic complaints. In the absence of systematic screening, usual care by primary care providers fails to detect between 30 and 50 percent of depressed patients. Practitioners frequently state that lack of time is an important obstacle to detection (see BATHE technique, p. 1155). In addition, clinicians cite their own emotional discomfort in dealing with depression and misplaced concern that patients may also be uncomfortable discussing depression as barriers to effective screening. Risk factors are presented in Risk Factors 17.1.

Estimates of comorbidity among the depressive and anxiety disorders are high. Data from the Epidemiologic Catchment Area (ECA) study indicated that 47 percent of patients with a history of major depression also meet criteria for comorbid anxiety disorder. An even higher percentage (59 percent) of patients who meet DSM-IV-TR criteria for MDD in the National Comorbidity Survey (NCS) had a history of comorbid anxiety disorder. MDD typically has a later age at onset than anxiety disorders, suggesting that MDD might be secondary to anxiety. This suggests that early identification and treatment of anxiety disorder may be an important intervention strategy for limiting subsequent development of depression.

RISK FACTORS 17.1

Major Depression

Age	Adolescent or older adult
Gender	Female
Ethnicity	
Family History	Strong family history of depression, suicide or attempt, alcohol abuse, or other substance abuse
History	History of migraine headaches, back pain, recent myocardial infarction, and/or peptic ulcer disease
Current Medical Condition	Current chronic disease (especially multiple diseases) Insomnia
Lifestyle	Stress Poverty Less than high school education Recent traumatic event Parent or caregiver of a child or children with behavioral disorders, especially hyperactivity Retired

Patients with depression have more impairment in overall quality of life compared with patients with most other chronic medical diagnoses. In addition, these patients are more apt to frequent health services in the primary-care setting than patients without mental disorders and they tend to be less satisfied with their overall care. Women suffer depression at twice the rate of men and depression is an independent risk factor for morbidity and mortality from cardiac disease. The World Health Organization (WHO) estimates that by the year 2020, depression will rank second only to cardiovascular illness in terms of disease burden and as a worldwide cause of disability.

The biological, genetic, and psychosocial factors in the etiology of depression have currently been identified

Pathophysiology

A number of studies have reported abnormalities in biogenic amines metabolites in blood, urine, and cerebrospinal fluid (CSF). The data reported are most consistent with the hypothesis that mood disorders are associated with heterogeneous dysregulation of the biogenic amines. Of the biogenic amines, norepinephrine and serotonin are the two neurotransmitters most associated with the pathophysiology of mood disorders. It is theorized that dopamine also plays a role. Although the data are not conclusive, other neurochemical factors have also been identified, including amino acid neurotransmitters such as GABA and neuroactive peptides, specifically vasopressin and endogenous opiates, and have also been implicated in the pathophysiology of mood disorders. The amino acids glutamate and glycine appear to be the major excitatory neurotransmitters in the central nervous system. The hippocampus has high concentrations of *N*-methyl-D-asparate (NMDA) receptors; thus it is possible that glutamine, in conjunction with hypercortisolemia, mediates the neurocognitive effects of chronic stress. There is emerging evidence that drugs that antagonize NMDA receptors have antidepressant effects.

The hypothalamus is central to the neuroendocrine axes. It receives many neuronal inputs that use biogenic amine neurotransmitters. Theoretically although it is possible that for a particular dysregulation of a neuroendocrine axis to be involved in the etiology of a mood disorder, it is more likely an underlying brain disorder. Other neuroendocrine abnormalities associated with mood disorders include decreased nocturnal secretion of melatonin, decreased prolactin release in response to tryptophan administration, decreased levels of follicle-stimulating hormones (FSH) and luteinizing hormone (LH), and decreased testosterone in men.

A correlation between the hypersecretion of cortisol and depression is one of the oldest observations in biologic psychiatry. Neurovegetative signs and symptoms of depression may be correlated to various neuroendocrine abnormalities. Specifically, these include (1) increased cortisol and corticotropin-releasing hormone (CRF), (2) an increase in adrenal size, (3) decreased inhibitory response of glucocorticoids to dexamethasone, and (4) a blunted response of thyroid-stimulating hormone (TSH) level to infusion of thyroid-releasing hormone (TRH). Anti-depressant therapy leads to normalization of these pituitary–adrenal abnormalities.

There have been recent advances in the evaluation of the hypothalamic–pituitary–adrenal (HPA) axis in depression. Depressed patients in one study had impaired function in the fast feedback loop; thus, for at least some of them, the functioning of cortisol receptors in the hippocampus may have been abnormal. Other studies demonstrate that hypercortisolemia can damage hippocampal neurons. This can lead to the conclusion that a cycle of stress, leading to increases in the release of cortisol, may result in increasing damage to an already impaired hippocampus.

Immunologic abnormalities have been reported in depressed persons, and in those grieving the loss of a significant other. The dysregulation of the cortisol axis may affect the immune status, meaning that there may be abnormal hypothalamic regulation of the immune system, specifically an upregulation of proinflammatory cytokines. This normalizes with antidepressant therapy.

Approximately 5 to 10 percent of all patients with depression have a coexisting thyroid disorder. About one-third of all patients with major depressive disorder who have an otherwise normal thyroid axis have been found to have a blunted release of thyrotropin, the thyroid-stimulating hormone. This abnormality has been reported in a wide range of psychiatric diagnoses, so the diagnostic implications are limited. Recent research has focused on the theory that a subset of depressed patients may have an unrecognized autoimmune disorder that affects the thyroid gland. Some depressed patients benefit from liothyronine (Cytomel). A thyroid level should be obtained on all depressed patients.

Sleep disorders are commonly associated with depression. Some studies have demonstrated a blunted sleep-induced stimulation of growth hormone release in depressed patients. In addition to inhibition of growth hormones and release of corticotropin-releasing hormone (CRH), somatostatin levels are lower in the cerebrospinal fluid (CSF) of depressed patients than in those with schizophrenia or in normal controls. Sleep electroencephalograms (EEGs) of many depressed persons show abnormalities, and in addition it is known that depressed patients complain of difficulties with sleep. Common abnormalities are delayed sleep onset, shortened rapid eye movement (REM) latency (the time between falling asleep and the first REM period), a longer first REM period, and abnormal delta sleep. The abnormalities associated with the sleep cycle of depressed persons have led researchers to theorize that depression reflects abnormal regulation of circadian rhythms. Animal studies indicate that standard antidepressant therapy are effective in resetting internal "biological clocks."

Increased ventricular size has been consistently correlated with schizophrenia. Positron emission tomography (PET) studies show decreased metabolic activity in the caudate nuclei and frontal lobes in depressed patients that returns to normal with treatment.

Other neuroanatomic considerations include support for the hypothesis that mood disorders involve pathology of the limbic system, the basal ganglia, and the hypothalamus. For example, patients with neurologic disorders of the basal ganglia and the limbic system (especially excitatory lesions of the nondominant hemisphere) may exhibit depressive symptoms. The limbic system and the basal ganglia are intimately connected, and the limbic system may well play a major role in the production of emotions. Alterations in sleep, appetite, and sexual behavior, as well as biologic changes in endocrine, immunologic, and chronobiologic measures in depressed patients all suggest dysregulation of the hypothalamus. The stooped posture of depressed patients, motor slowness, and minor cognitive impairments are similar to the signs of disorder of the basal ganglia, such as Parkinson's disease and other subcortical dementias.

Genetic factors are strongly implicated in the development of mood disorder, although it is impossible to rule out psychosocial factors, as well as other nongenetic factors. Adoption studies have also provided supporting data to the idea that there is a genetic basis for the inheritance of mood disorder. For major depression, the concordance rate in monozygote twins is about 50 percent, arguing strongly for a genetic disposition. A recent study indicated that a functional polymorphism in the serotonin transporter (*5-HTT*) gene may interact with stressful life events to markedly increase the risk for depression and suicide.

Psychopathology

Psychosocial factors also contribute to depression. Stressful life events have been demonstrated to precede first episodes of mood disorders. Some speculate that the stress accompanying the first episode results in long-lasting changes in the brain's biology. These changes, it is speculated, alter various neurotransmitter and intraneuronal signaling systems. This may involve the loss of neurons and reduction in synaptic contacts. Thus, the person is at high risk for subsequent episodes of mood disorder, unrelated to an external stressor. The external psychosocial factors most often associated with the onset of a major depressive episode is the loss of a spouse, or losing a parent, especially if it occurs before age 11. Another risk factor is unemployment; persons out of work are three times more likely to report symptoms of an episode or major depression than those who are employed. However, what may seem to be a relatively mild stressor from an outside perspective may be devastating to the person because of whatever idiosyncratic meaning that they assign to the event.

Patients with certain personality disorders—obsessive–compulsive behavior, histrionic, and borderline—may be at greater risk for depression than patients with antisocial or paranoid personality disorder. Projection and other externalizing defense mechanisms are used by the latter group to protect themselves from their inner rage. In psychodynamic terms, depression is viewed as anger tuned inward, toward the self. Most theories of mania view manic episodes as a defense against underlying depression. John Bowlby theorized that traumatic separations in childhood and damaged early attachments predispose to depression. Losses in adulthood are said to revive the traumatic childhood loss and so precipitate depression in the adult.

Other theories useful to the treatment of MDD is cognitive theory, which speculates that depression results from specific cognitive distortions. Referred to as "depressogenic schemata," these are cognitive templates that perceive both internal and external data in ways that are altered by early experiences. Aaron Beck, a well-known cognitive therapist/theorist, laid out a cognitive triad of depression that includes negative views about the self, about the environment (it is perceived as hostile and demanding), and negative expectations regarding the future. Much of cognitive therapy is aimed at disputing and restructuring these internal cognitive beliefs. (See Table 17.10 for information on cognitive behavioral strategies.)

The theory of "learned helplessness," based on classic research, internal causal explanations after adverse events are thought to produce a loss of self-esteem. Behaviorists who subscribe to this theory see improvement

Table 17.10 Cognitive Behavioral Strategies

Assumptions
- Alterations in content of underlying cognitive processes alter affective states and behavioral problems
- Correction of these faulty constructs can lead to clinical improvement
- Appraisal/perception of situations reflected in their cognitions (both thoughts and visuals)
- Through therapy, patients become aware of these dysfunctions and learn to alter them

Processes
- Identify and alter cognitive distortions that maintain symptoms
- Time-limited, usually 15–25 weeks, once weekly
- Collaborative empiricism
- Structured and directive
- Assigned readings
- Homework and behavioral techniques
- Desensitization in some patients
- Identification of irrational beliefs and automatic thoughts
- Identification of attitudes and assumptions underlying negative thoughts

Source: Adapted from Kaplan & Sadock's *Synopsis of Psychiatry,* 9th ed. Philadelphia, Lippincott Williams & Wilkins, 2003, pp 956–957.

of depression as predicated on the person's learning a sense of control and mastery over the environment.

Clinical Presentation

Assessment of major depression need not be overly complicated, but the focus of the assessment should include more than the presence or absence of significant sadness or apathy. As with other mood disorders, presentation of depression symptoms can vary greatly: Some patients may have little awareness of their symptoms, or may not recognize that their symptoms are in fact symptoms of major depression. The sadness and apathy that characterize major depression may be reported by the patient, observed and reported by significant others, or observed by the practitioner. Two quick questions that provide a preliminary screen for depression have been developed by the United States Preventive Services Task Force (see Advanced Assessment 17.4). The patient is first asked if he or she has felt down or hopeless over the past month and then asked if there has been little interest in doing things over the past month. A positive response to one or both questions in this screen indicates possible major depression but the test has a high false-positive rate. Thus, confirmatory testing should be performed using a validated screening instrument or a clinical interview.

The Patient Health Questionnaire-9 (PHQ-9) consists of a checklist of nine symptoms. The patient is asked to indicate the frequency with which these symptoms have

ADVANCED ASSESSMENT 17.4

Two-Question Depression Screen for Primary Care

1. Over the past 2 weeks, have you felt down, or hopeless?
2. Over the past 2 weeks, have you felt little interest in doing things?

A Yes to either question is a positive screen for depression.

SOURCE: U.S. Preventive Task Force.

occurred over the preceding 2 weeks. The test is scored based on symptom frequency. This instrument can be filled out quickly in the waiting room prior to a primary care visit and provides an effective supplementation to the two-question screening. A similar measure of symptom severity, the self-rated Quick Inventory of Depressive Symptomatology (QIDS-SR), can be used for the same purpose and has the additional benefit of including symptom severity and may thus provide a sensitive measure of change with treatment.

Programs aimed at enhancing public awareness of depression have been effective, in that more patients are likely to seek professional health care for major depression as a result of having accurately self-assessed their symptoms. Patients may bring in depression self-assessment surveys published in popular magazines or local newspapers. When patients have self-assessed their depression symptoms, practitioners can determine symptom intensity, symptom duration, and symptom impact on functioning. Is the patient distressed by some symptoms more than others? It can also be helpful to ask patients to identify which symptoms they consider treatment priorities.

Some patients with major depression may, as a result of the disorder, find it difficult to list their symptoms. In this case assessment, screening assessment tools such as the Zung Self-Rating Depression Scale (SDS) or Beck Depression Inventory (BDI), checklists, direct observations, or yes or no questions may be substituted. When yes or no assessment questions are used, all yes responses should be explored. Extremely depressed patients may not tolerate assessment in any form that requires effort on their part. They can become irritable and impatient with the practitioner for asking questions that, to the patient, seem unnecessary. This situation can sometimes be improved by indicating that the purpose of asking questions is to understand fully the patient's depression and not to qualify or disqualify the patient for treatment.

The Geriatric Depression scale (GDS) is a widely validated screening tool for use in older adults. Depression is one of the five major health problems confronted by older adults. The single most important thing to ask a patient with suspected depression is how she or feels in the morning. If a

Table 17.11 Components of Depression in Elderly Persons

- Vegetative—poor appetite, disrupted sleep, early morning awakening
- Somatic—pain thoughout body or out of proportion with underlying pathology
- Psychological—obsessive feelings of guilt and worry, ruminations throughout the night; suicidal ideation; memory problems
- Psychomotor—anxiety; psychomotor agitation
- Diurnal variation in symptoms—cannot "get moving" in AM, or specific time of day when depression is worst

patient reports that morning is the worst time and that it takes hours to get going, you can be sure this patient is depressed. Many patients diagnosed with dementia are acutally depressed. (See Table 17.11 for components of depression in older adults.)

Diagnostic Reasoning

DSM-IV-TR Symptom Criteria

The DSM-IV-TR symptom criteria for major depression state that five (or more) of the following symptoms have been present during the same 2-week period and represent a change from previous functioning. At least one of the symptoms are either (1) depressed mood or (2) loss of interest or pleasure:

- ▲ Depressed mood or decreased interest/pleasure (apathy)
- ▲ Five or more of the following present within the same 2 weeks:
  - Weight loss
  - Insomnia or hypersomnia
  - Observable behavioral agitation or retardation
  - Loss of energy nearly every day
  - Feelings of worthlessness or guilt
- ▲ Loss of concentration or indecisiveness
- ▲ Recurrent thoughts of death or suicide

Any depressed patient should be thoroughly evaluated for an unrecognized, bipolar illness.

In patients with comorbid anxiety and depression the symptom profile may be balanced or either symptom can predominate; in addition, some patients with so-called mixed anxiety and depression may demonstrate symptoms of both disorders but may not meet the full diagnostic criteria for either. Any patient who has symptoms of either depression or anxeity should be evaluated for current symptoms of both disorders. The range of DSM-IV-TR diagnostic categories must be considered before arriving at a final diagnosis. First rule out other medical conditions, and substance use. Then, it must be determined if the patient has ever experienced symptoms of mania, hypomania, or cyclothymia. Refer to DSM-IV-TR. There are useful paper and pencil assessment tools available also. Then the patients depressive symptoms must be assessed for severity, duration, recurrence, and the like to differentiate among the depressive disorders. Again, refer to DSM-IV-TR criteria. Then the range of other potential mental disorder must be sifted through, including uncomplicated bereavement.

Differential Diagnosis

All patients must be carefully evaluated for underlying medical conditions. Many medical and neurologic disorders and pharmacologic substances can produce symptoms of depression. Careful medical history and physical examination should be done on all patients, including a neurologic exam and routine blood work and urinalysis. Tests for thyroid and adrenal function should be included because disorders of both of these endocrine systems can mimic depression. Cardiac drugs, antihypertensive agents, sedatives, hypnotics, antipsychotics, antiepileptics, antiparkinsonian drugs, analgesics, antibacterials, and antineoplastics are all commonly associated with depressive symptomatology. A careful medication review, including over-the-counter drugs and herbal agents, is imperative. The most common neurologic disorders that may manifest depressive symptoms are Parkinson's disease (50 to 75 percent have depressive symptoms that do not correlate with physical disability), dementing illnesses (including Alzheimer type), epilepsy, cerebrovascular disease, and tumors. The interictal changes associated with temporal lobe epilepsy can mimic a depressive disorder, especially if the epileptic focus is on the right side. There is increasing evidence of linkages between depression and cardiovascular disease, not limited to sequelae but actually preceding the event. In brain tumors, depression is more common in cases of anterior lobe tumor as opposed to posterior lobe lesions, and in both cases it responds to antidepressants. The pseudodementia of MDD can be differentiated from true dementia related to onset (sudden in the case of pseudodementia), and guilt and self-reproach are common features of MDD, and not of the other dementias. Patients with depression will sometimes not answer questions whereas those with dementia may confabulate. Depressed patients may be "coaxed" into remembering during an interview; those with primary dementia cannot.

In terms of mental disorders, depression can be a feature of virtually any disorder listed in the DSM-IV-TR. It is a primary constellation of mood disorders, but has a high co-morbidity with the anxiety disorders, alcohol-use disorders, eating disorders, schizophrenia, schizophreniform disorder, and somatoform disorder, especially somatization disorder. Bereaved patients need assessment also in some instances (Table 17.11).

Management

Remission of symptoms should be the standard for successful treatment of depression. In clinical trails, only 25 to 35 percent of patients experience complete remission of depressive symptoms, suggesting that even fewer patients reach this goal in a real-world clinical setting. Achievement of remission is important because incomplete relief of symptoms may increase the risk of relapse and further impairment. The chance that any one treatment will result in complete remission, particularly in patients with mixed depression and anxiety, is very low. Depressed patients with a coexisting anxiety disorder tend to have a poorer outcome than those with depression alone. Treatment of a mood disorder such as major depression requires a Circle of Caring. Holistic approaches are especially important in the management of psychosocial disorders. Depression affects mind, body, and spirit. It is often impossible to determine whether the physiologic changes began before the psychological, or vice versa.

Pharmacologic Management

Pharmacologic therapy has become a mainstay for the treatment of major depression. About 7 out of 10 patients with severe major depression will obtain symptom relief by taking antidepressant medication. Prescribing antidepressant medication begins with patient education. Each patient should be given as much information as is necessary to ensure that he or she understands the hoped-for benefits of taking medication, the specific medication being prescribed, anticipated effects, possible adverse effects and how to handle them, and what to do in an emergency. When possible, this information should be made available in writing. Effective patient education makes it possible for patients to participate in their care and decreases the risks of having a patient agree to taking medications without being fully informed of the medication risks and benefits.

The process of prescribing medications begins with building a patient symptom profile. A comprehensive list of current and recent patient symptoms is developed. This symptom list includes the symptoms, their intensity, duration, and effects on day-to-day functioning and role performance. From this list, two to four target symptoms are selected. Target symptoms should be identified and used to determine the most appropriate antidepressant medication. These should be distinct symptoms of depression. For example, depressed patients often find themselves in conflict with their spouse or partner and may view improvement in this relationship a treatment priority. Relationship conflict is not a symptom of depression that can be treated with medication, however. In this example, a better target symptom might be irritability, the relief of which might lead to decreased relationship conflict.

Target symptoms are used to evaluate the effectiveness of medication during early stages of treatment and until full symptom remission is obtained. Reliable evidence of target symptom relief within 5 to 10 days tends to indicate that (in the absence of any serious adverse effects) the medication, dose, and schedule prescribed are appropriate. When the patient reports target symptom relief or the assessment indicates symptom remission has been achieved, the practitioner and patient develop a treatment and discontinuation plan. The duration of medication treatment for uncomplicated major depression is 6 to 12 months at the treatment dose. Longer treatment may be helpful for patients with complicated or multiple disorders, such as depression with comorbid anxiety. Patients who have a history of one or more years of untreated depression may require a longer period of treatment.

The side-effect profiles for the newer neurotransmitter receptor-specific antidepressant medications, for example, selective serotonin reuptake inhibitors (SSRI), are less severe than those for the tricyclic antidepressants (TCAs). The receptor-specific antidepressants also have a significantly lower risk of lethal overdose. The advantages of fewer adverse effects and greater patient safety are significant, but many patients will experience initial adverse effects from the newer antidepressants.

Patients who are sensitive to the powerful serotonin activity produced by the SSRIs may be better able to tolerate antidepressants that have both serotonin and norepinephrine (NE) activity, NE activity only, less specific serotonin activity, or an atypical antidepressant. Depressed patients who cannot tolerate SSRIs or the atypical antidepressants may be able to obtain excellent symptom relief from TCAs. TCAs are not less effective than newer antidepressant medications, but they can produce more side effects, take longer to work, and are lethal in overdose.

Antidepressant medications can be prescribed based on their half-life, neurotransmitter activity, side-effect profile, and clinical efficacy. The half-life for newer antidepressant medications ranges from hours to several days. Neurotransmitter activity accounts for the significant differences in medication effects, including sedation, activation, anxiolytic (anti-anxiety), and anticompulsive effects. Important common side-effect risks with serotonin-specific antidepressants include decreased sexual desire, decreased sexual response, headache, stomach upset, sedation, fatigue, or nervousness. Absolute medication-dose limitations have been defined for patients with seizure disorders, renal disease, and liver disease. Some newer antidepressants are contraindicated for persons with bulimia, and some drugs have significant liver P450-interaction effects. There appear to be fewer age-related dose limitations; thus, newer antidepressants tend to be well tolerated by depressed older adults and adolescents. Ongoing clinical trials with pregnant women suggest that for some women, antidepressant medication can be a safe option.

Individual reactions to antidepressant medications are unique, but in general, antidepressant medications with significant NE effects (e.g., bupropion) tend to be activating. Antidepressant medications with multiple neurotransmitter effects (e.g., venlafaxine) may be effective when serotonin-specific antidepressants are not. Patients who have difficulty adjusting to the short-term side effects of antidepressants with a short-half life (e.g., sertraline, paroxetine) may experience milder short-term side effects with longer half-life antidepressants (e.g., fluoxetine). For some

The Iceberg of Depression

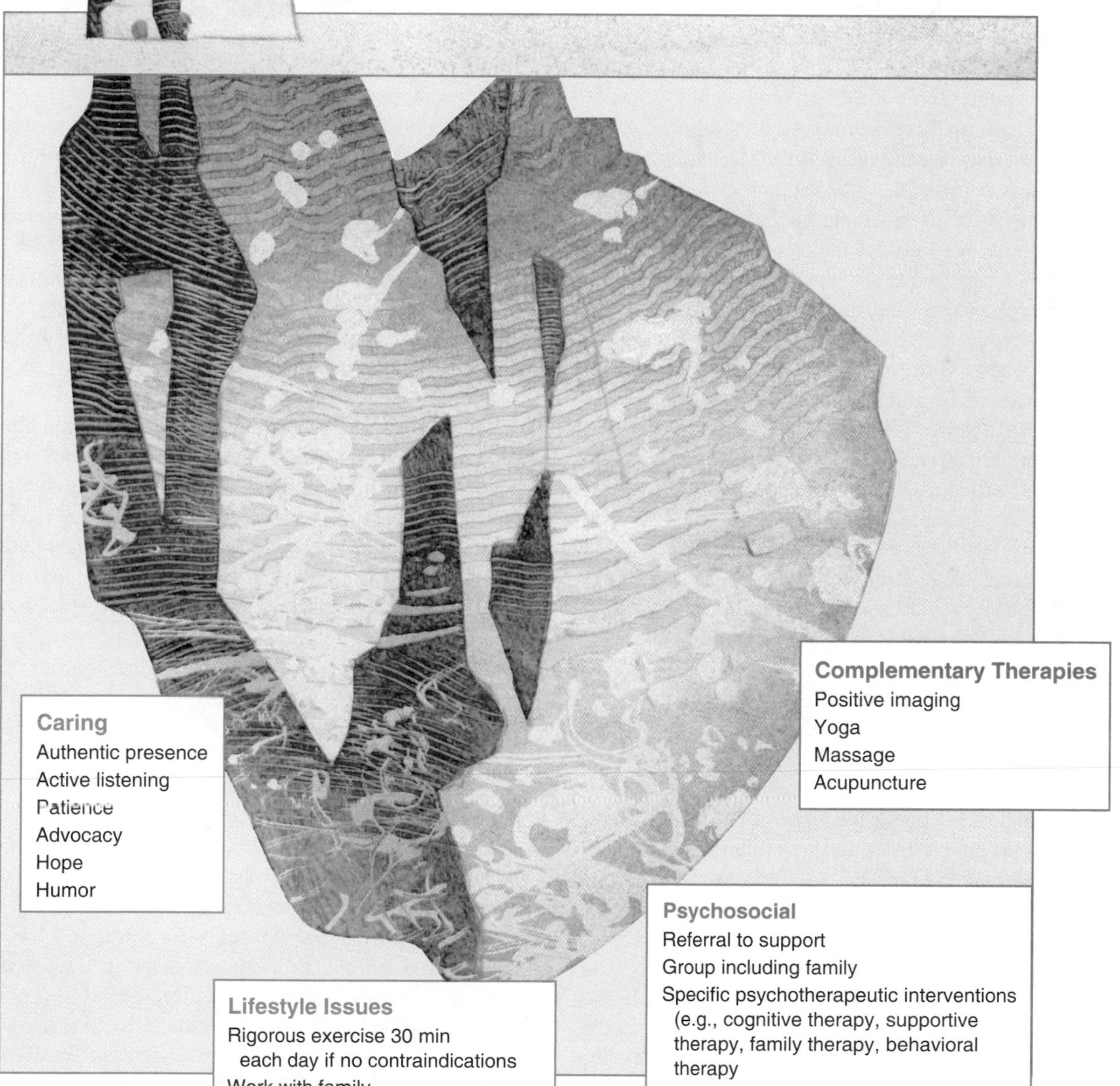

patients, dramatic decreases in adverse effects can be obtained by adjusting the time of day the medication is taken. Patients who are bothered by adverse effects when they take an antidepressant in the morning may experience only mild side effects if they take the same medication with dinner or at bedtime. Extremely low starting doses may be necessary when it is clear that a patient seems able to benefit from an antidepressant but cannot tolerate medication side effects during the early stages of treatment.

Cost should also be considered when prescribing antidepressant medications. A standard once-per-day dose schedule can range from $60 to $100 per month. Some managed-care organizations now limit the choice of antidepressant medications covered in their pharmacy benefits programs. Cost as an access to mental health care issue continues to be a major problem. Persons who might benefit from antidepressant medication may be unable to afford it. Leading pharmaceutical companies offer patient assistance programs that can be helpful. Practitioners can learn about the availability of these programs in their area by contacting the local pharmaceutical representatives.

Providers are advised to identify all compounds the patient is currently taking before starting an antidepressant medication, particularly if the patient has not taken a psychotropic medication before. This list should include all compounds—prescribed and self-administered. Many people now medicate themselves with over-the-counter (OTC) products that they may not consider medications. The high number of such products now available makes this information vital. Patient use of megadose vitamin and mineral supplements, weight-loss or weight-gain products, and nutritional supplements should also be noted. Presently, the standard of practice regarding the use of prescribed and herbal compounds is that the two treatments should not be used simultaneously.

For information on specific drugs for major depression, see Drugs Commonly Prescribed 17.1.

Nonpharmacologic Management

Both interpersonal and cognitive behavioral therapy have been shown to be effective for the treatment of depression and there is evidence that the combination of psychotherapy and pharmacotherapy may be more effective than either alone. Patients with major depression need hope and reassurance. Both are particularly important with patients who may have lived with untreated depression. Informing a person that his or her disorder is major depression and that the disorder can be treated sets the stage for patients to define goals for improvement and begin to combat the secondary demoralization that can develop after months of untreated depression. False reassurances and unrealistic expectations must be avoided, however. The support needs of patients with major depression can be significant. It is unlikely that, in a primary-care setting, practitioners will be able to meet all of a patient's support needs. For this reason, new sources of support should be identified. Friends, relatives, and spouse or partners are important potential sources of information, comfort, and assistance. Professional-led support groups and peer self-help groups are also highly effective.

Support is an important resource for all depressed patients, but patients who are anxious or irritable may require a great deal of practitioner patience. Anxious, irritable patients can be indecisive, critical, and demanding and can appear uncooperative or uninterested. Every effort must be made to avoid getting into a power struggle or challenging upset patients. In the long run, reassuring acceptance is easier and more effective.

Establishing a routine and focusing on activities and behaviors rather than feelings may be a constructive approach. Massage, relaxation therapies, exercise, good nutrition, and a variety of forms of self-care should be initiated and supported.

For some patients, the only important outcome of treatment for major depression is symptom relief. Normalized sleep, appetite, mood, energy, and concentration should, however, be viewed as minimal patient outcomes. Symptom relief and symptom remission are necessary patient outcomes, but if the patient's risk for future episodes of depression is to be significantly lowered, additional outcomes need to be addressed. Improved patient depression awareness is important. Patients treated for major depression should, as a stated outcome of treatment, increase their understanding of major depression and improve their personal methods of coping with depression. The most important outcome is that the patient will immediately seek help should symptoms of major depression return. Recurrent episodes of major depression or major depression that has continued unrelieved for months or is characterized by extremely high symptom levels requires referral and specialized care, sometimes in an inpatient setting.

Follow-Up and Referral

Follow-up during treatment of depression and/or anxiety is absolutely necessary to ensure adherence to therapy. The patient must be monitored to ensure that the prescription was filled and that the medication was taken. Treatment outcome should be assessed regularly using formal diagnostic assessment tools. Patients starting an antidepressant medication should be evaluated weekly for the first 4 weeks. This time period is used to assess medication impact on target symptoms, along with any side effects, and to provide support. For persons who can be treated effectively with antidepressant medication, satisfactory symptom remission often is achieved within 4 to 8 weeks. Many patients feel better in 2 to 3 weeks. Unless otherwise indicated, antidepressant medication should continue for 6 to 12 months. Inadequate dose and inadequate duration of treatment can significantly increase the risk of treatment failure and depression relapse. Short half-life antidepressants are discontinued gradually over a period of 2 to 3 weeks. Persons who experience significant serotonin withdrawal syndrome may report flu-like

Drugs Commonly Prescribed 17.1: Antidepressants

Drug	Mechanism of Action	Dose	Comments
MAOIs, older phenelzine (Nardil); tranylcypromine (Parnate)	Irreversible inhibition of MAO-A and MAO-B; enhance norepinephrine, serotonin, dopamine	Variable dependent on agent; orthostatic hypotension; use with caution in mania, suicidal, epilepsy; hypertensive crises; CNS overstimulation.	60%–70% remission rates; may be better in atypical depression; requires dietary restrictions.
Tricyclics (TCA) Amitriptyline (Elavil); desipramine (Norpramine); Nortriptyline (Pamelor); Doxepin (Sinequan); Imipramine (Tofranil, Tofranil-PM); protriptyline (Vivactil); trimipramine (Surmontil)	Block reuptake of norepinephrine, serotonin	Variable depending on specific drug *Wait 5 weeks after discontinuation of fluoxetine, MAOIs. Do not use with history of seizures, glaucoma, urinary retention. *Monitor for suicidality.	Response rates—43%–70% Remission rates—25%–60% Analgesic, anticholinergic, and antimuscarine actions; high side-effect burden *Risk of cardiotoxicity; narrow therapeutic index; high lethality with overdose
Tetracyclic Mirtazepine (Remeron)	Block reuptake of norepinephrine	Initially 15 mg once daily at bedtime; range: 15–45 mg/day Wait for 2 weeks after discontinuation of MAOIs.	Response and remission rates—53%–63% Similar to TCAs Risk of seizures at higher doses
SSRIs Fluoxetine (Prozac) Sertaline (Zolft) Paroxetine (Paxil) Citalopram (Celexa) Escitalopram (Lexapro)	Selectively block reuptake of serotonin	Variable depending on agent; no MAOIs for 5 weeks after discontinuing SSRIs; wait 2 weeks after discontinuing MAOIs to start; nausea, CNS stimulation *Administer in AM with food.	Response rates—60%–70% Remission rates—20%–35% Broad comorbidity coverage; less side effect burden than TCAs; safe in overdose; long half-life, monitor for drug interactions.
SNRIs Venlafaxine (Effexor, Effexor XL) Duloxetine (Cymbalta)	Blocks reuptake of serotonin and norepinephrine	Take with food. Effexor: 75 mg/day initially gradually (may start at 37.5 mg) average dose: 150 mg/day (maximum: 375 mg/day)	Response rate—65%–76% Remission rate—37%–45% Higher remission rates; less side-effect burden vs. TCAs; safe in overdose *Monitor B/P; taper slowly; increased sweating; monitor mental status, mood, affect, suicidality
NDRI Bupropion (Wellbutrin, Wellbutrin SR)	Blocks reuptake of norepinephrine and it is thought dopamine	Initial 50–100 mg/day; range—100–400 mg/day Take early in day to assess sleeplessness.	Response rate—52%–70% Effective in smoking cessation; less sexual dysfunction; safe in overdose *Increased risk of seizure
SA/SRI Nefazodone	Antagonist of 5-HT_2 receptors and blocks reuptake of 5-HT and NE	100 mg two per day initially; range: 300–600 mg/day increase dose gradually. Use with caution after MAOIs—wait for 2 weeks after discontinuation of MAOIs. Headache, nausea	Response rate—35%–67% Remission—35%–52% Modest antidepressant; used mainly for hypnotic and anxiolytic effects
Trazadone (Desyrl)		Initially 150 mg/day (maximum: 400 mg/day) Give at bedtime	Avoid ECT; do not give post-MI; potentiates alcohol, other CNS depressants; sedative effect; avoid use before or after discontinuation of MAOIs without adequate period

symptoms that last a few days. Consultation with a specialist should be considered if withdrawal symptoms appear to be significant or persistent. If this is a second episode of a MDD, the patient needs to be counseled that he or she in all probability will need to remain on medication indefinitely, or the remainder of his or her lives.

Patient Education

The person and his or her family need to understand that depression generates feelings of helplessness, powerlessness, and pessimism; major decisions should be delayed. The practitioner should reassure the patient that current feelings will change. All side effects of drugs should be clearly understood, and the provider should stress the importance of taking medication daily as ordered for maximum effect. The clinician should advise the patient and family that drugs to offset adverse effects are available, or that medication can be changed. Patients should be encouraged to maintain a schedule of activities. It is important to stress that feelings are not behaviors and to emphasize the importance of behaviors.

It is vital to teach the patient and family to report signs of increasing depression and suicidal thoughts. It has been known for some time that in some cases, starting a severely depressed patient on antidepressants may, after 1 to 2 weeks of treatment, provide the boost in energy needed for the patient to design and carry out a suicide plan. Danger signs and symptoms include:

- Hallucinations or delusions
- Severe adverse effects from antidepressant medications (e.g., severe urinary retention, fluctuation in blood pressure, seizures, cardiac complications)
- Suicidal thoughts
- Extreme self-care deficits (e.g., not able to care for basic needs).

Bipolar Disorder

Bipolar Disorder (BD) is commonly seen in the primary care setting and is frequently mistaken for other conditions, most commonly major depressive disorder (MDD). The DSM-IV-TR defines BD as a recurrent mood disorder featuring one or more episodes of mania, hypomania, or mixed episodes of mania and depression. The spectrum of BD includes type I (prior mania) and type II (prior hypomania only). The key difference between mania and hypomania is the degree of functional impairment. Patients with hypomania continue to function adequately—socially, academically, occupationally—although their behavior is significantly different from baseline. Clinicians must be able to distinguish between depressive episodes occurring in the context of unipolar and bipolar mood disorders, as patients suffering from BD require mood-stabilizing pharmacologic therapy, and their symptoms may worsen with antidepressant monotherapy.

Epidemiology and Causes

Bipolar disorder (BD) is the sixth leading cause of disability worldwide in patients 15 to 55 and the financial burden is higher than diabetes. This disorder can severely impact on a patient's quality of life; two-thirds of patients with BD are substantially adversely affected by their illness but the negative impact of BD goes beyond its morbidity rate. Thirty-four percent of patients with BD report a history of suicide attempt; 15 percent of patients will complete the attempt. Suicide attempts can occur in patients in the manic/hypomanic, depressive, and mixed phases of BD but are most likely to occur in patients in a depressive or mixed state.

BDI has a lifetime prevalence of 1 to 2 percent; when the entire spectrum of bipolar disorder is included the prevalence may approach 7 to 10 percent. Men and women are equally affected. The average age at onset usually occurs before adulthood but may develop up to the middle of the fourth decade. New onset of mania after age 50 is rare and should prompt consideration of secondary cause for symptoms. One-third of patients develop the disorder during childhood or adolescence. Over a 5-year period, 85 percent of patients will have a relapse after one affective episode. While most patients experience limited functional recovery despite successful syndrome treatment, early intervention is associated with improved outcomes. Unfortunately, although many patients present to a provider within 1 year from the onset of symptoms—usually to their primary-care provider—there is usually a 5- to 10-year delay from symptom onset to formal diagnosis. Many patients see up to four different clinicians before being properly diagnosed.

In a survey of 85,000 individuals from the general population, 3.4 percent screened positive for bipolar I disorder (BDI) or bipolar II (BDII). Among this group only 19.8 percent had been formally diagnosed with BD. About 31 percent of these patients had been misdiagnosed (and thus treated) for unipolar depression. Most commonly these patients present for treatment for dysphoria characteristic of a depressive episode than for the euphoria associated with a manic or hypomanic episode. Only one lifetime manic or hypomanic episode is required for a patient to be diagnosed with BD. Often patients, for a variety of reasons, may leave out this episode when reviewing their medical history. The majority of affective episodes in BD are depressed or mixed, which are much more disabling than manic episodes. Some patients may even identify periods of normal mood as depressed when compared with mania.

Patients with BD have a higher mortality rate, lower employment, greater interpersonal stressors, and more interactions with the criminal justice system than the general population. The majority have only limited functional recovery. Significant cognitive impairment is evident in 3 to 42 percent of patients with BD who are tested while euthymic. One large national insurance database indicated that claims for patients with BD yielded a 39.1 percent hospital admission rate, compared with 4.5 percent for all other behavioral health issues. When examining claims, out-of-pocket expenses were twice as high for patients with BD as for all other claimants. Treatment costs of bipolar disorder top those of diabetes.

The incidence of comorbid substance abuse is greater in patients who have BD than in any other psychiatric disorder except for antisocial personality disorder, with the majority of patients meeting lifetime criteria for a substance abuse disorder. Comorbid substance abuse is associated with greater relapse rates, poorer psychosocial outcome, slower recovery, increased hospitalization rates, and rapid cycling (defined as four or more affective episodes per year). The lifetime prevalence of anxiety disorders (e.g., generalized anxiety disorder, obsessive–compulsive disorder, panic attacks, social phobia, and PTSD) is 50 percent; the presence of a comorbid anxiety disorder is associated with worse functional outcomes. Common medical comorbidities in BD include migraine headache, asthma, and obesity.

An initial manic episode may be related to an adverse life event/stressor, however subsequent episodes may occur without an identifiable trigger. Patients with BD appear especially sensitive to sleep deprivation, which may occur in conjunction with stressors such as bereavement, childbirth, vacation, longer working hours, and shift changes. Seasonal changes may result in fall/winter depression and spring/summer mania. Light exposure may trigger manic episodes. Many women with BD report mood changes related to the menstrual cycle. Depressive episodes are typically followed by manic episodes.

Pathophysiology

Depression and mania are affective states on a continuum of mood disorder. As such, many current biologic theories of depression also apply to mania. Genetic components appear to play a more significant role in transmitting bipolar 1 disorder than MDD. Studies of families have demonstrated that first-degree relatives of bipolar 1 probands (the first ill subject identified in the family) are 8 to 18 times more likely than the are the first-degree relatives of control subjects to have bipolar 1 disorder and 2 to 10 times more likely to have MDD. In addition, first-degree relatives of probands with MDD are 1.5 to 2.5 times more likely to have bipolar 1 disorder than first-degree relatives of control subjects. The fact that about 50 percent of all bipolar 1 disorder patients have at least one parent with a mood disorder (most often MDD) further supports inheritability. If one parent has bipolar 1 disorder, the child has a 25 percent chance of developing mood disorder; if both parents have bipolar 1 disorder, the odds of the child developing a mood disorder is 50 to 75 percent.

Support of the genetic basis of mood disorder is also found in adoption studies, which show a strong genetic component for the inheritance of MDD; the only adoption study (as of this writing) for bipolar 1 disorder also supported a genetic basis. A concordance rate for bipolar 1 disorder in monozygotic twins is 33 to 90 percent; it is approximately 50 percent for MDD. In dizygotic twins, the concordance rate for bipolar I is approximately 5 to 25 percent, and 10 to 25 percent in MDD.

A variety of studies have reported, replicated, or failed to replicate various associations between specific genes or gene markers and mood disorder. Most genetic linkage studies in psychiatry have produced contradictory results. There does appear to be some possibility that an X-linked gene is a factor in the development of bipolar I in some patients and familes.

There are no specific associations between specific personality disorders and bipolar I; there is, however, some evidence that patients with dysthymic disorder and cyclothymic disorder are at risk for later development of MDD or bipolar I.

Psychopathology

As noted earlier, many theories view mania as a defense against underlying depression. Psychodynamic theorist Karl Abraham felt that manic episodes might reflect an inability of the patient to tolerate a developmental insult, such as the loss of a parent. Another psychodynamic view is that the euphoric self-satisfaction of the manic state is a reaction to intolerable self-criticism resulting from a tyrannical and rigid super-ego. Melanie Klein also viewed mania as a defense against depression, using manic defenses such as omnipotence in which the person develops delusions of grandeur. Bernard Lewin theorized that the ego of the manic patient was overwhelmed by fearful and uncontrollable impulses such as aggression, or pleasurable but overwhelming impulses such as sex.

Clinical Presentation

Routine screening for depression is advised in primary-care settings, but little attention has been focused on screening for past episodes of hypomania or mania. A study published in 2005 in JAMA reported positive screening results for lifetime bipolar disorder in 9.8 percent of patients ($n = 112$) between 18 and 70 years of age seen in a busy, urban medical clinic. This rate did not differ by sex, age, or race. These patients reported significantly worse health-related quality of life and increased social and family life impairment compared to those who screened negative. Only seven of the 112 patients who screened positive reported taking a mood-stabilizing agent in the past month. Primary care clinicians reported evidence of current depression in 47 of the 112 patients but did not record a bipolar disorder diagnosis in any of these patients. Current guidelines for BD caution against monotherapy with antidepressants because they may induce hypomania, mania, or a mixed depressive/manic episode. Clinicians need to recognize and screen for bipolar disorder along with depression in the primary care setting in order to appropriately diagnose and manage this common and unrecognized problem.

BD may be viewed as a disorder of "elevated mood" which may manifest itself as euphoria or irritability or dysphoria (mixed) characterized by a depressed mood, with or without irritability. Approximately 25 percent of all patients experience episodes of pure mania, 40 percent demonstrate mixed (dysphoric) mania formerly referred to as "manic–depression," and 10 to 25 percent are called "rapid cyclers" manifested as rapid shifts from mania to depression. The following mnemonic is useful for identifying BD:

- **D**istractibility
- **I**nsomnia (decreased need for sleep)
- **G**randiosity (inflated self-esteem)
- **F**light of ideas (racing thoughts, negative for rumination)
- **A**ctivities (increased, goal directed)
- **S**peech (pressured, increased talkativeness)
- **T**houghtlessness (pleasure-seeking activities that show poor judgment such as spending sprees, sexual indiscretions, reckless driving, arguments if irritable)

Either three of the above cardinal symptoms and euphoria **or** four of the above symptoms and irritability are defined as mania, a state in which the patient experiences functional impairment; psychotic symptoms may occur in as many as 50 to 80 percent of patients with delusional thinking that is mood-congruent. Hypomania may consist of some variations of all of the above without functional impairment or psychotic elements.

Manic episodes usually last 3 to 6 months if untreated. They begin rather abruptly and the first episode may be triggered by some external psychosocial stressor like the first year of college, although subsequent episodes may occur without a specific event. The symptoms typically escalate rapidly during a period of days. Older adult patients are more likely to manifest irritable rather than elated mood.

Hypomania "feels good" and is associated with "getting a lot done." Women are more likely to have hypomanic symptoms rather than full-blown mania and these are frequently not perceived as "abnormal."

Mania has been associated with changes in antidepressant therapy—either the addition, change, or even discontinuation, as well as the use of steroids, anticholinergic agents, and stimulants. A manic episode secondary to a pharmacologic cause is typified by history of common precipitant, later age at onset, and lack of BD in the family history.

Bipolar depressive states are manifested more as "atypical" unipolar depressive symptomatology such as hypersomnia, hyperphagia with carbohydrate cravings and weight gain, low energy, psychomotor retardation, and mood reactivity, such as excessive sensitivity to interpersonal rejection. Other ways that bipolar depression is different from unipolar is younger age at onset of the first depressive episode, family history of BD, higher frequency of suicidal thoughts, irritability, paranoia, and auditory hallucinations. Untreated depressive episodes may last 6 to 12 months, but often these patients have more recurrent and brief depressions of less than 3 months, and hypomania in response to antidepressant therapy. Many treatment-resistant patients suffering from depression may actually have BD.

The defining feature of BD is a lifetime history of at least one manic, hypomanic, or mixed episode. Depressive symptoms are typical but not required. Specific bipolar affective disorders according to the DSM-IV-TR are classified as follows:

- *Bipolar disorder I*— lifetime history of at least one manic or mixed episode
- *Bipolar disorder II*— lifetime history of at least one hypomanic episode with no lifetime history of a manic episode
- *Cyclothymia*— numerous episodes of depressed mood that do not meet full criteria for major depression *and* episodes of hypomania that occur over a period of two years. These patients have a 15 to 50 percent chance of developing BDI or BDII.

The criteria for manic, hypomanic, and mixed episodes are found in Table 17.12. Almost 90 percent of all BD experience depression and most BD patients present for treatment during a depressive episode. In ALL patients presenting with depression, clinicians should inquire specifically about symptoms of past manic or hypomanic episodes, past treatment and responses, and family history. The Mood Disorder Questionnaire (MDQ) is a validated screening tool for BD (see Fig. 17.1). The likelihood of underdiagnosis or a

Table 17.12 Criteria for Manic, Hypomanic, and Mixed Episodes*

Mania
A distinct period of abnormally elevated or irritable mood lasting at least 1 week (or any duration if hospitalization is necessary). Symptoms may include grandiosity, psychomotor agitation, high-risk behavior with adverse consequences, a decreased need for sleep, incessant talking, and distractibility. May include psychotic features and could be a danger to others. Marked impairment in occupational and/or social functioning

Hypomania
A distinct period of persistently elevated, expansive or irritable mood, lasting for at least 4 days, that is clearly different from the usual nondepressed mood. Symptoms, while similar to a manic episode, are not severe enough to cause marked impairment in occupational or social functioning and do not require hospitalization. No evidence of psychotic features.

Mixed Episode
Nearly every day for at least 1 week the criteria for a manic epsiode and a major depressive epsiode are met simultaneously. Severe occupational or social dysfunction is present and may necessitate hospitalization. Psychotic features may be present.

*Provided symptoms are not attributable to substance abuse or underlying general medical condition

Source: Adapted from APA, DSM-IV-TR, 2000.

1. Has there ever been a period of time when you were not your usual self and...	**YES**	**NO**
...you felt so good or so hyper that other people thought you were not your normal self or you were so hyper that you got into trouble?	❑	❑
...you were so irritable that you shouted at people or started fights or arguments?	❑	❑
...you felt much more self-confident than usual?	❑	❑
...you got much less sleep than usual and found you didn't really miss it?	❑	❑
...you were much more talkative or spoke faster than usual?	❑	❑
...thoughts raced through your head or you couldn't slow your mind down?	❑	❑
...you were so easily distracted by things around you that you had trouble concentrating or staying on track?	❑	❑
...you had much more energy than usual?	❑	❑
...you were much more active or did many more things than usual?	❑	❑
...you were much more social or outgoing than usual, for example, you telephoned friends in the middle of the night?	❑	❑
...you were much more interested in sex than usual?	❑	❑
...you did things that were unusual for you or that other people might have thought were excessive, foolish, or risky?	❑	❑
...spending money got you or your family into trouble?	❑	❑

2. If you checked YES to more than one of the above, have several of these ever happened during the same period of time? *Please circle one response only.*

YES **NO**

3. How much of a problem did any of these cause you — like being unable to work; having family, money, or legal troubles; getting into arguments or fights? *Please circle one response only.*

No problem **Minor problem** **Moderate problem** **Serious problem**

FIGURE 17.1 The Mood Disorder Questionnaire (MDQ). (*Source*: Hirschfeld, RM, et al: Development and validation of a screening instrument for bipolar spectrum disorder: The Mood Disorder Questionnaire. Am J Psychiatry 157:1873–1875, 2000.)

missed diagnosis is greatly lessened by the routine use of a screening instrument such as the MDQ. Use of the MDQ can identify 70 percent of persons with BD while eliminating the diagnosis for 90 percent of persons without the prediction. Bipolar Spectrum Diagnostic Scale is better for ruling out the diagnosis of BD than for giving a positive diagnosis. If a patient scores positive for BD on this scale, further clinical evaluation is necessary to make the diagnosis.

Corroborative information from (and involvement of) friends and family is particularly important in patients with BD, because patients with mania often lack insight into their symptomatology and do not report it. They feel euphoric during a manic episode and productive during an episode of hypomania. Family members and friends may be able to report suicidal ideation or personal factors associated with increased suicide risk that the patient has not revealed to any clinician.

As part of the history, ask specifically about the frequency, duration, seasonality, and other characteristics of a depressed patient's high and low moods, to help differentiate between bipolar and unipolar depression. Specific details about sleep–wake periods, including daytime naps, meal times, social activities, hobbies and other areas of interest, interpersonal attitudes and ability to work and perform household tasks are helpful. What is a typical day like? Patients with mania or depression usually do not report characteristic psychological descriptors (e.g., elation, grandiosity, racing thoughts, irritability) so activities may provide diagnostic clues. For example, grandiose thinking may manifest as reckless gambling, spending sprees, or sexual promiscuity. Comorbid alcoholism and/or substance abuse is common and needs to be identified. Conversely, increased productivity, enhanced perceptual ability, altered view on interpersonal relationships, and fluctuating symptomatology without substantial negative social or occupational consequences suggest hypomania.

Ask about suicide, ideation and intentions, and about extent of plans or preparations for, prior attempts at, family history of, and recent exposure to suicide. This is essential both at presentation and during subsequent mood episodes, because the lifetime risk for suicide in patients with BD is 10 to 15 percent. Most suicide attempts are associated with depressive episodes or during depressive features of mixed episodes.

Ask about chronic or recurrent physical nonspecific physical symptoms (e.g., fatigue, headache, or gastrointestinal distress) about depressive ("blues") and manic (e.g., driven, pressured, elated, irritable) feelings and behaviors. Vague bodily complaints often signal underlying depression or other emotional distress. Patients frequently present to their primary care providers with nonspecific somatic complaints, rather than the hallmark symptoms of mood disorder. The 5- to 10-year delay in diagnosis after symptom onset is not atypical because it may be only after years of exhaustive testing that has failed to reveal any causality, or after multiple treatment failures, that mood disorder is considered. This may also be related to cultural taboos and/or norms that affect the idiomatic language used to report distress. It is often more culturally acceptable to report physical rather than psychological distress.

On the other hand, many medical conditions may mimic or produce depressive or manic symptoms. Somatic disorder-induced mood symptoms generally resolve with the treatment of the underlying medical disease. Ask about recent medications and about treatment during prior episodes. Evaluate any suspected temporal association between drugs and symptoms, because many drugs can induce or exacerbate manic or depressive symptoms. Levodopa and corticosteroids are the most common causes of drug-induced mania; these agents can also cause depressive symptoms.

Assess the severity, frequency, and longitudinal course of depressive and manic episodes, and determine whether the symptoms meet the specific diagnostic criteria for mood disorder.

The patient's mental status should be assessed, including general appearance, attitude, behaviors, mood/affect, speech, thought processes and content, concentration, and memory. Focus the physical and neurologic exam (cranial nerves, reflexes, muscle tone, gait) on identifying/excluding a medical cause of the patient's symptoms, identifying comorbidity and/or possible precipitating factors (e.g., thyroid disorder, head injuries, substance abuse) establishing a baseline before initiating drug therapy.

A baseline complete blood count (CBC) with differential, platelet count, comprehensive blood chemistry panel (electrolytes, Ca, blood urea nitrogen [BUN], creatinine, hepatic panel, glucose), thyroxine (T4), thyroid-stimulating hormone (TSH), urinalysis, urine toxicology screen, pregnancy test, and EKG for patients over 40 should be done on all patients. Order brain magnetic resonance imaging (MRI) or computed tomography (CT) scans only if clinical findings suggest an underlying organic CNS disorder. Although brain imaging studies using single-photon-emission computed tomography (SPECT) and PET have reported abnormal blood flow and white matter abnormalities affecting certain brain areas of the brain in bipolar patients, these studies remain experimental and not applicable to clinical practice at the time of this writing.

> **THE PATIENT'S VOICE 17.2**
>
> **Bipolar Disorder**
>
> Depression, somehow, is much more in line with society's notions of what women are all about: passive, sensitive, hopeless, helpless, stricken, dependent, confused, rather tiresome, and with limited aspirations. Manic states, on the other hand, seem to be more the provenance of men: restless, fiery, aggressive, volatile, energetic, risk taking, grandiose and visionary, and impatient with the status quo.
>
> SOURCE: Kay Redfield Jamison: An Unquiet Mind: A Memoir of Moods and Madness. Vinatge Books, New York, 1995, p 122–123.

Diagnostic Reasoning/Differential Diagnosis

BDs have a 40 percent frequency of misdiagnosis. There are many reasons for this; lack of insight and poor memory on the part of the patients themselves when providing a history is but one part of the picture. Too many families are excluded, although input from friends and family may prove critical in getting an accurate picture of symptomatology. The current diganostic criteria in the DSM-IV-TR—due to be revised very shortly—is fairly unreliable for hypomania, which is a subtle phenomenon. There is a move to conceptualize bipolar as a "spectrum" disorder, meaning there is a broad range to the continuum of affective disorders. There may be a poor assessment of manic symptoms because often the patients present during a depressive episode. There tends to be overemphasis on symptoms rather than a careful and detailed history of course of illness in greater detail and specificity, a disregard for family history, and treatment response.

Based on the clinical and laboratory findings, exclude nonpsychiatric cause of mood disturbance, including general medical condition, alcohol or other substance abuse, or medication. After excluding a medical cause in a depressive patient (the mode of presentation of most BD patients) consider the following psychiatric disorders: major depressive disorder, bipolar, adjustment, anxiety, eating, personality, attentional deficit, schizophreniform, and somatoform.

Diagnose bipolar I disorder (BDI) if the patient has had at least one manic or mixed episode; diagnose bipolar disorder II (BPII) if the patient has had one hypomanic and one major depressive episode. Family history and premorbid function are important keys in distinguishing BD from other psychiatric disorders. The most robust finding during mania is the triad of manic mood, rapid and pressured speech, and hyperactivity. Patients with BD usually have good functioning prior to first affective episode and are asymptomatic during interepisode periods. While patients with schizophrenia might have negative symptoms such as alogia, avolition, and affective flattening, BD patients are more elated, euphoric, hyperactive and agitated. Psychotic symptoms tend to reflect the mood disturbance and are present only during affective episodes and are not as fixed and persistent as in schizophrenia. When present, delusions and hallucinations tend to have one or two predominate themes such as financial, religious, or sexual.

More difficult is making a distinction between a patient with borderline personality disorder (BPD) and a bipolar patient, especially with cyclothymia and when rapid cycling is present. Patients with BPD have symptoms that are continually present as they have a very reactive mood that can change rapidly in response to the environment. This greatly affects their interpersonal relationships. Patients with borderline personality have moods that may change rapidly throughout the day, in contrast to the moods of BD, which have a much longer period of duration—days or weeks—and are interspersed with interepisode stability. Borderline patients usually have a history of trauma, self-injury, chronicity of problems as opposed to state dependent problems, and subjective features of anger and countertransference. In the diagnostic hierarchy, mood disorder diagnosis precedes personality disorder.

Although the criteria for a bipolar depressive episode are the same as for a unipolar depressive episode, they manifest themselves in most cases with subtle difference (Table 17.13).

Comorbidities can further complicate the picture since the incidence of substance abuse and underlying anxiety disorders looms large in this population of patients.

Table 17.13 Distinguishing Between Bipolar and Unipolar Depressive Episodes

- Ask all depressed patients about history of mania and hypomania.
- Ask about family history of bipolar disorder—"loaded" family history is a clue to bipolarity in "unipolar" patients.
- Involve family member and/or significant other in screening process.
- Administer a screening instrument for bipolar disorder, such as the MDQ.
- Early age at onset (<25 years) is another clue for bipolarity in unipolarity.
- Psychotic features are another clinical clue for bipolarity in the unipolar patient as is seasonal pattern.
- Adverse and/or inadequate antidepressant response such as treatment-emergent hypomania or agitation, erratic or uneven antidepressant responses, multiple antidepressant failures, or "treatment-resistant depression."

Source: Adapted from Hirschfield, RM, and Vornik, LA: J Clin Psychiatry 2004 and Hirschfield, RM and Vornik, LA: In Bowden, CL (ed): Diagnosis and Management of Bipolar Disorder, 2004.

Management

The ideal treatment goal for patients with BD is complete remission of current symptoms, prevention of future affective episodes, and return to premorbid function. These patients need a Circle of Caring. They respond best to proactive, collaborative, and individualized treatment. BD is a chronic, lifelong problem that needs long-term management. Once BD is diagnosed in the primary care setting, consultation with a mental health specialist is important. This will provide assistance with managing pharmacologic regimens and acute crisis should it be necessary. The number one priority is to establish a therapeutic alliance with the patient to gain his or her trust and to identify a significant other who can provide timely and appropriate information as well as corroboration. Pharmacologic management, while a mainstay of therapy, can be difficult for the patient to accept and tolerate. A supportive relationship with the primary-care provider can help in monitoring the patient's overall status as well as adherence to the medication regimen. Data on psychotherapeutic interventions are strong also and patients should be referred for counseling. Cognitive–behavioral therapy (CBT) has proved efficacious, resulting in greater acute treatment response and supporting greater maintenance of treatment gains. It has been demonstrated that there are state-dependent effects and that what is learned on medication is different from what is learned off medication. Therefore, CBT should be reapplied when discontinuing medication.

Request an emergency psychiatric consultation and immediately hospitalize patients who pose an imminent danger to themselves or others, or are severely psychotic. Patients with mood disorders, particularly mania, are often unwilling to enter a hospital voluntarily and may require involuntary commitment.

Recent data suggest that one-third of patients completely recover with mood stabilizer monotherapy; two-thirds require polypharmacy. Approximately 50 percent experience partial recovery and 25 percent never recover (mostly rapid cycling). Predictors of good outcomes are euphoria mania, unipolar mania, late age at onset, and few episodes. Predictors of poorer outcomes are predominate depression, early age at onset, substance abuse, psychosis, mixed state, and many episodes (Table 17.14).

Pharmacologic Management

The mainstay of BD treatment is drugs with mood-stabilizing properties. Although most sources suggest beginning with a single agent, in reality, combination therapy is the rule, not the exception.

Treatment strategies in acute mania are the initiation of a mood stabilizer, usually lithium, which has proved effective in 60 to 80 percent of all hypomanic and manic episodes. Valproic acid is now usually preferred; however, for patients with multiple manic episodes, mixed episodes, and rapid cycling. Carbamazepine, another antiseizure agent, is a good alternative. Combinations of these agents may be used if patients do not respond to a single agent. If

Table 17.14 Management of Bipolar Disorder

Symptomatology—Manic/Mixed	Management Strategies
First-line	*Lithium plus an antipsychotic; *Valproate plus an antipsychotic; (Second-generation antipsychotics are preferable) Carbamazepine Electroconvulsive therapy (may be used if preferred by the patient, patients with severe illness, or if patient is pregnant) *For less ill patients, monotherapy with lithium, valproate, or an antipsychotic may be preferable.
Adjunctive treatments	Benzodiazepine Gabapentin Topiramate
Nonresponse	Optimize the initial medication dose Add or change mood-stabilizing drug Add or change antipsychotic Add lamotrigine
First-line	Lithium or lamotrigine Electroconvulsive therapy (for patients with life-threatening inanition, suicidality, or psychosis; severe depression/pregnancy)
Non-response	Optimize the initial medication dose. Add another mood stabilizer. Add an antipsychotic. Add an antidepressant. Electroconvulsive therapy

Source: Adapted from St. John, D: Bipolar affective disorder. Clin Rev 15(6):47 based on APA data, Am J Psychiatry, 2002.

the patient does not respond fully, atypical antipsychotics may be added to one or more mood stabilizer. Newer antiseizure agents, such as lamotrigine, topiramate, and gabapentin, although their efficacy has not been fully established, are promising. Lamotrigine has proved particularly effective for rapid cycling, particularly in patients with severe depression. Long-acting benzodiazepines, such as clonazepam and lorazepam, may be used for rapid treatment of manic symptoms and to calm and sedate patients until acute mania or hypomania has subsided and the mood stabilizer has taken effect.

In the case of psychotic symptomatology, antipsychotics may be added, or a benzodiazepine compound. For patients who do not respond to medication, electroconvulsant therapy may be helpful. When side effects become intolerable, or if the patient improves and recovery is sustained, or if the patient is still not responding to maximum doses, slowly withdraw the neuroleptic or benzodiazepine, and continue the mood-stabilizing agent. Some atypical antipsychotic agents have proved helpful in long-term treatment of BD.

Episodes of depression pose particular challenges. There are fewer approved treatments for bipolar depression. Overall, antidepressant medications do not control depression as effectively in bipolar as in unipolar depression, and may trigger mania. Mood stabilization is still the primary goal, however, and mood stabilization therapy (lithium, carbamazepine, and valproic acid) should be optimized (in the case of lithium, serum level of 0.8 mEq/L or above) before starting antidepressant therapy. If depression persists 2 to 4 weeks after optimization of the mood stabilizer, it is recommended that either bupropion (antidepressant), lamotrigine (anticonvulsant, mood stabilizer), or an SSRI (antidepressant) should be added. Venlafaxine may also be useful in some cases of severe depression that have not responded to other therapy. Any patient developing symptoms of hypomania while taking an antidepressant should stop taking them; in addition, they should be slowly tapered after a period of sustained remission. Severely depressed or delusional patients may benefit from an antipsychotic. Some studies have demonstrated that a subgroup of patients may respond to thyrotropin-releasing hormone, which regulates thyroid hormones. For depression unresponsive to all of the above strategies, consider ECT. Some sources recommend repetitive transcranial magnetic stimulation as effective and better tolerated.

Lithium remains the gold standard for treatment of BD. In addition, of all the therapies for BD, lithium has been shown to be uniquely effective in decreasing suicidal behavior. Lithium appears to be most effective early in the course of the illness, for classic manic symptoms, in patients in whom depression immediately follows mania, and in patients with a strong family history of BD. However, lithium also has a number of potential adverse effects, including a life-threatening neurotoxicity that can occur at serum levels higher than 2.0 mEq/L. Adverse drug interactions can occur with such commonly used drugs as thiazide diuretics, NSAIDs, angiotensin-converting enzyme inhibitors, and antipsychotics. Additional potential adverse effects include nausea, diarrhea, tremor, polyuria, and polydipsia. Lithium may exacerbate psoriasis and acne, cause hypothyroidism (5 percent to 35 percent), and in 20 percent of patients (usually after 15 or more years of treatment) lead to renal insufficiency. Lithium takes several weeks to become effective, and lithium may contribute to weight gain of at least 7 percent of baseline.

Because of the potential adverse effects, lithium therapy should be preceded by an evaluation of renal, cardia, and thyroid function, as well as a pregnancy test. Most patients demonstrate residual symptoms during maintenance therapy with lithium. If depression persists, the patient may need an adjunctive antidepressant.

Many patients do not stay on lithium. Some regret the loss of the exhilaration that occurs during a manic episode; some patients are concerned about weight gain, or tremor. In an earlier study, 50 percent of patients acknowledged some degree of medication nonadherence in the previous 2 years, and 32 percent reported only partial adherence in the preceding month.

Anticonvulsant medications are not mood stabilizers; however, some of these agents have proven effective for the treatment of mania and/or BD and/or maintenance. These agents have become alternative treatments for patients who need a mood-stabilizing agent but who do not fare well with lithium, although they also may be used in combination with lithium. Anticonvulsant agents work by enhancing the inhibitory activity of the neurotransmitter GABA.

Divalproex/valproate/valproic acid is considered first line pharmacologic treatment for acute mania or mixed episodes and maintenance. There is some evidence of antidepressant effect as well. Divalproex appears to be most effective for rapid cycling and mixed episodes, in patients who have had more than three manic episodes, and in patients with comorbid alcohol abuse. Valproic acid was comparable to lithium, and generally better tolerated, during the maintenance period. The most frequently observed side effects when valproic acid was used in the treatment of acute mania were nausea, vomiting, weight gain, tremor, dizziness, and sedation. Serious adverse effects include hepatotoxicity, pancreatitis, thrombocytopenia, and teratogenicity. Serum valproate levels, liver function tests, and complete blood cell counts should be monitored closely during treatment with valproic acid.

Valproic acid is a cytochrome 450 enzyme inhibitor and may engender metabolic interaction with other drugs. Valproic acid can induce menstrual irregularities and a higher risk for polycystic ovarian syndrome (PCOS) which affects 2 percent to 7 percent of women in their reproductive years, and is characterized by chronic anovulation and hyperandrogenism.

Carbamazepine has been used for maintenance therapy for bipolar depression since the 1980s, and also for treatment of bipolar mania. Some recent studies have suggested it may be effective for bipolar depression. Therapeutic serum levels for BD have not been established; usually concentrations used for seizure disorders are applied (4 to 12 μg/mL) are applied. Serum levels as well as CBC, platelets, and liver function must all be monitored as potential side effects include agranulocytosis, aplastic anemia, hepatic failure, Stevens-Johnson syndrome, and pancreatitis. It reduces levels of other drugs, however, such as oral contraceptives and dihydropyridine calcium-channel blockers.

Lamotrigine received approval as maintenance therapy for BD in 2003. This agent appears to have antidepressant effects as well as mood-stabilizing properties and has been found to be effective in rapid-cycling BD. The most significant adverse effects are Stevens-Johnson syndrome and toxic epidermal necrolysis, both of which can be fatal.

Conventional antipsychotic agents such as haloperidol have been frequently used to treat bipolar mania as a class; however, these antipsychotic agents have not proven reliable and antidepressant or prophylactic effects and extrapyramidal (EPS) symptoms are common (e.g., akathisia, dystonia, torticollis, parkinsonism, and tardive dyskinesia [TD]). Although these agents worked well in reducing symptoms such as paranoia, hallucinations, delusions and thought disturbances, they did little to improve overall social and occupational functioning.

Newer second-generation, or atypical, antipsychotics have a lower propensity to induce EPS. Both classes of drugs block dopaminergic transmission, but the newer drugs also act through various receptors such as dopamine, histamine, and alpha-adrenergic. These are standard agents for schizophrenia and are approved for use as monotherapy for mania and with mood stabilizers. Atypical antipsychotics include clozapine, olanzapine, risperidone, quetiapine, ziprasidone, and aripiprazole. Age, affective disorders, and diabetes predispose to TD so all patients still need to be closely monitored for EPS.

The atypical antipsychotics, however, induce metabolic changes and may induce or exacerbate obesity, diabetes, or both. Clozapine and olanzapine carry the greatest risk, quetiapine and risperidone have lower risks, and the newer agents, ziprasidone, and aripiprazole, have minimal risk for metabolic changes.

Patients at high risk for recurrence should consider lifelong therapy, generally with mood stabilizers. Lithium and the antiepileptic agent valproic acid are first-line agents used in maintenance therapy. Although there are some differences in side effects, the dropout rates are similar, and both agents demonstrate equal effectiveness. Carbamazepine and lamotrigine are also alternatives. The atypical antipsychotics have proved useful for maintenance, particularly in combination with mood stabilizers. ECT may be helpful for those who do not respond to medication.

In general, be prepared to change treatment modalities over time. Several weeks are required to assess the effects of new treatment. Optimization of mood stabilizers is of paramount importance and combination therapy is standard to achieve control. Antidepressants should be used with caution and only in cases of severe symptomatology, as there is still evidence that they may worsen disease course over time. Select drug regimens that are well tolerated and promote compliance.

Nonpharmacologic Management

Psychotherapy, while not effective as monotherapy, can significantly enhance treatment response and prevent relapse. Interpersonal, family-focused, cognitive–behavioral, supportive, and psychoeducational approaches increase illness awareness, improve collaboration with health-care professionals and supportive family and friends, and may assist in lifestyle regulation. There is good evidence that cognitive–behavioral therapy protects against relapse.

The onset of manic and depressive episodes is often associated with psychosocial stress. After discussing the patient's circumstances and needs, offer practical advice about ways to cope with stress and potential stressors. For example, encourage patients to pace their activities at work and to maintain a regular schedule. A change in sleep patterns often heralds the onset of a manic or depressive episode. Insomnia may be a precipitant or a prodromal warning sign. Maintenance of regular sleep habits helps prevent escalation of mood symptoms into a full-blown episode. Educate BD patients and their families about the risks of stress; substance abuse; and irregular and inconsistent sleep, meals, and other daily habits.

Follow-Up

Relapse rates for BD are high. Expect up to 90 percent of BDI patients who present with a single manic episode to experience a relapse, and approximately 40 percent to have multiple recurrences, approximately 5 to 15 percent to have rapid cycling (4 or more episodes a year), and only about 7 percent to have no recurrence. Generally, BDI has a less favorable prognosis than MDD. Between affective episodes, approximately 20 to 30 percent of BDI patients continue to have mood liability and interpersonal and/or occupational difficulties. As repeated mood episodes accumulate, BDI patients tend to follow a downhill course.

Persons with BDII have a better prognosis than BDI, although even BDII has a worse prognosis than MDD. Five to fifteen percent go on to develop rapid cycling, which has a very poor prognosis, and about 15 percent continue to have interepisodal mood liability and interpersonal and/or occupational difficulties.

Unfavorable risk factors include male sex, lower socioeconomic status, limited occupational functioning, alcohol dependency, psychotic symptoms, interepisode depression or persistence of symptoms, rapid cycling, and the switching of polarity within episodes (e.g., from mania to depression).

The therapeutic alliance, meaning a supportive relationship between patient and caregivers, is positively associated with good outcome. Education is a key component to effective adherence to therapy and family support. Open discussion of all treatment options, side effects, and their management is critical. Involving the patient in the decision-making is beneficial. Monitoring and managing symptoms over time is essential; self-monitoring and better symptom recognition are highly desirable goals. Prevalence of nonadherence with mood stabilizers ranges from 18 to 52 percent. Reasons include denial of diagnosis, unwillingness to take medication long term, perceived improvement in health, adverse side effects of medications. Patient adherence to medication regimen can make a difference in patient outcomes. In one 18-month study, 81 percent of partially adherent patients required hospitalization versus 9 percent of adherent patients. Patients may ask if they will need to continue taking the same medication for life. The specific medications prescribed may change as new agents are introduced and as the individual's treatment needs are reassessed. What will remain constant is the need to monitor the patient with BD over his or her lifetime.

Develop realistic treatment goals and promote confidence by actively listening and being responsive to patient needs. Regularly address mixed feelings about adherence to treatment. Patients with BD struggle with a variety of interpersonal and/or occupational issues. As stabilization management and supervision are lessened following an acute affective episode, patient attendance at follow-ups may decrease. During this postacute period, intensive collaboration with the patient and family can be invaluable for establishing the framework for long-term biopsychosocial interventions.

Involvement of family and friends is critical to successful follow-up as progression of BD may be difficult to validate via self-report. Sensitivity to early warning signs of potential mood destabilization is important. Many patients do not try to achieve treatment goals. Symptoms of illness often preclude sound judgment, and patient unwillingness to tolerate medication side effects are some of the causes of apparent nonadherence.

A frequent review of the relative trade-off between "quality of life" and "effects of treatment" and emphasizing the improved prognosis associated with maintenance mood stabilizer therapy with the patient may improve medication compliance. Cognitive–behavior therapy, family therapy, or interpersonal therapy should all target self-monitoring, treatment adherence, communication skills, and coping strategies to complement pharmacotherapy.

If a patient presents with early manifestations of relapse, promptly assess the clinical scenario and review the drug regimen. Investigate possible medication nonadherence, drug–drug interaction, and substance use. Do a drug level before initiating a change in the current regimen. If the cause of relapse is unclear or the symptoms fail to respond to standard treatment, consult with a psychiatrist.

Periodically reevaluate the patient for a known or new medical condition or medication use that may complicate management.

Patient and Family Education

Educate the family and patient about the nature of bipolar illness, and about the importance of medication compliance, regular visits for clinical and laboratory monitoring, and contacting their health-care provider before stopping or starting any medication. Avoid complementary therapies such as St. John's Wort as they interfere with some psychotropics.

Educate the patient and family as to the nature of bipolar illness and the importance of medication adherence, regular visits for clinical and laboratory monitoring, and contacting the health-care provider before starting or stopping any medication. Educate the patient and family as to potential side effects of all medications and inform them that many options are available to minimize or eliminate side effects. Discuss the importance of maintenance adequate blood levels in prevention of relapse, and of contacting the health-care provider in the event of experiencing unpleasant side effects rather than stopping the medication.

At follow up visits, regularly counsel the patient and family as to coping with stressors that may precipitate manic or depressive episodes, about maintaining a consistent lifestyle, about signs of relapse, and about medication adherence. Consider reinforcing recommendations with written patient instructions such as:

- ▲ Limit "everyday" stimulants such as coffee, alcohol and over-the-counter medications that contain these substances can trigger mood episodes.
- ▲ Maintain regular sleep patterns.
- ▲ Avoid alcohol and taking unnecessary or illegal drugs because they can trigger mood episodes and can prevent the benefits or increase the side effects of necessary medications.
- ▲ Try to maintain a regular work schedule. If necessary, take time off rather than "tough it out" if mood symptoms hinder ability to work.

As patients learn more about the stress of their illness on family members, it may help them reduce both their own stress and the disruption that it can cause. Patients may develop such insights by learning more about bipolar illness and by joining a bipolar support group or a mental health organization for lay people.

Educate patients and families to watch for early signs of relapse, including changes in sleep patterns, grooming habits, energy or sexual interest, concentration problems, mood instability, or changes in self-esteem. Most patients experience a change in sleep patterns early in the development of an episode of mania or depression. Even small amounts of stimulants may interfere with sleep patterns or mood and possibly trigger a relapse. Insomnia may be either a precipitant or a warning sign. Early recognition of these signals, promptly followed by contacting the health-care provider can help prevent relapse. Maintenance of regular sleep patterns (including a prescription for benzodiazepine to promote regular sleep patterns) may prevent escalation of early symptoms into full episodes.

There should be an individual action plan for coping and seeking assistance whenever the patient or family members suspect the patient is experiencing early manifestations of relapse. BD patients tend to minimize their limitations and vulnerabilities. They may decide to not continue treatment. Family members and friends who recognize signs of relapse need to know beforehand what their assigned roles are in the patient's action plan. In addition, family and friends may be an important resource when the patient is tempted to stop therapy.

Patients and/or family should feel free to contact their health-care provider for advice whenever necessary, especially in light of self-destructive, aggressive behavior, or any changes in daily routine that cause concern.

Acute Suicide Risk

Suicide, or intentional self-inflicted death, is the eighth leading cause of death in the United States and the second leading cause of death among children and adolescents. *Suicide* is derived from the Latin word for "self-murder." Given difficulties in reporting, it is clear that these numbers represent an underestimation. Completed suicide refers to self-inflicted death; attempted suicide refers to potentially lethal acts that do not result in death and nonlethal, attention-seeking gestures such as superficial cuts on wrists. Each person who attempts suicide is unique, but if there is a shared personal characteristic, it is likely to be a profound sense of hopelessness—hopelessness in the sense that the individual perceives there is no future, or that the future that he or she envisions is somehow unacceptable. Suicidal patients may be angry, sad, or confused. They may be quite honest about their suicidal plans or may refuse to disclose their true thoughts and feelings. Suicidal thoughts and feelings commonly are associated with mood disorders, principally BD, schizophrenia, and alcoholism. Persons who are overwhelmed by severe psychosocial problems and/or medical problems may also experience suicidal thoughts. Suicidal thoughts can have an acute onset, meaning that for a period of time, the person is at risk for acting on thoughts of suicide. Chronic suicidal thoughts are also common. In this case, the person never feels completely free of thoughts of taking his or her life. Impulsive suicidal behavior is the most difficult to assess, in that—by definition—this type of suicidal behavior is likely to occur without warning. Patients who are troubled by thoughts of suicide but are clear about their determination not to act on their suicidal thoughts may be appropriate candidates for primary-care management. For example, a patient who is in a great deal of pain associated with a serious physical illness may develop acute suicidal thoughts when overwhelmed by physical pain. Any suggestion of impulsive or chronic suicidal thoughts or evidence of actual suicidal behavior is an indicator for immediate evaluation by a specialist. (See The Patient's Voice 17.3.)

Epidemiology and Causes

Suicide was the 11th leading cause of death in the United States in 2000, with an age-adjusted rate of 10.6 per 100,000 people. There are approximately 30,000 completed suicides yearly in the United States, accounting for 2 percent of all deaths. The number of attempted suicides is estimated to be 650,000. About 10 to 20 percent of all persons who attempt suicide eventually take their own lives. Given the social stigma and pain associated with suicide, these numbers must be viewed as under-representing actual cases.

THE PATIENT'S VOICE 17.3

Suicide

Sylvia Plath was a poet and novelist (1932–1964), who at age 32 took her own life. She battled depression and mental illness for most of her life. She wrote *The Bell Jar* in 1963 after her first breakdown. The following is a quote from that book:

The silence drew off, baring the pebbles and shells, and all the tatty wreckage of my life. Then, at the rim of vision, it gathered itself, and in one sweeping tide, rushed me to sleep.

Older, white males who are widowed or unmarried have the highest suicide rate, as they are most likely to commit suicide with a firearm. Usually these men are living alone and lack social support. Unemployment, a fall in economic status, medical illness, family history, previous suicide attempt, and anniversary of a loss are all risk factors for suicide. Males are three times more likely than females to successfully complete a suicide, although elderly women (75 and older) account for 20 percent of the suicide deaths among those 65 and older and this number is expected to rise as this population of older women is growing. Single and widowed persons of both sexes have a higher incidence of suicide. Adolescent (15 to 24 years) and geriatric (65 years and older) populations are at highest risk, especially Native Americans and Caucasian males. Attempted suicide is 10 times more frequent than completed suicide. One study indicated that 91 percent of suicide acts involving firearms result in death, while drug overdoses – thought the most common method—lead to fatality only 2 percent of time. Fatality rates associated with drowning were found to be 84 percent; hanging (82 percent), and poisoning with gases (64 percent). The prime suicide site of the world is the Golden Gate Bridge in San Francisco.

Overall, the higher a person's social status, the greater the risk of suicide. A fall in social status may also trigger a risk of suicide. Special at-risk occupations include physicians (especially women and/or psychiatrists), musicians, dentists, law enforcement officers, lawyers, and insurance agents. Conversely, the suicide rate is higher among the unemployed than among the employed. Economic recessions and depressions, and times of high unemployment demonstrate increases in suicide rates; conversely, periods of high employment and war support decreased rates of suicide.

Thirty-two percent of persons who commit suicide have sought medical attention within the prior 6 months. Postmortem studies demonstrate a physical illness is present in 25 to 75 percent of all suicide victims and a physical illness is estimated to be an important contributing factor in 11 to 51 percent of suicides. The percentage increases with age. For example, 50 percent of men with cancer who commit suicide do so within 1 year of the diagnosis. Cancer of the breast or genitals is found in 70 percent of all women with cancer who commit suicide. A number of diseases of the CNS increase the risk of suicide, specifically, epilepsy, multiple sclerosis, head injury, cardiovascular disease, Huntington's disease, dementia, and acquired immune deficiency syndrome (AIDS). All these diseases are associated with mood disorders. Urogenital problems, specifically prostate hypertrophy treated with prostatectomy and renal disease treated with hemodialysis, are associated with increased suicide risk; both these conditions may have concurrent mood changes. Loss of mobility and disfigurement, as well as intractable pain, are all associated with increased risk of suicide.

Certain drugs such as reserpine (Serpasil), corticosteroids, antihypertensive agents, and some antineoplastic agents can produce depression which may lead to suicide.

Pathophysiology

There is reliable evidence that reduced central serotonin is associated with suicide. Recent studies also confirm some changes in the noradrenergic system of suicide victims. Neurochemical findings suggest some overlap between persons with aggressive and impulsive behaviors and those who complete suicide. It is thought that alcohol and other vasoactive substances may also play a role, perhaps by increasing the vulnerability of a person already so predisposed. Any linkage between low serotonergic function and aggressive or suicidal behavior is unclear, and it is thought that low serotonin may turn out to be a marker for, rather than a cause of, aggression and suicidal potential.

Suicidal behavior, like other psychiatric disorders, tends to run in families. This is well documented. A family history of suicide increases the risk of attempted suicide and that of completed suicide in most diagnostic groups. Twin studies suggest a genetic component in suicide. Over several studies, monozygotic twin pairs had a significantly higher concordance for both attempted and completed suicide then dizygotic twins. Danish-American adoption studies also yielded strong evidence that adoptees who had committed suicide had, on further investigations, strong family history in biological relatives compared to no evidence of suicide in the adopting relatives. A further study of adoptees with mood disorders demonstrated that adoptee suicide completers with a situational crisis or impulsive suicide attempt, or particularly both, had more biological relatives who had committed suicide than controls had. It was suggested that the genetic factors lowering the threshold for suicidal behavior may lead to an inability to control impulsive behavior. Environmental stress, or the presence of a psychiatric disorder, may be a potentiating mechanism that triggers or fosters the impulsive behavior in the direction of suicide. Molecular genetic studies have lent some consistent support toward genetic constellations that support lowered levels of serotonin, producing low serotonin turnover and thus a low concentration.

The risk for suicide in patients with mental disorders is highest for those diagnosed with mood disorder.

Sociologic Perspectives

The French sociologist Emile Durkheim made a major contribution to the study and understanding of suicide with his classic treatise on the subject at the end of the 19th century. He divided suicides into three social categories: (1) egoistic, (2) altruistic, and (3) anomic. According to Durkheim, egoistic suicide has to do with lack of integration into a social group. For example, unmarried individuals living singly are more likely to commit suicide than married couples are, and couples with children are the least likely. Urban areas have fewer social connections than rural communities, and thus higher suicide rates. Catholicism is seen as having more cohesiveness than Protestantism; Protestants have higher suicide rates than Catholics.

Excessive integration into a group can also lead to suicide, named by Durkheim "altruistic suicide." One has only to think of today's suicide bombers in Al Quada organizations to have an example; likewise, Japanese "Kamikaze" pilots of World War II are another example. Anomic suicide applies to persons who have disturbed integration into society; they do not follow—or cannot follow—customary societal and cultural norms. Anomie also refers to social instability, and a general breakdown of society's standards and values. A drastic change in financial circumstances, such as occurred against the social upheaval of the Great Depression on the 1930s, led some to suicide.

Psychological Theories

Sigmund Freud, in his paper *Mourning and Melancholia*, advanced the view that suicide is aggression turned inward against an introjected, ambivalently cathected love object. An earlier repressed desire to kill someone is a necessary antecedent to the act of suicide. Karl Menninger extended Freud's ideas. In his classic book, *Man Against Himself*, he theorized that suicide was inverted homicide predicated on the person's anger toward another person. He also described a self-directed death instinct (an extension of Freud's concept of Thanatos) with three components: the wish to kill, the wish to be killed, and the wish to die. More contemporary views focus on the suicidal patient's fantasies of what would happen if he or she committed suicide. These fantasies might include revenge, punishment, sacrifice, atonement, escape, new life, or control. Depressed persons are most likely to commit suicide as their depression appears to lift. Some suicidal patients use their preoccupation with suicide to ward off intolerable depression. A suicide attempt may cause a person's depression to lift, especially if it fulfills a person's need for punishment. Aaron Beck demonstrated that hopelessness was one of the most accurate indicators of long-term suicidal risk.

Clinical Presentation

Clinicians must assess an individual patient's risk for suicide on the basis of clinical examination. Acute risk factors include severe psychic anxiety, anxious ruminations, global insomnia, depression with delusions, and recent alcohol use.

Suicidal behavior is multidimensional, with complex factors contributing to the overall risk of a future suicide attempt. Suicide screening tools often focus on previous attempts or intent to commit suicide, with various supportive items such as demographic information, level of social support, and coexisting mental health disorders. Because the goal of a suicide scale is to prevent completion, the sensitivity of the scale must be high so as not to miss a potential suicide. The risk of high sensitivity is overidentification of potential attempts. The Modified SAD PERSONAS Scale (Risk Factors 17.2) has an administration time of 1 to 2 minutes, and the authors recommend this as a rapid screening tool for nonpsychiatrists to obtain the objective information necessary to make an initial assessment of suicidality.

Hopelessness about the future is a "red flag" for possible suicidal intent, as well as suicidal thoughts, especially if accompanied by a plan and intent. Giving away personal possessions, quitting a job, and an appearance of peace may all signal that the person has made the decision to commit suicide. Self-mutilation, suicide threats and attempts, hallucinations, and delusions all indicate high risk for suicide.

Patients who are suicidal may state their intentions, but many will find it hard to volunteer this information. The impulsive person will often appear to be so and will give information that shows a great deal of recent poor judgment. The determined person may refuse to answer questions or may give information freely, thinking that his or her plan cannot be interfered with. The confused patient is more likely to seem unable to protect him- or herself from harm. Confused patients include persons suffering from auditory hallucinations instructing him or her to commit suicide, and patients who are under the influence of drugs and alcohol. Suicidal patients may also express extreme anger and rage. Suicidal patients may also have thoughts of homicide, as though taking their own life permits them to consider taking someone else's life first. As this behavior becomes more common, clinicians have to keep in mind that a suicidal patient may also have thoughts of homicide.

Management

Suicide prevention is carried out at two levels—interpersonal and community. Interpersonal prevention includes risk assessment, intervention (e.g., medications, counseling, hospitalization), and referral to a specialist. Community prevention is based on the crisis model of 24-hour community hotline services and walk-in crisis counseling services. Crisis counseling services should include a crisis response team that is dispatched immediately to schools or locations where assistance may be need. These response teams can intervene to reduce the risk of suicide contracts among peers or "copycat" suicides. In 2001, the Surgeon General organized the National Strategy of Suicide Prevention, under the auspices of the National Institutes of Health (NIH).

RISK FACTORS 17.2

Acute Suicide Risk

The pneumonic "SAD PERSONAS" (Patterson, 1983; Campbell, 2004) may be used to evaluate a person's suicide risk. Consider RISK FACTORS within the context of the clinical presentation.

S = Sex
A = Age
D = Depression
P = Previous attempt
E = Ethanol abuse
R = Rational thinking loss
S = Social support loss
O = Organized plan
N = No spouse
A = Availability of lethal means
S = Sickness

The table below presents a detailed description of acute suicide risk factors.

Age	Males complete suicide (about one-half kill themselves using a gun) at a 3:1 ratio compared to female. Females are more likely to attempt suicide (usually by overdose) and act impulsively without warning than males.
Gender	The risk of suicide increases with age, with persons age 65 and older being more likely than younger persons to take their own lives (women peak at age 55; men at age 75). Older adults tend to use more lethal means and are less likely to voice their suicidal intent to others. Bereavement, social isolation, and deteriorating health status are thought to contribute to the high suicide rate in this group. Recent trends indicate that the suicide rate among young persons, aged 25–34, is increasing. Adolescents are a high-risk group, with suicide the second leading cause of death in this group. Gay adolescents who have been the victims of hate crimes, fear social rejection, or who are socially isolated can be at increased risk for developing suicidal thoughts.
Race and ethnicity	Caucasians are at the greatest risk for suicide; however, suicide is one of the leading causes of premature death in minority groups.
Employment status	Unemployed persons are at higher risk, although social class has not been shown to be strongly correlated with increased risk for suicide.
Marital status	Single, divorced, and widowed persons are at a significantly higher risk.
Immigration status	Persons who migrate within the United States are at higher risk for suicide, as well as those who immigrate to the United States. Social isolation appears to be a significant risk factor for immigrants.
Substance abuse problems	Persons with alcohol and drug problems are at extremely high risk for suicide, particularly when their substance abuse is complicated by other risk factors. Over one-third of persons who take their own lives were intoxicated at the time of their deaths. Alcoholism and substance abuse problems of a chronic nature account for 25% of all completed suicides.
Comorbidities	Major depression and bipolar disorders account for approximately 50% of all suicides. Schizophrenia and other psychotic disorders account for approximately 10% of completed suicides. Severe personality disorders, such as borderline personality disorder.
Medical conditions	Chronic, life-threatening, or painful physical illness is associated with increased risk for suicide. Specific high-risk illnesses include AIDS, Huntington's chorea, cancer, peptic ulcer, spinal cord injury, head injury, renal disease requiring dialysis, chronic intractable pain, uncontrolled diabetes with amputation, multiple sclerosis, multiple psychosomatic illnesses.
Medications	Certain medications increase suicidal risk: steroids, antihypertensives (reserpine, methyldopa, clonidine), corticosteroids, opiates, anti-tuberculosis drugs (isoniazid, ethionamide, cycloserine), anabolic steroid withdrawal, barbiturates, benzodiazepines, cocaine and amphetamine withdrawal.
Other	Additional suicide risk factors include recent bereavement, legal and financial problems, recent arrest or impending court dates, and being a victim of abuse or sexual assault.

Careful assessment of suicide risk factors, willingness to consult with other practitioners and specialists, and planning are the hallmarks of effective suicide risk management. The assessment should cover the patient's recent personal history and pay special attention to recent stressful life events and changes in mental status. Reports of recent losses, humiliations, demoralizing experiences, substance use and abuse, and relationship problems should be explored. Persons who have been abusing drugs and/or alcohol can suddenly become highly motivated to end their lives when they first realize that they are no longer in control of their substance use. Even a person who is recovering from substance abuse and has stopped using the substance can be at high risk for suicide when faced with the painful consequences of substance abuse, including withdrawal or severe drug cravings.

All suicidal statements should be considered *seriously,* but no one can predict the actual behaviors of a suicidal patient. One of the most valuable assessment tools for practitioners is the willingness to question a patient directly about his or her suicide risk. Two good general questions are "How long can you go on the way you are?" and "Are you feeling so badly that you sometimes wish you could go to bed and not wake up?" Examples of more specific questions are "What is your plan for suicide?" and "Have you assembled what you need?" Suicide plans are assessed on their *specificity, availability,* and *lethality* (SAL): The more specific and detailed the plan and the more available and lethal the method, the higher the risk of suicide.

Once it is determined that the patient is suicidal, the level of risk will determine the direction of the intervention. A major decision to be made is whether the patient needs to be hospitalized. The absence of a strong social support system, a history of impulsive behavior, and a suicidal plan of action are indications for hospitalization. If hospitalization is deemed necessary but the patient has no way of getting there, or if he or she refuses to go, it will be necessary to call 911 to dispatch someone from the police or sheriff's department to escort the patient to the hospital.

The primary goal of the intervention is to maintain the patient's safety. Therefore it is important to:

- ▲ Reduce or eliminate imminent danger.
- ▲ Never leave a patient alone who is actively suicidal.
- ▲ Involve family members or significant others who care so that they can stay with patient until the crisis has passed.

The best predictor of suicide risk is a history of previous suicide attempt. All persons with suicide gestures, attempts, and threats should be thoroughly screened for suicide risk factors and referred to a specialist for a full mental status exam, as well as psychiatric consultation. It is important to diagnose and treat any underlying psychiatric and/or substance-abuse disorders. The clinician and the patient's family or significant others should ensure the patient's safety by the least restrictive method, starting with removing potentially lethal objects and providing very close supervision. Some patients at acute high risk will require inpatient hospitalization for constant one-to-one supervision (including use of restraints, if indicated) and ongoing treatment. Electroconvulsive therapy (ECT) may provide rapid, safe, and effective treatment for severely depressed, acutely suicidal patients.

Sometimes a no-suicide contract can be initiated. In the case of an angry or manipulative patient, this is usually not advisable. If a patient who is considered seriously suicidal cannot make the commitment to abide by a no-suicide contract, immediate hospitalization is necessary. A no-suicide contract is not a guarantee that a suicide will not happen, nor is it a substitute for clinical judgment. A mental health professional should be the person to implement a no-suicide contract. When it is appropriate to use them, no-suicide written contracts should include the following components:

- ▲ An agreement from the patient not to harm him- or herself
- ▲ An agreement that the patient will contact a mental health professional if the patient's suicidal impulses become unmanageable
- ▲ An agreement from the mental health-care provider to be available to the patient for a specified period of time, usually until the patient returns for a follow-up visit or another part of the intervention has taken place (e.g., when the patient has met with a psychotherapist for evaluation or therapy)
- ▲ Contact numbers for the mental health-care provider
- ▲ Both the patient and mental health-care provider sign the contract. A copy is given to the patient and the original is kept in the agency records.

After this, it is essential to implement an ongoing program of help. This should involve:

- ▲ Treatment of the presenting symptoms
- ▲ Referral for individual or group therapy
- ▲ Referral for support groups
- ▲ Referral to a community program
- ▲ If the patient is not hospitalized and until treatment program is in effect, the clinician must continue to monitor the patient to ascertain his or her safety.

Appropriate documentation is critical. Follow the agency guidelines for documenting situations involving suicidal risk. Records should include statements made by the patient; the decision-making process followed; potential ramifications of nontreatment; what has been shared with the patient and the family; and the consultation process. Follow-up in the care of potentially suicidal patients includes care for self and knowledge of professional liabilities. Malpractice in patient suicides usually revolves around whether the relevant data were obtained—was the risk for suicide identified accu-

Table 17.15 Suicide Assessment and Management

Suicide Assessment

1. Psychiatric evaluation that includes:
   - Specific psychiatric signs and symptoms
   - Psychiatric history, including current treatment
   - Past suicidal or other self-injurious behaviors (including intent of such acts)
   - Family history of suicide, mental illness, and dysfunction
   - Current psychosocial situation and nature of crisis
2. Inquire about suicidal thoughts, plans, behaviors (elicit presence of suicidal ideation, suicide plan, intent and lethality of plan including access to weapons, pills)
3. Suicide risk estimation to include demographic factors, major psychiatric syndromes (primary and comorbid conditions), specific psychiatric symptoms, other aspects of psychiatric history and physical illness

Management

1. Attend to patient's safety.
2. Establish and maintain a therapeutic alliance.
3. Determine a treatment setting (e.g., involuntary hospitalization, partial hospitalization, and intensive outpatient programs, ambulatory settings).
4. Develop a plan of care.
5. Coordinate care and collaborate with other providers.
6. Promote adherence to treatment plan.
7. Provide education to the patient and the family.
8. Reassess safety and suicide risk (include suicide crisis and chronic suicidality).
9. Monitor psychiatric status and response to treatment.
10. Obtain consultation if needed.

Documentation and Risk Management

1. Documentation issues specific to suicide
2. Be aware of own emotions and reactions, particularly when responding to those with severe or recurring suicidality or self-injurious behaviors—for difficult-to-treat patients, consultation and supervision from a colleague, as well as documentation of same, is recommended.
3. Suicide prevention contracts: limitations and clinical usefulness—not recommended in patients who are psychotic, agitated, impulsive, or using intoxicating substances
4. Management of a suicide in one's practice
5. Mental health intervention for surviving family and friends after suicide

Source: Abstracted from http://www.guideline.gov—Practice Guidelines for the Assessment & Treatment of Patients with Suicidal Behaviors. American Psychiatric Association, 2003.

rately; and errors in judgment—after identifying suicidal potential, were appropriate precautions taken? A standard of care exists for assessment of suicide risk, but not for the prediction of suicide. Always document a complete suicide assessment and what actions ensued as a result (Table 17.15).

Follow-Up and Referral

Safety plans for patients who are not acutely suicidal include a follow-up appointment within 24 hours of assessment, and a follow-up telephone call for missed appointments. Patients should be given the local 24-hour crisis telephone number and information regarding access to emergency services. Family and friends who are participating in the safety plan are asked to participate. Practitioners must take responsibility to ask patients about weapons and pill stashes, and then take steps to have these items located and removed to safekeeping. If medications are prescribed, the amount should not exceed a 1-week supply, with no refills. Patients who are at risk should be seen at least weekly and social support systems must be mobilized. Be aware that caring for a patient with contemplating suicide can be very difficult (Table 17.16).

Patient Education

Patient and family education includes providing suicide crisis hot-line numbers to the patient and/or family members. Patients should be instructed to avoid alcohol. Encourage the patient to seek out adequate treatment for uncomfortable symptoms of physical illness, possibly including a prescription for analgesics to reduce suffering. Teach the patient that options appear narrowed when a person is feeling depressed and suicidal, and review alternative ways of thinking. Encourage the patient to reach out for support, and to reach out immediately when feeling the urge to harm him- or herself. Teach the patient to use specific, more constructive outlets for anger rather than self-destructive ones. Mobilize a social support system for the patient and educate significant others regarding suicidal risk and danger signs. Educate the patient and family that as the patient's mood "lifts" in response to antidepressant treatment, there is an increased risk of suicide related to increased energy. At these times, patients must be monitored closely for increased risk.

In the event that the patient does commit suicide, the clinician should prepare the family for a complex grief reaction that may follow. Suicide is particularly tragic because of the fallout that the death bequeaths to survivors.

Table 17.16 Support for Health-Care Providers Caring for Patients at Risk for Suicide

- Be aware of your personal and professional limits and honor them.
- Know the legal standards about suicide, duty to report, confidentiality, and liability.
- Consult with others so you are not the only decision-maker about the risk of the suicidal patient.

Edward Shneidman coined the term "post-vention," which refers to an intervention strategy that attempts to minimize the impact of patient suicide, and to assure that survivors of suicide have adequate services and support available to them. Post-suicide interventions by the clinician include:

- ▲ Educating the family members about suicide.
- ▲ Allowing the family members to share their grief, including any burdens or other factors that the family members may feel (e.g., guilt, shame, anger, inability to do anything, situation out of their control).
- ▲ Encouraging family members to attend support groups, such as Survivor of Suicide (SOS) groups, which are available in most communities.

The typical SOS group is sponsored by a mental health or social services agency and is facilitated by mental health professionals, survivor peers, or a combination of both. Referrals to such groups following a completed suicide are essential.

Anxiety Disorders

Anxiety disorders are the most prevalent psychiatric conditions in the United States. Data from the National Comorbidity Survey indicate a 24.9 percent lifetime and a 17.2 percent 1-year prevalence for any anxiety disorder. Although anxiety disorders were once thought to be of minor clinical significance, it is now clear that they are serious illnesses, responsible for substantial morbidity and, possibly, mortality.

The anxiety disorders, like the mood disorders, can also be viewed on a continuum. Anxiety disorders encompass diagnoses of Panic (with and without agoraphobia), Agoraphobia without Panic, Obsessive–Compulsive, Specific Phobia, Social Phobia, Posttraumatic Stress Disorder, Acute Stress Disorder, and Generalized Anxiety Disorder (GAD). The identification of comorbid depression in minimally 50 percent of patients with anxiety disorders is significant. Cases of MDD typically have a later onset than cases of anxiety, suggesting that MDD may be secondary to anxiety. The observation that anxiety poses a strong predisposition for depression also suggests that early identification and treatment of anxiety may be an important preventive intervention strategy for limiting the subsequent development of depression. Several of the more common anxiety disorders are discussed next.

Generalized Anxiety Disorder (GAD)

Generalized anxiety disorder (GAD) is characterized by excessive worry (over 6 months) about multiple concerns that are difficult to control. Persons with GAD experience a range of upsetting physical symptoms, along with hyperarousal and insomnia. A diagnosis of GAD requires evidence of disrupted or impaired occupational or social functioning. GAD is more disruptive than normal anxiety, which is characterized by apprehension and mild physical symptoms of upset such as headache. 50 to 90 percent of patients with GAD have another mental disorder, most commonly depression.

Epidemiology and Causes

Women tend to be diagnosed with anxiety disorders more often than men are. Individuals with a recent, childhood, or adolescent history of trauma can be more vulnerable to anxiety disorders, including panic disorder and specific phobias. Onset of GAD often occurs during childhood or adolescence. Prevalence in the general population is 5 to 6 percent, but this proportion rises to approximately 25 percent in primary care populations.

Persons with mixed anxiety and depressive disorder have become common enough that a new disorder—*comorbid anxiety and depression*—has been identified. Thirty to 50 percent of individuals diagnosed with GAD also have a current depressive disorder.

Physical health conditions can produce associated moderate to severe anxiety. For example, a person with GAD may also have concurrent coronary artery disease or respiratory disease. Individuals who present as anxious should always be evaluated to specifically rule out physical illness as a cause of their anxiety symptoms, or anxiety secondary to illness.

GAD is a persistent condition that can impact nearly every area of the affected person's daily life. Moderate to severe symptoms of anxiety can also develop, however, within the context of stressful circumstances, such as attending graduate school or finding infant care. Ongoing events, such as family violence, can become a source of generalized anxiety. An example of this would be an unemployed woman going through a bitter divorce who is living in a neighbor's guest room with her three children: During that time she develops mental, physical, behavioral, and emotional symptoms of GAD.

Decades of clinical research have resulted in improved psychological, behavioral, and physical models of anxiety disorders such as GAD. Generally speaking, the psychological models of anxiety disorders suggest that individuals who develop these disorders suffer from unconscious and semiconscious internal struggles that become mentally overwhelming. It has also been suggested that persons with anxiety disorders may have learned to respond to life experiences by becoming overwhelmed and anxious.

Biological models of anxiety disorder implicate biochemical dysregulation as the basis for anxiety disorders. The biochemical model suggests that anxiety symptoms are the result of overactive biochemical stress response and underactive calming biochemical responses. Under these biological conditions, mild situational anxiety can escalate or persist to the point of becoming difficult-to-control anxiety or GAD. Experts note that, like other mood disorders, anxiety disorders tend to run in families, suggesting that anxiety disorders may have a genetic basis in brain physiology. Anxiety disorders are also common as secondary disorders to substance-abuse disorders, and as noted above, commonly coexist with depression.

Pathophysiology

In discussing emerging biological models of etiology, it must be noted that there are different modes of thought. Do the biological events precede the psychological problems, or do the psychological discomforts trigger a complex cycle of biological response? The answer is as yet unclear. Nonetheless, the increasing knowledge of basic neuroscience as well as the actions of psychotropic drugs are shedding new light on longstanding human problems. It is well established that the autonomic nervous system of some patients with anxiety disorder, especially those with panic disorder, demonstrate increased sympathetic tone, adapt slowly to repeated stimuli, and respond excessively to moderate stimuli.

There are three major neurotransmitters associated with anxiety are norepinephrine, serotonin, and GABA. Much of the basic science research has been conducted on animals using behavioral paradigms and psychoactive agents. The general theory about the role of norepinephrine in anxiety disorders is that there is a poorly regulated nonadrenergic system with bursts of activity. The serotonergic antidepressants were noted to have therapeutic effect in certain anxiety disorders, which initiated research into the association between serotonin and anxiety disorders. The cell bodies of most serotonergic neurons are located in the raphe nuclei in the rostral brainstem and project to the cerebral cortex, the limbic system (especially the amygdala and the hippocampus), and the hypothalamus. It is theorized that certain drugs that stimulate these areas also stimulate anxiety. Thus, it is theorized, that other drugs may be developed that affect these areas that will quell the anxiety. The role of GABA in anxiety disorders is most strongly supported by the effectiveness of the benzodiazepines, which enhance the activity of GABA. Thus researchers hypothesize that some patients with anxiety disorder have abnormal functioning of their GABA receptors, although this connection has not been directly demonstrated.

There is solid evidence that at least some genetic component contributes to the development of anxiety disorders. Almost half of all patients with panic disorder have at least one affected relative. Although not as high as those for panic disorders, the figures for other anxiety disorders also indicate a higher frequency of illness in first-degree relatives of affected persons than nonaffected persons. Data from twin registries support the hypothesis that anxiety disorders are at least partially genetically determined. No anxiety disorders, however, are likely to result from a simple Mendelian abnormality. One recent study has attributed about 4 percent of the intrinsic variability of anxiety within the general population to a polymorphic variant of the gene for serotonin transporter, which is the site of action of many serotonergic drugs. Persons with the variant produce less transporter and have higher levels of anxiety.

The limbic system and the cerebral cortex are the focus of much hypothesis-building about the neuroanatomic substrates of anxiety disorders. In addition to receiving noradrenergic and serotonergic innervation, the limbic system also contains a high concentration of GABA receptors.

Two areas of the limbic system have received special attention: increased activity in the septohippocampal pathway, which may lead to anxiety, and the cingulate gyrus, which has been implicated particularly in the pathophysiology of obsessive–compulsive disorder. The frontal cerebral cortex is connected with the parahippocampal region, the cingulate gyrus, and the hypothalamus and thus may be involved in the production of anxiety disorders. Similarity in clinical presentation and electrophysiology between patients with temporal lobe epilepsy and patients with obsessive–compulsive disorder has implicated the temporal cortex as a pathophysiologic site in anxiety disorders.

Brain-imaging studies have typically been conducted with specific anxiety disorders. In one MRI study, for example, a specific defect in the right temporal lobe was noted in patients with panic disorder. Several brain-imaging studies have suggested abnormal findings in the right hemisphere but not in the left hemisphere, suggesting that some types of cerebral asymmetry may be important in the development of specific anxiety disorders. Structural studies (CT and MRI) have variously shown an increase in the size of cerebral ventricles, although in one study this was correlated with the length of time people had been taking benzodiazepines. Functional brain-imaging studies, including PET, single-photon emission computed tomography (SPECT), and electroencephalography (EEG), of patients with anxiety disorders have variously reported abnormalities in the frontal cortex, the occipital and temporal areas, and in one study of panic disorder, the parahippocampal gyrus. The caudate nucleus has been implicated in several functional neuroimaging studies in the pathophysiology of obsessive–compulsive disorder. Demonstrable functional cerebral pathological conditions appear to be causally relevant to their anxiety disorder symptomatology.

Psychodynamic Interpretations

According to classic psychoanalytic theory, anxiety was viewed as the result of psychic conflict between unconscious sexual or aggressive wishes and corresponding threats from the superego or external reality. In response, the ego mobilized defense mechanisms (Table 17.1) to quell unacceptable thoughts and feelings from emerging into conscious awareness. In a classic paper, "Inhibitions, Symptoms, and Anxiety," Freud states that "it was anxiety which produced repression and not as I formerly thought repression which produced anxiety." Interestingly, current neurobiologic understandings may be said to substantiate certain aspects of Freudian thought. The role of the amygdala, for example, which subsumes the fear response without any reference to conscious memory may be said to substantiate the idea of an unconscious memory system in response to anxiety.

Sadock and Sadock in Kaplan and Sadock's *Synopsis of Psychiatry*, 9th edition, note: "One of the unfortunate consequences of regarding the symptom on anxiety as a *disorder* rather than a *signal* is that the underlying sources of anxiety may be ignored" (2003, p 593), further substantiating Freudian views. They go on to note that from a psychodynamic perspective, the goal of psychotherapy is not to eliminate anxiety but to increase anxiety tolerance, that is, the capacity to experience anxiety and use it as a signal to investigate the underlying conflict that has created it. Just as pain lets one know that there is something amiss with the body, anxiety can alert that there is something amiss with one's emotional stability. Across the life cycle, anxiety appears in response to various new situations, such as going away from home for the first time, and at certain levels, can be energizing and mobilizing. For example, it is known that mild anxiety can improve performance on an exam; it is when anxiety veers above a certain level that it becomes counterproductive in a test-taking setting, causing the test taker to rush through the test and misread questions, for example, or to obsessively ruminate over certain choices. Critics of psychopharmacologic approaches to management of mental disorders see the eradication of anxiety through medication (and likewise depression, and other mental symptomatology) as counterproductive to addressing the underlying sources of the conflicts generating the uncomfortable emotions. Through conflict, it is theorized, comes growth.

Behavioral and learning theories of anxiety have fostered particularly effective treatments. According to this school of thought, anxiety is a "conditioned" response to certain environmental and interpersonal stimuli. The approach of desensitization to allergens provides a physiologic model for translation to behavioral models of treatment for anxiety. The person is gradually "desensitized" to the source of anxiety through gradually repeated exposures to anxiety-producing situations and the development of increasing mastery in handling the anxiety-producing stimuli. Cognitive approaches to anxiety have also proved effective. According to these models, faulty, distorted, or counterproductive thinking patterns accompany or precede maladaptive behaviors and anxiety responses. One school of cognitive thought sees those with anxiety as overestimating dangers and the probability of harm in a particular situation, as well as underestimating their own ability to deal with perceived threats to their physiologic and psychologic equilibrium. Cognitive-behavioral therapy evolved out of this model and has proven effective in dealing with a broad variety of psychological and physiologic symptomatology (e.g., fibromyalgia, see p 800; Table 14.10). Some studies suggest that effective psychotherapy and/or cognitive–behavioral approaches may alter abnormal patterns of brain activation although more work is needed in this area.

Existentialism arose as a school of philosophy in the mid-20th century. In a world newly devoid of religious meanings ("God is dead") and confronted with the repetitive human horrors of World Wars I and II, it was predicated that to be human was to be anxious, to be aware of the profound "nothingness" of life, and the vast void in existence and meaning. The critical consciousness of these underlying sources of one's anxiety would equip one to deal with them. One could either *choose* (another key concept in the Existential school of thought) to go on with life, regardless of this potentially crippling awareness, or succumb, and *choose* to commit suicide. This was seen as the most vital question for 20th century humans: to be or not to be. To be human is to be conscious. To be fully conscious is to be anxious. Otherwise, one would be living in an *inauthentic* state of denial. This would be "denying" aspects of human-ness and not participating fully in the human experience. The case could be made that current religious revivals in the United States, for example, could be seen as a regression to a world of certainty and a belief-based ethic as opposed to the relentless march of objective evidence. The rise of bioterrorism and nuclear weapons, and a post-9/11 consciousness, provide reinforcement of existential concerns for humankind as a whole.

Clinical Presentation

The primary symptoms of GAD are anxiety, motor tension, autonomic hyperactivity, and cognitive vigilance. The anxiety is excessive and interferes with other aspects of the patient's life. Shakiness, restlessness, and headaches are common manifestations of motor tension. Autonomic hyperactivity is commonly manifested by excessive sweating, various gastrointestinal symptoms (increased acidity, nausea, epigastric pain), palpitations, tachycardia, headaches, and shortness of breath. Irritability and a quick to startle response are typical of cognitive vigilance. Often these patients seek help with their somatic symptoms, and often will not accept a diagnosis of GAD.

DSM-IV-TR Symptom Criteria

The DSM-IV-TR symptom criteria for GAD are:

- Excessive worry or apprehension, more days than not, for at least 6 months, about a number of events and activities
- Anxiety causes clinically significant distress or impairment in social, occupational, or other important area of functioning
- Focus of the worry is not confined to features of other Axis I disorders (e.g., panic disorder, obsessive–compulsive disorder, social phobia)
- Difficulty controlling worrying
- At least three additional symptoms

- Restlessness
- Easily fatigued
- Difficulty concentrating
- Irritability
- Muscle tension
- Disturbed sleep

The distinction between GAD and normal anxiety is emphasized by the use of the words "excessive" and "difficult to control" in the criteria and by the specification that the symptoms cause significant impairment or distress.

A variety of questionnaires are available to assess anxiety. These include the Beck Anxiety Inventory, the Hamilton Anxiety Rating Scale, the Anxiety Disorder Interview Schedule, and the Primary Care Evaluation of Mental Disorders (PRIME-MD), which asks about somatic symptoms such as stomach, back, and chest pain; dizziness; and sweating; as well as mood-related symptoms such as depressed feelings and loss of interest in activities.

Aggressive measures to diagnose anxiety disorders and comorbid depression are essential as, left untreated, they can significantly disrupt an individual's life. Untreated anxiety can lead to depression.

Diagnostic Reasoning

The differential diagnosis of GAD includes all medical disorders that may cause anxiety and typically a medical work-up is necessary, including standard blood chemistry, EKG, and thyroid function tests specifically. Caffeine intoxication, stimulant abuse, alcohol, sedative, anxiolytic, and hypnotic withdrawal must all be ruled out. A complete list of all medications, both prescribed and over-the-counter, must be reviewed, including all herbal agents. An environmental/occupational assessment might also be called for as inhalation of volatile gases—such as gasoline, paint, insecticides, carbon monoxide and carbon dioxide—may all cause symptoms of anxiety.

The history and mental status exam should explore the diagnostic possibility of panic disorder, phobias, and obsessive–compulsive disorder. Patients with panic have tended to seek help earlier, as the disorder usually has a sudden onset of symptoms, is more disabling, and are less troubled by their somatic symptoms.

Distinguishing GAD from major depressive disorder and dysthymic disorder is difficult because of the frequency of co-occurrence. In patients with comorbid depression and anxiety, the symptomatic profile may be balanced or either symptom can predominate. Patients may meet all the criteria for one disorder and only partially those for the other; they may meet the criteria for both disorders; or they may demonstrate symptoms of both disorders but may not meet the full diagnostic criteria for either.

Any patient who has symptoms of anxiety or depression should be evaluated for current symptoms of both disorders. Both GAD and Social Anxiety Disorder (SAD) are commonly comorbid with MDD. Identification and treatment of depression in this group of anxious patients can lead to improved outcomes and quicker recovery.

Management

Education and Self-Care Management

Planning care for the patient with GAD begins with education. All too often, the person with GAD lacks sufficient general information about GAD and has little understanding about his or her personal GAD symptoms. Patient education includes symptom recognition, effective interpretation of physical symptoms, a decrease in the intake of stimulants such as caffeine and nicotine, and relaxation training. Changes in coping should focus on developing more effective self-awareness and relaxation skills. Patients who develop routine methods of preventing acute anxiety and promoting relaxation are more successful than patients who attempt to cope with their GAD on an as-needed basis.

Areas of patient functioning that have been affected by anxiety should be well defined, and clear goals of improvement should be developed for each area. Some areas of functioning may be less affected by anxiety than others; however, improvement in major areas of functioning, such as being able to function at work or to maintain personal relationships, should be included. Long-term negative outcomes associated with GAD often are the result of negative methods of reducing anxiety symptoms. Abuse of alcohol or marijuana is an example of the more common negative-symptom reduction methods used.

Pharmacologic Management

Benzodiazepines are the anxiolytics of choice in the acute management of GAD. They are almost immediately effective. Long-term daily use of benzodiazepines for GAD symptom relief or as sleep medication will cause more problems than it solves, however. Nonetheless, unrelieved GAD symptoms can lead to additional new problems, such as substance abuse, compulsive overeating or overspending, and severe social withdrawal. Antidepressants, usually an SSRI, can be efficacious for the long-term treatment of GAD. When a sedating medication is needed, moderately sedating TCAs can be considered.The goal of medication treatment for GAD should be to sufficiently reduce or relieve symptoms to enable effective self-care and to promote satisfactory levels of functioning. (See Drugs Commonly Prescribed 17.2.)

Follow-Up and Referral

Monthly follow-up appointments may be needed until the patient with GAD has established alternative resources for support and assistance. A clear follow-up plan decreases the problem of excessive appointments or appointments that do

Drugs Commonly Prescribed 17.2: Anti-Anxiety Agents

Drug	Dose	Comments
Alprazolam (Xanax; Xanax XR) — treatment of anxiety disorder; panic— benzodiazepine	Anxiety: 0.25–0.5 mg three/day; > at 3- to 4-day intervals to 4 mg/day in divided doses Panic: Xanax XR—begin at 0.5 mg dose up to 10 mg/day (maximum)	Schedule IV: Potential for abuse in abuse-prone patients; withdrawal syndrome; initially may experience sedation and ataxia; not effective for depression CNS depressant *Contraindicated acute narrow angle glaucoma
Clonazepam (Klonopin)—treatment of anxiety (GAD); panic—some favor as a help in sleep Benzodiazepine	0.25 mg two/day initially; increase to every 3–4 days by 0.125–0.25 mg two/day (maximum: 4 mg/day)	Schedule IV: Less sedating than other anxiolytics; onset of full anxiolytic effect can take 3–6 weeks; dizziness, nausea, headache; less dependence, withdrawal; CNS depressant – caution with alcohol
Lorazepam (Ativan) – treatment of anxiety Short-acting benzodiazepine	0.5- to 2-mg scored tablets Give in two to three divided doses, with largest dose taken at bedtime. Initially 2–3 mg daily; maximum: 10 mg/day Elderly: 1–2 mg/day	Schedule IV: CNS depression, especially sedation; use with caution with alcohol, suicidal tendencies; abuse potential. Not recommended for use in pregnancy, nursing mothers, psychosis, depression
Diazepam (Valium)—treatment of anxiety Benzodiazepine	2–10 mg two to four times daily; elderly: 2–2.5 mg one to two times/day Also injectable: 5 mg/mL	Schedule IV: CNS depressant; ataxia; paradoxical excitement; potentiated with alcohol; abuse potential; withdrawal
Azapirones (Buspirone)—treatment of anxiety (GAD)	Take consistently with regard to food; start at 7.5 mg twice/daily; increase by 5 mg/day every 3–4 days; usual range—20–30 mg/day (maximum: 60 mg/day)	*Onset of effect can take 3–6 weeks; less sedating; no dependence; dizziness, headache, nervousness initially; hypertensive crisis with MAOIs; avoid alcohol, grapefruit juice
	Newer Generation Antidepressants	
Fluoxetine (Prozac)—treatment of OCD; depression; bulimia; premenstrual dysphoric disorder	5–10 mg/day initially; usual dosage, 20–80 mg/day	GI side effects; sexual dysfunction; withdraw slowly; onset for depressive effects take 3–5 weeks
Paroxetine (Paxil)—treatment of panic disorder; social anxiety; PTSD Paxil CR	Controlled release formula—10 mg/day initially; usual dosage, 25–50 mg/day	As above
Sertraline (Zoloft)—treatment of panic; PTSD; social anxiety; OCD	25–50 mg/day initially; usual dose 50–200 mg/day	As above
Venlafaxine (Effexor)—treatment of GAD; social anxiety (immediate and extended release)	37.5 mg/day initially; usual dose 75–300 mg/day (maximum: 375 mg/day)	As above

not produce much progress. Practitioners may wish to make themselves available to anxious patients, but appointments that do not advance the patient's self-care development accomplish little. Referrals to patient education and support groups are critical for patients with GAD. The plan should include strict criteria for seeking emergency services. The goal is to protect the patient from unknowingly becoming overreactive to his or her GAD symptoms. Improvement can become more obtainable when a realistic understanding of the illness is maintained. Referral to a specialist is most useful when the patient needs this level of assistance in order to develop effective self-care skills.

Patient Education

Education about anti-anxiety medications should be reviewed with the patient and family members, including issues of overuse and dependency on medications, as well as potential adverse effects. The need to avoid combining anti-anxiety medications with alcohol should be addressed. The clinician should provide written instructions if the patient appears to have limited ability to concentrate. The practitioner should also discuss with the patient and family the causes and treatment of anxiety.

The provider may want to teach the patient and family complementary methods of anxiety management, such as relaxation techniques (see Complementary Therapies 17.1), guided imagery, music therapy, physical activity, yoga, acupuncture, and altering nutritional practices to a healthful diet.

GAD cannot be managed with medication alone. Consistent and active patient self-care is required. At the same time, the highly symptomatic patient, no matter how motivated, is unlikely to be able to engage in self-care when his or her GAD symptoms are poorly controlled. GAD symptoms can increase the difficulty of learning new information, including learning new self-care skills. Many primary-care settings now have access to comprehensive patient education programs that can give patients enough time to practice newly adopted self-care skills.

Panic Disorder

Panic disorder, which typically presents in young adulthood, is a disabling disorder. It can impair the social, family, and working lives of the patient suffering from it. *Panic disorder* symptoms are recurrent, intense, short episodes of panic-level psychological and physical symptoms of anxiety. The initial panic episode must be spontaneous and unexpected. A combination of sudden panic-symptom onset and panic-symptom severity creates secondary symptoms of fear. These secondary fear symptoms essentially define this disorder. Fear compels the patient with panic disorder to seek emergency health-care services repeatedly. To the patient, panic symptoms are life-threatening and signal a serious health problem or worse, impending nervous breakdown. Patients endure an unshakable sense of doom and danger that they cannot define. In theory, if the onset of panic symptoms were gradual instead of sudden or if the onset of symptoms could be anticipated, there would be little (if any) fear.

Patients who have lived with panic disorder for a while come to associate the onset of their symptoms with specific circumstances. They may or may not be accurate in their assessment, but they may nevertheless believe that a given situation or set of circumstances triggers their panic symptoms. When this is the case, the patient may then develop methods of avoiding the trigger situations and circumstances. Panic symptoms can be triggered by a wide variety of stimuli such as substance use, a change in daily routine, or exposure to feared situations, such as being in crowds or closed-in spaces. Panic triggers may or may not be easy to avoid. An episode of panic typically lasts about 10

COMPLEMENTARY THERAPIES 17.1

Relaxation Therapy for Anxiety

Step 1: Have the patient sit in a comfortable chair in a quiet location and minimize distractions; for example, turn off the telephone, hang up a "Do Not Disturb" sign.

Step 2: Have the patient close his or her eyes.

Step 3: Instruct the patient to breathe slowly using diaphragmatic breathing—in through the nose and out through the mouth, slowly and deeply, like blowing out a candle. (To help the patient with diaphragmatic breathing, have the patient keep their shoulders still and put his or her hand on their abdomen. The hand should move out while inhaling and in when exhaling.)

Step 4: Have the patient develop rhythmic breathing. Ideally, the patient should breathe in slowly for six counts, hold for 24 counts, then breathe out for 12 counts; then repeat ten times for at least three times a day.

Tell the patient that while breathing in and out to try some of the following:

Visualize a favorite, peaceful setting, such as a beach, forest, desert, or meadow.

Have peaceful music playing in the background.

Try autogenic relaxation, a technique where the patient imagines bodily sensations such as a feeling of heaviness or warmth spreading throughout all extremities.

Repeat a favorite phase, or mantra, with each breath.

Tense different muscles while inhaling and relax them while exhaling, starting with the feet and moving systematically up the body, muscle group after muscle group.

This breathing technique will help relax the patient as well as provide increased energy, health, and concentration. Have the patient try for at least 15 minutes each day. They are best done on an empty stomach; wait 1 hour after eating before starting. Also, advise the patient to not stand up suddenly after performing these exercises, as they can lower blood pressure, causing dizziness upon standing.

minutes or less; however, the secondary distress that follows a panic episode can last for hours.

The frequency and severity of panic episodes and the triggered emotional and behavioral responses to panic symptoms can vary from patient to patient. Individual patterns also may vary: A patient may change from having one or two episodes of panic in a year to experiencing daily episodes of panic; symptoms may vary from unconcerned recognition and acceptance of panic episodes to uncontrolled fear. Patients with panic disorder may have other anxiety disorders as well, such as PTSD or agoraphobia (fear of being in crowded, public places). More women than men are diagnosed with panic disorder.

Panic disorder differs from occasional *panic attacks.* The main distinction is that a diagnosis of *panic disorder* is based on a pattern of recurrent episodes of panic. The number of recurrent episodes used as a criterion for panic disorder ranges from six episodes in 6 weeks to four episodes in 4 weeks. There must be evidence of significant and persistent fear of a future panic episode. Because experts disagree on the recurrent criteria for panic disorder, the DSM-IV-TR does not specify a certain number of panic episodes over a specific period of time. Instead, the DSM-IV-TR criteria for panic disorder highlight the unexpected nature of panic episodes and the person's reaction to panic symptoms.

Persons with severe panic disorder become highly fearful of future panic episodes and may become preoccupied with searching for the "true meaning" of their panic symptoms. They are likely to make significant changes in their behavior and routines in the hope of avoiding future panic episodes. Without evidence of panic avoidance, it is difficult to confirm a diagnosis of panic disorder. Persons with panic disorder may become vigilant in their efforts to anticipate and thus avoid future panic episodes. Evidence of this anticipatory anxiety clarifies the diagnosis panic disorder.

Epidemiology and Causes

The prevalence of panic disorder is generally believed to be 1.5 to 3 percent; although perhaps 10 percent of the population has had at least one isolated panic attack. If agoraphobia is considered with panic disorder, the combined incidence is 3 to 5 percent. It is more common also in persons with medical conditions. For example, in pulmonary clinics (where patients with asthma and other conditions that cause shortness of breath seek treatment) 10 to 20 percent of patients may be affected by panic disorder. As many as 10 to 20 percent of patients who present to the emergency department (ED) with chest pain in actuality are suffering from a panic disorder.

Panic disorders typically appear in late adolescent or young adulthood, with a peak at 25 years of age. There is a second peak between 35 and 44 years. Panic disorder affects women approximately twice as often as men; panic disorder with agoraphobia affects women three times as often as men. Studies indicate that approximately 70 percent of patients with panic disorder have at least one major depressive episode during their lifetime. These patients also suffer from social anxiety or social phobia; they may also be generally anxious, chronic worriers, with high rates of post-traumatic stress disorder (PTSD) and obsessive–compulsive disorder (OCD).

Panic disorders appear to have a genetic component. Several studies have suggested that patients with panic disorder are at high risk for suicidal ideation and attempts. Comorbidity with major depression can increase the rate of attempted suicides. Further, panic disorder patients have a propensity to self-medicate with alcohol and drugs. These facts should alert the clinician to the serious nature of this disorder.

Individuals who suffer from recurrent panic episodes that are triggered by situational or circumstance factors can feel highly vulnerable. Repeated exposure to trigger experiences such as family violence, thunderstorms, or freeway traffic can impact the recurrence of panic episodes. Environmental factors can act as triggers by impacting the patient's perception of escape. For example, being in a large building without easy access to building exits, or in a violent household with no alternative housing choices can trigger panic symptoms when the patient perceives these experiences as situations where escape is difficult or impossible. Not being able to predict or control one's immediate circumstances can result in extreme feelings of susceptibility that may then trigger an episode of panic.

Pathophysiology

A number of studies have implicated peripheral and central nervous system dysregulation in the pathophysiology of panic disorder. In general, these studies have used biological stimulants ("panicogens") to induce panic attacks in patients diagnosed with this disorder, and then tracked the biological responses. Respiratory panic-inducing substances, such as carbon dioxide, sodium lactate, and bicarbonate, cause respiratory stimulation and a shift in the acid–base balance. It is theorized that these substances act initially at the peripheral cardiovascular baroreceptors and relay their signal by vagal afferents to the nucleus tractus solitarii and then onto the nucleus paragigantocellularis of the medulla. The hyperventilation in panic disorder, it is speculated, may be due to a hypersensitive suffocation alarm system that by increasing $P\text{CO}_2$ and brain lactate concentrations prematurely activates a physiologic asphyxia monitor. A number of other biological panicogens have stimulated, variously, multiple serotonergic effects, as well as activation of other noradrenergic and GABA receptors of the CNS directly.

The presynaptic alpha$_2$-adrenergic receptors appear to play a significant role, implicating the noradrenergic system. This response has been identified by pharmacologic challenges with the alpha$_2$-receptor agonist clonidine (Catapres) and the alpha$_2$-receptor antagonist yohimbine (Yocon), which works by stimulating firing of the locus ceruleus and elicits high rates of panic-like activity in panic disorder patients. Anxiety-like physiologic responses have been elicited by attenuation of local inhibitory GABAergic transmission in the basolateral amygdala, midbrain, and hypothalamus. Postsynaptic serotonin hypersensitivity is theorized to account for the serotonergic dysfunction observed in patients with panic disorder, as various studies with mixed serotonin agonist–antagonist drugs have demonstrated increased rates of anxiety and panic. The biological data related above have led to a focus on the brainstem (particularly the noradrenergic neurons of the locus ceruleus and the serotonergic neurons of the median raphe nucleus), the limbic system (possibly responsible for the generation of anticipatory anxiety), and the prefrontal cortex (possibly responsible for the generation of phobic avoidance).

Structural brain-imaging studies, such as MRI, have demonstrated pathologic involvement in the temporal lobes, particularly the hippocampus, in patients with panic disorder. One MRI study specifically reported cortical atrophy in the right temporal lobe of patients with panic disorder. PET, used for functional brain imaging, has implicated dysregulation of cerebral blood flow. These studies typically also use specific panic-inducing substances (such as caffeine, lactate, or yohimbine) to assess effects of panic on cerebral blood flow. Anxiety disorders and panic attacks are specifically associated with cerebral vasoconstriction. This in turn may cause CNS symptoms such as dizziness and peripheral nervous system symptoms such as hyperventilation and hypercapnia.

Genetic predisposition to panic disorders, especially in those with agoraphobia, a severe form of panic disorder, has been established in a number of studies. First-degree relatives of those with panic disorder have a four- to eightfold higher risk for the development of the disorder than first-degree relatives of other psychiatric patients. Twin studies have demonstrated a higher concordance for panic disorder in monozygotic twins than in dizygotic twins. No data exist indicating association between a specific chromosomal location or mode of transmission and panic disorder at this point in time.

Psychopathology

Although panic attacks are correlated neurophysiologically with the locus ceruleus, it is usually environmental or psychological factors that trigger the onset of panic, despite the fact that many of these patients describe the attack as "coming out of nowhere." Studies have shown that patients with panic disorder typically experience greater distress about life events than control subjects, and that in the months before the onset of panic, they demonstrate a higher incidence of stressful life events, specifically loss (>6 months). What was primarily a mild feeling of anxiety suddenly becomes an overwhelming feeling of apprehension and dread, replete with somatic symptoms.

Etiologically, from a psychoanalytic perspective, panic disorder is theorized to be the result of a breakdown of defense mechanisms against anxiety-provoking impulses, or "triggers." Agoraphobia is seen as being connected to loss of a parent in childhood and/or a history of separation anxiety. Unresolved childhood anxiety and fear of abandonment are aroused when alone in a public place, leading to a full-blown panic attack and establishing a "vicious" behavioral cycle. Defense mechanisms utilized may include repression, avoidance, and displacement. Traumatic loss in childhood may affect the developing nervous system, making it more susceptible to anxiety in adulthood. There may be a predisposing neurophysiologic vulnerability that interacts with environmental and psychosocial stressors to culminate in the development of panic disorder.

Studies of female twins support the above. Both parental separation and parental death before the child reached age 17 were strongly associated with panic disorder. Separation from the mother early in life had even higher correlates of resulting development of panic disorder than parental separation. A history of childhood sexual abuse was found in 60 percent of women with panic disorder, compared with 31 percent of women with other anxiety disorders. Interestingly, patients successfully treated with cognitive–behavioral therapy demonstrated a lack of panic response to lactate infusion; prior to this treatment, they had demonstrated panic response to lactate infusion.

Behavioral theories view anxiety as a learned response from parental behavior or through the process of classical conditioning. Classical conditioning supposes a noxious response (i.e., a panic attack) to a previously neutral stimuli, such as air flight. This results in avoidance of the neutral stimuli in the future. What exactly precipitates the first panic attack in this situation is less clear however. Nonetheless, behavioral–cognitive therapies (Table 17.10) have proved particularly successful in panic disorder.

Thus, the pathogenesis of the panic attacks may be related to neurophysiologic factors triggered by psychological reactions that are likely precipitated by the unconscious meaning assigned to stressful events. When assessing a patient with panic disorder a complete assessment of possible triggers should be done. Psychodynamic themes in panic disorder include:

- Difficulty tolerating anger
- Loss—physical or emotional—of an important person in early life or adulthood
- Internal representations of relationships involving sexual and/or physical abuse
- Parents perceived as controlling, frightening, demanding, and/or critical
- Typical defense mechanisms include reaction-formation, undoing, somatization, and externalization.
- Failure of signal anxiety function in relation to self-fragmentation and self–other boundary confusion
- A chronic sense of feeling trapped
- May be triggered by increased work responsibilities

Clinical Presentation

Ask the patient to describe the panic/anxiety episodes in detail, noting frequency, duration, and precipitating events.

Panic disorder is marked by recurrent and unpredictable panic attacks. The panic attacks come on unexpectedly, developing suddenly within 10 minutes and usually resolving within the hour. These attacks are distinct episodes of intense fear and discomfort associated with four or more specific physical symptoms. Frequency and severity attacks vary from once a week to clusters of attacks separated by months of well-being. The first attack usually occurs outside of the home.

Spontaneous panic attacks have no obvious stimuli, whereas situational panic attacks are in response to a phobic stimulus. Limited symptom attacks are spells manifesting one or two symptoms such as dizziness, tachycardia, or respiratory distress. Often limited symptom attacks occur early in the course of panic disorder or between panic attacks. Although panic disorder may occur without any obvious causative events, it can occur in early adult life after a loss, threat of a loss, physical illness, or an episode of drug abuse.

When describing their personalities during childhood, adults with panic disorder and agoraphobia frequently say they were shy and have histories of childhood separation anxiety, such as school phobia. Compared to control subjects, children of parents with panic disorder have a higher rate of behavioral inhibition in response to the unfamiliar.

After having several panic attacks, as many as 80 percent of patients begin to fear the next attack. They also experience phobic avoidance of circumstances associated with attacks. This is called anticipatory anxiety, which may become more disabling than the panic attacks themselves. Patients may become agoraphobic. This is an acquired irrational fear of being in places where one might feel trapped or unable to escape. Typically it leads to increasingly circumscribed lives; some patients eventually become homebound.

The risk factor with the best predictive power for panic disorder is a positive family history. Other types of mood and anxiety disorders often are comorbid in patients who experience panic disorder. It is important to look not only for panic disorders in the family history but also for other mental disorders.

Perform a comprehensive physical examination to rule out organic causes for the patient's symptoms, to identify a comorbid physical disorder that may affect the patient's health and therapeutic options, and if appropriate, to reassure the patient that there is nothing physically wrong. If the history suggests that significant organic disease is unlikely, the physical examination should be focused primarily on the organ system of most concern (e.g., the heart in a patient with chest pain). Consider laboratory tests to rule out physical causality.

DSM-IV-TR Symptom Criteria

The DSM-IV-TR symptom criteria for panic disorder are:

- ▲ A discrete period of intense fear or discomfort, in which four (or more) of the following symptoms developed abruptly and reached a peak within 10 minutes:
- ▲ Panic attack symptoms, including accelerated heart rate, pounding heart, sweating, shaking, sensations of smothering or being short of breath, choking sensations, chest pain, nausea or abdominal distress, feeling dizzy, lightheaded, or faint, de-realization (actual experiences seem unreal) or depersonalization (feeling detached or outside of oneself), fear of going crazy, fear of dying, numbness or tingling sensations, chills, or hot flushes.

The DSM-IV-TR symptom criteria for panic attack are:

During a panic attack (a discrete period of intense fear or discomfort), at least four of these symptoms will occur, reaching a peak within 10 minutes:

- ▲ Palpitations, pounding heart, tachycardia
- ▲ Sweating
- ▲ Trembling or shaking
- ▲ Sensation of shortness of breath or smothering
- ▲ Feeling of choking
- ▲ Chest pain or discomfort
- ▲ Nausea or abdominal distress
- ▲ Feeling of dizziness, unsteadiness, lightheadedness, or faintness
- ▲ Depersonalization ("out of body" experience)
- ▲ Fear of losing control or "going crazy"
- ▲ Fear of dying
- ▲ Paresthesias
- ▲ Chills or hot flushes

Diagnostic Reasoning

Consider medical conditions that may mimic symptoms/signs of panic disorder especially with the onset of an anxiety disorder after the age of 40. Consider that the use or withdrawal from therapeutic or recreational drugs may cause panic attacks. Therapeutic drugs include theophylline and steroids. Recreational drugs include cocaine, amphetamines, and caffeine. Drug withdrawal symptoms are typically associated with drugs such as alcohol, barbiturates, and benzodiazepines. The differential diagnosis of panic disorder is complicated by a high rate of comorbidity with other psychiatric conditions, especially abuse of alcohol and benzodiazepines, which patients may initially use in an attempt to self-medicate. Review patients' symptoms with other mental disorders that may overlap with panic disorder, such as PTSD, obsessive—compulsive disorder and the like.

Distinguish panic disorder from other anxiety disorders based on the patient's history as well as patient behavior and symptoms and the contexts in which they occur. The patient needs to satisfy the following four criteria:

1. A history of recurrent unexpected panic attacks
2. At least one of the attacks has been followed by 1 month (or more) of one (or more) of the following: (a) a persistent concern about having additional attacks, (b) worry about the implications of an attack or its consequences (having a heart attack, losing control, "going crazy," (c) a significant change in behavior related to the attacks.

3. The panic attacks are not due to any direct physiologic effects of a substance (e.g., drug abuse, medication) or a general medical condition (e.g., hyperthyroidism).
4. The panic attacks are not better accounted for by another mental disorder, such as social phobia, obsessive–compulsive disorder, PTSD, or separation anxiety disorder

Management

Pharmacologic Management

The pharmacologic treatment of panic disorder is relatively straightforward and effective. The major recent advances in the treatment of panic disorder has been the advent of SSRIs and their recognition as powerful antipanic drugs. Most cyclic antidepressants, monamine oxidase inhibitors (MAOIs), and high-potency benzodiazepines have strong antipanic activity as well. Successful treatments target spontaneous panic attacks. After panic attacks have ceased, patients are maintained on medication for a minimum of 6 months. Pharmacologic blockade of panic generally leads to a decrease in both anticipatory anxiety and phobic avoidance. A common approach is to use benzodiazepines for immediate relief. Other medications may be added, either concurrently or after symptoms are attenuated. Once these medications become effective, the benzodiazepine treatment may be tapered and discontinued. Although strong evidence is not yet available, preliminary experience suggests that some of the newer antidepressants, including mirtazapine, nefazodone, and venlafaxine, may be useful in patients with anxiety disorders, including panic disorder.

Nonpharmacologic Management

Consider recommending psychological treatments, especially cognitive behavioral therapy (CBT). CBT is aimed at altering the unproductive and dysfunctional thinking that helps to generate and maintain anxiety. Patients with panic disorder learn to decatastrophize their thinking so that attacks are avoided. CBT is effective in treating maladaptive behaviors associated with anxiety, mainly by gradual exposure to more adaptive situations. CBT encompasses a range of treatments, each consisting of several elements, including breathing retraining, psychoeducation, continuous panic monitoring, development of anxiety management skills, cognitive restructuring, and in vivo exposure. Some sources recommend a brief, highly focused behavioral and cognitive psychotherapeutic techniques for panic. When used in studies as the treatment modality, these interventions lead to reduction in panic, but other studies support a combination of CBT with medication. Hypnosis and alternative therapies (yoga, meditation) are sometimes useful as part of combined therapies, but not as effective as CBT. Some patients find relief in chiropractic treatment and acupuncture. (See Advanced Practice Nursing Interventions 17.2.)

Follow-Up and Referral

Patients with panic disorder can be managed in primary-care settings once a plan of care has been agreed to. Consider referring the patient to a psychiatrist if he or she fails to respond after 6 to 8 weeks of standard treatment. Consider referring patients to an appropriate medical specialist if an occult underlying organic disorder is suspected. A large variety of medical conditions can imitate anxiety and panic disorder.

> **ADVANCED PRACTICE NURSING INTERVENTIONS 17.2**
>
> **Panic Disorder**
>
> ***Management***
>
> Goal: Full remission, elimination of panic attacks, anxiety, phobias, and disability; restoration of well-being.
>
> Institute treatment with low-dose selective serotonin re-uptake inhibitors (SSRIs); increase dose as tolerated to target dose.
>
> Monitor closely for adverse effects.
>
> Continue treatment for 12–24 months; phase out treatment slowly (over 4–6 months).
>
> Refer to an anxiety disorder specialist if response is not satisfactory or if comorbid conditions are present.
>
> ***Patient and Family Education***
>
> Teach about panic disorder.
>
> Advise patient not to abruptly stop medication.
>
> **SOURCE:** Adapted from Ballenger, JC, et al: Consensus statement on panic disorder from the International Consensus Group on Depression and Anxiety. J Clin Psychiatry 59(suppl 8):47–54, 1998.

Patient Education

Cognitive therapeutic approaches include thought-stoppage techniques and desensitization. For treatment to be effective, the patient and family must understand the disorder and work together aggressively as active participants in the treatment plan. The patient and family must understand the potential adverse effects of any drugs prescribed and work toward using relaxation techniques, deep breathing, and the like to control panic.

Posttraumatic Stress Disorder and Acute Stress Disorder

Posttraumatic stress disorder (PTSD) is a syndrome that develops after a person witnesses, participates in, or hears of an extreme traumatic stressor. The reaction to this experience is typically fear and helplessness, relives the event over and over, and tries to avoid being reminded of it. The symptoms must be severe enough to last for more than a month after the event and must significantly affect critical areas in the person's life such as interpersonal relationships and occupational roles. The text revision of the DSM-IV-TR defines a disorder that is similar to PTSD but that is called Acute Stress Disorder, which occurs within 4 weeks of the event and remits within 2 days to 4 weeks. If symptoms persist after this period of time, then a diagnosis of PTSD is applied.

Both disorders are responses to experiences that are overwhelming, for example, war, torture, natural disasters, assault, rape, serious accidents, fires, and the like. Given the current Iraq War and the 2005 year that has seen a tsunami disaster in southeast Asia, a series of devastating hurricanes in the United States, as well as earthquakes in other areas, the state of the knowledge about both these responses will probably change as well as the prevalence of people affected.

Typically, persons reexperience the trauma in their dreams and daily thoughts, they try to evade anything that reminds them of the event (in some cases this is not possible), and they undergo a "numbing" of responsiveness along with a physiologic state of hyperarousal. This is usually accompanied by depression, anxiety, cognitive difficulties, and often substance abuse. Comorbid disorders make persons more vulnerable to developing PTSD. Nursing Situation 17.3 describes the case of Mr. B, a World War II veteran.

Epidemiology and Causes

Lifetime prevalence of PTSD in the community is approximately 8 percent, with a lifetime prevalence of 5 percent for men and 10.4 percent for women, although an additional 5 to 15 percent of the population may experience a subclinical form of the disorder. This estimation is thought to be far less than the actual numbers of people who meet the diagnostic criteria for PTSD.

Recent immigrants from areas of social and/or political instability can be highly susceptible to PTSD. However, for many reasons, immigrant patients may choose not to share their traumatic experiences with a practitioner. This reluctance may have to do with significant feelings of vulnerability that a recent immigrant may feel. Disaster survivors, such as those who have survived hurricanes, tornadoes, mass shootings, or fires, are susceptible to PTSD. Studies indicate that disaster survivors may develop symptoms anywhere from 1 week to 30 years after the event. Disaster survivors may seek primary health care for a physical illness that develops after the trauma. Survivors can become more vulnerable to physical illness without realizing why.

A national survey of more than 500 adults in the United States less than 1 month after the terrorist attacks on September 11, 2001 in New York City and Washington, DC to assess their reactions and their children to the attack found evidence of psychological sequelae. Forty five percent of adults reported one or more substantial symptom of stress, such as distressing recollections of the event, nightmares, insomnia, fearfulness, and irritability, among others. Ninety percent of those interviewed reported minor degrees of distress. Susceptibility to symptoms were associated with female sex, being nonwhite, having a history of psychological illness, and being close to the disaster site. More than 80 percent of parents reported that their children had one or more symptoms. One interesting finding was that the level of stress reported was associated with the extent of television viewing about the disaster.

A survey of Manhattan residents conducted 5 to 8 weeks after the World Trade Center collapse found that 9.8 percent, or an estimated 90,000 people, had PTSD or clini-

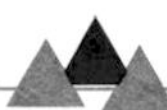

NURSING SITUATION 17.3

Posttraumatic Stress Disorder

Mr. B is a married 72-year-old salesman who came to the clinic seeking treatment for anxiety. He was referred by a veteran's service officer who felt he might be suffering from PTSD.

During World World II, Mr. B. was an infantry soldier stationed in Europe. In a major battle near the France-Germany border his company had been overrun by the Germans. His company lost 120 of 200 men, but Mr. B. was not injured. Three days after the battle, he had to return to the area to help retrieve the dead soldiers, many of whom had been his friends. Several days later, in another battle, Mr. B was injured and hospitalized; an injury he credits for saving his life as, when he was released from the hospital, he was given a noncombat job until his discharge.

Following his discharge, Mr. B drank heavily for many years and suffered sleep disturbances, including nightmares. He would also have vivid flashbacks of the war and his dead friends. During his twenties and thirties, he had problems with aggressive behavior. At age 49, he saw a psychiatrist when he began having phobic symptoms when crossing bridges. On and off for several years, he received various anti-anxiety medications.

SOURCE: Adapted from Buffman, MD, and Wolfe, N: Posttraumatic stress disorder and the WWII veteran. Geriatr Nursing 16(6):264–271, 1996.

cal depression. Another 3.7 percent met the criteria for both diagnoses. People who lived closer to Ground Zero had higher rates, as did those who had suffered personal losses, who had had another loss within the previous 12 months, or who had experienced extreme panic during or shortly after the attacks. Higher rates of disorders were found among Hispanic respondents than among whites, blacks, or Asians, and were higher among women than among men. Those in upper income levels had lower incidences. An additional study of more than 8000 children ages 10 to 13 at 9 months after the attacks found that 11 percent had symptoms compatible with a diagnosis of PTSD, and an additional 15 percent had signs of agoraphobia, such as fear of taking public transportation. Hispanic students and girls were disproportionally affected, as were those who had been exposed to prior unrelated traumatic events.

Other risk factors include female gender, age (the very young and the very old are especially susceptible), race, education, intelligence, socioeconomic status, education, family history, reported abuse in childhood, reports of other adverse childhood factors or trauma, extent of the trauma, poor social and/or family support, posttrauma life stressor may cause the emergence of PTSD, and comorbidities.

The prognosis for patients suffering from PTSD is influenced by multiple factors, including whether the disorder is acute, chronic, or delayed; the presence or absence of previous mental disorders; the patient's premorbid personality; available support resources; compliance with treatment; and the patient's ability and desire to learn new coping mechanisms. The adaptive person who suffers from acute PTSD after exposure to a traumatic event has a better chance for full recovery, especially if his or her family is supportive. Untreated, about 30 percent of patients recover completely, 40 percent continue to have mild symptoms, 20 percent continue to have moderate symptoms, and 10 percent remain unchanged or become worse. The National Comorbidity Study, for example, found that 60 percent of males and 50 percent of females had experienced some significant trauma but a much smaller proportion—as far as is known—go on to experience full-blown acute stress response and/or PTSD.

Pathophysiology

A number of biological variables have been implicated in PTSD. There is strong evidence, for example, for altered function in the noradrenergic system. Specifically, soldiers with PTSD-like symptoms may experience nervousness, high blood pressure, heart rate (HR), palpitations, sweating, flushing, and tremors—all symptoms associated with adrenergic drugs. Veterans with PTSD demonstrate increased epinephrine concentrations in 24-hour urine samples, and increased urine catecholamines in 24-hour urine samples in sexually abused girls. Lymphocyte beta-adrenergic receptors and platelet $alpha_2$—are downregulated in PTSD; it is theorized that this might be related to chronically elevated catecholamine concentrations. Flashbacks are reported in 30 to 40 percent of PTSD patients post-yohimbine (Yocon) administration.

A number of factors point to hypothalamic-pituitary-adrenal (HPA) axis hyper-regulation that is different from the neuroendocrine activity usually seen during stress and other disorders such as depression. There are low plasma and urinary free cortisol concentrations in PTSD, as well as more glucocorticoid receptors on lymphocytes. Challenge with exogenous corticotropin-releasing factor (CRF) demonstrates a blunted ACTH response. Suppression of cortisol by challenge with low-dose dexamethasone (Decadron) is enhanced in PTSD. Some studies have revealed cortisol hypersuppression in trauma-exposed patients who develop PTSD, compared with patients exposed to trauma who do not develop PTSD. Some studies of combat veterans with PTSD have shown lower average volume in the hippocampal region of the brain; and animal studies have demonstrated that changes in the hippocampus is correlated with stress. Some researchers feel that the hippocampus is not necessarily the only area of the brain to demonstrate structural changes in PTSD. Studies on depression have shown similar effects in the amygdala and prefrontal cortex.

Interestingly, combat veterans with PTSD show a naloxone (Narcan) reversible analgesic response to combat-related stimuli. This raises the possibility of opioid system hyper-regulation similar to the demonstrated hyper-regulation of the HPA axis. In general, there is a low plasma beta-endorphin concentration in PTSD. One study has shown that nalmefene (Revex), an opioid receptor antagonist, was useful in decreasing symptoms of PTSD in combat veterans.

Psychopathology

From a psychodynamic perspective, the (new) trauma is seen as reactivating a preexisting and unresolved childhood trauma. The defense mechanisms of repression, denial, reaction formation, and undoing are aroused by the precipitation of anxiety aroused by trauma, both new and preexisting. The ego "relives" and tries to "master" and reduce the anxiety. Other defense mechanisms activated may include minimization, splitting, dissociation, and guilt (as a defense against underlying helplessness). The mode of object relatedness involves projection and introjection of the following roles: omnipotent rescuer, abuser, and victim. The subjective meaning of the trauma may well determine its traumatogenicity and the traumatic event may resonate with childhood traumas. There may be an inability to regulate affect after the trauma, and subsequent somatization and alexithymia (inability to verbalize or identify feeling states).

From a behavioral perspective, the unconditioned stimulus (the trauma) that produces a fear response is connected, through classical conditioning, with a conditioned stimulus (physical or mental representations of the trauma—

sights, sounds, smells). Then, through instrumental learning, the conditioned stimuli elicit the fear response independent of the original unconditioned stimulus, and patients develop a pattern of avoiding both the conditioned stimulus and the unconditioned stimulus. "Secondary gain" may develop and reinforce the disorder and its persistence; these patients commonly receive financial compensation, possibly increased attention and/or sympathy, as well as the satisfaction of dependency needs.

From a cognitive model, the trauma that precipitated the disorder is unable to be processed by the affected person. The experience of stress continues and avoidance techniques develop as a way of distancing the discomfort. As patients attempt to integrate the trauma cognitively, it is alternatively acknowledged and blocked and avoided. (See Risk Factors 17.3.)

Clinical Presentation

The principal clinical feature of PTSD are painful reexperiencing of the event, a pattern of avoidance and emotional numbing. Typically, a combination of a trauma, the personal characteristics of the person experiencing the trauma, and a variety of posttrauma factors all must coalesce for the person to develop PTSD. A diagnosis of PTSD will rarely be made unless the patient exhibits at least one symptom from each symptom category.

- ▲ Intrusive Symptoms: The first category includes reexperiencing the traumatic event or having intrusive symptoms. The patient has frequent episodes in which the traumatic event is relived to the point that the trauma "intrudes" into current life. This experience can manifest itself as a nightmare, a flashback, or simply sudden, vivid memories that are accompanied by painful emotions or images related to the trauma. Each time the trauma is reexperienced, it can be so vivid that the patient suffers as though the trauma were literally happening again.
- ▲ Avoidance Symptoms: The second category includes avoidance symptoms. The patient avoids any situation or activity that might revive memories of the trauma. This symptom can severely impact the patient's relationships with others, because close emotional ties with family, friends, and colleagues may be included among the situations that the patient intentionally avoids. With avoidance, the patient may at first feel either nothing or numbness and is able to complete only routine or mechanical activities. Later, when trauma reexperiencing begins, the patient can alternate between episodes of excessive emotion and emotional numbness. Patients suffering from PTSD commonly complain that they cannot feel emotions, especially emotions toward those who are closest to them.
- ▲ Hyperarousal Symptoms: The third category includes hyperarousal symptoms. As a result of being hypersensitive or on edge, patients may experience episodes of unprovoked anger, jumpiness, and seem to be "on guard" most of the time. Patients may behave as though they are facing constant threats of danger or further trauma. They can become hyper-reactive to unexpected sounds or encounters. Problems with concentrating or remembering current information are common, and terrifying nightmares can lead to severe insomnia.

RISK FACTORS 17.3

PTSD

- Physical or sexual childhood abuse
- Sexual or other life-threatening assault/accident
- Combat exposure
- Being involved in fire, flood, hurricane, or other natural disaster
- Witnessing someone being badly injured or killed

Characteristic symptoms of PTSD include reexperiencing the traumatic event, recurrent dreams relating to the event, chronic anxiety and/or panic attacks, flashbacks, insomnia, difficulty concentrating, memory impairment, a sense of personal isolation, diminished interests in activities, avoidance of activities that recall memories of the event, irritability, restlessness, tremulousness, startle reactions, explosive outbursts, numbness of feelings, and atypical feelings of guilt. (See Nursing Situation 17.3.)

In addition to hearing the patient's complaints, the practitioner needs to assess other pertinent factors to help establish goals for the patient as part of the planning process. First, is the patient able to see the relationship between the traumatic event and the way he or she is feeling? What is the frequency of the intrusive symptoms? Who is available in the patient's environment to provide support? What coping mechanisms has the patient used successfully in the past? Is the patient suicidal or homicidal? What are the patient's sleep patterns? What is the concentration level? Can the patient complete tasks or perform on the job? Does the patient verbalize survivor guilt? Does the patient verbalize a desire to feel better? A short diagnostic tool can helps quickly assess if the patient is experiencing PSTD. (See Advanced Assessment 17.5.)

To meet the official DSM-IV-TR criteria for a diagnosis of PTSD, symptoms must have persisted for more than 1 month and must have caused clinically significant distress in social, occupational, or other areas of functioning. If the symptoms have been present for less than 1 month, the patient should be diagnosed with an acute stress disorder rather than PTSD. PTSD is considered *acute* if symptoms have been present for less than 3 months; *chronic* if the symptoms have been present for more than 3 months; and *delayed* if symptom onset occurs 6 months or longer after the trauma.

ADVANCED ASSESSMENT 17.5

PTSD Diagnostic Tool

In your life have you ever had any experience that was so frightening, horrible, or upsetting that in the past month, you: (answer Yes or No)

1. Have had nightmares about it or thought about it when you did not want to?
2. Tried hard not to think about it or went out of your way to avoid situations that reminded you of it?
3. Were constantly on guard, watchful, or easily startled?
4. Felt numb or detached from others, activities, or your surroundings?

Scoring: considered positive if there are two or more Yes answers OR the single hyperarousal item (no. 3).

Diagnostic Reasoning

DSM-IV-TR Symptom Criteria

The DSM-IV-TR symptom criteria for PTSD are:

- ▲ Exposure to a traumatic event or experience in which the person experienced, witnessed, or was confronted with actual or threatened death or serious injury to self or others.
- ▲ The person's response was intense fear, helplessness, or horror.
- ▲ The traumatic event is persistently reexperienced in one or more of the following ways:
  1. Intrusive, recurrent recollections
  2. Recurrent upsetting dreams of the event
  3. Reliving the event or flashback experience
  4. Intense psychological response when exposed to internal or external symbols of the event or elements of the event
  5. Intense physical response when exposed to internal or external symbols of the event or elements of the event
- ▲ Persistent avoidance or numbing response to stimuli associated with the trauma by three or more of the following:
  6. Efforts to avoid thought, feelings, or conversations associated with the trauma
  7. Efforts to avoid activities, places, or people that stimulate recollections of the trauma
  8. Inability to recall some important aspects of the trauma
  9. Marked loss of interest or decrease in participation in significant activities
  10. Feeling detached or disconnected from others
  11. Blunted feelings or limited range of feelings
  12. Sense of having a limited or shortened future
- ▲ Persistent symptoms of increased arousal indicated by two or more of the following:
  13. Difficulty falling or staying asleep
  14. Irritability or angry outbursts
  15. Difficulty concentrating
  16. Hypervigilance
  17. Exaggerated startle response
- ▲ Duration of symptoms is more than 1 month and related impairment.

A major consideration in the diagnosis of PTSD is the possibility that the patient has also incurred a head injury during the trauma. PTSD is commonly diagnosed as another mental disorder and is then inappropriately treated. In general, interviewing the patient about prvious traumatic experience can help identify this component in the patient's symptomatology. Borderline personality disorder, dissociative disorders, factitious disorders, and malingering may need to be considered.

Management

Crisis intervention immediately after the traumatic event may lead to avoidance of this disorder, although Critical Incident De-briefing (CID), previously thought to be a helpful approach, was found to increase symptomatology when used with survivors of 9/11, and is no longer recommended. Treatment that includes individual and/or group psychotherapy using psychodynamic principles has been proven helpful, hypnotherapy is a useful adjuvant treatment, and cognitive–behavior therapy (CBT) has proven particularly effective. Cognitive Processing Therapy (CPT), and Eye Movement Desensitization and Reprocessing (EMDR) are also helpful approaches.

CBT has been found to be particularly helpful. Several specific CBTs for PTSD include Prolonged Exposure (PE); Stress Inoculation therapy (SIT); and Image Rehearsal Therapy (IRT). PE was developed for women with rape trauma and is an effective first-line treatment with sustained benefit over time. One technique called "imaginal exposure" has the patient imagine and describe trauma and associated emotions and can be effective in reducing PTSD symptom severity. In vivo exposure uses systemic desensitization to triggers of trauma. With desensitization, the patient is exposed to his or her trauma "trigger" in a controlled environment. Improvement is achieved by gradually increasing the time of exposure to the trigger until the patient no longer reacts with panic.

SIT may be considered a "toolbox" for managing anxiety and focuses on correcting the patient's intrusive symptoms by teaching relaxation techniques such as breathing exercises that can be used to help self-manage intrusive symptoms when they occur. IRT is a brief approach—three sessions—which was found to decrease chronic nightmares and improve sleep quality. All of these approaches are specialized forms of care, but practitioners in primary-care settings can refer patients to providers who can provide these services.

Another intervention for PTSD is psychodynamic psychotherapy. This method focuses on helping the patient to examine personal values and how the experience of the traumatic event violated them. The goal is to resolve the conscious and unconscious mental conflicts that were created by the trauma. The patient works on strengthening his or her self-esteem as a way of increasing the ability to cope with the trauma.

Family therapy can be helpful when family relationships have been impacted by the patient's symptoms. When family members complain that the patient does not communicate and is difficult or unpredictable, a family therapist can help the family accomplish positive changes in their relationships and functioning, and help them learn to cope with their own feelings about the patient's experiences.

Group therapy or peer-counseling groups are also effective interventions for PTSD. Health groups can encourage members to share similar traumas and symptoms safely. Through participation in these groups, individuals with PTSD can learn that they are worthy and that they are not somehow guilty for their trauma. Patients may find it easier to learn new coping techniques from other group members.

Various medications can improve symptoms. SSRIs have been associated with the best results for the majority of patients with PTSD. They have been shown to improve ALL core PTSD clusters (numbing, intrusions, hyperarousal), and is effective in both genders, all trauma types, and in patients with comorbid disorders. For some patients, tricyclic antidepressants (Elavil, Norpramin, Tofranil) are effective. Anxiolytic medications are also used for acute or short-term symptom management only. Buspirone (Buspar) can reduce intrusive symptoms for some patients and is a safe anxiolytic. The gradual onset of effects can be a problem for some patients.

If response to SSRI is inadequate, and in the cases of severe symptomatology, other pharmacologic approaches may be necessary. Define realistic goals and individuate to the patient. In a patient with hyperarousal, an anti-adrenergic agents may be effective; an atypical antipsychotic might be called for in a paranoid and fearful patient (as many as 40 percent of patients may have comorbid psychotic symptoms); and with a severe comorbid depression, a TCA or MAOI may be necessary. With a patient with extremely labile/impulsive symptomatology, an anticonvulsant may be tried.

Relaxation therapy and other forms of complementary therapies are also helpful for persons with PTSD. Massage, positive imagery, meditation, and yoga have all been shown to be beneficial.

Follow-Up and Referral

Once a primary-care patient who has not fully recovered from a traumatic experience has been identified, the patient should be referred to a specialist. The symptoms of PTSD can be very disturbing, and most patients will require more time and support than is available in primary-care settings. Pharmacologic management may require specialized management, especially if an SSRI has been tried and the patient proves refractory to treatment. Patients will most likely wish to continue with their primary-care practitioner for some aspects of their care. Recovery from trauma is a slow process: Patients may stop and start treatment for years. When this is the case, their relationship with their primary-care practitioner becomes a stabilizing force.

Patient Education

It is important that the patient with PTSD and his or her family have a good understanding of the disorder, the chronic nature of PTSD, and the potential adverse effects of any medications prescribed. For some patients, interventions of a holistic nature may prove beneficial. Regular physical activity, good nutritional practices, and other self-care interventions can help to control symptomatology. Disease progression could lead to suicidal ideation and/or violence. The patient and family should be counseled regarding danger signs and the need for close follow-up and possible intervention.

Sleep Disorders

Insomnia, or difficulty sleeping, is an extremely common problem, yet one that is etiologically complex. It may be defined as difficulty in falling asleep or maintaining sleep, early morning wakefulness, intermittent wakefulness, or any combination of the above. It may be a transient phenomenon, associated, for example, with bereavement or a life crisis, or it may be a chronic problem. It may be associated with underlying psychosocial problems and/or stressors, medication usage, or substance abuse. *Primary insomnia,* as defined by the DSM-IV-TR, further specifies that insomnia involves some degree of daytime impairment or functional disturbance. Primary insomnia is that which cannot be traced to another medical or psychiatric disorder.

Epidemiology and Causes

It is estimated that insomnia, in some form or another, affects 35 percent (fully one-third) of the adult population, and a higher percentage of older adults. It is estimated that 10 percent to 17 percent of the population is affected by primary insomnia based on the criterion of sleep disturbance occurring every night for 2 weeks or more. Women appear to be slightly more affected than men are; however, men appear to nap more than women, perhaps because they suffer from sleep apnea or other conditions that cause excessive daytime sleepiness. Both men and women cite difficulty in staying asleep as the most common cause of their insomnia.

Acute insomnia may be precipitated by physical or emotional discomfort. Examples include pain, acute illness, and environmental disturbances such as noise, light, and temperature. Sleeping at a time that is inconsistent with daily biological (circadian) rhythms, because of plane travel across time zones (jet lag) or shift work, may also precipitate acute insomnia. Any number of underlying medical conditions may contribute to insomnia. Pain may contribute to wakefulness; indeed, often the question, "Does the pain awaken you at night?" is an important piece of information in determining the severity of pain. Examples of painful conditions that commonly affect sleep are arthritis and muscle cramps. Restless leg syndrome, which also occurs more commonly in elderly patients, may affect sleep. Insomnia is also associated with some types of delirium and dementias (e.g., "sundowning"). Acid reflux and duodenal ulcers may also cause insomnia. Fibromyalgia is closely associated with insomnia and is classified by some as a sleep disorder. An underlying metabolic disorder such as hyperthyroidism may contribute to insomnia. Sleep apnea may result in frequent wakefulness and insomnia. Insomnia related to discomfort in certain sleeping positions is common during pregnancy; it may also occur during the postpartum period because of caregiving that interrupts sleep, along with postpartum and hormonal shifts.

A variety of psychosocial problems may also contribute to insomnia: Anxiety, manic disorders, and schizophrenia specifically are associated with insomnia. Drug usage, including OTC drugs such as diet aids, decongestants, and cough syrup containing ephedrine, may aggravate or cause insomnia. A number of herbal products contain ephedrine, and in certain patients, ginseng may contribute to insomnia. Green tea, highly touted of late as an antioxidant, contains caffeine, and caffeine can contribute to insomnia, as can alcohol and smoking. In addition, a variety of prescription drugs may cause sleeplessness or frequent awakenings, specifically steroids, theophylline, phenytoin (Dilantin), and levodopa (Sinemet).

Additional risk factors for insomnia include chronic illnesses, obesity (also correlated with sleep apnea), and drug usage. It is important to consider cultural factors. For example, eating large meals late at night may interfere with sleep. Traumatic events can precipitate an acute, transient insomnia that may become chronic if not properly managed. Although alcohol is a depressant, there is a rebound stimulatory effect of alcohol, so drinking alcohol after 5 P.M. may contribute to insomnia. Smoking (because of the stimulatory effects of nicotine) also contributes to sleeplessness. Chronic stress, hyperarousal of the type associated with PTSD, poor sleep hygiene, and behavioral conditioning may contribute to primary insomnia—insomnia that cannot be related to any specific underlying factors.

Pathophysiology

Normal sleep is a periodic state of rest accompanied by varying degrees of unconsciousness and relative inactivity. It is normally an easily reversible, regular, recurrent state. The functions of sleep are restorative and hemostatic, critical for normal thermoregulation and energy conservation. Sleep disturbance is often an early symptom of impending mental illness.

Two physiologic states compose sleep: non-rapid-eye movement (NREM) and rapid eye movement sleep (REM). In NREM sleep most physiologic functions are markedly lower than in wakefulness although there may be episodic, involuntary body movements during NREM sleep. In contrast, REM sleep is characterized by physiologic activity level similar to those in wakefulness and a high level of brain activity, and is sometimes called *paradoxical sleep.* NREM sleep is composed of stages 1 through 4, with stages 3 and 4 being the deepest portions. Typically, NREM sleep is punctuated with a REM cycle typically every 90 to 100 minutes during the night. The first REM period tends to be the shortest, lasting less than 10 minutes; later REM periods may last 15 to 40 minutes each. Most REM periods occur in the last third of the night; most stage 4 sleep occurs in the first third of the night.

These sleep patterns change over the course of a person's life. In young adulthood, REM comprises about 25 percent of sleep, and NREM approximately 75 percent distributed as follows: (1) stage 1 = 5 percent; (2) stage 2 = 45 percent; (3) stage 3 = 12 percent; and (4) stage 4 = 13 percent. These figures remain fairly constant in normal sleep although there is a reduction in both slow-wave sleep and REM sleep in older persons. NREM sleep increases after exercise and starvation, and is thus thought to be associated with satisfying metabolic needs.

Different individuals seem to need different amounts of sleep. "Short sleepers" refer to persons who require fewer than 6 hours of sleep a night to function normally, whereas "long sleepers" refers to individuals who need to sleep more than 9 hours each night to function adequately. Long sleepers tend to be mildly depressed, anxious, and socially withdrawn; they also have more REM periods and more rapid eye movements within each period—known as *REM density*—than short sleepers. The latter tend to be socially adept, efficient, and ambitious. Physical work, illness, pregnancy, exercise, increased mental activity, and stress all may increase the need for sleep. Intense psychological stimuli, such as stress, may increase REM periods, as well as the use of chemicals or drugs that decrease brain catecholamines.

It is thought that there is not one simple sleep control center, but rather a number of interconnecting systems or centers that are located largely in the brainstem. These systems are thought to mutually activate and inhibit one another. Serotonin is thought to play a large role in sleep regulation, and destruction of the dorsal raphe nucleus of the brainstem, which contains nearly all the brain's serotonergic cell bodies, thus preventing serotonin synthesis, reduces sleep for a considerable period of time. The availability of amino acid precursors of serotonin, such as L-tryptophan, affects the synthesis and release of serotonin by serotonergic neurons. Essentially, serotonin has been implicated as the primary sleep-promoting neurotransmitter; catecholamines are considered responsible for wakefulness.

Normal sleep patterns are also controlled by norepinephrine-containing neurons located in the locus ceruleus. Electrical stimulation of the locus ceruleus, such as occurs in individuals with implanted electrodes to control spasticity, for example, profoundly alters all sleep patterns. Wakefulness is increased and REM sleep (REM-off neurons) markedly reduced by drugs and manipulations that increase firings of these noradrenergic neurons. Conversely, brain acetylcholine is also involved in sleep, particularly REM sleep. The injection of cholinergic–muscarinic agonists into pontine reticular formation neurons (REM-on neurons) in animal studies causes a shift into REM sleep from wakefulness. Patients who are depressed have been shown to have marked disruption of REM sleep patterns, such as shortened REM latency (60 minutes or less), a shift in REM distribution to the first half of the night rather than the last half, and an overall increased percentage of REM sleep. Drugs that reduce REM sleep such as antidepressants may produce beneficial effects in the depressed person; approximately 50 percent of persons with MDD evidence temporary improvement when their sleep is restricted or when they are deprived of sleep. Conversely, reserpine (Serpasil), which is one of the few drugs to increase REM sleep, also produces depression.

REM and slow wave sleep is reduced in patients with Alzheimer's dementia, theorized to occur related to the loss of cholinergic neurons in the basal forebrain. Melatonin secretion from the pineal gland is inhibited by bright light; it is secreted predominantly at night. It is thought that the anatomic site of a circadian pacemaker that regulates melatonin secretion is located in the suprachiasmatic nucleus of the hypothalamus, and that this is responsible for the largely self-regulating sleep–wake cycle. A variety of other sleep-promoting substances have been identified such as prostaglandin D_2, delta sleep-inducing peptide, interleukin-1, and fatty acid primary amines. The hypnotic effect of these substances is commonly limited to NREM or slow-wave sleep, although peptides that increase REM sleep have also been reported. A number of these putative "sleep factors," including interleukin-1 and prostaglandin D_2, are immunologically active as well, which suggests a relationship between immune function and the sleep–wake cycle.

Daily variations in a variety of physiologic functions affecting the endocrine, thermoregulatory, cardiac, pulmonary, renal, gastrointestinal, neurobehavioral, as well as sleep–wake cycles, are governed by the 24-hour rhythm in humans. Some of these variations are passively produced by periodic environmental or behavioral change, while others are driven by an endogenous oscillatory process, for example, the circadian variation in plasma cortisol that persists under a variety of environmental and behavioral conditions. The genetically determined period of this endogenous neural oscillator, which averages 24.2 in humans, is normally synchronized to the environmental light–dark cycle. The timing and internal architecture of sleep are coupled directly to the output of the endogenous circadian pacemaker. Misalignment of the output of the endogenous circadian pacemaker with the desired sleep–wake cycle can, therefore, induce insomnia, decreased alertness, and impaired performance of shift workers, and accounts for the phenomenon of jet lag.

Sleep deprivation for prolonged periods can lead to hallucinations, ego disorganization, and delusions. REM-deprived patients may exhibit irritability and lethargy. Debilitated appearance, skin lesions, increased food intake, weight loss, increased energy expenditure, decreased body temperature, and death are produced in studies of rats subject to intense sleep deprivation. Increased plasma norepinephrine and decreased plasma thyroxine levels are the neuroendocrine changes.

Clinical Presentation

Insomnia may not be the chief reason for an office visit. It may be detected, however, by incorporating sleep-related questions into the general review of systems. Direct inquiry is important, because patients with chronic insomnia often have never discussed their problem, or have lived with it for so long that they do not think that anything can be done about it. The primary consequences of acute insomnia are sleepiness, negative mood, and impairment of performance. The severity of the components is related to the amount of sleep lost on one or more nights. Patients with chronic insomnia frequently complain of fatigue, mood changes (e.g., depression, irritability), difficulty concentrating, and impaired daytime functioning.

The assessment should include questions about sleep as well as questions about daytime functioning, where the full effects of altered sleep are manifested. The actual number of hours of sleep required for each individual to subjectively feel refreshed varies markedly. Although the ability to maintain sleep alters with age, the individual's need for sleep does not change significantly. The patient's medical history and comorbidities are other important parameters that should be documented. Many medical problems, such as gastroesophageal reflux disease (GERD), worsen at night because they may be aggravated by recumbency.

It is necessary to rule out all underlying causes, for example, pain and the disease or condition that is the cause of the pain. A thorough drug history must be taken, including all OTC drugs such as decongestants and cough syrups, which often contain decongestants that act as stimulants. Additionally, a complete history of all herbal remedies used, especially teas that may contain caffeine or ginseng and a variety of other CNS stimulants, should be obtained. When patients buy products in health food stores, they often do not think of them as "drugs." Screen for any illicit drug and alcohol use. (See Focusing the History 17.2.)

It is also helpful for the patient to keep a sleep diary. A sleep diary is a useful tool to track exactly when and

FOCUS ON HISTORY 17.2

Insomnia

Questions to ask:

- How has the person been sleeping recently?
- How long has the problem existed?
- Does the person have any underlying psychiatric or medical conditions?
- Is the person's sleep environment conducive to sleep? For example, are there any problems that would make sleeping difficult, such as noise, temperature, light, or space?
- Does the person work shift work or odd hours? What time does the person usually go to sleep? Get up? Are these hours the same on the weekday as well as the weekend?
- Does the person travel frequently?
- Does the person use caffeine, alcohol, drugs, or tobacco? If so, how much, and what are the specifics concerning the patient's use?
- Does the person have difficulty staying awake or report dozing off during normal daily activities?
- Does the person report any daytime consequences of not sleeping?
- Does the person (or partner) report:
  - loud snoring, gasping, or stop breathing at night? (Suggests sleep apnea)
  - legs or arms jerking during sleep? (Suggests periodic limb movement)
  - creeping, crawling, or uncomfortable feelings in the legs that are relieved by moving them? (Suggests restless legs syndrome)

under what conditions the patient sleeps, as well as diet, exercise, and drug habits that may help reveal the underlying problem. In addition, a record of all exercise and physical activity may prove helpful. The sleep diary also helps to further define the nature of the sleep problem. The delayed sleep phase type of circadian rhythm sleep disorder, for example, manifests itself with difficulty falling asleep at the desired time, and difficulty waking at the desired time. The advanced sleep phase pattern, in contrast, is characterized by difficulty staying awake in the evening and by early awakening. Some persons awaken during the night and cannot fall back to sleep (Table 17.17).

Diagnostic Reasoning

DSM-IV-TR Symptom Criteria

There are three major categories of sleep disorders: (1) primary sleep disorders; (2) sleep disorders related to another mental disorder; and (3) other sleep disorders related to a general medical condition or substance-abuse. The American Sleep Disorders Association's International Classification of Sleep Disorders: Diagnostic and Coding Manual (ICSD) divides sleep disorders into four categories: (1) dyssomnias; (2) parasomnias; (3) sleep disorders associated with medical-psychiatric disorders; and (4) proposed sleep disorders. Certain specific psychiatric disorders, such as depression, mania, and schizophrenia, may present with insomnia, or as a sleep disorder. The APN should be alert to these possibilities and should question the patient regarding his or her personal and family history. The provider should screen for all these conditions, and other disorders such as GAD that may present with sleeplessness. Certain stressful situations, as well as traumatic events, may precipitate sleeplessness.

There may be objective corroboration by a family member of acute or chronic insomnia, but basically insomnia is a subjective complaint. In cases of suspected sleep apnea, it may be necessary for the patient to undergo polysomnography.

Management

Nonpharmacologic Management

First, all underlying causes of insomnia, such as pain, must be treated. Any drugs and/or herbals that may be contributory should be discontinued. In older adults, a "drug holiday" may be needed to assess further the underlying causes. Counseling regarding lifestyle changes should be instituted, including changing any dietary, drug, alcohol, or lifestyle issues (such as inactivity or smoking) that may be contributing to the sleeplessness. The patient should be encouraged to avoid daytime napping and to develop bedtime rituals that are conducive to sleep. An exercise schedule may prove beneficial, although evening exercise may be stimulating. Alcohol should be avoided after 5 P.M., as should heavy evening meals (a light evening snack may sometimes be conducive to sleep). Reassurance and supportive counseling are essential; insomnia is not a complaint that should be taken lightly. Issues of caregiving for young children or older adults living in the home may be a part of the clinical picture. Again, diversionary lifestyle changes and situational support may be more effective than pharmacologic measures for these patients. (See Advanced Practice Nursing Interventions 17.3.)

Pharmacologic Management

The first National Institute of Health "state of the science" conference on insomnia since 1983 was held in June 2005. One important finding was recognition of the tendency of insomnia to be a chronic, potentially lifelong illness. Given the chronic nature of this problem, long-term treatment is often advisable. The panel stated that evidence supports the efficacy of cognitive–behavioral therapy and of hypnotic medications for the treatment of chronic insomnia, but it noted that there is very little evidence to support the efficacy of other treatments (including antidepressants, antipsychotics, and antihistamines), despite their widespread use.

Table 17.17 Sample Sleep Diary

Name: ______________________________

	Sun	Mon	Tues	Wed	Thurs	Fri	Sat
Date							
Previous Night Bed time							
Today Rise time							
Previous Night Time needed to fall asleep (estimated)							
Previous Night Number of awakenings (estimated)							
Previous Night Total time awake (estimated)							
Previous Night Amount of sleep (estimated)							
Today Naps (time and duration)							
Today Alcoholic Drinks (number and time)							
Today Caffeinated Drinks (number and time)							
Today Medications (name and time)							
Today Stresses: (describe)							
Today Tiredness scale: 1 = very tired 2 = somewhat tired 3 = fairly alert 4 = alert							
Today Irritability scale 1 = very irritable 2 = somewhat irritable 3 = not irritable							
Today Other (describe)							

ADVANCED PRACTICE NURSING INTERVENTIONS 17.3

Insomnia

Behavioral Treatment	Relaxation therapy (progressive muscle relaxation therapy), autogenic training, EMG, biofeedback
Sleep Restriction Therapy	Poor sleepers often increase their time in bed. Sleep restriction therapy curtails this time. For example, if a person reports sleeping only 5 hours per night, they should be counseled to only stay in bed 5 hours per night. As sleep improves, increase time in bed in 15- to 30-minute intervals. It works best to alter bedtime and keep rising time constant. Do not reduce sleep to less than 5 hours per night.
Stimulus Control Therapy	Functions on premise that insomnia is a conditioned response to temporal (bedtime) and environmental (bed/bedroom cues). Objective is to re-associate the bed and bedroom with rapid sleep onset. Stimulus control therapy counsels: (1) Only go to bed when sleepy. (2) Use the bed only for sleep. (3) Get out of bed and go into another room when awake; only go back into the bedroom when sleepy. (4) Maintain a regular rise time, regardless of sleep deprivation during the night. (5) Avoid daytime napping.
Cognitive Therapy	Identify dysfunctional ideas about sleep and replace them with more functional approaches, e.g., 8 hours of sleep is not necessary for everyone; insomnia and less sleep does not have to destroy one's life. This approach helps minimize anticipatory anxiety around sleep.
Physical Therapy	Exercise: Regular physical activity will assist with sleep. Advise the patient not to exercise too close to bedtime. Massage: Weekly massage may assist with relaxation.
Pharmacologic Therapy	Hypnotics, antidepressants, antihistamines, melatonin
Reassurance and Support	Active listening and patience; encourage ventilation of feelings, especially if stress is a component of the insomnia.

Advantages of the sedative-hypnotics is that they hasten sleep onset, decrease the number of nighttime awakenings, increase in total number of sleep time (varies with medication duration of action), and make sleep more refreshing. Some of the disadvantages include that they may alter sleep architecture over time by decreasing slow-wave sleep and REM sleep, and cause residual sedation, psychomotor and cognitive impairment, psychological dependence in vulnerable individuals, as well as rebound insomnia. The eight agents with an indication for insomnia include five older benzodiazepines (estazolam, flurazepam, quazepam, temazepam, and triazolam) and three newer nonbenzodiazepine medications (eszopiclone, zaleplon, and zolpidem). The elimination half-lives of the sedative hypnotics (see Drugs Commonly Prescribed 17.3) vary tremendously, and as a result, so does their duration of action. The advantages and disadvantages of a given duration of action must be assessed in light of each patinet's individual needs. All agents in this class have some potential for abuse, although the newer agents may have less. All are classified as Schedule IV by the Drug Enforcement Administration (DEA). Clinical trials have provided some evidence that sleep can improve to some degree without the use of any medication, as patients receiving placebo often reported as much improvement during the study as those taking medication. In sleep studies, a placebo is not an "inactive" treament in that all study participants must adhere to nonpharmacologic regimens (such as going to bed and getting up at regular hours, not napping, avoiding caffeine and alcohol) that are recognized as effective remedies for insomnia.

Follow-Up and Referral

Transient insomnia may turn into chronic insomnia. For this reason treatment is essential. Insomnia should resolve with patience, counseling, and treatment. A concern is daytime sleepiness (sleep apnea, for example, is highly correlated with car accidents). The patient may need to be referred for supportive counseling, especially if insomnia is related to a traumatic event. The entire environmental situation of the patient and family should be assessed. Are there caregiver issues involved, and can external and additional support be provided or arranged for? Is there a need for diversionary activities, or a need to increase the individual's physical activity level? If sleep apnea is suspected, a polysomnography should be ordered.

Patient Education

The patient and family members need to be reassured and counseled regarding the transient nature of insomnia,

Drugs Commonly Prescribed 17.3: Sedatives and Hypnotics

Drug	Dose	Comments
Zaleplon (Sonata)—short-term treatment of insomnia (pyrazolopyrimidine hypnotic)	5 mg, 10 mg PO hs (maximum: 20 mg) Heavy meal can delay absorption	CIV—half-life 1 hour; take 4 hours before becoming active again; potentiates CNS depressants; behavioral changes
Zolpidem (Ambien)—short-term treatment of insomnia Zolpidem CR (imidazopyridine hypnotic)	6.25, 12.5 mg PO hs; start low with elderly; do not give to patients younger than 18 years of age	CIV—half-life 2.5–2.8 (CR) hours; take with liquid—food can delay absorption; CNS depression
Flurazepam (Dalmane)—short-term treatment of insomnia (benzodiazepine)	15 mg, 30 mg PO hs	CIV—**half-life 47–100 hours; potentiates CNS depression
Eszopidone (Lunesta)—insomnia (benzodiazepine)	2–3 mg PO hs; start with 1 mg in elderly	CV IV—half-life 6 hours; potentiates CNS depressants
Quazepam (Doral)—insomnia (benzodiazepine)	Initially 7.5 mg PO hs; increase to 15 mg after 1–2 days	CIV—*half-life approximately 39 hours; potentiates CNS depression
Triazolam (Halcion)—short-term (7–10 days) treatment of insomnia (benzodiazepine)	0.125, 0.25 mg PO hs; scored *Never give for more than 1 month.	CIV—half-life 1.5–5.5 hours; may aggravate suicidal tendencies, delusions; CNS depressant; paradoxical excitement; ataxia; abnormal behavior
Temazepam (Restoril)—short-term treatment of insomnia (7–10 days) (benzodiazepine)	7.5-, 15-, 22.5-, 30-mg tablets Elderly: begin with 7.5 7.5–30 mg PO hs *Never give for more than 1 month.	CIV—half-life 3.5–18.4 hours; CNS depressant; paradoxical excitement; precaution in drug and alcohol abuse; may have sleep disturbance after stopping drug
Estazolam (ProSom)—short-term treatment of insomnia (benzodiazepine)	1–2 mg PO hs; start with 0.5 mg in elderly; avoid abrupt cessation.	CIV—*half-life 10–24 hours; CNS depressant; paradoxical excitement; anxiety; incoordination
Pentobarbital sodium (Nembutal)—short-term treatment of insomnia when oral route not available (barbiturate)	150–200 mg IM/IV (maximum 5-mL/injection)—deep IM; inject slowly IV (no more than 50 mg/min); avoid abrupt cessation; short-term (< 2 weeks) use only	CII—*half-life 10–15 hours; numerous drug interactions, including pregnancy, nursing mothers (Category D); somnolence; respiratory depression; paradoxical excitement
Ramelteon (Rozerem)—sleep-onset difficulty (hypnotic—melatonin agonist)	8 mg PO within 30 minutes of bedtime; do not take with meal.	Avoid alcohol; somnolence Category C pregnancy; first non-scheduled agent (approved June 2005); NO CNS depression; caution in those with hepatic impairment
Diphenlhydramine (Nytol; Simply Sleep; Sominex; Unisom)—short-term treatment insomnia (< than 2 weeks) (anticholinergic—hypnotic)	Dosage depends on brand—basically 25–50 mg	OTC; potentiates CNS depression; caution with asthma, other respiratory disorders; glaucoma; hyperthyroidism; increased blood pressure

including the lifestyle measures that can be instituted to assist with sleep. The establishment of healthful sleep rituals, increasing physical activity and regular exercise, the need to refrain from alcohol consumption and smoking later in the day, and the need to eat lighter in the evening should be discussed. Care should be used with all pharmacologic therapies because of the possible adverse effects and their potential for drug dependency, especially in elderly patients.

Eating Disorders

Anorexia Nervosa, Bulimia Nervosa, Eating Disorder not otherwise specified (ED-NOS)

Eating disorders, which include both anorexia nervosa and bulimia nervosa, are not routinely assessed in primary care, although they are a significant health problem among women. Eating disorders occur on a continuum; the number of individuals with subclinical symptoms exceeds those with full disorder symptomatology. Being female is a risk factor for developing an eating disorder. At present the incidence of eating disorders among males is low, but there is evidence of persistent increases.

Anorexia Nervosa

Anorexia nervosa (AN) is characterized by a refusal to maintain a minimally normal body weight and an intense fear of gaining weight. In early adolescence, the patient may also fail to achieve expected weight and height gains.

There are two types of AN—restricting and binge-eating/purging. With restricting AN, weight loss is usually accomplished by reducing or restricting all food intake or restricting dietary fat. With binge-eating/purging AN, there is binge-eating followed by self-induced vomiting, and chronic and excessive use of laxatives or diuretics. Providers can expect patients to resist changes in their diet or weight. Angry patients may put a great deal of effort toward frustrating the practitioner's efforts to help.

Bulimia Nervosa

Recurrent episodes of binge eating, followed by compensatory methods to prevent weight gain, are the two essential features of *bulimia nervosa* (BN). Persons with BN undergo feelings of loss of control during bingeing episodes and their self-esteem is excessively influenced by their body shape and weight.

There are two types of bulimia—purging and non-purging. A person with BN who purges regularly will engage in self-induced vomiting, misuse of diuretics or laxatives, or enemas. With nonpurging BN, persons compensate for their food intake with excessive exercise or fasting. In extreme cases, individuals may abuse thyroid hormone replacement medication, or try other types of stimulant medication.

Some individuals with BN alternate between cycles of strict dieting or fasting and cycles of binge eating and purging, whereas others may compensate for binges with excessive (several hours every day) exercise patterns. Persons with BN who cycle between bingeing and fasting or extreme food restricting have a poorer prognosis. The daily number of times the person with BN purges tends to increase over time and can lead to serious medical complications. In the primary-care setting, it is not unusual for persons with BN to refuse to disclose their symptoms.

Eating Disorder Not Otherwise Specified

This classification describes patients who exhibit some, but not all, features of AN or BN. Examples are binge-eating disorder (BED), in which the patient engages in binge eating but none of the compensatory features of BN; female patients with regualr menses despite other AN symptoms; patients who purge after eating small amounts of food; and those who chew and spit out large amounts of food rather than swallow it. BED patients typically are middle-aged men and women with significant obesity. They typically have increased anxiety and depression compared to similarly obese individuals.

Epidemiology and Causes

In a culture dominated by images of extremely thin fashion models, the desirability of weight loss is pervasive. In the 2001 Youth Risk Behavior Surveillance Survey, 62 percent of girls and 29 percent of boys said they were trying to lose weight (although only 6.9 percent and 14.2 percent respectively were actually overweight). Although these disorders continue to be seen in predominantly adolescent girls, there is a spike in occurrences in women in their 50s, often related to a loss. Eating disorders have ben reported in up to 4 percent of adolescent and young adult students. Major mood disorders are more common in family members than the general population.

Recent research identified six core traits that have a genetic association with anorexia nervosa and bulimia nervosa: (1) obsessionality; (2) age at menarch; (3) anxiety; (4) minimum body mass index (BMI); (5) concern over mistakes; and (6) food-related obsessions. In a related study, the researchers were able to pinpoint the regions of the human genome responsible for those traits.

Anorexia Nervosa

One in 10 patients with AN dies suddenly from starvation, cardiac arrest, or suicide. The prevalence of AN is estimated at approximately 1 percent of the general population, and 90 percent of patients with AN are female. AN is associated with depression in 65 percent of cases; social phobia in 34 percent; and obsessive–compulsive disorder in 26 percent of cases.

AN is a serious medical disorder, beginning most frequently during adolescence and young adulthood, with estimates of mortality ranging from zero to 20 percent. Females are more vulnerable to developing an eating disorder as a result of Western cultural norms that overvalue petite female weight and size and thinness as a symbol of female competence, success, control, and sexual attractiveness. Studies have shown that persons with AN often have experienced a great deal of family conflict. Persons with AN who restrict their food intake tend to be perfectionists, whereas persons with AN who purge tend to be impulsive and rebellious. Individuals with AN who severely restrict their calorie intake report more obsessions and social awkwardness and are more isolated than those with the purging form of AN.

Bulimia Nervosa

Individuals with BN experience a profound loss of self-esteem, impaired social skills, poor coping techniques, and tend to have difficulties with interpersonal relationships. Persons with BN who use several compensatory measures to purge are more at risk than individuals who use only one purging method. Comorbidity with other psychological disorders is common, especially depression, anxiety, and substance abuse. Sociocultural ideals of extreme thinness and superfitness have increased the numbers of individuals—females and males—who restrict their dietary fat intake. It is estimated that 1 to 3 percent of the population have BN, and that 90 percent of persons with BN are female. Periods of food, calorie, and fat restrictions are often followed by bingeing and purging. The individual feels an intense sense of shame about this behavior and may go to great lengths to keep it secret from others, including health-care providers. It is important for primary-care providers to keep in mind Western cultural ideals in dieting and to screen for patients who may be affected by these eating disorders.

Eating Disorder–Not Otherwise Specified

In Western societies, it is estimated that 3 to 5 percent of the female population suffers from some variety of atypical eating disorder. Further, anorectic and bulimic behaviors not meeting DSM-IV-TR criteria (e.g., occasional fasting or bingeing/purging) have been reported in 10 to 20 percent of adolescent girls.

Pathophysiology

There appears to be a constellation of factors that include biological, social, and cultural forces that contribute to eating disorders. Recent studies point to some genetic differences in the major groups of eating disorders, AN and BN. When families of individuals with a high incidence of bulimia are examined, family members with an increased risk for obesity are found; however in families of individuals with the restricting subtype of anorexia, there is no increased risk for obesity. So although these are two genetically related, there clearly may be important differences between them. There is an increased frequency of BN in first-degree relatives of patients with this disorder. Some evidence points to higher concordance rates in monozygotic twins than in dizygotic. Sisters of patients with AN are more likely to be affected but the causality involved may be more social than genetic.

Some suggest a hypothalamic–pituitary axis (neuroendocrine) dysfunction. Serotonin, dopamine, and norepinephrine are all neurotransmitters shown to be involved in regulating eating behavior in the paraventricular nucleus of the hypothalamus, and some studies have suggested dysfunctions in these transmitters. Patients with BN often benefit from antidepressants supporting theories of serotonin dysfunction. Another school of thought speculates that endogenous opiates may contribute to the denial of hunger in patients with anorexia nervosa. When some AN patients are given opiate antagonists, they demonstrate dramatic weight gain. The state of starvation itself initiates dramatic physiologic changes in a variety of body systems leading to a cascade-like cycle that makes it difficult to discern which biologic change may have precipitated the process; nonetheless, it becomes self-perpetuating. Neurochemically, there are diminished norepinephrine turnover and activity.

Psychodynamics

Many theorize that eating disorders are culturally driven. Others view AN as a reaction to the demands of adolescence for increased maternal separation and differentiation, and these patients are viewed as having a lack of autonomy and selfhood. They may experience their bodies as under the control of their parents and so, they self-starve as a way of gaining control. Patients with AN appear to have close but troubled families, although no specific family constellation has been related to AN. Patients with AN and BN tend to be perfectionistic, high-achievers. Families of patients with BN tend to be less close and more conflicted; patients describe their parents as neglectful and rejecting. Patients with BN tend to be more outgoing than those with AN, but also they are more hostile and impulsive. They are more likely to abuse substances, shop-lift, and sexually act out. Their uncontrolled eating is experienced as ego-dystonic and they are more likely to seek help.

Psychoanalytically, the inability to separate from the mother is stressed in patients with AN and BN. In the case of BN, the struggle with food is viewed as manifesting their ambivalence toward separation from their caretaker (usually the mother); eating may represent a desire to "fuse" with the mother, and the regurgitation may be expressing an unconscious wish for separation. In the case of patients with AN, the mother may be perceived as intrusive and unempathetic, and the body may be perceived as though it were inhabited by an introject of this mother. Starving is seen as an unconscious attempt to "starve" the intrusive internal object—the mother. Patients with BN may lack the superego control of their counterparts with anorexia, and they have more difficulty controlling their impulses.

Clinical Presentation

Eating disorders are characterized by intense feelings of shame, guilt, and embarrassment. Providers can screen persons for an eating disorder by asking how satisfied the person is with his or her body weight and shape and by exploring any extremely negative responses. Expect resistance to change if an individual is not stable enough to make

FOCUS ON HISTORY 17.3

Anorexia and Bulimia

Anorexia Nervosa	
Warning Signs	To assess for warning signs of anorexia, it is important to obtain answers to the following questions: • Has the patient had any *substantial weight loss*? • Does the patient have signs or symptoms of *depression or mood swings*? • Does the patient have a *preoccupation with weight, calories, and food*? • Does the patient *wear baggy clothes*? • Does the patient have a history of *excessive exercise*?
Signs	Hypotension, hypothermia, dry skin, bradycardia, edema, lanugo
Symptoms	Amenorrhea, constipation, abdominal pain, hypothermia, lethargy or fatigue, anxious energy, headaches
Bulimia Nervosa	
Warning Signs	To assess for warning signs of bulimia nervosa, it is important to obtain answers to the following questions: • Has the patient had any significant *weight loss or gain*? • Does the patient have signs or symptoms of *depression*? • Does the patient have a *great concern for weight*? • Does the patient *visit the bathroom after meals*? • Has the patient alluded to *strict dieting/bingeing cycles*? • Does the patient have *marked criticism of one's body*?
Signs	Tooth enamel erosion, enlarged parotid glands, periodontal disease
Symptoms	Irregular menses, abdominal pain, fatigue or lethargy, peripheral edema, bloating, depression

major changes in his or her behavior. It is important to know key warning signs of eating disorders to provide care early in the disease process; early intervention has a better prognosis. (See Focusing the History 17.3.)

Assessment of people with eating disorders should be comprehensive and include physical, psychological, and social needs and a comprehensive assessment of risk to self. The primary care provider should take responsibility for initial assessment and the initial coordination of care. This includes the determination of the need for emergency medical or psychiatric assessment. Where management is shared between primary and secondary care there should be a clear agreement in writing as to who should be monitoring the patient on a regular basis. It should be shared with patient and family so all lines of responsibility are clear.

Screening for eating disorders may use brief screening methods such as questionnaires, and clinical presentation. Available screening instruments include the SCOFF Questionnaire, the Eating Disorder Screen for Primary Care (ESP), Eating Attitudes Test (EAT-26), and Eating Disorders Inventory–Second Edition (EDI-2). The SCOFF consists of five questions designed to assess the core features of anorexia nervosa and bulimia. It is a mnemonic, with each letter based on a key-word in each question of the screening tool: **S**ick, **C**ontrol, **O**ne, **F**at, and **F**ood. It was designed to be brief, to be administered in primary care, with yes and no responses. Two or more Yes answers are associated with potential for an eating disorder. Further study is recommended for this instrument. The Eating Disorder Screen is also a very short (four questions) screening tool; further study is recommended on this tool also. The Eating Attitude Test (EAT-26) is better validated but takes longer to administer and score. The Eating Disorder Inventory-2 (EDI-2) is a standardized measure of symptoms associated with anorexia, bulimia, and other eating disorders. Although reliable and valid with good psychometrics, it does not yield a specific diagnosis; it is to be used as a screening instrument to identify eating disorders in nonpatient and patient populations.

Assessment of body mass index (BMI), height, weight, and centile charts for age should be done on all patients. When AN or BN is suspected, a complete physical examination is needed to rule out other diseases or disorders that could produce severe weight loss. The patient must be undressed for any meaningful examination other than of the ears, eyes, and mouth. This might seem an unnecessary instruction, but research—often unpublished because no one wants to admit it—shows that half of cardiac auscultations in some teaching hospitals are performed through clothing.

Other physical assessments such as pulse, blood pressure, core temperature, examination of peripheries, cardiovascular examination, and sit-ups/squat test for muscle power should be done on all patients. Laboratory investigations include full blood count, erythrocyte sedimentation rate, BUN and electrolytes, creatinine, liver function tests, random blood glucose, urinalysis, and EKG.

Anorexia Nervosa

Assessment for AN should include a weight history, including highest and lowest weight, and the frequency with which the person experiences significant weight fluctuations. Ask about ideal weight goals. Persons with AN tend to have extremely unrealistic goals for a low ideal weight. Excessive weight loss is often the most obvious sign of AN, but individuals with AN rarely complain of weight loss. Persons with AN are likely to deny that a problem exists, although as they lose more weight, their fear of becoming fat intensifies. Severe weight loss eventually results in electrolyte imbalance and dehydration, with significant risks of serious medical complications such as cardiac arrhythmias. Individuals with AN who purge may experience electrolyte imbalances, edema, and enlarged parotid glands. Long-standing amenorrhea can leave females at risk for developing osteopenia and osteoporosis.

Individuals with AN may complain of hypothermia, constipation, lethargy, or excess nervous energy. APNs may find evidence of significant hypotension, dry skin, and dull hair. Hypertrophy of the salivary glands may be present if the person with AN purges. Chronic dehydration can result in impaired renal function, cardiovascular problems, and osteoporosis. Positive laboratory findings in AN include leukopenia, anemia, elevated BUN, elevated liver function tests, hypomagnesemia, hypophosphatemia, and elevated TSH. Hypercholesterolemia and sinus bradycardia are also common findings in patients with AN.

Bulimia Nervosa

Persons with BN vary in their weight and appearance but most have a normal BMI score. Many persons with BN have an extensive history of dieting. Assessment of dieting history, including both weight gain and loss as well as dieting, is important. BN is considered less life-threatening than AN; however, serious health complications can also develop with BN.

Dental erosion (from gastric acid) and periodontal disease are common in patients with BN, as are complaints of swollen salivary glands, especially the parotid glands, GERD, sore throat, and esophageal irritation. Persons who regularly engage in self-induced vomiting can develop scars or calluses on the backs of their hands from repeated trauma from the teeth.

Laboratory findings may indicate many abnormalities, including hypokalemia, hyponatremia, hypochloremia, increased serum bicarbonate, and/or elevated levels of serum amylase. In severe cases of purging, electrolyte imbalance and dehydration may lead to cardiac arrhythmias, which can lead to heart failure and sudden death. Esophageal bleeding, tears, and gastric rupture can also occur.

Diagnostic Reasoning

DSM-IV-TR Symptom Criteria

The three essential characteristics of AN are:

- ▲ Refusal to maintain body weight at or above a minimally normal weight—Abnormally low body weight (85 percent or less of the body weight expected for the individual's age and height)
- ▲ Intense fear of gaining weight or becoming fat
- ▲ Amenorrhea in postmenarcheal females (e.g., at least three consecutive missed menstrual cycles)
- ▲ Significant disturbance in the way one's body weight, size, or shape is perceived.

The essential features of BN include:

- ▲ Recurrent episodes of binge eating—A lack of control during the binge episodes
- ▲ Recurrent inappropriate compensatory behaviors to prevent weight gain

To meet the official (DSM) criteria for BN, both bingeing and purging must be experienced at least twice weekly (on average) for 3 months.

Management

If the patient's condition does not require hospitalization, outpatient treatment of eating disorders can be effective. A multidisciplinary team, including the primary-care practitioner, nutritionist, and a psychiatric nurse specialist, is needed. Good communication between team members is essential, because even motivated patients will have strong urges to resist treatment.

There are certain danger signals that mandate hospitalization. These include:

- ▲ Weight loss greater than 30 percent in 6 months.
- ▲ Signs that the person is suicidal.
- ▲ Evidence of physiologic instability such as hypokalemia or dehydration.
- ▲ Lack of response to outpatient treatment.

Evidence of psychotic thinking, hallucinations, or severe obsessions is also grounds for inpatient treatment, as are signs of other addictive behaviors, such as substance abuse. When there is severe family and or staff conflict over the proposed treatment plan, hospitalization might also be indicated, preferably at a specialty treatment center.

Inpatient Management

Goals for the patient who is hospitalized are fairly specific and include:

- ▲ Bedrest with supervised meals until the person has gained 21 pounds (9.5 kg).
- ▲ A 300-calorie stepwise gradual increase in calories consumed (as the calories consumed are increased and weight increases, there is a stepwise increase in activity as well).
- ▲ Work with the patient to establish the target weight.
- ▲ Weigh the patient daily at first; as the weight gain progresses, this may be reduced to three times per week.

- Medicate for symptom relief.
- For the patient with AN, the goal is to achieve a weight gain of 1 to 2 pounds (0.45 to 0.91 kg) per week, with tube feedings used only as a last resort.
- For the patient with BN, meals and bathroom privileges should be supervised, with no access to the bathroom for 2 hours after eating.

The patient's psychological and nutritional status should be continuously assessed. A supportive, structured environment and programs should be provided, preferably in a specialized center, or the patient should be admitted to a specialized eating disorder unit. If purging is involved, the clinician should identify the triggers and precipitants and help the patient work to establish alternative behaviors. There should also be a focus on playful rather than goal-oriented activities. Focused individual, group, and family therapies are also indicated.

Outpatient Management

On an outpatient basis, therapy revolves around building trust and a therapeutic alliance. The practitioner should involve the person with AN or BN in setting the target weight. The weight gain can be achieved gradually unless any danger signals surface.

The clinician should weigh the patient weekly at first and later monthly if progress is being made. The focus should be on overall indices of health, not just on weight. The practitioner should prescribe medication if necessary for symptom relief, and challenge any fear of uncontrollable weight gain. If purging is involved, precipitants should be identified and alternative behaviors should be established. A cognitive–behavioral approach combined with education is often effective. Family therapy (or in some cases, couple therapy) as well as individual therapy may be necessary; the person should be referred to specialists in these areas. These may be APNs who specialize in eating disorders and/or family therapy, and social workers, psychologists, or psychiatrists who have expertise in those areas. The primary-care provider can, however, continue to play an important role on the interdisciplinary team and should maintain contact with the person being treated for an eating disorder.

Activities for patients with eating disorders should be focused on playful activities as opposed to goal-directed activity, and it is important to monitor for excessive activity, especially with a patient with BN. The ultimate outcome is a diminished obsession with calories and eating, and weight stabilization on a balanced diet.

Pharmacologic therapy has been found to be effective in some cases; slightly more so with patients with BN. Antidepressant medications (especially SSRIs) have become mainstays of treatment of eating disorders. Fluoxetine (Prozac) 10 to 80 mg is the only FDA-approved drug for bulimia. It is sometimes necessary to use higher than normal doses for effective treatment of bulimia.

Follow-Up and Referral

Treatment of AN and BN requires specialized care. Providers play the key role in helping patients to accept referral to an eating disorders program. Making this decision is extremely difficult; patients may fail to follow through repeatedly before they actually accept treatment. Persons may appear to wish to have this decision made for them, but this is rarely the case. Involuntary treatment for an eating disorder is rarely effective. Persons who are dangerously malnourished and in need of emergency weight regain must be hospitalized.

The course of illness with an eating disorder is long. The course of the disease is highly variable. In a recent study of AN patients, about 50 percent achieved complete recovery, 21 percent had an intermediate outcome, and 26 percent had an outcome that was poor, with an overall mortality rate of 9.8 percent. Half of BN patients were reported to have recovered fully, 30 percent experienced occasional relapse, and almost 20 percent maintained the full criteria for BN. Relapse is common, especially during times of stress (e.g., marriage, childbearing). There is significant morbidity from cardiac arrest and eventual suicide. The speed of weight gain does not predict treatment success. Poor prognosis is indicated by repeated hospitalizations, initial low weight, being married, poor maturation. Depression is often a sequela of recovery. Both eating disorders are best approached as chronic conditions marked by improvement and relapse. Older women appear to reach a stage of development at which they have the psychological skill to establish control over their food- and weight-related behaviors. Recovered persons may continue to have complex feelings about food and their weight, but their self-care behaviors are more effective.

Patient Education

Information must be provided on the long-term effects of anorexia and/or bulimia. This may be especially important for the person with the disorder, as she (or he) may simply be unaware of some of the long-term health consequences. The provider can take the following steps: (1) Provide information on appropriate programs if dealing with addictions is involved in the treatment plan. (2) Review nutritional information and recommended dietary program. (3) Teach stress management and relaxation techniques for persons and families involved, especially at mealtimes, which are always tense. (4) Provide education on health effects of laxatives and diuretics. (5) Reinforce the long-term nature of these disorders and the need for long-term follow-up and treatment. (6) Point out that under stress, regressive behaviors occur. Involve the family in what symptoms to identify and report. For persons who have used self-induced vomiting, encourage better dental care. It is important to teach strategies for dealing with self-destructive behaviors in ways that do not reinforce them.

Attention-Deficit/Hyperactivity Disorder (ADHD)

ADHD is a persistent pattern of inattention and/or hyperactivity-impulsivity that interferes with social, school, and work functioning. The disorder typically manifests itself in childhood, but symptoms may continue into adolescent and adulthood. Adults must show a childhood onset of symptoms to receive a diagnosis of ADHD.

Inattentiveness in school and work activities is evidenced in difficulty following through on instructions as well as distractibility, performing work carelessly, not following instructions, and moving from one uncompleted task to another. In social activities, inattention is expressed as frequent shifts in conversation, not listening to others, not keeping one's mind on conversations, and not following details or rules of games or activities.

Hyperactivity is usually expressed through fidgetiness or squirming while seated, not remaining seated when expected to do so, and excessive running or climbing in situations where it is inappropriate. In adolescents and adults symptoms of hyperactivity take the form of feelings of restlessness and difficulty engaging in quiet sedentary activities. Impulsivity manifests itself as impatience, difficulty in delaying responses, blurting out answers before questions have been completed, difficulty awaiting one's turn, and frequently interrupting or intruding on others to the point of causing difficulties in social, academic or occupational settings. Impulsivity may lead to accidents and engaging in potentially dangerous activities without consideration of possible consequences.

Symptoms typically worsen in situations that require sustained attention or mental effort or that lack intrinsic appeal or novelty. Signs of the disorder may be minimal or absent when the person is under very strict control or in a one-to-one situation. The behaviors of ADHD are more likely to occur during group situations.

Epidemiology and Causes

The prevalence of ADHD is estimated at 3 to 5 percent in school-age children. The disorder is much more frequent in males than in females, with male–female ratios ranging from 4:1 to 9:1, depending on the setting. Although early onset is common (50 percent meet diagnostic criteria for ADHD by age 4), some patients have later onset, and it is not uncommon for the disorder to persist into adulthood. There is limited data on prevalence in adolescence and adulthood.

To date, no single etiology for ADHD has been identified. Data from biologic, environmental and psychosocial research suggest several risk factors or causes for the disorder. Data from family-genetic, twin, and adoption studies suggest a genetic origin for some forms of this disorder. Neuroimaging research suggests abnormalities in frontal networks as the underlying neural substrate (fronto-striatal dysfunction) and to catecholamine dysregulation as its underlying pathophysiologic substrate.

Recent work suggests that maternal smoking, alcohol abuse, and exposure to toxins during pregnancy is related to hyperkinetic-impulsive behavior in children. Perinatal influences that are thought to contribute to ADHD include prematurity, signs of fetal distress, precipitated or prolonged labor, and perinatal asphyxia. In addition, postnatal CNS abnormalities resulting from trauma, infections, or cerebral palsy have been linked to the development of ADHD in childhood. In addition, family history, comorbid conditions such as learning disabilities, mood disorders, Tourette's syndrome, oppositional defiant disorder, and conduct disorder are risk factors for ADHD.

Pathophysiology

At present, there is a lack of a specific neurophysiologic or neurochemical basis for the disorder. It is predictably associated with a variety of other disorders that affect brain function, such as learning disabilities. The suggested contributory factors for ADHD are prenatal toxic exposures, prematurity, and prenatal mechanical insult to the fetal nervous system. Food additives, colorings, preservatives, and sugar have at present no strong scientific evidence of being predisposing factors. September is the peak month for births of ADHD children with and without comorbid learning disorders. It is theorized that prenatal exposure to winter infections during the first trimester may contribute to the emergence of ADHD symptoms. Increasing evidence links a variety of prenatal insults across the entire pregnancy, not just the first trimester, to a variety of sequelae, previously unacknowledged. This includes birth traumas. This damage may be associated with circulatory, toxic, metabolic, mechanical, physical, infectious, inflammatory, and traumatic phenomenon. Children with ADHD may exhibit non-focal (soft) neurologic signs at higher rates than the general population.

A variety of neurotransmitters have been implicated in ADHD. The noradrenergic system, consists of the central nervous system (CNS) originating in the locus ceruleus and the peripheral sympathetic system. It may be the peripheral sympathetic system that is most implicated in ADHD. Theoretically, a dysfunction in peripheral epinephrine, which cause the hormone to accumulate peripherally, could "reset" the locus ceruleus through a feedback mechanism to the central system. The stimulant drugs, which affect both dopamine and norepinephrine, have been the most widely studied because of the effect they have in ADHD. Stimulants increase catecholamine concentration by promoting their release and blocking their uptake. Stimulants, as well as some tricyclics (specifically desipramine [Norpramin]) reduce levels of urinary 3-methoxy-4-hydroxyphenylglycol (MHPG), a metabolite of norepinephrine. Clonidine (Catapres) for example has been helpful in the treatment of ADHD, and it is a norepinephrine agonist. However, no overall evidence has supported the role of one neurotransmitter in the development of ADHD; it appears many transmitters may be involved.

CT head scans of children with ADHD showed no consistent findings. Studies using position emission tomography (PET) have found lower cerebral blood flow and metabolic rates in the frontal lobe areas of children with ADHD than in controls. It is theorized that the frontal lobes in children with ADHD are not adequately performing their inhibitory function in children with ADHD.

Clinical Presentation

Parents may be the first to note excessive motor activity (hyperactivity) during the toddler years. The disorder is not usually diagnosed during the toddler years, however, because that is the normative time for exploring and development of independent walking. Toddlers and preschoolers may have difficulty participating in sedentary activities, such as sitting still while listening to a story in preschool. Parents may describe the child as always on the go—the child may appear to constantly run, jump, and not sit still. A child with ADHD may appear to be "driven by a motor." There is excessive talking, interrupting others, difficulty following through, and poor organizational skills. ADHD is most often diagnosed during the childhood years (especially during elementary school) when the child's decreased attention span affects classroom work and academic performance. The school-age child with ADHD will usually have difficulty remaining seated; he or she will get up frequently, and squirm. Hyperactive behavior in these children also may include constantly tapping their hands, and shaking their feet or legs excessively. They may often get up from the table during meals; they may talk excessively and make excessive noise while watching television, doing homework, or other quiet activities.

In childhood and adolescence, impulsive symptoms associated with ADHD often lead the individual to break family, interpersonal, and educational rules. In adulthood, restlessness may lead to difficulty in participating in sedentary activities as well as to avoiding occupations, such as desk jobs, that provide limited opportunity for spontaneous movement. Adults with ADHD often complain of boredom and frustration with job and life routines.

No laboratory tests have been established that will detect ADHD. Although patients and family may report a history of a higher rate of physical injury (because of excessive motor activities and impulsivity), there are no specific physical features associated with ADHD. It is important for the APN to be able to distinguish symptoms of ADHD from developmentally age-appropriate behaviors in active children. Therefore, accurate knowledge of growth and development is essential. It is also important to differentiate ADHD from symptoms of inattention in children with low IQ or those with pervasive developmental disorders.

During a structured assessment in the practitioner's office, symptoms may not be evident, because they are most often seen in a less structured environment, such as school or work. Children with ADHD may not be able to report their own symptoms accurately because of their age; therefore, information should be gathered from parents or guardians and supplemented by reports from teachers. For an adult to receive the official (DSM) diagnosis of ADHD, some symptoms that caused impairment must have been present before the age of 7. It may be necessary to review early academic records or report cards for the presence of impulsivity, hyperactivity, and inattentive symptoms during the early school years. Additional questions related to family history of ADHD, including symptoms in children of a patient suspected of having ADHD, should be conducted. Adult patients may need to question their parents regarding ADHD behaviors that were evident from childhood. Key areas for questioning relate to complaints of boredom, disorganization or frustration in work, and a tendency for impulsive, impatient, and restless behavior.

Assessment of self-esteem and addictive behaviors in patients suspected of having ADHD is essential, particularly because the symptoms of ADHD can lead to feelings of despair and inability to form close lasting relationships. Several assessment tools exist for assistance in diagnosing ADHD. The majority of tools are designed for children and adolescents. One assessment tool—the Brown Adolescent and Adult Attention-Deficit Disorder Scale (a 40-item self-report scale)—is used for diagnosing the disorder in adults. Other tools include a learning disability evaluation (indicated when there is an apparent mismatch between IQ and achievement), a psychosocial evaluation of the home environment, and behavior rating scales. (See Nursing Research–Based Practice 17.3.)

Diagnostic Reasoning

DSM-IV-TR Symptom Criteria

Some hyperactive or inattentive symptoms must have been present before age 7 and some impairment from the symptoms is present in two or more settings (home or work [school]). In addition, there must be clear evidence of clinically significant impairment in social, academic, or occupational functioning. ADHD is characterized by 6 or more of the following symptoms of inattention that have persisted for at least 6 months to a degree that is maladaptive and inconsistent with developmental level:

Pattern of careless mistakes
Difficulty sustaining attention in tasks or play activities
Does not listen when spoken to
Does not follow through on instructions
Has difficulty organizing tasks and activities
Loses things necessary to complete tasks
Avoids, dislikes, is reluctant to engage in sustained mental activity

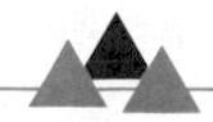

NURSING RESEARCH-BASED PRACTICE 17.3

Attention-Deficit/Hyperactivity Disorder

Lobar, SL, et al: Parent's, physician's, and nurse practitioner's perceptions of behaviors associated with attention deficit hyperactivity disorder. J Am Acad Nurse Pract 11(6):237–242, 1999.

This exploratory descriptive study conducted a survey to identify parents', nurse practitioners', and physicians' perceptions of behaviors most commonly associated with Attention-Deficit/Hyperactivity Disorder (ADHD). A convenience sample of 29 physicians, 23 nurse practitioners, and 41 parents who were members of a parent support group was obtained. The study utilized the ADHD Rating Scale, which highlights symptomatology consistent with hyperactivity, inattention, and impulsivity. In addition, qualitative data were collected from parents regarding their reasons for seeking health care for their children. This study arose in part because of the recurrent changes and revisions in nomenclature and defining criteria, and the use of multiple subjective observers in a child's behavioral evaluation that may confound the identification of ADHD. It was important to assess whether there was consistency in perceptions of ADHD in the varied reports.

This study found that there was no significant difference between nurse practitioners, parents, and physicians in their perceptions. All respondents were familiar with ADHD and were aware of the DSM criteria for the disorder. The researchers note that the similarity in responses may have been a function of shared knowledge. The parents in the support group were all well educated as to the definitions of ADHD. The addition of teachers, who are often involved in the observation of children with ADHD, might have been useful. The study supported the fact that collaboration between parents and health-care providers was important in enhancing the accurate formulation of a diagnosis of ADHD, which is based largely on subjective criteria.

Easily distracted by external stimuli
Forgetful

AND six or more of the following symptoms of hyperactivity–impulsivity have persisted for at least six months to a degree that is maladaptive and inconsistent with developmental level:

Hyperactivity	Often fidgets with hands, feet, squirms
	Leaves classroom or refuses to remain seated when it is expected
	Runs or climbs excessively
	Difficulty playing or engaging in quiet activities
	Acts as if "driven by a motor"
	Talks excessively
Impulsivity	Blurts out answers
	Difficulty awaiting turn
	Interrupts, intrudes

Management

Pharmacologic Management

Pharmacotherapy can help improve symptoms in the areas of school, work, and social and family life. However, many of the pharmacologic agents to treat ADHD are double-edged swords. Atomoxetine (Strattera) is a relatively new treatment for ADHD, a selective norepinephrine reuptake inhibitor. There can be some GI side effects and sedation initially, and it has a slower onset of efficacy. However, it falls into the nonstimulant category. It also can have significant interactions with paxil, Prozac, and quinidine. Psychostimulants are the most commonly used medications for the treatment of ADHD. The most commonly used medications include methylphenidate (Ritalin), D-amphetamine (Dexedrine, Adderall), and magnesium pemoline (Cylert). (See Drugs Commonly Prescribed 17.4.) Although these drugs are currently widely prescribed for ADHD, there are criticisms of the long-term nature of this therapy and the lack of longitudinal data. In addition, methylphenidate has become a drug of abuse and should be monitored carefully—20 mg of nongeneric have the highest street value; and the amphetamines have been long been known for their high addiction potential. Stimulants may increase levels of seizure drugs, SSRIs, tricyclics, and warfarin.

Nonpharmacologic Management

Treatment for ADHD primarily involves teaching time-management and organizational skills as well as pharmacologic interventions. Adolescents and adults often benefit from teaching time-management strategies to help with organization. Keeping a calendar, use of reminder cues, and preplanning techniques are helpful.

Follow-Up and Referral

Follow-up for patients diagnosed with ADHD includes performing a parent/teaching rating scale (e.g., Connor's scale) initially, again in 2 weeks, and then at regular intervals. Medications used for ADHD may cause headaches, abdominal pain (which can be avoided by taking medication with meals), and growth delay. Office visits should be scheduled

Drugs Commonly Prescribed 17.4: ADHD Medications

*Stimulants do not have an indication in adults and dosing guidelines are based on clinical studies rather than FDA-reviewed material. Doses of stimulants should advance slowly every several days until appropriate response is obtained

Drugs	Dose	Comments
Methylphenidate—available in short-acting and extended-release tablets (Concerta, Metadate CD, Ritalin LA)—Stimulant	5 mg bid to start; then three times per day (maximum: 2 mg/kg per day) Concerta—18 mg/day Metadate CD—20 mg/day Ritalin LA—10 mg/day	Swallow whole with liquid Insomnia, nervousness; headache, hypertensive crisis with MAOIs; Caution with anticonvulsants, anticoagulants
Amphetamine/*d*-amphetamine Adderall (available as 2.5, 5, 10, 20, 30 mg—short-acting) Adderall XR (extended-release)	2.5–5 mg/day (maximum: 1.5 mg/kg per day)—usually 40 mg/day in two to three doses Adderall XR—30 mg qd	Give on awakening Stop slowly, not suddenly May cause anorexia, insomnia, GI upset, emotional liability
d-Amphetamine (Dex Spansule) short-acting	2.5–5 mg/day (maximum: 1.5 mg/kg per day)	Hypertension, CNS overstimulation, tachycardia
Atomoxetine (Strattera) *FDA approved indication for adults	Weight $<$ 70 kg to $<$ 0.5 mg/kg per day (maximum: 1.4 mg/kg per day) Weight $>$ 70 kg to 40 mg/day (maximum: 100 mg/day)	Once daily in AM; interacts with MAOIs; GI upset; weight loss; mood swings

after 2 weeks (or sooner) and then monthly for 6 months to monitor blood pressure, insomnia, headache, abdominal pain, and alteration in growth. Also, a blinded trial with a Ritalin placebo may be performed. CBC should be monitored with methylphenidate (Ritalin, Concerta), and Focalin; monitor alanine aminotransferase (ALT) with Pemoline (Cylert). End point is improved grades, improved rating scales, acceptable family interactions, and improved peer interactions.

Children with ADHD are at increased risk for abuse, depression, and social isolation and should be monitored for these. Parents will need regular support and advice. The provider should establish contact with the child's teacher every school year. Parents, teachers, and advisors should encourage career choices that allow autonomy and mobility. There is no increased frequency of delinquency unless other comorbid features (such as oppositional defiant disorder or conduct disorder) exist.

Patient Education

There are a number of interventions that parents, family members, and teachers can do in addition to administering medication (Table 17.18). They must be educated to be aware of all potential adverse effects of medications, but also should be counseled extensively in behavioral techniques. Parents should be educated regarding realistic expectations, and should be made aware of support groups as well as child advocate groups. They must be helped to deal with whatever negative feelings may emerge as a result of the diagnosis of ADHD. Some families benefit from "anger training," "social training," and/or family therapy.

Sexual Assault

Sexual assault (SA) is defined by the National Crime Victimization Survey (NCVS) as forced sexual intercourse

Table 17.18 Patient Education: Attention-Deficit/Hyperactivity Disorder (ADHD)

Teach parents to:
- Have the child do one task at a time.
- Use "time out" periods for bad behavior.
- Make eye contact each time they are making a request.
- Reinforce good behavior or tasks the child does well with rewards and attention.
- Use behavior therapy such as token systems.
- Stop behavior before it escalates.
- Make use of parent support and advocacy groups.
- Deal with negative feelings and unrealistic expectations.
- Incorporate family therapy, anger training, and social training.
- Coordinate homework with teachers.
- Work closely with teachers for consistent behavioral plan.

Teach teachers to:
- Make sure child has a second set of books at home.
- Make work sessions short.
- Help child deal constructively with negative feelings.
- Provide immediate consequences for bad behavior.
- Reinforce good behavior.
- Coordinate homework with parents.
- Work closely with parents for a consistent behavioral plan.

involving physical force or psychological coercion, with vaginal, anal, or oral penetration by the offender(s), including the use of foreign objects. The three key components of sexual assault are:

- ▲ lack of consent;
- ▲ threat or use of force; and
- ▲ vaginal, anal, or oral penetration by body part or object.

Sexual assault is a violent act. The offender's intent is to dominate, humiliate, and degrade the victim. For the victim, sexual assault is a highly traumatic event that can have long-term effects on the physiologic and psychological well-being of the survivor.

Epidemiology and Causes

It has been estimated that every minute in the United States, an adult woman is sexually assaulted. According to the FBI, more than 100,000 forcible sexual assaults were reported to local police departments; however, most cases of sexual assault are not reported to the police. The United States study of sexual assault entitled "Rape In America" estimated that only one in six sexual assaults are actually reported to the police. With respect to prevalence, in 1994, the FBI has estimated that one out of three women and one out of seven men will be sexually assaulted at some point in their lifetime. In addition, it is estimated that one out of four females and one out of seven males will be sexually assaulted before the age of 18. The vast majority of sexual assaults occur before the age of 18.

According to the NCVS, women who are young, unmarried, and in a low-income group are the most frequent victims of sexual assault. The highest victimization rate for women is in the 16- to 19-year-old age group, with the second highest rate occurring in the 20- to 24-year-old age group. Divorced and single women experience higher rates of sexual assault than married or widowed women, and women in low-income groups experience higher rates of assault than women in moderate or high-income groups.

In addition, women of color report sexual assault twice as frequently as do white American women, with African American women reporting the highest rates of sexual assault. Sexual assault is more likely to occur in the survivor's home (43 percent) or in the home of a friend (15 percent). Most sexual assaults (65 percent) occur in the evening and during the summer months. Finally, most sexual assault survivors (78 percent) know their rapists. When the sexual assault is committed by a stranger, 31 percent of the time, the sexual assault takes place in the home of the survivor or a friend's home. In some cases, sexual assault is part of the larger picture of domestic violence.

Pathophysiology

Sexual assault, typically a rape, is an act of violence and humiliation that happens to be expressed through sexual means. Power and anger are expressed through rape; it is sexuality in the service of nonsexual needs. Male rapists are thought of in different categories: sexual sadists, who are aroused by the pain of their victims; exploitive predators, who use their victims as objects for gratification and in an impulsive ways; inadequate men, who believe no women would voluntarily sleep with them and who are obsessed with fantasies about sex; and men for whom rape is displaced anger and rage. Feminist theory sees women as an object for the displacement of aggression that a rapist cannot express directly toward other men. Women are considered men's property or vulnerable possessions. Rape is often part of another crime. Rapists typically threaten their victims with fists, a knife, a gun, and frequently harm them in other ways. Victims may be beaten, wounded, or killed. Men who commit rape, according to crime statistics, are typically between 25 and 44 years of age; 51 percent are white and tend to rape white victims; 47 percent are black and tend to rape black victims; the remainder are mixed. Thirty-four percent of all forcible rapes involve alcohol.

A rape is a life-threatening situation. During the rape itself, the primary motivation for the victim is to remain alive. The woman experiences shock and panic. Rapists may urinate or defecate on their victims, ejaculate into their faces and hair, force anal intercourse, and insert foreign objects into vaginas and rectums. After the rape, the women experiences shame, confusion, humiliation, fear, and rage. Many women become phobic about sex. Few women emerge from the assault completely unscathed. The degree of damage usually depends on the violence of the attack, the vulnerability of the woman, and the support system available to her immediately after the attack. Many victims go on to develop PTSD.

Clinical Presentation

Through their work with sexual assault survivors, experts have identified a set of immediate and long-term effects of sexual assault called the *rape trauma syndrome.* Rape trauma syndrome is considered a normal response to sexual assault. There are two identified phases of survivor responses—the *initial* or *acute phase,* characterized by a period of disorganization, and the *long-term phase,* characterized by a period of reorganization.

Initial or Acute Phase

During the initial or acute phase, many sexual assault survivors experience both physical symptoms as well as emotions such as fear, shock, and disbelief. Four major categories of physical symptoms have been identified:

- ▲ Physical trauma: Symptoms include soreness and bruising from the physical attack on the hands, throat, neck, breasts, thighs, legs, arms, back, buttocks, head, and face.
- ▲ Skeletal muscle tension: Symptoms include tension headaches, fatigue, and sleep disturbances.

- ▲ Gastrointestinal irritability: Symptoms include stomach pains, nausea, and a decreased appetite.
- ▲ Genitourinary disturbance: Symptoms include vaginal and/or anal bleeding and bladder and vaginal infections.

In the first few hours after the assault, survivors of a sexual assault often experience shock or disbelief. Several researchers have observed in their study of sexual assault survivors that survivors tended to have one of two emotional response patterns—expressed or controlled. The expressed style is the expression of fear, anger, and anxiety through behaviors such as crying, sobbing, paradoxical smiling, restlessness, and tenseness. The controlled style masks the psychological distress with a calm, composed, subdued affect. There were equal numbers of both expressed and controlled response styles among sexual assault survivors.

Long-Term Phase

In the long-term phase, psychological symptoms such as depression, anxiety, and fear are prominent. This phase has three components:

- ▲ Motor activity: Sexual assault survivors often exhibit an increase in motor activity with a range of activities, such as changing their residence and telephone number and adopting a variety of personal safety and security measures. They may turn to family and friends for assistance with these activities. Survivors may make special trips home or to some location that symbolizes safety and social acceptance.
- ▲ Nightmares: Nightmares following sexual assault are often upsetting and violent dreams can occur for months after the sexual assault. The nightmares may contain images that are clearly connected to the sexual assault, but nightmare content may also fail to be obviously related to the sexual assault.
- ▲ Trauma-phobia: As the term implies, *trauma-phobia* is a phobic reaction to trauma in which the phobia develops as a psychological defense against the sexual assault experience. The more common phobias are fear of being indoors, fear of being outdoors, fear of being alone, fear of being in crowds, fear of having people behind the individual, and sexual fears. Fear of sexually transmitted disease (STD), including HIV, is also a powerful source of psychological trauma. It has been estimated that 4 to 30 percent of sexual assault survivors are diagnosed with an STD as a result of the sexual assault.

Some victims of sexual assault have what has been called a "silent rape reaction"; these survivors have not reported the assault to anyone. These survivors experience psychological burdening and are not able to resolve their thoughts and feelings about the sexual assault. APNs have only recently started to consider unreported sexual assault as a basis for atypical psychological symptoms such as atypical anxiety, sexual relationship problems; significant changes in sexual behavior patterns; unexplained, sudden onset of phobias; and chronic low self-esteem.

Diagnostic Reasoning

DSM-IV-TR Symptom Criteria

The diagnosis of sexual assault is made by patient complaint and confirmed by forensic evidence.

Management

During the initial or acute phase, sexual assault survivors may be seen in emergency departments, rape crisis centers, primary-care offices, or police stations. If the sexual assault has occurred within the past few days, forensic physical evidence should be collected. The use of a Sexual Assault Nurse Examiner (SANE), if one is available, is highly recommended. These nurses receive special training in collecting forensic evidence and providing crisis intervention and offer a number of advantages over ER practitioners. For example, the survivor is seen by one specialist rather than by several practitioners, which decreases the time a sexual assault survivor spends in the ER and ensures that she (or he) receives sensitive, nonjudgmental care by a practitioner who is an SA specialist. Equally important, the nurse is skilled in the collection of forensic evidence, resulting in higher conviction rates of sexual assault.

Initial treatment for sexual assault survivors includes the sexual assault interview, physical exam for physical assessment and forensic evidence collection, and crisis intervention.

The Sexual Assault Interview

The sexual assault interview is performed in a room away from the waiting areas and exam rooms and while the survivor is still fully clothed, often with a police officer present. The sexual assault interview begins with general health information, including drug allergies, current medications, recent surgeries, major health problems, date of last menses, history of sexually transmitted diseases, use of contraception, and most recent consensual sexual contact.

Questions about the sexual assault follow the general health information questions. The sexual assault survivor is asked the date and time of the sexual assault and all events surrounding the sexual assault. This is important because accurate collection of forensic evidence requires that the examiner locate all points of physical contact and penetration as well as documenting the survivor's activity immediately following the sexual assault, such as bathing, douching, urinating, brushing teeth, and combing hair.

The physical exam is the final procedure of the interview. All physical exam and forensic evidence collection procedures should be explained to the sexual assault survivors. The physical examination can be traumatic for survivors; thus, survivors should be allowed to control the exam as much as possible. This can be accomplished by letting the survivors know they can refuse any part of the exam or stop the procedure at any time. Sexual assault survivors should also be encouraged to have a support person such as a friend, spouse, or parent with them during the exam. In addition to family and friends, a counselor from the local rape crisis center may also be available to support the sexual assault survivor during the exam. Although sexual assault survivors may decline such support, they should be encouraged to accept the support.

Physical Examination and Forensic Evidence Collection

The physical exam begins with the removal of all items of clothing. Each item of clothing worn at the time of the sexual assault is placed in a separate bag and then signed over to a law enforcement officer as forensic evidence. Physical forensic evidence that can be found on clothing includes hair, blood, semen, and saliva. If the clothing has not been washed, these items can be found up to a year later. A brief physical exam is performed to note the presence of any and all injuries (e.g., bruises, lacerations, teeth marks, swelling). Blood samples for pregnancy tests and tests for STDs are obtained.

The sexual assault kit, available in most states, should contain all materials needed. Forensic evidence includes samples of the individual's hair (head and pubic) and saliva, oral, vaginal, and rectal swabs, and fingernail scrapings. Information obtained during the interview will determine the forensic evidence collected. Pelvic, vaginal, and rectal exams are completed at the end of the exam. Semen can be found and collected up to 72 hours after the assault. Although forensic evidence should be collected as soon as possible, exams performed several days after the sexual assault can still produce findings.

Crisis Intervention

The final stage is to initiate crisis intervention. Crisis intervention with sexual assault survivors includes encouraging the survivors to talk about their feelings, validating these feelings, educating them about rape trauma syndrome, and identifying concerns related to the sexual assault. These concerns include prevention of pregnancy and/or STDs, physical safety, and the need for specialized sexual assault psychotherapy and community support groups. Physical safety becomes a focus of concern for anyone who has just been assaulted. Sexual assault survivors can become preoccupied with the fear that their attacker will try to hurt them again. This is especially true when the survivor knows the identity of the attacker or the assault occurred in the survivor's home. Clinicians can help survivors start to problem-solve safety concerns and help to meet the survivor's immediate needs for safety. Some individuals may elect to live with friends or family until they begin to feel safe again.

A supportive approach and focusing on restoring the victim's sense of adequacy and control over her life are the best means for supporting the victim provided there is no severe underlying pathology that might warrant a different treatment plan. Group therapy with homogenous groups have been found to be effective for many. A rape victim fares the best when she receives immediate support and can ventilate her feelings of rage and fear to loving family members, and supportive clinicians and law enforcement officials. Socially acceptable means of recourse, such as the arrest and conviction of the rapist, can help the victim. (See Advanced Practice Nursing Interventions 17.4.)

Follow-Up and Referral

Sexual assault survivors should be encouraged to use the support services available from community rape counseling centers, such as individual therapy, group therapy, and self-defense training. The majority of rape counseling centers offer 24-hour crisis hotlines. Many individuals may not feel they need this support, or that their family and friends are there for them. Survivors continue to be at risk for long-term problems, however, and to have long-term grief and mourning needs long after the immediate crisis has passed and significant others have come to believe that the crisis is over. Rape counseling centers personnel understand the long-term course of events of sexual assault. Some rape counseling centers are also able to provide advocates to support survivors as they deal with the legal and judicial systems. These services are often offered free of charge or at greatly reduced rates.

Patient Education

Education includes advising the patient about community support services as well as discussing the long-term effects of sexual assault.

The most common long-term effect of sexual assault is the development of PTSD. Recent research has indicated that sexual assault survivors may be the largest single group of PTSD sufferers. PTSD was originally defined to explain the set of symptoms observed in survivors of natural disasters and military combat and includes symptoms such as anxiety, depression, nightmares, flashbacks, and sleep disturbances. Researchers have found that 94 percent of the women who had been sexually assaulted met the criteria for PTSD 12 days after the sexual assault and that 46 percent of these women still met the criteria 3 months later.

In addition to having higher rates of PTSD, sexual assault survivors reported higher rates of drug and alcohol problems, depression, attempted suicide, anxiety, obsessive–compulsive disorder, and medical care use. Sexual assault survivors were 13.4 times more likely to have had alcohol-related problems and 26 times more likely to have had problems with drug abuse, as compared to nonabused women. Survivors were three times more likely to have had a major episode of depression, four times more

ADVANCED PRACTICE NURSING INTERVENTIONS 17.4

Crisis Intervention

Persons Amenable to Crisis Intervention	• History of recent, specific crisis situation (may be an event, e.g., sexual assault, natural disaster; or developmental, e.g., death, divorce, job loss) • Clearcut evidence of psychological incapacitation, specifically, severe anxiety related to the event • High motivation to overcome the crisis • Previously demonstrated ability to cope
Processes	• Practitioner must rapidly establish psychological rapport with the person and develop psychological insight on part of the person; speed is essential • Person must actively participate • Person and practitioner must work together to overcome the crisis
Methods	• Main task is to decrease anxiety through reassurance, suggestion, environmental manipulation, psychotropics • Review steps that have led to crisis and promote understanding of the maladaptive response to the crisis • Focus on developing more adaptive ways of coping with the crisis situation • Length of intervention may vary from 1–2 sessions to 1–2 months • Brief hospitalization may be part of the plan
Outcomes	• Patient better equipped to deal with future stressors • Intervention ended as soon as possible, hopefully at a higher developmental level than prior to crisis • Intervention may be viewed as both therapeutic and preventive

SOURCE: Adapted from Kaplan, H, and Sadock, BJ: Synopsis of Psychiatry, ed 8. Williams & Wilkins, Baltimore, Md., 2002.

likely to have had thoughts about suicide, and 13 times more likely to have attempted suicide as compared to nonabused women. Finally, survivors of sexual assault report more symptoms of illness across all body systems and perceive their health less favorably than do nonabused women. Symptoms that are diagnosed at a much higher rate in sexual assault survivors include chronic pelvic pain, gastrointestinal disorders, headaches, general pain, and premenstrual symptoms. Every effort should be made to encourage the patient to initiate long-term support for dealing with the trauma of sexual assault. The health-care provider, practicing within a Circle of Caring may be in the best position to maintain contact with the patient and facilitate growth and healing.

Bibliography

General

American Psychiatric Association: Diagnostic and Statistical Manual of Mental Disorders, ed 4, text revision (DSM-IV-TR). American Psychiatric Association, Washington, D.C., 2000.

American Psychiatric Association: Handbook of Psychiatric Measures. American Psychiatric Association: Washington, D.C., 2000.

Budman, SH, and Gurman, AS: Theory and Practice of Brief Therapy. Guilford Press, New York, 1988.

Erikson, EH: Identity, Youth, and Crisis. WW Norton, New York, 1968.

Glod, CA: Contemporary Psychiatric-Mental Health Nursing. FA Davis, Philadelphia, 1999.

Kaplan, HI, Sadock, BJ, and Grebb, JA: Kaplan and Sadock's Synopsis of Psychiatry, ed 9. Williams & Wilkins, Baltimore, 2002.

Kübler-Ross, E: On Death and Dying. Basic Books, New York, 1965.

Lazarus, RS, Averill, JR, and Opton, EM: The psychology of coping: Issues of research and assessment. In Coelho, G, Hamburg, D, and Adams, J (eds): Coping and Adaptation. Basic Books, New York, 1974.

Loretz, L: Primary Care: Tools for Clinicians. CV Mosby, St. Louis, Mo., 2005.

Maier, W, Buller, R, Philipp, M, et al: The Hamilton Anxiety Scale: Reliability, validity, and sensitivity to change in anxiety and depressive disorders. J Affect Disord 14:61, 1988.

Maruish, ME, ed: Handbook of Psychological Assessments in Primary Care Settings. Lawrence Erlbaum Associates, Mahwah, N.J., 2000.

Mechanic, D: Social structure and personal adaptation: Some neglected dimensions. In Coelho G, Hamburg, D, and Adams, J (eds): Coping and Adaptation. Basic Books, New York, 1974.

Oakley, LD, and Potter, C: Psychiatric Primary Care. Mosby-Year Book, St. Louis, Mo., 1997.

Selye, H: The Stress of Life. McGraw-Hill, New York, 1956.

Spitzer, RL, Kroenke, K, Linzer, M, et al: Health-related quality of life in primary care patients with mental disorders. Results from the PRIME-MD 1000 Study. JAMA 274:1511, 1995.

Spitzer, RL, Kroenke, K, and Williams, JB: Validation and utility of a self-report version of PRIME-MD: The PHQ primary care study. JAMA 282:1737, 1999.

Varcolis, EM: Psychiatric nursing clinical guide: Assessment tools and diagnosis. WB Saunders, Philadelphia, 2000.

Anorexia Nervosa and Bulimia Nervosa

American Psychiatric Association Work Group on Eating Disorders. Practice guideline for the treatment of patients with eating disorders (revision). Am J Psychiatry 157(1 Suppl):1, 2000.

Cotton, M, Ball, C, and Robinson, P: Four simple questions can help screen for eating disorders. J Gen Intern Med 18:53, 2003.

Crowther, JH, and Sherwood, NE: Assessment. In Garner, DM, and Garfinkel, PE (eds): Handbook of Treatment for Eating Disorders, ed 2. Guilford Press, New York, 1997, p 34.

Davison, GC, and Neale, JM: Abnormal Psychology, ed 6. John Wiley & Sons, New York, 1994, p 449.

Eliot, AO, and Baker, CW: Eating disordered adolescent males. Adolescence 361:143, 2001.

Mehler, PS: Diagnosis and care of patients with anorexia nervosa in primary care settings. Ann Intern Med 134:1048, 2001.

Morgan, JF, Reid, F, and Lacey, H: The SCOFF questionnaire: Assessment of a new screening tool for eating disorders. BMJ 319:1467, 1999.

National Collaborating Centre for Mental Health. Eating disorders: Core interventions in the treatment and management of anorexia nervosa, bulimia nervosa and related eating disorsers. Leicester (UK): British Psychological Society, 2004. Accessed May 20, 2005 from http://www.guideline.gov/summary/summary.aspx?doc_id=5295&nbr=003618&string="eating+disorders"

Spearing, M: Eating disorders: facts about eating disorders and the search for solution. NIH Publication No. 01-4901, 2001. Accessed December 20, 2005 from http://www.nimh.nih.gov/publicat/eatingdisorders.cfm

Tasca, GA, Illing, V, Lybanon-Daigle, V, et al: Psychometric properties of the eating disorders inventory-2 among women seeking treatment for binge eating disorder. Assessment 10:228, 2003.

Tobin, DL, Johnson, CL, and Dennis, AB: Divergent forms of purging behavior in bulimia nervosa patients. Int J Eat Disord 11:17, 1992.

Vitousek, KB, and Orimoto, L: Cognitive-behavioral models of anorexia nervosa, bulimia nervosa, and obesity. In Kendall, P, and Dobson, KS (eds): Psychopathology and Cognition. Academic Press, San Diego, Calif., 1993, p 191.

Walsh, T, and Garner, DM: Diagnostic issues. In Garner, DM, and Garfinkel, PE (eds): Handbook of Treatment for Eating Disorders, ed 2. Guilford Press, New York, 1997, p 27.

Anxiety

Baker, SL, Heinrichs, N, Kim, HJ, et al: The Liebowitz Social Anxiety Scale as a self-report instrument: A preliminary psychometric analysis. Behav Res Ther 40:701, 2002.

Greco, N, and Zajecka, JM: Evaluating and treating comorbid depression and anxiety in women. Womens Health Primary Care 3:5, 2000.

Hansen, S: Managing anxiety disorders in women. Female Patient 29:23, 2004.

Kim, SW, Dysken, MW, and Kuskowski, M: The Yale-Brown Obsessive-Compulsive Scale: A reliability and validity study. Psychiatry Res 34:99, 1990.

Kim, SW, Dysken, MW, and Kuskowski, M: The Symptom Checklist-90: Obsessive-compulsive subscale: A reliability and validity study. Psychiatry Res 41:37, 1992.

Kneepkens, RG, and Oakley, LD: Rapid improvement in the defense style of depressed women and men. J Nerv Ment Dis 184:358, 1996.

Lucki, I: Serotonin receptor specificity in anxiety disorders. J Clin Psychiatry 57:5, 1996.

Ninan, PT: Generalized anxiety disorder. Presentation at the Duke University Medical Center psychCME conference, Orlando, Fla, December 2005.

Palmer, BW, Jeste, DV, and Sheikh, JI: Anxiety disorders in the elderly: DSM-IV and other barriers to diagnosis and treatment. J Affect Disord 46:183, 1997.

Pollack, MH: Comorbid anxiety disorders in primary care. Therapeutic Spotlight, a supplement to Clin Rev June 2001.

Raj, BA, and Sheehan, DV: Social anxiety disorder. Med Clin North Am 85:711, 2001.

Robins, CJ: Psychosocial treatment of anxiety disorders. Presentation at the Duke University Medical Center psychCME conference, Orlando, Fla., Dec. 2005.

Singapore Ministry of Health, National Medical Research Council: Anxiety disorders guideline, 2003. Accessed May 20, 2005 from http://www.guideline.gov/summary/summary.aspx?ss=15&doc_id=5293&nbr=3616&string=anxiety

Stotland, NL: Social anxiety disorder. Female Patient 29:36, 2004.

Susman, JL, and Keller, MB: Diagnosing and treating depression and anxiety disorders in family practice. Accessed December 22, 2005 from http://www.medscape.com/viewprograms/3793_pnt

Vaillant, GE, Bond, M, and Vaillant, CO: An empirically validated hierarchy of defense mechanisms. Arch Gen Psychiatry 43:786, 1986.

Wise, TN: Anxiety disorders: Guidelines for effective primary care therapy. Consultant Mar. 2004.

Zung, WWK: A rating instrument for anxiety disorders. Psychosomatics 12:371, 1971.

Zung,WW: Prevalence of clinically significant anxiety in a practice family setting. Am J Psychiatry 143:1471, 1986.

Attention-Deficit/Hyperactivity Disorder

Alder, LA, and Chua, HC: Management of ADHD in adults. J Clin Psychiatry (Suppl 12), 2002.

Biederman, J, et al: Patterns of psychiatric comorbidity, cognition, and psychosocial functioning in adults with attention deficit hyperactivity disorder. Am J Psychiatry 150:1792, 1993.

Connors, K: ADHD: Recognition and Diagnosis. Presentation at the Duke University Medical Center psychCME conference, Orlando, Fla., Dec. 2005.

Farone, SV: Attention deficit hyperactivity disorder in adults: Implications for theories of diagnosis. Curr DirectPsychol Sci 9:1, 2004.

Goldman, LS, Genel, M, Bezman, RJ, and Slanek, PJ: Diagnosis and treatment of ADHD in children and adolescents. Council on Scientific Affairs, American Medical Association. JAMA 279:1100, 1998.

Lobar, SL, Waechter, ML, Oher, LE, and Phillips, S: Parent's perceptions' and nurse practitioners' perceptions of behaviors associated with ADHD. Nurse Pract 11:6, 1999.

McDonnell, MA, and Dougherty, M: Righting a troubled course: diagnosing and treating ADHD in adults. Adv Nurse Pract 53, Aug. 2005.

McDonnell, MA, Doyle, R, and Surman, C: Current approaches to the management of ADHD: Diagnosis in adults is often overlooked. Clin Rev 13:11, 2003.

National Institutes of Health: NIH Consensus Statement: Diagnosis and Treatment of Attention Deficit Hyperactivity Disorder. Nov. 1998. http://www.hlm.nih.gov/pubs/cbm/adhd.html.

Newcorn, JH: Treatment Options for ADHD. Presentation at the Duke University Medical Center psychCME conference, Orlando, Fla., Dec. 2005.

Spencer, T, et al: Is attention deficit hyperactivity disorder in adults a valid disorder? Harv Rev Psychiatry 1:326, 1994.

Bipolar Disorder

American Psychiatric Association: Practice guidelines for the treatment of patients with bipolar disorder, 2nd ed, 2002. Accessed December 22, 2005 from http://www.psych.org/psych_pract/treatgpg/bipolar_revisebook_index.cfm

Bowden, CL, Hirschfeld, RMA, and Shahady, EJ: Bipolar disorder: keys to diagnosis—strategies for effective management. Suppl to Consultant 45:14, 2005.

Das, AK, Olfson, M, Gameeroff, MJ, et al: Screening for bipolar disorder in a primary care practice. JAMA 293:5, 2005.

Delay, N, Stensland, MD, Viswanathan, S, and Ciaglia, M: Costs of polypharmacy, number of drugs, and switching for bipolar disorder: Presented at the ninth annual meeting of the International Society for Pharmacoeconomics and Outcomes research, Arlington, Va., May 2004.

Fagiolini, A: Battling bipolar disorder: Therapeutic approaches. Suppl to Clin Advisor 11, March 2005.

Frye, MA: Management of bipolar disorder. Presentation at the Duke University Medical Center psychCME conference, Orlando, Fla., Dec. 2005.

Ghaemi, SN: Overview of bipolar disorder. Presentation at the Duke University Medical Center psychCME conference, Orlando, Fla., Dec. 2005.

Goldberg, JF, Jackson, WC, Cohen, LJ, and Pomerantz, JM: 10 New multidisciplinary ways to look at bipolar disorder. Suppl to Consultant 2005.

Hirschfeld, RM: Development and validation of a screening instrument for bipolar spectrum disorder: The Mood Disorder Questionnaire. Am J Psychiatry 157:1873, 2000.

Jamison, KR: An Unquiet Mind. Vintage Books, New York, 1995.

Lingam, R, and Scott, J: Treatment non-adherence in affective disorders. Acta Psychiatr Scand 105:164, 2002.

Lynch, TR: Psychosocial treatments of mood disorders. Presentation at the Duke University Medical Center psychCME conference, Orlando, Fla., Dec. 2005.

Obrocea, G: Bipolar disorder: Best practice report. Best Practice of Medicine 2004. Accessed December 22, 2005 from http://merck.micromedex.com/index.asp?page=bpm_printmain&show_banner=no

St. John, DD: Bipolar disorder: Diagnosing a devastating illness. Suppl to Clin Advisor 3, Mar. 2005.

Depression

Alloy, LB, et al: The hopelessness theory of depression: Attributional aspects. Br J Clin Psychol 27:5, 1988.

Beck, AT, Rush, AJ, and Emery, G: Cognitive Therapy of Depression. Guilford Press, New York, 1979.

Blazer, DG: Depression in Late Life: An Update. Presentation at the Duke University Medical Center psychCME conference, Orlando, Fla., Dec. 2005.

Brigham and Women's Hospital: Depression: A guide to diagnosis and treatment, 2001. Accessed May 5, 2005 from **http://www.guideline.gov/summary/summary.aspx?doc_id**=3432&nbr=002658&string=depression

Brink, TL, Yesavage, JA, Lum, O, et al: Screening tests for geriatric depression. Clin Gerontol 1:37, 1982.

Brody, DW, and Serby, M: What you should know about adult depression. Clin Advisor, Sept. 2004.

Brown, GW: Genetic and population perspectives on life events and depression. Soc Psychiatry Psychiatr Epidemiol 33:363, 1998.

Brown, TA, Chorpita, BF, and Barlow, DH: Structural relationships among dimensions of the DSM-IV anxiety and mood disorders and dimensions of negative affect, positive affect, and autonomic arousal. J Abnorm Psychol 107:179, 1998.

Concrite, RC, et al: Life circumstances and personal resources as predictors of the ten-year course of depression. Am J Community Psychol 26:255, 1998.

Depression Guideline Panel: Depression in Primary Care, Vol. 1. Detection and Diagnosis: Clinical Practice Guideline. Agency for Health Care Policy and Research, Rockville, Md., 1992.

Hoyl, MT, Alessi, CA, Harker, JO, et al: Development and testing of a five-item version of the Geriatric Depression Scale. J Am Geriatr Soc 47:873, 1999.

Hypericum Depression Trial Study Group: Effect of Hypericum perforatum (St. John's wort) in major depressive disorder: A randomized controlled trial. JAMA 287:1807, 2002.

Institute for clinical Systems Improvement: Major depression in adults for mental health care, 2004. Accessed May 20, 2005 from **http://www.guideline.gov/summary/summary.aspx?doc_id**=5301&nbr=003624&string=major+AND+depression

Kelsey, JE: Pharmacotherapy of Depression. Presentation at the Duke University Medical Center psychCME conference, Orlando, Fla., Dec. 2005.

Kroenke, K, Spitzer, RL, and Williams, JB: The PHQ-9: Validity of a brief depression severity measure. J Gen Intern Med 16:606, 2001.

Moore, KM, Lapid, MI, Sampson, SM, Netzel, PJ, and Rummans, T: Depression in women. Womens Health Primary Care 8:8, 2005.

Roose, S: Overview of Depression, Presentation at the Duke University Medical Center psychCME conference, Orlando, Fla., Dec. 2005.

Schelde, JT: Major depression: Behavioral markers of depression and recovery. J Nerv Ment Dis 186:133, 1998.

Thase, ME: Depression, sleep, and antidepressants. J Clin Psychiatry 59:55, 1998.

The Office on Women's Health of the USDHHS: Achieveing remission in depression: Managing women and men in the primary care setting. Clin Courier 21:32, 2003.

Domestic Violence

Bergman, BK, and Brismar, BG: Can family violence be prevented? A psychosocial study of male batterers and battered wives. Public Health 106:45, 1992.

Brown, KB, Streubert, GE, and Burgess, AW: Effectively detect and manage elder abuse. Nurse Pract 29:8, 2004.

Family Violence Prevention Fund: National consensus guidelines on identifying and responding to domestic violence victimization in health care settings, 2004. Accessed May 20, 2005 from **http://www.guideline.gov/summary/summary.aspx?doc_id**=5529&nbr=003760&string=domestic+AND+violence

Feldhaus, K, et al: Accuracy of three brief screening questions for detecting partner violence in the emergency department. JAMA 277:1357, 1997.

Institute for Clinical Systems Improvement: Domestic violence, 2004. Accessed May 20, 2005 from **http://www.guideline.gov/summary/summary.aspx?doc_id**=6143&nbr=003971&string=domestic+AND+violence

Jensen, LA: The cycle of domestic violence and the barriers to treatment. Nurse Pract 25:5, 2000.

Jezierski, M: Abuse of women by male partners: Basic knowledge for emergency nurses. J Emerg Nurs 20(5):361, 1994.

Nicolaids, C: Intimate partner violence. Womens Health Primary Care 7:7, 2004.

Sherin, KM, Sinacore, JM, Li, XQ, et al: HITS: A short domestic violence screening tool for use in a family practice setting. Fam Med 30:5085, 1998.

US Preventative Services Task Force: Guide to clinical preventative services. Text revision. Ann Intern Med 140:5, 2004.

Grief

Joffrion, LP, and Douglas, D: Grief resolution: Facilitating self-transcendence in the bereaved. J Psychosoc Nurs Ment Health Serv 32:13, 1994.

Kübler-Ross, E: On Death and Dying. Basic Books, New York, 1965.

O'Gorman, SM: Death and dying in contemporary society: An evaluation of current attitudes and rituals associated with death and dying and their relevance to recent understandings of health and healing. J Adv Nurs 27:1127, 1998.

Periyakoil, V, and Hallenbeck, J: Identifying and managing preparatory grief and depression at the end of life. Am Fam Physician 65:5, 2002.

Rawlings, RM, and Kutner, JS: Helping women through grief and bereavement. Womens Health Primary Care 6:3, 2003.

Insomnia

Benca, RM: Diagnosis and treatment of chronic insomnia: A review. Psychiatr Serv 56:332, 2005.

Doghramji, K, and Neubauer, DN: Insomnia: Waking up to a significant problem. Consultant 45:13, 2005.

Krystal, AD: An Update on Sleep Disorders. Presentation at the Duke University Medical Center psychCME conference, Orlando, Fla., Dec. 2005.

Lader, M: Benefits and risks of benzodiazepines in anxiety and insomnia. Accessed December 22, 2005 from **http://www.benzo.org.uk/lader1.htm**

NIH State-of-the-Science Conference statement on manifestations and management of Chronic insomnia in adults. Accessed December 20, 2005 from **http://consensus.nih.gov/2005/2005InsomniaSOS026html.htm.**

Speilman, AJ, Saskin, P, and Thorpy MJ: Treatment of chronic insomnia by restriction of time in bed. Sleep 10:45, 1987.

Panic Disorder

Ballenger, JC, et al: Consensus statement on panic disorder from the international consensus group on depression and anxiety. J Clin Psychiatry 59:47, 1998.

Bourin, M, Baker, GB, and Bradwejn, J: Neurobiology of panic disorder. J Psychosom Res 44:163, 1998.

Edwards, S, and Uhlenhuth, EH: Panic disorder and agoraphobia: a sufferer's perspective. J Affect Dis 50:65, 1998.

Gorman, JM: Best practice of medicine—Panic disorder. Sept. 2000, modified on November 15, 2001. Accessed on December 22, 2005 from **http://merck.micromedex.com/index.asp?page**=bpm_viewall&article_id=BMP01PS09

Ninan, PT: Panic Disorder and Social Anxiety Disorder. Presentation at the Duke University Medical Center psychCME conference, Orlando, Fla., Dec. 2005.

Posttraumatic Stress Disorder

American Psychiatric Association. Practice guidelines for the treatment of patients with acute stress disorder and posttraumatic stress disorder. American Psychiatric Association, Arlington, Va., 2004. Accessed May 20, 2005 from **http://www.guideline.gov/summary/summary.aspx?doc_id**=2972&nbr=002198&string=PTSD

Baker, D: Relationship between posttraumatic stress disorder and self-reported physical symptoms in Persian Gulf veterans: Arch Intern Med 157:2076, 1997.

Butterfield, M: Posttraumatic Stress Disorder. Presentation at the Duke University Medical Center psychCME conference, Orlando, Fla., Dec. 2005.

Classen, C, Koopman, C, Hales, R, and Spiegel, D: Acute stress disorder as a predictor of posttraumatic stress symptoms. Am J Psychiatry 155:620, 1998.

Friedman, MJ: Postraumatic stress disorder. J Clin Psychiatry 58(Suppl 9):33, 1997.

Kaiman, C: PTSD in the World War II combat veteran. Am J Nurs 103:11, 2003.

Sego, S: Post-traumatic stress disorder: A real illness. Clin Advisor Oct. 2005.

Silva, C, et al: Symptoms of posttraumatic stress disorder in abused women in a primary care setting. J Womens Health 5:543, 1997.

Sexual Assault

Bachman, R, and Saltzman, L (eds): Violence against women: Estimates from the redesigned survey. U.S. Department of Justice, Washington, D.C., 1995.

Brownmiller, S: Against Our Will. Simon & Schuster, New York, 1975.

Burgess, A, and Holmstrom, L: Rape trauma syndrome. Am J Psychiatry 131:981, 1974.

Crime Victims Research and Treatment Center of the National Victim Center. Rape in America: At a glance. National Victim Center, Arlington, Va., 1992.

Goodman, L, et al: Male violence against women. Am Psychol 48:1054, 1993.

Rothbaum, B, et al: A prospective examination of posttraumatic stress disorder in rape victims. J Trauma Stress 5:455, 1992.

Winfield, I, et al: Sexual assault and psychiatric disorders among a community sample of women. Am J Psychiatry 147:335, 1990.

Substance Abuse

Allen, JP, Litten, RZ, Ferig, JB, et al: A review of research on the Alcohol Use Disorders Identification Test (AUDIT). Alcoholism Clin Exp Res 21:613, 1997.

Blow, FC, Gillespie, BW, Barry, KL, et al: Brief screening for alcohol problems in elderly populations using the Short Michigan Alcoholism Screening Test-Geriatric Version (SMAST-G). Alcoholism Clin Exp Res 22(Suppl):131A, 1998.

Bradley, KA, et al: Screening for problem drinking: Comparison of CAGE and AUDIT. Ambulatory Care Quality Improvement Project (ACQUIP). Alcohol use disorders identification test. J Gen Intern Med 13:379, 1998.

Caulker-Burnett, I: Primary care screening for substance abuse. Nurse Pract June:42, 1994.

Cocores, J: Nicotine dependence: Diagnosis and treatment. Psychiatr Clin North Am 16:49, 1993.

Ewing, JA: Detecting alcoholism. The CAGE questionnaire. JAMA 252:1905, 1984.

Fiellin, DA, Reid, C, and O'Connor, PG: Screening for alcohol problems in primary care: A systemic review. Arch Gen Psychiatry 160:1977, 2000.

Garbutt, JC: Alcohol use disorders: biology and pharmacology 2005 update. Presentation at the Duke University Medical Center psychCME conference, Orlando, Fla., Dec. 2005.

Gawin, FH: Cocaine addiction: Psychology and neurophysiology. Science 251:1580, 1991.

Graham, JD: Rock bottom: Recognizing alcoholism in your patients. Adv Nurse Pract 73, June 2000.

Hedlund, JL, and Vieweg, BW: The Michigan Alcoholism Screening Test (MAST): A comprehensive review. J Operat Psychiatry 15:55, 1964.

Julien, RM: A Primer of Drug Action. A Concise, Nontechnical Guide, to the Actions, Uses, and Side Effects of Psychoactive Drugs, ed 8. WH Freeman, New York, 1998.

Kopcha, J: Would you recognize a problem drinker? Clin Advisor 49, June 2005.

Knight, JR, Sherritt, L, Harris, SK, et al: Validity of brief alcohol screening test among adolescents: A comparison ot the AUDIT, POSIT, CAGE, and CRAFFT. Alcohol Clin Exp Res 27:67, 2003.

Maly, R: Early recognition of chemical dependence. Primary Care 20:33, 1993.

Pokorny, AD, Miller, BA, and Kaplan, HB: The brief MAST: A shortened version of The Michigan Alcoholism Screening Test. Am J Psychiatry 129:342, 1972.

McCaul, ME: Substance abuse vulnerability in offspring of alcohol and drug abusers. NIDA Res Monogr 169:188, 1998.

Pope, HG, and Yurgelun-Todd, D: The residual cognitive effects of heavy marijuana use in college students. JAMA 275:521, 1996.

Reinert, DF, and Allen, JP: The Alcohol Use Disorders Identification Test (AUDIT): A review of recent research. Alcohol Clin Exp Res 26:272, 2002.

Renner, JA, and Bierer, MF: Approach to the alcohol-abusing patient. In Stern, T, Herman, J, and Slavin, P (eds): The MGH Guide to Psychiatry in Primary Care. McGraw-Hill, New York, 1998.

Robins, LN: The intimate connection between antisocial personality and substance abuse. Soc Psychiatry Psychiatr Epidemiol 33:393, 1998.

VHA/DoD clinical practice guideline for the management of substance use disorders. Accessed May 20, 2005 from **http://www.guideline.gov/summary/summary.aspx?doc_id**=3169&nbr=002395&string=VHA%2fDoD

US Preventive services task force: Guide to clinical preventive services, ed 2. International Medical Publishing, Alexandria, Va., 1996.

Suicide Risk

Adamek, M, and Kaplan, M: Managing elder suicide: A profile of American and Canadian crisis prevention centers. Suicide Life Threat Behav 26:122, 1996.

Alper, BS: Suicide risk in patients on antidepressants. Clin Advisor, Aug: 143, 2004.

Beck, AT, Steer, RA, Beck, JS, et al: Hopelessness, depression, suicidal ideation and clinical diagnosis of depression. Suicide Life Threat Behav 23:139,1993.

Blumenthal, S, and Kupfer, D (eds): Suicide Over the Life Cycle: Risk Factors, Assessment, and Treatment of Suicidal Patients. American Psychiatric Press, Washington, D.C., 1990, p 177.

Center for Disease Control and Prevention: Suicide in the United States: Suicide fact sheet. Jan. 29, 1998.

Campbell, WH: Pearls: Revised 'SAD PERSONS' helps assess suicide risk. Curr Psychiatry 13:3, 2004.

Centers for Disease Control and Prevention: Suicide among older persons—United States, 1980–1992. MMWR 45:3.

Cochrane-Brink, KA, Lofchy, JS, et al: Clinical rating scales in suicide risk assessment. Gen Hosp Psychiatry 22:445, 2000.

Flavin, D, Franklin, J, and Frances, R: Substance abuse and suicidal behavior. In Kaplan, K, and Harrow, M (eds): Positive and Negative Symptoms as Risk Factors for Later Suicidal Activity in Schizophrenics versus Depressives. Suicide Life-Threat Behav 26:105, 1996.

Gaynes, BN, West, SL, Ford, CA, Frame, P, Klein, J, and Lohr, KN: Screening for suicide risk. Systemic evidence review No. 32. Rockville, Md., 2004. Accessed May 20, 2005 from **http://www.ahrq.gov/clinic/serfiles.htm**

Hockberger, RS, and Rothstein, RJ: Assessment of suicide potential by nonpsychiatrists using the SAD PERSONS score. J Emerg Med 6:99, 1988.

Holkup, P: Evidence-based protocol. Elderly suicide: Secondary prevention. University of Iowa Gerontological Nursing Interventions Research Center, 2002. Accessed May 20, 2005 from **http://www.guideline.gov/summary/summary.aspx?ss**=15&doc_id=3308&nbr=2534&string=suicide

Kessler, RC, Borges, G, and Walters, EE: Prevalence of and risk factors for lifetime suicide attempts in the National Comorbidity Survey. Arch Gen Psychiatry 56:7, 1999.

Lebowitz, BD, Pearson, JL, Scheider, LS, et al: Diagnosis and treatment of depression in late life: consensus statement update. JAMA 278:1186, 1997.

Li, G: The interaction effect of bereavement and sex on the risk of suicide in the elderly: A historical cohort study. Soc Sci Med 40:825, 1995.

Mackenzie, T, and Popkin, M: Medical illness and suicide. In Blumenthal, S, and Kupfer, D (eds): Suicide over the Life Cycle: Risk Factors, Assessment, and Treatment of Suicidal Patients. American Psychiatric Press, Washington, D.C., 1990, p 205.

Mann, JJ: A current perspective of suicide and attempted suicide. Ann Intern Med 136:4, 2002.

Patterson, WM, Dohn, HH, Bird, J, et al: Evaluation of suicidal patients: The SAD PERSONS scale. Psychosomatics 24:343, 348, 1983.

Quinnett, P: Suicide Intervention and Therapy: Undoing the Forever Decision. Classic Publishing, Spokane, Wash., 1992.

Resnick, PJ: Suicide Risk Assessment and Liability. Presentation at the Duke University Medical Center psychCME conference, Orlando, Fla., Dec. 2005.

Rubey, C, and McIntosh, J: Suicide survivors: Results of a survey. Suicide Life-Threat Behav 26:351, 1996.

Rudolph, ML, and Burt, VK: Suicide in elderly women: Addressing this growing concern. Womens Health Primary Care 6:6, 2003.

US Preventive Services Task Force: Screening for suicide risk: Recommendation and rationale. Am J Nurse Pract 9(3):46, 2005.

Resources

Academy of Child and Adolescence Psychiatry
http://www.aacap.org
Academy of Experts in Traumatic Stress
http://aaets.org
Alcohol Use disorders Identification Test: guidelines for use in primary care
http://www.who.int/substance_abuse/publication/alcohol/en/
American Psychological Association
http://www.apa.org
Association for Marriage and Family
http://www.aamft.org
Children and Adults with Attention-Deficit /Hyperactivity Disorder
http://www.chadd.org
Measuring Violence-Related Attitudes, Beliefs, and Behaviors Among Youths: A Compendium of Assessment Tools
http://www.cdc.gov/ncicp/pub-res/measure.htm
National Center on Elder Abuse
http://www.elderabusecenter.org/default.cfm
National Clearinghouse for Drug and Alcohol Information
http://www.health.org
National Institute on Alcohol Abuse and Alcoholism
http://www.niaaa.nih.gov
National Institute of Mental Health suicide facts
http://www.nimh.nih.gov/research/suifact.cmf
National Institute on Drug Abuse
http://www.nida.nih.gov
National Hospice and Palliative Care Organization
http://www.nho.org
Nursing Network on violence Against Women
http://www.nnvawi.org/assessment.htm
Partnerships Against Violence Network
http://www.pavnet.org/
Peace at Home
http://www.peaceathome.org/
Project Cork information on substance abuse
http://www.projectcork.org/
Sexual Assault Resource Service
http://www.sanesart.com/Default.asp
SleepNet
http://www.sleepnet.com
Treatment Improvement Exchange-Treatment Improvement Protocols (TIPs)
http://www.treatment.org/Externals/tips.html
US Dept of Justice Office on Violence Against Women
http://www.usdoj.gov/ovw/
World Health Organization
http://www.who.int/health_topics/en/

Emergency Problems

Jill E. Winland-Brown, EdD, MSN, APRN, BC
Brian O. Porter, MD, PhD, MPH
Edwin W. Schaefer, ND, RN, FNP

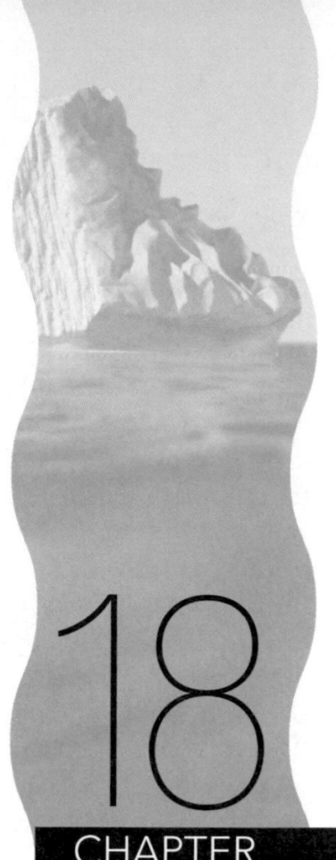

Common Problems

Pneumothorax and Hemothorax

Pneumothorax refers to the abnormal presence of air in the potential space between the parietal and visceral pleura in the thorax. *Hemothorax* refers to the abnormal presence of blood in the same region. For this potential space to become occupied by air or blood, there must be an injury to one of the pleura. A pneumothorax is described as *closed* if the chest wall is intact, or *open* if the chest is violated and communicates with the atmosphere.

Epidemiology and Causes

Pneumothorax and hemothorax are usually the result of a trauma that either penetrates the chest wall and violates the parietal pleura, or a blunt trauma that fractures ribs, which violates the parietal or visceral pleura. Most patients (60 percent) who have suffered a penetrating or high-energy blunt trauma to the chest will have a hemothorax and/or pneumothorax. A pneumothorax (in 25 percent of patients), or other extrathoracic injuries (in 13 percent) will usually accompany a hemothorax. The etiology of pneumothorax can be traumatic (ribs piercing the pleura as a result of a motor vehicle accident, for instance), iatrogenic (as a complication of a central-line insertion), idiopathic (spontaneous), or related to an underlying disease process (such as a ruptured emphysematous bleb in the lung apices).

A spontaneous pneumothorax occurs most often in tall, slender young men. It is usually the result of a rupture of a superficial bleb. A *bleb* is a defect on the lung surface that appears as an outpouching of the lung surface. Such defects may be inherited or related to forces placed on the lung during growth, development, and remodeling of inflammatory lung tissue. Cigarette smoking clearly predisposes to bleb formation and spontaneous pneumothorax with a clear dose–response relationship, likely due to repeated inflammatory insults to the lung parenchyma. Patients with weak connective tissue disorders, such as Marfan syndrome, as well as homocystinuria are also susceptible to primary pneumothoraces. In addition, women with thoracic endometriosis may suffer from recurrent catamenial pneumothoraces or hemothoraces, which are related to their menstrual cycles and bleeding from extrauterine endometrial implants. Rare heritable genetic conditions also exist that predispose to primary pneumothorax, such as the familial cancer condition characterized by renal cancer and benign skin tumors known as Birt-Hogg-Dube syndrome. However, such conditions are typically not suspected without a strong family history. Thirty to 50 percent of patients with a history of spontaneous pneumothorax will have a recurrence of this condition.

Secondary pneumothoraces are most often due to underlying emphysematous chronic obstructive pulmonary disease (COPD) or HIV-associated *Pneumocystis jiroveci* (formerly known as *Pneumocystis carinii*) pneumonia (PCP). Other common predisposing conditions include cystic fibrosis and other conditions that cause significant bronchiectasis, as well as any cavitary lung infection, such as tuberculosis (TB), in which cavities may rupture through the pareital pleura, leading to gas escape into the pleural space. Hemothoraces may similarly result when cavitary lung lesions invade both blood vessels as well as the parietal pleura; however, penetrating chest trauma remains the primary cause of hemothorax.

Pathophysiology

While the underlying etiology of pneumothorax and hemothorax varies widely as described in the preceding text, the collection of either gas or blood within the pleural space ultimately results from a similar pathophysiologic mechanism. The thorax contains the lungs, heart, and major blood vessels. A visceral pleural layer surrounds the outer surface of the lungs, while the chest wall is lined with a parietal pleural layer. The pleural space is a potential space resulting from the apposition of the two pleural membranes. The pleural cells that line the lungs and chest wall continually absorb any gas or fluid that collects in the pleural space, which maintains a negative pressure of –10 to –12 mm Hg. This thoracic pressure differential allows the lungs to expand during inspiration. Any trauma or membrane rupture that results in violation of either pleura can eliminate this negative pressure and allow fluid or air to collect in this space. In turn, this will negatively impact the ability of the lungs to expand effectively.

Clinical Presentation

Subjective

The most frequent presenting symptoms of patients with pneumothorax and hemothorax are dyspnea and chest pain. The severity of the symptoms depends on the size of the pneumothorax or hemothorax. Typically, these conditions are associated with other injuries, which may mask the dyspnea or chest pain. For example, a patient who has a head injury or is unconscious may have altered breathing patterns related to a cerebral event. If the clinician is not alert to the possibility of chest pathology, a pneumothorax or hemothorax may be missed. Fractured ribs may mimic the type of pain encountered with a pneumothorax or hemothorax. If rib x-ray studies are the only type (view) ordered, the technique used to correctly perform this type of x-ray exam will obscure the subtle radiographic findings of a pneumothorax. A chest x-ray film, with both posterior–anterior (PA) and lateral views, should be ordered for any patient who may have suffered chest trauma. A high index of suspicion is needed when considering a pneumothorax or hemothorax.

Objective

Because of decreased lung volume, patients with pneumothorax or hemothorax will usually have a lower than normal oxygen saturation, and may present with cyanosis and varying levels of tachypnea and tachycardia. Lung sounds can be used to help determine the presence of a pneumothorax or hemothorax: Auscultation of absent breath sounds on the affected side has a high-positive predictive value for these conditions, but a normal auscultation does not rule out the presence of pneumothorax or hemothorax. A patient with a large hemothorax can present with frank hypovolemic shock.

Diagnostic Reasoning

Diagnostic Tests

Any patient who has sustained blunt chest trauma and/or penetrating chest trauma must have an upright chest x-ray film to rule out pneumothorax or hemothorax. A supine chest x-ray film can miss many significant thoracic injuries and should not be relied upon to rule out these conditions. The clinician should review the x-ray film, comparing the lung fields bilaterally and looking for any differences in lung markings on one side. When a pneumothorax is present, a subtle light line will be noted—this is the edge of the lung tissue. Beyond that point, the pleural cavity will have absent lung marking. Depending on the technique used, the amount of fat, clothing, or other objects visible on the film, the difference in the pathologic and normal pleural cavity can be very difficult to visualize. It is helpful to use a bright viewing box, position the x-ray film horizontally, and focus on the lateral and lateral–superior aspects of the pleural cavity, where most pathology is found.

If a pneumothorax is suspected, but not found, on an inspiratory chest x-ray study, the APN should request an expiratory chest x-ray exam. During the expiratory phase, the thoracic volume is decreased; the relative size of the pneumothorax is increased and thus may be more easily detected.

If a hemothorax is suspected, the clinician should order a lateral decubitus view, which will reveal the shifting of blood to the lowest part of the pleural cavity. If doubt still exists or a more accurate determination of size of the defect is required, a computed tomography (CT) scan is the definitive test.

Differential Diagnosis

Differential diagnoses for pneumothorax and/or hemothorax include pneumonia, pulmonary embolism, myocardial infarction, angina, and intercostal muscle strain.

Management

Emergency Management

The patient with a pneumothorax or hemothorax is usually cared for and managed in the emergency department (ED); therefore, if the clinician suspects that a patient presenting to a primary-care setting has a pneumothorax and/or hemothorax, emergency medical services should be called, the patient's respiratory and cardiovascular status should be evaluated and supported as indicated, and then the patient should be transported to the ED immediately.

General Management

A pneumothorax is measured via percentage of thoracic volume. A mild pneumothorax is less than 15 percent, a moderate one is 15 to 60 percent, and a severe one is more than 60 percent. Most mild and some small to moderate pneumothoraces (fewer than 20 to 30 percent) can be treated conservatively with observation if the patient is not experiencing any untoward effects. The patient should be admitted for continuous observation and serial chest x-ray films. Patients should be placed on supplemental oxygen, even up to 100 percent for a significant pneumothorax, even if the O_2 saturation is normal on room air, as this helps resorption of the pneumothorax. If the size of the pneumothorax remains unchanged over 8 hours, it is usually safe to allow the body to absorb the air. Any patient with a larger, moderate, or severe pneumothorax will require a tube thoracostomy (chest tube).

A hemothorax of even mild to moderate size requires insertion of a chest tube. Any patient who presents with significant dyspnea, or who is too unstable for ancillary studies and has a high risk of having a pneumothorax or hemothorax, should receive a chest tube immediately. The tube should be inserted in the fourth to fifth intercostal space, at the anterior or midaxillary line. Directing the tube posteriorly and toward the apex can effectively remove both air and fluid. Because 2 to 20 percent of patients with chest tubes usually have infectious complications. antibiotic prophylaxis may be warranted in some patients.

Most pneumothoraces can be treated in a nonurgent manner. Patients with significant respiratory distress will respond quickly to insertion of a chest tube. Patients with a tension pneumothorax, however, require immediate stabilizing treatment (see Box 18.1).

Follow-Up and Referral

After a period of observation, patients with a mild pneumothorax who do not require a chest tube can be discharged with continued follow-up in 1 to 2 days. Patients with a large pneumothorax, a tension pneumothorax, or a hemothorax requiring a chest tube should not be discharged until the pleura has been drained of blood and the lung has been reexpanded for at least 24 hours. Strenuous exercise should be limited until the patient has fully recovered; it is possible to open and aggravate the pleural defect until it has fully healed.

Box 18.1 Tension Pneumothorax

Patients with a tension pneumothorax usually have some type of penetrating trauma such as a gunshot or knife wound. A *tension pneumothorax* develops when air in the potential space between the parietal and visceral pleura is under pressure. The defect in the pleura allows air to enter the potential space during inspiration, but because of a flap mechanism (which functions like a one-way valve), air does not escape. This type of mechanism increases the pressure on the affected lung and, if not corrected, will lead to a complete collapse of that lung. If the defect is left untreated, the pressure will continue to increase and force the mediastinum to the unaffected side. This will cause the major blood vessels to kink and restrict normal blood flow to and from the heart, which can cause death within minutes.

A tension pneumothorax is a true emergency and must be treated immediately. There is no time for x-ray exams to diagnose this condition. The emergent stabilizing treatment involves performing a needle thoracostomy. This is accomplished by inserting a large-bore (18-gauge or larger) needle into the chest. The needle should be inserted between the second and third rib intracostal space at the midclavicular line. The needle should be inserted just over the third rib, to avoid penetrating the neurovascular bundle that runs parallel to the rib on the inferior border.

Patient Education

Patients who have been diagnosed with a spontaneous pneumothorax should be counseled that up to 23 to 30 percent will have a re-occurrence at some point. An explanation of the signs and symptoms to watch for—such as dyspnea, persistent cough, and chest pain—should be given to all patients, regardless of the type of pneumothorax.

Poisoning

Because most adult poisonings are intentional and self-inflicted, the goal is to treat the immediate event and get the patient into counseling as soon as possible, to determine precipitating factors and prevent recurrence. During childhood, poisonings are most often due to accidental ingestions.

Epidemiology and Causes

It has been estimated that more than 2 million poisoning accidents occur each year. The majority of these involve children. More than 90 percent of all poisonings occur in the home. Children younger than age 6 account for approximately 60 percent of all poisonings reported. Adult poisonings account for 80 to 90 percent of all hospital admissions from poisoning. Most adult poisonings involve intentional ingestions, such as recreational drug exposures or suicidal gestures or attempts by overdose. Table 18.1 presents common poisonings. The American Association of Poison Control Centers has a Toxic Exposure Surveillance System (TESS), which is a database on detailed toxicological infor mation on more than 24 million poison exposures reported to U.S. poison centers. The Web address where annual reports are included is listed on the reference page 1130.

Pathophysiology

The pathophysiology of poisonings varies widely, depending on the substance inhaled or ingested. Discussion of a representative sample of potential toxins emphasizes this point. For example, with the inhalation of motor vehicle exhaust, the chemical binding of carbon monoxide (CO) to the hemoglobin component in blood results in the formation of carboxyhemoglobin (COHb) which prevents the binding of oxygen to hemoglobin with subsequent transport to bodily tissues. In contrast, with a tricyclic antidepressant overdose (e.g., amitriptyline, nortriptyline, imipramine), the toxic cardiovascular and central nervous system (CNS) effects are secondary to the anticholinergic effects of the medication

(Text continued on page 1078)

Table 18.1 **Common Poisonings**

Name/Type	Signs and Symptoms	Diagnosis	Management
Drugs			
Acetaminophen (Tylenol)	Nausea, vomiting After 24–48 h postingestion—hepatic necrosis with jaundice, hepatic encephalopathy, renal failure, possible death	Toxicology screen	Activated charcoal Acetylcysteine (Acetadote) for 36 h after ingestion
Barbiturates: Phenobarbital (Phenobarb) Pentobarbital sodium (Nembutal)	Decreased level of consciousness Drowsiness Confusion Ataxia Vertigo Slurred speech Shallow respirations Bradycardia Headache Cyanosis Hypothermia Cardiovascular collapse	Toxicology screen	Gastric lavage with activated charcoal and cathartic Airway maintenance Ventilatory assistance
Benzodiazepines: Clorazepate potassium (Tranxene) Diazepam (Valium) Alprazolam (Xanax)	CNS depression Drowsiness Dizziness Headache Ataxia Hypotension Memory impairment Salivation changes	Toxicology screen	Gastric lavage Symptomatic treatment
Central nervous system stimulants Used for hyperactivity attention deficit disorder (ADD), attention deficit hyperactivity disorder (ADHD) Methylphenidate (Ritalin, Concerta) Amphetamine mixture (Adderall)	Vomiting, emotional lability, nervousness, fever, dizziness, hypertension, tachycardia, psychosis, dyskinesias, Tourette's syndrome, seizures	Toxicology screen	
Cocaine	Nervous system stimulation Restlessness Hallucinations Tachycardia Dilated pupils Chills Fever Abdominal pain Vomiting Muscle spasms Irregular respirations, progressing to death	History of cocaine use Toxicology screen	Diazepam (Valium) IV Emetic Gastric lavage Oxygen Symptomatic treatment
Heroin	Euphoria Flushing Pruritus Miosis Decreased level of consciousness Bradycardia Shallow, slow respirations Hypotension Hypothermia	History of heroin use Toxicology screen	Maintain patent airway Oxygen Symptomatic treatment Naloxone (Narcan) 2 mg IV Nalorphine HCl IV Respiratory stimulant: 3–5 mL dexapram hydrochloride

Name/Type	Signs and Symptoms	Diagnosis	Management
Lithium (Lithobid, Lithotabs, Duralith)	Vomiting, diarrhea, slurred speech, decreased coordination, drowsiness, muscle weakness or twitching	CSF lithium level Toxicology screen	Induced emesis Gastric lavage Osmotic and saline diuresis (if renal function is normal) Urine alkalization Hemodialysis
Salicylates (aspirin, methylsalicylate)	Nausea, vomiting, gastritis, hypercapnia, tachycardia, tinnitus, agitation, confusion, coma, seizures, cardiovascular collapse, pulmonary edema, hyperthermia, possible death	Elevated prothrombin time Toxicology screen with a level > 100 mg/dL Arterial blood gases reveal respiratory alkalosis with an underlying metabolic acidosis	Activated charcoal Gastric lavage IV Nabicab Possible hemodialysis
Tricyclic antidepressants (SSRIs are relatively safe, even in overdose): Amitriptyline (Elavil) Imipramine (Tofranil) Nortriptyline (Pamelor)	Confusion Dizziness Decreased level of consciousness Hypotension Tachycardia Hyperthermia Mydriasis Dry mucous membranes Cardiac dysrhythmias Seizures	Toxicology screen	Gastric decontamination with activated charcoal and cathartic Symptomatic treatment
Foods			
General food poisoning Foods consumed with toxins present	Vomiting, afebrile, abdominal cramping	Toxins: *Staphylococcus aureus, Bacillus cereus, Clostridium perfringens, Shigella, Salmonella.* Toxin can be detected in food or stool specimens	Fluids and electrolyte replacement Ciprofloxacin (use with caution) Disease is usually self-limiting Antimotility drugs
Poisonous fish	Abdominal cramps Nausea Vomiting Diarrhea Paresthesia Hypotension Respiratory paralysis	History of ingesting fish	Supportive treatment for symptoms
Scromboid fish poisoning (bacteria producing scrombotoxin)	30 minutes to 2 hours after ingestion: Peppery sensation on tongue Pruritic rash Headache Dizziness Periorbital edema Nausea Vomiting	History of ingesting fish	Gastric lavage Antihistamines Symptomatic treatment
Other Substances			
Arsenic	Metallic taste Garlic odor to breath Burning pain throughout GI tract Vomiting Dehydration Shock Seizures	Order toxicology screen and/or attempt to discover type of material ingested by investigating all suspect containers	Gastric lavage Fluid and electrolyte management Treat shock and pulmonary edema Possible blood transfusions
Carbon monoxide	Deep respirations Pink (cherry red) tissues and skin (with COHb ↑ 30%) Initial bradycardia, progressing to tachycardia Pounding pulse Dizziness Paresis	Carboxyhemoglobin (COHb) ↑	100% oxygen, under hyperbaric pressure Symptomatic treatment

(continued)

Table 18.1 **Common Poisonings** (continued)

Name/Type	Signs and Symptoms	Diagnosis	Management
	Tinnitus Headache Faintness Nausea Dilated pupils		
Corrosive materials: Lysol, tincture of iodine, carbolic acid (phenol)	Burned tissues along GI tract Brownish stains on lips and tongue Stridor from laryngeal swelling Nausea Vomiting Abdominal cramps Hematemesis Watery, mucoid, or bloody stools Violet or black mucous membranes Carbolic acid—white or gray mucous membranes Hydrochloric acid—grayish mucous membranes Nitric acid—yellowish mucous membranes Sulfuric acid—tan or dark-stained mucous membranes	As above	Opiates for pain Possible tracheostomy Aggressive fluid and electrolyte resuscitation Antibiotics and corticosteroids
Iodine	Brown stains on lips and mouth Burning pain in mouth and throat Yellow emesis (blue if starch is present)	Diagnosis based on symptoms and open or empty container found at scene	Cornstarch or flour solution: 15 g in 2 cups of water given orally if patient is conscious, or gastric lavage if patient is comatose Morphine sulfate for pain
Lead Lead-based paints Lead-contaminated dust Hobbies (e.g., stained-glass windows)	Colicky abdominal pain, constipation, headache, irritability, coma, convulsions Chronic poisoning—learning disorders in children, motor neuropathy (wrist drop)	Blood levels: 10–50 μg/dL—mild toxicity 50–70 μg/dL—moderate toxicity 70–100 μg/dL—severe toxicity Microcytic anemia	*Up to moderate toxicity:* Edetate calcium disodium (EDTA) Oral chelator—succimer (dimercapto-succinic acid, DMSA) *Severe toxicity:* Edetate calcium disodium continuous IV, dimercaprol (BAL) IM
Strychnine	Sense of suffocation Cyanosis Dyspnea Tachycardia Muscle rigidity Contractions Seizures	As above	Gastric lavage Oxygen Sedatives

and the alteration in cardiac cells, which results in conduction disturbances such as QTc prolongation.

With a barbiturate overdose (e.g., phenobarbital), there is decreased neuronal activity, depressed central sympathetic tone, and inhibition of cardiac contractility. These medications act directly on inhibitory gamma-aminobutyric acid (GABA) receptors by increasing affinity of the GABA ligand to its cognate receptor and increasing the average opening time of chloride ion channels. Benzodiazepines such as lorazepam (Ativan), alprazolam (Xanax), and diazepam (Valium) are also CNS depressants that enhance GABA receptor activity but at a molecularly distinct portion of the receptor. Benzodiazepines increase ligand affinity and the frequency of ion channel opening, but not the duration of open channel time. Thus, given this difference in mechanism, benzodiazepines have less potential for toxicity than barbiturates, as their effects are saturable.

Clinical Presentation

Signs and symptoms of various types of poisoning are listed in Table 18.1.

Subjective

The history is an essential component of the diagnosis and treatment plan when a patient is being evaluated for a possible ingestion of a poisonous substance. Interviewing the patient, family, and significant others will give the practitioner valuable information regarding what may have been ingested, as well as the amount and time since the exposure. A lack of symptoms does not preclude the possibility that ingestion has occurred. The history may be very unreliable, because poison ingestion is usually associated with the pediatric population and suicidal gestures.

Objective

The physical examination should include an assessment for evidence of trauma and neurologic symptoms. The clinician should also assess for odors that may give a clue as to what was ingested. The neurologic examination should include a mental status examination, an assessment for seizure activity, and assessments of pupils, the gag reflex, and any focal signs. Additional cardiac, respiratory, gastrointestinal (GI), and renal assessment may be required, depending on the type of poison ingested.

Diagnostic Reasoning

Diagnostic Tests

The diagnostic tests ordered will vary depending on the poisoning situation. Laboratory testing should include toxicology screening. If the specific drug ingested is known, quantitative levels of that agent should be obtained (mg/kg of body weight), along with routine chemistry testing, which includes electrolyte levels. Carboxyhemoglobin (COHb) levels should be monitored to detect evidence of carbon monoxide poisoning.

Differential Diagnosis

Differentials for poisoning may range from manic–depressive disorder to a transient ischemic attack (TIA). Because many substances produce GI symptoms, GI tract disorders should also be ruled out. In addition, overdose of many substances produce CNS symptoms, so vascular and cerebral pathology must also be ruled out.

Management

Emergency Management

Poisonings are usually managed in the ED; therefore, if the patient presenting to a primary care setting has a complaint of poisoning, emergency medical services should be called, the patient's respiratory and cardiovascular status should be evaluated and supported as indicated, and then the patient should be transported to the ED immediately. Emergency management in this scenario includes the A, B, C, Ds, for airway control, breathing, circulation, and drugs.

Because aspirin and acetaminophen are commonly overdosed substances, many clinicians check ASA and acetaminophen levels with any overdose or potentially intentional toxin ingestion so as not to miss this diagnosis.

General Management

For management of common poisonings, refer to Table 18.1. If there is any question about treatment, the local poison control center should be consulted. The national poison control hotline (1-800-222-1222) can direct individuals to local control centers.

Management may also include gastric lavage and the administration of activated charcoal. Gastric lavage may be performed to prevent the poison from reaching the stomach or intestinal tract, where many chemicals are commonly absorbed. Gastric lavage is accomplished by the insertion of a large-bore orogastric tube and lavaging with normal saline solution. Gastric lavage should be performed only in a conscious patient, in order to avoid aspiration of stomach contents. Activated charcoal is often given after gastric lavage, especially after acute ingestions. Activated charcoal is given to absorb the toxins; however, it does not absorb heavy metals, alcohol, caustics, or cyanide. The dose of activated charcoal for children is 1 to 2 g/kg; for adults, the dose is 50 to 100 g/kg. The activated charcoal may be given with or without sorbitol. Sorbitol is a cathartic and may produce dehydration and electrolyte imbalance in young children; therefore, it should be used with caution.

Aside from gastric lavage and gastrointestinal decontamination, another method of eliminating toxins from the body includes a whole bowel irrigation by administering cathartic solutions such as "Go-Lytely." Forced diuresis and alteration of urine pH can be used to remove certain toxins. Acidic toxins can be trapped in alkaline urine and alkaline toxins trapped in acidic urine. Sodium bicarbonate administration can be used to alkalinize urine to a pH greater than 7.0.

Extracorporeal removal through dialysis, plasmapheresis, and exchange transfusion is capable of removing almost any toxin from the bloodstream. Chelation is used to remove heavy metals such as lead and hyperbaric oxygen is used for carbon monoxide poisoning.

Adults who are comatose should be given dextrose, thiamine, and naloxone. If hypoglycemia can be diagnosed, 50 to 100 mL of 50 percent dextrose should be given by IV bolus, as hypoglycemia can cause irreversible brain damage. In malnourished patients or patients with suspected alcohol abuse, 100 mg of thiamine should be given. 0.4 to 2 mg of naloxone given intravenously may reverse opioid-induced respiratory depression and coma. Additional doses may be required of up to 5 to 10 mg.

Follow-Up and Referral

Follow-up and referral will depend on the nature of the poisoning or overdose and the patient's response. If the poisoning or overdose was a suicide attempt or a call for attention, then a psychiatric referral is indicated.

Patient Education

When teaching the patient's family about poisonings, the clinician should advise the parents to call the national poison control hotline (1-800-222-1222) if a poisoning occurs. Historically, syrup of ipecac was used by parents to induce vomiting, but is not recommended by the American Academy of Pediatricians due to its potential for misuse and the regurgitation of corrosive ingested substances which may cause more damage.

General teaching points for preventing poisonings include:

- Keep all medications and hazardous products locked up and out of the reach of children.
- Keep all medications in child-resistant containers.
- Never call medication "candy."
- Dispose of all unused or old medications.
- Do not leave medications on countertops or tables, especially if children are present.
- Never transfer a hazardous material into another container.
- Do not mix chemicals.

Heat-Related Illnesses

Heat-related illnesses include heat cramps, heat syncope, heat exhaustion, and heat stroke. It is important to understand that heat-related illnesses are actually a continuum of conditions that range from mild to severe.

Heat cramps occur in hot weather when a person performs strenuous tasks and drinks large volumes of water, causing an electrolyte imbalance. Sodium chloride is lost from excessive perspiration.

Heat syncope is a heat-related fainting episode. This may occur because of vasodilatation and peripheral pooling of blood, volume deficit, and sluggish vasomotor tone. Venous return does not support the required cardiac output and syncope occurs. Heat syncope can result from inadequate cardiac output and postural hypotension. Recovery is immediate once the patient faints and lies flat.

Heat exhaustion occurs when there is a prolonged period of fluid loss (e.g., perspiration, diarrhea, or use of diuretics) and exposure to warm ambient temperatures without adequate fluid and electrolyte replacement. It is more common in young people and older adults.

A core body temperature of at least 104.9°F (40.5°C) characterizes *heat stroke.* Heat stroke occurs when heat production is greater than heat loss. There may be damage to multiple organ systems and mortality may be as high as 10 percent. Heat stroke may be classic or exertional and is a true medical emergency. It must be rapidly assessed and treated.

Epidemiology and Causes

It has been reported that on average, 300 persons die each year of heat-related illnesses. Heat stroke is ranked third—behind head and neck trauma and cardiac disorders—as a cause of death among high school athletes in the United States. Factors associated with an increased risk of heat-related illnesses include age (both very young children and older adults are at higher risk); a history of a chronic illness, such as a cardiovascular, endocrine, nervous system, or psychiatric disease; use of certain medications, such as antihistamines, beta-blockers, and diuretics, to name a few; fever or dehydration; a previous history of heat stroke; and heavy clothing. Many drugs possess anticholinergic side effects that may result in the inability to perspire. Individuals on beta-blockers may have a diminished inability to cope with heat, thus resulting in a heat-related illness. Autonomic neuropathy of diabetes can be causative of heat-related illnesses. As diabetes is prevalent within the population, this is an important cause of faulty heat dissipation. The conditions of autonomic neuropathy of diabetes, beta-adrenergic and cholinergic blockade are highly unrecognized contributors to heat-related illness that clinicians need to be alert to. Certain living conditions, such as living in an urban setting, living alone, and not using air conditioning during hot weather, are other risk factors. Exertion-related heat stroke may be a complication of unconditioned amateurs involved in strenuous athletic competitions.

Pathophysiology

Human beings are homeothermic, with a core temperature ranging from 97.5°F (36.1°C) to 99.5°F (37.5°C). Thermal regulation is controlled in the anterior hypothalamus, which receives information from the temperature of the circulating blood and from skin sensors. When the hypothalamus is stimulated, the respiratory rate increases to enhance heat loss via expired air; cardiac output is increased to facilitate cutaneous and muscular blood flow, which helps dissipate heat; and sweat glands become active in their role of sustaining evaporative heat loss.

Heat loss is dependent on radiation, convection, conduction, and evaporation. Radiation and conduction result in direct transfer of heat to the environment. When environmental temperatures reach 95°F, these mechanisms for heat transfer are no longer effective.

Convection is heat loss related to air circulation. This process relies on wind velocity. Evaporation of sweat is the only physiologic mechanism for eliminating heat in an environment hotter than 95°F. The body's ability to sweat is affected by skin conditions (such as sunburn), systemic diseases that affect sweating (such as cystic fibrosis), and drugs that inhibit sweating (such as phenothiazines). Increased core temperatures stimulate peripheral vasodilation and sweating. Venous return to the heart increases, resulting in increased cardiac output and heart rate. A concurrent sympathetic response that occurs simultaneously is decreased blood flow to the kidneys. The kidneys are damaged if this process continues; myoglobin is produced as a byproduct. If this condition is not aggressively treated, it will lead to rhabdomyolysis. Respiratory function may be compromised by pulmonary edema. Hepatic function is often decreased because of the general decrease in perfusion. Clotting abnormalities can range from thrombocytopenia to disseminated intravascular coagulation (DIC). This usually occurs in severe heat illness. The metabolic rate increases and sweat production can increase to 1.5 liters per hour (L/h), which may result in dehydration.

Acclimatization is a term that refers to the body's ability to adapt to heat stress. This adaptation primarily involves the sweating mechanism. In the unacclimatized person, each liter of sweat contains 30 to 50 mEq of sodium. This sodium level decreases to as little as 5 mEq/L in the fully acclimatized person, and the rate of sweating can be increased to 1.5 to 3 L/h. This means that the acclimatized person doubles sweat production, with one third to one fifth the loss of sodium. Potassium wasting compensates for sodium loss. Therefore, a fluid and electrolyte imbalance can develop quickly in an unacclimatized person. Cardiac output increases with acclimatization, as does muscle aerobic metabolism, which is more efficient. As the heart muscle responds, cutaneous circulation improves, and heat dissipation is augmented. The body develops a new, lower point at which sweating begins. Finally, increased secretion of aldosterone aids in sodium conservation by the kidneys and sweat glands. The additional sodium enhances extracellular fluid volume, which plays a part in the accelerated cutaneous blood flow and heat dissipation.

Clinical Presentation

Subjective

For any heat-related illness, a complete history of the circumstances preceding the incident should be obtained. Any past history that may assist with the differential diagnosis is crucial. Medications that the patient is currently taking should be reviewed.

Objective

A complete physical examination, including monitoring the patient's cardiac status, vital signs, and core temperature, should be performed.

The clinical presentation may include hot dry skin, decreased level of consciousness, tachycardia, tachypnea, decreased urinary output, hyperpyrexia of more than 104.9°F (40.5°C), hypotension, seizures, nausea and vomiting, decerebrate posturing, diarrhea, and dilated, nonresponsive pupils.

Table 18.2 describes the signs and symptoms and recommended management of the various types of heat-related illnesses.

Diagnostic Reasoning

Diagnostic Tests

There are no specific diagnostic tests performed. Management follows good assessment techniques (see Table 18.2).

Differential Diagnosis

The differential diagnosis of heat stroke should include CNS infections, cerebrovascular accident (CVA), and diabetic ketoacidosis. If the patient has recently traveled outside the country, the clinician should consider malaria or typhoid fever. In addition, the clinician should consider thyroid storm, meningitis, encephalitis, or brain abscess. Some toxicological issues to consider include salicylate, anticholinergic, PCP (phencyclidine), cocaine, or amphetamine toxicity.

Management

Emergency Management

Heat stroke is a medical emergency. If the patient presenting to a primary-care setting has heat stroke, emergency medical services should be called, the patient's respiratory and cardiovascular status should be evaluated and supported as indicated, and then the patient must be transported to the ED immediately.

General Management

Specific management of heat-related illnesses is presented in Table 18.2. General management includes cooling the patient. The safest and most practical method is to remove all clothing and spray warm water over the body surface. Evaporation can be increased with fans, which should circulate air over as much body surface as possible. If ice packs are used, they should be placed in the axilla and groin, with the skin protected from local injury by a wrapping over the pack. Extremities should not be packed in ice, especially in older patients, because this treatment is poorly tolerated in older adults. Cooling of the internal core temperature can also be achieved by gastric or peritoneal lavage with cold saline. In extreme cases, hemodialysis can be used to cool blood. The goal is to reduce the temperature to 102°F (38.8°C) within the first hour. Further active cooling should cease when a core temperature of 101°F (38.3°C) is achieved. Antipyretics are ineffective in lowering the temperature in heat-related illnesses. IV fluids, such as normal saline (NS) or dextrose and normal saline (D5/1/2NS) are usually given. Chlorpromazine (Thorazine) 25 to 50 mg IV or diazepam (Valium) 5 to 10 mg IV may be given initially to control shivering and then every 4 hours. In addition, the patient's urinary output, rectal temperature, and cardiac status should be monitored. Supplemental oxygen is also often administered.

Table 18.2 **Types of Heat-Related Illnesses**

Type of Illness	Signs and Symptoms	Management
Heat Cramps Heat cramps occur in hot weather when a person performs strenuous tasks and drinks large volumes of water, causing an electrolyte imbalance. Sodium chloride is lost from excessive perspiration.	Cramps, especially in the large muscle groups, such as shoulders, thighs, and abdominal wall muscles; weakness; nausea; tachycardia; pallor; profuse diaphoresis; cool, moist skin; and/or a history of ingestion of large amounts of hypotonic solution	• Sodium chloride PO or IV (depending upon the degree of discomfort and the clinical status of the patient). An oral saline solution of 4 tsp of salt per gallon of water may be used. Salt tablets are absorbed very slowly and should not be given. If IV therapy is indicated, 1000 mL 0.9% NaCl infused over 1–3 hrs is preferred. • Cool environment • Rest
Heat Syncope Heat syncope is a heat-related fainting episode. This may occur because of vasodilatation and peripheral pooling of blood, volume deficit, and sluggish vasomotor tone. Venous return does not support the required cardiac output, and syncope occurs. Heat syncope can result from inadequate cardiac output and postural hypotension. Recovery is immediate once the patient faints and lays flat.	Orthostatic syncopal episode, dizziness	• Place patient in a supine position • Oral fluid replacement • Cool environment • Rest
Heat Exhaustion Heat exhaustion occurs when there is a prolonged period of fluid loss (e.g., from perspiration, diarrhea, or use of diuretics) and exposure to warm ambient temperatures without adequate fluid and electrolyte replacement. Heat exhaustion is more common in young patients and older adults.	Thirst, anxiety, anorexia, cramps in muscles, malaise, syncope, headache, dehydration, tachycardia, muscle weakness, orthostatic hypotension, nausea and vomiting, cutaneous flushing and/or possible elevated temperature above 37.8°C	• Remove patient from the hot environment into an air-conditioned room or a shady or cool place • Treat symptomatically; for example, elevate legs for postural hypotension • Oral fluid replacement if no GI symptoms are present and if patient is alert and oriented; replace fluids and electrolytes at about 1 L per hour for several hours. Recovery should be rapid, within 2 to 3 hours. If not, patient may need additional interventions.
Heat Stroke Heat stroke occurs when heat production is greater than heat loss. Mortality rates from heat stroke may be as high as 10%. There may be damage to multiple organ systems. Heat stroke may be divided into classic and exertional. Heat stroke is a true medical emergency—it must be rapidly assessed and treated.	Core body temperature of at least 104.9°F (40.5°C), acute mental status changes, absent sweat, tachypnea, decreased urinary output, hypotension, seizures, nausea and vomiting, diarrhea, dilated nonresponsive pupils, decerebrate posturing	• Rapid cooling; if ice packs are used, place them in groin and axillary region. • Monitor rectal temperature. • Supplemental oxygen, including possible intubation, may be necessary. • IV fluids (usually 0.9% normal saline).

Follow-Up and Referral

A patient is discharged after a complete recovery. Other than teaching to prevent further episodes (see next section), no special follow-up or referral is necessary.

Patient Education

Heat-related illnesses, with their devastating effects, can be avoided or at least reduced in severity through simple preventive measures. These include becoming acclimatized; avoiding alcohol consumption during exposure in hot, humid areas; wearing protective, light-colored clothes and a hat when outdoors in hot weather, ingesting adequate amounts of balanced liquids (e.g., Gatorade) to maintain fluids, electrolytes, and homeostasis; and pacing personal activities. If a patient has suffered from a heat-related illness in the past, he or she will be more prone to heat-related illnesses in the future.

Patients should be taught to gradually build up time spent in hotter conditions (acclimatization). It should be stressed that the higher the temperature and greater the humidity, the greater the risk for heat injury. Fluids must be consumed before there is an urge to drink. If exercising, prehydration is important. The best fluids are simply water or a low-sugar electrolyte drink.

Education about heat-related illnesses should be a part of health maintenance. The clinician should remind parents not to leave children in cars unattended. Older adults should be cautioned about the increased risk of heat-related illnesses, especially if they have medical conditions or are taking medications that increase the risk of heat-related illnesses. Athletes should drink more fluids and exercise during the coolest part of the day.

Cold-Related Injuries

Because of the growing number of homeless persons and the increasing numbers of individuals participating in outdoor activities during cold weather, frostbite is becoming a growing concern.

Frostbite is freezing of an exposed area, usually the ears, cheeks, nose, fingers, and toes. If a previously frostbitten area becomes frostbitten again after it has healed, permanent tissue damage can occur, resulting in necrosis to that body part.

Epidemiology and Causes

The individuals at greatest risk for frostbite are adults age 30 to 49. The anatomic regions at greatest risk for injury are the hands and feet, which account for 90 percent of frostbite injuries. The ears, nose, cheeks, and penis are also prone to frostbite.

There are many predisposing factors that can contribute to frostbite. Cold is the most prevalent factor, but it is not the only factor. In addition, the duration of contact, humidity, wind, clothing, and preexisting medical conditions also contribute to the incidence of frostbite.

Prolonged contact with a cold object can produce frostbite. Humidity contributes to evaporative heat loss. Wet skin is more conducive to ice crystal formation. Wind (exposure in relation to the wind-chill factor) contributes to an increasing loss of heat. Inadequate clothing or overly constrictive clothing can contribute to an increased incidence of frostbite. Constrictive clothing can reduce circulation to extremities. Diseases such as atherosclerosis, diabetes, and previous cold-related injuries predispose individuals to frostbite. In addition, individual behaviors such as alcohol consumption and smoking increase the risk of frostbite.

Pathophysiology

The pathophysiology of frostbite occurs in several stages: tissue freezing, hypoxia, and release of inflammatory mediators. As tissues cool, the circulation slows, allowing ice crystals to form, first extracellularly and then intracellularly, which damages the cell membrane. Crystals that form extracellularly exert osmotic force and pull fluid from the intracellular space, resulting in cellular dehydration. As this process continues, the cell membrane is damaged. Intracellular crystals cause more damage to the cell as they expand within it.

Hypoxia results from cold-induced local vasoconstriction. This vasoconstriction leads to acidosis and increased local blood viscosity as well as hypoxia. Although the body has a natural defensive mechanism against the cold (called *cold-induced vasodilation*—the "hunting response," which prevents rapid freezing of the skin), prolonged exposure to cold eventually causes this response to fail, and freezing takes place. As capillary blood flow ceases, arterioles and venules thrombose, leading to the release of inflammatory mediators. The release of prostaglandins and thromboxane promotes vasoconstriction, platelet aggregation, and blood vessel thrombosis, which worsen endothelial damage. If left unchecked, this process will lead to cell death and widespread tissue necrosis.

Clinical Presentation

Subjective

Initially, the patient complains of a tingling sensation of the body part, followed by pain and eventual numbness.

Objective

Classically, the clinical presentation of frostbite has been categorized according to four degrees of injury. The classification should be applied after some rewarming has been done, because all victims of frostbite present similarly at first, with tingling and redness followed by pallor and numbness.

- First-degree frostbite (partial skin freezing): erythema, edema, hyperemia, no blisters or necrosis, occasional skin desquamation (5 to 10 days later), transient stinging and burning, and possible throbbing and aching; the patient may also have hyperhidrosis (excessive sweating).
- Second-degree frostbite (full-thickness injury): erythema, substantial edema, vesicles with clear fluid, blisters that desquamate and form blackened eschar, numbness, and vasomotor disturbances (in severe cases).
- Third-degree frostbite (full-thickness injury and subcutaneous freezing): violaceous/hemorrhagic blisters; skin necrosis and blue-gray discoloration; initially, no sensation (tissue feels like a block of wood) but shooting pains, burning, throbbing, and aching develop later.
- Fourth-degree frostbite (full-thickness injury and subcutaneous tissue, muscle, tendon, and bone freezing): Little edema is present. Initially, skin is mottled, deep red, or cyanotic; later, skin becomes dry, black, and mummified; possible joint discomfort.

Diagnostic Reasoning

Diagnostic Tests

There are no definitive diagnostic studies for frostbite, especially within the first week of injury. Doppler studies may be helpful to assess blood flow.

Differential Diagnosis

Differential diagnoses for frostbite may include:

- ▲ Frostnip—a mild form of cold injury
- ▲ Chilblain (erythema pernio)—tender red to red-blue itchy nodules on extremities triggered by cold weather and thought to result from chronic vasospasm. There is no actual freezing of the tissue.
- ▲ Immersion foot—hyperhidrosis (excessive perspiration) of the feet causing thickening, maceration, and tenderness of the skin due to prolonged submersion in water or cold (also called trench foot, as it affected soldiers camped for days in trenches during times of war)
- ▲ Hypothermia.

Management

Emergency Management

Frostbite is a medical emergency because of the potential for extensive tissue necrosis and loss of limb. If the patient presenting to a primary-care setting has frostbite, the area should be rewarmed as stated below. Hot liquids such as coffee, tea, or broth should be administered.

General Management

The basis of treatment for frostbite is reversing the pathologic effects of the ice-crystal formation, vasoconstriction, and the release of inflammatory mediators. Treatment should not be started if there is a possibility of refreezing. If it is suspected that the patient has second- to fourth-degree frostbite, hospitalization should be considered.

The first measure is to rewarm the affected area. Rewarming is accomplished by using warm water (104° [40°C] to 108°F [42.2°C]). Care must be taken not to rub the affected area. The affected part should be placed in water for 10 to 30 minutes until the tissue is pliable and red. This process can be very painful; therefore, narcotics should be administered and titrated for comfort.

Blister management in patients with frostbite is somewhat controversial. Blisters containing clear or milky fluid should be débrided and covered with aloe vera every 6 hours (q6h). Aloe vera is a potent antiprostaglandin agent. Hemorrhagic blisters should be left intact and covered with aloe vera. The affected area should be wrapped with a sterile dressing, splinted, and elevated. Silvadene and Bacitracin have proved to be effective as antibacterials; however, use of these topical ointments may interfere with aloe vera.

It is unclear whether prophylactic antibiotic use is warranted for frostbite. It has been demonstrated that the use of penicillin G, 500,000 units IV q6h for the first 72 hours, has proven effective. Ibuprofen 12 mg/kg/day should be administered for its antiprostaglandin activity. Ibuprofen is a potential inhibitor of thromboxane—more potent than other anti-inflammatory drugs. The patient's tetanus status should also be assessed. Patients who are being treated for frostbite should not be allowed to smoke.

Patients may need daily hydrotherapy to débride devitalized tissue. In some instances, referral to a surgeon for a fasciotomy or escharotomy may be needed if there is limited range of motion in an extremity or if the possibility of "compartment syndrome" develops. Compartment syndrome occurs when any structure such as a nerve or tendon is being constricted in a space. The sheath or tendon is enlarged due to the inflammation and no longer able to move freely in the compartment. This results in a cut-off of the circulation, a critical condition, and may result in loss of a limb. It may take up to 3 to 4 weeks for full demarcation of the tissue damage to occur; therefore, amputation should not be considered before this time.

Follow-Up and Referral

If dressings are in place, the patient should be monitored every 2 to 3 days to assess the healing potential. If débridement or grafting is necessary, the patient should be referred to a dermatologist or a vascular surgeon.

Patient Education

Patients should be taught to watch for signs of infection, to take medication as prescribed, and to use extreme care regarding further exposure to cold. The following preventive measures should also be recommended:

- ▲ Do not go outdoors for prolonged periods of time.
- ▲ Wear a hat or earmuffs, mittens, and dress in layers.
- ▲ Keep dry and change out of wet clothing.
- ▲ Dress in natural materials such as cotton or wool.
- ▲ Avoid caffeine, tobacco, and alcohol when going out in the cold, because these substances leave the skin more prone to thermal injury.
- ▲ Check the skin every 12 to 20 minutes for signs of frostbite.

Common Injuries

Wounds and Lacerations

Wounds and lacerations result in a break in the continuity of the skin. The mechanism and energy of the force causing the defect determines the type and severity of the wound. Wounds can range from trivial lacerations or abrasions, which occur at playgrounds on a daily basis, to more severe injuries requiring immediate surgical care. All wounds have the potential of becoming infected and should be evaluated for occult injury. Proper evaluation and care will reduce the morbidity associated with wounds.

Epidemiology and Causes

In one year, 12 percent of all visits to the ED—that is, 11.5 million visits to the ED yearly—were related to wounds. The average laceration seen in the ED is 1 to 3 cm in length; 13

percent of the wounds seen are considered "dirty." In one study, scalp and face lacerations accounted for 51 percent of wounds seen in the ED, upper extremity lacerations accounted for 34 percent, and lower extremity lacerations accounted for 13 percent. Adult wounds become infected about 5 percent of the time, whereas wounds in children become infected 1.2 percent of the time. Almost 75 percent of the patients with wounds were males averaging in their early 20s.

Wound care is a highly litigious area of health care. Missed fractures, missed foreign bodies, and wound infections are common reasons for medical practitioners to be named in a lawsuit. Although wound-care litigation is not associated with the highest payoffs, it is prudent in any case for the clinician to perform a thorough assessment and maintain complete documentation of wound care.

Pathophysiology

The skin is made up of several layers, which are divided into the epidermis and dermis. The skin acts as a barrier, regulates body temperature, aids in elimination of waste, and helps prevent dehydration. It also contains the cutaneous nerves, is a reservoir for nutritional stores and water, and is a source of vitamin D when exposed to sunlight. The ability of bacteria and other substances to penetrate the skin is related to the depth of the wound. Wounds that do not penetrate the stratum germinativum—the basement layer of the skin—do not leave scars.

The healing process is a complicated one and involves many processes that occur simultaneously:

- Injury Phase. This phase involves coagulation and platelet release. This process enhances the inflammatory response in the wound.
- Inflammatory Phase. This phase is characterized by increased capillary permeability, which allows white blood cells (WBCs) to migrate into the wound. Neutrophils and monocytes act as scavengers and rid the wound of debris and bacteria. In addition to providing wound defenses, inflammation stimulates other monocytes to promote fibroblast replication and neovascularization.
- Epithelialization Phase. This phase involves migration of fibrils across the wound. These fibrils are a result of collagen synthesis. This process requires tissue lactate and ascorbic acid and is directly related to local arterial Po_2. Of note, lacerations may heal by primary intention when the edges of the wound are approximated with sutures and allowed to heal together. Suturing techniques that allow for maximal eversion of the wound edges once approximated facilitate healing by primary intention. Alternatively, open wounds may heal by secondary intention, as granulation tissue fills in open lacerations whose edges are not approximated. Collagen synthesis in the healing wound peaks at day 7 posttrauma, and the tensile strength (which determines the ability of the wound to remain intact) increases rapidly at this stage. Typically, the wound will have only 15 to 20 percent of its normal tensile strength at 3 weeks and 60 percent by 4 months.
- Remodeling Phase. In this final phase, the process involves wound contraction and tissue formation. This process begins on the third day after the injury and continues for up to 6 months. The appearance of the wound can change during this period; that is why plastic surgeons will usually wait 6 months before considering revising a scar.

Clinical Presentation

Subjective

A thorough history of the injury must be obtained and documented. Information regarding how the wound occurred is important. The mechanism of wounding is useful in determining the likelihood of deep structure injury and likelihood of associated injuries. For example, a laceration that occurred when a glass shattered in the hand has a high likelihood of having a retained foreign body. A wound that occurred when a hand became caught in a machine has a high likelihood of having an associated fracture. The history must also include questions regarding medical history. For example, a patient with diabetes or a history of vascular problems has a higher possibility of infection (see Focusing the History 18.1).

FOCUS ON HISTORY 18.1

Wounds and Lacerations

History

- Mechanism of injury
- Potential for foreign body
- Potential for underlying injury
- Potential for infection
- Type of injury
- Age of wound
- Delayed or immediate presentation
- Tetanus immunization status
- Allergies
- Comorbidities (especially vascular problems)

Physical Examination

- Vital signs
- General examination
- Vascular injury
- Nerve involvement
- Located over joint
- Tendon damage
- Associated with fracture (open or closed)
- Range of motion
- Wound contamination
- Foreign body
- Avulsion injury
- Puncture

Objective

A description of any wound should include the length, depth, and type of defect found. The depth of the wound is described as *partial thickness* if all layers of the skin have not been violated. If any subdermal tissue can be seen in the wound, it is considered a *full-thickness* defect. Wounds this deep may involve injuries to deeper structures; further evaluation is necessary.

Different types of wounds are associated with specific types of associated injuries and special considerations. Refer to Advanced Assessment 18.1 for various types of wounds and special considerations associated with their assessment and treatment.

Any wound to an extremity should be evaluated for distal circulation and sensation. Circulation should be assessed by determining if the distal extremity has a strong pulse. For fingers or toes, the clinician should assess blanching. A normal blanch response (capillary refill time) is considered to be less than 2 seconds. Distal sensation should be checked to rule out nerve injury. A gross neurologic screening exam should be done on all patients who present with wounds to the extremities: This involves lightly touching the extremity or digit distal to the injury and comparing the response with sensation in uninjured extremities or digits. If the patient states that the sensation is similar, the clinician should document it. If the sensation is decreased, different, or if the patient complains of paresthesias, a two-point discrimination test should be performed to rule out nerve injury.

All wounds must be explored to identify any deep structure injuries or foreign bodies, and to help determine the type of closure required. After the wound is anesthetized, a bright light should be used to illuminate the wound. Wound edges should be retracted, but it is important not to cause trauma to the tissue that may impede normal healing. Blindly probing a wound can cause additional tissue destruction or nerve or vascular injury. Using an Adson forceps with teeth or tissue retractors, the clinician should hook the wound edge and retract it to expose deep structures. The clinician should probe the wound with gloved fingers only.

For large wounds, it is important to examine the full length of the wound, because only a small section of the wound may be deep enough to cause deep structure injury. The defect should be examined for any tendon injury. Exposed tendon will appear as a shiny white structure in the wound. Any wound that involves the extremities must be assessed for tendon and nerve injuries. The range of motion of the affected extremity or digit should be tested carefully against resistance in all planes in which the extremity can be moved. During the movement, the clinician should ask the patient if the resistance causes a pain in the wound. If a partial tendon laceration is present, movement against resistance will cause pain at the site. The wound needs to be explored and deep structures should be examined during the full range of motion to the involved extremity. A tendon injury may be hidden, because the defect may not be visible in the wound at the position in which it is being examined. The injury may have occurred at a different degree of flexion.

Examination for injuries to underlying muscular fascia is required. If a large defect is found, the fascia must be closed to prevent herniation of the muscle in the future.

If the wound is near a joint, violation of the joint capsule must be ruled out. The joint capsule is lined with a synovial membrane and contains synovial fluid, which lubricates the joint and also provides cushioning for the joint. If the synovial capsule is violated, the joint is seeded (contaminated) with bacteria and the possibility of developing a septic joint is likely. The joint capsule is a shiny white structure; if it has been penetrated, bone ends are palpable and can be visualized. Again, the joint must be examined through the full range of motion to look for a defect. If a joint violation is suspected but this cannot be confirmed by visualization, the clinician should order an x-ray film, which may show air in the affected joint. This is a rare finding, however, and should not be relied on to rule out the presence of joint violation.

A *saline-load test* can be performed to accurately determine if a joint violation has occurred. The practitioner should (using sterile technique) inject sterile saline in the joint, in a place away from the defect, and assess whether any saline escapes through the wound. The amount of saline to be injected is dictated by the size of the joint. Findings are considered negative when the saline injection causes distension of the joint without evidence of leakage, or, in a conscious patient, distends the joint capsule to the point of discomfort.

Diagnostic Reasoning

Diagnostic Tests

X-ray films should be taken of wounds that may be associated with a bony abnormality or that raise suspicion of a retained foreign body. Wounds that may have a retained foreign body should be assessed prior to anesthesia by palpating over the defect and margin of the wound to determine whether the patient can feel a foreign body in the wound. This sensation should be documented. X-ray studies can help to rule out foreign bodies, even fragments of glass down to 1 mm in size. Foreign bodies will appear either radiopaque (white) or radiolucent (black), depending on the substance. Some materials, specifically plant-type material (including wood and thorns), will not be visible on x-ray film. Reviewing the x-ray film in a dark room with only the view box illuminated improves the contrast on the x-ray film, making subtle findings easier to visualize.

The presence of a fracture near the wound defect must be treated as an open fracture. Treatment requires consultation with an orthopedic surgeon and close follow-up. Depending on the type of wound and its size and location, surgical irrigation and closure may be necessary. Prompt antibiotic prophylaxis is indicated—within 2 to 3 hours of injury, if possible.

ADVANCED ASSESSMENT 18.1

Wounds and Lacerations

Type	Special Considerations
Abrasion A partial-thickness defect to the skin, usually associated with an abrasive force being applied to the skin.	• Assure that the wound is thoroughly cleansed (this may require anesthesia). For cleansing larger areas of abrasion, consider using topical viscous lidocaine. Use caution with children, because the amount of medication applied to large wounds may cause lidocaine toxicity. Allow about 10–15 minutes after administration of lidocaine for sufficient absorption. • Remove all embedded dirt, because it can lead to "tattooing" of the skin. Tattooing can occur when the skin has healed and the epidermis has grown over the embedded dirt—the dirt is visible through the thin epidermis layer of skin. • Examine the entire area of the wound. Look for any deep lacerations, which may be hard to find because of the size of the wound. Any deep lacerations within an abrasion must be closed with sutures after thorough exploration, débridement, and irrigation. The goal of closure is to loosely approximate the edges. If the wound is deep, use a subcutaneous suture to allow the wound to heal without having to disturb the granulation tissue to remove the stitches later.
Stellar or Flap Laceration When the defect in the skin involves a flap or stellar defect; this usually occurs with a ripping mechanism or blunt trauma to a bony structure such as the skull.	• During exploration, fully retract the flap to allow for visualization to the base of the defect. Typically, this is the deepest part of the laceration. It is important to examine the area under the flap carefully for possible injuries to deeper structures. • Scalp lacerations should be explored for galeal injury. The galea is a fibrous fascia that covers the skull. If the galea has a large defect (more than 3 cm), it should be closed with deep sutures. • If a flap laceration has a nonviable portion, it should be excised. When closing these types of defects, the first suture should bring all the sections of the flap or star together. Following the initial stitch, closure of the remaining defect can be accomplished using normal interrupted sutures.
Linear Laceration Single linear or near-linear defect in the skin; usually caused by a sharp instrument.	• Thorough wound exploration is required to ascertain deep structure involvement. If tendons are involved, orthopedic consult is recommended. • If muscular fascia are violated, these defects must be closed with deep sutures. If these wounds are not repaired, the possibility of muscular herniation is increased. • If a joint is violated, an orthopedic consult is highly recommended. Depending on the mechanism of injury and how dirty the wound is, surgical exploration and irrigation may be necessary. • Wounds in regions with low cosmetic significance, such as the scalp, can be closed using staples, which are faster and easier to place and remove than conventional sutures. Staples have a lower tissue inflammatory response and are well tolerated. Staples must be removed with special instruments, however, so follow-up must be considered when the decision regarding type of wound closure is made. If the patient's primary-care provider is not familiar with staple removal or does not have the correct instrument, placement of stitches is recommended. • Wounds with low tension that do not cross a joint can be closed using tissue adhesive. This eliminates the need for suture removal and has been found to have similar or better cosmetic results than stitches. Using tissue adhesive to close wounds is much faster and decreases the amount of pain associated with wound closure. Before closing the wound, it is important to make sure that the wound has been thoroughly explored and cleaned. This may require infiltration with local anesthesia. Tissue adhesive can be used over wounds that have had subcutaneous sutures placed. Tissue adhesive can also be used to hold fingernails and toenails in place after nail-bed repair. • Wounds under high tension must be closed with subcutaneous stitches or mattress sutures to reduce the tension on the skin edge. High-tension wounds will produce a larger scar and have a higher risk of dehiscence. To avoid this, sutures should remain in place longer in these types of wounds.

(continued)

ADVANCED ASSESSMENT 18.1 (continued)

Wounds and Lacerations

Type	Special Considerations
Crush Injury A defect caused by a high pressure force, such as a dog bite.	• These wounds have diminished vascularization related to the tissue disruption and swelling. Debriding devitalized tissue is necessary to decrease the bacterial load and eliminate that potential nidus of infection. • The practitioner should consider whether delayed primary closure or allowing the wound to heal by secondary intention is appropriate. Consultation with the referring primary-care provider is recommended.
Tendon Injury A force applied that is great enough to cause a disruption to a tendon; this could be a penetrating or blunt force.	• All wounds near tendons must be explored for possible tendon injuries. If tendon damage is found, consultation with an orthopedist is recommended. • Extensor tendon injuries may be closed by the primary-care practitioner, providing he or she has been properly trained in the technique. Early antibiotic prophylaxis is indicated. • Flexor tendon injuries usually require primary wound closure by an orthopedic specialist. There is a high morbidity associated with flexor tendon injuries. Early antibiotic prophylaxis is indicated.
Joint Violation A force, usually applied by a sharp, penetrating injury, that disrupts the joint capsule.	• All wounds near joints must be explored for potential violations of the joint capsule. If any such injury is found, consultation with an orthopedist is recommended. • If the wound is near a joint and a violation of the joint capsule cannot be ruled out, the saline-load test can be used to assess whether penetration of the capsule has occurred. • If the metacarpophalangeal (MCP) joint is injured and any possibility of an injury from a bite (open mouth) exists, immediate follow-up by an orthopedist is needed. The area should be surgically irrigated to avoid joint morbidity.
Cellulitis An infection of deeper tissue, usually caused by a defect to the integrity of the skin that was inoculated by bacteria. The infection usually involves *Staphylococcus aureus* and/or *Streptococcus* bacteria.	• Placing patients with simple, noncomplex wounds on antibiotic prophylaxis does not affect the incidence of infection. Typically, 2–10% of wounds in adults will be infected. • Mild cellulitis should be treated with an oral course of a first- or second-generation cephalosporin. Although the infection can be treated on an outpatient basis, it is important to have the patient return for wound check within 24–48 hours, depending on the extent of cellulitis, to determine if the antibiotic therapy is effective. The region of erythema should be outlined with a tissue marker on initial examination; this demarcation can be used to assess treatment effectiveness or failure if the erythema continues to increase. Wounds that exhibit fluctuance (palpable fluid under the skin) should be incised and drained, to reduce the tension on the wound and decrease the bacterial load. • Patients with diabetes or other conditions that may involve vascular compromise need to be treated more aggressively. Treat the initial findings of cellulitis or wounds that appear dirty with parenteral antibiotics and place the patient on oral antibiotics. Close follow-up is required. These patients may need to be seen daily in the office, depending on the extent of cellulitis. • Patients who present with cellulitis should receive a thorough history and physical to determine the possible mechanism of injury. All hand and feet wounds that become infected should be x-rayed to rule out foreign bodies. Any wound that, based on the history and/or physical exam, has a high potential of having a foreign body should be x-rayed. • If fluctuance is felt, the wound should be incised and drained. The placement of a drain or packing is dictated by the size of the site and clinical judgment. • Patients with wound infections involving angioedema or accompanied by fever or chills should receive parenteral antibiotics. Inpatient treatment should be considered for these patients.

There is no indication for laboratory studies in the initial treatment of wounds and lacerations. If the patient presents with cellulitis or an abscess develops, a wound culture is indicated.

Differential Diagnosis

A differential diagnosis for wounds is usually not indicated because the diagnosis is usually obvious. Associated injuries include fractures, foreign bodies, sprains, and strains.

Management

Emergency Management

If the primary-care setting has suturing capabilities, a simple wound or laceration may be treated in the office. A patient with a large wound, however, especially one that needs major debridement or appears to be infected, should be referred to the ED. Patients with contaminated wounds should be asked about prior tetanus immunization. If more than 5 years have elapsed, a tetanus booster should be administered.

General Management

Wound Cleansing. Following a thorough history and physical examination, all wounds must be cleansed. The most effective way to lower the bacterial count in a wound is through irrigation with a high-pressure stream of solution aimed directly into the wound. The recommended solution is normal saline (NS). The amount of solution needed is dictated by the size and level of contamination of the wound. A good rule of thumb is to infuse 50 to 100 mL of saline per cm of wound length. Saline irrigation or even soapy water is preferred to a dilute povidone-iodine (Betadine) solution as Betadine can be irritating to lacerated tissue. Scrubbing, if employed, needs to be done gently to ensure that the mechanical force applied does not cause damage to the tissue. Scrubbing with an ionic polymer solution such as Shur Cleanse may also be used, because it has been shown to loosen up debris and remove superficial foreign bodies.

Wound Débridement. The wound needs to be débrided of devitalized tissue. Devitalized tissue is any tissue that is devascularized or extremely macerated. This type of tissue is a nidus for bacterial growth and disrupts tissue defenses. Débridement should be done using a sharp scalpel or scissors, so that the débrided edge will be clean and sharp. Using a sharp instrument will cause less tissue trauma and vascular damage at the wound margin. It is important to remove only devitalized tissue. A wound with jagged edges should not be débrided unless the edges are devitalized tissue. Jagged wound margins give the clinician landmarks to use when closing the defect. The jagged edges also increase the surface area of the wound edge and decrease the amount of tension on the wound margin, which can decrease the size of the scar.

Wound Closure. Wound closure is done to reduce the size of scarring and decrease the risk of infection or other morbidity. The closure technique used is dictated by the type of wound. To decrease tension in high-tension areas, subcutaneous stitches or a mattress technique will be helpful. To close a flap or stellar laceration, the half-buried horizontal mattress technique should be used. To avoid obvious scars and poor cosmetic results, landmarks must be meticulously aligned and skin layers placed in good alignment. Suturing techniques are illustrated in Therapeutic Procedures 18.1.

Wound Dressings. The wound should be kept clean, dry, and covered. For sites that are difficult to keep bandaged, a thin layer of antibiotic ointment should be applied to provide protection to the wound. The bandage should be changed daily or if it becomes wet or dirty. It is helpful to apply antibiotic ointment to the wound when the dressing is changed.

Antibiotic Therapy. Antibiotic prophylaxis for most wounds is not indicated. A clean, recently injured wound in a well-vascularized area has a very low chance (only 3 to 5 percent) of becoming infected. Antibiotic prophylaxis does not affect the infection rate. Dog, cat, or human bite wounds, however, have been shown to respond to antibiotic prophylaxis. Early antibiotic therapy, especially if initiated within 2 hours of wounding, has been shown to decrease the chance of infection from bite wounds. Grossly contaminated wounds or wounds that involve areas of diminished vascular supply, such as fingers, toes, and ears, may also benefit from prophylactic antibiotics. Wounds that have an increased risk of infection include:

- ▲ Crushing injuries
- ▲ Dirty wounds
- ▲ Jagged wounds
- ▲ Wounds with devitalized tissue
- ▲ Wounds that are more than 12 to 19 hours old
- ▲ Bite wounds, especially from humans and cats, and dogs (if they are meat eaters)
- ▲ Wounds with retained foreign bodies
- ▲ Wounds closed with subcutaneous stitches

Patients with diabetes or a history of vascular compromise should be started on antibiotics prophylactically. Parenteral administration of ampicillin/sulbactam (Unasyn), cephalexin (Keflex), or ceftriaxone (Rocephin) is the initial treatment of choice. This should be followed by oral therapy with amoxicillin/clavulanate (Augmentin), cephalexin (Keflex), or cefadroxil (Duricef). If the patient has allergies to penicillin or cephalosporins, the practitioner should consider prescribing doxycycline (Vibramycin), with or without clindamycin (Cleocin) or ciprofloxacin (Cipro).

When treating cellulitis or established infections, the clinician should consider initial parenteral therapy with ampicillin/sulbactam (Unasyn), cefoxitin (Mefoxin), cephalexin (Keflex), or ceftriaxone (Rocephin). If the patient has allergies to penicillin and cephalosporins, the cli-

(Text continued on page 1093)

THERAPEUTIC PROCEDURE 18.1

Suturing Techniques

Technique	Advantages	Disadvantages
Buried suture 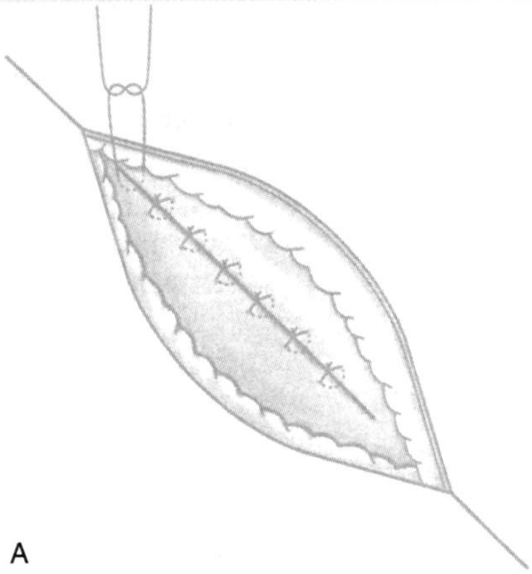 A	Allows good approximation of wound edges	Minimal eversion occurs
Buried vertical mattress suture 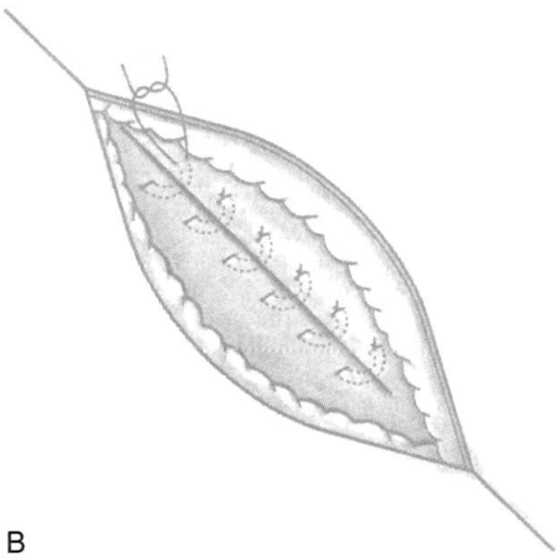 B	Has prolonged eversion; allows early removal of top layers of sutures	If too superficial, more likely to split
Running continuous suture 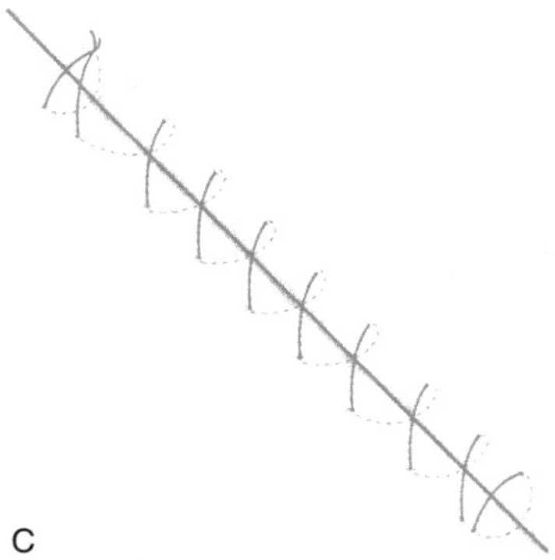 C	Quick; good for children; even tension	Entire suture must be removed

Suturing Techniques

Technique	Advantages	Disadvantages
Interrupted suture 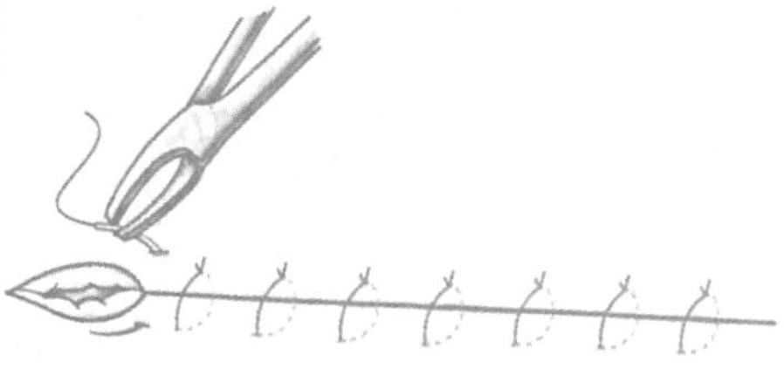 D	Permits precise adjustments between sutures; allows selection of sutures	Increased risk of uneven tension over the suture line; higher incidence of "railroad track" scarring
Vertical mattress suture 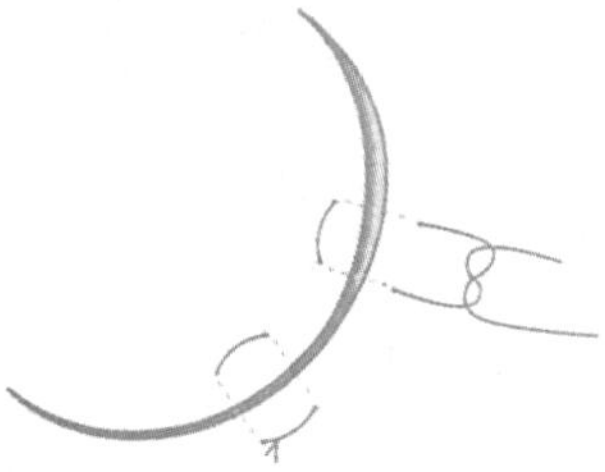 E	Good dead-space wound closure; increased wound eversions; increases wound strength	Time consuming; increased risk of suture marking; difficult to approximate wound edges
Corner (half-buried) suture 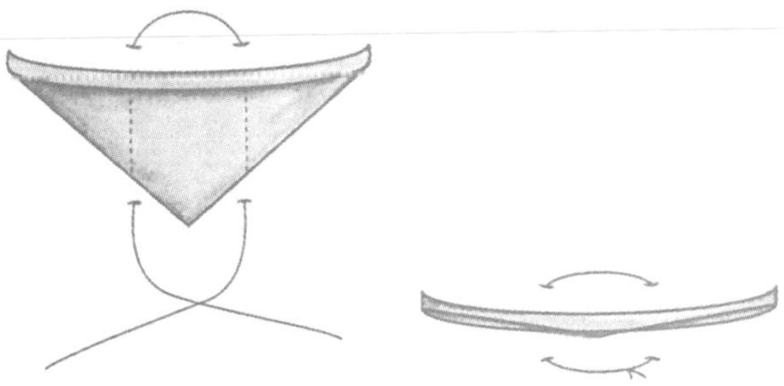 F	Used in skin-flap suturing; decreases risk of obstruction of blood supply to sutured skin flap	Edge approximation more difficult; risk of trauma to skin flap; increased risk of dead space

(continued)

Suturing Techniques

Technique	Advantages	Disadvantages
Subcuticular suture G	Lower incidence of scarring; best for edge approximation	Poor tensile strength; time consuming; poor wound eversion
Horizontal mattress suture H	Good dead-space closure; good wound eversion; some hemostasis occurs	Increased risk of scarring; increased risk of epidermal necrosis
Wound-closure strips 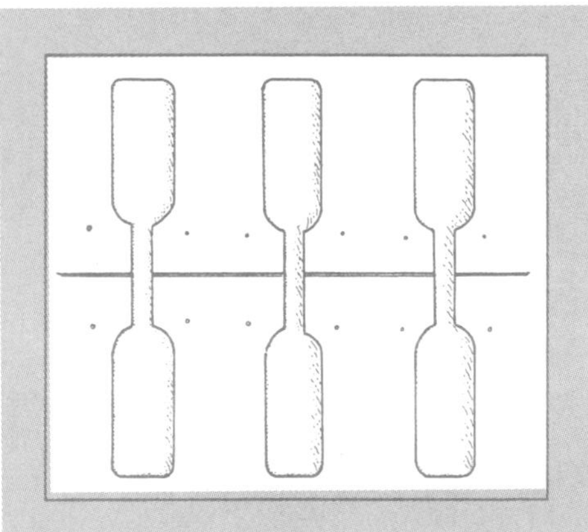	Minimal wound trauma; more resistant to wound infections	Poor wound eversion; more difficult wound-edge approximation

SOURCE: Colyar, MR, and Ehrhardt, CR: Ambulatory Care Procedures for the Nurse Practitioner. FA Davis, Philadelphia, 1999 pp 98–100, with permission.

Suturing Techniques

Suture Materials

<u>Nonabsorbable</u>	
Silk	Not recommended due to frequent tissue reaction
Nylon	Most common
Polypropylene	Best for subcuticular and continuous type suturing, Easiest to pull out
<u>Absorbable</u> (metabolized after about 3 weeks—used in inner tissues)	
Synthetic polymers	Synthetic for deep layers Absorbed by hydrolysis (not for skin)
Surgical catgut	Dissolves in an unpredictable time frame. Excites tissue reaction during its destruction

Tissue Adhesives

A "glue" type adhesive of *n*-butyl 2-cyanoacrylate monomers is used in combination with, or as an alternative to sutures in wound closure.

Suture Size

Smallest size — Largest size

10/0—9/0—8/0—7/0—6/0—5/0—4/0—3/0—2/0-0—1—2—3—4—5—6—7—8—9—10

6/0 is thinner than a human hair, use for example in eye surgery

Family practice clinicians use primarily 3/0 and 4/0

Suture Choices

Fine sizes	Plastic surgery Ophthalmic surgery Pediatric surgery Vascular surgery
Medium sizes	All other kinds of surgery
Heavy sizes	Retention Anchoring bone

nician should consider using doxycycline, clindamycin, or ciprofloxacin. All parenteral therapy should be followed with oral antibiotic therapy for 7 to 10 days. Appropriate choices for oral therapy include cephalexin or cefadroxil for most infections. Wounds that have a high chance of being infected with anaerobic bacteria (that is, wounds involving contamination with mucus or feces) need to have additional antibiotic coverage with clindamycin or amoxicillin–clavulanate. Close follow-up is important for the first 8 to 24 hours after therapy has been started. If the infection appears to be responding to the therapy, the clinician should continue oral therapy, with additional follow-up as indicated by the extent of the injury and infection. Severe infections require inpatient IV therapy. Outlining the area of erythema with a tissue marker during the initial visit will allow subsequent practitioners to assess treatment response more easily. Any extremity or digit that is infected should be immobilized, to reduce the inflammatory response related to mechanical movement of the cellulitic region.

Follow-Up and Referral

Patients should be followed up in the office every few days to check the status of wound healing. Home health care nursing is an effective mode of wound care follow-up in the outpatient setting

Suture Removal

Sutures must remain in place long enough to allow adequate tensile strength to develop during the healing process. The amount of time before suture removal varies with the location of the wound and the cosmetic importance of the wound site. Sutures that are left in too long can cause scarring; however, sutures over joints or areas of high skin tension must remain in longer.

The following are the recommended times for suture removal:

- Face: 4 to 6 days; after suture removal, reinforce wound closure with Steri-strips
- Scalp: 6 to 10 days

- Trunk: 7 to 10 days
- Arms and legs: 10 to 14 days
- Joints: 14 days

Patient Education

The patient may take a shower 12 to 24 hours after the initial wound repair. Studies have shown that wound healing has formed a protective barrier that will prevent bacterial invasion after as little as 8 hours. The wound should not be submersed in water, however, until after suture removal or scar formation.

The clinician should explain to the patient that up to 6 percent of wounds do become infected. Patients should watch for signs of infection, including redness surrounding the area (cellulitis), red streaks coming from the wound (angioedema), and any purulent discharge from the wound (wound infection). Other secondary signs of infection include increasing pain, fever, and chills. Patients with high-risk wounds should be instructed to follow up with the clinician who treated the wound or another provider in 1 to 2 days, so the wound can be evaluated for healing and signs of infection.

Patients may ask whether placing vitamin E ointment on the wound will promote healing. Topical vitamin E should be avoided because E is a weak steroid that can delay healing and cause dehiscence in high-tension wounds. Oral intake of vitamin E during the healing process is beneficial; a good diet will provide the needed amounts.

Aloe vera is a weak salicylate-containing gel. Patients may ask if applying this compound is useful to wound healing. Aloe vera may provide mild pain relief, but it does not improve wound healing or help reduce wound infections. Patients should be advised that taking ibuprofen (Motrin) or another nonsteroidal anti-inflammatory drug (NSAID) will serve the same function.

Box 18.2 presents discharge instructions for patients with wounds and lacerations.

Box 18.2 Discharge Instructions: Wounds and Lacerations

- Keep the injured extremity elevated above the level of the heart if possible.
- Cleanse the wound daily with warm, soapy water. Gently remove debris and any scab that is present.
- Lacerations over joints should be immobilized until the sutures are removed, to prevent further injury from mechanical irritation.
- Watch for signs of infection: redness, increased pain, swelling, fever, red streaks progressing up the extremity, any purulent discharge (pus) from the wound.
- Check wound as needed for any signs of infection. For high-risk wounds, routine checks every 24 hours are recommended.

Burns

In the United States, approximately 2 million patients each year suffer burn injuries. About 100,000 of these patients are hospitalized each year, and 12,000 die from burn injuries and their complications. Because the majority of patients with burn injuries are treated as outpatients, it is important for clinicians to possess the knowledge and skills to treat burn injuries. If a patient with a major burn is brought to an outpatient setting, it may be necessary to assess the patient so that stabilization can occur. Therefore, all practitioners should know how to perform a primary and secondary survey in the initial treatment of a burn victim.

While thermal injury is the most common etiology of burn wounds, several other etiologies of burns exist. Various agents that can cause burn injuries are listed in Table 18.3.

Chemical burns occur in industrial, military, home, agricultural, school, and research laboratory settings. For clinicians working in these settings, especially in a student health-care setting where there is a chemistry laboratory, it is important to have knowledge of the initial care of burn injuries.

People living in the United States spend increasing amounts of time outdoors, working, playing, and exercising, often in clothing that exposes a lot of skin to the sun. Few people know the degree of risk posed by overexposure to the sun and that the risks go beyond skin cancer. Overexposure to ultraviolet (UV) radiation not only results in painful sunburn, but also causes malignant melanoma, basal cell carcinomas, squamous cell carcinomas, actinic keratoses, premature aging of the skin, cataracts, immune-system suppression, sun poisoning (phototoxicity), and contact photodermatitis. *Sun poisoning (phototoxicity)*, also called *sun sensitivity,* is considered a systemic or allergic reaction to overexposure to the sun, usually in conjunction with sunburn. *Contact photodermatitis* is an acute or chronic inflammatory skin reaction resulting from the combined effects of a photosensitizing substance (drugs or chemical) plus UV light (immunologic/delayed hypersensitivity).

Epidemiology and Causes

The risk of all types of burns is highest in people 18 to 35 years of age. The male-to-female ratio is 2:1 for both injury and death. Burns are the second most common cause of accidental death in this country. The death rate in patients older than age 65 is three times greater than that of the overall burn population. Mortality rates from burns have significantly decreased over the last four decades. In the 1950s a 50 percent total body surface area (TBSA) burn was associated with a 50 percent mortality rate. Now, a young, previously healthy person can survive almost any size burn. This improvement in mortality rates is the result of a better

Table 18.3 Burn Injuries

Type of Injuries	Characteristics
Chemical	• *Damage:* Destruction of tissues from coagulation or dessication of tissue protein; action continues until agent is removed; skin penetration by many chemicals leads to systemic toxicity • *Effects:* Injury is generally deeper than it appears; small percentage of admissions to burn units
Cold Liquids/ Gases	• *Damage:* Frostbite (freezing of tissues) results in ice crystal formation, which draws water out of the cells into the extracellular space; crystals expand, causing mechanical destruction of cell walls and organelles • *Effects:* Cell destruction, electrolyte imbalances
Electrical	• *Damage:* Destruction of tissues from heat generated by electric current passing through tissues; arc burn or thermal injury • *Effects:* Injury is usually more extensive than it appears; cardiac conduction system may be affected, leading to sudden death or arrhythmias; severe muscle contraction can produce long-bone or vertebral fractures; severe muscle destruction leads to release of myoglobin, which can affect kidney function
Radiation	• *Damage:* Occurs primarily by gamma/x-ray particles; affects the reproductive mechanisms of tissue cells, leading to cellular death • *Effects:* Same as thermal
Thermal	• *Damage:* Destruction of tissues from flames, scalding liquids, or steam • *Effects:* Proportional to extent of injury and depth. Thermal burns account for highest percentage of admissions to burn units.

understanding of early resuscitation, metabolic support after the injury, early wound excision and closure, and control of infection.

More than 25,000 products are capable of producing chemical burns. About 40 percent of all reported occupationally related diseases concern the skin, and about 25 percent of these are caused by chemical burns. Common household chemical burns are caused by lye (drain cleaners, paint removers), sodium hypochlorite (disinfectants, bleaches), sulfuric acid (toilet-bowl cleaners), and phenols (deodorizers, sanitizers). The body sites most often burned by chemicals are the face, eyes, and extremities.

Health problems resulting from overexposure to sunlight are caused by UV radiation, which is commonly split into three bands: UVA, UVB, and UVC. UVA radiation is not absorbed by the Earth's ozone layer, which is in the atmosphere. The ozone layer protects the Earth by absorbing most UVB rays coming from the sun. UVB is particularly effective at damaging DNA. This damage is a cause of melanoma and other types of skin cancer. UVC radiation is extremely dangerous, but is completely absorbed by ozone and normal oxygen. Researchers have estimated that individuals get 80 percent of their lifetime sun exposure by age 18. Malignant melanoma is one of the fastest-growing forms of cancer in the United States. New cases of melanoma have more than doubled over the past two decades. There may be a link between childhood sunburns and malignant melanoma later in life.

Sunburn can alter the distribution and function of WBCs up to 24 hours after exposure to the sun. Repeated exposure to UV radiation may cause more long-lasting damage to the body's immune system. No matter what skin type or susceptibility to burns, sun exposure makes the body more vulnerable to infections and cancers. This is why diseases such as chickenpox, systemic lupus erythematosus, and herpes simplex become worse with sun exposure. Ultraviolet light therapy is used to treat psoriasis, however, because UV radiation decreases epidermal proliferation.

Overexposure to the sun can also change the texture of skin, giving it a tough, leathery appearance. The sun also causes discoloration in skin tone, including brown, red, yellow, or gray spots. Excess exposure to UV radiation can cause a painful burn of the cornea. Chronic eye exposure to UV radiation may increase the incidence of cataracts, pterygium (in which a fleshy membrane covers the eye), and possibly macular degeneration.

Risk for sun poisoning is increased in persons who take medications that cause photosensitivity, such as oral contraceptives, tetracycline antibiotics, amoxicillin, sulfa drugs, and thiazide diuretics. Risk of sun poisoning also increases with metabolic disorders such as diabetes mellitus or thyroid disease, and underlying infection. Patients who have had previous episodes of sun poisoning or use immunosuppressive drugs are also at increased risk. Other contributing factors include medical disorders such as discoid lupus erythematosus, systemic lupus erythematosus, or porphyria. Exposure to industrial light sources such as welding arcs places people at greater risk for phototoxicity.

Agents that may photosensitize the skin include oral antidiabetic agents, NSAIDs, antibiotics, phenothiazines, sulfones/sulfonamides, chlorothiazides, and griseofulvin. The PABA (*p*-aminobenzoic acid) in sunscreen lotion may also cause photosensitivity dermatitis.

Pathophysiology

Local Response

Cellular injury by heat results in the release of cellular enzymes and vasoactive substances, such as histamine, kinins, serotonin, prostaglandins, leukotrienes, and interleukin-1. The activation of complement also occurs. As a result, vascular permeability is altered and significant hemodynamic, metabolic, and immunologic effects occur locally and systemically. The magnitude of the response is proportionate to the extent of injury. At the capillary level, there is a significant shift of protein molecules, fluid, and electrolytes from the intravascular space to the extravascular space. Lymph flow increases initially but subsequently decreases or ceases because the lymphatic vessels become blocked by the serum proteins leaking through the walls of the damaged capillaries. In extensive burn injury (involving more than 25 percent TBSA), edema forms in both burned and unburned areas because of a generalized increase in capillary permeability and hypoproteinemia. The edema may also be caused by the volume and oncotic pressure effects of the large fluid resuscitation volumes. Maximum edema is seen 18 to 24 hours after burn injury. A decrease in cell transmembrane potential also occurs in extensive burns, causing a shift of extracellular sodium and water into the cell that results in cellular swelling. With adequate resuscitation, the membrane potential is restored within 24 to 36 hours.

Systemic Response

The response of all organ systems to burn injury occurs in a biphasic pattern of hypofunction followed by hyperfunction. The degree of physiologic change is proportionate to the extent of burn; it appears to reach a maximum response in the patient with burns over 50 percent of the TBSA. As the burn wound heals or is closed, organ function returns to normal.

The metabolic response is one of the most significant alterations after burn injury. Hypermetabolism begins as resuscitation is completed and is probably mediated by the secretion of catecholamines. The extensive healing process requires a rapid metabolic rate to support tissue anabolism and reaches its peak between the sixth and tenth days after burn injury. When the wound is closed, oxygen consumption slowly returns to normal. Protein wasting and weight loss are other elements of the metabolic response to a severe burn.

Wound Healing

When a burn injury disrupts the integumentary system, the body automatically responds with a series of overlapping physiologic changes to repair and restore epithelial continuity. The *inflammatory response* begins at the moment of injury and lasts from 3 to 4 days after injury. Localized edema, erythema, heat, and tenderness are characteristic signs of the inflammatory response. During the *fibroblastic phase,* which occurs approximately 4 to 20 days after the injury, cells needed for tissue repair and reconstruction proliferate. Fibroblasts at the wound site migrate over the new capillary network, laying down a bed of granulation tissue (collagen) to fill the wound space. During *wound contraction,* which occurs as granulation tissue forms, myofibroblasts cause the wound edges to pull toward the center. Epithelial cells from the burn margins, then migrate across the wound and eventually reproduce to form a protective barrier. This process is called *epithelialization.* Epithelial cells also migrate from the hair follicles and sweat glands, forming small islands of cells known as *epithelial buds.* Newly forming epithelial cells are easily damaged by mechanical trauma and desiccation. If allowed to dry, the wound will form neo-eschar, retarding the healing process. The epithelial cells must secrete enzymes to dissolve the eschar in their path. The *maturation phase* occurs when immature granulation tissue is highly organized and serves to restore tissue strength. This phase begins approximately 20 days after burn injury and continues beyond 1 year. Contractures can occur if a burn wound heals with extensive scar tissue formation over a joint. A *contracture* is the fixation of a joint or area of skin into a flexed or fixed position. This is caused by atrophy and shortening of muscle fibers or by scar formation and the loss of the normal skin elasticity.

Under optimum conditions, a partial-thickness burn heals in 2 to 6 weeks. The persistence of eschar on a full-thickness burn may delay healing; if the area involved is large, this will cause the patient to remain hypermetabolic. As bacteria proliferate beneath the eschar, there is a possibility of infection. Approximately 2 weeks after burn injury, the eschar begins to separate from underlying tissue as a result of microbial and leukocytic action on subeschar collagen fibers. Separation generally occurs from the wound margins inward but may occur in patches. Eschar may also be removed earlier by surgical excision.

Clinical Presentation

Sun poisoning may present with urticaria, a red rash accompanied by edema, fever, fatigue, dizziness, gastrointestinal symptoms, or malaise. Hematuria, casts, and proteinuria may occur. Contact photodermatitis results in pruritic papules with erythema and occasionally vesicles 24 hours or more after sun exposure. The skin rash will occur in the area where the chemical was applied and sun exposure occurred.

Burn injuries have been classified traditionally from first through third degree. Currently second- and third-degree burns are classified as either partial-thickness or full-thickness. Partial-thickness injuries can be further categorized as superficial or deep. The signs and symptoms of the various depths of burn are as follows:

- ▲ Superficial (first-degree) burns. These burns involve the epidermal layer only. The patient presents with pain, hyperemia, and erythema. The surface is dry, with no vesicles or blisters, and blanches with pressure. The wound heals in approximately 5 days, without scarring. The prototype of a first-degree burn is a mild sunburn. If it occurs over a large surface area, it can result in fever, weakness, chills, and vomiting.

- ▲ Superficial partial-thickness (second-degree) burns. These burns involve the epidermis along with the upper layer of dermis. Signs and symptoms include erythema, hyperemia, pain, moist skin, and hypersensitivity to touch. Vesicles and blisters appear several hours after injury. The healing time is within 21 days, with minimal scarring.
- ▲ Deep partial-thickness (second-degree) burns. These burns produce destruction of epidermis with most of the dermis. Epidermal cells lining hair follicles and sweat glands remain intact. This level of burn may convert to full-thickness injury. The burn wound may be pale, mottled, pearly white, mostly dry, often insensate, and difficult to differentiate from a full-thickness burn. The burn will heal by wound contraction and re-epithelialization within 3 to 6 weeks. Often excision and grafting are done to provide a better functional cosmetic result and to decrease length of healing time.
- ▲ Full-thickness (third-degree) burns. These burns result in destruction of all layers of skin down to or past the subcutaneous fat, sometimes involving fascia, muscle, and bone. The nerves are also destroyed. Hair pulls easily out of the follicles and the patient does not feel pain when this is done. The clinical picture is of thick, dry, leathery eschar; white, cherry red or brown/black in color; the tissue is insensate, with blood vessels thrombosed. The wound will require skin grafting.

Diagnostic Reasoning

Diagnostic Tests

Initial laboratory studies for a patient with a major burn should include a CBC, electrolytes, BUN, creatinine, and glucose. Pulse oximetry and arterial blood gas determinations should be done, including a COHb level to determine the percentage of hemoglobin bound to carbon monoxide.

The carboxyhemoglobin (COHb) levels listed below correlate with the following clinical symptoms:

- ▲ Less than 10 percent COHb: No symptoms
- ▲ 20 percent COHb: Headache, nausea, vomiting, loss of dexterity
- ▲ 30 percent COHb: Confusion, lethargy, ST-segment depression on ECG
- ▲ 40 to 60 percent COHb: Coma
- ▲ More than 60 percent COHb: Death

If the COHb level is less than 40 percent, treatment should consist of 100-percent oxygen administered by high-humidity flow mask. A patient who has a COHb level of 40 percent or higher should be considered for transfer to a hyperbaric chamber.

Differential Diagnosis

Photodermatitis must be differentiated from contact dermatitis that may develop from one of the many substances in suntan lotions and oils. Sensitivity to the sun's rays may also be part of a more serious condition such as erythropoietic protoporphyria, systemic lupus erythematosus, pellagra, or porphyria cutanea tarda.

Management

Emergency Management: Major Burns

A patient with a major burn should be taken immediately to a burn center. A *major burn* is defined as follows:

- ▲ Partial-thickness burn greater than 25 percent TBSA in a person 10 to 50 years of age, or greater than 20 percent TBSA in a child younger than 10 years of age or in an adult older than age 50
- ▲ Full-thickness burn greater than 10 percent TBSA in any individual
- ▲ Serious burn involving the hand, face, foot, or perineum
- ▲ A burn complicated by inhalation injury
- ▲ An electrical burn
- ▲ A burn in an infant, immunocompromised, or elderly patient

Primary Survey. Initial management of the patient with a major burn injury should include maintaining the patient's airway, breathing, and circulation. For airway management, the clinician should assess the patency of the patient's airway while maintaining the head and neck in a neutral position. If a spinal cord injury is probable, the APN should apply a cervical collar, sandbags, and backboard as appropriate.

For breathing management, while the clinician is maintaining the patient's breathing, the clinician should simultaneously observe the patient's skin color, monitor the oxygen saturation via pulse oximetry (SpO_2), and auscultate the lungs to ensure bilateral effective ventilation. The clinician should be alert for signs of smoke inhalation and thermal airway injury if the patient has a history of being in a fire in an enclosed space. Signs and symptoms include: facial burns; presence of soot around mouth and nose and in sputum; singed nasal hairs; coughing of carbonaceous black sputum; difficulty swallowing; signs of hypoxemia, such as tachycardia, dysrhythmias, anxiety, or lethargy; increased or decreased respiratory rate; increased use of accessory muscles for breathing; intercostal or sternal retractions; inspiratory stridor; hoarseness; and expiratory stridor. Once an airway injury has occurred, no measures can be taken to limit its progress and complete airway obstruction can occur. If signs of airway injury are present, the patient will need to be intubated. After extensive swelling has occurred, intubation will be very difficult. Humidified oxygen at 5 to 10 L/min should be administered by face mask along with a bronchodilator (albuterol 5 mg unit dose nebulized or 50 mcg/puff, four to eight puffs by metered-dose inhaler with a spacer, every 15 to 20 minutes as needed). If the patient has signs of carbon monoxide poisoning (headache, nausea, vomiting, dizziness, loss of manual dexterity, confusion, lethargy, unconsciousness, and cherry-red skin color), 100 percent oxygen should be administered via a non-rebreathing mask.

For circulation management, if the patient presents in the outpatient setting with thermal injuries that involve more than 20 percent TBSA, the patient will need to be transported to a hospital emergency department or burn center. If there is evidence of burn shock, the clinician should provide for oral rehydration using balanced salt solutions. The patient should be encouraged to drink enough fluid to keep the urine clear and copious. If this is not possible, a large-bore (16- or 18-gauge) IV catheter should be inserted in an upper extremity vein, preferably through unburned skin. The clinician should infuse lactated Ringer's solution at an initial rate of 500 mL/h. The specific hourly rate can be calculated later during the secondary assessment. Because the cell membranes leak even large molecules for the first 24 hours after a burn, the initial fluid of choice remains Ringer's lactate rather than protein solutions. If an indwelling urinary catheter is available, the clinician should insert a 16 French indwelling urethral catheter and measure the patient's urinary output. A urine output of 1 mL/kg per hour or 30 to 50 mL/h should be maintained. A patient with an extensive burn injury can be expected to develop an ileus, so, if an 18 French nasogastric tube is available, it should be inserted and connected to low, continuous suction to prevent aspiration.

Secondary Survey. The clinician should obtain a complete set of vital signs, including a rectal temperature. The airway and breathing should be continually reassessed and the oxygen administration adjusted as indicated. Signs of pulmonary injury can be delayed for 12 to 24 hours after the initial exposure to noxious gases. After the patient's airway, breathing, and circulation are under control, management should include a secondary survey. If there is time for a secondary survey before transportation to the hospital or burn center, the patient's clothing should be removed. Jewelry should also be removed and secured in a safe place. The patient should be placed on and covered with a clean, warm sheet and clean blankets with overhead warmers if available. No other wound care is required until the patient reaches the hospital or burn center.

At this point a head-to-toe systematic survey can be performed, checking for neurologic injuries and any fractures that need to be stabilized. The depth and extent of burn can now be estimated, using the "Rule of Nines," as shown in Figure 18.1. When the burns are scattered, a rule of thumb is that the size of the patient's palm is equal to approximately 1 percent TBSA.

The weight of the patient should be obtained, either from a scale or from the patient or family, and recorded in kilograms (kg). At this point, the volume of fluids required for resuscitation can be calculated. The clinician should administer 4 mL/kg of body weight per percent TBSA over a 24-hour period. One-half of the calculated amount should be administered during the first 8 hours after burn injury—not after the time the IV line was first established. The remaining half of the fluid should be administered over the next 16 hours. Patients transferred to burn centers from outpatient settings often arrive overloaded with fluids.

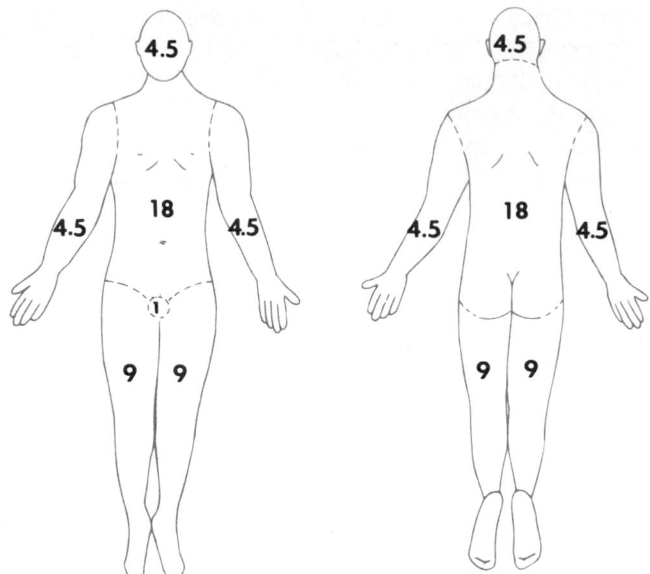

FIGURE 18.1 The rule of nines. (From Richard, RL, and Staley, MJ: Burn Care and Rehabilitation: Principles and Practice. FA Davis, Philadelphia, 1994, p 109.)

Pulmonary edema and hypoxia are exacerbated by overly vigorous fluid administration. Care must be taken to calculate the appropriate volume of fluids correctly and to monitor the patient's response to fluid resuscitation carefully.

During the secondary survey, the peripheral pulses should be evaluated every 15 minutes whenever patients have a burn injury over a large percentage TBSA. The clinician should observe the patient for edema formation as fluids are administered. There is the potential for the pressure of the edema fluid to obliterate arterial blood flow. This is especially true in extremities with circumferential full-thickness burns. The patient may need surgical removal or débridement of eschar to relieve the pressure. Blood pressure measurements should be taken every 15 minutes, although they are often somewhat misleading in this phase.

Pain medication should be administered. Prostaglandin inhibitors such as ibuprofen can be used to suppress or reduce the systemic inflammatory response that occurs with burns of all severity. A short-acting narcotic, such as IV morphine, can also be administered if not contraindicated. The patient will need tetanus immunization during the secondary survey, but administration of this medication and laboratory evaluations can be done once the patient reaches the hospital or burn center.

General Management: Minor Burns

A patient with minor burn injuries can usually be treated in an outpatient setting. Minor burn injuries include a burn of less than 15 percent TBSA in patients 10 to 50 years of age, or less than 10 percent in a child younger than age 10 or an adult older than age 50.

Superficial (First-Degree) Burns. These burns should be cooled with wet compresses. Ice should not be placed directly on the skin. Aloe vera gel can be applied topically to the burn. Remedies (anesthetic sprays) with benzocaine or lidocaine may provide relief from pain, but these medications produce sensitivity reactions in some people. The patient can be given ibuprofen (Motrin), 800 mg q8h, or aspirin or another NSAID. NSAIDs work by blocking the production of prostaglandins, which are thought to be important mediators of pain in sunburned skin. If sunburn is severe, the APN should administer oral prednisone in a rapid taper: day 1, 80 mg; day 2, 60 mg; day 3, 40 mg; day 4, 20 mg; day 5, 10 mg. There are no benefits to prescribing topical corticosteroid ointments or creams.

Superficial Partial-Thickness and Deep Partial Thickness (Second-Degree) Burns. These burns should be irrigated gently with cool water or saline solution to remove all loose dirt and skin. If the burn is chemical, the caustic agent should be washed off with large amounts of water. Any necrotic skin should be peeled off or trimmed. Small, thick blisters should be left intact. Thin, fluid-filled blisters, greater than 1 inch in diameter, should be drained and the dead skin trimmed off using aseptic technique.

There are at least three different methods for the outpatient management of superficial partial-thickness burns. The first method is to apply a topical antimicrobial to the wound. Agents commonly used are presented in Drugs Commonly Prescribed 18.1. Silver sulfadiazine (Silvadene) is the most frequently used topical agent, although it cannot be used in patients with sulfa allergies or on the face, because of silver staining. Alternative topical agents for burns on the face are ophthalmic gentamicin ointment, neosporin, or bacitracin. When these ointments are applied

Drugs Commonly Prescribed 18.1: Burns

Topical antimicrobial agents	Indications	Dosage and Comments
Bacitracin ointment	Antimicrobial, especially for sensitive areas (e.g., lips, eyelids)	Apply to cleansed area 2–3 times daily Does not penetrate eschar
Clotrimazole cream (Lotrimin)	Fungal infections of burn wounds	Apply thin coat to wound; wait 20 min before applying dressing Not for opthalmic use May cause skin irritation and blistering
Mafenide acetate (Sulfamylon)	Active against most gram-positive and gram-negative organisms Drug of choice for electrical and ear burns	Apply 1–2 times daily using sterile gloves; do not use dressings (may reduce effectiveness and cause maceration) Monitor for signs of acidosis; intake and output; and for signs of allergic skin reaction Penetrates eschar better than other agents Pain occurs on application to partial-thickness burns and for 30 min thereafter Allergic maculopapular skin rash may occur Use with caution in patients with impaired renal or pulmonary function Hyperchloremic metabolic acidosis may occur Superinfection with fungi possible
Silver nitrate	Active against wide spectrum of bacterial pathogens and fungal infections Used for patients with sulfa allergy or diseases such as Toxic Epidermal Necrolysis Syndrome	Apply 0.5% solution wet dressings 2–3 times a day; ensure dressings stay moist Preserve solution in a light-resistant container Protect area with plastic to prevent staining from solution spills and splashes; stains everything black (including unburned skin) Poor penetration of eschar Electrolyte imbalances may occur; methemoglobinemia may occur
Silver sulfadiazine (Silvadene)	Active against wide spectrum of microbial pathogens Most frequently used agent for partial- and full-thickness thermal injuries	Apply once or twice a day using sterile gloves; leave wounds exposed or apply gauze dressing over wound Do not use if cream is dark in color Transient neutropenia may occur after 2–3 days Only moderate penetration of eschar Bone marrow depression may occur Use with caution in patients with impaired hepatic or renal function

to the face, no overlying dressing should be used. If antibiotic creams are unavailable, such as in an outdoor setting or in the home, aloe vera gel can be applied to the burn.

Burn wounds on areas other than the face should be covered with a dressing, which should be removed twice a day at home. The burn should be washed with mild antiseptic soap and water, then more antibiotic ointment and a clean dressing should be applied. This regimen should continue for 7 to 10 days until the burn is healed. This particular method of therapy has some disadvantages in the outpatient setting. Some antimicrobial agents (such as Sulfamylon) encourage wound maceration and therefore cannot be used under a dressing. Also, most topical agents lose their potency in 6 to 24 hours following application, making frequent dressing changes necessary.

An alternative dressing for the superficial partial-thickness burn is to cover the burn with a fine-mesh gauze, such as Xeroform gauze, without a topical antibiotic. This gauze is covered with gauze pads, then a bulky absorbent dressing such as Kerlex is wrapped around the wound to provide some protective bulk. The clinician should inspect the wounds and change the dressings the following day, because the maximum amount of wound seepage occurs within the first 24 hours and the burn wound should be assessed for infection, which should be aggressively treated. The same type of dressing is reapplied and the burn is reevaluated after 4 days, and the bulky dressing removed. If a fluid collection has occurred beneath the Xeroform gauze, the dressing will need to be removed, the wound cleansed, and a new Xeroform gauze applied. If the Xeroform gauze is still in place, without any fluid collection, it should be left in place, and the burn rewrapped. Another follow-up visit should be scheduled for a reexamination in 5 days. At that time the Xeroform gauze, impregnated with the crust from the burn, should separate from the epithelium, revealing healed epithelium. Once the wound is left open, it must be kept clean and protected from extremes of temperature. The wound should epithelialize in approximately 3 weeks. Epithelialization, however, may not occur for 2 to 3 months if the wound is a deep partial-thickness burn in which the only skin remnants are the hair follicles or sweat glands.

A third method for outpatient burn-wound management is to place a semisynthetic occlusive dressing such as Biobrane, xenografts, Op-site, or DuoDerm over the wound. These dressings are less readily available and are expensive. They are most useful for the immunocompromised patient because they minimize the risk of infection. They can be used on flat-surface superficial partial-thickness burns of the extremities and trunk. The goal is for the dressing to adhere to the wound surface and for there to be no exudate or fluid between the dressing and the burn. The dressing is usually removed after 7 to 10 days, because the wound is typically healed by then. If there is leaking or nonadherence at any time, the dressing must be changed. Superficial partial-thickness burn wounds heal faster using this method, and patients find this method easier and more comfortable.

The clinician should administer oral antibiotics only if the burn becomes infected. Any partial-thickness burn will convert to a full-thickness burn if it becomes infected, especially with *Streptococcus* organisms; if infection occurs, the patient may have to be admitted for IV antibiotics. Signs of infection include pus, foul odor, cloudy blisters, increased swelling and redness in the normal skin around the burn, and fever greater than 101°F (38.3°C). Antibiotics prescribed for infections include cephalexin, dicloxacillin, or erythromycin. All patients with infected burns should receive tetanus prophylaxis.

Chemical Burns

Consultation from physicians at a burn center should be obtained for treatment of chemical injuries. When a patient with a chemical burn is assessed, the clinician should don protective clothing and gloves. The first priority is to stop the burning process. Any of the patient's garments that have become saturated with the chemical should be rapidly removed, and the patient should be transported rapidly to a shower irrigation area. All other garments should be removed from the patient before the irrigation is complete. If the agent is a powderlike material, such as lime, the clinician should brush off as much as possible before irrigating the burned area. The hair, the area under the nails, and between the toes should be checked for collections of the chemical. The patient may be more comfortable on a chair in a running shower, but any patient who is unstable should be kept horizontal during the irrigation. A chemical burn should be irrigated with water for no less than 30 minutes, and preferably for 60 minutes. Irrigation may need to be continued for hours in the case of alkali burns. Irrigation decreases the concentration of the chemical agent and physically removes it from the wound; the rate and amount of reaction between the chemical and the tissue will thus be decreased. Following irrigation in the outpatient setting, the clinician should place wet towels over the patient and arrange for transportation to the hospital. Although wet towels help to relieve pain and continue to dilute the chemical, caution is needed to prevent hypothermia if the burn (TBSA) is extensive. If possible, the clinician should take samples of the chemical agent with a product label to the ED. Use of pH litmus paper may help determine continued presence of alkali or acid in burn wounds. After irrigation and debridement of remaining particles and devitalized tissue, antimicrobial agents should be used and tetanus immunization updated as needed.

For moderate to large burns caused by hot tar or asphalt, the wound should be rapidly cooled with large volumes of water. The tar can then be removed using a petrolatum-based product such as Neosporin ointment. The wound can be dressed with a petrolatum-based dressing such as Xeroform gauze. The dressings can be changed and the wound should be washed with water every 6 to 8 hours until the tar dissolves. Tar can be removed from the cornea or conjunctiva with polysorbate-containing neomycin sulfate; consultation with an ophthalmologist is recommended.

If a patient presents with fingers that are adhered together with a fast-setting epoxy glue, the glue can be removed with acetone. If the glue is on the mucous membranes or in the eyes, the area can be swabbed with vegetable oil until the glue is removed.

If exposure to hydrofluoric acid (used in glass etching) or oxalic acid has caused a chemical burn, the affected area should be irrigated with water, then neutralized with subcutaneous injections of 10 percent calcium gluconate. This should be done only after consultation with physicians at a burn center.

If phenol (an acidic alcohol used in sanitizers and disinfectants) is the causative agent, the area should be irrigated with water only if a high-density shower is available. Phenol is more soluble in polyethylene glycol; therefore, a 50 percent solution of this agent should be used to irrigate the skin as soon as possible.

Follow-Up and Referral

Although dressing changes may not have been recommended until 5 to 7 days postinjury, all burn patients with a burn injury must still be reassessed in 24 hours for a burn check to reevaluate the depth and extent of the burn.

Patient Education

Patients should be advised to elevate the burned area, especially if it is an extremity, and to return to the clinician's office or the ED if signs of an infection appear. Patients should also be given a prescription for analgesic medication.

Patients with sunburns should be informed that sunscreens with PABA may cause photosensitivity dermatitis. Photoplex broad-spectrum sunscreen lotion not only provides protection for UVB radiation but also offers absorbent protection from UVA rays and may be beneficial for patients who experience photosensitivity activated by UVA. Other useful substitutes are sunshades that contain titanium dioxide, zinc oxide, or talc. The patient should notify the healthcare provider if pain and fever persist for more than 48 hours. Patients should be informed about the sunscreen protective factor index (SPF), a system of evaluating the effectiveness of various formulations for protecting the skin from the sun. Protective agents are rated 1 to 50 by the Food and Drug Administration (FDA). A sun-protective factor (SPF) of 15 means that the sunscreen provides 15 times the protection of unprotected skin.

The patient should also be informed about the Ultraviolet (UV) Index, which was developed by the National Weather Service (NWS) and the Environmental Protection Agency (EPA). The UV Index provides a forecast of the expected risk of overexposure to the sun and indicates the degree of caution individuals should take when playing, working, or exercising outdoors. The UV Index predicts exposure levels on a 0 to 10+ scale, where 0 indicates a low risk of overexposure, and 10+ means a very high risk of overexposure. A patient information sheet on sun safety tips should be given to patients, especially those who have sustained a sunburn severe enough to require treatment. See Table 18.4 for patient information for patients with sunburns.

Table 18.4 **Patient Information: Sunburn**

- Always wear sunscreen when outside on a sunny day. A sunscreen with a sun-protection factor (SPF) of at least 15 will block most harmful UV radiation. For the average adult, the recommended dose is 1 ounce, or one-quarter of a 4-ounce bottle, per application. Reapply every 2 hours, after being in the water, or after exercising and sweating.
- Use broad-spectrum sunscreens—those that contain active ingredients that absorb at least 85% of the UVA and UVB rays of the sun.
- Protect sensitive areas such as the nose and rims of the ears. Use a lip balm containing a sunscreen. This can help keep some people from getting cold sores.
- Minimize exposure to the sun during the hours when the sun is more directly overhead, when exposure is most damaging, from 8 A.M. to 4 P.M. Sun (UV) exposure at 8 A.M. or 4 P.M., when the sun is lower on the horizon, is typically only one-third than at midday. If your shadow is shorter than you are (around midday), you are being exposed to high levels of UV radiation.
- Wear sunglasses that block 99%–100% of UV radiation. Babies and children should also be protected with sunglasses in order to prevent cataracts that may develop later in life.
- Wear a hat with a wide brim to provide protection to your eyes, ears, face, and the back of your neck.
- Wear tightly woven, loose-fitting clothes during prolonged periods in the sun.
- Avoid sunlamps and tanning parlors.
- Watch for the UV index:
  - UV Index 0–2 (minimal): Precautions include wearing a hat.
  - UV Index 3–4 (low): Precautions include wearing a hat and using a sunscreen with an SPF of at least 15.
  - UV Index 5–6 (moderate): Precautions include wearing a hat, using a sunscreen with an SPF of at least 15, and staying in shady areas when outside.
  - UV Index 7–9 (high): Precautions include wearing a hat, using a sunscreen with an SPF of at least 15, staying in shady areas when outside, and staying indoors between the hours of 10 A.M. and 4 P.M.
  - UV Index 10+ (very high): Precautions include staying indoors as much as possible, and taking other precautions when outdoors.
- Be aware that UV radiation increases 5% for every 1000 feet of altitude. In North America, the sun is closest to the Earth on June 21, so spring skiing in the Rocky Mountains without protection is very dangerous. Snow and water can also reflect the sun's rays, making sun exposure more intense.

Animal and Human Bites

An animal bite is a bite wound to humans from dogs, cats, or other animals, including humans. In most cases bites result in puncture wounds, possible lacerations, and, in some cases, crush injuries. All bites, regardless of the source, are considered to be contaminated wounds and have a substantial risk for infection.

Dogs inflict over 80 to 90 percent of mammalian bites, with an overall infection rate of 15 to 20 percent. Risks of infection from dog bites are greatest for puncture wounds, crush injuries, and bites to the hand. Dog bites in general have a 5-percent infection rate, but a dog bite to the hand has a 40-percent infection rate. The most common infectious agents isolated from dog bites are *Staphylococcus aureus, Pasteurella multocida, Corynebacterium* species, and alpha-hemolytic streptococci.

Cats inflict 5 to 10 percent of mammalian bites. The needle-like teeth of the cat result in puncture wounds with a high incidence of infection—around 50 percent. In more than 50 percent of these wounds, *Pasteurella multocida* is isolated; this bacteria causes wound infections that develop within 24 hours of the bite, resulting in an intense inflammatory response. Serious bone and joint infections may be caused by *Pasteurella multocida.*

The third most common cause of mammalian bites is from human beings: These bites account for 3 percent of bites reported. Common infectious agents isolated from human bite wounds include *S. aureus,* streptococci, *Corynebacterium* species, *Bacteroides* species, and *Eikenelle corrodens.* Two percent of reported bites are from rodents.

Epidemiology and Causes

More than 1 million human and mammalian bites occur annually in the United States. Of these bites, 80 percent result in only minor injury. Researchers have reported that 1 percent of all patient visits to the ED are the result of bite wounds, and 1 to 2 percent of these wounds result in hospitalization. About 900 victims of dog bite injuries are treated in the ED everyday. Bite wounds occur in all age groups but are most common in children. Half of dog-bite victims are children younger than age 15. The majority of bite wounds are from a domestic pet known to the victim, with large dogs being the most common source of injury. Cat bites are more common in women; although, in general, men receive more bite injuries than women do. Human-bite injuries from fist-fights are common in teenagers and in alcohol-intoxicated men age 30 to 35. Accidental human bites occur most commonly in children, usually as a result of poorly supervised-interactions.

Some of the causes of animal bites include separating fighting animals; chasing wild animals; fist-fighting; disturbing a sleeping, feeding, unfamiliar, or injured animal; and kissing, teasing, or playing recklessly with an animal. Individuals who are more likely to be bitten by animals include those who work in animal control, mail delivery, farming, hunting, police work, and veterinary medicine. Some sick or injured wild animals—such as squirrels, skunks, or bats—will attack humans without provocation and may carry rabies. The clinician should be familiar with state laws and regulations regarding bite wounds from mammals and rabies prophylaxis, especially in areas where rabies is endemic.

Pathophysiology

The risk of bite-wound infection depends on the wound location, tissue damage, patient characteristics, time elapsed before treatment, and the type of animal that inflicted the bite. Wounds should be classified as low risk or high risk to facilitate decision making regarding antibiotic therapy and wound suturing. *Low-risk wounds* include lacerations involving the extremities, face, and body. Wounds at low risk for infection include bites on the face, ears, scalp, and mouth. Large, clean lacerations and bites by rodents are at low risk for infection. *High-risk wounds* include those in the hand, wrist, or foot; the scalp of an infant; a wound over a joint; or a penetrating wound of the cheek. Puncture wounds and nondébridable crush injuries are of high risk. Patients at high risk for infection are those older than age 50 and individuals with prosthetic joints or valves, asplenia, chronic alcoholism, diabetes mellitus, altered immune status, or peripheral vascular disease, or patients who are on chronic corticosteroid therapy. Bites from domestic cats, large cats, primates, pigs, or humans (especially hand wounds) present the highest risk of infection.

Human bites in locations other than the hand, if treated promptly, have no greater risk of infection than a dog bite. Most human bites are sustained in fights, but 15 to 20 percent of bites reported in one study were secondary to "love nips" (related to sexual activity). A closed-fist injury ("fight bite") occurs from a laceration over the metacarpophalangeal (MCP) joint caused by striking an opponent's tooth. When this occurs, infectious organisms from the mouth are inoculated directly into the bone or joint, which can lead to septic arthritis or osteomyelitis. Also, when the fingers of the closed fist are extended, the injured extensor tendons retract proximally, sealing off the tissues. This sets the stage for a rapidly progressive infection of the tendon and adjacent tissue layers.

Clinical Presentation

Subjective

The circumstances of the bite injury should be determined. These include the area(s) of the body injured, time elapsed since the injury, type of animal (including breed), current location of the animal, relationship of the animal to the victim, vaccination and health status of the animal, and whether the attack was provoked or unprovoked. The patient should be asked about his or her occupation, medication allergies, tetanus immunization status, any history of immunologic compromise, and any specific musculoskeletal, neurologic, or vascular complaints resulting from the bite. If the bite is on the patient's hand, the clinician should ask the patient which hand is the patient's dominant hand. Any comorbid conditions should also be determined.

Objective

Seventy-five percent of the bite wounds seen in the ED or practitioner's office will be located on the extremities where the victim handled or attempted to avoid the animal or another person. Injuries to the head and neck are the next most common bite wounds. The clinician should inspect the skin and soft tissues, noting the presence or absence of lacerations, punctures, scratches, abrasions, swelling, crush injuries, and/or devitalized tissue. All puncture wounds should be examined carefully and the likelihood of injury to structures beneath the skin must be considered. A vascular examination should be performed, noting skin temperature, capillary refill time, and relevant pulses.

The range of motion of all affected areas should be assessed, evaluating the functional status of potentially involved tendons. Motor and sensory nerve function should also be evaluated. To assess sensory function of the hand, the clinician must note sensation to light touch and two-point discrimination on the volar pads of the fingertips. The patient should be able to detect stimuli less than 5 mm apart in the axis of the digit; the response should be compared with the uninjured side. The patient should be evaluated for a skeletal injury and carefully assessed for neurovascular, joint, tendon, and osseous injury.

If the patient does not present with the bite wound until several hours to several days following the injury, the clinician should perform a careful search for evidence of local or systemic infection and regional adenopathy. Infection will be evidenced by increased pain, swelling, erythema, warmth, decreased range of motion at joints, or drainage from a puncture-wound site. A high index of suspicion should always be maintained for the possibility of a retained foreign body in the wound, especially when an infection develops at a puncture-wound site.

Diagnostic Reasoning

Diagnostic Tests

A radiograph of the affected area should be obtained if a fracture is suspected; if a foreign body is present (e.g., tooth fragment); if a bone, joint, or tendon has been penetrated; or if a puncture wound has become infected. In general, two-view x-ray films should be taken. A culture and Gram stain are not useful prior to the onset of clinically apparent infection. The examination of purulent material may show a predominant organism in an established infection, but culture is not warranted unless the results will change the treatment. If the patient presents with a localized wound infection several hours or days after the bite, the clinician should obtain a site Gram stain and both aerobic and anaerobic cultures after superficial decontamination of the wound but before débridement of devitalized tissues. Cultures of wounds are also indicated in cases in which an immunocompromised patient is infected, where there is sepsis, or when antibiotic therapy has failed. To obtain optimal cultures, the clinician should perform percutaneous or deep wound aspiration. If significant blood loss has occurred, it is important to obtain a CBC.

If the patient is seriously ill with a bite-wound infection, diagnostic tests should include a thorough laboratory evaluation (including CBC with platelets, electrolyte panel, glucose level, BUN, and creatinine levels, and prothrombin time/partial thromboplastin time [PT/PTT]), at least two blood cultures, wound-site Gram stain and cultures, and appropriate x-ray studies.

Differential Diagnosis

The diagnosis is typically straightforward by history; no differential diagnoses are indicated. However, to properly direct management, it is critical that the type (source) and extent of the bite wound be characterized as much as possible.

Management

Emergency Management

The clinician may treat bite wounds in the office using the protocol listed below.

General Management

Analgesia. Pain management is commonly provided with analgesic agents such as NSAIDs and acetaminophen (Tylenol). If non-narcotic oral agents are not effective and the patient is in severe pain, ketorolac (Toradol) 30 to 60 mg IM, or meperidine (Demerol) 1 mg/kg IM, with hydroxyzine (Atarax) 25 to 50 mg IM may be tried.

Wound Cleansing. Bites and scratches should be cleansed with mild soap and water or 1 percent povidone-iodine (Betadine) solution, removing the animal's saliva from the wound. Rid the wound of any particulate matter. If the bite was caused by a potentially rabid wild or domestic animal (e.g., skunk, raccoon), wearing protective gloves, thoroughly irrigate the wound with 1 percent benzalkonium chloride, which has been demonstrated to be capable of inactivating the rabies virus.

Local Anesthesia. Using a 25-gauge or smaller needle, the clinician should infiltrate the wound edges with a 1 percent lidocaine (without epinephrine). The maximum dose of lidocaine for local infiltration is 4 mg/kg (0.4 mL/kg of a 1 percent solution).

Wound Irrigation. The wound should be irrigated with 500 to 2000 mL of normal saline. For wounds considered to be at high risk for infection, the clinician can use a 1 percent povidone-iodine (Betadine) solution. For irrigation, a

30-mL syringe with an 18- to 20-gauge plastic catheter should be used to achieve an irrigation pressure of 5 to 8 psi. This method of irrigation has been shown to reduce wound infection.

Wound Débridement. The clinician should remove foreign material, devitalized tissue, and eschar. Margins of puncture wounds should be débrided to approximately a 1- to 2-mm rim, to allow for better drainage and improved cleansing.

Wound Closure. Fresh facial bites without signs of inflammation should be closed with sutures after thorough wound cleansing and preparation. Bite wounds of the hand should not be sutured. For bites to other areas in need of closure or bites greater than 24 hours old, one may consider using delayed primary closure. A layer of fine-mesh gauze can be applied to the wound, which should be packed open, dressed, and followed closely. If there is no purulence or wound-margin erythema at 3 to 5 days follow-up, then wound closure may be performed.

Tetanus Immunization. Bite wounds are tetanus-prone injuries. If the patient has received a primary immunization series but not a booster within the past 5 years, then a tetanus booster should be administered. For patients with absent or incomplete primary immunization, 250 units of tetanus immune globulin should be given in addition.

Antimicrobial Therapy. Patients should receive antibiotic prophylaxis for 3 to 5 days if the wound is a fresh bite wound; if they were bitten by a cat; have a hand bite; have moderate to severe tissue damage; have a wound that may involve a tendon, bone, or joint; have one or more puncture wounds; or have a suppressed immune system. Patients with infected wounds should be given antibiotic therapy based on the results of aerobic and anaerobic culture. The most common causative organisms isolated in wound infections after animal attacks are *Staphylococcus* or *Streptococcus*. Antibiotics prescribed should also cover the less common pathogens such as *Pasteurella* and *Eikenella*. Antimicrobial prophylaxis for cat bites, high-risk dog bites (to the hand, or bites with considerable tissue damage), and human bites can be provided with amoxicillin and clavulanate (Augmentin) 500 mg/125 mg PO tid (three times daily) for 3 to 5 days. An alternative that has fewer GI side effects would be cefuroxime (Ceftin) 250 to 500 mg PO bid for 3 to 5 days. Hospital admission and parenteral antibiotic therapy will be necessary for all significant human bites to the hand, especially closed-fist injuries and bites involving penetration of the bone or joint. Cefuroxime (Ceftin) 1 to 2 g IV q12 to 24h, or ampicillin-sulbactam (Unasyn) 1.5 to 3 g IV q6h, or ticarcillin–clavulanate (Timentin) 3.1 g IV q4 to 6h, should be used for these high-risk bites.

Positioning. The injured area should be elevated for several days postinjury. For bites located over joints, the joint should be immobilized for 3 to 5 days in proper position depending on the bite location: 20 degrees wrist extension, 70 to 90 degrees flexion for metacarpophalangeal joints, and 10 degrees flexion for proximal interphalangeal and distal interphalangeal joints.

Rabies Prophylaxis. Rabies is caused by a rhabdovirus that can be found in the saliva of many mammals. The rabies virus is highly neurotoxic and can be fatal. The clinician should refer questions about postexposure prophylaxis to the local health department or an infectious disease specialist. If a dog or cat is healthy and available for 10 days of observation, showing no development of rabies, no treatment of the exposed person is necessary. At the first sign of rabies in the dog or cat that has inflicted the bite, begin treatment. About 85 percent of all cases of animal rabies in the United States now occur in wildlife. A skunk, fox, bat, raccoon, coyote, bobcat, and other carnivores should be considered rabid unless proven negative by laboratory test. The risk of rabies in lagomorphs (rabbits) and rodents (e.g., mice, rats, chipmunks, and squirrels) is minute.

If postexposure rabies is indicated, both rabies immune globulin (RIG) and human diploid-cell rabies vaccine (HDCV) or rabies vaccine, adsorbed (RVA) should be given as soon as possible. The clinician should discontinue the vaccine if fluorescent-antibody tests for rabies of the sacrificed animal's neural tissue are negative. Dosing is as follows:

RIG: 20 IU/kg. If anatomically possible, one-half the dose should be infiltrated around the wound and the other half given IM (in the gluteal muscle).
HDCV: 1 mL IM in deltoid region on days 0, 3, 7, 14, and 28 if the patient has not been previously vaccinated.
RVA: 1 mL IM in deltoid region on days 0, 3, 7, 14, and 28 if the patient has not been previously vaccinated.

Individuals who have been previously vaccinated with either HDCV or RA should not receive RIG; they should, however, receive 1-mL "booster" doses IM of either HDCV or RVA on days 0 and 3.

The practitioner should also evaluate the potential for transmission of hepatitis B or C virus (HBV or HCV) in human bites. If HBV or HCV prophylaxis is indicated, hepatitis B immune globulin (HBIG), 0.06 mL/kg IM, should be administered immediately and repeated in 30 days. Also, the practitioner must consider whether the human bite was by a known HIV carrier.

Postexposure HIV Prophylaxis

Health-care workers working with combative HIV-positive patients who may be victims of human bite wounds, or those exposed to a needle stick or mucous membrane exposure involving an HIV-positive patient, should refer to the section on this topic in the chapter on Hematologic and Immune Problems which covers postexposure HIV prophylaxis which is an emergency problem.

Follow-Up and Referral

The patient should be discharged to home after thorough and meticulous wound management, with follow-up within 48 hours. Infection, cellulitis, abscess, osteomyelitis, septicemia, tenosynovitis, septic joint (suppurative arthritis), rabies, and the loss of an injured body part are all potential complications of bites. Other systemic diseases that can occur as complications are bubonic plague, cat-scratch disease, rat-bite fever, leptospirosis, tularemia, tetanus, and sporotrichosis.

Patients with severe cellulitis, systemic manifestations of infection, failure to respond to appropriate outpatient treatment within 48 hours, or bite-wound infections that involve a bone, joint, tendon, or nerve should be admitted. The practitioner should obtain early consultation with an infectious disease specialist if needed. Septic arthritis, osteomyelitis, and closed-fist injuries ("fight bites") will require orthopedic consultation.

Patient Education

If the bite was inflicted by a wild animal or in an unprovoked attack by a domestic animal, the practitioner should ask the patient to have the animal that inflicted the bite checked for rabies. The patient or his or her family should contact the local health department and consult with the animal control officer about the patterns of rabies among the animals in the local area. Individuals should be taught the importance of not petting or feeding strange or wild animals.

Patients will need to be reminded to elevate injured extremities to prevent swelling and to return for follow-up if signs of fever, redness, or swelling occur. The clinician should instruct patients to watch for red streaks, increased warmth at the wound site, increasing pain, foul odor, or increased drainage.

Arthropod Bites and Stings

Arthropods are members of Arthropoda, a large phylum of animal life characterized by an external body support structure known as an exoskeleton, which includes lobsters, crabs, as well as mites, ticks, spiders, and insects. Arthropod bites and stings involve penetration of the skin by some part of the animal accompanied by release of venoms that can cause local or systemic symptoms. Some arthropods, such as ticks, also transmit disease. The majority of disorders caused by bites and stings of arthropods are from spider bites; bee, wasp, and ant stings; caterpillar spine irritation; interactions with sucking bugs, beetles, flies and other winged insects; bites from lice, fleas, mites, and ticks; and stings from scorpions.

The venoms produced by venomous insects and other arthropods can be classified according to their effects:

- Vesicating toxins (e.g., from blister beetles, certain stinging caterpillars, and millipedes) produce blisters.
- Neurotoxins (e.g., from black widow spiders, bark scorpions, certain ticks, wheel bugs, and Hymenoptera [honeybees, bumblebees, wasps, hornets, yellow jackets, and fire ants]) attack the CNS.
- Cytotoxic and hemolytic toxins (e.g., from Hymenoptera, ground scorpions, mites, chiggers, wheel bugs, and the brown recluse spider) destroy tissue.
- Hemorrhagic toxins (e.g., from lice, fleas, ticks, mites, true bugs, and biting flies) prevent blood from clotting.

Of the Hymenoptera, the yellow jacket is the major cause for insect-sting reactions. The yellow jacket, hornet, and other wasps feed on sugary sources and are attracted to foods commonly found in garbage cans and at picnics. Yellow jackets, wasps, and hornets nest under logs, in the ground, or in walls; care should be taken to avoid disturbing them during gardening and lawn mowing. When a wasp stings, it injects a venomous fluid under the skin.

The imported fire ant is a small, light reddish brown to dark brown, nonwinged stinging insect that is responsible for increasing numbers of acute allergic reactions. This insect attaches itself to its victim by biting with its jaws; then it pivots around its head, stinging in multiple sites in a circular pattern with its stinger, which is located on its abdomen. The two species of imported fire ants (originally from Brazil) are found predominantly in nine southern states, particularly along the Gulf Coast, and are gradually spreading westward and northward. Fire ants inhabit loose dirt and make nests that produce up to 200,000 ants during a 3-year period. Fire ants swarm if provoked and may attack in great numbers. The fire ant's venom causes hemolysis, the depolarization of cellular membranes, activation of the alternate complement pathway, and general tissue destruction.

The brown recluse spider's (*Loxosceles reclusa*) natural habitat is along the Mississippi River Valley, especially in northwestern Arkansas and southern Missouri. Because this spider can live in old boxes and furniture, it is easily transported to other states. The brown recluse spider prefers warm, dry locations such as woodpiles, cellars, and abandoned buildings; it is generally nocturnal in activity. The "fiddleback" spider has a characteristic violin-shaped marking on the dorsum of its cephalothorax (head and body section). The spider's venom contains sphingomyelinase D; it is chiefly cytotoxic, causing local tissue destruction. The necrosis is caused by an aggregation of leukocytes and platelets that forms a hemostatic plug in venules and arterioles.

Black widow spiders (*Lactrodectus mactans*) are relatively aggressive. They are found throughout the United States, predominantly in the South. Around houses, the black widow spider is found in protected places such as garages, storage sheds, crawl spaces under buildings, and rainspouts. Female spiders of the genus *Lactrodectus* carry the characteristic orange-red hourglass-shaped marking on the ventral abdomen. Black widow spiders are the most feared of all spiders because they injure their victims by injecting one of the most potent venoms secreted by any animal. The *Lactrodectus* venom is a neurotoxin that acts on the myoneural junction and exerts its damage by releasing acetylcholine and norepinephrine.

Scorpions are found throughout the world. They are nocturnal and spend the day under rocks, logs, and floors. The only species that is particularly dangerous, *Centruroides exilicauda* (the bark scorpion), is found mostly in the southwestern United States. This small Mexican scorpion is usually less than 2 inches long, yellow to brown, and possibly striped. The last segment of the scorpion's tail-like structure contains the venom glands and stingers. Most scorpions are relatively harmless, producing only local reactions, but the venom of *Centruroides exilicauda* has effects similar to those of black widow spider venom, producing severe systemic toxicity. The venom is predominantly a neurotoxin that causes repetitive firing of axons by activation of sodium channels.

Some of the more common ticks in the United States are the brown dog tick and American dog tick. Ticks are frequently encountered by hikers and people who work outdoors. When feeding, ticks make a small hole in the skin, attach themselves with a modification of one of the mouthparts (which has teeth that curve backwards), and insert barbed, piercing mouthparts to remove blood. The American dog tick (*Dermacentor variabilis*) may transmit Rocky Mountain spotted fever (caused by the intracellular bacteria *Rickettsia rickettsii*), tularemia (caused by the coccobacillus *Francisella tularensis*), and other diseases from animals to people. This tick has also been reported to cause paralysis if it attaches at the base of the skull or along the spinal column. Paralysis is caused by a toxic secretion produced by the feeding tick. Lyme disease (caused by the spirochete bacterium *Borrelia burgdorferi*) is also transmitted by ticks. Most disease transmission occurs in the New England states, where the primary vector is the deer tick/black-legged tick (*Ixodes scapularis*). Species that are close relatives to the deer tick, such as the western black-legged tick (*Ixodes pacificus*), are also capable of transmitting the disease.

Fleas are wingless, blood-sucking insects, some species of which transmit arboviruses to humans by acting as host or vector for the organism. Certain species of fleas transmit plague, murine typhus, and tularemia. If a house has been previously occupied by pets that were infested with fleas, the abandoned hungry fleas may form a welcoming party for the newly arrived "human guests."

Chiggers, or "red bugs," are the larvae of harvest mites. Infestations due to chiggers are caused by mite larvae that feed on the host skin cells. In other parts of the world such as India, Central and Southeast Asia, and Australia, chiggers may transmit scrub typhus (caused by the rickettsial bacteria *Orientia tsutsugamushi*). Chiggers become active in the spring, although in southern states, such as Florida, they may be active all year. Chiggers attach themselves to the skin of humans or frequently to hair follicles or pores by inserting their piecing mouthparts. They prefer to attach themselves to parts of the host's body where clothing fits tightly or where the flesh is thin, tender, or wrinkled. During feeding chiggers inject digestive enzymes into the skin, which dissolves tissue. Chiggers feed by sucking up the liquefied tissues; they do not burrow in the skin. After 3 days, when the larva is engorged, it drops off. Chiggers are most often found in low, damp areas where vegetation is heavy, although some species prefer dry areas. They are most abundant in areas covered with shrubs and small trees where rodents are numerous.

Mosquitoes are blood-sucking arthropods attracted to hosts by moisture, carbon dioxide, estrogens, sweat, or warmth. They are vectors of many infectious diseases.

The species of blood-sucking flies that can produce allergic reactions are deerflies, blackflies, horseflies, and sandflies. Fly bites can also result in cutaneous myiasis in which parasitism by fly larvae occurs. When a fly, such as the human botfly, deposits an egg on human skin, the egg hatches immediately, and the larva enters the skin through the bite or through another small break in the skin. The larvae grow to 15 to 20 mm under the skin, as a growing red, pruritic papule develops into a tender furuncle, with eventual emergence of the fly larvae.

Some of the stinging caterpillars are the puss caterpillar, saddleback caterpillar, and the hag moth caterpillar. These caterpillars are found primarily in the southeastern states, especially in Texas and Florida. These caterpillars have spines that are hollow hairs containing poison sacs. When the spines break off, a toxin flows from the spines onto the victim's skin, causing a burning sensation.

Epidemiology and Causes

Millions of people in the United States are injured by venoms produced by insects and other arthropods each year, with a notable number of deaths. In one 10-year period, 65 deaths were reported to be caused by spiders in the United States. Of these, 63 deaths were from black widow spider bites. Bee and wasp stings cause more deaths than any other venomous animal (6 deaths per 100,000). These insect stings result in a rapid progression of toxic effects: 80 percent of the deaths result from anaphylactic shock less than 1 hour after the sting. Spider bites, however, have a longer time interval between bites and time of death, with 89 percent of victims dying more than 12 hours after being bitten. Ninety-five percent of all venomous animal fatalities occur from April to October, when animals and potential victims are most active. The risk of insect bites increases with lack of protective measures and in areas with heavy insect infestations. Previous exposure to venom can predispose the victim to anaphylaxis.

Pathophysiology

The normal or usual reaction following an insect sting is local erythema, pain, pruritus, and swelling. Insect stings always cause pain. This normal reaction should subside in 1 to 2 hours. The more significant reactions to insect bites can be categorized as large local reactions, toxic reactions, systemic or anaphylactic reactions, delayed reactions, and unusual reactions.

A *large local reaction* could spread more than 6 inches beyond the sting, consisting of prolonged and marked edema at the site of the sting injury, peaking at 48 hours and lasting as long as 1 week. This reaction may be accompanied by nausea, vomiting, and fatigue. A large local reaction can involve one or more neighboring joints and may even produce airway obstruction if the sting was in the mouth or throat.

A *toxic reaction* occurs when there is a history of multiple stings, often more than 10. Toxic reactions are caused by nonantigenic properties of Hymenoptera venom. They resemble systemic reactions, but have a greater frequency of gastrointestinal disturbances. Diarrhea, nausea, vomiting, light-headedness, and syncope are common signs. The patient may also have headache, drowsiness, fever, involuntary muscle spasms, edema without urticaria, and occasionally seizures. Urticaria and bronchospasm are not present and the symptoms usually subside within 48 hours.

Systemic or anaphylactic reactions may range from mild to fatal. The majority of such reactions occur within the first 15 minutes, and nearly all will occur within 6 hours after the insect sting, but may actually occur up to 24 to 36 hours. The shorter the interval between the sting and the onset of symptoms, the more severe the reaction. Fatalities that occur usually result from either hypotension or airway obstruction. The patient will present initially with generalized urticaria, itching eyes, dry cough, and facial flushing. These symptoms may progress rapidly to chest or throat constriction, dyspnea, wheezing, laryngeal stridor, frothy sputum, cyanosis, diarrhea, abdominal cramps, nausea, vomiting, chills and fever, vertigo, shock, loss of consciousness (LOC), and involuntary bowel and bladder function.

When an individual predisposed to Hymenoptera allergy is initially stung, there is an increase in the production of antigen-specific IgE antibodies. The antibodies become attached to mast cells and basophils, and the individual becomes sensitized to undergo an anaphylactic reaction following a subsequent sting. Anaphylaxis is a type I immediate hypersensitivity immune response to a triggering antigen/allergen found in insect venom. In this type of reaction, once introduced into the body, the circulating venom antigen binds to antigen-specific IgE molecules which are themselves bound to mast cells and basophils. Binding of two or more cell membrane-bound IgE molecules to the same antigen (a process known as antibody cross-linking) leads to the degranulation of mast cell and basophil cytoplasmic contents and the release of preformed vasoactive mediators including histamine and tryptase. These substances are potent systemic vasodilators, accounting for the immediate flushing and life-threatening symptoms of hypotension, angioedema, and mucosal swelling with potential airway compromise.

Infusion of histamine into normal subjects causes the following effects and can be diminished by antagonists of specific histamine receptors: flushing (H_1 plus H_2), hypotension (H_1 plus H_2), tachycardia (H_1), headache (H_1 plus H_2), pruritus (H_1), rhinorrhea (H_1), and bronchospasm (H_1). Honeybee venom contains histamine. Wasp venom contains histamine and serotonin. Hornet venom contains histamine, serotonin, and acetylcholine. The fact that histamine acts through both H_1 and H_2 receptors emphasizes the importance of administering both H_1 and H_2 antihistamines during allergic reactions. However, the only reliable method of countering the life-threatening hypotension and mucosal edema associated with anaphylactic histamine release is with immediate administration of epinephrine, a potent vasoconstrictor.

Following this immediate response, through complex lymphocyte (e.g., T cell) and granulocyte interactions, other inflammatory vasoactive cytokines begin to form several hours after exposure, including prostaglandins, leukotrienes, and bradykinin. These substances contribute to a second, later phase of anaphylaxis which typically occurs 6 to 12 hours following acute exposure to the triggering antigen. Leukotrienes and prostaglandins are responsible in part for vascular permeability, vasodilation, smooth-muscle contraction, and mucous secretion. Downregulation of the inflammatory response by these de novo-formed mediators is the goal of steroid treatment in anaphylaxis, since steroids such as hydrocortisone and methylprednisolone exert their peak effects 4 to 8 hours after administration and are ineffective against the immediate life-threatening anaphylactic response. In turn, steroids are more helpful for severe, prolonged allergic reactions and to manage delayed responses.

Another type of *delayed reaction* to insect venom can also appear 10 to 14 days after an insect bite or sting, which is also antibody-mediated but by IgG or IgM, rather than IgE. This type of reaction presents as a serum sickness-like illness, which is a type III antigen-antibody response in which immune complexes are deposited in the various tissues of the body. The patient's signs and symptoms include malaise, headache, fever, urticaria, lymphadenopathy, and polyarthritis. Additional unusual reactions may be neurologic or vascular in nature. They include nephrosis, vasculitis, serum sickness, encephalitis, and neuritis. Their etiology varies but may be due to an immunologic pathogenesis.

Clinical Presentation

Subjective

The clinician should determine the history of the sting or bite, including the exact time of injury, and an exact description of the arthropod or species of insect, if possible. As the skin is inspected for signs of the insect or spider bite, the patient should first be evaluated for any anaphylactic symptoms or signs of a systemic reaction. The clinician should also determine if the patient has had previous allergies to insect bites, a history of allergies or asthma, or any known allergies to horses or horse serum. A family history of anaphylaxis to bites or stings should also be elicited.

With stinging insects, the patient will usually remember the insult, because the sting induces immediate pain. For biting insects, there may be some delay between the actual bite and the itching that follows. The patient's history should be carefully pursued to identify the probable source of exposure. For indoor exposure, fleas are common offenders, although spider bites are also responsible for indoor bites. The clinician should inquire about whether pets have recently occupied the dwelling or if the patient has been to a home with pets.

Objective

Hymenoptera (bee and wasp) stings produce immediate pain and a red papule surrounded by a pale zone of edema, with varying amounts of local swelling. Large local reactions are common, spreading more than 6 inches (15.2 cm) beyond the sting, peaking at 48 hours, and lasting as long as 1 week. A mildly sensitive person will experience hives, malaise, wheezing, conjunctivitis, rhinitis, fever, and nausea. A severely sensitive person will suffer diffuse urticaria, facial swelling, laryngeal edema, bronchospasm, vomiting, cyanosis, abdominal pain, arrhythmias, and hypotension. Most fatalities occur within 1 hour of the sting.

Fire ant stings produce vesicles that become sterile pustules; these pustules subsequently become necrotic within several hours and may take up to 10 days to heal. If broken, the pustules may become infected. Systemic symptoms include nausea, vomiting, faintness, headache, fever, numbness, and muscle spasms.

Brown recluse spider bites are unusual in that persons bitten usually do not feel pain for 2 to 3 hours. A single necrotic lesion occurs, usually measuring 0.5 to 2 cm (less than 1/20 to almost 10) in size, self-limited in spread, and lacking adenopathy or sustained general toxicity. The typical bull's-eye lesion is created when the red blister is encircled by a pale, irregularly shaped and ischemic halo, which in turn is surrounded by extravasated blood. The pustule may gradually grow to a form a craterlike lesion over 3 to 4 days, with associated lymphadenopathy and low-grade fever. Rarely, there is a generalized systemic reaction 24 to 48 hours after the bite, with fever, malaise, arthralgias, rash, and hemolysis.

Black widow spider bites create an initial puncture wound that disappears rapidly, leaving a local swelling where tiny red spots appear. Symptoms of envenomation occur within 10 to 60 minutes, including severe pain in the bitten extremity and muscle spasms of the abdomen and trunk. Diffuse paresthesias, ptosis, and hyperactive deep tendon reflexes may be noted. Victims are in agonizing pain and may develop hypertension, headache, muscular rigidity and spasm, hyperreflexia, vomiting, abdominal pain, agitation, or psychosis. Symptoms peak at 2 to 3 hours after the bite and may last up to 24 hours.

Scorpion stings are immediately intensely painful, with little or no erythema or swelling. Generalized reactions may occur within 1 hour and progress to maximum severity in 5 hours. The reactions can be graded as follows:

Grade I: Local pain and paresthesias at the site of envenomation

Grade II: Pain and paresthesias remote from the sting bite, along with local findings

Grade III: Either somatic skeletal or cranial nerve neuromuscular dysfunction, including blurred vision, wandering eye movements, hypersalivation, difficulty swallowing, upper airway obstruction, slurred speech, jerking of the upper extremities, restlessness, arching of the back, severe involuntary shaking and jerking

Grade IV: Both cranial nerve and somatic skeletal neuromuscular dysfunction

Hypertension, nausea, vomiting, hyperthermia, tachycardia, and respiratory distress may also occur. Children under 10 years of age are more likely to have severe or prolonged reactions to scorpion stings. Older children and adults usually recover within 10 to 12 hours.

Tick bites can produce lesions that vary from small pruritic nodules to extensive ulceration, induration, and erythema. The lesions may be accompanied by malaise, fever, and chills. Tick-induced paralysis occurs more frequently during the spring and summer, when ticks are feeding. Symptoms occur 5 to 6 days after the adult female tick attaches and include irritability, restlessness, and paresthesias in the hands and feet. Over the next 24 to 48 hours, ascending, symmetric, and flaccid paralysis, with loss of deep tendon reflexes, occurs. Within 1 to 2 days, severe generalized weakness is possible, accompanied by respiratory paralysis.

Flea bites produce lesions that are so similar to those of lice and scabies that diagnosis is often difficult. Flea bites produce itching papules, found in zigzag lines, especially on the legs and in the waist area. The lesions present as central hemorrhagic puncta surrounded by erythematous and urticarial patches. Pruritus is intense. Once the lesions clear, dull red spots may persist. Impetigo may develop as a complication. If the fleas remain in the environment, new lesions continue to appear.

Itching from *chigger bites* is usually noticed 4 to 8 hours after chiggers have attached or have been accidentally removed. Initially, a papule develops and ultimately enlarges over 24 to 48 hours to form a nodule. Pruritus peaks on the second day. The fluid injection causes nodules to appear, which may last for 2 weeks. Patients who exhibit an allergic reaction to the fluid injected (saliva) will develop severe soft tissue edema, itching, and fever. Chigger bites usually occur around the ankles, waistline, knees, or in the armpits. Mite infestations may be associated with an erythema multiforme-like rash and fever.

An immediate skin reaction to *mosquito bites* includes erythema, wheal, and itching. A delayed reaction 12 to 24 hours later consists of redness, edema, and a burning pruritus. Blistering and necrosis can also occur. The immediate reaction is of short duration, whereas a delayed reaction may persist for hours, days, and even weeks. Some individuals have a history of allergy to mosquito saliva, consistent with an increasing reaction to seasonal exposures accompanied by progressively more pronounced edema and pruritus. The allergic response can be accompanied by fever, generalized malaise, nausea, vomiting, and necrosis, with resulting scarring.

Blood-sucking flies can cause pain and subsequent pruritus when they pierce the skin. Allergic reactions can occur; if flies inject their eggs under the skin, the patient can also develop myiasis. As the fly larvae hatch and grow under the skin, the initial pruritic papule becomes a furuncle with a central opening that exudes serosanguineous fluid. The tip of the fly larva may even protrude from the central opening, or bubbles produced by its respiration may be seen.

The *puss caterpillar's sting* causes intense immediate pain, often in spasms. This is followed by local edema, pruritus, and a rash of red blotches and ridges. The lesions consist of red or white papules and vesicles, often forming a perfect gridlike mark where the caterpillar made contact. Ordinarily no systemic manifestations occur; the localized symptoms typically subside within 24 hours. In some patients, however, the intense pain may cause nausea and vomiting, as well as headache, fever, and lymphadenopathy. The papular or urticarial rash usually subsides within a few hours to 1 to 2 days after contact, but it may persist for up to 1 week.

Diagnostic Reasoning

Diagnostic Tests

In an arthropod bite or sting that results in systemic involvement, the APN should order blood type and crossmatch, coagulation studies, CBC, electrolytes, BUN, creatinine, and urinalysis. Arterial blood gases and pulse oximetry may also be necessary. For suspected tickborne diseases such as Rocky Mountain spotted fever and Lyme disease, further laboratory studies are in order. For example, spirochetes can be seen in the blood smear in 70 percent of cases of tickborne relapsing fever. Lyme disease, Rocky Mountain spotted fever, and tularemia, which also occurs from tick bites, are diagnosed by antibody titer. However, results from these antibody titer assays are often not available for days to weeks, with empiric treatment often initiated prior to this. Thus, these tests are usually sent for confirmation only when a strong suspicion already exists and should not be sent indiscriminately.

Differential Diagnosis

Consultation with a regional poison control center may be indicated to correctly identify, diagnose, and/or treat arthropod bites and stings. It is very helpful to know which arthropods are indigenous to the local area, especially which ones have been causing recent infestations and injuries.

Bites of fleas, lice, and scabies mites produce lesions that are so similar that diagnosis is often difficult. Cercaria or nonhuman schistosomes cause similar lesions, which appear after the patient has been in infected water. Scabies has a more gradual onset but should also be considered in the differential diagnosis. The diagnosis of chigger infestation can usually be made on the basis of probable outdoor exposure and typical skin lesions. Patients who present with a "bull's-eye" rash following a suspected deer tick bite should be tested for Lyme disease.

When examining an urticarial reaction to an insect bite, other causes of urticaria should be considered, but if the hive has a central puncta, its cause is likely an insect bite. Other foreign bodies can produce pruritic papules in the skin. Dermatitis herpetiformis should be included in the differential diagnosis, particularly when only excoriations are found. Eruptions associated with other viruses or with atopic dermatitis, allergic or irritant contact dermatitis, and drug sensitivity must also be considered. An uncommon idiopathic disorder, Mucha-Habermann disease, also presents with scattered necrotic papules and vesicles, but this type of rash is usually more generalized and symmetric. Some of the other skin conditions that may be confused with local or systemic reactions to arthropod stings and bites include streptococcal necrotizing fasciitis, focal cutaneous necrosis, various infections, local thromboses, punctures, trauma, drug reactions, vasculitis, purpura, Arthus (type III, serum sickness) reactions, emboli to the skin, other bites that leave small puncture wounds, and artifacts.

Anaphylaxis from an insect sting may be confused with a vasovagal reaction, which is a disorder of central vasoregulation caused by increased parasympathetic tone mediated by the vagus nerve (cranial nerve X). A vasovagal reaction typically produces pallor, nausea, bradycardia, extreme diaphoresis, and hypotension that may result in syncope, whereas flushing, hypotension, tachycardia, and mucosal edema with severe bronchoconstriction are seen in anaphylaxis. Severe reactions to scorpion stings may present with symptoms similar to those of insecticide poisoning, with direct CNS effects.

Confirmation of stinging insect allergy is made by the detection of venom-specific IgE. This can be performed through an immediate reaction skin prick test, which measures the cutaneous histaminic response to dilute doses of allergen after scratching the skin surface with an antigen-coated needle tip, allowing for binding to IgE on skin mast cells with subsequent degranulation. Yellow jacket, honeybee, yellow hornet, bald-faced hornet, and wasp extracts are available for diagnosis and treatment of stinging insect allergies. A patient is considered sensitive if a skin reaction of 1+ or greater occurs at a venom concentration of 1 mg/mL or less, provided that the 1+ reaction is greater than that of the diluent control. This is the most sensitive test for picking up allergic states and is commonly used as an allergy screening tool. However, it lacks specificity and may thus overestimate allergic states.

IgE antibodies reacting with venom also may be measured by serum assay known as the radioallergosorbent test (RAST). In this test, a patient's serum is applied to a culture plate surface coated with the specific allergen of interest, allowing for specific antibody-binding to the plate. After excess serum is rinsed away, a second fluorescent-labeled antibody specific for the constant region of IgE is applied to the plate to reveal any of the patient's antigen-specific IgE which bound to the plate during the first step of the assay. Thus, the greater the amount of fluorescence, the higher the concentration of antigen-specific IgE in the patient's serum. The RAST is not as sensitive as the skin test, although it is more specific and is thus more effective in ruling out, rather than ruling in an allergic state.

Management

Emergency Management

Anaphylactic shock is a true emergency; the clinician should focus on stabilizing the patient while arranging for immediate transport to the ED if necessary.

Systemic or Anaphylactic Reactions. It should be stressed that anaphylaxis may be triggered by etiologies other than bites and stings. Anaphylactic reactions are extreme emergencies and may be a reaction iatrogenically by medications, environmental exposures, and especially food allergies, which are quite common. The treatment for anaphylaxis is standard and is included here.

The clinician should place a conscious patient in a comfortable position, ensuring unimpeded ventilation. Hypotensive patients should be placed supine or in a modified Trendelenburg position if respiratory status allows.

The clinician must maintain an adequate upper airway and give supplemental oxygen by mask or nebulizer with inhaled racemic epinephrine (0.5 mL of 2.25 percent epinephrine in 2 mL of NS), not to exceed three treatments in 60 minutes. In the case of impending upper airway compromise, inadequate oxygenation, or profound shock, the clinician must prepare for endotracheal intubation. Cricothyrotomy is to be performed if severe angioedema precludes intubation via the oral route.

In the situation of isolated cutaneous anaphylactic responses, early and minimal airway edema, and mild bronchospasm, the clinician should administer aqueous epinephrine 1:1000 subcutaneously (SC) in the deltoid region. The dose is 0.3 to 0.5 mg every 10 to 20 minutes as indicated. One can inject 0.1 to 0.2 mg of the epinephrine dose directly into the sting bite, causing vasoconstriction and reduction of swelling. If the reaction is limited to urticaria and pruritis, there is no wheezing or facial swelling, and the victim is more than 45 years old, one should reserve epinephrine for a worsened condition. Epinephrine maintains the blood pressure, causes bronchial dilation, and antagonizes adverse actions of the mediators of anaphylaxis. It also reduces the subsequent release of mediators through its action on mast cells and basophils.

In the setting of vasodilatory anaphylactic responses with hypotension, laryngeal edema, or severe bronchospasm, when there is no response to SC epinephrine, IV administration is a more appropriate route. Epinephrine is the single most life-saving treatment in the reversal of hypotension, airway edema, and bronchoconstriction associated with anaphylaxis. The clinician should place 0.1 mg (1 mL of 1:10,000 solution epinephrine) in 10 mL of normal saline solution (NS) and give it as a slow IV push over 10 minutes. This dose is to be repeated once or twice every 10 minutes as required. Alternatively, a continuous infusion of IV epinephrine at 1 to 5 mg/min can be started. This is constituted by adding 1 mg of 1:1000 aqueous epinephrine (1 mL) to 250 mL NS, creating a concentration of 4 mg/mL.

Excessive infusion rates may be associated with cardiac ischemia and arrhythmias. One-half of the above recommended doses should be used initially in elderly patients or those with cardiovascular disease, diabetes mellitus, thyroid disease, cerebral arteriosclerosis, or Parkinson's disease. Patients who are taking beta-adrenergic blocking agents may be refractory to treatment with epinephrine. Glucagon (5 to 15 mg/min IV) may be a useful agent in the treatment of anaphylaxis in the presence of beta blockade.

Antihistamines are included in the treatment regimen. With H_1-blocking antihistamines, the clinician may administer diphenhydramine (Benadryl) 50 mg to 75 mg IV or PO q6 to 8h as needed (in severe anaphylaxis, administer 100 mg IV initially); or hydroxyzine (Vistaril) 25 to 50 mg IM q6 to 8h as needed. The newer generation H_1 blockers such as cetirizine (Zyrtec, fexofenadine (Allegra), and desloratadine (Clarinex) are less sedating and may be just as effective if the patient may be treated with oral medications. For H_2-blocking antihistamines, the clinician may administer cimetidine (Tagamet) 300 mg IV q6h; or ranitidine (Zantac) 50 mg IV q6 to 8h. If available, cimetidine is the preferred H_2 blocker, because it has greater peripheral effects than does ranitidine, which is more GI-tract specific.

The clinician should treat bronchospasm as necessary with albuterol (2.5 mg in 3 mL of NS) 2.5 to 5 mg via nebulizer every 20 minutes as necessary. A loading dose of aminophylline 6 mg/kg IV (if the patient is not currently taking aminophylline or theophylline) may be administered over 20 to 30 minutes, followed by a continuous IV infusion (0.7 mg/kg/h) in otherwise healthy nonsmoking adults.

Circulatory support should be provided as necessary. The clinician can infuse 0.5 to 1 L of either NS or lactated Ringer's solution every 20 to 30 minutes as needed to support the blood pressure at a level above 90 mm Hg systolic. The need for further fluid resuscitation should be determined by monitoring blood pressure, cardiac rhythm, and urine output. Usually a total of 3 L can be given rapidly to an adult without ill effect. The clinician should be cautious with patients with CHF or the elderly, given the risk of pulmonary edema. Hypotension that is refractory to epinephrine and IV fluids may be treated with norepinephrine (Levophed) 1 mg/mL in 4-mL ampuls) 2 to 12 mg/min via IV infusion. Phenylephrine (Neo-Synephrine) 10 mg/mL in 1-mL ampuls) 0.1 to 0.5 mg IV bolus every 10 to 15 minutes as necessary, or 100 to 180 mg/min as a continuous IV infusion may also be used. The infusion should be decreased to 40 to 60 mg/min once blood pressure has stabilized; or treat with glucagon: place 1 mg in 1 L of 5 percent dextrose in water (D5/W) and administer IV at rate of 5 to 15 mg/min. Glucagon is useful in patients on beta-adrenergic blocking agents because it stimulates cardiac inotropic and chronotropic function independent of beta blockade. Patients taking beta-blockers may also benefit from terbutaline (0.25 mg SC, not to exceed 0.5 mg SC q4h).

If the allergic reaction is prolonged or severe, or if the patient is regularly medicated with corticosteroids, the clinician should administer hydrocortisone 200 mg, methylprednisolone (Solu-Medrol) 50 mg, or dexamethasone 15 mg IV, with a 10-day oral taper to follow. If the therapy is initiated orally, the clinician should administer prednisone 60 to 100 mg.

General Management

Normal Reactions. Normal reactions to arthropod bites and stings do not require treatment other than local applications of cold compresses (ice) and analgesics. Nonsteroidal anti-inflammatory drugs (NSAIDs) such as ibuprofen (Motrin) 800 mg PO are effective if given immediately, because they block prostaglandins. Secondary infections are common, therefore a topical antimicrobial ointment such as mupirocin 2 percent (Bactroban) ointment should be applied to the area.

Large Local Reactions. Large local reactions to arthropod bites or stings are treated with antihistamines, such as diphenhydramine (Benadryl) 50 to 75 mg IV or PO and cimetidine (Tagamet) 300 mg IV or PO. Intramuscular administration of diphenhydramine is not usually done because of the pain involved and the fact that the drug is absorbed very rapidly PO. A corticosteroid such as methylprednisolone (Medrol) 24 mg PO the first day, then tapered over 5 days, will hasten resolution of a large local reaction to a bee or wasp sting. Tapering slowly prevents a rebound flare-up of symptoms. Some clinicians also administer IV calcium gluconate (5 to 10 mL of 10 percent solution).

Delayed Serum Sickness-Type Reactions. Delayed serum sickness-type reactions in response to multiple bee, wasp, or fire ant stings can be managed with a corticosteroid such as prednisone (Deltasone) 60 to 100 mg, tapered over 2 weeks. The pruritus caused by insect bites can be controlled by a variety of oral antihistamines. Hydroxyzine (Atarax, Vistaril) is commonly prescribed, because its dosage is very flexible and it produces few anticholinergic adverse effects. If patients are driving and working during the day, they should reserve the hydroxyzine for nighttime use, to help with sleep. Treatment of urticaria may also require an antihistamine that is an H_2 blocker, such as cimetidine.

For arthropod bites, when topical steroids are needed, class I (e.g., betamethasone dipropionate [Diprolene ointment 0.05 percent]) or class II (e.g., fluocinonide [Lidex cream 0.05 percent]) topical steroids may be administered bid. Lesions may take weeks to resolve. Topical antipruritics include lotions with 0.25 percent menthol, 1 percent phenol, or both (Sarna lotion), and topical anesthetics such as pramoxine (Pramosone). Topical antihistamines and benzocaine are not recommended because of their potential for allergic sensitization. Topical doxepin (Zonalon) is now available and is effective. Infected insect bites can be treated with topical 2 percent mupirocin (Bactroban) or neomycin. Extensive impetigo will need treatment with oral antibiotics, dicloxacillin (Dynapen), or erythromycin (EES).

Hymenoptera Stings. When a patient is stung by a honeybee, the stinger should be removed by scraping it with a dull object. The stinger should not be grasped and pulled, because this contracts the venom sac, thus releasing more toxin. Wasps and other bees do not leave a stinger and are capable of stinging many times. One should cleanse the site and apply antiseptic. Blisters from fire ant stings should not be broken. Ice should be applied with a pack, with or without a paste of papain (unseasoned meat tenderizer), and the part should be elevated.

There is no specific antivenin for Hymenoptera stings. If the reaction is extensive, or if there is envenomation from multiple stings, more aggressive therapy may be indicated. This includes administering IV calcium gluconate (5 to 10 mL of 10 percent solution) with a parenteral antihistamine, diphenhydramine, 50 to 100 mg IV or orally. Oral prednisone, 40 mg daily for 2 to 3 days, can be very helpful in reducing the local swelling. Appropriate tetanus prophylaxis should be completed. In severe envenomations, an IV corticosteroid such as hydrocortisone, 2 mg/kg should be administered at the earliest opportunity (see also section on Systemic or Anaphylactic Reactions above).

Brown Recluse Spider Bite. The patient should apply cold compresses intermittently for the first 4 days after the bite, over a sterile dressing. Administer an oral antibiotic, such as dicloxacillin (250 to 500 mg q4 to 6h for 10 days), cephalexin (250 mg q4 to 6h or 500 mg q12h), or erythromycin (250 mg qid for 10 days). Ice and elevation may be beneficial. Drug treatment is controversial; many brown recluse spider bites are minor and heal without specific treatment other than tetanus prophylaxis. One current treatment for a severe wound is to obtain a glucose-6-phosphate dehydrogenase (G6PD) screen, and if negative, immediately give dapsone (Avlosulfon) 50 mg (adult dose) orally bid for 10 days. If G6PD enzyme deficiency is documented, the patient should discontinue dapsone to avoid hemolysis.

Black Widow Spider Bite. The natural course of the envenomation is to resolve completely after a few days, with pain persisting for a week or more. Ice should be applied judiciously to the bite wound. The clinician should administer a narcotic analgesic, such as morphine. All opioids may have a histaminic agonist effect, so these medications should be avoided in cases with significant histaminic responses.

Muscle relaxants such as diazepam (Valium) may also be given. The patient should be monitored for hypertension and administered a centrally acting or vasodilating antihypertensive if necessary. An alternative, more controversial treatment for black widow spider bites would be to add calcium gluconate 0.1 to 0.2 mL/kg IV given slowly to alleviate muscle spasm. Reserve antivenin for seriously ill infants and older patients and proceed with horse serum sensitivity testing. One vial of antivenin is sufficient for most patients; give 1 ampule (2.5 mL) in 10 to 50 mL NS by slow IV infusion.

Scorpion (Centroides exilicauda) Bite. The patient should apply ice for 30 minutes each hour to relieve local pain. Intense cooling should be avoided and the affected part should be immobilized. Do not apply a tourniquet. Opiate analgesics should be avoided because they potentiate the toxicity of the venom and may lead to apnea. The clinician should administer diazepam or phenobarbital to control seizures, along with sympathetic antihypertensive agents to control hypertension. Hyperthermia from uncontrolled muscular activity can be managed with cooling. The administration of antivenom (antivenin) is controversial because it is derived from horse serum and thus carries a risk of anaphylaxis. Horse serum sensitivity testing is done to screen against anaphylaxis which is a risk with many of the antivenin medications. Anti-venin should be administered only in a hospital critical care setting.

Tick Bite. The clinician should always remove ticks. The tick can be covered with alcohol, machine oil, mineral oil, salad oil, or gasoline on a tissue or gauze pad. This blocks the tick's breathing pores and causes it to withdraw from the skin. It may take 30 minutes for the tick to disengage its mouthparts. Ticks should not be removed manually because squeezing the tick's body may inject more viral or bacterial pathogens into the victim. The clinician should observe for a local reaction or infection at the site. Most victims of tick paralysis will show improvement within hours of tick removal and return to normal in several days. Patients with Rocky Mountain spotted fever or Lyme disease will require further treatment, including antibiotics, and follow-up monitoring for chronic health problems.

Flea Bites. The patient should clean the lesions well with soap and water and apply a topical antiseptic ointment. To relieve pruritus and discomfort, calamine lotion with phenol can be applied. A systemic antihistamine, such as hydroxyzine (Atarax), can be administered to control itching.

Chigger Bites. Chiggers are easily removed from the skin by taking a hot bath or shower and lathering with soap several times. The bath will kill attached chiggers. For moderate to severe cases, topical steroid creams and oral antihistamines may provide some relief. Systemic steroids will also provide relief for severe pruritus. Topical antibiotic therapy is indicated for secondary infection.

Mosquito Bites. Immediately after the person is bitten, he or she should apply a cold (ice) pack. A topical steroid ointment can be applied to the site. Oral steroids such as prednisone should be used only when the reaction is prolonged and severe, given their potential adverse effects.

Fly Bites. Fly bites are treated the same as mosquito bites. In addition, if the patient presents with cutaneous myiasis, the clinician should exert pressure to extrude the organism (fly larva). The larva may emerge if its breathing hole in the skin is occluded with heavy oil, nail polish, or bacon fat. Alternatively, the clinician can inject 2 mL of local anesthetic into the base of the lesion, thus extruding the larva by fluid pressure. Take care not to rupture the larva, because an inflammatory reaction may result.

Caterpillar Spine Irritation. Broken-off spines can be removed by applying adhesive tape, a commercial facial peel, or a thin layer of rubber cement. Then an oral antihistamine and/or NSAID can be administered. If the dermatitis is persistent and severe, the clinician should prescribe oral prednisone 60 to 100 mg for adults, to be tapered over 10 days.

Follow-Up and Referral

After a severe allergic reaction, further delayed reactions and recurrence of symptoms are possible, particularly as the effects of the medication decrease. Patients may benefit from repeated doses of antihistamines and glucocorticoids over the next several days. All patients with severe allergic reactions who are discharged home should have follow-up in 24 to 48 hours. All such patients should be referred to an allergy specialist.

Individuals who have experienced a serious anaphylactic reaction should be prescribed three kits for the self-administration of epinephrine by injection or nebulization (EpiPen or Ana-Kit) and instructed on its use. These patients should also keep in their kit some oral diphenhydramine and cimetidine. One kit should be kept in the glove compartment of the person's car, another in a bag or purse that is carried with the individual, and a third kit should be kept in the home.

Individuals with a history of an acute allergic reaction or a serum sickness-type reaction following an insect sting and who have positive venom skin tests are considered at risk for subsequent sting reactions. Venom immunotherapy to prevent such reactions may be recommended. Patients with large local reactions are not considered candidates for venom immunotherapy and do not require venom skin tests. Patients who have been treated for anaphylaxis and who use beta-adrenergic blocking agents should be switched to alternative medications.

Patient Education

Patient education information regarding arthropod bites and stings can be found in Table 18.5.

Table 18.5 Patient Education: Arthropod Bites and Stings

- Avoid mowing lawns or working with flowering ornamentals when bees and wasps are collecting nectar.
- Stand still if a stinging insect is near you. If it attacks, brush it off (do not slap at it) to prevent a sting.
- Do not walk in the yard in bare feet.
- Wear gloves when gardening.
- Keep garbage cans covered outdoors. Sweet items like soft drinks, ripened fruits, and watermelons attract bees and wasps.
- Avoid perfumes, hair sprays, and colognes.
- Pick fruit as it ripens or dispose of rotten fruits.
- If you are attacked by a swarm of bees, wasps, yellow jackets, or hornets, leave the area immediately, using your arms to protect your face.
- Control wasps by applying insecticides to the nest.
- Avoid areas where insect exposure is likely to occur and always wear shoes when outdoors.
- Avoid wearing perfumes, after-shave lotions, and brightly colored clothing, because these attract insects.
- If you are allergic to bee or wasp stings or to any medication, wear medical identification jewelry indicating the anaphylaxis-causing substance or event.
- Check bathrobes and bedsheets for spiders if you are about to use them after a long absence.
- When you enter an attic or storeroom to open cardboard boxes, give the brown recluse spiders a chance to vacate, as they will avoid you if they can.
- Have someone try to capture the spider for identification, immediately seek health care, and contact the local poison control center.
- Treat pets for ticks by using dusts, dips, or sprays.
- When you enter tick-infested areas, keep clothing buttoned, shirts tucked inside trousers, and trousers inside boots.
- Wear light-colored clothing, because this makes it easier to spot ticks; lighter clothing is also less attractive to biting flies.
- Do not sit on the ground or on logs in brushy areas.
- Keep brush cleared or pruned along frequently traveled areas. Use repellents to protect exposed skin; however, ticks will crawl over treated skin to untreated parts of the body.
- For treatment of flea infestations, treat not only the pet, but also professionally fumigate the house.
- If you are going into areas suspected of being infested with chiggers, wear protective clothing and use repellents.
- Apply a repellent containing *N,N*-diethyl-3-methylbenzamide (commonly known as DEET) and wear permethrin-impregnated fabric.
- Apply repellents to legs, ankles, cuffs, waist, and sleeves by applying them to clothing or directly to the body as directed by the label.
- Avoid unnecessary use of lights at campsites and camp in a site that is high, dry, open, and uncluttered.

Head Trauma

Head trauma that may be encountered by the clinician in a primary-care setting include cerebral contusions, concussions, skull fracture, epidural or subdural hematomas. In contrast, subarachnoid hemorrhage typically results from the spontaneous rupture of intracranial aneurysms (greater than 80 percent of cases), rather than a traumatic etiology.

Epidemiology and Causes

Head trauma is a leading cause of morbidity and mortality in the United States. It affects approximately 2 million persons per year, with about 1 head injury occurring every 15 seconds. About 30 percent of all visits to the ED are for treatment of head-related injuries. The vast majority of head trauma result from motor vehicle accidents (MVAs) in young adults 15 to 24 years of age. The next most common causes are football and wrestling in men and soccer and basketball in women. In people older than age 65, falls account for the majority of head injury deaths. Traumatic brain injury (TBI) may also be the result of drugs and alcohol, violence, and sports-related injuries.

Pathophysiology

Mild head trauma is usually the result of a sudden deceleration injury or rotation force that causes shearing forces within the brain. These forces cause axonal and blood vessel disruptions. Injury to small blood vessels can manifest themselves as petechial hemorrhages, or, if the bridging veins connecting the cortex to the venous sinuses are involved, acute subdural hematomas may occur, which are potentially fatal. In contrast, subarachnoid hemorrhages, with their resultant meningeal findings including extreme headache and neck stiffness, result far more commonly from ruptured intracranial saccular aneurysms, also called berry aneurysms (greater than 80 percent of cases), rather than from trauma.

The area of cerebral injury becomes ischemic and edematous. As edema increases, the autoregulatory control of intracranial vessels is lost. The blood-brain barrier breaks down, resulting in increased loss of fluid into the brain parenchyma, which in turn results in increased intracranial pressure (ICP). As ICP increases, cerebral blood flow decreases, leading to tissue hypoxia, a decrease in the serum pH level, and an increase in the carbon dioxide level. This process leads to cerebral vasodilation, and edema, which further increases the ICP (a vicious cycle). The increased ICP causes compromise in cerebral perfusion that, if not treated and reversed, leads to increasing hypoxia and secondary brain injury. If the condition remains untreated, the brain herniates downward toward the brainstem, causing irreversible brain damage. A summary of the clinical features of ICP and management guidelines is provided in Table 18.6.

Cerebral Contusion

A *cerebral contusion* is a focal brain injury involving cortical bruising and at times, vessel lacerations. This is one of the most common cerebral injuries; it is associated with hemorrhage, edema, and brain swelling. Contusions are

TREATMENT FLOWCHART 18.1
HEAD TRAUMA

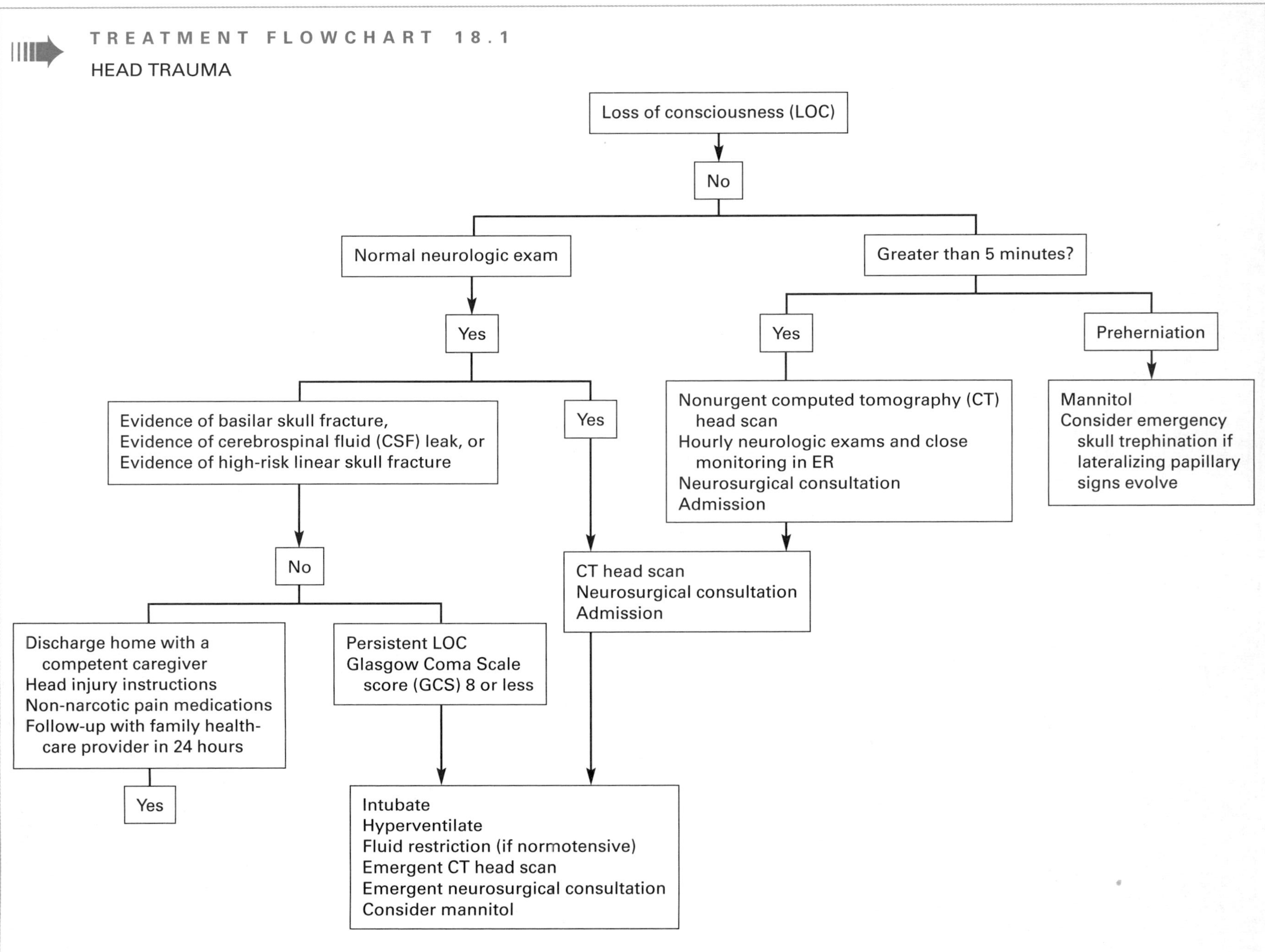

Table 18.6 Clinical Features and Management of Increased Intracranial Pressure (ICP)

0–15 mm Hg: normal
>15 mm Hg: increased

Clinical Features	Management to Reduce ICP
Decrease in level of consciousness (LOC) Headache Nausea Vomiting Amnesia Agitation, restlessness Increased BP with a widening pulse pressure Decreased pulse rate Changes in respiratory rate and pattern Papilledema, one or both eyes **Pupil Assessment** PERL—pupils equal and react to light PERRL—pupils equal, round, and react to light PERRLA—pupils equal, round, react to light and accommodation (All synonymous)	Elevation of head Restriction of fluids Acetazolamide (Diamox) 250 mg qid Induced hyperventilation Intravenous mannitol (Osmitrol) infusion Intravenous furosemide (Lasix) Possible surgical evacuation of hematoma

classified as *coup* (injury directly beneath the point of impact) or *contrecoup* (injury directly opposite the point of impact). Temporal and frontal lobes are the most common sites affected. Contusions are graded as mild or severe, and superficial or deep. Superficial contusions usually involve the cortical and subcortical tissue, whereas deep contusions penetrate the white matter.

Concussion

A *concussion* involves diffuse brain injury. It is associated with a transient loss of consciousness that occurs immediately following nonpenetrating blunt head trauma. Most patients with only a brief loss of consciousness (less than 5 minutes) are not admitted to the hospital if their subsequent neurologic exam remains within normal limits. However, close observation by a responsible adult educated in the warning signs of neurologic deterioration is critical for at least the next 24 hours.

A mild concussion is associated with a slightly longer loss of consciousness. It classically presents with confusion, disorientation, and at times, retrograde amnesia (inability to recall events surrounding the injury) or posttraumatic amnesia. The confusion and disorientation usually last only minutes, but recurrent dizziness, headache, and difficulty concentrating may last for months.

A classic concussion, resulting from a loss of consciousness of less than 6 minutes, typically produces retrograde and posttraumatic amnesia and mild neurologic impairment. The duration of amnesia can be a predictor of severity: The longer the amnesia, the more severe the concussion. Severe concussions usually have a normal head CT scan and neurologic exam; however, these patients are typically admitted to the hospital for close observation.

Postconcussion syndrome is usually associated with mild head trauma. The syndrome consists of the following signs and symptoms, which can start as early as 1 day posttrauma and persist up to 6 months post-injury—headaches, dizziness, fatigue, irritability, insomnia, anxiety, impaired concentration, and loss of memory. Loss of consciousness does not have to occur for postconcussion syndrome to develop, and it is estimated that up to 50 percent of patients who suffer mild head trauma will develop this syndrome.

Skull Fracture

Skull fracture may occur with a severe blow to the head. Skull fracture increases the risk of underlying epidural or subdural hematoma. Basilar skull fractures (fracture of the base of the skull) can occur as an extension of fracture in another area of the skull. Basilar skull fractures can cause leakage of cerebrospinal fluid (CSF), an entry point for bacteria leading to meningitis, or pneumocephalus (air entry into the CSF-filled spaces within the head). Key clinical manifestations associated with basilar skull fracture are hemotympanum (blood behind the tympanic membrane), ecchymosis over the mastoid process ("Battle's sign"), or periorbital ecchymosis ("raccoon sign"). Routine x-ray films may not reveal skull fracture; therefore, these clinical manifestations should be sought as evidence of basilar skull fracture. CSF may leak through the cribiform plate region of the skull causing nasal CSF rhinorrhea. Patients with suspected skull fracture require careful examination of the cranial nerves. Cranial nerves (CN) which are likely to be injured include the olfactory nerve (CN I), optic nerve (CN II), oculomotor nerve (CN III), trochlear nerve (CN IV), trigeminal nerve (CN V), abducens nerve (CN VI), facial nerve (CN VII), and acoustic nerve (CN VIII).

Epidural Hematoma

Severe head trauma can cause intracranial bleeding which can put pressure on the brain tissue. The brain is surrounded by the meninges: three layers of protective membranes. The layers from the cranial bone going interiorly consist of the dura mater, arachnoid membrane, and pia mater (see Fig. 18.2). Between each membrane is a compartment or space where blood from ruptured vessels can collect. Between the cranial bone and dura mater is the epidural space. The middle meningeal artery courses through this space and

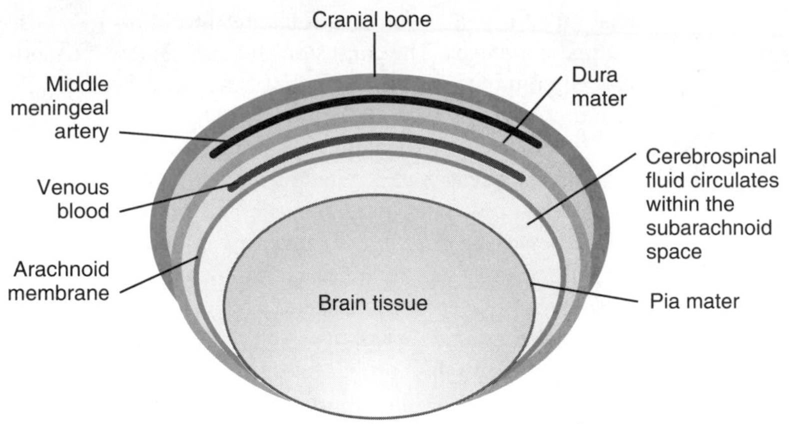

FIGURE 18.2 The layers of the meninges and cranial circulation. (Courtesy of Teri Capriotti, DO, MSN, CRNP.)

can rupture when the cranium (skull) is fractured. The middle meningeal artery runs tightly along the wall of the cranial bone forming grooves in the bone. With a skull fracture, this artery is easily ruptured and bleeds rapidly within the epidural space resulting in an *epidural hematoma*. The volume of blood may be large enough to displace the brain causing neurologic deficits and coma within hours after skull injury. Skull x-ray films reveal a fracture line that passes through a groove on the cranium. A head CT scan can visualize the region of the bleed, and brain dysfunction is due primarily to parenchymal compression, which can be relieved with evacuation of blood from the epidural space.

Subdural Hematoma

Head trauma can also cause a *subdural hematoma*, which is a venous bleed. Venous bleeding occurs within the subdural space—the compartment between the dura mater and arachnoid membrane (see Fig. 18.3). A venous bleed is slow and will clot off in a short amount of time. Thus, a subdural hematoma may develop slowly over days to weeks and can be due to relatively mild head trauma. Thus, subdural hematomas may be acute (less than 72 hours old), subacute (between 3 and 20 days old) or chronic (greater than 20 days old). Acute subdural hematomas most commonly result from traumatic rupture of the bridging veins, which span the cortex and the dural venous sinuses. If such acute bleeds require surgical intervention and are not rapidly treated within several hours postinjury, mortality rates are strikingly high (up to 90 percent in some series).

In contrast, chronic subdural hematomas pose less of a mortality threat. The majority originate from subdural hygromas, which are potential spaces formed between the dura mater and the brain surface following separation of the dura–arachnoid interface due to ischemic or traumatic brain injury of atrophy resulting in a loss of brain parenchyma. These spaces become filled with CSF. A neomembrane eventually forms which lines the space, becoming a site of neovascularization by fragile intracranial vessels prone to rupture and formation of the chronic subdural hematoma.

Neurologic deficits may not be noted until a large volume of blood is present. Brain dysfunction is primarily due to parenchymal compression, which can be relieved with evacuation of blood from the subdural space. CT scans and x-ray studies may not clearly reveal a subdural hematoma, making it difficult to diagnose. MRI can show displaced brain tissue away from the skull which is a key finding of subdural hematoma. Patients on anticoagulants, with coagulation deficiencies, or liver impairment are particularly susceptible to subdural hematomas. Alco-

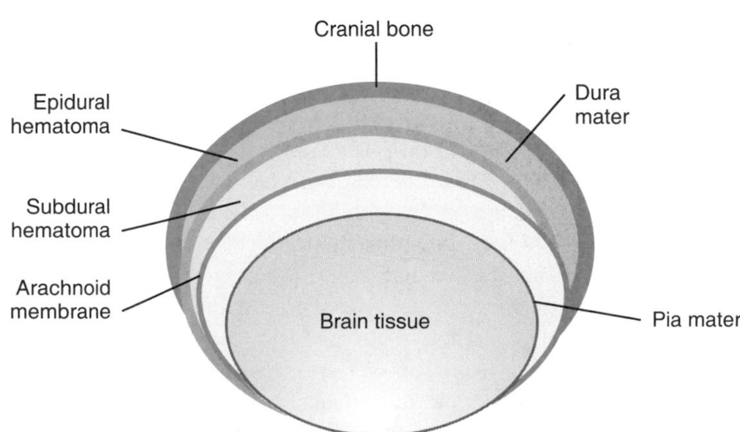

FIGURE 18.3 Location of epidural and subdural hematomas. (Courtesy of Teri Capriotti, DO, MSN, CRNP.)

hol abusers are also susceptible to subdural hematomas which may be a subacute as well as an acute condition. It can be a slowly evolving source of increased intracranial pressure.

Clinical Presentation

Subjective

A full history of the event causing the head injury is needed. This should include the mechanism of injury, an approximation of the amount of force involved with the trauma (if the event was witnessed), and whether the patient experienced loss of consciousness (LOC). Epidural hematomas are especially characterized by the patient losing consciousness briefly, then a brief 'lucid' moment when the patient may be awake and talking, followed by a momentary unconsciousness occuring minutes after the injury, then becoming increasingly symptomatic, possibly progressing to coma. If a family member or friend is with the patient, the clinician should ask that person if the patient appears normal; a person close to the patient can identify subtle changes that the clinician may not recognize. Patients may complain of headaches and confusion. When a patient complains of "the worst headache of my life," the clinician should suspect a subarachnoid bleed or subarachnoid hemorrhage.

Clinical presentation depends upon the structures involved. General symptoms include behavior, motor, and speech deficits. Intoxicated patients present clinical challenges. Signs and symptoms of cerebral injury can be masked by alcohol intoxication. These patients require a head CT scan, close monitoring, and serial neurologic exams until they are sober, because their history and initial physical exam will be unreliable. (See Table on Traumatic Brain Injuries 18.7.)

Objective

A patient presenting with a head injury should receive a rapid neurologic exam to rule out significant cerebral injury. This exam should include checking mental status, cranial nerves, extremity strength, deep tendon reflexes, and cerebellar function. Hypoactive reflexes may result from damage to the spinal cord.

The Glasgow Coma Scale (GCS) may also be used to rapidly evaluate the level of consciousness (see Advanced Assessment 18.2). The GCS establishes baseline data in each of three areas; eye opening, motor response, and verbal response. A numerical score is assigned according to the chart. A score of 15 represents normal neurologic function; a score of 7 usually indicates an unconscious patient, and a score of 3 represents a deep coma state. With any head trauma, the GCS should be done at least every two hours to assess for any changes.

The clinician may note bradycardia, hypotension, somnolence, seizures, and focal deficits. With a cerebral hemorrhage, these clinical features generally develop immediately after the trauma. These symptoms develop several hours after the injury with an acute epidural hemorrhage. An acute subdural hemorrhage may occur in a day, or may occur months after the head trauma.

All patients should be monitored for signs of an increased intracranial pressure (ICP). (See Nursing Research–Based Practice 18.1.) The early signs of increased ICP are headache, nausea and vomiting, amnesia, altered level of consciousness, changes in speech, drowsiness, agitation, restlessness, and/or loss of judgment. Any of these signs should prompt the caretaker to take the patient to the ED immediately.

Late signs of increased ICP are dilated, nonreactive pupils (from pressure on the oculomotor nerve), unrespon-

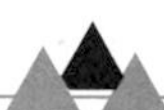

NURSING RESEARCH-BASED PRACTICE 18.1

Teasdale, TW, and Engberg, AW: Subjective well-being and quality of life following traumatic brain injury in adults: A long-term population-based follow-up. Brain Inj 19(12):1041–1048, 2005.

Primary Objective: To assess subjective well-being and quality-of-life in nationally representative samples of patients at long intervals following traumatic brain injuries.
Methods and Procedures: Patients with either cranial fractures or cerebral lesions were identified in a national computer-based register of hospital admissions and random samples were selected among those who had suffered the injury at 5, 10, or 15 years prior to the follow-up. Postal questionnaires were sent to them covering quality of life, for example, return to employment, family relationships, and current subjective well-being in terms of symptomatology, for example, somatic complaints, cognitive dysfunction. A response rate of 76% was obtained, comprising 114 patients with cranial fracture and 126 with cerebral lesions.
Main Outcomes and Results: The group with cerebral lesions had markedly poorer quality of life and subjective well-being than the group with cranial fractures and this did not vary across time. In both groups, the most common symptoms concerned cognition. Among the cerebral lesion group, quality of life outcome was fairly well predicted by severity of injury, but subjective well-being was less well predicted.
Conclusions: The negative consequences of traumatic cerebral lesions are marked and do not vary at long periods following injury.

ADVANCED ASSESSMENT 18.2

Rapid Neurologic Exam

Level of Consciousness

Glasgow Coma Scale

Motor Response	6	Follows commands
	5	Localizes pain on stimulus
	4	Withdraws from painful stimulus
	3	Shows abnormal flexion in response to pain
	2	Shows abnormal extension in response to pain
	1	No response
Verbal Response	5	Oriented
	4	Confused
	3	Inappropriate words
	2	Unintelligible sounds
	1	No responses
Eye-Opening	4	Spontaneous
	3	Opens eyes on verbal command
	2	Opens eyes on painful stimulus
	1	No response

Score: 14 = normal; <7 = coma

Mental Status

FOGS

Family story

Orientation

General information

Spelling

Calculations

Count backward from 100 by sevens or repeat a three-digit number

Recall

Recall two objects

Cranial Nerves

CNI	Olfactory	Smell (not usually assessed during acute exam)
CNII	Optic	Visual acuity, gross visual fields, fundoscopic exam
CNIII	Oculomotor	Pupillary response, eye movement (upward and medial gaze)
CNIV	Trochlear	Eye movement (downward and medial gaze)
CNV	Trigeminal	Teeth clenching, corneal reflex
CNVI	Abducens	Eye movement (lateral)
CNVII	Facial	Frown, smile, and puff cheeks; assess symmetry
CNVIII	Acoustic	Hearing
CNIX	Glossopharyngeal	Gag reflex
CNX	Vagus	Swallowing, gag reflex
CNXI	Spinal accessory	Shrug shoulders and turn head; assess strength and symmetry
CNXII	Hypoglossal	Articulation and tongue movement

Gross Motor Strength and Symmetry

Upper and lower extremities	Look for symmetry and strength

Cerebellar Function

Romberg's test	Look for stability and pronator drift
Coordination	Finger to nose and heel to shin
Reflexes	Biceps, triceps, patellar, Achilles, Babinski

siveness to verbal or painful stimuli, abnormal posturing patterns (e.g., flexion, extension, or flaccidity), increased systolic blood pressure resulting in a widening pulse pressure, decreased pulse rate, and changes in respiratory rate and pattern. The last three are known as the *Cushing response or reflex*. The late signs are usually observed in patients who are hospitalized and currently being monitored.

In addition, a patient with a basilar skull fracture should be assessed for:

- Hemotympanum—blood behind the tympanic membrane
- Battle's sign—ecchymosis over the mastoid process
- Raccoon sign—periorbital ecchymosis
- Rhinorrhea with CSF, or ear drainate with CSF
- Alterations with cranial nerve function:
  - CNI, olfactory nerve—anosmia, may experience loss of smell, or hyposmia
  - CNII, optic nerve blindness, field cuts
  - CNIII, oculomotor nerve—assess for PERL problems indicative of increased ICP, loss of eye movements, diplopia, ptosis, dilated or unreactive pupil
  - CNIV, trochlear nerve—impaired downward gaze, diplopia
  - CNV, facial nerve—loss of sensation, absent blink/ corneal reflex, muscle atrophy
  - CNVI, abducens nerve—eye fails to abduct, diplopia
  - CNVII, facial nerve—if lower motor neuron affected—ipsilateral (same side) weakness of entire side of face, loss of corneal reflex. If upper motor neuron affected—contralateral (opposite side)

    Weakness of lower half of face.

    Lost, delayed, or metallic taste
  - CNVIII, acoustic nerve—dizziness, hearing loss

Diagnostic Reasoning

Diagnostic Tests

For mild head injuries, if the patient did not have a loss of consciousness, and did not exhibit focal neurologic signs or have a history of significant mechanism of injury, close monitoring by a responsible adult is appropriate.

Patients with a history of LOC, significant mechanism of injury (which includes a fall that is equal to their height), a Glasgow Coma Scale score of 14 or less, impaired alertness or memory, a palpable depressed fracture, signs of increased ICP, positive findings on a rapid neurologic exam, or a documented skull fracture, should have a head CT scan. A plain CT scan is indicated; CT with contrast is not indicated for minor head trauma. If a cerebral hemorrhage is found, emergent surgery is indicated.

Electroencephalography (EEG) may be helpful when a posttraumatic seizure disorder is suspected. A lumbar puncture may be done for support in diagnosing subarachnoid hemorrhage as indicated by the presence of red blood cells, elevated proteins, and a moderate reduction in glucose. A lumbar puncture is contraindicated in an intracerebral hemorrhage as it may precipitate a herniation syndrome in patients with a large hematoma. MRI can show displaced brain tissue away from the skull, a key finding with a subdural hematoma.

Differential Diagnosis

Typically, a patient with a head trauma will present following an injury, making the diagnosis obvious. However, if a closed head injury occurred and the patient is comatose, other conditions that can result in coma must be ruled out, such as drug overdose, cerebral vascular accident (CVA), diabetic ketoacidosis, neuromuscular disorders, and so on.

Management

Emergency Management

A thorough history and physical exam is necessary for any patient who presents with a head injury. Immobilization should be maintained until the patient is fully awake and x-ray and/or CT findings are negative.

General Management

A patient with a minor head injury may be sent home with a competent caregiver who is able to follow the instructions listed under Patient Education. Management of patients with traumatic brain injuries is presented in Table 18.7.

Patients with temporal cerebral injury can be problematic, because these structures are close to the tentorium and midbrain. Progressive edema can lead to elevated ICP and herniation. It is important that the clinician repeat neurologic assessments often, to look for subtle changes that represent early signs of increased ICP. The earlier they are identified and treatment is begun, the better the prognosis for the patient. (See Nursing Research–Based Practice 18.1.)

An abstract on a complementary therapy used following traumatic injury is presented in Nursing Research–Based Practice Box 18.2.

Follow-Up and Referral

A patient with a mild head injury who is sent home with competent caregiver may not need any follow-up unless problems develop. The patient and caregiver must be alert to signs and symptoms of increased ICP (see Patient Education).

The patient with a severe head injury will be followed by a neurosurgeon. The patient may be discharged from the hospital directly to a rehabilitation facility and will be followed by their staff.

Research has shown that the prevalence of any psychiatric illness in the first year following moderate to severe traumatic brain injury approached 49 percent, and 34 percent followng mild TBI. Persons with a mild traumatic brain injury with prior psychiatric illness had evidence of persisting psychiatric illness. Patients with any TBI should be followed closely and monitored for any affective disorders to determine the need for early postinjury psychiatric intervention.

Patient Education

The patient with a mild head injury should be with a responsible adult for the first 24 hours after injury. Decreased activity and light diet are recommended for the first 24 hours. The patient should be awakened every 2 to 4 hours during the first 24 hours. The patient should report back if he or she develops vomiting, an inability to move their arms or legs

Table 18.7 Traumatic Brain Injuries (TBI)

Injury	Clinical Features	Diagnosis	Management
Concussion	Brief loss of consciousness (<5 minutes) Mild concussion—slightly longer loss of consciousness, confusion, disorientation, retrograde amnesia, recurrent dizziness, headache, dizziness, vertigo, difficulty concentrating, bradycardia, hypotension, transient neurologic deficits, visual disturbances	History MRI PET	Close observation for 24 h Non-narcotic pain medications
Cerebral contusion	Longer loss of consciousness Localizing personality, behavior, motor, and speech deficits Intracranial pressure (ICP) elevation	History	Monitor Glasgow Coma Scale (GCS) Neurologic consultant
Basilar skull fracture	Hemotympanum—blood behind tympanic membrane Battle's sign—ecchymosis over mastoid process Raccoon sign—periorbital ecchymosis CSF rhinorrhea Alterations in cranial nerve functioning CSF otorrhea	Cranial nerve examination Skull x-ray films CT	Monitor GCS Neurologic consultant Antibiotics if infection present Rare—intracranial surgical repair Monitor intracranial pressure
Epidural hematoma	Brief loss of consciousness→lucid moment→longer period of loss of consciousness Headache, confusion, somnolence, seizures, focal deficits, pupil abnormalities (unilateral and eventual bilateral pupil dilatation and decreased reactivity to light) Hemiparesis or hemiplegia, flexion or extension posturing	CT scan	Monitor GCS Monitor ICP Neurologic consultant With a significant mass effect—immediate surgical evacuation and ligation of bleeding vessels. If not possible, burr holes to evacuate hematoma
Subdural hematoma (SDH)	Extreme headache, neck stiffness Progressive decrease in level of consciousness, ataxia, seizures, incontinence, and eventual pupil and motor function alterations With severe SDH, GCS usually <8	MRI	Neurologic consultant Monitor ICP Monitor GCS Surgical intervention

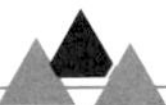

NURSING RESEARCH-BASED PRACTICE 18.2

Burr, JP: Jayne's story: Healing touch as a complementary treatment for trauma recovery. Holistic Nurs Pract 19(2):211–216, 2005.

Trauma recovery is a complex process. Present research acknowledges the difficulties of trauma recovery and limited conventional treatment options. Human biofield therapies are used successfully in a variety of settings for various patient complaints. The practices of human biofield manipulation; healing touch; and its predecessor, therapeutic touch, are effective holistic therapies that treat body, mind, and spirit to improve physiologic and psychological complaints, health perception, and well being. Jayne's story illustrates the beneficial integration of healing touch as a complementary therapeutic option in recovery from motor vehicle crash (MVC) trauma. Support for the incorporation healing touch therapy in the recovery regimen of individuals recuperating from trauma is suggested.

equally well, a temperature of about 100°F (37.7°C), a stiff neck, pupils of unequal size or shape, convulsions, severe headache that does not go away with acetaminophen (Tylenol) or ibuprofen (Motrin), confusion, disorientation, or a change in personality or behavior. These signs and symptoms are indicative of increased ICP and demand immediate attention in the ED.

Musculoskeletal Trauma

Musculoskeletal trauma refers to injuries involving the musculoskeletal system. These injuries may present as minor innocuous wounds or with obvious deformities. The clinician needs to resist the urge to treat the obvious deformity or fracture and neglect looking for the occult injury. Musculoskeletal sequelae can be associated with or caused by problems in other systems—neurologic, endocrine, nutritional, or psychological. A thorough history and physical examination are required to rule out other bodily system involvement. This section will discuss the musculoskeletal trauma of sprains, strains, and fractures.

Epidemiology and Causes

Musculoskeletal injuries are one of the most common injuries seen in the office and emergency/urgent care setting. Patients of all ages are susceptible to injury. The annual cost of caring for people with musculoskeletal system injuries is in the billions of dollars. The loss of productivity to industry is staggering. Musculoskeletal disorders as a frequent cause of work disability, account for productivity losses equivalent to 1.3 percent of the gross national product. There is an increase in the incidence of injuries among the younger population that can be attributed to a higher participation in sports and riskier recreational activities such as inline skating (rollerblading) and skiing.

Fitness classes and field sports are the most common culprits associated with musculoskeletal injuries in the younger population. Racket sports, walking, and low-intensity sports are associated with injuries in older adults. Usually the lower extremities are involved, especially the knees and ankles. Older patients tend to have more overuse injuries, such as metatarsalgia, plantar fasciitis, and menisceal knee injuries. Younger patients tend to have more patellofemoral syndromes and stress fractures.

Knees and ankles are the most common sites injured in high school athletes. Sprains and strains are by far the most common type of injuries. See Table 18.8 for considerations specific to knee and ankle injuries.

Occupational strains occur more often in the morning hours and in the first 4 hours of the work shift. Days earlier in the week, especially Monday, have a higher incidence of injury. Married workers age 30 to 50 are injured more frequently than other individuals. The occupations associated with a higher than average risk include nurses and truck drivers.

Americans have a fracture rate of approximately 21.1/1000 per year (23.5 per year per 1000 males and 18.8 per year per 1000 females), which is very similar to the rate in other industrialized countries. Males between age 15 and 49 were 2.9 times more likely to sustain a fracture than women were. There are three main peaks of fractures distribution—first among young adult males, second among older adults (affecting elderly men and women equally), and lastly, an increase in fractures, especially of the wrist, in women older than age 40.

Pathophysiology

Sprains and Strains

A *strain* involves micro- and macroscopic tears or stretching of muscle fibers. These injuries require more than just muscle contraction to occur; excessive stretching or stretching while the muscle is being activated is required. The injury usually occurs within the muscle's normal range of motion. The portion of the muscle that is typically injured is at the muscle–tendon junction. Research has shown that muscles that cross multiple joints or have a complex architecture are more susceptible to strains. Muscles most frequently injured include the hamstring, rectus femoris, gastrocnemius, and adductor longus muscles. A severe strain to the rectus femoris, hamstring, or abdominal wall muscles has been shown to have a poor prognosis for rehabilitation and may benefit from surgical repair.

A *sprain* is caused by stretching or twisting beyond the normal range of motion, of a joint or musculo–ligamentous unit. A sprain can be impossible to differentiate from a strain during the physical exam. Injuries involving joints are usually sprains, because ligaments are more prominent around joint capsules. A history of overuse and/or excessive force, as opposed to a fall, hyperextension, or twisting of a joint, is more likely related to a strain. If bony tenderness at the injury site is found during the physical exam, x-ray films are required to rule out fractures. A high suspicion of fracture is required, especially in the young and in older adults. The young are not able to provide an accurate history and full cooperation during the physical exam. Many minor fractures (such as a tarus fracture) are missed because the child does not complain and the parents or guardians are not aware of an injury. Older adults can have blunted pain sensation, especially to the extremities, related to neuropathies. The clinician should be aware of this and should be very astute when considering x-ray studies on these populations.

Fractures

A *fracture* is a break in the continuity of a bone; a fracture is usually associated with a blunt force. Fractures are classified as *open* or *closed,* depending on whether they communicate with the atmosphere. Open fractures have an increased incidence of infection and must be aggressively treated. Many need to be surgically irrigated. Fractures can be partial or complete. A *partial fracture* involves disruption

Table 18.8 Knee and Ankle Injuries

Knee Injuries

Assessment

A positive test is defined as increased laxity compared to the unaffected leg. Mild laxity with an end point reflects a positive test; this is considered a moderate or second-degree sprain. Significant laxity without an end point reflects ligament rupture and is considered a severe sprain or third-degree sprain.

- *Lachman's Test:* (Tests the patency of the anterior cruciate ligament.) Flex the knee to 40 degrees and, while stabilizing the upper leg, pull the lower leg just distal to the knee and attempt to distract the knee joint anteriorly. This tests the patency of the anterior cruciate ligament. This injury is typically (in 90% of cases) associated with a history of a popping sound or sensation when the injury occurred.
- *Posterior Drawer Test:* (Tests the patency of the posterior cruciate ligament.) Flex the knee to 40–45 degrees and stabilize the upper leg. Push the lower leg just distal to the knee and attempt to distract the knee joint posteriorly.
- *Varus Test:* (Tests the patency of the medial collateral ligament.) Flex the knee 5 degrees and place one hand on the distal lateral thigh and the other hand on the ankle. The knee joint is stressed medially; this causes distraction of the medial aspect of the joint.
- *Valgus Test:* (Tests the patency of the lateral collateral ligament.) Flex the knee 5 degrees and place one hand on the distal medial thigh and the other on the ankle. The knee joint is stressed laterally; this causes distraction of the lateral aspect of the joint.
- *Apprehension Test:* (Used to diagnose a patellar laxity.) With the knee fully extended and the patient relaxed, attempt to laterally displace the patella with mild pressure. During the procedure, the patient will become apprehensive to that maneuver. The patient will feel as though the patella will dislocate again. This is considered a positive test.

Radiology

Special attention should be directed to the tibial plateau. This region can show avulsion fractures. If a normal view of the knee shows no injury to that region and high suspicion still exists, the clinician should ask for a tunnel view, which will allow for a direct visualization of the plateau. The medial and lateral condyles must be closely examined for signs of avulsion. If a patella fracture is suspected, the clinician should ask for a sunrise view of the patella. This isolates the patella better and may show a fracture that would otherwise be missed.

Rehabilitation

If the patient has significant pain with ambulation, he or she should be placed on crutches and told to remain non-weightbearing for 24 hours, then to attempt partial weightbearing. If there is still pain, the patient should remain non-weightbearing until follow-up.

Quadricep and hamstring sets are recommended, to decrease the atrophy that occurs during immobilization. While the patient is in the immobilizer, have him or her lift the leg passively to contract the quadricep (anterior) muscles. Then the patient should actively push the leg posteriorly, to contract the hamstring (posterior) muscles.

For sprains and strains, the patient should remove the splint one to two times per day and passively fully flex and extend the knee.

Non-weightbearing is required for knee fractures until follow-up by an orthopedist.

Ankle Injuries

Assessment

- *Squeeze Test:* (Tests injury to the interosseous ligament.) Firmly squeeze the lower leg just distal to the belly of the calf. A positive test would elicit pain at the antero-lateral region of the ankle.
- *Tilt Test:* (Tests the patency of the calcaneo-fibular ligament.) Grasp the heel and medially manipulate the foot to stress the lateral aspect of the ankle. A positive test is defined as increased laxity compared to the unaffected leg. Mild laxity with an end point reflects a positive test; this is considered a moderate or second-degree sprain. Significant laxity without an endpoint reflects ligament rupture; this is considered a severe or third-degree sprain.
- *Drawer Test:* (Tests patency of the anterior talo-fibular and calcaneo-fibular ligaments.) Grasp the heel with one hand and the anterior shin with the other. Attempt to anteriorly distract the foot on the tibia. A positive test is defined as increased laxity compared to the unaffected leg. Mild laxity with an end point reflects a positive test; this is considered a moderate or second-degree sprain. Significant laxity without an end point reflects ligament rupture; this is considered a severe or third-degree sprain.
- *Ottawa Ankle Rules* (used to determine the need for x-ray exam): Following these rules has been shown to decrease the use of unnecessary radiographs and is nearly 100% sensitive for significant fractures to the ankle and foot.
  - (a) Determine if the patient was able to walk on the extremity just after the injury. If he or she was able to walk on it, then determine if the patient can still walk on it during the physical examination. Ability to walk on the injured extremity is defined as three to four steps with only a mild limp. If the patient answers no to either of these questions, an x-ray study is required.
  - (b) Palpate the lateral malleolus from the tip to 6 cm proximally (ankle x-ray film).
  - (c) Palpate the medial malleolus from the tip to 6 cm proximally (ankle x-ray film).
  - (d) Palpate the base of the fifth metatarsal (foot x-ray film).
  - (e) Palpate over the navicular bone (foot x-ray film).

  If pain is elicited over any of these bones, an x-ray is necessary. These rules have not been tested on patients older than age 60. Studies have shown that these rules do apply to pediatric patients.

Splinting

All sprains can be treated with a stirrup splint. This splint provides protection to the medial and lateral musculotendonous units. It does allow for plantar and dorsiflexion. This splint allows the injury to rehabilitate sooner and return to preinjury level much sooner.

Rehabilitation

For first-degree sprains, immediate weightbearing with the stirrup splint is appropriate. Avoid sports or high-exertion activities until the activity can be done pain-free. For grade II and III sprains, use crutches with non-weightbearing for 1–2 days, then progress as tolerated. If the activity being performed causes pain, the joint is not ready to progress to that level of activity yet. These injuries should be followed up by a practitioner in 3–5 days.

The patient should remove the splint two to three times per day and using the injured foot, spell out the alphabet in the air. The patient should plantarflex and dorsiflex the foot against no resistance.

of only a portion of the cortex, whereas a *complete fracture* involves circumferential disruption in the cortex. Complete fractures are unstable; inappropriate initial stabilization can lead to additional injuries to the muscles or neurovascular structures.

When assessing the patient, the clinician should ask about the mechanism of injury. Fractures can occur at locations other than the obvious site of injury. The force can be transmitted to other areas of the body, causing fractures. A person who fell off a roof and landed on his or her feet may have an obvious calcaneus (heel bone) fracture, but fractures of the hips, pelvis, and back must also be ruled out.

The goal of fracture management is to align the bones in a near-normal plane, to allow the fragmented ends to heal together and return to normal function. The initial phase of healing starts with hematoma formation. This bridges the fractured fragments. The inflammatory phase follows, and granulation tissue is formed on the fracture surfaces. During this process, the hematoma is reabsorbed, which provides the first continuity between the fragments. This takes place approximately 10 to 14 days after injury. During this time, the bone surrounding the fracture line becomes less dense. This makes the fracture line easier to identify. Callus is then formed on both the periosteal and endosteal surfaces of the bone; the callus acts as a biologic splint. The calcification of the bone then begins: First calcium phosphate is deposited, and then the bone undergoes osseous metaplasia. It takes approximately 2 to 3 weeks for the callus to be visible on x-ray film. The callus is then slowly reabsorbed, and the fracture surfaces develop a firm bony union. During this phase, the calcified region undergoes organization and the peripheral margins begin to smoothe. The process ends with remodeling, then consolidation.

In a healthy adult, the whole process takes approximately 2 months for smaller long bones (such as the humerus) and up to 4 months for large bones (such as the femur). Oblique fractures typically heal more quickly than transverse ones. Children tend to heal more quickly and older patients more slowly.

Radiologic (x-ray) evidence of abundant callus formation at the fracture site that is organized, and bone ends that have remained stable on serial films means the fracture should be stable enough to remove the cast. Limited activity is recommended until full strength is returned.

Clinical Presentation

Subjective

The signs of any musculoskeletal injury involve one or more of the following: pain, swelling, deformity, disability, abnormal motion, and tenderness. The history and mechanism of injury will help guide the physical exam. It will help one to focus on obvious and occult areas of injury. Documentation of the mechanism in the history is important. It is imperative that occult injuries are identified.

Objective

The importance of completing a thorough and complete physical exam cannot be emphasized enough. Life-threatening injuries must be identified quickly. This is facilitated by completing a quick primary survey, which can be accomplished in 90 seconds by an experienced practitioner. Following the primary survey, the more complete and thorough secondary survey can be completed. This is when fractures should be identified.

Diagnostic Reasoning

Diagnostic Tests

It is imperative that suspected sites of musculoskeletal trauma be radiographed to rule out fractures. Radiographic (x-ray) studies are the mainstay of orthopedic care. It is important that the clinician order the correct x-ray exam for the injury suspected. Many x-ray studies will include views of several joints and bones. The clinician must resist ruling out fractures in regions other than the area the specific x-ray exam ordered is intended to reveal. Each x-ray study has a specific technique that ensures that the correct angles, bony structures, and other information is included, to allow the practitioner to rule out pathology to that specific region. If a patient has pain in the foot and the ankle, an ankle x-ray film will miss foot pathology, and a foot x-ray film will miss ankle pathology. Advanced Assessment 18.3 presents tips on reading an extremity x-ray film.

ADVANCED ASSESSMENT 18.3

Reading an Extremity X-ray Film

- Conduct a thorough history and determine the mechanism of injury. This will help to determine the location and type of injury to expect. The area of injury should be examined. These procedures will focus your attention to the area of suspicion on the film. Always review the x-ray film after the exam, even if you viewed it before examining the patient.
- Using a well-lighted viewing box, follow the cortex of the injured area, looking for any defects. The cortex should be smooth and crisp; any area of haziness or any defect needs to be scrutinized using a bright (hot) light.
- Look at the soft tissue surrounding the area of concern. Injuries will cause soft tissue swelling. This may help focus your attention on the injured area. Scrutinize this region with a bright (hot) light.
- Several regions of the body, especially joints, have certain signs to look for that may reflect an occult injury. Confer with the collaborating physician or refer the patient to an orthopedic physician.

Differential Diagnosis

The goal of differential diagnosis in musculoskeletal trauma is to distinguish more serious bony fractures from strains and sprains, as these injuries are treated differently. As joint swelling and tenderness is a common presentation of such injuries, it is also critical to consider a variety of rheumatologic and infectious disorders, such as a septic joint, rheumatoid, or osteoarthritis. An appropriate history that seeks to characterize any preceding musculoskeletal trauma typically readily differentiates these conditions. However, if suspected, basic laboratory tests such as a CBC may also be helpful.

The differential diagnosis for fractures in addition includes *reflex sympathetic dystrophy*. Also known as Sudeck atrophy and causalgia, this is a posttraumatic syndrome with three clinical stages—*early, dystrophic,* and *atrophic*. Early in the condition, a constant aching or burning occurs in the affected limb. Motion or external stimulation increases the symptoms, usually out of proportion to the original injury. The dystrophic stage follows in which the skin of the affected extremity becomes glossy and cold and range of motion is limited. Finally, the atrophic stage is marked by skin atrophy and contracture. No correlation exists between incidence or symptom severity and the extent or type of the original musculoskeletal injury. Thus, early diagnosis of this syndrome is difficult, especially after an apparently trivial injury. Early diagnosis is extremely important, however, because the earlier treatment is initiated, the better the response. Treatment is aimed toward restoration of function through physical therapy. Antidepressant therapy may be beneficial, as well as prednisone.

Management

Emergency Management

Emergency management of the patient with musculoskeletal trauma initially consists of RICE therapy discussed below. If the patient can be seen immediately in the primary-care office, with radiographic capabilities, the patient may choose to see the clinician. If not, the patient should go directly to the ED.

General Management: Sprains and Strains

The principle of overtreating musculoskeletal injuries should be followed. After appropriate stabilization and 2 to 3 days of rest and elevation, the injury site can be more easily examined. The pain and swelling typically will be reduced, which will facilitate a better physical exam. Injuries that had negative x-ray studies initially but were extremely painful or were suspicious for fracture can be re-radiographed in 10 to 12 days. Because of the healing process, the fracture line can be more easily visualized at that time.

RICE Therapy. Rest, ice, compression, and elevation (RICE) are the mainstay of all musculoskeletal injury treatment. The amount of rest needed depends on the severity of the injury.

Rest means no use of the affected limb or joint, for minor injuries or sprains for 1 to 2 days, then slow progression as tolerated by the patient. If the activity being performed causes pain to the injury site, the level of activity needs to be reduced to levels that do not cause pain. Mild discomfort after activity is considered normal during the rehabilitation phase.

Ice, a potent anti-inflammatory, should be applied 30 minutes on and 30 minutes off, three to five times per day, to the injury site. Ice is also recommended during the rehabilitation phase if mild pain after activity is experienced. Ice therapy for 24 to 48 hours after the injury is recommended. After that period, warm, moist heat to the region is advocated to increase the circulation to the area, to promote reabsorption of blood and edema that has collected at the injury site.

Compression by elastic wrap or other splinting material is used to provide counterpressure at the site of injury, to help tamponade bleeding to the region. This will help decrease the amount of swelling and blood at the injury site. The influx of blood causes localized inflammation, which leads to leaking of plasma and other substances into the area.

Elevating the affected limb above the level of the heart will decrease bleeding into the tissue surrounding the injury and help to reduce the pain. After the first 48 hours, when bleeding into the area has stopped, elevation will facilitate reabsorption of blood and fluids at the injury site.

Pain Management. The use of a nonsteroidal anti-inflammatory drug (NSAID) for pain management is also recommended in conjunction with RICE therapy. Muscle relaxants such as cyclobenzaprine (Flexeril) may be indicated for the management of acute painful musculoskeletal conditions associated with muscle spasm. They reduce tonic somatic muscle activity at the level of the brainstem.

General Management: Fractures

Initial fracture care involves stabilization of the bone ends to avoid further injury or damage to neurovascular structures. During the secondary survey, when possible fractures are identified, immediate temporary splinting should be instituted. Severely angulated long bone fractures should be straightened before they are splinted. Splints should be applied in such a way as to immobilize the joints above and below the fracture site, to avoid motion of the bone ends involved. Commercially available metal and plastic splints are available for this purpose.

Following the x-ray and confirmation of a fracture, a more permanent splint should be applied. During immobilization, the clinician must consider the fact that fracture sites will continue to swell in the first 24 to 48 hours. Placing a rigid circumferential cast on the patient in the first 24 to 48 hours can lead to vascular compromise and compartment syndrome. To avoid this, the patient should be placed in a plaster splint. A plaster splint is placed on only half of the splinted limb and can be adjusted or molded to allow optimal stabilization of certain fractures. The skin should be padded to avoid local necrosis, and the splint should be secured by an elastic bandage. This type of splint allows the extremity to swell without affecting distal circulation.

Even with good technique, some fractures are not visible initially and will not appear until 7 to 10 days after the injury. At that time, the margins of the fracture absorb and will widen the radiolucent line at the fracture site. New bone will also be produced beneath the periosteum at the margins of the fracture, which will accentuate the fracture line. This will allow fractures that were not identified initially to be visualized. If a fracture is suspected but not visible at the initial visit, the injury should be treated as a fracture and reexamined clinically and radiographically in 7 to 10 days. The patient should be informed of the rationale for this treatment.

Follow-Up and Referral

The patient should be reexamined in 3 to 4 days following application of a cast or splint, to evaluate his or her neuromuscular status. In addition, the patient should be instructed to report any of the following signs and symptoms, which may reflect compartment syndrome—intense pain, hypoesthesia (a dulled sensitivity to touch), paresthesia (numbness, prickling, or tickling), muscular weakness, or paralysis. The patient with these signs should be referred to an orthopedic surgeon immediately. In 6 weeks to 2 months, a follow-up x-ray film will determine whether bone consolidation has occurred and if the cast can be removed.

Patient Education

Any site of a previous bony fracture will be weakened no matter how long after healing, and this site will always be more prone to a second fracture. Patients should always take this into account when deciding on what type of exercise or musculoskeletal activity to engage in.

In the future, it may be possible to predict which patients are at higher risk for fractures. Single bone mineral density measurement may be able to predict the risk of fragility fractures (distal radius, proximal humerus, hip, and vertebra) in women. This would help identify populations who would benefit from teaching and prevention strategies.

To avoid musculoskeletal injury, good physical conditioning is important. Consistent activity and exercise will strengthen muscles and reduce the chance of injury. See Chapter 14 for patient education about ways to prevent musculoskeletal injuries.

Table 18.9 provides a summary of risk factors, diagnostic considerations, and management of hip fractures.

Table 18.9 Hip Fracture

- By age 80, one in five women will suffer a hip fracture.
- There is a 30% mortality rate in elderly women within 1 year of injury.
- 50% of elders with a hip fracture do not return to independent living.
- Medicare costs for hip fractures approximate $3 billion/year.

Risk Factors
Elderly
Female
Falls, trauma
Osteoporosis

Types
Impaction or displacement
Dislocation
  Central
  Posterior
  Anterior

Assessment
Ecchymosis
Muscle spasm
Swelling
Five p's:
  Pain
  Pallor
  Paralysis
  Paresthesia
  Pulse

Diagnosis
History
Degree of mobility

Management
Possible Buck's traction prior to surgery
Surgical repair within 24 hours

Surgical Complications
Avascular necrosis (AVN)
Infection
Deep vein thrombosis

Follow-Up Treatment
Physical therapy
Diet: Adequate hydration, vitamin D, calcium
Medications: Calcium, bisphosphonates, calcitonin, synthetic PTH

Patient Education
Elevated toilet seat
Supportive chair
Avoid crossing legs
Fall precautions—no loose rugs

Lower Back Pain

Up to 80 percent of the population experiences lower back pain at some time in their life. A common problem in the workplace due to muscular or ligamentous strain, lower back pain accounts for one of the most frequent causes of days lost from work. Only about 15 percent of patients have a specific injury.

Pathophysiology

The most common causes of lower back pain are listed in Table 18.10. Disk herniation produces the deficits predictable for the site involved as listed in Table 18.10.

Clinical Presentation

Subjective

If no accident or trauma is involved, the patient will usually complain of a time-sequence history of symptoms which may be gradual or sudden and may be localized in the lumbosacral area or radiating. If a disk syndrome is present, the

Table 18.10 Most Common Causes of Lower Back Pain: Lumbar Spinal Nerve Impingement/Herniated Disc Signs

Spinal Nerve Affected	Dermatome; Sensory Deficit	Myotome; Weakness Shown	Reflex Affected
L4	Anterior thigh, medial shin	Quadriceps; knee extension weak	Patellar
L5	Great toe, dorsum of foot	Anterior tibial and extensor hallucis; dorsiflexion of great toe (walking on heels)	
S1	Lateral border of foot, small toe	Gastrocnemius; plantar flexion of foot (walking on toes)	Achilles

Any L4–S1 root irritation can cause "SCIATICA": pain from buttock down lateral leg; + straight leg raising sign; if pt. develops acute bladder, bowel problems, bilateral leg involvement = medical emergency.
Source: Teri Capriotti, DD, MSN, CRNP

patient may complain of radiation into the leg, sensory changes, motor weakness, or difficulties with bowel or bladder function.

Objective

The clinician should perform a neurologic examination of the lower extremities which will detect the small deficits reproduced by disk disease and the large deficits produced by such problems as cauda equina tumors. Performing a straight-leg-raising test may indicate nerve root irritation if radicular pain is produced when the leg is raised 60 degrees or less.

The disc herniation and radiculopathy of lumbar spinal nerves L4 to L5 and L5 to S1 are particularly common sources of acute back pain often due to trauma. L4 to L5 and L5 to S1 radiculopathy ("sciatica") may be objectively assessed in terms of dermatome sensory deficit, myotome muscle weakness, and deep tendon reflex deficits as depicted in Table 18.10. The clinician should assess for the inability to walk on toes, inability to walk on heels, and the inability to dorsiflex the great toe which may relate to specific lumbar spinal nerve involvement.

Classic lower back pain that is less serious involves pain in the lower back with or without pain radiating down one leg.

Diagnostic Reasoning

Diagnostic Tests

In the majority of cases, a precise diagnosis cannot be made. Usually the initial history and physical examination will lead to the diagnosis. The challenge is to identify patients who require more extensive or urgent evaluation. Diagnosis is usually not confirmed by palpation of the spine. Lumbar x-ray films are usually not indicated for patients with acute low back pain unless there is evidence of a possible fracture, or a possible tumor or infection. An MRI is reserved for patients who are surgical candidates or have evidence of systemic disease.

Differential Diagnosis

The differential diagnoses for lower back pain include muscular strain, primary spine disease such as disk herniation or degenerative arthritis; systemic disease, such as metastatic cancer; and regional diseases, such as aortic aneurysm. Patients with systemic disease such as vertebral osteomyelitis typically have a history of smoking, weight loss, age older than 50, diabetics, a history of recurrent urinary tract infections and cancer. Low back pain at night, unrelieved by rest of lying supine, may suggest a malignancy, either vertebral body metastasis, multiple myeloma, or a cauda equina syndrome, which is a serious complication of herniated disk and needs emergency medical treatment. Cauda equina syndrome, multiple lumbar nerve root compressions, is a medical emergency and the patient would present with leg weakness or of saddle area anesthesia, bowel or bladder incontinence, or impotence.

Low back pain that worsens with rest and seems to improve with activity is usually caused by ankylosing spondylitis or other seronegative spondyloarthropathies, especially with an incidious onset after the age of 40.

Patients with a penetrating peptic ulcer disease may present with back pain and this should be ruled out as a diagnosis. Patients with endocarditis may present with a cardiac murmur in addition to back pain and this should be further evaluated. In addition, referred back pain may be a result of renal stones.

Management

The majority of patients with lower back pain will improve in 1 to 4 weeks. Conservative therapy is indicated if all the differential diagnoses are ruled out. Treatment consists of NSAIDs unless severe pain requires opioids or muscle relaxants for 1 to 2 weeks. NSAIDs have proven to be as effective as opioids and muscle relaxants and the latter should be avoided if at all possible. The adage of "let pain be your guide" refers to keeping the patient mobile and ideally staying at work. Patients should not stay in bed for longer than 2 days, unless it is sciatica which may require a week in bed. A program of exercise should be developed that should allow the patient to return to a normal regimen as soon as possible.

Some patients benefit from heat therapy; some from ice therapy. It is individualistic. When heat is preferred, moist heat for 20 to 30 minutes at least four times per day may be effective. When cold therapy is preferred, ice over the affected area for 10 to 15 minutes every 1 to 2 hours may be effective. Some patients prefer heat alternated with ice.

Intensive rehabilitation for chronic back pain is more cost-effective and results in a reduction of disability and fewer complications than surgery although research shows that it is slightly less effective than spinal fusion surgery.

Follow-Up and Referral

If patients are not able to be managed by a general clinician, a specialist may be needed depending on the radiographic or MRI results. Physical therapy may be ordered by the general clinician or by a specialist. Patients should be followed up in 1 week to verify that the injury was in fact lower back pain and not more serious.

Patient Education

All patients should be taught good body mechanics. These include the following:

- ▲ Ask for help if one determines the weight is too great to lift by oneself.
- ▲ Keep back straight, lift with the legs.
- ▲ Push rather than pull objects.
- ▲ Do not twist sideways; face the object to be lifted.
- ▲ Use a footstool to lessen back strain.
- ▲ Do not sit or stand for prolonged periods of time, move or stretch at least every 1/2 hour.
- ▲ Sleep on a firm mattress, and sit in a supportive chair.
- ▲ Maintain good posture.
- ▲ Wear flat supportive shoes.

An exercise program should be developed to strengthen the back, relieve pressure on compressed nerves, and help protect the patient's back from reinjury. While most exercises should not be attempted until the episode of acute back pain is resolved, therapeutic exercises may relieve pain.

Foreign Body Obstructions

This section discusses ear, nose, throat, vaginal, and rectal foreign body obstructions. Common foreign body obstructions and their treatment are discussed in Table 18.11.

Epidemiology and Causes

Foreign body (FB) obstructions are common problems seen in the primary-care setting. Most of these problems involve children. FB obstructions most commonly result from the patient inserting a foreign body into a body orifice.

Pathophysiology

The pathophysiology of a FB obstruction depends on which orifice is obstructed. Otic (ear canal) occlusion may contribute to otitis externa or otitis media, especially if the tympanic membrane is ruptured. Nasal occlusion may predispose to rhinitis, sinusitis, or epistaxis (nose bleed). Moreover, nasal, pharyngeal, tracheal, or even esophageal occlusion may all result in varying degrees of respiratory compromise if the respiratory tract is at all obstructed either internally or via external compression on the airway.

A vaginal occlusion, if unattended, can lead to toxic shock syndrome (mediated by infection with *Staphylococcus aureus* or *Streptococcus pyogenes*) or pelvic inflammatory disease. A bowel obstruction may result from a FB occluding the rectum if the object inserted is high enough. Obviously, early diagnosis and intervention will best protect against adverse effects from prolonged obstruction.

Clinical Presentation

Subjective

The patient will present with a complaint of a FB, with signs and symptoms specific to the bodily orifice involved. However, if the individual is unaware of the presence of a FB, such as in the case of a forgotten tampon left in place, the patient may complain of a foul-smelling vaginal discharge. Alternatively, a nasal or otic occlusion may lead to a feeling of head fullness or headache. Of note, many of these affected patients are children who may or may not be able to fully express their discomfort or pain verbally.

Objective

Based on the patient's complaint and the orifice involved, the signs will vary. A rectal occlusion may cause abdominal cramping, an increase in bowel sounds, and abdominal distension. A vaginal occlusion may result in a foul-smelling vaginal discharge. An insect or piece of cotton caught in the ear may cause equilibrium problems, dizziness, tinnitus, and diminished hearing on the affected side. An FB in the nose of an adult is rare.

Diagnostic Reasoning

Diagnostic Tests

Diagnostic tests are usually not indicated, but radiologic studies may be appropriate if physical examination is insufficient to fully characterize the obstructing organism. However, as the majority of foreign bodies are not radiopaque, and x-ray findings may be quite subtle, requiring formal interpretation by a radiologist. In some cases, direct endoscopy of the nasopharyngeal, respiratory, or gastrointestinal tracts may be required to identify the obstructing object.

Differential Diagnosis

The diagnosis is usually obvious, because of the patient's complaint.

Management

Emergency Management

The clinician may attempt to remove the FB in the office. If the attempt is unsuccessful, the patient should be sent to the Emergency Department.

Table 18.11 Common Foreign Body Obstructions

Ears

Foreign bodies in the auditory canal are common problems, especially in children. Foreign bodies can be vegetative, inanimate, or animate objects. Foreign bodies in the ear are usually asymptomatic unless they are left in the ear for a prolonged period of time and an infection develops. The clinician should obtain a complete history to elicit whether there is a possibility of multiple foreign bodies. The practitioner should assess both ears to obtain a comparison view. It is important to try to ensure that there is no perforation of the tympanic membrane before trying to remove the foreign body.

A live insect trapped in the ear canal usually causes great distress. The patient will present with agitation, nausea, and tearing. The initial therapy is to immobilize the insect. This can be done by placing 2% lidocaine in the external ear canal, which will terminate the movement of the insect. The insect can then be removed.

Removal of inanimate objects is not always straightforward. If the patient is uncooperative or the foreign body is difficult to grasp, ear, nose, and throat (ENT) consultation is suggested. If the object becomes lodged too deeply, it will be difficult to remove and the patient may need general anesthesia for successful removal. If the object is small, irrigation is an option.

If the object is appropriately shaped and accessible, alligator or bayonet forceps may be used to grasp and remove it. Suctioning may also assist in the removal of an object. A Yankar suction catheter has a small orifice and a firm catheter tip that may facilitate foreign body removal.

After successful removal of the object, the ear canal needs to be checked for infections, superficial scratches, and tympanic-membrane perforation. If there is no evidence of infection, the patient may be discharged home. If an infection is present, it should be treated as an otitis externa.

Nose

Nasal foreign bodies are most commonly seen in children. They are usually discovered after purulent discharge is noticed. The history is important, but children are usually reluctant to admit to what or how much they have placed in their nose.

The diagnosis is made by direct visualization. If the patient or child is uncooperative, a restraining device or sedation may be needed. If the patient is cooperative, the following steps may be used to remove the foreign body:

- Help the patient to blow his or her nose, to see if the foreign object will come out.
- If the mucosa appears swollen, soak a pledget in Neo-Synephrine and insert it into the nare; care should be taken not to push the foreign body further into the nose.
- Using a nasal speculum and alligator or bayonet forceps, visualize the foreign body and gently remove it. Other methods include using an ear curette, single skin hook, or right-angle ear hook. Another method that has been used is to pass a small urinary catheter superior to (beyond) the object, inflate the balloon, and pull the object out.

All of these methods can be successful if the patient is cooperative. Care must be taken not to push the foreign body down the back of the patient's throat, where it may be aspirated into the trachea.

After successfully removing the object, the clinician should inspect the nares for other foreign bodies. No further treatment is necessary.

If removal is unsuccessful, a referral to an ENT specialist may be necessary.

Throat

Swallowed objects are commonly seen by the primary-care provider. Usually, they are not life threatening, but any object that becomes lodged in a position where it can obstruct the airway is a true emergency. Although most swallowed objects will pass spontaneously, up to 10 to 20% require some type of intervention. There are several physiologic narrow spaces in the esophageal-gastrointestinal tract that may restrict movement of objects. In the pediatric population, the cricopharyngeal area is the most common site for obstruction, followed by (in order of frequency) the thoracic inlet, aortic arch, tracheal bifurcation, and hiatal narrowing. The majority of obstructions in adults occur at the distal end of the esophagus. Usually once the object has passed through the pylorus, it will pass through the rest of the GI tract without problems. If the object has sharp edges, however, it can injure the intestines and/or become lodged anywhere in the GI tract. Ingested foreign bodies can also cause airway obstruction or perforation.

If the object becomes lodged in the esophagus, the adult patient may present with the feeling of something in the throat, pain, and the inability to swallow secretions. Pediatric patients may present with vomiting, gagging, choking, stridor, inability to swallow, increased salivation, and a sensation of a foreign body in the chest.

If there is a possible foreign body ingestion, a chest x-ray study should be ordered to see if the object is lodged in the esophagus. Foreign bodies will show up only if they are radiopaque. If the object is in the stomach, the patient should be monitored for passage of the object through the GI tract. The stool will need to be examined. If the object is not found, an abdominal flat-plate x-ray film can be used to determine the location of the object. Objects that fail to be expelled may have to be removed by invasive procedures such as colonoscopy or surgery.

A food bolus is usually the cause of ingested foreign bodies in the adult population. Typically, inadequately chewed meat is the main culprit. If the patient is unable to swallow saliva secretions, a chest x-ray film should be obtained. Glucagon, a smooth-muscle relaxant, may be administered intravenously to relax the esophagus. A 1-mg dose is given IV; the dose may be repeated after 20 minutes if the object has not passed. The patient will usually vomit, which causes the foreign body to be expelled; it is important to ensure that the patient does not aspirate the vomitus. If glucagon has not produced a successful effect, a GI consult should be obtained. Some references recommend a barium swallow to visualize where the obstruction is located; however, most GI specialists prefer that no barium be given because it can obstruct their view of the bolus during endoscopy.

If a coin becomes lodged in the esophagus, it should be removed by endoscopy. Two other methods that may be tried include passing an indwelling urinary catheter behind the object, inflating it, and pulling the object out. Objects that become lodged in the esophagus can be safely pushed into the stomach by a small urinary catheter.

Ingestion of button batteries can be a true emergency situation. The batteries can cause burns to the GI mucosa and must be removed quickly.

The treatment for ingestion of a sharp object is controversial. Most practitioners recommend that sharp objects be removed, so they do not cause a perforation before they pass into the intestine.

Vagina

Vaginal foreign bodies can be the result of children exploring their sexuality or an incident of child abuse; in adults, the foreign body may be a forgotten tampon or diaphragm. The only treatment necessary is removal of the foreign body. Most of the discharge and odor will disappear after the foreign body is removed. If the foreign body is lodged in the side wall of the vagina, the clinician should irrigate the area with normal saline to gently remove the object from the wall. If a foreign body is suspected in a small child, general anesthesia for exploration should be considered if the object is not visible and can be removed by gently pulling on the labia. Emotional support and reassurance is important to patients. Privacy must be maintained to avoid undue embarrassment.

Rectum

A variety of objects have been inserted into the rectum. They are usually found in the rectal ampulla and are usually palpable with digital examination. All patients presenting with the chief complaint of foreign body in the rectum need x-ray exams of the abdomen, to show the position, shape, and number of foreign bodies in the rectum. The x-ray film will also show if free air is present in the abdomen. This is indicative of a perforation of the bowel, which is the most serious potential complication.

Removal of the foreign body from the rectum requires that the rectal sphincter be relaxed. If a brief attempt at removing the foreign body is unsuccessful, the practitioner should consider conscious sedation to relax the sphincter muscle. Conscious sedation requires close monitoring and is best carried out in an inpatient or emergency setting. If there is any possibility of perforation, an emergency GI consult is needed.

General Management

See Table 18.11 for general management of ear, nose, throat, vaginal, and rectal foreign body obstructions.

Follow-Up and Referral

Follow-up is usually not indicated once the FB is removed. The patient should be alerted to signs and symptoms of an infection, should one occur after discharge. If a rectal perforation has occurred as a result of a FB, an emergency gastroenterology referral is indicated.

Patient Education

Because children are usually involved in FB incidents, prevention is essential. Parents should be encouraged to buy age-appropriate toys and to keep small objects out of the reach of children. Also, children should be taught not to put objects in the various orifices of their bodies.

Bibliography

General

Auerback, PS, Donner, HJ, and Weiss, EA: Field Guide to Wilderness Medicine, ed 2. Elsevier, Philadelphia, 2004.

Colyar, MR, and Ehrhardt, CR: Ambulatory Care Procedures for the Nurse Practitioner. FA Davis, Philadelphia, 1999.

Kasper, DL, Braunwald, E, Fauci, A, Hauser, S, Longo, D, and Jamison, L: Harrison's Principles of Internal Medicine, ed 16. McGraw-Hil, New York, 2004.

Marx, JA, Hockberger, RS, and Walls, RM: Rosen's Emergency Medicine: Concepts and Clinical Practice, ed 6. Elsevier, Philadelphia, 2005.

Newberry, L (ed): Sheey's Emergency Nursing Principles and Practices, ed 6. Elsevier, Philadelphia, 2003.

Rakel, RE, and Bope, ET: Conn's Current Therapy. WB Saunders, Philadelphia, 2005.

Head Trauma

Bond, MM, Viera, AJ, and Yates, SW: The "minor" head injury: Which patients need CT? Emerg Med April 48–64, 1999.

Fann, JR; Burington, B, Leonetti, A, Jaffe, K, Katon, WJ, and Thompson, RS: Psychiatric illness following traumatic brain injury in an adult health maintenance organization population. Arch Gen Psychiatry 61:53–61, 2004.

McQuillan, KA, Von Rueden, KT, Hartsock, RL, Flynn, MB, and Whalen, E: Trauma Nursing; Through Resuscitation Through Rehabilitation. WB Saunders, Philadelphia, 2002.

Ropper, AH: Concussion and other head injuries. In Kasper, DL, Fauci, AS, Longo, DL, Braunwald, E, Hauser, SL, and Jameson, JL: Harrison's Principles of Internal Medicine. ed 16. McGraw-Hill, New York, 2004, Chapter 357.

Musculoskeletal Trauma

Abasolo, L, Glanco, Ml, Bachiller, J, Candelas, Gl, Coilado, P, Lajas, C, Revenga, M, Ricci, P, Lazaro, P, Aguilar, MD, Vargas, E, Fernandez-Gutierrez, B, Hernandez-Garcia, C, Carmona, L, and Jover, J: A health system program to reduce work disability related to musculoskeletal disorders. Ann Intern Med 143(6):404–414, 2005.

Fairbank, J, Frost, H, Wilson-MacDonald, J, Yu, LM, Barker, K, and Collins R: Rehab as good as spinal fusion for chronic back pain. J Fam Pract 54(9):752, 2005.

Wounds and Lacerations

Phillips, N: Berry & Kohn's Operating Room Technique, ed. 10. .CV Mosby, St. Louis, Mo., 2004.

Resources

Pneumothorax/Hemothorax

American College of Chest Physicians—Improving Patient Care Through Education
http://www.chestnet.org

Poisonings

National Center for Injury Prevention and Control
http://www.cdc.gov/ncipc.org (through this site access TESS—Toxic Exposure Surveillance System)

Heat and Cold-Related Injuries

MEDDAC Preventive Medicine Climatic Injury Awareness and Prevention Site
http://iach.amedd.army.mil/departments/prevmed.asp

Burns

The Burn Resource Center
http://www.burnsurvivor.com

Insect Bites

West Nile Virus
http://www.emedicine.com/westnile.htm
Internet Sources on Inset Bites
http://www.lib.uiowa.edu/hardin/md/insectbites.html

Head Trauma

http://nlm.nih.gov/medlineplus/headandbraininjuries.html
American Association of Neurological Surgeons/Congress of Neurological Surgeons (AANS)
http://www.aans.org

Caring-Based Nursing: The Practice

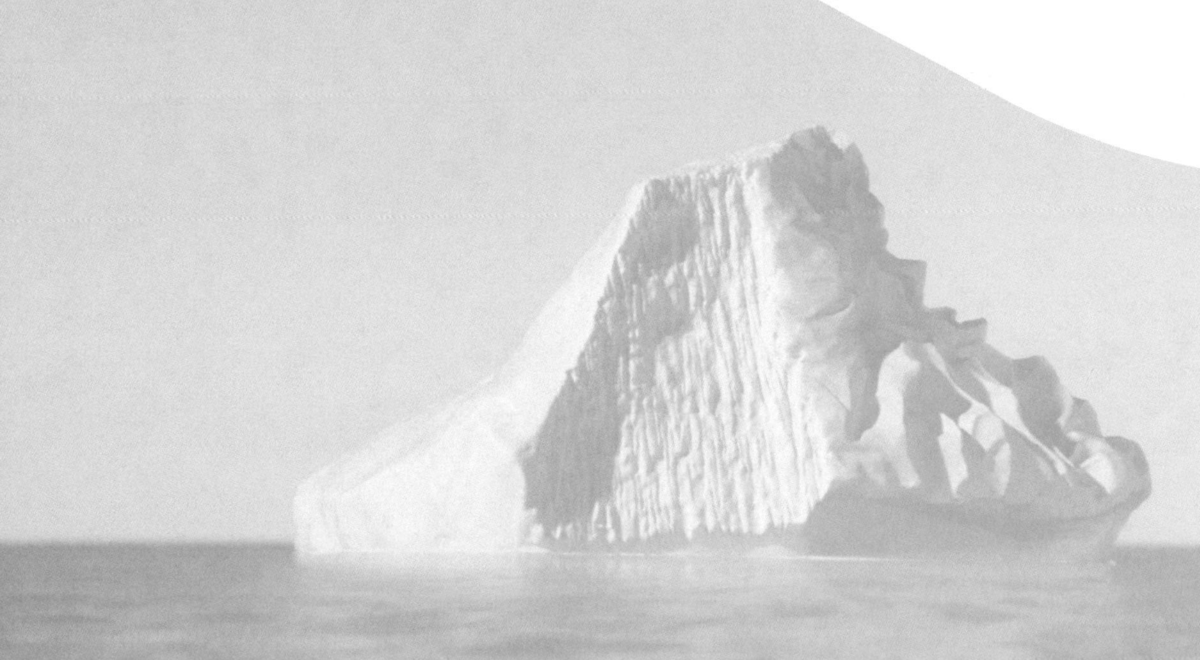

3 UNIT

"All segments of our profession need to work together toward a common goal, a future in which legal and professional regulation and education of nurses at the graduate level are aligned so that one educational product, the advanced practice nurse, is prepared to fill a variety of roles in the health care system."

–Linda R. Cronenwett: Molding the future of advanced practice nursing. Nursing Outlook 43:112–118, 1995.

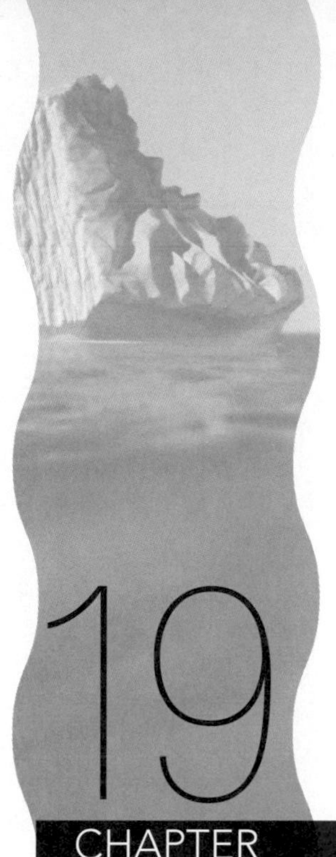

Palliative Care

Susan Derby, RN, MA, CGNP, ACHPN
Mary Layman Goldstein, RN, MS, APRN, BC

Death and Dying in America

Until the 20th century, most people died at home, cared for by family and close friends. Most people generally understood that doctors could not prevent illness or prolong life and the odds of reaching old age were essentially a matter of luck and good genes. Use of antimicrobials, improved sanitation, and technological advances have significantly improved life expectancy for the average American.

At present, in the United States, the total number of deaths from all causes is over 2 million per year. In 1900, the average life expectancy was about 45 to 50 years; by 1995, this had increased to approximately 75.8 years. The 10 leading causes of death in the United States are heart disease, cancer, accidents, cerebrovascular disease, chronic obstructive pulmonary disease (COPD), pneumonia and influenza, human immunodeficiency virus (HIV) infection, suicide, diabetes mellitus, and homicide. Heart disease, cancer, cerebrovascular disease, and COPD occur more frequently in older adults, accounting for more than 60 percent of all deaths. Cancer deaths may overtake heart disease within the next 10 years, as the population continues to age (Rosenberg, 1996; American Cancer Society, 2005).

Where Death and Dying Occurs

Discussions of where people die shed little light on how they die, how physical symptoms are managed, how psychological and spiritual issues are addressed, the level of training and education the staff has in end-of-life care management, and how suffering is relieved. The site where death occurs is influenced by many factors including age, marital status, family support, finances, reimbursement issues, cultural beliefs, and cause of death.

Over the past 50 years, death has become institutionalized with a shift from the home to the hospital or a health-care institution. According to the National Hospice and Palliative Care Organization for all Americans who died in 2003, about 25 percent died at home, about 25 percent in a nursing facility, and about 50 percent in a hospital—15 percent in the emergency room and 35 percent in acute care.

Hospice Care

Hospice care is often underutilized. In 1993 only about 11 percent of the population who died received hospice care; 2003 data from the National Hospice and Palliative Care Organization estimated that number to be about 28 percent. In one study of 6700 Medicare hospice patients from five states, the median survival after hospice admission was 36 days, 15 percent died within 7 days of admission, and 15 percent lived longer than 180 days. The mean age of the patients was 76.4 years, and 80 percent were cancer patients. There was substantial variation in survival; the most salient aspect was diagnosis. Patients with nonmalignant diseases, namely, dementia, chronic obstructive pulmonary disease (COPD), congestive heart failure, and stroke had longer survivals than patients admitted with a diagnosis of cancer. Terminal disease in cancer patients is easier to determine than in nonmalignant conditions and may account for their shorter survival under hospice care.

Barriers to utilization of hospice care include (1) difficulties in estimating prognosis, (2) criterion that the patient have a life expectancy 6 months or less, (3) primary management at home with intermittent respite care available for symptom control, (4) need for a caregiver in the home, (5) patient and family fear, (6) communication problems, (7) lack of knowledge and access to services, and (8) problems with funding mechanisms of insurers.

Prognosticating a life expectancy of 6 months or less in noncancer-related diseases has been especially difficult.

Guidelines have recently been developed by the National Hospice Organization to assist the provider in determining prognosis and eligibility for hospice care. Medicare hospice eligibility criteria are that (1) the patient be Medicare-eligible; (2) the patient must have a terminal illness with a physician-certified prognosis of less than 6 months; (3) the approach to care must be palliative, rather than curative; and (4) the patient must give informed consent to the hospice care.

A Paradigm Shift to Palliative Care

Both "hospice" and "palliative care," terms often used interchangeably, encompass skilled, compassionate care for people. Both provide supportive medical, social, emotional, and spiritual services to patients and their caregivers. Both services rely on the combined knowledge and skill of interdisciplinary teams of professionals. Hospice care provides care to patients at the end of life. Palliative care provides a support system to both the family and patient, integrating the psychological and spiritual aspects of patient care, throughout the trajectory of illness, from the time of diagnosis until death, and encompasses end-of-life care.

The continuum of care includes the offering of help to bereaved family members after the death of a loved one. The hospice movement in the United States has been greatly influenced by Dr. Elisabeth Kubler-Ross, who researched the dying process and advocated changes in the way society views death. In the United States, the first hospice opened in 1974 in New Haven, Connecticut. It was based on St. Christopher's Hospice, founded in Great Britain in 1967. Since that time, hospital-based programs have been primarily replaced by home-based and nursing home–based hospice programs.

Suffering and Spirituality

Receiving a diagnosis of an incurable disease can be one of the most frightening experiences for any human being. Fear of potential suffering, pain, and loss of control, of existence, and of relationships are some of the issues that confront the patient.

Suffering is an experience of the whole person and is highly personal and subjective. Cassell (1996) suggests that suffering is the state of distress by the threat of the loss of intactness or the disintegration of a person from whatever the cause. In serious illness, all aspects of the individual are affected: physical, mental, spiritual, emotional, and social. Suffering involves an eroding of the normal defenses that help to keep us intact, relate to others, and have purpose in life. Human suffering is a complex, multidimensional experience that often goes beyond physical pain.

When a life-threatening disease is first diagnosed, the individual may be terrified but often quickly shifts into a situation in which decisions regarding treatment must be made. During this phase the patient often seeks counsel, support, and advice from others including friends, relatives, and health-care professionals. Characteristic of this phase is an information-gathering period, in which the patient becomes knowledgeable about the disease, treatment, and adverse effects. The sense of involvement and exploration may extend to religion and spiritual aspects of being. After treatment, the patient may experience ongoing anxiety and depression related to fear of disease relapse. With disease relapse and progressive illness and disability, the patient may become more depressed and verbalize feelings of hopelessness. In one study (Fleming, 1995) that evaluated nurses' perspectives of patient suffering, four domains of suffering were identified: to bear it, to stay in control, to protect themselves, and to strengthen.

Spirituality is concerned with the transcendental, the inspirational, and existential way we live our lives. Victor Frankl, from his experience in Auschwitz, claims that suffering can be helpful if a meaning to suffering is identified. He used the terms "existential frustration" to define the confusion felt from a lack of meaning in one's situation and "existential vacuum" as the absence of meaning in one's life. When one is faced with unavoidable suffering, according to Frankl, the individual is free to choose how to respond and may either be master or victim. Finding meaning in suffering, says Frankl, comes from transcendence, or rising above the self and finding meaning. Meaning encompasses three domains: creativity, experience, and attitude. Meaning can be found in creating something or accomplishing a task, experiential meaning involves finding pleasure or nourishment of the soul in ordinary things, and attitudinal meaning involves finding courage or experiencing joy despite a terrible unalterable situation.

Providing care to people who are suffering is an awesome task that often challenges religious or spiritual beliefs. It calls for the highest level of knowledge, sensitivity, and empathy. Patients who are ill or dying report that they want nurses and doctors who are caring. We often hear stories from patients about "uncaring" health professionals who seem cold and indifferent to the suffering of their patients, and we all too frequently see some of these individuals in our daily practice. Palliative care encompass the basic tenets of caring including respect for the individual, empathy, and compassion. It calls for a Circle of Caring.

Medical and Nursing Education in Palliative Care

Education of health-care professionals in palliative and end-of-life care is not routinely a part of medical and nursing education. In most clinical settings, including both inpatient and ambulatory care, there are no established guidelines for pain and symptom management including terminal or end-of-life care. Even in settings in which guidelines do exist, there is variable support for or assurance that these guidelines are adhered to in practice. A study by an Institute of Medicine panel concluded that physicians and other caregivers in the United States fail to provide competent, palliative, and supportive care to dying patients. It also concluded that a significant number of terminally ill patients experience serious pain and other discomforting symptoms such as dyspnea.

Multiple studies document deficiencies in knowledge about pain and palliation of symptoms associated with progressive disease. In a survey in 1997 of medical residents in a university-based surgical program, a significant number of deficits existed in the knowledge of how to provide care for common symptoms of advanced cancer, including management of opioid-related nausea, vomiting, and terminal dyspnea. Another study surveyed physician knowledge and attitudes and reported prescribing practices among primary-care physicians and oncologists. Only 37 percent of primary-care physicians had formal training in pain management versus 91 percent of oncologists; both groups, however, were markedly deficient in knowledge of opioid equivalences. More than 50 percent of one group of oncologists surveyed related their own pain management practice as only "fair." Other surveys have documented deficiencies in physicians during their residencies in the areas of opioid selection, conversion, and management of opioid toxicities and addiction. In a recent survey of approaches of medical oncologists toward palliative care, for patients with advanced cancer, only a minority of physicians collaborated with a palliative care specialist, a palliative home service, an inpatient hospice, or a psychologist. Overall, 88.4 percent supported the belief that medical oncologists should coordinate the end-of-life care, but a substantial minority (42 percent) felt that they were inadequately trained for this task (Cherny, 2003).

Nurses' knowledge and attitude of pain and symptom management strongly parallels those of physicians, although there is some evidence that educational efforts have been beneficial. McCaffery and Ferrell (1997) compared the results from surveys in 1995 and 1998 of nurses' knowledge of pain assessment, opioid dosing, and likelihood of addiction. They found improvements in the nurses' assessment and titration upward of opioid dose as well as a decrease in concerns about addiction, although a clear association still existed between time on opioids and concerns about addiction. In another study of nurses' knowledge and attitudes of cancer-related pain, O'Brien and colleagues (1996) found that experienced nurses who have cared for cancer patients are more knowledgeable and have more liberal attitudes toward pain management than nurses who have not cared for cancer patients.

Educational Efforts to Improve the Practice of Pain and Palliative Care

The 1990s had seen major educational efforts by health-care professionals to improve knowledge deficits. A major directive in 1994 (Jacox, 1994) from the Agency for Health Care Policy and Research (AHCPR) issued clinical practice guidelines on the management of acute and chronic cancer pain, which have been implemented in many oncology settings. A variety of approaches and specific programs have been identified to address these knowledge deficits. The Joint Commission on Accreditation of Healthcare Organizations (JCAHO) standards on pain management has been helpful in making institutions accountable for assessment and management of pain across practice settings. Efforts at the academic and clinical level provide a framework for care of patients with advanced disease and for patients who are dying. Curriculum changes for both nurses and physicians in many schools now include comprehensive palliative care. In many hospitals, services of palliative care experts or pain and symptom management specialists are being incorporated into the routine care of oncology patients. Pain or palliative care services offering physician fellowships now exist in an increasing number of training centers. Many hospitals now provide programs for nurses offering education or clinical mentors. Quality assurance and improvement programs examining pain and symptom management now exist in many institutional settings.

Directives now exist from major professional organizations advocating pain and symptom management. These organizations include the American Nurses Association, American Pain Society, American Board of Internal Medicine, Oncology Nursing Society, American Geriatric Association, American Society of Pain Management Nurses, International Society of Nurses in Cancer Care, International Association for the Study of Pain, European Oncology Nursing Society, and the American Society of Clinical Oncologists. These clinical practice guidelines and directives, as well as major national professional educational efforts on end-of-life care (End of Life Nursing Education Consortium [ELNEC] and Education for Physicians on End of Life Care [EPEC]) are addressing the problem of inadequate control of pain and knowledge deficits.

Palliative Care

Palliative care focuses on the management of disease in patients with active, progressive disease. The focus of care is on the quality of life. Palliative care furthers the World Health Organization's definition of health, affirming dying as a normal life process. Palliative care as defined by the World Health Organization is an approach that improves the quality of life of patients and their families facing the problems associated with life-threatening illness, through the prevention and relief of suffering by means of early identification and impeccable assessment and treatment of pain and other problems—physical, psychosocial, and spiritual. The goals of care are to alleviate symptoms in a compassionate way, neither hasten nor postpone death, and to provide a support system to both the family and patient, integrating the psychological and spiritual aspects of patient care, throughout the trajectory of illness.

If we examine the characteristics of the most prevalent chronic illnesses, including coronary artery disease, chronic lung disease, cancer, cerebrovascular disease, and diabetes, similarities in the patterns of chronic illness are apparent. For all chronic illnesses, there is the initial diagnostic period when symptoms become present. This may be over a period of days, weeks, or months and is generally a highly stressful period, with disruption in function and routine. Once a treatment plan is initiated, symptoms may resolve, and the patient may enter a period of remission or stability lasting months or years. What follows are periods of exacerbation, often with hospitalizations, and periods of remission. During this time the patient usually experiences signs and symptoms of disease; alterations in lifestyle, role, family, and job relationships; and often psychological and spiritual distress. As time progresses, if the patient is not cured of the disease or stability is not long lasting, there comes a time of downward progression of disease with a decline in function and worsening symptoms. It is during this time most patients are referred for palliative care.

The goals of treatment for all chronically ill patients need to be clearly defined by the health-care provider, communicated to the patient and family at the time of diagnosis, and reinforced throughout the trajectory of illness. Broadly, these goals, which parallel the trajectory of disease, can be classified as curative, slowing progression of disease, and palliative control of symptoms or comfort care only. The terminal phase includes the management of symptoms at the end of life. Throughout all phases of illness, emphasis should be placed on palliative control of symptoms either from disease or treatment and maintaining optimum quality of life for the patient.

The Palliative Care Plan

The World Health Organization has indicated the need for integration of palliative care services throughout the trajectory of illness and stages of cancer from diagnosis to death. Devising a palliative plan of care should be part of the ongoing plan of care for the chronically ill patient. Appropriate care depends on several factors, including ongoing communication with the patient and family; assessment of the patient's and family's understanding of goals of care; religious, cultural, and spiritual beliefs; access to community agencies; psychological assessment and coping strategies; and preferences regarding advance directives. Dimensions of a palliative care plan for the health-care provider are outlined in Advanced Practice Nursing Interventions 19.1.

ADVANCED PRACTICE NURSING INTERVENTION 19.1

Dimensions of a Palliative Care Plan

1. Assessment of extent of disease documented by imaging studies, laboratory data
2. Assessment and interventions for physical signs and symptoms including pain, dyspnea, delirium
3. Assessment of coping strategies and psychological symptoms including presence and absence of depression, suicidal ideology
4. Level and quality of support provided by family and friends. Is additional assistance needed in the home and can it be put into place?
5. Coping strategies and psychological symptoms in family members or caregivers
6. Religious and spiritual assessment including degree of comfort from beliefs
7. Impact of disease on functional status. What can the patient do and what assistance is needed with bathing, dressing, ambulation, meal preparation?
8. Advance care planning. Have the patient's wishes and preferences for resuscitation, artificial feeding, and hydration been discussed? Has the patient identified a surrogate decision-maker who knows the patient's wishes? Is there documentation on advanced directives in the medical record?
9. Overall quality of life and well-being. Does the patient feel secure that all that can be done is being done? Does the patient feel physical and psychological symptoms are being satisfactorily addressed? Does the patient feel there is meaning to his or her life?
10. Family burden. Is attention being paid to support the caregiver so that burnout does not occur? What is the financial burden to the caregiver and can he or she manage bill paying and reimbursement issues?
11. Level of care needed in the home and provision for that care. What reimbursement issues affect obtaining the level of home care needed?
12. Is there a system in place for ongoing support and assistance to family members and caregivers after the death of the patient?

Palliative Cancer Care

In 2005 the American Cancer Society estimated that about 1,372,910 new cases of invasive cancer will be diagnosed in the United States in the next year. This does not include carcinoma in situ (noninvasive cancer). Among women, the most commonly diagnosed cancers are those of the breast, lung and bronchus, and colon and rectum. Among men, the most common cancers are cancers of the prostate, lung and bronchus, and colon and rectum. This year about 570,280 people are expected to die of cancer. Preliminary data suggests that overall cancer mortality has begun to decline; however, number of deaths have continued to increase because of the aging population. Cancer is a disease of aging and a prominent cause of overall morbidity and death. By the year 2020, the population will have increased an estimated 12 percent over that of 1990, but the total cancer incidence will have increased by 60 percent. In the United States, 60 percent of new cancer cases occur among those age 65 or older, with more than 50 percent of cancer deaths occurring among persons older than age 70.

The Role of the Primary Care Provider in Palliative Cancer Care

The health-care provider, as the primary-care provider of record, is critically important. There are a number of important points in the continuum of care for the patient with a chronic, irreversible disease process, most commonly a diagnosis of cancer, which call for a careful, comprehensive response. Often the primary-care provider is the first clinician to see the patient and because of this plays a crucial role. Although many patients are referred to specialists, the primary-care provider commonly provides a number of essential functions. Providing information on risk factors for many diseases, such as the use of sunscreens to prevent skin cancer, is an important role. Detecting occult disease in asymptomatic patients, or diagnosing disease in those with suspicious symptoms, is an essential responsibility of all health-care providers. In patients who have a strong family history of some malignancies the primary-care provider has a responsibility to educate and make appropriate referrals to specialists for genetic testing and/or counseling.

The discussion of the diagnosis, and the associated options, as well as arranging for specialty care is critical. This may be especially difficult in the diagnosis of cancer, a diagnosis most patient and families still perceive as a death sentence. It may be helpful to set a special appointment time for this discussion and encourage the patient to have a family member or advocate accompany the patient. A good understanding of the diagnosis and the potential prognosis is essential to the discussion, as well as awareness of the potential treatment options.

One must remember that the therapeutic window for treatment of certain cancers is small; thus, advice during this first discussion may be crucial in determining the patient's and family's course of action. Utilizing all of the caring processes during this time is important. It is essential to the subsequent care of the patient that as much information about the patient—biological, emotional, and spiritual—be provided to the specialty care provider. In this way, the primary care provider will remain an active and important component of the interdisciplinary team.

The patient should be referred for ongoing emotional and/or spiritual support at the time of diagnosis. Often the member of the health-care team who has had an ongoing relationship with the patient is in the best position to assess the psychological needs of the patient and their family. As a trusted care provider, the primary care provider is the ideal member of the team to recommend and implement this, and provide for ongoing follow-up care. This involves being knowledgeable of the appropriate time intervals for certain follow-up tests and knowing what to look for and when. The American Cancer Society is an excellent source for all health-care providers for state-of-the art information on cancer treatment.

The recognition and management of complications, either during or after treatment, is another role of the primary-care provider. Some of these complications may represent metastatic spread of the original cancer. Recognition is crucial. In some cases, complications may be life-threatening. A high index of suspicion must be vigilantly maintained: a manifestation of the caring processes of commitment, authentic presence, and courage. Advanced Practice Nursing Interventions 19.2 summarizes the role of the APN in palliative cancer care, although these interventions can be assumed by all primary care providers as well.

Principles of Palliative Care

The health-care provider who delivers primary care is often the one who provides care at the end of life; therefore, having a baseline knowledge of symptom management is crucial. Seriously ill patients with chronic disease and multiple comorbid medical conditions often cross practice settings from emergency room to home and from home to hospital. Because the Medicare hospice benefit is limited to patients with a 6-month prognosis, many patients with long-standing chronic illnesses, including cancer, are ineligible for hospice care, which for many patients has led to unrelieved suffering.

ADVANCED PRACTICE NURSING INTERVENTION 19.2

The Role of the Advanced Practice Nurse in Palliative Cancer Care

1. Teaching about risk factors for cancer and lifestyle change to decrease risk
2. Detecting cancer in asymptomatic patients or those with specific symptoms
3. Informing patient and family of diagnosis and prognosis. It is helpful if this is done in collaboration with the physician involved in the care of the patient.
4. Arranging for follow-up care, including psychosocial and spiritual support
5. Being an active participant of the interdisciplinary team
6. Providing follow-up care for ongoing symptom detection and management
7. Identifying and managing complications of care
8. Providing follow-up care and early detection of possible recurrences
9. Providing palliative care as necessary.
10. Referral to a palliative care specialist as indicated

Principles of palliative care useful for the primary-care provider include:

1. Careful evaluation of the patient's symptoms
2. A clear understanding of the pathophysiologic mechanisms involved
3. A judicious approach to diagnostic testing (with an aim of avoiding "overtesting" and testing that does not affect management)
4. Establishment of a treatment plan that is simple and subject to continual reevaluation
5. Determining what the patient's and caregiver's expectations are regarding their care at this stage of illness
6. Determining if the patient has special wishes regarding end-of-life care, including place of death and if advance directives have been discussed and documented
7. Referral to a pain and palliative care specialist for aggressive management of these symptoms if routine interventions are inadequate

Pain control is paramount. Pain is the symptom most feared by dying patients. While usually the manifestation of physical distress, pain may be exacerbated by anxiety, fear, loneliness, and depression. Patients differ vastly in the extent of clinical disease that yields pain, as well as in their ability to tolerate, accept, or cope with pain. Pain expected to be transient may be treated on an as-needed (prn) basis, but chronic pain needs to be treated via a scheduled regimen. The section of this chapter on pain discusses this in greater detail.

Clinical problems frequently seen in terminally ill patients include pain, dyspnea, fatigue, depression, anorexia, weight loss, constipation, and anxiety. Initial evaluation of symptoms must begin with determining the etiology of the symptom evaluating. This is usually done as part of the initial work-up. If the etiology of pain is secondary to the treatment, one should ask whether the treatment can be adjusted or whether it should be discontinued. Goals of care should be reviewed on a routine basis, especially at intervals when treatment decisions need to be made. Other challenges are the ethical dilemmas that may be faced by the health-care provider whose own beliefs may conflict or be different from the patient's family member's or caregiver's. It is important for the health-care provider to recognize that their beliefs are just that, and may frequently differ from that of the patient's. For example, one of the most common and controversial clinical issues at the end of life is the need for hydration. Differences of opinion may exist not only between health-care providers and the patient or caregiver, but between family members. When there are concerns about nutrition and hydration at the end of life, the amount of food or fluid given to a dying person should be guided by patients' desires and their ability to tolerate nourishment orally, rather than by calculated nutritional or fluid requirements. It is also important to understand that cultural differences often play a role and should be respected. At the end of life small amounts of fluids, ice chips, or mouth swabs, classic nursing interventions, are often beneficial.

THE PATIENT'S VOICE 19.1

Palliative Care

The Patient

"The pain was intolerable, every time I moved my back hurt. The morphine tablets made me sleepy and constipated. The pain of trying to have a bowel movement was almost as severe as the back pain. My doctor basically told me to bear it as these side effects were common."

The Son

"My father was clearly dying and was confused at times. The nursing staff gave him injections for pain but they did not seem to help. When I questioned the nurses, they told me they could not give him more because they did not want to slow his breathing. I thought, he's dying, make him comfortable."

Another frequent challenge is what is the best way to deliver medication, especially in the home or hospice setting when the patient is unable to swallow. Routes of administration to consider for the dying patient who cannot swallow include sublingual, intravenous, transcutaneous, subcutaneous, and spinal (e.g., intrathecal, epidural). Creativity is frequently called for, as well as the ability to work in concert with a team of providers, such as pharmacists, clergy, and homecare nurses. Close communication with patient and family, utilizing the processes of caring, courage, authentic presence, advocacy, patience, and commitment is crucial. This will enable the APN to truly "hear" the patient's voice.

Palliative Care of Symptoms in Dying Patients

Numerous studies have evaluated symptoms during the last weeks of life and indicate that patients experience a high degree of symptom distress and suffering. Portenoy and Ingham suggested in 1996 that symptom assessment should be multidimensional, involving determination of the incidence, duration severity, amount of distress, and impact on function and quality of life. A variety of symptoms in the last year and weeks of life have been identified in the literature including pain, weakness, fatigue, cognitive impairment, and dyspnea.

Seal and Cartwright (1994) studied the incidence of symptoms both in patients with cancer and noncancer the year before death and the effect of age on these symptoms.

Two populations in England were studied in the years 1969 and 1987. More than 80 percent of cancer patients in both groups experienced pain, whereas approximately 67 percent of noncancer patients experienced pain. The patients with cancer experienced more symptoms than those dying of nonmalignant diseases. There was an age-related difference in the incidence of mental confusion, loss of bladder and bowel control, and seeing and hearing difficulties. There was no age-related difference in patients reporting pain (72 percent), trouble breathing (49 percent), loss of appetite (47 percent), drowsiness (44 percent), sleeplessness (40 percent), constipation (36 percent), depression (36 percent), vomiting (33 percent), and dry mouth (33 percent).

Several studies have demonstrated that the most difficult end-of-life symptoms to manage are pain, respiratory distress, and confusional states. In a retrospective review of 100 patients in an inpatient palliative care unit, Fainsinger and colleagues (1991) identified 16 percent of the patients required sedation to control pain and delirium. In another evaluation of patients during the last week of life, Conill and colleagues (1997) assessed patients at two intervals, at their initial consultation and then during the last 7 days of life. Asthenia, anorexia, and dry mouth were the three most common symptoms in both periods, but the incidence of confusional states doubled during the last week of life (30.1 percent and 68.2 percent, respectively). Potter and colleagues assessed 400 patients referred to palliative care services and found the most prevalent symptoms in the cancer population overall were pain (64 percent), anorexia (34 percent), constipation (32 percent), weakness (32 percent), and dyspena (31 percent).

Needs of nursing home patients at the end of life have also been identified. In one study of nursing home residents during the last 3 months of life the most common symptoms include pain, dyspnea, fatigue, depressed mood, anxiety, and loneliness. In one nationwide study of terminally ill nursing home residents the terminal ill phase was identified with symptoms of anorexia, weakness, respiratory problems, and reflected a mainly noncancer population.

The suffering that patients experience at the end of life is not necessarily related to the severity of the symptom(s). Mild symptoms may cause severe distress, especially if the meaning of that symptom is frightening—if it signifies that death is near. Unrelieved symptoms at the end of life are extremely devastating, they can rob the patient and their loved ones of valuable time and meaningful interaction. During this time nurses have a responsibility as patient and family advocates to ensure that symptoms are addressed and treated appropriately.

Palliative management of three of the most difficult symptoms—pain, dyspnea, and delirium, will be discussed. Accurate assessment and diagnosis of these symptoms is assumed. The reader is referred to appropriate sections of this textbook for more information on assessment and diagnosis of these problems.

Palliative Management of Pain

According to the International Association for the Study of Pain, pain is identified as a subjective experience and is described as "an unpleasant sensory or emotional experience related to actual or potential tissue damage." Table 19.1 presents a review of the various types of pain.

Assessment

Pain management begins with accurate assessment of the patient's pain. This assessment should be incorporated into all routine bedside and ambulatory visits as well as when there is a report of worsening pain or new pain. Adequate assessment should enable the health-care provider to determine the cause of the pain, assist in determining treatment, and evaluating the effectiveness of therapeutic interventions and their impact on the quality of life. Assessment of pain is subjective and relies heavily on the patient's report. The use of an assessment tool can facilitate understanding and assist in determining treatment efficacy. Validated assessment tools include the Brief Pain Inventory and the McGill Pain Questionnaire. A 10-point (0 to 10) scale is commonly used and has been recommended in the AHCPR Clinical Practice Guidelines in the Management of Cancer Pain. If the patient cannot use a numerical scale, a categorical scale of none, mild, moderate, and severe is recommended. Pain assessment should include a detailed history of the pain including intensity and characteristics, a comprehensive physical examination, a psychosocial evaluation, and a thorough diagnostic work-up to determine the cause of the pain. Table 19.2 outlines the basic principles of pain assessment.

Management

Palliative management of the patient in pain includes pharmacotherapy, surgical management, and nonpharmacologic management.

Pharmacotherapy

The 1990 World Health Organization's Three-Step Analgesic Ladder provides an approach to the pharmacologic management of cancer pain. This approach advocates use of analgesics in a three-step analgesic ladder—nonsteroidal anti-inflammatory drugs (NSAIDs), opioids, and adjuvant drugs. The steps are as follows:

Step 1. Mild to Moderate Pain. Patients with mild to moderate pain should be treated with a nonopioid analgesic and, if indicated, an adjuvant drug. Examples of nonopioid analgesics are acetaminophen (Tylenol) and the nonsteroidal anti-inflammatory drugs (NSAIDs) such as aspirin, ibuprofen (Advil, Motrin), indomethacin (Indocin), ketorolac (Toradol), and naproxen (Naprosyn, Aleve, Anaprox). Examples of adjuvant drugs are tricyclic antidepressants

Table 19.1 Types of Pain

Pain may be described as an unpleasant sensory and/or emotional experience related to actual or potential tissue damage. The perception of pain is the result of tissue injury leading to the origination and conduction of pain signals by the central nervous system. Peripheral stimulation occurs when free nerve endings or nociceptors found in various parts of the body (e.g., skin, blood vessels, viscera, muscles) are stimulated, which in turn stimulates action potentials to be transmitted along afferent nerve fibers to the spinal cord.

Acute Pain

- Well-defined temporal pattern of onset
- Transient, may be associated with hyperactivity of the autonomic nervous system
- Increased blood pressure, pulse rate, respiratory rate, and perspiration.
- Patients may look like they are in pain and may cry or moan.

Chronic Pain

- Syndrome that is defined by a pattern of pain that persists beyond healing of the acute lesion or recurs over periods of months, or is associated with a lesion not expected to improve.
- Patients experience a decrease in observable signs of pain.
- BP and pulse rate are normal.
- Sleep disturbance, decreased appetite, depression and lassitude may be present.

Nociceptive Pain

Nociceptive (organic) pain results from activation and sensitization of nociceptors, or pain receptors, located throughout the body. Nociceptive pain may be further subdivided into somatic and visceral pain (Payne and Gonzales, 1998).

- Somatic pain
  - May be constant, aching, throbbing.
  - Examples include bone metastases, postsurgical incisional pain, musculoskeletal inflammation or spasm.
- Visceral pain
  - Results from inflammation, compression, distension, or stretching of thoracic or abdominal viscera (e.g., intra-abdominal metastases, liver metastases).
  - May be diffuse, gnawing or cramping.

Neuropathic Pain

Neuropathic pain refers to syndromes that may be related to damaged peripheral or central neural structures as a result of tumor progression or infiltration or from chemical injury to the peripheral nerve or spinal cord from surgery, irradiation, or chemotherapy.

- May be continuous or lancinating.
- May be burning, shooting, electric shock-like, squeezing, vise-like.

(TCAs) such as amitriptyline (Elavil), imipramine (Tofranil); anticonvulsants such as neurontin (Gabapentin), and lamotrigine (Lamictal).

Step 2. Moderate Pain. Patients who are opioid naive and present with moderate pain or who fail to have adequate analgesia from a nonopioid should be treated with an opioid (previously called weak opioids) and a nonopioid and adjuvant drug. Examples of these opioids are codeine, hydrocodone (Hycodan), and oxycodone with Tylenol (Percocet) or without Tylenol.

Table 19.2 Basic Principles of Pain Assessment

- Believe the patient's complaint of pain. The patient is the expert in determining the level of pain he or she is experiencing.
- Take a careful history of the pain complaint and incorporate into the overall plan and goals of care.
- If the patient has difficulty communicating because of cognitive or physical impairments, obtain a history from the family or caregiver.
- Observe for nonverbal cues (e.g., crying, grimacing).
- Assess for other symptoms (e.g., agitation, delirium, dyspnea) which may cloud the pain assessment.
- Assess for onset, timing, temporal characteristics, pattern of referral, aggravating and relieving factors.
- Assess for breakthrough or incident-related pain.
- Examine the site of pain on every patient encounter.
- Facilitate work-up which clarifies the etiology of the pain and extent of disease.
- Evaluate the psychological state of the patient and assess for depression, anxiety, delirium, or suicidal ideation.
- Determine appropriate opioid and route of administration. Consider cost of medications and economic burden on patient and family. Consider use of adjuvant analgesics especially if neuropathic pain.
- Assess and reassess response to treatment and monitor for presence of side effects. Treat side effects aggressively.

Step 3. Moderate to Severe Pain. Patients who present with moderate to severe pain or who fail to have adequate analgesia from the second level of intervention should receive an opioid (previously called strong opioids) and a nonopioid or adjuvant. Examples include morphine (MS Contin, Roxanol), hydromorphone (Dilaudid), levorphanol (Levo-Dromoran), methadone (Dolophine), and fentanyl (Duragesic). Opioids are frequently used in combination with an NSAID.

Figure 19.1 illustrates the WHO Clinical Ladder. Table 19.3 outlines common adjuvants for specific types of pain (e.g., neuropathic and bone pain).

Important considerations when providing pharmacotherapy for pain management include selecting the appropriate opioid, route of administration, and dosage schedule and determining an equianalgesic dose if switching to another opioid.

Selecting the Appropriate Opioid. When given properly, opioids are among the safest medications available, as adverse

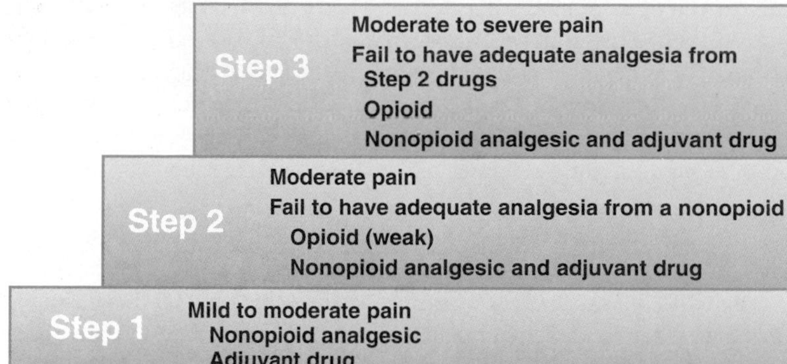

FIGURE 19.1 Three-step analgesic ladder.

effects are predictable and generally controllable. The potency of opioids varies, but they are generally interchangeable with appropriate dose and dosing interval adjustments.

Numerous factors, both patient and drug related, must be considered in the selection of an appropriate opioid. The opioid should be compatible with the patient's pain severity, age, and dosing and route of administration requirements. Often financial considerations need to be taken into account especially when the patient is receiving multiple drugs and the cost of medications needs to be limited. At the end of life, certain routes of administration may be preferable owing to ease of administration, need to titrate rapidly, patient comfort, and ability to swallow.

When evaluating an opioid for chronic use, renal and liver function should be assessed prior to initiation of the opioid. If patients have underlying renal or liver insufficiency they should be monitored for signs of toxicity. Opioids with long half-lives may not be tolerated in many elderly patients because of clearance or metabolism issues. For patients with moderate to severe pain who have limited prior treatment with opioids, begin with a short half-life agonist (morphine, hydromorphone, oxycodone). Morphine is the preferred drug because of availability of doses and

Table 19.3 Adjuvant Drugs for Specific Types of Pain

Neuropathic Pain

- Tricyclic antidepressant
  - Amitriptyline
  - Desipramine
  - Imipramine
  - Nortriptyline
- Antiepileptic drugs
  - Gabapentin (Neurontin)
  - Carbamazepine (Tegretol)
  - Oxcarbazepine (Trileptal)
  - Topiramate (Topamax)
  - Levetiracetam (Keppra)
  - Sodium valproate (Depacon)
  - Tiagabine (Gabitril)
  - Lamotrigine (Lamictal)
  - Zonisamide (Zonegran)
- Local anesthetics
  - EMLA (topical eutectic mixture of local anesthetics lidocaine and prilocaine)
  - Epidural and intravenous lidocaine
  - Oral local anesthetics
    - Mexiletine (Mexitil)
    - Tocainide (Tonocard)
  - Topical lidocaine 5 percent patches (Lidoderm)
- Glucocorticoids
- Alpha-2-adrenergic agonists
  - Tizanidine (Zanaflex)
  - Clonidine
- NMDA receptor antagonists
  - Ketamine
  - Dextromethorphan
  - Amantadine
- GABA agonists
  - Baclofen

Bone Pain

- Glucocorticoids
- Bisphosphonates
  - Pamidronate disodium (Aredia)
  - Zoledronate (Zometa)
- Other osteoclast inhibitor
  - Calcitonin
- Radiopharmaceuticals
  - Strontium-89
  - Strontium-153

Other

Skeletal muscle relaxants
- Tizanidine (Zanaflex)
- Benzodiazepines
  - Diazepam (Valium)
  - Clonazepam (Klonopin)
  - Lorazepam (Ativan)
- Antihistamines
  - Hydroxyzine (Vistaril)
- Antispasmodics
  - Baclofen

Topical agents
  - Capsaicin cream
  - Lidocaine 5 percent patch (Lidoderm)
  - EMLA cream

because it can be administered as a controlled-release tablet at 8- to 12-hour dosing intervals. Morphine should be used judiciously in patients with renal impairment because of the accumulation of morphine-3-glucuronide and morphine-6-glucuronide. It is also helpful to remember that in elderly patients, normal serum creatinine concentrations does not exclude renal impairment.

By beginning with a shorter half-life opioid the clinician can titrate the opioid easier than if beginning with a longer half-life opioid, such as levorphanol or methadone. It is also important to remember that the use of meperidine (Demerol) for the management of chronic cancer pain is not recommended because of its potential for central nervous system excitability, with possible tremors, myoclonus, and seizures.

Selecting an Appropriate Route of Administration. Begin with the most available, least invasive route. The oral route is generally preferred. In general, when drugs are administered orally, they have a slower onset of action, delayed peak time, and a longer duration of effect than drugs administered parenterally. Drugs administered parenterally have a rapid onset of action but a shorter duration of action.

If the oral route is unavailable, the rectal, sublingual, transdermal, or parenteral route may be used. Rectal suppositories containing morphine, hydromorphone, and oxymorphone are available, and controlled-release morphine sulfate may be administered rectally.

The transdermal fentanyl patch (Duragesic) is useful for patients who cannot tolerate oral drugs or for patients for whom compliance with an around-the-clock schedule is difficult to maintain. The fentanyl patch is contraindicated in the management of acute pain. Because steady state begins to be reached in about 12 to 24 hours after initiation of therapy, it is difficult to titrate using this delivery system. When the patch is removed serum concentrations fall slowly. The fentanyl patch is not recommended for use in patients who have varying levels of pain or who have severe effects such as sedation or confusion from opioids, as these effects may persist for long periods after the patch is removed. One must prescribe a short-acting opioid for breakthrough pain when using the fentanyl patch.

Parenteral routes of administration should be considered for patients who require rapid onset of analgesia or high doses of opioids that cannot be administered orally. Parenteral routes include intermittent IV, IM, or SC injections and continuous SC or IV infusions. Intermittent SC injections may be administered with the placement of an indwelling 27-gauge butterfly needle, which will eliminate the need for painful intermittent injections. Studies suggest that SC administration is equipotent to the IV dose. Continuous IV infusions include the use of patient-controlled analgesia (PCA), which can be administered at home. These infusion devices may also provide patient-controlled rescue doses as an adjunct to the continuous, or basal, rate.

Selecting a Dosing Schedule. Patients with continuous or frequent pain generally benefit from around-the-clock dosing, which prevents the pain from recurring. Continuous release formulations of opioids such as MS Contin, Kadian, OxyContin, and Fentanyl TSS® may improve patient adherence to opioid regimens. A "rescue," or prn dose provides a means to treat pain that breaks through the fixed analgesic schedule, or pain that occurs with specific activities such as changing position or ambulating. The drug used for breakthrough pain is usually the same drug, although a shorter, immediate release formulation, than is the continuous or sustained released opioid that is administered on a regular schedule. When using transdermal fentanyl a short half-life opioid is recommended (Hanks, 2004). Continuous or sustained release formulations should not be used as rescue doses or to rapidly titrate the opioid for patients with severe pain (Table 19.4). In these settings, short-acting opioids should be used; when analgesia is obtained and a stable dose has been determined, conversion to a continuous-release formulation can be made.

Switching to Another Opioid. If a switch to another opioid is required, the equianalgesic dose table should be used as a

Table 19.4 The Rescue Dose and Dose Titration

The Rescue Dose
The rescue dose is an additional dose of the opioid that is administered on an as-needed basis to treat breakthrough pain; a short-acting, immediate release opioid should be used. Oral rescue doses are usually administered on an every-1-to-2-hour schedule as needed. The dose of the oral rescue should be equivalent to approximately 50% of the dose administered every 4 hours. The dose of the parenteral rescue opioid should be 50% of the hourly infusion rate for patients receiving continuous infusion, administered on a 15- to 30-minute as-needed schedule. Another way of calculating the rescue dose is to administer 5%–15% of the 24-hour baseline dose. It is generally recommended that patients who require at least four to six rescue doses in a 24-hour period should have an escalation of the baseline dose.

Dose Titration
All patients with chronic cancer pain should be assessed regularly for pain intensity and relief and for the presence of adverse effects. A stepwise escalation of the opioid dose should be done until adequate analgesia or intolerable adverse effects develop. Generally, it is safe to titrate opioids 25%–50% every 24–48 hours. The severity of the pain should determine the rate of dose titration. Doses can become extremely large as a result of titration. It is important to remember that there is no ceiling to opioid doses and titration needs to be based on pain intensity and relief. Caution should be employed when titrating opioids with long half-lives, such as levorphanol or methadone, as accumulation of drug can occur with subsequent toxicity.

guide. For patients who develop unacceptable adverse effects that cannot be effectively managed, the opioid should be changed. Because of the existence of incomplete cross-tolerance between drugs, for patients on higher doses of opioids who require a drug switch, the alternative opioid should be reduced by one-half to two-thirds of the equianalgesic dose. If switching to an opioid with a long half-life, such as methadone, accumulation of the drug can occur, and the methadone dose should be decreased by 90 percent. Table 19.5 presents an equianalgesic dose table and guidelines on switching to another opioid.

Surgical Management

Anesthetic and neurosurgical approaches are indicated when conservative measures utilizing opioids and adjuvant analgesics have failed to provide adequate analgesia or when the patient is experiencing intolerable side effects. In evaluating patients for invasive approaches, it is important to clarify that all other conservative measures have been adequately tried and failed. Other factors to consider include presence of infection, coagulopathy or use of anticoagulant drugs, functional state, coexisting medical conditions, spinal cord disease, rapid progression of disease outside of site that is going to be blocked, or ablated (Cherny, Arbit, and Jain, 1996). Other factors to be considered include life expectancy, amount of support in the home, availablitity of local healthcare providers that can monitor and manage the intervention. These procedures include regional analgesia (spinal, intraventricular, and intrapleural opioids), sympathetic blockade and neurolytic procedures (celiac plexus block, lumbar sympathetic block, cervicothoracic [stellate ganglion] block), or pathway ablation procedure (chemical or surgical rhizotomy or cordotomy).

Nonpharmacologic Management

Physical and psychological interventions can be used as an adjunct with drugs and surgical approaches to manage pain. Referral to a professional who specializes in these modalities may be indicated as appropriate. Nonpharmacologic management may also include psychological therapy and/or use of peer-support groups. Physical modalities include cutaneous stimulation, exercise, immobilization, acupuncture, and transcutaneous electrical nerve stimulation (TENS).

Cognitive–behavioral interventions include relaxation, guided imagery, distraction, music therapy, and hypnosis. The major advantages of these techniques are that they are easy to learn and are safe and readily accepted by patients. Cognitive and behavioral interventions are helpful in reducing emotional distress, improving coping, and offering the patient and family a sense of control.

Relaxation exercises have been useful in the management of nausea and vomiting, dyspnea, pain, anxiety, and insomnia. Relaxation techniques are divided into deep and brief methods. Deep methods include autogenic training, meditation, and progressive muscle relaxation (PMR). Autogenic training consists of imagining a peaceful environment and comforting bodily sensations. Focusing techniques include heaviness in limbs, cardiac regulation, centering on breathing, warmth in abdomen, and coolness in the forehead. Meditation is a self-directed practice for relaxing the body and calming the mind. Transcendental meditation focuses on a suitable sound or thought (a mantra). Movement meditations include yoga and the walking meditation of Zen buddhism. PMR focuses on reducing muscle tone in major muscle groups by first tensing then relaxing the muscles. Brief methods include paced respiration, deep breathing, and self-control relaxation.

It may be helpful to consider the five major classifications or domains used by the National Center for Complementary and Alternative Medicine (NCCAM). These are alternative medical systems, mind–body interventions, biologically based therapies, manipulative and body-based methods, and energy therapies. Acupuncture, mind–body therapy and massage therapy are shown in the literature to have the strongest evidence for their role in the clinical management of pain.

Acupuncture is a treatment from traditional Chinese medicine, has been shown to effectively treat pain, depression, nausea, and other problems. In this holistic approach, thin disposable needles are placed in precise anatomical points to balance energy movement along the body's 12 meridians. Acupressure is the application of finger pressure to the acupuncture points. The NIH Consensus Development Panel on Acupuncture in 1998 found that the incidence of adverse effects from acupuncture is substantially lower than for many standard medical procedures or medications used for the same condition. Adverse effects include bruising at insertion site, mild discomfort, and rarely, at the insertion site, pneumothorax.

Acupuncture acts to promote the flow of chi or "Qui," vital energy, and is based on a holistic, energy-focused approach to individuals, not a disease-oriented approach, as seen in Western medicine.

Music has been shown to be an effective intervention for pain control through a variety of physiologic and psychologic effects. Music therapy, as defined by Spross and Wolff Burk in a 1995 study is the "scientific and systematic use of music to effect beneficial changes in physiological and psychologic processes that influences experiences of pain and illness." Physical effects may include increasing or decreasing the pulse rate and blood pressure. The use of music in the ill and dying can reduce mood disturbance and affect the suffering and total pain that patients with advanced cancer may experience.

Cognitive interventions such as relaxation, guided imagery, and hypnosis also fall under the NCAAM category of mind–body methods that may also be helpful in the management of chronic pain.

Energy Therapies

Therapeutic touch (TT) is the complementary technique based on systems theory of the multidimensional nature of

Table 19.5 Switching to Another Opioid

Equianalgesic Table

Drug	IV/IM/SC Duration	PO	IV:PO	Half-life
Morphine sulfate	10 mg 2–4 hours	30 mg	1:3	2–3 hours
Codeine	130 mg 2–4 hours	200 mg	—	2–3 hours
Hydromorphone	1.5 mg 2–4 hours	7.5 mg	1:5	2–3 hours
Levorphanol	2 mg 4–6 hours	4 mg	1:2	12–15 hours
Meperidine	75 mg 2–4 hours	300 mg	1:4	3–4 hours
Methadone	10 mg 4–8 hours	20 mg	1:2	12–15 hours
Oxycodone	— 2–4 hours	30 mg	—	2–3 hours
Oxymorphone	1-mg or 5-mg suppository 2–4 hours	—	—	2–3 hours
(i) Fentanyl	100-mcg patch/IV =	4 mg morphine sulfate	—	IV/hour

Switching from One Route of Administration to Another (Same Drug)

The following example illustrates how to switch from one route of administration to another using the same drug.

A 42-year-old woman with metastatic ovarian cancer is receiving morphine sulfate (MSO_4) 15 mg/h IV. She is going to be discharged in 2 days and would prefer to go home with an oral medication. Her parenteral morphine dosage needs to be converted to an oral morphine dosage, e.g., MSO_4 15 mg/h IV to MS Contin PO.

1. Calculate the 24-hour dose of the opioid (including around-the-clock [ATC] and prn rescue doses).
   MSO_4 15 mg/h IV = 15 mg × 24 h = 360 mg IV/24 h
2. Convert the 24-hour dose of the drug (at prior route of administration) to 24-hour dose of drug (at new route of administration) using the equianalgesic table.
   MSO_4 10 mg IV = 30 mg PO
   360 mg IV = 1080 mg PO
3. Determine the dosing interval of the new drug. Using sustained release morphine given q8–12h, the patient needs 1080 mg PO over 24 hours; therefore, 540 mg PO can be given q12h.
4. Calculate the prn rescue dose as 5%–15% of the total 24-hour mg dose of the drug. (It may be necessary to adjust the dose as it is commercially available.)
   5% of 1080 mg = 54 mg
   Therefore, the decision was made to give 60 mg PO q2h prn as a rescue dose.

Switching from One Oral Opioid to Another

A 65-year-old man with metastatic prostate cancer to bone is receiving sustained/controlled release oral morphine 60 mg PO q12h and is experiencing severe uncontrollable nausea and vomiting. The decision is made to switch him to oral hydromorphone.

1. Calculate the 24-hour dose of the prior opioid (including ATC and prn rescue doses).
   Sustained release morphine 60 mg PO q12h = 120 mg PO/24 hours
2. Convert the 24-hour dose of the prior drug to the 24-hour dose of the new drug using the equianalgesic table.
   Hydromorphone 7.5 mg PO = MSO_4 30 mg PO
   Hydromorphone 3 mg PO/24 h = MSO_4 120 mg PO/24 h
   30X = 900 mg PO
   X = 30 mg hydromorphone PO/24 h
3. Indicate the adjusted total 24-hour dose of the new drug.
   Adjust the dose of new drug as follows:
   a. Reduce the total 24-hour dose of new drug by 25%–50% to account for incomplete cross tolerance.
   b. If the patient has inadequate analgesia and no side effects from prior drug it may not be necessary to reduce the dose of new drug.
   c. Reduce the drug more if the patient has significant side effects from the prior drug.
   d. If the patient is frail, reduce the dose of the new drug more (75%).
   e. Reduce the dose of the new drug more if the dose of the prior drug is high (>75 mg IM morphine equivalent/day).
   f. If the new drug is methadone, reduce the total 24-hour dose by 90%.
   50% of hydromorphone 30 mg PO = 15 mg hydromorphine PO q24 hours
4. Determine the dosing interval of the new drug.
   Hydromorphone 15 mg PO/24 h = 2.5 mg PO q4h
   (It may be necessary to adjust the dose as it is commercially available. Hydromorphone 2 mg PO q4h)
5. Calculate the prn rescue dose as 5%–15% of the total 24 hour mg dose of the new drug. 2 mg PO q2h prn. (It may be necessary to adjust the dose as it is commercially available.)

the individual and the homeostatic concepts of balance and wholeness which work with energy fields in promoting relaxation and reducing pain. TT does not involve touching, it involves a conscious intention of the part of the healer to help the patient. The practitioner's hands are placed about 6 inches above the body, starting at the head, and moving down the body toward the feet. During the next phase, the treatment phase, the pracitioner channels energy to areas of the body.

Reiki is another energy therapy. It is defined as a vibrational or subtle energy facilitated by light touch whose use is thought to balance the biofield and assist the body to heal itself. The practitioner places his or her hands on the individual's head, back, front, or the site of discomfort to promote relaxation and decrease pain.

Complementary therapies are being offered more frequently to patients at the end of life. A recent hospice survey found that 60 percent of 169 hospices offered complementary therapies to patients. Massage therapy and music therapy were the most common.

Palliative Management of Dyspnea

Dyspnea may be one of the most frightening and difficult symptoms a patient can experience, and can be more difficult to treat than pain. Dyspnea is a subjective feeling of breathlessness, the sensation of labored or difficult breathing, which contributes to severe disability and impaired quality of life. It occurs before death in an estimated 20 to 70 percent of patients with advanced cancer. Patients often describe feelings of suffocation, tightness, congestion, air hunger, choking, or heavy breathing. A review of the literature on management of dyspnea at the end of life reinforces the growing recognition that dyspnea and fear of dyspnca

COMPLEMENTARY THERAPIES 19.1

Palliative Management of Pain

Diet and Nutrition

Macrobiotic Diet

The macrobiotic diet, often used as an anticancer treatment, derives 50–60% of its calories from whole grains, 25–30% from vegetables, and the remainder from beans, seaweed, and soups. Soybean intake, in the form of miso is advocated, and meats and processed foods are prohibited.

Genistein

Genistein, a substance in soybeans, is presently under investigation. Asian women have a lower rate of breast cancer than American women whose diet is substantially higher in fat, especially animal fat. The relationship between diet and breast cancer in Asian women needs further study.

Vitamins and Minerals

Megavitamins have been advocated as prevention for cancer. Orthomolecular therapy, or the treatment of large doses of vitamins and minerals, including vitamins A, C, and E, to treat disease including colds, influenza, and cancer can be associated with vitamin toxicity. Vitamins and minerals used in the treatment of cancer include selenium, beta carotene, chromium, and manganese.

Herbal Therapies

Herbal therapies have a long history in various cultures around the world. Those used for the treatment of cancer include iscador, Yin Chiao Chieh Tu Pein, chaparral tea, green tea, and soy proteins. Herbs used for pain management include chaparral tea, oil of flaxseed, or primrose for joint pain and fatigue, Jin Bu Han, willow tea, and capsicum cream topically. Management of insomnia may include passion flower, chamomile, and valerian (also used for anxiety and stress). Nausea and vomiting may be lessened by the use of lobelia and ginger, while cognitive functions may benefit from ginkgo (mental slowing, memory loss) and St. John's wort or licorice for depression.

Although many of these herbs are harmless, many can lead to serious toxicities, especially if taken in high doses. Ginger, gingko, garlic (colds, high cholesterol), and feverfew (migraine headache), when combined with aspirin or warfarin, can cause excessive bleeding. Comfrey (bruises) can produce liver toxicity. Lobelia, in high doses can produce coma and death. Jin Bu Han can produce hepatitis.

Metabolic and Detoxification Treatments

Metabolic therapies are based on the premise that cancer produces toxic substances that accumulate in the liver, leading to death. Tijuana, Mexico is the site of many clinics for many of these therapies.

Detoxification or cleansing therapies include ingestion of liver extract, massive doses of fruit and vegetable juices, and coffee enemas. These therapies can lead to dehydration, bowel rupture, and severe vitamin and mineral deficiencies.

Magnet Therapy

Bioelectromagnetics is the study of interactions between living organisms and their electromagnetic fields. Magnetic fields, created by low frequency magnets, have been claimed to treat a variety of conditions, including cancer and pain. Their use is under further investigation.

produce profound suffering for patients who are dying and their families. The causes of dyspnea are numerous and related to pulmonary disease, cardiac disease, cancer, metabolic abnormalities, radiation therapy, and surgery. Anxiety is always a component. Higginson and McCarthy (1989) reported that dyspnea prevalence increases in terminally ill patients and is the major uncontrollable symptom. The Hospice Nurses Association advocates aggressive assessment and therapeutic interventions for the management of dyspnea.

Assessment

Dyspnea is a multidimensional symptom, having both physical and psychological components. For most patients with organic disease, the respiratory distress gets worse with progression of disease. It is highly distressing for families and caregivers, who often feel helpless.

Various tools to measure dyspnea have been documented in the literature and include use of a visual analogue scale, structured interviews, self-report questionnaires, and numeric rating scales. Clinical assessment of dyspnea should include a complete history of the symptom, its onset and duration, precipitating and relieving factors; associated symptoms; and response to medications, oxygen, and behavioral interventions. A recent study has suggested that different ethnic groups use different words to describe dyspnea in the presence of airflow obstruction.

Data suggest that the frequency and severity of dyspnea increase with progression of disease and when death is approaching, and may be seen as a poor prognostic sign.

Management

Relief of dyspnea is aimed at treatment of the underlying disease process, whether malignant or nonmalignant in origin. Symptomatic interventions are used when the process is not reversible.

A variety of sources advocate the use of morphine to manage intractable dyspnea. Bruera's studies suggest that morphine can significantly improve dyspnea without significantly changing respiratory rate, oxygen saturation, or expiratory carbon dioxide. Management of dyspnea is based on the cause and includes pharmacotherapy (e.g., bronchodilators, steroids, diuretics, vasodilators, antibiotics, opioids, and sedatives), oxygen, nonpharmacologic therapies (e.g., relaxation and breathing exercises), and other appropriate therapies (e.g., transfusion, thoracentesis, and radiation therapy). Few random-controlled trails have been carried out in advanced cancer patients to evaluate the role of opioids and O_2 therapy in the management of dyspnea. For most dying patients, the pharmacologic use of benzodiazepines, opioids, and corticosteroids remains the primary treatment. There may be much resistance among primary-care providers to use opioids and sedatives because of unfamiliarity with these drugs, lack of experience in treating dyspnea in dying patients, low priority given to this symptom, and fear that these drugs may hasten death. Table 19.6 presents interventions commonly used for the management of dyspnea.

Table 19.6 Interventions for Dyspnea

Interventions	Comments
Pharmacotherapy	
Oxygen	3–5 L/min via nasal cannula
Morphine sulfate	SC: 50% higher than regularly scheduled dose SC: 5 mg bolus or 2.5 times regular dose q4h SC: 10 mg q4h IV: 5 mg/h Nebulized: 2.5–5 mg q4h Nebulized: 5–30 mg q4h
Bronchodilators	Nebulized: adrenergic and anticholinergic agents 4 times/day (ipratropium bromide [Atrovent], albuterol [Proventil], isoproterenol HCl [Isuprel], or metaproterenol sulfate [Alupent]) PO or IV: aminophylline PO: theophylline (Theo-Dur) 400 mg qd
Corticosteroids	Inhaler: beclomethasone (Vanceril) 1–2 inhalations 3–4 times/day PO or IV: dexamethasone (Decadron) 8–12 mg qd then taper PO: prednisone 10–30 mg
Anxiolytics	PO: lorazepam (Ativan) 0.5–2 mg bid–tid PO: diazepam (Valium) 2–10 mg bid–qid PO: chlorpromazine (Thorazine) 25–50 mg tid–qid PO: haloperidol (Haldol) 0.5–2 mg bid–qid
Diuretics	PO: furosemide (Lasix) 20–40 mg qd
Transfusions	
Nonpharmacologic Therapies	
Cognitive–behavioral	Relaxation therapy Guided imagery Music Distraction
Acupuncture	

The use of the mnemonic "BREATHES" may assist the health-care provider in the symptomatic management of dyspnea:

B: Bronchospasm. Consider nebulized albuterol and/or steroids.

R: Rales/crackles. If present, consider reducing fluid intake. If the patient is receiving IV hydration, reduce the fluid rate or discontinue. Consider gentle diuresis with furosemide 20 to 40 mg PO and spironolactone 100 mg PO daily.

E: Effusion. Consider thoracentesis or a chest tube, if appropriate. Consider intermittent pleural drainage with an indwelling thoracentesis tube.

A: Airway obstruction. If the patient is at risk or has had aspiration from food, puree solid food, avoid thin liquids, and keep the patient upright during and after meals for at least 1 hour. Keep patient NPO if end of life.

T: Tachypnea and breathlessness. Opioids reduce respiratory rate and feelings of breathlessness as well as anxiety. If patient is opioid naive, begin with morphine sulfate 5 to 10 mg PO q4h and titrate 25 to 50 percent daily, every other day as needed. Also consider an anxiolytic, such as Ativan 0.5 to 2 mg PO bid to tid.

H: Hemoglobin low. Consider a blood transfusion if anemia is contributing to dyspnea and fatigue.

E: Educate. Provide patient teaching and support to the patient and family during this highly stressful period.

S: Secretions. If secretions are copious, consider copalamine patch q72h, atropine 0.3 to 0.5 mg SQ q4h prn, or glycopyrrolate (Robinul) 0.1 to 0.4 mg IM/SQ q4 to 12h prn.

In the cancer population, two of the more common causes of dyspnea include airway obstruction from extrinsic compression or endobronchial tumor and malignant pleural effusion. Other options include therapeutic bronchoscopy with stent placement and the use of indwelling catheters for intermittent drainage of pleural effusions.

The use of breathlessness clinics using nonpharmacologic approaches have demonstrated their value in the treatment of breathlessness. This has been confirmed in a recent study of 30 outpatients with lung cancer who were referred to a breathlessness clinic. In this study, interventions were performed by a physiotherapist and outcomes included improvements in breathlessness, functional capacity, activity levels, and distress levels.

The Nursing Situation 19.1 presents an example of the palliative management of a patient with dyspnea.

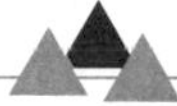

NURSING SITUATION 19.1

Dyspnea

Mr. Rather is a 70-year-old man with lung cancer that has metastasized to bone. The mediastinum and lung have persistent dyspnea. He has received radiation therapy to the mediastinum and completed his last course of chemotherapy 4 months ago. He is still at home receiving morphine sulfate 30 mg PO q4h around the clock for bone pain, which has been very effective. He is also receiving prednisone 30 mg PO bid for bronchospasm and had an albuterol inhaler, which he rarely used. He complains of feeling breathless and anxious. He is also very fatigued and cannot sleep at night. He refuses to go to the hospital and says he wants to die in his own bed. He refuses further aggressive intervention and has signed a home do-not-resuscitate (DNR) order. On physical exam, his breath sounds are decreased bilaterally, has occasional rhonchi, and no crackles are present. He has no distended neck veins, gallop, or peripheral edema. His respiratory rate is 24 per minutes at rest.

Assessment and Intervention

1. Determine the etiology of dyspnea. In the terminally ill patient, dyspnea often has multiple causes. A thorough history and physical examination should be performed and will assist in determining specific interventions. If excessive fatigue is present, consider obtaining a complete blood count (CBC) to determine if anemia is contributing to dyspnea. Rule out infection and congestive heart failure as contributing causes. If appropriate, determine pulse oximetry to determine benefits of oxygen therapy, or try nasal O_2 3 L/min prn. Mr. Rather is presently receiving morphine sulfate for pain. Increasing the opioids by 50% to a dose of 45 mg PO q4h should assist with tachypnea and anxiety. He will require assessments daily, and the opioids should be titrated daily or every other day by 25%–50%. Consider increasing his prednisone dose to treat the bronchospasm and a trial of nebulized morphine 2.5–5.0 mg q4h prn. Encourage use of an albuterol inhaler tid or qid for bronchospasm.
2. Consider the benefit versus burden of additional interventions that are employed. Mr. Rather has stated that no further aggressive interventions are to be used. As the goals of care have been identified by the patient, it is important that his family members understand them as well.
3. Assess functional status and reduce the need for physical exertion. Provide for assistance with daily activities, positioning techniques, and frequent rest periods. Use of a fan may assist with reducing feelings of breathlessness.
4. Address anxiety and provide support and reassurance. Determine level of support from family and significant others and from spiritual and religious beliefs. Reassure Mr. Rather that symptoms can be controlled. Consider a trial of an anxiolytic.
5. Provide for nonpharmacologic interventions (e.g., progressive relaxation, guided imagery), if appropriate, to reduce anxiety.

Palliative Management of Delirium

Delirium has been characterized as a global dysfunction of cognition, with associated disturbances in level of consciousness, attention, orientation, perception, thinking, memory, psychomotor function, sleep–wake cycle, and behavior. Symptoms develop over a short time and onset may be abrupt with waxing and waning of symptoms. Estimates of the prevalence of delirium range from 25 to 40 percent for patients with cancer at some point during their disease; in the terminal phases of disease, the incidence increases to 90 percent. The cause of delirium in the medically compromised and dying patient is often multifactorial and often nonspecific.

Assessment

Behavioral manifestations include a variety of symptoms that may be interpreted as depression, psychosis, and dementia. Symptoms include disordered cognition and alteration in arousal (attention), disturbance in consciousness and impaired attention, cognitive changes (memory deficit, disorientation, language disturbance, perceptual disturbance), nightmares, anxiety, restlessness and agitation, irritability, insomnia and daytime somnolence, hallucinations, delusions, and difficulty concentrating.

Delirium is often undertreated for several reasons including lack of assessment tools, inadequate knowledge of early signs of confusion, and inadequate time spent with the patient to determine cognitive function. Mental status questionnaires, such as the Mini–Mental State Exam and the newer Memorial Delirium Assessment Scale, are tools that are relatively easy to administer.

Diagnostic tests that may uncover physiological changes in the patient that correlate with decreased cognitive function include electroencephalography and brain imaging studies such as computed tomography and magnetic resonance imaging.

Management

Treatment of delirium usually includes identification of the underlying cause, correction of the precipitating factors, and symptom management. In the very ill or dying patient, however, there may be many causes, and the cause is often irreversible. The goal of palliative care of delirium is the promotion of comfort and relief of suffering.

Interventions that may be helpful include restoration of fluid and electrolyte balance, environmental changes, and supportive techniques such as elimination of unnecessary stimuli, provision of a safe environment, and measures that reduce anxiety. If the cause of delirium is pharmacologic, nonessential and central nervous system depressant drugs should be discontinued. Pharmacotherapy, using sedatives and neuroleptics, however, may be used to manage delirium. Table 19.7 lists drugs commonly used to manage delirium.

A variety of authorities advocate the use of sedation to manage symptoms at the end of life, including agitated delirium, that are refractory to aggressive measures. Symptoms that are refractory cannot be adequately controlled despite aggressive efforts to identify an acceptable therapy that does not compromise consciousness. When determining that a symptom is refractory, criteria that should be considered include that further interventions are incapable of providing adequate relief, are associated with excessive or intolerable morbidity, or are unlikely to provide relief in a timely manner. Inherent in this decision-making process is the informed consent of the patient, if possible, and the health-care proxy. As loss of interactional function will most likely occur, it is important that the patient understands the outcomes of this decision.

Table 19.7 Drugs Used to Manage Delirium

Drug	Dosage	Route
Haloperidol (Haldol)	0.5–5 mg q2–12 h For mild delirium, begin with 0.5 mg bid; for more severe symptoms begin with 1 mg bid–tid	PO, IV, SC, IM
Thioridazine (Mellaril)	10–75 mg q4–8h	PO
Chlorpromazine (Thorazine)	12.5–50 mg q4–12h	PO, IV, IM
Lorazepam (Ativan)	0.5–2 mg q1–4h	PO, IV May worsen a delirium and should not be used as monotherapy, always in addition to a neuroleptic when sedation is required
Midazolam (Versed)	30–100 mg/ 24 h	IV, SC
Risperidone	0.5–5 mg q2–12h	PO
Zyprexa	2.5–5 mg q12–24h	PO Use if sedation is needed to manage an agitated delirium

Bibliography

Agency for Health Care Policy and Research: Management of Cancer Pain. Clinical Practice Guideline No 9. US Department of Health and Human Services. Public Health Service. AHCPR Publication No. 94-0592. Washington, D.C., March 1994.

Aitken, RC: Measurement of feelings using visual analogue scales. Proc R Soc Med 62(10):989, 1969.

Alexander, HR Jr, and Fraker DK: Shunting procedures for malignant ascites and pleural effusions. In Lotze, MT, and Rubin, JT (eds): Regional Therapy of Advanced Cancer. Lippincott-Raven, Philadelphia, pp 271–280, 1997.

American Pain Society: Principles of Analgesic Use in the Treatment of Acute Pain and Cancer Pain, ed. 5. American Pain Society, Glenview, Ill.

American Thoracic Society: Standards for the diagnosis and care of patients with chronic obstructive pulmonary disease (COPD) and asthma. Am J Respir Crit Care Med 152(Suppl):S77, 1995.

Anderson, G, Christrup, L, and Sjogren, P: Relationships among morphine metabolism, pain and side effects during long-term treatment: An update. J Pain Sympt Manage 25(1):74, 2003.

APS Bulletin: NIH Consensus Development Conference on Acupuncture. 8(2):1, 1998.

Belman, MJ, et al: (Borg Rating of Dyspnea) Variability of breathlessness measurements in patients with chronic obstructive pulmonary disease. Chest 99:566, 1991.

Berenson, S: Complementary and alternative therapies in palliative care. In Ferrell, BR, and Coyle, N (eds): Textbook of Palliative Care Nursing. CV Mosby, St. Louis, Mo., 2005.

Berry, PE, and Dahl, JL: The new JCAHO pain standards: Implications for pain management nurses. Pain Management Nurses 1:3, 2000.

Bollinger, CT, et al: Silicone stents in the management of inoperable tracheobronchial stenoses: Indications and limitations. Chest 104: 1653, 1993.

Bookbinder, M, et al: Implementing national standards for cancer pain management: Program model and evaluation. J Pain Sympt Manage 12:334, 1995.

Booth, S, et al and Expert Working Group of the Scientific Committee of the Association of Palliative Medicine. The use of oxygen in the palliation of breathlessness. A report of the expert working group of the Scientific Committee of the Association of Palliative Medicine. Respir Med 98:66, 2004.

Brandt, HE, Luc Deliens, TH, Ooms, ME, van der Steen, JT, van der Wal, G, Ribbe, MW: Symptoms, signs, problems, and diseases of terminally ill nursing home patients. A Nationwide Observational Study in the Netherlands. Arch Intern Med 165:314, 2005.

Bredin, M, Corner, J, Krishnasamy M, Plant, H, Bailey, C, and A'Hern, R: Multicentre randomised controlled trial of nursing intervention for breathlessness in patients with lung cancer. BMJ 318:888, 1999.

Breitbart, W, Bruera, E, Chochinov, H, and Lynch, M: Neuropsychiatric syndromes and psychological symptoms in patients with advanced cancer. J Pain Sympt Manage 10:131, 1995.

Breitbart, WS, and Jacobsen, PB: Psychiatric symptom management in terminal care. Clin Geriatr Med 12:329, 1996.

Breitbart, WS, Rosenfeld B, Roth, A, Smith, MJ, Cohen, K, Passik, S: The Memorial delirium assessment scale. J Pain Sympt Manage 13:128, 1997.

Brock, DB, and Foley, DJ: Demography and epidemiology of dying in the United States with emphasis on deaths of older persons. In A Good Dying: Shaping Health Care for the Last Months of Life. Briefing book for symposium sponsored by the George Washington University Center to Improve Care of the Dying and the Corcoran Gallery of Art, Washington, D.C., April 30, 1996.

Bruera, E, Macmillan, K, Pither, J, and MacDonald RN: Effects of morphine on the dyspnea of terminal cancer patients. J Pain Sympt Manage 5(6):341, 1990.

Bruera, E, Schmitz, B, Pither J, Neumann, CM, and Hanson, J: The frequency and correlates of dyspnea in patients with advanced cancer. J Pain Sympt Manage 19(5):357, 2000.

Bruera, E, Miller, L, McCallion, J, Macmillan, K, Krefting, L, and Hanson, J: Cognitive failure in patients with terminal cancer: A prospective study. J Pain Sympt Manage 7:192, 1992.

Cancer Facts & Figures 2005. American Cancer Society.

Carrieri-Kohlman, V, et al: Differentiation between dyspnea and its affective components. West J Nurs Res 18:626, 1996.

Cassel, CK, et al: Caring for the dying: Identification and promotion of physician competency. Am Board Intern Med 1–26, 1996.

Cassileth, BR: Oncology Nursing Updates 5(4):1, 1998.

Cassileth, BR, Vickers, AJ, and Magill, LA: Music therapy for mood disturbance during hospitalization for autologous stem cell transplantation: A randomized controlled trial. Cancer 98:2723, 2003.

Cherny, NI, Arbit, E, and Jain, S: Invasive techniques in the management of cancer pain. Hematol/Oncol Clin North Am 10:121, 1996.

Cherny, NI, and Catane, R: Attitudes of medical oncologists toward palliative care for patients with advanced and incurable cancer. Report on a survey by the European Society of Medical Oncology taskforce on palliative and supportive care. Cancer 98(11):2502, 2003.

Cherny, NI, and Foley, KM (eds): Hematology Clinics of North America: Pain and Palliative Care. WB Saunders, Philadelphia, p 21, 1996.

Cherny, NI, and Portenoy, RK: Sedation in the management of refractory symptoms: Guidelines for evaluation and treatment. J Palliat Care 10(2):31, 1994.

Christakis, NA, and Escarce, JJ: Survival of Medicare patients after enrollment in hospice programs. N Engl J Med 335:172, 1996.

Cohen, MZ, Easley, MK, et al: JACHO: Cancer pain management and the JCAHO's pain standards: An institutional challenge. J Pain Sympt Manage 25:519, 2003.

Conill, C, et al: Symptom prevalence in the last week of life. J Pain Sympt Manage 14:328, 1997.

Cooper, RA, et al: Current and projected workforce of nonphysician clinicians. JAMA 280:788, 1998.

Cooper, RA, et al: Roles of nonphysician clinicians vs autonomous providers of patient care. JAMA 280:795, 1998.

Corner, J, Plant, H, A'Hern, R, and Bailey, C: Non-pharmacological intervention for breathlessness in lung cancer. Palliat Med 10:299, 1996.

Cowcher, K, and Hanks, G: Long-term management of respiratory symptoms in advanced cancer. J Pain Sympt Manage 5(5):320, 1990.

Coyle, N, et al: Character of terminal illness in the advanced cancer patient: Pain and other symptoms during the last four weeks of life. J Pain Sympt Manage 5:83, 1990.

Daut, RI, Cleeland, CS, and Flanery, ARC: The development of the Wisconsin brief pain questionnaire to assess pain in cancer and other diseases. Pain 17:197, 1983.

Demmer, C: A survery of complementary therapy services provided by hospices. J Palliat Med 7:510, 2004.

Deng, G, Cassileth, BR, and Simon, YK: Complementary therapeis for cancer-related symptoms. Support Oncol 2:419, 2004.

Dudgeon, DJ: Managing dyspnea and cough. Hematol Oncol Clin North Am 16:557, 2002.

Dudgeon, DJ, et al: Dyspnea in cancer patients: Prevalence and associated factors. J Pain Sympt Manage 21:95, 2001.

Dudgeon, DJ, Lertzman, M, and Askew, GR: Physiological changes and clinical correlations of dyspnea in cancer outpatients. J Pain Sympt Manage 21(5):373, 2001.

Eakin, EG, et al: Reliability and validity of dyspnea measures in patients with obstructive lung disease. Int J Behav Med 2(2):118, 1995.

Eisenberg, DN, et al: Trends in alternative medicine use in the United States, 1990–1997. JAMA 280(19):1720, 1998.

Escalante, CP, Martin, CG, Elting, LS, Price, KJ, Manzullo, EF, and Weiser, MA: Identifying risk factors for imminent death in cancer patients with acute dyspnea. J Pain Sympt Manage 20:318–325, 2000.

Fainsinger, R, Miller MJ, Bruera E, Hanson, J, and Maceachern, T: Symptom control during the last week of life on a palliative care unit. J Palliat Care 7(1):5–11, 1991.

Farncombe, M: Dyspnea: Assessment and treatment support care. Cancer 2:77, 1997.

Fishbein, D, Kearon, C, and Killian K: An approach to dyspnea in cancer patients. J Pain Sympt Manage 4(2):76–81, 1989.

Fleming, D: Patient suffering: A taxonomy from the nurse's perspective. J Adv Nurs 22:1120, 1995.

Frankl, VE: Man's Search for Meaning: An Introduction to Logotherapy. Beacon Press, New York, 1959.

Gomez, CF: Hospice and home care. Opportunities for training in caring for the dying: Identification and promotion of physician competency. Am Board Intern Med 27, 1996.

Graham, C, et al: Use of the McGill Pain Questionnaire in the assessment of cancer pain: Replicability and consistency. Pain 8:377, 1980.

Hanks, GW, Cherny, NI, and Fallon, M: Opioid analgesic therapy. In Doyle, D, Hanks, G, Cherny, N, and Calman, K (eds): Oxford Textbook of Palliative Medicine, ed. 3. Oxford University Press, Oxford, pp. 316–341, 2004.

Hardie, GE, Janson, S, Gold, WM, Carrieri-Kohlman, V, and Boushey, HA: Ethnic dfferences: word descriptions used by African-American and white asthma patients during induced bronchoconstriction. Chest 117:935, 2000.

Hatley, J, Laurence, V, Scott, A, Baker, R, and Thomas, P: Breathlessness clinics within specialist palliative care settings can improve the quality of life and functional capacity of patients with lung cancer. Palliat Med 17:410, 2003.

Hay, L, Farncombe, M, and McKee, P: Patient, nurse and physician view of dyspnea. Can Nurs 92(10):26, 1996.

Hall, P, Schroder, C, and Weaver, L: The last 48 hours in long-term care; a focused chart audit. J Am Ger Soc Mar 50(3):501, 2002.

Higginson, I, and McCarthy, M: Measuring symptoms in terminal cancer: Are pain and dyspnoea controlled? J R Soc Med 82:264, 1989.

Hospice Facts and Statistics. Hospice Foundation, 2002.

Ingham, JM, and Portenoy, RK: Symptom assessment. In Cherny, NI, and Foley, KM (eds): Hematology Clinics of North America: Pain and Palliative Care. WB Saunders, Philadelphia, pp 21–40, 1996.

International Association for the Study of Pain, Subcommittee on Taxonomy. Pain Trms: A list with definitions and notes on usage. Pain 6:249, 1979.

Jacox, A, et al: Management of Cancer Pain. Clinical Practice Guideline No. 9. AHCPR Publication No. 94-0592. U.S. Department of Health and Human Services, Public Health Service, Washington, D.C., March 1994.

Kennedy, BJ: Aging and cancer: Geriatric oncology. Keynote address to the integrating geriatrics into oncology education. Cancer 80:1270, 1997.

Kuebler, KK: Hospice and Palliative Care Clinical Practice Protocol: Dyspnea. Hospice Nurses Association, Pittsburgh, 1996.

Lawlor, PG, et al: Occurrences, causes, and outcome of delirium in patients with advanced cancer. A prospective study. Arch Intern Med 160:786, 2000.

Lawlor, PG, Fainsinger, RL, and Bruera, ED: Delirium at the end of life: Critical issues in clinial practice and research. JAMA 284:2427, 2000.

LeGrand, SB: Dyspnea: The continuing challenge of palliative management. Curr Opin Oncol 14:394, 2002.

LeGrand, SB, Khawam, EA, Walsh, D, and Rivera, NI: Opioids, respiratory function, and dyspnea. Am J Hosp Palliat Care 20(1):57, 2003.

Lethbridge-Cejku, M, Schiller, JS, and Bernadel, L: Summary health statistics for U.S. adults: National Health Interview Survey, pp 1–18, 2002.

Levin, ML, et al: Management of pain in terminally ill patient: Physician reports of knowledge, attitudes, and behaviors. J Pain Sympt Manage 15:27, 1998.

McCaffery, M, and Ferrell, B: Nurses' knowledge of pain assessment and management: How much progress have we made? J Pain Sympt Manage 14(3):175, 1997.

Mahler, DA, and Wells, CK: Evaluation of clinical methods for rating dyspnea. Chest 93:580, 1988.

Mercadante, S, and Arcuri, E: Opioids and renal function. J Pain 5(1): 2, 2004.

Miaskowski, C: The need to assess multiple symptoms. Pain Manage Nurs 3:115, 2002.

Morita, T, Tei Y, and Inoue S: Agitated terminal delirium and association with partial opioid substitution and hydration. J Palliat Med 6:557, 2003.

Mortimer, JE, and Bartlett, NL: Assessment of knowledge about cancer pain management by physicians in training. J Pain Sympt Manage 14(1):21, 1997.

National Hospice Organization: Medical guidelines for determining prognosis in selected non-cancer diseases. Med Guidelines Task Force, Arlington, Va., 1996.

NHO Hospice Facts and Figures, Alexandria Va., 2004

O'Brien, S, et al: The knowledge and attitudes of experienced oncology nurses regarding the management of cancer-related pain. Oncol Nurs Forum 23:515, 1996.

NIH Consensus Conference. Acupuncture. JAMA 280:1518, 1998.

NIH State-of-the-Science Statement on symptom management in cancer: Pain, depression, and fatigue. NIH Consensus State-of-the-Science Statements. 19:1, 2002.

Parker, SI, et al: Cancer Statistics 1997. J Am Cancer Soc 47(1):5, 1997.

Payne, R, and Gonzales, GR: Pathophysiology of pain in cancer and other terminal diseases. In Doyle, D, Hanks, GW, and MacDonald, N (eds): Oxford Textbood of Palliative Medicine, ed. 2. Oxford University Press, Oxford, pp 299–310, 1998.

Pereira, J, Hanson, J, and Bruera, E: The frequency and clinical course of cognitive impairment in patients with terminal cancer. Cancer 79: 835, 1997.

Portenoy, RK, and Bruera, E (eds): Topics in Palliative Care. Vol 1. Oxford University Press, New York, 1997.

Potter, J, Hami, F, Bryan, T, and Quigley, C: Symptoms in 400 patients referred to palliative care services: Prevalence and patterns. Palliat Med 17:310, 2003.

Potter, VT, Wiseman, CE, Dunn, SM, and Boyle, FM: Patient barriers to optimal pain control. Psychooncology 12:153, 2003.

Reynolds, K, Henderson, M, Schulman, A, and Hanson, LC: Needs of the dying in nursing homes. J Palliat Med 5(6):895, 2002.

Ripamonti, C: Management of dyspnea in advanced cancer patients. Support Care Cancer 7:233, 1999.

Ripamonti, C, and Fusco, F: Respiratory problems in advanced cancer. Support Care Cancer 10:204, 2002.

Ripamonti, C, and Bruera, E: Dyspnea: Pathophysiology and assessment. J Pain Sympt Manage 13(4):220, 1997.

Rosenberg, HM, et al: Births and Deaths in the US 1995. Monthly Vital Statistics Report, Preliminary Data from the Centers for Disease Control and Prevention, National Center for Health Statistics 45(3) Suppl 2, 1996.

Schonwetter, RE: Care of the terminally ill patients. Clin Geriatr Med 12:xi 1996.

Seale, C, and Cartwright, A: The year before death. Ashgate Publishing, Brookfield, Vt., 1994.

Sloan, PA, et al: Residents' management of the symptoms associated with terminal cancer. Hospice J 12:5, 1997.

Sykes, NP: The relationship between opioid use and laxative use in terminally ill cancer patients. Palliat Med 12:375, 1998.

Spross, JA, and Wolff Burke, M: Nonpharmacological management of cancer pain. In McGuire, DB, Henke Yarbro, C, Ferrell, BR (eds): Cancer Pain Management, ed 2. Jones and Bartlett, Boston, pp 159–205, 1995.

Thomas, JR, and von Guten, CF: Mangement of dyspnea. J Support Oncol May–Jun; 1(1):23; discussion 32, 2003.

Tuls Halstead, M, and Tuls Roscoe, S: Restoring the spirit at the end of life: Music as an intervention for oncology nurses. Clin J Oncol Nurs 6:332, 2002.

Twycross, R, and Lichter, I: The terminal phase. In Doyle, D, Hanks, GWC, and MacDonals, N (eds): Oxford Text on Palliative Medicine, ed 2. Oxford University Press, Oxford, pp 984–992, 1998.

Ventafridda, V, et al: Symptom prevalence and control during cancer patients' last days of life. J Palliat Care 6(3):7, 1990.

Von Roenn, JH, et al: Physician's attitudes and practice in cancer pain management: A survey from the Eastern Cooperative Oncology Group. Ann Intern Med 119:121, 1993.

Wong, NA, and Hones, HW: An analysis of discharge drug prescibing amongst elderly patients with renal impairment. Postgrad Med J 74:420, 1998.

World Health Organization: Cancer pain relief and palliative care. Report of a WHO Expert Committee (World Health Organization Technical Report Series, 804) WHO, Geneva, 1990, pp 1–75.

World Health Organization: Looking Forward to Cancer Pain Relief for All: International Consensus on the Management of Cancer Pain. WHO Collaborating Centre for Palliative Cancer Care, Oxford, 1996.

Resources

Academy of Pain Management
http://www.aapainmanage.com
Academy of Pain Medicine
http://www.painmed.org
American Botanical Council
http://www.herbalgram.org
American Cancer Society
http://www.cancer.org
American Holistic Nurses Association
http://www.ahna.org
American Pain Society
http://www.ampainsoc.org
Cancer Care
http://www.cancercare.org
Choices in Dying
http://www.choices.org
Food and Drug Administration
http://www.fda.gov
Hospice Foundation
http://www.hospicefoundation.org
National Cancer Institute
http://www.nci.nih.gov
National Hospice Organization
http://www.nho.org
National Institutes of Health
http://www.nih.gov
Oncology Nurses Society
http://www.ons.org
Physician's Drug Reference
http://PDRnet.com
US Pharmacopia
http://www.usp.org

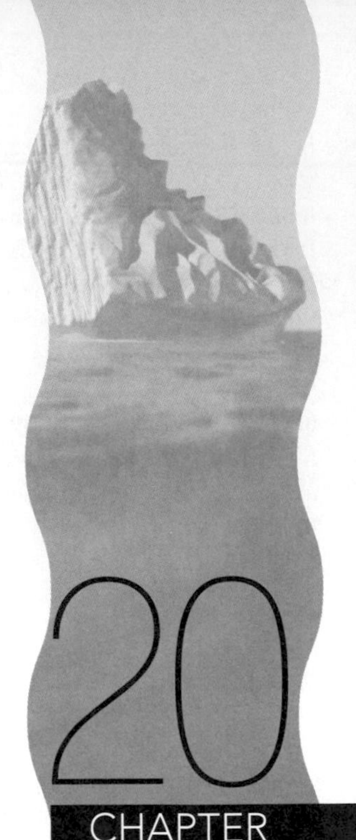

The 15-Minute Hour: A Short-Term Approach to Psychotherapy in Primary Care

Marian R. Stuart, PhD

Approaching the treatment of each patient as a unique entity having an individual history, cultural heritage, health belief system, educational level, behavioral style, vulnerabilities, and life stress and presenting with a specific problem can be experienced as a formidable challenge. Because there is little doubt about the role of psychosocial factors on the prognosis of disease, it is imperative that all health-care providers acquire the skills to effectively and efficiently address these issues during every clinical encounter.

Recent advances in science and technology have led to some marvelous discoveries in the biomedical field and have pushed back the frontiers of our understanding of physiology and pathology. As we continue to learn more and more about the functioning of the human organism at the cellular level, evidence is accumulating that clearly ties emotional events to biochemical expression in the body. The traditional separation of the mind and the body, for convenience in treatment and scientific investigation, creates invalid dichotomies. From this perspective, patients are considered either to have or not to have a given disease. Diseases are treated as independent entities amenable to categorization and presumed to have a specific cause. The clinician's task, in this model, is to diagnose and prescribe a cure to alter the natural course of disease. Among practitioners who adopt this limited approach, there is a disregard for critical lifestyle factors and the patient's perception of illness. This model also accounts for the loss of many of those human qualities that constitute the patient's total being or, as Engel in 1980 has so eloquently stated:

> The crippling flaw of the model is that it does not include the patient and his (or her) attributes as a person, as a human being. The biomedical model can make provision neither for the person as a whole nor for data of a psychological or social nature, for the reductionism and mind-body dualism on which the model is predicated requires that these must first be reduced to physiochemical terms before they can have meaning. Hence, the very essence of medical practice perforce remains art and beyond the reach of science.

Great strides are being made in disciplines such as psychoneuroimmunology that are scientifically investigating the relationship between the patient, stress, the environment, the patient's network of social support, and the development of disease. This chapter focuses on how accurate, timely identification of patients' stress and encouragement of constructive coping strategies can enhance clinical outcomes and contribute to more professional satisfaction for all health-care providers. In addition, this will aid the health-care provider in actualizing a circle of caring.

Epidemiology

It is a well-established fact that psychiatric illness is prevalent in populations that seek help in a primary care setting. A recent study by the World Health Organization (WHO) sampled 1500 patients in each of 15 sites all over the world, in cities such as Ankara, Athens, Rio de Janeiro, Shanghai, Bangalore, Seattle, Berlin, and Manchester. All continents, with the exception of Antarctica, were represented. The researchers found that, on average, one-third of patients presenting with medical problems could also be classified as having a psychiatric problem. Patients with mental health problems generally present to primary-care practitioners with somatic symptoms and are often not properly diagnosed. These are problems that are very amenable to treatment, but they must first be identified. In the real world, the distinction between psychiatric and medical illness is often blurred and mental and physical health are on a continuum. Psychological problems are often expressed as physical symptoms, and medical problems generally precipitate psychological distress. Health-care providers understand that medical illness is usually best treated if it is detected in an early stage. This is even more critical with psychological problems.

Ubiquity of Stress

Stress is the physical and mental response that results from having to adapt to demands from the external and internal environments. Managing life's complex issues presents a constant challenge. Distress is experienced when people's resources become overwhelmed and they feel out of control. When under stress, people cope differently than when they feel comfortable or pleasantly challenged. Our understanding of the relationships among stress, coping, and health has been enhanced by the long-term prospective studies of Vaillant published in 1979, whose findings include the following:

- People have persistent behaviors. Coping mechanisms that are adopted when young tend to persist into old age.
- Overwhelmed people regress functionally.
- Poor adaptation causes ill health. Stress does not cause disease, but disease may develop as a consequence of poor adaptation to stress.

Given this understanding, health promotion and disease prevention require teaching individuals constructive ways of coping with stress, whether the source of stress is a cataclysmic event, a daily hassle, or a personality characteristic. When people are overwhelmed by the circumstances of their lives, they often become sick and may visit their primary-care provider. It is important for the health-care provider to understand this to effectively screen for stressors and adopt techniques for providing effective support.

Social Support

Social support is a key element in stress management. When subjective perceptions of levels of control decrease, subjective feelings of stress increase dramatically. As the level of social support increases, an individual's subjective level of stress decreases. Lack of social support has been shown to be deleterious to a person's health. Health-care providers are in a position to provide essential social support, which means providing positive information about the person or the relationship or suggesting possible strategies for handling a particular problem.

The Importance of Feeling Competent and Connected

Feeling competent and connected to someone or something outside of oneself are basic human needs. Feeling competent involves a sense of being able to exercise one's autonomy. Feeling connected involves feeling valued by other people. When people are stressed, they often feel inadequate and isolated. The essence of social support is to reestablish a person's sense of competence and connection. The individual who is psychologically overwhelmed or medically ill does not feel a very high level of competence and is, therefore, even more in need of feeling connected. To feel healthy (and to have our bodies function optimally) we need to feel both competent and connected. By providing positive information about the person and the relationship, we enhance the patient's ability to function in a healthy way. Interventions the health-care provider may use to help the patient feel competent and connected are presented in Advanced Practice Nursing Intervention 20.1. While uniquely advanced practice nursing interventions they are of use to all health-care providers.

Types of Social Power

"Social power" implies the ability to influence another person. There are five specific kinds of social power, and

> **ADVANCED PRACTICE NURSING INTERVENTIONS 20.1**
>
> **Helping the Patient Feel Competent and Connected**
>
> ***The Person***
>
> "I can see how upset you are. This is a very difficult situation. I do know, however, that you have coped very successfully with similar incidents in the past. I have always been impressed with the way you come through in a crunch."
>
> ***The Relationship***
>
> "I care about you."
>
> "I want to know how this works out. I want you to call me or come back to see me and let me know what happened."
>
> The subtext here is that "You are going to work this out. I see you as capable and I care about you."
>
> ***Handling the Problem***
>
> "Read this book."
> "Call this agency."
> "Join a support group."
> "Do something really nice for yourself."
> "Keep a diary and keep track of when you get upset and what you are thinking at the time."

patients routinely attribute all of them to their primary-care providers. The types of social power and their sources are:

- Reward power: The provider can dispense prescriptions to alleviate pain, treat infections, or even induce sleep. Patients also need to have forms completed to legitimize their ability or inability to go to work, purchase life or disability insurance, or have the school or work environment modified.
- Coercive power: The provider is in a position to hospitalize patients, inflict all manner of uncomfortable treatments, perform invasive procedures, impose diets, and, under certain circumstances, even deny the ability to drive a car.
- Expert power: The patient considers the primary-care provider to be an expert in all aspects of human health and behavior. This includes subjects such as nutrition, human sexuality, and marital communications. The patient gives a lot of credence to the provider's views in these areas.
- Referent power: The patient values the relationship with the provider and wants to be both liked by the provider and to be like the provider. The connection inherent in the relationship helps to enhance the patient's self-esteem. This is the most potent type of social power. Referent power is what makes the establishment of rapport with the patient so important. The more the patient likes, respects, and wishes to feel connected to the provider, the more referent power is acquired by the clinician. The therapeutic relationship based on trust and rapport becomes a powerful tool to influence the patient. It enables the provider to become a healer.
- Legitimate power: The provider has power that is defined by the system. There is a contractual relationship that begins when the patient presents for a consultation. There is an exchange defined by monetary considerations, and the patient is expected to value the information dispensed by the provider.

Applying Social Power

Because the health-care provider possesses a great deal of social power, the way words are used has an impact that is often equivalent to performing a procedure. The placebo response has been shown to be one of the most widespread and powerful effects in medicine. Expectation of a positive response translates into an improved sense of physical well-being. Expectation of a particular effect actually precipitates cellular reactions that produce organic changes that can be quite dramatic. The health-care provider can learn to harness social power constructively by talking with patients with the intent of enhancing their ability to heal themselves. Practitioners are often not aware that their specific use of words is like a procedure that affects the patient's views of themselves, their options, and even their ability to fight disease.

Commonalities among Psychotherapeutic Techniques

Although many health-care providers feel more comfortable using the term "counseling", one must recognize that talking with patients about their concerns often has very therapeutic effects. As a result of the interaction, the patient often feels better and often becomes able to figure out problems that were formerly unsolvable. This is psychotherapy. Patients have a unique and distinct view of the world, and, although no one else can know precisely what someone else's view of the world may be, primary-care providers are uniquely positioned to assist their patients in coping with their problems, regardless of the nature of the specific problems. Skillfully employed, this professional attribute alone can decrease stress and enable patients to deal much more effectively with those things that are contributing to their misery. Frank in 1974 noted there are five common elements found in all schools of psychotherapy: (1) the expectation of receiving help, (2) participation in a therapeutic relationship, (3) obtaining an external perspective, (4) encouraging corrective experience, and (5) the opportunity for individual patients to test reality repeatedly.

The Expectation of Receiving Help

People seek psychotherapy because they are feeling helpless, hopeless, and demoralized in their inability to come to terms with a particular situation. In the overwhelming majority of cases, patients enter into a relationship with the practitioner truly believing that the practitioner is going to be able to help them with their symptoms. The expectation of receiving help improves the patient's outlook, in that hope is renewed.

Participation in a Therapeutic Relationship

The relationship between the practitioner and the patient exists for the sole purpose of fostering the well-being of the patient. The patient's ability to accept and incorporate the knowledge, skills, and attitudes of another individual in the resolution of a problem dictates a relationship based on mutual respect and caring. The practitioner's caring and concern is at the core of any therapy and becomes the therapeutic intervention.

Obtaining an External Perspective

When patients are feeling overwhelmed by the circumstances of their lives, it is hard for them to be objective or to evaluate a situation realistically. An essential part of any therapeutic relationship is the opportunity to talk things out with a respected listener who is able to present a more rational perspective. Practitioners can also provide an external perspective simply by asking questions that reveal unexplored options or lead to more effective problem solving. This has the added advantage of empowering the patient.

Encouraging Corrective Experience

The ultimate goal of all schools of psychotherapy is to lead patients to change their ineffective and self-defeating behaviors. As human beings, we have certain notions about how things should work, and when outcomes do not match our hopes and expectations, we tend to redouble our efforts without changing our strategies. This often leads to repeated defeats. Psychotherapy generally encourages the instigation of new and hopefully more effective patterns of behavior.

The Opportunity to Test Reality Repeatedly

Very often when people first start to change their behavior, no one notices. This can be very frustrating. Often the patient's perceptions are quite accurate, and it is extremely helpful to use the practitioner for repeated "reality checks." Follow-up visits to report on the effects of their efforts can help patients modify their expectations concerning various significant relationships. In all of these activities, the practitioner is the supporting listener and occasional commentator as the patient expresses feelings and concerns, explores ways of handling the situation, and ultimately works through the process of problem resolution.

The 15-Minute Hour

In this era of managed care, the primary-care provider has limited time to spend with individual patients. Nevertheless, the practitioner can learn to provide effective psychotherapy within the confines of the 15-minute visit. It is important to limit goals to solving "here and now" problems and to empowering patients. Because people develop persistent behavioral patterns through life and regress to them when overwhelmed by stress, support is the most crucial therapeutic tool. The practitioner's goal is to prevent poor adaptation to stressful circumstances and to enhance outcomes by encouraging effective problem solving. There are four specific therapeutic goals:

- ▲ Reestablishing the premorbid level of functioning. When people are overwhelmed, they go on "tilt," which means that they cease to function effectively, may act irrationally, or may even become abusive. They may not be able think clearly and appreciate details, and their problem-solving skills may be inadequate. They also feel a great deal of emotional distress. The provider's goal is to help the patient get off tilt.
- ▲ Preventing dire consequences. Because crises are generally time-limited, it is important to keep patients from making decisions that may have deleterious effects on their lives. Often, just slowing down the process can be very helpful.
- ▲ Expanding the behavioral repertoire. As a result of the therapeutic intervention, the patient may learn new ways to handle troublesome situations. The results will be reinforcing, and the patient may subsequently function at a more effective level.
- ▲ Enhancing the patient's self-esteem. Successful resolution of the crisis and the awareness of personal responsibility for having brought it about often allows the patient to feel better about him- or herself. Because this is generally a lasting effect, it represents the impact of the therapy.

The Technique: BATHEing the Patient

As with all skills in providing health care, the ability to incorporate appropriate questions regarding a patient's psychosocial situation is an acquired skill. The BATHE technique can be used as a quick screening test for psychiatric problems. It has become an established method to identify and address the psychosocial aspect of patients' problems during a brief office visit. It should be employed early in the interview, usually after elicitation of the chief complaint and history of present illness. BATHE has become the standard of primary care. The acronym stands for:

- ▲ **B**ackground: "What is going on in your life?" This determines the context of the patient's visit.
- ▲ **A**ffect: "How do you feel about that?" This allows patients to identify and report their emotional reactions.
- ▲ **T**rouble: "What troubles you about that?" This helps the practitioner and patient focus on the situation's subjective meaning.
- ▲ **H**andling: "How are you handling that?" This helps the practitioner assess the patient's level of functioning, helps the patient connect body and mind, and communicates the thought that the patient is handling the situation.
- ▲ **E**mpathy: "That must be very difficult for you." This legitimizes the patient's reaction.

Focusing the History 20.1 presents the BATHE technique.

Although BATHE is not the only technique the clinician can employ, it tends to bring order out of what is frequently a chaotic approach to a psychosocial assessment. In the process, it helps tie the biomedical model to the psychosocial in a way that is meaningful for both the healthcare practitioner of any disciplinary perspecitve and the patient. By asking pointed, focused questions, which lend themselves to brief but reasonably comprehensive answers, the clinician is able to incorporate this very necessary form

FOCUS ON HISTORY 20.1

The BATHE Technique

- Background
  A simple question, "What is going on in your life?" determines the context of the patient's visit. It answers the question "Why is the patient here now?"
- Affect (the feeling state)
  Questions such as "How do you feel about that?" or "How does that make you feel?" allows patients to identify and report their emotional reactions to the circumstances described.
- Trouble
  The question "What troubles you about that?" or "What about the situation troubles you the most?" helps both the practitioner and patient focus on the situation's subjective meaning. Even when the patient's affect is positive, this question should be asked. It is important to modify it appropriately: "Is there anything about it that troubles you?"
- Handling
  The answer to "How are you handling that?" helps the practitioner assess the patient's level of functioning, helps the patient connect body and mind, and communicates the thought that the patient is handling the situation.
- Empathy
  The statement "That must be very difficult for you," legitimizes the patient's reaction. Even when the patient is functioning suboptimally, it is important to reflect back the content of the circumstances and support the patient's attempts at resolution.

of assessment into a format that helps the patient express feelings, gain insight into the meaning of the situation, and become empowered. It also enhances rapport and saves unexpected and time-consuming revelations at the end of a visit. Most significantly, it satisfies all five elements of psychotherapy. Used during every visit, BATHE provides the expectation of help, a therapeutic relationship, an external perspective, the encouragement of new behavior, and the opportunity to test reality repeatedly.

Discipline must be exercised not to explore the circumstances of the patient's life to any depth, because this can be very time consuming. The therapeutic effect derives from focusing on the patient's feelings, the subjective meaning of the situation, assessment of how things are being handled, and support in the form of empathy.

Ownership

The health-care provider's inquiry into the patient's psychosocial status is designed to produce an enhanced comprehension of the overall dimensions of a patient's presenting problem. BATHE helps the practitioner assess the patient's situation so that therapeutic suggestions can be made and enable the patient to deal with his or her problem more effectively. It is crucial that the clinician not assume responsibility for resolution of the patient's particular situation. The patient continues to "own" his or her problem; however, the clinician is better able to assist the patient in the resolution of the problem by having a more comprehensive understanding of the situation and its effect on the patient. This is true whether the problem is predominantly biomedical or psychosocial, as one invariably has a component of the other ingrained in the patient's overall situation. Ownership of the problem remains with the patient, but what emanates from the therapeutic relationship is the patient's confidence that the practitioner is supportive and able to help. Trust in a relationship consists of an evaluation of a person's ability and willingness to provide necessary support.

Applying the BATHE Technique

Practitioners often worry, with good cause, that application of the BATHE technique may uncover unanticipated issues that cannot be adequately addressed within the allotted time. However, BATHE is a *screening tool*, and the practitioner must use judgment as to when and how extensively to explore what has surfaced. Often it is important to say, "I am glad that you have brought this up. Let me examine you to see if there is some physical problem that we need to be concerned about, and after that, we can talk some more." Although the clinician has an obligation to the patient to identify important, treatable conditions, it is not necessary that all of them be addressed immediately. In most cases, "BATHEing" the patient will take less than a minute and can prevent the all-too-frequent litany of complaints that suddenly emerge at the end of the interview.

The essence of therapy consists of making the patient feel competent and connected. There are many specific techniques that can accomplish this. Many cases, examples, and strategies can be found in the 15-minute hour. In most cases just BATHEing the patient helps to clarify the situation. Patients should always be given permission to feel what they feel. They should be provided brief information about the effects of stress, legitimizing their reactions to their situation. Specific suggestions can be made for managing stress or the circumstances and, if necessary, the patient should be encouraged to come back and explore the situation further. If serious problems emerge, referral is advised. Because it is vitally important to determine this, the clinician can take great pride in having uncovered any serious issues.

Psychological and physical health are intimately related. Physical illness causes psychological stress on patient and family. Psychological stress may result in functional symptoms and organic alteration. The mind–body is one entity. Patients' reactions to stress may result in decreased levels of functioning, a decreased sense of well-being, susceptibility to illness, and exacerbation of chronic conditions.

All effective psychotherapy is basically supportive: It helps the patient focus on strengths, raising self-esteem, and fosters the choosing of more effective behavioral options. The goal of the therapeutic intervention is to make the patient feel competent and connected. The practitioner should briefly explore the context of every patient's visit, which can be done quickly and efficiently by BATHEing patients. By doing so, the practitioner can help patients define their problems, express feelings, increase their understanding, and make them feel supported. Once the practitioner has helped patients define their problems, the practitioner's role is to accept patients' feelings, give permission for normal responses, and expect patients to handle their problems. Follow-up visits or referrals should be considered when problems seem to be serious.

Bibliography

Bartrop, RW, et al: Depressed lymphocyte function after bereavement. Lancet 1:834, 1977.

Cohen, SC, et al: Psychological stress and susceptibility to the common cold. N Engl J Med 325:606, 1991.

Engel, GL: The clinical application of the biopsychosocial model. Am J Psychol 137:536, 1980.

Frank, JD: Psychotherapy: The restoration of morale. Am J Psychol 131:271, 1974.

French, JPR Jr, and Raven, BH: The bases of social power. In Cartwright, D and Zander, A (eds): Group Dynamics: Research and Theory, ed 3. Harper and Row, New York, 1968.

House, JS, et al: Social relationships and health. Science 241:540, 1988.

Spiegel, D, et al: Effect of psychosocial treatment on survival of patients with metastatic breast cancer. Lancet 2:888, 1989.

Stuart, MR, and Lieberman, JA, III: The Fifteen Minute Hour: Applied Psychotherapy for the Primary Care Practitioner, ed 2. Praeger, Westport, Conn., 1993.

Vaillant, GE: Natural history of male psychologic health: Effects of mental health on physical health. N Engl J Med 301:1249, 1979.

Ustun, TB, and Sartorius, N: Mental Illness in General Health Care: An International Study. John Wiley & Sons, New York, 1995.

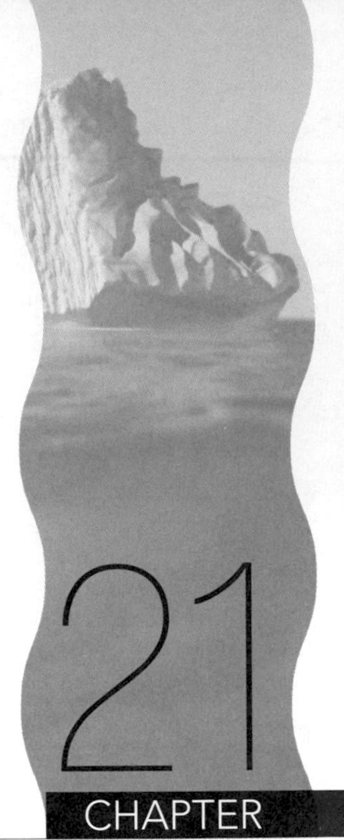

Evidence-Based Practice

Susan L. Folden, PhD, APRN, BC
Shawn Kneipp, PhD, APRN, BC

What constitutes evidence is a highly contested subject. In health care, evidence originates from research findings used to guide clinical practice, such as decisions regarding which diagnostic tests or treatment approaches are worthwhile. Although research findings are used to compile evidence for decision-making in practice, evidence-based practice and research-based practice are not necessarily the same. Both evidence- and research-based practice have strengths and weaknesses, which are largely determined by the context in which they are used. Generally, *evidence-based practice* refers to using research findings from several studies that are convincing enough to the majority of a community of scientists and clinicians to recommend that the findings be used for clinical decision-making and that, to some degree, they become a standard for care. Evidence-based practice also involves inclusion of patient and practitioner preferences and patient values in the clinical decision-making process. The key steps involved in implementing evidence-based practice are summarized in Table 21.1. *Research-based practice/research utilization* also incorporates research findings in clinical decision-making, but the research findings may not be endorsed by the clinical or scientific community as meeting the stringent criteria often used to evaluate findings that constitute evidence and may incorporate only findings from one study.

Arguments in biomedicine over which research findings do or do not constitute evidence are in some respects more limited than those occurring within the discipline of nursing. This does not mean that the conflicts over defining "evidence" in biomedicine are any less frequent or any less fervent than the arguments in nursing. It means the phenomena of interest to the discipline of nursing are more diverse on a human–environment–health-interaction scale when compared to the phenomena of interest to our colleagues in the medical sciences. Neither disciplinary perspective alone is sufficient when the goal is to provide humanistic, quality health care.

Although advanced practice nurses (APNs) function primarily from a nursing framework, they also incorporate aspects of the medical model into their practice. Thus, an understanding of the major research methods used in both disciplines and how to apply research findings to clinical practice situations are essential. This chapter focuses on evidence-based practice across disciplines and the predominant methods used to establish evidence for practice across disciplines.

The Aims of Nursing Research for Clinical Application

Despite the differences in perspective between nursing and biomedicine, the research conducted in each field has a common thread: the systematic pursuit of knowledge to answer questions of importance in the respective professions. Medicine relies heavily on a few methods to answer the majority of questions relevant to its practice, often drawn from epidemiology. This is not entirely so within nursing. As a discipline concerned with the human response to health and illness, the use of a few methods to study the complexities of being human is not only insufficient but is also considered by some nurse-scholars to be reductionist and dehumanizing with several scholars using the terms "cook-

Table 21.1 Key Steps in Implementing Evidence-Based Practice

1. Ask the burning clinical question.
2. Collect the most relevant and best evidence from a review of the literature including published literature reviews, meta-analyses, and clinical practice guidelines.
3. Critically appraise the evidence.
4. Integrate all evidence with one's clinical expertise, patient preferences, and values in making a practice decision or change.
5. Evaluate the change in outcomes after implementing into practice.

Source: Adapted from Melnyk, BM, and Fineout-Overholt, E: Evidence-Based Practice in Nursing & Healthcare: A Guide to Best Practice. Lippincott, Philadelphia, 2005. Box 1.1, p 9.

book care" and "menu-driven" to describe evidence-based practice guidelines. Because nursing focuses on the whole person, many of the questions that inform our practice are not easily answered using the highly controlled, experimental methods standard to the medical disciplines. Despite the inherent obstacles of our subjects of interest, there is a consensus within the nursing discipline to develop not only the scientific basis of nursing through conducting research but also to develop the understanding and utilization of research by nurses at all levels of practice.

A number of questions need to be answered with respect to health and nursing that are important for guiding clinical decision-making. Some answers are sought to understand better what the problem is from a conceptual perspective; others are sought to describe issues related to the problem. Still other answers are sought specifically for the purpose of determining the effectiveness of interventions to ameliorate the problem. All are relevant for practice and require a basic understanding of the various methodologic approaches used in nursing science.

The important question to be asked when using research for evidence-based practice is "What findings constitute evidence?" Perhaps the most useful way of addressing this question is with another: "How will the findings be used?" This approach assumes that it is better to answer the question with the method that fits best rather than applying a few select methods to all questions. This requires the ability to critically appraise findings in the literature. If the clinical situation requires a better understanding of what the experience of emergent cardiac catheterization is for postmenopausal women with acute myocardial ischemia, then clinicians need to look for the form of evidence (or findings) that best suits the situation. It will not be found in the results of randomized clinical trials: it will be found in studies specifically designed for understanding human experiences of health in a personal and meaningful way (such as phenomenologic studies or those using grounded theory). This requires that the question and the method fit and that the clinician intending to utilize findings in a practice situation critically appraise the merits and weaknesses of studies before applying the results to any particular situation.

Applying Research-Based Evidence to Clinical Practice

Being a primary-care practitioner in the current health-care climate is difficult. We are in the midst of a significant, and, at times painful transition of our entire health-care system. In the past, primary-care providers were able to determine which tests to order, which medications to prescribe, and what other treatments were necessary for patients without being questioned about their decisions or having to justify their actions to third parties. With the realization that health-care spending was spinning out of control (accounting for 15.3 percent of the gross domestic product [GDP] in 2003 with an expected rise to 18.7 percent of the GDP by 2014) and that funds were limited, the emphasis on expensive, high-technology care was tempered by a renewed interest in cost-effective practices. As a result, health-care providers are now subject to scrutiny by both insurance companies and other utilization review procedures.

Arbitrary or Informed Practice?

Wide variation in practice patterns within and across provider type, specialty practice, and geographic region has been a major impetus for establishing both federal and organization-specific guidelines. Studies of medical decision-making processes have revealed great variation between practitioners in their approach to diagnosing and treating the same conditions. Many of these studies have demonstrated that providers who observe the same clinical situation will disagree on the assessment findings with each other and that there is great variation in the medical management even when evidence-based guidelines exist.

This realization led to a search for a wider consensus on how to diagnose and treat a number of common health conditions and occurred on both national and local levels in the form of clinical practice guidelines, practice policies, and recommendations. Although some providers perceive that attempts to standardize aspects of clinical practice strip them of their decision-making power, the intent is to improve the clinician's ability to make better decisions that lead to better, more reliable outcomes for patients.

Practice Standards and Guidelines

Although the terms are often used interchangeably, clinical practice standards, guidelines, policies, and recommendations tend to originate from distinct processes and the purpose of each is somewhat different. In general, the term "policy" is used broadly and covers a spectrum of guidelines and standards. Practice policies are considered the foundation for improving the quality of health care and controlling costs. Several medical specialty societies and other agencies have either written policies or funded their development.

Practice Standards

Unlike guidelines, *practice standards* are inflexible and are intended to be used under all circumstances. Practice standards define correct practice rather than a framework that can be tailored to fit different contexts. The American Nurses' Association (ANA) has issued a definition of practice standards for nurses, which includes broad requirements for nursing practice in any setting and at any level of practice. As defined by ANA, practice standards are "authoritative statements that describe a level of care or performance common to the profession of nursing by which the quality of nursing practice can be judged." Two types of standards are delineated by the ANA: standards of care for clinical practice and standards of professional performance. Although considered requirements of professional practice, the ANA standards could be broadly interpreted. With respect to evidence-based practice, one obligation for nurses is to utilize research findings in practice, which may indirectly refer to the use of clinical guidelines, depending on the methods used to develop the guidelines.

Practice Guidelines

Guidelines allow for flexibility when making individual patient-care decisions. They are intended to provide a reference point and general direction for decision-making and are not to be interpreted as rigid criteria that must be followed regardless of the context in which they are being used. Nonetheless, guidelines should be followed in the majority of cases, unless there is a clear rationale for deviating from them to serve the particular needs of individuals. The usefulness of applying guidelines in clinical decision-making has become increasingly recognized over the past decade and is now an expectation in the delivery of health care.

Processes Used to Design Guidelines

Just as a clinician's practice is determined by current guidelines, the quality of the guidelines themselves is determined by the processes used to create them. In general, there are two approaches used to develop such guidelines: the traditional approach (also referred to as global subjective judgment) and a newer, evidence-based approach.

The traditional approach is based on the premise that "common" practice is "correct" practice, despite the scientific evidence available either to support or refute the outcomes of such practice. Under this approach, being common practice is sufficient evidence that the practice is appropriate. This method is dangerously repetitive, in that common practice is destined to reproduce itself. When this occurs, appropriate practices are determined by the collective actions of practitioners—whether or not there is evidence to support a practice—but the actions of practitioners are themselves based on guidelines that often have originated from common practice, not evidence.

This approach may have been appropriate in the past, when practice decisions were less complicated and fewer diagnostic tests or interventions were available as treatment options. Today, with the complexities involved in clinical decision-making, research-based evidence is required. Although there are still elements of the traditional approach, the majority of guidelines are now developed from available scientific evidence.

The Agency for Health Care Policy and Research (AHCPR) was instrumental in leading the way toward evidence-based practice, improving outcomes, and publishing national guidelines on a variety of health-care problems such as smoking cessation, early detection and treatment of Alzheimer's disease, and caring for HIV-infected patients. The Healthcare Research and Quality Act of 1999 reauthorized this agency and renamed it the Agency for Healthcare Research and Quality (AHRQ). The mission of the AHRQ is to improve the quality, safety, efficiency and effectiveness of healthcare for all Americans.

AHCPR clinical practice guidelines are being used not only as references for health care providers but also as the framework for insurance utilization review, quality assurance, and reimbursement. In addition, adherence or nonadherence to established guidelines (such as those published by the AHCPR) has played an increasing role in influencing medical malpractice litigation outcomes.

The implementation of AHCPR guidelines in clinical practice has not been without significant challenges. Originally, the Agency believed that clinicians would modify their practices to improve care if they were provided with clinically credible and useful information and that practitioner involvement in developing the guidelines would facilitate the use of guidelines in practice. Neither of these assumptions proved accurate: Studies indicated wide variation between a practitioner's knowledge of the recommended management of a particular health problem based on the guidelines and the practitioner's actions. With further studies, a number of barriers to implementing guidelines in practice have been identified and AHRQ's role in supporting evidence-based practice has been redefined to include keeping relevant information in the public domain; serving as an impartial, neutral broker; encouraging multidisciplinary input in all projects; advocating for patient's perspectives and needs; and protecting special populations.

Implementing Guidelines: AHRQ Program to Address Barriers

Structurally, the new AHRQ's role includes promoting initiatives focused on developing effective methods of implementing guidelines and analyzing the outcomes of care

Table 21.2 Criteria for Selection for Development of Clinical Practice Guidelines

A clinical practice guideline must meet all of the following criteria to be included in the NGC:

1. The clinical practice guideline contains systematically developed statements that include recommendations, strategies, or information that assists physicians and/or other health care practitioners and patients make decisions about appropriate health care for specific clinical circumstances.
2. The clinical practice guideline was produced under the auspices of medical specialty associations; relevant professional societies, public or private organizations, government agencies at the federal, state, or local level; or health-care organizations or plans. A clinical practice guideline developed and issued by an individual not officially sponsored or supported by one of the above types of organizations does not meet the inclusion criteria for the National Guideline Clearinghouse™.
3. Corroborating documentation can be produced and verified that a systematic literature search and review of existing scientific evidence published in peer reviewed journals was performed during the guideline development. A guideline is not excluded from the National Guideline Clearinghouse™ if corroborating documentation can be produced and verified detailing specific gaps in scientific evidence for some of the guideline's recommendations.
4. The guideline is English language, current, and the most recent version produced. Documented evidence can be produced or verified that the guideline was developed, reviewed, or revised within the last 5 years.

when clinical guidelines are widely disseminated and used. There are three parts to the initiatives. Evidence-based practice centers (EPCs) constitute the first part and involve a private–public partnership between the AHRQ and a variety of health-care organizations to produce evidence reports and technology assessments on several priority health-care topics. Topics to be the focus for EPC assessments are nominated by clinicians or others in the health-care industry and are chosen based on the selection criteria provided in Table 21.2. Final evidence reports are intended for use in practice guidelines, quality improvement programs, and the formation of policy at the state or federal level.

The second part of the AHRQ's initiative is the development of the online National Guideline Clearinghouse (NGC). The creation of the clearinghouse is a result of a private-public partnership between AHRQ, the American Association of Health Plans (AAHP), and the American Medical Association (AMA). It is an electronic repository for clinical practice guidelines and provides widespread access to a number of guidelines from various professional groups. A list of the guidelines can be found at http://www.guidelines.gov. Table 21.3 lists examples of organizations that have supported/published evidence-based practice guidelines. Guidelines published in the NGC are required to meet established AHRQ criteria and can be accessed through the Internet. Consistent reference to these guidelines have been used throughout this text.

A final aspect of the AHRQ's initiative involves product research and evaluation. This includes an array of research and evaluation activities aimed at the development of evidence for use in guidelines, implementation strategies, and the quality of practice when clinical practice guidelines are used (e.g., outcome-based research).

These initiatives reflect the new role the AHRQ has with respect to supporting evidence-based practice and are meant to improve the scientific basis of guidelines, decrease duplication efforts, distribute evidence on a national level, enhance uniformity, and reinforce public and private partnerships within the health-care sector.

Examples from the Field: Studies of Implementing Practice Guidelines

The clinician who uses clinical guidelines should evaluate their usefulness by examining the following major characteristics:

- Are the guidelines clinically important? To establish clinical importance, guidelines should convince you that following them will provide more benefits for your patients than whatever expected harms or costs are associated with applying them. In part, an examination of both the relative and absolute changes in an outcome is required to do this. Although relative risk (RR) is a frequently used measure of association in the medical and epidemiologic literature, it tells you nothing about the absolute impact of how many people are affected by a particular risk factor. For example, when the RR of death (or of developing breast cancer or some other outcome) is "2," that assessment is at times more meaningful if the risk is expressed in more explicit absolute values. That is, does a RR of 2 mean that 2 out of 10 patients will die when exposed to some risk factor, or is it 2 in 100,000? Each of these values provides different information regarding the clinical importance of the study findings used to develop guidelines. An understanding of the commonly used measures of disease frequency, measures of association, and other measures that assist with applying study findings in clinical practice is necessary to interpret and apply practice guidelines.
- How strong are the recommendations? This is largely determined by the strength of available evidence in making recommendations using clinical guidelines.

Table 21.3 Examples of Clinical Practice Guidelines/Evidence-Based Guidelines Developed/Published by Organizations and Agencies

Organization/Agency	Guideline	Website
Agency for Healthcare Research and Quality	Anemia in Oncology, Use of Epoetin	http://www.ahcpr.gov
American Academy of Neurology	Carotid Endarterectomy: An evidence-based review	http://www.aan.com
American Academy of Pediatrics	Treatment of the School-Aged Child with Attention-Deficit/Hyperactivity Disorder	http://www.aap.org
American College of Chest Physicians	Device Selection and Outcomes of Aerosol Therapy: Evidence–Based Guideline	http://www.chestnet.org/
American College of Physicians	Pharmacologic and Surgical Management of Obesity in Primary Care	http://www.acponline.org/
American College of Preventive Medicine	Healthy Diet	http://www.acpm.org
American Diabetes Association	National Standards for Diabetes Self-Management Education	http://www.diabetes.org
American Heart Association	ACC/AHA/ESC Guidelines for the Management of the Patient with Atrial Fibrillation	http://www.americanheart.org
American Medical Association	Roadmaps for Clinical Practice Series: Assessment and Management of Adult Obesity	http://www.ama-assn.org
Association of Rehabilitation Nurses	Practice Guidelines for the Management of Constipation in Adults	http://www.rehabnurse.org
Association of Women's Health, Obstetric and Neonatal Nurses	Continence for Women	www.awhonn.org
Gerontological Nursing Interventions Research Center: University of Iowa College of Nursing	Acute Pain Management in the Elderly	www.nursing.uiowa.edu
Indian Health Services	Evidence-based Practice: Maternal Child Health, American Indian and Alaskan Native	http://www.ihs.gov
National Heart, Lung and Blood Institute	Report 2: Guidelines for the Diagnosis and Management of Asthma	http://www.nhlbi.nih.gov
Substance Abuse and Mental Health Services Administration	Cultural Competence Standards in Managed Care Mental Health Services: Four Underserved/Underrepresented Racial/Ethnic Groups	http://www.samhsa.gov/

This list provides only a sample of such organizations and agencies and is not meant to include every group associated with the development of clinical guidelines, policies, or recommendations.

The quality of the study design, consistency of results, and the relative value of different outcomes must be equally considered. For example, even though the clinical outcomes associated with treating underlying causes of secondary hypertension may have been demonstrated repeatedly in several well-designed studies, the costs and risks of adverse outcomes associated with diagnostic tests to rule out a cause such as renal artery stenosis may be greater than the benefits when applied to the entire population. Thus, guidelines do not recommend that every person who develops hypertension undergoes extensive testing. Rather, specific characteristics of patients presenting with hypertension assist us in narrowing the population to those individuals who would reap the benefits of screening beyond any potential harm of the tests. Various grading systems for the strength of the evidence upon which recommendations are based have been used to assist practitioners in determining how "strong" the recommendations are, using clinical practice guidelines. For example, in the *Guide to Clinical Preventive Services* developed by the U.S. Preventive Service Task Force, a section describes the methodology for reviewing evidence and how the Task Force members "translated" the science into a five-point scale (with A through E ratings) that could be readily used by clinicians. Some guidelines use a Roman numeral scale to define the levels of evidence.

- Are the guideline recommendations applicable to your patients? Guidelines are developed for a variety of settings and for different practitioners. First, it is necessary to determine for what group the guidelines were written (e.g., primary-care providers, specialists, or quality assurance reviewers) and whether they suit the intended purpose. Second, a determination on whether patients served have the characteristics of patients for whom the guidelines were intended is needed. For example, if the patients you care for have a higher or lower prevalence of a disease or different set of risk factors for disease than those in the guidelines, the recommendations may not apply. The patient population for whom the guidelines are intended will likely be dictated by the sample characteristics of the studies used to develop them as evidence. Before applying recommendations to any one patient, first determine whether this patient's characteristics are consistent with those for which the guideline was intended and modify the guidelines when required (remember, they are meant to be flexible and adapted to individual needs when necessary).

Development of Evidence-Based Practice Guidelines

The process first adopted by the AHCPR to develop guidelines is outlined in Figure 21.1. This Framework has been adopted by numerous organizations/associations to develop evidence-based guidelines since its original publication.

The following are essential components of guideline development: (1) identification/clarification of the topic, (2) establishment of an expert panel, (3) a systematic review of the literature, (4) development of evidence-based tables, (5) writing a draft of recommendations based on the evidence, (6) external review of the recommendations, and (7) final acceptance of the revised recommendations by the panel. Panel members chosen to develop guidelines will depend on the focus of the guidelines and may include physicians, nurse practitioners, clinical nurse specialists, ethicists, pharmacists, therapists, and health-care consumers.

A crucial aspect of the development is the review of the literature and rating of the available evidence. An adaptation of one of the most common methods of rating evidence is listed in Table 21.4.

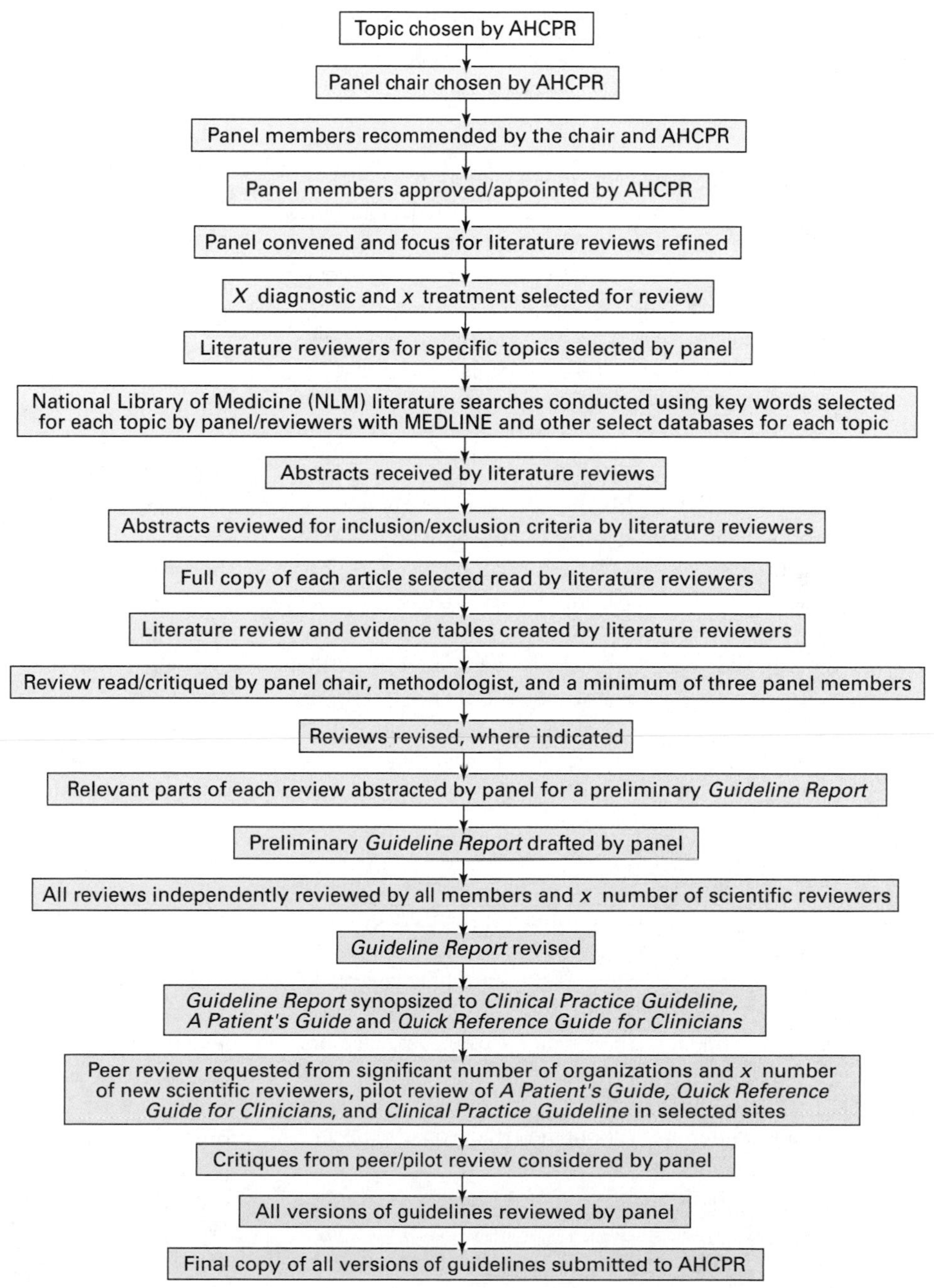

FIGURE 21.1 Guidelines development process for the Agency for Healthcare Policy and Research (AHCPR). (From Clinical Practice Guideline No. 5: Depression in Primary Care, Vol 2, Treatment of Major Depression, US Department of Health and Human Services. Agency of Healthcare Policy and Research, Rockville, Md., 1993, AHCPR publication 93-0551.)

Table 21.4 Quality of Evidence

I	Evidence obtained from at least one properly designed randomized controlled trial
II-1	Evidence obtained from well-designed controlled trials without randomization
II-2	Evidence obtained from well-designed cohort or case-control analytic studies, preferably from more than one center or research group
II-3	Evidence from multiple time series with or without the intervention. Dramatic results in uncontrolled experiments (such as the results of the introduction of penicillin treatment in the 1940s) could also be regarded as this type of evidence
III	Opinions of respected authorities, based on clinical experience, descriptive studies or reports of expert committees

Source: Evidence-based clinical practice guideline. Promotion of emotional well-being during midlife. Association of Women's Health, Obstetric and Neonatal Nurses (AWHONN).

An essential aspect in understanding the development and appropriate use of guidelines is to understand the foundations of the various research designs in medicine and nursing and how they contribute to practicing from an evidence or research base. Nursing uses a wide variety of study designs to inform practice. The medical disciplines, however, tend to use a few specific types of designs that are often given less attention in basic nursing research textbooks.

Research Designs for Level I Evidence

Randomized clinical trials (RCTs) are increasingly considered the most respected method for establishing the cause of disease or the efficacy of a treatment/intervention. For example, the Food and Drug Administration (FDA) requires evidence of a drug's efficacy from two independently conducted randomized trials before approving its use in the United States. The National Institutes of Health (NIH) are increasingly funding RCTs, and agencies or organizations developing clinical guidelines are now considering the evidence from RCTs to supersede the findings that exist from case-control or cohort studies.

The strength of RCTs to establish cause or efficacy lies in the ability of this design to maintain a high degree of control within experimental conditions. If there are different effects between the groups (e.g., blood pressure, the development of pressure ulcers, the prevention of pregnancy), the differences can generally be attributed to the intervention, exposure, or treatment rather than "extraneous" factors. Moreover, the random assignment of subjects into the treatment or control group allows for a high degree of confidence in making causal inferences about the effects of an exposure, intervention, or treatment.

RCTs also frequently employ the use of double-blinding to further strengthen the support for making a cause-and-effect relationship. When RCTs are double-blind, neither the principal investigators nor the participants know who is in the control or experimental group until either significant differences are noted in a (blind) analysis of the data or the study is complete. Its purpose is to eliminate the potential for participants in the experimental or control groups to either treat themselves or be treated differently.

Research Designs for Level II-1 Evidence

Quasi-experimental research designs evaluate the effectiveness of an intervention/treatment but subjects are not randomly assigned to either the treatment or control group. In these designs many of the other same methods to ascertain the internal validity of the study, such as control of extraneous variables and standardization of treatment, instituted in RCTs are implemented.

Research Designs for Level II-2 Evidence

Types of designs most often identified with this level of evidence are case-control studies and cohort studies. These types of studies are especially useful in answering clinical questions that address prognosis or causation. *Case-control studies* are unique in that they begin after a person has either developed or not developed a disease. ("Cases" are individuals who develop a disease and "controls" are those who do not.) Such studies go back in time to determine which factors are associated with the onset of disease and are thus generally considered retrospective, although they may be prospective. With this design, the study is generally initiated after the disease has developed. A group of individuals (cases) who have the disease and those (controls) who do not are selected and compared in terms of their prior exposures that are thought to be associated with the development of a particular type of disease. Case-control studies are also considered observational studies, because they do not manipulate the exposure (what may also be referred to as the intervention). The course of the disease is observed without interference. The lack of control over the exposure in case-control studies (along with other observational studies) risks introducing selection bias into the study, which may confound the results. This potential shortcoming of case-control studies has led to a significant degree of skepticism among a faction of researchers and clinicians alike, some of whom argue that case-control studies are essentially worthless because of the inherent potential for bias.

Despite the arguments against the value of the case-control design, it has contributed significantly to current understanding of the association between exposure and disease in many areas. In fact, it is the most commonly used epidemiologic design in the medical literature today. For example, the association between unopposed estrogen use in postmenopausal women and the development of endometrial cancer was established through several case-control studies. With the Women's Health Initiative study, the development of specific diseases in women using postmenopausal hormones is being studied extensively in an RCT.

The unique characteristic of a *cohort study* is that individuals are classified by their exposure status (exposed/unexposed) and then followed over time to see whether they develop a disease. Differences in disease frequency between the exposed and unexposed groups are then analyzed. Observation generally spans several years, because enough time must lapse for a significant number of individuals to develop the outcome, or disease. The time required for observation is generally less, however, if there is a high incidence of the disease in the population under study.

Although the majority of cohort studies are prospective, they may also be retrospective. The feature that distinguishes prospective from retrospective cohort studies is simply whether the outcome of interest (the disease) has occurred at the time the investigator initiates the study. If the disease has not occurred and only exposure status is known at the beginning of the investigation, the study uses a prospective cohort design. If both the exposure and disease have already occurred at the beginning of the investigation, then the study uses a retrospective cohort design.

The Nurses' Health Study at Harvard is an example of a well-known prospective cohort study. It is a large, ongoing cohort study that enrolled more than 120,000 married female nurses who were 30 to 55 years old in 1976. The nurses completed a baseline questionnaire about a number of demographic and health characteristics. Follow-up questionnaires at 2-year intervals asked about the development of disease and any new exposures. By comparing the exposed and unexposed groups on a number of variables (e.g., those who took hormone replacements and those who did not; those who ate high-fat foods and those who did not) and the onset of disease within each group, the study has provided important information about the relationships of these variables with the development of cancer and cardiovascular disease in women.

Perhaps the most renowned example of a prospective cohort study is the Framingham Heart Study. In this study, investigators identified and examined 5127 men and women from Framingham, MA, who were 30 to 59 years old in the 1950s. When the study was initiated, all 5127 participants were determined to be free from coronary heart disease. As in the Nurses' Health Study, information on demographic and health variables was gathered (such as cigarette smoking status and various clinical and laboratory parameters) at the onset of the study. Participants in the study have provided ongoing lifestyle and health status information and have been reexamined at regular intervals since 1952 for the development of coronary events. Prospective data from this study has been pivotal in identifying a number of major risk factors associated with coronary artery disease (CAD) and has been one of the sources of evidence for recommending lifestyle modifications to prevent CAD.

Research Designs for Level III Evidence

The purpose of descriptive research is to accurately portray the characteristics of a population or a clinical situation. Descriptive research can be quantitative or qualitative in design. In quantitative designs, the findings address the incidence, prevalence, or measurable characteristics of the population using descriptive statistics (frequencies, means, mode, etc.). In qualitative designs the population or clinical situation is displayed in a narrative format for the purpose of increasing the understanding of the various dimensions of the phenomena of interest. Common qualitative designs used in nursing research include phenomenology, ethnography, grounded theory, and historical analysis.

Study Design and the Degree of Evidence

Evidence-based health care in the form of rigorous data is widely supported as the new model for practice. As noted in the beginning of the chapter, what constitutes evidence and rigorous data is contested in the literature. Some suggest that the degree of evidence provided by a study is based on its method, or design. There is an increasing trend toward regarding evidence from RCTs as the only valid type of evidence appropriate for use in the practice setting. This perspective essentially disregards what we have learned and can continue to learn from observational studies such as case-control and cohort studies. Moreover, it has been suggested that learning an evidence-based perspective requires learning to ask only a few questions about the type of design used, which can be taught in a short course. Critics of an approach that parallels evidence-based practice with an RCT design point out what is absent from this point of view—a truly critical appraisal of the study in its entirety.

Some advocates of evidence-based medicine reject the notion that young clinicians learn how to practice from an evidence base in a matter of a few hours of lecture or in a crash-course setting. Such an approach to teaching evidence-based practice has been regarded as a grave error with serious consequences. The most sobering outcome of this approach is the failure to teach clinicians how to think or critically evaluate information. There are many circumstances in which randomization (and thus, evaluating the problem with an RCT) is impossible and where observational methods have provided invaluable information. Take, for instance, how we came to understand the relationship between alcohol use in pregnancy and fetal alcohol syndrome; smoking and cardiopulmonary disease; birth defects and thalidomide; the transmission of the human immunodeficiency virus (HIV) and viral hepatitis; and the development of endocarditis in intravenous drug use: Knowledge of these associations has come from observational studies. Randomizing women into experimental or control groups to either drink alcoholic beverages or not, or designing an experimental trial to determine how the transmission of HIV in humans occurs is not ethically possible (or desirable). The credibility of how we know what we know in practice must be determined through a critical appraisal of the information available. A framework for appraising the health science literature is needed, along with additional important issues to consider when considering applying research results to practice, and examples of how studies have provided a sufficient degree of evidence to change the standards of practice.

Using a Framework to Evaluate Health Science Literature

Critical appraisal of the health science literature can seem like an overwhelming and (perhaps) unimportant task, yet it is a professional responsibility within advanced practice nursing. Using a framework for guidance can assist APNs in taking the appropriate steps toward meeting this obligation. Some of the steps in applying the framework presented here are similar to those used for evaluating clinical practice guidelines. A framework for evaluating journal articles in the health science literature is presented in Table 21.5. This framework provides an organized approach to interpreting the information found in a variety of articles, be it a review of the current knowledge in an area or original research findings.

Evaluating the Evidence to Change Practice

For an example of evaluating evidence to change practice let's look at the use of angiotensin-converting enzyme (ACE) inhibitors in patients with congestive heart failure (CHF). In the early 1990s, several clinical trials demonstrated that the use of ACE inhibitors improved clinical outcomes in patients with CHF, not only with regard to mortality but also in exercise tolerance, symptom severity, progression to left ventricular dysfunction, and fewer hospitalization rates. The consistency of the findings and the fact that they came from well-designed RCTs provided unequivocal evidence that ACE-inhibitor use was beneficial for the majority of patients with CHF. As a result, the American College of Cardiology, the American Heart Association, and the AHCPR developed clinical guidelines for the treatment of CHF that strongly encourage ACE inhibitors as standard therapy. The use of ACE-inhibitors is now considered a standard of care and should be incorporated into the care of persons with CHF.

Table 21.5 A Framework for Evaluating Health Science Literature

1. Look at the title to determine whether it reflects your specific interest.
2. Validate that the content is relevant to your original interest and the title by reading the abstract.
3. Evaluate and determine what is being studied:
   What are the study questions or hypotheses?
   What are the specific study variables under study?
   How are the variables defined and measured?
4. Evaluate and determine who is being studied:
   What are the characteristics of the study sample or subjects?
   How were subjects elected for the study?
   Is there an adequate sample size?
5. Evaluate and determine the type of study design and assess its validity:
   Do the designs of the studies support the statements made?
   Have other studies in similar (or different) samples found consistent results?
6. Evaluate and determine how data have been analyzed:
   What are the descriptive statistics used to describe the sample characteristics?
   Could the degree or pattern of missing data influence the results?
   Were the inferential statistics used appropriate for the study question and design?
   Remember that statistical tests of significance do not determine causation or clinical significance.
7. Evaluate what you have determined thus far:
   Have you been skeptical?
   Have you judged the quality of the literature based on the journal in which it was published?
   Do you realize that there is no such thing as a "perfect" study?
   How have you judged the author's treatment of contradictory results?
   Remember that validity and reliability are crucial aspects of the study.
8. Discuss your evaluation with colleagues and seek other opinions (such as in a journal club):
   Do your colleagues agree with your evaluation?
   Do the results or recommendations suggest a change in your clinical practice? If so, what change is suggested and how will it be implemented?

Outcomes

Distinguishing between intermediate and clinical outcomes is also critical before applying research findings to practice. Outcome research has been increasingly funded in recent years. An outcome is generally considered the dependent variable of the study. Intermediate outcomes include things such as bone mineral density (BMD) measurement, hemoglobin levels, and an eosinophil level. Clinical outcomes include measures such as the number of hip fractures, a person's functional status, peak flow values, or the number of acute asthma exacerbations experienced.

Improvement in intermediate outcomes does not necessarily lead to improvements in clinical outcomes. For example, in early studies of using fluoride to treat osteoporosis, BMD values improved greatly when given to osteoporotic women, but the number of fractures over time did not differ from those in women who were given placebos. Thus, intermediate outcomes, although important to study to gain an understanding of disease processes and treatment, should not be substituted for clinical outcome data.

Nursing Science: Building the Evidence for Practice

Historically, nurses have been increasingly involved in conducting research. Essentially, the inception of the National

Center for Nursing Research (NCNR), which would later become the National Institute for Nursing Research (NINR), marked a new era by aligning nursing science with other respected institutes within the NIH. This increased both federal funding for nursing research and the visibility of nursing science on a national level. Investment in nursing research continues to grow in terms of resources, funding, training, and the expectation for using research as the basis, or evidence, for practice.

Methodologically, nursing science has evolved from the predominant methods of acquiring human knowledge. Many methods of knowing contribute to our knowledge or understanding of the world. The scientific method, however, is a specific approach used to answer questions in an orderly and systematic manner. Qualities of the traditional scientific method, such as achieving the greatest degree of control over the study, are present in case-control, cohort, and RCT designs. The scientific approach has been defined over hundreds of years of debate and has included competing ontologies (what we ought to know) and epistemologies (how we ought to know). In textbooks of nursing research, maximizing order and control are frequently acknowledged as *the* aim of well-done scientific inquiry. Although a full explanation of the history of the philosophy of science is beyond the scope of this chapter, a perspective embracing order and control is adopted from a logical-positivist philosophy, which has greatly influenced the way science is conducted today. The more recognized concept of empiricism was also borne out of the logical-positivist philosophy of knowing. Empiricism refers to the process whereby "evidence rooted in objective reality and gathered directly or indirectly through the human senses" is used as the basis for generating knowledge. Clinicians tend to be more familiar with the notion of empiricism than logical positivism, because it is the root for the term "empirical evidence" so often seen in the scientific or clinical literature. Note the use of the term "objectivity" in the definition of empiricism. The goal of objectivity (via methods that promote order and control) has largely established the hierarchy of nursing research that shapes science within the discipline.

The notion of objective science being the epitome of science, however, has been contested within nursing and other disciplines. Harding, for example, calls into question the purity of objectivity and provides a cogent argument for redefining "objectivity," "rationality," and "the scientific method" in both the social and natural sciences. In a related critique, Keller suggests the traditional scientific method is not as much objective as it is masculine and uses examples from her work as a mathematical biophysicist. The feminist analyses of science that Harding and Keller contributed have to some degree been adopted by a community of nurse-scientists who believe that control, objectivity, and traditional scientific rationale are antithetical to the goals of nursing research and practice. Other nurse-scientists, however, believe an empirical approach is the best method for understanding clinical phenomena and developing nursing interventions. Still others believe a combination of methods (or various ways of triangulating) provides a more clear, encompassing answer to questions asked within the discipline.

The dialogue surrounding what standard to use in evaluating the degree of evidence required from nursing research for use in practice continues. As noted previously, much of this discussion centers around the question that is asked and the methods used to answer it. An example of using evidence-based guidelines and nursing research to care for a family with a child with diabetes in presented in Box 21.1.

There are numerous other examples of nursing research that have contributed to the knowledge base of nursing. Familiarity with nursing research findings is as important for advanced practice as familiarity with medical research findings. Critically appraising studies regarding the appropriate use of results is one of the most important skills APNs will be required to use in practice.

Clinical Decision-Making and the Patient's Health-Care Decisions

The decisions APNs make in practice are fundamental to the quality of care given. Eddy expresses the importance of critically evaluating the components of clinical decision-making. He states, "In general, the goal of a decision regarding a health practice is to choose the action that is most likely to deliver the outcomes that patients find desirable." He identified two main steps of a decision: (1) collecting and analyzing evidence (or data) on the benefits, potential harms, and costs of various options, and (2) making a judgement about how to use the available evidence to achieve the health outcome desired.

Applying analytic procedures for determining the credibility or reliability of data to be used as evidence is only one aspect of the decision-making process, however. An equal challenge in making practice decisions lies in the second part of the process, which involves making a judgment about how to use the evidence available. This second step is not a question of facts but of patient values or preferences. One of the most substantial qualities of advanced practice nursing is establishing a relationship with our patients, providing them with the most current information we can, and allowing them to make health-care decisions they determine are best for themselves. In this respect, Eddy further reminds us that it is not entirely important what you as a clinician prefer for your patients, "it is the patient's preferences, not ours, that count."

Box 21.1 Example: Integration of Evidence-Based Practice and Nursing Research–Based Practice

The management of the child with type 1 diabetes requires a multidisciplinary approach of which the family is an integral part. Below are two resources available to the APN to assist in the management of the child with diabetes.

Evidence-Based Practice Guidelines

The American Diabetes Association-Professional Association supports the development of clinical guidelines for the mangement of diabetes. The foundation of the guideline for the management of diabetes is the recommendations made as to glycemic control. These include:

1. Lowering A1C has been associated with a reduction of microvascular and neuropathic complications of diabetes. (A)
2. Develop or adjust the management plan to achieve normal or near-normal glycemia with an A1C goal of <7%. (B)
3. More stringent goals (i.e., a normal A1C, <6%) can be considered in individual patients and in pregnancy. (B)
4. A lower A1C is associated with a lower risk of myocardial infarction and cardiovascular death. (B)
5. Aggressive glycemic management with insulin may reduce morbidity in patients with severe acute illness, preoperatively, following myocardial infarction, and in pregnancy. (B)
6. Less stringent treatment goals may be appropriate for patients with a history of severe hypoglycemia, patients with limited life expectancies, very young children or older adults, and individuals with comorbid conditions. (E)

The panel rated the strength of the evidence supporting the first recommendation as "A." An "A" indicated that there was clear evidence from well-conducted, generalizable, randomized controlled trials that were adequately powered, or at the least supportive evidence from well-conducted randomized controlled trials that were adequately powered, including evidence from a well-conducted trial at one or more institutions. Evidence supporting the second through fifth recommendations were rated as "B." An evidence rating of "B" indicated that there was supportive evidence from well-conducted cohort studies. The final recommendation was given an evidence rating of "E." Evidence rated as E indicated that support for the recommendation was from expert consensus or clinical experience.

The guidelines also addressed nutrition and psychosocial assessment and care. The recommendations listed under psychosocial assessment and care are:

1. Preliminary assessment of psychological and social status should be included as part of the medical management of diabetes. (E)
2. Psychosocial screening should include but is not limited to attitudes about the illness, expectations for medical management and outcomes, affect/mood, general and diabetes-related quality of life, resources (financial, social, and emotional) and psychiatric history. (E)
3. It is preferable to incorporate psychological treatment into routine care rather than to wait for identification of a specific problem or deterioration in psychological status. (E)

Nursing Research

Sullivan-Bolyai et al conducted a study to describe the experiences of parents managing their child's type 1 diabetes with the use of continuous subcutaneous insulin infusions (CSII), commonly referred to as the insulin pump. In this qualitative study, 14 mothers and 7 fathers were interviewed and asked to describe the day to day experience of managing their child's diabetes. The children ranged in age from 2 to 11 years and their mean age was 7.2 years of age. Parents in this study agreed that the pump was very effective in managing their child's diabetes and believed that their child's glucose was under much better control with the pump as compared to using multiple daily injections (MDI). The results of Sullivan-Bolyai and associates' research indicated that some parents are reluctant to change to an alternative method of achieving glycemic control for their child. But all of the parents in their study, once familiar with the device, were very satisfied with the results and reported a better quality of life since they changed methods. Another important finding was that parents reported more freedom and flexibility in their lives once their child was switched from MDI to the insulin pump. Some parents reported that once the child was placed on the insulin pump they often were tempted to impose stricter controls on their child's glucose levels.

Impact on Advanced Practice Nursing

The ADA guidelines indicate that there is strong, reliable evidence to support interventions that assist the child with diabetes to maintain normal to near-normal glycemic levels, with less convincing evidence given to support less strigent control in very young children. Two methods currently used to achieve control are multiple daily injections (MDI) and continuous subcutaneous insulin infusions (CSII), commonly called the "insulin pump."

These guidelines also include a mandate for the primary-care provider to provide psychosocial assessment and care. One assessment needed is the parents' comfort with technology and resources. Technology once limited to secondary and teritiary health-care settings is now available in the community and is often managed by lay persons and caregivers.

The method used to achieve glycemic control of the child is ultimately the parents' decision. However, APNs who care for these children and families will be influential in the education and support of these families as they make complex health-care decisions for their child. Using the guidelines as the goals for management, APNs can provide parents with evidence-based rationale for glycemic management of their child and assist them in their choices.

Relaying information to parents based on nursing research, such as the research conducted by Sullivan-Bolyai and colleagues, may relieve some initial hesitancy in parents about switching from MDI to SCII to manage their child's diabetes.

One important consideration in using this research in practice is that the sample for the above research was described as Caucasian and well-educated. Will these same experiences be similar in other samples? However, perceptions of parents that their child's diabetes is under better control with the insulin pump and that this method has improved their quality of life can be useful to APNs in their care of families managing this complex health condition.

Sources: American Diabetes Association-Professional Association. Standards of Medical Care in Diabetes. V. Diabetes Care. (2005). Retrieved September 22, 2005 from http://www. guideliines.gov.

Sullivan-Bolyai, S, Knafl, K, Tamborlane, W, and Grey, M: Parents' reflections on managing their children's diabetes with insulin pumps. J Nurs Scholar 36:316–323, 2004.

Bibliography

Agency for Healthcare Policy and Research: AHCPR: Overview. Vol. 1998: Agency for Healthcare Policy and Research, Washington, D.C., 1998.

Agency for Healthcare Research and Quality: Reauthorization Fact Sheet. Retrieved September 22, 2005 from http://www. ahcpr.gov/about/ahrqfact.htm.

American Diabetes Association-Professional Association: Standards of Medical Care in Diabetes. V. Diabetes Care.(2005). Retrieved September 22, 2005 from http://www.guideliines.gov.

Boberg, EW: Comprehensive Health Enhancement Support System (CHESS): In-Home, Computer-Based Patient Education and Support, Translating Evidence into Practice. Agency for Healthcare Policy and Research, Washington, D.C., 1997.

Borbas, C: Implementing Changes in Healthcare Organizations: Lessons Learned and Future Challenges., Translating Evidence into Practice. Agency for Healthcare Policy and Research, Washington, D.C., 1997.

Brennan, TA: Practice Guidelines and Malpractice Litigation: Collision or Cohesion? Translating Evidence into Practice, Agency for Healthcare Policy and Research, Washington, D.C., 1997.

Carr, CA, and Schott, A: Differences in evidence-based care in midwifery practice and education. J Nurs Scholar 34:153–158, 2002.

Dean-Baar, S, et al: Standards of Clinical Nursing Practice. American Nurses' Association, Washington, D.C., 1991.

Eddy, DM: Clinical Decision-Making: From Theory to Practice. Jones and Bartlett, Boston, 1996.

Feinstein, A: A bibliography of publications on observer variability. J Chronic Dis 38:619–632, 1985.

Frantz, RA, and Xakellis, GC: Implementing Pressure Ulcer Guidelines in Long-Term Care, Translating Evidence into Practice. Agency for Healthcare Policy and Research, Washington, D.C., 1997.

Green, L: Using evidence-based medicine in clinical practice. Primary Care 25:391–400, 1998.

Harding, S: Whose Science? Whose Knowledge? Thinking from Women's Lives. Cornell University Press, Ithaca, N.Y., 1991.

Hennekens, CH, and Buring, JE:. Epidemiology in Medicine. Little, Brown, Boston, 1987.

Kamerow, DB: Clinical Evidence: Creation, Assessment, and Implementation, Translating Evidence into Practice: What Do We Know? What Do We Need? Agency for Healthcare Policy and Research, Washington, D.C., 1997.

Kanouse, DE: Overcoming Barriers to Implementation, Translating Evidence into Practice. Agency for Healthcare Policy and Research, Washington, D.C., 1997.

Keller, EF: Reflections on Gender and Science. Yale University Press, New Haven, Conn., 1995.

McCall, J, and Culpepper, L: How to read medical journals. In Rakel, R (ed): Essentials of Family Practice. WB Saunders, Philadelphia, 1993.

Melnyk, BM, and Fineout-Overholt, E: Evidence-Based Practice in Nursing & Healthcare: A Guide to Best Practice. Lippincott, Philadelphia, 2005.

Mitchell, GJ: Research issues: Questioning evidence-based practice in nursing. Nurs Sci Q 10,154–155, 1997.

National Institutes of Health Consensus Conference: Acupuncture. JAMA 280:17, 1998.

Polit, DF, and Beck, CT: Nursing Research: Principles and Methods, ed 7. Lippincott, Philadelphia, 2004.

Rosoff, AJ: Evidence-based medicine and the law: The courts confront clinical practice guidelines. J Health Polit Policy Law 26:327–368, 2001.

Sackett, DL: Clinical Epidemiology: A Basic Science for Clinical Medicine. Little, Brown, Boston, 1991.

Slowther, A, Ford, S, and Schofield, T: Ethics of evidence-based medicine in the primary care setting. J Med Ethics 30:151–155, 2004.

Sullivan-Bolyai, S, Knafl, K,Tamborlane, W, and Grey, M: Parents' reflections on managing their children's diabetes with insulin pumps. J Nurs Scholar 36:316–323, 2004.

U.S. Preventive Services Task Force: Guide to Clinical Preventive Services, ed 2. Williams & Wilkins, Baltimore, 1996.

Vandenbroucke, JP: Observational research and evidence-based medicine: What should we teach young physicians? J Clin Epidemiol 51:467–472, 1998.

Veeramah, V: Utilization of research findings by graduate nurses and midwives. J Adv Nurs 47:183–191, 2004.

Wilson, MC, et al: Users' guides to the medical literature. VIII. How to use clinical practice guidelines. What are the recommendations and will they help you in caring for your patients? JAMA 274:20, 1995.

Zir, L, et al: Interobservervariability in coronary angiography. Circulation 53:627, 1976.

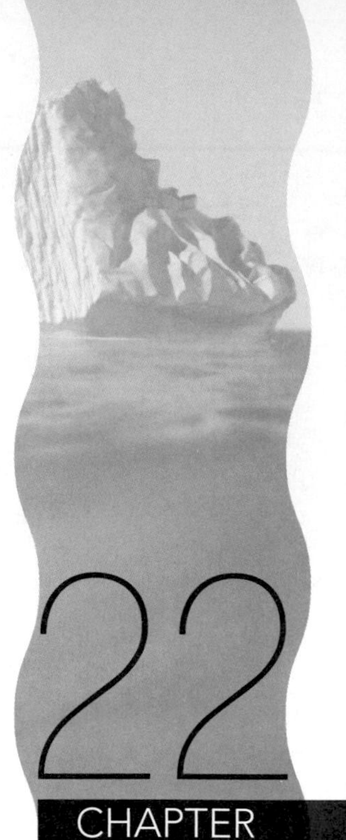

Ethical and Legal Issues of a Caring-Based Practice

Jill E. Winland-Brown, EdD, MSN, APRN, BC

Ethical Issues

With economic, social, and legal constraints present in our everyday practice, it is no wonder that health-care providers face ethical dilemmas daily. This section begins with an overview of what ethics is, what constitutes an ethical dilemma, different theoretical approaches to analyzing dilemmas, and a description of ethical principles. Each of us lives by a moral code, whether or not we have taken the time to reflect on what this means. Some people live by the simple code of "an eye for an eye"; others use the "Golden Rule" that forms the core of major religions (see Table 22.1).

It is more and more difficult to practice ethically in health care today for many reasons, including dehumanizing procedures, technological advances that affect the quality of life, and the potential for unauthorized sharing of confidential information and violations of privacy because of easy access to data banks. Patients and providers must contend with these and many other problems. Historically, the "virtuous" man or woman who faithfully followed rules that were largely etiquette could be termed *ethical.* Even the early Code for Nurses of the American Nurses Association in 1950 dealt with issues of etiquette as being synonymous with ethics. Today, in view of the questions posed by modern health-care practices, those rules seem simplistic.

Table 22.1 Golden Rules

Whatsoever ye would that men should do to you, do ye even so to them.	*Christianity (Jesus)*
What is hateful to yourself, don't do to your fellow man.	*Judaism (Rabbi Hillel)*
What you don't want done to yourself; don't do to others.	*Confucius*
Hurt not other with that which pains thyself.	*Buddhism*
May I do to others as I would that they should do unto me	*Plato*
Do naught to others which if done to thee would cause thee pain.	*Hinduism (Mahabharata)*

Ethics

Ethics is a branch of philosophy that considers what is right and what one ought to do when confronted with moral choices. It is termed *bioethics* when those moral choices involve health care. Personal and professional values influence our daily professional lives. Many of these values are known and explicit; others are hidden and unknown. When involved in a professional practice, providers cannot escape the need to clarify their own values. Many excellent books on values clarification (see Resources) are available that can assist health-care providers in exploring their own values and in deciding what is meaningful or valued to them to facilitate self-understanding.

Ethics is integrally related to nursing, because nursing is a practice with an inherent moral sense. Nursing ethics attempts to articulate that moral sense, to assess its fulfillment, to explore new possibilities for its fulfillment, and to appraise its adequacy. A classic saying is that "a patient doesn't care what a nurse knows until he knows a nurse cares." This could not be truer than in any situation with a health-care provider and a patient involving life and death choices. The patient wants to know that the provider is an advocate, a friend, and a trusted expert, not someone who is consumed with billing practices or always watching the clock.

The Skill of Ethical Action

Ethics are the standards or principles governing one's actions in professional practice. It is what the professional "ought" to do. Ethical behavior serves to protect the rights of human beings; a code of ethics is characteristic of all professions. To apply ethics, there are three basic philosophical skills that clinicians need to foster or acquire. First, the clinician must develop an ability for in-depth questioning, not just taking information at face value. Next, the clinician must develop the ability to understand different points of view and make a reasonable, empathetic effort to understand another person's opposing viewpoint. Finally, the clinician must not be afraid to argue a point logically. A dialectic exchange occurs when both parties learn something; it is a win–win situation. It is similar to a more formal debate in that those who do not know their opponent's arguments do not completely understand their own.

Professional Codes

The American Nurses Association (ANA) has a Code of Ethics for Nurses, the American Medical Association (AMA) has a code of ethics entitled the Principles of Medical Ethics, and the American Hospital Association has a Patient's Bill of Rights, which delineates the hospital's code of conduct owed to patients. There is also a Code of the International Council of Nurses (ICN). The ANA's Code of Ethics for Nurses (the Code) was first adopted in 1950. It helped to legitimize nursing as a profession, because one of the components of a profession is having a code of conduct that governs its actions. The Code was formulated by nurses, for nurses, and was voted on at a national ANA convention that had delegates representing all the ANA members. The Code serves as a contract between society and the nursing profession: It explicitly sets forth the values and ethical principles that guide the clinical decisions of all practicing nurses. The Code provides a framework within which nurses and advanced practice nurses can make ethical decisions and be held accountable to the public for those decisions. It also provides guidance for carrying out the professional role and aids in justifying differences between personal and professional values.

The primary purpose of the Code of Ethics is promotion of high-quality nursing care and protection of the public from incompetent or unethical nursing practice. The Code, revised in 2001, continues to indicate that the recipient of care is the primary consideration in any conflict of interest. The Code sets the ethical standards for nursing, whereas the Nursing Practice Act of each state establishes the legal standards. The requirements of the Code may often exceed, but are not less than, those of the law.

One of the provisions of the Code states that part of being a professional, and one who is ethical, is to advance the profession by being a member of the association that represents the professionals. For nurses, this is the ANA. Although there are many "splinter" organizations, the ANA is the umbrella organization that speaks for all nurses. Yet only about 10 percent of nurses belong to the organization. Increasing membership, particularly among advanced practice nurses, is one of the challenges facing nurses who need to become active to effect legislative change. Nineteen nursing organizations served on the Call to the Nursing Profession and Nursing's Agenda for the Future Steering Committee to identify strategic areas of concern that need to be addressed to bring about positive changes for nursing and the health-care system by 2010. Many of these will affect advanced practice nurses (Table 22.2).

Ethical Dilemmas

Ethical dilemmas may stem from conflicts regarding what is "right" and other duties and obligations. These conflicts may be between two ethical principles one holds, between two possible actions that both seem right in some way, between the demand for action and the need for reflection, and between two unsatisfactory alternatives. Socrates said that we "must let reason determine our ethical decisions rather than emotion." This is why nursing students are taught to use ethical dilemma resolution guidelines to assist them in the process. Before we can resolve a dilemma, however, we must explore different theoretical approaches and discuss ethical principles.

Ethical Issues for Health-Care Providers

While there are endless ethical issues for providers in the health-care arena, the most common facing practitioners today include:

1. End-of-life issues: do not resuscitate (DNR) orders, advanced directives, artificial nutrition, and hydration

Table 22.2 Areas of Focus Needed to Effect Positive Changes for Nursing and Health-Care System

Leadership and Planning
Delivery Systems
Legislative/Regulation Policy
Professional/Nursing Culture
Recruitment/Retention
Economic Value
Work Environment
Public Relations/Communication
Education
Diversity

Source: Nursing's Agenda for the Future—A Call to the Nation, April 2002. http://www.nursingworld.org

2. Cost-containment issues
3. Breaches of patient confidentiality
4. Incompetent and/or unethical conduct of other health-care professionals
5. Pain management
6. Informed consent
7. Access to care
8. HIV and AIDS issues
9. Issues surrounding genetics

Theoretical Approaches

There are many different ethical theories, from developmentalists such as Kohlberg, with an ethic of justice, to a feminist perspective of Gilligan, with her ethic of caring. Many studies have been done to examine the ethical reasoning of males and females. At least one study comparing the decision making regarding dilemmas between medical students (mostly male) and nursing students (mostly female) found no difference in reasoning abilities. We all face dilemmas with different value systems. Because each individual may use different ethical theories as a basis for his or her decision making, it is necessary to understand where someone else is coming from. These ethical theories suggest how and what to think about in dealing with conflicts that require choices. They do not solve dilemmas but suggest ways of structuring and clarifying the process.

Two of the most common approaches to analyzing ethical dilemmas are *deontology* and *teleology.*

Deontology

- ▲ Principle of universalizability: act the same in similar situations.
- ▲ Consider the nature of the act itself and the principles or rules involved.
- ▲ "Duties" are based on "rights."
- ▲ The means justify the ends.
- ▲ "Do unto others as you would have others do unto you."

Teleology

- ▲ Utilitarianism: the greatest amount of happiness or the least amount of harm for the greatest number
- ▲ Considers consequences; calculates benefits
- ▲ Theories that focus on goals or ends
- ▲ Ends justify the means
- ▲ Community-oriented theory; also thinks of future generations

These two approaches to analyzing dilemmas may be further explained by comparing the ways both could be applied in several situations. In the first situation, the same outcome may occur even though two different approaches are taken. Consider the patient who has just found out he is HIV-positive and does not want his partner to be told. A clinician using the deontologic approach would act the same in any similar situation and would never tell a lie: The clinician would tell the partner that the patient was HIV-positive. A clinician using the teleologic approach would focus on the ends justifying the means: The clinician would feel that the partner has a right to know because he could become infected. The clinician also would calculate the consequences of telling or not telling and would feel that it is best for everyone involved in this situation to know the truth about the patient's condition. In this situation, both the deontologist and the teleologist came to the same decision.

Another example of a situation in which these two different approaches are used, but with different outcomes, is a situation involving a terminally ill patient who is on life support. The deontologist would consider the nature of the act itself (the sanctity of life), the uniqueness of each individual, and the high SENSE of duty, and would keep the patient on the ventilator. The teleologist, on the other hand, would consider the consequences of maintaining the dying patient on life support, would recognize and consider the suffering of the patient and family, both now and after long-term ventilator treatment, and would support the family in withdrawing the life support. It is imperative that health-care providers look at both sides of ethical dilemmas and at both approaches to analyzing dilemmas so that they may effectively communicate with someone who is approaching the situation from a different viewpoint. If the clinician is unable to "speak the language" of others involved in the dilemma, there is no communicating, and the dilemma may remain unsolved. Communication among all parties is essential.

Communication

At the Spring 2005 meeting of the National Organization of Nurse Practitioner Faculties (NONPF), Dr, Marilyn Chow stressed the effects of miscommunication. Of almost 3,000 sentinel events reviewed by JCAHO from 1995 through 2004, 74 percent resulted in patient deaths. Of these, 65 percent were the result of communication problems. More than 60 percent of medication errors are the result of miscommunication. In ethical dilemmas, effective communication is the key. Lawyers assert that most malpractice and liability cases are the result of poor communication. Nurse practitioners usually excel in the area of communication, which has been cited as one reason that nurse practitioners are sued less often than physicians are.

Ethical Principles

Just as we use principles of physics, biochemistry, psychology, and body mechanics in our everyday functioning as clinicians, we must incorporate principles of ethics in our everyday reasoning (Table 22.3). These bioethical principles (relating to health care) help us respond to specific dilemmas despite the diversity of the moral traditions from which they are derived. Each ethical conflict that a clinician faces may call for the application of different principles. A dilemma may occur that requires one principle to be sacrificed in favor of another, depending on the situation. Just because the

Table 22.3 Ethical Principles

Autonomy	Confidentiality
Beneficence	Fidelity
Nonmaleficence	Justice
Veracity	

clinician may be clinically competent does not necessarily mean that he or she has expertise in dealing with ethical dilemmas. Reasoning at a principled level is a skill that each individual must practice in order to become morally competent.

Autonomy

The first ethical principle is *autonomy,* which deals with personal liberty of action and self-determination, along with respect for all persons as individuals. It is one of the most frequently mentioned moral principles in contemporary biomedical ethics. Autonomy, sometimes defined as "free will," is a principle deeply rooted in the liberal Western tradition emphasizing the importance of individual freedom and choice. Mayeroff (1971) suggests that autonomy is living the meaning of one's life. A truly autonomous person freely chooses actions that are authentic and in concert with basic values. Clinicians as well as patients are autonomous. Professional autonomy includes control over the terms of practice, content of the discipline, and the regulation of standards.

This principle of autonomy in bioethical contexts is the basis for medical decisions and informed consent, along with access to health care. The principle of autonomy involves giving patients options and allowing them to choose their own course of action, thereby nurturing the wholeness of the person. Informed consent addresses the strong advocacy component of the health-care provider role and is a large component of autonomy (Table 22.4). Lack of informed consent accounts for about 10 percent of all lawsuits against providers.

Table 22.4 Elements of Informed Consent

Informed consent has two elements:

I. Informed: information given to the patient about procedure or treatment

II. Consent: the patient's autonomous agreement

To be informed, the patient must receive in terms that he or she can understand all the information that would affect a reasonable person's decision to consent or to refuse the procedure or treatment. The information should include:

1. Description of proposed procedure or treatment
2. Name and qualifications of person performing the procedure
3. Explanation of the potential for death or serious harm or for the discomforting side effects during or after the treatment
4. Alternative treatments available
5. The effects of not having treatment

Situations requiring informed consent include invasive procedures; treatment with significant risks, such as chemotherapy; clinical trials; and research. Situations that do not require informed consent include those involving therapeutic privilege, in which the provider anticipates harm from the knowledge that would be shared during the consent process, in an emergency situation, or with the therapeutic use of placebos. Informed consent at its best helps to ensure that the patient takes an active role in dealing with the medical uncertainties and potential problems associated with any procedure to be performed.

A potential ethical behavior that restricts autonomy is paternalism. Health-care providers assume that they know what's best for the patient and many times order what they deem to be appropriate, thus acting in a paternalistic manner toward patients that restricts their autonomy. The overall term is *parentalism,* that is, acting as a parent would toward a child and assuming that one knows what is best. An example of parentalism is the clinician who orders a medication for a patient without obtaining his or her consent and says, "Take this, it's essential." Although that may be true, to respect the patient as a person, we should involve him or her in the care and get the patient's approval for treatment. By giving the patient a vested interest in the outcome of care, he or she may be more likely to adhere to the prescribed regimen.

Parentalism involves both paternalism and maternalism. *Paternalism* is the way a father would act toward a child, a more stern approach. A clinician who says, "Cigarettes will kill you. If you're not going to stop smoking, I can't care for you anymore," is using a paternalistic approach. *Maternalism* is the way a mother would react to a child. The end result is the same as paternalism, but it usually involves gentle coercion. A clinician addressing the same patient in a maternalistic manner might say, in effect, "Please don't smoke; it hurts my feelings when you don't follow my recommendations. I don't want to go to your funeral." The best way a clinician can respect a patient's autonomy is to give him or her all the facts, and let the patient choose.

Parentalistic behavior, regardless of benevolent motives or the magnitude of the benefit to be secured or the harm to be avoided, overrides the right of each adult to be treated as a person. To respect another as a person and maintain his or her autonomy is to take full account of the patient's values. To disregard these values and act paternalistic toward a patient shows contempt for the individual as a person. It regards the person as a mere object rather than one's equal as a person, even if the provider is trying to do something to benefit the patient or protect the patient from harm.

It is within this principle of autonomy that the patient's competence and capacity are considered when dealing with patients who exhibit mental status changes.

Competence is a legal status; all adults older than age 18 years are assumed to be competent unless a judge specifically declares otherwise. *Capacity* is judged clinically and has to do with whether or not the patient is capable of understanding the options presented. Substituted judgment is a different approach to maintaining someone's autonomy, because the patient's own value system is used in making a decision: One seeks to decide what the patient would have decided, if the patient had been able to do so.

There are some instances in which the principle of autonomy may be overridden by the state. These situations include an emergency procedure that is necessary to protect a life, such as a blood transfusion for a child of a Jehovah's Witness, or an intervention when the potential for suicide exists. A provider can legally treat a patient without getting his or her consent if the patient needs immediate treatment to save his life; to prevent loss of an organ, limb, or function; if the patient is unconscious; or in the case of a minor, if the family cannot be reached. In such situations, the law assumes that if a patient could decide, he would choose to receive treatment. This exception is limited. It does not apply if the provider knows the patient had previously said he would refuse such treatment if and when offered, or if the provider can wait for consent to be obtained. In only two instances is it legal to have a consent form signed by someone other than the patient: (1) in the instance of a minor, and (2) when the patient has been declared legally incompetent.

Another exception to the need for informed consent is when a patient waives the requirement to be informed. A patient may not want to know the details. Nonetheless, the provider still has two responsibilities. The provider must make sure the patient understands that risks and alternatives do exist, and then the provider must clearly document the patient's waiver of his right to receive information. Some facilities assume no responsibility for obtaining informed consent and supply no forms for doing so. Their premise is that even with detailed consent forms, it is impossible to provide all the relevant information and that completing the forms actually lessens the communication between the provider and the patient. The actual process of informed consent is what should be aimed for, rather than the completion of forms.

Beneficence

The second ethical principle is *beneficence,* which is mentioned in the Nightingale pledge. It is the provision of benefits and a balancing of harms and benefits and requires positive action. One must purposefully choose the right action, not merely by omission, and do what is in the best interest of the patient. Positive beneficence requires personal risk-taking. For example, clinicians who care for persons with AIDS are acting beneficently toward those patients by caring for them. Beneficence encompasses the principle of utility or proportionality when one weighs the probability of benefits and harms in order to produce the maximal net benefit (utility).

Nonmaleficence

The third ethical principle is *nonmaleficence,* the idea that a health-care provider should, above all, "do no harm," which is mentioned in the Hippocratic oath. This principle, the foundation on which health care rests, forms the basis for most medical and nursing codes of ethics. It usually involves omissions and does not require taking positive action; the emphasis is on not taking the wrong action and doing something to harm the patient. Several moral rules, such as the prohibition of killing, are derived from nonmaleficence. It must be stressed, however, that it is almost always impossible to ensure someone's benefit without risking some harm. Consider the patient with cancer who is receiving chemotherapy. Chemotherapy may be considered a positive benefit, but the side effects are definitely deleterious. Paternalism is also deeply imbedded within this principle, because it is extremely difficult to respect a patient's autonomy while wanting to resolve the conflicts between beneficence and nonmaleficence. Most clinicians "want" the patient to choose the "right" decision. Consider the situation in which we know a patient would benefit from chemotherapy, yet the patient refuses because of a bad experience that a relative had with similar therapy. The patient's autonomy overrides our beneficent wish in this situation.

Veracity

The fourth principle is *veracity,* or truth telling. There are many half-truths or omissions that health-care providers do or do not tell patients because they feel that the patient cannot "handle" the news. Using the principle of autonomy, it is the right of the patient to know and to decide if he or she wants any further information or not. As practitioners, we cannot make that decision for our patients.

Confidentiality

The fifth principle is *confidentiality,* which involves respecting privileged information. This is becoming more and more of a problem, because computers can provide access to all kinds of personal information. Consider the situation of the patient who requests a breast cancer gene test to see if she is a candidate for prophylactic care, and the insurance company cancels her policy because she might develop breast cancer in the future. Confidentiality, as well as veracity, are extremely important components of the provider-patient relationship.

Health-care providers need to be aware of the Health Insurance Portability and Accountability Act (HIPAA) which has been fully implemented since 2003.

All health-care providers are responsible for maintaining secure electronic files and for ensuring confidentiality when sharing information between health-care providers and third-party organizations.

Fidelity

The sixth ethical principle is *fidelity,* or keeping promises. How many times have we heard providers say that if treatment A does not work, they will try another drug, or treatment B? When the time comes, however, they change their minds because the referral is not indicated, or it would make a negative impact on the audit that the insurance company will do shortly, or the insurance company will not pay for it. We promise that we are going to do all we can to help a patient, and then, when care is futile, the type of care is changed to custodial caring rather than curative caring.

Justice

The principle of justice or fairness involves weighing individual rights. Justice is the most complex and difficult principle to apply to health care. We frequently must use this principle to allocate scarce resources. The decision must be based on principles rather than emotion; to be fair to patients, like cases should be treated alike. For example, if there are only so many patient-controlled analgesia pumps available and several candidates need one, who will get the last one? Who should get the liver transplant, and how many times should it be done before it is considered futile? One of the goals of *Healthy People 2010* is to eliminate health disparities. The principle of justice employed in all situations will help to achieve this goal.

If these ethical principles are applied deliberately and consistently in practice, fewer mistakes will be made, less harm will be done to patients, autonomy will be respected, and decisions will be based on ethics. Changes in the health-care system are a challenge to health-care providers. Do these changes present ethical dilemmas? Definitely so! An ethical dilemma is a situation in which there is no satisfactory answer, and, although many options are available, one seems to conflict with another. Nursing Situation 22.1 presents an ethical dilemma.

Resolution Guidelines

Although there is no blueprint for analyzing dilemmas, the mnemonic ETHICAL is a framework that can be used to provide a systematic method for acting consistently in ethical dilemmas, thus allowing reason rather than emotion to guide one's actions.

E Examine the data.
T Think about which person(s) should be making the decision.
H Humanize the options by constructing a decision tree.
I Incorporate the ethical principles, legal statutes, standards of care, etc.
C Choose an option.
A Act.
L Look back and evaluate.

Consider the following situation and use ETHICAL as a framework to guide your actions:

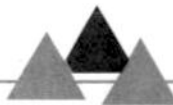

NURSING SITUATION 22.1

Ethical Dilemmas

Situation 1

Shelly has been a clinician for a number of years and has been frustrated with the change in the health-care system and the resultant care that patients receive. When Joseph Harms, one of her patients, was cut back to part-time hours, he and his wife lost their health insurance. Mrs. Harms has been treated by Shelly for several years now for type 2 diabetes mellitus and has been very erratic in glycemic control. They cannot afford to come in as frequently as they did in the past and now must pay the office bill and for medications out of their own pockets. Shelly gives them free samples whenever possible and feels like she is not giving the best quality care when they insist they cannot afford any blood work—only the Accu-Chek in the office. Each office visit costs $60. Shelly has no control over billing.

1. What may happen if a fasting blood sugar, glycohemoglobin, and urinalysis are not routinely ordered?
2. What may happen if Mrs. Harms cannot afford to see the ophthalmologist and podiatrist this year?

Situation 2

Jessica is 16 years old and is on birth control pills. Her relationship with her mother is precarious. Jessica's mom accompanies her to the nurse practitioner's office because of symptoms of bronchitis. Samantha, the NP, wants to order an antibiotic as her birth control pills will not be effective during that time. Samantha is not sure whether or not Jessica's mom knows she is taking BCPs or not. Jessica's mom won't leave the room.

1. Jessica's mom already stated she would not leave Jessica alone in the room. Should Samantha insist?
2. Should Samantha go ahead and tell Jessica about the interactions between antibiotics and BCPs and the need to use precautions when/if engaging in sexual activities with her mom present?
3. How far does the principle of confidentiality extend? Does the fact that Jessica is a minor play any part?

Sylvia is an 86-year-old woman who presents with a massive suspicious breast lump and a new cough. She has not had a well-woman exam in years, nor has she done a monthly breast self-exam. The clinician explains that she wants Sylvia to get a mammogram. Sylvia refuses, stating that she does not want to know the results. What if the test is positive? Sylvia does not want surgery at her age. After a lengthy discussion, the clinician broaches the subject of advance directives. Sylvia states that, as a widow, she has nothing to live for, but she does not want to sign "a death sentence." She states that, "When God wants me, he'll take me." This implies that she does not want extraordinary measures taken to keep her alive.

When applying the resolution guidelines in this situation, the first aspect to consider is **E**, examine the data. The clinician has detected a breast mass and recommended a mammogram as the next step in the diagnostic process. Sylvia has refused. In this step, all the information should be collected and the key participants identified. When interpreting the data, the conflicts presented in the situation should be identified. Are there conflicting rights and obligations? Is there a conflict between two unsatisfactory choices of action? The clinician should enter the world of the person involved and look at the situation from that perspective. The Circle of Caring model is definitely utilized in ethical dilemmas. The clinician should delineate the scope of responsibility and authority of each person. Factors should be identified that could limit each person's ability to participate in the decision making, such as fear, coercion, and pain.

The second step, **T**, refers to thinking about and identifying the person(s) who should be making the decision. We do not know if other family members are involved in Sylvia's care, but because she is coming to the office by herself, the clinician assumes that she is independent, competent, and certainly capable of making her own decisions. Even if there were a daughter nearby, the decision would still be Sylvia's to make, although the clinician might ask Sylvia if he or she could discuss the situation with her daughter and share his or her perspective. In most instances, there are other persons or ethical agents involved in the decision making, such as the patient's family, physician, institution, clergy, social worker, and various therapists and consultants. The rights, duties, and responsibilities of each participant must be clarified and analyzed. In addition, because health-care ethics is a complex subject, there will always be difficult cases that will require consultation with people who have special training in relevant fields.

The third step, **H**, is to humanize the options by constructing a decision tree as shown in Table 22.5. This allows all the options to be considered along with all the consequences of those options. Visualizing the results in this fashion can help narrow down acceptable options.

Table 22.5 Resolution Guidelines: Constructing a Decision Tree

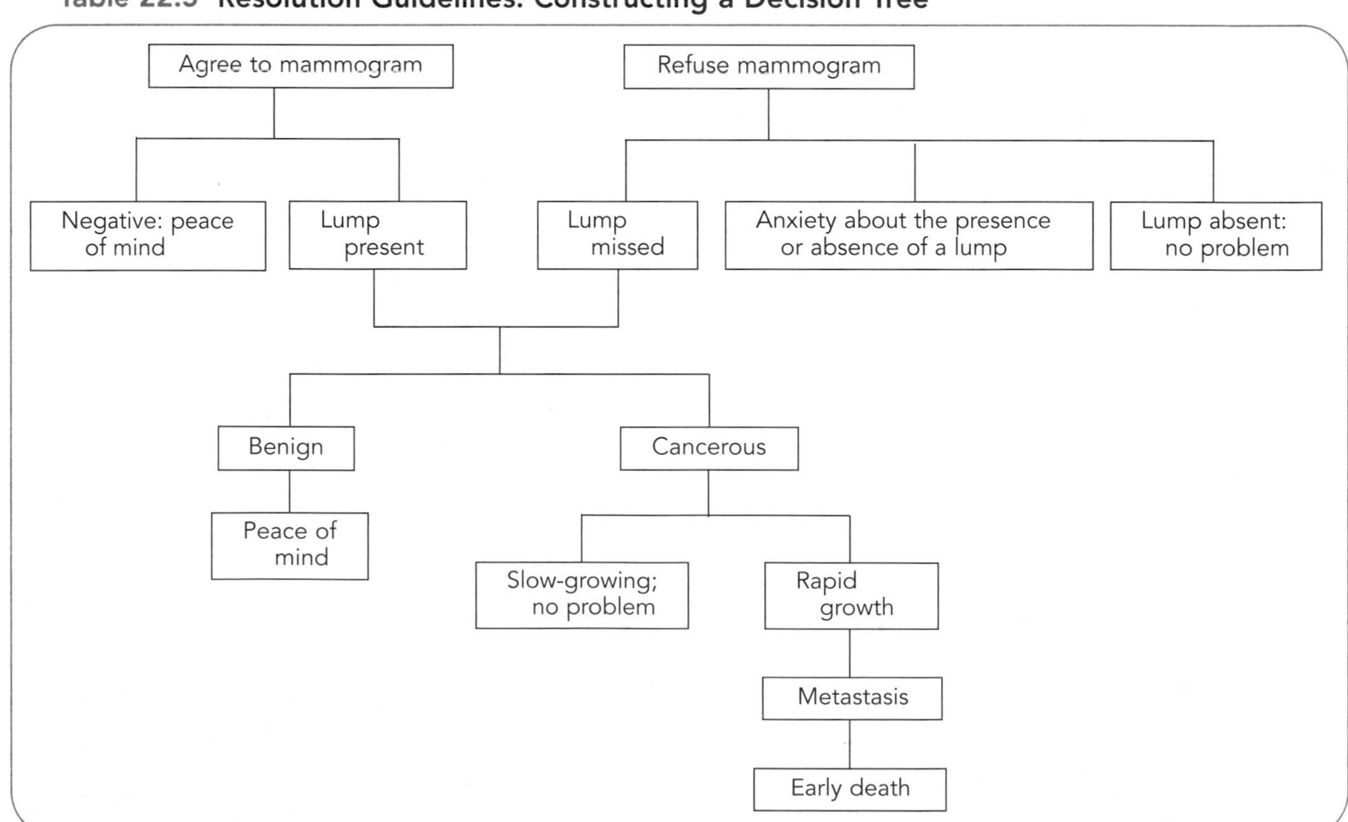

Each state defines the scope of practice within the state Nurse Practice Act. Every state has a Nurse Practice Act.

The fourth step, **I**, stands for incorporating all the extraneous data that must be considered when making ethical and/or legal choices. Certainly the clinician is reflecting on his or her ethical principles. By allowing Sylvia the right to make her own choice, even though it is in disagreement with her own recommendation, the clinician is maintaining Sylvia's autonomy. If the clinician were to be beneficent in his or her actions, he or she might strongly urge (coerce) Sylvia to have the mammogram. But then what? Why pursue the mammogram if Sylvia has already stated that if it shows a problem, she will not consider any further action, for example, a biopsy, or more invasive surgery? Does Sylvia have the right to choose an option that might essentially be signing a "death warrant"? Yes, she does, as long as she is competent and has all the information presented to her. The decision tree allows Sylvia to see all the options and the resulting consequences. Although we cannot predict which branch of the tree this particular scenario will take, Sylvia considers all branches. In this step in the ethical inquiry, all the basic principles should be considered. How does each ethical principle relate to the decision? The Code of Ethics for Nurses should help guide the action. Although codes by definition are brief and general, when used in combination with exploring the relationship of all the ethical principles to the proposed decision, the outcome will be ethical. This step usually points to the most ethical course of action. The ultimate goal of laws is to protect individual rights without jeopardizing the welfare of the general population. Laws must be considered in directing action, seeking consultation, and requesting necessary assistance in selected patient-care situations.

The next step, **C**, involves choosing an action, and the following step **A** refers to actually acting on the decision. Sylvia has known all along what her choice would be—taking no action, which is actually choosing an action. The final step, **L**, stands for looking back or evaluating the situation, so that if the clinician were faced with a similar situation in the future, he/she might consider more choices and thus have more "branches" in the decision tree for consideration, or be aware of more legal precedence, and so forth. Especially when we are acting in the role of the primary moral agent, we need to keep abreast of the consequences of our own actions as well as those of others who are acting on behalf of the patient. Previous experience in similar situations can provide a frame of reference for comparisons and assist the clinician in making quality decisions. Although a decision tree is not meant to "lead" the patient to action, it does allow the patient and provider to consider more choices than may have been thought available. Brainstorming should be used; all choices proposed should be taken under consideration, even if they seem unrealistic at the time. Sometimes the first "irrational" choice ends up being the best choice for the patient and his or her family.

Nursing Research-Based Practice 22.1 describes a study in which caregivers are responsible for health decisions for an elderly relative.

Institutional Ethics Committees

When health-care providers have difficult and unclear choices to make, the best course of action is to consult the local Institutional Ethics Committee (IEC). The Joint Commission on Accreditation of Health Care Organizations (JCAHO) includes a patient's rights chapter. The Standards of JCAHO state that "the organization has in place a mechanism for the consideration of ethical issues arising in the care of patients and to provide education to caregivers and patients on ethical issues in healthcare." Although this mandate may be applied loosely and does not mean that the organization will have an ethics committee in place, there is

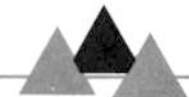

NURSING RESEARCH-BASED PRACTICE 22.1

Hansen, L, Archbold, P, and Stewart, B: Role strain and ease in decision-making to withdraw or withhold life support for elderly relatives. J Nurs Scholars 36(3):233–236, 2004.

An exploratory descriptive study of family caregivers' role in making end-of-life decisions for elderly relatives was conducted. The study focused on role strain and the ease in decision making before, during, and after the actual process. Role strain was defined as the difficulty in making the end-of-life decision. Ease in decision was defined as being comfortable in making the end of life decision and being content with the decision made. Role strain resulted from having the role and not being prepared or ready to make the decision. After the decision was made, role strain was secondary to being unsure that the right decision was made, guilt, regrets, anger, and feeling distant from other family members. Ease in decision making resulted from the caregiver feeling as if they made the correct decision, parted peacefully from the deceased, had become closer to family and was better suited to make future life support decisions. Comments made by participants included "I felt like I was doing the right thing" and "We kind of drifted apart as adults. We have become closer."

The study notes that life support decision making is part of the continuum of the family caregiving role and has both short and long term effects on the individuals making the decision. Nurses should recognize their role in providing support to caregivers at this time. The resultant decrease in role strain and increased ease in decision making will facilitate the end of life decision by the caregiver.

always some help available. A parish nurse may be available for consultation, a bioethicist may be available, or there may be an IEC in place. The purposes of IECs are to serve as a forum for health-care professionals' ethical concerns as well as for conflict resolution between any of the parties involved. IECs provide advice, education, and consultation to the staff and patient and possibly to the community on actual and potential questions of ethics. They also provide recommendations for and help develop institutional policy, procedure, and guidelines in areas of bioethical concern; develop formal policies and procedures for identifying, reporting, and resolving ethical questions and conduct retrospective reviews of decisions on ethical questions; and offer recommendations for improving policies and procedures used to resolve ethical issues.

IECs are usually multidisciplinary in nature because of the varied amount and type of health-care workers involved in any patient situation. They are comprised of physicians, nurses, social workers, clergy, administrative personnel, legal counsel, a patient representative, and someone from the community. The patient representative must actively advocate for the patient and in doing so, subordinate his or her own needs, opinions, and moral positions to those of the patient or family member. The patient representative works to focus and refocus the committee on the welfare and rights of patients. The ANA, as well as the AMA, have developed many position statements (see Table 22.6 for selected ANA position statements available), such as those on referrals to the most appropriate provider, sexual harassment, and so forth, to assist practitioners to consider when drafting policies. Health-care providers should not hesitate to use their professional organizations as resources.

Table 22.6. American Nurses Association Position Statements

Bloodborne and Airborne Diseases
- 19 different statements including one on Guidelines for Disclosure to a Known Third Party About Possible HIV Infection

Ethics and Human Rights
- 16 different statements including: Cloning (2005); and Assisted Suicide (update due 2006)

Social Causes/Health Care
- 16 different statements including: Home Care for Mother, Infant and Family Following Birth; and Nutrition Screening for the Elderly

Drug and Alcohol Abuse
- 5 different statements including Polypharmacy and the Older Adult

Nursing Education

Nursing Practice
- 5 different statements including a National Nursing Database to Support Clinical Nursing Practice

Nursing Research

Consumer Advocacy
- 2 different statements including one on Referrals to the Most Appropriate Provider

Workplace Advocacy
- 9 different statements including one on Sexual Harassment

Unlicensed Assistive Personnel
- 2 different statements

Joint Statements
- 8 different statements including a Paper on Computer-Based Patient Record Standards

Full text position statements available at www.nursingworld.org

Table 22.7 Relationship Between Ethical and Legal Issues*

	Legal	Illegal
Ethical	Assisting an older patient to complete an advance directive	Assisting in the death of a 99-year-old terminally ill patient
Unethical	Ordering emergency contraception in a Catholic-Church-affiliated clinic	Billing for a treatment that was not done

*Although one may not agree with the choices of situations explaining ethical and legal issues, they are presented here for demonstration purposes—to explicate the intricacies of the ethical and legal relationship. Laws represent the minimum ethic governing behavior; compliance with them is mandated. Ethics operate at a higher level; they offer guidelines for resolving ethical dilemmas.

Relationship Between Ethics and Law

Although clinicians strive to be ethical in all their actions, they must also think of legalities. Actions that are ethical are not always legal, whereas actions that are illegal are sometimes ethical (Table 22.7). Advance practice nurses should always strive to practice within the ANA Scope of Practice, their State Practice Act, and the Code of Ethics for Nurses, in addition to being cognizant of individual state laws on prescribing authority, signing death certificates, authorizing disabled parking permits, etc. The circumscribed actions and duties that are allowable in the profession are termed the *scope of nursing practice,* which are defined and guided by each state in the Nurse Practice Act and by common law. Common law principles govern many interactions affecting nursing and are based on a traditional justice perspective. The state Nurse Practice Act, however, is the single most important piece of legislation for nursing because it is the Practice Act that affects all facets of nursing practice. The Nurse Practice Act cannot grant exceptions, waive the Act's provisions, or expand practice outside the Act's specific provisions.

Legal Issues

Scope of Practice

The scope of practice defines the duties and responsibilities of the advanced practice nurse and delineates the permissible boundaries of the professional practice. It is defined by statute, rule, or a combination of the two. A major legislative task for the future is for advanced practice nurses to define a separate scope of practice within each Practice Act that enables them to act autonomously without barriers to practice, such as limitations on prescriptive authority.

Overview of Nurse Practitioners

There are more than 106,000 licensed nurse practitioners in the United States and numbers continue to expand annually. In 2004, the typical NP:

- Was female.
- Was 47 years old.
- Practiced as a family NP.
- Had at least 12 years of experience as an RN prior to her NP license.
- Practiced in a primary care ambulatory setting.
- Was satisfied with his or her practice.
- Had no plans to retire.

Licensure and Certification

Many non-nursing individuals assume that licensing and credentialing are synonymous. It is the responsibility of the clinician to educate other providers and consumers regarding what they can and cannot do. Legal authority for all nursing practice, including advanced practice nursing, rests with the individual Board that administers the legal statutes that define nursing practice in each state. In some states, for advanced practice nurses, it is the Board of Nursing; in others, it is the Board of Medicine; and in a few states, it is the Board of Pharmacy. Legal authority for professional practice was delegated to the states and territories by the U.S. Constitution and is not regulated by federal statutes.

An individual is permitted to practice basic or advanced practice nursing by licensure. *Licensure* protects the public from unsafe practitioners by ensuring a minimal standard for competency. Basic licensure as a registered nurse (RN) is a legal status granted by each state's Board of Nursing. The National Council Licensure Exam that licenses RNs (NCLEX-RN) does not ensure high nursing standards. Passage of the NCLEX is designed to assess minimum competency to practice safely. The curriculum of a nursing program, although providing a foundation of nursing knowledge that will graduate a safe and competent practitioner, is not specifically geared to the NCLEX exam. Nursing programs retain autonomy over their own curricula.

Similarly, the nurse practitioner curriculum is under the control of the graduate faculty and is geared to advancing nursing-based knowledge. On graduation, each prospective advanced practice nurse applies to the appropriate state board for an advanced nursing license. In some states, the graduate must pass a national certification exam to be eligible for this license. Although the licensing statutes may spell out prescriptive privileges for advanced practice nurses, they do not necessarily do that, nor is that the primary purpose of professional licensure. Prescriptive authority for nurse practitioners varies from state to state. Some states mandate the filing of a protocol that documents physician oversight, but other states do not. (Table 22.8 shows a sample protocol.) Laws in most states do not mandate physician supervision of nurse practitioners. Protocols are similar to standing orders; they can be used as evidence to establish breach of the standard of care if they are not adhered to. The ability to prescribe controlled substances varies from state to state.

Credentialing means that the practitioner has met certain criteria through licensure, education, and certification. Criteria for credentialing vary, depending on the credentialing body. A hospital, for example, may use credentialing to grant hospital privileges. The granting of clinical privileges to practice in an institution is influenced by many factors. The primary factors governing the ability of a nurse practitioner to obtain clinical privileges are the institutional policy, medical staff by-laws, state law, and JCAHO accreditation standards. Other factors include the desire of the collaborating physician, the nurse practitioner's education, certification, and continuing education credits, along with his or her eligibility for third-party reimbursement and prescriptive privileges.

Certification is a voluntary process with no legal authority. The primary purpose of certification is to document excellence and specialization. Certification by a nongovernmental agency or association certifies that an individual has met certain predetermined standards for competency and specialization in a particular area. Although some states mandate that a nurse practitioner pass a national certification exam before granting licensure to practice at an advanced level, this is not the case in all states. National certification may be necessary to obtain third-party reimbursement; however, that is not the primary purpose of certification. Although certification at the national level does provide the public with information about the skills of the practitioner; that is the realm of licensure, not the primary purpose of certification. Other than the specialty organizations, there are two groups that certify advanced practice nurses in adult or family practice: the ANA and the American Academy of Nurse Practitioners (AANP).

Prescriptive Authority

Since the mid-1970s, advanced practice nurses have had some type of prescriptive authority. Prescriptive authority is an integral component of advanced nursing practice and is regulated from state to state. It is important for advanced practice nurses to know the extent of the prescriptive authority they have in the state in which they are practicing and what restrictions, if any, there may be. Restrictions may range from collaborative or supervisory requirements to a need for countersignatures, formulary restrictions, specific protocols, and/or site restrictions. Most states grant statutory independent prescribing authority to advanced practice nurses, although a limited number of those states exclude

Table 22.8 Sample Advanced Practice Nursing Protocol

I. Requiring authority: Nurse Practice Act, Specific State—list Statutes, Chapters, Administrative Code. Administrative policies pertaining to certification of Advanced Registered Nurse Practitioners (ARNP).
II. Advanced Registered Nurse Practitioner Certification: __________(name, home address, phone number) is certified as an ARNP #__________ by the (list State) Board of Nursing.
Supervising Professional: Name, address, license number, and DEA number of physician.
III. General Area of Practice: __________ may manage the health care for those patients for which he or she has been educated. His or her master's degree is in __________.
List practice address, including primary and satellite sites.
IV. Specific Management Areas:
- A. The following measures may be initiated by the ARNP:
  1. Conduct a history and physical on patients.
  2. Take medication history, review medication profiles, and suggest necessary revisions.
  3. Order and interpret diagnostic tests necessary to treat, including, but not limited to lab work, x-ray exams, pulmonary function tests, electrocardiograms.
  4. Diagnose and treat conditions within the scope of practice of a family nurse practitioner.
  5. Instruct patient and families in treatment and medications.
  6. Refer to other providers as appropriate.
- B. The following medications to include but not limited to, may be prescribed, initiated, monitored, altered, or ordered by the nurse practitioner in accordance with education: antibiotics, antihistamines, antihypertensives, anti-inflammatory agents, anti-gout agents, anticonvulsants, antimicrobial agents, antifungals, antiarrhythmics, antiparasitic agents, antianginals, antidepressants, antianxiety agents, antipsychotics, beta-blockers, calcium-channel blockers, cathartics, laxatives, contraceptives, diuretics, expectorants, muscle relaxants, nonsteroidal anti-inflammatory drugs, optical agents, otic agents, over-the-counter agents, steroids, stimulants, vasodilators, vaccines.

Controlled substances may be initiated by the ARNP only within the facility in which he or she practices, after appropriate federal and state guidelines have been followed by the supervising physician. (Will vary according to state.)
- C. Admit, initiate visits, and discharge patients in hospitals that have granted visiting privileges. Conduct histories and physicals, order diagnostic tests, treatments, and prescribe medications.
- D. Any other measures within the scope of preparation and experience of the ARNP.

V. All of the above functions may be performed under the general supervision of the physician.

Signed: ____________________ ARNP Date: __________

Signed: ____________________ MD Date: __________

the authority to prescribe controlled substances. Some states require that advanced practice nurses have additional training to gain prescriptive privileges. These differences severely limit the mobility of nurses who anticipate moving to another state. This is another legislative challenge facing advanced practice nurses today.

Unfortunately, medication errors accompany prescriptive privileges. Because most patients are taking three or more medications in a 24-hour period, drug–drug interactions are a common medication error. Advanced practice nurses and anyone prescribing medications must ask each patient what medications he or she is taking before ordering a new one and must always consider the potential interactions. It is the clinician's responsibility to empower the patient with knowledge regarding any adverse effects of the medications. The clinician must educate the patient about signs and symptoms to watch for and should provide guidelines regarding when to notify the clinician if a problem arises. (See Nursing Research–Based Practice 22.2.)

Reimbursement

Payment standards in the United States are set by Medicare and Medicaid. Advanced practice nurses have made great strides in this area and now receive third-party reimbursement in many settings. Payment by private insurance companies is contract-specific and varies with each state's insurance commission. Reimbursement has long been a controversial issue. Should advanced practice nurses receive equal pay for the same work as physicians? In some areas, these practitioners are reimbursed at 80 percent of the physician rate. Does this mean they only did 80 percent of the work, or did it only 80 percent as well as a physician would have? If one asks the recipient of care, the patient will most likely state that the advanced practice nurse gave at least 100 percent of care compared to the level of care provided by or expected from the physician. This is a moot point, however, in managed care contracts, in which a fixed predetermined rate is given to all providers, whether advanced practice nurse or physician. Reimbursement issues are another legislative challenge facing these nurses. When reimbursement issues and practices are addressed, advanced practice nurses will be able to practice independently and truly autonomously.

Malpractice

There are three components that must all be present to establish malpractice. (1) The provider must have a duty to the patient, (2) the standard of care must be deviated from or

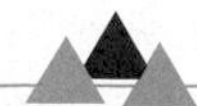

NURSING RESEARCH-BASED PRACTICE 22.2

Greider, L: The pulse of the news: Medical mistakes. AARP Bulletin 41(1): January, 2000.

The Pulse of the News: Medical Mistakes

Dr. Lucian Leape, MD, of the Harvard School of Public Health, contributed to the National Academy of Sciences report on medical errors in hospitals. It is estimated that between 44,000 and 98,000 deaths every year are the result of medical errors. In addition, more than 7000 patients die every year as a result of medication errors. Leape believes that medical mistakes generally result from bad systems, not bad people. He recommends that patients take charge of their own bodies; that might help cut down the number of medical mistakes.

We should empower patients to:

1. Think of providers as partners in care, not persons on pedestals.
2. Do research at the library or on the Internet.
3. Ask questions about every procedure, test, and medication.
4. Make a list of all medications being taken, including dosage. Share this list with every health-care provider.

Providers should be accustomed to patients asking a lot of questions and should actually encourage this. If the provider is "put off" by a lot of questions, the patient should go elsewhere.

breached, and (3) harm or damages must occur as a result of the duty and a breach of the standards of care. A plaintiff must prove duty, breach of the duty, damages or injuries, and causation. *Duty* means that a relationship has been established between the defendant and the plaintiff. *Breach of the duty* is the failure to do what the reasonable and prudent person would have done in the same or similar circumstances. *Damages or injuries* include medical expenses; pain and suffering, both physical and mental; lost wages and lost earning capacity; loss of companionship, society, affection, and sexual relations; hedonic damages; and punitive or exemplary damages. *Causation* means that the plaintiff must prove a direct causal connection between the act of negligence and the alleged injuries.

Take the situation of Sally, a clinician caring for Mr. B., who is suffering from congestive heart failure. Sally increases his diuretic but makes no note of his potassium level and orders no replacement potassium. When Mr. B. returns a week later for routine lab testing, his potassium level is found to be low. Sally orders a potassium supplement to begin immediately and a follow-up potassium-level measurement. Is Sally guilty of malpractice? No. Although Sally did have a duty to Mr. B., and she did deviate from the standard of care (which would have been to order a potassium supplement at the beginning), no harm came to Mr. B. Because all the components were not met, malpractice was not established. If patients were aware of this, many false claims would not be filed. If Mr. B. had died from a fatal arrhythmia due to his low potassium level, however, then Sally could be held liable.

In the outpatient office setting, the most common reason for a malpractice suit is failure to diagnose correctly. Approximately one-third of the malpractice cases brought against general practitioners involve cases of failure to diagnose in a timely manner. These cases usually involve cancer, particularly cancer of the breast. Failure to diagnose promptly accounts for the highest number of liability cases. After cancer of the breast, cancers of the lung, colon, and testes are the highest number of cases of failure to diagnose cited in lawsuits. Failure to refer and failure to manage fractures and trauma are also among the top allegations in malpractice cases. Failure to obtain informed consent accounts for approximately 10 percent of the cases.

APNs must carry liability insurance to protect themselves and their assets. Each APN should have a lawyer who will represent him or her rather than someone who is looking out for the employer's best interests. There are typically two reasons why nurses are told that they should not carry their own insurance. The first is that a policy will encourage a lawsuit. There is no evidence to support this, and lack of coverage does not discourage a lawsuit, should there be a legitimate claim. The other reason is that nurses are told that their employer carries liability insurance that will also protect them. Although it is true that employers may provide insurance coverage for their employees, that coverage is subject to the provisions of the insurance agreement, and the employer is the client, not the nurse.

There are several different types of policies available. One type, called the claims made policies, covers only situations in which the incident occurred and the claim was made while the policy was in effect. Clinicians must review the policy to see if they are to be protected for past incidents, or they should purchase a tail policy that covers future claims. The best type of policy to get is an occurrence policy, which covers liability arising from all acts or omissions during the period the policy was in effect, no matter when the claim is brought. This is the ideal policy, because a claim can be made several years after an incident occurs.

Professional liability policies may be expensive, so the clinician may want to negotiate payment of the policy as part of the employment contract, if he or she is working in a group practice.

Collaboration

Collaboration is a form of interaction among and between providers during their delivery of care. The term implies that there are shared values and that the goal must be directed to what is in the patient's best interest. There is a constructive commitment to work toward that end. There is also mutual trust and understanding and respect of what each has to offer in this interdependent relationship. Both the nurse and physician must respect the boundaries of their disciplines and value what the other has to offer and bring to the relationship.

The Institute of Medicine emphasizes the importance of collaboration in the relationship of high quality and safe patient care and suggests that five core competencies be incorporated in all health professionals' education. These include:

- ▲ Provide patient-centered care.
- ▲ Work in interdisciplinary teams.
- ▲ Use evidence-based practice.
- ▲ Apply quality improvement.
- ▲ Use informatics.

The curricula of advanced practice nursing programs have included these competencies and the Circle of Caring Model in addition emphasizes the essential nature of collaboration between advanced practice nurses and all physicians and health-care professionals they work with.

In addition, advanced practice nurses must collaborate with physicians, because there are many situations they will encounter that are outside their scope of practice. The problem arises when the nurse practitioner–physician relationship is one of supervision rather than collaboration. Different state Boards of Nursing delineate the role in different ways. Some states require that physicians supervise or sponsor advanced practice nurses, which limits the nurse's scope of practice. Other states require that there be a collaborative relationship. A major challenge for the advanced practice nurse is to assert his or her autonomous being and maintain a professional, collegial, and collaborative relationship with physicians.

In 1997, when the Oxford Health Plan allowed members to choose nurse practitioners as their primary-care providers and pay them the same rate as physicians for the same care, advanced practice nurses were finally recognized as independent practitioners who could provide quality care. In a situation such as this, collaboration is key, because advanced practice nurses are the first to recognize that they are not expert in all areas.

Prior to being hired, it may be difficult to foresee whether a practice will be truly collaborative or not. There are tools available to assist a new nurse practitioner in learning the skills of contract negotiation. One such comprehensive tool used to evaluate one's needs and desires in an employment or contractual arrangement is published by the American Academy of Nurse Practitioners, titled "Contract Negotiation for Nurse Practitioners."

Health-Care Reform

The United States is the only industrialized nation in the world without a national health insurance plan in place. Issues of limited access to care and the high number of uninsured Americans mandate that this situation change. The push for the government to get involved is more and more being recognized as a medical necessity. Because insurance companies do not think it is economically viable to construct a national plan, it is up to the American public to promote such action. In the early 1990s, the ANA and more than 40 organizations endorsed a broad initiative to open the door for a national health policy and developed "Nursing's Agenda for Health Care Reform" by which the organization hoped to create a health-care system that assured access, quality, and services at affordable costs. The plan called for a basic "core" of essential health-care services that would be available to everyone. Although this plan eventually was not successful it showed that the American public was ready for drastic action regarding insurance reform. The ANA has been very active in supporting programs that have been politically unpopular such as Medicare when it was first introduced. Oregon is the only state to have made a successful attempt toward a unified health-care program. They accomplished this by rank ordering the community values of persons in the state. Their number-one value is prevention, followed by quality of life. Many meetings were necessary to accomplish this, but the result has proved quite successful. If one state can accomplish this, it surely must be possible for the rest of the nation. Because nurses are the advocates for patients and persons, it is our role to be involved in the development of public policy that will effect change in all aspects of health care.

All health-care providers have an ethical duty to actively engage in legislative efforts that will ensure the best possible conditon to optimize the health of the nation. As advocates, providers need to know their state legislators and governors. Information on how to contact each governor is located at the American Academy of Nurse Practitioner's Web site at www.aanp.org and the link to Congressional Legislative Committees.

Bibiography

American Academy of Nurse Practitioners Committee on Practice: Contract Negotiation for Nurse Practitioners. American Academy of Nurse Practitioners, Washington, D.C., 2003.

American Nurses Association: Code of Ethics for Nurses. American Nurses Publishing, Washington, D.C., 2001.

American Hospital Association: Patient's Bill of Rights,1992.

Beauchamp, TL, and Childress, JF: Principles of Biomedical Ethics, ed 5. Oxford University Press, New York, 2004.

Burnard, P, and Chapman, CM: Professional and Ethical Issues in Nursing, ed 3. Elsevier, Philadelphia, 2004.

Chow, MP: From a presentation on Transforming the Future: Opportunities and Challenges in Health Care at the 31st Annual Meeting of the National Organization of Nurse Practitioner Faculties (NONPF), April 14–17, 2005, Chicago, Ill.

Ethics Committees: Bioethics Forum 10(4). The Bioethics Development Group, Kansas City, Mo., 1994.

Friedson, E: Professional Dominance. WW Norton, New York, 1970.

Gilligan, C: In a Different Voice. Harvard University Press, Cambridge, Mass., 1982.

Goolsby, MJ, and Towers, J: From a presentation on NP Characteristics & Practices: 1989–2004 at the 31st Annual Meeting of the National Organization of Nurse Practitioner Faculties (NONPF), April 14-17, 2005, Chicago, Ill.

Kohlberg, L: Philosophy of Moral Development, Harper & Row, San Francisco, 1981.

Long, KA: The Institute of Medicine Report—Health Professions Education: A Bridge to Quality. Policy Politics Practice 4(4): 259–262, 2003.

Mayeroff, M: On Caring. Harper & Row, New York, 1971.

Winslow, R: Nurses to take doctor duties, Oxford says. The Wall Street Journal, Feb 7, 1997, p A3.

Resources

American Academy of Nurse Practitioners
http://www.aanp.org
National Alliance of NPs
325 Pennsylvania Ave. SE
Washington, DC. 20003
(202) 675-6350
American College of Nurse Practitioners
http://www.acnpweb.org
American Nurses Association
http://www.nursingworld.org
National Organization of Nurse Practitioner Faculties
http://www.nonpf.com
Web site for NPs
http://www.webnp.net
National League for Nursing
http://www.nln.org
NP Central
http://www.npcentral.net
End of Life Nursing Education Consortium Project (ELNEC)
http://www.aacn.nche.edu/elnec

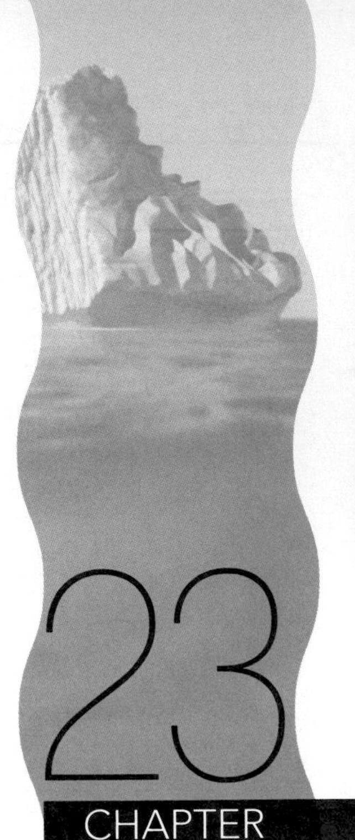

The Business of Advanced Practice

Marcie Rutherford, PhD(C), MBA, RN
Patricia Welch Dittman, PhD(C), RN, CDE
Lynne M. Dunphy, PhD, MSN, APRN, BC
Carolyn Zaumeyer, MSN, ARNP, BC

The business of a clinical practice has become more and more daunting for health-care providers and their office managers. The complexity of billing, management, medicine, and the law present formidable challenges. With the health-care industry constantly changing, providers attempt to reduce the costs and provide services more efficiently. Medicare reform, government regulations, and the growth of managed care have created a highly competitive market.

Advanced practice nurses (APNs) are working in both rural and urban areas and in various settings, including community health centers, public health departments, hospitals and hospital clinics, school and college student health clinics, business and industry employee health settings, physician offices, independent APN offices, health maintenance organizations (HMOs), nursing homes, hospices, home health agencies, the Armed Forces and Veteran's Administration facilities, and schools of nursing. No matter what the setting, the APN needs to be aware of how the practice is financed and managed. This awareness will assist APNs to increase their value as an important part of "the team" and provide the knowledge required to "grow" the business or organization. This awareness will also assist the APN pursuing independent practice. Now, more than ever, a health-care provider's financial success depends on the ability to anticipate change and respond appropriately.

Planning for Success

Having success in business does not just happen; it is a result of research, planning, and a great deal of hard work. At one time, just being a good health-care provider would practically guarantee bountiful financial rewards; however, it is not enough any more. There are many excuses for not planning: "It's difficult." "It's too expensive." "I don't have the time." "I don't need to plan because my practice is doing just fine." Good planning usually produces good results. There are many benefits of good planning. Planning forces you to examine issues such as "Where are we now?" "Where do we want to go?" and "Can we get there from here?" These questions become critical whenever the environment of a marketplace is undergoing change. Asking "How do we get there?" begins the process of evaluating opportunities and making choices regarding future directions. The benefits of planning become readily apparent when comparing what actually did happen with what was anticipated. By monitoring your performance, you can adjust your plans and increase the probability of achieving your goals and objectives. The APN today must be business savvy. Business courses were not part of the curriculum at traditional medical schools and nursing schools until recently. But now many business courses are being integrated into educational curricula for health-care professionals.

Introduction to the Business of Primary-Care Practice

The practitioner faces a health-care system in crisis. The cost of health care is still increasing despite more than two decades of aggressive changes in reimbursements aimed at curbing this trend. What has been the impact of the cost control efforts? The CMS Office of Actuary in 2005 reported Medicare costs increased from $113.9 billion dollars in 1990 to $308.9 billion dollars in 2004 and Medicaid costs increased from $76.9 in 1990 billion dollars to $276.8 billion dollars in 2004. Economists continue to call for changes.

Managed care carriers have proclaimed their intentions as aimed at improving the quality of health care, preventing illness, screening for disease, and maintaining health by properly managing the health-care system. In reality, time and actions have proven that managed care carriers are focused on the reduction of health-care spending while the costs of their premiums are rising. Medicare, quite different in concept, was designed to assist those older than 65 and the disabled. It was designed to reimburse health-care costs when episodes of symptomatic illness occurred. Only in the last few years, and under pressure from the public, have a handful of screening and health promotional services been included as a paid Medicare benefit.

It is predicted that in less than 10 years time Medicare trust funds will no longer cover the payouts needed by the "baby boomer" generation. A study conducted by the *New England Journal of Medicine* in the 1990s indicated that 24.1 percent of insurance premiums go to the complex billing and administrative services versus medical services. Providers become frustrated with the complicated billing and paper maze that is required for payment. Managed care carriers base their billing edits and rules on Medicare policies and tweak the rules to reduce payouts. Claim rejection by both Medicare and private insurance cause frustration for the provider and increased payment responsibilities for the patient. All members—hospitals, physicians, nurses, vendors, and administrators—have been affected and have altered their businesses and practices to adapt to the changes. Most members see a terribly mismanaged health-care system that shows no sign of healing.

So how are economic changes in the health-care system impacting APNs? Practitioners are changing the rules that determine how health care is delivered. In 1992 Barbara Safriet summarized a study involving 501 physicians and 298 APNs which demonstrated APN-directed health care enhanced the ability of the system to deliver quality and cost-effective care. Safriet (1998) identified that nurse practitioners face educational, political, and economic challenges and must seize the opportunities to become leaders in the reform of health care and demonstrate the need for a full range of providers to ensure a better health-care system. Practitioners are trained in advanced assessment skills that prepare them to determine differential diagnosis and identify possible treatments to meet the need of the patient. They often, however, lack a clear understanding of their business and are ill prepared to handle this aspect. Statistics of the state of the health-care system brings the message home:

- ▲ In 2004, more than 45 million people in the United States, including 9 million children, were without health insurance coverage (Kaiser Commissions on Medicaid and the Uninsured, 2005).
- ▲ In 2003, 14 million Americans could not afford to buy all of their prescription medications (Tu, 2005).
- ▲ In 2005, 52 percent of Americans put off accessing care for serious conditions (Gallop Poll, 2005).
- ▲ The United States is the only industrialized country not offering universal health care.

A foundation of knowledge is needed by all practitioners to allow them to participate in both the clinical and business aspects of their profession. This chapter provides the following information: an overview of key business concepts needed to become financially savvy, a review of health-care billing and payment rules, a look at current technology as an important tool needed to manage a business, an exploration of the personal decisions practitioners make that affect job satisfaction, a discussion of ethical business concerns, and an overview of business strategies required for success.

Financial Savvy

Financial "savvy" means to have an understanding and to be knowledgeable in the monetary affairs of the business. The business of health care has been described as complex, tricky, confusing, frustrating, and resource intensive. Money has become an important focus as the health-care industry is increasingly challenged to provide health care in a cost-sensitive environment. Quality health care and maintaining financial health at times appear in competition. As money has become an important focus the premiums and out-of-pocket expenses began shifting the risk back to the consumer. The number of underinsured and uninsured has risen to the point that the system is now in crisis. Politically, health care is a project that few politicians want to touch. Costs are still increasing despite more than two decades of aggressive changes in reimbursements aimed at curbing the trend.

Nursing often views economic issues in opposition of caring for the patient. In today's health-care environment of cost limitations and rationing of resources providers should realize that to sustain the ability to provide care to their patients they must manage the funding. The funding will allow them to grow the business of caring for their patients and allow them to care for more patients tomorrow. Keeping a health-care business in the black is not an easy task. Being ill-prepared in business management creates a no-win situation for both the provider and the patient.

Understanding the rules of business empowers providers. With business knowledge, providers will be able to impact and improve their business. One significant change the health-care profession faced in the last few decades was the impact of managed care in care delivery. Medicare, Medicaid, Workers' Compensation, and Champus programs also impact health-care delivery and make up the balance of the agencies that formulate the rules that govern how health-care providers are paid. Medicare billing rules lead the way and managed care follows in their footsteps. To understand the business aspects of health care, the provider must have exposure to and understand the basis of both the Medicare and managed care programs. To become financially savvy, a practitioner should understand the impact of ensuring consistent cash flow, know the importance of managing their accounts receivables, actively work to control expenses and overhead, utilize the budget as a valuable management tool, and periodically analyze operational reports and financial statements.

The Importance of Maintaining Cash Flow

Maintaining optimum cash flow is a basic fundamental concept in all businesses. Without adequate capital a business will not grow or survive. Health care in the 1970s and 1980s was created on a foundation of increasing payments for increased services. Slowly but continuously since the mid-1980s to early 1990s initiatives were put in place by the government, public, employers, and insurance carriers to reduce the money paid out per episode of medical care. Payment is predetermined and services must be clinically indicated and justified by the pateint's presenting symptoms. Cash flow is the amount of money received and available for disbursement. In today's health-care industry providers are aware that payment is not guaranteed based solely by delivering services.

Today's health-care payments have been reduced to the point that the profit margin is very slim. As the margin between expenses and receivables narrows, the importance of continuous cash flow becomes more critical. Health care is in a downward trend and further cost cutting is predicted. The physician payment fee is predicted to be reduced more than 4 percent in each of the next several fiscal years. In 2006, CMS established 19 (as of now) quality indicators that physicians will be able to track and document outcomes to CMS. In 2007, physicians who have tracked these outcomes will have the opportunity to increase their Medicare fee rate. Physicians who fail to report outcomes will receive the full payment reduction each year.

Commercial carrier contracts are based on the Medicare fee and the carriers "allowed amount" is therefore reduced relative to the Medicare fee. In addition, the patient out-of-pocket expenses are becoming a larger portion of the insurance payment. Many patients do not understand their insurance policy and payment responsibility, and refuse or are unable to pay their portion. To maintain a fluid cash flow attention must be paid to the accuracy of the biling process which starts when patient demographics are collected and continues until the bill is collected. If payments are not maintained as a continuous stream, expenses of the practice (accounts payables) continue to build, and the business will be strained. The slower the collection of the cash the less money is available for enhancement of services. Issues that affect steady and continuous cash flow include:

- "Unclean" claims—Claims with missing patient, medical coding, and data elements
- Inability to utilize electronic file submissions—reduces the cash cycle by 20 days
- Slow processing of carrier payments
- Delay in addressing bill denials and carriers requests for additional documentation
- Failure to identify when payments are inaccurate (low)
- Changes in software, data fields, and interfaces by providers and/or carriers

Providers who ensure claims are complete, accurate, and comply with the carrier's guidelines will benefit by timely payment (within 30 days) for the services they provided.

Outstanding Accounts Receivables

Accounts receivables is the money that has been billed to patients for services rendered but has yet to be collected. Accounts receivables are monitored by financial managers to ensure that the outstanding billings are collected in a timely manner. The longer money goes uncollected the less likely that the money will be able to be collected. When money goes uncollected beyond 120 days it is very difficult to obtain payment and it should be anticipated that a percentage of this money will go uncollected. Accounts greater than 30 days old should be "worked," identifying why payment has not been received and making efforts to seek payment. Knowledgeable medical billers and billing software that allows for claim tracking are essential for success.

Controlling Costs and Managing Overhead

How do business managers get the most out of their money? Managers emphasize the control of costs and leaders look to maximize the effectiveness of the services provided. To control overhead costs managers must identify the costs related to services. Reducing costs must be evaluated as to the impact on outcomes. Alternative strategies to increase efficiency and reduce costs should be continuously evaluated. Analyzing costs often presents interesting challenges and dilemmas. In most business decisions if the outcome choices are considered equal, the least cost service would be chosen. Health-care outcomes are often difficult to measure and until recently little emphasis was placed on measuring outcomes. Health care generates voluminous amounts of data but it is rare and often difficult to link the data to meaningful information aimed at measuring how treatments benefited the patient. Economic analysis, to be valid, must evaluate the costs and benefits of services.

Cost analysis involves understanding the resources needed to provide a service. Direct cost—labor time, supplies used, and equipment needed—are easy to identify and should always be evaluated before adding a new service. Indirect costs—administrative costs, cleaning costs, electricity costs, etc.—may be harder to review and allocate directly to individual services. In addition, costs can be fixed or variable depending on whether they fluctuate with activity. The mortgage payment of the practice is fixed and the supply expenses of the company are variable—or fluctuate based on service activity. It is important, however, for a provider to review the cost impact of services before adding new services. Payments must cover direct costs to avoid a loss. To realize a profit; payment dollars must also offset a portion of the indirect expenses.

The impact of cost analysis has an important impact on the practitioner's practice. Some practices encourage and stress the need for practitioners to treat patients in a shorter and shorter time frame. The normal visit is commonly seen as a 15-minute block of the office day. This time frame is an average—some visits take 30 minutes while others last only 5 minutes. When a nurse practitioner sees a Medicare patient reimbursement is set at 85 percent of the physician fee schedule. Physician overhead costs commonly can run as high as 50 percent of net revenue. Table 23.1 demonstrates the Medicare fee for South Florida, Local 3, offset by the overhead. The APN's salary is paid out of the profit so it becomes clear why 15-minute visits work best.

APN must realize the importance of maximizing the use of their time and obtaining a complete assessment of the patient's health status so that the medical recommendation can be made. Intermingling established patient's visits could offset extended time spent with new patient visits. Follow-up care can be treated in a shorter window of time but a good mix of new and established patients is important to ensure a profit. In the examples given in Table 23.1, assuming the nurse practitioner takes 4 weeks' vacation, 1 hour for lunch, all visits being Medicare patients at level 3 Evaluation and Management (E&M) lasting 30 minutes, the breakeven point would be realized after approximately 300 days into the year. If half of their patients are not able to pay for services, it will dramatically impact when the practice breaks even. Reality will impact this analysis, however, as factors such as the number of new patients, the number of commercial patients (contracted rate being approximately 70 percent in General Practice Specialty of Medicare fee), the length of the visit, the number private pay patients, the services the physician provides, and so forth. The economic reality of providing patient care is obviously important and grows in importance as the margin shrinks.

Financial Statements

Accounting is a system that keeps track of the financial state of a business. Financial statements keep track of every business transaction that occurs monthly in the practice. The performance of a business can be reviewed in four financial statements:

- ▲ Balance sheet—quantifies the net worth of the business at a set time (month, quarterly or yearly).
- ▲ Operating or Income Statement—Compares revenue to expenses in a period of time.
- ▲ Cash Flow Statement—Details the movement of cash in and out of the business.
- ▲ Net Income Statement—Demonstrates whether assets grew as a result of the year's business activities.

By reviewing these documents, the health of the company can be assessed. For example, if the revenue of the company increases dramatically but the costs also increase significantly the company may not realize any additional net gain. These statements also provide an overview of the company assets as well as their corresponding liability or debt.

Budgeting Skills

All businesses need direction and boundaries within which decisions can be made. It is important not only to state what needs to be done, but also to indicate the resources needed to provide the services. Developing and following a yearly budget communicates to the entire organization anticipated spending and revenue projections by itemizing the resources allocated to their product.

Budgeting has several very important purposes and is a key tool in managing a business. Budgets help planning, improve communication, facilitate coordination, improve motivation, help control expenses, and contribute to assessing performance. Budget preparation should involve all parties. By gathering all of the facts a manager can gain a realistic guideline for resource consumption, maintain targeted allocation for these resources, and help ensure that all employees of the business remain motivated toward staying within budgeted boundaries. A successful practitioner

Table 23.1 Break-even Analysis

CPT	Visit/h	FEE	85%	Overhead	Profit (Loss)
99211	2	$ 43.82	$ 37.25	$ 21.91	$ 15.34
99211	1	$ 21.91	$ 18.62	$ 10.96	$ 7.67
99212	2	$ 79.04	$ 67.18	$ 39.52	$ 27.66
99212	1	$ 39.52	$ 33.59	$ 19.76	$ 13.83
99213	2	$107.12	$ 91.05	$ 53.56	$ 37.49
99213	1	$ 53.56	$ 45.53	$ 26.78	$ 18.75

Note: NP Salary based on $65,000/year.
Benefits based @ 25% = Resulting Salary + Benefits = $81,250 ($39.06/hour)
*NP Salary paid from profit.

demonstrates the skill of goal setting and planning and for efficient allocation of resources.

Analytical Skills

Yogi Berra stated, "I don't want to make the wrong mistake." Unfortunately medical errors are not rare, and occur at a rate greater than acceptable to the public and medical community. According to the Institute of Medicine (2000) study *To Err Is Human*, which identified a high number of medical errors occurring in the medical environment, leadership must be challenged to decrease the number of errors. The task of reviewing existing medical practices using a systems approach is daunting; however, the benefits are worthwhile. Unfortunately the initial investment needed for major changes may be hard to sell. Turbulent times and financial pressures may entice providers to resort to an economic survival mode. Much may be lost if the proper financial analysis is not performed. Taking shortcuts in the area of monitoring and analysis could result in an increase in medical errors, increased health-care costs, and a reduction in revenue.

A practitioner must be prepared to meet the challenges of these tumultuous times. Kerfoot (2003), who authors an ongoing article, "On Leadership," in *Nursing Economics* stated, "Clinicians are highly valued for their ability to recognize familiar patterns and to use their gut in times of complexity to come to conclusions and options for interventions." Not only must a practitioner think through a diagnostic clinical problem, but also provide input on the economic impact of the care delivered in this clinical episode. Practitioners are stakeholders in this rapidly changing health-care structure.

Insurance Carriers Set the Rules

Rising health-care costs were the main reason that private health insurance came to be. By the early 1900s many citizens could no longer afford to pay for their health-care services. Between 1910 and 1915 Workers' Compensation laws were designed and implemented to first cover any lost wages for employees injured on the job, and later to compensate for medical expenses and death benefits. The Depression set the stage, as the thought of lost wages due to illness as well as the debt from medical care became an overwhelming concern for all citizens. In the late 1920s, Baylor University, Texas conceived of the first model for private health insurance. This concept became the Blue Cross plan. The plan was rapidly implemented nationwide and employers offered plans as an employee benefit. The retired, aged, and disabled population were not to gain health benefits until 1965 under Medicare. Although most citizens today believe in universal health coverage, the most recent attempt at a national program, in 1992 by the Clinton administration, failed miserably. Americans struggle with knowing, on the one hand, that all citizens should be able to acquire needed health care, but on the other realizing that higher taxes to pay for the high costs of such a system would impact their income. Practitioners struggle to understand the various types of health-care plans and find it difficult to remain abreast of the variety of coverage restrictions unique to each. In addition they must also confront the growing number of uninsured and underinsured patients. To be successful in health-care practitioners look for the knowledge needed to sustain practice and to improve delivery results.

Cash Private Pay

According to the *American Medical News* in 2004 more than 45 million Americans have no health insurance. These patients delay seeking health care and often enter the system in acute need of care and resources. It is important to determine how your practice will accommodate these patients and determine a fair payment program that will foster autonomy, responsibility, and facilitate health-care delivery.

Private pay patients should be identified and counseled as to their payment options regarding needed health-care services. It is easier and fairer to determine a standard discount for patients demonstrating a true need. Unless the practice mission is to serve underserved populations, it becomes important for practice success to decide the level of nonpaying patients the business can afford to service. Patients able to make some contribution toward their health services must be held to their responsibility for payment. Precollection prior to services rendered is the safer means to ensure gaining payment and prepayment for services may be worth a higher discount. Patients may be offered a payment plan (over time) option but they should understand their fee responsibilities. Patient pay billing increases practice expense and private pay fees are the hardest fees to collect.

The underinsured patient account may end up in the private pay category of the Accounts Receivables. These accounts are often several months old (aged) by the time the insurance carrier pays their portion and leaves a balance that becomes the "patient responsibility." These fees are often copayment and/or deductible and a contracted provider has a legal responsibility to collect these fees. Again the best time to collect payment is at the time of service. A call to the telephone number on the patient's insurance card will validate eligibility for the plan (card is not expired) and will confirm the co-insurance and deductible rates that the patient must pay.

Medicare

Participating providers in the Medicare program are assigned a provider number and unique physician identifying number (UPIN) by completing a Medicare 855 Form (2005) and indicates they agree to perform services for payment equal to 100 percent of the Medicare fee. The Centers for Medicare and Medicaid (CMS) policy payment of 100 percent of the physician fee schedule stipulates that 80 percent of the allowed rate will be paid by CMS and 20 percent is the responsibility of the patient. Most patients on the traditional Medicare plan contract a secondary insurance plan, for a monthly premium, that pays for the 20 percent co-insurance fee and the yearly deductible of $110 dollars (2005). Nonphysicain practitioners are paid at a rate of 85 percent of the Medicare fee schedule with 65 percent of the fee paid by Medicare and 20 percent due from the patient or their secondary. All participating Medicare providers must, by law, make a documented good faith effort to collect all copayments and deductibles from the patient. No Medicare beneficiary may be billed additional rates for covered Medicare benefits and must be informed in writing if the services provided are not covered under their Medicare plan.

To ensure full payment Medicare patients should be queried as to their contracted secondary insurance plan. For patients without a secondary plan the 20 percent of the fee should be collected at the time of services. The yearly deductible should be collected in the beginning of the calendar year. These fees, if not precollected, will convert to patient responsibility and will increase the burden of collecting the private pay fee at a later date.

All providers have the option to elect to be a "nonparticipating" provider or to "opt out" of the Medicare program. As a nonparticipating physician the practitioner can set his or her charge rate at 115 percent of the Medicare rate but can collect only 95 percent of the Medicare fee. The Medicare program will pay 75 percent of the Medicare fee schedule and the patient must pay the remaining 20 percent of the allowed (fee) amount. The physician can elect to be in the Medicare program only one time per year and must provide notice to patients and referring physicians if he or she elects to be nonparticipating. Patients also must be informed of the physician's status prior to rendering services. "Opting out" of the Medicare program limits the ability of participating physicians to utilize referral services. No participating Medicare physicians can refer to physicians who have opted out of the Medicare program. An APN working for an "opting out" physician will not be able to bill for Medicare services.

Medicaid

Medicaid is a program that pays for medical assistance for individuals and families with low incomes and resources. This program became law in 1965 and is jointly funded by federal and state governments and assists states in providing medical and long-term care assistance to people who meet the program's eligibility criteria. Medicaid is the largest funding source of health assistance of low- and limited-income patients. Medicaid payments are made directly to the participating providers who in turn must accept the Medicaid payment as payment-in-full. Two exceptions are the different limits for disproportionate share hospitals (DSH) and for hospice care. States may impose nominal coinsurance and deductible rates. Emergency and family planning services must be exempt from the copayment responsibility. The federal program has no set state rate but rather must match the individual states' contribution as mandated by law. Reimbursement rates must remain sufficient to enlist enough providers willing to perform services and ensure that care is available to the general population in the region.

Guidlelines are included in the Medicaid Web site (http://www.cms.hhs.gov/medicaid/). There are limitations and criteria for APN services outlined in each state's guidelines. It is critical that the receptionist in all practice areas verify the eligibility status of the patient before the time of treatment.

A significant trend has been the rapid growth of managed care enrollment in the Medicaid program. In 1995 almost a quarter of all Medicaid recipients were enrolled in managed care plans and the trend continues to grow. Many states are putting increased pressure on Medicaid beneficiaries to elect into a managed care plan. Managed care plans offer states greater flexibility to manage health-care spending and alternative services to control costs. Patients electing coverage through a managed care plan follow the guidelines set by the managed care carrier.

Contracted Insurance Carriers (Commercial)

Patients with insurance coverage, either through their employer or from individual contracting, receive guaranteed coverage of health according to the guidelines and restrictions of their plan. As mentioned earlier, starting in the 1920s employers included insurance as a benefit to their employees. The rising costs of insurance premiums over the last decade (20 percent increases in premiums yearly is not uncommon), however, have forced many employers to eliminate insurance premiums as a covered employment benefit. The majority of employers still offering insurance have increased the out-of-pocket expenses or the employee portion of the monthly premium. Forty-seven percent of all Americans find it difficult to pay for health care (Gallup Poll, 2004) and make up the growing number of underinsured citizens. Out-of-pocket responsibilities create financial burdens that cause many to delay care.

Managed care functions on the premise of limitations of services. Managed care is a market-driven entity and financial incentives become the driving force in health-care changes. Managed care insurance carriers require authorization or referrals before agreeing to cover services. Medical necessity must be documented and provided to the carrier. It is important to realize that if a plan requires authorization for evaluation and/or treatment the provider must have the authorization before rendering services. It is also a reality that many patients either do not understand their plans' criteria or do not wish to make the effort to seek authorization. Practitioners who function as specialists or who refer patients to a specialist must understand the referral process. Most plans refuse to retrospectively grant authorization after services are provided—even when the servcies are clearly medically needed.

Managed care plans are often tailored by employers who limit covered benefits to reduce the cost of the premiums. Health Maintenance Organizations (HMOs) have a higher number of limitations than Preferred Provider Organizations (PPOs). Point of Service (POS) plans and Open Access plans are considered HMOs. These plans may not require referral from a primary care physician to access specialist care but if the patient goes to a provider out of network the patient will either incur higher copays or have no insurance coverage from their plan. Network restrictions include laboratory, radiology, and therapy treatments. Pharmacy formularies are predetermined and treatment physicians are often limited to the brand and generic drugs that can be prescribed. Patients who receive unexpected medical bills often blame the practitioner for failing to warn them of their options or financial results of the recommended plan of care. Patients expect their providers to offer more than good medical care, they expect them to understand the business aspects of health care and to be their advocate.

To be included on managed care contracts the APN should contact the plan, submit credentialing information, and request a formal contract for review. Without contracting for services the APN cannot bill with a provider number. Many states do not contract APNs and require the APN bill services with the physician's provider number. While this allows the APN to obtain 100 percent of the bill rate it does not allow the APN to document the services or patient outcomes related to their services. APNs should actively work with the managed care plans to gain credentialing categories and once they are a provider category they will be able to document how they benefit the plan. Many speculate, as they seek alternative ways to provide health care more economically, that APNs seem a perfect fit for managed care, meeting the health needs of their patients at a lower rate than physician care, when indicated by their scope of practice.

Noncontracted Insurance Carriers (Commercial)

Patients with insurance coverage must seek care from a provider who is directly contracted and included in the provider network on their plan. All plans provide a listing of providers by specialty at the time of enrollment and maintain an up-to-date listing on the Internet. Patients at times do not understand their insurance plan restrictions or simply wish to access care from a physician of their choosing. When patients seek care out of network the provider has the responsibility to inform the patient before rendering services. The exception to this criterion is in the event of an emergency care or in the event no network providers are available to the beneficiary. If the eligibility of the patient is verified at the time of treatment the patient should be forewarned of the additional out-of-pocket expense they will be required to pay. Out-of-network payment should be collected at the time of service to avoid future billing and collection activity. Patients unable to pay the out-of-network expenses may be able to gain authorization for in-network eligibility if the need for services can be demonstrated.

Other Insurance Plans

Auto Liability, Workers' Compensation, and Champus are additional plans that function in most states under the managed care plan environment. It is important that the plan responsibility is identified at the time of service (i.e., auto accident injury, injury sustained while on the job, services provided to a veteran, etc.). All of these plans have provisions, billing criteria, and reporting criteria. Auto liability patients in the Medicare program will be denied payment for medical services billed to the Medicare program. Managed care contracting will direct payment to Workers' Compensation and require documentation for coverage. Traditionally these plans limit use of APNs for care delivery but this should not deter a practitioner from seeking coverage. New prepayment insurance plans and discount cards (resembling and often misinterpreted as insurance cards) must be carefully reviewed with the patient. Discount cards are noncontracted agreements and the practitioner should be aware of and agree to fee reductions prior to rendering services. Patients trust in their provider and this trust is fostered when the practitioner is knowledgeable in the billing rules of his or her business.

Understanding the Codes

The provider is an important aspect to the success of the business operation, directing the use of costly health-care resources. To become a strong business partner, each practitioner can optimize the billing rules and criteria required for payment. The foundation of the billing for all payers are the CPT, HCPC, ICD-9-CM coding and documentation that matches and supports code selection.

CPT Coding and Modifiers

Current Procedural Terminology, Fourth Edition (CPT) is a listing of descriptive terms and identifying codes for reporting medical services and procedures performed by physicians and nonphysician practitioners. This reference should be obtained yearly and remains an important reference that should be kept readily available when procedural issues arise in the care of patients. Two resources to obtain CPT manuals and other coding references are:

http://www.ama-assn.org/ama/pub/category/3113.html.
http://www.ingenix.com

It is important to understand the history and use of this reference when billing for CMS services as well as managed care and other insurance carriers. Code usage may vary according to the guarantor.

In 1977, the Health Care Administration Financial Administration (HCFA) was developed within the Department of Health and Human Services to rein in the spiraling costs of health care related to the Medicare program that had been enacted in 1965 and implemented in 1967. Originally in 1965 Medicare was the responsibility of the Social Security Administration (SSA) and the federal assistance to the Medicaid program was administered by the Social and Rehabilitation Service (SRS). The Department of Health, Education, and Welfare (HEW) oversaw the SSA and SRS. HCFA was created to coordinate Medicare and Medicaid. HCFA was challenged with controlling costs, monitoring that the services billed were delivered, adopt codes to describe medical procedures, and assign reimbursement rates for each service code. HCFA selected Current Procedural Coding (CPT) codes that were developed by the Editorial Board of the American Medical Association. In the early 1990s commercial insurance carriers began using these codes. The Resource-Based Relative-Value Scale (RBRVS; Hsiao, 1987) was authorized by Congress to be used to set reimbursement rates. This RBRVS scale is discussed later in the chapter.

CPT Coding Design

Beginning in the 1980s physicians have been paid according to office or surgical procedure based on calculated resource costs which are designed to reflect the costs needed to provide the services. These costs were calculated based on three components:

- ▲ The physician's work or medical expertise—approximately 54 percent of RVU
- ▲ The practice overhead expense—approximately 41 percent of RVU
- ▲ Professional liability and malpractice expense—derived from a formula

This resultant relative value (RVU) is multiplied by the conversion factor—which is a monetary value determined yearly by HCFA/CMS and is adjusted for geographic region. RVUs are assigned by CMS based on recommendations from the Relative-Value Update Committee (RUC) of the American Medical Association (AMA). Each specialty society in AMA presents work and practice expenses that are sent to CMS and published in the Federal Register for comment.

According to the AMA, the purpose of CPT terminology is to provide a "uniform language that will accurately describe medical, surgical, and diagnostic services, and will thereby provide an effective means for reliable nationwide communications among physicians, patients, and third parties." Nomenclature provides a uniformity to assist in management reporting, medical review, education, outcome measurement, and medical research. CPT is the most uniformally accepted nomenclature utilized by all health-care facilities, providers, and vendors. In 2000 the CPT Code Set was designated by the Department of Health and Human Services as the national coding standard for physician other health-care professional services and procedures under the Health Insurance Portability and Accountability Act (HIPAA). As of 2005 all Medicare and Medicaid billing must be sent electronically and the CPT Code Set is mandated for use. To improve cash flow and minimize claim denials based on untimely submission, most providers are implementing electronic billing to all insurance carriers. Each service or procedure code is represented by a five-digit code. The coding was created to simplify the medical documentation and reporting. CPT code inclusion or exclusion does not indicate an endorsement by AMA of the procedure, nor does it indicate that payment will be considered. Inclusion of a CPT occurs when a procedure is submitted to the AMA and is found to be a practice from many practitioners in different locations. CPTs are published once a year and implementation occurs in January each year. CPT (2005) contains six sections:

Section	CPT Code
▲ Evaluation and Management	99201–99499
▲ Anesthesiology	00100–01999, 99100–99140
▲ Surgery	10021–69990
▲ Radiology (includes Nuclear Medicine and ultrasound)	70010–79999
▲ Pathology and Laboratory	80048–89356
▲ Medicine	90281–99199, 99500–99602

Practitioners should select the code that provides the most specific and accurate match to the services performed. If no code exists that accurately identifies the services, an "unlisted" service code in the designated section of CPT should be used.

CPT Modifiers and Add-On Codes

Specific guidelines are presented at the beginning of each section and should be reviewed before selecting a code. "*Add-on* codes" are indicated that accompany a primary procedure code and are indicated in the CPT manual. Examples of add-on codes are CPTs that indicate additional time spent with the patient such as "prolonged service" codes. These codes should never be used alone and must be used with the appropriate primary or E&M code. A *modifier* provides a means to report that a service or procedure has been altered by the circumstances of its use. It is important that modifiers are understood and the use of each modifier be reviewed. Modifiers assist the practitioner in getting paid. The following is an example of the proper use of modifiers:

> *Separately Identifiable Service on the Same Day as an E&M- Modifier-25* A previously treated patient is referred to a gynecologic specialist's office following abnormal Pap test results. The patient's pathology is reviewed and a vaginal exam is performed. From the examination it is determined that a colposcopy is warranted. The colposcopy is performed on the same day

as the Evaluation and Management (E&M) examination of the patient. The practitioner will bill a 99213 for an established patient visit of Expanded focused complexity and a -25 modifier will be added. The colposcopy is also billed on the same day of service and was ordered as a result of the E&M findings. Without the -25 modifier the E&M visit would not be paid.

The CPT and payment fee values are applicable only to Medicare services and are regulated and paid by the regional carriers. Private commercial carriers can independently determine whether to utilize CPT codes and/or the reimbursement values for the payment year. Physicians contract individually with each private carrier and the payments by most carriers are based on the Medicare CPT's and a reimbursement value that may or may not be the current year's. Commercial carriers alter CPT to benefit their company and/or to match the capabilities of their software programs. Medicare providers must use CPT codes to legally obtain payment, and the level of service documentation must substantiate the billing code.

New CPT Requests

The accuracy and effectiveness of CPT coding depends on the coding being updated so it reflects the changes in medical practice. It is important that practitioners participate and provide information directly or through professional organizations. The CPT manual provides instructions on requesting updates to the CPT nomenclature. The effectiveness and accuracy of CPT relies on its ability to reflect practice. Practitioners should communicate changes in practice and request coding changes that match these changes. Providers can provide valuable information by actively participating in this process. It is important for providers to realize that as profit margins shrink accurate coding becomes essential to maximizing the viability of the business. When requesting a new code the practitioner should provide supportive information from research articles and medical journals, specific cost information related to the uniqueness of the code, and specific recommendation concerning the new or existing codes. Suggestions should be submitted to:

CPT Editorial Research & Development
American Medical Association
515 North State Street
Chicago, Illinois 60610

Code changes can also be submitted online at:
AMA/CPT Web site: http://www.ama-assn.org/ama/pub/article/3866-3846.html.

HCPC Codes

CPT Category II and Category III (also called Level II and Level III) coding are commonly referred to as HCPC coding. HCPCS procedures are established by CMS's Alpha-Numeric Editorial Panel, and represent primarily items and supplies and nonphysician services not covered by CPT Level coding. Drug administration, pharmaceuticals, and durable medical equipment supplies are located in this file. New codes often are assigned a HCPC II code and are tracked for a year before a permanent CPT level code is assigned. Demonstration codes used for data collection are also assigned an alphanumeric code. It is important, however, that the provider realizes that the presence of an HCPC code, as well as a CPT code, does not mean that payments will be made on that code. There is limited payment allowed in Medicare B physician billing for HCPC II and III level coding.

The Health Insurance Portability and Accountability act (HIPPA, 1996) requested an alternative coding system. Category I coding is currently identified as the current procedural codes. HCPC codes include Category II codes that are optional codes designed to track and determine quality of care and good outcomes. The Health-Plan Employer Data and Information Set (HEDIS) is a set of standardized performance measures identified as indicators for consumers so they can evaluate the quality aspects of the care delivery in addition to costs. Indicators are selected based on current health issues such as cancer, diabetes, asthma, heart disease, etc., and monitor such indicators as immunization age, mammography frequency, urinary tract infection occurrence, cervical cancer screening, etc. HEDIS is supported and overseen by the National Committee of Quality Assurance (NCQA) and oversees that patients are obtaining adequate care.

ICD-9-CM Codes

CMS and the National Center for Health Statistics (NCHS), two departments within the federal government, provide guidelines for coding and reporting using the International Classification of Diseases, 9th Revision, Clinical Modification (ICD-9-CM). These guidelines have been approved by the American Hospital Association (AHA), the American Health Information Management Association (AHIMA), CMS and NCHS. These guidelines are required under the Health Insurance Portability and Accountability Act (HIPAA) for all health-care settings. Volume 3 codes are exclusively used by hospitals for procedural reporting, and Volumes 1 and 2 are used by all providers. These codes are intended to identify the diagnosis of the patient and to ensure that consistent, complete documentation in the medical record is maintained. ICD-9-CM coding is used by all insurance carriers as the specific reason for the encounter, to indicate procedures performed (CPT codes), and the conditions treated. The health-care practitioner is legally accountable for indicating the patient's diagnosis. Medicare and many commercial carriers have implemented medical policies that allow computer editing on CPT/ICD-9-CM code matches. For example, a chest x-ray exam will not be paid as a preoperative screening test unless the patient has a diagnosis indicating respiratory symptoms. It cannot be overemphasized that a provider should not select a diagnosis code based on the ability of the code to obtain payment for the care provided.

The National Center for Health Statistics (NCHS) is the federal agency responsible for the use of the International Statistical Classification of Diseases and Related Health Problems and has been challenged with the implementation of a revised ICD-10-CM that will replace ICD-9-CM Volumes 1 and 2. This version was originally presented for a comment period in December of 1997. After the 60-day comment period, the version draft of the ICD-10-CM was removed from the NCHS homepage. A new draft version has been available for public viewing since 2003 and the American Hospital Association (AHA) and the American Health Information Management Association (AHIMA) is conducting a joint testing. On completion and publication in the Federal Register, a 2-year implementation period will be implemented. This change in diagnosis code options will make a significant practice and documentation change for all practitioners.

Fee Schedule

Each year CMS publishes the *Physician and Non-Physician Practitioner Fee Schedule* (Medicare fee). As of January 1, 2005 the fee schedule took effect promptly on all billing submitted after January 1st. This schedule provides a payment rate based on a state local base rate multiplied by the RBRVS. The RBRVS is calculated for each CPT and is based on:

- ▲ Practice overhead costs
- ▲ Malpractice costs
- ▲ Facility and nonfacility RVU

The fee provided for every CPT becomes the payment rate for all Medicare services provided for that year. When procedures occur that have no CPT code reflecting the care, the new code will be paid as a percentage of charge (managed care plans) or at a rate similar to the closest CPT code. To submit the code the provider will use the unlisted and unspecified codes for each body system. Payment for unlisted codes may be delayed, requiring the provider to send medical documentation to detail the services provided. Unfortunately manual billing with the supporting documentation delays payment beyond 45 to 60 days.

Commercial insurance plans negotiate contracts based on a payment at a percentage of charges or at a percentage of the Medicare fee. Carriers may pay some specialists higher than Medicare, however, in Florida, most primary-care physicians and internists are paid at a percentage lower than Medicare. General practitioners' and internists' practices are comprised of a high percentage of employed/managed care covered patients. To maintain their patient base they must compete for their patient base within a large network of similar specialty trained providers. Collusion prohibits physician specialties from secretly and collectively sharing rates for the purpose of monopolizing or maintaining a higher payment rate. Commercial insurance plans market their plan to employers and clients by demonstrating the large network availability. To maintain their patient volume internists are often forced to sign contracts at rates lower than the Medicare fee. In addition, managed care providers adjust the Medicare fee and often develop their own RVU rate. Many also bundle CPT services (i.e., when an E&M service is performed with a needed office procedure code for treatment, only the procedure CPT fee is paid). Denials from commercial insurance companies are less predictable and claim rules are implemented and altered by the plan at any time. Claim processing guidelines should be reviewed on each contracted plan.

Encounter Form and Medical Documentation

The encounter form is the tool that prompts the clinician to provide proper documentation to support billing. The coding not only supports the billing but also provides invaluable data for identifying patient trends and becomes the foundation for planning future community needs. The following quote from CMS in 2005 provides broad overview of Evaluation and Management coding.

> Medical record documentation is required to record pertinent facts, findings, and observations about an individual's health history, including past and present illnesses, examinations, tests, treatments, and outcomes. The medical record chronologically documents the care of the patient and is an important element contributing to high quality care. Consistent and accurate documentation of the E&M codes provides reliable data, demonstrates the appropriateness of the services, and creates a legal document to verify care to an insurance carrier.

See Figs. 23.1 and 23.2 for sample encounter forms with ICD-9-CM and CPT codes.

Providers must accurately document all aspects of patient care. The CPT codes most frequently utilized are the E&M codes. These codes should relate to documentation in the medical record that details the reason for consultation, the history of the present illness, the review of body systems, the physical examination, and the recommendations for testing and treatment. If a procedure is performed at the same time as an E&M visit the procedure should be separately documented. The practitioner performing a consultation must document the finding back to the referring physician, offering a medical opinion based on the patient findings. In addition, payment guidelines in 2006 require the provider to produce (if audited) the referring physician's request for consultation from his or her patient medical record. The nature of the presenting problem will often indicate the level of history taking and support the degree of examination that results in the medical decision-making required to care for the patient. Complicating and comorbid conditions in the medical history of the patient, as well as the review of testing

ENCOUNTER FORM

Last Name Patient: ____ First Name Patient: ____ Middle Init.: ____ Sex: M ___ F ___

Married ____ Single ____ Other ____

Last Name Insured: ____ First Name Insured: ____ Middle Init.: ____ Relation to Insured ____

Address: ____ Social Security: ____

City: ____ State: ____ DOB: ____

Zip Code: ____ Phone: ____ Cell: ____ Email: ____

Insurance ID: ____
Applied HCD; Date ___ Approved_ Denied ___ Expir._
Medicaid: ________ Student: ________
Medicare:_______ Uninsured: ______ Self Pay: _______
HCD II:_______ Others: _______

EVALUATION/MANAGEMENT MEDICAL

New Patient	Established Patient	Description
___ 99201	___ 99211	Nurse Visit
___ 99202	___ 99212	Focused
___ 99203	___ 99213	Expanded
___ 99204	___ 99214	Detailed Hx./exam
	___ 99271	Phone Mgmt-Brief
	___ 99272	Phone Mgmt-Intermed
	___ 99273	Phone Mgmt-Complex
	___ 99361	Team conf-30 min
	___ 99262	Team conf-60 min

School Health

___ School Health Screeing
___ School Health Episodic Visit
___ School Health Physical Exam

PREVENTATIVE MEDICINE

New Patient	Established Patient	Description
___ 99381	___ 99391	under 1 yr Well Child
___ 99382	___ 99392	1-4 yr Well Child
___ 99383	___ 99393	5-11 yr Well Child
___ 99384	___ 99394	12-17 yr Well Child
___ 99385	___ 99395	18-39 yr Well Adult
___ 99386	___ 99396	40-64 yr Well Adult
___ 99387	___ 99397	65+ yr Well Adult

Individual Risk Counsel	Grp. Risk Reduction
___ 99401 (15 min.)	___ 99411 (30 min.)
___ 99402 (30 min.)	___ 99412 (60 min.)
___ 99403 (45 min.)	**Health Risk Tool**
___ 99404 (<10 min.)	___ 99420 Admin & Assess
___ 99405 (60 min.)	___ 99429 Unlisted Prevent.

IMMUNIZATIONS

___ 90701	DTaP (v06.1)
___ 90718	Td-DT (.065) Tetanus
___ 90713	IPV (V0.0)
___ 30645	HIB (V03.81)
___ 30707	MMR (06.4)
___ 30744	Hepatitis B,3 dose
___ 30743	Hepatitis B,2 dose
___ 30716	Varicella (V05.5)
___ 30733	Meningococcal (03.9)
___ 30658	Flu vaccine (V04.810)
___ 90663	Pneumovax, Adult
___ 90657	Pneumovax, Child
___ 86580	PPD Plant (74.10)
___ 90471	Injection 1st.
___ 90471	Injection 2nd x ___.
___ 90782	Injection therapeutic-IM or SC
___ 90783	Injection IM Antibiotics

OFFICE LABS

___ 82270	Fecal Occult Blood
___ 36416	Finger or Heel Stick
___ 94439	Free T4
___ 82962	Glucose
___ 85018	Hemocue
___ 82270	Hemocult (1-3)
___ 86677	*H. pylori*
___ 87210	HOH/Wet mount
___ 86308	Monospot
___ 84152	PSA
___ 87220	Skin KOH prep
___ 87880	Quick Strept
___ 84443	TSH
___ 81000	Urine Dipstick
___ 81025	Urine Pregnancy
___ 36415	Venipuncture

LABS SENT OUT

___ 88074	Acute Hepatitis Panel
___ 86038	ANA
___ 80048	Basic panel
___ 85025	CBC with Diff
___ 88053	Comp. Panel
___ 82552	CRP**/CRF**??
___ 88051	Electrolyte Panel
___ 84233	ESR

LABS SENT OUT-CONT.

___ 83001	FSH
___ 87800	GC/Chlamydia
___ 83020	Hgb Electrophoresis
___ 83036	HgbA1c
___ 83002	LH
___ 80061	Lipid Panel
___ 80076	Liver Function Panel
___ 88155	Pap Smear
___ 84146	Prolactin
___ 84152	PSA
___ 88069	Renal Function Panel
___ 86430	RF**
___ 84702	Serum HCG
___ 85660	Sickle Cell Screen
___ 88142	Thin Prep
___ 87070	Throat Culture
___ 82465	Total cholesterol
___ 84443	TSH
___ 84430	T4
___ 84550	Uric acid
___ 87086	Urine Culture
___ 87081	Wound Culture

Cedar 1-6_Surgical Cedar PROCEDURES

Code	Description	Code	Description
___ -76	Repeat Procedure (modifer)	___ 34640	Nebul. W/o instruct.1st
___ 95115	Allergy Shots	___ 34640	Nebul. Repeat
___ 92551	Audiometry (V72.1)	___ 34150	Peak flow
___ 82607	B12 shot	___ 54050	Penile Lesion Destruct.
___ 16000	Burn tx. Initial (V58.3)	___ 94760	Pulse Ox (Single)
___ 16020	Burn tx. Subsequent (58.3)	___ 94010	Spirometry
___ 51701	Catherization (593.9)	___ 94060	Spirometry Pre/p-Bronchodil.
___ 29130	Finger Splint Applied	___ 92567	Tympanogram
___ 69200	Foreign Body_Ear (931)	___ 57061	Vaginal Lesion Destruct
___ 65205	Foreign Body_Eye	___ 99173	Vision (Snelling)(V72.0)
___ 28190	Foreign Body_Foot	___ 56501	Vulvar lesion Destruct.
___ 30300	Foreign Body_Nose	___ 17003	Wart/Skin Destr.(2-14 lesions)
___ 26010	I&D Finger Abscess Single	___ 17000	Wart/Skin Destr. 1st.
___ 10120	I&D Foreign Body, Simple subQ	___ 12001	Wound Repair-body simple <2.5cm
___ 10060	Impact.Cerumen Removal (380.4)	___ 12011	Wound R epair-head, 2.5 cm
___ 34664	NDI/Nebul. Initial & Demo		

Diagnosis codes: Most important first, top 4 are reported to insurance company (*confidential codes)

a. __________ b. __________ c. __________ d. __________ e. __________ f. __________ g. __________

FIGURE 23.1 Sample encounter form.

Adult Health		DIAGNOSIS			
EXAMS		**DISEASE**		**ABDOMINAL AND PELVIC**	
796.4	Abn. Clinical Findings NEO	716.99	Arthritis Multiple Sites	709.00	Abdominal Pain NOS Site
V65.40	Counseling NEO	716.94	Arthritis Hand	709.01	Abdominal Pain R-Upper Quad.
V65.44	Counseling HIV	716.97	Arthritis Ankle Foot	709.02	Abdominal Pain L-Upper Quad.
V65.45	Counseling Sex Transmit Disease	716.95	Arthritis Pelvic Region	709.03	Abdominal Pain R-Lower Quad.
V72.6	Laboratory Exam	466.00	Bronchitis	709.04	Abdominal Pain L-Lower Quad.
V70.0	Routine Exam	010.25	Cerumen Impacted	709.05	Abdominal Pain Epigastric
		575.11	Cholecystitis, Chronic	709.07	Abdominal Pain Generalized
		564.0	Constipation	709.9	Abdomen/Pelvic Sympt. NEC.
		250.01	Diabetes Type 1	535.5	Gastritis
		250.02	Diabetes Type 2	550.3	Gastroenteritis, Colitis Allergic
		530.01	GERD	530.01	Gord
INFECTION		535.5	Gastritis	553.3	Hiatal Hernia
372.00	Conjunctivitis	611.1	Hypertrophy of Breast, Gynocomart	550.1	Inguinal Hernia, Unilateral
692.01	Dermatitis due to cosmetics	244.9	Hypothyroidism	550.2	Inguinal Hernia, Bilateral
692	Dermatitis due to detergents	242.9	Hyperthyroidism		
692.3	Dermatitis due to drugs	406	Pneumonia		
692.5	Dermatitis due to food contact skin	601.9	Prostatitis unspecified		
692.03	Dermatitis due to metals	795.5	TB Tart Reaction-Par. PPD	**SIGNS**	
692.9	Dermatitis NOS	454.9	Varicose Veins NOS	205.9	Anemia NOS
692.6	Dermatitis due to plants			624.1	Atrophy of the Vulva
692.71	Dermatitis due to sunburn			300.4	Depression Anxiety
601	Cellulitis and abscess finger			707.91	Diarrhea
602.3	Cellulitis and abscess arm, forearm			700.4	Dizzines/Vertigo
602.4	Cellulitis and abscess hand			705.6	Enlargement of Lymph Nodes
602.6	Cellulitis and abscess leg			704	Headache
602.0	Cellulitis and abscess foot			455.6	Hemorrhoids
601.10	Cellulitis and abscess toe			272.4	Hyperlipidemia
692.90	Eczema			401.90	Hypertension Unspec.
492.0	Emphysema, NOS			724.2	Low Back Pain
000.0	Enteritis, NEC	**URINARY TRACT**		270.01	Morbid Obesity
700.6	Fever	595.0	Acute Cystitis	707.01	Nasuea/Vomiting
604	Impetigo	595.2	Chronic Cystitis	523.0	Periodental, Gingival Disease Unspec.
407.1	Influenza with other resp. symptoms	700.37	Continuous Leakage	V22.2	Pregnancy State, Incidental
407.0	Intestinal flu	700.1	Dysuria	706.05	Shortness of Breath
462.0	Pharyngitis	599.7	Hematuria	473.9	Sinusitis
472	Rhinitis	610.0	Prolapse Vaginal Wall	700.5	Sleep Apnea/Sleep Disturb Unspec
477.9	Rhinitis, allergic	700.20	Retention of Urin NOS	465.9	URI
133	Scabies	700.41	Urinary Frequency	79.19	Viral Syndrome
706.2	Sebaceous Cyst	700.31	Urge Incontinence	564	Constipation
473.9	Sinusitis	700.39	Urinary Incontinence		
692.76	Sunburn Second Degree	599.0	Urinary Tract Infection NOS		
704.1	Sore throat				
463	Tonsilitis				
465.90	URI				
070.10	Viral Warts NOS				
	Other		**Other**		**Other**

FIGURE 23.2 ICD-9-CM diagnosis codes.

required because of these conditions, will increase the level of the patient visit. Documentation is often requested by the carrier to justify the level of care provided and billed. All practitioners should develop formats that support and provide the key elements of information for medical record documentation.

Many software programs are available to assist the provider to achieve optimal documentation. It is important for the provider to evaluate the software to ensure the format meets the needs of the providers, improves documentation, and includes aspects to prevent "canned" documentation from being imbedded inaccurately in a document. Always proofread transcribed and electronic medical documentation to ensure accuracy of the information and resulting coding. It is important to realize the billing criteria required for insurance payment on delivered health services are based on complicated rhetoric and create delays in the billing process, making billing a game in which the rules are continually changing. All practitioners need to learn the game.

Playing the Insurance Payment Game

The practice is impacted by the efforts adopted to control health-care spending. It may seem fundamental but it is important for practitioners to not only bill for the services they provide but also to review their payments obtained for services. The payment environment in today's health-care system functions as a game and the goals often appear to focus on carriers keeping their money or paying as slowly as possible. CMS billing guidelines are predicated with rules that require complicated coding, a specific bill format, computer edits designed to deny or delay payment, and medical necessity criteria required to justify the level of services. The claim form—HCFA 1500—is complicated with specific fields that must be populated with data and as of 2005 this form must be transmitted on an electronic file without field errors. The reality is that with knowledge and luck 50 percent of the claims will be paid within 30 to 45 days and the remainder of the claims will trickle in over the next several months, with a percentage of the claims going unpaid.

Medicare audits and probes randomly sample medical documentation to ensure new practitioners and those that billing falls outside the "normal" trends are reviewed. The practitioner must learn how to code and document E&M and procedural services included in their scope of practice. By learning what the payers are seeking to support treatment and systematically including this information when applicable in their visit documentation, providers will ensure payment for their services. Practitioners must determine what their fair billing rate will be, develop collection policies to support collecting the expected payment, and continually monitoring as to the status of their net revenues. Reviewing documentation rules and practices will be required to gain full payment. By billing correctly the first time practitioners enhance their cash flow and their financial picture.

Setting Your Fees

Setting your fees (charge) is not just a process of guessing "what seems fair." What you bill the patient must be higher than the insurance carriers' allowed amount, as the insurance carrier pays the lesser of the charge or the fee. Ideally all patients should be billed the same amount. The resulting fee schedule provides a fee for a CPT performed in the physician's office (global rate), fee for procedures performed in the hospital (professional component only as the hospital carries the facility expense), or the fee for the facility, other than the physician's or provider's (technical component of the fee schedule). These fees are created and intended to reflect the costs of the services provided as well as include a practice mark-up to ensure a profit.

The Medicare fee schedule is a standardized fee setting tool mandated by the CMS and is the foundation of the contracted payment rate used by commercial carriers (i.e., United Healthcare, Blue Cross, Aetna, Humana, etc.) reimbursement for services provided to their patient. It is important that the practitioner realizes that there is no profit included in these fees. These fees should be the base used in setting a charge rate for all patients. In addition, providers should do their homework and shop around to verify the office charges (Medicare fee plus an increase for profit) and to determine what patients are willing to pay. Because managed care contractors' rates are often negotiated below the Medicare fee, providers must know their cost threshold before agreeing to a contracted rate. The office should validate their direct and indirect costs, as well as their fixed and variable costs, related to the services provided and determine how closely the Medicare fee mimics costs. Cost efficiencies will be needed to ensure that money will be available to maintain optimal services and grow future services.

Collections Policies

Income is not keeping up with rising health-care costs. It was reported by Ginsburg (2004) that between 1999 and 2003, the per capita spending for services covered by private health insurance increased by 39 percent. Given that the average hourly earnings of United States workers increased by only 14 percent during that period, affordabiltiy is an acute and growing concern. With health-care costs increasing faster than incomes, many people are not able to afford insurance coverage. With a growing percentage of patients falling into the private pay category, practitioners must determine how they will fairly pursue payment for services rendered. Good collection policies begin with determining a fair bill rate and communicating this rate to the patients before rendering services. Collecting out-of-pocket payments prior to providing services is the most effective collection policy, however the financial status of the patient and the need for medical care does not always make this possible. Patients must feel satisfied with the level of care provided and able to fulfill their financial responsibilities in a way that maintains their autonomy.

Insurance billing and the patient responsibility post insurance payment, will need follow-up review to track the claim status. If claims are denied or additional medical or claim information is requested from the payer, the provider should be diligent about responding to the payer in order to obtain payment. All practitioners should know who is doing their billing and routinely ask the status on their billed claims. Adequate and knowledgeable medical billers are necessary to ensure payment of more than 50 percent of your expected payment. Insurance carriers benefit when providers do not take the time to pursue appeals on denied billing. With the assistance of educated medical coders the practitioner can successfully demonstrate that the services provided were clinically needed, medically justified, and covered under standard medical policy. The knowledge and billing follow-up effort will be worth the return. Once a practitioner becomes knowledgeable in the game of billing the process

Table 23.2 Common Policies and Procedures

- Do not agree to patient's requests for the provider to accept what the insurance pays or "I'll pay after my insurance."
- Collect copayments and deductibles at the time of the visit.
- Implement frequent billing cycle (e.g., every 15 days).
- Accept credit cards.
- Establish patient plans for patients not able to pay in full.
- Collecting money, posting money, and depositing money should be done by different employees.
- Verify that billers make daily bank deposits and that receipts are matched daily to the posted payments of that day.

will become less frustrating and more predictable. The best provider learns the rules, thereby increasing the percentage of billed claims that are paid in the first billing.

Because many providers cannot collect cash at the time of service, patient billings are required. Policies and procedures must be implemented for handling and collecting payments for services. Common topics to address in practice policies and procedures include the items contained in Table 23.2.

Billing procedures should identify how to process private pay payments, Medicare, Medicaid, commerical contracted payers, and noncontracted commercial insurance payments.

Knowing Your Financial Picture

Change is constant in the health-care business. Because of the rapidly changing extenal environment, it is increasingly important to understand how leaders anticipate and implement change. Practitioners should monitor their net revenues monthly as they relate to their charges and patient activity. Payments should also be periodically reviewed relevant to the payer source. Today's provider is challenged to meet not only the practical workforce needs of the health-care system, but also produce work that will be authorized and generate payment. Practitioners should know how to structure their job to function in the most cost-effective way and find avenues to generate reimbursement, which will allow the practitioner to remain financially viable. To be effective the practitioner should attend to financial details as well as remain knowledgeable of pathophysiology to participate fully in today's health-care industry. Software programs make it possible to collect and document all of the care provided to the patient and this information supports the provider's ability to justify the recommendation for health-care services and technology.

Technology or Bust

The information collected in health care is used to establish reimbursement, plan for access to health care, identify service needs, and monitor the quality of care. The initial motivation for the development and implementation of computerized information systems was financial and administrative. More recently nursing has made strides in medical data collection and analysis, but nursing lags behind medicine in developing data support mechanisms. This lag has been linked to a lack of agreement about how nursing knowledge should be represented and on how nurses make decisions. Nursing should move forward in this area as data must be generated, stored and retrieved electronically to allow for comparisons. The computer allows the practitioner to collect large quantities of data; however, these data can be converted to useful information only if a common data set has been agreed upon and analyzed.

Working within an established system enhances the provider the ability to enter, access and trend patient information across the health-care continuum. Starting January 1, 2006 hospital settings will require medication management across the continuum. The health-care continuum will include the inpatient and outpatient hospital settings, as well as hospital-based clinics, home health, long-term care, and physican-based practices. The rationale for this decision is based on the belief that to manage patients across their disease episode, all practitioners must be diagnosing from the same current information. The patient's memory is not always a reliable source of information in an acute health-care episode.

Advances in information technology and the need for better data and information management converged to create controversy about electronic medical and client health records. In 1991 the Institute of Medicine (IOM) of the National Academy of Science released their study and recommendations regarding the development of the computerized medical record. Today legislation and professional groups are encouraging initiatives on Clinical Patient Records (CPR) which would provide the following benefits:

1. Provide a longitudinal account of care, since more and more care is being given outside the hospital.
2. Meet the need for an information system that allows tracking of care to nursing home, retirement home, or clients' private residences.
3. Move away from an emphasis on episodes of care and toward measurement of care across settings and times.

The ideal electronic medical record should have a system that would make available complete and accurate data, practitioner alerts and reminders, clinical decision support, cost-effective options, interconnectivity linking carrier eligibility and authorization requirements, a clean and accurate electronic bill, and link to evidence-based bodies of knowledge. Why do practitioners need to know this? They are the advocates who will assist patients to gain access to needed services. Practitioners become problem-solvers who help patients navigate a confusing and frustrating system that appears to frequently put up roadblocks in the effort to reduce health-care spending. To be effective problem-solvers practitioners must understand the computer system impacting care delivery and provide input as the system is being built.

A Good Business Fit

To be effective, practitioners select the environment that meets their clinical skills and interest. APNs select a specialty based on past clinical experience and through networking. It is important that they feel comfortable with the physicians with whom they will be practicing. The physician–nurse practitioner relationships should be cordial, based on mutual respect, collaboration, and trust. Collaboration is supported by developing a clear scope of practice where the practitioner's professional expertise and avenue for appropriate supervision is fostered and where protocols are defined by law and regulation. It is important for the practitioner to understand the expectation of the practice as to the number of daily patient visits and resulting net payment. This business arrangement should be mutually beneficial for both parties. It is important that everyone is clear on the business arrangements and clinical expectations. Negotiations should include a frank discussion to arrive at salary, benefits, hospital privileges, and call expectations. In addition, the practitioner should understand the inherent risks with the selected specialty and the insurance coverage contracted to mitigate these risks.

Negotiating Salaries and Benefits

Before negotiating an agreement with a selected physician or office a practitioner can develop a desired scope of practice and draft a practice agreement as required by your state. Each state had defined criteria as to the use of collaborating physician and prescriptive authority granted to the practitioner. This information should be reviewed and understood.

The practitioner should network and research the practice that is being considered. Key areas to examine prior to entering a provider relationship would include reviewing the practice setting (i.e., office, hospital rounds, clinic, nursing home, procedures, on-call time, etc.).

The physician specialty, personality, practice setting, patient population, and style of practice all should be evaluated. Important to the practitioner will be the degree of autonomy associated with the practice. The physician should be interviewed and the practitioner questions may include:

- ▲ Any current or pending malpractice claims against the physician and/or practice
- ▲ Medicare and Medicaid status
- ▲ Number of hospitals with whom the physician(s) have privileges
- ▲ Number and type of managed care contracts and research how these carriers reimburse for NP services
- ▲ Number of support staff available to assist the NP
- ▲ Expectations for net revenue generation

Salary and Benefits

Salary

Carolyn Buppert (2005), a nurse attorney, suggests that nurse practitioners get involved in deciding important economic questions regarding their practice and compensations. There are four methods by which a practitioner can negotiate payment:

- ▲ Straight salary
- ▲ Salary based on percentage of payments.
- ▲ Salary plus a percentage (bonus) based on payments.
- ▲ Hourly rate

There are positives and negatives to each method. The *straight sala*ry is the easiest method of payment. The practitioner is paid a set amount weekly, biweekly, or monthly and can plan for the income stream but if the hours or work increase dramatically—that is, call time, rounds, discharge summaries, dictation, and so forth—there is no additional compensation.

Payment based as a *percentage of payments* is a harder dollar amount to predict and calculate. A practitioner's salary is calculated based on the percentage of payments typically collected the month prior. Many factors can affect net payment and often changes in the practice are not within the practitioner's control, for example, computer system, billing staff, managed care contracts, referral sources, and so forth. This payment method has the largest possibility for error and fluctuation in cash flow.

The *salary plus percentage (bonus) based on payments* would allow the practitioner to profit from the higher volume of patients seen and the work hours needed to provide the care but this method often is created at a predetermined rate that is difficult to achieve. In this case, the practitioner would be paid a set amount weekly, biweekly, or monthly and, when the payments generated by the practitioner reached a certain predetermined milestone, additional bonus payments would be provided.

The last method of payment—*hourly payment*—is often well understood as it is similar to how hospital employees and nurses are paid. In this method the practitioner provides time information as to hours worked and this method allows for fluctuations in patient flow and changes in job responsibilities. This method, however, requires the nurse to essentially punch a time card and will reduce the amount of autonomy the practitioner has in movement and flexible office time.

Benefits

When interviewing for a position the practitioner should make a list of benefits that are a necessity versus those that are desired. The benefits that fall into the must-have category include health, dental, retirement, disability, life insurance, vacation, malpractice insurance, call time, and sick time. Optional benefits may include short-term disability, education allowance, car allowance, investment options, professional meetings, and so forth. Each practitioner should survey other APNs to verify what the standard benefit packages are in the area. Do your homework and make sure your needs and wants are put in writing.

Seeking and Negotiating Hospital Privileges

All hospitals have credentialing approval processes that require the practitioner to submit and validate their educational preparation, licensing, certifications, and clinical competencies. Credentialing usually falls under the allied health validation process established by Joint Commission on Accreditation of Healthcare Organizations (JCAHO). Credentialing falls under Medical Staff Hospital Bylaws set up by the Specialty Departments within the Medical Staff rules and regulations. Credentialing committees usually meet quarterly, so it is important to have your information complete and submitted before the time when the practitioner needs to be able to see patients. Practitioners can obtain a copy of the hospital's rules and regulations and familiarize themselves with these regulations, ensuring they will be able to meet the guidelines of the facility.

Practice Insurance

Insurance policies are critical for every business to meet the states' requirements for incorporation. The practitioner should be aware of the insurances needed to start and maintain a successful business. Some insurance plans are required to obtain the tax identification number (TIN or EIN), and these must be obtained in order to apply for a city, state, and county business license. Table 23.3 provides an overview of manditory and optional insurance plans carried by businesses.

These insurance options offer protection for an employer against unforeseen events that could put the practice at risk. As an owner, practitioner, or administrative employee of the business these policies should be reviewed annually. As the practice grows and changes, these policies must remain current. For example, significant growth in computers and software in the practice should be added to the practice liability policy, as these purchases increase the value of the practice significantly.

Two of these insurance plans require some additional comments. Workers' compensation insurance had become very expensive over the last few years. Coverage and available premiums may become limited and very costly with only one or two employee claims. High-risk businesses often must resort to the Joint Underwriting Association (JUA), considered the state's providers of last resort, and premiums may impact the financial health of a business. All practitioners should be aware of the practice policies as to

Table 23.3 Corporation Insurance Plans

Types of Plans	Coverage
Workers' compensation	Medical expenses resulting from on-the-job injury, illness, and death
Unemployment insurance	State and federal coverage; provides payment for loss of employment.
Liability insurance	Covers structure, furniture, equipment in the event of a disaster.
Business interruption	Covers loss payments/income in the event of a disaster.
Employee fidelity bonds	Verifies employee honesty and deters theft.
Life insurance	Many types and should be investigated. Covers practitioners.
Disability insurance	Risk of disability greater than death and creates financial hardship.
Malpractice insurance	Covers defense of practitioner in the event of lawsuit. Many types

drug screening, background verification, employment screening, and yearly inservicing on workplace safety that will protect from avoidable claims. The other insurance that impacts medical businesses is malpractice insurance.

Malpractice premiums have doubled and tripled for physicians over the last few years. The number of frivolous lawsuits is increasing and practitioners feel at risk of an environment encouraging patients to join a litigation lottery. Many physicians are opting to "go bare," whereby they declare they will meet the minimum payment requirements of the state and demonstrate an ability to meet liability claims up to a payment limit. Practitioners without malpractice coverage create a greater risk for all other providers required to maintain malpractice insurance—that is, hospitals, practitioners, and so forth. If the provider desires to carry insurance protection, he or she should purchase the highest amount of coverage affordable. The ideal coverage is an occurrence policy for a 1 million per claim and 3 million in aggregate coverage. Because failure to have proper coverage can be catastrophic, or at least very expensive, it makes good sense to understand the product being purchased and the exposures that are not covered. Several states require that practitioners carry malpractice insurance or post a bond. When investigating the purchase of a malpractice insurance policy, the practitioner should review and compare several different carriers for limits of coverage, whether the policy covers the business and employees, extent of coverage for legal defense, how long the insurance company has been in existence, and the differences between claims-made policies and occurrence policies. The rates can vary greatly, and the stability of each carrier should be examined. It is important to calculate the price of tail coverage when shopping policies and understand the definition of disability for automatic tail provisions. Tail coverage is an insurance policy that ensures coverage for malpractice claims reported after a claims-made policy lapses. The status of the malpractice crisis for practitioners will impact how practitioners practice in the future.

Doing the Right Thing

To maintain a business profits are needed and this basic premise must be understood. Health-care costs appear to be rising as reimbursements appear to be in a downward spiral. Health-care providers are forced to compete for patients and the higher paying type of patient or the insurer pool that offers the highest fees are in greater demand. Competition is causing health-care providers to make previously unacceptable decisions, providing treatment based on the resulting fees. Lucrative procedures may suddenly be offered in a greater proportion, while patients who consume a large proportion of resources suddenly find themselves underserved, or unable to gain access to care. In this competitive environment values and ethics are tested. Practitioners should review common policies implemented to control and support practice decision-making, which fall under Fraud and Abuse/Compliance Plans, HIPAA, Risk Management, Compliance Plans, and Performance Improvement.

Fraud and Abuse/Compliance Plans

The ANA Board of Directors in 1995 developed a statement that outlines nursing's contract with society for safe and ethical practice. This Code of Ethics for Nursing provides a foundation to build standards of conduct that the practitioner should abide by. In 1996 the ANA developed a Task Force to interpret, review, and revise the code. In 2001 the ANA House of Delegates approved the nine provisions that revised the code and offered the revised *Code of Ethics for Statement.*

As health care has evolved and become more sophisticated, the area of ethics has grown. Economic pressures have created ethical issues. Ethical conflicts arise when nurses balance competing pressures from the professional values systems and the financial pressures within their employer organizations. An example of this is the investigations that the United States Department of Justice has pursued when dealing with Medicare fraud allegations. Medicare fraud is estimated to cost $30 billion annually and has caused the federal government to levy high fines and determine, in the false claim act, the need for whistleblower protection.

Why is this information on business ethics so important to practitioners? The practitioner is asked to document in the medical record diagnoses, treatment, and modalities. The health-care industry has not always been honest or accurate about its billing practices, and in response Medicare requires audits of a certain percentage of charts or medical records to prove that the charges and proper codes were used. Examples of health-care fraud include upcoding reimbursement claims, billing for medically unnecessary therapy, and billing Medicare for physician services provided by the nurse practitioner. As of 1996 to willfully and knowingly utilize deceptive billing is a legal violation. Reckless disregard for the rules is auditable and subject to corrective audits and fines. Fines and damages are up to three times the claim amount, with mandatory penalties of $5000 to $10,000 per claim. One of the themes of the targeted audits includes the review of physician's billing using their provider number when the APN performed the services. Table 23.4 shows typical audit forms ensuring practitioners follow billing guidelines and standard practices for E&M billing.

Compliance plans are recommended for all health-care practices. By identifying a compliance officer and developing a compliance plan for the practice safeguards are put into place that may prevent episodes of fraud and abuse. Anti-kickback efforts, conflict of interest disclosure, and identification of questionable business practices should be fostered as the responsibility of all employees to assure business practices discourage fraud and abuse.

Other issues that affect the provider–patient relationship are depersonalization, shorter care delivery time, denial of coverage, and restriction of health-care choices. Many health plans, authorizing policy changes, have been linked to an increase in malpractice liability claims. The nurse practice act holds the nurse directly accountable for the quality and safety of patients within their care. The practitioner should be aware that developing and maintaining the patient's trust is one of the key defenses against malpractice claims.

HIPAA

Policy concerns that are on the forefront involving patients are Health Insurance Portability and Accountability Act of 1996 (HIPAA) and the 1998 Patient Bill of Rights. The eroding partnership between the patient and the providers of health care will affect whom the patient will trust. Nursing has consistently rated the highest in the Medical Practitioners top list of trusted professionals as reported in the annual Gallup Polls. Nursing has a responsibility to utilize this position and voice their suggestions and perspectives.

HIPAA can mean different policy concerns to different people. The act was separated into two Titles.

- Title I of the *Health Insurance Portability and Accountability Act of 1996* (HIPAA) protects health insurance coverage for workers and their families when they change or lose their jobs.
- Title II addressed administrative simplification and required the Department of Health and Human Services to establish national standards for electronic health-care transactions and national identifiers for providers, health

Table 23.4 **E & M Chart Audit Tool**

CPT	Focus	Elements		
New Visits		History	Exam	Medical Decision
99201	New patient, level 1	HPI – 1 – 3 elements ROS – N/A PFSH – N/A	Single-system – 1–5 elements Multi-system – 1–5 elements	Straightforward
99202	New patient, level 2	HPI 1 – 3 elements ROS – 1 PFSH – N/A	Single-system – 6+ elements Multi-system – 6+ elements	Straightforward
99203	New patient, level 3	HPI – 4+ elements ROS – 2–9 PFSH – 1	Single-system – 12 elements Multi-system – 12 elements, 2 systems or 2 elements, 6 systems	Low complexity
99204	New patient, level 4	HPI – 4+ elements ROS – 10 PFSH – 3	Single-system – All elements Multi-system – 2 elements, 9 systems	Moderate complexity
99205	New patient, level 5	HPI – 4+ elements ROS – 10 PFSH – 3	Single-system – all elements, +1 each system Multi-system – 2 elements, 9 systems	High complexity
Established Visits				
99211	Established patient, level 1	Minimal/RN visit	Minimal exam	
99212	Established patient, level 2	HPI – 1 – 3 elements ROS – N/A PFSH – N/A	Single system – 1–5 elements Multi-system – 1–5 elements	Straightforward
99213	Established patient, level 3	HPI – 1 – 3 elements ROS – 1 PFSH – N/A	Single system – 6 + elements Multi-system – 6 + elements	Low complexity
99214	Established patient, level 4	HPI – 4+ elements ROS – 2–9 PFSH – 1	Single system – 12 elements Multi-system – 12 elements 2 system or 2 from 6 systems	Moderate complexity
99215	Established patient, level 5	HPI – 4+ elements ROS –10 PFSH – 3	Single system – all elements, + 1 from each System Multi-system–2 elements from 9 systems	High complexity

Note: NEW PATIENTS - need all three criteria – history, exam, medical decision
ESTABLISHED PATIENTS - require two out of three criteria - history, exam, medical decision

Additional information on history criteria:

History of present illness (HPI): Location, quality, severity, timing, context, modifying factors, associated signs or symptoms.

Pertinent family and social history (PFSH)

Review of systems (ROS)

plans, and employers. It also addresses the security and privacy of health data. These standards were implemented to improve the efficiency and effectiveness of the nation's health-care system by encouraging the widespread use of electronic data interchange in health care.

HIPAA legislation is important to the daily management of the practitioner practice setting. HIPAA legislation implemented in April 2005 focused on password management, work station security, e-mail and Internet use, and facility/physical security. Password protection is emphasized to ensure the privacy of patients' health-care information. With increased mandatory submission of electronic files for billing the patient data, the provider must take precautions to protect the patient's personal information. This responsibility should be taken seriously. HIPAA court cases involving infringements are currently active in the court system. In the least the practitioner is expected to demonstrate an understanding of the regulation and be an example of HIPAA compliance in personal practice.

Risk Management

Risk management is an extension of performance improvement. This program should be organization-wide with a focus on identifying risks, control occurrences, prevent damage, and control legal liability. The goal of a risk management program is to prevent undesirable events from happening and minimize the impact of financial loss due to malpractice claims. There are eight areas of responsibilities for risk management programs:

1. Risk identification
2. Loss prevention and reduction, including incident reports and investigations
3. Insurance claims management
4. Administration of workers' compensation and handling medical/legal issue
5. Liability assessment of contracts
6. Risk management education
7. Handling product recall and Safe Medical Device Act issues
8. Ensuring compliance with accreditation standards and state and federal rules or laws

Practitioners can be involved with any of the above-mentioned areas of risk management. Depending on the location of their practice, they may oversee many or all of these issues. An example of risk-prone area in health care is the needle stick injury. Most health-care systems have assessed and taken action to minimize the potential for an occurrence to a health-care worker. Disclosure is an additional area of concern when dealing with patients or their families. When a negative outcome happens, the patient and their family have a right to know what occurred. To protect the safety of the patient, reporting and remediation must occur as quickly as possible. With the rising number and costs of malpractice claims risk management becomes a powerful tool to demonstrate prudent care is monitored to ensure appropriate care.

Performance Improvement

Performance improvement initiatives should be part of the day-to-day routine of the medical practice setting. In some medical offices, the practitioner is the only professional nursing caregiver and needs to feel comfortable with setting the patient outcome indicators. The practitioner should take the lead to encourage office personnel in the importance of ongoing improvement. Ultimately the goal of performance improvements should lead to a demonstrated improvement in quality. Data analysis of quality monitoring requires the ability to derive trends from statistical data. Once a negative trend is determined a corrective action plan to address the trend is imperative for demonstrating and monitoring a successful turnaround and improvement. One clear demonstration of performance improvement is the continual reduction length of stay in hospitals. The average length of stay was reduced by almost 50 percent in the last ten years, with all clinical members focused on ensuring the patient's needed therapy and treatment proceeds uninterrupted.

Business Strategies

To compete in the business of health-care, practitioners must plan and develop business strategies. Creating a business plan that fits the practice will provide a guide to maintain, develop, and manage the company. This information should be used to market the efforts of the company to future patients.

Business Plan

Simply put, the business plan helps the business get organized. This document provides an organized picture of how you and your coworkers judge whether your business is succeeding or not. This plan should be developed to guide current and future growth of the business. Your business plan will support the needs for funding and will allow lenders to assess the risk involved in investing. It is important that the practitioner review the practice's financial statements. Table 23.5 provides items to include in the business plan.

This information will be invaluable as the business grows and will assist with marketing services and attracting partnerships with other providers. Good information is invaluable, and ongoing review of your business health will allow your services to be expanded. This expansion will allow your business to offer care to those in need.

Marketing Plan

Despite the growth in the numbers of APNs over the last several decades, the profession remains one of the best-kept secrets in health care. Why is this the case? It may be because practitioners are poor at marketing their services to

Table 23.5 **Business Plan**

Inclusions	Description
Company objectives	Summary of company key ideas
History of the company	Idea that started the company
Company goals	Short- and long-term goals, as well as identify the customer
Management team	Background and responsibilities of the managers
Mission statement	Unique aspects of your service
Capital and operating expenses	Costs of doing business
Marketing strategy	Convincing lenders and contributors of potential for the business
Financial projections	Balance sheet, income statements, cash flow, and units of service
Exit strategy	Benchmarks used to indicate success and failure

the public and media. Practitioners tend to share their successes and inroads with each other and within the profession only—through their journals, conferences, and other APNs. The consumer media and the general public have been largely overlooked. News media seeking information target physicians to get their answers. APNs have not done a good job marketing their contributions to health care.

So what decisions need to be made by a new practitioner regarding marketing? First, practitioners can explore opportunities that will inform their patients and the public on the role of the practitioner. Second, practitioners may reach out to the media. Practitioners can seek out local news and broadcasting media that specialize in health. Third, practitioners should share the news regarding faculty, new office, public health issues, and so forth. This important information regarding their practice should be shared with local media via press releases. Fourth, practitioners can make themselves available to news media for commentary and interviews. Being proactive with the media is critical to opening a positive dialogue and educating the media on their profession. Small inroads into public relations will lead to role clarity and realized health-care benefits. In a qualitative study, Torn and McNichol (1998) found that even though there was a demonstrated role of high-level clinical judgment, autonomy, and decision-making, the misuse of the APN title and the discrepancies in the skill, knowledge, and educational level makes the role vulnerable at a national level. Marketing decisions should be made with the understanding that all efforts should focus on clearly displaying, communicating, and defining the nurse practitioner role.

Patients within a practitioner's own practice should be educated regarding the role of the nurse practitioner in the office. There is an awareness gap that exists in the general public and among nurses about the practitioner's role. The waiting room is an ideal spot to offer educational material to a captive audience. All new patients should receive information regarding the role of practitioners in the office and inform the patient how they may be contacted by the practitioner. In an exploratory descriptive design study, Donohue (2003) measured the congruency of expectations to actual services received during a practitioner's visit in an ambulatory clinic setting based on health information, trust, self-disclosure, time, acceptance, and respect. The actual receipt of services was found to be similar to their patient's expectations. The practitioner must realize the importance of selling his or her services to the customer. The customer must learn how they will benefit from the practitioner relationship and partnership.

Last but not least, practitioners need to market their role to physicians based on their practical experience and the benefits they can provide. Depending on the setting, the practitioner can free up the physician to focus on the acutely ill patient, while assuring that the chronically ill patients are not shortchanged. The number of patients receiving medical care on a daily basis will increase by adding the practitioners to the practice. The practitioner can assist hospitals by performing rounds, history and physicals, reviewing test results and counseling with the family. The practitioner will gain the respect and become valued by the physician, and a mutually beneficial partnership will evolve.

Conclusion

APNs must demonstrate their vision, voice the fiscal impact on resources, demonstrate flexibility, and provide creative means to create a successful business. If practitioners remain limited or one-dimensional in their own focus as a medical profession and ignore their role in the business of health care, their voice will go unheard. Communication becomes the key to success for the practitioners and they can become knowledgeable in the business of health care so they can articulate their needs in relation to the benefit to the business. Key business skills that practitioners should seek include skills needed to become financially savvy, the knowledge of basic business concepts, an understanding of how health care is paid, and strategies aimed at enhancing and growing future business. A nurse must not only be able to think through a diagnostic clinical problem, but also must be able to provide input on the economic impact of the care delivered in this clinical episode. Practitioners provide excellent health care for the patient but they should also feel fluent in business concepts. As stakeholders in the business they play an essential role in overseeing health-care change and assuring the ongoing health of a health-care delivery company.

Practitioners are a welcome addition to the care setting that physicians monopolized for decades. They offer an alternative option to the patient who understands and connects with the role of the practitioner. They are an available addition to the physician practice and enhance the health-care team's ability to become a cohesive group that can focus on providing medical care and ensuring optimum patient outcomes. Utilizing practitioners in health-care delivery will improve the health-care system—but practitioners must be able to articulate how. A motivation that drives the practitioner quest for knowledge is to become the more powerful ally of the uninsured and underinsured. To become leaders in health-care delivery they must speak the language of economists, accountants, administrators, and lawmakers. A study by Green (2005) on patient satisfaction with nurse practitioners' care included 817 patients who indicated the highest satisfaction score for APNs on their questionnaire, commenting "My nurse practitioner treats the whole person." This is a powerful business mission. To treat their entire patient, however, the APN must be imaginative and develop rational strategies based on a knowledge of finance and the allocation of scarce resources. It is clear that nursing needs to have a basic understanding of how the business of health care works. Only then will nurse practitioners be able to become visionary leaders in the fiscal planning essential to create a quality health-care system.

Bibliography

Aguilar, A, Aguilar, D, Anaya, A, and Ortiz, G: Public awareness of the nurse practitioner role. New Mexico Nurse 48(3):5–6, 2003.

American Medical Association CPT: Physicians Current Procedural Terminology. American Medical Association, Chicago, 2005.

American Medical Association International Classification of Diseases, revision 9, Vols. 1 and 2, Chicago, 2005.

American Nurses Association: Code of ethics for nurses with interpretive statements. American Nurses Publishing, Washington, D.C., 2001.

American Medical News, September 13, 2004.

Bates, D, and Gawande, A: Error in medicine: What have we learned? Ann Intern Med 132(9):763–767, 2000.

Buppert, C: Capturing reimbursement for advanced practice nurse services in acute and critical care: Legal and business considerations. AACN Clin Issues Adv Pract Acute Crit Care 16(1):23–35, 2005.

Center for Medicare and Medicaid Services: Health Insurance Portability and Accountability (HIPAA). Retrieved March 26, 2005 from http://www.cms.hhs.gov/hipaa.

Centers for Medicare and Medicaid Services: ARNP/PA/CNS guidelines. (First Coast Service Options, Inc.) Medicare Education and Training, Jacksonville, Fla., 2005.

Centers for Medicare and Medicaid Services: Year 2005 Medicare Part B physician and non-physician practitioner fee schedule. First Coast Service Options, Inc., Jacksonville, Fla., 2005.

Centers for Medicare and Medicaid Services: Medicaid: A brief summary. Retrieved on April 30, 2005 from http://www.cms.hhs.gov/publication/overview-medicare-medicaid.

Chase, SK: Clinical Judgment and Communication in Nurse Practitioner Practice. FA Davis, Philadelphia, 2004.

Contino, DS: Leadership competencies: Knowledge, skills, and aptitudes nurses need to lead organizations effectively. Crit Care Nurse 24:52–64, 2004.

Donohue, RK: Nurse practitioner-client interaction as resource exchange in a women's health clinic: An exploratory study. J Clin Nurs 12(5): 717–725, 2003.

Dunham Noonan, MD, Weiss, K, Stichler, JF, Looker, P, and Jones, ML: The bottom line. AWHONN Lifelines 6(2):123–134, 2005.

Gallup Poll: Costs hurt those who need healthcare most. Retrieved on July 30, 2005 from http://www.gallup.com/poll/content/login.aspx?ci=16114.

Gallup News Service: Honesty and ethics poll. Retrieved April 12, 2005 from http://www.globalethics.org/newsline/members/issue.tmpl?articleid=11219922225391.

Ginsburg, PB: Election 2004: Controlling health care costs. N Engl J Med 351(16):1591–1593, 2004.

Green, A: Patient satisfaction with nurse practitioner care/caring. Retrieved on April 17, 2005 from http://www.asbn.org.

Goodacre, S, and McCabe, C: An introduction to economic evaluation. Emerg Med J 19:198–201, 2002.

Hannah, K, and Shamian, J: Integrating a nursing professional practice model and nursing informatics in a collective bargaining environment. Nurs Clin Am 27(1):31–45, 1992.

Hoffman, ED, Klees, BS, and Curtis, CA: Brief summaries of Medicare and Medicaid. Centers for Medicare and Medicaid Services, Department of Health and Human Services, Baltimore, Md., November, 1, 2005.

Hsiao, WC: The resource-based relative value scale: An option for physician payment. Inquiry 24(4):360–361, 1987.

Huber, D: Leadership and Nursing Care Management, ed 2. WB Saunders, Philadelphia, 2000.

Institute of Medicine: To err is human: Building a safer health system. Retrieved on July 2002 from http://www.iom.edu/iom/iomhome.nsf.

JONA: Panel urges nurses to take active role in information systems decisions. J Nurs Admin 23(2):7–8, 1993.

The Kaiser Commission on Medicaid and the Uninsured: Threadbare: Holes in America's health care safety net. The Henry J. Kaiser Family Foundation, Menlo Park, Calif., November, 2005.

Kerfoot, K: On leadership: Learning or intuition?—less college and more kindergarten: The leaders challenge. Nurs Econ 21(5):253–255, 2004.

Light, DW: Universal health care: The conservative perspective. Massachusetts Nurse 72(3):1–5, 2002.

Mackey, TA, McNiel, NO, and Klingensmith, K: Outsourcing issues for nurse practitioner practices. Nurs Econ 22(1):21–26, 2004.

Marquis, B, and Huston, C: Fiscal Planning, Leadership Roles and Management Functions in Nursing Theory and Application, ed 4. Lippincott, Williams & Wilkins, Philadelphia, 2002.

Safriet, BJ: Health care dollars and regulatory sense: The role of advanced practice nursing. Yale J Regul 9(407):417–489, 1992.

Safriet, BJ: Still spending dollars, still searching for sense: Advanced practice nursing in an era of regulatory and economic turmoil. Adv Pract Nurse Quart 4(3):24–33, 1998.

Schroeter, K, Derse, A, Jukerman, C, and Schiedermayer, D: Ethics and managed care. In Practical Ethics for Nurses and Nursing Students. University Publishing Group, Hagerstown, Md., pp 98–101, 2002.

Torn, A, and McNichol, E: A qualitative study utilizing a focus group to explore the role and concept of the nurse practitioner. J Adv Nurs 27(6):1202–1211, 1998.

Tu, HT: More Americans willing to limit physician-hospital choice for lower medical costs. Centers for Studying Health System Change, Retrieved July 25, 2005, http://hschamge.org/CONTENT/735/?topic=topic09.

Updegrave, W: Can Medicare be cured? Money Fall:73–78, 2003.

Yandle, CE: How to write a business plan. Microsoft Small Business Center. Retrieved May 2, 2005 from http://www.microsoft.com/smallbusiness/issues/business_startups/business_plans_entities/.

Putting Caring into Practice: Caring for Self

Karilee Halo Shames, PhD, RN, HNC

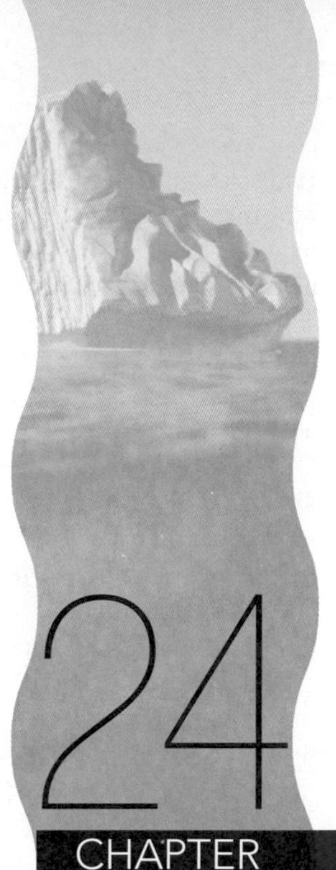

A review of the processes introduced in the Circle of Caring model provides a valuable starting point for the discussion of self-care of the advanced practice nurse (APN), and indeed any health-care provider. Caring for others makes it incumbent on us all to care for "self." The goal is to actualize the model by directing health-supporting maneuvers toward oneself first, enabling the practitioner to experience and integrate the value gained from self-care, and to use this strength as a source of replenishment in helping others. This chapter provides an introductory historical overview, a theoretical context for self-care maneuvers, and suggestions for practical application in advanced practice nursing and primary-care practice in general.

Historic Overview

The caring processes include patience, courage, advocacy, authentic presence, commitment, and knowing. To understand the value of these processes in advanced practice nursing, consider a model of health promotion through the human energy field as introduced by nurse theorist Martha Rogers and further systematized by Delores Krieger. This basic introduction provides a rationale for the necessity of self-care in advanced practice nursing.

Martha Rogers: Theories and Implications for Self-Care in Nursing

Martha Rogers presented a system of applying the principles of quantum physics to human health and well-being. Her theories used the principles of resonance, helicity, and integrality, each of which describes interaction between atoms and molecules, whereby the movement of one has an impact on the movement of others nearby. Just as these principles operate in the laws of physics, Rogers extrapolated to explain how the same interactions occur within and around the human body. This understanding of energy-field interactions opened a new avenue for nurses to demonstrate their unique art and science, providing a rich contextual framework within which we can expand our awareness of health and vitality.

Basic Energy Field Theory

According to energy field theory, human beings are more than simply a body. The body is the densest part of the human energy field. Extending beyond the physical body is a more subtle aspect of the person, a series of interconnected layers of being, progressing outward from the most dense to more subtle layers. People with highly developed perceptive skills can readily detect subtle levels of being. Some see auras of light and color around the human body, such as we see in early paintings of Jesus and Christian mystics showing a halo around the head. Others perceive energy fields through other senses, including a kinesthetic way of knowing. Intuition, long considered to be one of nursing's greatest strengths, might be more easily understood and appreciated as an alignment of the five senses, allowing for a synergy commonly referred to as the "sixth sense."

Presumably the human energy field serves as a template, storing information about the person in its various layers, progressing from the physical to the emotional layer and then to the mental and spiritual layers. These layers are overlapping and interconnected, consistent with Rogers' concepts that human beings are irreducible, unitary, and whole. Healers with highly developed intuitive skills can read the information surrounding the body, thereby assisting people in understanding their life challenges more completely. Most people perceive through sensory awareness, though it is often a less than conscious process. Nurses and healers can learn to develop these intuitive skills through practice.

Delores Krieger: Therapeutic Touch

Touch, used in all cultures for thousands of years, is an ancient art form that has been and continues to be researched to establish its credibility and efficacy. Modern science is beginning to establish a method for measuring the biofield; yet, at this time, it has not fully quantified its effects. Although much information is anecdotal, there continues to be vast interest in research on the value of touch therapies, with a number of well-known names working in this area such as Depek Chopra, Larry Dossey, the Shames, and Delores Krieger.

Delores Krieger, a former student of Rogers, further applied the principles of energy-field interaction, creating a sequential process whereby nurses and caregivers could direct their intentionality toward the patient's well-being, frequently resulting in a sense of relaxation and restoration for both caregiver and recipient. This gentle caring maneuver, known as therapeutic touch, originated in the nursing doctoral program at New York University in the 1970s and has been taught in major universities across the world.

In developing this practice, Krieger quickly realized that if a nurse were to provide adequate restoration for the patient, the nurse must first find a way to replenish his or her own energy field, restoring its integrity and fullness. The rationale for this initial step, which Krieger referred to as "centering," was simply that in finding a calm, peaceful place within, the nurse could use the resulting state of relaxation to focus his or her intentionality on behalf of the patient. The beauty of this particular model is that not only does the patient derive benefit from the application of therapeutic touch, but the nurse benefits as well. The nurse's presence extends to the patient through field interaction.

Centering, the first step in therapeutic touch, provides a way of calming the mind, releasing one's ability to affect another through gentle touch or nontouch. To touch another without using hands has long been an unspoken aspect of nursing, which has been further explored since the scientific application of energetic interventions. This process, currently referred to as "intentionality," or presence, became a part of the centering step.

When the health-care provider, centers and sets his or her intention toward reestablishing balance in the patient, the nurse is preparing to have an impact on the flow of energy through the patient, using his or her own energy field as a tool. The nurse then proceeds with the nursing process, using innate sensing abilities to assess, followed by other gentle interventions in the field. These steps allow the patient to experience greater flow of energy through the body, resulting in increased vitality for life. Other disciplines can find their own perspectives enriched by work in this area.

An Expanded View of Healing

To move into a more comprehensive view of human existence, we can start by expanding our concepts of health and healing. We are at present witnessing an explosion of information supporting a more holistic, or multidimensional, paradigm. We can further explore this paradigm by examining relevant terminology.

In modern medicine, the goal has been geared toward curing. Curing can be measured as a reflection of decreased symptomatology. Medicine is largely concerned with outcomes, whereas nursing is concerned with process. As nurses, we have seen patients "cured" again and again; the symptoms are assuaged, but the recidivism rate is high. A patient who presented with superficial symptoms initially is treated, and the presenting symptoms are alleviated; however, we may see the same patient again and again with varying symptoms. Some of the newer symptoms might even be more serious than the initial presenting symptoms. Have we helped the patient to heal?

Health is a dynamic process, not a state of being. The Greek root word is *halos,* meaning "hale, hearty, whole, holy." As nurses, we may see many instances of patients being cured, yet not achieving health, a sense of being whole. To heal, one must do more than eliminate symptoms; one must address the root cause. Healing is a process that implies "making whole." Why does a patient return again and again with the same or different symptoms? What can we as nurses do to decrease this seemingly never-ending cycle? What might be the role of healing compared with curing? People can be cured, yet they may return many times for healing. People can be healed until death. These concepts take on new meaning when we understand the fine yet powerful distinction between curing and healing.

Another distinction reflects different views of curing and caring. Traditionally, medicine has been concerned with curing whereas nursing has focused on caring. As we approach a healthier system, the lines between caring and curing blend. APNs can serve as a bridge between these models, allowing for both to be integrated and applied. As APNs are enriched in their nursing practice by a biomedical perspective, biomedicine is increasingly recognizing its need to embrace a more holistic perspective. It is here that we can learn from one another for the mutual health of all our patients and all of us.

Expanding Caring

Caring has long been considered the domain of nursing, though many health providers care in their own ways. The Circle of Caring model presented in this textbook helps us to deepen our conceptualization of the ways nursing contributes to the process of healing. This model provides for conceptualization instead of simply skills and techniques, and it expands the traditional medical model. The principles presented by Rogers and further developed by Krieger become actualized. The emphasis is on caring, not only for the patient, but also for self and each other. In any healing environment, the importance of knowing self becomes the basis for all caring interventions. We can now explore how this concept becomes even more apparent when working with energy.

Introduction to Energetic Approaches in Healing

To establish a framework for the concept of energetic healing, Fig. 24.1 demonstrates a correlation between a model familiar to nurses, Maslow's Hierarchy of Needs, and the ancient Sanskrit system of *chakras,* or energy vortices in the human energy field.

Abraham Maslow, a psychologist, developed a model that conveys a hierarchy of needs. Inspired by his life experiences to search for a comprehensive theory of human behavior, Maslow sought a synthesis in art and science, incorporating poetry, philosophy, religion, art, values, and scientific principle.

According to Maslow's 1969 model, individuals must first tend to the basic physical needs (air, water, food, safety, security, physical comfort) before being able to meet intermediate goals (acceptance, approval, recognition) and even loftier goals (self-fulfillment, realization of one's potential). Because Maslow's expertise was in psychology, this model naturally largely represents a map for progression in the mental realm. We might, at this point, expand our conceptualization to entertain the notion that humans are more than physical beings, more than mental beings, having the capacity to move beyond the physical and mental to a realm considered to be spiritual.

On the right of Fig. 24.1, we see the representation of the seven major *chakras,* or energy centers. According to

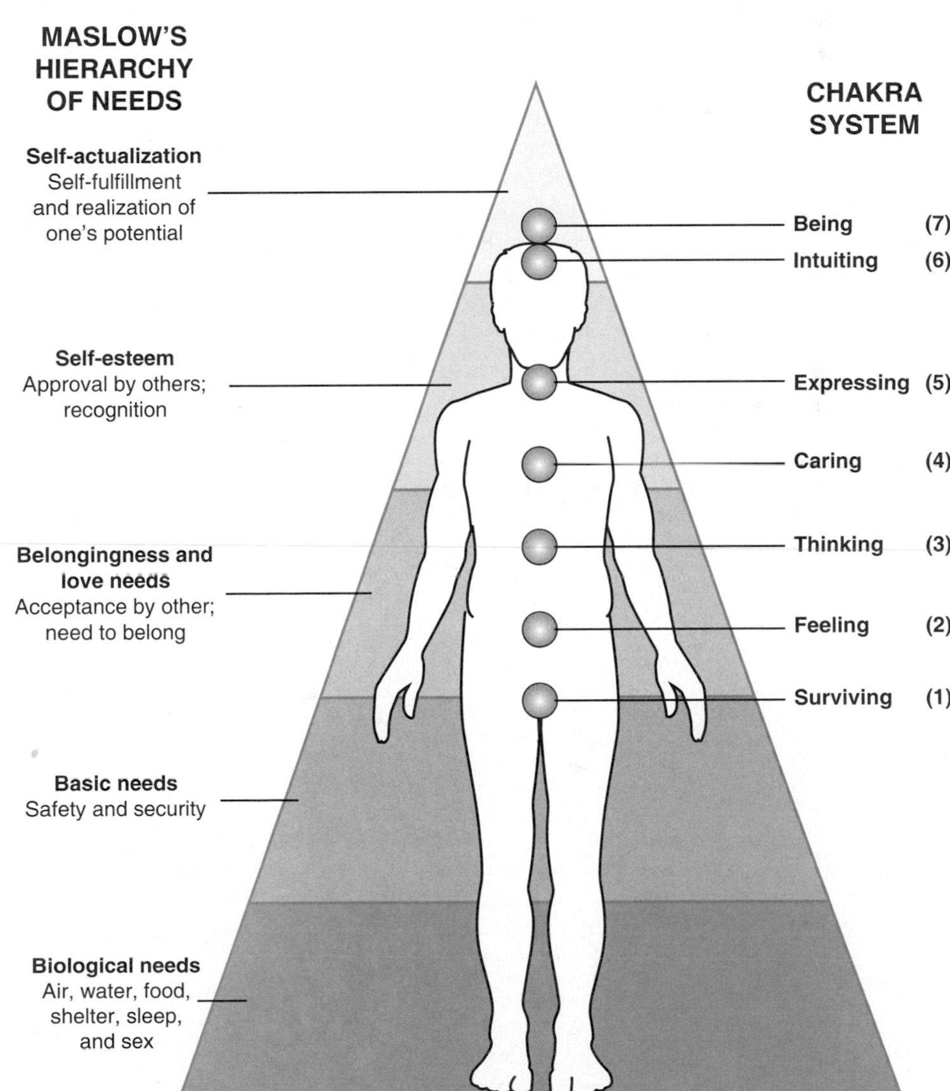

FIGURE 24.1 Actualizing our healing potential. (© Copyright, Karilee Halo Shames, RN, PH, HNC. Nurse Empowerment Workshops and Services, PO Box 2398, Mill Valley, Calif. 94942, with permission.)

Eastern philosophy, human beings have hundreds of energy vortices, most notably where there are articulations (joints). Just as acupuncture works with the unseen energy flow through meridians, so do the *chakras* represent centers of energy flow that cannot, to date, be easily seen or measured. *Chakras* are depicted as vortices, swirling in a clockwise direction like tornadoes from the body in both front and back, serving to pull in energy from the universal energy field surrounding us.

According to this energetic framework, the human being is much more than the body. We consist of physical, mental, emotional, and spiritual realms, all of which interact and interface. There is a continuous flow of energy in, through, and out of us. It could be envisioned by considering the person as having the capacity to plug in electrically to an outlet allowing energy to flow in, filling the body, and allowing him or her to do something that requires this energy. As long as we are plugged into the source of energy, we have an infinite supply.

In the psychological realm, Carl Jung in 1971 described a similar ability to tap into something larger, which he referred to as the collective unconscious. As energetic beings, we operate through our ability to "plug in" to the universal energy field, surrounding us in all directions. As long as our energy centers are open and flowing, we have input, throughput, and output in a continuous flow. When one or more *chakras* become blocked, however, there is a diminished flow, which eventually can result in lack of energy, decreased capacity to produce and be effective, and ultimately, in disease. Our challenge, as nurse-healers, is to actualize our potential, to allow energy to flow freely through us, enabling us to work not only with the physical but also with the emotional, mental, and spiritual aspects of being.

The Major Energy Centers

The *chakras* seem to correlate rather closely with Maslow's Hierarchy of Needs. The lower *chakras* relate to physical needs, which, when nourished, provide a solid foundation for an expansion into the mental and spiritual realms.

Each *chakra* reflects an aspect of being, which is concerned with some condition of our life. The first *chakra* relates to survival and vitality, the second to sexuality, creativity, and emotions. The third speaks of fear and power issues and our ability to make decisions and think clearly. The heart is known as "the great transformer," pulling energy from the lower three centers (primarily physical) into the upper *chakras* (spiritual). The fifth *chakra* relates to communication and self-expression; the sixth (known in Eastern philosophy as the "third eye") has to do with clear-seeing, or clairvoyance; and the seventh, at the center at the top of the skull, the crown, is where we interface with the universal energy field, or God, depending on one's frame of reference.

When all *chakras* are open and fully flowing, energy pours through and nourishes us. As this occurs, we are revitalized and restored. We are fully participating in life, interacting with the world and environment around us, restoring and rejuvenating. The breath helps energy to circulate, as does drinking water and nourishing our bodies with natural (unprocessed) food. We can further support our well-being through exercise and the use of imagery and meditation. All of these serve to enhance our flow of energy, enabling us to be most vital—our fullest expression of who we are.

When a *chakra* is blocked, however, it impedes the flow of energy through our entire system. Just as debris can build up in a creek, so that little by little, more debris accumulates until eventually there may be no water flowing through at certain points, the flow of energy can become blocked. Depending on which *chakra* is diminished, a variety of physical and emotional symptoms may result. Nursing Situation 24.1 provides an example.

Use of Self as a Healing Instrument

The multidimensional paradigm suggests that healing can occur on many levels. We may heal from a traumatic injury on the physical level but experience recurrent emotional residue as a result of the trauma. An excellent example of this frequently occurs postoperatively when the wounds are closed but the patient continues to have fear or to sense other remnants of trauma.

Many of us have heard patients remark, "I haven't felt right since that operation." That operation could have been many years ago. In these instances, there may be lingering emotional trauma that can be accessed and alleviated through gentle healing maneuvers.

Similarly, many nurses carry wounds from their work-related trauma. These wounds are sometimes physical and at times emotional. When we have had negative experiences, we tend to store them in the body or in the energy field, and these can accumulate with time, resulting in a diminished flow of vitality and life force.

The Inner Healer

In most cultures, there is a concept of the inner healer, or inner advisor. This relates to an aspect within each person, perhaps a place where the will to live exists. Our work as caregivers is to inspire each patient's "will to be well," to strengthen and reinforce it so our patients can effectively use their own self-healing skills.

Just as our immune system automatically sends white blood cells to fight infection when we get a cut, so does our inner healer intuitively know the medicine that is needed for each injury and situation we experience, no matter which level. What is needed is simply to keep the "germs" out.

"Germs" can exist on the mental level as well as the physical. Consider the body–mind connection in the role of healing. When we think negative thoughts, we are filled with fear, which weakens our response to that which challenges us. Much has been done to clarify the importance of keeping

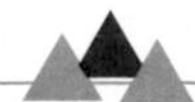

NURSING SITUATION 24.1

Caring for Self

Mary M. is an advanced practice psychiatric nurse working at a county hospital on a locked ward. Recently divorced, Mary is a full-time caregiver for her 9-year-old son. She used to be diligent in her daily exercise program, but now she is finding that she has no time for self-care. In addition, she feels increasingly less patient and compassionate in her caretaking role with disturbed patients. What used to be enjoyable work now seems draining.

Mary has been feeling tired lately and is uncertain if there is a physiologic reason or simply emotional stress as a result of the ongoing struggles and legal challenges from her divorce. She consults with a physician, who tests her for low thyroid activity and other possible causes. He gives her a clean bill of health.

Mary then decides to consult with a colleague, an APN who works holistically. The APN talks with Mary for a while, ascertaining more about the challenges she is facing in her daily life and how she is coping emotionally with the difficult changes. After recommending a return to her daily exercise program, some stress reduction techniques, and a review of her diet, the APN suggests energetic intervention (therapeutic touch).

Mary rests on the table while the APN moves her hands through Mary's energy field. An initial assessment reveals diminished energy flow in the second, fourth, and fifth centers. These centers correlate to emotions, forgiveness issues, and communications.

The healer helps Mary balance her energy through gentle movements of the hands and setting her intentionality toward making energy available to Mary. When she has completed the balancing work in Mary's energy field, she then asks how Mary is feeling about the issues uncovered. Mary recognizes that she has more healing work to do to complete and integrate the experience of her divorce. Based on this interaction, Mary arranges to consult with a nutritionist, resume her regular exercise program, and seek temporary counseling support, in addition to attending several more therapeutic touch sessions.

Within a couple of weeks, Mary is feeling much restored and is coping better with the demands of her life, both personal and professional. She no longer feels irritable with her patients and is enjoying this new phase of her life with her son. She feels much more closure with her divorce, having restored self-esteem and forgiveness for both herself and her ex-husband. Mary is now free to move on and grow. Certainly her patients will receive better care.

a healthy mind in a healthy body. As caregivers, we simply cannot afford to diminish our life force through negativity.

Consider the energetic model of interaction, and we can easily ascertain why it is critical that we maintain positive thinking. If we are fearful and anxious, we are not breathing fully; oxygen exchange can be compromised as a result. Emotionally and mentally, when we are fearful, we also diminish our ability to see all options clearly, which can result in poor decision-making.

All health-care providers in direct patient care cannot afford to have compromised clarity of thought. Many times, the lives of our patients depend on our mental acuity, on our ability to assess quickly and accurately and to act appropriately. For these reasons, it becomes imperative that nurses maintain an open, flowing system of energy.

Energetic Transference

In psychology, the term "transference" relates to an energy exchange, not particularly healthy or desirable, between patient and therapist. In the holographic model of healing, considering the human being as multidimensional, it becomes even more important for the healer to maintain an open, flowing system of energy. If the nurse or healer is not free of constrictions, he or she can affect the patient in undesirable ways. There is an old saying in psychotherapy circles: "Either the patient gets better or the therapist gets worse."

When the health-care provider and patient interact, their fields connect. The provider who is not grounded and centered can be more easily pulled off balance, making inappropriate statements and decisions about the patient's care. Many patients are quite ill and energetically depleted. Without being centered, the nurse can be pulled more easily into the patient's distress, reacting with sympathy instead of the healthier response, empathy.

Sympathy connotes a second *chakra* connection, which is based on emotions. Empathy is more a form of compassion, coming up through the more balanced space of the heart. When we work empathically, we empower our patients. When we come from sympathy, we can be giving them messages that undermine their self-healing endeavors and confidence. Our work is largely to remind our patients of how powerful they are and how well prepared they are to heal themselves. When we support them in activating their own inner healer, we are planting seeds that last a lifetime. We are also undoing messages they may have received that made them believe they are incapable of healing themselves.

The Health-Care Provider as a Laboratory

For many years, Albert Bandura, a psychologist at Stanford University, has studied mechanisms governing empowerment and self-efficacy. Bandura (1997) found that what was most effective in empowering others is what he called "mastery modeling." This term simply relates to the ability to have a positive impact on others through our example.

One of the best aspects of this energetic model is the understanding we gain that as we become models of health and wholeness, we affect others through our being. There is a consistency and authenticity between who we say we are and who they see us as. That is very beneficial because it eliminates the confusion that arises with mixed messages.

Health-care providers therefore must work with the concepts of the Circle of Caring and the circle of energy flow. We can learn to use situations from our everyday practices to advance our self-care skills and our sense of wellness and wholeness.

Challenges Inherent in Advanced Practice Nursing

Nursing as a profession has multiple inherent challenges. To further complicate matters, those in advanced practice nursing must deal with even more confusion about the boundaries and unique aspects of nursing.

The relationship between physicians and APNs requires even more delicacy and sensitivity than that of registered nurses, who do not have diagnostic and prescriptive authority. Managed care has changed the expectations for physicians rather abruptly, leaving many to abandon their chosen work and others to accept significant financial loss.

The changing face of health care dictates an incredible need for flexibility as we approach a new era in medicine. APNs have a greater opportunity to work independently, yet they experience increased risk and legal action. Hospital politics have made strange bedfellows of a variety of practitioners, all working in various ways against the fragmentation of care that can result in increased iatrogenic illness. Patients are more critical, more frightened, and more confused.

In addition, APNs may feel squeezed between the conflicting values. Physicians may both respect and reject them. Job insecurity plagues the health professions, as does role confusion and massive dysfunction of a system in chaos. Nurses want to advocate for their patients in a system that does not appreciate or, at times, even allow them to do their job appropriately and effectively.

Journey to Health

The greatest challenge in this major transition is to balance caring for self with care for others to be most efficacious. This balancing act is often a result of a deep conviction and understanding of the principles of self-care. In addition to pharmacologic and physiologic knowledge, APNs add instinctive knowledge to daily problem solving. These diverse skills can be blended for extremely successful outcomes in patient care.

The APN can experiment with holistic tools and modalities, starting with self. Only when the nurse explores and learns to find this middle ground will he or she be able to maintain the excellent degree of health needed to be useful consistently in service to those entrusted to him or her.

According to the Standards of Holistic Nursing Practice of the American Holistic Nurses Association, holistic nurses are committed to personal development to ensure expertise in practice and interventions. This journey includes the necessity for setting clear intentionality, maintaining a positive attitude for healing endeavors, using crisis as opportunity, and mentoring others toward their personal goals. In addition, professional holistic nursing care demands that nurses help patients to identify patterns that put them at risk and to employ preventive measures. All of these are possible as the nurse expands his or her awareness and foundations of practice and caring.

Where to Begin

Some nurses find themselves suffering from maladies that are physical, mental, emotional, or even spiritual. They feel they are in crisis, facing burnout, or they are increasingly despondent about their work options. These nurses begin to explore holistic modalities out of their need for greater ease in their lives.

For others, the call to experiment arises from the patients. Many health-care consumers are interested in pursuing more natural, less invasive therapies, having heard about them from friends or seen evidence of their efficacy in journals and news media reports. Patients report successful or extremely pleasant encounters with new ways to treat their conditions, and nurses become curious.

Some nurses are exposed to new ways of healing through their universities or in-service education departments. Increasingly, universities are adopting holistic curricula, introducing classes in holistic nursing, and seeking integrated models of practice. APNs in private practice are introducing expanded concepts of nursing care with natural therapies that are less costly and invasive.

There is no right place to start. Any health-care provider can seek courses in holistic practice or find a practitioner in their own community who practices modalities that are more natural. The nurse may wish to experience various types of body massage, energy therapy, and exercise and may want to learn from books that describe how to practice in certain ways. The practitioner may want to try a more hands-on approach first, with experiential classes that allow him or her to feel his or her own body's response to certain treatments, and then to practice these tools using personal skills.

The important thing is to remain open-minded. Healthy skepticism is a valuable tool; the skeptic within us allows us to be discerning, to make appropriate choices, and to ascertain what makes sense to us and what does not.

Nursing is an art and a science; therefore, our care requires that we balance both. The art of nursing is gentle, compassionate, and caring. Practicing this art requires, as Florence Nightingale (1859/1950) said, "as exclusive a devotion, as hard a preparation, as any painter's or sculptor's work; for what is the having to do with dead canvas or cold marble compared with having to do with the living body, the temple of God's spirit? It is . . . the finest of the fine arts."

Modalities

Holistic nursing does not require the use of alternative treatment modalities. It is a philosophy, a way of life that embraces healing of the whole person, including the nurse as well as the patient. However, a great variety of tools can be tapped in exploration of the more natural realm. Many of these modalities are currently taught in classes, some offering continuing education for nurses. Others might be taken for pure enjoyment and learning.

Touch therapies are an increasingly popular way to share. There are various systems of touch therapies, including many forms of massage and energy therapy. Nurses are increasingly studying systems for healing through touch, taking classes to learn therapeutic touch, Reiki, Shiatsu massage, polarity, Touch for Health, and others. Some nurses are even attending advanced educational programs, receiving certificates in specific treatment modalities including chiropractic, acupuncture, and oriental medicine, which combines acupuncture with knowledge of herbs used in the East.

Other tools that nurses are finding useful include aromatherapy, which is widely used in England and gaining popularity in the United States, and imagery, which combines beautifully with hands-on therapies to assist in relaxation and deep inner healing. Imagery, related to hypnosis, refers to use of the senses to access one's inner healer, creating a safe place from which one's healing attitudes and commitments can be fortified and enhanced. Homeopathy is another modality that some nurses have chosen to investigate.

In addition to these tools, many providers are studying to learn more about the use of exercise programs, and particularly nutritional supplementation, to enhance their patient's overall health.

A recent addition to the healing modalities is aquatherapy, a process of using the healing properties of water to restore balance and well-being. The concepts presented by Keegan and Keegan in 1998 help nurses and other health-care professionals to understand the importance of caring for self and the connection between self-care and other-care.

Once again, these modalities all work together for the benefit of health promotion, stress reduction, and health education. Nurses can learn more about natural, noninvasive ways to support the body's innate healing abilities. Florence Nightingale reminded us that nursing's work is to put the patient in the best position for nature to act upon him or her.

Psychoneuroimmunology: Contributions to the Body–Mind Concept

In considering Nightingale's thoughts, we might ask ourselves how we can put the body in the best position for nature to act upon us. A major contribution to healing helps us to understand the importance of thoughts, emotions, and attitude on our health and wholeness.

In the 1970s, Candace Pert, a researcher at the National Institutes of Health, made a discovery that defined her career as a scientist. While attempting to help our society understand the importance of psychosomatic illness, Pert explored receptors that initiate physiologic changes. These receptors function as scanners on the cellular level waiting to pick up messages. Binding occurs when the right chemical appears (Pert refers to this as sex on the molecular level). She identified ligands—chemical keys that cause receptors to activate. Three types of ligands include neurotransmitters, steroids, and peptides. Researchers later discovered that every peptide, no matter where it was found, was made in various parts of the organism, including the brain. Pert began looking for peptide receptors in the brain and found them in all parts, including the hypothalamus, cortex, and limbic system. She then mapped the distribution of chemicals in the brain, facing the contempt of her colleagues as she attempted to explore the body–mind connections. She concluded that the core structures (amygdala, hippocampus, and limbic cortex) within the limbic system, considered to be the seat of emotions, contained the largest percentage of neuropeptide receptors. Through many years of diligent research, she concluded that the body is actually the unconscious mind.

Pert's work helps us to comprehend the interconnectedness between mind and body; the link between emotions and immunity. She found that molecules of emotion run every system of our body, demonstrating an enormous body–mind intelligence, one that is wise enough to seek wellness and help us to keep ourselves healthy. In learning to keep ourselves well, we can inspire healthier attitudes in our patients.

Nursing Diagnoses: Changing the Way We Think

As nurses change the way we think and care for ourselves, we are changing the way we view our patients, leaning more and more toward a whole-person approach to health care. Reflecting our deeper and more complex understanding of humans, we are evolving nursing diagnoses that support the multidimensional aspects of our being. These "nursing diagnoses" are helpful conceptual tools for all health-care professionals working with patients in multidimensional ways.

Several nursing diagnoses are relevant to our exploration of self-care and caring for others as whole beings. One of these is "spiritual distress," considered to be a disruption of the life principle pervading a person's entire being, transcending one's biological and psychological nature. Providers are afflicted with this as well as patients. It is characterized by concern with belief systems, suffering, inner conflict, and interconnections. People with spiritual distress can exhibit sleep disturbances, dramatic alterations in mood, and other similar symptoms. Providers who are helping patients with spiritual distress to cope support them in their endeavors to reconnect with inner resources, a sense of being connected to something greater, and to one's purpose and meaning. To be effective caregivers, providers also need to tend to these issues within themselves. In fact, all health-care professions can achieve a greater sense of wholeness and well-being through learning to care for onself first.

Another related nursing diagnosis is energy field disturbance. This involves a disruption of flow surrounding the person, resulting in disharmony of body, mind, and spirit. Many subtle changes can be detected through use of hands and intentionality to ascertain whether this is present, including temperature, sight, and movement. Providers who are aware of these subtle needs, in themselves and others, are likely to be most effective in their assessment, planning, and interventions.

The Health-Care Challenge: Actualizing Our Potential

For health-care providers to actualize ourselves and to claim our proper place in the emerging paradigm, we must return to our roots; we must remember what it is that makes us unique, valuable, and necessary. The system is changing in ways we cannot even imagine, and the new era will feature a new image for us all.

That new image has not yet been formed. As healers look back to our past, contemplate our present, and anticipate the future, we are in the process of defining and refining the art of caring. As we capitalize on that which makes nursing unique, we will usher in new visions for our profession, as well as all of the health-care professions.

A review of ethical considerations for holistic nursing practice reminds us that we are here to facilitate healing and to alleviate suffering, within a context of body–mind–spirit awareness. The nurse has a responsibility to model healthy behaviors, striving to achieve harmony and balance in his or her own life while assisting others to do the same. Nurses have the right to use all appropriate nursing interventions and research findings to support the health of their patients and to share their unique knowledge with other members of the health-care team.

Our work presently is to heal from within, individually and collectively. As we honor our multidimensional existence and experiment with healing modalities, we are strengthening our core. As each health-care provider cares for self, the seeds of a brighter, more effective future are planted.

We will move from a sick-care system to another model of caring, one that promotes greater access to more gentle methods. People will learn from the nursing profession about caring for themselves and the benefits of nurturing self. Nurses will be the models for a healthier future for consumers, and consumers will support the evolution of the healing arts as demonstrated through the nursing model. One missing ingredient in today's health-care system is actualized nursing.

Nursing is the art of human caring. It includes health promotion, health education, and patient advocacy. In honoring these various aspects of nursing practice, APNs direct their skill and intentionality toward creating a peaceful, harmonious environment, sharing that approach with others. As Nightingale (1859/1980) reminded us, "Nature alone cures . . . and what nursing has to do is to put the patient in the best position for nature to act upon him."

The new era provides fertile ground for us to experiment, to plant seeds, and to reap a future that empowers consumers and providers alike. Nursing can assume a leadership role in the transformation of health care across the planet, with an expanded and global perspective on health and healing. In addition to caring for our patients, we can move into caretaking the environment and all aspects that are interconnected in the ecosystem of health. This vision promotes nurturing as the essence of healing and APNs as viable leaders of the movement. The foundation is self-care; the result is health care that nourishes self and others simultaneously.

Bibliography

Bandura, A: Self-Efficacy: The Exercise of Control. Freeman, New York, 1997.

Carpenito, L (ed): Nursing Diagnosis: Application to Clinical Practice, ed. 5. Lippincott, Philadelphia, 1993.

Chopra, D: Quantum Healing. Bantam Books, New York, 1990.

Dossey, L: Healing Words: The Power of Prayer and the Practice of Medicine. HarperSanFrancisco, San Francisco, 1993.

Dossey, B, Keegan, L, and Guzzetta, K: Holistic Nursing: A Handbook for Practice, ed 3. Aspen, Gaithersburg, Md., 1995.

Dossey, B (ed): Core Curriculum for Holistic Nursing. Aspen, Gaithersburg, Md., 2000.

Hover-Kramer, D, and Shames, K: Energetic Approaches to Emotional Healing. Delmar, New York, 1996.

Jung, C: In Campbell, J (ed): The Portable Jung. Penguin Books, New York, 1971.

Keegan, G, and Keegan, L: Healing Waters: The Miraculous Health Benefits of Earth's Most Essential Resource. Berkley Books, New York, 1998.

Krieger, D: Accepting Your Power to Heal: Personal Practice of Therapeutic Touch. Bear & Company, Santa Fe, N.M., 1993.

Nightingale, F: Notes on Nursing: What It Is, and What It Is Not. Churchill Livingstone, London, 1980 (1st ed. 1859, Harrison & Sons).

Pert, C: Molecules of Emotion: Why You Feel the Way You Feel. Scribner, New York, 1997.
Rogers, M: Introduction to the Theoretical Basis of Nursing Practice. FA Davis, Philadelphia, 1970.
Shames, K: Creative Imagery in Nursing. Delmar, New York, 1995.
Shames, K: The Nightingale Conspiracy, revised ed 2. Enlightenment Press, Montclair, N.J., 1993.
Talbot, M: The Holographic Universe. HarperPerennial, New York, 1991.

Resources

American Holistic Nurses Association
P.O. Box 2130, Flagstaff, AZ 86003-2130
1-800-278-AHNA
http://www.ahna.org

Holistic Alliance for Professional Practitioners, Entrepreneurs, and Networkers
P.O. Box 90177, Gainesville, FL 32607
1-888-8HAPPEN
E-mail: happen@mindspring.com
http://www.happen.org

Holistic Nursing Programs and Organizations, Advanced Practice Nurses: Certificate Program in Holistic Nursing
P.O. Box 307, Shutesbury, MA 01072
E-mail: cphn@th.net.
http://www.cyberc.com/cphn

Nurses Certificate Program in AMMA Therapy
The New York College
6801 Jericho Turnpike, Suite 300, Syosset, NY 11791-4413
E-mail: AYoung@nycollege.edu

Nurses Certificate Program in Interactive Imagery: Beyond Ordinary Nursing
P.O. Box 8177, Foster City, CA 94404
E-mail: ncpii@aol.com
http://members.aol.com/NCPII/NCPII.html

Nurse Healers Professional Associates
1211 Locust St., Philadelphia, PA 19197
E-mail: nhpa@nursecominc.com
http://therapeutic/touch.org

Transformational Pathways: The Challenge of Self Healing Program
Presented by H.A.P.P.E.N., Inc.
P.O. Box 90177, Gainesville, FL 32607
1-888-8HAPPEN
E-mail: happen@mindspring.com
http://www.happen.org

Index

Note: Page numbers followed by the letter b refer to boxed material. Page numbers followed by the letter f refer to figures; those followed by t refer to tables.

C

J

K

L

P

Q

R

S

W

X

Y

Z